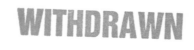

September 11, 2001

Dedication and Prayer

The calamitous events of September 11, 2001, occurred during the final days of this book's production. Some of these tragic events took place in full view of the staff working at Weill Cornell Medical Center and in The Empire State Building. It is to the victims of the terrible events of that day in New York, Washington, D.C., and Pennsylvania that we dedicate this book. It is offered with the prayer that humankind will one day learn to live in peace so that we may all enjoy life's blessings.

Inaugural Volume of the Weill Cornell Health Series
Antonio M. Gotto, Jr., M.D., D.Phil. General Editor

FROM

WEILL MEDICAL COLLEGE

OF CORNELL UNIVERSITY

The CORNELL

Illustrated

Antonio M. Gotto, Jr.

M.D., D.Phil.

General Editor

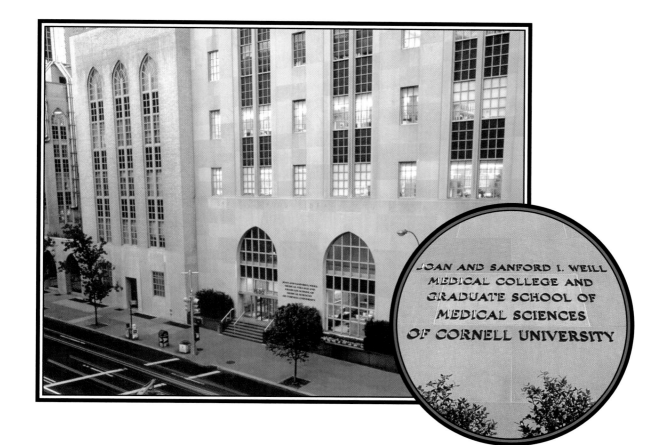

Encyclopedia

of HEALTH

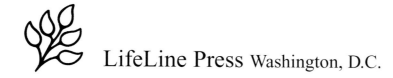

LifeLine Press Washington, D.C.

DISCLAIMER

All health and health-related information, including the descriptions and images contained in this book, are intended for informational or educational use only and not as a substitute for the diagnosis of a competent healthcare professional or treatment by a physician. This information is intended to offer only a general basis for individuals to discuss their medical conditions and concerns with a health-care provider. As medical science is advancing continually, and since medical conditions and needs vary considerably from person to person, this book is not to be considered complete or current in any way. Every effort has been made to make the content and presentation of information in this work accurate and comprehensive, but that does not preclude the possibility of errors or of the omission of relevant medical information.

No product or treatment method included in this book is to be considered endorsed or recommended by Weill Medical College, Cornell University, medical advisors and consultants, or the publishers, producers, and distributors of this work; nor should the omission of any product or treatment be interpreted as disapproval of that product or treatment method. Readers are advised that they should consult a competent and qualified healthcare professional and physician in determining their medical condition and needs, and that is the only means of treating health-care problems or situations recommended herein.

Correspondence regarding this book should be addressed to the Publisher: LifeLine Press, a division of Regnery Publishing, Inc., One Massachusetts Ave., N.W., Washington, D.C. 20001

First Edition

Library of Congress Cataloging-in-Publication Data

The Cornell illustrated encyclopedia of health: the definitive home medical reference /
Antonio M. Gotto, Jr., General editor.
p. cm.
Includes bibliographical references and index.
ISBN 0-89526-186-3
1. Medicine, Popular-Encyclopedias. 2. Health-Encyclopedias.
I. Gotto, Antonio M.
R125.C674 2001   616'.003—dc21

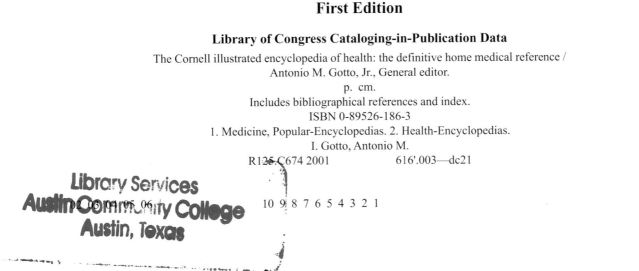

Produced by
The Reference Works, Inc.
Harold Rabinowitz, Director

Jenna Bagnini, Managing Editor
Stephen P. Smith, Rachel Soltis, Editors
Noam Levy, Mara Naaman, Associate Editors

Writers
Ed Edelson
Jan Erikson
Lee Gillette
Richard Kopf
Richard Harth
Jan Hutchinson
Ed Lucaire
Ilana Rabinowitz
Rachel Teitz

Bibliographies
Sonia Lin

Index
Bill Todd

Editorial
Colin Enriquez
Cassandra Heliczer
Sherry Holder
Niel Vuolo

Line Editing
Connie Buchanan
Heather Fenby
John House
Dee Ito
John Lazar

Copy Editing
Betty Richman
Diane Lane Root
Bob Sommerville

Images
Troy Schremmer
Rachel Soltis
Norman Curry, Corbis, Consultant
Carlos Tenorio, ADAM, Consultant
Maggie Bartlett, NCI, Consultant

Editorial Assistance
Virginia Reiff
Jamie L.D. Wurdinger
Alonzo Cox, Intern
Noreen Shaput, Intern

IT Consulting
Mitchell G. Pessin, MP Services

Designed by
Bob Antler, Antler DesignWorks
with Pam Kagyama and Todd Miller

For LifeLine Press
Thomas L. Phillips, Chairman, Eagle Publishing
Jefferey L. Carneal, President, Eagle Publishing
Alfred Regnery, President, Regnery Publishing
Michael Ward, Associate Publisher
Marjory G. Ross, Vice Pres. & General Manager
Jed Donahue, Editorial
Steve Owen, Art Director
Fred Gearhart (in memoriam), Manufacturing

For Weill Medical College of Cornell University
Alan Arellano, Chief Medical Photographer, WMC
Leslie Greenberg, Assistant to Dr. Gotto
Jesse Jou, Editor for Dr. Gotto
Myrna Manners, Vice Provost, Public Affairs
Felicia Narvaez, Director, Publications
Ron Phillips, Manager, Biomedical Communications, WMC
Jonathan Weil, Director, Communications
Annette Williams, Assistant to Dr. Gotto

How To Use This Book

The Cornell Illustrated Encyclopedia of Health represents the combined efforts of the publishing professionals of The Reference Works and the LifeLine Press imprint of Regnery Publishing; the medical experts of Weill Medical College of Cornell University and the physicians of New York-Presbyterian Hospital and Cornell Physicians Organization; and the image resources of ADAM, the Corbis-Bettmann Archives and a number of other image archives and illustrators. The result is a home medical reference that is easy to use, comprehensive and authoritative, and illuminating in its illustration and design.

The challenges posed in producing a work such as this are formidable: the information is presented alphabetically for easy access by the reader, but when all the articles in a given area of health and medicine are collected, they constitute a complete and comprehensive presentation of that area. For this reason, much attention has been paid to the cross-referencing apparatus of the work. Following the directions of the cross-references and the "Signpost" boxes that appear at the end of many articles gives the reader the opportunity to survey an entire area of medicine and health without losing the facility offered by alphabetical presentation of succinct elements of information.

Special Features

A number of special features have been incorporated into this book that we hope will make it easier and more useful to the reader.

Titles. The Encyclopedia is arranged alphabetically—the headers on each page indicate the first article beginning on that page for left-hand pages and the last article that begins on that page for right-hand pages. Nearly all titles are followed by a brief definition; some articles contain a line under the main title indicating alternate names and terms for that subject.

Papilledema
Also known as choked disk or swollen optic nerve

A swelling of the optic nerve that causes increased intracranial pressure.

Titles of articles in the area of first aid or emergency medicine are in red when used in the page headers.

Alert Boxes. Readers will find two kinds of sidebars in the articles: regular sidebars (in blue) contain material that is related to the main subject of the article or relevant tables; and red "Alert" sidebars, which contain information of particular importance and highlight material that require special caution by readers. In all instances, readers are reminded that seeking competent medical assistance and attention is the most advisable course in addressing a health problem.

Resource Boxes. Many entries contain a "resource box" at the conclusion of the entry which contains several print references and, in many instances, the names of relevant organizations, with telephone contact information and web site addresses.

Signposts. Also at the end of many articles are blue boxes that refer readers to other arti-

Below, a sample Resource Box; at right, a sample title with an alternate name for the entry's subject, followed by a definition box. On the opposite page, top left, a sample Signpost

Resources on Bereavement

Byock, Ira, *Dying Well: Peace and Possibilities at the End of Life* (1998); Callanan, Maggie, and Patricia Kelly, *Final Gifts: Understanding the Special Awareness, Needs, and Communications of the Dying* (1997); Kubler-Ross, Elisabeth, *On Death and Dying* (1997); McWilliams, Peter, *How to Survive the Loss of a Love* (1993); National Mental Health Association, Tel., (800) 969-NMHA, Online: www.nmha.org/infoctr/factsheets/42.cfm; www.nycornell.org/psychiatry/index.html.

cles in the Encyclopedia. These cross-references are layered, insofar as they indicate first the articles that provide background information, then the entries that deal with the subject

> *Background material on AIDS can be found in* IMMUNITY AND AUTOIMMUNITY. *Related information is contained in* INFECTIOUS DISEASES, PUBLIC HEALTH AND ENVIRONMENTAL HEALTH, ONCOLOGY *and* PHARMACOLOGY. *See also* ALTERNATIVE MEDICINE *for more on rehabilitation and therapies.*

in greater detail, and finally the articles that contain material related to the entry.

The Emergency Medicine and First Aid Appendix. Many articles on emergency medicine and first aid appear twice in the book: once in their proper place alphabetically and a second time at the back of the book, on pages bordered in red. This was done to facilitate finding this material in the event of an emergency.

A work of this kind faces another challenge: how to produce a print product that is current in a field that changes as rapidly as medical science. Readers will note that the time between the editorial production of the book and its manufacture has been very short—a matter of weeks for a process that ordinarily takes nine months to a year. Revisions were made virtually up to the moment the book went to press.

Yet, even this was unsatisfying to the editors. In what may prove to be a landmark project in health publishing, the producer and the publisher have, in concert with Weill Medical College, created A "Living Encyclopedia," in which the work is to be continually updated online. Readers will then be able to use the Encyclopedia as a "print portal"—a virtual catalog to the on-line versions of the Encyclopedia, which will be appearing as part of the Weill

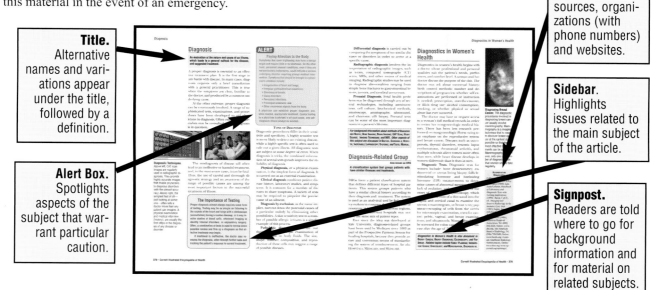

Title. Alternative names and variations appear under the title, followed by a definition.

Alert Box. Spotlights aspects of the subject that warrant particular caution.

Resource Box. Provides print sources, organizations (with phone numbers) and websites.

Sidebar. Highlights issues related to the main subject of the article.

Signpost. Readers are told where to go for background information and for material on related subjects.

The material contained in the Emergency Medicine and First Aid Appendix is also available on-line, and is downloadable to a PDA (Palm Pilot, Visor, and others)—at the Weill-Cornell website (http://www.med.cornell.edu) and at the NewYork-Presbyterian Hospital website (http://www.nyp.org).

The Index. A sizable Index appears as the final section of the book. In it, article titles appear in **blue bold type** and article titles that deal with first aid and emergency medical situations appear in **red bold type**. The index entries on symptoms appear in plain red type.

Medical College website, as well as on other internet sites.

The organization of these sites will follow the organization of the Encyclopedia, and updates will be based on and will refer to material in the entries as they appear in this book. Medical editors and physicians will be updating the articles on-line continually, so that readers will be able to access the ongoing development of the Encyclopedia as it is improved, enhanced, and updated. Look for this at:

http://www.med.cornell.edu

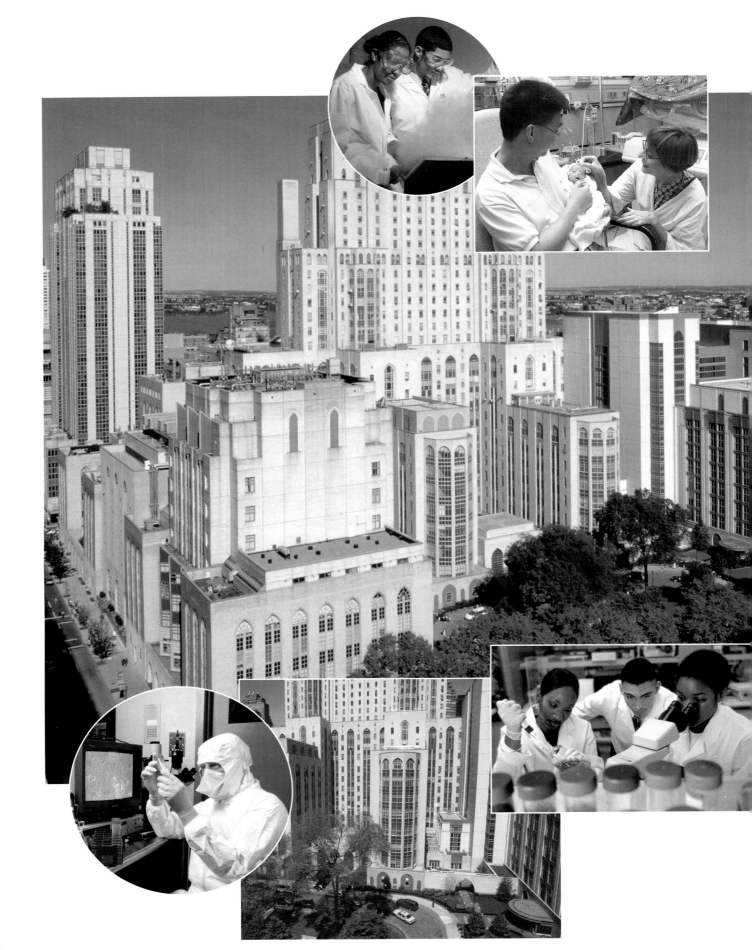

The Greatest Instruments

Antonio M. Gotto, Jr., M.D., D.Phil.
The Stephen and Suzanne Weiss Dean and Professor of Medicine
Weill Medical College of Cornell University

"You do solemnly swear, to that which you hold most sacred, that into whatsoever house you shall enter, it shall be for the good of the sick to the utmost of your power."—from the Hippocratic Oath

Every year in August, I welcome bright and enthusiastic young men and women who hear me recite the Hippocratic oath before entering their study of medicine at Weill Medical College of Cornell University. On that first day, my faculty and I do not expect them to understand the full weight of Hippocrates' charge. By the time they take the oath at their graduation ceremony, however, we hope our students have taken a few core values to heart: a trust that their strong scientific foundation will prepare them to critically evaluate and apply the latest medical developments; an enduring curiosity so that they may make their own contributions to the advancement of medical science; keen powers of observation so that their clinical judgment will stand them in good stead; and, most importantly, a deep sense of compassion so that they will appreciate the unique history of every patient.

The young physician of today has seen the field of medicine progress with incredible speed as new technologies have been applied to health problems that previously withstood even the most assiduous research efforts. And the role of medicine in maintaining the quality of life we all hope for has grown as the population has aged and as the assaults on our environment and, of late, our safety have mounted. At the same time, there is pressure from government and private insurers to keep costs down, which may lead physicians to overlook the personal elements in patient care. However, the sacrifice and heroism of health-care workers following the events of September 11 remind us of the crucial role played by the personal element. For in the final analysis, health care involves one person attending to the needs, the pain, the life of another person. A caring and compassionate doctor at one end of a stethoscope will do much for the caring of the patient at the other end.

The positive relationship between a doctor and a patient remains one of the greatest instruments for ensuring quality health care. We have seen a dramatic shift as patients move away from viewing themselves as passive recipients of medical care toward taking an increasingly active role in their own treatment. Physicians must welcome this development, because well-informed and actively involved patients are likely to be better patients—more apt to follow instructions, be alert to symptoms, follow up with their physicians, and cooperate with the physician—something every doctor needs—in the medical recovery and treatment process.

The volume in your hands reflects this theme by providing a broad survey of the latest information. Our goal is to help you become a better-informed and more savvy patient, guided by the expertise of some of the best doctors in the United States. We hope that this will enable you to talk openly with your physician and not feel intimidated by what may seem to be an overwhelming body of knowledge.

Like all medical reference books for the general reader, this book contains a disclaimer designed to protect the university and the publisher. Although many readers may look upon the disclaimer as an unfortunate artifact of modern life, it contains one aspect that would be saluted by every health-care provider: there is no substitute for direct contact and consultation with a physician. This applies to doctors no less than to patients. A physician seeking counsel of a colleague is as vital to the practice of medicine as is a patient seeking the advice and attention of a physician. Listening to others and hearing a diversity of opinion is an essential part of daily life; why would that be any different in a field as complex and important as health care? As the medical school of a great university, we are dedicated to the free exchange of information and opinion on medical science around the world, and that is a second great instrument of medicine: the sharing of ideas—between researchers and practitioners, between physicians and their colleagues, between patients and health-care providers, and, ultimately, all peoples and nations on the small planet we share.

Anchored by the principle that "into whatsoever house it shall enter, it shall be to the good of the sick," we hope The Cornell Illustrated Encyclopedia of Health will prove to be a valuable resource to begin your investigation of the many medical issues that affect you, your household, and the world around you.

New York City
October 2001

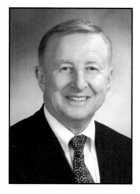
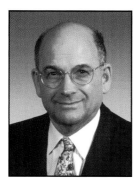
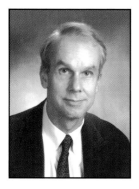
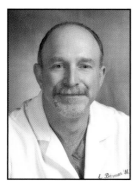

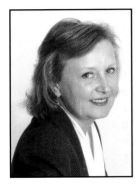
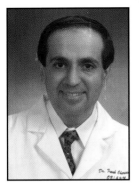
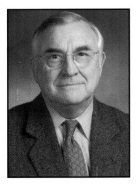
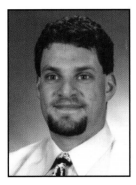

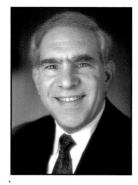

Genetics, Genetic Diseases, Gerontology and Geriatrics, and Respiratory Medicine

Dr. Ronald G. Crystal is creator of the FDA-approved augmentation therapy that is used around the world to treat patients with emphysema. He currently serves as the Bruce Webster Professor of Internal Medicine, Professor of Genetic Medicine, Director of the Institute of Genetic Medicine, and Director of the Belfer Gene Therapy Core Faculty at Weill Medical College of Cornell University. Dr. Crystal earned his B.A and M.S. in physics from Tufts University and his M.D. from the University of Pennsylvania. Prior to joining Cornell, he served at the National Institutes of Health as Chief of the Pulmonary Branch of the National Heart, Lung and Blood Institute. Dr. Crystal's early research focused on the pathogenesis and therapy of inflammatory disease of the lung, including fibrotic lung disorders and emphysema. He is currently conducting research on in vivo gene therapy.

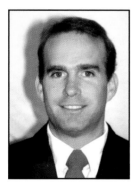

Surgery

Dr. John M. Daly is the Lewis Atterbury Stimson Professor and Chairman of the Department of Surgery at Weill Medical College of Cornell University. He is also the Surgeon-In-Chief at Weill Cornell Medical Center of NewYork-Presbyterian Hospital. Dr. Daly served as Program Director of the General Surgery Residency Program from 1993 to 2000. He is a member of many scientific boards and societies. Additionally, he is the principal investigator of several projects, author of more than 95 book chapters and 200 peer-related articles, and an editor of four publications. His expertise in surgical oncology has been recognized by his listing in the "Best Doctors in America" (Castle Connolly), the "Best Doctors in New York" (Castle Connolly), and the "318 Top Cancer Specialists for Women" (Good Housekeeping magazine). Dr. Daly has lectured worldwide. He is a graduate of Temple University School of Medicine, with clinical and research interests in surgical oncology, metabolism, and nutrition. Dr. Daly was assisted in his review Patricia A. Sullivan.

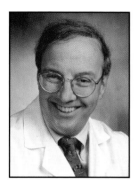

Ophthalmology

Dr. Kip W. Dolphin specializes in ophthalmology, orbital tumors, and cosmetic and reconstructive eye surgery. He received his M.D. from Thomas Jefferson University Medical College and is a member of the Alpha Omega Alpha Medical Honor Society. Dr. Dolphin completed his fellowship in oculoplastics and reconstructive surgery at the Manhattan Eye, Ear & Throat Hospital prior to his appointment at Weill Medical College of Cornell University where he is Associate Professor of Clinical Ophthalmology. In addition, he serves as the Residency Director of Ophthalmology at Weill Cornell Medical Center of NewYork-Presbyterial Hospital.

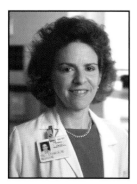

Women's Medicine

Dr. Orli Etingin has been on the faculty of Weill Medical College of Cornell University since 1983. She is Vice Chairman of the Department of Medicine, Professor of Clinical Medicine, and Professor of Medicine in Clinical Obstetrics and Gynecology. In 1980 she graduated from the Albert Einstein College of Medicine of Yeshiva University as a member of the Alpha Omega Alpha Medical Honor Society, and received the American Medical Women's Association Award and Edward Weinstein Award. Since then she has served on numerous committees, developed and led a multidisciplinary program in women's health at the Weill Cornell Medical Center of NewYork-Presbyterian Hospital, and counseled patients in coagulation disorders in pregnancy. She is the founder and director of The Center for Women's Healthcare at Weill Cornell Medical Center and Editor-In-Chief of two nationally distributed newsletters.

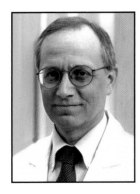
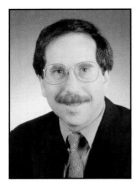
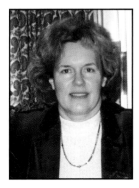
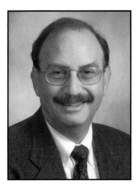

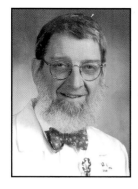
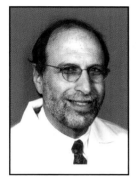
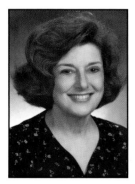
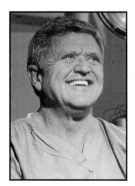

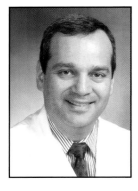
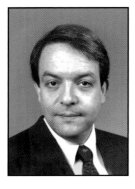
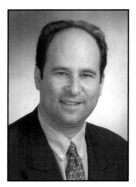
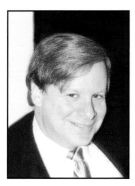

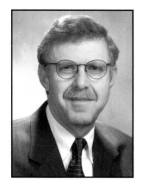

Preventive Medicine, Public Health and Environmental Health

Dr. Alvin I. Mushlin is the Nanette Laitman Distinguished Professor and Chairman of the Department of Public Health at Weill Medical College of Cornell University. In addition, he is the Physician-In-Chief of Public Health at Weill Cornell Medical Center of New York-Presbyterian Hospital. Dr. Mushlin is a Robert Wood Johnson Clinical Scholar and received his M.D. from Vanderbilt University School of Medicine and a master's degree in public health from the Johns Hopkins School of Hygiene and Public Health, with an emphasis on epidemiology and medical care. His research activities include diagnostic testing and screening for breast cancer, magnetic resonance imaging, and developing approaches for detecting coronary artery disease. Dr. Mushlin's publications encompass more than 75 papers, book chapters and editorials. He serves on several state and national committees and is a member of the New York State Cardiac Advisory Committee.

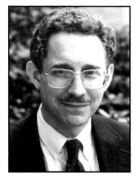

Immunology and Autoimmunity

Dr. Carl F. Nathan, a noted authority in the field of immunology, is Chairman of the Department of Microbiology and Immunology at Weill Medical College of Cornell University. He is also the R.A. Rees Pritchett Professor of Microbiology and author or co-author of more than 200 publications. Dr. Nathan has served as Acting Dean of Weill Medical College, Senior Associate Dean for Research, Director of the Tri-Institutional MD-Ph.D. Program, and Co-Chairman of the Immunology Program at Weill Graduate School of Medical Sciences of Cornell University. He has conducted research on the molecular mechanisms of innate immunity, studying the process by which macrophages and neutrophils kill microbial pathogens, tumor cells and host cells. Dr. Nathan received his B.A. from Harvard College and his M.D. from Harvard Medical School, specializing in immunology.

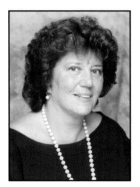

Pediatrics

Dr. Maria I. New is one of the world's leading pediatric endocrinologists and children's advocates. A graduate of the University of Pennsylvania School of Medicine, she has conducted pioneering research on disorders of adrenal steroidogenesis. Her most noteworthy contributions include the discoveries of apparent mineralocorticoid excess (AME) and a second form of low renin hypertension called dexamethasone suppressible hyperaldosteronism (DSH). Dr. New is Chairman of the Department of Pediatrics, Chief of Pediatric Endocrinology and Metabolism, and Director of the Children's Clinical Research Center at Weill Medical College of Cornell University, where she holds the Harold and Percy Uris Professorship of Pediatric Endocrinology and Metabolism. She is also Pediatrician-in-Chief at Weill Cornell Medical Center of New York-Presbyterian Hospital. Author of more than 500 articles and papers, Dr. New was appointed to the National Academy of Sciences in 1996, and is also a member of the New York State Public Health Council.

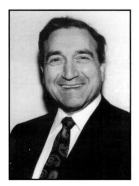

Nutrition

Dr. Richard S. Rivlin serves as the American Health Foundation's Vice President, Medical Affairs and Naylor-Dana Chair of Nutrition. In addition, he is the Program Director of the NIH-funded Clinical Nutrition Research Unit and a Professor of Medicine at the Weill Medical College of Cornell University. Educated at Harvard Medical School, he has worked as an educator, physician, and scientist at Cornell since 1979. He introduced the first required courses in nutrition at Weill Medical College, and treats a wide variety of nutritional and endocrine disorders. His research centers on vitamin metabolism, thyroid hormone control and nutrition in cancer prevention. His numerous awards include the Lifetime Achievement Award, American College of Nutrition, 2001. He is past president of the American Society of Clinical Nutrition.

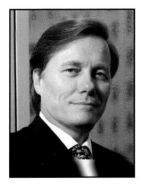
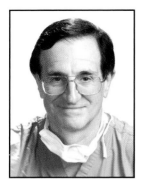
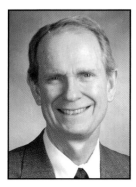
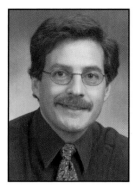

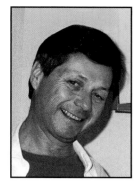

Immunology and Autoimmunity

Dr. Kendall A. Smith is the Rochelle Belfer Professor in Medicine at Weill Medical College of Cornell University, Professor of Immunology at Weill Graduate School of Medical Sciences of Cornell University, and Attending Physician at Weill Cornell Medical Center of New York-Presbyterian Hospital. He received his B.S. at Denison University and his M.D. from Ohio State University College of Medicine. His current research focuses on developing cytokines to treat infectious diseases, immunodeficiency diseases, and cancer. He is responsible for discovering and identifying the Interleukin-2 molecule (IL-2), an immune-stimulant protein that has been used to treat cancer patients for more than 10 years, and its receptor. His past positions include Director of The Norris Cotton Cancer Center's Immunology Program, Co-Chairman of the Cornell Graduate School of Medical Sciences Immunology Program, and Chief of the Division of Immunology.

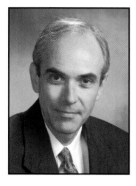

Diagnostics and Imaging

Dr. H. Dirk Sostman is the Senior Associate Dean for Clinical Affairs and Professor and Chairman of Radiology at Weill Medical College of Cornell University. In addition, he is Radiologist-in-Chief of the Weill Cornell Medical Center of New York-Presbyterian Hospital and Associate Chief Medical Officer of Weill Cornell's Physician Organization. A graduate of Yale Medical School, he is an authority in cardiovascular and pulmonary imaging. He has received many awards and honors, including the Fales Prize and has been cited as one of the Best Doctors in New York by New York magazine. In the past, he served as an Associate Professor and Chief of MRI at Yale and a Professor and Vice Chairman of Radiology at Duke University. Dr. Sostman is a member of the Society for Cardiovascular Magnetic Resonance, the Fleischner Society, and the Society of Thoracic Radiology. He is an international lecturer and author of more than 100 research papers.

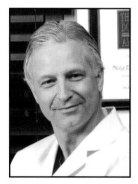

Anatomy and Neurosurgery

Dr. Philip E. Stieg is Professor and Chairman of the Department of Neurological Surgery at Weill Medical College of Cornell University and Neurological Surgeon-in-Chief at the Weill Cornell Medical Center of New York-Presbyterian Hospital. He headed the first laboratory to develop and characterize primary cultures of astroglial cells. He has studied the mechanisms of injury in the central nervous system and membrane transport after traumatic brain injury. Dr. Stieg received a B.S. from the University of Wisconsin, a Ph.D. in anatomy and neuroscience from Union University, and an M.D. from the Medical College of Wisconsin. His was previously Associate Professor of Neurosurgery at Harvard Medical School. Dr. Stieg has accrued numerous honors and awards, including "Who's Who In Health & Medical Services." He has a strong interest in cerebral protection, restorative function, neural transplantation, and neuronal regeneration.

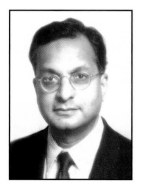

Nephrology

Dr. Manikkam Suthanthiran has made groundbreaking discoveries regarding organ transplants. His laboratory is currently involved in studies funded by the National Institutes of Health, one of which will help physicians to predict organ rejections in transplants more accurately. He is the Stanton Griffis Distinguished Professor of Medicine at Weill Medical College and Chief of Nephrology and Transplantation Medicine at New York-Presbyterian Hospital. Dr. Suthanthiran received his medical education at the University of Madras in India and did his internship, residency, and fellowship training in nephrology at Wayne State University in Michigan, followed by fellowships in nephrology and renal transplant immunology at Peter Beent Brigham Hospital and Harvard Medical School in Boston. He is a past president of the American Society of Transplant Physicians. Dr. Suthanthiran's primary research is in human transplantation immunobiology.

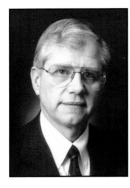
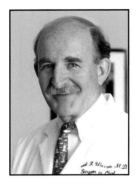
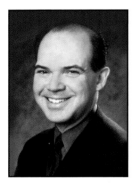
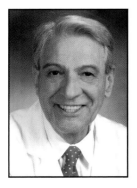

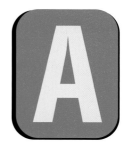

Abdomen

The part of the body between the chest (thorax) and the upper thighs.

The abdomen consists of the abdominal cavity and the pelvic cavity. The abdominal cavity is separated from the chest (thoracic) cavity by the diaphragm muscle; it contains the organs of the digestive and urinary systems. In the lower abdomen is the pelvic cavity, which is surrounded by hip bones (pelvis) containing the internal reproductive organs. The peritoneum, a thin, two-layered membrane that covers the stomach and intestines, lines the inside of the upper abdomen. Other abdominal structures include the liver, spleen, gall-

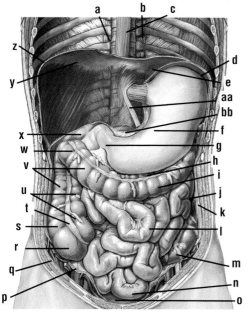

bladder, pancreas, inferior vena cava, duodenum, bile and pancreatic ducts, appendix, colon, and rectum. The lower ribs and spine shield these organs from behind, while the front of the abdomen is covered only by muscle, skin layers, connective tissue, and varying layers of fat.

> *Information about the organs in the abdomen is contained in* Stomach; Intestines; Gallbladder; Appendix; Colon; Pancreas; *and* Liver. *See also* Abdominal Pain *and* Abdominal Swelling *for information on disorders affecting the abdomen.*

Abdominal Pain

Discomfort in the abdominal region.

Abdominal pain consists of irritation, soreness, tenderness, or cramping in the abdominal and pelvic cavities, which are located below the ribcage (the thoracic cavity) and above the thighs. The thoracic cavity is separated from the abdominal cavity by the diaphragm muscle. However, no structure separates the abdominal cavity from the pelvic cavity. The abdominal cavity and its organs are covered by a thin membrane known as the peritoneum.

Causes

Abdominal pain may have numerous causes, ranging from harmless to quite serious. Perhaps the simplest and most common causes of abdominal pain arise from an individual's lifestyle: an excess of alcohol, spicy or fried foods, or foods high in fat, as well as late, heavy meals, may cause pain or nausea. Stress, anxiety, and tension can cause abdominal pain in both adults and children.

Abdominal pain may also be caused by a number of underlying physical conditions, which may require medical attention. These may include:
- injury to abdominal organs;
- food allergy, intolerance or poisoning;
- menstrual cramps;
- colic in infants;
- stomach flu;
- urinary tract infection (cystitis);
- ulcer;
- ruptured esophagus;
- gallstones;
- appendicitis;
- irritable bowel syndrome;
- hernia;
- pelvic inflammatory disease (PID);
- uterine fibroids;
- ovarian cysts;
- a fetus developing outside the uterus (ectopic pregnancy);
- diverticulitis;
- bowel obstruction;
- cancer of the stomach or colon;

The Abdominal Cavity. At left, the organs of the abdominal cavity are surrounded by the peritoneum, either entirely or in part. **a.** inferior vena cava; **b.** descending aorta; **c.** esophagus; **d.** spleen; **e.** left lobe of the liver; **aa.** falciform ligament; **bb.** lesser ormentum; **f.** the stomach body; **g.** stomach pylorus; **h.** the gastro-omental artery and vein; **i.** the transverse colon; **j.** the greater omentum (over the descending colon); **k.** transversalis facia; **l.** jejunum; **m.** the sigmoid colon; **n.** the ileum; **o.** urinary bladder (covered by peritoneum); **p.** the parietal peritoneum; **q.** inguinal ligament; **r.** the cecum; **s.** the ascending colon; **t.** tenia coli; **u.** omental appendages; **v.** haustra coli; **w.** tenia coli; **x.** the gallbladder; **y.** the right lobe of the liver; **z.** the diaphragm.

TYPES OF ABDOMINAL PAIN

Based on the patient's description of the severity, type, and location of the pain, as well as any correlations between the pain and eating, urinating, and bowel movements, a physician can determine if the pain is likely to indicate a serious condition and if it requires further testing or treatment.

• **Gas pain** (flatulence) is a bloated, distended feeling in the lower abdomen. It can usually be controlled with lifestyle changes, such as a healthy diet, maintenance of a healthy weight, and exercise.

• **Heartburn** is a burning sensation in the upper abdominal area. It is usually harmless and can be controlled by changes in lifestyle and eating habits.

• **Menstrual Pain.** In women, cramp like abdominal pain that occurs just before or during menstruation or that occurs during ovulation is usually normal and requires no special treatment other than over-the-counter pain relievers.

• **Peptic ulcer pain** is felt in the breastbone at the point where the ribs meet (the sternum). It may be eased temporarily with antacid medication and food. A doctor will prescribe a course of medication, possibly including antibiotics and antacids.

• **Kidney pain** is recurring and intermittent. It may begin below the rib cage and travel to the groin area, and is generally felt toward the back. Further testing is usually

---

Abdominal Pain in Children

More than 10 percent of school-aged children develop abdominal pain. In 90 percent of the cases, the discomfort is caused by stress and anxiety. If the child is depressed or exhibits mental health problems, he or she should see a mental health professional, such as a social worker or psychologist. The closer the pain is to the navel, the more likely it is that the pain is caused by a physical disorder. Children with abdominal pain should be examined for signs of hepatitis, parasite infestation (worms), sickle cell anemia, and lead poisoning.

---

done to determine the underlying cause.

• **Pelvic organ inflammation** is a less centrally located pain. It can spread to the entire abdominal region. There may be a vaginal discharge. Further testing is usually needed to determine the exact cause.

• **Appendicitis pain** is a sharp pain that may begin at the navel and travel to the lower right side of the body. Acute appendicitis requires immediate surgery.

• **Gallbladder pain** is a constant, cramp-like pain that begins below the right set of ribs. It may be accompanied by fever and vomiting. Gallstones can be surgically or nonsurgically removed.

WHEN TO CONTACT A PHYSICIAN

Contact your physician if:
• You experience severe pain.
• You have had an abdominal injury within the last 72 hours.
• Pain occurs during pregnancy.
• Pain is prolonged and persistent.
• High fever and nausea, sometimes in conjunction with constipation and bloating, accompany the pain.
• You cannot keep food or liquid down for a period of more than 72 hours.
• Pain is accompanied by bloody stools or vomit.

ALERT
Emergency Abdominal Pain

You may have a medical emergency and should contact your physician immediately if you experience acute abdominal pain with fever and nausea. This may indicate appendicitis, a bowel obstruction, or complications of diverticulitis, a disease in which small pouches form in the lining of the intestines, become inflamed, and may bleed. A rigid abdomen may indicate peritonitis. Blood in stools or in vomit can be a symptom of gastrointestinal bleeding and requires immediate attention.

If abdominal pain is accompanied by chest, back or jaw pain, excessive sweating, anxiety, or a sense of impending doom, it may indicate a heart attack. Immediate emergency medical care is required.

Background material on abdominal pain can be found in ABDOMEN. Information about related symptoms is contained in ABDOMEN, SWELLING; CONSTIPATION; DIARRHEA; and NAUSEA. See also APPENDICITIS; DIVERTICULITIS; GALLSTONES; HEARTBURN; IRRITABLE BOWEL SYNDROME; KIDNEY DISORDERS; PELVIC INFLAMMATORY DISEASE; PERITONITIS; and PREMENSTRUAL SYNDROME for more on specific causes of and treatments for abdominal pain.

Resources on Abdominal Pain

Thompson, W. Grant, *The Ulcer Story: The Authoritative Guide to Ulcers, Dyspepsia, and Heartburn* (1996);National Institute of Diabetes and Digestive and Kidney Diseases, Tel. (301) 496-3583, www. niddk.nih. gov; www.nycornell.org/ medicine/digestive/index. html.

Abdominal Swelling

Increase in size of the abdomen that may be accompanied by unusual firmness and a sensation of tenderness.

Abdominal swelling can occur for a variety of reasons. The abdomen may be enlarged due to pregnancy, obesity, gas in the intestines, or water retention before menstruation. More dangerous causes include: accumulation of fluid in the abdominal cavity (ascites); heart or kidney failure; reduced thyroid activity; cancer; liver disease; tuberculosis; inflammation of the abdominal lining (peritonitis); and inflammation of the pancreas. If the abdomen becomes enlarged for no known reason, especially if it is hard or painful to the touch, medical attention should be sought. *See* THYROID.

Abdominal X-Ray

A radiological test used to find abnormalities in organs of the abdomen.

In basic abdominal x-ray analysis, the patient's abdomen is x-rayed with no special preparation on the patient's part. Basic x-rays can reveal paralysis or obstruction of the stomach and intestines, and possibly enlargement of organs such as the liver, kidney, and spleen. Basic analysis is the most convenient method, but it does not result in as detailed an image as other, more sophisticated x-ray techniques.

Barium X-Ray. Further information concerning the abdomen and digestive tract is often obtained through the use of barium. Barium is a chalky liquid that appears white on an x-ray image. After a patient swallows a mixture containing barium, the interior and exterior outlines of the esophagus, stomach, and small intestine can be seen more clearly as can abnormalities such as tumors, polyps, and ulcers. Barium, either swallowed or administered by enema, can be used to visualize the intestines, though it may cause some mild cramping and discomfort.

CAT SCAN. A more sophisticated x-ray known as Computer Tomography (CAT scan) uses multiple x-ray scans to create a highly detailed, three-dimensional image. With this technique, the diagnostic range of abnormalities and diseases of the abdominal region is greater. *See also* BARIUM X-RAY; *and* CAT SCAN.

Abducens Nerve

The sixth cranial nerve, a small motor nerve.

The single task of the abducens nerve is to link the muscle that moves the eye outward (lateral rectus) to the brain. Paralysis of or damage to the abducens nerve results in the eye turning inward, which causes double vision. *See* STRABISMUS.

Similar to all 12 pairs of cranial nerves, the abducens nerve emerges from the brain stem; in contrast, the spinal nerves emerge from the vertebrae. The abducens nerve originates in the brain stem, the lowest section of the brain, and travels through the skull to the back of the eye socket. Due to the lengthy route that the nerve travels inside the skull, the abducens nerve is especially susceptible to damage, resulting from a skull fracture or a brain tumor. The damage usually causes double vision.

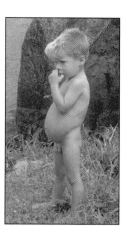

Abdominal Swelling. A boy with a swollen abdomen from the parasitic infection schistosomiasis. In underdeveloped countries, such sights are often the result of malnourishment.

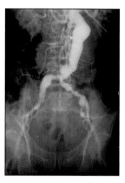

Abdominal Angiogram. Above, a picture of an angiogram of the abdomen, showing an aortic aneurysm.

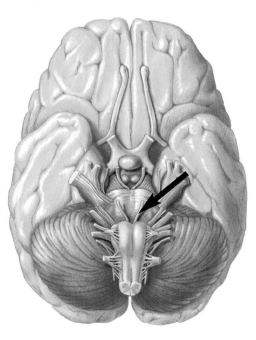

The Cranial Nerves in the Brain. Left, the abducens nerve (arrow) emerges from the medulla before traveling to the eye.

Ablation

The surgical removal of diseased or dead tissues.

Tissue can be cut away (excision), burned (cauterization), frozen (cryosurgery), exposed to radiation, or removed with a laser. Radioactive iodine may be used in the ablation of portions of the thyroid. *See also* CRYO-SURGERY; DIATHERMY; *and* LASER.

Abortifacient

Chemical administered to pregnant mothers for the purpose of inducing delivery of a fetus during the early weeks of its development and thereby terminating pregnancy (abortion).

A recently developed drug, RU-486 (mifepristone), induces abortion when it is administered before the ninth week of pregnancy. The drug is usually used in conjunction with prostaglandins, substances that are found in menstrual fluid and semen and that cause contractions in the muscle wall of the uterus. Mifepristone blocks the action of the hormone progesterone on the lining of the uterus; this strengthens the effects of the prostaglandins that have been administered.

SIDE EFFECTS

Side effects of prostaglandins include nausea, vomiting, flushing of the face, and fainting. They have also been linked to asthma attacks in asthmatic women.

OTHER ABORTIFACIENTS

Other types of abortifacients include saline and urea. These are injected into the sac containing the fetus (amniotic sac) in order to stimulate uterine contractions. Sometimes oxytocin, an otherwise naturally ocurring hormone that stimulates contractions during birth, is administered intravenously.

High doses of oral contraceptives are sometimes used to prevent pregnancy after unprotected sex. They must be taken within 72 hours of intercourse. Side effects include nausea and vomiting. *See also* ABORTION; CONCEPTION; CONTRACTIONS; FETUS; *and* PREGNANCY.

Abortion

The termination of a pregnancy before a fetus can survive on its own.

A miscarriage is referred to medically as a spontaneous abortion. An elective abortion is a surgical procedure performed to end the pregnancy. Elective abortion procedures vary depending upon what time in the pregnancy they are performed.

METHODS

First Trimester. During the first trimester, methods of abortion include menstrual extraction, suction curettage, and non-surgical abortion.

In menstrual extraction, the contents of the uterus are suctioned out without dilation of the cervix. This method is best performed in the first five to seven weeks of pregnancy. It is sometimes performed before positive confirmation of pregnancy, in a procedure known as a preemptive abortion. Menstrual extraction can be done without anesthesia; however, the failure rate of menstrual extraction is higher than that of other methods.

Suction curettage is similar to menstrual extraction, except that the cervix is first dilated. This is usually necessary after the sixth week of pregnancy. Different means

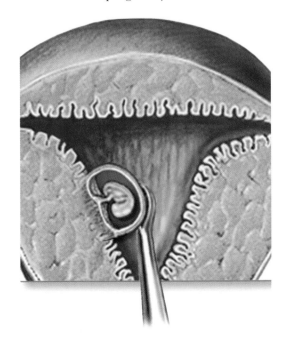

Abortion. At right, an abortion procedure performed during early pregnancy known as a "D&C"—dilation and curetage—in which the fetus is removed surgically from the uterus wall.

may be used to evacuate the contents of the uterus: suction, vacuum aspiration, or either of those combined with curettage, in which the uterine lining is gently scraped.

A non-surgical abortion involves the use of drugs to terminate a pregnancy before the ninth week. Mifepristone, known more commonly as RU-486, is taken in combination with contraction-inducing chemicals known as prostaglandins. Sometimes, however, this method is unsuccessful and must be followed by a conventional suction curettage.

Second Trimester. Most abortions are performed before the 13th week of pregnancy. During the second trimester, abortion becomes more complicated and carries a higher risk of complications. Second-trimester abortions can be performed by dilatation and evacuation, but the procedure takes longer and almost always requires anesthesia.

After the 16th week, saline or prostaglandins can be injected into the amniotic sac. Saline causes fetal death and stimulates mild contractions. Prostaglandins result in stronger contractions. The woman then undergoes labor and delivery. Prostaglandins can also be administered vaginally to induce abortion.

AFTER THE ABORTION

Some women may receive medication to control bleeding and help the uterus contract. The patient may feel cramps for a few days afterward and may also be more tired than usual. Regular activities can be resumed almost immediately, but more strenuous pursuits should be delayed for a few weeks.

After a late second-trimester abortion, the breasts may start producing milk, as they normally would after childbirth. The milk will dry up within a few weeks. In the meantime, ice packs and a firm supportive bra can alleviate discomfort.

LONG-TERM PROGNOSIS

Provided that there were no complications or postoperative infections, a previous abortion should not impair a woman's ability to carry a pregnancy to term.

When Contemplating Abortion

No one should have to decide all alone whether or not to have an abortion. For some, hearing the opinions of family, friends, or clergy is essential for the best possible outcome; others may feel they have no one to turn to for advice, or that they need a fresh perspective from someone who is not a friend or family member. Counselors at the National Abortion Federation Hotline (1-800-772-9100) are trained to listen, advise, and help. The number is toll-free and callers need not give their name, age or any other personal information.

Making the decision requires knowing your state's abortion laws. Some state laws restrict abortions after the 12th week of pregnancy.

In addition to any physical discomfort or pain, aborting a fetus for whatever reason can be emotionally traumatic. Ambivalence and grief are often part of the recovery process. Patients should give themselves time to cope, lean on able friends or family, or consult a trained counselor or psychotherapist.

Anatomical information on reproduction may be found in EMBRYO; FEMALE; *and* REPRODUCTION SYSTEM, FEMALE. *For more information on abortion procedures, see* ABORTIFACIENT; *and* INTRAUTERINE GROWTH RETARDATION. *Counseling issues are discussed in* BIRTH DEFECTS; FAMILY THERAPY; INCEST; PREGNANCY COUNSELING; *and* SAFE SEX.

Resources on Abortion
Stotland, Nada Logan, *Facts and Feelings: A Handbook for Women and the People who Care about Them* (1998); Sears, William, et al., *The Pregnancy Book* (1997); Maternity Center Association, Tel. (212) 777-5000, Online: www.materni ty.org; www.nycornell.org/obgyn/.

Abrasion, Dental

Rubbing or scratching that causes erosion of outer layers of tooth.

Dental abrasion arises when the covering of the tooth is worn away (especially the enamel, the outermost layer, but also the dentin and cementum). Areas around the base and front of the two pointed teeth (canines) and the two grinding teeth just behind (premolars) are most often affected. One of the most common causes of dental abrasion is brushing too vigorously or using a toothbrush with hard bristles.

Dental abrasion can cause sensitivity and pain, particularly upon chewing or exposure to cold or hot foods and liquids. The gums may recede, resulting in increased sensitivity, as well as an appearance of abnormally large teeth.

Abrasion is treated with a desensitizing dentifrice, bonding, or filling. To prevent abrasion, brush with a soft toothbrush in a circular motion to loosen food and plaque, then in an up-and-down motion to brush away residue, rather than from side to side. *See also* BONDING; DENTIFRICE; FILLING; GUMS; PLAQUE; *and* TEETH.

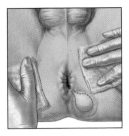

Anal Abscess. An abscess just under the skin will form a tender, painful lump. It may rupture naturally, or a doctor may drain it, clean it and possibly prescribe antibiotics.

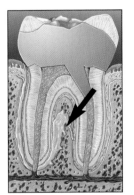

Dental Abscess. An abscess in a tooth causes sensitivity and pain upon chewing. If untreated, it may rupture, further damage the tooth, and possibly spread to the bloodstream. If a tooth abscess is suspected, it is best to see a dentist

Abscess

A pocket of pus, usually the result of a localized bacterial infection.

When bacteria invade a part of the body, the immune system sends white blood cells to destroy them. Over time, an accumulation of dead white blood cells, dead bacteria and other cells destroyed by the bacteria forms a pocket of pus. The body builds a wall around the pus to keep it contained, creating an abscess. If the abscess ruptures, the bacterial infection may destroy nearby tissue and spread to other tissues, organs, or the bloodstream.

SYMPTOMS

Symptoms of abscess include extreme sensitivity, swelling, redness, and fever. Blood tests may show a high white blood cell count. If the abscess is near the skin, a noticeable lump will appear. If the abscess is in a tooth, sensitivity and pain upon biting or chewing may occur. An abscess in the brain may cause headaches, loss of sensation, or seizures.

If the abscess is deep in the body it may produce no symptoms and may grow very large undetected. Recent advances in the development of x-ray machines, such as Computerized Transaxial Tomography (CTT or CAT), ultrasound, and Magnetic Resonance Imaging (MRI) can reveal the abscess, but it will have the same appearance as a tumor, so a biopsy with cultures and pathology is often necessary.

TREATMENT

If an abscess is near the skin it will usually rupture, expel its contents, and heal naturally. If the pain is intense, a physician may puncture the wall of the abscess to drain its contents. Antibiotics may be prescribed to protect against infection, particularly if the abscess ruptures internally. If the abscess is deep in the body, a radiologically guided drainage procedure may be performed using indwelling drainage tubes. Occasionally, the abscess must be drained surgically. *See also* ANTIBIOTIC DRUGS *and* BLOOD CELLS.

Acanthosis Nigricans

A disorder in which skin on the back, the sides of the neck, under the arms, or in the groin thickens and becomes darker.

Skin affected by acanthosis nigricans may have a rough or velvety texture, can vary from gray to black, and may itch. Acanthosis nigricans can occur at any age.

CAUSES AND TREATMENT

Acanthosis nigricans may be of unknown cause, or it may be associated with malignant disease, various endocrine disorders, obesity, or side effects of certain drugs. Treatment involves correcting any underlying causes, if possible. Medications such as Retin-A may cause some improvement in the appearance of affected areas. *See also* PIGMENTATION *and* SKIN.

Access to Care

The ability of an individual to obtain medical care when it is needed.

Access to care measures the ability of an individual to obtain satisfactory health care. The determinants of access are many, including financial, technological, and geographic factors.

Access to care has two main components, process and outcome. Process refers to the procedural aspects of obtaining care, such as whether or not a facility is available, how difficult it is to schedule an appointment, etc. Outcome refers to the care received. This includes aspects such as whether care was actually obtained, how long it took, and the quality of care.

In the United States, socioeconomic factors play a major role in determining access to care. The ability to obtain adequate health insurance is an important factor. Forty million Americans have no health insurance. In addition, poverty, unemployment, and location also affect access to care. *See also* HEALTH INSURANCE; HEALTH MAINTENANCE ORGANIZATION; HOSPITALS; MEDICADE; *and* PUBLIC HEALTH.

Accidents

Unexpected and undesirable events, often resulting in injury.

Many accidents are preventable. For instance, helmets, shatterproof lenses and other protective equipment is available for activities from biking to woodworking. Utilizing safety measures that can be easily implemented while driving, in the workplace, and at home is very important.

QUESTIONS TO ASK

Some general questions important in assessing the severity of an accident include:

• **Is the victim breathing?** Are the air passages clear? If a victim is not breathing, artificial respiration may be necessary.

• **Is the victim's heart beating?** Is there a pulse? If the victim is unconscious and there is no easily detectable pulse, cardiopulmonary resuscitation (CPR) should be performed.

• **Is the victim bleeding?** A pressure pad on the site of the bleeding—not a tourniquet above it—should be used to control blood loss. In cases involving a broken bone or a foreign object embedded in the wound, pressure may not be advisable.

• **Is the victim fully conscious?** Are there obvious causes for loss of consciousness, such as injury or drug overdose?

In the case of a serious accident, trained emergency personnel should be called immediately. If the victim appears to be suffering from shock, the best course is generally to try to keep the person warm, without attempting to move the victim.

Accidents in the Home

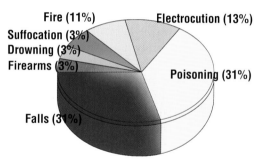

Fire (11%)
Electrocution (13%)
Suffocation (3%)
Drowning (3%)
Firearms (3%)
Poisoning (31%)
Falls (31%)

Keeping Children Safe

In the home. Store all cleaners, chemicals, medicines, appliances, and matches out of children's reach or in locked cabinets. Cap or tape over unused electrical outlets. Use only shatterproof glass for doors or tabletops and safety locks on windows. Install safety gates in front of stairways.

In the car. Use weight-specific child car seats; never acquire one second-hand. Never put a child in a seat with an airbag. Keep windows closed.

Outdoors. Children should cross streets with adults. Never leave children alone near water; warn them against eating berries; teach them not to talk to strangers; and help them memorize their address and telephone number.

TYPES OF ACCIDENTS

Burns. Fire, hot water, chemicals, and electricity all can cause burns. Second and third-degree burns must be treated by medical personnel. Minor burns with unbroken skin should be immersed in cool water, cleaned carefully with soap and warm water, and covered lightly by gauze. If the skin is blistered and broken, immediately contact a physician.

Electrical Injuries. It is crucial to disconnect the source of electricity without endangering the rescuer. Use a nonconductive material, such as wood or plastic, to separate the current-carrying conductor from the victim. Treat for burn or shock.

Drowning. Water damage to the lungs and lack of oxygen are two of the most serious dangers in drowning. Time under water, the temperature of the water, whether it is salt or fresh, and the age of the victim all may affect the likelihood of recovery. CPR may be necessary.

Poisoning. A general approach, coupled with identifying the toxic substance, is the best approach for successful treatment. Do not induce vomiting without advice from a physician or assistance from a regional poison control center.

> *Background material on safety may be found in* AUTOMOBILE SAFETY; HEALTH HAZARDS, PUBLIC; *and* WATER SAFETY. *Further information regarding types of accidents may be found in* BURNS; ELECTRICAL INJURY; EYE EMERGENCY; *and* SHOCK.

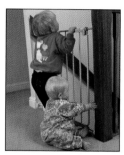

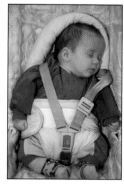

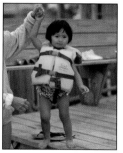

Safety Devices. Adults must be certain that children under their supervision are protected from injury by such measures as guard rails for stairs (top); car seats for travel in cars or any other conveyance (middle); and life jackets for swimming, boating, or any activity near water.

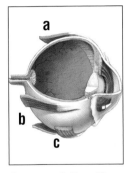

Accommodation. The Mechanism that allows the eye to focus on distant objects is among the most sensitive and sophisticated in nature. The muscles that manipulate the shape of the eye include: the superior rectus (a); the medial rectus (b); the inferior rectus (c); and the lateral rectus (on the far side of the eye).

Accommodation

Adjustment of the lens of the eye to see objects at different distances.

Accommodation is the process by which the lens of the eye is able to automatically change to enable both distant and near vision. When the eye is at rest, the lens is flat, thin, and focused for distance vision. In order to focus on a nearby object, the ciliary muscle contracts, and the lens becomes thicker and more convex.

With age, the lens becomes less elastic and cannot change shape as rapidly or as much. As a result, older people have difficulty refocusing the eye from distant to near objects, resulting in an inability to focus on close objects (presbyopia). *See also* MYOPIA *and* PRESBYOPIA.

Accreditation

The process of certifying, usually by a national review board, that an institution meets certain predefined standards.

Many medical institutions, including hospitals and medical schools, must undergo a process of accreditation, in which an official review board certifies that the institutions meets predefined standards.

The accreditation process provides important information indicating that the hospital has procedures in place to assume adequate physical plants, safety regulations, and quality services.

The Liaison Committee on Medical Education accredits medical schools in the United States. Accreditation allows enrolled students to qualify for federal loans and take licensing exams to practice clinical medicine.

The National Joint Commission on the Accreditation of Healthcare Organizations establishes hospital standards and accredits American hospitals. Residency programs and physicians also undergo an accreditation process in the United States. *See also* BOARD CERTIFICATION; CERTIFICATION; HOSPITALS; PHYSICIANS; *and* SPECIALISTS.

Acetic Acid

Clear, pungent liquid with many uses in medicine and industry.

Acetic acid is used in the manufacturing of dyes, plastics, photographic chemicals, insecticides, and cellulose acetates. Pharmaceutical uses include vaginal jellies and solutions for treating ear infections. In developing countries where the cost of routine cervical cancer screening is prohibitive, acetic acid is used to swab the cervix, which makes precancerous changes more visible to the naked eye.

Achalasia

Impairment of the ability of the esophagus to move food to the stomach, resulting in difficulty swallowing, as well as pain and regurgitation after eating.

In achalasia, the wave-like motion of the esophagus is reduced; the lower esophageal sphincter spasms and does not relax. Causes include heredity, nerve damage, and infection. Treatment involves dilating the esophagus with either a balloon catheter, a series of graduated cylinders (bougies), or the prescription of nitrates, calcium channel blockers, or botulinum toxin. *See also* ESOPHAGEAL DILATATION.

Achlorhydria

The absence of hydrochloric acid in the stomach's digestive juices.

Hydrochloric acid contributes to the acidity of the digestive juices and aids in the digestion of proteins. Generally, achlorhydria causes no symptoms and remains undiagnosed. A lack of hydrochloric acid may affect the absorption of vitamin B_{12} and may contribute to food sensitivities. It may be associated with pernicious anemia, advanced age, or the presence of a gastric ulcer, with the latter indicating an increased probability of stomach cancer. Specific treatment is not necessary unless it is accompanied by another condition.

Achondroplasia

Formerly known as dwarfism

Shortness of stature due to a bone growth disorder.

Caused by a single gene, achondroplasia is characterized by shortened limbs, especially in the upper arms and thighs. Other bones in the body reach a normal length. The symptoms of achondroplasia are apparent at birth; they include short limbs, a prominent forehead, and an arched back. People born with achondroplasia have a 50 percent chance of passing the gene to their children, but it can also occur spontaneously.

Acid Reflux

Also known as gastroesophageal reflux

Regurgitation of the stomach contents into the esophagus.

Acid reflux occurs when the lower esophageal sphincter relaxes, allowing acidic material from the stomach into the esophagus. About 10 percent of adults experience reflux once a week; one in three once a month. Nearly 25 percent of pregnant women experience acid reflux daily. Many babies are born with an incomplete lower esophageal sphincter, which results in the "spitting up" often seen in infants. The sphincter usually matures by 12 months.

SYMPTOMS

The most common symptom of acid reflux is heartburn, a burning in the chest that occurs because the esophagus does not have the stomach's protective lining. Heartburn usually occurs after meals or while lying down; it may be accompanied by vomiting or excess salivation.

COMPLICATIONS

Infrequent acid reflux is not dangerous. Frequent reflux may lead to inflammation of the esophageal lining, which may make swallowing painful and difficult and may cause ulcers or bleeding. It may also lead to Barrett's esophagus, a condition that is characterized by precancerous changes to the lining of the esophagus. Infants may develop pneumonia from the aspiration of the stomach contents into the lungs.

TREATMENT

Liquid antacids can alleviate heartburn. Acid production can be blocked by various medications such as cimetidine, ranitidine, famotidine, and omeprazole. The esophageal sphincter can be strengthened with drugs such as bethanechol and metoclopramide. Surgery for very severe cases of acid reflux involves a procedure called fundolication, which creates a high pressure zone in the lower esophagus to prevent reflux. *See* BARRETT'S ESOPHAGUS; DIGESTIVE SYSTEM; ESOPHAGUS; *and* ULCER.

Treating Heartburn

Acid reflux can be minimized through fairly simple lifestyle changes, such as:
- Avoiding foods that trigger reflux. These may in clude spicy, acidic , and high-fat foods, such as tomatoes, chocolate, caffeine, and alcohol.
- Stopping smoking.
- Maintaining a healthy weight.
- Eating smaller portions.
- Avoiding lying down immediately after eating.
- Sleeping with the head slightly elevated.

Acidosis

An overacidity of body fluids.

Fluids in the body are either acidic or alkaline. In order for the the body to operate healthily, there must be a balance between these two substances. Acidosis occurs when there are too many acids or too few alkalis in the blood. This may happen as a result of errors in how the body processes food into energy or an impairment in breathing, which causes a build-up of carbonic acid.

Symptoms of mild acidosis include fatigue, nausea and vomiting, and headache. In severe acidosis, blood pressure drops, resulting in shock, coma, or even death.

Treatment involves diagnosing and treating the underlying cause. In emergency situations, dialysis or treating the blood with bicarbonates may be necessary. *See also* KETOSIS *and* ALKALOSIS.

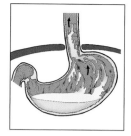

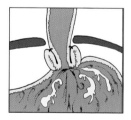

Acid reflux, above, results when the lower esophageal sphincter muscle fails to keep gastric juices in the high-pressure area of the stomach, allowing acid into the esophagus. A surgical procedure called **fundoplication** (below) can be used to treat the disease and relive the discomfort of heartburn. The procedure involves folding the stomach lining so as to reinforce the barrier between the esophagus and the stomach.

Acne

Also known as acne vulgaris, cystic acne, and pimples

An inflammatory skin condition characterized by superficial skin eruptions that are caused by clogged skin pores.

Acne is caused when the lubricating (sebaceous) glands in the skin pores become plugged when secretion occurs faster than oil and skin cells can leave the pores.

Acne occurs in males and females of all ages and seems to run in families. However, adolescent boys are the most affected segment of the population. Acne usually begins in puberty and may persist through the 30s and 40s. Three out of four teenagers have some degree of acne, but most cases clear up by adulthood.

Acne is not caused by eating fatty foods or chocolate, contrary to popular opinion. However, dirt and oil on the face may aggravate existing breakouts. Other factors that increase the chances of acne developing are hormonal changes, stress, weather extremes, endocrine disorders, certain tumors, and hormones such as cortisone, testosterone, progestersone, and estrogen.

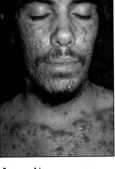

Acne. Above, severe acne on the face and chest. Though commonly associated with adolescence, acne can afflict adults at any age.

How Acne Forms. Acne results from the accumulation of oil (sebum), bacteria, and the pigment that gives skin its color (called melanin). The excess material builds up around the hair follicle as a pimple, until it bursts through the skin, creating a blackhead.

Resources on Acne

Chu, Tony C., *The Good Skin Doctor* (1999); Turkington, Carol A. and Jeffrey S. Dover, *Skin Deep : An A-Z of Skin Disorders, Treatments and Health* (1998); National Psoriasis Foundation, Tel. (800) 723-9166, Online: www.psoriasis.org; www.nycornell.org/dermatology/.

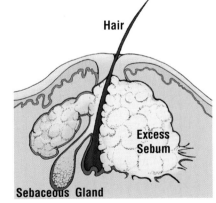

Hair

Excess Sebum

Sebaceous Gland

SYMPTOMS

Symptoms of acne include skin rash, whiteheads, blackheads, pustules, cysts, redness, inflammation, and scarring. Acne normally appears on the face and shoulders, but may also occur on the trunk, arms, and legs.

When clogged skin causes the follicle to bulge, whiteheads develop. When the top of the follicle darkens, blackheads occur. If the plug causes the wall of the follicle to rupture, the oil and bacteria that are nor-

mally found on the skin can enter and form infected areas, called pustules. If these infected areas are deep within the skin, they may enlarge and form cysts. A cyst develops when the sebaceous glands keep producing oil, and the lining of the pore grows and produces dead cells and debris. Instead of rupturing, the hair follicle enlarges and forms a firm lump under the skin. Cysts are normally not painful.

Home Remedies for Acne

Home treatment of acne may lessen its effects. Skin should be washed with soap and water at least once or twice a day. Hands should be washed before and after treatment of the outbreak. Touching or rubbing acne aggravates the condition and should be avoided, as should oil-based lotions and cosmetics.

TREATMENT

There are numerous treatments for acne, aimed at preventing new acne and healing old skin eruptions. Topical medications, including those that contain benzoyl peroxide, sulfur, resorcinol, tretinoin, and retinoic acid, may dry excess oil and promote healing. Antibiotics such as tetracycline or erythromycin may be prescribed, as they kill bacteria in the pores and have antiinflammatory properties. Synthetic vitamin A analogues are used to control severe cases. Cortisone may also be used. Surgical methods of treating acne include chemical skin peeling, dermabrasion, and removal and drainage of cysts.

Oral tetracycline is usually not prescribed for children until they have all of their permanent teeth, as it can permanently discolor teeth that are still forming.

Acne is a chronic condition that will eventually lessen. Uncomplicated acne is not dangerous. Untreated, severe acne can result in scarring. Complications can include cysts, skin abscesses, skin pigment changes, and psychological damage.

Basic information on skin anatomy may be found in CYST; DERMATOLOGY; FOLLICLE; *and* HAIR. *More information on skin care is contained in* CHAPPED SKIN; DRY SKIN; HIVES; MOLE; *and* RASH. *Related material on dealing with acne is found in* ADOLESCENCE; BIRTHMARK; *and* SCAR.

Acoustic Nerve

Also known as auditory nerve

The nerve that conducts sound impulses from the ear to the brain.

The acoustic nerve, a sensory nerve, is part of the vestibulocochlear nerve. It contains the cochlear nerve, which transmits sound impulses from the cochlea, a snail-shaped part of the inner ear, to the brain, where the nerve impulses are perceived as sounds. *See also* AUDITORY NERVE; EAR; HEARING; NERVE; *and* NERVOUS SYSTEM.

Acoustic Neuroma

A benign tumor surrounding the acoustic nerve.

Acoustic neuromas originate in the supporting cells of the eighth cranial nerve. They extend into the skull where the nerve enters into the inner ear (auditory meatus). Acoustic neuromas are rare, accounting for five to seven percent of all brain tumors. They are more common in women and between the ages of 40 and 60.

SYMPTOMS
Acoustic neuromas may put pressure on nearby nerves, leading to discomfort, hearing loss, dizziness, ringing in the ear (tinnitus), and loss of balance (ataxia). If the tumor continues to grow, it may reach the fifth cranial nerve (the facial nerve), causing severe facial pain. It can also spread to the sixth cranial nerve, causing double vision.

DIAGNOSIS
Diagnosis is based on hearing tests, balance tests, CT scanning, MRI, and auditory brain stem response, a test that analyzes the nerve impulses traveling to the brain.

TREATMENT
Surgeons can perform microsurgery to remove small tumors very close to the facial nerve. Larger tumors may require more comprehensive surgery. After surgery, some patients may experience additional hearing loss or facial numbness due to damage to nearby nerves. *See also* BRAIN TUMORS.

Acrocyanosis

A condition causing chronic blue coloring of the hands or, less frequently, the feet, particularly upon exposure to cold.

Acrocyanosis is thought to be caused by constriction of arteries that take blood to the extremities; it is not related to diseases of the arterial walls. It is more prevalent among women than among men. Acrocyanosis is painless, but sufferers complain of coldness, excessive sweating, and swelling of the hands or feet. Heat seems to relieve the symptoms; cold exacerbates them. The pulse is normal, and there is no concomitant damage to the skin. To date, there is no effective treatment. *See* CIRCULATION.

Acrodermatitis Enteropathica

Also known as Danbolt-Closs and Brandt syndromes

A disorder resulting from a zinc deficiency.

Acrodermatitis enteropathica can be caused either by a lack of zinc in the diet or by the body's inability to absorb it properly.

Symptoms of acrodermatitis enteropathica appear in infancy immediately following weaning. They include a characteristic scaling of the skin (psoriasisform dermatitis), hair loss, infection around the edge of a finger or toenail (paronychia), diarrhea, and growth retardation.

Diagnosis is based on the symptoms, and the disorder is easily treated with oral zinc supplements. *See* NUTRITION *and* ZINC.

Acromegaly

A hormonal disorder that causes excessive growth of the skull, jaws, hands, and feet.

The pituitary gland, located at the base of the brain, is responsible for, among other functions, the release of growth hormone. Excessive secretion of this hormone, as may be caused by a benign tumor in the gland, can lead to growth disorders. If this type of tumor occurs before a person reaches puberty, the result may be gigantism, or excessive growth. If the tumor appears

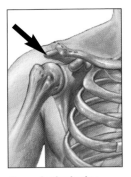

Acromioclavicular joint, beneath the muscle connecting the collar bone and the shoulder blade.

later in life, the result may be acromegaly.

Symptoms. Symptoms of acromegaly include enlarged hands and feet and a broadened or elongated face. The ears, nose, and jaw may grow bigger. The voice may deepen. Headaches or vision problems may also occur.

Diagnosis may be made through hormone testing procedures, as well as a CT scan or MRI to locate the tumor. Once the tumor is diagnosed, treatment options may include removal through surgery, radiation therapy, and drugs that will shrink the size of the tumor. *See also* CAT SCAN; GROWTH HORMONE; HORMONES; GIGANTISM; GLANDS; PITUITARY GLAND; PITUITARY TUMORS; SKELETON; SKULL; *and* TUMOR.

Acromioclavicular Joint

The joint between the end of the collarbone and the bony top of the shoulder blade called the acromion.

Injuries to the acromioclavicular joint, though rare, are often caused by a fall and direct impact on the shoulder. Usually, injuries result in a partial dislocation (subluxation). The joint becomes inflamed, the ligaments and joint lining become stretched and bruised, and the bones feel misaligned. In the rare event of total dislocation, the ligaments are torn, the inflammation is more severe, and the bones are noticeably out of joint. In either partial or full dislocation, symptoms include pain, tenderness, and restricted movement.

Treatment for subluxation is rest and immobilization of the shoulder in a sling, plus a corticosteroid injection and local anesthetic if pain persists. Complete dislocation requires a strap around the collarbone (clavicle) and elbow to force the clavicle back into place. The strap is removed after three weeks. Successive injuries can cause the joint to degenerate and can result in osteoarthritis, a chronic inflammation of the joint that makes movement painful. *See also* DISLOCATION, JOINT *and* JOINT.

ACTH
Abbreviation for adrenocorticotrophic hormone

A hormone produced by the pituitary gland that directs the release of hormones from the adrenal gland.

Adrenocorticotropic hormone is one of the hormones secreted by the pituitary gland. ACTH causes the outer layer of the adrenal gland (the adrenal cortex) to secrete the corticosteroid hormones, hydrocortisone and corticosterone. These hormones combat tissue damage caused by inflammation and influence glucose, fat, and protein metabolism in almost every area of the body.

ACTH production can increase in response to stress, intense emotion, injury, infection, or a drop in blood pressure. This increase leads to greater production of corticosteroids, which then affects the immune system and other functions.

Usually, an increase in levels of corticosteroids triggers a drop in ACTH production, and vice versa, thus keeping an overall balance of the hormones in the body. However, sometimes a disorder may cause a chronic overproduction or underproduction of ACTH.

Overproduction. Overproduction of ACTH may be caused by a tumor in the pituitary gland. This leads to a condition known as Cushing's syndrome, characterized by a rounded face, humped upper back, weakened bones, weakened immune system, and psychological changes. This can be treated by removing the tumor with surgery or radiation. *See also* CUSHING'S SYNDROME.

Underproduction. ACTH levels may become too low if the pituitary gland is not active enough. The result of this may be failure of the adrenal glands to produce glucocorticoids, which is characterized by fatigue, low blood pressure, low blood sugar, and low tolerance for physical stress. *See also* ADRENAL FAILURE.

For background information on the role of ACTH in bodily functions, see ADRENAL GLAND; HORMONES; PITUITARY GLAND; *and* PITUITARY TUMORS.

Acting Out

Expressing a feeling, wish, fantasy, or memory through behavior rather than acknowledgement.

Older children and teenagers may act out for reasons ranging from seeking independence to responding to abuse.

In the context of psychotherapy, acting out refers to a situation in which a patient's behavior is used to express feelings, memories, or conflicts that cannot be acknowledged or put into words.

In its broadest sense, acting out refers to any situation in which a person's behavior serves to express fears, imaginings, feelings, memories, or fantasies and may be self destructive.

A person who continuously quits jobs or leaves relationships may be using behaviors to express unconscious fears of success or inadequacy. The most serious forms of acting out include substance abuse, delinquency, and self mutilation.

Examining these behaviors in psychotherapy may provide valuable information about the patient's inner life. *See* ADOLESCENCE *and* CHILD BEHAVIOR.

Actinic

Sun-induced—used to refer to skin changes.

Sunlight may cause cancerous and precancerous skin conditions, especially in individuals with fair complexions. Sunlight plays a key role in the development of basal cell carcinoma, the most common form of skin cancer. Actinic keratosis, a precancerous skin thickening caused by sun exposure, can lead to squamous cell carcinoma, one of the three most common forms of skin cancer. Sunlight exposure is also believed to be an important factor in the development of malignant melanoma, the most deadly form of skin cancer. Exposure to sunlight is also the major factor contributing to wrinkles and brown spots, changes recognized as aging of the skin.

Prevention. To avoid excessive sun exposure, protective clothing should be worn, such as hats, long-sleeved shirts, or pants. Exposure to the sun at midday, when the sun's rays are the most direct, should be avoided. A sunscreen with an SPF of 15 or higher should be used regularly. *See also* CANCER *and* SKIN.

Actinomycosis

Infection caused by *Actinomyces israelii* bacteria.

Actinomyces israelii bacteria commonly can be found in the nose and throat, where they do not cause disease. Rarely, injury may allow them to penetrate under the skin, where they multiply and create an infection.

Types. There are four types of actinomycosis. depending on where the bacteria grow. The cervicofacial form; which is most common, affects the face; the thoracic form affects the lungs; the abdominal form affects the gastrointestinal tract; and the generalized form affects many organs.

Symptoms. Infection on the face is characterized by hard, reddish lumps (abscesses), usually along the jaw, that eventually rupture and drain through the skin. In other types, lumps also form and may also result in a draining cavity. Pulmonary actinomycosis is accompanied by cough.

The cervicofacial form is the most easily treated, but all types of the disease require months of treatment with antibiotics, including penicillin, erythromycin, or tetracycline. Surgical drainage of the abscesses caused by the disease may also be necessary. *See also* ABSCESS *and* ANTIBIOTIC DRUGS.

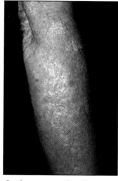

Actinomycosis. Arm tumors associated with actinomycosis are generally treated by a long regimen of antibiotics.

Acupressure

An ancient Chinese technique in which pressure is applied to the body for the purpose of alleviating pain or treating other symptoms and maladies.

Like acupuncture, the technique of acupressure developed out of the ancient Chinese view that applying pressure on parts of the body can improve the functioning of internal organs. This view differs significantly from that of Western medicine, although Chinese physicians often call upon both bodies of knowledge in their work.

The theory (in simple terms) behind acupressure is that the body requires a free flow of its life force energy—known as ch'i (pronounced "chee")—to function properly. Ch'i travels through the body in channels known as meridians, which surface at several key points on the body. Constriction of muscles and consequent pressure on organs and body fluids disrupts the natural balance and flow of ch'i through the body. This disruption is believed to result in a number of symptoms and diseases. Applying pressure on the meridians is believed to "unclog" the passageways and allow the body to naturally repair itself.

Acupressure may be applied by a professional acupressurist or be self-applied. The pressure may be applied by the fingertips or knuckles, or by a blunt-tipped instrument called a tei shin. A deep massage technique is applied to these points to stimulate and release the flow of energy.

The approach to physiology and medicine implied in acupressure is different from Western approaches. Meridians are not equated to nervous, lymphatic, or circulatory systems, or ch'i to blood, hormones, or nerve impulses. However, acupressure may stimulate the release of endorphins, the body's own pain killers.

Ch'i may be an appealing intuitive notion, but it is a very difficult concept to define or measure in the context of Western medicine. The wealth of practical experience gathered over centuries and the support of Western medicine indicates that acupressure techniques can be of great benefit for treating certain conditions.

Applications. Acupressure techniques have been used in the treatment of headaches, back pain, muscle pain and spasms, insomnia, and gastrointestinal and gynecological problems. In most cases there are no known risks associated with the procedure, but pregnant women should be aware that some acupressure techniques have been known to cause premature contractions. These techniques should be applied by a licensed acupres-

Acupuncture. The ancient art and science of acupuncture has been developed over centuries of practice and observation. At right, a chart over 600 years old of acupuncture points and meridians.

surist or at least under the supervision and guidance of a trained practitoner. *See also* ACUPUNCTURE; ALTERNATIVE MEDICINE; BODYWORK; CHINESE MEDICINE; SHIATSU; *and* THERAPEUTIC TOUCH.

Acupuncture

An ancient Chinese technique in which designated points on the body are stimulated by the insertion of needles, along with massage and the application of heat, for the purpose of treating specific ailments or inducing anesthesia.

Acupuncture came to wide Western attention in 1972 when a respected columnist for the *New York Times*, James Reston, traveling with President Nixon to China, was treated with acupuncture for the relief of postoperative pain following an emergency appendectomy. Although the techniques had been known in the West for well over a century and were respected, they were still part of an ill-understood medical tradition brought to the United States by Chinese

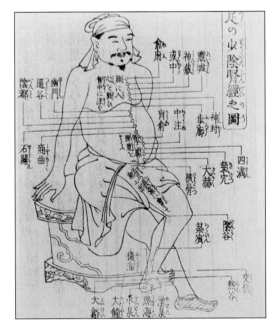

immigrants in the 1800s. Further interest was stimulated with Dr. Isadore Rosenfeld's reports in the late 1970s of witnessing Chinese doctors performing open heart surgery without western anesthesia, but with the benefit of acupuncture.

Theory. Acupuncture is embedded in the Chinese view of the human being and, ultimately, of the universe. While some of these ideas may be translated into approximations of traditional Western concepts, they are, in large part the product of a unique world view and a particular appreciation of the human body. For example, the ancient Chinese concept of ch'i (pronounced "chee") is often likened to the Western concept of energy. However, such a comparison is on shaky ground because it oversimplifies one of the most central ideas in the Chinese healing arts.

The human "circuitry" of ch'i through the body is comprised of twelve "meridians"—intangible lines that connect points into which the insertion of needles can alter the flow of ch'i and ameliorate certain conditions. One meridian, for example, relates to the stomach and runs from the top of the head to the soles of the feet. There are many acupuncture points along this meridian; great skill and a vast amount of training and experience is required to apply acupuncture technique effectively for a stomach ailment. The same is true for the meridian associated with the heart, which runs along the inner surface of the arm. There are 365 acupuncture points on the body; their exact location, however, often varies with individual body type.

Some believe that there may be a physical basis for the effectiveness of acupuncture. Many of the meridian points correspond to areas where nerves surface from a muscle or are located between a muscle and bone or between a bone and a joint. At these points, the nerves are believed to be particularly sensitive to stimulation provided from outside the body.

Technique. Needles ranging in diameter from a hair thickness to that of a sewing needle, are inserted directly into the skin. The skin and the needles are cleansed with alcohol before the treatment, and infection is rare. Needles should not be used for more than one patient unless they are thoroughly sterilized between uses.

The precise location of the needles and the angle at which they are inserted is de-

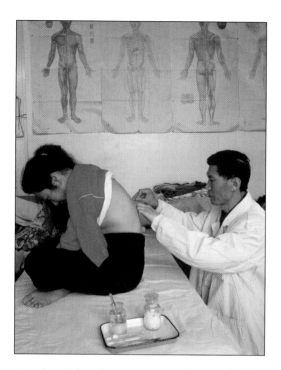

termined by the acupuncturist, as is the depth of penetration and the exact method of insertion. The needles may be inserted by a tapping motion or by a twirling motion. Typically, treatments are administered once a day for ten days, followed by a respite of three to seven days, following which they resume. Acupuncture thus requires a an instinctive feel for the patient and the way the body is responding to the therapy.

Applications. Acupuncture has been used to treat ailments as diverse as allergies, skin rashes, gastrointestinal disorders, muscular pains, and emotional and psychiatric disorders; it has often been applied as a way of controlling pain.

See ALTERNATIVE MEDICINE; CHINESE MEDICINE; HOLISTIC MEDICINE; *and* OSTEOPATHIC MEDICINE *a discussion of the foundations of acupuncture. More on alternative therapies is found in* BIOFEEDBACK; MANIPULATION; SHIATSU; *and* THERAPEUTIC TOUCH. *Details on pain management will be found in* ANESTHESIA; HYPNOTHERAPY; *and* PAIN.

Acupuncture in Practice. In the Far East, acupuncture is a routine element of medical practice. Acupuncturists appear no different from Western health practitioners and there is nothing especially "alternative" about this treatment in that culture. Below, a detail showing the many acupuncture points of the ear. A thoroughly trained acupuncturist will see the body in the same complexity as any Western trained health care professional.

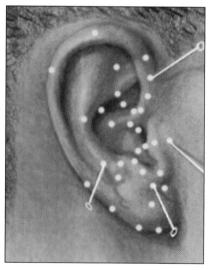

Resources on Acupuncture

Pizzorno, Joseph E., et al., *Clinician's Handbook of Natural Medicine* (2001); Wiseman, Nigel, *Fundamentals of Chinese Acupuncture* (1991); www.nycornell.org/ medicine/gim/index.html.

Addison's Disease

Condition caused by the underproduction of adrenocortical hormones.

The hormones hydrocortisone and aldosterone, secreted by the adrenal glands, help to control the use of the body's intake of fats, proteins and carbohydrates. The hormones also help maintain a balance of sodium and potassium. The rate and amount of hydrocortisone secreted are dictated by the hypothalamus and pituitary gland, found in the center of the brain. Aldosterone secretion is controlled by renin secreted by the kidney. When a disease affects the release of these hormones, the systems they operate can fail, causing the condition known as Addison's disease. The disease can either be chronic, in which the onset is slow and gradual, or acute, in which case adrenal crisis can be brought on by infection, injury, or stress; in these cases, the body is not able to produce the hormones necessary to handle a psysiologic stress.

CAUSES

The most common causes of Addison's disease are autoimmune disorders, in which the body's own immune system attacks itself. A less common cause of the disease is an infection that affects the adrenal glands, such as tuberculosis or fungal infections.

SYMPTOMS

Symptoms of Addison's disease include unexplained weight loss, weakness, fatigue, some abdominal pain, lightheadedness, and darkening of the skin on the palms, knees, elbows, and skin creases.

DIAGNOSIS

The symptoms are the primary clue for Addison's disease, as well as knowledge of any existing autoimmune conditions. Blood tests for the disease may not reveal any problems until symptoms become severe. At that point, tests may show a decrease in sodium, due to the low production of the hormone aldosterone, low blood glucose, or high potassium. Tests can determine whether the cause of the problem is located in the adrenal or the pituitary gland.

TREATMENT

Treatment should be aimed at the underlying cause, if possible. Hormonal replacement therapy is the most basic part of treatment, through daily doses of cortisone and sometimes flurocortisone. Self-treatment includes careful attention to fluid intake and replacement, especially after situations that cause extra loss of fluid, such as exercise or any minor illnesses that may cause vomiting or diarrhea. Addisonian crises—the severe condition brought on by adrenal failure—are emergencies that are treated through rapid infusions of saline solutions and hydrocortisone.

Information on adrenal functions may be found in ADRENAL GLANDS; ENDOCRINE SYSTEM; *and* HORMONES. *More on Addison's Disease is found in* ADRENAL FAILURE; AUTOIMMUNE DISORDERS; FUNGAL INFECTIONS; *and* TUBERCULOSIS. *See also* HASHIMOTO'S THYROIDITIS.

Adenitis

Also known as lymphadenitis

Swelling of a gland, especially of a lymph node.

Lymph, a milky body fluid that contains infection-fighting white blood cells called lymphocytes, flows outside blood vessels through intercellular spaces known collectively as the lymphatic system. Lymph nodes strain the lymph for viruses and bacteria. In doing so, the nodes nearest a site of infection often swell and become tender.

For example, streptococcal tonsillitis or mononucleosis affect the lymph glands in the neck, a condition called cervical adenitis. In mesenteric lymphadenitis, lymph glands in the membrane surrounding the intestines (peritoneum) swell.

Painkillers, hot compresses, and antibiotics are used to treat adenitis. Swelling can persist after the infection has been brought under control, but typically recedes in a few days. *See* BACTERIA; LYMPH NODES; TONSILLITIS *and* VIRUS.

Resources on Acupuncture

Greenspan, Francis S., *Basic & Clinical Endocrinology* (2000); Shin, Linda M., *Endocrine and Metabolic Disorders Sourcebook* (1998); www.nycornell. org/medicine/edm/index.html.

Adenoidectomy

A surgical procedure to remove the adenoids.

The adenoids, located in the upper throat (pharynx), may be surgically removed if they become too enlarged. Typically, the adenoids enlarge during early childhood and disappear by puberty. Oversized adenoids can cause recurring infections of the middle ear and sinuses, which, in turn, can impair hearing and language development. Often performed in with a tonsillectomy, the operation rarely has any complications, and the patient is usually allowed to eat the following day. *See also* THROAT.

Adenoma

Noncancerous tumor arising from epithelial tissue.

An adenoma is a benign growth in the tissue that lines the inner surface of a gland or organ (epithelium). An adenoma will not invade neighboring tissue, but it can grow enough to compress adjacent structures. While an adenoma is not malignant, it can cause problems. For example, an adenoma of an endocrine gland, which secretes a hormone into the blood stream, can cause overproduction of the hormone. An example is Cushing's syndrome, in which an adenoma of the pituitary gland causes an excess production of corticosteroid hormones. *See* CUSHING'S SYNDROME.

Adenomatosis

Overgrowth or tumors that affect the glands.

Adenomatosis is a general term used to describe overgrowth (hyperplasia) or the development of benign tumors on one or more of the endocrine glands. Glands that may be affected include the adrenal glands, pituitary gland, parathyroid glands, thyroid gland, and pancreas.

Tumors on a gland often cause excess secretion of that gland's hormones, which can lead to a variety of malfunctions in the systems run by those hormones. For example, a tumor on the parathyroid gland can cause overproduction of parathyroid hormone, which results in high calcium fatigue and weakened bones. A tumor of the pituitary gland might cause an overproduction of growth hormone, leading to accelerated growth in children or enlarging of the hands, feet, and face in adults. *See* ADRENAL TUMORS; HORMONES; PANCREAS; PARATHYROID TUMORS; PITUITARY TUMORS; THYROID TUMORS.

ADH

Acronym for antidiuretic hormone

Hormone that helps regulate the amount of water in the blood.

ADH is one of the hormones released by the pituitary gland. When the hypothalamus, a part of the brain that regulates the pituitary gland, detects an incorrect level of water in the body, it sends a message to the pituitary, which releases the amount of ADH needed to correct the situation.

Water is taken into the body every day through water, food, or chemical reactions in the cell. When water levels are too high and the blood becomes diluted, ADH production is reduced, and the kidneys act to dispose of the excess. Water is also constantly being lost—through urine, sweat, feces, and breath. When too much water has been lost production increases.

ADH disorders are caused by abnormalities in the hypothalamus, either inherited or due to tumors, infections, or other conditions. Some types of very rare tumors in the pituitary gland also cause excess secretion of ADH and lead to water retention. These can be treated with surgery or radiation. Diabetes insipidus can cause the pituitary gland to release too little ADH, resulting in excess production of urine. Alcohol can inhibit ADH secretion and results in excessive urine production. *See also* DIABETES INSIPIDUS *and* PITUITARY GLAND.

Adenoidectomy. The adenoids, when enlarged, can cause middle ear and sinus infections. The adenoids are generally removed with the tonsils.

Adipose Tissue

Specialized connective tissue, located just under the skin, that functions as the major storage site for fat.

Adipose tissue has three functions. It acts as heat insulation, a mechanical cushion to absorb shock, and a source of energy. Subcutaneous adipose tissue, found directly below the skin, is an important insulator. Fat is the major form of energy storage in the body and provides a buffer for energy imbalances if the body's intake differs from its output. Adipose tissue also surrounds and protects the body's internal organs. *See* METABOLISM *and* SKIN.

Adolescence

The period from the onset of sexual maturation until early adulthood, beginning in girls as early as eight and in boys as early as ten, and continuing until the late teen years.

Humans undergo remarkable changes in the years between childhood and adulthood. They develop adult bodies and begin to make adult decisions. Each person's experience of adolescence is unique, and the challenges an adolescent faces can range from terrifying to exhilarating. While there is no simple way for a teen's loved ones to make the process of adolescence easier, loving support, open communication, balance between flexibility and firmness, and setting a good example can help an adolescent learn to make healthy choices and reach adulthood prepared and balanced.

PHYSICAL CHANGES

Physically, adolescence begins with puberty, the onset of adult physical development. The timing of when a child's body begins to mature and the specific changes that occur are determined by several factors, including genetics, environment, nutrition, and overall health.

Boys. In boys, changes begin around the ages of 10 to13, when the testes and scrotum begin to grow, and pubic hair appears. Between ages 11 and 14, boys grow rapidly; the larynx enlarges, causing deepening of the voice accompanied by occasional "cracking." The sweat glands mature, causing sweat to have a stronger odor. By this time, teens should develop habits of bathing or showering regularly and may choose to use a deodorant.

Around ages 13 to 14, boys experience their first ejaculation (spermarche), as a result of masturbation or during sleep. In over half of boys, tenderness and swelling around the nipples occurs; this condition is normal and disappears within a few months to two years.

Following spermarche, pubic hair becomes darker, coarser and curlier, and the testes grow. The greatest growth spurt often occurs during this time. extremities enlarge, the voice deepens, and the body changes from a child to an adult form. Body and facial hair appear.

Boys usually reach adult physical development by age 17, although some continue to grow into their early twenties.

Girls. Adolescence begins earlier in girls than in boys—possibly as early as eight. The first noticeable changes are generally swelling and tenderness around the nipples and the development of pubic hair. Girls experience a dramatic growth spurt in the initial stages of adolescence. The hips broaden, and the percentage of body fat becomes higher. A clear or white odorless vaginal discharge may be noticed. The sweat glands mature, causing sweat to have a stronger odor. Girls should by this time develop habits of regular showering and may choose to use deodorant.

Between the ages of 10 and 16 girls experience their first menstruation (menarche). It may take several years for menstruation to become regular. Cramps may accompany menstruation. Non-asprin pain relievers help. If bleeding is heavy, painful or lasts for more than eight to 10 days, a doctor should be consulted.

After menarche, girls continue to grow and develop an adult body shape. Breasts grow for about four or five years after they first start to develop. Generally, physical development is complete by age 16 or 17.

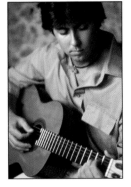

Coming of Age. As young people grow, their interests also mature—from toys to personal appearance; from cartoons to the arts and other more adult activities.

PSYCHOLOGICAL CHANGES

Adolescence is a time of great psychological and emotional growth. During this time, a teen begins to question what he or she had previously assumed, develops skills of abstract reasoning, and learns to make choices about how he or she wants to live.

Relationships with Family. During adolescence, an individual begins to transition from a child who identifies strongly with his or her family into an adult who has a sense of self-identity and self-reliance. This process varies greatly between individuals. Often the transition is not easy and can be confusing and even hurtful to both the adolescent and his or her family.

A young teenager often begins to rebel against family rules. This may be as minor as protesting a curfew or choosing clothing that parents think is inappropriate, or it may be dangerous, such as experimenting with drugs or alcohol. As an adolescent becomes older, he or she may start to question the family's values, such as religion and politics.

While adolescents need space to establish a separate identity, they are not always able to make mature decisions. Parents can help adolescents by maintaining a balance in rules—allowing harmless, if bizarre, behavior but providing firm, clear rules when the adolescent's health or safety could be at risk. Talking openly, honestly, and lovingly about any concerns an adolescent raises can help parents and teens make better informed and more reasonable decisions.

Relationships with Peers. While separating from their parents, adolescents often look to a peer group to provide support and role models. Adolescents are often concerned with fitting in and with being attractive to each other, and they may go to great lengths to do so.

Parents can monitor an adolescent's safety within a peer group by getting to know his or her friends and the families of those friends. Suddenly changing a peer group, stopping talking about or to friends, or any sudden change in mood or behavior can be warning signs that an adolescent is having problems with peers.

HEALTH AND SAFETY

During adolescence, teenagers establish many of the foundations of adult health, from hygiene to eating habits to exercise. Developing healthy patterns during this time is difficult—teenagers often are preoccupied with other issues—but can establish a basis for lifelong healthy practices.

It is particularly important for adolescents to eat well, sleep enough, and exercise. Adolescents tend to eat a lot of "junk" food and tend not to sleep enough. While some adolescents engage in sports, others lead very sedentary lifestyles.

Teens also begin to make choices about their safety. Motor vehicle accidents are the leading cause of death among adolescents. Teenagers may also make poor decisions about drugs and alcohol. While some experimentation is normal, teenagers are particularly vulnerable to developing substance dependence. For example, nearly all smokers begin smoking in their teens.

Parents can help adolescents make good decisions about health and safety by providing a good example and speaking frankly about possible consequences of their decisions.

ALERT

Adolescent Depression and Suicide

Suicide is the third leading cause of death among adolescents. Generally, teenagers commit suicide because they feel alone, overwhelmed, and trapped in a situation. Recognizing and speaking with an adolescent about these feelings can often help prevent this act of desperation. Counseling can also help a depressed teenager learn about and cope with his or her emotions.

Some signs of suicidal feelings include:
- Loss of interest in friendships, activities, or personal appearance.
- Sudden change in behavior or personality.
- Withdrawal and isolation.
- Substance abuse.
- Self-mutilation or violent behavior.
- Giving away possessions, saying good-bye to family and friends, or talking about suicide.

Never ignore an adolescent who talks or hints about committing suicide. Most adolescents who kill themselves give warning signals before acting.

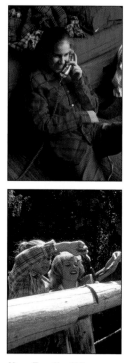

New Family. When children enter into their teen years, friends may replace family as their confidants and companions. While friendships between friends of the same gender remain important (bottom), an increased emphasis in intergender relations is seen (top).

Resources on Adolescence

Burg, Fredric D., ed., *The Treatment of Infants, Children, and Adolescents* (1990); Chan, Paul D., Family Medicine (2001); Goldstein, Mark A., and Myrna Chandler Goldstein, *Boys into Men: Staying Healthy through the Teen Years* (2000); www.nycornell. org/medicine/edm/index.html.

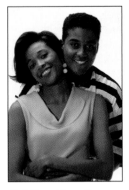

Relationships. Some teens struggle to mature emotionally, even though they have matured physically. Teens who receive strong peer and parental support will be able to better handle issues of safe sex and substance and sexual abuse.

ADOLESCENT SEXUALITY

One of the most complicated aspects of adolescence is sexuality. Teenagers become physically mature before they are emotionally able to handle sexual relationships. They may want or feel pressured to have sex for reasons ranging from their body's urges to peer pressure to simple curiosity.

The more a teenager knows about sex and his or her body, the more he or she will be able to make informed decisions. Adolescents who are not educated are less likely to have good reasons not to have sex and are more likely to engage in unsafe sexual practices. Teens who understand the development of their bodies, know about contraception and the risks of pregnancy and sexually transmitted diseases, and have discussed the emotional implications of having sex are more likely to be able to stand up for their beliefs and their safety.

Sexual Orientation. Especially in the early teen years, sexual experimentation with members of the same sex is common. This does not necessarily mean that a teenager is homosexual or bisexual; however, neither does it mean that he or she is not. People may be aware of their sexual identity from birth or may discover it later in life. Becoming aware of a homosexual or bisexual orientation can be difficult, and adolescents may be afraid to talk about it with friends and family members. Love and acceptance can go along way toward helping a teen accept and live healthily with his or her sexual identity.

Date Abuse. While most adolescent relationships are more or less healthy, adolescents—especially girls—may find themselves in relationships that are damaging, emotionally or physically. A boyfriend (or, more rarely, a girlfriend) is abusive if he is possessive, controlling, belittling, or violent, or if he tries to manipulate or force someone into engaging unwillingly in sexual activity. A person in an abusive relationship may be ashamed, believe that she somehow deserves the treatment, be afraid that the abusive person will hurt her if she talks, or fear that the adults in her life will not believe or support her.

For parents, warning signs of an abusive relationship may include a loss of interest in school or social activities, depression, a sudden or gradual drop in self-esteem, or seeing one boyfriend to the exclusion of all other friends. For a person who feels he or she is in an abusive relationship, it helps to talk to a parent or trusted adult. The phone book has numbers for domestic violence and rape crisis hotlines, which may be a safe way to discuss a situation and learn about options for changing it.

Basic physiological information on human development may be found in CHILD DEVELOPMENT; GROWTH; *and* PUBERTY. *Further information regarding adolescent health may be found in* ACNE *and* DEPRESSION.

Adrenal Glands

A pair of glands, located on top of the kidneys, that release hormones into the bloodstream.

The adrenal glands are each composed of two parts; the adrenal cortex and adrenal medulla. The adrenal cortex releases corticosteroids, which affect metabolism, some physical characteristics, and chemicals in the blood. The adrenal medulla releases epinephrine and norepinephrine, which help the body respond to stress.

As with many other glands, the adrenal glands release their hormones under the direction of the hypothalamus and pituitary gland, located in the center of the brain. The hypothalamus uses information from other parts of the body to trigger the pituitary gland to release adrenocorticotropic hormone (ACTH), which affects the timing and amount of hormones released by the adrenal glands.

ADRENAL CORTEX

The adrenal cortex is composed of three areas. The outer layer releases the hormone aldosterone, which regulates sodium levels in blood and urine. The amount of sodium affects blood volume and pressure. The inner and middle areas of the adrenal cortex produce androgens, hydrocortisone, and corticosterone. Androgens are responsible for developing some male sexual characteristics. Hydrocortisone combats damage caused by inflammation throughout the body. This hormone also influences some functions of the immune system.

Hydrocortisone is the hormone that has the greatest effect on the body's daily operations. It governs the way the body uses new nutrients and its stores of fats, proteins, and carbohydrates. The amount of hydrocortisone is directly controlled by secretion of ACTH. The levels of ACTH rise and fall through a daily cycle: the highest amount is produced in the early morning, then falls throughout the day until it reaches its lowest level at about midnight. Hydrocortisone levels follow those of ACTH. Stress or intense emotions can also affect the release of ACTH and hydrocortisone, which help the body manage and recover from stressful situations. If the level of hydrocortisone gets too high, then the release of ACTH is reduced, until balance is restored.

Adrenal Gland Disorders

Surplus or under-production of the adrenal hormones can occur because of several different disturbances; some are found in the following list.

• *Autoimmune disorder.* This disorder, in which the body attacks the adrenal gland, usually results in the reduced production of the adrenal hormones. A type of this disorder is called Addison's disease.
• *Congenital defects.* Birth defects of the adrenal glands usually result in the adrenal cortex being unable to produce enough hormones, which affects the baby's development.
• *Infection.* Infection can destroy the adrenal glands, causing a condition known as adrenal insufficiency. The most typical culprit was once tuberculosis, but that illness has been in decline. Autoimmunity is now the most common cause of adrenal insuffieiency.
• *Tumors.* Cancer in the adrenal glands is likely to cause overproduction of hormones. Tumors in the tiny glands are very difficult to detect, but they may be found by a CT scan, radionuclide scanning, a process which analyzes the amount of radioactive iodine taken in by the thyroid, or through specialized urine collection assays.

ADRENAL MEDULLA

The smaller interior region of the adrenal gland works in close association with nerve tissues. It releases two hormones, epinephrine and norepinephrine. The sympathetic nervous system, which controls involuntary responses, becomes activated during stress, fear or exertion. During these times, the nerves trigger the release of epinephrine and norepinephrine, which work to help the body handle stress. They increase heart rate, allowing more blood to work through the system. The blood flow is redistributed so that the muscles that operate some of the organs receive less blood, and more support is sent to the active, skeletal muscles. The hormones also work to increase lung capacity and make breathing easier by widening the airways.

ADRENAL FAILURE

In instances of damage to the adrenal gland itself or to the pituitary gland, the adrenal glands may be unable to produce enough steroid hormones, resulting in adrenal failure.

Over time, adrenal failure results in weakness, weight loss, and patchy darkening of the skin. People with adrenal failure are at risk for acute adrenal crisis, a sudden drop in blood pressure accompanied by weakness and dehydration, that can be triggered by injury, infection, or stress. If not treated immediately, this may lead to seizures, shock, or coma.

Adrenal failure is treated by administration of corticosteroids. Acute adrenal failure should be treated with an injection of hydrocortisone and intravenous glucose and saline solutions to treat the low blood pressure. Generally, people with Addison's disease or another form of adrenal failure learn to recognize possible trigger situations and give themselves an increased dose of hydrocortisone to ward off a crisis.

Background material on adrenal physiology may be found in BLOOD PRESSURE; ENDOCRINE SYSTEM; KIDNEYS; METABOLISM; *and* PITUITARY GLAND. *For additional material on adrenal hormones, see* ACTH; ANDROGEN; EPINEPHRINE; CORTICOSTEROID HORMONES; *and* NOREPINEPHRINE.

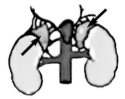

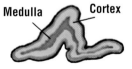

Adrenal Glands. Top, the adrenal glands (arrows) sit atop the kidneys, just one of the organs the hormones they secrete control. Bottom, the structure of the adrenal gland. The medulla secretes epinephrine and norepinephrine, which activates the autonomic nervous system, stimulating the heart in times of stress. The cortex produces corticosteroid hormones which affect metabolism and blood pressure.

Resources on Adrenal Glands

Nuland, Sherwin B., *The Wisdom of the Body* (1997); Greenspan, Francis S., et al., *Basic & Clinical Endocrinology* (2000); Shin, Linda M., et al., *Endocrine and Metabolic Disorders Sourcebook* (1998); www.nycornell. org/medicine/edm/index.html.

Adrenal Hyperplasia

A rare birth defect that causes underproduction of hydrocortisone and aldosterone and overproduction of androgen hormones.

Adrenal hyperplasia is usually caused by a genetic defect. It affects the hormones of the adrenal cortex: hydrocortisone, which directs the use of fats, proteins, and carbohydrate; aldosterone, which helps maintain sodium levels in the blood; and androgen hormones, which cause development of male sexual characteristics.

In adrenal hyperplasia, an enzyme necessary for making hydrocortisone is missing. This prevents the production of hydrocortisone, and the resources usually used to make that hormone are used instead to make androgens, creating an excess.

In the most extreme cases, what appear to be a penis and scrotum will be part of a female baby's anatomy, although signs of abnormality may not appear until puberty, when menstruation does not occur or is irregular with pronounced acne or body hair. Males may also be born with the condition, but their sexual organs appear normal; the condition may lead to early puberty. The loss of hydrocortisone and aldosterone can cause vomiting and dehydration. With hormone replacement therapy, normal development and fertility can occur. *See* ADRENAL GLANDS; ANDROGEN HORMONES; *and* CORTICOSTEROIDS.

Adrenal Tumors

Abnormal growths affecting the adrenal gland.

Adrenal tumors can be benign or cancerous. They may cause medical problems by increasing output of adrenal hormones. For example, excess hydrocortisone can cause Cushing's syndrome, while excess production of epinephrine and norepinephrine causes hypertension and sweating attacks. Adrenal tumors include pheochromocytoma and neuroblastoma. They are generally removed surgically. *See also* ADRENAL GLANDS *and* TUMORS.

Adrenalectomy, Laparopscopic

Surgical removal of the adrenal glands using a flexible tube known as a laparoscope.

A physician may decide to remove the adrenal glands if they become diseased or if the adrenal hormones exacerbate another illness, such as breast cancer. Laparoscopy is a minimally invasive surgical technique used to examine abdominal organs and perform minor surgery. A laparoscope is a rigid tube that contains fiberoptics, a video camera, and provides access for surgical instruments. Images from the camera are sent to a video monitor.

Procedure. The patient must fast for twelve hours prior to surgery. The surgeon makes four small (up to three-quarters of an inch) incisions in the side of the abdomen and inserts a laparoscope through an incision. Air is passed through the tube to inflate the abdominal cavity, and instruments are passed through the tube. The glands are located, removed, and put into a tiny pouch that is pulled out of an incision.

After Surgery. The patient may be discharged as soon as the next day or even hours after surgery, with a return to normal activity within one to two weeks. Oral supplements replace the hormones once provided by the adrenal glands.

Benefits. Laparoscopy avoids the need for long incisions across the abdomen and thus minimizes tissue damage. The risk of infection is reduced because of the decreased amount of time tissues are exposed to air. The average hospital stay is two to three days, as opposed to the five to seven days that previous, more highly invasive surgical techniques required.

Limitations. Laparoscopic removal is not appropriate for adrenal glands affected by cancerous tumors or that show characteristics of malignancy. Only benign tumors less than 10 centimeters in diameter qualify, since larger ones are more likely to be cancerous and are harder to view. *See also* ADRENAL TUMORS *and* LAPAROSCOPY.

Aerobics

Exercise in which the body is able to meet the muscles' increased need for oxygen while active at a level higher than normal.

Aerobic exercise is characterized by repetitive movement of muscles at submaximal intensity, but for sustained periods of time. During aerobic exercise, the energy for muscular contraction is released from body stores of fats and sugars that are burned in the presence of adequate levels of inspired oxygen. Aerobic exercise can be sustained when the oxygen requirements of the contracting muscles are matched by the available oxygen supply.

An aerobic exercise program can improve mobility, coordination, and strength for anyone, including the elderly. Aerobic exercise encourages the growth of capillaries, which improves the supply of blood to the cells. It also conditions the heart by slowing its rate during rest or exercise. Regular exercise can reduce the incidence of heart attack and lower high blood pressure. *See* ANAEROBIC; EXERCISE; *and* OXYGEN.

Aerodontalgia

Also known as dontalgia

A sudden and temporary pain in a tooth due to a change in air pressure.

Aerodontalgia occurs when the air pressure in the chamber housing the nerve of a tooth changes. It is common among pilots and divers because they are subjected to frequent and often rapid changes in air pressure. Underwater pressure can cause the chamber to contract, while the low air pressure of high alltitudes has the opposite effect. Both conditions are accompanied by considerable pain and irritation.

Aerodontalgia is usually the result of improper dental work, such as fillings or root-canal treatment, or inflammation of the pulp of the tooth Treatment consists of treating the pulpitis, possibly through antibiotics or a root canal, or by replacing damaged or ill-fitting fillings. *See* DENTISTRY.

Aerophagia

Swallowing air during the course of eating.

Small amounts of air are normally swallowed while eating. However, large amounts of swallowed air, which may be a result of anxiety or eating too quickly, may make a person feel full and lead to excessive belching or flatulence. *See* FLATULENCE.

Aflatoxin

Naturally occurring cancer-causing (carcinogenic) mixture of elements produced by the mold *Aspergillus flavus*.

Aflatoxin is a carcinogen that grows mainly on almonds, peanuts, cottonseed, and animal feed corn in hot, humid areas, where crops have been stored in damp places. Aflatoxin is a greater health threat in developing countries with fewer regulations than in the United States. Animal feed crops, however, are less strictly regulated, and meat and milk can become contaminated. *See also* CANCER *and* CARCINOGEN.

Afterbirth

Another name for the placenta.

During pregnancy, the placenta is attached to the wall of the uterus and serves as the filter through which the fetus receives blood, nutrients, and oxygen. After labor and delivery, it detaches from the uterine wall and is expelled through the vaginal canal, often referred to as the afterbirth. *See* CHILDBIRTH *and* PLACENTA.

Afterpains

Abdominal cramps occurring after labor.

After the delivery of a baby, uterine contractions continue as the uterus shrinks back to its pre-pregnant size. Occasionally, abdominal cramps accompany these contractions. They may intensify during breastfeeding. *See also* PREGNANCY.

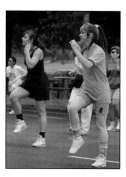

Aerobic Exercise. Low impact aerobics provides the benefit of exercise to the cardiovascular system without causing damage to bones and muscles. For many, the biggest hurdle is to find ways of making the exercise fun so the regimen will be one to which one may adhere.

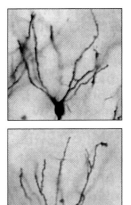

Cellular Memory Loss.
Brain cells produce and store memory by making connections with each other. Any time the brain is stimulated, the brain cells make new connections. Above, top, youthful nerves. Above, bottom, as the body ages these connections can break down unless they are properly stimulated; with this comes the onset of memory loss.

Resources on Aging

Hayflick, Leonard, *How and Why We Age* (1997); Medina, John J., *Clock of Ages* (1996); Schneider, Edward L. and John W. Rowe, *Handbook of the Biology of Aging* (1996); Weiss, Robert, et al., *Complete Guide to Health and Well-Being After Fifty* (1988); American Association of Retired Persons, Tel. (800) 424-3410, Online: www.aarp.org; American Geriatrics Society, Tel. (212) 308-1414, Online: www.americangeriatrics.org; National Council on Aging, Tel. (800) 424-9046, Online: www.ncoa.org; www.nycornell.org/medicine/geriatrics/index.html; www.cornellaging.org/.

Agent Orange

A herbicide used as a defoliant in the Vietnam war.

The toxic element in Agent Orange is dioxin, an herbicide by product known for its extreme toxicity. Exposure to Agent Orange has been linked by the National Academy of Sciences to increased incidence of various diseases, including: non-Hodgkin's lymphoma, Hodgkin's disease, soft-tissue sarcoma, respiratory cancers, prostate cancer, chloracne (a persistent acne like skin condition), multiple myeloma, transient peripheral neuropathy, porphyria cutanea tarda, and the birth defect spina bifida. Recent research has also associated it with adult-onset diabetes. *See also* CANCER; DIABETES; HODGKIN'S DISEASE; LYMPHOMA, MULTIPLE MYELOMA; NEUROPATHY; NON-HODGKIN'S; PROSTATE, CANCER OF; PORPHYRIA; SARCOMA; *and* SPINA BIFIDA.

Aggression

An expression of hostility or anger directed at oneself or at others.

Aggressive behavior is often directed at those with whom a person has the most contact, such as family members or close friends. Aggression can be physical or verbal. In childhood, aggressive behaviors may include biting, temper tantrums, or fighting. In adolescence, aggressive behavior may be a way to test the limits of authority, or it may be a sign of a deeper underlying problem. As people age, their ability to express themselves and become self-sufficient may alleviate some of the frustrations and anger that led to earlier aggressive acts.

Aggression may have both innate and learned aspects. Infants may experience rages with no apparent model or unusual provocation. On the other hand, aggression often is a response to external stimuli, such as frustration or exposure to abuse. Also, aggression may result from physiological, but not inborn, causes, such as substance abuse, brain damage, or illness.

Aging

The process by which the body changes over time, a process that continues throughout life.

Every living thing grows old and dies, although genetics and environment can greatly affect how each individual ages and how aging affects quality of life. While there is a great many things we don't know about aging, it is known that, over time, cells lose their ability to replace themselves and function. Some cells, such as red and white blood cells that are replaced constantly, have very short life spans; while other cells, such as brain and heart muscle cells, have long life spans.

Theoretically, the mechanism of cell replication should allow cells to duplicate themselves indefinitely. In practice, however, cells replicate only a finite number of times (some not at all) before their genetic material becomes corrupted. This leads to a general breakdown in the cells' ability to function, as well as an increased risk for certain diseases, such as some cancers.

The process of aging varies from person to person, and even within a person, but some physiological effects are commonly indicative of aging:

• **Skin and Hair.** The skin becomes thinner, drier, and wrinkled. Hair loses pigment and may become thin and fragile, or some or all of it may fall out.

• **Body Fat.** There is a depletion in lean muscle mass. Changes in body fat can influence the effectiveness of many medicines.

• **Bone Density.** Bones tend to become less dense because the production of sex hormones leads to lessened metabolism of calcium. Osteoporosis can become a major problem for both men and women, although women are generally at greater and earlier risk.

• **Cartilage.** The cartilage thins, erodes, and becomes less resilient, and thus more prone to injury. The joints become stiff and movement becomes more difficult; arthritis may develop. Similar changes in the cartilage between rib and breastbone make breathing more difficult. Deterioration in cartilage between vertebrae causes compression of the spine and consequent pain in the neck and lower back.

• **Cardiovasular System.** The smaller blood vessels throughout the body become less flexible and less able to supply blood to the various tissues and organs. Buildup of plaque in the arteries to the heart reduces blood flow, raises blood pressure and may cause varicose veins. Heart disease is the major cause of death, although it affects women later in life than it does men.

• **Respiratory System.** Lungs lose flexibility and capacity. The ribs and breast bone can fuse and reduce lung capacity. The lungs become less efficient at absorbing oxygen and releasing carbon dioxide.

• **Digestive System.** The digestive system is not greatly affected as a person ages, but good diet is even more important than in younger years. Most organs have more than enough capacity to perform their functions in youth, so that with age their diminished capacity is still adequate for the body's needs. Though the kidneys lose up to half of their filtering structures (glomeruli) by age 75, they can still purify the blood.

• **Reproductive System.** In women, follicle cells in the ovaries produce lower levels of estrogen and progesterone, leading to the cessation of the menstrual cycle (menopause). Some women may experience hot flashes, discomfort, and irritability during menopause. Lower levels of hormones can result in fat accumulation below the waist, sagging of breast tissue, and thinning and drying of the vagina. Estrogen is believed to play a large role in many bodily functions, such as heart function, calcium metabolism, and mental acuity, so that a drop in estrogen may impact on a woman's total health.

In men, deterioration of the testes results in lower levels of testosterone, reducing muscle strength and accelerating deterioration of the skin and bones. The penis becomes smaller, erectile tissue becomes rigid, and fewer sperm are produced. The prostate gland may enlarge to twice its normal size, constricting the urethra and making urination difficult.

• **Nervous System.** Most nerve cells that die are not replaced, and loss of neurons in the brain results in a decline of certain elements of cognition, such as the ability to learn, memory, and perceptual processing, as well as in balance, coordination, and sensory perception.

Contemporary society has seen two conflicting trends with regard to aging. On the one hand, increased technology, mobility and greater economic opportunity have all but dissolved the extended family, making older people less an integral part in the life of the young. Those same forces have also provided older people with increased opportunities for second careers and more chances to lead fulfilling, active lives in their later years.

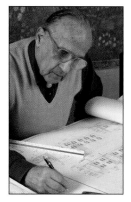

Keeping Mentally Fit. Mental, intellectual, and emotional fitness is often as important as keeping physically fit, especially for retired individuals and the elderly. Pursuing educational opportunities and hobbies, will keep the mind active and sharp while "exercising" the brain.

Maintaining Quality of Life in Old Age

Loss of muscle and bone mass is not an inevitable part of aging; it can be reversed or even halted by hormone replacement therapy, calcium supplementation, and exercise. Exercise is paramount to a high quality of life in old age. A physician can tailor a program to an individual's needs and interests. Exercise can include walking, bicycling, swimming, jogging, or even dancing. Even if a person is bedridden, exercise is necessary: this can be as simple as lifting and turning the limbs and the head, or can be as involved as using a pull-up bar installed over the bed.

Keeping mentally fit is as important as, and often linked to, the maintenance of physical health. Those who discover new interests, places, and friends seem healthier than those who do not. Attending classes, reading, working on puzzles, and volunteering are all ways to maintain mental agility and renew and form social bonds. Staying involved with people and daily activities can improve mood and health.

Preventive medicine can often find health problems before they become serious. A hearing test should be taken every few years after the age of 65; a mammogram every year after age 40 (earlier if there is a family history of breast cancer); a stool test for blood yearly after age 50; a test for thyroid disease every few years after 60 (if a woman); an eye exam every one to three years after 65; and a sigmoidoscopy (examination of the rectum and sigmoid colon) every few years after age 50.

See CELL; GERIATRIC MEDICINE; HEART; NERVOUS SYSTEM; REPRODUCTIVE SYSTEM; *and* SKIN *for a discussion of the foundations of aging. Further information on specific aging subjects may be found in* CANCER; DE MORGAN'S SPOTS PROSTATE, ENLARGED; MENOPAUSE; *and* STROKE.

Agnosia

An inability to identify familiar objects, although the brain receives sufficient sensory information.

Agnosia occurs when a person has normally functioning senses but is unable to properly interpret sensory information. Although sensory information may be properly stored, the brain must recall a similar object in order to identify it. For example, in order to recognize a red balloon, the brain needs to have stored sensory information about a similar item. Agnosia is caused by a failure in the parietal or temporal lobes of the brain, in which memory of familiar objects, uses, and sounds are stored. Damage to these areas reduces the brain's recall ability. The most common cause of agnosia is head injury and stroke.

Generally, agnosia affects only one of the senses. Thus an individual may be able to recognize an object by sight and sound but not by touch.

Visual agnosia is the inability to recognize objects in spite of normal vision.

Auditory agnosia is the inability to recognize sounds despite normal hearing.

Tactile agnosia is the inability to recognize familiar objects by touch, despite normal tactile sensation in all the fingers.

No specific treatment exists for agnosia. Some patients recover spontaneously. *See* BRAIN *and* STROKE.

Agoraphobia

A fear of being in public or open places.

Agoraphobia often begins with a panic attack in a situation that might not have caused anxiety previously. The symptoms of a panic attack are a racing heart, hyperventilation, and fear of impending doom. The attack appears suddenly with an apparent lack of warning.

After a panic attack, a person often assumes that the situation in which it occurred, such as driving on a highway, riding in a train, or being in a crowded mall, was the cause. A person developing agorapho-

bia may then attempt to avoid any situations from which it would be difficult to escape or which would be embarrassing to be in during a panic attack.

Agoraphobia involves varying degrees of avoidance, but in the most severe cases the disease may become totally disabling; as the world that the agoraphobic considers safe becomes smaller and smaller, he or she becomes totally housebound. People with agoraphobia may be more comfortable venturing into situations they determine risky if they are with a trusted companion.

TREATMENT

Agoraphobia can be treated in different ways. One or more methods may be combined, including desensitization, which treats agoraphobia by facing the fearful situations in the presence of a therapist; talking therapy, in which a person tries to understand the cause of the panic attacks; and drugs such as antidepressants.

Therapies for Phobias

Anyone can have a phobia. People with phobias do not simply "snap out of it," and such advice usually only worsens the condition. Treatment becomes necessary when the cause of a phobia is encountered regularly and severely impairs day-to-day functioning. Psychotherapy is the most effective treatment and may be combined with anti-depressant drug therapy. Cognitive-behavioral strategy is the most effective approach to treatment. The patient learns to take an active step-by-step approach and use positive feedback to cope with stressors. Systematic desensitization involves using relaxation techniques and gradually increasing exposure to the object or situation causing the phobia until the fear lessens or disappears. For example, a fear of flying may be treated with deep-muscle relaxation, videotapes designed to reduce fear of flying, and tranquilizers and a beta-blocker to help reduce the physical manfiestations of fear. Hypnosis may also help.

Background material on agoraphobia may be found in ANXIETY; DEPRESSION; PANIC DISORDER; STRESS; *and* UNCONSCIOUS. *More information on treatment options is contained in* ANTIANXIETY DRUGS; BEHAVIOR THERAPY; COGNITIVE-BEHAVIORAL THERAPY; RELAXATION TECHNIQUES; *and* PANIC ATTACKS.

Resources on Agoraphobia

Scrignar, C.B., *From Panic to Peace of Mind : Over-coming Panic and Agora-phobia* (1991; National Alliance for the Mentally Ill, Tel. (800) 950-6264, Online: www.nami.org; National Depressive and Manic-Depressive Assoc., Tel. (800) 82-NDMDA; www.ndmda.org; ww.ny-cornell.org/psychiatry/.

AIDS

Acronym for Acquired Immune Deficiency Syndrome

A disease that destroys the immune system, caused by a virus known as Human Immunodeficiency Virus (HIV).

Two main strains of the HIV virus, HIV-1 and HIV-2, cause AIDS. HIV-1 is more common in the Western Hemisphere, Europe, Asia, and most of Africa. HIV-2 is more prevalent in West Africa; it is transmitted less easily and progeses less quickly to AIDS than HIV-1. In both strains, the virus may persist at low levels for years in a host without causing disease. The only sign of infection will be the presence of antibodies against the virus. Once immunodeficiency occurs, if left untreated, death usually follows within two to three years of the first onset of symptoms.

The HIV virus itself does not kill the patient. Instead, it destroys the immune system, leaving the patient susceptible to other diseases, especially certain types of cancers and pneumonia. These diseases are the immediate causes of death.

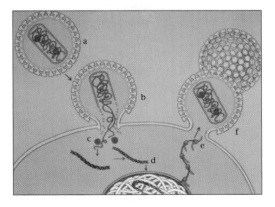

HISTORY

Although evidence existed in the 1970s of a mysterious syndrome in which previously rare cancers and infections were commonly seen, AIDS was first identified as a disease in 1981, at which time the initial "at risk" groups were defined. The first population group in the United States deemed to be at risk was homosexual men, primarily those who lived in major cities, such as New York and San Francisco. Over time, it became clear that all segments of the population are

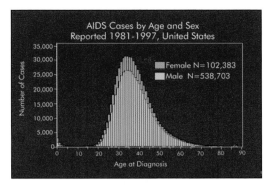

affected by AIDS. For example, of the 34.7 million adults worldwide now living with HIV or AIDS, 47 percent are women.

A blood test for the disease did not become available until 1985. By that time, guidelines for preventing transmission of the disease had been developed, but AIDS had grown into a full-blown epidemic, particularly in Africa, where it is believed to have originated.

The exact origin of HIV is unknown. There is evidence that AIDS has actually been around for about 50 years, as HIV has been detected in frozen tissue samples. The most common theory is that it is a mutated form of Simian Immunodeficiency Virus (SIV) that somehow crossed the species barrier, most likely when hunters came into contact with the blood of contaminated chimpanzees.

THE COURSE OF THE DISEASE

HIV infects a specific type of white blood cells (lymphocyte) called a T helper cell. More specifically, it attacks T helper cells that have a protein known as CD4 on the outer membrane. This kind of cell is essential in triggering the immune response to infection or other foreign materials. The HIV virus invades CD4 cells and inserts its own genetic material into them. There it uses the cell's resources to create more copies of the virus and eventually kills the CD4 cell. After enough CD4 cells are destroyed, the body is no longer able to fight off infection or destroy cancerous cells.

Because symptoms appear only after CD4 levels are very low, the progress of HIV infection is followed not by tracking symptoms, but by CD4 levels. The normal range

Disabled Immune Cells. Below, the HIV-1 virus, as it proliferates, causes immune system cells to fuse into giant, but ultimately ineffective cell clusters.

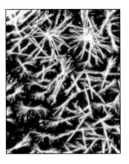

HIV Life cycle. Far left, the virus (a) binds to the cell membrane (b) and deposits its genetic material (c) into the cell. This does not trigger an immune response; the cell "believes" the viral material belongs there. An HIV enzyme then transcribes viral RNA onto the cell's DNA (d), creating a provirus. Another enzyme, HIV protease attaches the provirus onto the cell's DNA, and the cell begins to manufacture new viral particles (e). Eventually the viral particles fill the cell, exhausting and killing it, but not before budding from the cell (f) to find new cells to infect.

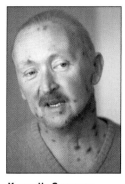

Kaposi's Sarcoma.
Above and below, Kaposi's sarcoma is a type of malignant tumor that is a common complication of AIDS but is otherwise rare. The lesions of Kaposi's sarcoma appear on the skin as slightly raised, purplish nodules, below. Bottom, lesions after treatment with AZT. Right, a micrograph of malignant cells in an individual with AIDS.

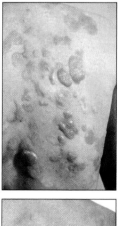

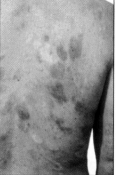

is 800-1,300 per microliter of blood. In the first few months following infection, the count decreases by 50 percent. The immune system forms antibodies against the virus and continues to fight it but is unable to rid itself of the infection permanently. Within six months of the initial infection, the amount of virus in the blood (viral load) stabilizes. However, the CD4 cells continue to be affected. Symptoms of AIDS may not occur for another few years, but by

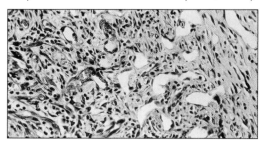

then there will be high viral levels and CD4 counts of below 200.

The blood test for AIDS identifies the presence of antibodies against HIV. However, it is important to note that there is a time lapse of a few months between infection and antibody formation. During this time, viral particles are in circulation, and a person can unwittingly pass the infection on to others. Once the presence of HIV antibodies is detected, the individual is said to be HIV positive.

Signs of AIDS Infection

Symptoms associated with HIV infection include unexplained fever, chills, or night sweats lasting many weeks; a general and persistent feeling of fatigue; an unexplained weight loss; swollen glands; and recurring diarrhea.

As the illness progresses, the person with HIV infection becomes susceptible to various opportunistic infections. These include pneumonia, thursh, tuberculosis shingles, herpes simplex, meningitis, and encephalitis.

The most common infection is Pneumocystis carinii pneumonia (PCP). Kaposi's sarcoma (KS), a rare tumor, is also common in people with AIDS. The onset of one of these infections can be the first sign of the presence of AIDS, the patient having never developed any of the warning signs. The virus can even infect the brain, causing various mental disorders.

TRANSMISSION

The AIDS virus is transmitted in body fluids such as blood, breast milk, semen, and vaginal secretions. There does not seem to be a high concentration of the virus in other fluids, such as urine or saliva. Casual contact with an infected person does not result in the transmission of the virus. However, oral sex can transmit the virus.

The most efficient methods of HIV transmission include having sexual intercourse in which there is an exchange of body fluids, sharing needles for IV drugs, and receiving transfusions of contaminated blood or blood products. The virus can also be transmitted through organ or tissue transplants. An infected mother may pass the virus on to her newborn child. A person who does not exhibit any symptoms of AIDS may still be HIV positive and therefore capable of transmitting the virus.

Susceptibility to HIV infection increases if there is a break in the skin or mucous membranes, which allows the virus to enter the bloodstream. The presence of another sexually transmitted disease in the body also increases chances of HIV infection.

SYMPTOMS

The earliest symptoms of HIV infection include a low-grade, intermittent fever, a rash, swollen lymph nodes, weight loss (wasting), and fatigue. A person who is infected, however, may not experience any of these symptoms. After initial infection, several years may pass without any symptoms.

As the immune system is affected and CD4 levels fall, the body becomes prey to various diseases, referred to as opportunistic diseases.

Opportunistic Diseases. AIDS patients often see other illness manifest with their weakened immune systems: a type of skin cancer called Kaposi's sarcoma; a fungal infection called thrush, caused by the fungus *Candida albicans*; a fungal infection in the lungs, caused by *Pneumocystis carinii*; tuberculosis or atpical mycobecterial infections; cryptosporidium, a gastrointestinal infection; a viral infection in the brain called progressive multifocal leukoencephalopathy; a virus, cytomegalovirus, that affects the retina and causes blindness; and, in women, cervical cancer.

TREATMENT

Various drugs have been developed to fight the AIDS virus. The oldest of these drugs is AZT. Another medication is called ddI (didanosine). These drugs work by attempting to disrupt key chemical reactions in HIV's metabolic cycle, including those controlling its reproduction. However, the virus mutates rapidly, and the drugs lose their effectiveness after a while.

Recently, newer and more effective drugs have been developed in the fight against AIDS. The most promising new medications include a class of drugs known as protease inhibitors. These include the drugs called saquinavir, ritonavir, and indinavir. Protease inhibitors prevent the virus from being able to break down proteins in the host cells, which it needs to do in order to make new, properly developed copies. Protease inhibitors can reduce viral loads to undetectable levels, enabling patients to live normal lives. However, patients must continue to take these drugs indefinitely. The regimen is complicated, and the medications are expensive. There are some unpleasant side effects associated with their use and some indication that the drugs may lose their effectiveness after an extended period of time. Nonetheless, protease inhibitors go a long way in converting AIDS from a fatal disease to a chronic condition.

Although there have been several attempts at developing a vaccine against AIDS, there has been little recent success to date. However, the most recently developed drugs can greatly prolong the lives of patients infected with HIV. The National Institutes of Health (NIH) recommends that patients begin a course of drug treatment only when the CD4 and T-cell concentration in the blood falls below 350 cells per cubic millimeter, because of the dangers inherent in the long-term toxicity of the antiviral drugs.

Recently, clinical trials have been initiated exploring immune-based therapies

(IBTs), designed to augment the immune system reaction to HIV. Agents such as interleukin 2 (IL-2) are being tested to boost immunity to HIV.

PREVENTION

The transmission of HIV can be sharply reduced or eliminated entirely by a few basic practices. Intravenous needles should be safely disposed after each use and should not be shared; safe sex should be practiced in which there is no exchange of bodily fluids; and every sexual partner's history should be determined. The chances of contracting AIDS from a blood transfusion has been minimized, as blood products are routinely tested for HIV before use. (Donated blood is screened for other viral anti-

---

ALERT

HIV TESTING

The HIV test consists of two tests. The first test is very sensitive: it finds anything that looks at all like HIV antibodies. This test is used to screen blood and blood products. If the first test is positive, that is, if antibodies to HIV appear to be present, another test is done. The second is specific and is called a confirmatory test. It separates the false positives from the true positives of the first test. A person is HIV-positive only if the second test is positive for HIV antibodies.

The standard HIV test performed in the United States only detects antibodies for HIV-1; a person who is infected with HIV-2 will test negative. If a person has reason to believe that he or she may have been exposed to HIV-2 in endemic countries in West Africa, he or she should receive a test specifically designed to detect HIV-2.

---

bodies as well, including those for hepatitis.) It has been found that taking the drug AZT (zidovudine) during pregnancy reduces the chances of passing HIV to the fetus to just 25 percent.

Background material on AIDS can be found in IMMUNE SYSTEM; AUTOIMMUNE DISEASES AND VIRUS. *Related information is contained in* HIV, INFECTIOUS DISEASES; PUBLIC HEALTH; SEXUALLY TRANSMITTED DISEASES; *and* SAFE SEX. *See also* ANTIVIRAL DRUGS; DIET AND NUTRITION; *and* ALTERNATIVE MEDICINE *for more on treatment options.*

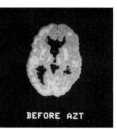

BEFORE AZT

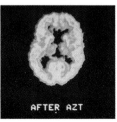

AFTER AZT

The Effects of AZT on the Brain. AZT is a medication that reduces the amount of HIV in the body. AZT can cross the blood-brain barrier, substantially reducing damage to the brain and central nervous system. Top, an MRI scan showing the brain before AZT was prescribed. If brain function is reduced, as in this case, then dementia can ensue. Below, after AZT is prescribed there is often a slowing or even a regression of HIV in the brain.

Resources on AIDS

Petrow, Steven, ed., *HIV Drug Book* (1995); Shilts, Randy, *And the Band Played On* (2000); Stine, Gerald J., *AIDS Update 2001: An Annual Overview of Acquired Immune Deficiency Syndrome* (2001); American Foundation for AIDS Research, Tel. (212) 806-1600, Online: www.am-far.org; AIDS Action Council, Tel. (202) 986-1300, Online: www.aidsaction.org; Gay Men's Health Crisis, Tel. (212) 807-6664, www.gm-hc.org.

Air

A combination of gases and particles that provides a protective layer for the Earth and sustains life.

The air we breathe is composed of nitrogen, oxygen, carbon dioxide, and trace amounts of other gases. Air also contains varying amounts of water vapor (humidity), and dust and ash (from storms and combustion). The central factor in respiration, air plays an important role in the existence of almost all life on Earth. Animals use oxygen and produce carbon dioxide as a waste product; plants use carbon dioxide and produce oxygen as waste, thus creating a cycle that sustains both forms of life.

Extending 600 miles from the surface of the Earth, the air around the planet (the atmosphere) shields its inhabitants from the harmful rays of the sun.

Though not noticeable, air has weight and mass. In fact, the friction caused when objects, such as meteors, enter the atmosphere is usually enough to disintegrate the object.

Most man-made air pollutants are introduced into the atmosphere through the burning of fossil fuels. Primary pollutants include sulfur oxides, nitrogen oxides, carbon oxides, volatile organic compounds, and particulate matter. These pollutants interact with chemicals in the air to create secondary pollutants.

The balance of oxygen and carbon dioxide in the atmosphere is now at risk. Continued and increased deforestation and burning of fossil fuels are increasing carbon dioxide levels and removing the protective layer of ozone, threatening the future of life on Earth. *See also* POLLUTION.

Air Conditioning

Artificial means of cooling that can, under some improper conditions, spread disease.

Air conditioning is a process in which an apparatus called an air conditioner is used to control, and usually lower, the temperature and humidity in an enclosed space. Air conditioning systems are designed to maintain a comfortable environment inside buildings, but, if maintained improperly, they can contribute to poor air quality and "sick building syndrome."

Inadequate cleaning of air conditioners allows dust and dirt to accumulate in fans, which impairs filter performance. Contaminants accumulating inside air-conditioning systems may include dust, hair, skin, soot, dead insects, fungi, mold, and bacteria. As a result, the use of air conditioning may cause discomfort for people and contribute to the spread of disease. *See* AIR *and* LEGIONAIRRES' DISEASE.

Airway Obstruction

Blockage of the respiratory passages resulting in difficulty or cessation of breathing.

Most deaths caused by a foreign body in the air passages occur in children under the age of five, two-thirds of whom are infants. Adults are acutely aware of a foreign body in the airways, but children may show no symptoms unless the air passages are almost entirely obstructed. The Heimlich maneuver for children over the age of one is the same as that for adults, except that the compression should be gentler. Do not use the Heimlich maneuver for children under the age of one. Instead, lay the infant face down with its chest on one open hand tapping firmly between the shoulder blades with the heel of your other hand. *See also* CARDIOPULMONARY RESUSCIATION (CPR); CHOKING; *and* HEIMLICH MANEUVER.

Akinesia

Complete or partial loss of movement.

Akinesia is a condition in which an individual experiences either a limited or total loss of movement. It may be caused by a nerve injury that results in paralysis, as in the case of stroke. It can also be caused by diseases, such as Parkinson's disease, in which the muscles become rigid. *See also* PARKINSON'S DISEASE.

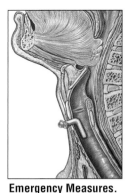

Emergency Measures. In some cases of airway obstruction an emergency tracheotomy, technically referred to as a cricothyroidotomy, may be necessary. This procedure is only performed when a person is not breathing and there are no gasping sounds after the Heimlich maneuver has been tried repeatedly. When possible, this should only be performed by emergency medical technicians (EMTs). A careful 1–2 inch horizontal cut is made in the center of the neck below the Adam's apple and a tube is inserted. The patient is instructed to breathe twice through the tube every 5 seconds until emergency personnel arrive.

Albinism

A group of inherited conditions in which there is little or no pigment in the eyes, skin, or hair.

In the United States, one in 17,000 people has some type of albinism, with varying amounts of pigment produced. In most cases, skin and hair are very light, and eyes are blue, hazel, or brown. Red or pink eyes are rare. Albinism affects all races.

TYPES

Most people with albinism have very light hair and skin, but this is not universal. Oculocutaneous albinism involves lack of pigment in the eyes, hair and skin, whereas ocular albinism involves light-colored eyes but skin and hair comparable to that of other family members.

There are two main types of oculocutaneous albinism. Type 1 albinism, or tyrosinase-related albinism, results in almost no pigmentation. Type 2 albinism is characterized by slight rather than no pigmentation.

CAUSES

Albinism is caused by a recessive gene that leads to a failure to form melanin. In Type 1 albinism, the gene results in a lack of the enzyme tyrosinase, which plays a key role in melanin production. In Type 2 albinism, a different gene is affected.

Most children with albinism have normal parents, who carry one normal gene and one gene for albinism. The child must inherit the gene from both parents.

SYMPTOMS

Other than light coloration, vision problems are the major symptom of albinism. These may include astigmatism, farsightedness, nearsightedness, crossed eyes (strabismus), sensitivity to bright light, and irregular rapid eye movements (nystagmus). Some individuals are legally blind.

The vision problems result from abnormal development of the retina and patterns of nerve connections between eye and brain. If albinism is suspected, an eye exam will provide a definitive diagnosis.

Hermansy-Pudlak syndrome, an uncommon form of albinism, involves problems with abnormal bleeding, as well as lung and bowel disease. It should be suspected if a child with albinism shows unusual bleeding or bruising.

TREATMENT

The lack of pigment cannot be corrected, but associated problems can be treated or compensated for. Vision problems can be alleviated with the use of corrective lenses and surgery to correct weak or defective eye muscles. A person with albinism can compensate for sensitivity to light by wearing tinted lenses outdoors. There is no need for someone with albinism to be kept indoors, but sunblock should be used to prevent melanoma and other skin cancers. *See* EYES *and* PIGMENTATAION.

Albuminuria

The presence of albumin in the urine, indicating failure of the kidney's filtering system.

Albuminuria can be a sign of a kidney disorder. Albumin, a protein made in the liver, is the most common protein in the body, playing several important roles. Albumin helps the body retain certain substances, such as calcium, some hormones, and certain types of drugs, by attaching to them and preventing them from being filtered from the body. Albumin is normally prevented from being excreted in the urine by the filtering activity of the kidney. The presence of albumin or other proteins in the urine can be detected by a simple test using commercially available dipsticks.

Albuminuria may be brought on by exertion or fever, in which case it should resolve on its own. It may indicate a failure of the filtering mechanism of the kidney, the glomerulus (glomerulonephritis). Albuminuria can also be caused by damage to the kidney resulting from high blood pressure or diabetes. Treatment involves dignosing and treating the underlying cause. *See also* DIABETES; HYPERTENSION; MELLITUS; NEPHRITIS; *and* PROTEINURIA.

Alcohol Dependence

A disorder in which a person is unable to control his or her intake of alcohol.

Alcohol dependence is characterized by a craving for alcohol, inability to moderate the amount of drinking, physical dependence on and tolerance for alcohol, and withdrawal symptoms when drinking stops.

While over half of all Americans drink socially, about 15 million are dependent on or abuse alcohol. This impacts much of the American population, either through their own dependence or abuse or that of immediate family members. Alcoholism is more common in families in which other members also abuse alcohol. It is most likely caused by a combination of both genetic or environmental factors.

DEVELOPMENT OF DEPENDENCE

Early in use, cravings for alcohol tend to be psychological in origin. They may result from the sedative effect that alcohol provides: numbness and relief from uncomfortable feelings.

Over time, the dependence becomes physical. An individual develops a tolerance, and it becomes necessary to increase consumption to achieve the same "high."

Drinking increasing amounts of alcohol on a daily basis results in physical addiction. If intake suddenly stops, blood pressure rapidly increases and withdrawal occurs. Symptoms of withdrawal include insomnia, sweating, anxiety, rapid pulse, nausea, and vomiting. In severe cases, withdrawal includes delirium trements, which involves delusions, hallucinations, and extreme agitation; severe withdrawal can be life threatening. Withdrawal from alcohol takes three to five days and should be supervised by a physician or within an alcohol treatment program.

COMPLICATIONS

The human costs of alcohol abuse and dependence can include problems with family, such as physical and emotional abuse and neglect, increased risk of homicide and suicide, and work-related problems, such as accidents and lost time at work.

Strictly economic costs, resulting from medical problems, lost productivity, legal proceedings, and increased incidence of crime, are roughly $100 billion each year and increasing. Further, alcohol abuse and dependence can be fatal. Alcohol-related accidents can injure or kill the intoxicated person or those around him or her. Consumption of a large amount of alcohol in a short time can result in unconsciousness, coma, or even death. Long-term drinking can result in serious health complications, such as cirrhosis of the liver.

DIAGNOSIS

One of the greatest impediments to diagnosing and treating alcohol dependence is denial. The alcohol-dependent person may not recognize or be willing to admit that there is a problem. This may result from the guilt and shame associated with continued drinking in the face of interpersonal, legal and financial problems. One way to determine if moderate social drinking has progressed into full-fledged alcohol abuse or dependence is by a questionnaire with specific questions (such as the Michigan Alcoholism Screening Test—see Alert box.)

CODEPENDENCE OR ENABLING

Ironically, family members, who would benefit the most by having an alcohol-dependent person become sober, often support a person's dependence on alcohol. It is difficult—and may be emotionally or

ALERT

Are You at Risk?

If two or more of these apply, alcohol abuse or dependence may be present. A physician can help assess and provide treatment options for problem drinking.
- Are you spending a great deal of energy keeping your drinking a secret, including hiding liquor and organizing your day around drinking?
- Do you have difficulty getting along with others because of hostile behavior, rages, lack of interest in others, or grandiose behavior?
- Does it annoy you when people criticize your drinking?
- Do you ever feel guilty about drinking?
- Have you tried to stop drinking for a week but only lasted for a couple of days?
- Have you ever had a drink in the morning to help you stop shaking?
- Has your drinking caused problems with coworkers and family members?

physically dangerous—to demand that an alcoholic confront his or her behavior, so family members often end up by providing protection, as opposed to true help, to an alcohol-dependent individual. This enabling can come in the form of making excuses for absences from work or social obligations; lending money or paying bills; and even drinking with the person.

Because loved ones tend to enable an alcohol-dependent family member, family treatment options are an important part of treatment for alcohol dependence.

TREATMENT

The only treatment known to be effective is complete abstinence. Moderate drinking is not possible after a person has developed alcohol dependence. Recovery can only begin when a person recognizes his or her dependence and is motivated to change; help from a treatment professional vastly improves chances of recovery.

There are a number of treatment options, and it is often best to use a combination of methods. Treatment may be provided on an outpatient basis, in a hospital, or in a residential treatment center. Association with a support group, such as Alcoholics Anonymous, may supplement it.

Detoxification, in which alcohol is safely eliminated from the system in a way that minimizes withdrawal symptoms, is necessary in severe cases of alcohol dependence. Doctors may prescribe medication that helps prevent a relapse, such as disulfiram (Antabuse) or naltrexone (ReVia). Community programs may provide training in work and parenting skills, job placement, and legal assistance.

Alcoholics Anonymous is used in combination with many treatment plans and has proven highly successful in providing the support and structure to help people stop drinking, although its approach does not appeal to everyone.

TREATMENT FOR THE FAMILY

It is important for family members to seek treatment, even if the dependent person does not. Approximately one in four chil

---

Alcoholics Anonymous

Alcoholics Anonymous (AA) is an informal society of more than 2,000,000 recovered alcoholics in the United States and other countries. It is founded on the principle that recovering alcoholics are best equipped to help others overcome the struggle with alcohol addiction. Members meet in local groups ranging from a handful to hundreds of people. The organization is informally organized—there are no governing officers, regulations, or dues—an office in New York supports worldwide activities.

AA offers a twelve-step recovery program that forces the alcoholic to confront the addiction and overcome it. The steps begin with the recognition that the person is powerless to control the drinking and a willingness to accept help from a spiritual power. The process continues with recognizing and taking responsibility for past actions, making amends, and working with fellow AA members to help each other maintain abstinence. Meetings provide peer support and a social activity that emphasizes abstinence; members also have contact members from whom they can seek support during times when meetings are not scheduled.

---

dren are affected by alcohol abuse. The basic function of a family—to provide a nurturing, secure environment—may be missing, and most children of alcoholics suffer lifelong deficits. Many children of alcoholics suffer from neglect and abuse.

Al-Anon is a support group for spouses and significant others of alcohol-dependent adults. Alateen offers support to children of alcoholics. Family therapy may also be appropriate as part of a treatment plan.

PREVENTION

Multiple intervention strategies should be aimed at the social, cultural, economic, and individual influences that can result in alcohol consumption. School-based education programs, including clubs such as SADD (Students Against Drunk Driving), utilize peer pressure, instruction on the negative impact of alcohol, and activities that improve self esteem and problem-solving skills. Social attitudes about drinking, such as laws limiting or banning advertising of alcohol in certain venues, the enforcement of laws against serving and selling to underage drinkers, and education about the health effects of alcohol, reduce the incidence of alcohol consumption.

Background information on alcohol dependence may be found in ALCOHOL INTOXICATION; DEPRESSION; *and* SUBSTANCE ABUSE. *More information on alcohol-related disease is contained in* ALCOHOL-RELATED DISORDERS; FETAL ALCOHOL SYNDROME; HANGOVER; *and* LIVER DISEASE.

Resources on Alcohol Dependence

Knapp, Caroline, *Drinking: A Love Story* (1997); Ketcham, Katherine, *Beyond the Influence: Under-standing and Defeating Alcoholism* (2000); Knott, David H., *Alcohol Prob-lems: Diagnosis and Treat-ment* (1989); Alcoholics Anonymous (local chapters in the phone book); Al-Anon: (800) 356-9996, On-line: www.al-anon.alateen.org; Mothers Against Drunk Driving: (800) 438-MADD, National Council on Alcoholism and Drug Dependence, (800) 622-2255, www.-ncadd. org/-problems.html www.nycornell.org/psy-chiatry/.

Alcohol Intoxication

Also known as drunkenness

Drinking excessive amounts of alcohol, which impairs the central nervous system and results in physical, mental, and emotional deficits.

When a person drinks alcohol, it is absorbed into the bloodstream, where it affects the central nervous and other body systems. The legal blood-alcohol level of intoxication is generally determined to be .08 to 0.1 percent. Before reaching that level, people may experience limited functioning, judgment errors, irritability, limited self-control, and reduced reaction time and coordination.

As blood alcohol levels increase, physical and mental abilities decrease. Gait becomes unsteady and speech slurs. Mental impairment progresses from disorientation to drowsiness to coma. Risk of death occurs at levels of over 0.3 percent.

The degree of impairment with a given intake of alcohol is subject to a number of factors. Lower weight and higher body fat result in faster absorption of alcohol. Drinking on an empty stomach increases intoxication, since food in the stomach absorbs alcohol. Those who have developed a tolerance to alcohol must imbibe a greater quantity of alcohol to become intoxicated.

The combination of alcohol and certain medications can increase the effects of both drugs, as well as the risk of life-threatening reactions. This is particularly true of sleeping pills and opioid painkillers, since their action on the body, like alcohol, is to depress the central nervous system. *See* ALCOHOL DEPENDENCE *and* SUBSTANCE ABUSE.

Alcohol Related Disorders

A wide range of physical and emotional health problems, either as a result of consumption of large amounts of alcohol at one time or as a result of chronic, long-term use.

An individual intoxicated by alcohol experiences impaired judgment, reduced reaction time, and impaired memory. Even one or two drinks can impair judgment and physical ability; increasing amounts of alcohol lead to further loss of physical and mental ability and can be life threatening.

ALCOHOL POISONING

Consuming extremely high quantities of alcohol (a blood-alcohol level higher than 0.3 percent) poses a risk of death due to alcohol's toxicity. Indications of alcohol poisoning include unconsciousness, shallow breathing, and possibly a bluish tinge to the lips. In this state, the body's vital functions are severely impaired, and emergency medical help is required. The person should be turned on the side to prevent possible inhalation of vomit.

CHRONIC ALCOHOL CONSUMPTION

Chronic alcohol consumption affects almost every system of the body, particularly the nervous, gastrointestinal, and cardiovascular systems. It affects the liver, impairs sexual functioning, causes birth defects, and is associated with emotional disorders.

Alcohol damages the immune system and can lead to reduced ability to fight disease. Because alcohol is high in calories but has minimal nutritional value, people who chronically consume alcohol are more likely to be both obese and malnourished.

Nervous System. Alcoholic neuropathy—damage to nerves throughout the body—is an early nervous system disorder arising from chronic alcohol use. Symptoms include tingling, numbness, and pain in the arms and legs. This damage is reversible with the cessation of drinking.

A very serious disease resulting from long-term alcohol abuse is Wernicke-Korsakoff syndrome, caused by a deficiency of vitamin B_1 (thiamine). Symptoms include memory loss, confusion, inability to learn new tasks, unsteady gait, and blurred vision.

The disease is treatable in the early stage with injections of thiamine, resumption of a normal diet, and abstention from alcohol. Advanced, untreated stages may progress to coma and possibly death.

Other brain and nervous system disorders include the potential for blackouts, seizures, mild dementia, and insomnia.

Gastrointestinal System. Consumption of alcohol over a long time can lead to impaired ability to absorb nutrients, inflammation of the stomach lining (gastritis), and ulcers. Chronic alcohol use also has been linked to inflammation of the pancreas (pancreatitis). Acute attacks involve severe abdominal pain that radiates to the back; chronic inflammation can lead to weight loss and symptoms of diabetes.

Risk for cancers of the mouth, throat, esophagus, stomach, and intestines increases. This risk is greatly increased when alcohol use is combined with smoking.

Cardiovascular System. Chronic alcohol use can lead to elevated blood pressure (hypertension), which causes stress on the heart and the blood vessels. Hypertension may be indicated by headache, fatigue, confusion, nausea, or tremors, or it may be "silent" and have no symptoms.

Alcohol has a toxic effect on the heart muscle and can lead to weakening and thinning of the heart (cardiomyopathy). Symptoms of alcoholic cardiomyopathy include rapid or irregular pulse, shortness of breath, fatigue, and swelling. If untreated, cardiomyopathy may lead to heart failure and arhythmias, and can be fatal.

Liver. The liver is particularly susceptible to damage, as it is key in breaking down alcohol. Liver disease may arise from the toxic effects of alcohol itself and as a result of malnutrition. Compromised liver function limits the body's ability to process impurities, alcohol itself, and medications. Severe liver disease can be fatal.

There are three stages of liver damage that result from chronic alcohol consumption: fatty liver, hepatitis, and cirrhosis. In its early stages, alcohol places increased demands for oxygen on the liver and causes an accumulation of fat that impairs the liver's ability to absorb oxygen.

Inflammation of the liver (hepatitis) may develop after years of excessive drinking. Symptoms include loss of appetite, abdominal discomfort, and yellowing of the skin (jaundice).

If untreated, hepatitis may progress to cirrhosis. The liver shrinks as scar tissue and abnormal cells replace healthy tissue.

All stages of liver disease may be improved by a healthy diet, vitamin supplements, and cessation of drinking, although earlier intervention leads to greatly improved prognosis. Cirrhosis is irreversible; a liver transplant may be a last resort.

Chronic alcohol use can lead to an increased risk of liver cancer. Because the immune system and liver are impaired, other cancers are more likely to spread to the liver and develop into secondary tumors.

Psychiatric Problems. Because alcohol is a depressant, chronic alcohol dependence is often associated with depressive illnesses and suicide. Other psychiatric disorders, such as anxiety disorders, psychoses, and psychotic episodes are typical of alcohol withdrawal and the later stages of Wernicke-Korsakoff's syndrome.

Sexual Dysfunction. Alcohol use is associated with a greater likelihood of sexual dysfunction, such as impotence or lessened enjoyment of sex. This may result from poor health, physical impairment of the reproductive system, or psychological effects of alcohol use, such as depression or lack of trust and communication.

Because intoxication impairs judgment, people who abuse alcohol are more likely to have unplanned, unprotected sex, leading more often to sexually transmitted disease and unwanted pregnancy.

FETAL ALCOHOL SYNDROME

Alcohol use during pregnancy can result in a variety of birth defects, often grouped under the term fetal alcohol syndrome. These occur because of the immediate effects of alcohol and because alcohol compromises the absorption of nutrients during crucial stages of development. Disorders that may arise in fetal alcohol syndrome include cleft lip and palate, cardiac defects, vision and hearing problems, poor coordination, mental impairment, and attention-deficit hyperactivity disorder. Children born of mothers who abuse alcohol during pregnancy may have lifelong mental, emotional, and physical problems. *See* CIRRHOSIS *and* FETAL ALCOHOL SYNDROME.

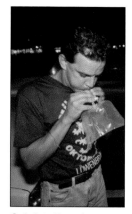

Sobriety Test. Law enforcement agencies across the nation use either an Intoxilyzer or an Intoximeter to test sobriety, especially of drivers. Above, an individual will have to breathe into such a device to measure blood alcohol levels.

Aldosterone

Hormone released by the adrenal glands that regulates sodium and potassium levels in the blood.

Sodium and potassium help regulate the water balance in the body, as well as heart rhythm, direction of nerve impulses, and muscle contraction. Sodium and potassium levels are maintained by the kidneys. When sodium levels drop below normal, the kidney releases the hormone renin, which trigers the production of angiotensin II. This, in turn, causes the secretion of aldosterone, which signals the kidneys to retain sodium and water.

ALDOSTERONISM

Excess production of aldosterone is usually the result of a tumor in the adrenal gland (Conn's syndrome) or hyperplasia of both adrenal glands. It can also be due to a disease that impairs blood flow, such as heart failure or cirrhosis of the liver. A tumor causes secretion of extra aldosterone with low renin. Reduced blood flow to the kidneys causes the kidneys to release renin, which stimulates production of aldosterone. Aldosteronism causes high blood pressure (hypertension) because the body retains too much sodium. Potassium levels drop, resulting in fatigue and weakness.

If a tumor is causing the condition, it can be surgically removed. In other instances low-salt diet may be recommended, and a diuretic, spironolactone, that blocks the action of aldosterone may be prescribed.

HYPOALDOSTERONISM

Insufficient production of aldosterone can be caused by Addison's disease, a disorder resulting in the destruction of the adrenal gland resulting in weakness, weight loss, darkening of the skin in patches, and a vulnerability to acute adr-enal crisis, in which the blood pressure drops dangerously and shock and coma may set in. Addison's disease can be treated with hormone supplements. *See* ADDISON'S DISEASE; CIRRHOSIS; CONN'S SYNDROME; POTASSIUM; *and* SODIUM.

Alexander Technique

A technique of bodywork therapy that emphasizes the importance of posture and balance in an effort to relieve tension.

The Alexander Technique was originated by Frederick Matthias Alexander (1869–1955), a Shakespearean actor born in Tasmania, who developed his regimen in an effort to treat problems he was having with his voice projection on stage. Noticing that his body tensed whenever he was about to speak, Alexander cured his voice problems through a rigorous program of balance and posture training. His technique calls for training in the proper and balanced way of walking, standing, sitting, and getting up from a seated or prone position. He termed this alignment the "Primary Control Mechanism."

The training has been used (especially in England) to relieve stress and stress-related disorders: fatigue, insomnia, anxiety, depression, chronic pain and muscle tension, and, on occasion, digestive and respiratory ailments. *See also* ACUPRESSURE; BODYWORK; SHIATSU; *and* THERAPEUTIC TOUCH.

Alkalosis

When bodily fluids are too alkaline (basic).

The body functions normally when the amount of acids and alkalis, also called bases, are in balance. Alkalosis occurs when the body loses too many acids or retains too many alkalis. It may be the result of two types of errors. Metabolic alkalosis occurs when the acid is severely reduced, such as when a person has taken too much of an antacid or lost a large amount of stomach acid through vomiting. Respiratory alkalosis is caused by breathing out too much carbon dioxide. This may occur when a person breathes too rapidly (hyperventilates), such as during a panic attack or if the person is at higher altitudes. Symptoms of alkalosis include confusion, tremors and muscle spasms, nausea and vomiting, and numbness or tingling in the face or extremities. Treatment involves treating the underlying cause: ceasing to use the drug that caused the condition, controlling loss of fluids, calming breathing, etc. Most cases of alkalosis respond well to treatment. *See also* ANTACID DRUGS; HYPERVENTILATION; *and* METABOLISM.

Allergen

A foreign particle or substance that provokes a special type of immune reaction, an allergic reaction, in sensitized individuals.

Allergens are not harmful in nature but cause unfavorably strong immune reactions among certain individuals. The first contact with an allergen does not cause a reaction, as the body has not yet developed antibodies against it; subsequent exposure to the allergen is required. Common allergens include pollen, mold, animal dander, legumes, nuts, and insect venom.

While many allergic reactions are unpleasant but not harmful, in some cases, exposure to an allergen can result in a life-threatening condition known as anaphylactic shock, in which the circulatory system fails and blood pressure drops rapidly. Allergens that have been known to trigger anaphylactic shock in some individuals include bee and other insect bites, certain foods and drugs, and some dyes used in diagnostic imaging. *See also* ALLERGY.

Allergy

The immune system's reaction to a foreign particle or substance as if it were a disease-causing agent.

The first exposure to an allergy-causing material, known as an allergen, does not result in an allergic reaction. For unknown reasons, the immune system becomes sensitized to the substance and responds to subsequent encounters with an immune reaction. In a normal immune response, the body recognizes a foreign material, such as a virus or a toxin, as dangerous and develops antibodies to locate and destroy it. When the body again encounters that type of particle or substance, the immune system is easily mobilized to destroy it. In an allergic response, the body responds to a particle, which is normally harmless, such as dust, pollen, or certain types of foods.

The specific antibodies produced in an allergic reaction are known as Immunoglobulin E (IgE). These antibodies trigger the release of histamine and other chemicals when exposed to an allergen. Histamine is a chemical transmitter that can cause various changes in the body. For example, in the nose it causes blood vessels to dilate and become more permeable. In the lungs, histamine causes swelling of the airways that, if severe, can block breathing.

TYPES
A particle or substance that triggers an allergic response is known as an allergen. Common allergens include dust, mold, pollen, drugs, animal dander, insect venom, poison ivy, food, heat, and cold. Heat and cold are not particles themselves, but it is thought that exposure to heat or cold triggers chemical changes in the body that the immune system responds to as if they were invading particles. Foods most likely to provoke an allergic response include cow's milk, egg whites, peanuts and other legumes, nuts, and wheat.

SYMPTOMS
Symptoms of an allergic reaction vary depending on the type of allergen, how it entered the system, and the location in the body at which contact occurred. An inhaled allergen can cause sinus congestion, runny nose, watery eyes, or wheezing and impaired breathing. An allergic reaction caused by contact between an allergen and the skin can result in itching, rash, or hives, raised itchy bumps on the skin. An allergic reaction to a food or a drug can vary greatly and may affect the entire body; reactions may include abdominal pain or upset, hives, swelling, or inability to breathe.

Symptoms vary greatly from person to person. Some allergic reactions may cause only minor distress, such as a runny nose or itchy eyes, while others may result in life-

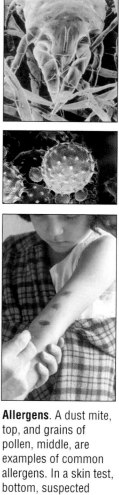

Allergens. A dust mite, top, and grains of pollen, middle, are examples of common allergens. In a skin test, bottom, suspected allergens are applied over small scratches in the skin; if the skin becomes reddened, itchy or inflamed, it is likely that the patient is allergic to that substance.

Allergy

Resources on Allergy

Mims, Cedric A., *The War Within Us: Everyman's Guide to Infection and Immunity* (2000); Kendall, Marion D., *Dying to Live : How Our Bodies Fight Disease* (1998); Ravicz, Simone, *Thriving With Your Autoimmune Disorder : A Woman's Mind-Body Guide* (2000); American Academy of Allergy, Asthma & Immunology, Tel. (800) 822-2762, Online: www.aaaai.org; American Autoimmune Related Diseases Association, Tel. (800) 598-4668, Online: www.aarda.org.

Allergic Reaction. After the body is first exposed to an allergen, it develops antibodies against it. Left, when the body is later exposed to the same allergen (a), the antibodies (b) bind to the surface of a mast cell (c), which contains histamine (d), a substance responsible for many allergic symptoms. Right, after the antibodies attach to the mast cell, the allergens bind to the antibodies, linking two or more and causing the mast cell to burst and histamine to be released.

threatening conditions, such as an asthma attack or anaphylactic shock.

ANAPHYLACTIC SHOCK

Anaphylactic shock is a severe and often life-threatening allergic reaction. It can be triggered by bee or other insect stings or bites, certain drugs or foods, dyes used in diagnostic tests, or even a blood transfusion. Shock occurs when the allergic reaction triggers the blood vessels to dilate, causing circulatory failure and a drastic drop in blood pressure. Swelling of tissues in the throat may result in a blocked air passageway. Loss of consciousness may follow. Like other allergic reactions, anaphylaxis does not occur upon the first exposure to an allergen but only after prior sensitization.

If a person appears to be entering into anaphylactic shock, seek medical help immediately. Individuals who have a known allergy that can induce anaphylactic shock should carry an emergency kit that contains injectable epinephrine.

Asthma is a disorder in which certain situations trigger the airways to close up and mucus production to increase, resulting in partial or total impairment of breathing. Triggering conditions vary from person to person but include exposure to allergens as well as respiratory infections, exposure to cold, stress, and other situations. Asthma attacks range from fairly mild to life-threatening. People with asthma usually carry inhalers to limit the symptoms of an attack, but an asthma attack can be an emergency that requires immediate medical attention.

DIAGNOSIS

Determining the cause of an allergic reaction often takes time and patience. Tests usually involve trial and error to see if a given possible allergen triggers a reaction. In a skin test, small amounts of a suspected allergen are placed on the skin of the upper arm or back. Either the skin is scratched to allow entry of the allergen or the allergen is injected. Swelling and redness at the test site are considered a positive result. Several allergens are usually tested at the same time. Skin tests have a wide margin of error, however. They are most reliable for airborne allergens.

The Radioallergosorbent Test (RAST) measures the amounts of specific IgE antibodies in the bloodstream. The results are not immediately available.

If a food allergy is suspected, one food at a time is eliminated from the diet and then added back to determine if it is triggering an allergic reaction.

TREATMENT

Antihistamines are the drugs most often used to control symptoms of allergic reactions. A shot of epinephrine is given in the case of anaphylactic shock, and anti-inflammatory drugs are given in the case of an asthma attack. Either of the two situations may require hospitalization and more intensive treatment. The most effective treatment is avoiding the allergen altogether.

Immunotherapy. Allergy shots, or immunotherapy, can be administered to eliminate the allergy entirely. In immunotherapy, a small amount of an allergen is injected in order to stimulate the body to produce an antibody to neutralize it. This, in turn, blocks the IgE antibodies from reacting with the allergen and provoking the allergic response. The allergies for which shots are most effective include pollen, mold, insect bites and animal hair.

Immunotherapy must be carried out on a regular basis, with doses increasing until the allergic response is eliminated. The frequency of the shots declines afterwards, but treatment must be continued for an extended period of time, often for years.

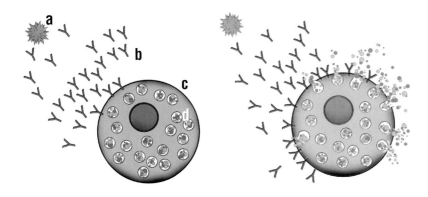

PREVENTION

The best way to prevent an allergic reaction is to avoid contact with the allergen, if at all possible. This may involve not eating certain foods or avoiding animals. Air conditioning may be helpful for some respiratory allergies. A more drastic step is moving to another climate; however, even though the offending trees or plants have been left behind, the new environment may contain different allergens.

> *Basic biochemical information on allergy may be found in* ALLERGEN; B CELL; FOOD INTOLERANCE; IMMUNE RESPONSE; IMMUNOLOGIC MEMORY; *and* T CELL. *Further information regarding allergy is contained in* ANTIGENS; CELLULAR IMMUNITY; FOOD ALLERGY; HAY FEVER; *and* HISTOCOMPATIBILITY. *Treatments for allergies are discussed in* ANAPHYLACTIC SHOCK; HYPERSENSITIVITY; IMMUNIZATION; *and* SENSITIZATION.

Allopurinol

A drug used to treat gout.

Allopurinol is an organic compound used to treat gout, a metabolic disorder that causes joint inflammation. Allopurinol interferes with the formation of uric acid, a substance present in abnormal quantities in the blood of people who suffer from gout. The painful inflammation experienced by gout sufferers occurs when uric acid in the blood forms crystal deposits in the joints, kidneys, and other areas of the body.

Allopurinol is normally used to treat only severe forms of gout. Generally, allopurinol treatment is continued for many years, if not indefinitely. The substance causes the uric acid deposits to be reabsorbed and prevents the formation of uric-acid kidney stones. *See also* GOUT; KIDNEY STONES; *and* URIC ACID.

Alopecia Areata

A common disease that results in the loss of hair on the scalp and elsewhere on the body.

Alopecia areata develops when an unknown stimulus causes the immune system to suppress the functioning of a number of hair folicles. The hair folicles become small and hair production slows; hair ceases to grow above the skin. The hair follicle remains alive; regrowth is possible if the appropriate signal is received. In one out of five persons with the condition, someone else in the family is also affected by the disease, indicating a possible genetic link. The condition is also more likely to occur in families whose members have asthma, hay fever, atopic eczema, thyroid disease, diabetes, rheumatoid arthritis, lupus erythmatosus, pernicious anemia, or Addison's disease, all of which may be connected to the immune system. People with alopecia are usually healthy otherwise.

SYMPTOMS

The first signs of alopecia areata are usually one or more small, round patches in which hair ceases to grow. The condition may stop after only slight hair loss, or it may continue until complete baldness occurs. If all the scalp hair is lost, the disorder is called alopecia totalis. If all of the scalp and body hair is lost, the disorder is then called alopecia universalis.

TREATMENT

There is no cure for alopecia areata, but there are various treatments. Most treatments work best on mild cases, and none are universally effective. Cortisone injections into and around the bald patches are the most common treatment for mild cases. Other treatments include topical minoxidil and anthralin cream. For more extensive cases, cortisone pills, minoxidil, and topical immunotherapy treatment are available. People with severe alopecia may wish to wear a wig to conceal the condition.

> *Background material on Alopecia may be found in* HAIR; HAIR GROWTH; RASH; *and* SCALP. *Further information regarding hair loss may be found in* ELECTROLYSIS; HAIR REMOVAL; *and* HEREDITY.

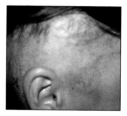

Alopecia Treated. The brownish tinge indicates onthreslin treatment.

Infected Alopecia. Below, in rare instnaces, alopecia can become infected, giving rise to prestules (pus-filled lesions).

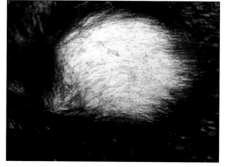

Alpha-fetoprotein

Protein produced by the liver and yolk sac of a fetus.

Alpha-fetoprotein (AFP) is a protein found in a fetus but is not usually produced by healthy adults. It seems to keep substances like calcium and hormones in the body, as well as to monitor the flow of water between tissues and into the bloodstream. Alpha-fetoprotein leaves the fetus through urination to become part of the amniotic fluid. As the fetus swallows the fluid, AFP is returned to the digestive system. At that point, some AFP goes into the intestines, while the rest flows into the fetus' circulatory system.

Between the 15th and 20th weeks of pregnancy, it is possible to test the levels of AFP in the mother's bloodstream as an indicator for a variety of birth defects. An abnormal level of AFP may indicate any of a number of complications. However, the test should not be considered a reliable diagnosis, but rather an indication of risk that may call for further testing. Ultrasound scans can often resolve many of the questions raised by an abnormal AFP level.

UNDERSTANDING AN AFP TEST

Normal AFP levels in a fetus allow only a small amount to flow into the mother's bloodstream. Abnormal amounts of AFP in the maternal blood test may indicate an abnormality in the pregnancy. Some reasons for abnormal AFP include:

- **Multiple Pregnancies.** Often a high AFP level means that more than one fetus is present, each releasing a normal amount of AFP.
- **Incorrect Age of Fetus.** A high level of AFP may simply mean that the initial date of conception was incorrect.
- **Down's Syndrome.** A low AFP level may indicate Down's syndrome.
- **Neural Tube Defects.** High levels of AFP may point to the presence of spina bifida, a condition in which the vertebrae do not cover the spinal cord.

Amniocentesis, or a removal of some of the fluid surrounding the fetus, can confirm the presence of high AFP.

AFP IN ADULTS

Levels of AFP are virtually nonexistent in healthy adults who are not pregnant, but AFP may be produced as a result of some liver diseases. Liver cancer, viral hepatitis, and cirrhosis of the liver may all lead to increased AFP levels. In these cases, the level of AFP may be used to monitor progress of the disease and effectiveness of treatment. *See also* BIRTH DEFECTS; DOWN'S SYNDROME; FETUS, HEPATITIS; *and* Liver.

Alternative Birth Methods

Methods of giving birth wit physician assistance in a nontraditional manner.

In recent years, there has been a growing trend for women to to be more actively involved in the process of giving birth; to some individuals, it is no longer a passive medical procedure. Alternative birth methods include delivery at birthing centers (which are often associated with hospitals or recognized health-care facilities), use of a midwife or a labor coach (doula) assisted by a trained physician, and the use of clinically supervised hypnosis or acupuncture for pain relief. Some couples have even opted for a "water birth."

BIRTHING SETTINGS

Birthing centers, designed to facilitate alternative births, combine the relaxed feel and supportive environment of a home setting with the necessary medical facilities and resources specifically designed to facilitate the birth process.

Even within a traditional hospital setting, there is are specific trends toward a more "home like" feel. Many hospitals are increasingly replacing labor, delivery, and recovery rooms with a single birthing room. Additional family members are sometimes invited to be present at delivery. Birthing rooms provide a more comfortable environment along with conventional facilities if necessary.

ALTERNATIVE HEALTH CARE PROVIDERS

A midwife is a professional, licensed individual who has received training in obstetrics and gynecology; he or she provides basic medical guidance during the birth process. In the absence of any complicating factors or emergencies, midwives can deliver with appropriate physician's assistance or backup.

A doula does not work in the same role as a midwife. Rather, he or she acts as a labor coach, assisting the mother through the stages of labor and delivery. Her function varies according to what the mother requests.

NATURAL METHODS

Natural Childbirth refers to labor and delivery without medications. Most women use Lamaze or a similar program of controlled breathing to help them relax and deal with contractions, although anesthesia is available if necessary. Occasionally, women are finding alternative methods of pain management, such as hypnosis or acupuncture.

Water Birth. A controversial procedure is the water birth, in which the mother gives birth in a pool of warm water. This is intended to provide a soothing environment for the mother and ease the transition for the newborn. The baby receives its oxygen from the mother through the placenta and the umbilical cord. A complex physiological mechanism inhibits the baby from taking a breath until it is lifted out of the water. Afterwards the parents can spend their initial bonding time, with the baby, in the warmth of the water.

High-Risk Pregnancy. In the case of a pregnancy in which there is a high risk for complications, most health-care providers agree that the mother should opt for a conventional labor and delivery in a hospital setting with adequate medical supervision.

See ALTERNATIVE MEDICINE; CHILDBIRTH; FETUS; and MIDWIFERY for a discussion of the foundations of alternative birthing. More information on alternative birth methods is contained in CESAREAN SECTION; CHILDBIRTH, COMPLICATIONS OF; and DELIVERY.

Alternative Medicine

Also known as complementary and integrative medicine

Medical and health practices considered outside traditional Western medical practices.

The practices associated with the term "alternative medicine" represent a wide variety of approaches to health, the human body and the world. This variety is reflected in the many terms that are used to refer to these practices, each implying an underlying ideology, as well as a set of practices.

Complementary medicine implies an association with traditional Western medical practices, perhaps even supportive (or mutually supportive) of them.

Integrative medicine implies a combination of traditional and non traditional techniques that utilizes the best aspects of different techniques and accounts for the inter relatedness of the systems of the body.

Natural healing implies an aversion to pharmaceuticals and a use of substances and techniques that are available without assistance from a physician.

UNDERLYING CONCEPTS

The rise of interest in alternative medical practices—by the year 2000, half of Americans sought an alternative therapy or product, spending nearly 20 billion dollars on alternative medicine annually—may be explained by a growing realization that some of the underlying concepts of the field have merit, such as the following:

• The body's defense and healing mechanisms are formidable, and a significant goal of medicine should be to stimulate and direct these capabilities.

• The human body functions in a complex way. Systems affect one another, requiring an approach that treats inter relationships in addition to isolated parts.

• The environment, particularly as altered by industrial civilization, can have a significant impact on health.

• The role of the brain and mind are still not understood in health and healing processes. Experience and anecdotal evidence indicate that the connection may

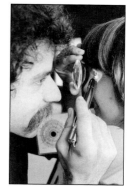

Iridology Diagnosis. Above, an alternative medicine practitioner uses iridology (iris diagnosis)—the practice of observing bodily changes by visualizing the iris—to diagnose an individual. Iridology was developed by Ignatz von Peczely, a Hungarian physician, in the middle of the 19th century, and popularized in America by Bernard Jensen. This practice has yet to find clinical support.

Resources on Alternative Medicine

Ditchek, Stuart H., et al., *Healthy Child, Whole Child Integrating the Best of Conventional and Alternative Medicine to Keep Your Kids Healthy* (2001); Pizzorno, Joseph E., et al., *Clinician's Handbook of Natural Medicine* (2001); Robbins, Jim, *A Symphony in the Brain: The Evolution of the New Brain Wave Biofeedback* (2001); Swenson, David, *Ashtanga Yoga* (1999); National Center for Complementary and Alternative Medicine, Tel. (888)644-6226, On-line: nccam.nih.gov; http://www.nycornell.org/medicine/gim/index.html.

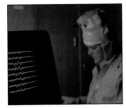

Biofeedback. Above, a biofeedback machine monitors such body functions as breathing, heart rate, blood pressure, and body temperature. Practitioners of biofeedback believe that one can learn to control such body functions through concentration and relaxation as a form of relaxation therapy. It can treat stress-related conditions and some kinds of pain.

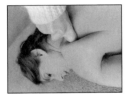

Deep Massage. Above, deep tissue massage releases chronic tension throughout the body. Slow strokes and deep finger pressure are used to soothe the tightest muscles and tendons. This form of therapy focuses of deep layers of muscle tissue. This therapy is generally used to relieve a stiff neck and painful shoulder or back muscles.

have enormous implications for preventing and healing disease and disorder.

• A patient's attitude plays a significant role in the healing process. Individuals participate in their own health by learning about and maintaining healthy lifestyle practices and by complying with medical regimes prescribed by a physician.

• Alternative approaches often involve spirituality in a health and medical regime, broadening options for care without necessarily compromising the effectiveness or acceptance of conventional treatments.

BASIC ALTERNATIVE THERAPIES

The therapies that fall under the rubric of alternative medicine can be divided into six areas: diagnostics; physical therapies or bodywork; natural healing; stimulation; detoxification; and stress management. A seventh category, unconventional alternative therapies, consists of therapies that have little to no scientific support.

Diagnostics. Several alternative diagnostic methods, based on foundations of Eastern religions and philosophies, have a basis in scientific medical research. These include examination of the pulses around the body; examination of the abdomen; observation of skin color and quality of posture and movement; examination of the tongue; listening to the quality of voice and bodily sounds; detailed questioning about habits and family history; examination of bodily fluids; and examination of the patient's sensory experiences.

Among diagnostic methods for which a scientific basis is either absent or tenuous are: psychic methods involving clairvoyance or dowsing; analysis of hair, nails, or other parts of the body with instruments that have no relevance to health; diagnosis based on "auras" (Kirlian photography and polycontrast interface photography); diagnosis based on "readings" of crystals; and faith healing. *See* AYRUVEDIC MEDICINE; CHIROPRACTIC, CHINESE MEDICINE; HOMEOPATHY, *and* OSTEOPATHY.

Physical therapies or bodywork involve manipulation of the body through movement, massage, stretching, or correction of

posture and movement. Chiropractic therapy involves manipulation of the spinal column. Osteopathy involves a combination of traditional medicine and correction of alignment and movement. Other therapies are associated with such names as Alexander, Feldenkrais, Rolf, Rosen, Aston, Heller, Trager, Prudden (myotherapy), and Fitzgerald (reflexology). These methods can help make the individual aware of and feel responsible for his or her own body. They may be of benefit as a complement to traditional therapies. They can be harmful, however, if they discourage an individual from seeking necessary conventional therapies. *See* BODYWORK, CHIROPRACTIC, *and* OSTEOPATHY.

Natural healing involves the use of substances from the "natural" world, although the term may be misleading. Some herbal remedies from various natural healing methods have been used effectively, and often a remedy is produced and marketed, after many years in use as a folk remedy, as a pharmaceutical. *See* AROMATHERAPY, CANCER, DIET THERAPY FOR, HERBAL REMEDIES HOMEOPATHY, *and* NATUROPATHY.

Stimulation denotes therapies that attempt to stimulate the defense and healing mechanisms of the body. This includes acupuncture and acupressure, important methods in Chinese medicine that have been used for anesthesia, treatment of back pain, spasms, and headaches, and controlling addictions. Acupuncture involves the introduction of thin needles into the body and acupressure involves external pressure on critical points. *See* ACUPUNCTURE; ACUPRESSURE; CELL THERAPY; *and* SHIATSU.

Detoxification focuses on ridding the body of toxins and disease-causing agents (real or supposed). These include: chelation therapy, in which a chemical solution is introduced intravenously; colon therapy, in which enemas are used to cleanse the large intestines; fasting; and hydrotherapy, which uses immersion and steam baths. Detoxification should not be used as a substitute for needed medical attention. Some methods can be dangerous.

It is important to realize that detoxifying enzymes are present in virtually every organ system of the human body. They are responsible for breaking down the cancer-causing chemicals in our environment (carcinogens) as well as in drug metabolism. Many nutrients and foods, such as vitamin E, omega-3 fatty acids, garlic, and green tea, increase the levels of the body's detoxifying enzymes. *See* CHELATION THERAPY; COLON THERAPY; FASTING; *and* HYDROTHERAPY.

Stress Management. The connection between stress and health is a matter of ongoing investigation, but there is little doubt that managing stress is important to a healthy life.

Therapies devoted to stress reduction include meditation, in which relaxation is achieved by emptying the mind, biofeedback training, in which electronic devices are used to train an individual to relax, and movement therapies, such as qigong, yoga, and t'ai chi chuan, in which controlled movement or relaxation induce a calm state. *See also* BIOFEEDBACK TRAINING; MEDITATION; T'AI CHI CHUA; *and* YOGA.

UNCONVENTIONAL THERAPIES

For some therapies, there are no data about effectiveness, and some have been used unscrupulously in the past. Extreme caution is advisable when dealing with such therapies. Included in this category are: energy medicine, which uses electronic devices to monitor radiation from the human body; light therapy, which uses colored lights as a form of stimulation; crystal therapy, which uses crystals to "focus" energies; magnetic therapy, in which magnetic fields are applied to relieve pain (some evidence supports this, but not to the extent claimed by proponents); oxygen therapy, in which concentrated oxygen is applied to affected areas; and sound therapy, in which sounds and tones are administered.

In all cases, an alternative therapy should not be pursued without consulting a competent physician. Many physicians are open to the possible effectiveness of alternative therapies, so asking a doctor will most likely result in a thoughtful assessment of which therapies and practitioners the patient should consider.

BEFORE SEEKING ALTERNATIVES

The Office of Alternative Medicine of the National Institute of Health offers the following guidelines:

- Discuss the matter with your physician. You may wish to consult the Office of Alternative Medicine (888-644-6226).
- Investigate the safety and effectiveness of the considered treatment.
- Investigate the credentials and record of any practitioner you consider.
- Inquire how treatments are going to be administered and verify that they conform to accepted safety standards.
- Consider the cost of the alternative treatment and be certain it is not preventing you from seeking competent standard medical treatment.

Altitude Sickness

A condition caused by insufficient intake of oxygen at high altitudes.

Altitude sickness is a common problem among climbers who ascend rapidly to high altitudes. Decrease in air pressure as altitude increases can cause altitude sickness. The concentration of oxygen is 21 percent at sea level and higher altitudes, but air pressure decreases as elevation increases, resulting in less total air inhaled with each breath. Thus, there is less oxygen available from each breath. This lack of oxygen can impair the functioning of the lungs, muscles, heart, and nervous system.

SYMPTOMS

At altitudes above 8,000 feet, over 20 percent of people report symptoms such as dizziness, fatigue, shortness of breath, nausea, and headaches. More severe symptoms include pronounced shortness of breath, mental disorientation, and disturbed balance.

In the most severe form, fluid builds up in the lungs (pulmonary edema) and the brain swells, which may lead to coma.

TREATMENT AND PREVENTION

The simplest treatment is returning to a lower altitude. If symptoms of altitude sickness persist and are severe, the individual may benefit from the prescription medication Diamox, which promotes faster, deeper breathing, and helps more oxygen to the bloodstream.

To prevent altitude sickness, climbers should progress slowly to higher altitudes. Mountain climbers should rest for a day or two after reaching an altitude of 8,000 feet and rest for a day or two for every 2,000 feet thereafter. At altitudes of over 10,000 feet, supplemental oxygen may be needed. Climbers should drink plenty of fluids, eat foods high in carbohydrates, and avoid alcohol or any drugs that interfere with respiration, such as sleeping medications. Good cardiovascular health also reduces the likelihood of altitude sickness. *See also* RESPIRATION *and* RESPIRATORY SYSTEM.

Aluminum

A soft, lightweight metal used in antacids and various materials; it may have toxic effects.

Aluminum is a naturally occurring element found in earth and in most bodies of water. It is found in body tissue, but its function is not understood. It is used in some antiperspirants and in many antacids.

When used in antacids, aluminum can neutralize high levels of acid in the stomach. However, long-term use of antacids containing aluminum can result in a deficiency of phosphorus (hypophosphatemia), which causes weakness and possibly confusion and can result in excretion of elevated amounts of calcium, eventually leading to a loss of bone density (osteoporosis).

There is some speculation that ingested aluminum (from cooking utensils to antacids) has some association with Alzheimer's disease. Increased levels of aluminum have been found in the brain tissue of people who have died from Alzheimer's disease, but these deposits are thought to be a consequence of the disease rather than its cause. *See* ALZHEIMER'S DISEASE.

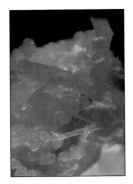

Alveolitis. Above, a microphotograph of the air sacs where the transfer of gases in and out of the blood takes place.

Alveolitis

An inflammation of the air sacs in the lungs (alveoli), caused by an immune reaction or microbes.

Alveolitis is one aspect of hypersensitivity pneumonitis, in which the body becomes sensitized to particular foreign bodies, resulting in immune reactions that damage lung tissue. Foreign bodies that the immune system reacts to can include fungi, chemicals, bacteria, and organic dust. Damage from alveolitis is irreversible in a small percentage of cases.

Types. In the subacute form of alveolitis, coughing and shortness of breath develop over the course of several days. The condition may grow severe enough to require hospitalization.

Chronic hypersensitivity results from repeated exposure to the allergen on a regular basis. Scar tissue may form in the lungs. Shortness of breath, coughing, fatigue, and weight loss become progressively worse. Respiratory failure may ultimately result.

Symptoms can appear within hours to days of exposure. They include fever, chills, cough, shortness of breath, loss of appetite, nausea, and vomiting. Symptoms usually subside within a few hours if no further contact with the antigen occurs, although complete recovery may take longer and may require antimicrobial treatment.

Diagnosis is primarily made by listening to the sounds of chest; alveolitis produces a characteristic crackling sound. X-rays or lung function tests may also be performed.

Treatment is aimed at alleviating symptoms. Corticosteroids can help reduce inflammation. If the damage to the lungs severely compromises pulmonary function, supplementary oxygen may be needed.

Prevention. Identifying the antigen that causes alveolitis is often difficult. Once that is accomplished, the best prevention is to avoid all future contact with the antigen. However, that may not be feasible.

Prognosis is good if exposure to the antigen can be limited, although the chronic form is often progressive. *See also* ALLERGY *and* RESPIRATORY SYSTEM.

Alveoplasty

Surgical reshaping of the bone structures in the mouth being fitted for dentures.

The bony structure of the alveolar ridge lies under the gums. When a person receives dentures, the dentures must be fitted to the form of the alveolar ridge. Dentures are painful and do not successfully stay in place if there are large irregularities in the bone. Alveoplasty contours the bone so the dentures will fit securely and comfortably. *See also* DENTURES.

What to Expect. The procedure can be done with a local anesthetic, possibly with some sedation. The gum is opened to reveal the irregular area of bone, which is shaped and smoothed. The gum is then closed and stitched. The incision, bruising, and swelling heal in about two weeks.

Alveolus

One of 300 million air sacs in each lung.

The exchange of oxygen and carbon dioxide between the blood and the lungs occurs in the alveoli. The alveoli make up most of the lungs' volume, and they create a vast surface area for gas exchange.

Air travels through the trachea, which divides into two branches called bronchi. The bronchi further subdivide into bronchioles, which become narrower and branch out. At the tip of each branch is a balloon-like alveolus. Clusters of alveoli form alveolar sacs, which are shaped like bunches of grapes and cobwebbed with capillaries. The alveolar and capillary walls form the respiratory membrane—gas flows on one side and blood flows on the other. Alveoli walls are much thinner than tissue paper. Carbon dioxide diffuses from the blood into the alveoli, and oxygen diffuses out of the alveoli and into the blood. Oxygen molecules are captured by red blood cells and carried to the heart, which pumps blood through the body. Carbon dioxide in the alveoli is exhaled. *See* RESPIRATION; LUNG; BLOOD; OXYGEN; CARBON DIOXIDE.

Alzheimer's Disease

A degenerative disease in which the nerve cells of the brain deteriorate, resulting in impaired memory, thinking, and behavior.

Twenty-five to fifty percent of all people over the age of 85 are likely to have Alzheimer's disease—a common cause of dementia among the elderly. Named after the German neurologist Alois Alzheimer who discovered the disease in the early 1900's, Alzheimer's disease has been diagnosed in over 4 million people in the United States. It is most prevalent among the elderly but should not be considered a natural consequence of the aging process.

CAUSES

It is generally thought that Alzheimer's disease is probably not caused by just one factor, but by a combination of genetic and environmental factors. Genetic predisposition is probably present in more than half of the cases of Alzheimer's disease. Some researchers believe Alzheimer's disease is caused by a virus; if this is the case, identifying the virus could lead to the development of a vaccine.

SYMPTOMS

Alzheimer's disease predominantly affects the parts of the brain that control thought, memory and language ability, resulting in a loss of cognitive ability known as dementia. Symptoms, which become progressively more severe, may include:

- **Memory Loss.** Short term memory is lost first. In later stages, the person may cease to recognize familiar places, objects, friends, and family members.
- **Disorientation,** such as getting lost in a familiar neighborhood.
- **Impaired ability to perform skilled tasks**, progressing eventually to an inability to perform self-care tasks, such as putting on clothing and washing.
- **Language Impairment**, such as the inability to find the appropriate words in a conversation.

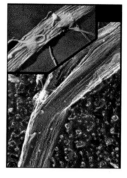

Aging Dendrites. Both the axons, bottom, and the dendrites , top, of the neurons in the brain of an Alzheimer's sufferer show signs of wear and plaque not found in the normal brain.

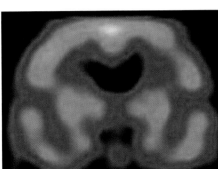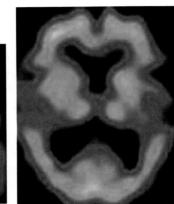

Brain Scan of an Alzheimer's sufferer. Though it is believed Alzheimer's disease is caused by local neural damage, MRI scans of the brain reveal that blood flow to the brain of an Alzheimer's sufferer, above right, is restricted compared to normal blood flow, above left.

- **Impaired social functioning;**
- **Irritability**, aggression, and paranoia;
- **Sleeplessness**;
- **Depression**.

Despite cognitive impairments, Alzheimer's patients can retain remarkable physical capability until very late in the disease.

Progression of the disease is usually characterized by three stages. In the first stage, signs of memory loss, such as forgetting words or misplacing objects, may be so subtle that they are not easily identified. Some researchers believe that the onset of Alzheimer's is so slow that it begins to develop decades before recognizable signs appear. In the second stage, deterioration of cognitive abilities becomes more apparent. By the third stage, the disease usually has become so severe that the person is unable to care for him or herself.

DIAGNOSIS.

Diagnosis is based on symptoms and on ruling out other possible causes of dementia. Blood, urine, and spinal fluid tests should reveal no other causes for the symptoms. Imaging tests such as magnetic resonance imaging (MRI), positron emission tomography (PET) scanning, and computerized tomography (CT) scanning reveal that the brain tissue has shrunk, cavities within the brain have enlarged, and protein deposits have formed. However, the diagnosis can only be absolutely determined (confirmed) by autopsy and microscopic examination of the brain cells.

TREATMENT

No treatment can cure Alzheimer's disease. However, if it is identified early, medications—including aricept, reminyl, and exelon—can be prescribed to delay the progress of the disease in some patients.

Some underlying health disorders that may contribute to congnitive impairment, if untreated, include:

- thyroid disease;
- anemia; and
- nutritional disorders.

Medications can be prescribed to treat symptoms such as sleeplessness, aggression, anxiety and depression. Many new drugs and experimental procedures are currently being studied by researchers around the globe.

Alzheimer's Disease in the Family. Initial care of the Alzheimer's patient is usually performed in the home by family

---

Additional Information and Assistance

Alzheimer's can be a difficult disease for family members and other caregivers. Knowing about the course of the disease, treatment options, and where to find emotional support can make caring for a person with Alzheimer's less difficult.

Alzheimer's Association
919 N. Michigan Avenue. Suite 1000
Chicago, IL 60611-1676
800-272-3900
This organization supports caregivers and families. There are chapters in many major cities that can offer referrals to local services and resources.

Alzheimer's Disease Education and Referral Center
PO Box 8250
Silver Spring, MD 20907-8250
800-438-4380
This division of the National Institute on Aging is funded by the federal government. It offers information on diagnosis, treatment, and patient care, and referrals to resources and services nationwide.

Eldercare Locator
1112 16th Street NW, Suite 100
Washington, DC 20036
800-677-1116
This is a division of the National Association of Area Agencies on Aging. It provides information and referrals to home and local services offered by state agencies.

members. As the disease progresses, families may become unable to care for their loved one at home and may choose a nursing facility better equipped to monitor the needs of someone with severe dementia. This choice is difficult and many choose to research possible alternatives before selecting this option, such as adult day care.

At present, Alzheimer's disease cannot be cured, although it can be delayed somewhat. The disease is progressive, and death usually occurs, on average, about 10 years after the original diagnosis, though it greatly varies.

Basic physiological information on Alzheimer's Disease may be found in BRAIN; DEMYELINATION; NERVE; *and* SYNAPSE. *For additional information on symptoms of the disease, see* AGING; DEGENERATIVE DISORDERS; MEMORY; *and* SENILITY.

Amalgam, Dental

An alloy used in dental repair.

Dental amalgam is informally called silver fillings. It is an alloy of silver and other metals, chosen for their durability. After a cavity is prepared, the amalgam is packed in and shaped while it hardens. Silver fillings as we know them have been used successfully for more than a century and can last for decades.

There has been concern in the last decade or so because many amalgams contain traces of mercury. The American Dental Association has approved amalgam as safe, citing numerous studies and its long history of use. Still, some people have had their silver fillings removed and replaced with other substances. There have been reports of allergic reactions to amalgam, but these are extremely rare. *See also* ALLERGY, CARIES, DENTAL; *and* DENTISTRY.

Amaurosis Fugax

Temporary partial or total loss of vision.

Amaurosis fugax is a condition in which there are brief periods of vision loss varying from seconds to minutes. The vision loss is usually in one eye only. It may occur rarely or it may recur frequently throughout the day. Amaurosis fugax occurs as a result of a momentary blockage of the eye's blood vessels by particles of clotted blood and cholesterol, which are dislodged from the walls of the arteries of the neck and heart region. Temporary vision loss, whether it occurs once or many times a day, indicates a high risk for coronary disease or stroke. These symptoms should not be ignored. *See also* ARTERIES; BLOOD VESSELS; CHOLESTEROL; CORONARY DISEASE; EYES; HEART; NECK; *and* STROKE.

Amaurotic Familial Idiocy

A range of inherited disorders of progressive deterioration of the nervous system.

Amaurotic familial idiocy is an outdated term for a number of degenerative nervous system disorders, the most well-known of which is Tay-Sachs disease. The name refers to three features of the disorders: blindness (amaurotic), a genetic cause (familial), and severe retardation (idiocy).

The disorder is passed on through a recessive gene; a child must receive a copy of the defective gene from each parent in order to have the disease. If both parents are carriers, each child has one in four chance of inheriting the disorder. If only one parent is a carrier, a child has a 50 percent chance of also being a carrier but will not have the disease. The symptoms results from the excessive storage of a compound called lipofuscin that, when present in large amounts, damages nerve tissue.

Symptoms. The disorder usually becomes apparent sometime after the first year or during adolescence or early adulthood. Children develop difficulty with muscle coordination (ataxia), as well as walking abnormalities, vision problems, retardation, and seizures. Later onset of the condition exhibits less severe symptoms. *See also* AGING; BLINDNESS; BRAIN; CHROMOSOMES; GENETICS; GERONTOLOGY; MUSCLES; *and* TAY-SACHS DISEASE.

Resources on Alzheimer's Disease
Gruetzner, Howard, *Alzheimer's: A Caregiver's Guide and Sourcebook, 3rd Edition* (2001); Shenk, David, *The Forgetting: Alzheimer's: Portrait of an Epidemic* (2001); Terry, Robet D., ed., *Aging and the Brain* (1988); West, Robin L. and Jan D. Sinnott, eds., *Everyday Memory and Aging* (1992); Alzheimer's Disease Education and Referral Center, Tel. (800) 438-4380, On-line: www.alzheimers.org; www.nycornell.org/medicine/neurology/index.html ;www.nyp.org/css/.

Ambidexterity

The ability to use both hands equally well.

Handedness, a preference for using one hand over the other, is determined by the structure of the brain. The cerebrum is divided into two hemispheres. The left hemisphere controls the right side of the body, and the right hemisphere controls the left side. In the vast majority of the population, one hemisphere is dominant. In two-thirds, the left hemisphere is dominant—thus most people are right-handed.

Ambidexterity refers to a state in which neither hemisphere is dominant; and therefore an individual is able to use one hand as well as the other. True ambidextrous individuals are exceedingly rare.

Most people can be "trained" to use their weak hand. For example, a person who breaks the preferred arm may learn to write with the other hand. Also, left-handed people used to be "encouraged" by their families and schools to use their right hands instead. This is not the same as natural ambidexterity.

Infants start out ambidextrous and rarely show a preference before the age of one year, due to the fact that their brains are still rapidly developing. A clear preference before that time may be an indication of a problem. *See* CEREBRUM *and* HANDEDNESS.

Amblyopia

Loss of sight caused by a failure of the nerves to properly transmit images to the brain.

Amblyopia is a permanent reduction of vision, usually resulting when the vision in one eye is significantly weaker than in the other eye. It appears to result from a failure of the nerve fibers between one or both eyes and the brain to successfully link up. For development of proper vision, it is necessary that each side of the brain receive a clear visual message from each eye. In infants and small children, if vision is blocked or an eye is not used, the nerves do not develop in a way that enables normal sight.

Causes. The most common cause of amblyopia is misalignment of the eye (strabismus), a defect in which one of the eyes has weaker vision and deviates too far to the right or left. The eyes receive significantly different pictures and thus send different messages to the brain. Usually the brain ignores the message emanating from the weaker, deviated eye. Prolonged suppression of the use of the eye can result in complete loss of visual ability in that eye.

Another cause is congenital cataracts, in which the lens of the eye is clouded, prevent successful formation of clear images. Infants born with cataracts do not develop the nerve pathways necessary for sight. Although cataracts can be removed, if they are not caught and treated early enough, vision loss may persist.

Treatment. Young children are the best candidates for correction. If the condition is not corrected early enough, vision in the affected eye may be permanently reduced. Strabismus can be corrected with special glasses, eye exercises, a patch worn over one eye, or surgery on the eye muscle. Congenital cataracts can be surgically removed. *See also* CATARACT SURGERY *and* STRABISMUS.

Ambulance

Vehicle carrying life-support equipment designed to transport victims of illness or accident.

Ambulances are far more varied in function, design, and staffing than most people realize. In a simple emergency, emergency medical technicians (EMTs) trained in basic life support (BLS) are dispatched. In a severe emergency that requires highly trained personnel and soph- isticated equipment, skilled paramedics trained in advanced life support (ALS) are sent.

EQUIPMENT
Some ambulances contain stretchers with collapsible legs so that a victim can be transported from the home or an accident site to an emergency treatment center. A fully equipped advanced life support emergency ambulance will have a cardiac moni-

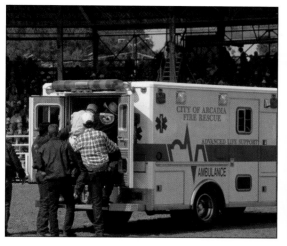

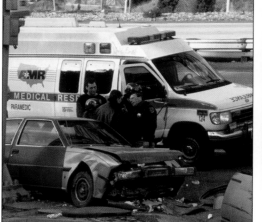

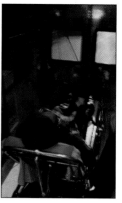

Ambulance. Frequently the most important element in a medical response to an accident or an emergency is the ambulance service. Getting patients to medical facilities quickly and administering initial emergency procedure en route, above, can make an enormous difference in the outcome. Above, left, a larger ambulance may have more room for equipment, but a smaller vehicle, above middle, may be better able to negotiate urban traffic.

tor and defibrillator, oxygen and oxygen monitoring equipment as a well as intravenous fluids and medications that may be needed in medical emergencies.

In addition to these vehicles, there are also various types of non-emergency ambulances, which are used primarily for transport. These can include medicars and vans that deliver people to hospitals and daycare clinics. Chair cars are non-emergency ambulances designed to lift a wheelchair and hold it firmly in place. *See also* FIRST AID; HOSPITAL; PREVENTATIVE MEASSURES *and* STRETCHER.

Ambulatory Care

Also known as outpatient care

Medical services provided to individuals on an outpatient (nonhospitalized) basis.

Ambulatory health care consists of services provided to patients who are neither hospitalized nor institutionalized. It may include a wide variety of medical services, including diagnosis, observation, treatment, and rehabilitation.

There are many types of outpatient care. Hospitals often have outpatient clinics. Communities often have neighborhood health centers and walk-in clinics. Physicians may offer some forms of treatment, including minor surgery, in their offices. Ambulatory surgery is usually an operation that does not require an overnight hospital stay. Examples of ambulatory surgery include laser vision correction, some types of endoscopy, and plastic surgery. *See also* OUTPATIENT TREATMENT.

Amebiasis

Infection of the large intestine caused by a parasite.

The parasite *Entamoeba histolytica* lives on other bacteria and on the lining of the intestine. It produces cysts that are passed with the stool and spread to others by contact with infected stool, unsafe sexual practices, and through contaminated food or water. Fruits and vegetables fertilized by human waste or washed in polluted water can carry the parasite. People contract amebiasis by swallowing the cysts.

Symptoms of amebiasis are chills, fever, and diarrhea, which may be bloody and produce cramps. Symptoms may be delayed for weeks or months after infection.

Diagnosis. Amebiasis is diagnosed by microscopic examination of the stool, which reveals the parasite or the cysts. If the parasite attacks the intestinal wall a lump may be formed; this lump can be misdiagnosed as cancer.

Treatment. Amebiasis is treated with drugs aimed at destroying the parasite, including iodoquinol, paromomycin, metronidozole, and diloxanide. Early treatment is usually successful, but the disease can be fatal if not treated. *See also* PARASITE.

Amelogenesis Imperfecta

Insufficient enamel in the outer layer of the teeth.

Amlegenesis imperfecta is an inherited disorder in which the enamel of the tooth is extremely thin and brittle, resulting in discoloration and greater susceptibility to disease and decay. The teeth appear yellowed, because dentin, the second layer of the teeth, shows through the enamel.

Treatment usually involves capping the teeth with artificial crowns. This makes the teeth look better and protects them from bacteria. *See also* CARIES, DENTAL *and* DISCOLORED TEETH.

Amenorrhea

Absence of menstrual periods in women who are not pregnant and have not undergone menopause.

Amenorrhea is classified into two categories: primary amenorrhea, which indicates a delay in reaching first menstruation (menarche), and secondary amenorrhea, which indicates a cessation of menstruation in someone who has previously menstruated. Amenorrhea is distinct from the condition known as oligomenorrhea, in which menstruation is irregular or infrequent but not entirely absent.

Primary amenorrhea is diagnosed in girls if they have not begun menstruating by age 16. Menarche can be delayed in athletic or very thin girls whose body fat level is below a certain percentage. A doctor should be consulted if, in addition to delayed menarche, a girl has not yet undergone other sexual changes, such as breast development and the growth of pubic hair by age 14.

Secondary amenorrhea is defined as the absence of menstruation for six months or longer in adult women who are not pregnant.

Causes of secondary amenorrhea vary widely. It can be a result of losing a lot of weight very quickly or intense, prolonged bouts of exercise. Stress and a very high or very low level of body fat can prevent the ovaries from producing estrogen in a normal cyclic manner. Taking oral contraceptives can affect a woman's monthly cycle, even a few months after she has quit taking them. Women who are breast-feeding often fail to menstruate for several months. As women approach the age of menopause, it is normal for the number of menstrual periods to decrease, and for the duration between them to grow longer. Menopause is established when a woman has not had a period for at least 12 months and her hormonal levels are consistent with that diagnosis.

It is important to note that amenorrhea may or may not indicate a lack of ovulation; even if a woman is not menstruating, she may still ovulate.

Serious causes of secondary amenorrhea include tumors and disorders of the pituitary gland. Postpartum pituitary necrosis occurs when the pituitary gland fails, either partly or completely, at the time of childbirth. This results in a failure to resume menstruating, as well as an inability to produce milk.

Diagnosis. The doctor will perform a physical exam, check to see if the ovaries are producing a normal amount of estrogen, and determine if ovulation is occurring. In general, any woman who is sexually active, has been menstruating regularly, and whose period is two or more weeks late should undergo a pregnancy test.

Treatment for amenorrhea depends on determining and correcting the underlying cause. If amenorrhea is a result of having lost or gained a lot of weight, regaining normal weight is the first step to resuming menstruation. Exercise should be moderate rather than excessively strenuous. If estrogen levels are low, estrogen therapy may be recommended; in any case, a sufficient level of estrogen is needed for the prevention of osteoporosis later in life. If amenorrhea is caused by a pituitary tumor, the tumor can be surgically removed.

Unless it is caused by a serious disorder, the biggest difficulty with secondary amenorrhea may be lack of ovulation. Amenorrhea may or may not be accompanied by a failure to ovulate. If ovulation is affected, a woman who wishes to get pregnant may need to see an infertility specialist.

American Medical Association

Organization of American physicians.

The American Medical Association (AMA), founded more than 150 years ago, is the main organization of physicians in the United States. It serves as a voice for American physicians .

The AMA promotes standards in medical practice, research, and education. It publishes *The Journal of the American Medical Association* and other specialized medical journals. It works as an active advocate of patients' rights, health insurance reform, and many other issues in public health. The seat of AMA policy making is the AMA House of Delegates, where state, local, and other representatives set policy for the organization. *See also* ACCREDITATION *and* BOARD CERTIFICATION.

Amino Acids

The basic building block of protein; essential in maintaining muscle and tissue in the body.

Amino acids are organic compounds that can be joined together in chains to form proteins. They are either produced by the human body (non-essential) or acquired through protein in the diet (essential) if not produced by the body in sufficient amounts. Amino acids can be converted into a sugar (glucose) by the liver, but most are necessary to maintaining connective tissues, blood, skin, organs, and muscles. Amino acids also play a major role in healing wounds, fetal development, milk production, and the growth of hair and nails.

Dietary sources of amino acids include animal and plant proteins. Animal proteins are more complete in providing essential amino acids, while vegetable protein sources usually lack one or more essential amino acids. For a vegetarian diet to be ad-

equate, complementary vegetable sources (in which one source provides amino acids missing in the other) should be combined. *See also* PROTEINS *and* PROTEIN SYNTHESIS.

Amnesia

Partial or total loss of memory caused by shock, brain injury, or mental or physical illness.

There are two types of memory: long-term and short-term. Long-term memory stores information for long periods of time, while short-term stores information only briefly. Most amnesias are a result of impaired functioning of long-term memory, either in the process of information storage or in the recall of the information.

Types of amnesia include:
- **Anterograde Amnesia**—the inability to learn new information.
- **Amnestic Syndrome**—the loss of all memory except short-term memory.
- **Post-Traumatic Amnesia**—the loss of memory of a traumatic event.
- **Retrograde amnesia**—memory loss of events prior to onset of brain damage.
- **Wernicke-Korsakoff Syndrome**— memory loss and other neurological impairments caused by thiamine (vitamin B_1) deficiency, usually a result of excessive intake of alcohol.
- **Transient Global Amnesia**—a confusion of time and place that may be caused by excessive alcohol, barbiturates, or benzodiazepine drugs.

Causes. Memory disorders may occur as a result of a head injury, a stroke, or a brain tumor. Amnesia may also be caused by diseases, such as Alzheimer's disease, dementia, encephalitis, and thiamine deficiency. They may also have a psychological cause, in which memory of a traumatic event is suppressed.

Treatment. In amnesia caused by thiamine deficiency, treatment consists of administering thiamine. In posttraumatic amnesia, psychotherapy may help. There is no known treatment for other amnesias, although some may self-correct over time. *See also* DEMENTIA *and* MEMORY.

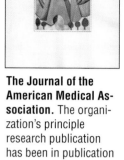

The Journal of the American Medical Association. The organization's principle research publication has been in publication since 1883.

Resources on Amnesia
Damasio, Antonio R., *Descartes' Error: Emotion Reason and the Human Brain* (1994); Herman, Judith, *Trauma and Recovery* (1992); Restak, Richard, *The Secret Life of the Brain* (2001); Schachter, Daniel L., *Searching for Memory: The Brain, The Mind, and the Past* (1996); West, Robin L. and Jan D. Sinnott, eds., *Everyday Memory and Aging* (1992); National Mental Health Association, Tel. (800) 969-NMHA, On-line: www.nmha.org; www.nycornell.org/medicine/neurology/index.html ;www.nyp.org/css/.

Amniocentesis

A prenatal test for detecting congenital defects in which a sample of fluid from the amniotic sac is removed and analyzed.

Amniocentesis is one of the most commonly performed prenatal tests for detecting congenital defects. The procedure is done early in the second trimester of pregnancy, usually between the 16th and 18th weeks. A small amount of amniotic fluid is drained from the sac surrounding the fetus. The fluid contains cast-off fetal cells, which are then cultured and analyzed for the presence of chromosomal anomalies,

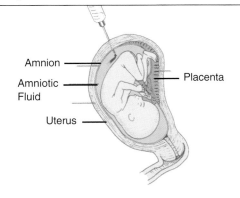

Amnion

Amniotic Fluid

Placenta

Uterus

such as the presence of the extra chromosome that causes Down's syndrome. Additionally, amniocentesis can determine the presence of spina bifida or other neurological disorders, kidney disease, and various metabolic problems. The test also reveals the baby's gender, but it is not performed solely for that purpose.

Amniocentesis is recommended for all women age 35 or older, as the chances of

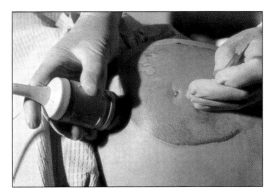

Amniocentesis. Amniocentesis has become more common as the risk to mother and fetus has gone down; it is generally performed when the benefits of detecting a problem outweigh the risks of the procedure. Below, left, an ultrasound wand provides a clear view (far right) of the fetus as a needle is inserted into the amniotic sac. It may soon become possible to retrieve the fetus' genetic information from a blood test of the mother, but the immunological barrier between the fetus and the mother may make complete prenatal diagnosis from maternal blood difficult.

giving birth to a child with a birth defect increases with age, those who have a family history of conditions such as Down's Syndrome or spina bifida, and those who have previously had children with birth defects. The test can also be performed later in pregnancy to see if there is a chance of blood (Rh) incompatibility or to determine if the baby's lungs are mature enough for an early delivery.

Procedure. Prior to amniocentesis, an ultrasound is done to examine the fetus and determine its exact location. A long, thin needle is inserted into the abdomen; the needle is aimed at a part of the amniotic sac that is not near the placenta or the fetus' face. This process should be monitored continuously with ultrasound, so that the location of the needle and of the fetus are known at all times. About two tablespoons of amniotic fluid are withdrawn through the needle.

Usually the woman's partner is present during the procedure. Afterwards there may be some slight cramping; this is normal and should dissipate within a day or so. Any fever, fluid leakage, or severe cramping should be reported to a physician.

There is a waiting period of a few weeks between the time when the procedure is performed until the results are available, due to the necessity of growing the cells in a culture medium.

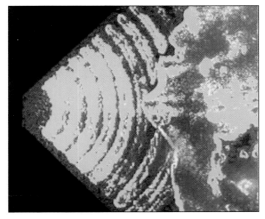

Risks. Amniocentesis is generally safe, but it does carry a very minor risk of miscarriage, however, this risk is usually out weighed by the potential benefits of this procedure.

Chorionic Villus Sampling. Recently, another test, chorionic villus sampling, has been developed. This test can detect many of the same genetic abnormalities as amniocentesis, but it can be performed much earlier, between 10 and 12 weeks. This is a more invasive procedure; a catheter is inserted into the uterus through either the cervix or the abdominal and a small sample of placental tissue is removed by suction. Chorionic villus sampling is not as effective as amniocentesis in determining the presence of certain disorders, and occasionally both procedures must be performed to make a correct diagnosis. Chorionic villus sampling may carry a higher risk of miscarriage and uterine infection than amniocentesis. *See also* PREVENTIVE SCREENING.

Amphetamine Drugs

Stimulant drugs that also act as appetite suppressants, but which can be addictive.

Amphetamine drugs operate by stimulating the production of neurotransmitters, chemicals that transmit messages between nerve endings (for example, norepinephrine). Nerve activity in the brain increases, making a person feel awake and alert. Amphetamines were once prescribed as a method of weight loss, but they are now rarely used for that purpose because of the dangers of addiction and abuse.

Amphetamines are primarily prescribed to treat attention deficit hyperactivity disorder and narcolepsy, a sleeping disorder that results in suddenly falling asleep in the course of normal activity.

Abuse. Amphetamines are addictive and continue to be used illegally. Improper use can cause tremors, palpitations, anxiety, hallucinations, high blood pressure, and seizures. An overdose of amphetamines can lead to cardiac arrest. Signs of overdose include anxiety, agitation, sweating, constricted pupils, aggressive or violent behavior, and palpitations. If a person has overdosed on amphetamines (or is suspected of having taken a large dose of amphetamines), emergency medical help is needed.

Basic biochemical information is contained in ANTIANXIETY DRUGS; NEUROTRANSMITTERS; *and* SYNAPSE. *Further information regarding amphetamines may be found in* EATING DISORDERS; NARCOLEPSY; *and* WEIGHT LOSS. *Details on abuse of these drugs will be found in* DRUG DEPENDENCE; FAMILY THERAPY; *and* SUBSTANCE ABUSE.

Amputation

Surgical removal of part or all of a limb or appendage, usually to prevent the spread of gangrene.

Body parts that may be amputated include arms, legs, hands, feet, fingers, toes, and, on rare occasion, penises. An amputation may also occur accidentally (traumatic amputation), or a limb may be missing from birth (congenital amputation).

Reasons for Surgery. The primary reason for most amputations is an interrupted blood supply to the body part, which results in tissue death (gangrene). The interruption can be caused by injury to blood vessels or by impaired blood circulation due to diabetes mellitus, atherosclerosis, obstructions in the arteries, and other circulatory disorders. Severe infections, frostbite, malignant tumors, and bone cancer may also require amputation.

Complications from diabetes are easily the largest single cause of amputations. High levels of blood sugar can cause the walls of small blood vessels to thicken (arteriosclerosis), which can impair circulation in the legs and feet and subsequently cause gangrene. About 800,000 diabetic patients in the United States develop chronic foot ulcers, which lead to approximately 55,000 limb amputations each year.

Procedure. The site of amputation must contain healthy tissues and be above the site of the gangrene in order to ensure proper healing. A circular incision is made around the part to be amputated; skin and muscle are cut below the level at which the bone is cut in order to create flaps that will later provide a stump. Tissue, muscles, blood vessels, and nerves are severed. The surgeon makes an effort to sever the nerves above the stump in order to minimize pressure pain when the patient is eventually fitted with a prosthesis. The blood vessels are tied off, and the bone is severed and then rounded off and covered with connective tissue. The muscles and skin flaps are then sutured. Tubes are inserted in each side of the wound to allow for drainage.

Recovery. The average hospital stay following amputation lasts from two to seven days. The recovery period is approximately six weeks, during which physical therapy begins and after which a prosthesis is fitted. Recent innovations in prosthetics are so effective that most patients can resume quite normal lives and participate in sports and other activities.

Background material on amputations may be found in CIRCULATORY SYSTEM; DIABETES; *and* GANGRENE. *More information on the procedure is contained in* ANESTHESIOLOGY; RADICAL SURGERY; *and* SURGERY. *Coping with amputations is discussed in* DISABLED, *and* PROSTHESIS.

Amyloidosis

A rare condition in which a substance called amyloid, made up of protein and starch, accumulates in different tissues and organs.

Amyloidosis usually occurs after age 40 and is most common in men over the age of 60. Primary amyloidosis is of unknown cause, and secondary amyloidosis occurs as a complication of another condition, such as malignant myeloma, Hodgkin's disease, rheumatoid arthritis, cystic fibrosis, tuberculosis, or an inflammatory ailment.

Symptoms of amyloidosis include weakness, fatigue, breathlessness, numbness and swelling of the hands and feet, and weight loss; patients may also experience lightheadedness. The tongue may appear enlarged and rubbery. Other symptoms depend on the extent and location of amyloid deposits. Extensive deposits can severely impair the functioning of affected organs. Deposits in the kidneys can cause impairment of their filtering mechanisms, result-ing in an increase of protein in the urine, swelling of the ankles, and changes in appetite. Deposit in the heart can cause an abnormal heartbeat or a reduced ability to pump blood as the accumulation of amyloid reduces the flexibility and contractility of the heart muscle. Deposits in the skin can produce waxy bumps, often around the face and neck. Deposits in the stomach and intestines can result in diarrhea or constipation.

Diagnosis. Amyloidosis is diagnosed by taking a tissue sample from an affected tissue or organ and examining it under a microscope, revealing an excess of protein.

Treatment. Primary amyloidosis cannot be cured, but treatments can relieve some of the major symptoms. When deposits build up in the lungs or bladder, surgery can bring relief. Anti-inflammatory medications such as methotrexate or cyclophosphamide may be prescribed. Secondary amyloidosis can be alleviated by treatment of the underlying condition, with additional therapy aimed at relief.

Prognosis. The long-term prognosis is often not favorable, since progression of the disease can result in kidney or heart failure. If the kidneys fail, dialysis or a kidney transplant may be performed. *See also* CYSTIC FIBROSIS; GENETIC DISORDERS. HODGKIN'S DISEASE; *and* RHEUMATOID ARTHRITIS.

Amyotrophy

Wasting away or shrinkage of a muscle.

Amyotrophy is a reduction in size of muscles fibers. It is usually caused by inadequate nutrition, decreased use of a muscle, or disturbance to a muscle's blood or nerve supply, as in diabetes mellitus or poliomyelitis. In diabetes, weakening and deterioration of the muscles is usually accompanied by pain. Neuralgic amyotrophy involves pain in the shoulders and upper arms, with muscle atrophy and paralysis across the shoulders. Amyotrophic lateral sclerosis (Lou Gehrig's Disease) is a well-known cause of progressive amyotrophy. *See also* MOTOR NEURON DISEASE.

Anaerobic

Requiring no oxygen.

Certain organisms, energy processes (metabolic processes), and forms of exercise do not require the presence of oxygen. Anaerobic exercise focuses on muscle building and bone strengthening. Short, strenuous forms of exercise, such as sprinting, are also primarily anaerobic, since the muscles work faster than they can be supplied with oxygen. During anaerobic exercise, a byproduct of exertion known as lactic acid builds up in the muscles. Lactic acid buildup disrupts muscle activity and may result in cramping of the muscles and exhaustion. Lactic acid has to be broken down in order for muscle function to return to normal. Therefore, anaerobic exercise cannot be sustained for a long period of time, because of the inevitable buildup of lactic acid in the muscles.

Anaerobic metabolism is far less efficient than aerobic metabolism, yielding only one-fifth of the amount of energy-producing chemicals generated by aerobic metabolism. Aerobic cardiovascular exercise is extremely beneficial in many ways, and it makes the body more energy-efficient. *See also* ADP; AEROBIC; ATP; CRAMP; EXERCISE; FITNESS; FITNESS TESTING; LACTIC ACID; METABOLISM; *and* MUSCLE SPASM.

Anal Dilation

A procedure for enlarging the anus.

The anus can be dilated by a physician using a special instrument called an anal dilator, or by using the fingers. A patient can also use an anal dilator with the help of lubricating jelly. Anal dilation is usually performed for conditions in which the anus becomes too tight, such as anal stenosis, a congenital condition in which the anus is too constricted to allow the normal passage of feces. The anus can also be dilated to relieve hemorrhoids. *See also* ANUS, CANCER OF; ANUS, DISORDERS OF; COLON CANCER; *and* HEMORRHOIDS.

Anal Discharge

Passage of pus, blood, or mucus through the anus.

Anal discharge can be caused by hemorrhoids—abnormally enlarged veins in the lining of the anus that are prone to bleed. It can also be due to an anal fissure—a tear extending upward into the anal tract—or proctitis, inflammation of the rectum. The discharge of mucus from the anus can irritate the skin around it, causing intense itching. The symptoms of anal discharge can be relieved by taking warm therapeutic baths for 10 to 15 minutes after each bowel movement and by a diet rich in fiber. *See also* ANUS, DISORDERS OF; ANAL FISSURE; HEMORRHOIDS; *and* PROCTITIS.

Anal Fissure

A visible tear or laceration near the anus.

An anal fissure can be caused by an injury, a small ulcer resulting from chronic infection, passage of rough stools, severe diarrhea, or damage during childbirth. The condition causes severe pain, which can be accompanied by the passage of some blood. While many fissures heal on their own, treatment to relieve the pain can include an anesthetic ointment or warm, therapeutic baths after bowel movements. Minor surgery may be needed in severe cases. Preventive measures include a diet rich in whole grains, fruits, and vegetables to increase the intake of fiber. *See also* ANAL DILATION; ANUS, CANCER OF; *and* ANUS, DISORDERS OF.

Anal Fistula

An abnormality in the passage from the inside of the anal canal to the external skin around the anus.

The most common cause of an anal fistula is an abscess that discharges pus into the anus and the surrounding skin. Other possible causes include diseases such as Crohn's disease, intestinal cancer, tuberculosis, and damage during childbirth. Symptoms include severe pain in the rectum or abdomen and fever lasting more than two days. Most fistulas are treated by a surgical procedure, done under general anesthesia, called a fistulotomy, in which the passage is opened, the fistulous lining removed, and the pus drained. *See also* ANUS, DISORDERS OF; CROHN'S DISEASE; *and* TUBERCULOSIS.

Analeptic Drugs

Medications that stimulate breathing.

Analeptic drugs are used for conditions in which normal breathing stops, such as apnea in a newborn child or respiratory failure in an adult. They can also be given to help restore normal breathing for a patient who has been under general anesthesia. Breathing is controlled by the respiratory center of the brain, which regulates the rate and volume of respiration. Breathing can stop when the brain stops sending signals to the respiratory system. Analeptic drugs, such as doxapram and nikethamide, act on the respiratory center, restoring more normal function. *See also* ANESTHESIA, GENERAL *and* APNEA.

Analgesic Drugs

Drugs to relieve pain, ranging from relatively mild painkillers, such as aspirin, to powerful and addictive drugs, such as morphine.

Analgesic drugs may be used for a number of reasons. Weak analgesics, such as aspirin, acetaminophen, and ibuprofen, are used to relieve mild pain. More potent analgesics, such as morphine, are used to relieve the severe pain that follows injury, surgery, or is associated with life-threatening diseases, such as Acquired Immunodeficiency Syndrome (AIDS) and cancer. There are two main types of analgesics: nonopioid and opioid.

Nonopioid analgesics include aspirin, acetaminophen, and ibuprofen (which is a nonsteroidal anti-inflammatory drug, or NSAID). These drugs are often available over the counter and are used to treat minor pain, and to reduce fever and inflammation.

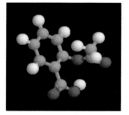

Analgesic Drugs.
Aspirin, above, and NS-AIDs inhibit proteins called COX-1 and COX-2. A new type of NSAID, available with a prescription, only inhibits the COX-2 proteins. This can reduce side effects on the stomach. These new drugs are used to prevent joint pain in patients with osteoarthritis. There have also been signs that these drugs may prevent colon cancer.

Opioid analgesics include codeine, morphine, and methadone. They block the transmission of pain signals to the brain. Opioid analgesics are potent and often addictive, and they must be used under the supervision of a physician. Analgesics may also be combined with each other. For example, some drugs combine acetaminophen with codeine. *See also* OPIATE.

Anaphylactic Shock

A severe, often life-threatening, allergic reaction.

Anaphylactic shock can be triggered by an allergic reaction to bee or other insect stings or bites, certain drugs or foods, dyes used in diagnostic tests, or even a blood transfusion. Shock occurs when the allergic reaction is so severe that it triggers the blood vessels to dilate, causing a sudden drop in blood pressure and circulatory failure. The allergic reaction may also trigger swelling of tissues in the throat, which can result in blocked air passageways. Loss of consciousness may follow.

Symptoms. Symptoms of anaphylactic shock may occur at any time within two hours of exposure to the specific allergen. They include a rapid pulse; difficulty breathing; pallor; cold, clammy skin; very low blood pressure; nausea and vomiting; and convulsions. If left untreated, the patient will lapse into a coma.

Treatment. Anaphylactic shock necessitates immediate medical intervention. If the patient's breathing ceases, mouth-to-mouth resuscitation should be performed at once. *See also* ALLERGY.

ALERT

Treatment for Anaphylactic Shock
In cases of anaphylactic shock, emergency services (911) should be called immediately. Lay the victim down and elevate the legs. Persons with a history of anaphylactic shock may have a syringe of epinephrine on their person; this should be injected. If the victim possesses a device called an "EpiPen," remove the cap and firmly strike the victim's thigh. If the victim stops breathing, it is important to perform CPR until medical help arrives.

Anastomosis

A natural or man-made connection in the body.

An anastomosis usually occurs between blood vessels or between tubular organs (such as the intestines). Normally separate, the vessels or organs may be joined because of injury or through surgery.

An example of a natural anastomosis is a joined artery and vein (arteriovenous fistula). Small arteriovenous fistulas can be cut during surgical procedures using lasers. Surgical anastomosis may be required to bypass blockages or obstructions. Bypass surgery may be performed when an artery is blocked by a clot or by deposits of fat. In instances in which a part of the intestine is blocked or diseased, as in Crohn's disease and ulcerative colitis, the healthy surrounding tissue may be surgically severed and joined in order to bypass the diseased portion. *See also* CROHN'S DISEASE.

Anatomy

The science of the structure of organisms.

Knowledge of the body and its functions, acquired primarily from the dissection of corpses, is the basis of all medicine. The study of the structure of the human body dates back to ancient Egypt, where it was studied with the naked eye, known as gross anatomy. A sound and complete text of human anatomy was not compiled until 1543 by the Flemish scientist Andreas Vesalius (1514-1564). The science of anatomy includes several branches: comparative anatomy (the study of differences between human and animal anatomies); surgical anatomy (the knowledge of internal organs and blood vessels required for surgery); systematic anatomy (the study of body systems, such as the circulatory system); embryology (the study of the embryo and fetus); and cytology and histology (the microscopic study of cells and tissues). *See also* CIRCULATORY SYSTEM; CYTOLOGY; DIGESTIVE SYSTEM; EMBRYO; FETUS; HISTOLOGY; *and* NERVOUS SYSTEM.

Androgen Drugs

Synthetic forms of male sex hormones (androgens) used to treat testosterone deficiency in men.

Androgens, including fluoxymesterone may be used to treat delayed puberty or in adult males. They may also be used to treat testosterone deficiency in the adult male, which can cause lowered sex drive and impotence in adult men. In women, the androgen danazol may be used to slow production of estrogen to treat the growth of abnormal breast tissue.

ANDROGEN ABUSE

Androgens have often been abused by athletes, since high dosages of these drugs can lead to increased muscle mass and strength. The effects are greater among women and are enhanced when combined with exercise and a high-protein diet. At these high levels of use, androgens are very dangerous. Side effects can include liver dysfunction and jaundice, as well as psychological effects, such as irritability and aggression. Women experience enlargement of the clitoris, male pattern baldness, hair growth, deepening of the voice, irregular menstrual cycles, and reduction of breast size.

ANTI-ANDROGENS

Anti-androgens (including flutamide and others) are medications that are used to treat prostate enlargement and cancer in men. *See* BREAST CANCER; CANCER; DANAZOL; PROSTATE, CANCER OF; *and* PROSTATE, ENLARGED.

Regions of the Body.
Each region of the body has a specific name, which is used by physicians and other medical professionals during surgical procedures and laboratory studies. Right, the major regions of the body, each labeled with its name and location.

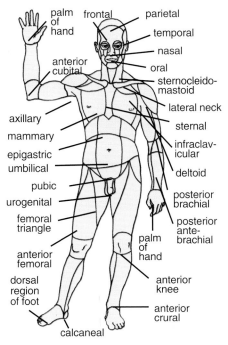

Androgen Hormones

Hormones that help to develop male secondary sexual characteristics.

The adrenal glands produce androgen in both sexes, but in men androgens are also produced in the testes. In women, the ovaries produce a small amount of testosterone until menopause sets in. Production of androgen hormones is controlled by the pituitary gland; in the testes it is dictated by pituitary hormones called gonadotropins, while the hormones in the adrenal glands are regulated by the release of ACTH from the pituitary gland.

EFFECTS OF ANDROGENS

During adolescence, an increase in the production of androgen hormones from the testes, especially the hormone testosterone, causes the development of such adult male characteristics as growth of facial and body hair and a deepened voice. Androgen hormones also stimulate the process of protein synthesis, while slowing the breakdown of proteins. This change in metabolism accounts for the increase in muscle bulk, especially across the shoulders and chest, as well as growth in the long bones, adding to height. Androgens increases sebum secretion, which can cause acne, and also heighten aggression. Androgens released by the adrenal glands generally have little masculinizing effect.

DISORDERS

Too much, not enough, or a total lack of androgen can lead to a variety of physical disorders and conditions.

Excess Androgen. Overproduction of androgen hormones can cause early sexual development in males, as well as rapid early growth. In women, excess androgen will lead to some masculinization, including deepened voice, increase in body hair, and lack of menstrual periods. Excess androgen is usually related to tumors in the pituitary or adrenal glands, or in the case of women, the ovaries.

Androgen Deficiency. If the testes fail to function, or if the pituitary glands fail to release enough gonadotropins, men may lack typical secondary sexual characteristics. The voice may not deepen, body hair will not grow, and there may be a lack of sexual drive.

Androgen Insensitivity Syndrome. This rare, congenital disorder occurs when an infant born with the genetic makeup of a male instead displays all the external characteristics and psycosexual characteristics of a female, due to an inability of the cells to respond to testosterone due to defects in the androgen receptors. The child will grow up female, at puberty estrogen production allows the development of breasts. When menstrual periods do not occur, investigation will lead to the discovery of this condition. *See also* ADRENAL GLANDS; GONADOTROPIN HORMONES; HORMONES; PITUITARY GLAND; *and* SEXUAL CHARACTERISTICS, SECONDARY.

Anemia

A condition that occurs when there are too few red blood cells in the blood, resulting in an insufficient amount of hemoglobin for healthy oxygenation of body tissues.

Hemoglobin is made up of heme, an iron-rich compound, and globin, a protein. Each molecule of heme (there are millions in each red blood cell) attaches to a molecule of oxygen in the lungs—a process called oxygenation. This turns the blood a bright red color. When a red blood cell travels to oxygen-poor tissues of the body, the oxygen molecule in the hemoglobin is exchanged for a molecule of carbon dioxide, and the blood turns a dark purple

Resources on Anemia
Mazza, Joseph J., *Manual of Clinical Hematology* (1998); Seeman, Bernard, *The River of Life: The Story of Man's Blood from Magic to Science* (1961); Starr, Douglas, *Blood: An Epic History of Medicine and Commerce* (1998); The National Hemophilia Foundation, Tel. (800) 42-HANDI, On line: www.hemophilia.org; www.ny-cornell.org/medicine/hematology/index.html;www.nyp.org/css/.

Androgen-Deprivation Therapy

Androgens, such as testosterone, are hormones that stimulate the growth of both healthy and cancerous cells in the prostate gland. Reducing these hormones, though not a cure, can slow the progression of prostate cancer. Orchidectomy, the surgical removal of the testicles, is the most reliable procedure, but it limits libido and is often rejected by the patient as a deprivation of manhood. Alternatively, the medications leuprolide and buserelin limit the pituitary gland's production of luteinizing hormone, which spurs testosterone production, while flutamide, cyproterone, and bicalutamide block testosterone from attaching to its cell receptors.

color. The amount of hemoglobin in the blood is controlled by the body, within limits. When the total amount drops below 14 to 18 grams per 100 milliliters in healthy men or 12 to 16 grams per 100 milliliters in women, the bone marrow will normally go into production mode to generate more red blood cells and more hemoglobin. When this process is disrupted, and the blood contains too few red blood cells or too little hemoglobin, the result is anemia.

CAUSES

The most common cause of anemia is a deficiency of iron. Iron is necessary for the function of hemoglobin, the carrier of oxygen to the tissues of the body. Another cause is bone-marrow malfunction. Red blood cells are produced in the bone marrow; when the bone marrow is diseased and unable to function, the red blood cell levels will drop and the person will experience symptoms of anemia.

During surgery, or in accidents when blood vessels are broken or cut, the body senses reduced levels of blood in the system and draws fluids from other body tissues to keep the blood vessels filled. Along with the loss of blood, the red blood cell count is diluted, resulting in the symptoms of anemia. If the amount of blood loss approaches one-third of the total blood volume, a person is at severe risk of death.

Other causes of anemia include situations where red blood cells themselves are destroyed or distorted. This may occur because of exposure to excessive x-rays, nuclear radiation, and certain chemicals and drugs, or by diseases, including inherited genetic abnormalities, in which there are too few healthy red blood cells to carry oxygen to the tissues of the body. Deficiency of B vitamins, such as B_{12}, can also cause a drop in red blood cell levels.

SYMPTOMS

The body initially responds to anemia by reducing blood flow to the skin and kidneys. The anemic person exhibits a characteristic pallor, but kidney function is not affected since the kidneys normally receive much more blood than necessary.

Lacking adequate levels of hemoglobin, people with anemia become tired, weak, short-winded, and often lightheaded or dizzy. They may experience headaches, ringing or roaring in the ears (tinnitis), chest pain (angina pectoris), and muscle cramps in bed at night. These symptoms are likely to be more severe when the loss of hemoglobin is rapid, as in an accident, or during surgery when copious bleeding reduces the blood volume dramatically in a short period of time. Severe anemia can result in heart attack or stroke, particularly if it occurs rapidly or if it is associated with a drop in blood pressure.

When red blood cell loss is more gradual, symptoms are likely to be compensated for by other body functions and are therefore less noticeable.

TREATMENT

Replacement of red blood cells by blood transfusion is the recommended treatment when the loss of blood is rapid and severe. Obviously, the source of the blood loss must first be established, and the loss stopped as quickly as possible. If blood loss is slower and controlled, the anemic person may be treated with iron supplements and shots of vitamin B_{12} or folic acid, so that the bone marrow will be assisted in building up the supply of red blood cells. For the long term, the best treatment is determining and, if possible, treating the underlying cause of the anemia. *See also* BLOOD COUNT; HEMOGLOBIN; TRANSFUSION, AUTOLOGOUS; *and* VITAMIN B COMPLEX.

Anemia, Aplastic

A condition caused when the bone marrow does not produce enough stem cells—the earliest form of red blood cells, white blood cells, and platelets—resulting in a lack of these cells.

Aplastic anemia often has no obvious cause. It may appear after taking certain prescription drugs, such as phenylbutazone, sulfonamides, and anticonvulsants, or after exposure to toxic substances, such as benzene, arsenic, and insecticides. It

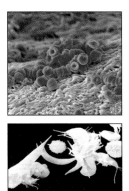

Anemia. Above, top, hemoglobin is essential for the oxygenation of body tissues. A lack of hemoglobin results in anemia, as does the production of misshapen (sickle) red blood cells, such as those that are pictured above, bottom.

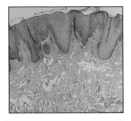

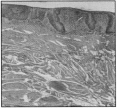

Red Blood Cells. Above, top, malformed red blood cells from the tongue, such as those found in people with pernicious anemia, are unable to properly oxygenate the body. Normal blood cells from the tongue, above, bottom, can perform this function well.

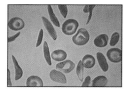

Sickle Cell Anemia.
Sickle cell anemia is a type of hemolytic anemia, in which red blood cells are malformed, or "sickle." Sickle cells are pictured above. The red blood cells of individuals with sickle cell anemia cannot adequately oxygenate body tissues. Cells collect in capillaries and clog the flow of blood to the tissues of the body.

may also be caused by chemotherapy or radiation treatment. Aplastic anemia sometimes appears after a bout of viral hepatitis or during pregnancy. Occasionally, the body's immune system is compromised; it then begins to produce antibodies that attack and destroy stem cells.

SYMPTOMS

The symptoms of aplastic anemia are typical of all anemias, and include fatigue, weakness, dizziness, and headache. In addition, normal blood clotting is compromised by a low platelet count, so the patient bruises easily and bleeds excessively. The lack of enough white blood cells leaves the patient vulnerable to upper respiratory infections, skin infections, and inflammation around the anus. Patients must be especially careful about personal cleanliness, and infections should be treated immediately with antibiotic, antifungal, or antiviral drugs.

TREATMENT

If the condition is mild and the onset slow, no particular therapies are required. If the cause of the aplastic anemia was exposure to drugs or other toxins, the anemia may subside naturally. If the condition is severe and the onset rapid, aplastic anemia can be fatal. Transfusions may be necessary but should be used sparingly, as a person suffering from aplastic anemia may already have a tendency toward autoimmune reactions. Drug therapies include medications to suppress the immune system. A combination of drugs seems to work better than any drug alone. If the bone marrow has been seriously compromised, bone marrow transplantation may be necessary. Young adults generally have a good survival rate with such transplants. In general, however, prognosis for individuals with severe aplastic anemia is limited.

Background material on aplastic anemia can be found in BLOOD and BLOOD COUNT. Related information is contained in HEMOGLOBIN; STEM CELL; and TRANSFUSION, AUTOLOGOUS. See also FANCONI'S ANEMIA and PERNICIOUS ANEMIA for more information on other types of anemia.

Anemia, Hemolytic

A condition that occurs when red blood cells produced by bone marrow are destroyed more quickly than they can be produced.

When the number of healthy red blood cells in the body is reduced, the bone marrow attempts to compensate by producing more of these cells. If increased production is not enough to make up for the loss, or if the bone marrow is not capable of producing an adequate amount of healthy red blood cells, the person becomes anemic.

Causes. Hemolytic anemia can be triggered by environmental factors, or can be the consequence of inherited abnormalities of the hemoglobin or other red blood cell components. Sickle cell anemia is a hemolytic anemia in which misshapen red blood cells are produced. These cells are fully incapable of oxygenating body tissues and may clog smaller capillaries. Hemolytic anemia may also result from autoimmune problems, in which the immune system attacks healthy red blood cells.

Symptoms. Symptoms of hemolytic anemia are similar to those of all anemias: fatigue, exhaustion, shortness of breath, dizziness, and headache, to which is added jaundice (yellowing of the skin and eyes). Untreated hemolytic anemia may swell the spleen or liver, as these organs must clean the blood of deformed or destroyed red blood cells. The heart works harder to make up for inadequate oxygenation, and the patient may experience chest pains.

Treatment. Hemolytic anemias can be difficult to control, but they can be treated. If there is an autoimmune problem, steroids may be prescribed. Surgery may be recommended to remove the spleen if it is destroying red blood cells. Autoimmune hemolytic anemias in particular respond well to removal of the spleen.

Background material on hemolytic anemia can be found in BLOOD and BLOOD COUNT. Related information is contained in AUTOIMMUNE DISORDERS; CHEST PAIN; JAUNDICE; LIVER; and SPLEEN. See also AUTOIMMUNE DISORDERS and LEUKEMIA for more information on possible causes.

Anemia, Iron-deficiency

A condition caused by insufficient iron in the body.

Iron is essential to the creation of hemoglobin. When red blood cells die, iron is reclaimed in the bone marrow and used to make new red blood cells. If there is a chronic deficiency of iron in the body, however, too few red blood cells will be created and the person will become anemic.

CAUSES

Iron-deficiency anemia may occur as a result of blood loss from an accident or from chronic internal bleeding, caused by ulcers, colon cancer, or hemorrhoids. Women who bleed heavily during menstruation may become anemic, and pregnant women must provide iron for the developing fetus, which may draw from a limited supply. When children experience growth spurts, they need extra iron. Genetic conditions that prevent absorption of iron can also lead to iron-deficiency anemia. Finally, people in developing countries are vulnerable, because they often become infected with parasites that cause slow, chronic blood loss from the gastrointestinal tract.

SYMPTOMS

The red blood cell count of patients declines, lowering the hemoglobin concentration. The red blood cells become small, a typical sign of iron-deficiency anemia. When fully advanced, the symptoms include: chronic fatigue; shortness of breath; pallor; a reduced immunity to infection; a craving for non-foods, such as ice or dirt; irritation of the tongue; cracks at the corners of the mouth; and cracks in the fingernails.

TREATMENT

Iron-deficiency anemia responds well to dietary treatment, and the symptoms are quickly eliminated. Changes in the diet take three to six weeks to become effective. If the iron deficiency is the result of chronic blood loss, it is very important to determine the source of that loss. *See also* COLON CANCER *and* HEMORRHOIDS.

Anemia, Megaloblastic

A condition caused by a lack of folic acid or vitamin B_{12} in the blood.

If red blood cells are enlarged and misshapen, the condition may be megaloblastic anemia.

CAUSES

Although it may be caused by drugs used to control cancer or by anticonvulsant medications, megaloblastic anemia is usually caused by an inadequate supply of vitamin B_{12} or folic acid, resulting either from the body's inability to process the vitamins (more common with B_{12}) or from a dietary lack (more common with folic acid). Folic acid is found in green leafy vegetables, citrus fruits, liver, and kidneys. Vitamin B_{12} is found in liver, chicken, pork, beef, eggs, and dairy products. B_{12} deficiency, also called pernicious anemia, results in a chronic, slow-developing disease caused by the inability of the body to digest and utilize B_{12}.

Alcoholics who get most of their calories from alcohol are at risk for megaloblastic anemia. Long-term alcoholics actually lose the ability to absorb folic acid, which further promotes the incidence of this form of anemia. Pregnant or breast-feeding women are also vulnerable to megaloblastic anemia because of their bodies' extra demands for folic acid for the growing fetus.

SYMPTOMS

In mild cases, there may be no physical symptoms. In more extreme cases, the person will experience fatigue, pallor, shortness of breath, rapid heartbeat, weight loss, and a sore tongue.

TREATMENT

As with any other anemia, identifying and treating the underlying cause is key. The treatment for megaloblastic anemia is often dietary. In the case of pernicious anemia, the vitamins must also be regularly injected. *See also* ALCOHOL DEPENDENCE *and* ANTICONVULSANT DRUGS.

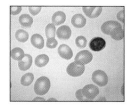

Megaloblastic Anemia. Enlarged and misshapen red blood cells, pictured above, are seen in patients with megaloblastic anemia. This condition often results from dietary or metabolic problems, such as a deficiency of vitamin B_{12} or folic acid.

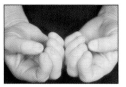

Sign of Anemia. Anemic individuals may demonstrate physical symptoms, especially if the disease is in an advanced stage. Above, the skin on the hands of an anemic patient is jaundiced (yellow) and pale, and the fingernails are cracked. **In Older Individuals**, pernicious anemia (B_{12} deficiency) is associated with a neurological condition that can cause tingling sensations in the arms and legs and problems with balance.

Anencephaly

A condition in which a large area of the brain does not develop.

Anencephaly, like spina bifida, is a type of neural tube defect, usually caused by abnormalities in several genes. The condition can be diagnosed prenatally by amniocentesis and ultrasound. It is invariably fatal, resulting in a stillbirth, or death within a few days after birth.

Couples who give birth to a baby with anencephaly or spina bifida have a two to three percent chance of having another child with the condition. Ninety-five percent of all instances of neural tube defects occur in families with no previous history. *See also* GENETIC DISORDERS *and* SPINA BIFIDA.

Anesthesia

The loss of normal feeling or sensation, especially the sensation of pain.

The term anesthesia commonly refers to an artificially produced loss of awareness or feeling resulting from the administration of an anesthetic drug. Anesthetic drugs are medications that are used during surgical operations or other painful procedures, such as childbirth. Anesthesia may also occur as a result of nerve damage, certain psychological disorders, or states of extreme stress or excitement.

Types. The two main types of surgical anesthetics are general and local. Both types of drugs produce anesthesia. General anesthetic drugs affect the brain and produce unconsciousness, while local anesthetic drugs simply block the nerve supply in a particular area of the body. Some local anesthetics, such as spinal blocks and epidural anesthetics used in Cesarean births and other procedures performed on the lower part of the body, are sometimes described as regional anesthetics. Anesthetics may be administered by inhalation, injection, or suppository, or the drugs may be applied topically. *See also* ANESTHESIA, GENERAL *and* ANESTHESIA, LOCAL.

Resources on Anesthesia
Cottrell, James E. and Stephanie Golden, *Under the Mask : A Guide to Feeling Secure and Comfortable During Anesthesia and Surgery* (2001); Rushman, G.B., et al., *A Short History of Anesthesia* (1996); Rutkow, Ira M., *Surgery: An Illustrated History* (1993); American College of Surgeons, Tel. (312) 202-5000, Online: www.facs.org; www.med.cornell.edu/surgery/;www.nycornell.org/medicine/gim/index.html; www.nycornell.org/medicine/anesthesiology/index.html; www.nycornell.org/medicine/emergency/index.html.

Anesthesia, Dental

An induced loss of sensation for dental purposes.

The nerves and roots of teeth are extremely sensitive. For this reason, most dental work on the teeth, gums, or supporting bone is performed with a local anesthetic. This type of anesthetic enables the treatment to be performed painlessly, or with a minimum of discomfort.

The most common local anesthetic used by dentists is lidocaine, which is injected around the tooth or jaw and quickly numbs the surrounding area. Depending on the nature of the dental work, the dentist may administer several doses. Local anesthetics are very effective, although they make most people feel as though they have a swollen lip or tongue. Local anesthetics last for 30 minutes to several hours depending on which type is used. Discomfort after the dental procedure can usually be controlled with aspirin, acetaminophen, or similar pain-killing drugs.

Adjuncts to local anesthetics are sedation and general anesthetics. The administration of an antianxiety medication can be used in conjunction with a local anesthetic for nervous patients. Simple sedation procedures involve nitrous oxide or oral tranquilizers. General anesthetics or intravenous sedatives are occasionally used for dental surgery. General anesthesia usually consists of a number of drugs in combination. Under general anesthesia, patients are totally unconscious. *See also* ANESTHESIA; ANESTHESIA, GENERAL; ANESTHESIA, LOCAL; *and* NSAIDs.

Anesthesia, General

The use of medication to induce a reversible loss of consciousness and sensation in a patient to prevent pain and movement during major surgery.

Until the 1840s, when ether was first used as a general anesthetic, surgeons used substances such as alcohol, opium, and cannabis to provide patients with pain relief during surgery. The development of chloroform was the first in a long process of the development of drugs that could effectively produce a controlled, reversible state of unconsciousness, lack of sensation, and muscle relaxation for surgery.

TYPES

Currently, general anesthesia consists of using a combination of drugs, administered by inhalation or injection to produce a maximum effect while minimizing complications. The types of drugs used consist of premedications, induction agents, anesthetic gases and volatile agents, analgesics, muscle relaxants, and reversal agents. The anesthesiologist is responsible for choosing the best combination of drugs, administering them, monitoring the patient during unconsciousness, and bringing the patient back to consciousness after surgery.

Premedications include benzodiazepines (midazolam, diazepam, and lorazepam), droperidol, atropine, and morphine. They are administered intravenously before surgery to relax the patient, ease anxiety, eliminate pain, and reduce saliva and mucus production. Midazolam acts rapidly and has a short duration; it is favored for short operations. Diazepam and lorazepam act slower but last longer; they are used for longer operations.

Intravenous induction agents induce unconsciousness. They include thiopental sodium (or sodium thiopentone), methohexital, etomidate, ketamine, and propofol. One of the newest intravenous induction agents, propofol, acts rapidly (within one to three minutes) and for a short duration (twelve minutes). Propofol is therefore used for short surgical procedures. Its anti-nausea (anti-emetic) qualities makes it a good option for patients who are prone to nausea and vomiting. However, propofol can cause slowing of the heart rate (bradycardia) and lowered blood pressure (hypotension) and therefore should be used with care on patients with coronary artery disease.

Anesthetic gases and volatile agents include halothane, ether, nitrous oxide, isoflurane, sevoflurane, desflurane, enflurane, and xenon. The latter agents induce

or maintain unconsciousness. Halothane also acts as a bronchodilator, causing the airways to expand, and is therefore appropriate for patients with lung disease. These agents are administered via a mask or breathing tube. When muscle relaxants are also used, artificial respiration is needed to ensure that breathing is maintained.

Analgesics or painkillers are given to prevent pain during surgery and to reduce the need for further anesthesia during the operation. These analgesics include morphine, meperidine (Demerol), fentanyl, and sufentanil. Fentanyl and sufentanil are opioids that act quickly (30 to 60 seconds) but only for short periods of time (20 to 60 minutes). Since fentanyl and sufentanil can depress the respiratory function, causing the patient to stop breathing, patients given this drug must be closely monitored. Fentanyl, sufentanil, and morphine can cause slow heartbeat, and meperidine can sometimes increase the heart rate.

Remifentanil is a promising, relatively new analgesic (approved by the FDA in 1996) that lacks the side effects of other opioids. It is safely broken down (metabolized) by enzymes in the bloodstream within minutes, unlike many drugs that have to be broken down by the liver and kidneys, which can take hours. Thus remifentanil takes effect more quickly and loses its effect more quickly, and so it is easier for the anesthesiologist to control.

Muscle relaxants (neuromuscular blockers) inhibit muscle function. These are selected based on the length of surgery and the patient's medical status. Mivacurium is used for short procedures (lasting 10 to 30 minutes), and rocuronium, vecuronium, cisatracurium, or atracurium are usually selected for intermediate-length procedures (40 to 80 minutes). Rocuronium is preferred when the onset of effect is needed within 60 to 90 seconds. Vecuronium and cisatracurium are favored for patients with cardiovascular problems. Atracurium and cisatracuriam are appropriate for patients with kidney or liver dysfunctions.

Reversal agents counteract muscle relaxants, re-establishing muscle function.

The anesthesiologist chooses various drugs based on the patient's condition, medical history, and needs, and on the drug's effects. For example, etomidate is often used in emergency surgery on patients with low blood pressure. Ketamine can increase heart rate, blood pressure, and intracranial pressure; it therefore should not be used on patients with severe cardiac conditions or brain trauma.

COMPLICATIONS

Because complications are always possible during and after major surgery, an important part of the anesthesiologist's job is to monitor the patient's general progress and reactions to the combination of drugs and to the operation itself.

Possible complications under anesthesia include: low blood pressure (hypotension); irregular heart beat (cardiac arrhythmia); extremely slow heart beat (bradycardia); heart attack (myocardial infarction); inhibited respiration; airway obstruction (bronchoconstriction); high fever; allergic reactions; nausea; vomiting or inhalation of vomit into the lungs; reduced oxygen supply (hypoxia); muscle cramps; brain damage; and possibly even death in rare cases. Drug dosage and the patient's reactions to the drugs must be continuously monitored in order to prevent or quickly reverse complications. Drugs such as atropine or glycopyrolate are sometimes used to counteract some of these complications, as they raise blood pressure and speed up heartbeat.

A significant recent advance in anesthesia has been the laryngeal mask airway, which consists of an elliptically-shaped cuff connected to a tube. This device can be easily inserted into the patient's mouth without the aid of a laryngoscope, freeing the anesthesiologist's hands and maintaining the airway.

> *Background material on general anesthesia can be found in* ANESTHESIA; PHARMACOLOGY; *and* SURGERY. *Related information is contained in* ATROPINE; BRADYCARDIA; BRONCHOCONSTRICTION; HEART ATTACK; HYPOXIA; NITROUS OXIDE; *and* PREMEDICATION.

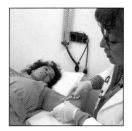

Anesthesia.
Patients are given anesthetic drugs before surgery or childbirth to prevent movement or to block painful sensations. Above, an anesthesiologist administers a local anesthetic drug to a patient prior to the implantation of a subdural (beneath the skin) contraceptive device.

Anesthesia, Local

A loss of normal sensation in a limited part of the body, induced by a physician in order to eliminate pain during surgery or other medical procedures.

Local anesthesia is produced by the use of drugs that temporarily block the transmission of pain-carrying impulses along nerve fibers. Unlike general anesthesia, local anesthesia does not cause loss of consciousness. It has fewer side effects and complications than general anesthesia; it is often used in minor surgical and diagnostic procedures, and during childbirth.

Local anesthetics desensitize the area around the site of application. Local anesthetics include benzocaine, bupivacaine, ropivacaine, lidocaine, procaine, tetracaine, and cocaine. They may be injected or topically applied in a liquid, spray, cream, ointment, or gel form.

Benzocaine is a drug used to relieve the pain of skin irritations, mucous membranes (such as the gums), and hemorrhoids, and is usually applied in ointment, cream, gel, lozenge, spray, and liquid forms. Bupivacaine is a frequently used local anesthetic for pain relief during and after operations. The onset is quick (in a few minutes), but the duration of action is comparatively long. Ropivacaine is a relatively new variation of bupivacaine, possibly with less potential central nervous system and cardiovascular toxicity. Procaine (Novocaine), lidocaine, and tetracaine are examples of synthetic local anesthetics often used in dental procedures.

Regional Anesthesia. When a local anesthetic is injected near a major nerve, it produces what is called regional anesthesia, or nerve block. This type of anesthesia affects a relatively large area of the body while allowing the patient to remain conscious.

Injection of an anesthetic drug into the cerebrospinal fluid around the spinal cord is called a spinal or intrathecal anesthesia; it is used during surgery of the lower extremities and abdomen. Frequently used during Cesarean sections, spinal anesthesia is also used during childbirth, although since it prevents the woman from being able to push the baby out, it may increase the likelihood of a forceps delivery.

Injecting a local anesthetic into the space between the two membranes surrounding the spinal cord (the durae) is known as epidural anesthesia or an epidural. It is often used during childbirth, as it allows for more sensation and movement. Epidurals take effect within 15 to 30 minutes. A catheter is inserted to allow delivery of the epidural throughout the procedure. Mobile epidurals use a lower dose of local anesthetic in combination with an opioid, such as fentanyl, to permit mobility with a strong pain-killing ability.

Another example of a regional nerve block is the blocking of the ulnar and median nerves by injecting anesthetic near the elbow in order to perform surgery on the hand or palm.

> *Background material on local anesthesia can be found in* ANESTHESIA. *Related information is contained in* LIDOCAINE; PROCAINE; *and* TETRACAINE. *See also* CESAREAN SECTION; CHILDBIRTH; CHILDBIRTH, COMPLICATIONS; CONTRACTIONS; *and* DELIVERY *for more on the use of epidural anesthesia.*

Anesthesia, Spinal

Also known as intrathecal anesthesia

A specific type of anesthesia in which a local anesthetic is injected into fluid around the spinal cord.

Spinal anesthesia provides pain relief during surgery on the lower extremities or abdomen. Spinal anesthesia may be prescribed for patients whose condition makes them unsuitable for a general anesthetic. In addition, it may be used for older patients, those with diabetes, and those with sickle cell disease. Spinals are sometimes used when a skilled anesthetist is not available to administer general anesthesia.

Spinal anesthesia takes effect in about the same time frame as general anesthesia and usually lasts one to three hours. In some patients it can cause a rapid drop in blood pressure. About one to two percent of patients develop headaches after the spinal anesthesia wears off. *See also* AGING.

Aneurysm

The ballooning of the wall of an artery, caused by disease, injury, or a congenital weakness of the blood vessel.

There are two major kinds of aneurysm: degenerative and dissecting. A degenerative aneurysm occurs when the middle wall of the artery, the tunica media, has been weakened and the force of blood pressure causes the artery to become distended. A dissecting aneurysm occurs when a tear develops in the artery wall, allowing blood to enter. This tear can be caused by inflammation, disease, or a congenital defect. The split can grow in size and more extensive regions of the artery are damaged.

Other Causes. Less common causes of aneurysms include diseases, such as Marfan's syndrome or inflammation of blood vessels. More than 20 percent of persons with Marfan's syndrome develop dissecting aneurysms.

While aneurysms can form anywhere in the body, they are most often seen in the aorta, the main artery carrying blood from the heart; in the region of the abdomen below the kidneys; in the chest cavity; or in the vessels supplying blood to the brain.

Degenerative aneurysms may be the result of atherosclerosis—the thickening and narrowing of arteries caused by increasing deposits of plaque along the blood vessels—but may also be caused by abnormalities in the arterial wall. Dissecting aneurysms often are associated with hypertension, since abnormally high blood pressure can weaken the artery wall over time. Cigarette smoking can also cause aneurysms.

INCIDENCE

At least 70 percent of persons with dissecting aneurysms have hypertension. Age is also a factor in causing aneurysms, since the aorta can grow weaker as a person ages. Dissecting aneurysms of the aorta are rarely seen in persons under the age of 40, with the notable exception that such aneurysms can occur during pregnancy,

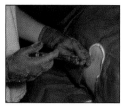

Spinal Anesthesia.
Above, a spinal anesthetic is injected into the fluid surrounding the spinal cord. Spinal anesthesia can be used to prevent movement and block sensations of pain during surgery of the lower abdomen or extremities; it is also used in some cases of childbirth (such as during a Cesarean section), though the procedure known as an epidural (in which the anesthesia is applied further from the spinal column) is more commonly used during delivery. Below, a diagram illustrating the administration of a spinal anesthetic.

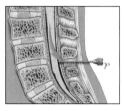

Resources on Aneurysm
Berne, Robert M., *Cardiovascular Disease* (2001); Burch, George E., *A Primer of Cardiology* (1993); Debakey, Michael, and Antonio Gotto, *The New Living Heart* (1997); Yao, James S.T., et al., *Aneurysms: New Findings and Treatments* (1994); American College of Surgeons, Tel. (312) 202-5000, On-line: www.facs.org; www.med.cornell.edu/surgery/; www.nycornell.org/medicine/cardiology/index. html; www.nycornell.org/medicine/emergency/index.html

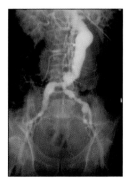

Aneurysm.
Above, ballooning of an artery, called an aneurysm, can be seen with an angiogram, an x-ray image of the arteries. Before the angiogram is taken, a contrast dye is injected into the artery to be studied through a catheter, making the artery and the aneurysm visible on the x-ray. Below, a diagram of an aortic aneurysm, which affects the aorta, located in the heart.

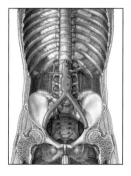

apparently because of the increase in blood pressure that occurs at that time.

DIAGNOSIS

Because atherosclerosis and hypertension increase the risk, persons with either of these conditions should be examined regularly for aneurysms. During a physical examination, the physician may feel for a pulsating lump in the abdomen to detect an abdominal aneurysm or listen for an unusual murmur in the aortic valve to detect a thoracic aneurysm, but should be assessed on a regular basis.

TREATMENT

Small aneurysms generally do not call for immediate treatment, since they do not pose a direct threat to health. But aneurysms can grow and possibly rupture, creating a condition that can be life-threatening if it occurs in the aorta, the heart wall, or the brain. When an aneurysm is two to three inches in size, surgery may be performed to remove the damaged part of the artery. When the ballooning region is cut out, it is replaced by a patch or artificial graft. If the aneurysm is close to the aortic valve, which controls blood out of the heart, the valve may be replaced by a mechanical valve or one made of animal or human tissue. Open-heart surgery may be needed to repair an aneurysm in the chest.

OUTLOOK

Statistics show that the five-year death rate for persons who undergo surgery for an aneurysm is about 40 percent, while it is 80 percent for those who do not undergo surgery. The mortality rate is higher for emergency surgery when an aneurysm ruptures in the aorta or heart wall, but the risk of death or serious damage without surgical intervention is much higher.

Background material on aneurysm can be found in AR-TERIES, DISORDERS OF. *Related information is contained in* ARTERY; ATHEROSCLEROSIS; HYPERTENSION; INFLAMMATION; MARFAN'S SYNDROME; *and* OBESITY. *See also* HEART VALVE, ARTIFICIAL *and* OPEN HEART SURGERY *for more on rehabilitation and therapies.*

Angel Dust

A drug abused for its hallucinatory properties and reduction of pain perception.

Angel dust, also known as PCP (phencyclidine), was initially developed in 1958 as an intravenous general anesthetic. It was discontinued after symptoms of agitation, hallucinations, delirium, and disorientation were observed in patients after anesthesia. Since then, PCP has been used as a recreational drug. It is manufactured in illegal laboratories. The effects of the drug appear almost immediately and generally last from four to six hours. Symptoms can include both physical and mental manifestations, including toxic psychosis similar to schizophrenic behavior, hallucinations, violent and bizarre behavior, vomiting, convulsions, agitation, anxiety, catatonic rigidity, fast heartbeat (tachycardia), hypertension, and kidney malfunction. *See also* DRUG DEPENDENCE; DRUG OVERDOSE; PSYCHOSIS; TACHYCARDIA; *and* HYPERTENSION.

Angina Pectoris

A pain or pressure in the chest that lasts for several minutes and can radiate into the neck or arm.

Angina pectoris results from a decreased supply of oxygen to the heart muscle. It is caused most often by coronary artery disease, the narrowing of the arteries of the heart that results from atherosclerosis (the buildup of fatty deposits in those blood vessels). Angina may also be triggered by a coronary artery spasm, the sudden temporary narrowing of the coronary arteries; by aortic stenosis, the narrowing of the aortic valve through which blood flows from the heart; or by an arrhythmia, an abnormal heart rhythm.

Angina pectoris generally occurs in times of physical exertion or emotional stress, although there is a variant form, Prinzmetal's angina, that usually occurs while a person is at rest. Angina can occur in men in their 30s, but it usually does not make itself evident until the 50s. It starts later in life in women. It is often accompanied by feelings of suffocation and impending death, as well as pain radiating into the left arm.

TREATMENT

After angina is diagnosed, the initial goal of treatment is to remove any underlying cause of the condition. An obese patient should lose weight to reduce the workload of the heart. A smoker should stop smoking, since the nicotine, carbon monoxide, and other elements in cigarette smoke accelerate the progression of heart disease. If the patient has hypertension, a drug can be prescribed to lower the blood pressure. Medications can be prescribed for arrhythmia or for high blood-cholesterol levels. Attacks of angina can be prevented or treated with nitrate medications, such as nitroglycerin, or with other medications that increase the flow of blood to the heart muscle and the rest of the body. Examples of such drugs include beta-blockers, angiotensin-converting enzyme (ACE) inhibitors, and calcium channel blockers.

LONG-TERM TREATMENT

Weight reduction, diet, and drug treatment may reduce and control the symptoms of angina in many cases, but cannot cure the disorder. The cardiologist will monitor an angina patient closely to determine if the attacks occur more often, are more severe, or last longer. These indicate a worsening condition that increases the risk for a heart attack (also called a myocardial infarction).

If angina attacks are brought on by even mild exertion or stress, the condition may have progressed to unstable angina, in which the risk of a heart attack is increased considerably, and which is not well controlled by medications. An individual with unstable angina may be hospitalized, often in a coronary intensive care unit, and treated with heparin and aspirin to improve blood flow, decreasing the risk of a heart attack while further treatments for the angina are determined.

In some cases, narrowing of the arteries can be determined to be the cause of unstable angina. If this narrowing is not widespread, it can be treated by balloon angioplasty, a procedure in which a balloon is inserted into a narrowed area of a blood vessel to widen it, improving blood flow. A tube called a stent may be implanted to help keep the blood vessel open. More severe cases, in which artery disease is widespread, require surgery in the form of a coronary artery bypass operation, which is performed under general anesthesia. In this operation, a segment of a vein is removed from the leg and is attached to the artery or arteries where blockages are found, looping around the narrowed areas to restore better blood flow.

> *Background material on angina pectoris can be found in* CIRCULATION, DISORDERS OF. *Related information is contained in* ACE INHIBITOR DRUGS; ARRHYTHMIA; ATHEROSCLEROSIS; BETA-BLOCKER DRUGS; HYPERTENSION; *and* OBESITY. *See also* ANGIOPLASTY, BALLOON *and* CORONARY ARTERY BYPASS *for more on specific treatments.*

Angioedema

Also known as angioneurotic edema

An allergic reaction limited to skin and underlying tissues; it may be accompanied by hives.

Angioedema may be precipitated by a sudden allergic reaction, most often to a particular food, but also to medications, insect bites or stings, pollens, molds, and animal dander. The disorder causes swelling in the skin or in mucous membranes in the mouth, throat, or gastrointestinal tract. Swollen areas are painful but not itchy. The disorder can be accompanied by nausea, vomiting, and cramps. Swelling of the upper airways is a life-threatening complication of the disorder.

Angioedema can often be prevented by avoiding the triggering allergen or, if this is not possible, by plasma transfusions. Angioedema is sometimes treated with antihistamines, and aminocaproic acid can end an attack. Corticosteroids are also often administered to treat angioedema. *See also* ALLERGY *and* HIVES.

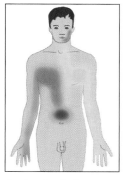

Angina Pectoris. Above, angina pectoris is a pain or pressure that is felt in the chest and sometimes in the arm or neck as well (colored areas). Angina results from a decrease in the amount of oxygen supplied to the heart.

Resources on Angina
Bellenir, Karen, *Heart Diseases and Disorders Sourcebook* (2000); Burch, George E., *A Primer of Cardiology* (1993); Debakey, Michael, and Antonio Gotto, *The New Living Heart* (1997); Gould, L.K., *Heal Your Heart* (2000); American Heart Association, Tel. (800) 242-8721, online: www.amhrt. org; www.nycornell.org/ medicine/cardiology/index.html; www.nycornell.org/medicine/emergency/index.html

Angiography

Also known as arteriography

A diagnostic procedure that uses x-rays to examine arteries for defects or blockages.

Angiography can be used to create an image of any artery in the body. The arteries most often viewed are those within the brain, kidneys, legs, or heart. A contrast material ("dye"), which contains iodine and shows up clearly on an x-ray image, is injected into the relevant blood vessels while the x-ray is performed.

Coronary angiography is an x-ray of the arteries of the heart. A flexible plastic tube (catheter) is threaded into an artery in the arm or groin toward the heart and into the coronary arteries. The catheter's progress in the direction of the arteries may be monitored through the use of x-rays. Once the catheter's tip has reached the desired point, the physician injects a dye visible on x-ray through the catheter into the coronary arteries, allowing the arteries to be seen on a monitor. A diagnosis of coronary artery disease (atherosclerosis) can be made with this technique, because diseased arteries have narrowed or irregular inner walls. After a diagnosis is made, a balloon angioplasty may then be performed to unblock the artery.

Pulmonary Angiography. A similar procedure is used to view the blood supply to the lungs through the pulmonary artery, particularly if the doctor suspects a blood clot (pulmonary embolism).

Cerebral angiography detects blood vessel abnormalities in the brain by injecting a control material ("dye") into the arteries that supply it. Abnormalities that may be detected by cerebral angiography include: bulges in arteries (aneurysms); inflammation of arteries (arteritis); and stroke.

Alternatives. Computed tomography (CT) and magnetic resonance imaging (MRI) scanning are replacing conventional angiography by enhancing images produced from dilute quantities of dye injected into a peripheral vein, rather than directly into the artery. Complications from conventional angiography may include damage to injected vessels and surrounding organs, reactions to the radiopaque dye, and sometimes bleeding. The noninvasive CT and MRI angiography methods avoid many of these complications. They can be substituted for catheter angiography in many, but not all, patients.

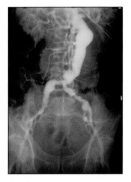

Angiogram.
Above, an angiogram demonstrating the presence of an aneurysm (ballooning of an artery wall). An aneurysm is only one of the many conditions that can be diagnosed through the use of angiography. Below, an angiogram of the liver shows a mass of blood vessels.

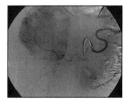

Background material on angiography can be found in DIAGNOSTICS. *Related information is contained in* ARTERIES, DISORDERS OF; CATHETER; CT SCAN; *and* MRI. *See also* ANEURYSM; ARTERITIS; ATHEROSCLEROSIS; *and* PULMONARY EMBOLISM *for more on these conditions.*

Angioma

Also known as a birthmark

A collection of unusually dense blood vessels located on or just below the skin, which cause red or purple discolorations.

Angiomas often appear at birth, and for that reason are sometimes called birthmarks. There are several types of angiomas. Strawberry marks appear on the face, chest, or back. They are raised, bright red stains that may grow larger very rapidly in the early years, but will usually shrink and disappear by ages seven to nine. Port-wine stains are flat with colors that range from pink to purple. They appear on the face, neck, arms, or legs. Small angiomas may disappear in time, but they can cover very large areas of skin and may last a lifetime. Laser surgery can remove these discolorations, but scarring is possible. *See also* PORT-WINE STAIN *and* STRAWBERRY NEVUS.

Angioplasty, Balloon

A procedure performed to widen a blocked artery.

Balloon angioplasty attempts to widen a partially blocked artery; it is done when lifestyle changes and medication have not been effective in controlling the pain of angina. It can also be used, in some cases, as first-time treatment for a heart attack. It is accomplished under local anesthesia and sedation. When a site for insertion is chosen and anesthetized, the cardiologist inserts a long, slender catheter into an artery of an arm or leg and moves it to the location of the blockage, guiding it into place by using a continuous x-ray video image. A second, thinner catheter with a deflated balloon at its tip is then inserted through the first catheter. When it reaches the blockage, the balloon is inflated for one to two minutes to break up the plaque formations that have narrowed the artery, forcing the walls of the blood vessel outward to restore more normal blood flow. In most procedures, the balloon is inflated and deflated more than once. After the procedure, the balloon and catheter are removed.

In many cases, balloon angioplasty is followed by the insertion of a stent, a flexible wire mesh tube designed to prevent restenosis, the narrowing or closing of the artery. For implantation, the collapsed stent is positioned over a balloon catheter and moved to the site of the blockage. The balloon is inflated to open the stent. The stent is then locked in place and the balloon is removed.

Precautions. Anticoagulant agents are used to prevent the formation of clots near the blockage, but clots sometimes do occur, requiring immediate treatment. Other, more common complications are developments of an irregular heartbeat or a spasm of the artery. Close monitoring of the patient usually ensures quick detection and treatment of these problems.

While platelet blockers or blood-thinning agents are prescribed after angioplasty, restenosis occurs within six months in 15 to 25 percent of cases. It is most likely to occur in patients with an underlying condition, such as diabetes, or those who continue to smoke or do not follow the guidelines for a low-fat diet. When restenosis takes place, a second angioplasty may be performed to try to reopen the artery. If a stent was not used in the first procedure, one may be implanted during the second operation.

Angioplasty is most often performed when a patient has a single blockage, but it can be done when there are several

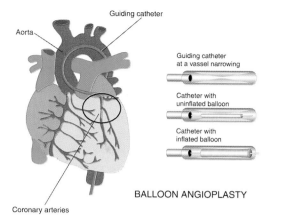

Guiding catheter

Aorta

Guiding catheter at a vassel narrowing

Catheter with uninflated balloon

Catheter with inflated balloon

BALLOON ANGIOPLASTY

Coronary arteries

blockages in more than one artery. It is sometimes an emergency procedure used after a heart attack. More than a half-million angioplasties are done in the United States annually. *See also* CORONARY ARTERY DISEASE *and* HEART, DISORDERS OF.

Angiotensin

General name for two proteins involved in the regulation of blood pressure, in what is called the renin-angiotensin-aldosterone (RAA) system.

Renin is an enzyme released when there is a lack of blood flow to the kidneys. The release of renin by the kidneys stimulates the release of angiotensin I, which itself is inactive and is changed to an active protein, angiotensin II, by a converting enzyme. Angiotensin causes small blood vessels to narrow, raising blood pressure. It also stimulates the outer part (cortex) of the adrenal glands to release the hormone aldosterone, which acts to raise blood pressure. The RAA system can be mistakenly activated by the narrowing of a kidney artery or a kidney disorder, causing hypertension.

A class of medications called angiotensin-converting enzyme (ACE) inhibitors is commonly used to treat hypertension. These medications lower blood pressure by preventing the conversion of angiotensin I to angiotensin II. ACE inhibitors not only allow the arteries to remain wider, but also promote the release of salt by the kidneys. ACE inhibitors are also used to treat congestive heart failure, in which the heart weakens and loses its ability to pump blood. *See also* HEART FAILURE.

Balloon Angioplasty. Above, a visual depiction of a balloon angioplasty. Such a procedure is used to clear a blockage from an artery when diet and medication have not been successful in controlling the chest pain of angina. In most cases, a stent is implanted after the procedure to ensure that the artery does not collapse or become blocked again.

Resources on Angioplasty

Berne, Robert M., *Cardiovascular Disease* (2001); Brammell, H.L., et al., *Cardiac Rehabilitation* (1999); Burch, George E., *A Primer of Cardiology* (1993); Debakey, Michael, and Antonio Gotto, *The New Living Heart* (1997); American Heart Association, Tel. (800) 242-8721, online: www.amhrt.org; www.nycornell.org/medicine/cardiology/index.html; www.nycornell.org/medicine/emergency/index.html

Anisometropia

The inability to focus both eyes equally.

Anisometropia is usually caused by a difference in the size or shape of the lens of the eyes, causing light to refract differently in each eye, resulting in blurred vision in one or both eyes. This may occur when one eye is normal and the other is nearsighted, farsighted, or has an astigmatism (a malshaped cornea).

Substantial anisometropia often results in permanent visual defect (ambylopia). It is often difficult to rectify this condition. Even though glasses can improve vision, the images on the retinas will not be alike. Although there is no cure, contact lenses are a better option than glasses because they can minimize the perception of uneven images. *See also* Eye, Disorders of.

Ankylosing Spondylitis

An inflammatory disease that affects the joints, most often between the vertebrae and the pelvis.

Ankylosing spondylitis is characterized by pain in the lower back and hips. Chest pain, loss of appetite, fatigue, pain and redness in the eyes, and pain in other joints may follow the initial pain. Pain is generally worse after inactivity; exercise can relieve some of the stiffness. This joint inflammation can lead to ankylosis, a permanent stiffness of the joint.

There is no definitive known cause for ankylosing spondylitis, though there seem to be indications that it is hereditary. It occurs in less than one percent of the population, and it is generally more common in men than women. The onset of the disease is usually between the ages of 20 and 40. Blood tests and x-rays reveal abnormalities that indicate the disease.

No cure exists for this condition, but much can be done to relieve the symptoms. Exercise will help by strengthening the muscles. Breathing exercises, proper posture, and sleeping on the stomach can also help to reduce the inflammation, as can anti-inflammatory drugs.

If treated, most people only suffer from a minor curvature of the spine, which does not usually affect quality of life. If the disease is progressive in nature, it may lead to increased curvature of the upper spine (thoracic kyphosis) and inability to elevate the head. In especially severe cases, surgery may be required to relieve the problem. *See also* Anti-Inflammatory Drugs.

Anorgasmia

The inability to achieve sexual satisfaction (orgasm), despite normal desire and excitement.

Anorgasmia is one of several, often overlapping, sexual disorders. The term is usually used in reference to women. A man's difficulty with reaching orgasm is termed erectile dysfunction (ED).

Causes. As in any sexual disorder, the causes may be complex, often involving both physical and psychological components. There are a number of diseases, disabilities, and surgical procedures, as well as various medications, that may interfere with the ability to achieve orgasm.

Psychological factors contributing to anorgasmia may be a poor relationship with a partner, or a feeling of exhaustion or distraction. In addition, there may be poor communication between the partners in relation to fulfilling each other's needs.

Insufficient foreplay is a major contributing factor to anorgasmia. Women require more time to achieve orgasm than men, and need adequate clitoral stimulation. At least 30 to 40 percent of women require direct clitoral stimulation in order to climax and cannot achieve orgasm through intercourse alone. Between five and eight percent of women are unable to have an orgasm even with clitoral stimulation. Some women are able to achieve orgasms during masturbation but are unable to achieve orgasm with a partner. Some women are unable to relax sufficiently to achieve orgasm, either through feelings of fear or vulnerability, or due to guilt about sex.

A decreased interest in having sex (low libido) is often found together with anorgasmia, but some women can have orgasms even though they have little desire for sex.

Treatment. Once any underlying physical causes have been treated, counseling for both partners is often helpful.

With therapy, approximately 30 to 50 percent of women can "learn" to have orgasms. Of these, 70 to 80 percent will be able to achieve orgasms with their partners, but not necessarily during intercourse.

Many women and men have unrealistic expectations surrounding orgasm—that it must occur during sexual intercourse or else it "doesn't count," that it must occur simultaneously with a partner's climax, or that orgasm must be reached every time. These concerns are not included under anorgasmia; however, they may require therapy due to the resulting stress of not meeting those expectations. *See also* ERECTILE DYSFUNCTION; ORGASM; SEXUAL DYSFUNCTION; *and* SEXUAL INTERCOURSE.

Anoxia

A condition in which the tissues of the body receive too little oxygen.

Anoxia is a term used to describe the absence of oxygen in body tissue. This condition is often the consequence of cardiac arrest, smoke or carbon monoxide inhalation, reduced oxygen levels, or strangulation. Anoxia commonly results in muscle spasms, seizures, or coma. It is a life-threatening emergency. If anoxia persists for more than four to six minutes, permanent brain damage or death is likely.

Anoxia is marked by a total lack of oxygen to body tissues. It is a severe condition and is very rare. In contrast, hypoxia is a deficiency of oxygen. It is more common than anoxia, and often occurs at higher altitudes among people who have climbed too quickly to become accustomed to reduced levels of oxygen.

If anoxia is not due to cardiac arrest, treatment is to make sure air passages are open to oxygen administration, possibly followed by respiratory assistance and supplemental oxygen, if available. *See also* CARBON MONOXIDE *and* OXYGEN THERAPY.

Antacid Drugs

Medication used to relieve symptoms of indigestion or disorders caused by excess acid.

Over-the-counter antacids include compounds containing magnesium and aluminum or calcium carbonate. They neutralize acids in the stomach and are used to treat fairly infrequent, mild to moderate cases of heartburn, indigestion, and reflux, and to help peptic ulcers to heal. For patients with frequent acid-related symptoms, two classes of acid-suppressive drugs are available: histamine H2 receptor antagonists, including cimetidine, ranitidine, or famotidine; and the more potent proton pump inhibitors, including omaprazole, lansoprazole, and rabeprazole.

Antacids can interfere with how other medications are absorbed into the body. A physician should be consulted if a person is taking any medications and wishes to also take an antacid; in general, antacids should not be taken within one or two hours of another medication. *See also* HEARTBURN.

Antepartum Hemorrhage

Any bleeding during the second half of pregnancy.

There are several possible causes of antepartum hemorrhage, including a low placenta and premature separation of the placenta from the uterine wall. Bleeding may be light or heavy and may also be accompanied by abdominal pain. Both the source and the amount of blood are important in determining if there is a threat to the pregnancy. *See also* ABDOMEN.

Mild bleeding may cease on its own, but a doctor should be notified immediately about *any* prenatal bleeding. Heavier bleeding can be dangerous and requires immediate attention. Treatment may include close monitoring and bed rest in an attempt to postpone labor; hospitalization may be necessary. When the hemorrhage poses a major health threat, a decision may be made to induce labor or to perform a Cesarean section. *See also* PREGNANCY.

Resources on Anthrax

Biddle, Wayne, *Field Guide to Germs* (1995); Grist, Norman R., et al., *Diseases of Infection: An Illustrated Textbook* (1992); Payan, Gregory, *Chemical and Biological Weapons: Anthrax and Sarin* (2000); Shaw, Michael, ed., *Everything You Need to Know About Diseases* (1996); Centers for Disease Contol and Prevention, Tel. (800) 311-3435, Online: www.cdc. gov; Infectious Disease Society of America, Tel. (703) 299-0200, Online: www.idsociety.org; Office of Rare Diseases, Tel. (301) 402-4336, Online: rarediseases.info.nih.gov; www.nycornell.org/medicine /cardiology/index.html; ww.nycornell.org/ medicine/emergency/ index.html

Anthracosis

Also known as black lung disease

A chronic lung disease caused by the inhalation of coal dust.

Anthracosis turns the normal pink color of the lungs to a dark black; it is diagnosed through an x-ray. Once a common disorder primarily found in coal miners, anthracosis is now also diagnosed in city dwellers.

Symptoms. In the early stages of the disease, the symptoms of anthracosis resemble those of bronchitis, characterized by coughing and shortness of breath. If the cause is not removed, the coughing gradually worsens over a period of years.

Treatment. The lung damage caused by inhaled dust cannot be repaired or treated directly. Breathing clean air halts the progress of anthracosis and may help to reduce the severity of symptoms. Patients with this condition should avoid further exposure to dust particles.

Risk Factors. Anthracosis is aggravated by cigarette smoking. *See also* LUNG.

Anthrax

A disease caused by Bacillus anthracis, a spore-forming bacterium that infects the skin, lungs, and gastrointestinal tract.

Cause. Anthrax is a highly contagious disease that is usually transmitted to humans from animals. The spores can lie dormant in the earth for many years and then infect animals or humans when inhaled, ingested, or exposed to an open wound. It is considered a possible bioterrorism agent.

Symptoms. Symptoms of anthrax become evident between 12 hours and a week after exposure to the bacteria, depending on the location of the infection. A skin infection starts with a bump on the skin that resembles an insect bite. The bump ruptures, leaving an ulcer and then a black, hardened center of dead tissue with swelling around it. Nearby lymph nodes become infected and the disease spreads to the lungs, bringing on symptoms similar to

influenza. Fever rises and difficulties in breathing soon lead to shock and possibly death. Gastrointestinal anthrax produces inflammation of the gastrointestinal tract, abdominal pain, vomiting of blood, and severe diarrhea. This infection can spread to the blood and result in death.

Prevention and Treatment. Those who are exposed to animals or animal products on a daily basis can be vaccinated for anthrax. Skin infections related to anthrax are treated with penicillin injections or with oral antibiotics, such as doxycycline or ciprofloxacin (Cipro). Intravenous penicillin is required to treat lung infections caused by the disease. *See also* ANTIBIOTIC DRUGS *and* ANTIBIOTIC RESISTANCE.

Antianxiety Drugs

Drugs used to treat symptoms of anxiety.

Beta-blockers, benzodiazepines, antidepressants, and barbiturates may be used as antianxiety drugs. These medications temporarily relieve the anxiety that hinders a person from coping with everyday life, and that may be caused by any of a number of underlying disorders.

Antianxiety drugs have a calming effect. Beta-blockers treat the symptoms of anxiety by reducing shaking, tremors, heart palpitations, and sweating. These medications achieve their calming effect by acting on various neurotransmitters. These chemicals help the body deal with stress by automatically increasing heart beat, air flow to the lungs, and blood pressure. By keeping the chemicals from binding with beta-receptors, unusually high blood pressure and rates of heartbeat and breathing are reduced. Benzodiazepines decrease nerve activity in the brain by influencing gamma-aminobutyric acid, a chemical implicated in sleep, alertness, and anxiety. Examples are alprazolam, clonazepam, and diazepam.

Benzodiazepines are an effective short-term treatment that may, however, be physically addictive in some people. *See also* ANXIETY *and* BETA-BLOCKERS.

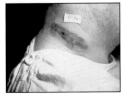

Anthrax. One of the first symptoms of anthrax is a cutaneous (skin) lesion on the skin, as seen above. As the disease progresses, the lymph and respiratory systems are also eventually affected. As a military or terrorist weapon, anthrax spores can be produced so that they may enter the lungs; this is inhalation anthrax and it is often fatal.

Antiarrhythmic Drugs

Medications prescribed to treat irregular heartbeat (arrhythmia).

The type of antiarrhythmic drug that is prescribed depends on the type of irregular heartbeat, the cause of the arrhythmia, and the patient's response to different medications. The oldest drug in this class is digitalis, which strengthens the contractions of the heart, making it pump more blood. Digitalis also slows transmission of electrical pulses through the atrioventricular node, slowing the heart. Although digitalis has classically been used to treat congestive heart failure, it can also be prescribed for atrial fibrillation, in which the atria, the upper chambers of the heart, beat very rapidly, up to 300 to 400 times a minute.

Beta-blockers or calcium channel blockers also reduce the ventricular heartbeat by slowing the conduction of atrial beats through the atrioventricular node. Beta-blockers act by preventing epinephrine and norepinephrine, molecules that control the heartbeat, from acting on receptors in heart cells. Calcium channel blockers act to relax the heart muscle by reducing the flow of calcium into the heart tissue. These and other antiarrhythmic drugs may be used alone or in combination. *See also* BETA-BLOCKER DRUGS; CALCIUM CHANNEL BLOCKERS; *and* DIGITALIS DRUGS.

Antibiotic Drugs

A family of drugs used to treat bacterial infections by destroying the bacteria or impairing their ability to reproduce.

When bacteria invade the body, they reproduce very quickly; some produce toxins that are harmful to the human host. The immune system sends white blood cells to surround and destroy the bacteria, releasing proteins that counteract the effects of the toxins. But if the bacteria become too numerous or the immune system is compromised, an infection results. This may range from a minor, localized infection, such as a urinary tract infection, to a systemic and severe infection, such as blood poisoning (septicemia).

Until World War II, doctors had no medications to fight bacterial infections. But in the early 1940s, a number of "miracle drugs" were developed, beginning with sulfa drugs, then penicillin and its derivatives. Since then, a number of groups of antibiotics have been developed.

Types of Antibiotics. Antibiotics are classified according to their chemical makeup and how they act on bacteria. Some can affect a broad range of bacteria, while others are effective against very specific bacteria.

Penicillin antibiotics prevent bacteria from building cell walls, thereby destroying them. Tetracycline antibiotics act by interfering with the bacteria's internal functions, such as protein synthesis. Newer antibiotics, such as cephalosporins and fluoroquinolones, are considered broad spectrum antibiotics, because they attack a number of different bacterial types. Cephalosporins act by blocking cell wall synthesis, and fluoroquinolones act to block bacterial DNA synthesis.

Side Effects. Antibiotics can have side effects, including intestinal inflammation, diarrhea, abdominal pain, nausea, and vomiting. Sensitive individuals can have severe, potentially life-threatening allergic reactions to antibiotics. *See also* ALLERGY.

Antibiotic Resistance

The ability of bacteria to evolve so that they can continue to multiply and thrive despite the administration of antibiotic drugs.

Bacteria live on the skin and mucous membranes, and abound in the intestinal tract. Many types of bacteria are benign or even helpful, because they compete with disease-causing bacteria and limit their proliferation. Although antibiotics destroy disease-causing bacteria, they also kill benign bacteria, and dangerous bacteria may be able to mutate and develop resistance to the antibiotics.

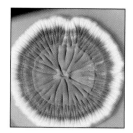

Penicillin Mold. Above, the penicillin mold is used to make penicillin antibiotics, which are commonly used to fight bacterial infections. Penicillin antibiotics prevent the invading bacteria from building cell walls, causing them to die. Recently, bacteria resistant to common antibiotics have appeared.

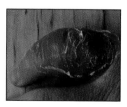

Sealer's Finger. Above, sealer's finger is a bacterial infection thought to be transmitted through a small cut in the finger of those who handle seals. Within a few days, extremely painful swelling of the finger occurs. Sealer's finger is difficult to treat, as the bacteria that causes the infection does not respond to antibiotics.

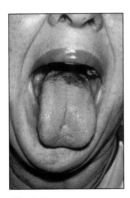

Black Tongue.
Above, if bacteria have invaded the mouth and built up on the rough surface (papillae) of the tongue, the tongue may appear black. Black tongue is also a possible side effect of antibiotic drugs.

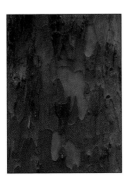

Yew Tree.
Above, the bark of the yew tree is often used in the manufacture of anticancer drugs. The type of drugs produced prevent cancerous cells from dividing and, thus, from multiplying.

If physicians prescribe broad spectrum antibiotics when there is no fever or other sign of bacterial infection, or if the drugs are not taken for the full term, bacteria in the body may mutate, and drug-resistant strains can appear. Antibiotics are not appropriate to combat flu or the common cold. Antibiotics do not affect viruses; indeed, they can expose the body to bacteria, such as *Clostridium difficile*, which causes digestive problems, and fungi, such as Candida, which causes a yeast infection of the vagina. *See also* CANDIDIASIS.

Antibody

> A protein produced by certain white blood cells that identifies foreign invaders in the bloodstream for other white blood cells to attack.

Antibodies, also called immunoglobulins, are essential components of the body's immune system. Five different types of antibodies have been identified: IgA, IgD, IgE, IgG and IgM. When a foreign, infectious substance (antigen) enters the body, antibodies bind to that substance and signal the white blood cells to find and destroy the antigen.

Infusion of Antibodies. If a person has a weakened immune system, he or she may need to receive a transfusion of antibodies into the bloodstream. This will provide the patient with antibodies, produced in the circulatory system of another human, that will help mobilize the body's defenses against bacterial attack. *See also* ANTIGEN *and* GAMMA GLOBULIN.

Anticancer Drugs

> Medications to treat cancer.

A large number of drugs are available to treat cancer, and new medications are constantly being developed. All have the same purpose: to stop the uncontrolled reproduction of malignant cells or to destroy those cells with the fewest possible ill effects on the body's normal cells and tissues. That goal is not entirely achievable, since some normal cells grow as rapidly as cancer cells. These normal cells include the follicles from which hair grows and the tissue that lines the intestinal tract. Hair loss and nausea are thus almost inevitable side effects of many anticancer drugs.

Nevertheless, chemotherapy with anticancer drugs is part of the treatment of many cancers. Chemotherapy may be given before, after, or during surgery or radiation therapy. The drugs may be given singly or in combination. They may be taken orally, be injected, or be infused into the bloodstream. They may be aimed specifically at a region of the body or at the entire body. They may be accompanied by drugs that reduce the side effects of chemotherapy. *See* CHEMOTHERAPY *and* RADIATION THERAPY.

CLASSES

There are several broad classes of anticancer drugs. The first class of drugs that were developed are the alkylating agents, which interfere with rapid cell growth by binding to DNA, the genetic molecule in the nuclei of cells. Development of the alkylating agents began with the observation that nitrogen mustard gas, used as a weapon in World War I, interfered with the reproduction of white blood cells and thus might be a weapon against leukemia. Commonly used alkylating agents include cyclophosphamide and busulfuran.

Another class consists of the plant alkaloids, which also act on the genetic material of cells. They interact with the chromosomes, the bodies that carry the genes, in a way that prevents cell division, which is an essential part of multiplication. Commonly used plant alkaloids include vincristine, vinblastine, etoposide, and taxol.

A third class of anticancer drugs is the antimetabolites, which act by preventing cancer cells from obtaining the nutrients they need to reproduce. Fluorouracil and methotrexate are examples of some widely used antimetabolites.

Antibiotics are a fourth class of anticancer drugs. These differ from the medications used to treat bacterial infections, as the drugs do not act against foreign invaders but against the body's own cancerous cells, disrupting the process by which DNA governs cellular reproduction. *See also* ANTIBIOTIC DRUGS.

Another class of anticancer drugs acts against the hormones that various kinds of cancers need to reproduce. One prominent example is tamoxifen, which blocks the activity of estrogen and thus disrupts the growth of breast cancer cells; it is used both to treat breast cancer and to prevent it. Various kinds of hormones can also be use to treat cancer, since they interfere with cell reproduction. Hormones used in cancer treatment include estrogens and progestins (female sex hormones), androgens (male sex hormones), and corticosteroids.

ADMINISTRATION

Anticancer drugs are administered in a number of ways. One basic method is by mouth. Oral chemotherapy can be done at home, but careful attention must be paid to details. Some drugs should be taken with food, others on an empty stomach. The exact dose that is prescribed must be taken, since an overdose can be toxic and an underdose can be ineffective.

Another method is to infuse medication into a vein. Often this is done by inserting a catheter, a thin tube, into a vein, and injecting medication through the catheter. The injection may be done with a syringe or by a drip method, in which the medication flows out of a bag connected to the syringe. The catheter is taken out after the medication is delivered. *See also* CATHETER.

One problem with this method is that some patients have veins so small that repeated insertion of a catheter is difficult or impossible, because the veins become scarred. These patients may receive their intravenous medication through a more permanently implanted catheter called a vascular access device. A port is an access device implanted under the skin, most often on the chest, so that medication can be injected. Minor surgery is required to implant these devices.

All methods of intravenous infusion deliver anticancer drugs to the entire body. In some cases, a more effective treatment is to aim the chemotherapy directly at the cancer, which allows an attack by larger doses. This can be done by pumping the medication into the artery that carries blood to the cancer. Another method is intraperitoneal chemotherapy, or targeting the drugs at the abdominal cavity. This method is used for cancer of the ovary. Bladder cancer can be treated by giving medication through a catheter placed in the bladder. Cancer of the brain or spinal cord can be treated by injecting drugs into the spinal cord.

SIDE EFFECTS

The most common side effects of anticancer drugs result from their action on normal cells that reproduce rapidly in the gastrointestinal tract, the mouth, and hair follicles. Not all anticancer drugs act on the follicles to cause hair loss, but this side effect is possible; it can have serious effects on the morale of cancer patients. Some patients handle this problem by shaving their heads or wearing a wig. Techniques for minimizing hair loss include handling the hair very gently, avoiding possible harsh chemicals in hair dyes and permanent wave products, and using a smooth pillowcase to minimize the friction on hair. In almost every case, hair loss caused by anticancer drugs is temporary.

Severity of nausea and vomiting vary according to the drugs administered and the size of the dose. Some patients experience only mild problems, but others become nauseated for hours. Gastrointestinal effects can now be easily controlled in most patients by drugs given at the same time as the chemotherapy. Training in relaxation techniques can help many patients.

Anticancer drugs can have many other side effects, including persistent fatigue, weight loss, anemia, and reduced resistance to infection. Drugs, such as growth factors, are available to treat some of these complications. All these side effects can affect mood, emotional status, and mental function. Psychological counseling can be helpful, as can the knowledge that the side effects will be temporary in most cases.

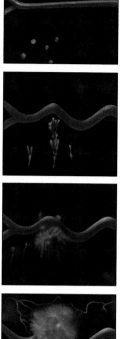

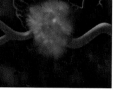

Anticancer Drugs.
Anticancer drugs make it impossible for cancerous cells in the body to reproduce. Top, implanted cancer cells glow green with a fluorescence protein. Second from the top, three of the original cancer cells have survived to begin replicating. Third from the top, the cancer cells have reached the existing blood vessel. Bottom, even though there are only about a hundred cancer cells, they have already created new, fully-functioning blood vessels.

Anticholinergic Drugs

Drugs used to prevent the reception of acetylcholine at nerve endings.

Acetylcholine is a neurotransmitter, a chemical that assists nerve cells in communication with other nerve cells, muscles, and glands. Among other functions, acetylcholine slows down and weakens the heart beat, constricts blood vessels in the muscles, constricts the pupils in the eyes, and increases muscle spasms in the intestines. Anticholinergic drugs block the effect of acetylcholine, thus strengthening the heart beat, opening blood vessels, and relieving intestinal spasms.

Uses and Examples. Anticholinergic drugs are used to treat patients with Parkinson's disease, irritable bowel syndrome, urinary incontinence, asthma, and slow heartbeat (bradycardia). Examples of common anticholinergic drugs are atropine, benztropine, and dyphenohydramine.

Side Effects. Side effects of these drugs may include confusion, blurred vision, dry mouth, constipation, lightheadedness, and loss of bladder control. *See also* ACETYL-CHOLINE *and* BRADYCARDIA.

Anticoagulant Drugs

Drugs that reduce the formation of blood clots.

Coagulation, an essential protective process of the blood to stop bleeding after an accident or from disease, can be life-threatening if it stops or impedes the flow of blood to the brain, heart, or other critical organs. In this case the physician will most often prescribe heparin, warfarin, or aspirin—drugs that thin the blood and reduce its clotting ability.

Heparin is usually administered by injection. It may dissolve early clots and protects the patient from clots that have formed within the blood vessels, which can break off and flow to the rest of the body.

Warfarin, also known as Coumadin, is administered orally. It counteracts the effects of vitamin K, a vitamin essential for production of the main blood-clotting agents. Vitamin K is found in plants, especially in green leafy vegetables. Warfarin acts more slowly than heparin, and its effects linger for a day or two after the patient stops taking it.

Aspirin. Small daily doses of aspirin (about 81 mg) are now known to provide protection from heart attack or stroke. Aspirin acts directly on the platelets that would normally clot. Its effects are slow to develop and may last for days.

The major side effect of all anticoagulant drugs is the danger of uncontrolled bleeding. Patients who are taking anticoagulants should be regularly monitored by their doctors. *See also* ASPIRIN; COAGULATION; *and* HEMOPHILIA.

Anticonvulsant Drugs

Drugs used to prevent seizures.

Anticonvulsant drugs are effective in preventing seizures in more than half of epilepsy patients. These drugs greatly reduce the frequency of attacks in another third of these patients. Anticonvulsant drugs are also administered to victims of head injury to prevent seizures.

Cause. Seizures are a result of exceedingly high electrical activity in the brain. Anticonvulsant drugs neutralize the overload of electrical activity.

Use and Examples. There is no single drug that is effective for all types of seizures. Some individuals need more than one type of anticonvulsant drug to control their condition. Commonly used anticonvulsant drugs include carbamazepine, clonazepam, diazepam, and phenobarbital. Proper dosage is critical to the drug's success. Possible adverse reactions to anticonvulsant drugs include drowsiness, impaired memory, fatigue, damage to the kidneys and liver, and high blood pressure.

It is important not to abruptly stop taking an anticonvulsant drug. The dosage must be gradually reduced, or the seizures may reappear. *See also* EPILEPSY; HYPERTENSION; *and* PHENOBARBITAL.

Antidepressant Drugs

Medications that treat symptoms of clinical depression by correcting brain chemical imbalances associated with these disorders.

Antidepressant drugs are used to treat depression. These drugs regulate an imbalance in an individual's brain chemistry. They take approximately two to three weeks to become effective. Although antidepressant drugs may be required for a long period of time to manage depression and prevent a relapse, typically, they are not physically addicting.

TYPES

Several types of antidepressants are available on the market.

Selective Serotonin Reuptake Inhibitors (SSRIs) decrease the inactivation of serotonin by the brain, making it more available and thus increasing its effects. Serotonin is a chemical in the brain (a neurotransmitter) that is involved in mood and thinking. SSRIs are safe and generally have few side effects. SSRI trade names in the United States include Zoloft, Paxil, Prozac, Celexa, and Luvox. These drugs are indicated for a variety of conditions beyond depression, including obsessive-compulsive disorder and panic disorder. Side effects of SSRIs include sexual disinterest or dysfunction, headaches, nervousness, insomnia, and weight gain.

Anecdotal reporting of the effects of SSRIs, including increased comfort in social situations and mood-brightening, has led to the increased use of SSRIs in recent years. As a result, there are concerns about overuse of SSRIs for people who are not suffering from an illness but who are simply experiencing the normal worries or disappointments of life.

Tricyclics decrease inactivation of the neurotransmitters norepinephrine and serotonin. These drugs, which have been used for over 40 years, are less popular than the more recently developed SSRI drugs because they are unsafe in overdose and they have undesirable side effects, including

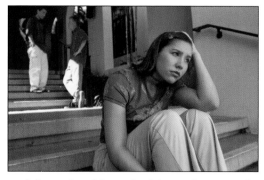

weight gain, blurred vision, dry mouth, constipation, drowsiness, dizziness, and excessive sweating.

Monoamine-Oxidase Inhibitors (MAO inhibitors, or MAOIs) affect the enzyme monoamine oxidase, which inactivates many neurotransmitters, such as serotonin, dopamine, and norepinephrine. For some patients, MAOIs are effective antidepressants, though side effects can be severe.

Side effects of MAOIs include weight gain, headaches, dizziness, and low blood pressure. A dangerous blood pressure reaction may be triggered by eating certain foods (such as cheese), by consuming alcohol, or by taking some types of cough, cold, and pain-killing medications. For this reason, MAOIs are generally prescribed only after other medications prove ineffective, and they must be prescribed with close consultation from a physician, as well as attention to the diet and other medical requirements of the patient.

Newer Antidepressants. In an effort to develop safe and tolerable antidepressants with a broad spectrum of effectiveness, several new drugs have been brought to the market in recent years. All of these drugs affect the neurotransmitters serotonin and norepinephrine in some way. Some of the newer drugs, which include the trade names Serzone, Effexor, and Remeron, are free of some of the undesirable side effects of SSRIs and MAOIs.

Background material on antidepressant drugs can be found in DEPRESSION. *Related information is contained in* NEUROTRANSMITTER; PANIC DISORDER; *and* PHARMACOLOGY. *See also* ACNE; HYPERTENSION; INSOMNIA; *and* SEXUAL DYSFUNCTION *for more on specific side effects of the drugs.*

Antidepressant Drugs. At left, constant feelings of hopelessness or despair may be signs of clinical depression, a mental disorder that is sometimes caused by an imbalance in brain chemistry. Antidepressant medications, including selective serotonin reuptake inhibitors, monoamine-oxidase inhibitors, and newer varieties, can help correct this imbalance.

Resources on Depression
Beckham, E. Edward and William R. Leber, eds., *Handbook of Depression: Treatment, Assessment, and Research* (1985); Greist, John H. and James W. Jefferson, *Depression and Its Treatment* (1992); Solomon, Andrew, *The Noonday Demon: An Atlas of Depression* (2001); Wender, P.H., and D.F. Klein, *Mind, Mood, and Medicine: A Guide to the New Biopsychiatry* (1981); National Alliance for the Mentally Ill, Tel. (800) 950-6264, Online: www. nami.org; National Depressive and Manic-Depressive Association, Tel. (800) 82-NDMDA, Online: www.ndmda.org; National Mental Health Association, Tel. (800) 969-NMHA, Online: www.nmha.org; www.ny-cornell.org/psychiatry/.

Antidiarrheal Drugs

Medications given to treat persistent diarrhea.

Two major classes of antidiarrheal drugs are narcotics, such as codeine, and bulking agents, such as psyllium. These drugs are usually prescribed if diarrhea persists for two days or more. Narcotic drugs act on the muscles in the intestinal wall, slowing the passage of feces, and allowing more water to be absorbed by the intestine. Bulking agents reduce the volume of feces by absorbing fluid from the stool. Antidiarrheal agents should be used with care. Overuse of these medications can lead to constipation; if the diarrhea is due to an intestinal infection, taking such drugs may delay recovery. *See also* CONSTIPATION *and* DIARRHEA.

Antidote

Drug or other substance given to counteract the effects of a poison.

Antidotes may work in several ways, depending on the type of poisoning being treated. They may function by chemically neutralizing the toxin, by preventing its absorption by the body (rendering it insoluble), by coating the stomach to prevent absorption, or by absorbing the poison themselves. *See also* ANTITOXIN.

Antiemetic Drugs

Medications used to treat nausea and vomiting.

Severe vomiting can lead to dehydration and a serious drop in blood pressure. It can also lead to a serious electrolyte imbalance, due to the loss of potassium and sodium. In situations in which vomiting is severe or recurrent, antiemetic drugs may be prescribed. They may be used to treat nausea and vomiting caused by motion sickness, vertigo, inner ear disorders, radiation therapy, and chemotherapy.

Most antiemetics work by suppressing the central nervous system (phenothiazine drugs) or the nerve pathways (antihista-

mines) or by inhibiting the passing of nerve impulses (anticholinergics), all of which tend to suppress the vomiting reflex. Recently, marijuana has been used as an antiemetic for people undergoing chemotherapy, although its use is controversial because of its history as an illegal recreational drug.

Antiemetics should be used with care. Regular use can mask potentially serious underlying conditions. The most common side effect is drowsiness. *See also* CHEMOTHERAPY; MÉNIÈRE'S DISEASE; MOTION SICKNESS; VERTIGO; *and* VOMITING.

Antifreeze Poisoning

Adverse physical effects resulting from the ingestion of antifreeze.

Antifreeze is usually made of a type of alcohol, either methanol or ethylene glycol. Both are extremely toxic if ingested, and a few swallows can be lethal.

Symptoms of poisoning include cramps, headache, depressed breathing, and convulsions. Methanol has the potential to damage the optic nerves and cause permanent blindness; ethylene glycol can result in kidney failure.

Both of these alcohols are processed (metabolized) by the kidneys into highly toxic substances. Therefore, a rapid response is essential in treating antifreeze poisoning. The slightest suspicion of antifreeze poisoning is cause for seeking immediate medical help. *See also* POISONING.

Antifungal Drugs

Drugs used to treat diseases caused by fungi.

Antifungal drugs destroy the cell walls of fungi. However, because fungal cell walls are relatively thick, antifungal drugs tend to be more powerful than antibiotic drugs, which destroy bacteria.

TYPES

There are two major categories of antifungal drugs: topical drugs, which are used on the skin, and systemic drugs, which are taken by injection or swallowed.

Topical Antifungal Drugs. Fungi prefer warm, moist places, so most fungal skin infections are in the mouth, armpits, groin, between the toes, and in the genital area. The most familiar infections are athlete's foot, jock itch, yeast infections of the vagina, and ringworm (which is not a worm but a fungus that makes circular rings on the skin). Topical antifungal drugs can be very successful in relieving the itching and scaling of these infections, as well as in combating the infections themselves.

Topical antifungal drugs are available over the counter as ointments, creams, powders, sprays, and vaginal suppositories. Amphotericin B is probably the most widely prescribed medication for fungal infections, especially for people with compromised immune systems. The azole family, including fluconazole, itraconazole, and ketoconazole, offers many alternatives if amphotericin B is ineffective. These have fewer side effects than amphotericin B.

Most topical antifungal drugs must be used for periods of between two to four weeks, depending on the specific infection. Vaginal yeast infections (also called candidiasis) call for topical medications in the form of suppositories, tablets, or creams inserted with an applicator. These include clotrimazole, lotrimin, miconazole, and monistat. Symptoms should clear up within seven days, but it is important to finish the full course of treatment.

It is important to wash the hands before and after application of the drug, and contact between the drug and the eyes should be carefully avoided. If there is swelling, blistering, or other irritation, treatment should be stopped at once.

Systemic antifungal drugs are similar to those used topically, and are taken orally or injected. They are sometimes used to treat candidiasis, which can appear in the nose or throat as well as the vagina, or other infections that can be found in the lungs and other organs. Amphotericin B, fluconazole, and ketoconazole can be relatively toxic if taken orally. They may cause drowsiness, dizziness, chills, fever, headache, vomiting, or damage to the kidneys.

Alcohol should be avoided during the use of antifungal medications. There are also several medications that may interact with systemic antifungal drugs, including acetaminophen, birth control pills, antidepressants, antihistamines, muscle relaxants, and warfarin. Consult a physician about possible drug interactions.

> *Background material on antifungal drugs can be found in* FUNGAL INFECTIONS *and* INFECTIOUS DISEASE. *Related information is contained in* ATHLETE'S FOOT; CANDIDIASIS; *and* RINGWORM. *See also* ANTIDEPRESSANT DRUGS; ANTIHISTAMINE DRUGS; MUSCLE-RELAXANT DRUGS; *and* ORAL CONTRACEPTIVES *for more on possible drug interactions.*

Antigen

A "marker" that identifies an invader as foreign and therefore elicits an immune response.

Foreign particles or substances are recognized by the immune system as antigens, including toxins (biologically produced poisons) and microorganisms, such as fungi, bacteria, or viruses. Almost any foreign molecule in nature can be recognized as foreign and therefore can be an antigen, even if it is not intrinsically harmful. *See also* ALLERGY *and* IMMUNE SYSTEM.

Antihelminthic Drugs

Drugs used to combat intestinal parasites.

Helminths are intestinal parasitic worms that cause disease. These organisms have the ability to inhabit even the most hostile region of the body—the highly acidic stomach and intestines. They are also resistant to the body's defenses (immune system). These special abilities make intestinal parasites especially difficult to treat.

Antihelminthic drugs are used to combat intestinal worms. They include such medications as diethylcarbamazine, mebendazole, niclosamide, praziquantel, pyrantel, pamoate, albendazole, and ivermectin. These drugs both eliminate and prevent complications of worm infestations. Complications may include anemia, vitamin deficiency, and intestinal obstruction. Antihelminthic drugs work by incapacitating the worms' ability to latch onto the intestinal walls or simply by killing the worms.

Worms may also inhabit the lungs, liver, or other organs. Antihelminthic drugs make these worms more vulnerable to the immune system. After the immune system kills the worms, they and the damage they have caused may require surgical removal.

Today's antihelminthic drugs are generally safe, inexpensive, and effective in a single-dose treatment, depending on the severity of infestation. Treatment of school-age children is of critical concern, as children of this age experience the greatest prevalence of helminth-related diseases, some of which are believed to affect learning and to pose serious health risks. *See also* ASCARIASIS; FLUKE; PARASITE; ROUNDWORM; SCHISTOSOME; SCHISTOSOMIASIS; TAPEWORM; *and* WORM INFESTATION.

Antihistamine Drugs

Allergy drugs that block the effects of the body chemical histamine.

Histamine is a chemical in cells of the body that is released during an allergic reaction; it is responsible for many of the symptoms of allergy. It causes the airways to the lungs (the bronchi) to become abnormally narrow. The effect produces cramping and congestion in the upper respiratory tract and itching and hives in the skin. Histamine also stimulates itching, sneezing, and coughing.

Antihistamine drugs work to block the effects of histamine in the skin, eyes, nose, bronchial passages, and other tissues. They reduce itching by preventing histamine from irritating nerve fibers, and suppress nerve centers in the brain responsible for coughing. This type of drug suppresses the symptoms of an allergy but does not cure it.

Antihistamine drugs have other uses. They can be given to stop persistent vomiting, which can be caused by histamines,

and they may also be given by injection in emergency situations to treat anaphylactic shock, a rare but extremely severe allergic reaction that can be life-threatening.

A number of antihistamine drugs are available without a prescription. These over-the-counter drugs include diphenhydramine, chlorpheniramine, and clemastine. In combination with other ingredients, these drugs are used in formulations to treat the common cold, sinus problems, and allergies. Many over-the-counter sleep aids also contain antihistamines. All of these over-the-counter medications can cause drowsiness in a large percentage of people who take them; their other side effects may include nervousness and excitability, dizziness, dry mouth, constipation, difficulty in urination, loss of appetite, ringing in the ears (tinnitus), and blurred vision.

Newer antihistamines are generally available only by prescription and do not cause drowsiness. They include loratadine, fexofenadine hydrochloride, astemizole, terfenadine, and cetirizine. But these antihistamines can have their own serious side effects. Terfenadine and astemizole have been linked to serious disturbances of heart rhythm in persons with liver diseases, including those caused by alcohol abuse, occupational exposure to substances that damage the liver, and other liver toxins. Patients who are prescribed astemizole or terfenadine are advised not to take a number of other medications, such as antibiotics, including erythromycin, clarithromycin and troleandomycin; and oral antifungal drugs, including ketoconazole, fluconazole, and micronazole, because the combination can be toxic. Patients who are prescribed these antihistamine medications should carefully read the labels and leaflets included in the package to avoid potentially dangerous drug interactions.

Background material on antihistamine drugs can be found in ALLERGY. *Related information is contained in* ALCOHOL DEPENDENCE; ANAPHYLACTIC SHOCK; ANURIA; *and* TINNITUS. *See also* ANTIBIOTIC DRUGS *and* ANTIFUNGAL DRUGS *for more on possible drug interactions.*

Antihypertensive Drugs

Medications prescribed for the treatment of high blood pressure (hypertension).

High blood pressure (hypertension) sustained over long periods of time causes damage to the heart and to blood vessels in the kidneys and eyes. Hypertension is one of the major causes of death in industrialized countries.

Antihypertensive drugs are used when non-drug methods of reducing high blood pressure, such as a program of moderate exercise combined with a low-salt diet, are not effective. This is the case for 75 percent or more of patients with this serious condition. Physicians have a number of antihypertensive drugs at their disposal.

DIURETICS

Among the oldest agents are the diuretics, which have been used in the United States for more than 40 years. A diuretic, commonly called a water pill, lowers blood pressure by encouraging the kidneys to reduce the amount of water in the body, thus reducing the volume of blood. There are several kinds of diuretics. Thiazide diuretics, the most commonly used, act in the tubules, the structures that carry urine in the kidneys. Loop diuretics are named for their site of action, the loop of Henle, where the kidney filters waste products from the blood. Potassium-sparing diuretics prevent the excess loss of potassium sometimes caused by thiazide diuretics.

BETA-BLOCKERS

Beta-blockers act on the beta nerve receptors in the autonomic nervous system, which controls heart rate. Beta-blockers reduce the rate at which the heart beats, thus lowering the pressure that the blood exerts on the arteries. They also act on some of the hormones that regulate blood pressure, such as epinephrine (adrenaline).

CALCIUM CHANNEL BLOCKERS

Calcium channel blockers lower blood pressure by reducing the flow of calcium into the muscle cells that constrict the diameter of blood vessels. With less calcium, the muscles are less active and the blood vessels become wider, allowing blood to flow more easily, thereby reducing the patient's blood pressure.

ACE INHIBITORS

Angiotensin-converting enzyme (ACE) inhibitors prevent the formation of angiotensin II, a molecule that causes arterioles, small blood vessels, to constrict; they also stimulate the release of aldosterone, a hormone that is important in the regulation of blood pressure.

ALPHA-BLOCKERS

Alpha-blockers act on a different kind of receptor in the autonomic nervous system than beta-blockers. Their target is the alpha receptors, which control constriction of the arteries. They also inhibit the effect of norepinephrine, an adrenal hormone that acts to raise blood pressure.

OTHER DRUGS

Vasodilators are drugs that cause blood vessels to open wider. Peripheral adrenergic antagonists inhibit the activity of norepinephrine but are not widely used because they have a sedative effect.

WHAT A PHYSICIAN MIGHT CONSIDER

In choosing a drug, the patient's age is an important factor, as is the presence of any underlying medical condition, such as diabetes, kidney disease, or heart disease. Side effects must also be considered. For example, beta blockers can cause impotence, thus it would not be advisable to prescribe these drugs to a man with erectile dysfunction (ED). Sometimes several medications must be tried in order to select the drug or combination of drugs that is best for a given patient at that time.

Background material on antihypertensive drugs can be found in HYPERTENSION. *Related information is contained in* ACE INHIBITOR DRUGS; BETA-BLOCKER DRUGS; CALCIUM CHANNEL BLOCKERS; *and* DIURETIC DRUGS. *See also* SEXUAL DYSFUNCTION *for more on physicians' considerations.*

Resources on Hypertension

Berne, Robert M., et al., *Cardiovascular Physiology* (2001); Debakey, Michael E. and Antonio M. Gotto, *The New Living Heart* (1997); Gould, Lance K., *Heal Your Heart* (2000); American Heart Association, Tel. (800) 242-8721, Online: www.amhrt.org; Heart Information Network, Tel. (973) 701-6035, Online: www.heartinfo. org; National Heart, Lung, and Blood Institute, Tel. (301) 496-4236, Online: www.nhlbi.nih.gov; www.nycornell.org/cardiothoracic.surgery/; www.nycornell.org/medicine/cardiology/index .html;www.nycornell.org/ medicine/cp/index.html.

Anti-Inflammatory Drugs

Drugs that reduce swelling and inflammation.

Inflammation is caused by an increase of blood supply to an injured or infected area. White blood cells move freely into the inflamed location. Inflammation produces tenderness and even pain if the tissues are in an area that is constrained by the skin. There are many kinds of anti-inflammatory drugs. Two of the most common types are nonsteroidal anti-inflammatory drugs (NSAIDs) and corticosteroids.

NSAIDs

NSAIDs include aspirin, ibuprofen, and other anti-inflammatory drugs. They may be used to treat mild conditions, such as a headache or a muscle strain, or chronic conditions, such as osteoarthritis and rheumatoid arthritis.

NSAIDs block the production of prostaglandins. Prostaglandins are substances whose release is triggered by injury or infection. They enlarge the blood vessels, encourage inflammation, raise the temperature of the body, and reduce the ability of the blood to clot. Thus, by blocking prostaglandins, NSAIDs prevent inflammation from occurring.

Side Effects. NSAIDs may trigger allergic reactions or increased sensitivity to sunlight; they also may worsen asthma and kidney disorders. They should not be taken in conjunction with anticoagulant drugs, diuretics, diabetes medication, or steroids.

Aspirin can be irritating to the stomach, and prolonged use may lead to peptic ulcers. Aspirin reduces the ability of the blood to clot, so people who bruise easily or have blood-clotting problems should avoid aspirin. Aspirin should also be avoided in the last trimester of pregnancy and for children under 12 with a viral infection, as it may increase the risk for Reye's syndrome in the fetus or child. Reye's syndrome is a rare but serious disease of the brain and liver.

Ibuprofen, like aspirin, can irritate the stomach. Further, it may cause drowsiness, dizziness, and nausea; it reduces the clotting ability of the blood as well. It should not be taken by people with kidney problems, liver problems, high blood pressure, or heart failure.

Aspirin is often prescribed in small doses over long periods of time to reduce the clotting ability of the blood and to protect against heart attacks. Otherwise, the use of NSAIDs should not be continued for more than ten days to reduce pain or for more than three days to reduce fever.

CORTICOSTEROIDS

Corticosteroids are synthetic versions of hormones produced by the body. They include cortisone, prednisone, and hydrocortisone, and are used to treat inflammatory conditions ranging from rashes to irritation of the joints or digestive tract, to prevent asthma attacks, as a replacement for corticosteroids that the body cannot produce on its own, and as a long-term treatment after an organ transplant to prevent rejection. Like NSAIDs, they work by blocking prostaglandin production, and also by suppressing the immune system. They may be taken orally, used as a topical cream, injected, or inhaled.

Side effects generally occur only over long-term use. As a result, doctors try to prescribe corticosteroids only for a short period of time to avoid the side effects.

Over the long term, side effects include:
- skin damage from topical corticosteroid use;
- raised blood pressure;
- mood changes;
- swollen ankles;
- slowed growth in children;
- osteoporosis;
- increased risk of infection due to immune suppression;
- characteristics of Cushing's syndrome (a round, puffy face; acne; easy bruising; and fat deposits on the torso).

Long-Term Effects. Use of synthetic corticosteroids blocks the production of natural corticosteroids. Thus, long-term use of corticosteroids should be ceased slowly and under the supervision of a physician, so that the body is able to start gradually producing its own corticosteroids.

> *Background material on anti-inflammatory drugs can be found in* INFLAMMATION. *Related information is contained in* CORTICOSTEROIDS; CUSHING'S SYNDROME; NONSTEROIDAL ANTI-INFLAMMATORY DRUGS; *and* PROSTAGLANDIN. *See also* REYE'S SYNDROME *for more on possible serious side effects of anti-inflammatory drugs..*

Antipsperspirant

A lotion, cream, or spray applied to the skin to reduce excessive sweating.

Body odor occurs when sweat remains on the skin, allowing the growth of bacteria that breaks down chemicals in sweat. Antiperspirant works by reducing the production of sweat, as well as blocking the ducts that drain sweat onto the skin. Deodorants may contain antiseptics to destroy odor-causing bacteria or perfume to conceal odor, but do not block sweat production.

A high concentration of antiperspirant may cause burning, itching, and irritation of the skin. A deodorant may be preferable if antiperspirants are clogging pores. If irritation occurs, use of the antiperspirant should be stopped and a dermatologist should be consulted. *See also* BODY ODOR.

Antipsychotic Drugs

Also known as neuroleptics

Drugs prescribed to eliminate psychotic symptoms, such as incoherence, delusions, hallucinations, bizarre behavior, and severe agitation.

Antipsychotic drugs do not cure patients, but in the majority of cases they will reduce psychotic symptoms with continued use. Commonly prescribed antipsychotic drugs include halperidol (Haldol), chlorpromazine (Thorazine), thiothixene (Navane), risperidone (Risperdal), olenzapine (Zyrexa), quetiapine (Seroquel), ziprasidone (Geodon), and clozapine (Clozaril).

Function. Antipsychotic drugs work by blocking dopamine receptors in the brain. Dopamine is a neurotransmitter, a chemical that carries signals between nerve cells in the brain. Too much dopamine is associated with psychotic symptoms, such as delusions, hallucinations, disorganized thinking, and aggression. Antipsychotic drugs block dopamine receptors, thus helping to relieve psychotic symptoms. The drugs are most commonly prescribed in the treatment of schizophrenia, though they are also used to treat other disorders, such as mania and dementia.

Side Effects. In general, all antipsychotics are relatively safe. Side effects of antipsychotics may be unpleasant but are rarely dangerous. However, patients occasionally discontinue use of these drugs—and thus lose their benefits—in order to alleviate side effects.

Early side effects may include drowsiness, dry mouth, blurred visions, tremors, or restlessness. Patients may also report a general slowed-down feeling. A side effect, resulting from long-term use, is tardive dyskinesia, in which tics, tremors, and involuntary movements develop in the face and sometimes in other parts of the body. In addition, the newer antipsychotic drugs have been noted to cause weight gain, blood sugar regulation problems, and bone marrow suppression in some patients.

Careful monitoring of these drugs by a physician is important, to check for possible adverse reactions and to determine the optimum dose, since side effects are reduced with lower doses. These medications do not, however, result in dependence.

Administration. Antipsychotics are usually administered daily by pill or liquid. In the case of Polixin and Haldol, they may be given by injection, which acts for one to four weeks.

Innovations. Some newer antipsychotic drugs block the receptors for both dopamine and serotonin, which is another neurotransmitter. In some patients, these drugs are particularly effective, though they are not without side effects. *See also* AGGRESSION; DELUSION; DEMENTIA; DOPAMINE; PSYCHOSIS; *and* SEROTONIN.

> **Resources on Psychopharmacology**
> Barchas, Jack D., *Psychopharmacology: From Theory to Practice* (1977); Hardman, Joel G., and Lee E. Limbird, *Goodman and Gilman's The Pharmacological Basis of Therapeutics* (1996); Wender, P.H., and D.F. Klein, *Mind, Mood, and Medicine: A Guide to the New Biopsychiatry* (1981); National Alliance for the Mentally Ill, Tel. (800) 950-6264, Online: www. nami.org; Nat. Depressive & Manic-Depressive Association, Tel. (800) 82-NDMDA, Online: www. ndmda.org; National Mental Health Association, Tel. (800) 969-NMHA, Online: www.nmha.org; www.ny-cornell.org/psychiatry/.

Antirheumatic Drugs

A class of drugs used for rheumatoid arthritis, as well as for types of arthritis related to other autoimmune diseases.

There is no clear-cut single cure for rheumatoid arthritis, so the goal of antirheumatic drugs is to alleviate pain; prevent damage to bones, joints, and tissues; and preserve mobility. Rheumatoid arthritis is a condition in which the body's immune system attacks the joints.

Antirheumatic drugs suppress the production or activity of white blood cells, which minimizes damage by the autoimmune system. They reduce inflammation and prevent the deterioration of cartilage lining the joints. Antirheumatic drugs are considered second-line therapy, which means they are put into use if nonsteroidal anti-inflammatory drugs are ineffective. They are also called disease-modifying antirheumatic drugs or slow-acting antirheumatic drugs. *See also* AUTOIMMUNE DISORDERS *and* RHEUMATOID ARTHRITIS.

Antiseptics

Preparations used to cleanse and disinfect minor wounds or scrapes.

Antiseptics are used to prevent or stop the growth of the bacteria that invade an open wound, thus preventing infection. Antiseptics are intended for application to the skin or mucous membranes of the area around the victim's wound; they are therefore milder than disinfectants, which are intended for the disinfection of inanimate objects, such as knives or medical instruments. In hospitals or nursing homes the preferred antiseptics are chlorhexidine for general skin application and iodophor for genital areas. These are available in liquids, ointments, and creams.

Hexachlorophene and iodine are not recommended for use as antiseptics. Hydrogen peroxide is not particularly effective as an antiseptic either. *See also* BANDAGE *and* FIRST AID.

Antisocial Personality Disorder

A personality disorder characterized by deceitfulness, disregard for the rights and safety of others, irresponsible behavior, and lack of remorse for these violations.

A person with antisocial personality disorder may also be known as a sociopath or a psychopath. The disorder is several times more common in men than in women, and it affects approximately two to three percent of the population.

CAUSES
There may be a genetic component to antisocial personality disorder, although there is substantial evidence that it tends to develop in those who were raised in abusive or neglectful homes. There may be genetic and neurobiological components to antisocial personality disorder..

CHARACTERISTICS
Antisocial personality disorder is generally preceded by conduct disorder, a behavioral disorder in children characterized by aggressive and destructive behavior. It begins before age 15, reaches a peak from the mid-20s to the mid-40s, and may diminish as the individual gets older.

People with antisocial personality disorder have difficulty maintaining relationships due to their disregard for others and their lack of feelings of remorse or guilt. They tend to be unfaithful, intolerant of frustration, and irresponsible with respect to financial obligations. Aggressive, impulsive, hostile, and promiscuous behaviors, as well as criminal activities and substance abuse, are common in individuals with this psychological condition.

Antisocial personality disorder does not respond well to treatment, because individuals tend to be noncompliant, lack motivation, and distrust authority, including those who are trying to treat them. *See also* ANXIETY DISORDERS; BEHAVIORAL DISORDERS; *and* PERSONALITY DISORDERS.

Antispasmodic Drugs

Medications that relieve spasms of the digestive system, bladder, and urethra.

Antispasmodic drugs, such as dicyclomine and belladonna, relax bowel and bladder spasms. These drugs are used in the treatment of conditions such as irritable bowel syndrome and irritable bladder, in addition to prescribed dietary measures. They block the activity of acetylcholine, a nerve chemical that causes muscle contraction. Side effects include headache, dizziness, dry mouth, blurred vision, and difficulty urinating. They should be used with caution by patients taking other drugs, such as antacids, antihistamines, and antidepressants, and by persons with medical conditions, including heart disease, bronchitis, and glaucoma. *See also* IRRITABLE BLADDER *and* IRRITABLE BOWEL SYNDROME.

Antitoxin

A naturally or artificially made protein and blood solution that eliminates a bacterial toxin.

When exposed to harmful bacteria, the body creates an antitoxin to neutralize the poison of that particular bacteria.

The body cannot produce the appropriate type or amount of antitoxins for the treatment of diseases such as diphtheria, tetanus, botulism, and dysentery. In these instances, the antitoxin must be manufactured artificially.

Artificial antitoxins are created in laboratories by repeatedly injecting a healthy animal with small doses of the toxin until high levels of antitoxin accumulate in its blood. Samples of the animal antitoxin are stored for the purpose of future administration into the blood of human sufferers.

Antitoxins are used cautiously because of potential patient allergies to animal antitoxins. The "borrowed" state of immunity may be either temporary or long-term, depending on the type of bacterial illness.

Antivenin. Similar in function to an antitoxin, antivenins also serve as an antidote to venom. Antivenin is made with infection-fighting chemicals (antibodies) developed in an animal, usually a horse. Small amounts of venom are injected over time into the animal's bloodstream, and the antibodies are collected.

The antivenin is administered to the patient by injection, either into a vein (intravenously) or into a muscle (intramuscularly), in order to neutralize the venom present in the body. As with antitoxins, the potential of an allergic reaction to animal products is a concern in treating a poisonous bite. *See also* ANTIBODY; POISON; TOXIN; *and* VENIN.

Antiviral Drugs

Drugs used to treat viral infections.

Viruses are much more difficult to combat than bacteria or fungi, because they penetrate healthy cells and use the cell's own life mechanisms to multiply. Thus damaging or destroying viruses within cells can also damage or destroy the cells.

The immune system handles many viruses successfully. Common colds, flu, measles, mumps, and chicken pox are self-limiting diseases that the body can successfully eliminate in short periods of time. However, certain viruses are more dangerous, and others can remain in the body throughout an individual's life.

Generally, more severe viral infections are prevented by immunization rather than treated after infection. Polio and smallpox have been essentially eliminated as a result of vaccinations for these diseases. However, with the appearance of viruses like AIDS, hantavirus, and ebola, and the spread of the herpes and hepatitis B viruses, efforts to produce new antiviral drugs have intensified.

To combat viruses, a drug must be lethal to the virus without harming healthy cells. Antiviral drugs act by interfering with the process viruses use to reproduce or by stimulating the immune system to attack the virus directly.

TYPES OF ANTIVIRAL DRUGS

The list of available antiviral drugs is still very short in comparison to antibiotics. Acyclovir and famcyclovir are used against herpes simplex, herpes zoster (shingles), and chicken pox. Gancyclovir is also effective against herpes simplex and herpes zoster, as well as against cytomegalovirus, but it can reduce resistance to bacterial infection and can cause excessive bleeding. Valacyclovir is used to treat herpes zoster and genital herpes, but it should not be taken by anyone with a compromised immune system, such as an HIV patient, or anyone who has just had a bone marrow or kidney transplant. AZT (zidovudine) is well known for its use against AIDS, as are drugs called protease inhibitors, which include the drugs ritonavir, nelfinavir, and indinavir. Ribavirin is a broad-spectrum antiviral drug that may be used against measles and mumps, and if used in combination with interferon against hepatitis C. Amantadine is prescribed for influenza A and interferons for hepatitis B and C.

Administration and Dosage. In most cases, antiviral drugs should be taken as early as possible after the onset of the disease, or even before, if a person is known to have been exposed to a source of infection.

Some antiviral drugs function best when they are kept at a constant concentration in the bloodstream throughout the day. This usually requires taking the medication at spaced intervals. Most antiviral drugs are taken with a glass of water, while others are taken with food. The effects of the drugs should be noticeable within a couple of days of first use.

Side effects of antiviral drugs may include dizziness, confusion, lightheadedness, and blurred vision. Elderly people may experience more extreme side effects when taking antiviral drugs, and alcohol may exacerbate the side effects.

> **Background material on antiviral drugs can be found in** VIRUSES **and** VIROLOGY. **Related information is contained in** AIDS; AZT; CHICKEN POX; COLD, COMMON; HEPATITIS, VIRAL; HERPES SIMPLEX; HERPES ZOSTER; INFLUENZA; MEASLES; MUMPS; POLIOMYELITIS; PROTEASE INHIBITORS; **and** SMALLPOX.

Resources on Viral Diseases
Fettner, Ann Guidici, *The Science of Viruses* (1990); Fields, Bernard, et al., *Fields' Virology* (1996); Garrett, Laurie, *The Coming Plague* (1994); Radetsky, Peter, *The Invisible Invaders: The Story of the Emerging Age of Viruses* (1991); Ryan, Frank, *Virus X* (1997); Centers for Disease Contol and Prevention, Tel. (800) 311-3435, Online: www.cdc.gov; Infectious Disease Society of America, Tel. (703) 299-0200, Online: www.idsociety.org; Office of Rare Diseases, Tel. (301) 402-4336, Online: rarediseases.info-.nih.gov/ord; www.nycornell.org/medicine/infectious/index.html.

Antral Irrigation

Surgery to drain nasal passages.

Antral irrigation is a type of surgery for cases of serious or chronic inflammation of the lining of the sinuses (sinusitis). Sinuses are the hollow cavities in the bones surrounding the nose. When a sinus infection is present, the membranes in the sinus passageways become inflamed, and fluids cannot pass through to the nose. Symptoms of sinusitis include sinus headaches and tenderness and swelling of the nasal passages. If sinusitis recurs, surgery may be recommended by a physician.

During an antral irrigation, a small flexible tube is inserted through the nose or above the teeth into the sinus, creating a temporary additional opening through which the sinus cavity is irrigated. A syringe may be used to draw out the infected fluid, which can be tested to determine the nature of the sinus infection.

Antral irrigation usually cures sinus infections. If the infection is severe and remains after a few weeks, surgery can be performed to create a larger opening through which the sinuses can be drained. *See also* SINUSITIS.

Anuria

A suppression of urine production by the kidneys.

A lack of urine production points to a serious underlying problem with the functioning of the kidneys; it should be viewed as a medical emergency requiring immediate treatment. Anuria can be caused by severe damage to the kidneys, which can result in acute kidney failure. It can also be due to rapidly progressing inflammation of the filtering units of the kidneys (glomerulonephritis). Other causes include a blockage of the flow of urine due to an enlarged prostate gland (in men) or a bladder tumor (in both sexes).

Without treatment, anuria can cause uremia, retention of excess waste products in the blood, which can be fatal unless treated. Blockage of urine flow can be corrected by surgery, while kidney failure may require artificial kidney treatment (dialysis). *See also* DIALYSIS; GLOMERULONEPHRITIS; OLIGURIA; PROSTATE GLAND, ENLARGED; TUMOR; *and* UREMIA.

Anus, Cancer of the

Cells that grow abnormally in the anus.

Cancer of the anus is uncommon and usually is unrelated to other cancers of the intestinal tract. The anus is about 1.5 inches long and is surrounded by muscles called the anal sphincters, which open during defecation to allow feces to exit. Symptoms of cancer of the anus include bleeding, discomfort, and swelling. The usual treatment is surgery, which is most effective if the cancer is detected at an early stage. After surgery, the anal sphincters can continue to function. *See also* COLON CANCER.

Anus, Disorders of the

Conditions affecting the canal at the end of the digestive tract.

The anal canal, the last stop for waste matter before it leaves the body, is encircled by two rings of muscles, the anal sphincters. Most disorders affecting the anus are not serious, although they can be painful and irritating. The most serious disorder is cancer of the anus, which is fortunately rare. Anal cancer causes swelling, bleeding, and discomfort, and is usually treated by surgical removal of cells in the affected area. Imperforate anus, a birth defect in which the end of the anus is not fully open, is also treated surgically.

Hemorrhoids are large varicose veins just below the layer of cells lining the anal canal. They cause burning, itching, bleeding, and discomfort during bowel movements. They can be removed by sclerotherapy, banding, or surgery.

Anal stenosis, a narrowing of the anus that prevents the normal passage of feces,

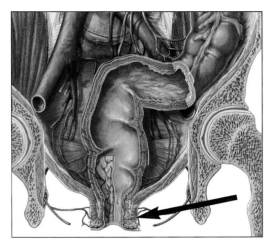

Anal Canal.
The anal canal, left (arrow), is the canal through which waste matter (feces) leaves the body. Two rings of muscle, called the sphincters, encircle the anal canal and control the evacuation of the feces.

can be a birth defect or the result of scarring after surgery for another anal condition. Constipation and pain during bowel movements are symptoms of anal stenosis, which can be corrected by anal dilation.

An anal fissure is a tear caused by an injury or an ulcer that extends upward from the anal sphincters, causing pain and bleeding. Many anal fissures heal on their own, but some require surgery.

An anal fistula is an opening in the anal wall that can be repaired surgically. *See also* ANAL FISSURE; ANAL FISTULA; ANUS, CANCER OF; *and* ANUS, IMPERFORATE.

Anus, Imperforate

A birth defect in which one end of the anal tract is not open.

Imperforate anus can occur at either end of the anal canal, at the point where the rectum meets the anus, or where the normal anal opening should exist. The upper congenital defect is more serious, resulting in the failure of many essential structures surrounding the anus to develop, and often with malformations of the urinary tract. While major surgery is required to repair it, the results are usually good. A defect to the lower end of the anus is simpler to treat, involving a minor surgical process to remove the tissue covering the opening, sometimes accompanied by the widening of the anus (anal dilation). *See also* ANAL DILATION *and* ANUS, DISORDERS OF.

Anxiety

A combination of emotional and physical states that mirror the fight-or-flight response.

Normal anxiety occurs at all stages of life with varying levels of intensity. Excessive levels and occurrences of anxiety may interfere with an individual's ability to cope with the stresses of everyday life. Anxiety may include a sense of impending doom, apprehension, or dread. Occasionally, anxiety may attach itself to something concrete, such as fears for the safety or health of family members, even though there is no objective reason to believe that these problems exist.

CAUSES

There are three theories about the causes of anxiety; it most likely results from a combination of causes and requires a combination of treatments.

• Those who feel that anxiety is biologically based believe that anxious people have a more easily triggered "fight-or-flight" response, leading to the physical and emotional symptoms that occur in stressful situations.

• Psychological theory views anxiety as an impulse that is kept out of awareness because the sufferer finds it unacceptable or fears a loss of control.

• Behavior psychologists believe people are sometimes conditioned to respond with fear as a means of improving performance, but it becomes a habit that is inappropriate and counterproductive when practiced on a broad scale.

SYMPTOMS

Symptoms may include tension, feelings of dread, and sharp pains in the heart or a racing heart. Diarrhea, nausea, vomiting, and dry mouth may occur. Feelings of agitation may be manifested by an inability to sit still, by pacing, by nail-biting, or by chain-smoking. Anxiety will often interfere with the ability to concentrate and will cause accelerated breathing, lightheadedness, trembling hands, or excessive sweating.

TREATMENT

Insight psychotherapy may help to treat relatively mild cases of anxiety. In insight psychotherapy, the patient develops a supportive, stable relationship with a therapist and thus has an opportunity to express otherwise unspeakable thoughts or feelings and to learn to recognize the source of the anxiety. Medication may be necessary, especially when anxiety is accompanied by acute panic attacks, in which an individual has a sudden overwhelming sense of impending doom and suffers severe physical symptoms of anxiety. Anxiety and panic attacks often respond to antidepressants or antianxiety medications. Desensitization (exposure to fears) is sometimes used when the anxiety is caused by a specific trigger (as in the case of phobias or some panic attacks). Other techniques such as meditation, relaxation exercises, and hypnosis may also be combined with psychotherapy and medication to alleviate feelings of anxiety. *See also* ANTIDEPRESSANT DRUGS; PANIC DISORDER; PHOBIA; *and* PSYCHOTHERAPY.

Anxiety Disorders

A number of disorders characterized by a feeling of anxiety that seriously interferes with daily activities and relationships.

Generalized anxiety disorder is a chronic state in which feelings of worry dominate a person's life, even when a solution is at hand or the person knows that worrying will not change the situation. The worrying and feelings of dread disturb sleep, feelings of well-being, and the ability to cope with normal daily stress.

Panic disorder is an acute form of anxiety that involves sudden severe attacks of anxiety in which a person experiences symptoms such as shortness of breath, an increased heart rate, or feelings of impending doom and other anxiety symptoms.

Phobias occur when excessive fear is attached to a specific situation or object, such as flying, spiders, or closed spaces, and negatively affects day-to-day life.

Posttraumatic stress disorder is caused

by highly stressful events such as war, witnessing a murder, or surviving a catastrophic event. Symptoms may occur immediately or years later and may include flashbacks of the event, nightmares, insomnia, depression, and agitation.

Obsessive-compulsive disorder is a condition in which people are troubled by uncontrollable, repetitive thoughts (obsessions). They perform repetitive actions (compulsions) to ease their discomfort. *See also* OBSESSIVE-COMPULSIVE BEHAVIOR.

Aorta

The main artery of the body carrying oxygenated blood out of the heart.

The aorta supplies all the other arteries with the exception of the pulmonary artery, which transports blood from the heart to the lungs to pick up oxygen. The aorta is a tubelike vessel with a diameter of about one inch at its point of origin, the upper surface of the left ventricle, one of the blood-pumping chambers of the heart. From there, the aorta curves upward before turning down toward the rest of the body. Arteries that supply the head and neck radiate from the arch of the aorta before the downward curve.

The diameter of the aorta and the thickness of its walls are greatest near the heart, allowing it to manage the high volume of blood that flows through it and the higher blood pressure at that point. As the aorta runs downward through the chest and the abdomen, a succession of smaller arteries branch off from it. In turn, they branch into smaller vessels, the arterioles. The aorta terminates in the abdomen, feeding into two iliac arteries that carry blood to the lower part of the trunk and to the legs.

Aortic Aneurysm

A widening or bulging of the main blood vessel that carries blood from the heart.

An aneurysm is a bulge in a blood vessel, similar to a bulge in an overinflated inner tube. An aortic aneurysm affects the aorta, the main artery leading away from the heart. An aneurysm may burst, severely disrupting the circulation of blood.

Causes. In many cases, the cause of an aortic aneurysm is arteriosclerosis, a hardening of the arteries. The condition may also be caused by an inherited disease such as Marfan's syndrome, a rare genetic disorder that affects connective tissues.

Diagnosis. An aortic aneurysm can be detected by x-ray, or it can be detected by imaging techniques, such as magnetic resonance imaging (MRI).

Treatment. Aortic aneurysms are generally repaired surgically. If the surgery fixes the aneurysm before it breaks, 80 percent to 90 percent of patients survive. If the aneurysm is distended or has burst, emergency surgery is always necessary, and the outlook is poor. *See also* ANEURYSM.

Aortic Dissection

A tear in the inner wall of the aorta.

An aortic dissection is a tear in the inner layer of the aortic wall, which allows blood to enter the arterial wall and create a separation between the inner and outer layers of the wall. Aortic dissection can lead to a weakening of the outer wall of the aorta and can cause an aortic aneurysm, a heart attack (myocardial infarction), a stroke, or kidney failure.

Symptoms. Severe pain in the front or back of the chest is the most common symptom of aortic dissection. Typically the pain is between the shoulder blades and in the upper abdomen. The pain is described as ripping or tearing in nature.

Treatment. An aortic dissection is a medical emergency and must be treated as soon as possible. The initial treatment for aortic dissection is surgery to repair and rebuild the aortic wall. After surgery, a combination of diet, exercise, and medication is prescribed in order to lower blood pressure and prevent further injury to the aorta. *See also* CARDIOVASCULAR SYSTEM; HEART ATTACK; *and* HYPERTENSION.

Resources on Anxiety Disorders

American Psychiatric Association, *Diagnostic and Statistical Manual of Mental Disorders, 4th Edition* (1994); Greist, John H. and James W. Jefferson, *Depression and Its Treatment* (1992); Solomon, Andrew, *The Noonday Demon: An Atlas of Depression* (2001); Wender, P.H. and D.F. Klein, *Mind, Mood, and Medicine: A Guide to the New Biopsychiatry* (1981); Nat. Depressive & Manic-Depressive Association, Tel. (800) 82-NDMDA, Online: www.ndmda.org; National Mental Health Association, Tel. (800) 969-NMHA, Online: www.nmha.org; www.ny-cornell.org/psychiatry/.

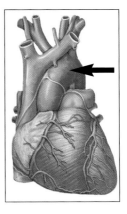

Aorta. The aorta, marked by the black arrow, carries oxygenated blood out of the heart to the rest of the body. Disorders affecting the aorta include aneurysm (bulging), dissection (a tear in the aortic wall), inflammation, and stenosis (narrowing of the aortic valve).

Aortic Insufficiency

Leakage of blood through the aortic valve.

The aortic valve controls the flow of blood out of the heart into the main artery, the aorta. Aortic insufficiency results in blood flowing backwards into the left ventricle, where the valve is located. The heart must work harder to pump blood to the body, and the extra effort can lead to abnormal dilation of the heart muscle with ballooning of the wall of the left ventricle. The result can be heart failure, a progressive weakening of the ability of the heart to pump blood, causing breathing difficulties and abnormal fluid retention in tissues, which can be life-threatening.

Causes. Aortic insufficiency can be due to a congenital abnormality of the aortic valve. It can also be caused by a variety of diseases, including inflammation of the aorta resulting from bacterial infection of the aortic valve, ankylosing spondylitis, and rheumatic fever.

Diagnosis. There are often no noticeable symptoms in the early stages of aortic insufficiency. It is detected when a physician hears a murmur, the sound resulting from abnormal blood flow. A chest x-ray and echocardiography confirm the diagnosis. Heart failure caused by aortic insufficiency is treated with drugs, but surgery is needed to repair a damaged valve. *See also* Congestive Heart Failure.

Aortic Stenosis. Aortic stenosis affects the aortic valve, the valve that leads to the left ventricle. The aortic valve is marked above by a black arrow.

Aortic Stenosis

A narrowing of the aortic valve that obstructs the flow of blood out of the left ventricle.

An obstructed ventricle must work harder; it slowly becomes thicker and less able to pump blood, leading to heart failure.

Causes. Aortic stenosis can be caused by a congenital abnormality of the valve, but it is often due to atherosclerosis. Other causes include rheumatic fever, which leads to inflammation of the valve, and calcification. The condition may result from an autoimmune disease, such as rheumatoid arthritis. Many cases are described as idiopathic, meaning that there is no known cause. Idiopathic aortic stenosis is more common in men than in women.

Diagnosis. Aortic stenosis can be picked up on routine physical examination. Echocardiography uses ultrasound to show the detailed structure of the valve; it often includes a Doppler echocardiography test that measures the flow of blood through the valve. A chest x-ray can show abnormal enlargement of the heart caused by aortic stenosis. Cardiac catheterization, in which a thin tube is threaded through a blood vessel to the heart, can help establish whether surgery is necessary. In some cases, the patient may undergo a stress test, which measures heart performance during exercise.

Treatment. Many patients suffering from aortic stenosis will require surgery to repair or replace the aortic valve. In most cases, the valve is replaced by a mechanical valve or one made of human or animal tissue. Mechanical valves last longer, but the patient must take an anti-coagulant drug to prevent formation of blood clots. An animal or human valve will have to be replaced eventually. While aortic stenosis was once a life-shortening diagnosis, surgery now allows most patients to lead normal lives. *See also* Atherosclerosis; Autoimmune Disorders; Rheumatic Fever; *and* Rheumatoid Arthritis.

Aortitis

A rare condition causing inflammation of the aorta, the main artery carrying blood from the heart.

Aortitis can be caused by untreated syphilis or by ankylosing spondylitis, an inflammatory disease that affects the joints of the spine. It is also seen in persons with arteritis—inflammation of the arteries in any part of the body.

The inflammation caused by aortitis can produce undue widening of the artery and thinning of some segments of the arterial wall. These abnormalities can result in the formation of an aneurysm, the ballooning out of the aortic wall. The weakened part of the aorta may eventually burst, and the resulting loss of blood can be fatal. Aortitis can also damage the ring of tissue around the aortic valve, which controls the flow of blood from the left ventricle, resulting in aortic insufficiency, a backflow of blood into the ventricle that can lead to heart failure and the diminished capacity of the heart to pump blood.

The heart failure caused by aortitis can be treated by drug therapy or surgery; aneurysms resulting from the condition can be repaired surgically. *See* ANEURYSM *and* AORTIC ANEURYSM.

APGAR Score

A tool for evaluating the health of newborn infants.

The health of a newborn baby is evaluated according to a scale devised by Dr. Virginia Apgar. The APGAR score rates each of five signs: **a**ppearance or color; **p**ulse or heart rate; **g**rimace or reflex irritability; **a**ctivity and muscle tone; and **r**espiration.

A score of two is given for every sign that is normal. If the signs are absent, a score of zero is given. If the signs are below normal, they are given a score of one. A normal APGAR score five minutes after birth is eight or greater.

A total score of ten indicates an infant in the best possible health. The heart rate is more than 100 beats per minute; the baby is breathing well, is active, and responds to stimuli. The skin is completely pink.

If the score is zero to four, the heart rate is slow, the reflex response is severely limited and the skin is a pale blue. These infants require immediate assistance.

> **For background information on APGAR score, see** PEDIATRICS. **Further information can be found in** BIRTH WEIGHT **and** CHILDBIRTH. **See also** BREECH DELIVERY **and** FETAL DISTRESS **for more on possible causes of low APGAR scores.**

Aphakia

The loss of the lens of the eye.

Aphakia can occur as a result of cataract surgery in which the lens is intentionally removed, or when it is destroyed as a consequence of injury. The damaged lens is later absorbed by the fluid within the eyeball (aqueous humor). People with aphakia are unable to properly focus their eye. This condition is corrected by lens implants, contact lenses, or glasses. *See also* CATARACT *and* EYE, DISORDERS OF.

Aphasia

The impairment or loss of the ability to understand or communicate through speech, signs, or writing.

Aphasia is the inability to use language as a result of damage to the language areas of the brain. Individuals with aphasia have difficulty expressing themselves or understanding others. They have difficulty with writing, reading, speaking, and sometimes comprehension. A person with aphasia can see, hear, and produce noise; the process of communication in the brain is impaired.

Types. There are two main types of aphasia, caused by damage to different areas of the brain that govern language. Patients with Broca's aphasia understand the meaning of speech, but cannot reply appropriately. Speech is hesitant, sluggish, and lacks natural rhythm. In Wernicke's aphasia, patients have difficulty comprehending their own speech. Their words are garbled and grammar is incorrect.

Causes. Stroke, tumor, and head injury are the most common causes of aphasia. The loss of speech is caused by damage to the Broca's area or Wernicke's area, which are primarily responsible for speech.

Treatment. The main treatment for aphasia is speech therapy. Following head injury or stroke, there may be variable amounts of spontaneous recovery, although the more severe the aphasia, the smaller the chance of recovery. *See also* BRAIN DISORDERS.

Aphonia, Hysterical

The sudden loss of the voice.

Hysterical aphonia differs from other throat disorders, such as laryngitis and dysarthria, in that there is nothing wrong with the larynx, vocal cords, or nerve and brain mechanisms required for speech. Hysterical aphonia is usually caused by a severe attack of emotional distress; there is nothing physically wrong with the patient.

To diagnose hysterical aphonia, a physician will test the vocal cords. If they operate normally while coughing, but not while speaking, that is evidence of the condition. Treatment for hysterical aphonia consists of psychotherapy and other emotional support. The voice usually returns quickly. *See also* LARYNX; SPEECH DISORDERS; SPEECH THERAPY; VOCAL CORDS; *and* VOICE, LOSS OF.

Apnea

An involuntary, temporary stoppage of breathing.

Apnea can result from any disorder affecting the nerve center in the brain stem that controls breathing. Usually, there is a disruption of the impulses sent to the chest muscles that expand and contract the lungs. An episode of apnea can last for a few seconds, or it can last for as long as several minutes.

One common form of apnea, sleep apnea, causes brief interruptions of breathing during sleep, waking the affected individual repeatedly throughout the night. Sleep apnea is not life-threatening, although it can disrupt normal living by causing extreme sleepiness during the day.

More dangerous forms of apnea result from damage to the brain stem respiratory center, head injury, and temporary or permanent interruption of blood flow to the brain (known as transient ischemic attack and stroke, respectively). Prolonged apnea is the cessation of breathing long enough to be life-threatening. Blockage of the airways by food, drink, or an inhaled object is another cause of prolonged apnea.

The treatment of apnea depends on the underlying cause, such as removal of any object that obstructs the airway. In cases where the nerve center in the brain stem that controls breathing is affected, medications that stimulate breathing (analeptic drugs) may be prescribed. *See also* ANALEPTIC DRUGS; SLEEP APNEA; *and* STROKE.

Appendectomy

The surgical removal of the appendix to treat acute appendicitis, which is an inflammation or infection of the appendix.

The appendix is a small outgrowth at the place where the small and large intestines meet. It has no apparent function in humans. An inflamed appendix, if untreated, can burst and cause infection of the abdominal lining (peritonitis) or an abdominal abscess.

Symptoms of appendicitis include abdominal pain, tenderness in the right lower abdomen, mild fever, elevated white blood cell count, vomiting, and loss of appetite.

Diagnosis. To diagnose acute appendicitis, the doctor will use a laparoscope (a thin telescope and video camera) to probe the abdomen. Even if the appendix is determined to be healthy during this procedure, it is usually removed to eliminate the possibility of appendicitis in the future.

Procedure. An appendectomy is performed with the patient under general anesthesia. The surgeon makes a small incision in the abdomen, removes the appendix, and joins the intestine. If the appendix has burst, the abdominal cavity is washed out with a salt (saline) solution, and a flexible drainage tube is inserted into the infected area to siphon off pus.

An appendectomy may be performed in as little as 10 minutes or in as long as an hour, depending on the problems encountered. Postoperative infection is the most common complication of an appendectomy, which is why the patient is given antibiotics as soon as possible, even preceding the operation. The average hospital stay is two to four days. *See also* APPENDICITIS.

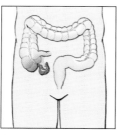

Appendix.
The appendix, shown above in red, is located at the junction of the small and large intestines. It has no known function, but may become inflamed, resulting in further infection if it is not removed promptly.

Appendicitis

The infection and inflammation of the appendix.

The appendix is a small, worm-shaped structure attached to the cecum, where the small and large intestines meet. It has no known function. It can become infected as a result of blockage by a piece of feces or other foreign body, or by a tumor. Often, however, the cause of the infection is unknown. Appendicitis most commonly occurs in individuals between the ages of 10 and 30, although it can occur at any age.

Symptoms. The classic symptoms of appendicitis are a cramplike abdominal pain beginning around the navel and migrating to the lower right side. The pain may be accompanied by severe nausea and vomiting, as well as a low-grade fever. If the appendix ruptures, the pain may disappear for a time. The abdominal lining becomes infected, however, and pain and progressive illness return.

Diagnosis. Diagnosis of appendicitis follows from an abdominal exam, which may reveal tenderness. A blood test will show an increased white blood cell count in response to the infection. Computed tomography (CT) scans are often performed to confirm a diagnosis postoperatively.

Treatment. Appendicitis is treated by the surgical removal of the appendix. In the case of a burst appendix, intravenous antibiotics are administered to prevent peritonitis, an infection of the abdominal cavity lining. *See also* APPENDECTOMY.

Appetite, Loss of

A diminished desire to eat.

Loss of appetite occurs for various reasons and can be a symptom or indicator of many illnesses, including depression, cancer, and gastrointestinal problems. Diminished appetite is normal in the case of minor illnesses. However, in the case of chronic illness, appetite loss can be serious.

Conditions that may diminish the desire to eat include kidney disease, various cancers, liver disease, emphysema, parasitic infections, traveler's diarrhea, viral gastrointestinal infections, and vitamin deficiency, among others. A relative decrease in appetite occurs frequently in older adults. Often, side effects of a particular medication may include nausea and loss of appetite. Loss of appetite may also occur in people who are grieving or lonely.

Diagnosing and treating the underlying cause of appetite loss remains the most successful approach. If loss of appetite is associated with nausea, a doctor may prescribe anti-nausea medications. A doctor should remain informed of all side effects of medications so the doses can be regulated to minimize adverse effects. If the loss of appetite continues, a doctor or a registered dietician may recommend ways to increase caloric intake, and may also suggest a nutritional drink as a supplement to solid food. Rarely, drugs may be administered to stimulate appetite. *See also* ANTIEMETIC DRUGS.

Appetite Stimulants

Drugs given to improve appetite in cases of illness in which body weight has been lost.

Illness, injury, depression, and other causes can result in weakness and weight loss. During and after treatment, building strength and regaining body mass is important. Appetite stimulants can aid in the process by fostering weight gain; some, however, have been suspected ov causing heart disease.

Appetite stimulants come in a variety of forms. Megase, cyproheptadine, corticosteroids, and antidepressants are sometimes used to stimulate appetite and foster weight gain. Patients who suffer the wasting syndromes associated with chemotherapy or AIDS have found that the medical use of marijuana, or drugs synthesizing the active ingredients in marijuana, may help increase appetite. Thalidomide may also be prescribed, although its use is strictly regulated because it causes birth defects. Doctors may recommend nutritional supplements to increase caloric intake.

It is important to note that appetite

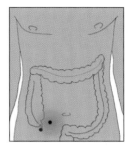

Appendicitis Pain Areas. The pain of appendicitis is usually felt around the navel, spreading toward the lower right side of the abdomen. Above, areas of the body in which appendicitis pain may be felt.

Resources on Appetite

Groff, James L. and Sareen S. Gropper, *Advanced Nutrition and Human Metabolism* (1999); Heimburger, Douglas C. and R. L. Weinsier, *Handbook of Clinical Nutrition* (1997); Mahan, Kathleen L. and S. Escott-Stump, *Krause's Food, Nutrition & Diet Therapy*(2000); Shils, Maurice E., et al., *Modern Nutrition in Health and Disease* (1999); American Dietetic Association, Tel. (800) 366-1655, Online: www.eatright.org; Center for Nutrition Policy and Promotion, Tel. (202) 418-2312, Online: www.usda. gov/cnpp; Food and Drug Admin., Tel. (888) INFOFDA, Online: www.fda.gov; www.nycornell.org/medicine/nutrition/index.html.

stimulants do not always work; they can cause significant side effects, including jaundice, acne, and liver disease.

The use of appetite stimulants should be combined with a vigorous exercise and strengthening program to prevent the accumulation of fat that often occurs with weight gain of this kind. *See also* EXERCISE; JAUNDICE; LIVER; MARIJUANA ; NUTRITION; *and* THALIDOMIDE.

Appetite Suppressants

Drugs that reduce the desire to eat.

Some appetite suppressants can be acquired without a prescription as diet aids. However, there are a number of these drugs that require a prescription because of the significant potential for abuse. Common appetite suppressants include benzocaine and various amphetamines. While most appetite suppressants affect the portion of the brain that regulates body functions (the hypothalamus), drugs like benzocaine incapacitate the taste buds.

The effects of appetite suppressants are temporary. These drugs are meant to be taken for two months or less. Their purpose is to aid in changing eating habits and energy processing (metabolism). They are not meant to become a long-term substitute for a low-calorie, balanced diet.

Side Effects. Although advances in pharmacology are developing safer forms of these drugs, taking appetite suppressants beyond two months can result in habituation. Some nonprescription appetite suppressants can cause elevated blood pressure or irregular heartbeat. Beyond two months, increased dosages may be required in order to achieve the same effect. These increased dosages may be accompanied by increased risks of side effects, such as dizziness, headache, insomnia, nervousness, restlessness, and irregular heartbeat.

Appetite suppressants should be used on a strictly short-term basis, and only in combination with a low-fat, reduced-calorie diet and increased exercise. Any weight loss will be temporary unless diet and exercise are maintained. Fiber-based appetite suppressants should be used with great caution as well, since they can cause nutritional imbalances, gastrointestinal upsets, and, potentially, could lead to obstruction of the digestive tract.

This is not to say that fiber is detrimental to health. On the contrary, replacing high-calorie foods with those high in fiber is a valid weight-loss strategy. Modifying eating habits, together with increasing energy expenditure through a regular exercise program, is a healthier, long-term way to achieve and maintain weight loss. *See also* WEIGHT *and* WEIGHT REDUCTION.

Apraxia

A loss of ability to perform coordinated movements.

Apraxia is the inability to execute deliberate movements despite normal muscle coordination and strength. It is caused by injury to the nerve tracts in the cerebrum, which controls voluntary muscle movement. Apraxia patients usually know what they want to do but have difficulty recalling the required sequence of actions to produce the desired action or movement. Cerebral damage may be a result of a head injury, stroke, infection, or brain tumor. Recovery from apraxia is variable. Some skills may return spontaneously, while others must be relearned. *See also* BRAIN TUMOR *and* STROKE.

Arachnoiditis

An inflammation of the arachnoid, one of the membranes that cover the brain and spinal cord.

As a result of inflammation of the arachnoid, fibrous tissues (adhesions) form, causing pain and nerve damage. Arachnoiditis may be caused by trauma or by an infection such as syphilis or tubercular meningitis, although it often arises from an unknown cause. Arachnoiditis is a disabling condition. As the disease progresses, the symptoms increase and become permanent. Paralysis may occur.

There is no cure for arachnoiditis. The goal of treatment is to return the patient to a level of functionality. Pain management is imperative for patients whose condition is progressive. Surgical removal of the adhesions is only minimally effective, as scar tissue continues to develop, and the surgery itself may cause additional trauma. Research is ongoing to develop new treatments for pain and nerve damage. *See also* Nerve Injury *and* Paralysis.

Arcus Senilis

A yellowish, grayish band that encircles the cornea with advancing age.

Arcus senilis is commonly seen in older people. A yellowish, grayish band forms toward the front of the eye. This band overlies the outer tip of the pigmented part of the eye (iris). Surrounding it is an area of normal cornea. Arcus senilis does not spread and does not affect eyesight.

Arcus senilis is caused by the decay of fatty substances within the cornea. It develops slowly, beginning with a band at the lower part of the cornea and then reaching the upper part of the cornea. The sides of the cornea complete the band.

When the band is seen in children it is called arcus juvenilis. The juvenile condition may be related to a metabolic disorder called hyperlipidemia. *See also* Eye, Disorders of *and* Hyperlipidemia.

Aromatherapy

A therapy regimen that uses aromatic herbal oils, inhaled or applied topically by massage.

Plants, herbs, and the oils extracted from them have been used medicinally for thousands of years in many cultures. The modern resurgence of interest in the healing properties of these "essential" oils dates to 1937, when a French chemist, Réne-Maurice Gattefossé, burned his hand while working in the laboratory of his family's perfume business and relieved the pain by immersing his hand immediately in a vat of

ALERT

Not to be Taken Internally

Aromatic oils should not be consumed, as they may be toxic even when diluted. In addition, the oils should not be applied near the eyes; even the fumes of many oils can be highly irritating.

lavender. Gattefossé coined the term aromatherapy and proceeded to investigate the restorative properties of many of the oils and products that were central to the perfume and culinary industries. A great deal of additional research was conducted by a French physician, Jean Valnet, who used herbal oils (when conventional medications and antibiotics were unavailable) as an army surgeon during World War II. Valnet was among the first to suggest that aromatherapy might also be effective in treating some psychological problems.

Today, essential oils are used for a number of purposes, including the alleviation of stress, the relief and lessening of pain, the prevention of disease and infection, and the induction of sleep.

The "Essential Oils." Among the most widely used essential oils, along with their popular uses, are:
- chamomile and spikenard—two substances used to treat stress and anxiety;
- eucalyptus—used especially to alleviate mild congestion;
- everlast—used topically in concentrations of not more than two percent, to treat scars and bruising;
- geranium—a fragrant agent, used to treat fungal infections;
- lavender—used for burns and insect bites;
- mandarin—a highly fragrant oil used to ease anxiety;
- niaouli—used to treat oily skin and hemorrhoids;
- peppermint—used to relieve nausea and motion sickness;
- rosemary—particularly rosemary verbena, a variety used widely for skin care and cell regeneration.

See also Alternative Medicine; Holistic Medicine; *and* Massage.

Arrhenoblastoma

A rare noncancerous tumor of the ovary.

Although an arrhenoblastoma is not malignant, it can cause problems in women because it increases the production of male sex hormones, which normally are secreted in very small amounts by the ovaries. This overproduction causes a development of male sex characteristics, such as male pattern baldness and unusual deepening of the voice; it can also disrupt the menstrual cycle and cause enlargement of the clitoris. These problems can be solved by surgical removal of the affected ovary. *See also* ANDROGEN HORMONES.

Arrhythmia, Cardiac

An abnormality of the heart rate or rhythm.

Arrhythmias are caused by interference with the generation or transmission of the electrical impulses that govern the heartbeat. These impulses originate in the sinoatrial node, located in the right atrium, an upper chamber of the heart. From there, they are conducted to the atrioventricular node, a transmission center in the middle of the heart. After a brief delay during which the two atria contract, an impulse goes to the bundle of His and Purkinje fibers, a group of fibers that travel to both ventricles. When the muscle cells of the ventricle receive an impulse, they contract to cause a heartbeat.

The heart generally beats between 60 and 100 times a minute in a healthy adult at rest. Children have faster heartbeats, 90 to 120 per minute. A healthy heartbeat has a regular, even rhythm. This orderly process can be altered by a variety of conditions, including a heart disorder, anemia, thyroid abnormalities, fever, and even stress.

TYPES

The two general classes of arrhythmia are tachycardia, an abnormally fast heartbeat (usually more than 100 beats per minute), and bradycardia, an abnormally slow heart-

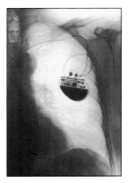

Pacemaker.
One of the possible treatments for cardiac arrhythmia is a pacemaker, shown in the x-ray above. This device is implanted under the skin and maintains a normal heart rhythm by sending an electrical impulse to the heart.

beat (usually less than 60 beats a minute). Arrhythmias are also classified by the region of the heart that is affected. For example, if the upper chambers, the atria, are affected, the condition is called atrial or supraventricular. If the lower chambers are affected, the condition is called ventricular.

The most common arrhythmia causing a slow heartbeat is sinus bradycardia, which originates from a failure of the sinus node to generate or conduct electric impulses properly. The problem can be caused by damage to the sinus node due to age or disease, or a failure of the body's nervous system to control the electrical pulses. In some cases, the heart can alternate between bradycardia and tachycardia, a condition called sick sinus syndrome. A slow heart rhythm can also result from improper transmission of electric impulses through the atrioventricular node or the pathways leading from it, a condition called heart block. This form of bradycardia is generally caused by damage to or inflammation of tissue due to the aging process, or to high blood pressure or coronary artery disease. Lyme disease can sometimes result in heart block.

DIAGNOSIS
The presence and nature of an arrhythmia can be diagnosed by a variety of methods. The most basic procedure is the electrocardiogram, a record of the heart's electrical activity made by attaching electrodes to the chest and limbs. An electrocardiogram is often done during an exercise test, and now may be enhanced and processed by a computer. Some patients may wear a Holter monitor, which gives an ECG reading for 24 to 48 hours. In special cases, an electrophysiology study may be done, with cathodes carrying electrodes threaded into the heart to get detailed information.

TREATMENT
Once diagnosed, an arrhythmia may be treated by one of a number of medications. Depending on the condition, the cardiologist may prescribe digitalis, a beta-blocker, a calcium channel blocker, or an antiar-

rhythmic drug. Some patients will receive an implanted pacemaker or defibrillator in addition to or instead of drug therapy.

Background material on cardiac arrhythmia can be found in HEART; HEART BEAT; *and* PALPITATION. *Related information is contained in* INFECTIOUS DISEASES; ONCOLOGY; *and* PHARMACOLOGY. *See also* ALTERNATIVE MEDICINE *for more on rehabilitation and therapy options.*

Arsenic

A naturally occurring chemical mineral, existing in both gray and yellow crystalline forms.

Though people are exposed to minute quantities of arsenic in food and water without injury, it is deadly in greater amounts. It is especially dangerous in its processed white form, because it is odorless, tasteless, and colorless in solutions. Arsenic is commonly used in insecticides, herbicides, fungicides, wood preservatives, in the electronics industry, and in smelting. Inhaling arsenic on a long-term basis (occupationally or by living near an ore smelter) can cause lung cancer, and dermal contact causes skin cancer. Arsenic has been linked to liver cancer as well. Symptoms of exposure include abdominal pain, vomiting, diarrhea, headache, memory loss, convulsions, tremors, and paralysis.

Arteries, Disorders of

Conditions affecting the arteries.

Arteriosclerosis is a thickening and loss of elasticity of the artery walls that is most often caused by atherosclerosis, narrowing of the blood vessel due to the formation of plaques, deposits consisting primarily of low-density lipoproteins. The buildup of these plaques or the formation of blood clots arising from the plaques can reduce blood flow, resulting in a variety of problems, depending on what part of the body is affected. For example, reduced flow to the legs can produce the pain called intermittent claudication. Complete blockage of a heart artery can cause a heart attack

(myocardial infarction); blockage of a brain artery can result in a stroke.

Arteritis is an inflammation of the arterial wall that can also cause partial or complete blockage of blood flow. It can occur in the scalp (temporal arteritis) or in the limbs (Buerger's disease, named after American physician Leo Buerger, which occurs mostly in male cigarette smokers).

Periarteritis nodosa is an autoimmune condition that can affect arteries all over the body. *See also* IMMUNITY.

Raynaud's phenomenon causes excessive constriction of the small arteries of the fingers and toes, triggered by exposure to cold weather or a number of other factors, such as smoking or emotional stress. *See* ARTERITIS *and* RAYNAUD'S PHENOMENON.

Arteriosclerosis

The thickening and decreased elasticity of the arterial walls.

The most common form of arteriosclerosis is atherosclerosis, a condition in which the inner linings of the arteries become thick and irregular due to a buildup of plaques—deposits that are comprised of fatty material, fibrous tissue, and calcium. The buildup of the plaques can reduce the amount of blood flowing to a given area, resulting in pain and cramping. Atherosclerosis is a leading cause of illness and death in most industrialized countries, including the United States.

Arteriosclerosis is most common in older people, because arteries tend to thicken with age, but the condition can be accelerated by lifestyle factors such as cigarette smoking and a diet high in saturated fat, or by genetic disorders.

Arteriosclerosis of heart arteries can lead to partial blockage that causes chest pain (angina) and other symptoms, or to the complete blockage that results in a heart attack (myocardial infarction).

Arteriosclerosis of the arteries of the neck and brain can result in complete blockage of arteries, leading to a stroke. *See also* ATHEROSCLEROSIS.

Resources on Cardiac Arrhythmia
Berne, Robert M., et al., *Cardiovascular Physiology* (2001); Debakey, Michael E. and Antonio M. Gotto, *The New Living Heart* (1997); American Heart Association, Tel. (800) 242-8721, Online: www.amhrt.org; Heart Information Network, Tel. (973) 701-6035, Online: www.heartinfo.org; National Heart, Lung, and Blood Institute, Tel. (301) 496-4236, Online: www.-nhlbi.nih.gov; www.ny-cornell.org/cardiothoracic.surgery/;www.ny-cornell.org/medicine/cardiology/index.html; www.nycornell.org/medicine/cp/index.html.

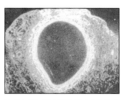
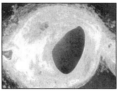

Atherosclerosis.
Atherosclerosis, the most common type of arteriosclerosis, is pictured above, bottom. Plaque deposits in the artery, which restrict the passage of blood, are clearly visible. Above, top, a normal artery. Below, the Rubor test involves checking for poor circulation in the feet.

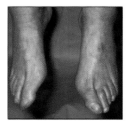

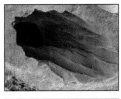

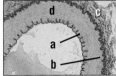

Artery.
Arteries are the blood vessels by which blood travels from the heart to the rest of the body. Above, top, the inside of a normal artery is elastic, allowing for the passage of blood. Above, bottom, a cross-section of a normal artery, magnified 100 times. Lining each artery is the lumen (labeled *a*), the outside of which is called the epithelium (*d*). Surrounding the epithelium is the tunica intima (*b*), which in turn is surrounded by the tunica media (*c*).

Arteriovenous Fistula

An abnormal direct connection between one or more arteries and veins.

Normally, arteries and veins are connected through a web of tiny blood vessels, called capillaries. With an arteriovenous fistula, this connection is bypassed.

An arteriovenous fistula can be congenital, or it can be caused by an accident or injury. The fistula is only treated if it causes symptoms. The problems caused by an arteriovenous fistula depend on its location. A fistula in vessels close to the skin can produce a swollen, pulsating bump. Fistulas in a lung can interfere with the intake of oxygen by the blood, resulting in cyanosis, a bluish skin color indicating lack of oxygen; breathing difficulties at times of exertion; and coughing up blood. A fistula in the brain can cause tiny hemorrhages or can shunt blood from its normal course.

If a fistula that produces symptoms is in a reachable location, it can be removed by surgery that restores the normal path of blood flow. Arteriovenous malformations in the brain can be treated surgically, by proton-beam radiation, or by a technique that sends small pellets of glue to the affected area, blocking blood flow within the fistula and in the vessels leading to it. *See also* ANASTOMOSIS.

Arteritis

An inflammation of the wall of the artery that can cause partial or total blockage of the blood vessel.

Polyarteritis affects a number of arteries in different areas of the body, most often the skin, intestines, kidneys, and heart. The cause of the condition is unknown. The symptoms include fever, weight loss, weakness, and fatigue. If the lungs are affected, asthma may result. Bloody diarrhea and abdominal pain are symptoms of intestinal arteritis. Polyarteritis most often occurs in middle-aged men. The treatment is to control the symptoms with corticosteroid and immunosuppressant drugs.

Cranial arteritis most often occurs in persons over 50, more often in women than in men. Its cause is unknown, and it affects arteries in the scalp, causing headaches and tenderness. It can cause vision problems. If the retinal artery is inflamed, there is a risk of total blindness without treatment. Most patients recover in one to two years when treated with corticosteroid drugs or aspirin.

Buerger's disease, also called thromboangiitis obliterans, affects the legs and sometimes the arms. It occurs mostly in men who are heavy smokers. They must stop smoking to stop the progression of the disease, since smoking constricts the blood vessels, increasing the chance for blockage. Otherwise, gangrene may develop, making amputation of a limb, toes, or fingers necessary. *See also* BUERGER'S DISEASE.

Artery

A tubelike vessel that carries blood from the heart.

Arteries have thick walls made of a fibrous outer layer, a muscular middle layer, and a thin inner layer. They withstand pressure and regulate flow to the smaller vessels. The ventricles pump blood through two pulmonary arteries to the lungs and the rest of the body. *See also* ARTERIOSCLEROSIS.

Arthralgia

Pain or stiffness in a joint.

Arthralgia refers to intense pain and stiffness in one or more joints, which is generally accompanied by arthritis (inflammation of the joints).

The elderly are especially susceptible to arthralgia. It can be present for years with no inflammation before it develops into an inflamed, arthritic condition.

Anti-inflammatory drugs, such as ibuprofen, can ease pain and reduce swelling. Warm baths, massage, and stretching exercises sometimes provide relief. *See also* AGING; ARTHRITIS; BURSITIS; OSTEOARTHRITIS; *and* RHEUMATISM.

Arthritis

Inflammation of a joint with pain and stiffness.

Without the cushioning provided by cartilage, the joints of the human body would not be able to withstand the kind of pounding they are put through daily. When this cushion wears out, the joints have no more protection, and arthritis can develop.

Arthritis is not a specific disease but rather a condition that results from various disorders. Symptoms, treatment, and prognosis vary with each type. Some of the most common arthritis disorders include:

Osteoarthritis. The most common arthritis by far is osteoarthritis. It is caused by simple wear, tear, and use that breaks down the cartilage. It may begin in middle age, but the likelihood of this kind of arthritis increases with age. An injury that damages the cartilage in an area or places the joints in a position where they have less cushioning may also lead to arthritis. Osteoarthritis is typically found in the fingers, hips, knees, and spine. Up to 90 percent of the population experiences some kind of osteoarthritis once they reach their 60s. Women are more likely to feel it in the fingers, and men tend to have osteoarthritis in the hips and knees.

Rheumatoid Arthritis. This type of arthritis is the result of the body's immune system attacking itself, damaging its own joints and cartilage. The pain and swelling is usually found through peripheral joints, as opposed to osteoarthritis, which affects smaller areas at a time. Hands, feet, and arms may become swollen and deformed; in some cases, organs may be affected. Rheumatoid arthritis affects about 2.5 million people per year, and usually sets in between the ages of 40 and 50. It is three times more common in women.

Seronegative Arthritis. Disorders of this type show the symptoms of arthritis but do not test positive for rheumatoid arthritis or show the signs of osteoarthritis. They are usually related to skin disorders, such as psoriasis, intestinal disorders, and autoimmune disorders not associated with rheumatoid arthritis.

Infective Arthritis. This disease may occur when bacteria from an infected wound or infection in the bloodstream invades a joint. It may also be caused by an illness in another location of the body, such as chicken pox, mumps, rubella, rheumatic fever, or gonorrhea. Infective arthritis leads to pain, swelling, and the feeling of heat in the infected area.

Gout. This arthritis is caused by the accumulation of waste products of the body in its crystal form (uric acid) in the blood. It typically affects one joint at a time, most commonly the large toe.

Symptoms vary according to the kind of arthritis, but common to all are pain, swelling, and stiffness. With osteoarthritis, stiffness in the morning may last less than half an hour, while in rheumatoid arthritis it may last significantly longer. Swelling may be minor, but in some forms of arthritis it may develop to the point of deformity. In rheumatoid arthritis, small lumps may develop under the skin from swollen blood vessels, or fluid (such as Baker's cysts) may accumulate in some areas.

Diagnosis. The symptoms usually indicate the type of arthritis, but further diagnosis may include blood tests, x-rays, or fluid drawn from the affected joint to test it for microorganisms.

Treatment. The type of arthritis determines the treatment. For example, infective arthritis requires antibiotics or surgical drainage. For osteoarthritis and rheumatoid arthritis, anti-inflammatory drugs can help to relieve pain and swelling. Acupuncture and massage may reduce pain as well. Exercise can help reduce the instance of deformity. Maintaining a healthy weight can take some pressure off the affected joints. In cases where the pain and swelling have become unmanageable, arthroplasty (joint replacement) may be performed.

> *Background material on arthritis can be found in* JOINT. *For further information, see* OSTEOARTHRITIS *and* RHEUMATOID ARTHRITIS. *See also* ANTIRHEUMATIC DRUGS *for more on treatment therapies.*

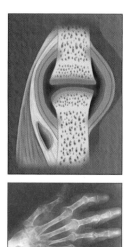

Arthritis.
Arthritis is not a single disease, but a general term that is used to refer to joint inflammation from various other disorders. Above, top, a joint demonstrating the inflammation characteristic of rheumatoid arthritis. Above, bottom, an x-ray of a hand of a patient with osteoarthritis. Disintegration of the cartilage in the joints is clearly visible.

Resources on Arthritis
Lorig, Kate, and James F. Fries, Maureen R. Gecht, *The Arthritis Helpbook: A Tested Self-Management Program for Coping with Arthritis and Fibro-myalgia* (2000); Costill, David L., *Inside Running: Basics of Sports Physiology* (1986); American Physical Therapy Association, Tel. (800) 999-APTA, Online: www.apta.org; Arthritis Foundation, Tel. (800) 283-7800, Online: www.arthritis.org; Nat. Osteoporosis Found., Tel. (800) 223-9994, On-line: www.nof.org; https://public1.med.cornell.edu/cgi; www.nycornell.org/medicine/cp/index.html.

Arthrodesis

Surgery in which bones are fused together to prevent the movement of a diseased joint.

When pain and deformity in a diseased joint cannot be alleviated by drugs, splinting, or physical therapy, or if an injury has caused a joint to become unstable, then surgery becomes an option. Arthrodesis is a surgical procedure that is usually employed when a joint cannot be replaced with an artificial joint, or when such replacement fails, particularly after infection.

Arthrodesis is a procedure in which cartilage is removed from the ends of two bones, as well as the surface layer of each bone. The two ends are then joined so that the fresh bone cells fuse together. Plates, rods, or screws may be temporarily inserted to keep the bones in place. Bone grafts may also be performed. Knees and ankles may also require pins to promote stability until healing is complete.

The fusion process can take up to six months. Bones may fail to fuse, but tough fibrous tissue may fill in the gap between them, providing as much strength as actual fusion. A benefit of arthrodesis is that it rarely requires further care or surveillance. *See also* ARTHRITIS.

Arthroplasty

The replacement of an extremely diseased or deformed joint or part of a joint with a metal or plastic substitute.

The most common types of artificial joint replacements are for the hip, knee, finger, elbow, and shoulder joints. Hip replacement operations were first performed in the 1930s, but the procedure was vastly improved in the 1960s. Improved metal and plastic have led to artificial parts that increase mobility and can self-lubricate. Cement is the common means of attaching the joints to the bone. Improved methods of hygiene in the operating room, such as filtered air, help to prevent joint infections that were previously a serious problem.

Arthroscopy

A means of examining and performing surgery directly on the interior of joints.

Arthroscopy not only helps in diagnosing joint diseases and abnormalities, but it can be used as a surgical tool in treating them, in a process known as arthroscopic surgery.

DESCRIPTION
An arthroscope consists of a thin fiberoptic tube with a miniature camera at the end. The device may be fed through small incisions in the tissue in order to permit direct viewing of a joint. Very small surgical tools can be passed into the joint through the flexible tubing, allowing an orthopedic surgeon to perform a variety of procedures. Since the arthroscope examines the joint directly, it is the most accurate means of diagnosing and treating joint problems. This is especially useful in knee surgery, where less precise surgery often injures soft tissue.

SURGERY
Major joint surgery of ankles, knees, hips, shoulders, elbows, and wrists, as well as the repair of smaller joints, can be accomplished arthroscopically. It is even possible to examine and treat tiny joints in the jaw by this method.

The arthroscope has proven especially effective in the reconstruction of the knee ligament. Before arthroscopy, this procedure required the surgeon to open the knee completely in order to replace the knee ligament with a tendon extracted from around the knee. Such surgery typically required months of recovery and disability. Using arthroscopy, procedures such as this can now be performed on an outpatient basis. The doctor inserts a pencil-sized arthroscope into a one-quarter-inch cut. The arthroscope is attached to a video camera, allowing the patient to watch the procedure if he or she desires. Patients undergoing arthroscopic knee ligament reconstruction are often able to begin walking unaided in a week to 10 days. *See also* JOINT *and* KNEE JOINT REPLACEMENT.

Artificial Insemination

The implantation of healthy sperm into a woman's uterus in order to enable pregnancy.

In artificial insemination, semen is collected and placed into a woman's uterus at the time of ovulation. The partner's semen is usually used if it contains sufficient healthy sperm.

However, if there are not enough sperm for successful fertilization, donor sperm is used. Semen from a donor is usually obtained from a sperm bank. Donor semen is frozen and stored for later use while the donor is tested for various diseases.

Artificial insemination usually has a higher success rate when donor semen is used instead of the partner's semen, particularly if the partner does not have healthy sperm. However, the overall success rate is greater when fresh semen rather than frozen is used.

"Washed" sperm indicates a semen sample in which only the most active sperm have been selected for use. This may increase the chances for conception.

For background information on artificial insemination, see CONCEPTION *and* FERTILIZATION. *Further information can be found in* INFERTILITY. *See also* FERTILITY DRUGS AND IN VITRO FERTILIZATION *for more on the procedure used in artificial insemination.*

Artificial Sweeteners

Chemicals used as low-calorie substitutes for sugar.

Used appropriately, artificial sweeteners in such foods as diet sodas may be helpful for weight reduction. Other authorities believe that their overall impact on weight control in the general population is relatively minor.

Sorbitol is sometimes used by people with diabetes as a sugar substitute. However, it contains about 140 calories per serving and thus is not effective for weight reduction. Sorbitol is not absorbed well by the intestines; therefore, prolonged use may cause diarrhea.

Saccharin has no calories and is 500 to 600 times sweeter than sugar. Animal tests have indicated that saccharin may be cancer-causing (carcinogenic); however, the amount of saccharin that is required to produce tumors in rats is enormously greater than the amount of the sweetener that is consumed by humans. Because of this fact, saccharin was recently removed from the federal government's list of possible carcinogens.

Aspartame has almost no calories and is about 200 times sweeter than sugar per gram. Aspartame is safe for most people in normal quantities, but it may be dangerous to people who have a liver-enzyme deficiency known as phenylketonuria (PKU). Products containing aspartame are labeled with a warning for phenylketonuronics. *See also* CARCINOGEN *and* PHENYLKETONURIA.

Asbestosis

A progressive, potentially fatal condition caused by the inhalation of airborne particles of asbestos.

Asbestos is a group of mineral fibers mined for its resistance to heat and electricity. The modern asbestos industry began in 1868, when asbestos was still considered a miracle fiber and was widely used in insulation and concrete construction materials for residential and commercial buildings. The practice was continued until the confirmation of the serious health hazards of asbestos in 1989.

Asbestos dust is highly cancer-causing (carcinogenic), greatly increasing the risk for lung cancer, cancer of the membranes lining the chest and abdominal cavity (mesothelioma), and gastrointestinal cancer. Asbestos also increases the risk for contracting tuberculosis.

Asbestosis results from long-term asbestos dust exposure. It may take as long as 30 years to develop. Chronic exposure to asbestos dust results in inhaled fibers lodging in the small passages of the lungs (bronchioles). The body tries to isolate the fibers by surrounding them with scar tissue, resulting in the thickening and diminished

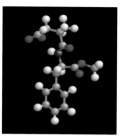

Aspartame.
Above, a chemical model of aspartame, an artificial sweetener often found in diet soft drinks. Labels on such soft drinks warn individuals with the enzyme deficiency phenylketonuria that beverages containing aspartame should be avoided.

Resources on Fertility Treatment
Adashi, Eli Y., John A. Rock, Zev Rosenwaks, *Reproductive Endocrinology, Surgery, and Technology* (1996); Noble, Elizabeth, *Having Your Baby by Donor Insemination: A Complete Resource Guide* (1998); Vercollone, Carol Forst, Heidi and Robert Moss, *Helping the Stork: The Choices and Challenges of Donor Insemination* (1997); The Weill-Cornell Ctr. for Reproductive Medicine & Infertility, Tel. (212) 746-1762, www.ivf.org/home.html.

elasticity of the lungs. Over time, the air sacs (alveoli) in the lungs that are connected by the bronchioles are broken down, making it increasingly difficult for the body to receive enough oxygen.

Early symptoms of asbestosis include shortness of breath and coughing. In the advanced stages, symptoms include fatigue and chest pain occurring after the slightest exertion. Respiratory failure may eventually occur. No effective treatment for asbestosis exists. *See also* BRONCHIOLITIS; CARCINOGEN; *and* MESOTHELIOMA.

Ascariasis

A parasitic infestation by the roundworm called *Ascaris lumbricoides*.

Ascariasis is the most common parasitic infection in the world, affecting some one billion people worldwide. While ascariasis may affect any age group, children are especially susceptible and may be affected more severely than adults. The human roundworm that causes ascariasis (*Ascaris lumbricoides*) is transmitted through contact with contaminated fecal matter. This can occur as a result of poor hygiene and lack of sanitation, and through the use of human feces as fertilizer.

Cause. Ascariasis infection results when roundworm eggs are ingested. These eggs hatch, producing a larval stage in the intestine. Larvae soon migrate through the bloodstream to continue development in the lungs, eventually exiting through the bronchial tree. Larvae are then swallowed and returned to the small intestine, where they complete their maturation into adult roundworms. Mature roundworms live in the intestine; their eggs are expelled with the feces.

Symptoms. Symptoms of ascariasis may include wheezing; shortness of breath; skin rash; persistent cough; passing of worms in feces, or from the nose or mouth; stomach pain; diarrhea; and vomiting.

Diagnosis and Treatment. Ascariasis is diagnosed through a stool and parasite exam or through abdominal x-ray. Treat-

ment for ascariasis employs antihelminthic drugs, which kill the parasites. *See also* ABDOMINAL X-RAY; ANTIHELMINTHIC DRUGS; FECES, ABNORMAL; INFECTIOUS DISEASE; PARASITE; *and* TROPICAL DISEASES.

Ascites

An accumulation of fluid in the abdominal cavity.

In ascites, large amounts of fluid accumulate in the peritoneal cavity, the space between the lining of the abdominal organs and the lining of the abdominal wall. The amount of accumulated fluid may be more than two gallons.

Causes. Ascites can occur as a result of any disorder that results in fluid retention and swelling (edema) in the body. The condition usually occurs due to chronic conditions—such as liver disease (for example, cirrhosis or chronic hepatitis), kidney or heart failure, inflammation of the pancreas, reduced thyroid activity, or cancer—rather than from an acute disorder. Most cases of ascites are caused by liver disease. Ovarian cancer is the cancer that most commonly causes ascites.

Symptoms of ascites usually do not become apparent until large amounts of fluid have accumulated. Once that occurs, the patient experiences abdominal distention, discomfort, and shortness of breath. The abdomen may be taut, the navel may protrude, and the ankles may swell.

Diagnosis. Tapping the abdomen produces a characteristic sound. A small amount of abdominal fluid may be removed to examine its chemical and cellular composition and determine the cause.

Treatment for ascites includes bed rest and a low-salt diet. If possible, the underlying condition should be treated. Diuretics are administered to eliminate much of the excess fluid. If necessary, a large amount of fluid may also be removed (aspirated) through a needle in a procedure known as therapeutic paracentesis. If an infection develops, a condition known as spontaneous bacterial peritonitis, it is treated with antibiotics. *See also* PERITONITIS.

Aspergillosis

A disease caused by a fungus that is usually only dangerous for people with compromised immune systems.

The spores of the Aspergillus fungus are found in fermenting compost piles and damp hay. It attacks people with immune systems that are already weakened, such as by AIDS, burns, chemotherapy, or drugs to prevent rejection of organ transplants.

Symptoms of aspergillosis include wheezing, shortness of breath, cough, chest pain, and fever. The fungus may form a ball in the lung or cause a form of pneumonia. Aspergillosis is treated with antifungal agents, such as Amphoterecin B. Allergic symptoms may occur from aspergillosis; these respond to corticosteroids. *See also* AUTOIMMUNE DISORDERS.

Asphyxia

A lack of oxygen or an excess of carbon dioxide in the body.

Every organ in the body depends upon a constant supply of oxygen, taken in by the lungs and carried by the blood to every part of the body. Anything that interferes with this process can lead to asphyxia. Causes of asphyxia include abnormally low levels of oxygen in the air (such as in mines or at very high altitudes), obstruction or closing of the breathing passages (as in asthma), trauma to the chest or lungs, or certain poisons. Sufferers usually breathe more rapidly and deeply to overcome the lack of oxygen. If the problem is not corrected, loss of consciousness and death can result.

If the airway is obstructed, the object causing the obstruction must be cleared. Victims who are in a place that lacks adequate oxygen, such as a mine shaft or an area of high altitude, must be immediately transported to a location with higher oxygen levels, but only if the rescuer's breathing will not be compromised. If poisoning is involved, a trained medical professional should be contacted. *See also* ANOXIA.

Aspirin

A popular drug used to relieve pain, lower fever, and reduce swelling and the chance of a heart attack.

Aspirin (acetylsalicylic acid) reduces pain by blocking the production of prostaglandins, hormones that cause inflammation. Taken regularly in small doses it reduces the danger of heart attack by reducing the ability of the blood to clot.

Aspirin may aggravate stomach ulcers, since it irritates the stomach lining. It can also trigger an asthma attack in those who suffer from asthma. Aspirin may also adversely affect people with liver or kidney problems. Children should not take aspirin, since it increases the risk for Reye's syndrome—a rare, potentially deadly disease that affects the brain and liver. Pregnant women should avoid aspirin in their last trimester, because it may harm the fetus. *See also* ANALGESIC DRUGS; ANTICOAGULANT DRUGS; *and* BLOOD CLOTTING.

Astereognosis

An inability to identify objects by touch.

Astereognosis is a rare disorder, in which people are not able to recognize an object by handling it. The patient does not have difficulty holding an object or a loss of sensation in any fingers; rather, the area of the brain that deals with touch is unable to interpret the incoming signals.

Astereognosis can affect one hand or both hands, in which case it is referred to as tactile agnosia. If it is centralized in one hand, the ability for touch recognition is normal in the other hand.

Astereognosis and tactile agnosia most often result from a stroke or from an injury to the area of the cerebrum responsible for touch recognition. There is no specific treatment for these conditions. Although some patients can improve or even recover suddenly and seemingly without cause, most will need to make adjustments in their daily routines to deal with their disability. *See also* AGNOSIA *and* STROKE.

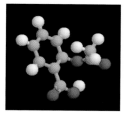

Aspirin.
Above, a chemical model of acetylsalicylic acid, or aspirin. This medication may be taken regularly (in small doses) as part of physician-initiated endeavors to reduce a patient's chances of suffering a heart attack.

Asthma

A respiratory disorder causing attacks of breathlessness and wheezing.

Asthma can occur at any age, but about half of all cases strike children under the age of ten. Childhood cases often become less severe or clear up entirely with age. There appears to be a genetic factor—overall incidence in the American population is about five percent, but someone with a child or parent who has asthma runs a 20 to 25 percent risk of developing the disorder.

Asthma attacks are unpredictable. They can occur often or seldom, with variations in severity, and can happen at any time, although they are slightly more likely to take place at night. In addition to breathlessness and wheezing, asthma attacks can cause coughing and chest tightness.

CAUSES

In about five out of six asthmatics, the attacks are triggered by an allergic response to something in the air. When a substance capable of causing an allergic reaction (antigen) is breathed in, its presence is recognized by the immune system. An immune system molecule (immunoglobulin E—abbreviated IgE) and an immune system cell (mast cell) work together against infection. The presence of an antigen causes the mast cell to release a number of substances that act on the smooth muscles that line the airway and lungs. These substances (histamine, leukotrienes and prostaglandins) cause the muscles to contract. They also cause the lining of the airway to become inflamed, as well as thick mucus that blocks the airway to be released. The combination of inflamed, narrowed airways and clogging mucus makes breathing more difficult. Breathing difficulties may continue for hours after the initial attack. Antigens that can cause this reaction differ from person to person and include natural substances such as pollen, insect droppings, and animal dander, and fragments of hair and skin.

For a minority of patients, asthma attacks are triggered by something other than an allergic reaction. Cigarette smoke can cause an attack and can increase the severity and frequency of asthma episodes resulting from other causes. Air pollution can set off an attack, and so can the fumes of kerosene, natural gas, or a wood fire. A common cold or other viral respiratory infections can have the same effect.

Some drugs can initiate an asthma attack for individuals who are sensitive to aspirin or nonsteroidal anti-inflammatory drugs. A drug-related asthma attack can be severe enough to cause respiratory failure.

ALERT

Preventing Asthma Attacks

It is possible to prevent asthma attacks by testing for and avoiding the allergens that cause them. For instance, parks and the countryside may be avoided due to pollen; mattresses can be wrapped in plastic, and the house kept dust free to minimize dustmites. Cromolyn sodium and corticosteroid drugs can prevent asthma attacks; they are most effective when inhaled many times a day. It is often not possible to build up immunity through injections of an allergen, as can be done with some other allergies.

Physical activity can also set off an attack by causing a bronchospasm, a contraction of the muscles that line the airways of the lung. Such an asthma attack is more likely to occur on a cold day. But exercise is not necessarily forbidden for people with asthma. The kind of exercise, the amount of exercise, and where it is done must be chosen with care. For example, running outdoors on a winter day may set off an attack, but swimming in a heated pool is much less likely to, since breathing warm, moist air has a beneficial effect. Sometimes anxiety or stress can also set off an attack. In some cases, no specific underlying cause of asthma can be defined.

TYPES

Asthma can be categorized as either intrinsic or extrinsic. Extrinsic asthma can be traced to a specific cause, while there is no apparent external cause for intrinsic asthma. The extrinsic form of the condition tends to develop earlier in life than intrinsic asthma.

Asthma can also be categorized by the frequency and severity of the attacks. Definitions set by the National Institutes of Health establish four categories of asthma. The first category is mild intermittent asthma, in which symptoms occur less than twice a week and attacks are brief. The second category is mild persistent asthma, with more frequent attacks. Moderate persistent asthma is a category in which attacks are more severe, and the final category, severe persistent asthma, describes attacks that occur almost continually, with crises that limit physical activity, and lung function less than 60 percent of normal.

DIAGNOSIS

A large part of asthma management relies on early diagnosis and treatment. Diagnosis is based first on the symptoms: breathing difficulty, coughing, and wheezing. The diagnosis can be confirmed by pulmonary function tests, chest x-rays that detect lung abnormalities, and allergy tests to determine sensitivity to various allergens. Such tests are advisable for anyone with a close relative who has asthma, because of possible genetic vulnerability.

TREATMENT

Treatment of an asthma attack starts with the earliest possible detection of the onset of the attack. In most cases, warning signs begin hours before the onset of symptoms. Deterioration of breathing that signals an oncoming attack can be monitored by a device called a peak flow meter, which indicates the efficiency of breathing. A reading below 80 percent of maximum effectiveness is an indication that preventive measures should be taken, such as increasing the dose of asthma medications. A reading below 50 percent is a clear sign of trouble needing medical attention. The symptoms of an asthma emergency include severe breathing difficulty, blue-tinted lips and nails because of a shortage of oxygen, and an abnormally fast heartbeat.

Management. Because asthma is a chronic condition, treatment must be a continuing process, with specific measures taken based on the severity of the condition and on individual sensitivity to triggers. If specific allergens are identified as asthma triggers, steps should be taken to limit exposure to them. In general, the breathing environment should be kept as clean as possible.

Medication. Medications can be taken on a daily basis to reduce the inflammation that causes asthma attacks. Among these medications are cromolyn sodium and corticosteroids. Their use should be supervised by a physician because of the possibility of side effects, such as loss of appetite and severe acne. They can be taken by inhaler, through a nebulizer, or in pill or liquid form, depending on the medication and the dose required.

Most asthma attacks do not require emergency measures. Their severity can be reduced by bronchodilators, medications that widen the airways by relaxing the muscles around them. There are a variety of bronchodilators in different families, such as beta agonists, anticholinergics, and methylxanthines. They can be taken in different ways. For example, beta agonists, such as albuterol, can be taken through a metered dose inhaler or a nebulizer, pills or liquids, or by injection. The inhaled forms of the drugs work fastest, most often within five minutes. Pills or liquids take up to 30 minutes to work, but are effective for as long as six hours. Injections usually are an emergency measure given under a doctor's supervision.

Living with Asthma. Asthma is a highly personal condition. Asthmatic patients should work closely with doctors to develop the most effective measures of preventing attacks and minimizing their effects when they occur. For the great majority of patients, asthma can be kept under control well enough to permit near-normal living.

> *Background material on asthma can be found in* BREATHING DIFFICULTY. *Related information is contained in* BRONCHODILATOR DRUGS; EMPHYSEMA; INFLAMMATION; STEROIDS, ANABOLIC; *and* X-RAY.

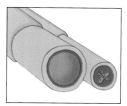

Asthma.
The breathing problems characteristic of asthma occur when the airways become inflamed and clogged with mucus. Above, on the right is an inflamed airway, while on the left is a normal airway through which air can pass easily.

Resources on Asthma
Crystal, Ronald G., *The Lung: Scientific Foundations* (1997); Kittredge, Mary, *The Respiratory System* (1989); Parker, Steve, *The Lungs and Breathing* (1989); Perry, Angela R., *Essential Guide to Asthma* (1998); American Lung Association, Tel. (800) 586-4872 (LUNG-USA), Online: www.lungusa.org; Lung Line Information Service, Tel. (800) 222-5864, Online: www.nationaljewish.org; American Academy of Allergy, Asthma and Immunology, Tel. (800) 822-2762; www.aaaai.org/; www.nycornell.org/pediatrics/pedallergy.html

Astigmatism

A structural defect of the cornea.

The normal cornea is round. The astigmatic cornea is oval-shaped; this may cause blurred vision, eyestrain, headache, or squinting, because the eye cannot focus light at a single point on the retina. Astigmatism is common, and it may be hereditary. In many cases it is unnoticeable or mild. Astigmatism afflicts half of all nearsighted people and is sometimes acquired due to other disorders or diseases, such as keratoconus, chalazion, lenticonus, and drooping eyelid. Glasses, some contact lenses, or surgery can correct the problem. *See also* CORNEA, DISORDERS OF.

Aston Patterning

A technique of movement and bodywork therapy derived from Rolfing.

Aston patterning was developed by Judith Aston, a UCLA-trained dancer who was involved in two serious car accidents in the 1960s. After working with Ida Rolf (renowned for her research on the structural alignment of the body), Aston's condition improved significantly. Eventually Aston developed her own version of Rolf's technique that focused on body movement and deep-tissue massage (Rolf focused primarily on the body's static alignment). The technique was more completely developed by Aston in 1977.

In contrast to Rolf's theory, Aston patterning in its most contemporary variation emphasizes the asymmetrical quality of all movement. Her technique focuses on four main areas: fitness training, massage and soft-tissue bodywork, movement reeducation, and environmental design. Aston patterning also places emphasis on the ergonomics of an individual's environment, from clothing to furniture to living arrangements. It is widely used for the treatment of postural dysfunction. *See also* ACUPRESSURE; ALTERNATIVE MEDICINE; ROLFING; *and* THERAPEUTIC TOUCH.

Astrocytoma

A malignant tumor of the brain.

Most astrocytomas develop in the cerebrum, the major part of the brain, but they can also occur in the brain stem and spinal cord. Their name is derived from the observation that the tumors develop from star-shaped cells called astrocytes. About half of all brain tumors are gliomas, which arise from the supporting (glial) cells of the nervous system, and astrocytomas are the most common type of glioma.

Astrocytomas are classified into four categories, ranging from grade one, a slow-growing tumor that may not cause symptoms for years, to grade four, a rapidly growing tumor that quickly causes major symptoms. Astrocytomas cause symptoms common to all brain tumors, including frequent headaches, nausea, vomiting, blurred or double vision, loss of smell and hearing, memory disturbances, and changes in personality.

Astrocytomas are diagnosed by neurological examination and tests, including magnetic resonance imaging (MRI) and computed tomography (CT) scanning. Magnetic resonance imaging studies are also used to guide the surgery that is the first line of treatment, usually followed by radiation therapy or chemotherapy.

The prognosis for most astrocytomas is limited, but some patients can survive for years with advanced treatments. *See also* BRAIN TUMOR *and* CANCER.

Asymptomatic

Lacking symptoms of illness.

Symptoms are often the most reliable means for a doctor to diagnose illness in a patient. Some illnesses, however, are asymptomatic—particularly in their early stages. Infectious diseases, for example, require varying incubation periods, during which the person may feel normal and appear asymptomatic. *See also* AIDS; INFECTIOUS DISEASE; *and* INFLUENZA.

Ataxia

The loss of coordination.

Ataxia is the inability to coordinate voluntary movement of the muscles. This can affect limb or eye movements, speech, balance, poise, and gait.

CAUSES

Ataxia is caused by injury to the cerebellum, the region of the brain that is responsible for coordination. Damage may also be a consequence of damage to the nerve pathways that carry information to and from the cerebellum. It may be caused by a stroke, a brain tumor, or a spinal cord injury. The most common cause of ataxia in adults is intoxication from alcohol or drugs. Ataxia may also be a symptom of inner ear disease or of a degenerative nervous system disorder, such as multiple sclerosis or Parkinson's disease. It is also sometimes seen in syphilis patients who have not been treated.

SYMPTOMS

Most ataxia patients walk in a clumsy manner. They lack natural rhythm and are unsteady on their feet. Other symptoms depend on the specific nerves or impaired areas of the brain.

Patients with Parkinson's disease usually experience tremor (shaking) due to a degeneration of cells in the basal ganglia, a part of the brain located in the cerebellum, which is responsible for smoothing out movements. People with sensory ataxia have difficulty moving with their eyes closed. This occurs because of injury to the nerves that carry sensory information to the muscles. People with nystagmus have difficulty controlling eye movements, and people with dysarthria have mispronounced and garbled speech.

DIAGNOSIS

CT scanning and MRI are used to detect the cause of the ataxia. If possible, the underlying cause of the ataxia is treated. *See also* PARKINSON'S DISEASE *and* NYSTAGMUS.

Atelectasis

A slow or sudden collapse of a segment of a lung.

Atelectasis occurs when the clusters of tiny air sacs of the lung (alveoli) become filled with fluid or collapse, usually because the airways of the lung become obstructed. Most commonly, the obstruction is caused by a plug of mucus, although a tumor, an enlarged lymph gland, or an inhaled object may be responsible. Persons who are most vulnerable to atelectasis include heavy smokers and people with cystic fibrosis disease. In children, the condition can occur at birth or be caused by whooping cough in an older child.

Symptoms. A collapsed lung can no longer supply the blood with oxygen and remove carbon dioxide from the blood. Atelectasis usually is not a life-threatening condition for adults, since the uncollapsed part of the affected lung may retain enough function to meet the body's needs.

Even if an entire lung is obstructed, the other lung can function well enough to compensate for the damage. But atelectasis in a child can be a much more serious matter. The major symptom of atelectasis is difficulty breathing, sometimes accompanied by coughing and chest pain.

Diagnosis. A chest x-ray can detect atelectasis and the cause of the blockage. If only a small part of a lung is affected, the x-ray will show horizontal lines in that area. A larger affected area will appear as a dense shadow on an x-ray.

Treatment. Frequent coughing, deep breathing, postural drainage, and chest percussion often are effective as treatment for atelectasis. For postural drainage, the patient lies on a bed, with the head and chest hanging over the edge, so that gravity will drain the mucus into the upper part of the lung, where it can be coughed out. Surgery may be needed if a tumor is responsible for the blockage. Once the flow of air is restored, the lung may gradually return to normal, although some part of the lung may suffer permanent damage or scarring. *See also* CYSTIC FIBROSIS.

Atherosclerosis

A condition in which the inner layer of the arterial walls thickens, causing the blood vessels to lose elasticity and become narrower, impairing the flow of blood.

Atherosclerosis, often called hardening of the arteries, can occur with age. In younger and middle-aged persons, it is due to the buildup of plaque (raised patches containing fatty deposits, decaying muscle cells, fibrous tissue, and fats) inside the artery wall. These plaques are especially likely to form in the arteries of persons with high blood levels of low-density lipoproteins. As the artery narrows, the smooth lining of the blood vessel becomes rougher and can rupture, increasing the risk that blood clots will form. Such a clot, or thrombus, can break away to block blood vessels.

RISK FACTORS

Hereditary factors play a role in atherosclerosis, as do other medical conditions. It is more likely to develop in persons with hypertension, elevated blood cholesterol levels, or diabetes. It is also more prevalent among those who are obese and smokers. Lifestyle is important in the development of atherosclerosis. The major risk factors include cigarette smoking, high cholestorol, and a lack of physical activity.

The condition is more common in men than in women until the middle years of life, but that changes at about age 60, when the difference is greatly reduced. Since 1984, more American women than men have died of cardiovascular disease, much of it related to atherosclerosis.

DIAGNOSIS

Atherosclerosis is first diagnosed with a general medical history and examination. The physician may feel the carotid artery in the neck or pulses in the feet to detect signs of arterial narrowing. The degree of narrowing of a blood vessel can be determined by angiography, an x-ray examination of the arteries, or by echocardiography, which uses high-frequency sound waves to obtain images of the vessel. A patient may take a stress test, during which an electrocardiogram is taken while the individual walks on a treadmill or rides a stationary bicycle.

TREATMENT

If the blood vessels have become dangerously narrow, balloon angioplasty may be performed to widen them. A catheter with a balloon at its tip is threaded to the narrowed area, where the balloon is inflated to open the artery and then removed. Angioplasty is often followed by insertion of a stent, a thin tubular mesh device that helps keep the narrowed portion of the blood vessel open.

Several experimental techniques are also being tested to treat atherosclerosis. Laser ablation uses the high-powered light from a laser instead of a balloon to perform angioplasty. In atherectomy, a high-speed drill mounted on a catheter is used to cut plaque off the wall of the artery.

Coronary artery bypass surgery may be done when these measures are not effective—for example, when the left main branch of the coronary artery is dangerously narrowed by atherosclerosis, or when all three coronary arteries are in danger of becoming blocked, conditions that create a high risk of fatal heart attack (myocardial infarction). In bypass surgery, another blood vessel, often a vein from the leg or an internal mammary artery, which supplies blood to the chest wall, is sewn into place to provide an alternate route for blood flow around the blocked region. Bypass surgery is most effective when accompanied by medical treatment and lifestyle changes aimed at limiting atherosclerosis.

Atherosclerosis is relatively easy to prevent. Smokers with the condition should stop smoking cigarettes. A low-cholesterol, low-calorie diet, rich in fiber, fruits, and vegetables, can reduce blood levels of cholesterol and promote weight loss in overweight individuals. Medication may be prescribed to help lower blood cholesterol levels and to reduce blood pressure. *See also* ARTERIOSCLEROSIS; CORONARY HEART DISEASE; HEART ATTACK; *and* OBESITY.

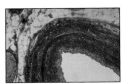

Atherosclerosis. Above, a cross-section of an artery affected by atherosclerosis. This condition can lead to an increase in blood pressure, as the artery narrows to the point where the blood has difficulty getting through.

Resources on Atherosclerosis

Berne, Robert M., et al., *Cardiovascular Physiology* (2001); Debakey, Michael E. and Antonio M. Gotto, *The New Living Heart* (1997); Gotto, Antonio, *HA Patient's Handbook of Cholestorol Disorders (2000)*; American Heart Association, Tel. (800) 242-8721, Online: www.amhrt.org; National Heart, Lung, and Blood Institute, Tel. (301) 496-4236, Online: www.nhlbi.nih. gov; www.nycornell.org/ cardiothoracic.surgery/; www.nycornell.org/medicine/cardiology/index.html; www.nycornell.org/medicine/cp/index.html.

Athetosis

Slow, involuntary movements of the fingers, hands, toes, feet, face, and head.

Athetosis is a symptom of any of a number of nervous system disorders. It is characterized by slow involuntary movements, such as twitching and grimacing. The affected individual has difficulty maintaining balance, and walking is accompanied by twisting and turning movements. Athetosis can occur together with chorea, which is characterized by uncontrolled, repetitive movements (choreothetosis).

Causes. Individuals with athetosis and chorea have damaged basal ganglia. The function of the basal ganglia, located in the cerebellum of the brain, is to produce smooth and controlled movements. An excess of the neurotransmitter dopamine in the basal ganglia prevents this area from functioning properly .

The most common disease that causes athetosis and chorea is Huntington's disease. In children, athetosis can be caused by brain injury at the time of birth or by infection affecting the brain. Athetosis can also be drug induced by phenothiazines or levodopa derivatives.

Treatment. Antipsychotic medications that block the action of dopamine are effective in controlling athetosis. If athetosis is drug-induced, involuntary movements may subside when the drug is stopped.

For background information on athetosis, see NERVOUS SYSTEM. *Further information can be found in* BASAL GANGLIA; CEREBELLUM; CHOREA; DOPAMINE; HEAD INJURY; HEMIPLEGIA; HUNTINGTON'S CHOREA; NEUROTRANSMITTER; PARKINSON'S DISEASE; *and* SPASM. *See also* ANTIPSYCHOTIC DRUGS *for more on treatment.*

Athlete's Foot

Also known as tinea pedis

Fungal infection in which the skin between the toes cracks, peels, and blisters.

Athlete's foot is a condition usually caused by a fungus that grows in warm moist places. The most common place for the fungus to grow is on sweating feet in enclosed shoes. The infection can also be picked up in dirty areas, such as locker-rooms or pools, where others may carry the bacteria. Athlete's foot is primarily experienced by adolescent and adult males; about 80 percent of all men may have had the infection at some time in their lives.

Athlete's foot is usually cured by keeping the affected area clean and dry. Antifungal creams, such as tolnaftate, miconazole, or compound undecylenic acid may help as well. If self-care does not clear up the infection within two to four weeks, a doctor may prescribe a course of oral antifungal medications.

Prevention or minimization of athlete's foot is possible through such precautions as keeping the feet dry and well-ventilated. Keeping the feet clean with antibacterial soap can also help to prevent the growth and spread of the infection, as can wearing sandals in public showers or pools. *See also* ANTIFUNGAL DRUGS; DERMATOLOGY; FUNGAL INFECTIONS; HYGIENE; INFECTIOUS DISEASE; *and* TINEA.

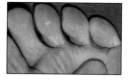

Athlete's Foot.
The fungus causing athlete's foot, above, favors warm moist conditions. If these conditions are minimized, it is possible to prevent athlete's foot.

Atony

The lack of normal muscle tone (tonus).

Atony is a condition in which the muscle has lost tone and tension; it lacks firmness and becomes flaccid and weak. Atony may follow a nerve injury or may be caused by a nervous system disorder. Damage to a main nerve center (plexus) causes damage to every part of the body supplied by that nerve center. For example, any damage to the brachial plexus, located in the neck, may cause atony in the arms. Damage to the lumbosacral plexus, which is located in the lower back, could cause muscle atony in the lower back, pelvis, and legs.

Treatment depends on the cause of the disorder. Doctors may prescribe corticosteroids for plexus disorders. If there was physical injury to a plexus, muscle tone may improve with time, as the injury heals. *See also* CEREBRAL PALSY; MULTIPLE SCLEROSIS; MUSCLE; *and* NERVE.

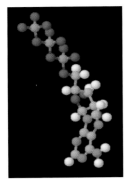

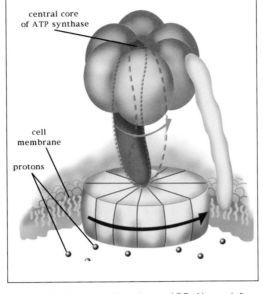

central core
of ATP synthase

cell
membrane

protons

ATP.
At right, ATP catalysis begins when protons that are passing through the transmembrane protein —ATP synthase—cause the enzyme's core to rotate. This rotation brings about a change in the synthase that allows the enzyme to attach a phosphate ion to ADP. Above, left, a chemical model of ATP. ATP is made of (from bottom) adenine, ribose, and three high-energy phosphate groups. It is popularly known as the "cell's power source."

ATP

Also known as adenosine triphosphate

A natural substance essential for short-term energy storage and transport throughout the body.

ATP, or adenosine triphosphate, works in conjunction with ADP, or adenosine diphosphate, to generate the energy needed by cells to carry out their various functions. ATP is the main chemical that stores and carries energy in the blood. This energy is then released in localized areas of the body when ATP degrades to ADP. In order to release energy to fuel metabolic processes, the ATP molecule is broken down so that the energy of one of its bonds can be released, yielding the combination of ADP and a phosphate ion. Later, with energy from the oxidation of food compounds, cells recombine ADP and phosphate ions to form ATP, ready for the next expenditure of energy.

Background material on ATP can be found in METABO-
LISM. *For further information, see* ADP; AEROBIC; ANAERO-
BIC; BIOCHEMISTRY; BLOOD; DIGESTIVE SYSTEM; ENERGY; ENERGY
REQUIREMENTS; GASTROINTESTINAL TRACT; *and* METABOLISM, IN-
BORN ERRORS OF.

Atrial Fibrillation

An irregular heartbeat (tachycardia) in which the upper chambers of the heart, the atria, beat very rapidly, up to 300 to 500 times a minute.

When atrial fibrillation occurs, the atrioventricular node, a structure that conducts impulses between the atria and the lower chambers of the heart (ventricles), cannot respond to every beat. It will block the atrial impulses so that the ventricles contract less frequently—only 125 to 175 times a minute.

Causes. Atrial fibrillation usually occurs when the left atrium is enlarged, commonly because of chronic heart disease, such as rheumatic heart disease or atherosclerosis, but it can also occur in the absence of heart disease. The conditions that can bring it on include overactivity of the thyroid gland, lung disease and pericarditis—inflammation of the membrane that covers the heart. Excessive consumption of alcohol or caffeine, or the use of street drugs, such as cocaine, are also associated with an increased risk of atrial fibrillation.

Symptoms. As the atria fail to pump blood effectively, symptoms include fatigue, shortness of breath, palpitations and chest pain caused by reduced blood supply (angina). Atrial fibrillation causes the ventricles to lose 20 to 30 percent of their ability to pump blood to the lungs and the rest of the body, but the pumping capacity usually remains sufficient for the body's needs.

**Atrial Fibrillation:
Visiting the Doctor**

Any fatigue, chest pain, ankle swelling, faintness, sudden limb weakness, or vision or speech loss should be reported to a doctor. The physician may examine the heart rate, breathing, pulse, blood pressure, neck veins, ankles, and legs. Tests may include: thyroid function tests; tests of blood levels of digoxin, potassium, and magnesium; tests of the kidneys; prothrombin time tests, if warfarin (Coumadin) is being taken for blood-thinning; an electrocardiogram; and a Holter or an event monitor, if the atrial fibrillation is periodic.

Diagnosis. Atrial fibrillation is diagnosed when the pulse rate is irregular and does not keep time with the heart rate, since many of the beats that can be heard through the stethoscope do not push blood out to the wrist, where the pulse is measured. Diagnosis is confirmed by an electrocardiogram, which records the electrical activity of the heart.

Treatment. Drugs such as digitalis and beta-blockers can be prescribed to lower the heart rate, with anticoagulants given to prevent formation of blood clots. Radiofrequency ablation may be performed when drug treatment is ineffective, or as first-line therapy to maintain normal (sinus) rhythm. *See also* BETA-BLOCKER DRUGS.

Atrial Flutter

A condition in which the upper chambers of the heart beat too rapidly, at a rate of 200 to 300 beats a minute. The lower chambers, the ventricles, beat more slowly—once for every two or three beats of the atria.

Atrial flutter is different from but related to atrial fibrillation, in which the atria beat irregularly 300 to 400 times a minute. Some individuals alternate between periods of atrial flutter and fibrillation.

Often occurring after open-heart surgery, atrial flutter can cause the ventricles—the lower chambers of the heart—to beat too rapidly, resulting in a diminished ability to pump blood. The cause for the condition sometimes cannot be found, but it is often the result of heart disease, high blood pressure, coronary artery disease, an overactive thyroid, or alcohol abuse. Symptoms of atrial flutter, which can be more severe in persons whose ventricles are affected, include fatigue, lightheadedness, dizziness, palpitations, shortness of breath, weakness, and fainting. Atrial flutter is five times more common in men.

Cardiologists distinguish between Type I and Type II flutter; Type II has a faster heartbeat and is more difficult to treat. Treatment of atrial flutter is similar to that for fibrillation. *See also* ATRIAL FIBRILLATION *and* CORONARY ARTERY DISEASE.

Atrial Natriuretic Peptide

A naturally occurring protein molecule, produced in the wall of the upper chambers of the heart, that lowers blood pressure.

Atrial natriuretic peptide is produced in response to an increased tension of the heart muscle that can be caused by high blood pressure or by a reduced ability of the heart to pump blood (heart failure). Atrial natriuretic peptide induces the release of large amounts of sodium into the urine. It also significantly increases the production and excretion of urine. The result is a reduction in the volume of fluid in the blood, which lowers blood pressure.

Atrial natriuretic peptide also lowers blood pressure by acting on the angiotensin system and preventing the formation of angiotensin II, a naturally occurring substance that constricts blood vessels. This causes the blood vessels to widen, allowing the blood to flow more easily.

High levels of atrial natriuretic peptide are found in children with congenital heart disorders that cause heart failure. The levels of the protein have been found to fall to normal in children when surgery succeeds in correcting a heart abnormality. *See also* ANGIOTENSIN *and* HEART DISORDERS.

Atrophy

A condition in which a tissue or organ shrinks or wastes away, usually because of reduction in size or number of cells.

Limbs, organs, or tissues atrophy when they fall into disuse, usually because of injury or disease. Atrophy may also be caused by poor circulation, which can prevent adequate cell nutrition, as well as by the use of protein reserves by the body, which inhibits the growth of body tissues. Nerve damage causing immobilization, or a missing enzyme or hormone, may also inhibit the proper growth and maintenance of a cell.

Exercise, adequate nutrition, and treatment of the underlying condition can help rejuvenate the area. *See also* STROKE.

Attention Deficit/Hyperactivity Disorder

Also known as ADHD or ADD

A behavior disorder characterized by an inability to focus involving excessive motion and activity.

Although the cause of ADHD is not known, there are probably several different factors that can result in hyperactivity and an abnormally short attention span. It is theorized that there is a genetic predisposition to ADHD, because it often tends to run in families. Recent research suggests that abnormal function of neurotransmitters such as dopamine may be a possible cause of the disorder. In addition, there is a possibility that prenatal or natal brain injury may cause the disorder; there may also be a connection between attention deficit disorder and fetal alcohol syndrome.

SYMPTOMS

Symptoms of ADHD include hyperactivity, impulsive behavior, short attention span, learning problems, difficulty concentrating, disorganization, and difficulty in completing projects. It begins in childhood, is often diagnosed during the first few years of school, and often continues throughout the individual's life.

INCIDENCE

ADHD affects three to five percent of children in the United States, afflicting boys about four times more often than girls. The prevalence of prescriptions for stimulant medications (such as Ritalin) have resulted in concerns that ADHD is overdiagnosed and medications are given to normal, active children to make them easier to control. This might be the case in classrooms in which as many as 25 percent of the children are medicated. However, children who do not meet full criteria for ADHD, but are distractable in association with learning disabilities, often focus better when given stimulants. Thus, the benefit of stimulant drugs is not limited to ADHD.

DIAGNOSIS

The fact that many of the symptoms of ADHD, including a short attention span or difficulty sitting still, are present in most children makes it difficult to diagnose this disorder. Distinguishing between normal childhood activity or distractability and ADHD depends upon a number of criteria. The symptoms must begin before age seven, be present continuously for at least six months, and be observable in many different situations, whether in school, at home, or in peer relationships. The level of distraction and hyperactivity must interfere significantly with the ability to function in school, with friends, and at home. When a diagnosis was missed in childhood, ADHD is often difficult to detect in adults. Distractibility and agitation in adulthood without a history of childhood ADHD could be due to chronic depression, alcohol or drug dependence, or other causes.

TREATMENT

Treatment may include medication, behavior therapy, individual tutoring for associated learning weaknesses or disabilities, individual and family therapy to reduce conflict and stress, or a combination of several approaches. Behavior modification includes creating a structured, stable, and consistent environment. In addition, a program of rewarding good behavior may also be indicated. Most children need help with developing stronger organizational skills.

Medications prescribed to treat ADHD include the stimulants methylphenidate (Ritalin), amphetamine (Dexedrine), and pemoline (Cylert), although the latter is rarely used due to the risk of liver toxicity. Low doses of stimulants help both children and adults to concentrate better, while high doses cause agitation and excessive motor activity in both age groups. Although stimulant medications often improve the symptoms of ADHD, they may also have side effects, such as sleep difficulty, irritability, loss of appetite, stomachaches, and headaches.

Nonstimulant medications used to treat ADHD include the antidepressant bupro-

Resources on Attention Deficit Disorder (ADD)
Alexander-Roberts, Colleen, *The Adhd Parenting Handbook: Practical Advice for Parents from Parents* (1994); Barchas, Jack D., *Psychopharmacology: From Theory to Practice* (1977); Barkely, Russell A, *Taking Charge of ADHD* (2000); National ADD Association, Tel. (847) 432-5874 (ADDA); Online: www.add.org; Federation for Children with Special Needs, Tel. (800) 331-0688, Online: www.fcsn.org; www.nycornell.org/pediatrics/; www.nycornell.org/psychiatry/.

pion (Wellbutrin) and the antihypertensive medications clonidine (Catapres) and guanfacine (Tenex).

Some children outgrow attention deficit disorder, and others find ways of adjusting to the disorder and improving their ability to cope with it as they grow older; ADHD continues into adulthood in 60 to 70 percent of cases. *See* ANTIDEPRESSANT DRUGS.

Audiology

The study of hearing with an emphasis on the deterioration of hearing and deafness.

Audiology is the science that studies how hearing works, how it is lost, and ways to treat hearing loss. The auditory or acoustic nerve (the eighth cranial nerve) is the neurological center responsible for hearing.

Causes of Hearing Loss. Hearing loss is a symptom of an underlying disorder. It can be caused by a mechanical problem in the middle or inner ear, or a blockage preventing the conduction of sound. It may also be caused by damage to the auditory nerve pathways in the brain. This form of hearing loss can be inherited, or it can be caused by exposure to very loud noise or by viral infection of the inner ear. Brain tumors and childhood diseases such as mumps, rubella, meningitis, and untreated inner ear infections can also cause hearing loss. In addition, natural and gradual hearing loss is part of the aging process.

The Audiologist's Role. Hearing tests can be performed with a simple tuning fork. Usually an audiologist uses an electronic device (an audiometer), which tests a patient wearing earphones in a soundproof room. The patient responds to a series of beeps and tones by pressing a button. Each ear is tested separately, and the results are then plotted on a graph.

Treatment of hearing loss depends on the cause. If there is an infection or fluid in the middle ear, the ear can be treated with antibiotics and drained. Usually, however, there is no cure for hearing loss. The patient is fitted with a hearing aid specific to his or her particular form of hearing loss. A person who cannot hear sounds even with the assistance of a hearing aid may receive a cochlear implant. *See also* HEARING AID.

Aura

A "warning" sensation before the onset of a seizure or migraine headache.

An aura is a "warning" symptom, in which an individual may see lights, smell a strange scent, or hear a peculiar sound. An aura may be a precursor to a migraine attack or an epileptic seizure.

Auras experienced before a migraine attack may include a feeling of satisfaction or fatigue. A craving for sweets or an intense feeling of thirst may develop. Other warning signals include flashing lights in the visual field, obscured vision, and speech complications. As the "warning" symptoms dissipate, the migraine pain intensifies.

An epileptic aura may be a hallucinatory sound or smell. Abdominal pain or a "heavy" feeling in the head may also occur.

Auscultation

The process of listening, either directly or with a stethoscope, to sounds produced by the body.

Auscultation is one of the oldest and simplest means of assessing the health of the cardiovascular system. A doctor simply listens—either unaided or with the use of a stethoscope—to the sounds produced by different parts of the body. The inexpensiveness and ease of the technique, as well as the amount of information that can be gathered, have made auscultation the most routine of examination procedures.

Cardiac Auscultation. The most common form of this procedure, in which the doctor listens to the sounds of the heart, is known as cardiac auscultation. This allows a doctor to monitor the heart rate and rhythm, identifying irregularities in the pace or spacing of heartbeats, as well as skipped heartbeats or those occurring in

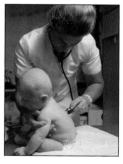

Auscultation Exam. Above, a doctor performs an auscultation examination on an infant. During auscultation, the doctor listens to and evaluates sounds in the patient's body. This type of diagnostic exam is so simple, it is very commonly used during physical examinations, though proper interpretation of the sounds is something of an art.

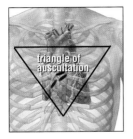

Auscultation Points.
Above, the location of the various auscultation points in the body. The functioning of the lungs, the heart, or the intestines can all be evaluated by auscultation, depending on where the stethoscope is placed. The area in which the auscultation points are located is referred to as the "triangle of auscultation."

sudden flurries or runs.

Also of critical concern is the proper functioning of the heart valves. Malfunctioning creates various forms of turbulence in the patient's blood flow, producing "murmurs" of the heart. Such murmurs may be due to seepage of blood from heart valves that do not thoroughly seal, causing a characteristic "whooshing" sound that is clearly audible through the stethoscope. Narrowed valves produce different sounds.

It is important to note that heart murmurs may occur in patients that do not have a significant heart abnormality. Pregnancy, for instance, can often produce a type of heart murmur associated with increased blood flow, and nonthreatening murmurs may also occasionally be detected in infants and children due to the rapidity of blood flow within tiny structures of the developing heart.

Auscultation of Blood Vessels. The doctor may also place the stethoscope over an artery or vein, listening for sounds of turbulent blood flow, which can result from the narrowing of blood vessels or from abnormal connections between an artery and a vein. These characteristic sounds are known as bruits—a French word meaning "noise." Such bruits are often the result of partial blockages of arteries in the leg or neck, which disturb the smooth passage of the blood.

Auscultation of the chest may sometimes produce sounds known as rales, rhonchi, or wheezes. These noises occur when the airspaces in the lungs are partially blocked by mucus or other fluids, or when there is a spasm or a thickening of the bronchial walls.

Further Testing. If abnormalities of heart function, lung function, or blood flow are detected through auscultation, the doctor may wish to refine the diagnosis through a variety of further tests. These tests may include echocardiography, Doppler examination, x-ray, CT, MRI, cardiac catheterization, and ECG (electrocardiography), as well as other tests. *See also* CIRCULATORY SYSTEM; HEART DISORDERS; PERCUSSION; *and* STETHOSCOPE.

Autism

A developmental disorder characterized by an inability to relate to other people socially.

Autistic children do not develop normal social skills or relationships. They behave in ways that are often ritualistic and may be self-damaging. Autism is often, but not always, accompanied by mental retardation. The disorder is rare, occurring in three out of 10,000 children; it affects two to four times more boys than girls. Typically the disorder becomes evident before the age of three. Previous to onset, the child may develop normally, but then will start to regress in social skills and interactions.

CAUSES
The cause of autism is unknown. However, research indicates that there is probably a biological cause, because it is often accompanied by various central nervous system disorders. Scientists have linked autism to a viral infection (congenital rubella), an inherited enzyme deficiency (phenylketonuria), and a chromosomal disorder (fragile X syndrome).

SYMPTOMS
One of the earliest symptoms of autism can be when an infant or toddler violently objects to being picked up or held. Autistic children do not form social relationships, even with parents and siblings. They avoid eye contact, do not like physical closeness, and do not learn to behave according to social standards.

These children are often highly dependent on routine, reacting with tantrums to deviations from their normal schedules. They may obsessively play with toys or other objects, lining them up or arranging them rather than playing imaginatively. It is often difficult to teach them new skills because the children thrive on familiarity.

Autistic children have difficulty learning to speak and gesture like normal children. They may shriek, rock, or inflict self-injury through behaviors such as headbanging or biting.

Most children with autism are mentally retarded, although this is difficult to diagnose accurately, as children with autism do not communicate in a way that is easily gauged by tests that measure intelligence. Some autistic children, such as those with Asperger's syndrome, have normal or above-average intelligence, and some have a remarkable capacity in one specific intellectual area, such as music or rote calculation.

One out of five autistic children begin to develop seizures before adolescence.

DIAGNOSIS

There is no specific diagnostic test for autism; thus the diagnosis is usually based on a description of behavior and the observation of the symptoms by a trained professional. The evaluation may also test the affected individual for other brain disorders that may, in some cases, accompany autism. These tests may include computed tomography (CT) or magnetic resonance imaging (MRI).

TREATMENT

There is no cure for autism; the goal of treatment is to teach adaptive behaviors and minimize destructive and self-destructive behaviors. Children with closer to average intelligence can benefit from speech, physical, behavioral, occupational, and various other type of therapies. Medication can control seizures and can limit violent behavior and other symptoms, but it is not a cure and is not a treatment in itself. The vast majority of autistic children need more intensive care than can be provided at home and are often institutionalized.

Regardless of the therapy options pursued, counseling for all family members can help the family learn about the disorder and assist them in coping with the difficulties of raising an autistic child.

Background information on autism can be found in BRAIN, DISORDERS OF. *For further information, see* CHILD DEVELOPMENT; CT SCANNING; MRI; *and* NERVOUS SYSTEM. *See also* DOPAMINE; NEUROTRANSMITTER; *and* SEROTONIN *for more on brain chemistry involved in autism.*

Autoimmune Disorders

Diseases in which the immune system begins attacking the body's own tissues.

Normally, cells of the immune system can distinguish other body cells from foreign cells, but in people with autoimmune diseases this mechanism has gone awry. It is unknown what stimulates the immune system to react in such an abnormal manner.

Types. Rheumatoid arthritis, myasthenia gravis, Eaton-Lambert syndrome, Goodpasture's syndrome, Graves' disease, Hashimoto's thyroiditis, dermatomyositis, Guillain-Barré syndrome, lupus, scleroderma, and Sjögren's syndrome are examples of autoimmune diseases.

Symptoms. Immune reactions normally result in inflammation. In the case of autoimmune diseases, the inflammation is chronic and results in long-term damage. The most common targets of autoimmune disease are connective tissues. The muscles can also become inflamed, as can the membrane coverings around the heart and lungs. The brain can be affected as well.

Diagnosis. Each autoimmune disease has a particular set of symptoms, but sometimes these overlap, making it difficult to diagnose a precise autoimmune disease. Analyzing the abnormal antibodies can be helpful in making a diagnosis.

Treatment. Anti-inflammatory drugs, particularly NSAIDS, such as aspirin and ibuprofen, can be used to treat mild inflammation. Corticosteroids, such as prednisone, are more effective for more severe symptoms but have more side effects. Immunosuppressive drugs can be used to suppress the immune system response altogether. However, these drugs increase the body's susceptibility to infection and have potentially dangerous side effects.

Recently, there has been considerable success in treating some cases of autoimmune arthritis and intestinal disease with biological agents that block a protein produced during inflammation, called TNF. *See also* IMMUNE SYSTEM *and* IMMUNITY.

Resources on Autism
Andron, Linda, et al., *Our Journey Through High Functioning Autism and Asperger Syndrome: A Roadmap* (2001); Baron-Cohen, Simon, and Patrick Bolton, *Autism* (1993); Maurice, Catherine, *Let Me Hear Your Voice: A Family's Triumph over Autism* (1997); Autism Society of America, Tel. (800) 657-0881, (800) 3AUTISM, Online: www. autism-society.org; Federation for Children with Special Needs, Tel. (800) 331-0688, Online: www.fc-sn.org; www.nycornell.org/pediatrics/; www.nycornell.org/psychiatry/.

Resources on Autoimmune Disorders
Desowitz, Robert S., *The Thorn and the Starfish* (1987); Granstein, Richard D., *Mechanisms of Immune Regulation* (1994); *Life, Death, and the Immune System: Articles from* Scientific American (1994); Nilsson, Lenhart, *The Body Victorious* (1987); American Autoimmune Related Diseases Association (AARDA),Tel. (810) 776-3900, Online: www. aarda.org; www.nycornell.org/immunology.

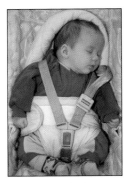

Automobile Safety. Above, automobile safety is especially important for children under the age of five, who should be secured in a car seat whenever they are in a car. Most states legally require this precaution.

Autonomic Nervous System. At right, the autonomic nervous system controls the cardiac muscles, the smooth muscles, and the glands.

Automobile Safety

Precautionary measures in order to prevent accidents and injuries.

Motor-vehicle accidents are a major cause of death among healthy Americans, killing 45,000 people each year. Many deaths can be prevented by the use of seat belts, which should be used even if state law does not demand it. Precautions that prevent accidents include: sober, defensive driving; obedience to speed limits; alertness to other cars and road and weather conditions; use of turn signals; and looking both ways at train crossings.

Most states require child safety seats for children under the age of four or five. Never use a child safety seat in the front seat, especially a rear-facing seat. Small children and the elderly should sit in the safest place, the back seat; neither they nor anyone under five feet tall should sit in a seat equipped with an airbag, as the inflation can cause injury or death. Otherwise, install an airbag on/off switch.

Dispose of potentially distracting loose debris inside the car. Keep hair and loose clothing clear of open windows. Do not overload the vehicle with luggage or cargo that could obstruct views. Ensure windshield wipers, washers, defrost and defoggers, and headlights and taillights function.

Never drive under the influence of alcohol or illicit drugs. In addition, avoid driving when taking prescription or over-the-counter medications that cause drowsiness.

Teenagers should not be allowed to drive until they pass all tests required by state law, accumulate sufficient experience practicing driving in safe areas, and understand precautionary ground rules, which are enforced by parents. *See also* ACCIDENTS.

Autonomic Nervous System

The nerves that control vital functions.

The autonomic nervous system begins in the hypothalamus, a tiny structure in the center of the brain that sends messages to all the regions in the body to control hormones that control various internal functions. The main chemicals involved in the nervous system include adrenalin, epinephrine, and norepinephrine. The autonomic nervous system consists of the sympathetic and parasympathetic nervous systems.

The sympathetic nervous system controls the body's response to stress—the

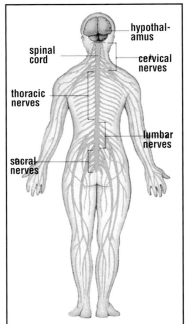

fight-or-flight response. The reaction of the sympathetic system is for the most part involuntary; it cannot be consciously controlled. The main chemical involved in sympathetic nervous system response is called adrenaline or epinephrine, and is released by the adrenal glands. The sympathetic nerves reduce blood flow to the stomach and intestines, increasing blood flow to the heart, lungs, and muscles. The heart pumps faster and the bronchial tubes widen to increase air flow.

The parasympathetic nervous system causes responses nearly opposite to those caused by the sympathetic nervous system. The parasympathetic nervous system can be controlled voluntarily. Acetylcholine, a neurotransmitter, is the chemical by which impulses are transmitted in the parasympathetic nervous system; once activated, blood flow increases to the internal organs, and heart and breathing rates decrease. The parasympathetic nervous system thus allows the body to recover from stress; it is dominant when the body is resting or digesting food.

Autopsy

The examination and dissection of a deceased person to determine the cause or causes of death.

When death is by homicide or suicide, of a suspicious nature, or due to an accident, an autopsy is generally required. It is performed by a county coroner or a medical examiner (a physician with qualifications in pathology). Consent forms for next of kin to sign usually offer two options: a limited autopsy or a complete autopsy. Sometimes, life insurance policies require an autopsy to ascertain that the insured did not mischaracterize any conditions. Once performed on about half of all deaths, autopsies are currently performed on only around 10 percent of deaths.

Aviation Medicine

The branch of medicine that studies the effects of air travel on the human body and treats aviation-related illnesses.

Aviation medicine is a specialized branch of medicine that studies the effects of flight on the human body. The goals of aviation medicine are to understand the physics of aviation, to assess the health risks encountered during flight, and to develop treatments for aviation-related illnesses.

Aviation medicine focuses primarily on the health of pilots and their crew, though this branch of medicine has also identified numerous problems encountered by passengers on civil aircraft, such as altitude sickness. The ultimate aim of aviation medicine is to promote the safety of humans while they are exposed to the physical and psychological rigors of flight, which can include extreme temperatures, low atmospheric pressure, oxygen deprivation, the strong forces of acceleration and deceleration, and the psychological pressures of making quick decisions under substantial environmental stress.

History. As aviation has developed, so has the study of its effects on the human body. Altitude sickness was first identified almost three thousand years ago by the Greek philosopher Aristotle. The ailment was described in detail by Aristotle, who observed the breathlessness suffered by those scaling Mount Olympus. In 1588, the Spanish missionary Joseph de Acosta wrote the first scientific history of altitude sickness from his observations of the natives of the Andes.

The 19th-century French physiologist Paul Bert is generally regarded as the father of modern aviation medicine. He described in detail the effects of high and low air pressures on balloonists. His observations spurred a broad program of research early in the 20th century. During World War I, the United States established the first physical standards for pilots, cutting the rate of pilot error due to physical impairment. Research into the psychological stress of flight also began at that time. In 1953, the American Medical Association first recognized aviation medicine as a preventive medical specialty.

Since World War I, new research has increased our knowledge of the physics of flight. Aviation medicine has kept pace with innovations in flight technology, such as the jet engine and space travel. Much effort has centered on the development of a safe ejection seat. Oxygen equipment has improved, cabin pressurization has become the norm, and the need for new cardiovascular standards for pilots and crew has received serious attention.

Effects of Flight. Certain aspects of flight exert effects on the human body. The force inflicted on the body during acceleration and deceleration, changes in atmospheric pressure, the rapid and turbulent movement of the aircraft, and the disruption of environmental time cues all have the potential to affect the human body in serious ways.

Recently, aviation-medicine specialists have turned their attention to the loss of consciousness caused by changes in the force of gravity during acceleration and deceleration. During rapid acceleration and deceleration, the force of gravity on the body can increase dramatically.

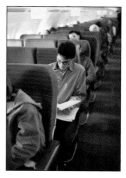

Passenger Health. Passengers on an airplane, above, are subjected to stresses on the body during flight. These stresses include the disruption of the body's clock, changes in air pressure, and the turbulent movement of the aircraft. Specialists in aviation medicine study the effects of these stresses on the bodies of passengers, flight attendants, and pilots, and treat aviation-related illnesses.

Reduction in air pressure is also a serious health risk. Air pressure may drop during ascent, reducing the amount of oxygen taken into the body with each breath. The muscles can only function temporarily without oxygen, and the brain and eyes are also extremely sensitive to a lack of oxygen in the environment.

The speed at which an aircraft moves can disturb the semicircular canals of the inner ear, which detect motion. This can result in the dizziness and nausea characteristic of motion sickness.

The internal biological clocks of pilots and passengers moving across many time zones may be disrupted. The presence of light, activity levels, and the consumption of food are signals used by the body to adjust its internal rhythms to time. When environmental stimuli clash with the internal rhythms of the body, jet lag results.

Symptoms. The symptoms of flight-related illness can range from the nausea and lightheadedness characteristic of motion or altitude sickness to more severe symptoms. Mild flight-related sickness can result from any of the environmental conditions mentioned above. In general, severe flight-related illness results from the extreme gravitational force on the body during acceleration and deceleration, or from a lack of oxygen. Loss of consciousness and even death may occur in extreme cases of flight-related illness.

Treatment. The simplest treatment for flight-related illness is to align the body, especially the head, with the plane of the aircraft. This requires reclining the body. Several prescription medications, such as antihistamines, also help prevent and treat motion sickness. Other more severe flight-related conditions, such as those that result from gravitational force on the body or a lack of oxygen, are not treatable and should be prevented.

> *Background material on aviation medicine can be found in* PUBLIC HEALTH. *For further information, see* JET LAG *and* RESPIRATORY SYSTEM. *See also* DEATH; FAINTING; *and* NAUSEA *for more on particular symptoms of flight-related illness.*

Avoidant Personality Disorder

A personality disorder characterized by extreme timidity and discomfort in social situations, fear of rejection and judgments of others, and hypersensitivity to criticism that goes beyond shyness.

While the cause of avoidant personality disorder is unknown, symptoms begin in childhood and often begin with an assumption by the patient that people are predisposed to be negative and judgmental. This may be based on an individual's childhood experience, or it may be the result of a genetic predisposition to this psychological disorder.

Symptoms. The primary fear of an individual with avoidant personality disorder, of judgment by others, leads to a socially isolated lifestyle where new acquaintances are avoided. Situations such as job interviews and social gatherings, where judgments may be made or where social interactions take place, will be avoided, as will any situation that involves a risk of failure or of rejection by others.

Extreme self-consciousness manifests itself in excessive concern and apprehension about appearance, as well as hypersensitivity to even the most diplomatically presented constructive criticism.

Treatment. A variety of treatments are available for avoidant personality disorder, including psychotherapy and behavior therapy. In all cases the goal is to help the patient face difficult social and interpersonal situations. Much like treatment for phobias, behaviorally oriented treatments attempt to desensitize patients by helping them approach feared situations in a controlled manner. Supportive psychotherapy is also used and may be combined with group therapy, where the opportunity exists to develop social skills.

> *For background information on avoidant personality disorder, see* PSYCHIATRY. *Related information is contained in* ADDICTION; ALCOHOL DEPENDENCE; DRUG DEPENDENCE; *and* PERSONALITY DISORDERS. *See also* PSYCHOTHERAPY *for more on treatment.*

Avulsion

Tearing of body tissue from its normal attachment.

The term avulsion is most commonly used to refer to an avulsion fracture, in which an overstretched ligament tears off a fragment of the bone to which it is attached. The tear may be small or quite large, depending on the severity of the injury and the size of the affected bones or joints.

Elevation of the damaged area or the use of a splint to hold the torn area together in a neutral position are common treatments. In less severe cases, a compress may suffice to treat the injury. *See also* EXCISION *and* SURGERY.

Ayurvedic Medicine

A system of medicine developed in India over the past 5,000 years, typified by a holistic and highly individualized approach to the patient.

Ayurveda, meaning "science of life," refers to the system of medicine that has been developed in India over the past 5,000 years, based on the sacred scriptures of the Vedas known as the Samhitas. The system blends Hindu spiritual concepts, such as reincarnation, with Eastern teachings regarding the efficacy of massaging pressure points (akin to the Chinese method of acupressure), and a highly structured view of the human body. Dr. Deepak Chopra is largely responsible, through his various writings and lectures, for the surge of interest in Ayurvedic concepts in the West. The various therapies that are applied in Ayurvedic medicine include: dietary adjustments; fitness training; yoga; meditation; massage; herbal tonics; herbal baths; enemas; and medicated inhalation.

BODY TYPES

Ayurvedic medicine is based on the concept of metabolic body types, known as *doshas*: there are three—*vata, pitta,* and *kapha,* corresponding roughly to slim, average, and heavy. A person is actually a complex combination of all three. Each individual's health and physical well-being, from susceptibility to certain diseases to personality and attitudes about life, are the result of the interplay of the doshas. Generally, one dosha predominates and dictates the health profile of the individual throughout life.

The *vata* type tends to be thin with prominent joints and cool dry skin; hyperactive, moody, and energetic; erratic, intuitive, and unconventional. This person eats and sleeps at irregular hours, is prone to nervous disorders and cramps, and is beset with anxieties and dramatic mood swings.

The *pitta* type tends toward a medium build and warm, moist skin; an orderly approach to life marked by intense efficiency; punctual, deliberative, and loving, yet short tempered; articulate, intelligent, and logical. This individual is prone to ulcers and gastrointestinal disorders, as well as hemorrhoids, acne, and dermatological (skin) disorders. He or she is often compulsive and driven.

The *kapha* type is heavyset, with thick hair and pale, oily skin; tends to be slow but graceful and coordinated; and is even-tempered, relaxed, and slow to anger. This type of person needs long periods of sleep and a social environment, often procrastinates, moves with great deliberation, and is tolerant and forgiving. He or she is prone to obesity, allergies, and respiratory illnesses; as well as high cholesterol and cardiovascular problems.

The healthy individual has his or her *doshas* in balance, and the goal of Ayurvedic medicine is to assist an individual in promoting the activity of a weak or deficient *dosha* within the body.

AYURVEDIC DIAGNOSTICS

Ayurvedic practitioners pay special attention to observing parts of the body believed to be the seats of the *doshas* and that indicate the balance of *doshas* within the body. Most prominent in Ayurvedic diagnostics are the pulse, the tongue, the eyes, and the nails. An Ayurvedic practitioner will listen to several pulses around the body (not just the several on the wrist) for slight and

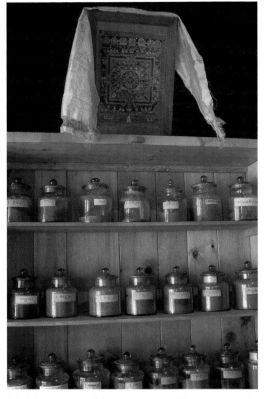

Ayurvedic Medicine. Right, various herbs are used in the rejuvenation (*rasayana*) phase of Ayurvedic treatment. The types of herbs used differ depending on the needs of the individual who is being treated.

highly nuanced fluctuations. The tongue is especially important in this approach. Practitioners also pay close attention to the eyes, looking for small irregularities signalling problems elsewhere in the body; the nails and the cuticles; and the urine, relying on both visual observation and its odors over a period of time.

PROCEDURES

After a diagnosis has been made and the imbalance in the body has been determined, treating the disease or condition involves four stages: cleaning and purification; palliation; rejuvenation; and mental and spiritual healing.

Purification involves the removal of toxins from the body. This may be achieved through a variety of methods, including techniques that induce vomiting, bowel purging, enemas, etc. These methods, known collectively as Pancha Karma, are designed to remove toxins from the body, considered to be the origin of disease and bodily imbalance.

Palliation, called *shaman*, strives to bal-ance the *doshas* of an individual. This step engages the spiritual dimension of healing, through the integration of fasting, chanting, yoga stretches, breathing exercises, and meditation. This combination of techniques may be tailored to treat a particular condition, or it may be used as a form of preventive therapy for a healthy individual as well.

Rejuvenation, called *rasayana*, aims to improve the body's ability to function. In this phase, an individual undergoes a process of tonification, which is designed to revitalize the body's reproductive system, to enhance the individual's sexual performance, and to slow down the aging process. *Rasayana* treatments may require the ingesting of herb tablets and special mineral preparations, in conjunction with yoga stretching and exercise.

The final phase in an Ayurvedic treatment plan is known as *satvajaya*, which focuses on the overall condition of the mind. *Satvajaya* attempts to enhance mental and spiritual functioning by relieving psychological and emotional stress. Releasing unconscious negative thoughts is also strongly encouraged. Different forms of meditation, sound therapy, and crystals are used toward this goal.

OUTLOOK

Ayurvedic medicine is most commonly taught and practiced in India; however, this type of medicine has gained broader appeal in Europe, Japan, and North and South America in recent years.

> *Background material on ayurvedic medicine can be found in* ALTERNATIVE MEDICINE. *For further information, see* AROMATHERAPY; AUSCULTATION; FASTING; *and* HOMEOPATHY. *See also* HOLISTIC MEDICINE *and* MEDITATION *for more on specific practices.*

Babesiosis

Infection transmitted by a microscopic parasite in ticks.

Babesiosis is a rare, potentially fatal, illness that occurs mainly in coastal areas in Europe and the northeastern United States. The single-cell microorganism known as *Babesia* is transmitted by infected ticks. Deer, meadow voles, and mice are animals that may carry such ticks.

The babesia parasite attacks the red blood cells. Infected individuals may feel tired and experience a loss of appetite and a general malaise. Fever, drenching sweats, muscle aches, and a headache usually ensue. Symptoms will last from several days to several months. For severe cases, intensive hospital care will be necessary, and patients are treated with quinine and clindamycin or atovaquone.

Deer ticks also transmit Lyme disease, and bitten individuals are at risk of acquiring both diseases. Prevention involves taking the general precautions regarding tick-infested areas, including wearing long sleeves and pants and using an appropriate insect repellent. *See also* BITES; BLOOD; FEVER; LYME DISEASE; *and* PARASITE.

Bacilli

Rod-shaped bacteria.

Bacteria are classified by shape (either spiral, spherical, or rod-like) and by whether they stain blue (gram-positive) or pink (gram-negative) in laboratory testing. These categories are caused by differences in the cell walls of the bacteria.

Gram-positive bacilli cause the disease named diphtheria. The antibiotic penicillin is used to treat it. Gram-negative bacilli have a second outer membrane, which makes them more difficult to treat. They are responsible for gastroenteritis, cholera, and *E. Coli.* They are treated with antibiotics. *See also* ANTIBIOTIC DRUGS; BACTERIA; CHOLERA; DIPHTHERIA; GASTRITIS; GASTROENTERITIS; *and* PENICILLIN.

Back Pain

Pain or stiffness in back muscles, either temporary or chronic.

The back does an astonishing amount of the work of everyday living. The spine supports the body while it is standing, sitting, lifting, and walking. It contains the spinal cord, the nerve center responsible for all movement from the neck down. Because of the heavy responsibilities borne by the spine, almost everyone experiences back pain at some point in life.

The most common kind of back pain is a lower-back strain, caused by such things as carrying or lifting improperly, long periods of sitting or bending or sitting awkwardly, poor posture, and even sleeping on the stomach or on a mattress that does not provide enough support. This kind of back pain generally does not require any kind of testing or x-rays, and usually clears up with minor treatment.

Treatment. Common lower back strain usually disappears with the help of rest, anti-inflammatory drugs, or painkillers. Treatment of chronic pain may include an

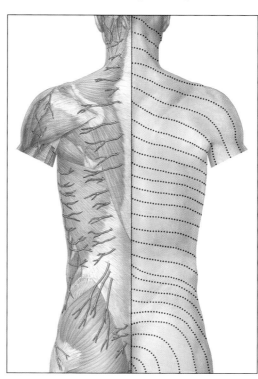

Back Dermatomes. Left, a diagram of the back's dermatomes. Dermatomes are described as any area of skin that is enervated by the sensory fibers from a single spinal nerve— they cover the entire body. In some of the extremities, dermatomes overlap. The shoulders, upper back, lumbar, and buttocks are all covered by different sets of dermatomes. Abnormal back dermatomes provide vital information about nerve damage that may cause pain.

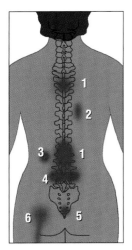

Back Pain. Above, specific areas of the back that are most often, and most severely affected by equally specific kinds of pain include (1) osteoarthritis that occurs along the spine; (2) fibrositis in the large back muscles; (3) kidney infections, which are marked by pain on the sides of the back; (4) damaged joints, ligaments, muscles, or disks often cause lower back pain; (5) falls usually cause coccyx pain and; (6) sciatica is marked by pain radiating down below the back and into the leg.

extended regimen of physical therapy—exercises to strengthen the affected area. Supports or braces may also help, and in some cases, such as with compression fractures, crutches can help relieve the weight and pressure of walking while the fracture heals. Electric stimulation, ultrasound, or occasional injections of anesthetics may help to relieve the pain and stiffness. Treatment should include measures to stop the strain from recurring, such as exercise or a change in routine.

More severe disorders, including spondylolisthesis, may require surgery to stabilize the spine. Injuries often require immediate medical assistance. Disk surgery may be performed to relieve pain from bulging disks by removing all or part of the disk. This procedure is risky and may not relieve all the pain. It is best used for injuries where an acute rupture of a disk causes a clear loss of nerve function that may lead to permanent damage.

Kinds of Back Pain

Other kinds of back pain include:

- **Osteoarthritis:** pain and stiffness located in the upper back, due to deterioration of joints;
- **Spondylolisthesis:** slippage of vertebrae because ligaments are not holding them in place; usually caused by a bone fracture or abnormality;
- **Spondylosis:** loss of flexibility in spine as disks between vertebrae wear out;
- **Pyelonephritis:** pain caused by kidney stones or infection, usually located in the back, near where the rib cage ends;
- **Compression fracture:** injury caused by sudden stress on the causing vertebrae to collapse on one side, distorting the curve of spine; may compress nerve-root as well, causing numbness, tingling, or weakness in affected areas;
- **Ruptured disk:** failure of spacing disks between vertebrae, causing the gel in the disk to bulge or rupture, which may lead to compression of the spinal cord; usually caused by age or excess strain;
- **Sciatica:** pain that runs from the buttock down the back of the leg into the foot, from pressure on the sciatic nerve as it leaves the spinal cord; usually caused by disk prolapse or damage to a spinal facet joint;
- **Coccygodynia:** pain and tenderness at the base of the spinal column; occurs after childbirth or a fall in which the coccyx strikes the ground.

Natural Therapy. There are a number of alternative therapies that some individuals find effective in the treatment of back pain. Regular massage treatment, with a licensed and trained professional, can relieve the ordinary stresses that are often the result of repetitive muscular stresses. Acupressure, shiatsu, and reflexology are also effective treatments for some cases of back pain, although results vary.

Prevention. Common types of back pain are easily prevented. Good posture while sitting and standing keeps the spine properly aligned, which makes it less vulnerable to ordinary injuries. Heavy objects should be lifted correctly, by using the legs and stronger upper back muscles, rather than the muscles in the lower back. A mattress should provide the proper support and sleep on the stomach should be avoided. Simple practices such as these can relieve unnecessary stress. A lifelong exercise program and proper nutrition will help keep the bones in the back strong so they will be able to withstand the wear and tear of age.

Related anatomical information can be found in Osteoporosis; Spine; *and* Vertebra. *Information regarding back pain and treatment may be found in* Occupational Medicine; Sprain; Whiplash Injury; *and* Pain Relief.

Bacteremia

The presence of bacteria in the bloodstream.

Normally, bacteria in the bloodstream are removed by the white blood cells. When bacteria are particularly virulent or numerous, the condition progresses to cause septic shock, which can be life-threatening.

Causes. Surgical procedures involving infected parts of the body may introduce bacteria into the bloodstream, which is why antibiotics, such as penicillin, are administered to patients immediately after most operations. Drug users who use infected needles are at risk of sepsis, as are cancer patients who are taking drugs that may inhibit the immune system, people with AIDS and all other individuals who have compromised immune systems. *See also* Blood.

Symptoms. Small infestations of bacteria cause few if any symptoms, since the immune system clears them away quickly; if sepsis becomes more extreme, however, the person may suffer chills and fever, weakness, nausea, vomiting and diarrhea. Sepsis can spread quickly to organs such as the brain, the heart, and the bone marrow, and produce abscesses, so immediate treatment with antibiotics is indicated even before the specific bacteria are identified. *See also* BACTERIA *and* URINARY SYSTEM.

Bacteria

One-celled organisms that account for many diseases, but are also at the bottom of the food chain on which humans depend for sustenance.

A bacterium differs from a human cell because it has no nuclear membrane It has only a cell wall and a single strand of DNA.

TYPES

The three primary types of bacteria have been categorized based on how they react to oxygen environments:

- Aerobic bacteria need an atmosphere of free oxygen to thrive;
- Anaerobic bacteria cannot tolerate free oxygen, and live in places like mud and the large intestine;
- Facultative anaerobes live with free oxygen, but do not need it to thrive.

In unfavorable conditions, bacteria form endospores that can survive in outer space, the pressure of the deepest ocean, and, recently, the attack of antibiotics.

REPRODUCTION

Bacteria reproduce by fission (mitosis), in which the cell divides in two. Bacteria can, however, exchange nucleic acids and DNA without dividing. This is how they learn from each other and, more importantly, how they propagate a resistance to antibiotic medicines. There are so many bacteria on Earth that attempts to count them have yielded incredible numbers. Scandinavian researchers have found at least 4,000 species of bacteria in a single gram of soil.

FUNCTION

Bacteria have many useful purposes, both for humans as well as for the ecology of the planet. Bacteria make oxygen through the chemical process known as photosynthesis. They also enrich the soil, turn specific fruit sugars into alcohol, ferment cheese, decompose organic waste, and can also clean up some kinds of toxic wastes. Among the totality of bacterial organisms, most are completely harmless to people.

Bacteria that cause disease are called pathogens. These are responsible for an incredibly wide range of diseases, most notably pneumonia, cholera, plague, syphilis, septic shock, and tetanus.

BACTERIA AND DISEASE

The battle against disease is primarily a battle against bacteria. Viruses, fungi, and parasites are all disease-causing organisms, but bacteria are the prime cause of most infections. These pathogens invade the body through the skin and mucous membranes, by touch, by ingestion, and even through the air we breathe.

Open cuts or bruises are virtual invitations for bacteria to invade, occupy, multiply, and produce the toxins that cause what we know as disease. Most infections are successfully dealt with by the immune system with white blood cells, gamma globulin, and lymph fluid.

For example, staphylococci are found in quantity on everyone's skin, but a cut, bruise, or blemish on the skin permits the bacteria to invade the bloodstream. If the immune system is functioning well, the staph is neutralized quickly and the body avoids infection. However, if the bacteria are allowed to multiply and spread to other organs of the body, the person experiences rash, fever, increased heart rate and blood pressure, headache, nausea, vomiting, and diarrhea.

See ALCOHOL INTOXICATION; CEREBELLUM; *and* EAR *for a discussion on the foundations of balance. More on balance problems is found in* DIZZINESS; POSTURE; *and* SYNCOPE. *Material on balance problems is found in* ANXIETY; EAR, DISORDERS OF; *and* ELECTRONYSTAGMOGRAPHY.

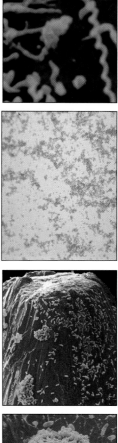
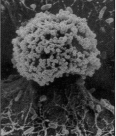

Bacteria. Above, microscopic images of various types of bacteria. Spherical (coccus), rod-like (bacillus), and curved (vibrio, spirillum or spirochete) shapes mark different kinds of bacteria that are found in all environments. At the bottom is a colony of cocci and bacilli feeding. Bacteria are the unicellular organisms that cause diseases and infections.

Bacteriuria

Bacteria in the urine.

The presence of a small number of bacteria in the urine is not uncommon in many healthy persons. Bacteriuria is especially common in women because the female urethra, the tube through which urine is passed, is shorter and opens close to the anus, which is normally colonized by bacteria from the vagina, rectum, and skin. Bacteriuria is a cause for concern only when the bacterial count is high and when pus cells are also found in the urine. Symptoms of an infection of the bladder, urethra, or kidneys requiring antibiotic treatment include frequent urgent urination accompanied by pain or a fever. *See also* BACTERIA; KIDNEY; *and* URINARY TRACT DISORDERS.

Baker's Cyst

A cyst that forms behind the knees.

A Baker's cyst is an accumulation of joint fluid that forms behind the knee. The cysts are most commonly found in patients with rheumatoid arthritis, and are usually harmless and, in most cases, painless. Larger cysts may become irritated due to normal activity of the knee.

A Baker's cyst usually clears up on its own, though ice and anti-inflammatory medication can help reduce swelling. In some cases, a doctor may drain the cyst. Baker's cysts tend to recur, but strengthening the muscles around the knee may help reduce the incidence. *See also* ARTHRITIS.

Organs of Balance. The organs within the inner ear (labyrinth) control balance through a set of intricate measurements that are taken and relayed to the reflex centers of the brain. The vestibule (a) and the semicircular canals (b) produce and send these signals through the vestibular nerve (c) to the cerebellum, which is constantly reacting to maintain balance.

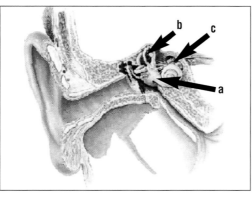

Balance

The body's state of equilibrium, which reinforces stability, allowing it to remain upright.

A region in the brain, named the cerebellum, collects information from the eyes; sensory receptors in the skin, muscles, and joints; and three semicircular canals in in the inner ear to assess the body's position. It uses this information to direct the muscles to contract or relax and thus maintain the body's upright position.

Balance problems and dizziness are experienced from time to time by 40 percent of the adult population. Dizziness can appear as light-headedness, a sense of motion when a person is still, or a sense that the room is spinning.

The loss of balance and a sense that everything is spinning around is called vertigo. Dizziness may be accompanied by nausea, hearing loss, pressure in the head or ears, ringing in the ears (tinnitus), and anxiety. *See also* ANXIETY.

Problems with Balance. Loss of balance is generally a symptom of another, often more serious, disorder. It is frequently caused by injury or disorder in the inner ear, which detects the position and movements of the head and is essential for a sense of balance. Balance problems may also arise as a result of injury or disorder in the nerves that receive information about the body's position. Dizziness can also be caused by alcohol or drug use, brain injury, anemia, high or low blood pressure, infection, and hypoglycemia.

Diagnosing Balance Problems. To evaluate balance disorders, a series of tests called electronystagmograms are used. These tests check for specific types of eye movements that characterize a balance disorder. Once the underlying cause of a balance disorder is diagnosed, it can be treated.

> *Background information related to the anatomy of* BALANCE *can be found in* BLOOD PRESSURE; BRAIN; EAR; EYE; *and* MUSCLE. BALANCE *related disorders include* ANEMIA; DIZZINESS; HEAD INJURY; HYPOGLYCEMIA; *and* VERTIGO. *Also see* EAR ACHE; MIDDLE-EAR EFFUSION, PERSISTENT; *and* TINNITIS.

Balanitis

Inflammation of the head of the penis.

Balanitis can be caused by a bacterial or fungal infection, such as thrush, which is sometimes contracted from a sexual partner or a result of an allergic or irritant reaction to soaps, detergents, or a number of various other chemicals. It can also occur as the result of a failure to keep the penis in a clean and sanitary condition.

Men with diabetes are more likely to contract balanitis. It is particularly uncommon among men who have been circumcised. Symptoms include pain, itching, redness, and a whitish discharge. Balanitis in diabetic individuals can often be a sign that sugar regulation is poorly controlled.

Balanitis can be prevented by a routine that incorporates good hygiene, washing the penis carefully, and the use of an antibacterial soap or ointment.

If an underlying infection exists, that must be treated as well. The use of a soothing cream will help relieve the itchiness and irritation. Any chemical agents that could possibly cause an allergic reaction must also be eliminated. *See also* BACTERIA; INFECTION; PENIS; *and* THRUSH.

Balloon Catheter

A type of catheter (a flexible hollow tube) with an inflatable sac or balloon at its tip, which is used primarily in urinary or arterial procedures.

A catheter is a flexible tube that is inserted into an opening or small incision in the body in order to observe a specific organ and perform delicate treatment.

When the balloon in a balloon catheter is inflated, it keeps the catheter in place while at the same time expanding the desired area. The two most common types of balloon catheters are urinary catheters and embolectomy catheters.

URINARY CATHETERS

The urinary catheter, which is sometimes referred to as a Foley catheter, is the oldest type of balloon catheter. It is used to drain the bladder of patients who are incapacitated or those who cannot leave their hospital beds due to their condition.

The catheter is pressed into the bladder through the urethra. One line in the catheter tube injects water into the balloon while another line drains urine and water into a special bag that hangs at the side of the patient's bed. Balloon dilation is also used to enlarge the urethra when prostate enlargement causes urinary obstruction.

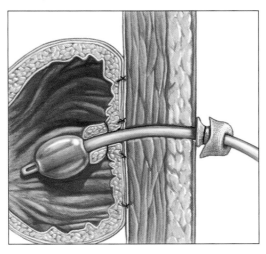

EMBOLECTOMY CATHETERS

EMBOLECTOMY CATHETERS

Embolectomy catheters expand and unblock narrow arteries. They are used to expand blocked arteries of the heart, in a procedure called a coronary angioplasty, and to repair heart valves, which is also called a valvuloplasty. They may also be used to monitor blood pressure in specific areas of the heart and arteries.

Balloon catheters may be used to help close or stop up blood vessels to control bleeding or to starve a tumor of its blood supply. A balloon catheter is used to treat bleeding or enlarged veins (varices) in the esophagus or stomach. The balloon compresses the veins and stabilizes bleeding until surgery can be performed.

Balloon Catheter. Doctor E. B. Foley and Charles Russell Bard developed the balloon catheter in 1934 and it has improved the quality of hundreds of thousands of lives since. Balloon catheters have proven effected for people of both sexes; they are also effective for short- and long-term usage.

Related articles include BLEEDING; CATHETER; STOMACH; *and* VEIN. *Other vital information about this topic can be found in* PROSTATE; URETHRA; *and* URINARY SYSTEM. *See also* BED, HOSPITAL *for information about long term care that may require the use of a balloon catheter.*

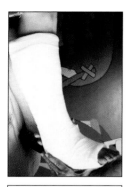

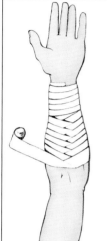

Types of Bandages.
Top, a plaster cast is a type of bandage used to set broken bones so that they heal in the proper position. Plaster casts limit motion at the joints adjacent to the break, facilitating the healing process. At the bottom, a drawing of a wrist that is bandaged firmly but not too tightly; this type of bandage would be effective to treat a sprain or a strain. Near the wrist, this bandage is wrapped as a spiral; the cross-over pattern that lines the forearm is called a reverse spiral.

Bandage

A gauze or adhesive covering used to protect a wound or control bleeding.

Bandages are an essential element of any health-care device or institution, from the family first aid-kit to the local hospital. For minor cuts or bruises, strips of adhesive tape with a folder of sterile gauze in the center protect a wound from infection and permit the blood to clot.

If the wound is bleeding profusely, a gauze pad must be pressed firmly against the would in order to control the bleeding. Adhesive bandages come in many sizes, and a variety should be kept on hand for minor emergencies.

The adhesive bandage should be removed no more than one or two days later so that the wound can be examined for any signs of infection such as redness, swelling or the presence of pus. A fresh bandage can then be applied.

Joint sprains and strains are often treated with elastic bandages that restrain movement and provide some support.

Triangular bandages should be kept in every first-aid kit so that temporary splints can be made or injuries can be wrapped.

Plaster casts, another sort of bandage, can be put in place only by a health care professional. They treat broken bones that have been set back into place. Fiberglass bandages, which set faster, weigh less, and resist water, are also coming into regular use. *See also* BLEEDING *and* SPRAINS.

Barbiturate Drugs

Any of a group of organic compounds that come from barbituric acid; they are potentially addictive sedative-hypnotic drugs that are used occasionally as a sleep aid and an anticonvulsant.

Barbiturates, which include such drugs as amobarbital (Amytal); secobarbital (Seconal); and phenobarbitol (Nembutal), are depressants that act on the central nervous system and the respiratory system. Barbiturate use will affect the heart rate, blood

pressure, and body temperature, as they cause a feeling of relaxation, calm, and sleepiness that may relieve strong tension, intense anxiety, or temporary insomnia. Barbiturate drugs, such as secobarbital, will also slow signals in the brain and thus may prevent seizures.

Prolonged use of barbiturates may lead to an addiction or to an increased tolerance, in which an individual needs an increasingly larger dose in order to achieve a similar effect. When used in conjunction with alcohol or other sedatives, barbiturate drugs can render a person unconscious, cause a coma, or even be fatal.

Barbiturates are particularly dangerous for senior citizens. The side effects are likely to be more severe, and there is a possible interaction with other drugs. The elderly should avoid barbiturates except when prescribed to control seizures.

Pentothal sodium may be used as an intravenous anesthetic for brief operations. Its reputation as a "truth serum," however, has been exaggerated. Barbiturates may cause drug habits; a doctor's prescription and his or her advice must always be followed closely.

Further information about topics related to BARBITURATE DRUGS *can be found among* BREATHING DIFFICULTY; NERVOUS SYSTEM; RESPIRATORY SYSTEM; *and* SLEEP. *More information can be found in* DOSE *and* DRUG OVERDOSE.

Barium X-Ray

Any diagnostic test using barium sulfate, a chalky substance that is opaque to x-rays.

Because barium is opaque to x-rays, it appears white on an x-ray image. When it is introduced into the gastrointestinal (GI) tract, it reveals the outlines (and any abnormalities) of the esophagus, stomach, and intestines. *See* DIGESTIVE SYSTEM.

Upper GI Series. Examination of the upper gastrointestinal tract, the esophagus, stomach, and duodenum, may be accomplished with a barium sulfate drink. A person takes the drink and the doctor follows the progress of the barium using a series of x-rays. The health of the swallowing mechanism may also be observed using a form of radiography that can image the process in real time (fluroscopy). An upper GI series may be completed in half an hour, though some preparation by the patient is required. If the small intestine is also studied, a barium test may require several hours. An upper GI series is used to diagnose:

- foreign bodies within the GI tract;
- tumors or polyps;
- ulcers;
- constrictions or strictures;
- fistulas—abnormal connections between parts of the GI tract;
- reflux;
- achalasia—an inability of the esophagus to move food into the stomach;
- hiatal hernia— a part of the stomach protruding into the esophagus.

ALERT

Emergencies and Barium X-Rays

Irregular bowel movements, vomiting blood or bile, upper or lower abdominal pain or blood, mucus, or pus in the stool, could indicate a serious condition, particularly if symptoms appear suddenly or are accompanied by weight loss. Similarly, persistent difficulty swallowing may indicate an esophageal disorder of benign or malignant origin. Medical attention should be sought immediately. A complete diagnostic workup of the GI tract—barium studies followed by more direct means of viewing affected areas—will allow for a definitive diagnosis.

Barium Enema. The lower intestine may be examined using a barium sulfate enema. In this procedure, the large bowel is filled with a barium solution. Two methods exist. The first, known as single contrast, fills the bowel with barium alone. The second, known as double contrast, includes air with the barium, to further distend the bowel. The radiologist examines the results with respect to the filling and passage of barium through the colon.

A barium enema is used to diagnose:

- tumors;
- polyps;
- ulcers;
- obstructions;
- twisted loops of intestine;
- diverticulitis—inflamed sacs or pouches in the walls of the colon;
- ulcerative colitis—inflammation of the colon with patches of ulceration;
- irritable colon;
- damage to the veins of the colon.

RISKS

Several health conditions may prevent the safe use of barium studies, including severe ulcerative colitis, perforation of the gut.

PREPARATION

While both the barium swallow and barium enema are simple, relatively painless procedures, their success depends on proper preparation. For a barium swallow test, the patient should not eat or drink after midnight on the evening before the test.

The barium enema requires a low-residue diet for one to three days preceding the test. The patient should drink as much water as possible 12 to 24 hours before the test, and take laxatives on the afternoon before the test. Patients should obtain the specific preparations preferred by the radiologist performing the test and follow those instructions carefully.

Related information about other diagnostic techniques can be found in CAT SCAN; MRI; PET SCANNING; SCANNING TECHNIQUES; ULTRASOUND SCANNING; *and* X RAY. *Disorders that barium x-bays are used to diagnose include* COLITIS; DIVERTICULITIS; POLYP; TUMOR; *and* ULCERATIVE COLITIS.

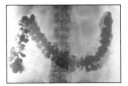

Barium X-Ray. Since it is opaque to x rays, barium sulfate is a helpful tool in diagnosing digestive system disorders. Patients drink a solution and then a doctor follows its passage through the body in a series of x rays, helping to identify trouble areas and abnormalities. Above, the barium solution is coursing though the large intestine.

Barotrauma

Injury to the middle ear due to change in atmosphere or water pressure.

Barotrauma is a condition in which a sudden change of air or water pressure causes damage to the middle ear. This may advance to a ruptured eardrum. It often occurs when a person with an ear, nose, or throat infection travels on a plane.

Cause. The inner ear and outer ear are separated by the eardrum, a thin membrane that vibrates in response to sound. The ear drum will often become damaged if there is a sudden change in the air pressure or water pressure. The eustachian tube maintains equal air pressure at all times. If the outside air pressure suddenly increases or decreases, air must move rapidly through the eustachian tube in order to maintain equilibrium.

Aircraft always depressurize before takeoff. This process lowers the air pressure in the ear as well. The aircraft is later repressurized for landing, which causes a sharp rise in air pressure in the ear canal. In healthy people, air then rushes in through the eustachian tube and balances the pressure difference. This process can be hastened if a person chews, swallows, or breathes out lightly while holding the mouth and nose closed.

Normally, a person will not suffer barotrauma as a result of a regular airline flight. However, a person with congested sinuses may not be able to equalize pressure inside and outside the ear and may suffer some damage. Scuba divers also are in danger of barotrauma; their risk is more serious than with airline passengers.

Symptoms. Symptoms of barotrauma include pain in the ear and some degree of hearing loss. Some people may also experience ringing in the ear (tinnitus); pain in the sinuses (barosinusitis); and a pus-filled or bloody discharge from the ear. Usually these symptoms disappear by themselves in a few days. If the pain persists or if there is sign of infection, a health care professional should be consulted.

Prevention. It is best not to fly with congested sinuses. If flying is necessary, a physician may prescribe a decongestant nasal spray to be used before the airplane takes off or lands. *See also* AVIATION MEDICINE; EAR; SPACE MEDICINE; *and* TINNITUS.

Barrett's Esophagus

A condition in which the normal lining of the esophagus is damaged and replaced by a layer of cells similar to those lining the intestines.

In Barrett's esophagus, the esophageal lining is initially damaged by persistent acid reflux from the stomach, eventually causing a transformation from esophageal to intestinal cells, called intestinal metaplasia. The new layer of cells can resist further effects from exposure to the acid, but inflammation may cause the interior passageway of the esophagus to narrow. New linings may also develop ulcers that may cause bleeding or trouble swallowing.

There is no cure for Barrett's esophagus, but further damage can be prevented by stopping acid reflux. Lifestyle changes, such as eating small meals, losing weight, and taking antacid drugs such as ranitidine are recommended. Barrett's esophagus is associated with an increased risk of cancer. Periodic endoscopy is recommended to increase the chances of early detection and treatment. *See also* ESOPHAGUS.

Barrier Methods of Contraception

Any method of contraception that prevents sperm from entering the uterus during sexual intercourse.

The various types of barrier methods of contraception include condoms, both male and female, diaphragms, cervical caps, and vaginal creams and jellies.

Vaginal creams and jellies can be used separately or in conjunction with either a diaphragm or cervical cap. Used alone, they are not as effective as any of the other types of barrier contraceptives.

Condoms. Today, condoms come in male (below) and female varieties. Female condoms are still relatively new on the market, especially when compared to the male condom, which can be traced back to the 13th century. The more popular male type of condom, which is usually made of latex, is rolled over the tip of the erect penis before intercourse begins. A reservoir at the end is designed to catch and hold sperm and prevent it from entering the partner's body. Condoms can effectively prevent the transmission of sexually transmitted diseases as well as prevent conception.

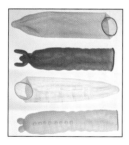

The **male condom,** sometimes called the male prophylactic, is used to prevent semen from entering the vagina. Often made of latex, a type of rubber, it is rolled over the erect penis and contains a reservoir—a space in the tip—to hold the sperm upon ejaculation. Condoms can also be made of materials such as lamb intestine, but those are more porous and therefore not as effective as their latex counter- parts. Most condoms also contain a spermicide. If used correctly, condoms are 99 percent effective in preventing pregnancy.

Condoms can be used with additional lubricant, but only water-based substances should be used, as petroleum-based materials may weaken the condom and lead to breakage. A fresh condom must be put on prior to each incident of intercourse.

The **female condom,** which lines the vagina, has a similar construction to its male counterpart. It is larger and is held in place with a ring. The failure rate of the female condom is higher than that of the male condom, however, these two methods can be used at the same time.

The **diaphragm** is a dome-shaped rubber cup that fits over the cervix and prevents sperm from entering into the uterus. It is filled with a contraceptive cream or jelly that contains a spermicide. The diaphragm, which must be fitted by a medical practitioner, should cover the entire cervix without causing any discomfort. If it causes any discomfort at all, a gynecologist should be contacted immediately. Neither the woman nor her partner should be able to feel it if it is properly positioned.

The diaphragm must be inserted prior to intercourse and should remain in place for at least 8 hours afterwards but not more than 24 hours. If more than one instance of intercourse occurs while the diaphragm is in place, additional spermicide must be inserted into the vagina.

The diaphragm needs to be refitted after a woman gives birth, has an abortion, or a miscarriage, or if a woman has gained or lost more than ten pounds. Some doctors recommend refitting every year, whether or not any of these events have taken

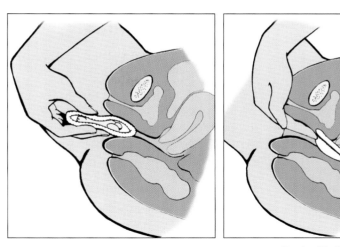

place. The diaphragm has an effectiveness rate of between 80 and 90 percent when it is used properly.

The **cervical cap** is a smaller and more rigid version of the diaphragm. It fits directly over the cervix and, just like the diaphragm, it must be fitted by a health care professional. A contraceptive cream or jelly must be used as well. The cap should be inserted before intercourse and left in place for at least 8 hours afterwards, but not longer than 48 hours. It is comparably effective to a diaphragm.

The **contraceptive sponge**, as its name implies, is a small sponge filled with spermicide. It is inserted into the vagina, near the cervix, prior to intercourse. Unlike the diaphragm or cervical cap, it does not need to be fitted by a medical practitioner. It is 80 to 90 percent effective, but is currently unavailable in the United States.

Contraceptive creams, foams, and jellies contain spermicide. They are usually used in conjunction with diaphragms or cervical caps, but can also be used alone. When placed in the vagina, they both physically block sperm from entering the reproductive tract and also kill any sperm that they come in contact with. They have an effectiveness rate of about 60 percent.

Barrier Methods. Any device that prevents sperm from entering the uterus during intercourse falls under the category of a barrier method of contraception. There are many different options, including the diaphragm (above), a dome shaped rubber cap that is inserted into the vagina before sex. A diaphragm covers the cervix and stops sperm from penetrating the uterus, where it could, potentially, fertilize an egg. Other barrier methods include the cervical cap, which works much like the diaphragm; the contraceptive sponge; and the condom, which is available for males and females.

Background information about specific Barrier Methods of Contraception *can be found in* Contraception; Condom; *and* Sponge, Contraceptive. *Articles about other methods of contraception include* Natural Contraception; Oral Contraceptives; *and* Pregnancy. *For more information about* Pregnancy, *see* Delivery *and* Pregnancy Counseling.

Bartholin's Glands

Small glands that secrete a lubricating fluid in the vagina during sexual arousal.

Bartholin's glands, named for the Danish anatomist Kasper Bartholin, are located to the left and right of the entrance of the vagina. Usually, these glands are only noteworthy if they become blocked or infected, as with gonorrhea. Any blockage of the gland opening will result in the formation of an abscess. Sometimes a cyst may form afterwards and need to be removed surgically. As with any infection, the condition is treated with antibiotics. An abscess may need to be lanced. *See also* GONORRHEA.

Basal Cell Carcinoma

Skin cancer originating in the basal cells, the innermost layer of the skin.

Basal cell carcinoma is the most prevalent form of skin cancer in the United States, accounting for 75 to 90 percent of the more than one million nonmelanoma cancers diagnosed each year.

TYPES

About half of all cases of basal cell carcinoma are nodular cancers that are flesh-colored or translucent nodes. These can form crusts or ulcerate. Less common are superficial lesions, red and scaly patches with the appearance of psoriasis. A smaller percentage of cases are morpheaform lesions, which are off-white or yellow areas that resemble scar tissue. Least common are pigmented lesions, which are darker than the skin surrounding them.

INCIDENCE AND CAUSES

Skin cancer is rarely found in persons with dark skin. Persons at highest risk are those over the age of 50 with fair skin who live in very sunny or tropical regions. The risk is believed to be directly related to the amount of exposure to ultraviolet radiation, partly from home sun lamps or tanning salons, but mostly from solar radi-

Basal Cell Carcinoma. The skin cancer known as basal cell carcinoma can appear as a ruptured skin sore. These lesions can appear anywhere on the skin, including the face, ears, lips, arms, legs, or torso. The above image shows a lesion characteristic of basal cell carcinoma that is about one and a half millimeters long.

ation. Chronic, unprotected exposure to sunlight early in life causes a significant increase in the risk of basal cell carcinoma and other skin cancers in adulthood. Basal cell carcinoma occurs in several forms—each produces a distinctive lesion.

SYMPTOMS

About 80 percent of basal cell carcinomas occur on the head and neck, although they also can occur on the chest, back, hands, or other parts of the body. The warning signs of basal cell carcinoma are a sore or mark on the skin with an appearance, size, shape, or thickness that changes with time; a new growth that does not heal in a few weeks; a sore or spot that itches, hurts, erodes, or bleeds persistently; or a persistent skin ulcer of unknown cause.

TREATMENT

Basal cell carcinomas can be treated with surgical removal or with radiation therapy, and a complete cure is quite common. Left untreated, basal cell carcinoma will gradually grow into the underlying structures. Such growths usually are not life-threatening, as they rarely spread to any other parts of the body. They can, however, be very destructive locally. The risk of additional skin cancers is high in people who do not take preventive measures, most notably protecting themselves against exposure to the sun. This can inconvenience those living in tropical regions.

PREVENTION

The most obvious protective measure against basal cell carcinoma is to stay out of direct sunlight. Those who cannot avoid exposure should wear protective clothing, especially hats, and should use sunscreen products, with a sun-protective factor (SPF) of 15 or higher, and coverage reapplied every few hours.

Articles vital to an understanding of Basal Cell Carcinoma include AGING; CANCER; CARCINOMA; CARCINOMATOSIS; SKIN; SKIN CANCER; SQUAMOUS CELL CARCINOMA; and TUMOR. For related information about the effects of the sun see SUNBURN; SUNLIGHT, ADVERSE EFFECTS OF; and SUNTAN.

Basal Ganglia

The large collection of nerve cells in the cerebral cortex of the brain that are responsible for the movement of the body.

The basal ganglia work with the cerebellum to produce smooth, coordinated movement. The nerves in the cerebellum cause excitation of nerve signals, while the nerves in the basal ganglia cause inhibition of signals. When the two structures work together in a balanced fashion, controlled movement is possible. Studies of neurological disorders suggest that the basal ganglia are extremely important to the first stages of initiating movement. *See* BALANCE.

Degeneration or injury to the basal ganglia can result in trembling, shaking, physical weakness, and involuntary movements. Parkinson's disease and Huntington's chorea are neurological disorders that affect the basal ganglia. *See also* BRAIN.

Basal Metabolic Rate

The amount of energy required to sustain the operations of the body at rest.

The basal metabolic rate, BMR, is the caloric expenditure of an organism at rest. It is measured in calories, or joules, per square meter of body surface per hour, and represents the minimum amount of energy required to maintain life at normal body temperature. The basal metabolic rate is usually calculated by measuring the oxygen and carbon dioxide exchange of the resting body at room temperature 12 to 14 hours after a meal. The more oxygen consumed per unit of time, the higher the individual's body metabolism.

The basal metabolic rate is controlled mainly by hormones. The endocrine hormones that control the basal metabolic rate include epinephrine, norepinephrine, insulin, and corticosteroid hormones. Thyroid hormones also control the basal metabolic rate, and these hormones regulate many of the chemical processes that occur in the body.

In the past, the BMR was widely used to assess thyroid function because thyroid hormones are the prime regulators of tissue oxygen consumption and metabolism. However, new procedures for thyroid measurement have made the BMR obsolete as a test of thyroid function. *See also* HORMONES *and* METABOLISM.

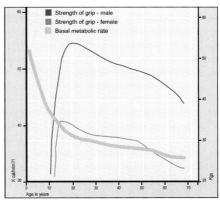

Baseball Elbow & Finger

Overuse of the forearm muscles, resulting in tissue inflammation around the elbow (baseball elbow) or an injury in which a heavy blow bends the finger out of position (baseball finger).

Baseball Elbow. This condition occurs when the cartilage lining the elbow joint is damaged by the over extension of the forearm, so that spurs may form in the tissue, limiting motion or breaking off and forming loose flakes. Repeated pitching or hitting may cause such an overextension. This leads to friction between the exposed areas of bone and loose cartilage, which can inhibit motion. Baseball elbow can also be caused by a single extreme action that tears the cartilage. Surgery can repair the torn tendon and remove loose flakes of cartilage. Baseball elbow can be avoided, and damage reduced through strength training and warm-ups. Learning proper mechanics will also reduce the risk of injury. Also, this condition is not limited to baseball; any activity that leads to an overextension may bring about this condition.

Baseball Finger. Usually a sports-related injury, baseball finger occurs when a baseball—or a ball from any sport such as basketball, football, or stickball—hits the tip of the finger at a very high speed. The finger is bent, tearing the tendon or possibly pulling off a fragment of bone. The affected finger may be splinted while it is healing, or a wire may be inserted through the bones to keep the finger straight while it heals. *See also* SPORTS MEDICINE.

Basal Metabolic Rate. There are a number of formulas that will calculate basal metabolic rate with varying degrees of accuracy; the outcome depends on height, weight, and age. Strength development in males is slightly greater than in females but, regardless of sex, the body's basal metabolic rate declines with age. Sometimes, dieters will go below their suggested basal metabolic rate; this is always a poor health decision.

B Cell

Also known as B lymphocyte

A type of lymphocyte, or white blood cell, that binds to antigens and produces antibodies.

When stimulated by an invading substance—an antigen—B cells differentiate into plasma cells. The plasma cells then produce antibodies against the antigen. *See also* BLOOD *and* IMMUNE SYSTEM.

BCG

Also known as Bacillus Calmette-Guerin vaccination

A vaccination against tuberculosis that is routinely administered in many countries, but not the U.S.

The BCG vaccination against tuberculosis is not recommended in the United States because it is an imperfect preventative. It is also used to treat some forms of bladder cancer. The vaccine is derived from a bovine microbe that is similar to the human microbe, but not exactly the same. There is still some risk of TB infection.

The Center for Disease Control recommends that the BCG vaccine be given only under specialized circumstances—namely to children with negative tuberculin skin-test results who are at very high risk for TB but who cannot be given newer vaccines or therapies. *See also* VACCINATIONS.

The BCG vaccination is not recommended for people with an impaired immune response or people who had had their immune system supressed.

HIV infection should be ruled out before the vaccine is given. Although no harmful effects of BCG on the fetus have been observed, the vaccine is generally not administered to pregnant women. The BCG immunization itself may cause a positive reaction to the skin test for TB. However, a person who was given the vaccine is still more likely to exhibit a positive result due to an authentic TB infection for a number of reasons, including:

- if the person was vaccinated a long time ago;
- if there was recent contact with someone with infectious TB;
- if the person comes from an area where TB is common; and
- if a chest radiograph findings show evidence of previous TB.

The BCG vaccination is still recommended for travelers in areas where there is a high rate of TB. *See also* TUBERCULOSIS.

Bedbug

Blood-sucking insect, whose saliva produces irritation and small ulcerations to the skin.

Bedbugs are small insects belonging to the family Cimicidae. The common species known to prey on humans in temperate regions, *Cimex lectularis*, mostly feeds at night, while spending the day in crevices in walls or in bedding. Bedbugs are reddish brown, oval, flat, wingless, and a little less than a quarter of an inch long.

The bedbug bite is not known to transmit disease, although it may cause a raised temperature. Normally, the bites cause skin irritation and occasionally infection. When a human host is unavailable, the parasite may prey on other mammals or poultry and may live for up to a year without feeding. Bedbugs mature from eggs over the course of two months in warm climates, and several generations per year may be produced. Control includes proper hygiene and spraying, steaming, or fumigating infested furniture. *See also* PARASITE.

Bed, Hospital

A bed with three sections used in hospitals for a prescribed period of time as part of the recuperation process.

A traditional hospital bed is designed to meet the needs of hospital patients and other sick people. The bed has a frame with three sections, each of which can be raised. The design allows caretakers to elevate the patient's head, legs, or midsection. Hospital beds also have guard-rails that can be raised or lowered. New beds often have modified the traditional design.

Bedbugs. These crawling insects will invade the home, suck blood, and cause skin ulcerations. They generally feed at night, while spending their days in the walls or in the bed's crevices. Proper hygiene and regular fumigation will rid a house of these pests.

Hospitals are often compared by the number of beds they contain. The bed-occupancy index is the percentage of available beds per unit and is a useful measurement used for many purposes.

Bed rest is an essential treatment for illnesses such as rheumatic fever, diseases with infectious periods (measles and chicken pox), and various injuries such as fractured vertebrae or ruptured disks.

Prolonged rest may subject a patient to bedsores, muscle deterioration, back soreness, weakness, lethargy, and depression. Bed rest can cause some calcium loss and bone demineralization, and it can foster development of calculi (stones) in the urinary tract. Postoperative bedridden patients may develop blood clots due to slow blood flow (deep vein thrombosis), and elderly patients are susceptible to gravity-induced (hypostatic) pneumonia. Patients are encouraged to be physically active as soon as possible in order to prevent complications from prolonged bed rest. *See also* Bedsores *and* Hospitals, Types of.

Bedsores

Lesions or sores caused by unrelieved pressure by an external object and resulting in damage to underlying tissue.

A bedsore, or pressure ulcer, goes through four stages. The first stage involves redness, which disappears on pressure. In stage two, swelling, redness, induration, blistering, or opening occurs. The skin starts to die (becomes necrotic) in stage three, and the necrosis extends through the tissue into the bone in stage four. Unrelieved pressure can affect the superficial tissue, the muscles, and the bone. Often bedsores result in prolonged hospitalization.

Causes. Bedsores may be caused by pressure from infrequent turning, friction or the irritation that comes from uncomfortable supports or wrinkled bedding, trauma to the skin, moisture on or near the skin, disuse atrophy (wasting away of muscle or tissue), infection, malnutrition, anemia (condition marked by low amounts of hemoglobin in the blood) spasticity (a rigidity in a group of muscles), and the loss of pain and pressure sensations due to spinal cord injury. The most commonly affected areas are the sacrum—a bone in the lower spine— the buttocks, and tissue over the heels.

Treatment for bedsores consists primarily of preventive techniques: increased circulation; adequate nutrition; increased activity; and relief of pressure. Physical therapy, keeping the skin clean and dry, and making sure the bony prominence do not rub together will also help patients to avoid the condition. Wheelchair patients should change position every 15 minutes to prevent bedsores. *See also* Bed, Hospital.

Behavior Therapy

Therapeutic approach that attempts to alleviate symptoms by addressing them directly rather than analyzing their cause.

Behavior therapy is one aspect of the more comprehensive study of cognitive behavior therapy. This sort of therapy is appropriate and has proven effective for two types of problems.

When specific symptoms are present, such as a phobia or obsessive-compulsive disorder or, in the case of sexual problems like premature ejaculation or impotence, an approach that addresses these symptoms may have a more immediate effect than one that analyzes them. An additional reason to treat these symptoms with the direct behavioral approach is that there may be an urgency to alleviating a symptom that interferes with a patient's ability to function. Self-destructive behaviors, including nail biting, smoking, and alcohol abuse, respond well to behavior therapy. In these situations, operant conditioning is the preferred treatment approach.

TYPES

Desensitization is the process of exposing a patient to a feared situation or object in a controlled manner that allows the individual to understand the association between

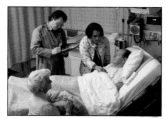

Modern Hospital Beds. Above, a modern hospital bed that can reduce the incidence of bedsores, such as those below, will also provide easy access for doctors to treat patients.

Bedsore Sites. The use of modern hospital beds (such as the one pictured above) will reduce the incidence of the lesions and sores caused by unrelieved pressure. When incapacitated, people lie in one position for long periods, lesioning the underlying tissue on the back of the head, top of the back, and at the lumbar region near the buttocks.

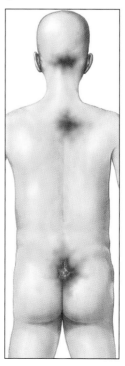

the feared situation (stimulus) and their anxiety reaction. In this way it can be treated and alleviated. For example, the process may begin by having a person afraid of flying start by imagining being in an airport and eventually progress to taking a flight. Flooding, a related treatment, is a process in which the patient is immediately forced to endure her or his greatest fear and remain in that situation until the fear subsides. This is risky, however, and may have undesirable consequences.

Operant conditioning is a therapy that attempts to change behavior by rewarding an individual's positive behaviors and punishing self-destructive or problematic behavior. These procedures tend to reward rather than punish, especially with children, who are often treated with token economy. For example, tokens are given to children who respond appropriately to a certain stimulus; these tokens can be traded in at a later time for rewards.

Biofeedback, often used in treating migraine headaches and other types of intractable pain, helps a patient control unconscious physiological responses by monitoring them. For example, a patient hooked up to a biofeedback monitor will hear sounds that indicate an increase in muscle tension, heart rate, and blood pressure. By becoming aware of the process by which the pain develops and progresses, a patient may learn to short circuit the process. *See also* ALTERNATIVE MEDICINE; BIO-FEEDBACK; *and* PSYCHOTHERAPY.

Behcet's Syndrome

Chronic, multisystem disease that causes inflammation of small blood vessels throughout the body.

Behcet's syndrome is a disease with many symptoms, and is most common in the Middle East and Japan. It can affect all organs, as well as the nervous system.

Primary symptoms of the disorder include recurrent mouth ulcerations, genital ulcers, eye lesions, skin lesions, fatigue, fever, arthritis, and pain. If the disease affects the nervous system, it can lead to

speech problems, impaired balance, movement and memory loss, blindness, stroke, meningitis, spinal cord swelling, and intestinal complications. The cause of the disorder is unknown. Treatment for Behcet's syndrome is aimed at reducing pain and inflammation with antiinflammatory and immunosuppressive agents. *See* BLOOD.

Belching

Also known as burping

The release of swallowed air through the esophagus and mouth.

The main causes of belching air include eating too fast, wearing dentures, and chewing gum. It can also be a nervous habit. Drinking carbonated beverages can also contribute to gas in the stomach. Belching is a response to the bloated feeling in the stomach and may temporarily relieve indigestion or nausea, but it may in turn result in yet more air being swallowed. *See* STOMACH.

Belladonna

A plant of the nightshade family with leaves that are used for medicinal purposes.

Belladonna is a member of the nightshade family and is found in wooded areas across Europe and Asia. Its leaves are crushed and pressed and made into infusions or other preparations to treat a number of ailments from the common cold, flu, and high fever to dry mouth, nausea, and delirium. It contains two extremely potent substances—atropine and hyoscyamine, which act on the central nervous system, the smooth and cardiac muscles, and the secretory glands. These belladonna alkaloids are extractable from other plants in the nightshade family; the substances are used to treat the respiratory and cardiac system, as well as functioning as an antispasmodic.

Belladonna is also a highly toxic plant that, if ingested regularly, or in large amounts, may cause poisoning, resulting in glaucoma, esophageal reflux, prevention of stomach contractions, dry mouth, inability to urinate, fever, and memory loss. Children are particularly sensitive to atropine, and even low doses can be lethal. If belladonna poisoning is suspected, seek medical help immediately. Many homeopathic practitioners still prescribe belladonna; it is available over- the-counter in both liquid and tablet form. *See also* HOMEOPATHY.

Bends

Also known as decompression sickness

A life-threatening condition in which nitrogen bubbles form in the blood and body tissues, obstructing circulation.

The bends is a painful, sometimes life-threatening, condition. It is caused by the formation of nitrogen bubbles in the blood-stream and body tissues, resulting from a rapid reduction in the pressure of the air surrounding the body. It is most often experienced by divers who return too quickly to the surface of the water.

Causes and Symptoms. When the pressure outside the body decreases rapidly, nitrogen and other gases collect in bubbles in the blood vessels. These bubbles block the blood vessels and deprive the body of essential nutrients. As a result, during the 24 hour period following the dive, the individual may experience a tingling of the skin and alternating hot and cold sensations, followed by a loss of muscular control and pain that begins in the joints and spreads to other body areas. If the illness is sufficiently severe, the bends can lead to unconsciousness and even death. The condition may also lead to brain damage and possibly to bone destruction.

Treatment and Prevention. Apart from the most severe cases, the bends will subside if the affected person returns to a higher-pressure, lower-altitude environment. If necessary, a person can be treated with recompression in a sealed pressure chamber. The pressure in the chamber is raised and then lowered slowly, allowing the person to adjust to the reduction in air pressure. To avoid the bends, divers will sometimes breathe pure oxygen before and during their ascent. *See also* BLOOD.

Benign

Term designating a mild form of a disease or a nonmalignant growth.

A benign medical condition is one that does not pose a threat to life. In oncology, growths are designated as benign if they do not multiply rampantly. A benign growth is distinguished from one that is malignant. A malignant growth will grow without restraint and pose a danger to health and life. Determining whether a growth is benign or malignant is an essential element of medical diagnosis. Because benign growths may become malignant, they may be removed surgically, as is often done when a benign tumor on the mucous membrane of the intestinal tract is detected. *See also* CANCER; DIAGNOSIS; MALIGNANT; *and* ONCOLOGY.

Benzodiazepine Drugs

Also known as tranquilizers

A group of medications used to counteract anxiety and as a sleep aid.

They include chlordiazepoxide, better known as Librium; alprazolam (Xanax); diazepam, (Valium); clonazepam (Klonopin); temazepam(Restoril); and triazolam (Halcion); among others. They work by reducing signals passed between brain cells, thus slowing mental activity.

Benzodiazepine drugs may be prescribed as a short-term treatment for insomnia or anxiety. However, treatment of both these ailments should be aimed at the underlying cause rather than just at alleviating the symptoms.

These drugs are highly addictive both psychologically and physically and therefore should be taken with care. Mild withdrawal symptoms include nausea, anxiety, irritability and insomnia. If the addiction has progressed further, withdrawal can include convulsion, delirium, and seizures.

Drug interactions with alcohol, some antibiotics, and the heart drug digoxin are possible and extremely dangerous. *See also* ANXIETY; BRAIN; *and* INSOMNIA.

Bereavement

Feelings of loss and sadness experienced after the death of a loved one, beloved object, or body part.

Although much has been written about the emotional stages that one experiences after a loss, these stages are not universally the same. On first hearing of the loss, one may experience shock and denial, amplified in situations where the death followed an accident or brief illness. The initial numbness eases the difficulty in handling the arrangements involved in planning and organizing a funeral. At this stage, the bereaved may pick up a phone to call someone who has died or may even imagine seeing the person. The next stages involve a complex of emotions, including protest, anger at the loss or at the loved one for abandonment, and fear. Finally, in a healthy process of grieving, the loss is accepted and one will be able to move on with normal activities, utilizing the support of friends and family.

Danger Signs. To show no emotional reaction for some time after the loss of a loved one should be cause for concern, because in some way the grief will manifest itself later, and one cannot recover from a loss without mourning. Other signs to be concerned about include serious depression, an inability to make decisions, loss of appetite, giving away possessions, and an expression of wishes to die. If these reactions occur, outside help from a therapist or support group can prove valuable in ac-

cepting loss. Inappropriately intense or long-lasting grief that includes depression may require psychotherapy and perhaps even medication. *See also* DEATH.

Beriberi

Disease resulting from a deficiency of thiamine (vitamin B₁), which affects the nervous system.

Beriberi is a disease caused by a deficiency of thiamine, a nutrient essential to the metabolism of carbohydrates and proteins. Symptoms include muscular atrophy, anemia, leg muscle spasms, and paralysis.

Three main forms of the disease exist: wet beriberi, characterized by heart failure and tissue swelling; dry beriberi, which causes central nervous system manifestations, peripheral nerve dysfunction, and numbness in the hands and feet; and infantile beriberi, a leading cause of death in infants between two and five months old who live in rural areas where polished rice is a staple food. Beriberi is found all over the world, but in the U.S., it is most common among alcoholics; alcohol affects the nutrient absorption and displaces a healthy diet. Large doses of vitamin B₁ have proven beneficial for the prevention and tratment of beriberi. *See also* VITAMIN B.

Berylliosis

An occupational disease caused by inhalation of beryllium dust or fumes.

Beryllium is a metal used in the aerospace, electronics, and nuclear industries. Workers breathe it in because of improper ventilation. Short-term exposure may cause lung inflammation that results in coughing and loss of breath. Long-term exposure to small amounts of beryllium results in severe lung damage, leading to chronic breathing difficulties, and liver damage. Corticosteroid drugs can relieve some of the symptoms of berylliosis but can do nothing about damage to the lungs and liver, indicating the importance of preventive measures to keep beryllium out of the air in workplaces. *See also* LUNG.

How to Help When Someone You Care For Is Grieving

No one can completely understand the feelings of loss that another person experiences; everyone has a unique emotional makeup, nature of the relationship of the bereaved to the loved one, prior losses that may effect the bereaved's emotions, and life situation at the time of the loss. For this reason, telling someone that you "understand" is not a helpful response to grief. Being present while allowing the bereaved to express uncomfortable emotions, such as anger, pain, and anguish, is helpful. Remaining calm and not feeling embarrassed in the face of crying or bitterness is also a helpful way of accepting and sharing the pain of the bereaved. It is not helpful, however, to deny the person's grief with comments that suggest he or she will feel better soon or that it is best to move on now. Helping with chores around the house or cooking meals without waiting to be asked (except when specifically requested not to do so) will also be useful.

Beta-Blocker Drugs

A family of drugs that block adrenaline effects.

Beta-blockers reduce the impact of adrenaline, which responds to stress by narrowing blood vessels and increasing the heart rate. These drugs prevent the narrowing of the blood vessels and reduce the demands on the heart, lowering blood pressure. Beta-blockers control migraine headaches, angina, the effects of anxiety, irregular or rapid heartbeat, and high blood pressure.

These drugs are not addictive, but do need to be taken for relatively long periods of time before they are effective. In addition, since high blood pressure does not produce symptoms, the effect of beta-blockers may not be noticed except in lowering blood pressure. These drugs are very effective in reducing repeat heart attacks.

Side Effects. There are few side effects but they vary from person to person. They include nausea and vomiting, dizziness and light headedness, diarrhea, lowered libido, slowed heart rate, low blood pressure, cold hands or feet, depression, fatigue or weakness, sleep disturbances, and dizziness if the person rises from a prone position too rapidly. Less frequently, blurred vision and difficulty in breathing have been reported. People with asthma, slow heart rates, congestive heart failure or certain cases of diabetes should not use beta-blockers.

Since beta-blockers lower blood pressure and induce weakness and fatigue, those over 50 may find it hard to maintain exercise routines. If this last side-effect occurs adjust exercise levels accordingly. *See also* BLOOD *and* BLOOD PRESSURE.

ALERT

A Dangerous Combination

The combination of beta-blockers and injections of epinephrine can be extremely dangerous, since it may raise the blood pressure to very high levels. Also, nonsteroidal anti-inflammatory drugs like Tylenol or aspirin can negate the effects of beta-blockers. Do not stop taking beta-blockers abruptly, since that can cause a spike in blood pressure and result in a heart attack or a stroke.

Betamethasone

A synthetic corticosteroid used to treat swelling allergic reactions, asthma, and arthritis.

Corticosteroids are hormones produced in the adrenal glands that control inflammation, maintain blood-sugar levels, and control blood pressure and water balance in the circulatory system. Synthetic corticosteroids are prescribed to replace corticosteroids that the body is not producing, to prevent rejection of transplanted organs, or to treat some inflammatory diseases. This drug can be taken orally as a pill or a liquid; it is also available as a lotion. Short-term use is unlikely to produce side effects, but long-term use can result in bloody stools, confusion, eye pain, ulcers, fever, sore throat, urinary frequency, thirst, irregular heartbeat, and depression. *See* HORMONES.

Bezoar

Foreign matter in the stomach or intestine.

There are several types of bezoars. Lactobezoars are formed out of clumps of undigested milk; they are often found in infants fed on formula high in calcium. A bezoar made of vegetable matter is called a phytobezoar. Trichobezoars are composed of ingested hair (hairball). This disorder is more common in emotionally disturbed and mentally retarded children. Bezoars are also found in adults who have had part of their stomach removed.

Symptoms. Often, with small bezoars, there are no symptoms. Large bezoars may completely fill the stomach and cause indigestion, upset stomach, and vomiting. Persistent vomiting may lead to dehydration.

Treatment. A small bezoar may pass naturally, it can be removed with drugs that break it down, or it can be removed by endoscopy. A large bezoar may require surgery. If a child tends to pull or chew on hair, keep the hair trimmed short so the ends do not reach the mouth. Limit access to other fiber-filled materials. *See also* DEHYDRATION *and* STOMACH.

Bifocals

A lens that is split into two so that it treats both near and far-sightedness.

Usually, the top half of a bifocal lens lens is for distance viewing and the bottom half is for near objects. Progressive addition lenses (PALs) are becoming a favorite alternative to bifocals. PALs provide a progressive change in lens strength from top to bottom. They are easier to use because there is no line of image shift and they permit focus in the middle range. *See also* EYE.

Bile

A digestive substance that contributes to the digestion of fats, cholesterol, and fat-soluble vitamins.

Bile is secreted by the liver and is stored in the gallbladder. It is released through a duct to the first portion of the small intestine (duodenum), where it is used in the process of digestion. Its primary purpose is to break down (emulsify) large droplets of fats into smaller droplets, enabling digestive enzymes to work on them more efficiently. *See also* DIGESTIVE SYSTEM.

Bile is also responsible for the removal of some waste products from the body, including hemoglobin from degraded red blood cells and excess cholesterol. Bile salts increase the solubility of cholesterol, fats and fat-soluble vitamins, making it easier to absorb them. It also stimulates the small intestine to secrete water, thereby helping the contents move along more rapidly. Bile is excreted slowly from the body in the feces, giving them their characteristic color and odor. *See also* BILIARY SYSTEM; BILE-DUCT OBSTRUCTION; KIDNEY; *and* LIVER.

Bile-Duct Obstruction

Blockage in the duct that carries bile from the gallbladder to the small intestine.

Bile is produced in the liver, stored in the gallbladder, and released into the small intestine. The flow of bile may be impaired at any point along the way, resulting in an accumulation of bile in the liver and a lack of bile in the digestive tract. Impairment of bile flow is known as cholestasis.

Causes. Bile-duct obstruction is caused most often by the presence of gallstones in the bile-duct. In addition to gallstones, obstruction can also be caused by inflammation or scarring of the duct or the presence of a tumor. Problems with the pancreas, such as inflammation or cancer, may also obstruct the flow of bile.

Hemobilia is the presence of blood in the bile-duct, usually a result of trauma to the liver, which may form an obstructing clot. The clot may dissolve on its own or require surgical removal.

Primary sclerosing cholangitis is a disorder that hardens and thickens portions of the bile-duct walls, partially blocking the duct. It is often associated with other disorders such as chronic inflammatory bowel disease and ulcerative colitis.

Symptoms. The most common symptoms of this disorder include jaundice, chills, high fever, pain in the upper right portion of the abdomen, tea-colored urine, and light stools. The stool may also contain fat because the lack of bile interferes with fat digestion. Bone loss and a tendency to bleed easily may occur due to impaired absorption of several important nutrients.

Diagnosis. The presence and, often, the cause, of bile duct obstruction can be ascertained with noninvasive studies such as an ultrasound or a CT scan. Cholangiography is a contrast x-ray procedure used to provide images of the bile-duct by injecting contrast dye directly into it.

Treatment. In the case of gallstones, bile-duct obstruction is usually treated by an endoscopic procedure, followed by surgical removal of the gallbladder when the obstruction is still present—this prevents future problems. For obstructions caused by tumors, surgical removal is preferred, but in cases where the lesion is considered unremovable, a stent or drainage tube may be placed across the obstruction by a gastroenterologist or a radiologist. *See also* BILIARY CIRRHOSIS, PRIMARY; *and* HEPATITIS.

Biliary Atresia

A congenital condition in which the bile ducts fail to develop normally.

Bile, a fluid involved in digesting fat, is secreted by the liver and carried to the intestines through the bile-ducts. If the ducts are only partially developed or missing entirely, bile accumulates inside the liver, eventually entering the bloodstream and causing jaundice (yellowing of the skin).

Symptoms. The first symptoms of biliary atresia become noticeable when a newborn is approximately two weeks old. The urine becomes progressively darker, and feces are pale. The skin appears jaundiced, and the liver enlarges. By the time the infant is three months old, the symptoms have expanded to include stunted growth, itchiness, irritability, and high blood pressure in the portal vein. If left untreated, biliary cirrhosis—progressive and irreversible scarring of the liver—can occur.

Treatment. Surgery is performed to relieve the pressure of the bile accumulation in the liver and also to construct new bile-ducts. However, this procedure is possible in only 5 to 10 percent of infants with biliary atresia. The prognosis is good following this form of surgery. Other surgical procedures that may be performed involve repositioning the liver so its surface directly touches the intestine, enabling the bile to travel without ducts. In these cases, the prognosis is not as good. *See also* BILE.

Biliary Cirrhosis, Primary

Inflammation of the bile ducts in the liver, leading to eventual scarring and obstruction.

The cause of biliary cirrhosis is unknown, but the condition occurs frequently in people suffering from an autoimmune disease such as rheumatoid arthritis, scleroderma, or autoimmune thyroiditis. Women between the ages of 35 and 60 make up the majority of patients with biliary cirrhosis. In some cases, biliary cirrhosis is not a primary disease, but occurs as a result of prolonged bile-duct obstruction or congenital malformation of the bile-ducts.

Symptoms. Itching and fatigue are the initial symptoms, and it can be months or years until further symptoms appear. Later symptoms include an enlarged liver or spleen, fatty deposits in the skin or eyelids, pale or fatty stools, and abnormalities in the bones, kidneys, and nerves. Later, symptoms of liver cirrhosis develop. Many cases are discovered through blood testing before symptoms occur.

Treatment. There is no known cure for biliary cirrhosis, although the drug ursodiol has been shown to lessen the progression of the disease. Treatment is generally aimed at controlling the symptoms and reducing complications. The drug cholestyramine can be taken to control itching. Supplements of calcium and vitamins A, D, and K are needed, as they cannot be absorbed without adequate amounts of bile. Liver transplants are the best—and sometimes the only—option for patients in the most severe stages of the disease.

Prognosis. The progression of biliary cirrhosis varies among patients. Some patients experience a slowly worsening condition, while others develop severe cirrhosis in just a few years. Treatment can slow progression of the disease, prevent or delay complications, and prolong survival. *See also* BILE; BILIARY SYSTEM; KIDNEY; *and* LIVER.

Biliary Colic

Pain resulting from an obstructed flow of bile from the gallbladder.

Biliary colic may be caused by gallstones or inflammation. The pain may be intermittent, rising and then subsiding. Attacks usually begin 30 to 60 minutes after a meal, especially a meal high in fat content. The location of the pain may vary, but it is felt most often in the central upper abdomen. The pain may extend to the right shoulder blade. Other symptoms may include nausea, vomiting, chills, fever, and jaundice. Treatment involves the removal of the gallbladder. *See also* BILE; *and* BILIARY SYSTEM.

The Gallbladder. The gallbladder (top right) stores and concentrates bile before it is emptied into the the common bile duct and the duodenum (which is the first part of the intestine). Here, it is shown during surgery.

The Biliary System. The biliary system (shown at right) is a complex system of organs and ducts—connecting those organs to others—that breaks down the body's fats while producing and storing major bodily fluids, including, but not limited to, bile. Bile is stored in the gallbladder (a) and the liver (b), before traveling through the common bile duct (c) to the duodenum (d). The other four ducts include the cystic, hepatic, common, and pancreatic.

Biliary System

The liver, gallbladder, pancreas, ducts, and secretions that remove waste products from the body and break down fats.

The biliary system's role in the digestive process is to remove waste products from the liver and then render fat into a form that is suitable for processing by the lower digestive tract.

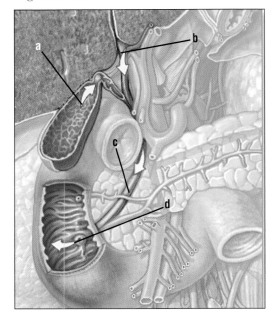

Bile. The biliary system's primary digestive product is bile (gall), a secretion from the liver that flows through the hepatic bile-ducts to the pear-shaped gallbladder. In the gallbladder, bile is concentrated to as little as ten percent of its original volume and stored one gram at a time. Bile in the gallbladder is much thicker, denser, and darker than the bile that comes from the liver. If the gallbladder is surgically removed, due to the formation of solid deposits called gallstones for example, then bile concen- tration decreases. This is not serious, however, since in a single day, the adult liver produces about three grams of bile, which contains water, cholesterol, a dark brown pigment called bilirubin, proteins, electrolytes, and salts.

Bile is effective in the breakdown of fats. With a pH of between 5 and 6, bile is acidic.

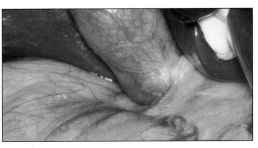

DIGESTION

After leaving the stomach, large drops of fat enter the the first part of the intestine, the C-shaped, foot-long duodenum. This triggers the pancreas to produce hormones that contract the gallbladder, squeezing out the bile into the common bile-duct, and to open the papilla of Vater that leads from the bile-duct into the duodenum. There the bile breaks down the fat into microscopic milky globules that are further broken down by a pancreatic enzyme (lipase) and easily absorbed by the intestinal walls. The duodenum receives partially digested materials from the stomach and bile from the gallbladder (via the bile-duct) so that it can begin absorbing nutrients before entering the next section of the intestine, the jejunum.

ABSORPTION

When no more bile is required, the gallbladder relaxes and returns to its regular activities of collecting bile. Approximately 5 percent of the bile exits the body in the feces, while the remaining 95 percent is absorbed by the intestines, passed into the bloodstream, and circulated back to the liver. Any minor amount of bile that is lost can easily be replaced by the liver, if it is functioning normally. Women, obese individuals, and people over the age of 60 are at particular risk of the bile crystallizing into stones while in the gallbladder. Gallstones are painless at first but may cause blockage and extreme pain. They often require surgical removal.

Background information about organs vital to the BILIARY SYSTEM *include* BILIRUBIN; GALLBLADDER; INTESTINE; LIVER; *and* PANCREAS. *Related topics of interest include* DIGESTIVE SYSTEM; ENZYME; *and* PROTEINS. *See also* JAUNDICE.

Bilirubin

A by-product of the process in which enzymes break down hemoglobin in dead or aging red blood cells. Excessive bilirubin is a strong indicator of liver malfunction.

Produced in the bone marrow, spleen, and elsewhere in the body, bilirubin is a product of hemoglobin, the substance that carries oxygen in the blood. When red blood cells age and die, the white blood cells break the hemoglobin into its component parts, heme and globin. The heme is converted into bilirubin, which is filtered out in the liver and excreted through the bile-ducts to the gallbladder. By this time, bilirubin is a dark brown pigment that turns the bile yellow and the feces brown.

Bilirubin in the Blood. Normally, only a small amount of bilirubin is present in the blood at any given time. The level rises when red blood cells are destroyed or, more often, when the liver does not process bilirubin as rapidly as it usually does. Starvation, stress, or an underlying illness can also cause such an increase. The excess bilirubin is deposited in the skin and whites of the eyes, resulting in the jaundice characteristic of liver disease. Bilirubin is also excreted by the kidneys, imparting a dark color to the urine.

Jaundice. Fetal hemoglobin is broken down around the time of birth. The relatively immature liver of a newborn often cannot process the bilirubin, resulting in a very mild and temporary form of jaundice. Most infant jaundice is resolved on its own as the baby's feeding schedule and bowel functions improve. Very high levels of bilirubin can lead to kernicterus, a type of brain damage.

Bilirubin Diagnostics. Measuring the amount of bilirubin in the blood is one of a number of diagnostic tests for liver function. Elevated bilirubin levels may be an indication of an obstruction in the bile-duct, liver damage, or the breakdown of an excessive number of red blood cells (hemolytic anemia). *See also* ANEMIA; BLOOD; DIAGNOSIS; JAUNDICE; *and* SPLEEN.

Billings' Method

A method of family planning that may be used to avoid or induce pregnancy, based on natural cycles of fertility and infertility.

Devised by a pair of Australian physicians, the Billings' Ovulation Method of Family Planning has been encouraged by some as a low-cost method of contraception, particularly for those whose religious convictions prohibit other forms of birth control. The Billings' method requires a detailed log to be kept at the end of each day, recording cervical mucus leaving the vagina and the condition of the vulva. By this means, the condition of fertility is evaluated. Some critics of the procedure question the level of protection it affords, particularly if instructions are not properly understood or faithfully observed. *See also* OVULATION.

Billroth's Operation

The surgical removal of the lower part of the stomach; it is the same as a partial gastrectomy.

This type of gastrectomy was originated by the Prussian born Viennese surgeon Theodor Billroth (b. 1829–d. 1894) in 1881. Billroth was a strong proponent of using antiseptics in surgical practice to prevent infections, a practice that permanently changed how operations were henceforth performed.

Considered a founder of modern surgery, Theodor Billroth was the first person to successfully remove the bottom half of the stomach and reattach the remaining piece to the first portion of the intestine (duodenum). A similar treatment is still used today for peptic ulcers and some gastric tumors. If the duodenum is also damaged, that too may be removed and the jejunum attached to the stomach. *See also* GASTRIC TUMOR *and* STOMACH.

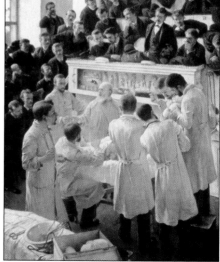

Billroth's Operation. Pictured below is an illustration of Theodor Billroth performing a partial gastrectomy in front of a classroom full of eager students. While such teaching procedures have been common since the middle of the 19th century, Theodor Billroth made surgical history when he successfully developed this operation and many talented students were eager to learn from him.

Biofeedback. This form of relaxation therapy involves concentrating on one's own body functions while they are monitored by a machine. The device aids people in learning how to regulate breathing, heart rate, and blood pressure. Pioneered in the 1930s, the method gained popularity in the 1960s when Dr. Barbara Brown began using it in her research. Today, it is used for stress-related conditions and to monitor chronic pain.

Biofeedback/Biofeedback Training

A form of relaxation therapy where the client's vital functions are monitored by a biofeedback device.

The objective of biofeedback training is to teach a person to regulate his or her unconscious bodily functions (breathing, heart rate, blood pressure) to treat a specific condition, and to improve an individual's health. Pioneered in 1938 by O. Hobert Mowrer, biofeedback gained widespread attention when, in the late 1960s, Dr. Barbara Brown used it to regulate the "altered states" of a number of yogis.

METHOD

"Biofeedback training" is based on the premise that an individual may learn to consciously regulate his or her own biological systems when immediate information about how that system is functioning is available. When an individual is relaxed, he or she will tend to have warm skin, produce little sweat, and have a fairly slow and even heart rate. A biofeedback device can detect the slightest alteration in a person's vital signs and will offer an accurate reading of this information. A skilled biofeedback practitioner will help the patient with analysis of the readings and assists the patient in stabilizing these functions. For example, to regulate an individual's heart rate, a person would work with a biofeedback device designed to display a blinking light or beep for each heartbeat. Over time, the client learns to alter the rate of the signal by consciously controlling her or his heart beat in order to achieve a state of physical relaxation.

There are a number of different kinds of monitoring devices used to measure the

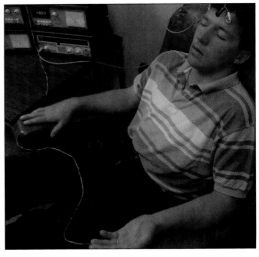

body's functions. They include an ST device to monitor skin temperature, a GSR to monitor galvanic skin response, an EMG (electro-myogram) to gauge muscle tension, and an EEG (electroencephalogram) used to measure brain-wave activity.

Biofeedback and Back Pain

For back pain, many people turn to biofeedback techniques. Many new clinics that deal with pain management, both in the private sector and those affiliated with hospitals, have an experienced staff of psychiatrists and psychologists teaching the methods of biofeedback. The process may take many weeks to learn, but patients come out of the classes with new knowledge about how they experience pain and, more importantly, how to transform their perception of it. Learning to control pain and heat to regulate bodily functions improves the quality of life and lifestyle of many patients.

Patient Participation

Biofeedback is an active treatment that requires the patient's participation. During a biofeedback session, an individual will first be asked some questions about family history and general health, then sensors that monitor body function will be applied to various places on the body, depending on the disorder that is being treated. A therapist will work with the patient to develop mental exercises to treat their specific disorder. Once a patient learns the most affective mental patterns, they can be practiced without the aid of a biofeedback device.

APPLICATIONS AND TREATMENT

Biofeedback has proven beneficial in treating a number of disorders, especially stress-related conditions. Upon completion of treatment, most biofeedback patients are able to recognize the symptoms of their condition and may alleviate them through their learned methods of regulation and relaxation.

See ALTERNATIVE MEDICINE; BRAIN; *and* MIND-BODY MEDICINE *for further discussions. Information may be found in* MEDITATION; *and* YOGA. *Details on applications will be found in* BACK PAIN; EPILEPSY; PAIN RELIEF; *and* STRESS.

Bioflavonoids

Color pigments and antioxidants in nutrients.

There are about a thousand different bioflavonoids, which act as coloring pigments, throughout the plant kingdom. Bioflavonoids also work as antioxidants against environmental toxins. Their potential role in cancer and heart disease prevention is currently under investigation. The most popular bioflavonoids include rutin, quercetin, and hesperidin; dietary supplements are available in both powdered and pill forms. A diet high in certain fruits and vegetables will provide large amounts of bioflavonoids. *See also* ALLERGIES; ALTERNATIVE MEDICINE; DIETARY FIBER; VITAMIN A; *and* VITAMIN C.

Biomechanical Engineering

The use of engineering principles to understand biological systems.

Biomechanical engineering applies the principles of mechanical engineering to the study of the human body. The goals are to understand the body from a mechanical standpoint and to use that knowledge to help treat human disease. Artificial organs, medical instrumentation, and pacemakers were all developed as a result of the study of biomechanical engineering.

Application to Medicine. Biomechanical engineers study a diverse range of health-related topics, which include gait and locomotion, the cardiovascular system, sports medicine, prosthetics, orthopedics, and neural control over locomotion. Generally, biomechanical engineers integrate biology, clinical medicine, and mechanical engineering. Clinical and biological data provide the starting point for biomechanical inquiry. Once biological data and engineering knowledge are used to develop a theoretical framework, mathematical modeling, biological experimentation, and computer simulations are often used to test the applications of the theory. The design

and evaluation of medical devices is a common aspect of biomechanical research.

In the study of prostheses, for example, a biomechanical engineer might evaluate the mechanical and chemical properties of the materials used in a prosthetic device and monitor whether or not the device has the desired effects. In order to develop an internal device, the engineer might study how the cells of the skin or blood vessels adhere to the compounds in the device. Biomechanical engineers also design drug delivery systems, study the properties of muscle contractions, and model the human skeletal system during movement.

History. As an academic discipline, biomechanical engineering has grown rapidly in the past few years. It is part of the larger discipline that is called bioengineering, which includes the study of the chemical properties of biological systems (biochemical engineering) and the use of living organisms or parts of living organisms for health purposes (biotechnology). In the 1960s, American universities first began developing advanced bioengineering departments. There are now dozens of accredited universities that offer doctoral degrees in the field of biomechanical engineering.

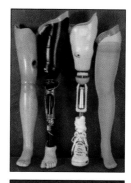

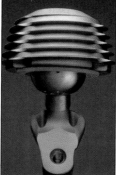

Devices of Biomechanical Engineering. Prosthetic legs (top right) come in many different shapes, sizes, and weights for various activities; they can be specialized for athletic participation and for daily use. The prosthetic titanium hip replacement (below right) is one of the finest achievements of biomedical engineering, but it pales in comparison to the replacement heart valve (at left). The most recent advance in biomechanical engineering includes a completely self-contained heart that will last for years with only minor upkeep.

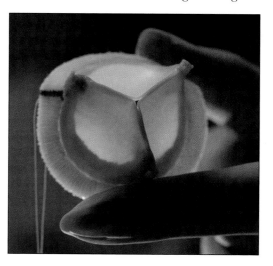

Background information on biomechanical engineering may be found in ERGONOMICS; ORTHOPEDICS; *and* PROSTHESIS. *For additional material on prosthetic devices, see* DISABLED, AIDS FOR THE; LIMB, ARTIFICIAL; HIP FRACTURE; WALKING AIDS; OCCUPATIONAL MEDICINE; *and* ORTHOPEDICS.

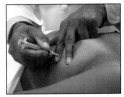

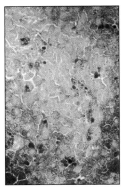

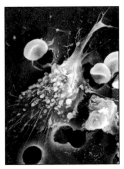

Biopsy. Top, a physician's hand taking a needle biopsy in order to determine the nature of a cyst or tumor. Middle, a microscopic image of a pretreatment biopsy showing test-animal cells before they are treated with tumor necrosis factor—a tumor killing agent. Bottom, cancer is often a battle between the body's immune system cells and cancerous cells.

Biopsy

A diagnostic test in which a sample of tissue is removed for study.

The term biopsy refers both to the surgical procedure that removes the tissue and the tissue sample itself. Such tissue samples are examined under a microscope in order to diagnose a variety of abnormalities, to track the progress or spread of disease, or to evaluate the success of treatment. Most notably, biopsies are used to determine if body tissue is cancerous.

Biopsy serves a great variety of uses, and many kinds exist—some requiring more specialized techniques than others, both in terms of tissue extraction and subsequent study. Biopsied material may, under light or occasionally electron microscopy, betray signs of tumor and malignancy, inflammation, infection, or other abnormalities.

TYPES OF BIOPSY

A recent technique for biopsy, known as fine-needle aspiration, involves inserting a slender needle into the tissue to be examined and withdrawing a tiny sample, which is then processed to be viewed under a microscope or electron microscope. For some biopsies, such as a liver biopsy, a larger-bore needle is required to extract a core of tissue. In other biopsies, a hollow punch is used to pull out a small piece of tissue.

While a biopsy may be examined by the pathologist for a variety of abnormalities, the technique has proven most indispensable for the diagnosis of a variety of cancers. Of the numerous forms of biopsy, three examples are described below:

Breast. Lumps in the breast tissue are often initially evaluated through biopsy. A lump of tissue is removed either through surgery (surgical-excision biopsy) or with a needle. If the lump is fairly small, the procedure may be done with local anesthetic. Another form of biopsy for breast lumps is beginning to replace the surgical-excision biopsy. Known as core biopsy, it uses a needle to extract breast tissue to be studied under the microscope.

Liver. Liver biopsies are sometimes carried out during exploratory surgery. Usually, however, liver tissue is biopsied by a needle inserted through the skin (percutaneous liver biopsy). An alternative method (transvenous liver biopsy) is performed by inserting a catheter into a neck vein and threading the device through the heart and into one of the veins emanating from the liver. This strategy is often used in patients where liver bleeding is a concern. Generally, the patient will remain in the hospital for several hours to be monitored as bleeding or other complications may sometimes occur. Liver biopsy helps the diagnostician assess liver damage or disease and, when necessary, plan a course of treatment. Liver biopsy is also common following liver transplant, to gauge the success of the treatment.

Bone Marrow. Bone marrow samples are usually taken from the hipbone, and occasionally from the breastbone. The pathologist may use biopsy to study the shape, proportion, and balance of blood cells, as well as their production within the bone marrow. Two types of bone-marrow biopsies are performed: bone-marrow aspiration and bone-marrow core biopsy. They are often performed at the same time.

With bone-marrow aspiration, a small amount of soft marrow is drawn into a needle and spread on a microscope slide for study. A diagnosis may be made solely on the basis of the bone-marrow aspiration examination, though the procedure breaks up the delicate arrangement of cells, which is often difficult to reconstruct. When the arrangement of the cells needs to be seen, a bone-marrow core sample is taken using an internal coring device on the biopsy needle. The core is subsequently prepared to be viewed under a microscope. The test takes only a few minutes and causes very little discomfort for the patient.

Basic information may be found in in BREAST CANCER; CANCER SCREENING; *and* ELISA TEST. *More on biopsy is contained in* BLADDER TUMOR; CONE BIOPSY; LIVER BIOPSY. DEVELOPMENTAL DELAY; MENSTRUATION, IRREGULAR; *and* PROGERIA. *See also* DIAGNOSTICS IN WOMEN'S HEALTH.

Biorhythms

According to the controversial theory, biorhythms are rhythmic cycles, overlooked by science, that affect human behavior.

The theory of biorhythms states that each person is significantly influenced by personalized cycles, beginning the day of their birth, that affect intellectual, emotional, and physical behavior. Unlike biological theories that posit the existence of daily rhythms shaped by exposure to light and biologically set clocks, biorhythmic theory holds that everyone is subject to cycles that broadly influence daily living, each of which governs a complex but important domain of behavior (e.g., emotion, intellect, and intuition).

BIORHYTHMIC THEORY

According to the most popular version of biorhythmic theory, which has several forms, a given biorhythmic cycle can affect mood, endurance to diseases, mental capability, learning ability, critical and analytical abilities, judgment, and, more generally, all important aspects of the operations of an individual's mind and body.

There are three cycles, which correspond to intellectual, emotional, and physical state. Each cycle begins at birth and repeats until death. The cycle has several parts. In the first part, ability related to the domain—whether it is intellectual, emotional, or physical—reaches a peak. After the peak, the cycle goes through a period of a similar length during which it decreases until it reaches a minimum.

The day that the cycle switches from increasing to decreasing is called the critical day, while the day during which the cycle reverts from negative to positive is the neutral day. During critical and neutral days, the cycle is unstable.

The three cycles, however, do not coincide. Each one is a different length, though all three begin at birth. Some versions of biorhythmic theory include a fourth cycle, the intuitional, which influences intuition, instinct, and subconscious behavior.

HISTORY

Biorhythmic theory originated in the study of numerology. It began in the 19th century with Wilhelm Fliess, a Berlin physician, numerologist, and close friend of Sigmund Freud. Fliess championed an early version of the theory, according to which men are governed by a 23-day cycle while women are influenced by a 28-day cycle.

Many skeptics have challenged the scientific validity of biorhythmic theory. While dozens of studies have claimed to provide scientific evidence for the theory, critics counter that these studies suffer from methodological or statistical errors.

ALTERNATIVE MEDICINE; COGNITIVE-BEHAVIORAL THERAPY; and MIND BODY MEDICINE; discuss the foundations of BIORHYTHMS. Related topics include AROMA THERAPY; HERBAL MEDICINE; HOMEOPATHY; and YOGA. Also see the discussions on ACUPRESSURE and WITHDRAWAL, EMOTIONAL.

Bipolar Disorder

Also known as manic-depressive illness

Mood disorder characterized by alternating periods of depression and mania.

An individual suffering from bipolar disorder usually experiences the first episode in the teens or twenties. A first occurrence is unlikely after age 50. If the symptoms of bipolar disorder first appear at a late age, other causes for the mood swings, including brain illness or injury, problems with prescription medications or substance abuse, or endocrine disturbances should be considered.

Incidence. About 1 to 2 percent of the population is estimated to suffer from bipolar disorder. Men and women are equally affected. There seems to be a higher rate of incidence among family members; the likelihood of developing this disorder increases to 10 to 15 percent when an immediate relative has been diagnosed.

Mania. The manic phase of bipolar disorder involves a feeling of euphoria and it is often accompanied by elevated mood, decreased need for sleep, and reckless behaviors such as out-of-control spending and irresponsible and unprotected sex. A manic phase typically involves an inflated sense of self-esteem, believing that one is more powerful and important than is accurate or realistic.

The mind races with ideas, and thoughts bounce from one topic to another without any meaningful focus or depth. Judgment tends to be impaired, and decisions made in this phase can have lasting detrimental effects on one's personal well being. In some types of manias, the individual may also become irritable and impatient. A person experiencing a manic episode may talk incessantly and loudly and and impose on others, often overstaying a welcome. New interests may suddenly present themselves, requiring purchases and a whirlwind of activity to pursue. When in this phase, the body is in a constant state of motion.

Depression. The depressive phase of this illness is characterized by feelings of sadness and hopelessness, often accompanied by guilt, shame, and an extremely low sense of self-esteem. There is less interest in sex or any activity that is satisfying. It is difficult to feel any satisfaction or pleasure in activities, family, or friends. Thinking is slow, there is difficulty concentrating and remembering, and dark thoughts pervade the conscious mind. The person tends to be extremely tired and suffer from sleep disturbances, particularly insomnia, although some people feeling depressed may sleep for excessive amounts of time, at times from 12 to 14 hours per night. The risk of suicide is high during a depressive period.

TYPES

Bipolar I Disorder. In this form of bipolar disorder, the ups and downs of mood are extreme and feel out of control. The wildly elevated moods and crippling depressed moods may cause serious problems with the ability to work, get along with others and maintain a stable family life.

The relative periods of mania and depression vary from person to person. Peri ods of mania typically alternate with periods of depression, but it is possible that one type of mood predominates over the other. Manias can also occur simultaneously with depressions (this is known as "mixed states"). About 40 percent of patients are affected by mixed states. Manic periods tend to last a few weeks to a few months before the mood dips into a depression. Depressive episodes are more likely to last longer.

A problem to watch for is rapid cycling, where extreme highs and lows alternate quickly, or when discrete manic or depressive episodes occur four or more times per year, giving an individual little respite from an emotional roller-coaster ride.

Bipolar II Disorder. This mood disorder involves unstable moods, varying from elevated to depressed, but the intensity of the manic phases is not as severe as in bipolar I disorder. A less intense manic phase is known as hypomania. Depressive states, however, can be extreme and long lasting, and the risk of suicide may be high.

Cyclothymic Disorder. Although unstable moods swing from up to down quickly, they are not as intense or long-lasting as with either of the bipolar mood disorders. It is important, however, to be aware if mood is chronically unstable and to seek treatment, because it is likely that cyclothymic disorder will develop into full blown bipolar disorder.

TREATMENT

Bipolar disorders are chronic. A doctor will attempt to manage the symptoms, keeping moods from changing quickly and from

---

ALERT

A Difficult Diagnosis

Bipolar disorder must be diagnosed by a psychiatrist and requires both medication and psychotherapy to be effectively managed. Antidepressant medications alone are dangerous to someone suffering from a bipolar disorder and may initiate a manic episode or accelerate the rate and intensity of mood swings. A prescription of antidepressants alone is particularly hazardous with bipolar II disorder, where most of the moods may be depressed and those moods last for long periods of time.

reaching extreme highs and lows. The most effective treatment combines medication and psychotherapy. Medication consists of a mood stabilizer such as lithium, Tegretol, or Depakote. Lithium use must be carefully monitored by a physician because it can build up in the blood. The side effects of lithium tend to be increased thirst, weight gain, trembling, and hair loss. Lithium can diminish mood swings and help even out and stabilize feelings and thoughts. Mood stabilizing drugs generally take a few weeks to build up effectiveness, and other drugs may be prescribed in the interim for acute anxiety or depression.

Psychotherapy helps to ground the patient in reality and allow for the chance to manage life decisions and activities. Because manic episodes of bipolar disorders can be so pleasing, without psychotherapy, a patient is more likely to stop taking medication, so as to "enjoy" elevated moods.

> *See* DEPRESSION; HISTRIONIC PERSONALITY DISORDER; *and* PERSONALITY DISORDER; *and* SUICIDE. *for a discussion of this subject. Treatment options are discussed in* ANTIANXIETY DRUGS; ANTIDEPRESSANT DRUGS; *and* PSYCHOTHERAPY.

Birth Control

> **Various methods of contraception, used to prevent or control the number of births.**

Family planning refers to methods used to plan the number and time between births, whereas contraception refers specifically to methods of preventing pregnancy. Various birth control methods are used for both purposes. Types of birth control used involve barrier (including such devices as condoms, both male and female, the diaphragm, and spermicidal jellies) and hormonal methods (including "the pill"), the calendar method (a plan for scheduling sexual intercourse around the days that it is least likely to bring about pregnancy), and surgical methods such as sterilization, (vasectomies and tubal ligations) and abortion(both surgical and with prescript- ion medications, such as RU-486). *See also* BARRIER METHODS *and* SPERM.

Birth Defects
Also known as congenital abnormalities

> **Disorders that are apparent at or before birth, or that develop shortly afterwards.**

Birth defects usually occur as a result of developmental "errors" during pregnancy. Approximately 3 percent of newborns have a major birth defect. The severity of birth defects ranges from relatively minor to quite serious. Very severe defects often result in a stillborn delivery or the death of a baby within a few days of birth. Of the remaining abnormalities, many conditions are correctable surgically or in some cases will resolve on their own.

Causes. The cause of most birth defects is unknown, but the following factors have been shown to play a role in increasing the risk of birth defects: lack of proper maternal nutrition, exposure to caustic levels of radiation, consumption of certain drugs and alcohol, infection, trauma, and inherited conditions.

Chromosomal Abnormalities. A woman over age 35 has an increased chance of giving birth to a child with a chromosomal abnormality. The resulting syndromes are caused by the presence of an additional chromosome or, in rare cases, by the absence of one of the regular chromosomes. Down's syndrome, which results from the presence of an extra chromosome in the 21st pair, is a gastrointestinal, urogenital and central nervous system (the brain and spinal cord) abnormality.

Heart defects include:
- Atrial and Ventricular Septal Defects—holes in the walls separating the right portion and left portion of the heart;
- Patent Ductus Arteriosus—an abnormal connection between the aorta and the pulmonary artery, which is normally present before birth but fails to close off afterwards;
- Aortic Valve Stenosis—a narrowing of the aortic valve, obstructing blood flow;
- Pulmonary Valve Stenosis—a narrowing of the pulmonary valve that obstructs blood flow;

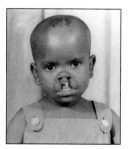

Corrective Plastic Surgery. Above, a child with a birth defect that twisted her mouth prior to corrective surgery, later performed by plastic surgeons. Many disfiguring birth defects are corrected in this way.

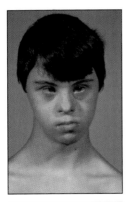

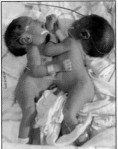

Birth Defects. Pictured at top is a boy with Down's syndrome, a birth defect caused by an extra copy of chromosome 21; there is no cure yet, but individuals living with this disorder can lead fulfilling and successful lives. Below, a pair of twin boys who are connected at the abdomen (siamese twins, properly called conjoined twins); each has his own set of vital organs, but they share their livers and their hearts. The surgery to separate conjoined twins is often complex, and many times they cannot both be saved.

- Coarctation of the Aorta—narrowing of the aorta that reduces blood flow to the lower half of the body;
- Transposition of the Great Arteries—a reversal of the normal connections of the aorta and pulmonary artery with the heart;
- Underdeveloped Left Ventricle Syndrome—also called hypoplastic left heart syndrome, the left side of the heart is severely underdeveloped or absent. This condition is usually fatal;
- Tetralogy of Fallot—a combination of defects, including a large ventricular septal defect, displacement of the aorta, narrowing of the outflow passage from the right side of the heart, and an abnormally thick wall in the right ventricle.

Gastrointestinal defects include the following disorders:

- Esophageal Atresia—an incompletely developed esophagus that is not connected to the stomach;
- Tracheosophageal Fistula—an abnormal connection between the esophagus and the trachea;
- Diaphragmatic Hernia—a hole in the diaphragm that allows the abdominal organs to protrude into the chest;
- Hirschsprung's Disease—also called congenital megacolon, in which part of the large intestine lacks the nerves that control rhythmic contractions;
- Omphalocele—a hole in the central abdominal wall that allows the abdominal organs to protrude;
- Anal Atresia—incomplete development of the anus;
- Biliary Atresia—bile ducts that fail to develop properly.

Bone and muscle defects commonly affect the skull, spine, hips, legs, and feet. Most of these are correctable surgically.

- Facial Abnormalities—cleft lip or cleft palate, which may occur together;
- Spinal Abnormalities—torticollis, in which the neck is twisted to one side and the head is tilted;
- Hip, Leg, and Foot Abnormalities—dislocation of the hip or knee.

Clubfoot means the foot is twisted into an abnormal shape or position;

- Missing Limb—either part or an entire arm or leg are missing at birth;
- Osteogenesis Imperfecta—abnormally fragile bones which break easily;
- Arthrogryposis Multiplex Congenita—one or more joints are fused together;
- Muscle Abnormalities—usually due to a defect in the pectoralis major muscle of the chest, or a similar defect involving the abdominal muscles.

Brain and spinal cord defects, many of which are detected before birth, include:

- Anencephaly—most of the brain fails to develop. This condition is fatal;
- Microcephaly—a small head. Infants survive, but are usually mentally retarded and have other related disorders;
- Encephalocele—a skull defect allows a portion of the brain to bulge outward;
- Porencephaly—the presence of a cyst or cavity in the cerebrum. It is evidence of brain damage, but some children with the condition exhibit normal intelligence;
- Hydranencephaly—an extreme form of porencephaly: the cerebrum is almost completely absent. Children with this condition are severely retarded;
- Hydrocephalus—used to be called "water on the brain." The ventricles, or spaces, found in the brain are much larger than normal and produce excessive amounts of cerebrospinal fluid. Failure of this fluid to drain results in severe pressure inside the brain;
- Spina Bifida—one or more of the vertebrae fail to develop properly, leaving a portion of the spinal cord exposed.

Urogenital abnormalities often include ambiguous genitals. In hermaphrodism (which is rare), a baby is born with both ovaries and testicles. After doctors study the infant's chromosomes, it is "assigned" gender based on the results, and surgery is performed for cosmetic purposes.

Basic information is contained in CHROMOSOMAL ABNORMALITIES; DEFORMITY; GENETIC DISORDERS; HEREDITY; GENETIC COUNSELING; NEONATAL CARE; *and* TAY-SACHS DISEASE.

Birth Effects

The effects that occur during labor and delivery.

Between two and seven out of every 1,000 newborns will experience a birth effect, regardless of the quality of obstetric care. The likelihood of a birth effect increases with either pre- or post-mature infants, breech or other abnormal presentation, and an unusually large fetus and small pelvis of the mother.

Forceps and vacuum extraction are procedures in which devices assist in the delivery process; these can also be a source of birth effects. However, these methods are often necessary to ensure the health, and continued life, of both mother and child.

TYPES

The most common birth effects are:

- **Caput Succedaneum**: swelling of the scalp and face due to pressure against the birth canal. It may also include mild discoloration or distortion of the face and usually disappears within a few days.
- **Cephalohematoma**: a collection of blood under the scalp, sometimes accompanied by a skull fracture. It usually goes away on its own in 2 weeks to 3 months and rarely requires treatment.
- **Fractured Collarbone**: may occur when there is difficulty in delivering the shoulder or during a breech birth. It is sometimes accompanied by a dislocated shoulder.
- **Facial Nerve Palsy**: results from pressure over the facial nerve during a difficult labor or due to the use of forceps. It may involve an entire side of the face. If no nerve injury was incurred, improvement is immediate once the pressure is relieved. Micro surgery may be required to repair torn nerve fibers.

Basic information is contained in CHILDBIRTH; CHILDBIRTH, COMPLICATIONS OF; DELIVERY; CEPHALOHEMATOMA; *and* CESAREAN SECTION. *Related material on birth complications is found in* INFANT MORTALITY; *and* MATERNAL MORTALITY.

Birth Weight

The weight of a newborn infant, an important indicator of the infant's health.

The average newborn weighs between 5.5 and 10 pounds and is between 18 and 22 inches in length. Due to fluid loss and initially small feedings, babies lose 6 to 10 percent of their weight during the first few days of life. However, once their appetite increases, most babies rapidly make up for this loss and at the end of the first month weigh an average of 2 pounds more than they did at birth.

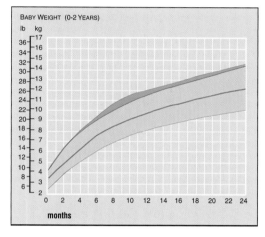

BABY WEIGHT (0-2 YEARS)

months

Premature babies, those born before 35 weeks, weigh less than full-term infants. Low birth weight (less than 5.5 pounds), along with a short time of development in the womb (gestation), is a risk factor for neurological or developmental problems.

Babies with a birth weight over 10 pounds are more likely to have complicated deliveries or require a Cesarean section, and they may be too large to fit through the birth canal. Diabetic mothers tend to have larger babies as excess blood sugar crosses the placenta, raising the fetus' own glucose levels. As a result, extra fetal insulin is released and acts similar to a growth hormone.

See APGAR SCORE; DELIVERY; NEONATAL CARE; *and* PREMATURITY. *More information is contained in* BIRTH INJURY; INTRAUTERINE GROWTH RETARDATION; PREMATURITY. BLUE BABY; CHILDBIRTH, COMPLICATIONS OF; *and* POSTMATURITY.

Birth Weight and Average Baby Weight for the First Two Years of Life. Within the first eight to ten months of life, a newborn will often grow quite rapidly. The red and blue areas show the average weights for boys and girls, respectively. Due to physiological reasons, girls weigh very slightly less than boys throughout the first two years of life. The discrepancy is, however, nearly statistically irrelevant.

Birthmark

A raised or flat discoloration that appears on the skin shortly before or after birth.

Birthmarks are usually painless, and any concern is more cosmetic than medical.

TYPES

Milia are small white cysts found on the face that resemble whiteheads. They disappear without treatment.

Salmon patches, also known as stork bites, are small, flat, pale, pink spots found in up to 50 percent of all newborns. They are collections of tiny capillaries and are found most often on the eyelids, upper lip, between the eyebrows, and on the back of the neck. Their color deepens with temperature changes or crying spells. The facial spots eventually fade. *See* SKIN.

Hemangiomas are benign tumors made of newly formed blood vessels. They are usually bright red in color and may appear anywhere on the skin.

Strawberry (or cheery) hemangiomas appear primarily on the face, back, or chest and are more commonly found in girls. They usually appear within the first two months. Most strawberry hemangiomas grow rapidly and then remain at a fixed size for a while before they disappear. Usually no treatment is necessary. More than half of them disappear by age 5; over 90 percent are gone by age 9. Sometimes a faint discoloration or puckering of the skin persists after the mark has disappeared.

Cavernous hemangiomas are more deeply rooted than the strawberry variety. They are typically red-blue in color with a spongy texture. Some disappear on their own; others require treatment with corticosteroid medications such as prednisone.

Port-wine stains are flat hemangiomas consisting of dilated capillaries. They are usually found on the face. Size is highly variable; a mark may cover half of the face. They do not disappear on their own and are usually treated with laser surgery, which has a higher success rate in adolescents and adults than in small children. *See* DELIVERY.

Bisexuality

Sexual interest toward males and females.

People who feel attracted to both sexes, although not necessarily to the same degree, are called bisexual. Sexual orientation appears to be present from childhood. What causes an individual to have a particular preference is unknown; no hormonal, biological, or psychological influences have been identified. *See also* HERMAPHRODITISM; HETEROSEXUALITY; HOMOSEXUALITY; SEX; SEX CHANGE; SEX HORMONES; SEXUAL CHARACTERISTICS, SECONDARY; SEXUAL INTERCOURSE; SEXUAL RESPONSE; *and* SEXUALITY.

Bites

The wounding, piercing or stinging of the flesh by an animal, insect or another person.

Animal Bites. Depending on the region of the world, some animal bites are more likely than others. In Pacific coastal areas, attacks from sharks, jellyfish, and other aquatic creatures are not uncommon. In regions of Central and South America, crocodile attacks are serious. Bites from cattle, horses, and pigs can also be fatal. However, in totality, dogs are responsible for the greatest number of animal attacks.

Any bite from an animal that breaks the skin presents the danger of infection. The mouth of an animal contains many bacteria and viruses, many of which can cause infections. Rabies, from dogs, cats, bats, and other animals is a major risks. Superficial bites and scratches can be treated the same as minor wounds. In all other cases, professional treatment must be sought.

Treatment of a severe animal bite begins with cleaning and examination of the wound. Instead of stitching a wound, the physician may choose to bandage it to avoid enclosing bacteria from the bite in the wound. To reduce infection, a course of antibiotics or an antitetanus injection may be administered as a preventive measure. An antirabies vaccine or immunogloublin may also be administered.

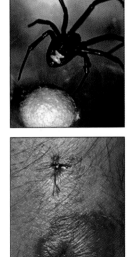

Spider Bites. Top, the bite of a black widow spider may produce severe symptoms, but it rarely kills except in the cases of the very young and the very old. Black widow spiders can be identified by the red hourglass marking on their abdomen. Insect bites can cause tissue death and the formation of bullae. Below is a two to three millimeter wide sore caused by a poisonous bite.

Emergency rooms report far more human bites than most expect. The human mouth contains many bacteria and viruses that can infect a wound. Human bites rarely cause significant tissue damage and thus are deceptive in appearing more benign than they are.

Most human bites can be treated by washing the area with soap and warm water and applying a cold compress to reduce swelling and pain. At times infectious antibiotics are necessary to adequately heal a developing bacterial infection. *See also* BACTERIA; BITES; *and* SPIDER BITES.

Black Eye

The bruised appearance of the skin around the eye following an injury.

A direct blow to the eye causes damage to the small blood vessels under the skin, causing blood to collect in the injured area. Because the skin around the eye is loose and relatively transparent, bruising is darker in this area than in other body parts. This bleeding is usually minor. A cold compress, held over the eye reduces inflammation and relieves pain. *See also* BRUISE.

Blackwater Fever

A complication of one of the more dangerous forms of malaria, caused by the rupture of many red blood cells.

Malaria is a parasitic infection spread by female mosquitoes. After infection, the parasites migrate to the liver where they multiply and periodically release parasites into the blood that attack the red blood cells. The symptoms of the various types of malaria differ slightly, but the most dangerous—falciparum malaria—produces fever, chills, headache, and muscle aches. Blackwater fever is a complication of falciparum malaria that appears in people who have taken quinine to treat the disease. In patients with blackwater fever, large numbers of red blood cells rupture and darken the urine. Blackwater fever is treated with completion of an appropriate malaria therapy as well as hydration. *See also* BLOOD; MALARIA; INFECTION; *and* PARASITE.

Bladder

The organ that stores urine.

The bladder is a round, hollow muscle behind the pubic bone. The inner lining is called the urinary epithelium. The kidneys feed urine into the bladder through tubes called ureters. The neck of the bladder is at the bottom and opens to the urethra. A sphincter muscle keeps it closed until urine is passed. Infants urinate reflexively when the bladder swells and sends messages to the spinal cord to relax the urethral sphincter, releasing urine. The child gradually learns how to control the urethral sphincter by recognizing the discomfort of a full bladder and countering the release impulse with a conscious constriction of the urethral sphincter. *See also* URINE.

Bladder Control

The ability to control the organs—particularly the ring of muscle tissue at the outlet of the bladder—that regulate urinary flow.

Various disorders may block regular urinary activities, including bladder-neck contracture, an enlarged prostate, and a urethral obstruction. A surgical treatment for the loss of urinary control is known as bladder-neck suspension. The stress of age, weight gain, and childbirth stretches the pelvic-floor muscles, causing the neck of the bladder to drop. From a lower position, the bladder neck will open whenever abdominal pressure increases. Nearly anything, from coughing to physical activity, increases abdominal pressure. Bladder neck suspension is now performed laproscopically, with three small incisions that are made at the abdomen. Sutures are then used to create a mesh that restores the bladder-neck to its natural position. *See also* BLADDER; INCONTINENCE; KIDNEY; URINE; URINARY DIVERSION; *and* URINARY SYSTEM.

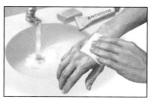

Treating Bites. First aid for treating bites includes immediate cleaning and disinfection of the wounded site, as well as applying pressure and the proper kind of bandages. If possible, the animal should also be quarantined for examination.

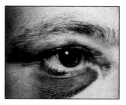

Black Eye. A black eye is caused by bleeding in the tissue surrounding the eye. This is usually seen after trauma. Although unsightly, a black eye is much like a bruise and can be treated similarly. A cold compress will relieve swelling.

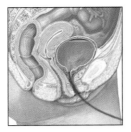

Cytoscopic Bladder Biopsy. A cytoscope is a thin flexible tube used for viewing internal structures. Many surgeons prefer cytoscopy because it is a minimally invasive procedure. The flexible cytoscope is inserted through the urethra into the bladder so that doctors can see these organs and diagnose any disorders. Images can also be recorded for evaluation at a later time or by a specialist.

Bladder Tumors

Growths on the inner lining of the bladder.

A large percentage of reported bladder tumors are simply superficial growths (a growth on the surface of the organ; it has not grown into the bladder wall). Growths often recur—they can also become highly invasive and quite dangerous.

INCIDENCE

Bladder cancer is the fourth most common sort of cancer in males and the eighth most common cancer in females in the United States. It is a cancer that usually affects older individuals, with an average diagnostic age of about 65.

Chronic exposure to carcinogens and an inherited inability to block the activity of cancer-causing agents are major risk factors for bladder cancer. Thus, cigarette smokers are at four times the risk of non-smokers, and workers in some industries that involve exposure to certain chemicals are also at risk. Individuals who work with aniline dyes, benzidine, and other compounds used in rubber, leather, and paint production also have a higher than normal incidence level of bladder cancer.

The risk is also increased for people undergoing radiation therapy for other cancers of the pelvic area and for patients receiving some anticancer drugs, such as cyclophosphamide.

TYPES

Many bladder growths are papillomas (a specific type of malignant tumor) that are easily treated, but some invade the muscular wall of the bladder.

The most prevalent form of bladder cancer is called a transitional-cell carcinoma. This type of bladder cancer accounts for more than 90 percent of all reported cases. About eight percent of bladder cancers are squamous cell cancers (referred to as as squamous cell carcinomas), which are malignant, and approximately two percent are diagnosed as adenocarcinomas, which are also malignant.

SYMPTOMS

The most prominent symptom of bladder cancer is blood in the urine; this gives the urine a reddish tinge. In the majority of cases, bloody urine is the only symptom, although some people may experience urinary urgency, a burning sensation while urinating, inability to control urinary function, and chronic pain. Diagnosis usually is done by cytoscopy, in which a doctor can view the interior of the bladder by passing a tube through the urethra. A biopsy may also be done in to obtain a tissue sample.

TREATMENT

Tumors can be removed or destroyed through the cytoscope, by surgery, with chemotherapy, or by laser vaporization. If a cancer has spread through the bladder lining, a partial or total cystectomy can be done to remove some or all of the bladder. If the tumor spreads beyond the bladder, chemotherapy can be used Radiation therapy may also be used in some cases. Survival rates depend on the stage at which the tumor is detected and how much of the bladder is already involved.

Background material is in URINARY SYSTEM. *For additional material see* CANCER; CANCER SCREENING; CYTOSCOPY; *and* PROSTATE, CANCER OF THE. *Treatment options are discussed in* CHEMOTHERAPY; RADIATION THERAPY; *and* SURGERY.

Blastocyst Transfer

Transferring a fertilized egg into a woman's uterus.

After removing eggs from a donor, a reproductive endocrinologist will fertilize these eggs and leave them to incubate in a laboratory for about three to six days; about five days after fertilization, human embryos are called blastocysts.

A blastocyst transfer is an in vitro fertilization option for assisted reproduction. By waiting for five days, a doctor is able to recognize which embryos are growing the fastest and therefore which ones are most likely to implant and create a full and healthy pregnancy. *See* INFERTILITY; PREGNANCY; *and* PREGNANCY COUNSELING.

Blastomycosis

An infection caused by soil-dwelling fungus.

Blastomycosis results from the inhalation of yeast-like fungus—*Blastomyces dermatitidis*—found in the soil of the eastern part of the United States and Canada. The infection causes a red skin rash, cough, chest pain, fever, chills, night sweats, fatigue and weight loss. Those symptoms can develop weeks or months after exposure to the fungus. The condition most often occurs in men between the ages of 30 and 50 and farmers. It is diagnosed by detecting the fungus in sputum or skin tissue samples. The infection is treated with amphotericin B, an antifungal medication. *See also* SKIN.

Bleaching, Dental

A procedure used to whiten discolored teeth.

Dental bleaching consists of applying chemical compounds to teeth to whiten them. The simplest, least expensive method is the use of over-the-counter whitening toothpaste. These are minimally effective and can take many weeks. Professional bleaching is an at-home as well as in-office procedure. A dentist first ensures that the teeth are healthy, are not hypersensitive, and do not have crowns. The dentist molds a tray in which a bleaching gel solution bathes the desired teeth. The at-home bleaching requires several days or weeks. The in-office process can be done in as little as an hour and a half. *See* DENTISTRY.

Bleb

Large blister, greater than 10 millimeters in diameter, that forms on the lungs and is filled with air.

Blebs on the lungs are most common in people who also have emphysema. They are usually discovered in a chest x-ray. If a bleb ruptures, however, air may come into contact with the pleural space between the chest and the lung, causing the lung to collapse. Blebs that occur on the skin and are filled with clear liquid are called bullae. *See also* BLISTER; EMPHYSEMA; LUNG; *and* X-RAY.

Bleeding

Losing blood from the circulatory system when blood vessels are torn, cut or, damaged.

The body has an elaborate system of safeguards to control bleeding and repair injury. The basic system of repair is based on the platelets in the blood. These are small, round disks that stick to each other and clog the opening in the blood vessel to limit blood loss. On the other hand, blood clots in the circulatory system are extremely dangerous if they clog blood flow. They can cause heart attack, if the blood cannot reach the heart, or stroke, if it cannot reach the brain.

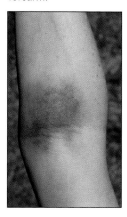

Bleeding. Blood from injured tissue accumulates near the skin's surface, causing bruising such as that seen below in an image of bruising on the inside of the forearm.

ALERT

The Danger of Internal Bleeding

It often takes several days or weeks for the symptoms of internal bleeding to show up in a patient, if they appear at all. If there is blood coming from any bodily opening—if an individual is coughing, vomiting, urinating, or defecating blood—that is a sign of internal bleeding. If any of these conditions is present, medical help should be sought immediately. Visit a health care professional after any traumatic injury, no matter how insignificant it may seem. Someone who is bleeding internally may also react with a tense or a spasming abdominal muscle to the touch or the abdominal region may just be tender in general. Internal bleeding is potentially life-threatening and professional care must be sought as soon as possible.

The fluid (known as plasma) that carries red blood cells, white blood cells, and platelets also contains proteins called procoagulants, which promote coagulation, and anticoagulants, which inhibit coagulation. It is the balance among the factors that determines whether the blood starts the coagulation process and whether the clots dissolve after healing has taken place.

The life span of platelets is about ten days, so new platelets must be produced in the bone marrow to replace those that are dead or in use. This is an ongoing process in healthy bone marrow; if it is interfered with by disease or poor nutrition, a major health risk can result. *See also* BLEEDING DISORDERS; BLEEDING, TREATMENT OF; BLOOD; BRUISE; EMERGENCY MEDICINE; *and* TRAUMA.

Bleeding Disorders

Any of a number of disorders in which a person bleeds too easily. These can be caused by defects in the components in blood plasma that control the clotting process, or by defects in the number or condition of the platelets.

The blood-clotting process is complex, involving the production of coagulant and anticoagulant factors in the plasma and platelets (cells in the blood). If there are too few platelets in the blood, or if the coagulant and anticoagulant factors are balanced improperly, clots will not form and bleeding will not cease. When a blood vessel break has healed, it is critical that the blood clots dissolve and do not recur, or else they can block blood flow to the brain, the heart, the lungs, and other organs.

PLATELET DYSFUNCTION

Platelet dysfunction describes a number of diseases arising from platelets that do not clot properly or, conversely, clot too easily.

Thrombocytopenia is the condition involving a reduced level of platelets in the blood. The symptoms include easy bruising of the lower legs (often with many tiny purplish dots), nosebleeds, and blood in the stool or urine. In extreme cases there may be bleeding from the intestinal tract. Thrombocytopenia may be caused by a problem in the bone marrow where the platelets are produced—either a reduced level of production or a production of short-lived platelets. Platelets can also collect in an enlarged spleen, thus not circulating to the rest of the body.

Thrombocytopenia may be caused by an auotimmune disease or by drugs like he-parin or sulfa antibiotics, or as a complication of other diseases such as viral or bacterial respiratory infection, particularly in children. The chronic form of this disease appears frequently in young to middle-aged women. It is also found in alcoholics and those with leukemia and lymphoma. People with severe cases of this disease are advised to stay in bed to avoid accidents that might be fatal when bleeding cannot be stopped. Transfusions of platelets or of gamma globulin may be prescribed to replace platelets and increase their lifespan.

Thrombocytosis, another platelet dysfunction, is a condition caused by a high platelet count. The symptoms include blood clots and painful burning or throbbing of the hands or feet. It is most often a complication of some other disease or illness, such as cancer, leukemia, or rheumatoid arthritis. Small blood vessels may be blocked, and the reduced blood flow can result in brain damage, retinal damage, or heart attack. Aspirin is the treatment of choice for this condition, but at the risk, however, of producing intestinal bleeding. Other drugs such as alpha interferon have been successful in controlling this disease.

COAGULATION DYSFUNCTION

Coagulation dysfunction is a term used to describe a number of diseases arising from a lack or malfunction of one or more of the factors necessary for blood clotting. Causes include hereditary factors and medications used to treat other diseases.

Von Willebrand's disease is the most common of the inherited forms. When the von Willebrand factor in the bloodstream is not functioning properly, platelets do not become sticky and thus do not cluster at the broken blood vessel wall.

Hemophilia is also a deficiency in one of the clotting factors necessary for proper coagulation. It is caused by a gene inherited from the mother, but affects male children almost exclusively. Hemophiliacs must be particularly careful to avoid injury and to warn their doctors preceding surgery or dental extractions, where bleeding may become uncontrollable. Another serious con-

Bleeding In Older Individuals

Older people have more bleeding problems than younger ones. They are more likely to have cancers that destroy platelets, or they may be taking one or more of a long list of drugs that interfere with platelet function. Older people often have a lowered level of vitamin K, which works in the liver to produce procoagulant factors, or they may have other liver diseases that destroy the available platelets.

cern is bleeding and bruising at the joints —knees, ankles, and elbows—and in the muscles and intestines. Internal bleeding can result in permanent nerve damage as well as damage to the cartilage and joints, causing pain and stiffness. Hemophiliacs must avoid drugs like aspirin and heparin. Treatment is most often a lifestyle that carefully avoids the risk of injury. When severe, doctors may prescribe transfusions to replace the missing clotting factors.

Disseminated Intravascular Coagulation. Normally, blood clots only at the site of a broken blood vessel, but when the clot encouraging factors predominate, blood may start clotting in the smaller blood vessels. When blood clots appear in the bloodstream in the absence of injury, they may clog the smaller blood vessels. This condition is called disseminated intravascular coagulation. Symptoms include pallor, fatigue, fever, bruises, and excessive bleeding during surgery or dentistry. Usually this condition is a complication of another disease, such as an infection or cancer. The body tries to dissolve these clots, which increases bleeding even from minor punctures or wounds. The clots may kill tissue, which can turn gangrenous.

See BLOOD; CARDIOLOGY; CIRCULATORY SYSTEM; *and* HEART *for basic information.* CARDIOVASCULAR DISORDERS; HEMOPHILIA; *and* SICKLE CELL ANEMIA *contain related details.*

Bleeding, Treatment of

Measures used to stop bleeding. These vary according to the nature and severity of the wound.

Blood pressure in the veins is lower than that in the arteries. Bleeding from the veins tends to be slow and steady while bleeding from the arteries may be copious and pulsating. Any bleeding should be controlled as quickly as possible, but bleeding from the arteries is particularly dangerous.

Ascertaining the Severity of a Wound. The amount of blood lost is not a good indicator of the seriousness or severity of the trauma. Bleeding from head wounds can be heavy even from minor cuts or scrapes,

because the blood vessels are close to the surface. Bleeding from a deeper wound elsewhere on the body might seem less dangerous, while a large share of the bleeding is internal.

It is best not to come into direct contact with the blood, since this is one of the ways of contracting AIDS or other infectious diseases. Immediately after treating a bleeding wound, a person should wash her or his hands in hot, soapy water.

Pressure Points & Severe Bleeding

Besides direct pressure, indirect pressure should be applied to the most severe wounds and to wounds that have foreign objects embedded in them. There are several specific arterial pressure points throughout the body that will slow the supply of blood to the wound. They are located at the ankles, behind the knees, at the point where the thigh meets the trunk, on the inside of the arm just below the shoulder, below the wrist, and just above the collarbone. After finding the arterial pressure point nearest the wound, hold it tightly with two or three fingers. Pressure should only be maintained long enough to control the bleeding. If direct pressure is also being applied to the wound, it should be maintained for the duration or until medical professionals arrive.

Pregnancy. Some amount of bleeding or spotting is not unusual during pregnancy, particularly in the first trimester. Vaginal bleeding, however can signal the start of a serious problem. A physician should be contacted immediately.

Home Treatment. The first rule in bleeding treatment is to put pressure on the wound and hold it until the bleeding stops or more specific remedies can be applied. However, this is not true if there is a possible skull fracture or some other broken bone near the wound or if there is an object embedded in the wound. If the wound is to one or both eyes, a light clean dressing must be applied to both eyes, since any eye movements may damage the wounded eye. If the wound is to the nose and it is unbroken, a cold compress should be applied.

Tourniquets. Once, a common treatment, tourniquets are now considered a dangerous means of stopping bleeding.

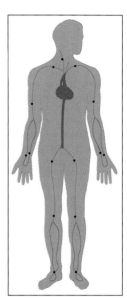

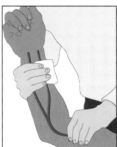

Treating Bleeding. Pressure points are marked with black dots (top). Pressure should be applied at these points to manage rapid bleeding. Even though these points may be a distance from the bleeding itself, the arteries bringing blood to the wound are supplied from blood vessels at these points, thus, pressure will slow the bleeding. Below, pressure applied directly to the trauma site will also slow bleeding. Whenever possible, the injury should be elevated.

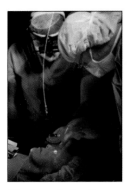

Blepharoplasty. Above, surgeon prepares for a blepharoplasty operation, more commonly known as eyelid surgery. This procedure is often done for cosmetic purposes, as it reduces some of the most visible signs of aging; however, sometimes this surgery is done for medical reasons. Drooping eyelids can impair a person's field of vision.

ALERT

Shock

When the word "shock" is used, very often it is meant to convey a sense of psychological trauma that does not have medical significance. However, in medical terminology shock results when there is not enough blood flow to the vital organs. If there is a danger of shock, stop any ongoing blood loss by applying direct pressure to the wound. Have the patient lie flat on his or her back. Keep the patient covered and warm and call emergency medical service (EMS) personnel as soon as possible.

Wrapped tourniquets can cause gangrene, making an injury worse. The only time a tourniquet can even be considered is when an extremity has been amputated in an accident. Tourniquets are made of straps or fabric folded to about two inches wide; a belt or strap of fabric is best. It should be wrapped just above the wound and knotted at the pressure point. A bandage and properly applied pressure is preferred.

Types of Injuries. Bruises are the result of blows that do not break the skin. They may cause tissue damage appearing as discolorations under the skin, as well as internal bleeding if the blow is severe. Internal bleeding should be treated only by a doctor.

Scrapes or other abrasions should be washed in warm, soapy water. If there are loose foreign objects in the wound, try to rinse or pluck them out. After cleansing, an antibiotic ointment and bandage with sterile gauze can be applied.

Puncture wounds may be as mild as a splinter or as serious as a gunshot wound. Any penetrating wound offers serious danger of infection, since the foreign object carries bacteria through the protective layer of skin. Tetanus shots are usually recommended if the puncture wound is relatively deep, since the bacteria that cause tetanus are likely to have contaminated most puncturing objects. Tetanus prophylaxis may be needed so a medical professional should be contacted to assess the appropriateness of such a treatment.

Further information may be found in BLEEDING DISORDERS; BLOOD TRANSFUSION; *and* INTERNAL BLEEDING. *Details may be found in* ANTICOAGULANT DRUGS; *and* OCCULT BLOOD.

Blepharoplasty

Plastic surgery performed on the upper or lower eyelids to remove wrinkled or sagging skin or to correct a drooping eyelid.

Blepharoplasty is usually done for cosmetic reasons, but the operation is sometimes performed for practical reasons (drooping eyelids can cause reduced visibility for drivers) and may therefore be covered by some medical insurance policies.

The operation is usually done in a doctor's office under a local anesthetic. The operation takes around one to two hours, and the patient almost always goes home the same day. Extra skin on the upper or lower eyelid is cut away, and the remaining skin is stitched together. Incisions are made—either with a scalpel or, as is becoming increasingly common, with lasers—along the natural folds of the eyelids so that scars are not noticeable. Stitches are removed after a week. Swelling may last for several days, and bruising for up to two weeks. *See also* PLASTIC SURGERY.

Blind-Loop Syndrome

A condition in which a loop of the intestine is blocked off from the rest of the organ so that nothing may pass through.

Blind-loop syndrome may occur after the removal of part of the stomach (partial gastrectomy), or as a complication of inflammatory bowel disease or scleroderma. Food becomes trapped in the blocked section of intestine, and new food bypasses the loop. The trapped food leads to increased bacterial growth, which may spread to the rest of the intestine and cause abdominal distension. Food passes through a shorter section of the intestine, possibly leading to ineffective digestion and absorption of fats and fat soluble vitamins. Vitamin B_{12} deficiency may occur due to bacterial uptake of the vitamin. Treatment includes surgery to remove the blockage, as well as treatment of any underlying condition. Antibiotics may also be helpful. *See* ABDOMEN *and* INTESTINE.

Blind Spot

A tiny area located where the retina meets the optic nerve, devoid of the receptors necessary to capture light.

Everyone has a blind spot. It affects peripheral vision and is particularly noticeable when looking at an object up close. Draw an X on a sheet of paper and a dot six inches to the right. Hold the paper in an outstretched hand, close the left eye, focus on the X with the right, gradually pull the paper closer—the dot vanishes when it enters the blind spot of the right eye. The blind spot goes unnoticed because the brain automatically "fills" it with compensatory neural information that "assumes" the continuity of appearance when the image falls into the blind spot. *See also* EYE.

Blindness

The inability to see or see clearly.

Blindness usually means a drastic loss of vision that glasses or contact lenses cannot correct. Partial vision loss is more common and limits everyday living severely enough that it requires either complete or partial correction. Blindness in the United States is technically defined as the corrected sharpness of vision that is 20/200 or less in the better eye; meaning the visual field is diminished to 20 degrees or less. Loss of central or peripheral vision, or both, can happen slowly or quickly. Central vision loss will be apparent to the victim, but loss of peripheral vision may be undetected until it causes a loss of coordination.

About 40 million people the world over are partially or totally blind. Vitamin A deficiency causes blindness in millions of children in poor regions of Africa, Asia, South America, and other areas. The number of legally blind in the U.S. is approximately 214 people per 100,000.

Causes. Injury, disease, or degeneration of the eyeball, brain, or nerve pathways linking the eye to the brain, or anything that blocks light on its way to the retina may

cause blindness. For example, Sjögren's syndrome prevents the eye from tearing and can cause keratoconjunctivis sicca, which clouds the transparency of the cornea, the convex front of the strong outer shell of the eyeball. Vitamin A deficiency, chemical damage, and injury can also cloud the cornea. Infections such as ophthalmia neonatorum, or swelling of the conjunctiva in newborns, trachoma, herpes simplex, and bacterial ulcers cause corneal ulcers that, when healed, leave scars that can impair vision.

Infections such as tuberculosis, sarcoidosis, syphilis, toxocariases, or toxoplasmosis are among the known potential causes of uveitis, an inflammation of the iris, ciliary body, or choroid. Though it is sometimes a birth defect or occurs during childhood, cataract usually develops in old age owing to a deteriorating lens that clouds and causes blindness.

Most of the eyeball contains a clear fluid that clouds with bleeding caused by diabetes mellitus, hypertension, hyphema (in which blood seeps into the watery substance in the front of the lens, the aqueous humor), and vitreous hemorrhage (in which blood enters the vitreous humor, the gelatinous substance behind the lens).

Retinal Damage. Blindness can also be caused by damage to the retina: retinal hemorrhage, bleeding into the retina caused by diabetes, hypertension, vascular disease

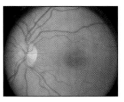

Blind Spot. Above, an image of the retina of the human eye. This structure is only about 200–250 micrometers thick, but its multilayer design is highly light-sensitive. At its periphery is a type of unnoticed "vanishing line" where it can no longer see because no visual messages are sent to the brain.

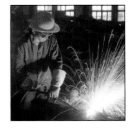

Protective Eyewear. People working in laboratory and industrial situations, such as the welder seen above, often wear protective eyewear. This will protect their eyes from harmful situations and chemicals.

Protective Eyewear

Parents should consider protective eyewear for their children who play sports. Annually, emergency rooms treat over 15,000 children for sports-related eye injuries. Anyone who works in an industry where there is a potential for eye damage should also wear protective lenses. Industrial-strength glass, plastic, or polycarbonate lenses meet or exceed standards, and each has its advantages. Glass resists scratching and can accommodate prescription lenses, but often glass lenses are heavy and uncomfortable while plastic and polycarbonate lenses are light and fog-resistant. If abrasive chemicals come into contact with the eyes, they must be flushed out immediately with copious amounts of water and 911 should be called as soon as possible.

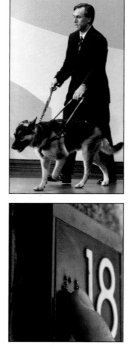

Living With Blindness. There are a number of lifestyle aids that help individuals who are blind go about their daily business. Top, visually impaired mountain climber, Erik Weihenmayer and his seeing eye dog walking across a stage to make an address. Below, numbers and letters in public places and at home can be written with raised dots known as braille. This can be helpful in elevators, on the front door of houses, and in other places. Also, most books have been converted into braille so that they can be enjoyed by everyone, regardless of visual ability.

or injury; retinopathy due to diabetes or hypertension; retinal artery occlusion, the blockage of blood supplying the retina; retinal vein occlusion; retinal detachment; tumors such as retinoblastoma and malignant melanoma; and macular degeneration, an old-age deterioration of the central retina. All can impair vision severely.

There are many different types of glaucoma, a degeneration of the nerve fibers constituting the optic nerve, causing blindness. Loss of peripheral vision, often detected after the disease is in an advanced stage, is the most common result.

Amblyopia. Another form of abnormal vision is amblyopia ex anopsia, known commonly as lazy eye, which results from one eye's lack of use in childhood and often occurs in tandem with misalignment of the eyes (strabismus) or unequal focus between the eyes (anisometropia). This condition is common among children in the U.S., but treatable if detected early.

The optic nerve and nerve pathways transmit impulses of electrochemical energy received by the retina to the brain. A tumor lodged in the bony cavity around the eyeball, called the orbit, or in the brain may apply pressure that blocks the impulses from traveling through the nerve or pathways. Similar blockages may result if blood flow to the optic nerve is impeded by diabetes mellitus, hypertension, tumors, injuries, or temporal arteritis; by an inflammation of the optic nerve (optic neuritis) that occurs in multiple sclerosis; or by the poisonous effects of chemicals or lack of nutrients that cause nutritional-deficiency amblyopia or optic neuropathy.

Nerve impulses travel from the retina to the visual cortex, a region in the brain that translates the messages into images. A brain tumor or hemorrhage that presses against the visual cortex, or a stroke that constricts blood flow, may cause blindness.

TREATMENT

Vision loss should be treated at once. The cause can be determined by an eye exam: ophthalmoscopy, slit-lamp examination, perimetry, or tonometry. Visual evoked potentials can measure electrical activity in the brain produced by visual stimulation.

Other Symptoms include the patient's description of when and how quickly vision loss occurred, age, and medical history may help determine a precise diagnosis. Ultrasound, CT scanning, or MRI may be used to detect damage or deficiencies in the eyes, orbits, optic nerves and surrounding structures, or the brain. The retina and choroid may be examined by a technique of photographing the inside of the eye called fluorescein angiography. The cause will determine the treatment. Depending upon an organization's definition of blindness, services may be available to those with irreparable vision loss. *See also* BLIND SPOT; CORNEA, DISORDERS OF; EYE; VISION; VISION, DISORDERS OF; *and* VISION, LOSS OF.

Blister

Also known as a bulla (large) or vesicle (small)

A raised fluid-filled bump just under the outer layer of the skin.

Blisters can be caused by burns or by the friction, such as with a shoe, against the skin. Blisters can also be caused by certain viral infections. Herpes simplex type I invades the mouth and causes blisters. One out of 1000 people may be infected with this form of the virus. Most people come into contact with it before age 20. Herpes simplex type II causes genital herpes and infections in babies. Other viruses and certain bacteria can also cause blisters.

Both herpes viruses are very contagious. The first symptoms occur about one to two weeks after the initial exposure. Blisters in the mouth usually heal in seven to ten days. The virus then becomes latent, and recurrences are usually less severe. In the case of blisters caused by viral infection, antiviral medications, such as acyclovir, are used to treat the symptoms and help reduce pain. Blisters caused by burns or by friction should be allowed to heal on their own, unless they are particularly severe, in which case medical attention should be sought. *See also* SORE; SKIN; *and* VIRUS.

Blood

The fluid that circulates throughout the body, acting as a transportation system.

Blood carries oxygen and nutrients to the cells and tissues, and collects carbon dioxide and waste products for delivery to the lungs, liver, and kidneys for excretion.

The blood is one of the best measures of the health of a human body. Its functions are so wide-ranging and critical that one of the first diagnostic procedures a doctor does is to draw blood and submit it to a number of tests to determine the most probable cause and progress of a illness.

There are about 10 to 12 pints of blood in an average adult male, and about 8 to 9 pints in an average adult female. If a person's blood loss comprises more than 20 percent of their total amount, then the individual is in grave danger of dying, since the brain needs a regular and adequate supply of oxygenated blood in order to function properly for any duration of time.

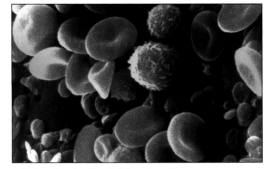
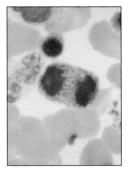

of the body. Red blood cells carry oxygen from the lungs to the tissues and other organs and take carbon dioxide back. White blood cells clean the blood of bacteria and other dead or dying cells. Platelets circulate in the blood to plug holes in the veins or arteries that would otherwise drain blood from the body's systems.

Blood Cells. Above left, the biconcave shape of red blood cells allows for maximum surface area as they transport oxygen throughout the body. Above right, immature red and white blood cells at 500 times magnification.

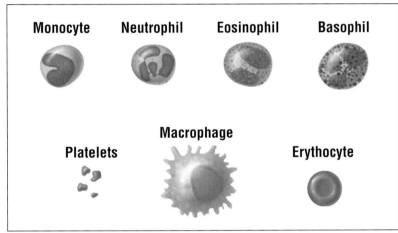

Monocyte   Neutrophil   Eosinophil   Basophil

Macrophage

Platelets   Erythocyte

Blood is the main regulator of the body's core temperature. If the body temperature is too high, blood moves to the surface of the skin in order to it cool down. If the body temperature is dangerously low, the blood tends to pool in the most critical internal organs around the abdomen, and especially in the heart.

The blood is also the main protection against disease. It carries molecules called antibodies that are designed to kill specific bacteria or viruses.

Basic information on this subject is contained in BLOOD CELLS; BLOOD PRODUCTS; HEMOGLOBIN; *and* LEUKOCYTES. *More specific articles on circulation are contained in* BLOOD PRESSURE; CIRCULATORY SYSTEM; THROMBOSIS; *and* TRANSFUSION. *Details on disorders are in* BLOOD DISORDERS; HEMOPHILIA; *and* HYPERTENSION.

Blood Constituents. At the left are some of the constituents of blood. Monocytes are white blood cells that make up 3 to 8 percent of the blood. A neutrophil is a granular white blood cell that is especially fatal to foreign antigens. Eosinophils are also granular. Basophils are granular white blood cells. Macrophages are often the largest of the white blood cells; these cells "ingest" bacteria. Platelets activate to stop bleeding. Erythrocytes are the most common of the blood cells, they are better known as red blood cells. They carry oxygen to the body's various tissues.

ALERT

Blood and the Rhesus (Rh) Factor

Blood is divided into four main types, which are determined by hereditary factors. Blood is also typed by whether or not the Rhesus factor is present in the blood. Eighty-five percent of Americans are Rh positive. The Rh factor is particularly important to pregnant women, because if a fetus inherits a conflicting Rh factor from its father, the mother's body may produce antibodies against the fetus's blood. The Rh factor is also important for those who receive blood transfusions because the recipient may reject donor blood that matches in type, but not in Rh factor.

Components. Plasma is the name of the blood fluid that is mostly water but also contains a myriad of chemicals and hormones that regulate the various functions

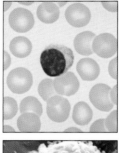

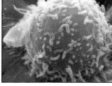

A Red Blood Cell and White Blood Cells. Top, a lymphocyte, or white blood cell, among a number of red blood cells. Below, a B lymphocyte covered with an infectious invader triggers a response by the immune system.

Red Blood Cells.
Below, red blood cells, produced in the bone marrow, are not always completely mature when they are first produced; immature blood cells are often called blast cells. Far right, red blood cells will develop in to their final form before long. Sometimes, the biconcave shape of red blood cells, the shape that increases the cell's surface area, may also cause cellular stacking; this is where red blood cells adhere to one another in small stacks.

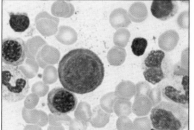

Blood Cells

Components of the blood that transport gases, fight disease, and stop bleeding.

Blood cells, along with chemicals and hormones that regulate the functions of the body, are carried in the plasma. There are three main types of blood cells: red blood cells, white blood cells, and platelets.

Red Blood Cells. The most numerous of the cells in the blood are red blood cells, or erythrocytes. They are produced by the bone marrow and move oxygen from the lungs to the cells of the body. They also move carbon dioxide back to the lungs to be exhaled.

The key element in this process is hemoglobin, a molecule in red blood cells that, when enriched with oxygen, gives them a distinctive scarlet color. On the return trip to the lungs, hemoglobin carries carbon dioxide and is a much darker red. Red blood cells also help manage the balance of the blood's relative acidity.

Red blood cells have a lifetime of about 120 days; then they wear down and must be replaced. The dying cells are washed from the bloodstream in the liver, spleen, and bone marrow, but the proteins and iron are reclaimed and used in the production of new red blood cells.

White Blood Cells, known as leukocytes, are mostly produced in the bone marrow, but their function is very different from that of red blood cells. The leukocytes play a critical role in the body's immune system. They are usually larger than the red cells, but they vary in size and shape.

There are five main types of white blood cells: neutrophils, lymphocytes, monocytes, eosinophils, and basophils. All of these protect the body against disease. When bacteria, viruses, fungi, or parasites attack healthy tissue, chemicals are released into the bloodstream to attract neutrophils (a granular white blood cell) and monocytes, which will "swallow" the small bacteria and then clean up any foreign debris.

The red swelling and pus that may collect in an infected site is actually an accumulation of neutrophils that have functioned well and died in the process.

Lymphocytes produce toxins and antibodies that protect against the substances generated by bacteria, viruses, and chemicals that would harm the body.

Monocytes, a type of white blood cell, are produced in the bone marrow and the spleen. They attack foreign bacteria and ingest and break down dead or damaged cells, including red blood cells, that have reached the end of their life. Monocytes make up 3 to 8 percent of white blood cells.

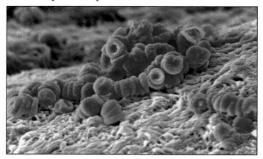

Platelets are tiny cells that plug holes in the arteries or veins where blood may be escaping. Platelets are made in the bone marrow, and there are literally trillions of them in a healthy body, so they are always readily available. Normally, the walls inside veins or arteries are a smooth layer of tissue. When there is a break in the wall, the platelets change in character: they stick to the broken edges of the break, build a web across the opening, and then collect in a plug or clot to stop the loss of blood—all this in a matter of seconds, for a small break. They also release chemicals that attract more platelets and promote clotting.

The danger of overactive clot formation is that if one breaks loose from the wall of the blood vessel and makes its way to the heart, lungs, or brain, it can plug the passageway completely and cause a heart attack, pulmonary thrombosis, or a stroke.

Basic information regarding Blood Cells *can be found in* B Cell; Cardiology; Lymphocyte; *and* Plasma. *Advanced topics can be found in articles on* Blood; Rh Incompatibility; Surgery; *and* Transfusion, Autologous.

Blood Clotting

The process in which parts of the blood thicken into a solid mass in order to stop bleeding.

Inevitably, of the millions of blood vessels in a body, at least some are damaged or break open every day. The body's response is a complex system called hemostasis.

Normal Blood Clotting. (See diagram sequence at the right) When a blood vessel (a) is ruptured, it almost immediately constricts to stop or slow the blood loss (b). This spasm is caused by chemicals released (c) from the platelets and the blood vessel wall—blood cells whose primary function is to protect the circulatory system. A plasma protein called the von Willebrand factor is released; it changes the chemical nature of the platelets so that they become large and sticky, with a spiny surface. The platelets stick to the rough edges of a broken blood vessel and construct fibrous strands that form a mesh across the opening. This attracts more platelets and gives them a structure on which to build a sort of net. The blood loss is stopped, and the body can then begins healing and repair.

If there is a large break in a blood vessel, a more drastic process occurs. The blood becomes thick and clings to the blood vessel walls. The formation of a blood clot is called coagulation. After the clot has been formed and the rupture sealed, the blood clot shrinks and draws the edges of the break together to start the process whereby the opening is healed and scar tissue built. The clot itself slowly dissolves under the control of blood factors and is replaced in a process called fibrinolysis.

Coagulation Problems. When the blood clotting system is not correctly balanced, an individual may bruise easily. When tiny blood vessels under the skin break, they release small amounts of blood that collect and darken the skin to a blue or purplish color. Normally this is not a dangerous condition, but if it persists or grows more extreme, it may indicate a serious problem that can become life-threatening.

Conversely, an incorrect balance may produce clots that travel through the bloodstream or do not successfully control the loss of blood. If free-floating clots block the blood vessels of the brain, heart, or lungs, they can produce strokes, heart attacks, or pulmonary embolisms, all of which are life threatening. Even clots lodged in the smaller blood vessels can restrict the flow of blood to those areas and may cause severe damage to any of the adjacent tissues.

Anticoagulant Medications. Because excessive blood clotting can be quite dangerous, a large number of different medications are used to control blood clot production. Aspirin is now recommended in small daily doses for people with heart disease because it thins the blood and reduces the likelihood of blood clots forming on plaque in the coronary arteries.

Heparin is administered by injection and it treats and prevents acute blood clots, especially after surgery. It may produce skin staining, as damaged blood vessels leak blood into the surrounding tissues.

Warfarin works by blocking the function of vitamin K, which is essential to the production of blood clotting factors. Dosage of this and other anticoagulants must be monitored closely, since too much promotes bleeding, and too little provides no protection against the formation of clots.

More recently, a new group of drugs has been developed that actually dissolve the clots. These are called fibrinolytic drugs, and they can prevent death when a blocked artery is starving the heart muscles, or when a person has suffered a stroke and may be in danger of severe brain damage. Again, the effect of these drugs must be monitored closely because they frequently cause excessive bleeding.

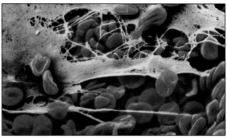
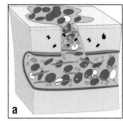
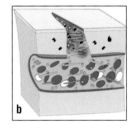
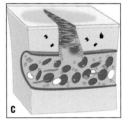

Blood Clotting. Top, a fibrin mesh forms around a wound (specifically, a break in a blood vessel) trapping blood cells, and stopping bleeding. The stages of wound repair are also detailed above—from the wound (a), to the formation of fibrin threads (b), to the formation of a clot (c).

Background material on BLOOD CLOTTING *may be found in* BLOOD CELLS; HEMATOLOGY; *and* THROMBOSIS. *For additional material on clotting, see* ANTICOAGULANT DRUGS; FIBRINOLYSIS; *and* HEMATOMA. *Clotting problems are discussed in* BLEEDING DISORDERS; HEMOPHILIA; *and* LEG ULCERS.

Blood Clotting Tests

Tests performed on blood to measure how quickly it clots.

Blood clotting (coagulation) is a complex process that is measured through a variety of tests. One common test, prothrombin time, is used to assess the effects of an anticoagulant medications known as coumadin. Another, called activated partial thromboplasmin time, evaluates the proper dosage for heparin, an anticoagulant drug.

Coagulation depends on a number of substances (coagulation factors), which must be present in the correct quantities for the coagulation process—which involves various parts of the blood—to occur normally. Blood clotting halts the flow of blood from a wound and it simultaneously with the constriction of the wounded blood vessel. The absence of clotting factors in the blood produces the uncontrolled bleeding associated with hemophilia, a hereditary blood disorder. These same blood factors control when and how a clot from a larger wound will dissolve and they need testing.

Background material on Blood Clotting Tests can be found in the articles detailing BLOOD; BLOOD CELLS; BLOOD CLOTTING; *and* THROMBOSIS. *Related information is contained in* B CELL; BLOOD DISORDERS DIAGNOSIS; HEMOPHILIA; *and* HEMATOLOGY. *See also* BLOOD DONATION; ELECTROCOAGULATION; *and* PHOTOCOAGULATION *for more information.*

Blood Count

Also known as complete blood count or CBC

A test that measures six critical factors in a sample of whole blood.

Blood count is taken to diagnose anemia, infections, or if a person's blood-clotting function is impaired. The red blood count (RBC) measures the number of red blood cells per cubic microliter. It is normally between 4 million and 5.2 million. The hemoglobin (HGB) and hematocrit (HCT) counts, both measure the blood's ability to carry oxygen from the lungs to the body. If the values are low, the diagnosis is anemia.

A white blood count (WBC) of between 4,000 and 10,000 cells per cubic millimeter is normal. Higher counts may indicate that the individual is fighting an infection. Lower counts suggest that a person may be taking certain kinds of medication, undergoing chemotherapy, or have an autoimmune or other blood disorder.

The mean corpuscular volume (MCV) is an indication of what kind of anemia a person may have. A high count may indicate a need for vitamin B_{12}, while a low count may indicate an iron deficiency.

The platelet count (PLT) measures the number of platelets in the blood and indicates the ability of the blood to clot. *See also* BLOOD; BLOOD CELLS; BLOOD CLOTTING; VITAMIN B_{12}; CHEMOTHERAPY; DIAGNOSIS; INFECTION *and* VITAMIN B COMPLEX.

Blood Disorders

Diseases arising from a malfunction in any of the components of the blood.

The blood is a complex mixture of fluids and cells that assist in the metabolic process and serve the critical functions of protecting the body from infection and promoting healing. A malfunction of any blood component will lead to a blood disorder.

Blood consists of a water-based plasma that contains essential proteins and salts. The blood serves as a carrier of red blood cells, whose primary function is to take oxygen from the lungs and deliver it to the cells and tissues of the body. On the return trip, the red blood cells pick up carbon dioxide and deliver it to the lungs, where it is exhaled. The blood also carries white blood cells, whose function is to attack invading bacteria and viruses, and to scavenge the blood for dead or deformed cellular material. Finally, the blood carries platelets, which are tiny cells that plug leaks in the vascular system.

RED BLOOD CELLS

The most common blood disorder is anemia, a disorder marked by a lack of red blood cells. This results in insufficient amounts of hemoglobin, which carries oxygen to the body.

Anemia can be caused by mechanical factors, such severe blood loss in an accident or during surgery. Anemia can also be the result of inadequate iron, vitamin B_{12}, or folic acid in the blood, an imbalance among the various hormones, or a disease of the bone marrow. Some chemotherapy drugs can induce anemia by interfering with the bone marrow function, or by reducing the ability of the red blood cells to carry oxygen.

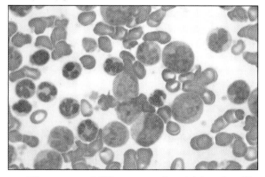

The normal life span of red blood cells may be decreased when disease invades the bone marrow. Their life will also be shortened when the immune system does not recognize the body's own red blood cells and attacks them as foreign bodies. Red blood cells can be damaged as they flow through a mechanical heart valve or they can be hurt by high blood pressure. Deformed red blood cells are unable to carry oxygen or carbon dioxide in the body.

A person suffering from anemia exhibits a characteristic pallor, is chronically fatigued, and is made breathless by the slightest exertion. An individual who loses blood rapidly will experience dizziness and a sharp drop in blood pressure. Some forms of anemia are associated with jaundice, in which case the urine turns dark orange. The spleen may also become enlarged as it struggles to strain out dead or damaged red blood cells.

The most common type type of anemia is iron-deficiency. Inherited forms, such as sickle cell, are significantly less common and there are few cases of aplastic anemia. When the normally disk-shaped red blood cells are more spherical in nature, the disorder is called spherocytosis. When the cells are elongated and curved, the condition is called sickle cell anemia. Inherited forms of anemia cannot be cured, but the symptoms can be controlled. Anemic individuals are advised to avoid activities that make great demands on the oxygen supply (such as intense workouts from sports), to treat even minor viral infections seriously, and to get flu shots. In an emergency, an anemic patient is given transfusions.

WHITE BLOOD CELLS

White blood cells constitute the body's basic immune system. Over 70 percent of white blood cells are neutrophils, whose primary function is to attack bacteria or fungi. Neutrophils scavenge dead cells and foreign objects that may embed themselves in the body tissues. It is the neutrophils that gather at the site of an infection and make the area red, hot, and tender to the touch. Neutropenia is a disorder marked by a lack of neutrophils, leaving the body vulnerable to infection. Aplastic anemia can cause neutropenia, as can certain drugs; a tendency for the disorder may be inherited.

Lymphocytes protect the body against viral infections. They also work with the neutrophils to eliminate bacteria and fungi and assist in the healing process. Lymphocytopenia is a disorder marked by a low number of lymphocytes circulating in the body. It is frequently seen when a person suffers from cancer (or when a person undergoes some forms of cancer treatment), leukemia, rheumatoid arthritis, HIV, or AIDS, among other conditions.

Platelets are blood cells that become sticky when they detect a break in a blood vessel. They slow or stop bleeding by building a plug at the rupture. In Von Willebrand's disease, a critical factor for blood clotting is missing, and the platelets do not stick to the edges of broken blood vessels.

See ANEMIA; BLOOD CELLS; HEART; BLEEDING DISORDERS; CARDIOVASCULAR DISORDERS; *and* SICKLE CELL ANEMIA. *Related material on blood problems is found in* BACTEREMIA; HEMOPHILIA; HYPOVOLEMIA; *and* THROMBOSIS, DEEP VEIN.

Leukemia Cells. Left, a blood smear showing leukemia cells. Young blood cells, called blasts, as pictured at the left, are often present in the bone marrow (where blood cells are produced) and in the blood. Myelogenous leukemia is diagnosed when there are too many white blood cells circulating in the body.

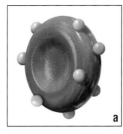

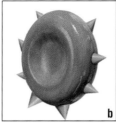

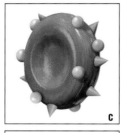

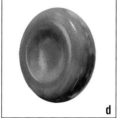

Blood Groups. The various blood groups are differentiated by the antigens found on the red blood cells. Above is an illustrated rendering of red blood cells and representations of surface antigens. (a) Type A blood has A antigens on its surface. (b) Type b blood has B antigens on its surface (c) Type AB blood has both type A and type B antigens on the surface. (d) Type O blood has no antigens on the surface.

Blood Donation

The process of giving whole blood or blood components to patients who need transfusions.

More than 12 million people donate blood every year, through organizations such as the Red Cross. A total of 14 million pints of blood are stored according to rules established by the Food and Drug Administration (FDA), and are later used in transfusions for patients in need of blood.

Procedure. The blood donation process is safe, and quite easy; only sterile equipment is used. Blood is collected from the donor through a needle inserted into a vein in the arm. Usually, one of the larger veins near the inside of the elbow is used. A tourniquet is placed on the upper arm to facilitate needle insertion.

Precautions. Most people experience no adverse effects after giving blood, but donors are still advised to avoid strenuous exercise for the remainder of the day and drink adequate fluids. *See also* BLOOD; BLOOD CELLS; BLOOD CLOTTING; HEMODIALYSIS; HEMOGLOBIN; *and* HEMOPHILIA.

Blood Gases

Critical gases present in the blood, specifically oxygen and carbon dioxide.

The concentration of oxygen and carbon dioxide in blood gives a measure of the capacity and efficiency of the lungs and the acidity of the blood. Low oxygen levels in the blood indicate a problem with red blood cells and hemoglobin. It is the hemoglobin that removes the oxygen from the lungs and carries it to the cells of the body, where it is exchanged for carbon dioxide. If oxygen levels are low, a person will be anemic—a disorder marked by a shortage of red blood cells.

While oxygen is necessary for human body functioning, it is also a toxic element, since it combines with almost any carbon-based molecule. The balance is a delicate one, since too much oxygen can damage the lungs and the eyes. *See* LUNG.

Blood acidity is regulated by the kidneys and lungs. Too much carbon dioxide will make the blood acidic. This can be caused by certain diseases, by extreme exercise (long-distance running, for example), or by certain medications used to control diabetes. Kidney and liver disease can also produce overly acidic blood. *See also* KIDNEY.

Blood Groups

Categories into which blood is divided, (mostly for transfusion purposes) depending on the presence or absence of certain molecules.

Before 1900, transfusions did more harm than good because the recipient would often react violently to the new blood and would sometimes actually die. Blood from all humans is not interchangeable and has to be further categorized into a number of different groups. These groups need to match if the transfusion is to be successful.

Blood is divided into four main groups, which are determined by hereditary factors. Early in the twentieth century, Karl Landsteiner found two different molecules on the surface of red blood cells. He called them type A and type B. If a person has only type A molecules on their red blood cells, his or her blood is called type A. If there are only type B molecules, the blood is called type B. If he has both kinds, it is called type AB, and if it has neither, it is called type O blood. Type A donors can give blood to type A and AB recipients. Type B donors can give to type B and AB recipients. Type AB can give only to other type AB recipients. Type O can give to any recipients but can only receive blood from others with type O blood.

Blood is also categorized based on whether or not the Rhesus (Rh) factor is

Population By Blood Group			
Percentages and the Rh Factor			
Blood Group	A	B	AB	O
Rh Positive	34%	8%	3%	35%
Rh Negative	8%	2%	1%	9%

present. This antigen was discovered by Landsteiner and Weiner in 1940. If blood contains the Rhesus factor, it is Rh positive. If not, it is Rh negative.

The Rh system is very complex, as it is determined by a combination of at least three genes, and maybe more. The Rh factor is particularly important to pregnant women because of the potential for incompatibility of the mother with a fetus that inherits a conflicting Rh factor from the father. If an Rh-negative mother conceives a child with Rh-positive blood, her body may form antibodies against the fetus's blood, resulting in hemolytic disease of the newborn (erythroblastosis fetalis).

> *Basic biochemical information on blood groups may be found in* BLOOD; BLOOD CLOTTING; BLOOD COUNT; *and* BLOOD GROUPS. *More on blood constituents is contained in* HEMOGLOBIN; LYMPHOCYTE; PLASMA; *and* RH INCOMPATIBILITY;

Blood Poisoning

Also known as septicemia

A disease caused by bacteria from an infected part of the body entering the bloodstream.

Blood poisoning—or septicemia—occurs when a disease-producing organism (pathogen) enters the bloodstream. It may result in life-threatening septic shock.

Septic shock differs from septicemia because septic shock is not an infection, but is rather the response of the body to the existence of large quantities of bacteria in the bloodstream.

CAUSES

Blood poisoning occurs as a result of a contaminated blood transfusion or from an infection that is already present in the body. As recently as the 1940s, nearly one-quarter of all transfusion patients contracted blood poisoning, but the introduction of disposable, sterilized containers and effective refrigeration procedures have reduced this occurrence to a virtual rarity. Today, about 90 percent of cases of blood poisoning are caused by infectious bacteria. Almost all others arise from fungal or viral infections.

The bacteria that infect the blood can come from various sources. An open wound can serve as a point of entry, or the patient may already be suffering from a disease involving bacteria in the bloodstream, such as listeriosis. Some unpasteurized dairy foods contain the bacteria *Listeria monocytogenes*, which causes listeriosis. Septic shock is the major cause of mortality in burn patients because certain bacteria associated with sepsis (bacterial infection) thrive on burned flesh. Septicemia is a risk for hospitalized patients, who may develop infections during the course of their stay. Especially at risk are those who already have a compromised immune system, such as those with cancer or AIDS.

> **ALERT**
>
> ### Septic Shock and Blood Poisoning
>
> Septic shock is very hard to diagnose because its symptoms are common to those of so many other disorders, including blood poisoning. Symptoms of blood poisoning include fever, chills, diarrhea, nausea, headache, vomiting, and abdominal pain. Septic shock is indicated by: thirst, weakness, lethargy, confusion, dilated pupils, fever, low blood pressure and weak pulse, extreme pallor or bluish skin, rapid or shallow breathing, nausea or vomiting, and loss of consciousness.
>
> If left untreated, multiple organ failure can occur. While sepsis (a bacterial infection) alone can cause death in 30 to 40 percent of cases, if three or more organs fail, septic shock is fatal in over 90 percent of cases. If septic shock is suspected, place the victim in the shock position; lay the victim on his or her back with the feet elevated above the heart. The head should lie flat. A blanket may be used for warmth.

DIAGNOSIS AND TREATMENT

A blood culture can determine the nature and amount of the organisms that have invaded the bloodstream, and what course of treatment to pursue. Patients suffering from septicemia are often given antibiotics.

> *Basic biochemical information is contained in* BACTERIA; BLOOD; *and* INFECTION. *More advanced subtopics are contained in* BLOOD TRANSFUSION; SEPSIS; *and* SEPTIC SHOCK. *Blood Poisoning treatment options are discussed in* PENICILLIN DRUGS; SHOCK *and* TOXIC SHOCK SYNDROME.

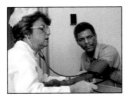

Blood Pressure. Above, a nurse tests a man's blood pressure. If necessary, he may have to change his diet and his lifestyle habits in order to reduce his blood pressure. In some cases, people are given medication for the same purpose. Far right, a digital blood pressure machine measures both blood pressure and pulse rate. These are useful for home monitoring of blood pressure. Some physicians will recommend this device for patients who wish to monitor their own blood pressure throughout the day.

Blood Pressure

The force exerted by the blood against the arteries as the heart beats.

Blood pressure is expressed through the use of two distinct numbers. The first number is for systolic pressure and the second is for diastolic pressure. Systolic pressure is the pressure at which blood is forced out of the heart, and diastolic pressure is the pressure of the blood between heart beats.

Blood pressure is measured in millimeters of mercury, which is marked as mm/Hg. The millimeters of mercury measurement is an expression of the height to which a column of mercury is raised in a sphygmomanometer, the standard device for measuring blood pressure.

Classically, blood pressure has been measured by placing a soft cuff around the patient's upper arm. The cuff is then inflated until it is tight enough to stop the normal flow of blood. Then it is gradually deflated until the health care professional taking the measurement can hear the beat of the pulse as blood flow resumes, then deflated again until the beat is no longer heard. This technique results in two numbers: the systolic pressure, the higher number recorded as the first beat is heard, and the diastolic pressure, when the blood is flowing freely enough that the beat can no longer be heard.

ALERT

Hypertension

Hypertension, or high blood pressure, is a major risk factor for cardiovascular conditions such as heart attack and stroke. It is defined as a blood-pressure level of 140/90 or greater that is found in several measurements over a period of time. There are variations among individuals, however.

Some persons may have systolic pressure within normal limits but an elevated diastolic pressure of from 110 to 115 mm Hg.

Older persons are more likely to have a form of hypertension in which the diastolic reading is below 90 but the systolic reading is abnormally high—160 mm Hg or higher. This systolic hypertension increases the risk of heart attack, stroke, or heart failure.

NORMAL LEVELS

A healthy young adult at rest will have a systolic pressure ranging from 100 to 130, with diastolic pressure ranging around 60 to 80. Blood-pressure changes with age and with activity. A baby may have a normal blood pressure reading of 70 over 50 (70/50). The systolic pressure is always expressed first. Blood pressure in an adult will be lowest during rest or sleep and highest during intense physical activity that increases the body's demand for oxygen. Generally, pressure begins to rise when a person awakens from sleep, remains at a steady level during the day, and begins to decrease at bedtime.

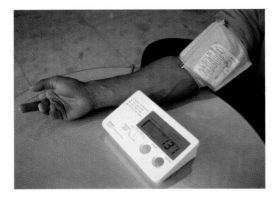

RISK FACTORS

Blood pressure can change because of environmental factors affecting the body. For example, caffeine or cigarette smoke can raise pressure, so it is advisable not to have coffee or other caffeine-containing beverages before a blood-pressure measurement is taken.

Stress, either emotional, physical, or both, also has the potential to raise blood pressure. Anger and fright can cause the adrenal glands to produce epinephrine, which is a hormone commonly known as adrenaline. This hormone will act to make the heart beat more often and harder, causing blood vessels to constrict and increasing blood pressure drastically.

Background material may be found in DIASTOLE; HEART BEAT; PLAGUE; PULSE; *and* SYSTOLE. *Further information regarding blood pressure problems may be found in* CONGESTIVE HEART FAILURE; PORTAL HYPERTENSION; *and* STRESS.

Blood Products

A term used to describe all the various forms in which blood is modified and sold or distributed for medical or research purposes.

The chief concern regarding the distribution of blood products is that they not carry any viruses or bacteria that will harm the recipient. Blood is made up of four major components: red blood cells (RBC), white blood cells (WBC), platelets, and plasma. When blood is donated, it may be separated into its component parts and distributed as is deemed necessary. Blood and its components are produced and used in many different forms.

ANTICOAGULANT FACTORS

An anticoagulant factor is added to whole blood to keep the blood fluid. It can be stored for five weeks, although certain factors deteriorate after a week. Freezing plasma preserves coagulant factors for a longer period. "Fresh" blood is less than 24 hours old and treats people with bleeding disorders, however, it is used rarely to resuscitate people with massive blood loss.

RED BLOOD CELLS

Red blood cells remain when most of the plasma is removed, so that they take up about 70–80 percent of the volume of the blood. A preservative may be added, which also reduces the thickness of the material and allows it to flow more freely. This type of blood is used during surgery as well as to assist people suffering from anemia, as well as those who have bone marrow disease or are being treated with chemotherapy.

Platelets are said to be "stunned" when in storage, and may take four hours after transfusion to be fully functional. They are transfused into patients with severe loss of clotting ability due to a very low platelet count. Platelet concentrate has a shelf life of five days.

Fresh frozen plasma is administered when there is a problem with coagulation or when there is serious bleeding. The plasma contains coagulation factors that may be helpful in these cases. Frozen plasma has a shelf life of one year. Plasma is also separated into its various components of albumin and immunoglobulins, which are useful in immunotherapy. *See* BLOOD.

Basic information may be found in BLOOD; BLOOD CLOTTING; BLOOD COUNT; BLOOD GROUPS; HEMOGLOBIN; LYMPHOCYTE; *and* PLASMA. *Blood transfusion is discussed in* BLOOD TRANSFUSION; *and* TRANSFUSION, AUTOLOGOUS.

Blood Smear

Also known as peripheral smear

A droplet of blood smeared on a microscope slide for examination.

A blood smear uses a drop of blood taken from either the patient's fingertip, the back of the hand, or the inside of the elbow. The blood is then dripped onto a carefully cleaned slide. A second slide is used to spread the droplet of blood across the first slide, creating an even smear suitable for microscopic examination and analysis. The different types of blood cells are then examined for any abnormalities in number, shape, appearance, or proportion.

USES

A blood smear may be used to test for a variety of disorders, including:

- osmotic fragility, a condition in which red blood cells are shaped in such a way that they are likely to rupture easily;
- iron deficiencies;
- liver diseases, including jaundice;
- uremia; a toxic condition existing with severe kidney disease;
- anemia, including the sickle-cell variety; and
- lukemia.

If anything abnormal is diagnosed from the test, a health-care professional will direct treatment.

Background material on blood testing may be found in BLOOD COUNT; BLOOD GASES; BLOOD COUNT; *and* INTRAVENOUS INFUSION. *Related material on blood disorders is found in* BLOOD DISORDERS; *and* BLOOD POISONING. *See* \Pap Smear.

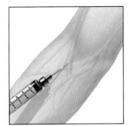

Drawing Blood. Above, in order to draw blood, an area of skin must first be cleaned, and a needle inserted. After a quantity of blood is drawn, the needle is removed and the blood can be taken to a laboratory for testing and analysis. Blood is regularly drawn to facilitate a diagnosis.

Blood Tests

Tests designed to evaluate the properties of blood and its components.

Because of the wealth of information blood tests supply, they are part of almost every routine physical examination.

In addition to its intrinsic functions of carrying oxygen and fighting disease, blood transports a vast array of ingredients essential to a healthy body, including electrolytes (such as sodium, potassium, and phosphorus) fats and cholesterol, uric acid, creatinine (a substance that reflects kidney function), proteins, hormones, and a wide variety of other vital substances.

Testing the blood can often provide detailed information on the quality of organ function without the need to directly sample organ tissue.

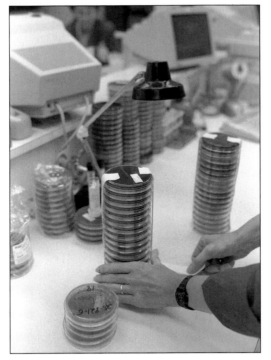

Blood Tests. Right, blood samples in petri dishes go to a hematology lab for various types of testing. Blood tests are of central importance because of the great amount of information that comes from such an examination.

One common blood test is the complete blood cell count, or CBC, which measures the total number of red blood cells (erythrocytes), and white blood cells (leukocytes), and platelets, present in a sample of blood. Today the process is generally performed with sophisticated machines, which require only a small blood sample. These diagnostic devices can test the blood sample in under a minute.

For males, normal blood contains about 5 million red blood cells; for females, blood contains about 4.5 million red blood

Additional Blood Tests

Among the many other blood tests available, ESR (erythrocyte sedimentation rate), Coombs' antiglobulin test, and blood coagulation tests are among the more common. ESR measures the rate at which red blood cells settle to the bottom of a vial of blood. Rapid sedimentation rate can indicate inflammation, anemia, infection or cancer. Coombs' test examines the blood for the presence of antiglobulins on cell surfaces. These irregular antibodies are often produced through a condition known as autoimmune hemolytic anemia. Coagulation tests measure the rate of blood clotting; they can identify clotting disorders such as hemophilia and assess the efficiency of anticoagulation therapy.

cells per microliter. On average, and across gender, there are 5,000 to 10,000 white blood cells per microliter and about 450,000 platelets.

In addition to the cell count, a complete blood count test reports the percentage of each type of white blood cell (differential), measures hemoglobin (the iron-carrying molecules that supply tissue and organs with oxygen) content, and evaluates the size and shape of red blood cells—this is a general marker for the health of blood and, by extension, an individual.

Abnormalities in size and shape of red blood cells can indicate disease. For example, sickle-cell anemia and spherocytosis are characterized by, respectively, crescent-shaped and spherical red blood cells. Iron deficiencies produce red blood cells of reduced size, while oversized oval red blood cells may indicate pernicious anemia due to deficiencies in vitamin B_{12} or folic acid.

Technical information on blood tests may be found in BLOOD; BLOOD COUNT; BLOOD SMEAR; *and* HORMONES. *Further information can be found in* ANEMIA; BLOOD DISORDERS; LIPID DISORDERS; *and* TUBERCULOSIS. *Related material is discussed in* DIAGNOSIS; HYPERGLYCEMIA; IRON; KIDNEY DISORDERS; LIVER DISORDERS; *and* VITAMIN B.

Blood Transfusion

The transfer of blood or blood components, usually by pint, directly into another person's bloodstream through a vein.

Blood transfusion compensates for significant blood loss during a major operation or after a hemorrhage, bleeding peptic ulcer, wound, burn, or other life-threatening forms of trauma. Different components of blood may be transfused to treat various disorders such as:

- chronic anemia: consistently low levels of red blood cells;
- hemophilia: deficient clotting factor, leading to uncontrolled bleeding;
- leukemia: production of too many white blood cells; and
- thalassemia: inability to properly produce hemoglobin.

Types of Whole and Partial Blood-Transfusion Products and Their Uses

The different types of blood products have various uses, including:

- Whole blood: to treat acute blood loss.
- Packed red blood cells: for chronic anemia.
- Washed red blood cells: for allergies induced by frequent transfusions.
- Platelets: for severe bleeding caused by a deficiency in platelets.
- White blood cells: for infected patients who have a low white blood cell count.
- Plasma: for shock without blood loss.
- Fresh-frozen plasma (freshly drawn plasma, or concentrates of the antihemophilic factor of plasma): for bleeding hemophiliacs.
- Albumin (concentrated from the plasma): for shock or for chronic low albumin disorders and the severest forms of malnutrition.
- Gamma globulin (an antibody concentrate) — for prevention of viral hepatitis and protection against or modification of measles after exposure.
- Fibrinogen (a concentrated clotting factor) — for bleeding that is caused by a deficiency or an absence of fibrinogen.

Newborn babies with disease affecting the red blood cells (such as osmotic fragility, spherocytosis, sickle cell anemia, and thalassemia) and with abnormally high levels of bilirubin in the blood need a transfusion directly from donor to recipient. This is called an exchange transfusion, in which nearly all of the recipient's blood is replaced by donor blood in order to avoid jaundice or severe brain damage.

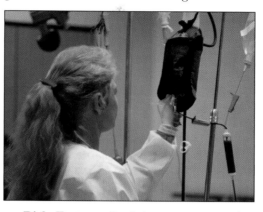

Risk Factors. Recipients must receive their own blood type (A, B, AB, or O) with the proper Rh factor. The only exception is if donor blood is type O, Rh-negative because anyone can receive O-negative blood. If blood has not been matched properly, antibodies in the recipient's blood may cause incompatible donor blood cells to burst (hemolyze), resulting in fever or chills, shock, or kidney failure. It is also possible for a patient to have an allergic reaction to transfused white cells, plasma proteins, and platelets.

Contracting a life threatening infection, such as HIV, hepatitis B or C, syphilis, toxoplasmosis or malaria, was a major risk of blood transfusions in the past. However, donated blood is well-screened for disease today. Other risks include heart failure or liver damage in the elderly due to iron overload. Patients with chronic anemia who have had regular transfusions over many years may accumulate excess iron in their systems, which can cause damage to organs such as the heart, liver, and pancreas. A drug like deferoxamine can counteract this accumulation.

Testing Blood for Transfusion . Left, each individual has unique blood, so the best transfusion match is always one's own. There are more than 100 subgroups of blood types and, although it is generally safe, blood from a random donor even of the same type may cause a transfusion reaction. Blood from a close relative or a family member also has a greater chance of matching closely and causing the least reaction.

Background material on may be found in BLOOD CELLS; HEMATOLOGY; INTRAVENOUS INFUSION *and* TRANSFUSION; AUTOLOGOUS. *Details on applications will be found in* BLEEDING; CHEMOTHERAPY; DEHYDRATION; *and* TREATMENT OF, ANEMIA.

Blue Baby

A newborn whose skin tone is a pale or dusky blue, indicating poor respiration and insufficient oxygen intake. Immediate assistance is required.

The bluish complexion is typically caused by low oxygen levels in the blood from a defect in the heart or arteries. Specific causes include the transposition of the great arteries, hypoplastic left heart syndrome, or the tetralogy of Fallot. Such a defect permits some oxygen-poor blood arriving in the heart to skip its oxygen-gathering circulation of the lungs. This can be a life threatening condition for newborns. The blood remains bluish (cyanotic), oxygen-poor, and colors the infant's skin. A surgical procedure called the Blalock-Taussig Shunt that connects a blood vessel leaving the heart to one entering it usually corrects the problem. *See also* CIRCULATORY SYSTEM.

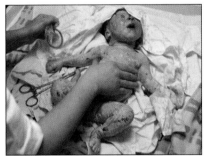

Blue Baby. The first Blalock-Taussig shunt, the procedure that treats the condition known as blue baby, was performed in 1944 by Dr. Alfred Blalock—it was suggested by Dr. Helen Taussig. This procedure corrects the disorder that makes a baby actually turn blue, as seen above.

Blue Cross/Blue Shield

A national association of locally operated health insurance organizations.

Blue Cross/Blue Shield is the association for the oldest and largest group of health insurance companies in the United States. There are 47 independent, locally operated Blue Cross/Blue Shield companies. The plans are located in the 50 states, the District of Columbia, and Puerto Rico. These companies offer a variety of health insurance plans to individuals, small businesses, and large employer groups.

Blue Cross covers hospital care and Blue Shield supports physician services. In 1982, the Blue Cross Association merged with the National Association of Blue Shield Plans. Collectively, the Blue Cross and Blue Shield companies provide medical coverage for about one quarter of the U.S. population. *See also* BED REST, HOSPITAL; HEALTH MAINTENANCE ORGANIZATION; HOSPITAL; INSURANCE; *and* MEDICARE.

Blurred Vision

Images that appear blurry, fuzzy, or foggy; or an otherwise impaired ability to see clearly.

Appearing suddenly or over time, blurred vision can occur in one or both eyes or in a particular visual field. Glasses, contact lenses or an updated prescription are among the usual solutions, but abnormalities caused by damage or disease of the nerves behind the eye, the retina, the aqueous or vitreous humor, the lens, the iris, or the cornea can also cause blurred vision, and demand different treatment. Old age may also cause blurred vision. Many people over the age of 40 encounter blurred vision when reading or trying to focus on something close, but the ability to see far away, typically does not decline. Refractive errors are the leading cause of blurred vision, and include nearsightedness, farsightedness, and a discrepancy in the curvature of the cornea called astigmatism. *See also* EYE.

Blushing

An involuntary physical response to feelings of modesty, embarrassment, or shame, characterized by a reddening of the face or neck.

Blushing is caused by the widening of blood vessels just under the skin's surface. Given the nature of the emotions that give rise to it, blushing is usually involuntary. It may be accompanied by a flush of warmth and light sweating. It may also occur as a side effect of corticosteroid drugs such as prednisone, or in association with a rare disorder. During or after menopause, a drop in the production of estrogen can cause a flushed face, neck, and chest, also called a hot flash. The same can happen to men after a testicle is removed. Either cause can be treated with hormone therapy.

Blushing is typically tolerable, but in rare individuals it does occur severely and frequently. Such individuals may undertake psychotherapy or alternative therapies in order to relieve their nearly constant blushing. *See also* ALTERNATIVE MEDICINE.

Board Certification

Approval process in a medical specialty.

Physicians who practice a medical specialty such as cardiology often undergo a process of board certification. Certified physicians must pass an extensive examination in their specialty and must also meet certain educational requirements.

Although specialists can practice without board certification, it represents an official stamp of approval for a physician. Certification indicates that the physician has made a commitment to meet the professional standards. Most American hospitals require certification of their specialists. *See also* ACCREDITATION *and* AMERICAN MEDICAL ASSOCIATION.

Body Contour Surgery

Surgical procedures performed to improve body shape by removing fat and skin.

In body contour surgery, fat and skin are cut away or suctioned out (liposuction) to remove unwanted or unsightly deposits of fat. Surgery alone, however, is not an effective form of weight reduction; proper diet and exercise are necessary to maintain a healthy weight. In some cases, excess skin or localized deposits of fat may remain after a person loses a significant amount of weight; body contour surgery may be appropriate in these instances.

Abdominoplasty is the removal of excess fat and skin from the lower abdomen and may include tightening muscles of the abdominal wall. It is usually recommended for people who are unable to lose significant weight through dieting or for people who have lost weight through dieting, but need to reduce the surface area of skin.

The surgeon makes a horizontal incision in the skin over the lower part of the abdomen. If fat is excessive, an additional vertical incision is made higher up. If necessary, excess skin is removed. Drains are then inserted into the wound to prevent infections from the collection of blood.

Full recovery may take several weeks. There should be minimal stress on the abdomen to reduce scarring.

Liposuction, developed in the 1970s, is the most commonly performed cosmetic surgery procedure. Excess fat is removed with a tube (cannula) attached to a vacuumlike machine that sucks out the tissue. Because large amounts of body fluid and blood are also sucked out, they must be replenished to prevent shock.

Tumescent liposuction is the most common type of liposuction performed because it involves minimal blood loss. In this technique, the surgeon injects a saline solution beneath the skin containing small amounts of a local anesthetic, usually lidocaine, and the hormone epinephrine, or adrenaline. The anesthetic numbs the area and reduces postoperative discomfort, while the epinephrine reduces bleeding, bruising, and swelling. This solution is then suctioned out along with fat cells.

Ultrasound-assisted liposuction (also known as UAL), a newer technique used since 1996, is an emulsification process in which fat is "melted" and suctioned out. Ultrasound is especially appropriate for dense, fibrous areas such as the buttocks, back and, breast (in males). In this form of liposuction, the surgeon inserts a small, heated probe that produces vibrations at ultrasonic frequencies, causing fat cells to rupture and release their oily contents, which are then vacuumed out.

ALERT
Complications

Body contour surgery is an invasive procedure that carries the same risks as any other type of major surgery involving general anesthesia. People at greatest risk for complications from liposuction are those with diabetes, heart disease, lung disease, and poor blood circulation.

Background information on body contour surgery may be found in ANATOMY, SKIN; PLASTIC SURGERY; *and* SKELETON. *Further information regarding plastic surgery may be found in* COSMETIC SURGERY; FACE LIFT; LIPOSUCTION; *and* RHINOPLASTY. *Techniques are discussed in* Z-PLASTY; SILICONE; SKIN GRAFT; *and* SKIN GRAFT.

Body Odor

Odor caused by the deterioration of body sweat.

Sweat does not have an odor, but the bacteria in it can proliferate and decompose, causing an unpleasant odor. The areas most susceptible are the armpits and genitals, owing to the presence of glands that promote the growth of bacteria. On other parts of the body, sweat is composed mainly of salt and water, and does not harbor as much bacteria.

Body odor is most easily prevented by good hygiene. Regular washing will remove sweat before bacteria can grow. Antiperspirants and deodorants can reduce the production of sweat and mask the odor. *See also* ANTIPERSPIRANT; BACTERIA; *and* SWEAT.

Bodywork

A variety of techniques that manipulate the body to prevent and treat disease.

Bodywork refers to a number of therapies designed to improve body functioning through better alignment and balance. Various forms of physical manipulation were practiced by ancient civilizations throughout the world and by healers during the Middle Ages before the advent of Western medicine.

In the late nineteenth century, American doctor Andrew Taylor Still devised a manner of bone-setting called osteopathy, based on the notion that an individual's physical health can be restored through the manipulation of the skeleton and muscles. Later, Canadian healer Daniel David Palmer laid the groundwork for chiropractic medicine with his discovery of the relationship between the skeletal frame and the nervous system. By "adjusting," or re-aligning, the spinal column back, Palmer believed he was able to treat any number of physical ailments.

Modern Era. In the twentieth century, many new therapies were developed based on the principles of osteopathy and chiro-

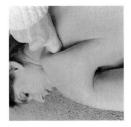

Bodywork.
Deep tissue massage (above) is a method of manipulating the body's energy in an effort to relieve pain and stress.

practic. The best known schools of bodywork include the Alexander Technique, the Feldenkrais Method, Rolfing, Aston-patterning, Hellerwork, the Trager Approach, and Reflexology. The energetic systems of bodywork, which encourage the free flow of energy in the body, include acupressure, shiatsu, myotherapy, and therapeutic touch. Many of these therapies use methods such as massage, deep tissue manipulation, and energy balancing in an effort to reduce aches and pains, stimulate the flow of blood, and relax the body.

Because physical therapy and relaxation are the primary aims of many of these techniques, practitioners often use more than one. Today, bodywork techniques have become increasingly popular.

See ALTERNATIVE MEDICINE *for a discussion of the foundations of bodywork. More information is contained in* ACUPRESSURE; MIND-BODY MEDICINE; *and* SHIATSU. *Eastern methods are discussed in* CHINESE MEDICINE *and* YOGA.

Boil

Also called furuncle

The result of an infection—usually involving staphylococcus bacteria—that has developed around a blocked hair follicle or oil gland.

Boils are usually caused by a staph infection that enters the body through a break in the skin. Immune problems, diabetes, overuse of corticosteroids, and poor health can cause a predisposition to boils.

A boil is red and tender for about four to seven days, after which pus collects inside, turning the boil white. The pus, a collection of white blood cells, fights the infection. A boil may be painful until the skin breaks and the pus drains.

Treatment for boils involves applying hot compresses and, usually, oral antibiotics. If the pain is severe, a doctor can lance the boil. Boils should not be lanced at home, as this can lead to the spread of infection. A boil on the eyelid is called a stye. *See also* ANTIBIOTIC DRUGS; CARBUNCLE; CORTICOSTEROID DRUGS; DIABETES; INFECTION; LANCE; PUS; *and* STYE.

Bonding

The development of an emotional attachment between parents and a newborn.

The process of bonding begins before a baby is born, with the plans made for the baby before birth, with the mother sensing the movement of the fetus, and during visits to the obstetrician when the heartbeat is heard and the ultrasound is seen.

Bonding helps ensure the emotional health of a child. It is achieved through touching, eye contact, and exchanges of physical contact, between parent and child. Parents and children bond in individual ways, at their own pace, and according to their culture.

Certain situations may present challenges to bonding. Postpartum depression, for example, can inhibit bonding and should be treated as soon as possible. When an infant is born prematurely and is kept in the hospital on machines, steps should be taken to ensure that the parents still spend time touching and talking to the infant. If a parent's family life did not provide an adequate model for parent-infant interaction, the parent may need counselling to learn ways of interacting with the infant. *See also* POSTPARTUM DEPRESSION.

Bonding, Dental

Application of synthetic material to teeth.

Bonding treats dental abnormalities such as fractured and malformed teeth, stains, chips, and spaces. It has been used to restore decayed areas as well as protect exposed roots. Bonding can be used to attach orthodontic appliances.

Procedure. Bonding materials include plastics, porcelain, and acrylic. There is generally no need for anesthesia. A solution is applied to teeth to create a rough surface to which the bonding material can bind easily. The bonding material can be molded or may act as a base for another applied surface. *See also* DENTURES *and* TEETH.

Bone

Hard connective tissue of the body consisting of collage, calcium, and phosphate crystals.

Bone supports and protects the body. Its hardness comes from collagen, calcium, and phosphorus, and its resilience from the arrangement of its cells in columns called haversian canals. The periosteum, a network of blood vessels and nerves, covers the dense outer layer of bone that contains a spongy red matter called bone marrow, which produces blood cells that have a major role in the circulatory system.

The long, short, flat, and irregular types of bones that comprise the skeleton anchor the body's muscles; joints complete the body's system of locomotion.

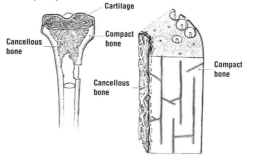

Cartilage — Cancellous bone — Compact bone — Cancellous bone — Compact bone

Hormones ultimately manage bone growth by controlling the activity of two types of cells: osteoblasts attract calcium phosphate onto the protein framework of the bone, while osteoclasts remove it. Growth hormones from the pituitary gland, the adrenal hormones, the sex hormones estrogen and testosterone, parathyroid hormone, and the thyroid hormone thyrocalcitonin also control the amount of calcium in the blood.

Bones begin as cartilage in the fifth or sixth week of pregnancy. Ossification—the hardening of cartilage into bone—begins a week or two later and continues into early adulthood.

Basic anatomical information is contained in BONE MARROW *and* SKELETON. *For more on bone injuries, see* DISLOCATION *and* FRACTURE. *Details on bone disorders are found in* ARTHRITIS; BONE, DISORDERS OF *and* BRITTLE BONES.

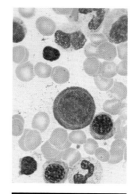

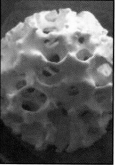

Bone.
Bone is a hard tissue that functions as support and protection for the human body. Above, top, red blood cells are produced in the bone marrow. Bottom, bone tissue. Left, diagrams of bone structure.

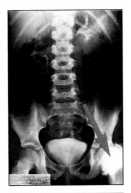

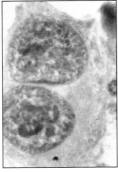

Bone Cancer.
Bone cancers can occur anywhere in the body. Most are metastases, which originate from cancer in another part of the body. Above, top, an x-ray that reveals a bone tumor on the hip. The tumor can be seen as a white spot in the lower right-hand corner. Osteosarcoma is a type of bone cancer common in older patients. Above, bottom, osteosarcoma cells taken from a leg mass.

Bone Cancer

A malignant tumor of the bone.

Most bone cancers are metastases, colonies originating from cancer in another part of the body. Cancer rarely originates in bone. The most common kind of primary bone cancer is osteosarcoma, which occurs primarily in children and young adults. In older patients, osteosarcoma is most often a result of Paget's disease, a condition that disrupts the normal process of bone formation. This kind of bone cancer can occur anywhere in the body. In younger people, bone cancers generally arise in a long bone of a leg or an arm, although they can also occur in the knee, hip, or shoulder.

The second most common primary bone cancer is chondrosarcoma, which arises in the cartilage that forms a protective layer around the bone, usually in the shoulder, upper leg, or pelvis. A rare form of bone cancer is Ewing's sarcoma, which occurs in the legs or pelvis. Aside from Paget's disease in older patients, there is no known cause of bone cancer.

SYMPTOMS

As a bone cancer grows, it can cause distortion of the bone if it is near the surface and extends into the surrounding tissue. The result is a visually evident swelling, usually accompanied by pain as the tumor presses on nearby nerves. A deeper-lying bone cancer may not cause swelling, but is painful. Other symptoms of bone cancer include tenderness or stiffness in the affected area and an increased risk of fractures, even under slight stress, as the bone is weakened by the tumor.

DIAGNOSIS AND TREATMENT

The tests used to diagnose bone cancer include x-rays of the bone, computerized tomography or magnetic resonance imaging scans, and biopsies. Bone cancers may be graded as G1 and G2, which are less likely to form metastases, or G3 and G4, more aggressive cancers that tend to grow rapidly and spread into neighboring tissue and other parts of the body. Less aggressive bone cancers can be treated with radiation and removal of a small segment of bone, or by curettage, a procedure in which the tumor is scraped off the bone. Aggressive bone cancers, which are more common, require surgical removal of a large segment of bone. Amputation of a leg or arm in which a bone cancer has developed is often necessary.

Amputation can be avoided in certain cases of bone cancer by limb-sparing surgery, in which the affected bone is replaced by a metal prosthesis or a graft of cadaver bone. Limb-sparing surgery usually is preceded by chemotherapy, sometimes with radiation therapy. It is possible only when the cancer has not invaded neighboring soft tissue and nerves.

See BONE MARROW; CANCER; *and* CANCER SCREENING F*or a discussion of the foundations of bone cancer. Further information may be found in* BONE TUMORS; LEUKEMIA; OSTEOSARCOMA; *and* RADIATION THERAPY. *Related material is contained in* BONE IMAGING; *and* BONE MARROW TRANSPLANT.

Bone Cyst

An opening in the bone that is filled with fluid.

Bone cysts tend to develop at the end of long bones. They may be present at birth, or may occur as the result of injury or a tumor later in life. Cysts often go unnoticed, unless the bone is examined because of a fracture. An operation to empty the fluid from the cavity and refill it with bone chips can remedy the condition. *See* BONE.

Bone, Disorders of

Disease or injuries that affect the normal growth or function of the bones.

Bones can suffer from the same problems as other tissues or organs, but of course react and respond in their own unique way. Most bone disorders can be detected through x-rays, scans, or blood tests. Each is treated in the way that will provide the best remedy for the condition.

TYPES OF BONE DISORDERS

- Fractures occur when a bone is hit with a heavy direct blow, twisted, or is repeatedly stressed. *See* FRACTURE.
- Osteomyelitis is an abscess due to an infection in the bone. *See* OSTEOMYELITIS.
- Autoimmune disorders, such as rheumatoid arthritis, are the result of the immune system attacking its own body.
- Degenerative disorders occur with age. The best known is osteoarthritis, in which the bones around joints wear down from use. Osteoporosis causes decreased bone density. *See* OSTEOPOROSIS.
- Genetic disorders include bone problems that are inherited, such as achondroplasia (dwarfism). *See* GENETIC DISORDERS.
- Hormonal disorders (i.e., gigantism) are caused by excess growth hormones, resulting in larger than average growth.
- Nutritional disorders occur as the result of a poor diet. Nutritional deficiency can lead to soft, weak bones. Rickets and osteomalacia are examples of this.
- Bone tumors, such as osteoma or chondromatosis, occur as benign or malignant swellings of bone and cartilage. *See also* BONE; CHONDROSARCOMA; *and* TUMOR.

Bone Graft

A surgical procedure in which a fragment of healthy bone is attached to injured or diseased bone in order to promote new growth.

Bone grafts are generally used to restore bone lost through injury or surgery, promote healing of a fracture, or fuse together parts of a diseased or disabled joint. Bone grafts are also sometimes used in cosmetic surgery to reshape the face, skull, or other disfigured parts of the body.

In a bone transplant, healthy bone is attached to injured or diseased bone, providing a protein that stimulates growth. Rejection of the transplanted bone is rare.

The most common sources of bone material are the upper hip bones (iliac crests), which contain much spongy bone; the ribs, which are used when curved bone is needed; and the forearm (ulna), which is often used to fuse joints together. Generally, the bone is taken from a person's own body, a donor, or a cadaver.

Alternatives. A new glue made of calcium phosphate is now being used as a substitute for bone grafting and to connect shattered bones until they bond together, sparing patients the risk of complications from bone-graft surgery. Bone graft substitutes are currently being tested in conjunction with fusion devices, in the hopes of reducing the pain and long recovery associated with spinal fusion procedures.

Procedure. The procedure may be performed in a doctor's office, but is often painful owing to the thick needle required for removing a segment of the bone (trephine biopsy). *See also* LEUKEMIA.

Bone Imaging

A variety of techniques used to create an image of a bone for diagnosis and treatment planning.

Standard x-rays expose bone to a beam of x-rays, which easily penetrates surrounding soft tissue but is absorbed by the bone, yielding an image on x-ray film. This method is used to detect, arthritis, as well as fractures and bone dislocations, and to follow the course of their healing.

CT, Computed Tomography, is a form of x-ray that allows more precise definition of soft tissue. A computer guides the x-ray, markedly improving resolution and allowing the identification of bone erosions, infections of bone, loose material within the joint, tumors and complicated fractures of the bone.

MRI, Magnetic Resonance Imaging, is used to compose a detailed three dimensional image of bone and associated soft tissue. It has proven especially useful in the diagnosis of herniated disks; injuries of joints, such as the knee, shoulder, or wrist; tumors of the bone or soft tissue; and bone death (avascular necrosis) associated with insufficient blood supply.

Radionuclide bone scanning requires radioactive substances to be injected into the bloodstream. A scanner sensitive to ra-

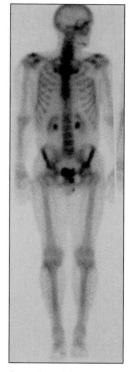

Bone Imaging.
Advanced bone imaging techniques, such as radionuclide bone scanning, aid physicians in the diagnosis of a variety of ailments. Above, a bone scan of an entire human body.

diation tracks its movement and concentration. Abnormal areas of bone absorb higher amounts of the substance. This imaging may provide detailed information concerning inflammation, infection, or bone cancer. *See also* COMPUTERIZED TOMOGRAPHY; MRI; *and* RADIONUCLIDE SCANNING.

Bone Marrow

The soft tissue inside bones.

Bone marrow's primary responsibility is the production of red blood cells, platelets, and white blood cells. During childhood, all of the bone marrow is red marrow, which produces red blood cells. In adults, however, most of the red marrow is converted to yellow marrow, which is composed mostly of fat and connective tissue. Red marrow in adults is usually centered in the spine, skull, ribs, and pelvis, with yellow marrow responsible only for the production of some white blood cells. However, in situations where an increased number of blood cells is necessary, the legs and arms of an adult may begin to produce red blood cells to fulfill the need.

Bone marrow disorders may include aplastic anemia, in which the marrow does not produce enough red blood cells. It is usually caused by an injury or suppression of marrow. Once the primary cause is determined, treatment may include the transfusion of healthy blood cells or immunosuppressive therapy. Leukemia occurs when the marrow has been replaced by cancerous cells. Transplants of compatible, healthy marrow may cure the disease. *See also* LEUKEMIA.

Bone Marrow Biopsy

Removal of bone marrow cells for analysis.

A bone marrow biopsy is done to help diagnose leukemia and other cancers as well as blood disorders such as anemia. The tissue removed in the biopsy is examined microscopically by a pathologist or a hematologist, a specialist in blood disorders. In addition to its use in diagnosis, a bone marrow biopsy may be performed to monitor the effects of treatment on a cancer or other disease.

Process. The usual sites of a bone marrow biopsy are the pelvis or breastbone. The skin and tissue that surround the area to be penetrated is anesthetized, and a long, thick needle is inserted into the bone until it reaches the marrow, the soft substance at the center of the bone where blood cells are produced. Fluid from the marrow is extracted, in what is called aspiration, and a small piece of tissue is also often removed.

Procedure. The procedure takes a few minutes and can be performed in a doctor's office. Patients usually experience very little pain. *See also* ANEMIA; BIOPSY; BONE MARROW; CANCER; *and* LEUKEMIA.

Bone Marrow Transplant

A surgical procedure in which healthy bone marrow is used to replace defective marrow in order to treat life-threatening diseases of the blood and of the immune system.

A bone marrow transplant is a dangerous procedure that is used to treat potentially fatal diseases such as leukemia, cancer, and congenital disorders of the blood or immune system, such as thalassemia and severe combined immunodeficiency. It is also used to replace bone marrow lost through aggressive radiation and chemotherapy treatments used to fight cancer.

In these diseases, a person's bone marrow is unable to produce healthy red or white blood cells. A bone marrow transplant can allow the person to begin producing healthy blood cells.

PROCEDURE

Bone marrow transplants are generally performed at special transplant centers, which have a staff experienced with the procedure and the facilities necessary for both the surgery itself and the recovery period afterwards.

Healthy donor marrow can be taken from another person or from the patient's

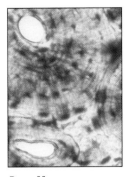

Bone Marrow.
Bone marrow makes up the inside of all bones and is responsible for the production of red blood cells, platelets, and white blood cells. Above, an image of compact bone marrow.

own marrow. If bone marrow is transplanted from a donor (allogeneic bone marrow transplantation), the donor's tissue type must be compatible to that of the patient. A person has a 25 percent chance of having the same tissue type as that of a sibling; thus, the greater the number of siblings, the greater the chance of finding a match. In addition, a national program provides listings of over 700,000 potential bone marrow donors for patients without matching family members.

If a person uses his or her own bone marrow—known as an autologous transplant—the marrow is generally removed when the patient is in remission or prior to radiation or chemotherapy. This marrow is then frozen and stored until it is needed.

The chief sources of donor marrow are the top of the hip bones (iliac crests) and the breastbone (sternum). Bone marrow is removed through biopsy when the donor is under general anesthesia.

In the recipient, all of the existing bone marrow is first destroyed through radiation. The donated bone marrow is then transfused into the vein. It circulates through the blood system and quickly finds its way into the gaps in the bones, ultimately fostering growth of new, healthy marrow in the bones.

COMPLICATIONS

The major complications of bone marrow transplant are infection and graft-versus-host disease (GVHD). After a transplant,

the bone marrow takes several months to grow before it functions fully and effectively. In that time, the blood lacks the white blood cells instrumental in fighting off infection. Thus, the patient is likely to be susceptible to any number of infections during the post-transplant period.

Graft-versus-host disease occurs when the white blood cells from the donor marrow recognize the cells in the patient's body as foreign and attack them. This can be treated with immunosuppressant drugs such as cyclophosphamide or cyclosporine. However, the drugs must be used indefinitely, which weakens the body's ability to fight infection.

PROGNOSIS

The younger the patient, the more likely a bone marrow transplant will be successful. The long-term survival rate of a relatively young patient is more than 80 percent.

Background on bone marrow transplant may be found in BONE; BONE MARROW; TISSUE TYPING; *and* TRANSPLANT SURGERY. *For more information see* GRAFT-VERSUS-HOST DISEASE *and* IMMUNE RESPONSE. *Details contained in* BONE MARROW BIOPSY; CHEMOTHERAPY; *and* RADIATION THERAPY.

Bone Tumors

Section of abnormal growth developing out of healthy bone.

Bone tumors can disrupt the normal functioning of bones if they prove to be cancerous (malignant). A benign tumor, such as an osteoma (a growth that afflicts the skull and long bones of the body), can be left untreated if it does not produce adverse affects. In instances of pain, blood flow obstruction, or disfigurement, the tumor should be removed surgically.

Malignant bone tumors normally occur when cancer travels (metastasizes) through the body. Cancer originating in bone is rare (only two to four percent of all tumors). Bone cancer is divided into two categories: a bone generating type (osteosarcoma); and a cartilage generating type (chondrosarcoma).

After diagnosis with tomography, or CT scanning, the two malignant types require surgical removal of the entire bone and connecting joints. This is followed by radiation and chemotherapy. If diagnosed and treated early, there is a 60 to 65 percent survival rate. The percentage drops to between 25 and 50 percent for later stages. *See also* BENIGN; CANCER; MALIGNANT; METASTASIS; *and* TUMOR.

Booster

Supplementary immunization administered after the original vaccination to "boost" the immune system.

Boosters maintain the level of antibodies against a particular antigen (a substance that triggers an immune system response). For example, a booster shot for tetanus is recommended every 10 years for adults and children over the age of 12. If the shot is not administered following this schedule, the individual may regain susceptibility to tetanus infection. *See* IMMUNIZATION.

Borborygmi

A rumbling or gurgling noise in the abdomen produced by intestinal activity.

Borborygmi is a normal effect of intestinal activity. It may indicate hunger or be a result of indigestion or anxiety. It may also be accompanied by belching. Borborygmi occurs as the result of air and different fluids moving through the intestines and is a natural part of the digestive process.

Diseases of the intestines may affect the noises produced by the intestines; thus a physician may listen to abdominal noises as a part of diagnosing ailments.

Borderline Personality Disorder

A personality disorder characterized by volatile moods and self-destructive behavior.

An individual may be diagnosed with borderline personality disorder between late adolescence and early adulthood. Characteristic behavior includes stormy, unstable relationships, difficulty adjusting to change, and wide swings in attitude toward oneself and others.

Cause. Borderline personality disorder, like other personality disorders, may result from a complex array of circumstances. However, the primary cause of this behavior is believed to be an intense fear of abandonment. The fear generates a sense of instablity in the person, resulting in hypersensitivity and low self-esteem.

People with borderline personality disorder may suffer from a fragile self-image, so that mild slights, real or imagined, provoke extremely volatile reactions. Typically, relationships are often begun with inappropriate intensity and prove to be unstable over time.

In addition, an individual with borderline personality disorder may engage in self-destructive behavior such as substance abuse, uncontrolled spending, or unsafe sex. Also common is self-defeating behavior, including quitting a promising job, leaving school, or ending a relationship because of a minor disagreement.

Underlying causes seem to be a mixture of inborn tendencies and environmental influences. Many people with borderline personality disorder grow up in unstable families and are exposed to alcoholism, abuse, or neglect. The precariousness of a child's situation in a constantly changing and threatening environment contributes to the uncertainty and instability that results in an intense fear of abandonment.

Treatment. Long-term psychotherapy may be useful in controling impulse behaviors and regulating a person's temperment, although a successful therapeutic relationship is often extremely difficult for an individual with borderline personality disorder to establish. Short-term therapy may be appropriate to manage crises.

Basic psychological information is contained in PERSONALITY DISORDERS. *For information on treatment, see* ANTI-DEPRESSANT DRUGS; *and* PSYCHOTHERAPY. *Related disorders are discussed in* DEPRESSION *and* SUICIDE.

Bornholm Disease

Also known as pleurodynia or epidemic myalgia

An infectious disease characterized by pain in the lower chest and abdomen.

Bornholm disease, named after a Danish island where an outbreak occurred, causes sudden extreme pain in the lower chest or upper abdomen. Children are particularly susceptible, but Bornholm disease can strike at any age. Coxsackie B virus causes the disease, which may recur several times over a few weeks, although it typically lasts only a few days.

Symptoms. Symptoms include fever, headache, sore throat, and fatigue. The condition often spreads during epidemics.

Complications. Complications may include meningitis (swelling of the lining of the brain and spinal cord), pericarditis (swelling of the heart lining), or orchitis (swelling of the testes).

Treatment consists of relieving the symptoms whenever possible. No cure is known at present. *See also* ABDOMINAL PAIN; EPIDEMIC; FATIGUE; INFECTIOUS DISEASE; *and* MENINGITIS.

Bottle-Feeding

Using milk—whether expressed breast milk or formula—in a bottle to feed a baby.

Bottle-feeding can be a healthy and practical alternative to breast-feeding. Some mothers opt not to breast-feed their babies due to the time and energy it involves. Others nurse for only a few weeks or months, or decide to combine bottle and breast feeding from the outset.

There are many reasons for choosing not to breast-feed. Each woman must make the decision she feels most comfortable with. Some mothers are uncomfortable with the idea of breast-feeding; others may wish to return to work or share the responsibilities of morning and nighttime feedings with a partner. All medications taken by the mother are passed on to her baby through the breast milk, as are diseases such as AIDS; bottle-feeding is the only al-

ternative for mothers who find themselves faced with these circumstances.

Bonding. Regardless of the reasons for bottle-feeding, it is important for a parent to use the feeding time as an opportunity to bond with the baby. Holding the baby, perhaps speaking softly to him or her, is just as essential as providing nutrients. It is important to hold the bottle at the correct angle and to minimize the amount of swallowed air. Burping after each feeding, or during mid-feeding, is also necessary.

Breast Discomfort. Whether a mother chooses to breast-feed or bottle-feed, the breasts of non-nursing mothers will fill with milk a few days after delivery. The milk will gradually "dry up" over the course of the next several weeks. Any discomfort can be alleviated by ice packs and by wearing a well-fitting supportive bra.

Formulas. There are a variety of formulas available today, made of soy or modified cow's milk. They come in ready-to-feed containers, or in condensed or powder form. Parents should read the package instructions carefully and prepare the formula properly to ensure that the baby's nutritional needs are being met. Some babies, when exposed to the amino acids found in cow's milk, may experience allergic reactions later in life. If there is a history of this allergy in the family, parents should choose a soy milk alternative for their infants.

Benefits. Studies have shown that bottle-fed babies have less frequent and firmer stools than breast-fed babies. They also tend to go for longer periods between feeding sessions.

Weaning a baby from a bottle to a cup may be done as early as six months. It is important to make sure the baby's fluid intake does not lessen during the transition as is possible if the baby is weaned too soon.

Background information on infant feeding may be found in CHILD DEVELOPMENT; FEEDING, INFANT; *and* POSTNATAL CARE. *Further information regarding breast feeding may be found in* BONDING; DEHYDRATION IN INFANTS; INFECTION, CONGENITAL; *and* WITCHES' MILK. *Related material on breast care is found in* BREAST, DISORDERS OF; BREAST TENDERNESS; *and* NIPPLE.

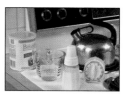
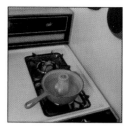
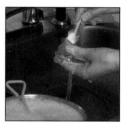
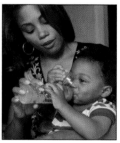

Bottle Feeding.
Bottle feeding requires careful preparation. Formula powder, a measuring cup, sterile water, a tea kettle, and a timer (shown above, top) are some of the items needed when preparing baby formula. Formula should be slowly warmed in a pan on the stove (second from top) or in a microwave oven. The bottle's nipple must always be cleaned thoroughly with soap and a brush (second from bottom). Above, bottom, a mother bottle-feeding her child.

Braces

There are many types of braces used to correct or treat a wide range of disorders. Below, top, an x-ray showing a brace designed to repair a fractured hip. Middle, a woman uses a wrist brace to relieve symptoms of carpal tunnel syndrome. Bottom, a war veteran is shown wearing a neck brace that stabilizes the neck firmly, allowing it to heal.

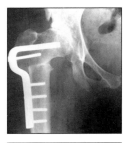

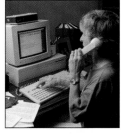

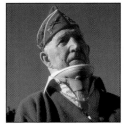

Botulism

Rare and potentially fatal food poisoning.

Botulism is an extremely serious and potentially fatal form of food poisoning resulting from a toxin generated by an anaerobic bacillus. *Clostridium botulinum* is usually found in improperly preserved food, although it rarely appears in commercially produced foods. The bacillus also lives in soil and can infect an open wound through contact with the infested soil.

ALERT | **Prevention**

Bulging cans of food should be thrown away. As a precaution, home-preserved food should be boiled for ten minutes before serving. Babies under the age of one year should not be fed honey or corn syrup, since both may contain spores of *Clostridium botulinum*, which, though harmless to adults, can cause botulism in infants. The illness may lead to paralysis, dehydration, pneumonia, or death.

If botulism poisoning is suspected, seek medical help immediately and notify health authorities, especially if the source of infection is thought to be a restaurant or a commercial product. Symptoms of botulism poisoning can appear between six hours and eight days after eating tainted food, and include blurred or double vision; paralysis of limbs, chest muscles, throat, and eye muscles; dry mouth and difficulty swallowing; breathing difficulty; vomiting; and abdominal pain. Treatment involves administration of an antitoxin as well as rehydration fluids. *See* FOOD POISONING.

Bougie

A slender, flexible rod used to dilate narrow passages in the body.

Bougies are most commonly used in the urethra and esophagus to remove obstructions or permit better flow of blood, urine, or other fluids. Medicine-soaked bougies that melt at body temperature are sometimes used as a delivery system for drugs.

Bowed Leg

An outward curve of the legs.

Young children often have bowed legs, which straighten out as they grow, usually by age two or three. If the condition does not correct itself, surgery may be required to eliminate the curve. Bowed legs may also result from a nutritional deficiency, such as the lack of vitamin D, which causes rickets, or from a developmental disorder, such as Blount's disease. *See also* NUTRITIONAL DISORDERS *and* RICKETS.

Bowen's Disease

A skin disorder evident as a bright red or pink scaly patch located on sun-exposed skin.

Bowen's disease is a form of squamous cell carcinoma that is limited entirely to the epidermus, or upper layer, of the skin. If left untreated, the skin disorder can become invasive.

Treatment for Bowen's disease involves surgery to remove the diseased area of skin. Since the affected cells can extend beyond the red areas, liquid nitrogen treatments and scraping and burning procedures are not recommended. *See also* SKIN CANCER *and* SQUAMOUS CELL CARCINOMA.

Brace

Device that holds parts of the body in place to correct or heal a deformity or an injury.

Orthopedic braces may support a weakened limb, such as the wrist, or help an injured joint remain stable while maintaining normal movement, as in the case of a knee with torn ligaments. A brace can help relieve chronic lower back pain by taking some of the load from the lower spine. In adolescents, a brace may be a means of correcting scoliosis by preventing the back from curving further while growing. Braces may consist of plastic, metal, or other elastic materials. *See* BONE, DISORDERS OF.

Orthodontic Braces. A dentist installs braces to correct tooth placement and encourage precise growth. Metal bands are attached to anchor teeth. Metal or strong synthetic brackets are then attached to each tooth to direct growth. Arch wires are attached to each bracket and connected to the anchor teeth. Correction and eventual removal of braces may take several years. *See also* COSMETIC DENTISTRY.

Brachial Plexus

A major nerve center that conducts signals from the neck to the spine.

The brachial plexus is responsible for distributing nerves to the arms and hands. A plexus is similar to an electrical junction; it is a central hub for nerves extending to different sites in the body.

Injury. A brachial plexus injury is a nerve injury that affects the muscles in the shoulder, arm, and hand. Most often, the brachial plexus is injured because of an accident or a tumor in the lungs. An autoimmune reaction, in which the body produces antibodies that attack the brachial plexus, can also cause it to malfunction. A brachial plexus injury can occur at birth if a baby's neck or shoulders are stretched too far, resulting in the tearing of nerves (brachial plexus palsy).

Symptoms. Symptoms include pain, immobility, and weakness in the arm. Depending on the severity of damage, the impairment may range from minor weakness to complete paralysis.

Diagnosis. A physician may use an electromyogram (EMG) and nerve conduction studies to determine the extent of injury. Computed tomography (CT) or magnetic resonance testing (MRI) may be used to establish whether a cancerous tumor or other growth is causing the injury.

Treatment. Treatment depends on the cause. Surgery, involving nerve grafting and muscle or tendon transfer, may be necessary, followed by physical therapy. *See also* CAT SCAN; EMG; *and* MRI.

Bradycardia

An abnormally slow heartbeat.

Bradycardia originates in the sinoatrial node, the heart's natural pacemaker, which sends out the electrical impulses that control the rhythm of the heartbeat. This node can malfunction if the fibrous tissue in it hardens or if there is an imbalance of the hormones controlling its function.

An abnormality in the sinoatrial node can result in sinus bradycardia, in which the heart rate remains below 60 beats per minute, even during exercise. Another condition causing bradycardia is sinus arrest—also called sinus pause—in which the pacemaker cells of the sinoatrial node fail to activate, so that the heart might not beat for three seconds or longer. Bradycardia can also be caused by sinoatrial block, in which the electrical impulses fail to leave the node. These conditions can be corrected by implanting a pacemaker. *See also* SINOATRIAL NODE *and* SINUS BRADYCARDIA.

Normal Bradycardia

Bradycardia is usually defined as a heart rate under 60 beats per minute, but this rate may be normal in a trained athlete, and heart rate often decreases to 40 beats or less in young, well-conditioned persons during sleep. It is when a slow heart rhythm decreases blood flow enough to cause symptoms such as fatigue, shortness of breath, or even fainting spells that bradycardia requires treatment.

Braille

A system of writing for the blind that uses raised dots to represent letters.

Braille is an alternative system of writing that makes the written word accessible to blind people. Raised dots are used to represent letters of the alphabet, punctuation marks, and other symbols. Each character is represented by a unique arrangement of dots which, when used in combination, create words. Braille provides blind persons

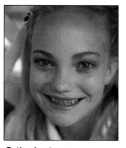

Orthodonture. Orthodontic braces are used to correct tooth placement or encourage proper growth. Above, a girl shows off her smile and her orthodontic braces.

Braille.
Braille is a system of raised dots that represent letters. Blind people may use Braille to read and write. Above, a finger is used to "read" the number 18.

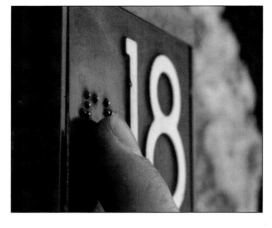

with access to a wide range of educational and recreational reading materials.

Description. Unlike printed text, Braille is read by moving one or both hands from left to right along each line of text, allowing the finger to feel the arrangement of rounded bu-mps. On average, Braille is read at a speed of 125 words per minute. Experienced Braille readers can read as fast as 200 words per minute.

History. The Braille alphabet was invented by Louis Braille (1809-1852), a French inventor and teacher. Braille, who was blind, encountered an alphabet for the blind that was invented by Charles Barbier, in which simple messages coded in dots were embossed on cardboard. Braille modified this system for more general use. *See also* BLINDNESS; SIGHT; *and* TOUCH.

Brain

Located in the skull, the brain is the body's command center.

Weighing about three pounds and housing 100 billion neurons, the jelly-like brain controls thought, movement, and speech, sending messages to all parts of the body and deciphering replies as the major organ of the central nervous system (CNS). Its partner in the CNS is the spinal cord, and together they control breathing, heartbeat, and body temperature.

REGIONS AND FUNCTIONS OF THE BRAIN
Sections. The brain has three main parts: the brain stem (an extension of the spinal cord), the cerebellum, and the forebrain. In evolutionary terms, the brain stem and cerebellum are the oldest sections; the former controls vital functions such as blood pressure, breathing, sleeping, and digestion, while the latter handles coordination, balance, and posture. Powered by unconscious reflex impulses, these two sections interpret sensory messages received from nerves throughout the body and reply with commands that stimulate the necessary changes—for instance, to increase the rate of breathing during strenuous exercise.

The third and largest section of the brain, the forebrain, consists mainly of the egg-shaped cerebrum, which accounts for 70 percent of the entire nervous system's weight. Its winding, crinkled, bunched appearance conceals about two-thirds of its actual surface area. These folds (gyri) and fissures (sulci) are visibly divided into four surface areas called lobes, which control speech, vision, thought, and memory. The frontal, occipital, parietal, and temporal lobes are named after the skull bones that cover them.

Hemispheres. Underneath this outer membrane, the cerebrum is divided into two hemispheres, right and left, each of which has an outer layer called the cerebral cortex. The cerebral cortex is comprised of gray matter and six layers of nerve cells that are the realm of movement, sensation, and conscious thought. While the cortex functions much like the older parts of the brain, it can perform tasks of extreme complexity, such as writing and speech, and manage the conscious processes of perception, memory, and decision-making.

Much of the cerebrum beneath the cortex is made up of bundles of nerve fibers. This "white matter" forms connections between different swaths of the cortex and the other, smaller part of the forebrain. The basal ganglia are clusters of cells connected to the cerebellum and brain stem that convey motor signals from the cortex to skeletal muscles.

The dominant hemisphere, which is typically the left in right-handed people, controls language, arithmetic, and logic.

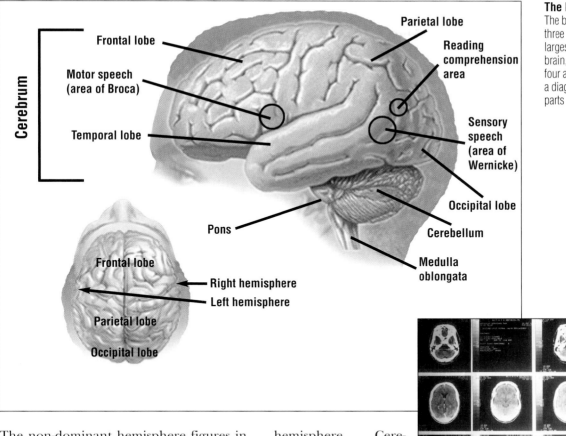

Frontal lobe

Motor speech
(area of Broca)

Temporal lobe

Cerebrum

Parietal lobe

Reading
comprehension
area

Sensory
speech
(area of
Wernicke)

Occipital lobe

Cerebellum

Pons

Medulla
oblongata

Frontal lobe

Right hemisphere

Left hemisphere

Parietal lobe

Occipital lobe

The Brain.
The brain is divided into three main regions. The largest section, the forebrain, is subdivided into four areas, or lobes. Below, a diagram depicting the parts of the brain.

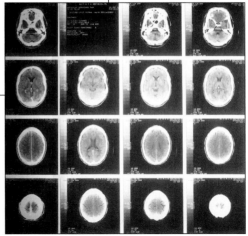

Brain Regions.
The brain is a complex organ comprised of many structures that perform specialized tasks. Above, X-ray images from a CAT scan of the brain. The scanner is rotated to provide as many different views of the brain as possible.

The non-dominant hemisphere figures in visual and spatial orientation and may be the realm of creative thought and artistic appreciation. Most people whose right hemisphere is the dominant one are left-handed and male.

Central Structures. Acting as intermediaries between the brain stem and cerebrum, the central structures include two oval-shaped relay messengers called thalami; a tiny regulator of appetite, thirst, and body temperature called the hypothalamus, which also affects sleep, aggression, and sexual behavior; and the hormone-producing pituitary gland, which maintains metabolism, growth, fluid balance, sexual development, and other physiological factors by influencing other glands. The limbic system of nerves surrounds the thalami and deals with additional memory functions, smell, and possibly emotions.

Ventricles. The brain also has four ventricles; one in the center of the forebrain, one in the brain stem, and one in each hemisphere. Cerebrospinal fluid circulates through the ventricles, nourishing the brain and serving as a cushion to prevent injury from a sudden movement or blow. The fluid also circulates between two of the three layers of membrane, the meninges, which surround the entire brain and spinal cord. The brain maintains a large supply of blood. The carotid arteries of the neck feed a network of arteries at the base of the skull and two more arteries parallel to the spinal cord. Twenty percent of the blood pumped by the heart goes to the brain.

Basic physiological information on the brain is contained in BRAIN STEM; CENTRAL NERVOUS SYSTEM; *and* CEREBELLUM. *For additional material on brain functions, see* MEMORY; SENSATION; *and* SLEEP. *Details on brain disorders are found in* AUTISM; BRAIN DISORDERS; COMA; *and* EPILEPSY.

Brain Abscess

An accumulation of pus in the brain.

Pus can accumulate between the skull and the membranes that cover the brain (the dura mater), or inside the brain. Brain abscesses usually occur in younger people between the ages of 10 and 35; abscesses are rare in seniors. *See* ABSCESS *and* PUS.

Causes. Forty percent of all infections that cause a brain abscess originate in the sinuses, ears, or teeth. In some cases, bacteria from another infected part of the body may also be the cause. For instance, bacteria in the heart or lungs may be carried to the brain by the blood. The resulting body of pus, often surrounded by inflamed tissue, puts pressure on neighboring regions.

Symptoms. Symptoms can include persistent headaches, nausea, vomiting, disturbances of vision, and seizures. Depending on where the abscess forms, it can cause partial paralysis, loss of muscle coordination, difficulty in understanding speech, and impairment of thinking.

Diagnosis. Diagnostic tests such as computed tomography (CT) and magnetic resonance imaging (MRI) are used to locate the abscess and rule out the existence of a tumor. A sample of the abscess may be removed and examined under a microscope to assess possible malignancy.

Treatment. An antibiotic, such as penicillin or cephalosporin, is usually prescribed. An antibiotic is often unsuccessful in draining the abscess and surgery is required. If an abscess is pressing against the brain or spinal cord, surgery is essential to prevent permanent damage.

Prognosis. Ninety percent of brain abscesses are not fatal, although some impairment may remain owing to brain damage.

Brain Death

Irreversible cessation of all functions of the brain.

Brain death is determined by use of an electroencephalogram, which measures brain activity. The individual is declared brain dead if an EEG (electroencephalograph) shows flat tracings for a period of twenty-four hours. This indicates that the entire brain has ceased to function. During this time, the patient's circulation and breathing may continue through artificial means, making the diagnosis of death—through the cessation of breathing and heartbeat—impossible.

The use of brain death to determine the moment of death raises many medical, religious, and ethical questions. If the notion of brain death is accepted, physicians are able to remove vital organs and use them in transplants before the heart has stopped beating. Critics of the idea of brain death question when the cessation of brain activity actually becomes irreversible. *See also* BRAIN *and* ELECTROENCEPHALOGRAPH.

Brain Disorders

A defect or disease that is centralized or dispersed throughout the brain.

A brain disorder involves two complications that other organ disorders do not have. First, the brain is encased in a hard skull that does not allow room for any added growth. Thus, a brain tumor, abscess, or hemorrhage that swells increases pressure on the brain. A localized disorder can affect the operation of the entire brain. Second, brain cells are not replaceable, so their destruction can result in an irreversible loss of function.

Causes. Two main causes of brain disorders are impaired oxygen and blood supply. Brain cells cannot survive longer than a few minutes without oxygen. Oxygen deprivation can occur at birth, resulting in cerebral palsy, or later in life as a result of choking or drowning. Most adult brain disorders are caused by decreased blood supply. A stroke, for example, can result from a blocked artery or a hemorrhage.

Babies may be born with brain defects as a result of a chromosomal disorder, as in Down's syndrome or Tay-Sachs disease. These diseases impair brain function.

Some brain disorders are caused by infections. Encephalitis, a viral infection, and meningitis, a bacterial infection, are examples of infections that cause brain disorders. Ear, tooth, and sinus infections can lead to a brain abscess. Some disorders are caused by brain tumors. Tumors are either primary—born in the brain tissues themselves, as in acoustic neuroma—or secondary—resulting from cancer cells originating in other parts of the body.

Brain disorders are prevalent in older persons. The elderly have a higher risk of stroke owing to a higher incidence of high blood pressure, coronary disease, and diabetes. Alzheimer's disease and Parkinson's disease are two forms of degenerative brain disease common in the elderly.

Symptoms. Symptoms associated with brain disorders include:

- Headache;
- Dizziness;
- Loss of balance;
- Numbness;
- Memory loss (aphasia); and
- Seizures.

Diagnosis. A neurologist will perform a physical examination and look for signs of muscle degeneration, lack of sensation, mental confusion, and slow reflexes. He or she may ask the patient to push or pull, using resistance to test muscle strength. The physician examines the functioning of the sensory nerves by using a pin or a blunt object to apply pressure to the area in question. The patient's reflexes are tested using the knee-jerk reflex. An electroenchephalograph (EEG) is used to measure the electrical activity in the brain. Additional tests are often administered, such as computed tomography (CT), magnetic resonance imaging (MRI), and Doppler ultrasound scanning.

Treatment. Treatment varies depending on the underlying cause. For some degenerative brain diseases such as Alzheimer's, no cure is presently available.

See BRAIN; and NERVOUS SYSTEM for a discussion on the foundations of brain disorders. More information is contained in AUTISM; EPILEPSY; and STROKE. Treatment is discussed in ANTICONVULSANT DRUGS and NEUROSURGERY.

Brain Hemorrhage

Bleeding in or around the brain.

A hemorrhage can be caused either by injury or by rupture of a blood vessel. Brain hemorrhages account for about one-quarter of all strokes; the rest are caused by blockage of a blood vessel. Brain hemorrhages are classified by the site where the bleeding occurs.

An extradural hemorrhage occurs underneath the skull but above a membrane called the dura.

A subdural hemorrhage occurs below the dura but above a second membrane called the arachnoid. Both extradural and subdural hemorrhages are usually the result of injury.

A subarachnoid hemorrhage occurs on the outer surface of the brain below the arachnoid, resulting in a flow of blood into the space between the brain and its lining.

An intracerebral hemorrhage occurs within the brain. The common cause of subarachnoid and intracerebral hemorrhages is a ruptured aneurysm—the blood vessel balloons, weakening the vessel wall.

ALERT

Stroke Symptoms

The symptoms of a stroke caused by a brain hemorrhage include loss of consciousness; a sudden, severe headache; sudden weakness or numbness of an arm, leg, or one side of the face; and loss of the ability to speak or to understand speech. These symptoms call for immediate emergency treatment.

In brain hemorrhages, brain cells die because they lose their supply of oxygen. Cells also die as blood accumulates in the brain, or between the brain and the skull, putting excess pressure on brain cells. Because the skull allows little room for tissue to expand, any bleeding that occurs there increases the pressure to dangerous levels.

Basic anatomical information is contained in BRAIN and CAROTIC ARTERY. For further information on brain hemorrhage see CEREBROVASCULAR ACCIDENT; EMBOLISM; and STROKE. Details will be found in BLOOD PRESSURE.

Brain Imaging

Any means of creating an image of the brain or the chemical processes within the brain.

MRI, or magnetic resonance imaging, of the brain uses magnetic fields and pulsed radiowaves interpreted by computer to produce precise images. An MRI scan is performed with the patient lying horizontally within a tube-like unit for 30 to 45 minutes. Because the process uses magnetic fields rather than x-rays, as in CT scanning and angiography (described below), it is among the safest of procedures. MRI provides stunning detail of soft tissue, which may be visualized in three dimensions with the aid of a computer. MRI is an effective means of detecting tumors of the brain or brainstem, abscesses, stroke, nerve damage, swelling or bleeding, and other nervous system disorders, including those of the spinal cord.

CT, or computed tomography, employs computerized x-ray scans to create an image of the brain. Radiation is caught by detectors opposite the x-ray source, which record the unabsorbed x-rays passing through the skull. The x-ray source and detector rotate around the skull during the CT scan, and the resulting data is processed by computer. Like MRI, CT scanning results in thin, sliced images of brain tissue. When put together, these images provide a three-dimensional picture of the brain. A contrast dye injected into a vein may be used to enhance the image.

Cerebral angiography uses dye injection to develop a picture of the brain's circulatory system. A thin catheter is fed through the body's blood vessels and into the brain. Then a dye, visible on x-ray, is injected. The procedure requires local anesthetic and takes one to two hours to complete. Cerebral angiography is particularly useful in the detection of aneurysms, arterial blockages, and narrowing or swelling due to an inflammation of the blood vessels.

SPECT (single-photon emission computerized tomography) and PET (positron emission tomography are used to study where and how quickly the brain uses its blood supply and nutrients. Following the injection of radioactive isotopes into the bloodstream, emissions from the isotopes can be followed in the brain by means of specialized scanning. A computer then makes a map of how the isotopes are distributed. The more active an area of the brain, the greater the concentration of radioactive material. The techniques are a powerful tool for studying the brain.

> *Background material may be found in* BRAIN; IMAGING TECHNIQUES; MEDICAL TESTS; *and* RADIATION. *Further information regarding brain imaging techniques may be found in* ANGIOGRAPHY; CAT SCAN; MRI *and* X-RAY. *Related material is contained in* BRAIN ABSCESS; BRAIN DISORDERS; BRAIN HEMORRHAGE; *and* BRAIN TUMOR.

Brain Stem

Portion of the spinal cord that leads into the brain.

The brain stem is a three-inch-long column of nerve cells and fibers that serves as the message highway between the brain and the spinal cord. Owing to its connection to ten of the twelve pairs of cranial nerves, the brain stem controls basic functions, such as breathing, eye reflexes, and vomiting.

Three sections comprise the brain stem: the medulla, pons, and midbrain. The spinal cord merges with the wider medulla, the container of the ninth to twelfth cranial nerves that communicate taste and signal muscles integral to speech and movement of the tongue and neck; the tenth cranial nerve is called the vagus nerve, which relays messages regarding vital functions such as heartbeat, blood pressure, breathing, and digestion. The stem widens with the pons. Sensory messages from the eyes, ears, and teeth, and motor signals to the jaw, face, and eyes, pass through the nuclei of the fifth to eighth cranial nerves bundled together in the pons. It also houses thicker tracts of nerves that join the cerebellum where it attaches to the rear of the brain stem. The nuclei of the third and fourth cranial nerves are located in the top and smallest part of the brain stem, the mid-

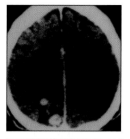
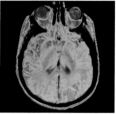
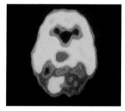

Brain Imaging.
The diagnostic tools now available for brain medicine have made marked strides in the past two decades. Above, top, a CAT scan of a brain shows a lesion in the hindbrain. Second from the bottom, an MRI. Bottom, PET scan of a brain shows the malignant tumor.

brain. These control additional eye movements and the pupil. Red nuclei and the substantia nigra—cell groups that help control movement of the arms and legs—are also located there. *See also* BRAIN; NERVE; *and* SPINAL CORD.

Brain Tumor

An abnormal growth in the brain.

Brain tumors differ from most other tumors because the distinction between a benign growth, which grows slowly, and a malignant—cancerous—growth is less important in the brain than elsewhere in the body. Because a brain tumor can dangerously compress brain tissue within the limited area of the skull, even a benign tumor can cause serious problems.

Incidence. Primary brain cancers—those that develop in the brain rather than being formed as colonies from other cancers—are the second most common form of cancer among children, and rank eighth among adults. The incidence of brain tumors is highest between birth and the age of five and reaches another peak between ages 15 and 24. The incidence begins to rise again after age 50.

Types. The two major types of brain cancer are gliomas, which arise in the glial cells—the supporting tissue of the brain—and nonglial tumors, which arise in nerve cells and other brain tissues. Most brain cancers are gliomas. Their subtypes include astrocytomas, brain cell gliomas, and ependymomas—named for the type of glial cells affected—and mixed tumors, which involve more than one type of glial cell. Nonglial tumors include acoustic neurinomas, which affect the acoustic nerve; meningiomas, which affect the brain lining, and medulloblastomas, which arise in the nerve cells of the cerebellum.

Symptoms. The general symptoms of all brain tumors include headache, usually severe and persistent; vomiting (not always accompanied by nausea); seizures; and changes in mental attitude and function. Other symptoms depend on the site of the tumor; for example, a tumor of the optic nerve can cause double or blurred vision.

Diagnosis. Brain tumors are diagnosed by magnetic resonance imaging (MRI) or computerized tomography (CAT) scans, which can show the location and size of the growth. Neurological tests may be performed to assess the effect of a tumor on brain and body function, and blood tests can be performed to detect tumor markers, such as the overproduction of hormones caused by a pituitary tumor. Specialized tests such as an x-ray of the blood vessels in the head (cerebral arteriogram), or a brain scan using an injected traceable substance, may be ordered.

An advanced development in brain tumor diagnosis and treatment is the use of stereotactic techniques that give a three dimensional view of the brain. A combination of computerized tomography and magnetic resonance imaging offers a precise picture of the size and location of a tumor. The picture is used to guide stereotactic radiosurgery, in which beams of radiation are delivered with precision to the cancer site deep in the brain, reducing or eliminating damage to normal brain tissue.

Treatment. Surgery is a primary treatment for a brain tumor. Surgical removal of the tumor is usually followed by either radiation therapy or chemotherapy. Radiation therapy is not generally administered to young patients because of the risk of permanent damage to the brain. Survival rates have greatly improved over recent decades, and nearly half of all brain tumors now can be cured.

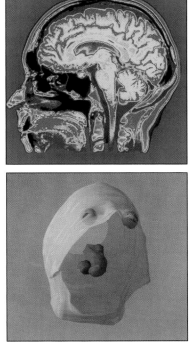

Brain Tumor.
Brain tumors can now be detected using sophisticated imaging techniques. Above, top, a CAT scan of a human head. Above, bottom, a computer-generated image of a brain with a tumor. This method, known as Sterrotactic Radiosurgery, maps the brain and allows for direct delivery of radiation therapy to tumors that were once considered inoperable. In this image, the tumor can be seen in red.

Background material on brain tumors may be found in BRAIN; CANCER; MALIGNANT; *and* TUMOR. *For additional information, see* ASTROCYTOMA; EPENDYMOMA; GLIOMA; *and* MENINGIOMA. *Diagnosis and treatment is discussed in* BRAIN IMAGING; CAT SCAN; CHEMOTHERAPY; MRI; RADIATION THERAPY; *and* SURGERY.

Branchial Disorders

Disorders involving the neck area, usually resulting from a developmental anomaly in a fetus.

Branchial cysts are small swellings located on either side of the neck. The swelling contains a pus-like fluid that has a high cholesterol content. Generally, branchial cysts appear in early adulthood.

A **branchial fistula** is an abnormal passageway between the back of the throat and the external neck surface; usually it is a small hole in the neck of an infant. It is referred to as a branchial cleft sinus if it extends only partway toward the throat.

A branchial fistula, whether partial or complete, may discharge mucus or pus. The fluid may appear externally on the surface of the neck or internally, resulting in a chronic cough. This condition may be congenital or develop later in life owing to a ruptured branchial cyst. Branchial cysts or fistulas are treated with surgery. *See also* CYST *and* FISTULA.

Brash, Water

Sudden filling of the mouth with saliva.

Normally, saliva flow is stimulated by feelings of hunger or by the smell or sight of food. With water brash, the production of saliva is not caused by such stimuli. Water brash is frequently accompanied by abdominal pain and may occur before a meal. It is usually indicative of a disorder of the upper gastrointestinal tract, such as a duodenal ulcer.

Water brash is often confused with acid reflux, the regurgitation of gastric juices, but it is an entirely different phenomenon. Gastric juices have an unpleasant, sour taste, whereas the liquid here is tasteless.

Braxton-Hicks Contractions

Irregular uterine contractions experienced between the fourth and ninth months of pregnancy.

Braxton-Hicks contractions are generally not painful and are experienced more often in a second or third pregnancy. These early contractions help the uterus grow and aid in blood circulation from the uterus to the placenta. They may be caused by fatigue, as they generally occur late in the day, or after physical exertion.

Braxton-Hicks contractions usually intensify and occur more frequently toward the end of pregnancy, and are sometimes mistaken for labor pains. What distinguishes false labor from true labor pains is that these contractions do not cause the cervix to dilate. In addition, Braxton-Hicks contractions are concentrated in the abdomen, whereas true labor contractions begin in the lower back and radiate to the front. *See also* PREGNANCY.

Breakthrough Bleeding

Any blood spotting or staining in the middle of the menstrual cycle.

Breakthrough bleeding is most commonly associated with the first few months of taking birth control pills, occurring in 10 to 30 percent of users. Gradually, the incidence of breakthrough bleeding decreases to between one and 10 percent. It may take a few months for the body to adjust and for the bleeding to stop. Bleeding does not mean the pill is not working effectively.

To avoid or minimize of breakthrough bleeding, it is important to take the pill every day and at roughly the same time each day. A seven-day course of additional estrogen, like that used for postmenopausal hormone replacement, may be given during episodes of breakthrough bleeding. Also, a pill containing a higher dosage of estrogen can usually solve the problem. Otherwise, abnormalities of the reproductive system, such as fibroids, polyps, or infection, should be ruled out.

Basic information on breakthrough bleeding is contained in BIRTH CONTROL; BLEEDING; *and* MENSTRUAL CYCLE. *For additional information, see* FIBROIDS; INFECTION; *and* POLYPS. *Related material available in* ESTROGEN; HORMONE REPLACEMENT; *and* PREGNANCY.

Breast

Also known as the mammary gland

An organ consisting of specialized tissues and fat whose primary function is to provide milk for a newborn infant.

Structure and Function. The primary function of the breast is to provide milk for a newborn infant. Within the breast, several tiny sacs called alveoli produce milk when stimulated by estrogen and progesterone hormones during pregnancy. The alveoli are arranged in clusters called lobules. Several lobules, in turn, form a lobe, of which there are 15 to 20 within each breast. In females, layers of fat separate the lobes from each other. A single milk duct extends from each lobe to carry the milk to the openings at the tip of the nipple.

The size and the shape of the breast depend upon the amount of fat present. Other contributing factors are age, climate, health, and the time of the month in relation to the menstrual cycle. Slight swelling is common prior to menstruation.

The skin covering the nipple has several nerve endings, making it highly sensitive. Stimulation of these nerves causes the uterus to contract. The nipples also contain erectile tissue, which becomes engorged with blood when stimulated. The skin of the nipple contains several oil and sweat glands to help keep it soft.

The pigmented area surrounding the nipple is called the areola. The color is usually paler in women who have never been pregnant. The areola enlarges and darkens during pregnancy and when the breasts are producing milk. Montgomery's glands are small glands located in the areola that enlarge during pregnancy.

Development. Approximately one to two years before the onset of puberty, the amount of estrogen and progesterone produced by the ovaries increases, causing the breasts to begin to fill out. When menstruation begins, the hormone levels increase further, stimulating the continued development of the breasts. Layers of fat are deposited, giving the breasts their size and shape. The amount of glandular tissue increases slowly. In most women, the milk glands are fully developed by the early teens. By the late teens or early twenties, the breasts reach their final form; there are no further changes until pregnancy.

Five to six weeks after pregnancy begins, the breasts gradually become larger and more sensitive. This is due to increased hormone production by the ovaries, pituitary gland, and placenta. The breasts continue to enlarge until midway through the pregnancy. After delivery, their size increases even more with the onset of milk production.

The milk glands begin secreting small amounts of a thin, watery fluid called colostrum from about the fourth month of pregnancy on. Colostrum production increases in the first 12 to 24 hours after giving birth; true milk production does not begin for a few more days. The breasts return to their prepregnant state within a few weeks of giving birth, if the mother does not nurse. If she does breast-feed, the breasts will return to their former state after weaning.

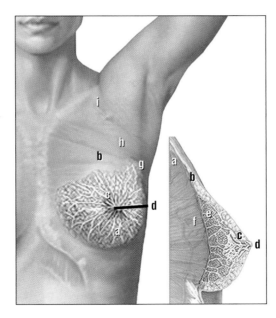

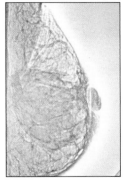

The Breast.
The primary function of the breast is to provide milk for a newborn infant. Above, a mammogram image of a breast. Left, diagrams illustrate both the front and side views of a woman's breast: (a) fatty tissue; (b) the suspensory ligaments; (c) the areola; (d) the nipple; (e) grandular tissue; (f) the chest wall; (g) the axillary tail of the breast; (h) pectoralis major muscle; (i) location of the collar bone.

Background material on breast may be found in REPRODUCTIVE SYSTEM, FEMALE. *For additional information, see* BREAST FEEDING; BREAST SELF-EXAMINATION; ESTROGEN; *and* MILK. *Related disorders are discussed in* BREAST CANCER; BREAST DISORDERS; *and* BREAST LUMP.

Breast Cancer

Malignant tumor of the breast.

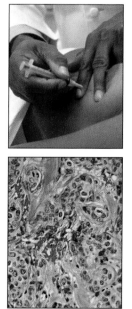

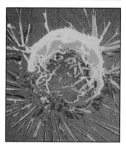

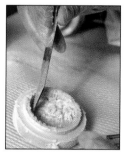

Breast Cancer Biopsy. If a physician has reason to believe that a patient has developed breast cancer, a tissue sample, or biopsy (top) must be taken. The sample will be placed in a culture dish (bottom) and examined for evidence of cancer cells (middle images).

Breast cancer is the most common cancer among women in the United States. One out of every 14 American women will develop breast cancer, and one of every 20 will die of it. According to the American Cancer Society, 172,000 cases of invasive breast cancer were anticipated in 1999. Over 182,000 cases were anticipated for the year 2000. Men can also develop breast cancer, although it is rare; fewer than one percent of all breast cancer cases occur in men. The incidence of breast cancer increased stead-ily starting in the 1970s. Many experts believe the increase was due to earlier detection through self-examination and x-ray examination of the breast (mammography). Lending support to that view is a steady increase in the survival rate for breast cancer patients, an indication that the malignancy is being detected in its earlier, more treatable stages.

Estrogen, the female sex hormone produced by the ovaries, plays an important role in the growth and spread of breast cancer. The precise effects of estrogen on breast tissue are, however, still unclear. Women who experience prolonged exposure to estrogen—because they started menstruating at an early age, had children after the age of 30, or had a late menopause—have a higher incidence of breast cancer.

Antiestrogen drugs, such as tamoxifen and raloxifene, block the effect of estrogen on breast tissue and are widely used in treatment and prevention. But the major

Early Detection of Breast Cancer

Three measures are recommended for early detection of breast cancer. One is self-examination every month to detect lumps or other changes in the breast. A second is an examination by a physician or trained nurse practitioner every three years from ages 20 to 40 and every year after that. The third is mammography, a breast cancer screening x-ray, every two years from age 40 to 49 and once a year after that.

risk factor for breast cancer is age. A 60-year-old woman is 14 times more likely to develop breast cancer than a 30-year-old woman. The risk increases for any woman with a first-degree relative—sister, mother, or daughter—who has had the disease. Obesity also increases risk, because fat cells convert estrogen to estradiol, a more powerful version of the hormone. A woman who has had cancer in one breast has at least a threefold increased risk of developing it in the other breast.

SYMPTOMS

The symptoms of breast cancer start with a change in the physical appearance of the breast—an alteration in size or shape, a lump in or near the breast or under the arm, or an ulcer or other lesion of a nipple. Irritation of the skin on a breast, a swollen and reddened breast, and persistent pain in the breast may also be indicators of an underlying cancer.

When breast cancer is suspected, diagnostic measures include a small tissue sample taken either through a fine needle, or a large tissue sample (biopsy). The biopsy sample may be tested for the presence of receptors for estrogen and progesterone. Surgical examination of the axilla (armpit) is an essential part of the evaluation of breast cancer. If such receptors are found, drugs that block the growth-stimulating effects of those hormones may be prescribed.

TREATMENT

The treatment of breast cancer depends in large part on the stage at which it is detected, but many other factors are involved: the hormone sensitivity of the cancer, the woman's age and menopausal status, her family history, and her general health.

For a small, early-stage cancer that has not spread beyond the breast, breast-conserving surgery such as a lumpectomy followed by radiation therapy may be sufficient. Larger cancers may require mastectomy—removal of the entire breast. Postoperative treatment with hormones or chemotherapy is often prescribed to prevent the spread of tumor cells.

Several drug combinations are routinely used, while others are being tested. One in current clinical use combines cyclophosphamide, methotrexate and fluorouracil. Doxorubicin and taxol are also often used. The types of drugs that are prescribed and the length of time over which they are given vary widely, depending on individual circumstances. Tamoxifen and other drugs block the effects of the estrogen hormone and may be helpful in prevention and treatment of breast cancer.

PROGNOSIS

After treatment, a woman may be placed on continuing tamoxifen treatment to prevent recurrence of the cancer. The drug does increase the risk of endometrial cancer slightly, but its benefits are believed to far outweigh that risk. Tamoxifen therapy is continued for no more than five years, since no benefit has been demonstrated for a longer period of treatment.

The field of breast cancer treatment is still changing. Despite ongoing clinical trials, controversies still arise over the value of different treatment combinations and how to use them. Early detection remains essential for the best results. The five-year survival rate for a woman whose breast cancer is detected at the earliest stage is over 95 percent, compared to about 10 percent for a cancer detected much later. Overall, the five-year survival rate for all breast cancer patients is over 83 percent.

MAMMOGRAPHY

Mammography is a screening technique for early detection of breast cancer. The procedure is painless and requires the use of low-level x-rays to examine breast tissue for possible signs of malignancy.

Many physicians recommend regular mammogram tests for women after age 40. Between the ages of 35 and 40, women are encouraged to have a mammogram to help establish a baseline to evaluate later examinations. Detection of an abnormality may be followed up with a variety of further tests, including ultrasound, thermography, and removal of tissue for analysis (biopsy).

A Genetic Predisposition to Breast Cancer?

Some breast cancers are the result of an inherited genetic mutation. Two genes that increase the susceptibility to breast cancer have been identified; they are designated BRCA1 and BRCA2, Breast Cancer One and Two, respectively. BRCA1 is associated with an increased risk of cancer of the breast and ovary, while BRCA2 is associated with breast cancer alone. Tests for the presence of these genes can be done for women from families with a history of the cancer.

High-Risk. Women belonging to high-risk groups should maintain strict vigilance against breast cancer through frequent self-examination and regular mammography. High-risk groups include women who have first-degree relatives with cancer, are of African-American descent, over 50, and those who give birth after the age of 30.

Procedure. The x-ray equipment used for mammography is specifically designed for examination of the breasts, which are examined individually. The procedure is noninvasive, and the radiation dose is not believed to pose significant long-term health risks. The technique of mammography involves compressing the breast between a film plate and a special paddle, which helps record an accurate reading onto a slide that is very similar to an x-ray or photo negative. Normal breasts appear in the slide as dark gray, with white areas corresponding to glandular and fibrous tissue.

Effectiveness. Mammography can reduce breast cancer deaths by 25 to 35 percent among women who have the examination at one and two year intervals. However, mammography should serve to supplement regular breast self-examinations, which should be performed once a month on the same day, preferably several days following menstruation, when menstrual hormones are less active. Self-examination may be performed at home and is an ideal preventative method for detecting lumps or irregularities of the breast.

Background material on breast cancer may be found in BREAST; CANCER; MALIGNANT; *and* TUMOR. *For further information see* BREAST LUMP; ESTROGEN; *and* LYMPH NODES. *Diagnosis and treatment is discussed in* BIOPSY; BREAST SELF-EXAMINATION; BREAST SURGERY; CHEMOTHERAPY; CYCLOPHOSPHAMIDE; MAMMOGRAPHY; *and* RADIATION THERAPY.

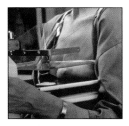
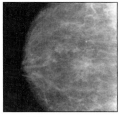
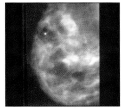

Breast Cancer Screening.
Mammography (top) is the most effective means of screening for breast cancer. Middle, a mammogram of a normal breast. Bottom, a mammogram of a breast in which the white areas may indicate an abnormality.

Breast Disorders

Any disease or injury related to the breast.

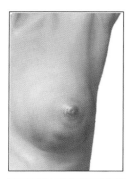

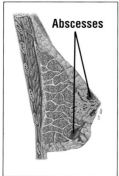

Abscesses

Breast Disorders.
Breast infections (above, top) are most common in women that breast-feed their children. When a breast becomes severely infected, abscesses (bottom) may develop .

There is a variety of breast disorders, ranging in seriousness from mild to severe.

Breast Tenderness. Premenstrual tenderness and mild swelling are common in most women. These are caused by changing hormone levels in the body preceding the onset of menstruation.

Breast Lumps. The vast majority of lumps are not malignant but should still be investigated. Lumps may or may not be painful and may be accompanied by a greenish or straw-colored discharge. Cysts are benign fluid-filled sacs, caused by abnormal activity of fluid-forming tissue, and range in size from very tiny to egg-size. They may disappear or decrease in size a few days after menstruation. Cysts generally disappear after menopause. If fluid can be withdrawn from a lump, it is just a cyst.

Lumps that are not cysts and are not cancerous are usually fibroadenomas—benign tumors found mostly in young women. These have a firm, smooth, rubbery feel, and can be easily moved under the skin. Other lumps can be caused by an infection or severe injury to the breast tissue. A lipoma is a tumor of fatty tissue. A blocked milk duct can also result in the formation of a lump. Lumps in the areola are usually cysts formed by blocked oil glands. They may form boils if infected. If a breast lump appears malignant, a mammogram or ultrasound test is necessary for a definitive diagnosis.

Breast Infections. A breast infection, called mastitis, is a red, tender, or painful swelling or lump in the breast. It may accompany fever and the presence of a lump in the armpit, caused by a swollen lymph node. Breast infections are common in women who are or have recently stopped nursing. The infection is usually caused by bacteria that have entered through a cracked nipple. If the infection is severe, a pus-filled sac (abscess) may develop.

Breast infections are treated with antibiotics, along with a mild analgesic for pain and fever. If an abscess is present, it will need to be drained. Breast infections can be prevented by keeping the nipples clean between feedings. A nursing mother is advised not to express milk from the infected breast until it is completely healed.

Nipple Problems. Discharge from one or both nipples is usually breast milk, especially in women who have recently been breast-feeding. Breasts may continue to produce milk in small amounts even several months after weaning.

Galactorrhea—the term for a discharge from the nipple other than milk—may be accompanied by missed menstrual periods. It may be a side effect of medication, a symptom of a disorder of the pituitary gland, or perhaps a tumor. A large pituitary tumor needs surgery, and tends to recur, necessitating long-term treatment with medication or radiation. Galactorrhea may also be due to hypothyroidism, in which the thyroid gland is not producing enough of the hormone thyroxin. The discharge is usually white in color. A dark red or black discharge containing blood may be due to a benign tumor in a milk duct, or it may be an indication of cancer.

Indented or retracted nipples are normal—unless they had not been that way previously. A sudden change in the nipple's appearance could be a sign of cancer. Scaling of the nipple is usually not serious but should examined for signs of cancer.

Prevention. Breast self-examinations are the easiest way to ensure early detection of breast disorders. An exam consists of gently massaging the breast in a circular motion to check for lumps or other abnormal tissue. The exam should be performed during the same time each month to account for week-to-week variations in size and shape. If an abnormality is suspected, the woman should consult a physician.

See ABSCESS; BREAST; CANCER; NIPPLE; *and* INFECTION *for a discussion on the foundations of disorders of the breast. Details on specific disorders will be found in* BREAST CANCER; BREAST LUMP; BREAST TENDERNESS; GALACTORRHEA; *and* JOGGER'S NIPPLE. *Prevention is discussed in* BREAST SELF-EXAMINATION *and* MAMMOGRAPHY.

Breast-Feeding

Also known as nursing or lactation

Feeding an infant with breast-produced milk.

Breast tissue contains several tiny sacs, called alveoli, where milk production occurs. The alveoli are arranged in clusters called lobules. Several lobules in turn form a lobe, of which there are from 15 to 20 within each breast. A single milk duct extends from each lobe to carry the milk to the openings at the tip of the nipple.

During pregnancy, the pituitary gland produces a hormone known as prolactin, which stimulates the breasts to produce milk. Beginning in the fourth month of pregnancy, the breasts produce a thin, sticky liquid known as colostrum. This is the forerunner to milk. For the first few days after delivery, the breasts produce increasing amounts of colostrum; actual milk is produced on the third or fourth day.

If the mother chooses to breast-feed, the baby's sucking stimulates the breasts to increase production. If nursing does not occur, the breasts eventually "dry up" over the course of a few weeks.

The milk's appearance is signaled by an increased heaviness in the breasts. They will feel much firmer than normal and may even become engorged, especially in the beginning, before the amount of milk has adjusted to the baby's needs. More frequent feedings, or perhaps some manual expression, will help the mother feel more comfortable, as will wearing a well-fitting supportive bra. The "let-down" reflex stimulated by the infant's sucking causes the release of milk from the breast. There may be a certain amount of leakage between feedings; many women use disposable pads to absorb the flow.

ADVANTAGES TO BREAST FEEDING

• Breast-feeding is convenient. There is no need to measure formula or sterilize bottles and nipples. Breast milk is always available and at the proper temperature.

• Breast-feeding helps restore the body to its prepregnant state—as the baby sucks,

the uterus is stimulated to contract, thus helping it to return more quickly to its normal state. The breasts also produce a hormone called oxytocin, which helps the uterus contract.

• Women who breast-feed have been shown to have less chance of getting breast cancer.

• Breast milk is an almost perfect food, having exactly the right proportion of nutrients needed for proper infant development. No formula as yet has been devised that exactly duplicates mother's milk.

• Breast milk is more easily digestible, and babies who are breast-fed have less colic and stomach upsets, as well as fewer rashes and allergies.

• Breast milk contains antibodies from the mother, which help to protect the infant from disease during the first few months of life.

The majority of women are capable of breast-feeding, regardless of the size of their breasts. In the early stages, many women experience discomfort from engorged breasts and sore or cracked nipples. Breasts pumps may relieve excess milk, and nipple shields may be used during feeding to alleviate soreness.

Getting Started

Some women prefer to nurse lying in bed, others sitting up. Regardless of the position, the mother should cradle the baby's head gently and guide his or her mouth to the nipple. The entire areola (the pigmented area surrounding the nipple) should enter the baby's mouth; otherwise the nipple will become sore and irritated. Sucking is instinctive, and the baby will do the rest with little or no help from the mother. During the first few days, women are advised to keep feedings relatively short to avoid sore nipples. Most women find it is best to offer both breasts to the baby at each feeding and to alternate which breast is offered first. At the end of a feeding, slide a finger between the baby's lips and the nipple to break the suction.

Background material on breast feeding may be found in BREAST; NIPPLE; MILK; *and* POSTNATAL CARE. *For further information see* COLOSTRUM; OXYTOCIN; *and* PROLACTIN. *Related material is available in* BOTTLE-FEEDING; BREAST PUMP; LACTOSE INTOLERANCE; *and* PREGNANCY.

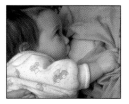

Breast Feeding.
Breast feeding has been shown to be healthier for both the child and the mother. Above, an eight-month-old child being nursed by her mother.

Mastectomy.
There are several procedures used for the removal of a breast lump. In a segmental lumpectomy (below, top) the lump and a wedge of the breast are removed. A radical mastectomy (middle) is a procedure in which the entire breast and chest muscles are removed along with lymph nodes in the underarm in an effort to treat breast cancer. The breast and a sample of lymph nodes from the underarm are removed in a mastectomy procedure (bottom).

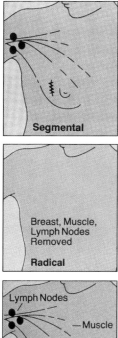

Segmental

Breast, Muscle, Lymph Nodes Removed

Radical

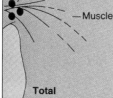

Lymph Nodes

—Muscle

Total

Breast Lump

A cyst, tumor, or infection found in the breast tissue.

Breast lumps result from many different phenomena and may be life-threatening. Over 80 percent are benign, but any breast lump should be examined by a doctor.

Fibrocystic Breast Disease. This is a common cause of breast lumps. The disease characteristically appears in women after age 30 and generally subsides before or during the onset of menopause. The lumps are the result of dilated tissue in and around the milk duct, forming cysts. Lumpiness in one or both breasts tends to follow the menstrual cycle and is usually most severe at the start of menstrual bleeding. These cysts may be diagnosed by taking a small sample of fluid from the breast with a needle, or by using ultrasound.

Benign Fibroadenoma, another type of breast lump, is composed of fibrous breast tissue. Unlike fibroplasic cysts, a fibroadenoma is solid rather than fluid-filled, firm, moveable, and generally not tender to the touch. Benign fibroadenomas usually range in size from one and one-half to two inches in diameter and are non-threatening, though occasionally they may be mistaken for breast cancer, particularly during pregnancy when they tend to grow larger.

Fat Necrosis, or the death of fatty tissue within the breast, causes another form of breast lump. Bruised skin over the region of the lump and tenderness are common. Such lumps generally heal without incident and are non-threatening.

Breast Cancer. Fewer than 20 percent of breast lumps prove to be cancerous. Those of a cancerous nature usually appear as a single lump, which may not cause any pain when touched or pressed. The vast majority of breast lumps are not cancerous. However, a clinical breast exam is essential if a lump is detected through self-examination.

> *Background material may be found in* BREAST; CANCER; MALIGNANT; *and* TUMOR. *For addition information on breast lump see* BREAST CANCER. *Related material in* BIOPSY; BREAST SELF-EXAMINATION; *and* MAMMOGRAPHY.

Breast Pump

A mechanical device, hand or battery-operated, used to expel milk from the breasts.

Pumping is a useful way to ease breast engorgement or to obtain breast milk for later use. The pump consists of a rubber bulb and a tube of either plastic or glass that empties into a container for storing the milk. After the pump is cleaned and sterilized, it may be placed over the nipple for use. Manual pumps are squeezed, stimulating the flow of milk from the breast; electric pumps generate their own squeezing motion. *See also* BREAST FEEDING.

Breast Self-Examination

A simple at-home procedure used to check the breast for lumps.

While the technique of breast self-examination is not a substitute for a doctor's analysis or a mammogram, self-examination is an extremely useful early warning system, and is the method responsible for identifying over 90 percent of all breast masses. Every breast differs somewhat in structure and feel. The self-exam seeks to identify changes in breast tissue, unfamiliar sensitivities, swellings, or lumps.

Because the breasts vary in size and consistency over the course of the menstrual cycle, it is best to pick the same day each month and use it consistently as the day for for the breast self-examination. It is recommended that the test be carried out several days following menstruation, when menstrual hormones are less active.

While breast self-examinations are an important aspect of prevention and detection of breast cancer, they are not a substitute for regular clinical checkups. Women over the age of 50 should have a check-up and mammogram performed yearly. If any lumps or other abnormal signs appear during self-examination, they should receive the immediate attention of a doctor, who will most likely examine the breasts and recommend further diagnostic testing.

HOW TO PERFORM A BREAST SELF-EXAM

Breasts should be checked while lying flat on your back. Raising your left arm above your head, use your right arm to check the left breast. Press on the breast with the flattened fingers of your right hand. Begin the test in the nipple region, using a circular motion, gradually checking the entire breast for signs of tenderness or lumps. Avoid using the fingertips, which will interpret the natural breast tissue as lumpy.

Most cancerous breast lumps occur under the nipple or in the portion of the breast leading toward the underarm, so these areas are of particular concern. Repeat this procedure with the right breast and left hand.

After carefully feeling each breast for irregularities or lumps, examine them visually, standing before a mirror. Note any changes in color or texture of the skin, or unevenness between the two breasts in terms of size, contour, or shape.

Squeeze the nipple of each breast firmly (though not painfully), and note if there is any discharge.

Finally, repeat the test of palpating each breast, as you did while lying down—but this time standing in the shower so that any lumps will be in a different position. The water will increase your sensitivity to anything unusual. *See also* BREAST LUMP.

Breast Surgery

Surgical repair or alteration of one or both breasts.

Breast enlargement, also called augmentation mammoplasty, is a cosmetic operation for women who feel that having larger breasts will improve their appearance. The individual is usually administered a short-duration general anesthetic. The surgeon makes a small incision under the existing breast lines or under the armpits, pushes the implant—a plastic sac containing a saline solution—under the breast tissue, and closes the incision. Internal scar tissue often forms near the implant, altering shape and giving the breast a rigid feel. Typically, the result is satisfactory, but

sometimes a second operation is required to further accommodate the implant.

Women with exceptionally large breasts may desire breast reduction, also known as reduction mammoplasty, because of back, neck, and shoulder pains, or because they are not pleased with the shape of their breasts. The patient is usually given a general anesthetic. The surgeon makes small incisions positioned to make tissue-removal easier and to minimize scarring. Skin and fatty tissue are removed, the remainder contoured to achieve the desired cup size, and the nipple relocated to a higher position. Most women are usually satisfied, but scarring may necessitate a second operation.

Breast reconstruction is performed either at the same time as a mastectomy or when the site of removal has healed. The operation differs from enlargement because there is little existing breast tissue; fat and muscle may have to be transplanted from other body areas. When only a tumor and immediate surrounding tissue are remove, an implant is inserted; this technique produces less scarring. *See also* COSMETIC SURGERY.

Breast Tenderness

A feeling that may be accompanied by swelling, and is usually related to premenstrual syndrome.

Breast tenderness occurs as the result of hormonal changes that take place near the end of the menstrual cycle. Different women experience varying degrees of pain and many find that their breasts become larger than normal. Usually no treatment is necessary other than taking a painkiller (analgesic) for mild pain relief. A supportive bra may also alleviate some discomfort.

As a preventive measure, some women find it helpful to avoid caffeine, sugar, and alcohol, as well as to limit their salt intake, which prevents fluid retention.

During the first trimester of pregnancy, there may also be a feeling of tenderness in the breasts as they respond to increased hormonal levels. *See also* MENSTRUATION.

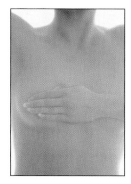

Breast Self-Examination. A breast self-examination is not a substitute for a mammogram or visit to the doctor's office. It is a simple and effective early detection method, however, and should be performed regularly. Above, a women performs a breast self-examination.

Breast Surgery. Women who have undergone a mastectomy usually choose to have reconstructive breast surgery as well. Below, top, a reconstructed breast. Bottom, a silicone breast implant.

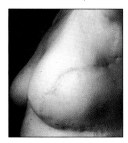

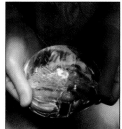

Breathing Difficulty

An abnormal change in depth and rate of breathing.

Breathing difficulty can be a symptom of many different diseases, or it can be a general physical and lifestyle characteristic. It results from any condition that affects airflow into or out of the lungs, the ability of the lungs to infuse the blood with oxygen, or the ability of the brain stem to regulate breathing.

Breathing difficulty can be either labored breathing or pain related to breathing movements. Whether a person is asleep, resting, or exercising, breathing difficulty can occur.

ALERT
Allergy and Shock

Persons with allergies can experience extreme breathing difficulty during an unusually strong response—anaphylactic reaction—to an allergy-causing agent such as peanuts, fish, eggs, bee stings, or medications such as penicillin. The reaction causes a severe drop in blood pressure, constriction of the airways of the lungs, and swelling of the throat or tongue. An anaphylactic reaction requires immediate treatment with epinephrine or other medication and emergency resuscitation. Individuals prone to anaphylactic shock are advised to carry their own medication and wear a medical identification bracelet warning of the potential problem.

Anemia or a similar blood problem can lead to breathing difficulty. Anemia is a shortage of oxygen-carrying red cells in the blood. The body does not get enough oxygen, so the lungs must work harder. The end result is continued breathlessness.

Anxiety. Times of stress or tension can bring on abnormally rapid or deep breathing (hyperventilation) that causes faintness and a feeling of being unable to breathe adequately, sometimes accompanied by muscle spasms or numbness of the hands and feet. These symptoms are caused by an excess loss of carbon dioxide from the blood and can be lessened by breathing into a paper bag, which helps to restore normal carbon dioxide levels.

Altitude Sickness. Breathing difficulty can occur at high altitudes, where the air is thinner and less oxygen is taken in with each inhalation. It is often experienced by individuals who are unaccustomed to high altitudes and can worsen with activity for those who are less physically fit. As the lungs work harder to supply the body with oxygen, there is a feeling of breathlessness. Eventually, the individual's system becomes accustomed to the thinner air. Problems can be lessened by a reduction in physical activity while this change occurs.

Obesity and Pickwickian Syndrome

One form of breathing difficulty that can occur in overweight persons is the Pickwickian syndrome or obstructive sleep apnea. In Pickwickian syndrome, obesity leads to the narrowing of the upper air passageway, causing periodic obstruction of breathing during sleep. The result is repeated episodes of obstructive choking and startled awakening accompanied by gasping. The complications of Pickwickian syndrome include excessive daytime sleepiness, morning headaches, and loss of concentration. The condition can eventually result in serious heart abnormalities such as ventricular tachycardia—an abnormal heartbeat.

Breathlessness is the inability to breathe at the rate required by the body. It is most commonly associated with exertion (intense exercise) and panic attacks. This is normal for those in good health and not a cause for concern. Other more serious causes of breathlessness include heart problems, regular or repeated exposure to poor air quality (as in smoky or dusty workplaces), allergies, and smoking. Treatment of these problems will help to remedy the symptom of breathlessness.

Circulation Disorders. Chronic heart conditions, such as impaired ability of the heart to pump blood—heart failure—can cause breathing difficulty. Other heart conditions that cause breathing difficulty include a blood clot in the lung (pulmonary embolism) and abnormally high blood pressure in the arteries of the lung (pulmonary hypertension).

Lack of Fitness. Many physically inactive people do not have the heart and lung capacity needed to respond to the body's increased demand for oxygen at times of exertion. The increased demand causes discomfort and pain. The remedy is to cease the physical activity. The long-term solution is regular fitness training.

Lung Damage. Conditions that cause temporary or permanent damage to the lungs inevitably result in breathing difficulty. Emphysema (chronic breathing difficulty) damages the lungs by destroying the sensitive tissue where oxygen enters the blood and carbon dioxide is removed from blood. Breathing difficulty can be due to inflammation of the lungs (pneumonia) or inflammation of the airways of the lung (bronchitis). In these cases, breathing difficulty may be temporary, easing when the infection that causes the inflammation yields to treatment. Physical damage, such as a collapsed lung (pneumothorax) or excess fluid around the lung (pleural effusion), also causes breathing difficulty.

Smoking and Breathing

The damage that smoking does to lung tissue is a major cause of breathing difficulty, and smoking exacerbates the difficulty resulting from any other cause. For someone who smokes, the first step in treating breathing difficulty is to quit smoking. For someone who does not smoke, an essential preventive measure is not to start.

Obesity. An obese person may have trouble breathing during even mild exertion because of the extra effort required by excess body tissue. In addition, extreme obesity may have an affect on the breathing control center of the brain stem, aggravating the problem. Painful breathing, chest tightness or pain, and wheezing may occur as the result of this condition. Gradual weight loss and regular fitness training can reduce or eliminate any accompanying breathing problems.

Basic anatomical information on breathing difficulties is contained in BLOOD CELLS; HEART; *and* LUNG. *Further information may be found in* ALLERGY; ALTITUDE SICKNESS; ANEMIA; ANXIETY; BRONCHITIS; EMPHYSEMA; HEART, DISORDERS OF; OBESITY; PNEUMONIA; *and* SHOCK.

Breech Delivery

Term used when a baby is born leading with his or her feet or buttocks.

Most babies are born head-first, a position known as occiput anterior. Approximately four percent of all babies are born in breech position.

A breech baby lies in the uterus with its feet or buttocks near the cervix. As a result, these are the first body parts to emerge from the birth canal. Breech presentation can be a cause for concern, as it may interfere with the newborn's first attempts to breathe. Doctors can usually tell in advance that a baby is in breech position and may attempt to turn the baby around. If the attempts are unsuccessful, the baby may be delivered via Cesarean section to avoid complications.

Breech births are very common in premature infants, because the fetus does not assume the head down position until the end of pregnancy. Other conditions associated with breech presentation include multiple pregnancy, uterine abnormalities, tumors, hydramnios, and placenta previa.

Other abnormal presentations include occiput posterior, in which the baby is positioned head down but its face is turned toward the mother's front. This makes it particularly difficult for the body to pass through the birth canal and usually necessitates the use of forceps or even a Cesarean section.

Transverse Presentation. In transverse presentation, the baby is positioned sideways in the uterus, with its head on one side of the mother's abdomen, its feet on the other. The shoulder often blocks the birth canal, making vaginal delivery impossible and raising the possibility that the umbilical cord will become obstructed, interfering with the baby's oxygen supply. A Cesarean section must be performed as soon as possible after active labor begins. Transverse presentation may result in prematurity and placenta previa. *See also* EMERGENCY CHILDBIRTH; HYDRAMNIOS; PLACENTA ; *and* PREMATURITY.

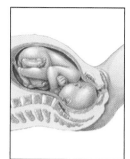
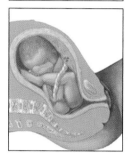

Breech Delivery.
Breech delivery is the term used when a baby is born leading with its feet or buttocks. Above, top, a baby being born in the normal, head-first position. Bottom, a baby in the breech position.

Bridge, Dental

A permanent or removable substitute for a missing tooth or teeth.

Bridges improve the speech and bite for people with missing teeth. Consisting of false teeth connected by a metal frame, a bridge also prevents the shifting of remaining teeth. A bridge differs from a denture, a false-tooth appliance attached by suction through an artificial gum or baseplate.

Crowns are often used to anchor the bridge to healthy teeth, since it is impossible to link a bridge to a piece of gum. Occasionally, the supporting tooth is further built-up or reinforced with a metal or plastic post cemented into place after a root canal is done. If a bridge is anchored using crowns, it becomes a permanent part of the mouth.

In general, dentists fit bridges to make use of existing healthy teeth. When a bridge is poorly fitted, it can cause pain and discomfort and should be replaced. *See also* DENTURE *and* TEETH.

Brittle Bones

Loss of bone density, resulting in bones that are fragile and easily fractured.

Bones constantly go through the process of breaking down and rebuilding in order to facilitate growth, repair injury, and maintain strength for everyday activity. With age, the ability to rebuild bone slows down and cannot keep up with the dissipation of the bone. Calcium helps to create new bone. As part of the normal aging process, calcium levels in the body decrease, causing bones to lose their density and become brittle. Brittle bones may also be a symptom of osteoporosis or a genetic defect, such as osteogenesis imperfecta. *See* OSTEOGENESIS IMPERFECTA *and* OSTEOPOROSIS.

Bronchiectasis

Respiratory disorder caused by damage to the airways (bronchi) of the lung.

Bronchiectasis usually develops early in life, either as a congenital condition or as the result of an infection, such as pneumonia, measles or tuberculosis. The condition has become less common as the incidence of those infections have declined. In bronchiectasis, the bronchi become rigid, distorted, abnormally wide, and filled with stagnant fluid. This fluid is a breeding ground for bacteria and other infectious agents, so the condition leads to periodic lung infections and a persistent cough that produces large quantities of green phlegm.

Treatment aims to control chronic symptoms; this includes taking antibiotics to fight infections and regularly lying in a position conducive to coughing up fluid from the affected area of the lung (postural drainage). In severe cases, surgery may remove a damaged area of the lung. *See also* POSTURAL DRAINAGE.

Bronchiolitis

An acute viral infection of the lower portions of the lungs that is common in babies.

Bronchiolitis occurs primarily in babies two to eight months old, although it can occur in some adults suffering from bronchitis. Breathing problems occur due to inflammation in small airways of the lungs, called bronchioles. Bronchiolitis is often caused by the respiratory syncytial virus (RSV).

Symptoms. The first signs of bronchiolitis are symptoms of a common cold, followed by wheezing, a persistent cough and rapid, shallow breathing, often accompanied by a fever. The baby's skin may have a bluish tinge because of a lack of oxygen.

Treatment. Parents must wait for the viral infection to clear, although respirator inhalers may be recommended for some cases. Severe cases require hospitalization for administration of oxygen and respiratory treatment to clear the bronchioles. Although antibiotics are not effective against a viral infection, they may be given to help prevent an accompanying bacterial infection. *See also* BRONCHITIS; OXYGEN THERAPY; *and* RESPIRATORY THERAPY.

Bronchitis

Inflammation of the airways (bronchi) of the lungs.

Irritation of the bronchi causes persistent coughing and produces large quantities of sputum. There are two types of bronchitis, determined by the duration and regularity of inflammation. Acute bronchitis is often sudden, but of short duration. Chronic bronchitis is more gradual, continuing over a long period and recurring over many years. Smoking and air pollution are major contributors to both types.

ACUTE BRONCHITIS

Acute bronchitis most often occurs in the winter months, when the incidence of colds and influenza is high. Older people, infants, and people with chronic respiratory diseases are most vulnerable.

Cause. The condition is usually a complication of a viral infection, such as the common cold or influenza. The underlying cause of acute bronchitis is the inflammation of the mucous membrane of the bronchi. This inflammation causes swelling, which reduces air-flow, and congestion, which makes breathing difficult.

Symptoms. An attack of acute bronchitis results in breathlessness, fever, wheezing, a cough that brings up discolored phlegm (yellow or green), and chest pain that may be worsened by the cough.

Complications. Although complications, such as pneumonia or pleurisy, are uncommon, a doctor's advice should be sought if a bout of bronchitis lasts for more than three or four days, if a sufferer's temperature stays over 101°F, or if blood is found in the sputum. The doctor may prescribe an antibiotic to treat any possible accompanying bacterial infections. Regular bouts of acute bronchitis could be a sign of chronic bronchitis, which requires close medical attention.

CHRONIC BRONCHITIS

Chronic bronchitis is diagnosed when a cough that produces sputum lasts for at least three consecutive months during two consecutive years. It may be accompanied by or contribute to the development of emphysema, a lung disease that damages the tiny air sacs (alveoli) of the lung, while oxygen enters blood and carbon dioxide is removed from blood. The combination of these two conditions is called chronic obstructive pulmonary disease.

Incidence and Causes. Chronic bronchitis generally occurs in people over 40 and is twice as common in men than in women. It is believed to affect one American in 20. The major cause of chronic bronchitis is the progressive damage done to the respiratory system by smoking. Air pollution can be a major contributing factor; workers exposed to dust and irritating fumes from sources such as coal mining and metal working are at high risk.

Chronic bronchitis causes the same symptoms as acute bronchitis—coughing, breathing difficulty, and fever—but these symptoms do not go away. Unless progression of the disease is stopped—by giving up smoking and taking protective measures against air pollutants, for example—damage to the lungs can cause abnormally high blood pressure in the arteries of the lung (pulmonary hypertension).

Diagnosis and Treatment. Diagnosis of chronic bronchitis may include chest x-rays, sputum analysis, and pulmonary function tests. Those tests help distinguish bronchitis from asthma, another chronic condition in which the airways of the lung become abnormally narrow. Asthma can be distinguished from bronchitis because the symptoms it causes—wheezing and breathlessness—can vary from hour to hour or day to day, unlike those of bronchitis. Bronchodilator drugs may be prescribed to widen the airways and, in especially severe cases, oxygen therapy may be provided through a ventilator.

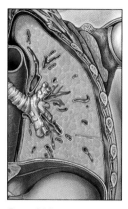

Bronchitis.
Bronchitis is an inflammation of the air sacs, or bronchi (above), of the lungs.

Background material on breathing difficulties is contained in INFLAMMATION *and* LUNG. *Further information may be found in* BRONCHODILATOR DRUGS; CHEST PAIN; CHEST X-RAY; COUGH; EMPHYSEMA; FEVER; *and* SPUTUM. *Related material can be found in* BRONCHIOLITIS; COLD, COMMON; INFLUENZA; *and* SMOKING, PASSIVE.

Bronchoconstrictor

Medications that narrow the airways in the lungs.

Doctors may want to induce temporary bronchoconstriction, either to aid in the diagnosis of asthma or to test the effectiveness of a bronchodilator, a drug that increases oxygen flow by widening the airways of the lung. Bronchoconstrictors that can be used for these purposes include a natural body chemical that causes allergic reactions (histamine), or the medication dinoprost (a prostaglandin). Narrowing of the lung airways—the bronchi—is generally undesirable because it reduces the amount of oxygen reaching the tissues of the body. *See also* HISTAMINE; LUNGS; *and* PROSTAGLANDIN.

Bronchodilator Drugs

A family of drugs that relax the muscles around the air passages to the lungs (bronchi), making it easier to breathe.

Diseases that inflame the bronchial passages make it difficult to breathe and restrict the amount of oxygen provided to the tissues of the body. Some common diseases that bronchodilators are used to treat are asthma, emphysema, and bronchitis. Asthma is usually an allergic reaction, while the vast majority of people with emphysema and chronic bronchitis developed the condition from smoking.

Most bronchodilators relax the passageways to the lungs, while others, such as epinephrine, constrict blood vessels, which can reduce inflammation, slow or stop bleeding, and increase blood pressure. In larger doses, bronchodilators also affect heart function and may be used as a treatment for heart-rhythm problems. When used to treat bronchial diseases, bronchodilators are taken either orally or as an inhalent.

Short-term bronchodilators are intended for fast, temporary relief and are effective for about four hours. The relief should be evident within two or three minutes. These include albuterol, pirbuterol, metaproterenol, terbutalin, and bitolterol, among others. They are administered through an inhaler and take effect within twenty to thirty minutes. Side effects may include quickened heartbeat, nervousness, shakiness, nausea and dizziness.

Long-acting Bronchodilators include beta-agonists and methylxanthines, which help people breathe more easily over a long period. The beta-agonists include salmeterol (used in an aerosol inhaler or powder inhaler), albuterol (taken orally), and theophylline (taken orally). Salmeterol is not recommended for use in acute attacks of bronchitis. It is intended for long-term control of asthma symptoms, especially at night. It is usually taken with an anti-inflammatory drug, is longer acting, and has fewer side effects, though the patient may experience nervousness, trembling, dry mouth, and rapid or irregular heartbeat. Theophylline may cause nausea, nervousness, and insomnia. *See also* ASTHMA; BRONCHITIS; EMPHYSEMA; OXYGEN THERAPY; *and* RESPIRATORY THERAPY.

ALERT

Caffeine and Bronchodilator Drugs

Caffeine should be avoided when taking any bronchodilator drugs. If the patient experiences a change in blood pressure or heartbeat, trembling, lightheadedness, chest pain, or vomiting, a physician should be consulted immediately.

Bronchopneumonia

Pneumonia that affects the entire lung.

Bronchopneumonia gets its name from the fact that the inflammation starts in the small airways of the lung (bronchi), then spreads throughout the lungs. Bronchopneumonia is the most common form of pneumonia, which is an inflammation of the lungs caused by a viral or bacterial infection. It is distinguished from lobar pneumonia, which affects only one lobe. Symptoms consist of a cough, fever, and green or yellow sputum. Treatment of viral bronchopneumonia includes bed rest, drugs to relieve coughing and pain, and antibiotics to defend against possible bacterial infection. *See* LUNG *and* PNEUMONIA.

Bronchoscopy

A diagnostic technique used to view the bronchi, the small airways of the lungs.

The bronchoscope is a fiberoptic device designed to pass through the patient's trachea, allowing a doctor to view the larynx, trachea, and associated airways—the tracheobronchial tree. A bronchoscope is a flexible tube five to seven millimeters in diameter. A larger, more rigid form of the device is generally used in removing airway obstructions. Specialized tools can be passed through the bronchoscope to extract sample tissue from the throat and deeper in the airway for biopsy.

Preparation and Procedure. The patient must fast for six to 12 hours before bronchoscopy. The test may be performed under either local or general anesthetic and requires 45 to 60 minutes to complete. The slender fiber of the bronchoscope is inserted into a nostril, fed through the trachea and into the bronchial tree. The anesthetic dulls the gag reflex, and the patient should feel nothing more than a tugging sensation. A few patients feel as if they are being suffocated; however, there is no risk of suffocation.

Following the test, food should be avoided for several hours until the gag reflex returns. Though complications are rare, sore throat and temporary hoarseness are not uncommon. If the doctor has used bronchoscopy to perform a biopsy, the patient may cough up small amounts of blood for a day or two.

Unless absolutely necessary, bronchoscopy is not to be performed on patients with severe oxygen deprivation (hypoxia); asthma; recent heart attack (myocardial infarction); or severe, progressive heart pain (unstable angina pectoris).

Bronchoscopy is an effective means of diagnosing a number of respiratory ailments including tuberculosis, interstitial lung disease (in which the lung tissue is scarred and thickened), sarcoidosis (in which the lungs and other organs are inflamed), benign tumors, lung cancer, fungal lung infection, and conditions such as hemoptysis (coughing up blood). *See also* BIOPSY; LUNG IMAGING; *and* TUBERCULOSIS.

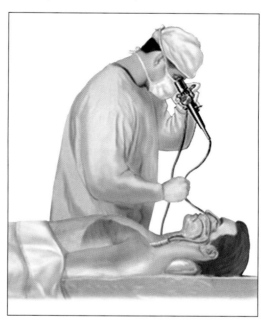

Bronchoscopy.
A bronchoscopy is a fiberoptic device used to view the small airways of the lungs. The device can also be used to obtain tissue samples for further examination. Left, an illustration of a bronchoscopy being performed on a patient.

Bronchospasm

Temporary, abnormal narrowing of the airways of the lungs.

The airways (bronchi) leading to the lungs contract and relax in response to orders sent from the autonomic nervous system. When muscles in the walls contract improperly, or when the lining of the lungs is inflamed, the bronchi may experience spasms that cause them to narrow. Wheezing or coughing will occur owing to the reduced flow of air out of the lungs.

Bronchospasms can be caused by an allergic reaction or an infection of the respiratory tract. Chronic diseases such as asthma and emphysema can also cause bronchospasms. *See also* ASTHMA; COUGHING; EMPHYSEMA; LUNGS; *and* RESPIRATORY TRACT INFECTION.

Brown Fat

A type of fat used to store triglycerides and generate heat.

Brown fat more closely resembles glandular tissue than "regular" fat (white adipose tissue). It ranges in color from dark red to tan, depending on its lipid content. Unlike white fat, brown fat also contains vascular tissue and nerves. Brown fat is seen most prominently in newborn animals. Comprising up to five percent of body weight in human infants, it slowly decreases with age. While all infants are born with brown fat, by adulthood virtually none of it is left. Brown fat is important in small mammals and all hibernating animals because of its ability to dissipate stored energy as heat. Brown fat also appears to play a role in the control of body weight. *See* FATS AND OILS.

Brucellosis

Also known as Malta, Mediterranean, undulant, or Gilbraltar fever

An infection contacted from the Brucella bacteria.

Brucellosis is a bacterial illness found primarily in livestock. The disease spreads to people through contact with infected farm animals or by consumption of unpasteurized dairy products, particularly cheese.

Incidence. Brucellosis is rare in the United States, except in some Western states and among visitors from locations where the disease is more common, such as Spain, Mexico, and South America. There are about 100 to 200 cases of brucellosis in the United States each year. People who contract the disease are usually slaughterhouse workers, farmers, or veterinarians.

Symptoms. Often a chronic illness, brucellosis may persist for years, causing malaise (a generalized feeling of illness), recurring fevers, chills, excessive sweating, weight loss, headache, and pain in a variety of locations. Acute brucellosis generally begins with mild flu-like symptoms. In the undulant form, the patient suffers from a fever that peaks in the afternoon at levels around 104° Fahrenheit, rising and falling throughout the day. One of its alternate names, undulant fever, derives from the undulating or up-and-down nature of its symptoms.

Diagnosis. The presence of the brucella bacteria that cause brucellosis is diagnosed through a blood culture, a urine culture, a bone marrow culture, or a serology test.

Treatment. Doctors use antibiotic therapy to treat the disease and to prevent relapse. Tetracycline or an aminoglycoside is often prescribed.

Prevention. To prevent brucellosis, it is most important to avoid unpasteurized milk and to limit cheese consumption to aged cheeses. In addition, people who handle meat should wear protective glasses and clothing and should protect skin breaks from contact with potentially infected animal products. A vaccination against brucellosis is available for cattle, but is not suitable for human use.

Complications. The complications of brucellosis include bone and joint lesions, infective endocarditis (infection of the lining of the heart chambers and heart valves), encephalitis (inflammation of the brain), and meningitis (inflammation of the tissue surrounding the brain).

Prognosis. Although a patient may appear to recover from brucellosis, there is a great likelihood that the illness will recur a few months later. In this instance, a physician should be consulted so treatment can be readministered.

See BACTERIA; INFECTION; *and* FOOD CONTAMINATION *for a discussion on the foundations of brucellosis. For additional material on brucellosis, see* ENDOCARDISIS; ENCHEPHALITIS; LESION; CANCER; *and* MENINGITIS. *Diagnosis and treatment is discussed in* ANTIBIOTIC DRUGS; BLOOD TESTS; TETRACYCLINE DRUGS; *and* URINALYSIS.

Bruise

Injury-related skin discoloration.

Everyone experiences bruises—from mi-nor bumps to sprains—in the course of a normal life. The purple discoloration appears when the blood from small ruptured vessels leaks into tissue and under the skin. Bruising typically occurs from a blow, but it can also result from a twisted ankle, a strained muscle, or a scrape that removes parts of the skin. People who have blood clotting problems bruise easily, because the blood continues to leak into the skin.

Bruises in the Elderly

Because of thinner skin and more fragile blood vessels—particularly if they have been exposed to a lot of sun—the elderly bruise easily even from what might seem normal hand pressure. Often, bruises will appear on the forearms and the backs of the hands. No treatment is necessary, though reabsorption of the blood may take a long time.

Other than applying a cold compresses on the bruised site for ten to fifteen minutes every hour to reduce swelling and pain, there is no specific treatment for bruising. Most bruises will eventually heal on their own as the blood is reabsorbed into the body.

Background material on bruises may be found in BLOOD; CIRCULATORY SYSTEM; *and* SKIN. *Further information is contained in* COMPRESS; PURPURA; *and* SPRAIN. *Related material can be found in* ELDERLY, CARE OF THE; FIRST AID; *and* SWELLING.

Bruits

The sound produced by the turbulent flow of blood in the body.

A number of causes of bruits exist, and they can all be generally observed simply by listening to the body (auscultation), usually with the aid of a stethoscope. Bruits are often indicative of turbulent blood flow, which may be due to obstruction by arterial plaque (particularly in the arteries of the leg or neck), or disorders in the functioning of valves. However, bruits are not always associated with irregularities of blood flow. Fetal circulation, for example, creates a bruit within the mother's uterus. *See also* AUSCULTATION; BLOOD; BLOOD DISORDERS; *and* CIRCULATORY SYSTEM.

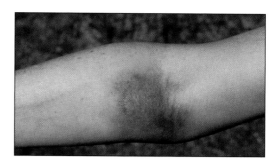

Bruxism

Unconscious grinding or clenching of teeth.

Bruxism usually occurs during sleep, but can even take place while awake. Although the exact cause of grinding, or clenching, is not known, it is possibly related to the release of tension, teething, or even a poor bite. Bruxism erodes the surface of teeth and can damage the temporomandibular joints. As they wear down, teeth become more sensitive and prone to decay. Fillings and crowns may also be damaged.

If the cause can be identified, the problem can be eliminated or controlled. If not, the patient can be fitted with a biteplate that fits over the teeth and is worn at night (or whenever the grinding occurs). This device does not prevent the grinding, but rather takes the brunt of the wear and protects the teeth. *See also* TEETH.

Buck Teeth

Term used for varying degrees of abnormally protruding upper teeth.

Buck teeth is a common term used to describe large front teeth and a severe overbite, a condition in which the top teeth extend beyond the bottom teeth and jut out. Like underbite, overbite is a form of malocclusion, in which the teeth do not fit properly together when a person bites down. Orthodontics can often correct this problem by reshaping the dental arch. Sometimes, one or more teeth have to be extracted to create space for other teeth to move into. *See* ORTHODONTIC APPLIANCES .

Bruise.
A bruise usually appears as a purple discoloration. This occurs when blood from ruptured vessels leaks into tissue under the skin. Left, a bruise appears on the arm of a woman who had a blood test.

Budd-Chiari Syndrome

A rare condition in which the liver becomes swollen because the veins draining blood from the organ are blocked.

Budd-Chiari syndrome can lead to portal hypertension (increased pressure in the portal vein, the large blood vessel that carries blood from the stomach, intestine, and spleen to the liver) and also to liver failure (impairment of liver function that can result in brain damage). The condition can develop in patients with polycythemia vera, in which there is overproduction of red blood cells by the bone marrow, and other conditions in which there is excess production of blood cells. Budd-Chiari syndrome can also develop in sickle-cell disease. It sometimes occurs during pregnancy.

Symptoms include jaundice and abdominal pain (ascites) from an excess accumulation of fluid in the peritoneal cavity (the space between the membranes that line the abdominal wall and organs).

Treatment. The syndrome is treated by surgery to remove whatever is obstructing the veins, such as a blood clot, a tumor, or a congenital malformation of the veins. Corrective surgery is of limited value, with fewer than one third of patients surviving for more than one year and almost all dying within two years. The only life-saving procedure for most patients is a liver transplant. *See also* LIVER FAILURE; LIVER TRANSPLANT; *and* PORTAL HYPERTENSION.

Buerger's Disease

A disease in which the blood vessels become thick and narrow, blocking the flow in arteries and veins, particularly in the hands and feet.

Early symptoms of Buerger's disease are pain in the extremities, numbness, or tingling. Later, the fingers and toes may develop ulcerations and gangrene owing to inadequate blood flow. Many other diseases show similar symptoms, but treatments that would normally be prescribed for these diseases have no effect on Buerger's disease, which is almost certainly associated with cigarette smoking—all reported cases are among moderate to heavy smokers. The only treatment known to be effective is immediate and total cessation of smoking. *See also* DRUG; DRUG DEPENDENCE; *and* GANGRENE.

Bulla

Thin walled blisters greater than five millimeters in diameter.

Bulla are large blisters that form on the skin and contain clear fluid. Occasionally bulla may form on the lungs, where they can rupture and cause spontaneous pneumothorax, in which air enters the pleural cavity between the lungs and the inside of the chest cavity. Bulla that form on the lungs and contain air are called blebs. Bullas are commonly caused by allergens and irritants, physical trauma, sunburn, insect bites and viral infections, such as herpes simplex and herpes zooster. *See also* BLEB.

Bunion

Deformity that occurs at the top of the first metatarsal bone.

When shoes that are too tight force the big toe against the other toes, the metatarsal bone, which joins the arch to the toe, begins to rub against the side of the shoe. The underlying tissue becomes inflamed, and a bony growth develops. As this bump continues to grow larger, the big toe is forced, creating a bunion.

The most common cause of bunions is the regular wearing of narrow-toed, high-heeled shoes, which squeeze the toes and put the front of the foot at an unnatural angle. Flat feet, gout, and arthritis also may increase the risk of bunions. Some ballet dancers who dance in pointe shoes also develop bunions. A bunionectomy is surgery that repairs the deformed joint and bone. Splints or pins may be inserted to hold the toe in place during the healing process. *See also* ARTHRITIS; CALLUS; *and* GOUT.

Bunion
A bunion (below) is a deformity of the metatarsal bone, which joins the arch and the toe. Shoes that fit poorly are the most common cause.

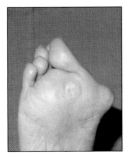

Burkitt's Lymphoma

A cancer of the lymph nodes that occurs primarily in children in Africa and New Guinea.

Burkitt's lymphoma is believed to be caused by an abnormal response to the Epstein-Barr virus, which causes mononucleosis and is also associated with nasopharyngeal cancer.

The disease is rarely seen in adults. Most patients have large masses of cancer tissue in the abdomen, often accompanied by tumors of the jaw. Some suffer anemia resulting from deterioration of the bone marrow, which produces red blood cells. A variant of Burkitt's lymphoma is sometimes seen is patients with AIDS.

Without treatment, the disease progresses rapidly. Intensive administration of anticancer drugs such as cyclophosphamide, methotrexate, and vincristine can result in long-term survival in about 80 percent of patients. Radiation therapy may reduce the severity of or eliminate symptoms, if not cure the disease.

See Bone Marrow; Cancer; Epstein-Barr Virus; Lymphoma; Mononucleosis; *and* Virus *for a discussion of the foundations of this subject. Further information may be found in* AIDS; Anemia; *and* Radiation Therapy. *Related material is available in* Anti-Cancer Drugs; Cyclophosphamide; *and* Radiation Therapy.

Burns

Destruction of the skin or deeper tissues from excessive heat.

Burns result from direct dry heat, fire, wet heat as from scalding, chemicals such as acids, and electric current. Burns are divided into three categories.

First-Degree Burns damage only the outer surface of the skin. After a burn, the skin becomes red, extremely sensitive to the touch, wet, and swollen.

Second-Degree Burns are deeper. Blisters form and are filled with a clear, thick liquid. The area is painfully sensitive to touch and is swollen.

Third-Degree Burns go deeper still. The immediate surface may be charred and leathery or white and soft; observers may not realize that a burn has taken place. There may be some blistering. The area may be extremely painful to the touch or, if nerve endings have been destroyed, there may be no pain at all.

Inhalation and Chemical Burns. Inhalation burns occur when hot gases enter the mouth, air passages, or lungs. Chemical burns of the throat and esophagus can be the result of drinking acid, alkali, mustard gas, or phosphorus.

Treatment depends on the source and depth of the burn. Extensive second-degree burns and all third-degree burns should be treated by trained medical personnel.

Doctors will first make sure the victim can breathe properly. Oxygen will be supplied if carbon monoxide poisoning is suspected. Lost fluids will be replaced intravenously; this method also serves as a preliminary response to treating shock.

The site will be carefully cleaned of dirt and other debris. If necessary, doctors may administer an anesthetic so that the area can be scrubbed with a soft brush. An antibiotic cream may be applied and the area covered with a loose bandage. The burn area will be vulnerable to infection, so it must be kept clean and covered with sterile bandages.

Skin Grafts. More extensive burns often require a section of skin to be taken from an unburned part of the body, from another person or even from a pig, since pig skin most resembles human skin. Grafts from the victim will integrate well with the surrounding skin. Grafts from other sources will serve to protect the area for ten days to two weeks; the grafts are sloughed off as the person heals.

Besides being painful, burns take a long time to heal, can be disfiguring, and require extensive physical therapy. Victims of extensive burns can be depressed and may need psychiatric assistance to see them through.

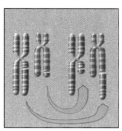

Translocation of Genes.
The mechanism of Burkitt's lymphoma on the cellular level is believed to involve a genetic mishap in which chromosomes do not replicate properly, resulting in cancerous cells.

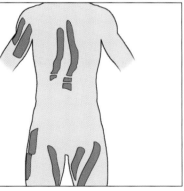

Skin Grafts.
Extensive burns may require skin grafts (above), which involve removing skin from an unburned part of the body and using it to replace the skin on the severely burned area.

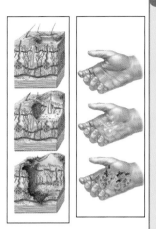

Burns.
Classified by the extent of damage to the skin, burns can be first (top), second (middle), or third (bottom) degree.

Bursitis.
Bursitis is caused by inflammation of the bursa (arrow).

Bursitis

Inflammation of the bursae.

The bursae are fluid-filled sacs located where tendons or muscles pass over bony protrusions. They lessen friction and help to maintain smooth movement. Bursitis occurs when these sacs become inflamed, usually because of chronic overuse, infection, injury, rheumatoid arthritis, or gout. Bursitis is most commonly found in the shoulder, but other high-risk areas include the knees, elbows, Achilles tendon, and first metatarsal of the foot.

Pain or swelling in the affected area is the usual indicator of bursitis. Examination by a physician will confirm the condition. Most cases of bursitis can be healed by resting the affected area, along with nonsteroidal anti-inflammatory drugs to relieve pain and reduce the inflammation. If that approach does not work, draining the fluid (aspiration) or the injection of corticosteroids may be necessary. If the bursitis is caused by an infection, antibiotics should be administered, and minor surgery may be performed to drain the infected bursa.

Proper mechanics and movement, as well as being aware of overuse, can help to

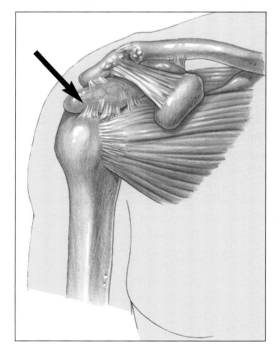

avoid bursitis. Most bursitis cases heal themselves with sufficient rest over the course of a few weeks, and individuals may resume their normal activities or sports.

Background material on bursitis can be found in INFLAMMATION; MUSCLES; *and* TENDON. *Related information is contained in* GOUT; INFECTION; RHEUMATOID ARTHRITIS; *and* SWELLING. *Details on treatment are available in* ANTIINFLAMMATORY DRUGS; *and* CORTICOSTEROID DRUGS.

Bypass

An operation performed to reroute blood or digestive fluids around a portion of a blood vessel or a part of the digestive system in an effort to remedy a blockage that has been caused by a disease or progressive condition.

Coronary Bypass. The most common form of this procedure is coronary artery bypass graft (CABG) surgery, which restores blood flow to the arteries around the heart.

CABG may be performed to relieve a dangerous narrowing of the left main artery, the major vessel supplying blood to the heart muscle to relieve severe angina— chest pain that cannot be treated effectively by medications or angioplasty—or to bypass blockages of the coronary arteries.

CABG surgery may be performed by cutting open the breastbone (sternum) with a vertical incision up to 10 inches long, spreading the sections apart with a vise-like instrument, then cutting away the tissues around the heart to make it visible to the surgeon. This technique requires that the heart be stopped and the patient's blood routed through a machine to maintain the body's oxygen supply. After surgery, an electric shock is given to restart the heart.

Once the chest is opened, blood vessels that will be used to create the bypass are harvested. The most commonly used vessels are the internal mammary artery, taken from the chest wall, or the great saphenous vein, taken from the inside of the calf or the thigh. Incisions are made in the arteries to be bypassed, and the surgeon sews the harvested vessels into place. Typically, the operation takes three to four hours,

after which the patient spends 24 hours in an intensive care unit and several more days in the hospital.

More recently, a technique called minimally invasive surgery has come into use. It allows CABG surgery to be performed while the heart is still beating, through an incision no more than four inches long. Minimally invasive surgery is being performed more and more in select cases as surgeons and their staffs undergo the necessary training. This technique also poses less risk to the patient.

Other Types of Bypass. Patients suffering from portal hypertension (liver disease causing increased blood pressure in the veins of the intestinal tract) or from esophageal varices (enlarged veins in the esophagus) may have surgery to reroute blood through a shunt. A patient with an intestinal cancer that is too large to be removed by surgery may have a bypass procedure that joins sections of the intestine on either side of the tumor. These bypass operations are less common than CABG surgery, which is performed on hundreds of thousands of patients in the United States each year.

Blocked or narrowed arteries in the legs may lead to a condition known as lower limb ischemia. If lifestyle changes do not solve the problem, a femoral artery bypass may be attempted. In the operation, the blocked artery is bypassed via a portion of vein from the same leg or an artificial device. Through the graft, blood supply to the limb is increased.

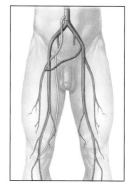

Femoral Artery Bypass.
When blocked arteries cut off bloodflow to the legs, lower limb ischemia results. A bypass procedure may be performed in order to reroute the blood through a vein in the same limb.

See CIRCULATORY SYSTEM; DIGESTIVE SYSTEM; ESOPHAGUS; HEART; LIVER; *and* TENDON *for a discussion of the foundations of bypass. Further information is contained in* ANGIOPLASTY; ARTERY; HEART DISEASE; HYPERTENSION *and* ISCHEMIA. *Related material can be found in* GRAFTING.

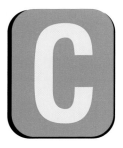

Cachexia

A condition in which the body wastes away, characterized by major weight loss and severe illness.

Cachexia is a profound wasting of the body that occurs primarily in people with advanced cancer, particularly of the lung, pancreas, liver, and digestive tract, as well as with widespread malignancies. It is also an end stage of many serious illnesses.

Causes. Although the causes of cachexia are not entirely understood, one factor in wasting seems linked to the release of tumor necrosis factor (TNF or cachectin) and is also influenced by metabolic changes induced by the tumor(s). In cancer-related cachexia, the wasting afflicts muscle tissue, bone, and fatty tissue.

Symptoms of cachexia may be aggravated by the side effects of cancer treatment, such as the nausea and vomiting associated with chemotherapy and radiation, which can also intensify nutrient loss and appetite reduction. Cachexia itself is a state of metabolic imbalance.

Treatment. The most successful treatment for cachexia is to remove the tumor or treat the underlying disease. Research is addressing treatments from cautious refeeding and enteral and parenteral nutrition, to dietary supplements and ways of maintaining appetite and the use of appetite stimulants and experimental drugs such as thalidomide. *See also* CHEMOTHERAPY.

Cadmium Poisoning

Poisoning caused by the inhalation of fumes or dust from cadmium.

Cadmium is a metal widely used in industry and may be inhaled from cadmium-emitting factories. It may be present in contaminated water, soil, air, and food. Toxic levels may be ingested via contaminated foods or liquids from vending machines soldered with cadmium compounds. Ingestion can cause vomiting, diarrhea, head-ache, aching muscles, salivation, and chills. At risk for poisoning are painters, welders, ce-

ramic workers, and photographers. Inhalation can result in metal fume fever and, over time, shortness of breath, loss of smell or sensation, cough, weight loss, fatigue, yellow rings on the teeth, bone pain, and kidney damage. Continuous exposure causes accumulation in the body, resulting in kidney failure and lung inflammation, eventually leading to emphysema or death. *See also* POISONING.

Café au Lait Spots

Tan colored birthmarks, similar in color to coffee with milk.

A café au lait spot is a congenital, pigmented mark on the skin. It may be a normal birthmark. However, several large spots together may occur in neurofibromatosis, a genetic disorder that causes abnormal cell growth. In the case of neurofibromatosis, there will also be multiple small lumps in the skin and possibly in affected organs. There is no known way to prevent cafe au lait spots. *See also* BIRTHMARK *and* NEUROFIBROMATOSIS.

Caffeine

Stimulant and diuretic obtained from certain natural substances.

Caffeine is a substance that occurs naturally in coffee beans, tea leaves, cacao trees, and kola nuts. It is added to soft drinks (cola and non-cola) and is a component of many over-the-counter and prescription drugs, including diet pills, stimulants, pain relievers, and allergy medicines.

Caffeine stimulates the central nervous system. It can be used to increase alertness, and to treat migraine headaches. It also acts as a diuretic. Too much caffeine can result in negative side effects. The amount of caffeine that is "too much" varies from person to person. Possible effects of caffeine toxicity include cardiac arrhythmia, diarrhea, vomiting, heartburn, and convulsions, as well as anxiety, tremors, and insomnia. Chronic consumption may cause agitation, irregular heartbeat, fever, hyperventilation, and respiratory failure.

Under certain conditions, caffeine can be addictive. Withdrawal may occur in heavy coffee drinkers who abruptly stop their intake of caffeine. Symptoms of withdrawal include headaches, tiredness, and irritability. Withdrawal symptoms can be prevented by reducing intake gradually.

Calcaneus

The heel bone.

The largest bone of the foot, the heel bone juts backward from under the ankle. Attached to the back of the heel bone, the Achilles tendon dictates the foot's vertical movement. Muscles necessary for arch support are attached to tendons in the sole of the foot that meet under the heel bone.

The impact from a jump or fall can break the heel bone; the fracture is usually treated by placing the leg and foot in a cast. If the fracture is severe, joints involved in the foot's lateral movement may be seriously or irreparably damaged. Mere walking may result in stiffness and pain.

The bond between the heel bone and the Achilles tendon is placed under considerable stress in sports that require a lot of running. Since this part of the bone is not fully developed in children, they may experience swelling. Pain felt in the bone when walking or standing may come from swelling of the tendons that control the arch-supporting muscles. *See* BONE *and* FOOT.

Calcification, Dental

Calcium accumulation in preparation and maintenance of developing teeth.

Dental calcification is the process by which teeth absorb calcium, an important element that makes them hard and durable (as it does with bone). Other substances in addition to calcium are incorporated into the teeth before and during their growth.

The mineral fluoride plays an important role in the process of tooth growth, strengthening the calcium composition of enamel and preventing decay. However, too much fluoride can cause fluorosis, a condition in which fluoride pits the tooth enamel. Problems with calcification and other forms of mineralization can be addressed by dentists or dental specialists. *See also* CALCIUM *and* TEETH.

Calcinosis

A condition in which small, white calcium bumps form on the fingers and other body parts, usually as a result of scleroderma and other diseases.

Scleroderma is an autoimmune disease, in which, for an unknown reason, the immune system attacks the body. Calcinosis may also be caused by other autoimmune diseases. Bumps come through the skin surface and leak a chalky, white fluid. Although found most often on the fingers and near joints, the bumps may appear anywhere. Calcinosis may range from mild—involving only one bump—to more serious—involving clusters of bumps. Usually there is no treatment for calcinosis, although sometimes bumps can be removed surgically if they are numerous or painful. In some cases, the drug colchicine is used to reduce swelling. *See also* AUTOIMMUNE DISORDERS; CALCIUM; *and* SCLERODERMA.

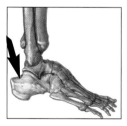

Calcaneus.
The heel bone is the largest bone of the foot. Its location makes it the bone that has to bear the heaviest weight and the strongest impact.

Calcitonin

A hormone that controls blood calcium levels.

The thyroid gland produces the hormones thyroxine, tri-iodothyronine, and calcitonin. The parathyroid glands, located on each side of and behind the thyroid gland, produce parathyroid hormone. Calcitonin works with parathyroid hormone (PTH) to maintain correct levels of calcium in the blood. If too much calcium is in the blood, increased thirst, urination, or changes in mental status may occur; if calcitonin is produced, it causes calcium to be absorbed by the bones, reducing blood calcium levels to normal. Low levels of calcium results in decreased production of calcitonin. The release of calcitonin relies mainly on blood calcium levels.

Synthetic injections of calcitonin can be used to treat Paget's disease, which causes abnormal bone growth and deformity. Calcitonin may also be used to treat hypercalcemia, a condition in which an overactive parathyroid gland, bone cancer, or certain tumors can cause excess levels of calcium in the blood, which may result in nausea, loss of appetite, vomiting, and excessive urination. The use of calcitonin as a drug usually causes few side effects. *See also* BONE, CANCER OF; CALCIUM; HYPERCALCEMIA; *and* PAGET'S DISEASE.

Calcium

A mineral essential for the maintenance of several body tissues and functions.

Calcium is the most plentiful mineral in the body, 99 percent of which is located in the skeletal tissues. The remaining one percent is located in the body's soft tissues and fluids and is essential to functions such as hormone secretion, nerve signal transmission, and muscle contraction. It is crucial that the proper balance of calcium in the body's fluids be maintained.

Blood levels of calcium are maintained by intestinal absorption of dietary and secreted calcium, deposition and release of calcium in the bones, and urinary excretion. If dietary calcium is insufficient, skeletal calcium stores are released into the bloodstream. Sustained release of calcium from the bones may lead to osteoporosis.

Supplements. A normal blood calcium level is essential to a healthy life. Calcium supplementation is strongly advised for individuals of all ages, particularly pregnant and lactating women and older adults who do not consume enough dairy products regularly. The United States Recommended Daily Allowance for calcium is 1000 milligrams and higher for adults; women who are pregnant, lactating, or postmenopausal have a higher requirement. Rich sources of dietary calcium include milk and milk products, oysters, broccoli, and tofu. Green leafy vegetables often contain high levels of calcium, although large amounts of phytochemicals in some of these sources may limit their absorption. *See also* BONE *and* MINERAL.

Calcium Channel Blockers

Drugs that act to relax arteries and slow the heart in order to reduce blood pressure and angina.

Calcium ions must move through cell membranes for proper functioning of the heart muscles and arteries. Calcium channel blockers stop the movement of calcium into cells. This relaxes the muscles of the heart and the walls of the arteries, allowing them to enlarge, reducing blood pressure and decreasing strain on the heart.

Side Effects. Calcium channel blockers may have some serious side effects, especially when taken in conjunction with other drugs. Drugs that may interact with calcium channel blockers include—but are not limited to—other heart medications, diuretics, anti-seizure medications, and some immunosuppressants. Side effects may include heart problems, such as irregular rhythms, congestion or heart failure, and dangerously low blood pressure. It is important to discuss possible drug interaction side effects with a physician. *See also* ANGINA PECTORIS *and* VASODILATOR DRUGS.

Calculus, Dental

Deposits of hardened plaque on the crown and roots of teeth.

Plaque consists of the sticky remains of food and bacteria left by inadequate brushing. Minerals from saliva can accumulate in areas of plaque, forming a hardened layer known as calculus or tartar. Teeth near saliva ducts—the lower front teeth and upper back teeth—are especially susceptible to this condition. The concentration of mineral and organic material and bacteria progressively inflames and irritates the gums, resulting in gum disease.

During a routine dental examination, the dentist or hygienist will take an instrument and remove the calculus from each tooth (scaling). Some people develop plaque and calculus more frequently than others. Proper care of the teeth, including brushing and flossing, is the best means of preventing serious calculus problems. *See also* PLAQUE; SCALING, DENTAL; *and* TEETH.

Calculus, Urinary Tract

A stone that forms in the kidney, ureter or bladder.

Calculi (stones) form from minerals that are by-products of metabolism. For example, leafy vegetables and coffee have a high content of a chemical called oxalic acid. The body transforms this into oxalate, which is found naturally in urine. Oxalate can combine with calcium to form a compound that dissolves poorly and can form calcium oxalate stones. Stones can range in size from tiny grains to stones as large as golf balls. Nearly 75 percent of stones found in the kidney and the ureter, which leads from the kidneys to the bladder, consist of calcium oxalate. Another 20 percent are associated with infections of the urinary tract that cause a buildup of calcium, magnesium, and ammonium, while about five percent occur in persons with gout, some forms of cancer, and chronic dehydration.

Stones can form in the bladder as a result of chronic urinary tract infection, enlarged prostate or some bladder disorders.

Symptoms. Small stones in the kidney may cause no problems. But when a stone lodges in the ureter, it can cause severe pain and bleeding, as it lodges in a narrow part of the ureter and blocks the flow of urine. The pain may be intermittent or severe enough to cause vomiting. Bladder stones can also interfere with the flow of urine, resulting in difficult urination.

Diagnosis. The size and location of calculi can be determined by x-rays, pyelography—in which a dye is injected into the urinary tract—or computerized tomography (CT) scanning. Ultrasound scanning can capture images of the urinary tract; blood and urine tests may be performed to detect high levels of calcium and other minerals involved in stone formation.

Treatment. Small stones may pass through the ureter on their own; increasing water intake may encourage stones to pass. Techniques for removing stones that remain lodged in the ureter or kidney include ureterorenoscopy, in which an endoscope with a basket-like device is used to capture the stone; lithotripsy, in which a shock wave is used to break up the stone; percutaneous nephrolithotomy, in which a tube is inserted through the skin into the urinary tract to break up the stone and remove the pieces; and lithotomy, a major surgery that involves opening the kidney. The acute pain caused by calculi can be eased by pain relievers (analgesics).

Urinary Calculi After Age 30

The incidence of calculi in the urinary tract is highest between the ages of 30 and 50, with men in that age group four times more likely than women to develop stones. While the incidence lessens with age, so does the gender difference; over 60, women and men are at equal risk. The most basic preventive measures are drinking a lot of water and limiting foods that contain oxalic acid and other substances associated with stones.

Basic anatomical information on urinary tract calculus is available in URINARY SYSTEM. *Additional material can be found in* BLADDER *and* KIDNEY. *Related subjects include* CALCIUM; CAT SCAN; *and* LITHOTRIPSY.

Caliper Splint

An orthopedic leg brace.

A deformity or disorder of the leg that causes difficulty standing and walking may be partially remedied by wearing a caliper splint around the limb. A caliper splint is usually made of leather, fiberglass, or metal rings joined to one or two metal rods. The splint exerts pressure on deformed or weakened muscle, so that the weight is supported mainly by the hip bone rather than by the leg. It needs only to reach below the knee to help support the injured ankle; longer splints may be jointed to accomodate knee flexion.

Muscle disorders that may be aided by a caliper splint include Osgood Schlatter's disease (inflammation of the bone and cartilage of the shin) and Perthes' disease (which affects the growth plate of the thighbone in children). *See also* OSGOOD SCHLATTER'S DISEASE *and* PERTHES' DISEASE.

Callus

A hardened, thickened area of dead skin formed from keratin, caused by friction or pressure.

Calluses are most commonly found on the soles of the feet. The skin there is about 40 times thicker than on any other part of the body; calluses on the feet actually act as an extra layer of protection.

General wear and tear of the feet can lead to callus formation; babies have smooth feet, while adults who walk, run and perform other activities inevitably build up calluses. Wearing poorly fitting shoes or going barefoot frequently adds to the likelihood of the formation of calluses. Dancers and musicians may develop calluses in highly used areas, such as on their toes or fingers.

Calluses are rarely harmful, unless they become infected or inflamed or put excessive pressure on another body part. People with diabetes should pay particular attention to calluses in order to prevent the formation of ulcers. The simplest treatment is to remove the source of friction, for example, by switching to shoes that fit better. Medications and ointments will soften and destroy calluses; if necessary, minor surgery can be performed to remove them.

Bony Callus. After a bone breaks, bone gradually grows to fill in the fracture site. This gap is first filled by a blood clot, which is then replaced by a fibrous tissue known as fibrocartilage, forming a cartilaginous callus. Spongy bone then replaces the fibrocartilage, forming a bony callus. Eventually, strong bone grows to replace the temporary growth. During the healing process, the bony callus may show up on x-rays or be felt, but it will disappear when the permanent bone is in place. *See also* DIABETES *and* SKIN.

Caloric Test

A diagnostic test performed to measure functioning of the inner ear.

A caloric test may be performed to help determine the cause of dizziness, vertigo, or hearing loss, or if a person has had a negative reaction to certain antibiotics. The procedure tests reflexes arising from stimulation to the inner ear.

In a caloric test, a measured amount of cold water is inserted into the patient's ear, followed by a measured amount of hot water. With cold water, the patient's eyes should move rapidly away from the irrigated ear (rotary nystagmus), while with hot water, the eye should move toward the irrigated ear. If these reflexes fail to occur, nerve damage is indicated.

No special preparation is necessary for the caloric test, although sedatives and medication for motion sickness should be avoided prior to the test.

Results of a caloric test may help diagnose disorders such as a benign tumor of the inner ear (acoustic neuroma), localized tissue damage (infarction), tumors of the brain stem or cerebellum, or tumors or inflammation of the inner ear regions. *See also* ACOUSTIC NEUROMA; BALANCE; BRAIN; DIZZINESS; EAR; *and* HEARING.

Calorie

A measure of energy; specifically, a unit used to express the heat output of an organism and the energy value of food.

A calorie is a unit of measurement that refers to the amount of heat derived from the combustion of a fuel. In exact terms, it is the amount of heat necessary to increase the temperature of one gram of water 1° Celsius. Most food and the physical expenditure of energy is measured in kilocalories, which are equal to 1,000 calories.

Human caloric requirements vary depending on activity level, age, and state of health. In devising an individual's caloric requirements, it is important to include two components: calories necessary to fulfill the body's basic metabolic needs even when the person is asleep or resting, called the resting metabolic rate; and calories burned up in physical activities. In general, if a person takes in more calories than he or she expends, weight is gained; if intake is less than expenditure, weight is lost.

Calorimetry

The study of the loss and gain of heat, due to the body's absorption of nutrients.

The term calorie is often used as a unit of heat. Measurements of heat can be made and studied with the aid of a calorimeter, which records the heat exchanged in the body under specific conditions.

In human nutrition, however, the kilogram calorie or kilocalorie is generally used as the primary unit of measurement. Two common types of calorimeter exist: the calorimeter bomb measures potential food energy, while the respiration calorimeter measures the heat produced from respiratory gases. Proper caloric intake is essential to good health. For adult men and women, between 1800 and 2900 kilocalories (commonly referred to simply as calories) should be consumed daily; the exact amount depends on the person's age, health, and level of physical activity.

Counting Calories

Below is a list of common foods and the number of calories yielded from a serving.

Grain products

White bread	65/slice
Whole-wheat bread	70/slice
Bagel	200
Bran muffin	140
Chocolate chip cookie	45
Oatmeal raison cookie	61
Egg noodles	200/cup
Spaghetti	190
Toasted wheat germ	431
Cooked brown rice	232
Cooked white rice	186

Beverages

Coffee (Black)	2/cup
Tea	2
Lemonade	100
Cola	100
Club soda	0
Beer	49
Light beer	33
Gin, vodka, whiskey	73/oz.

Dairy products

Whole milk	150/cup
Skim milk	86/cup
Half-and-half	20/tbsp
Heavy cream	51/tbsp
Sour cream	30/tbsp
Shredded cheddar cheese	455/cup
Cream cheese	99/oz

Eggs

Raw egg	79
Egg white	16
Egg yolk	63
Butter-fried egg	95

Fish

Fish sticks	77/ea
Tuna in oil	56/oz
Tuna in water	37/oz
Smoked salmon	33/oz
Fried shrimp	68/oz

Spreads and oils

Butter	100/tbsp
Regular margarine	100
60% fat margarine	75
Corn oil	125
Sunflower oil	125
Olive oil	125
Italian dressing	80
Mayonnaise	100

Meat and poultry

Ground beef	82/oz
Steak	78
Bacon	36/strip
Ham	69/oz
Pork chops	90/oz
Sausage	40/link
Hot dogs	145/ea
Fried chicken thighs	238/ea
Roasted chicken thighs	153/ea
Roasted white meat turkey	44/oz

Vegetables

Cooked black beans	227/cup
Cooked garbanzo beans	269
Cooked string beans	44
Broccoli	24
Cabbage	16
Cauliflower	24
Carrot	31/ea
Celery	6/stalk

Fruits

Apple	80
Orange	60
Banana	105
Grapefruit	39/half
Grapes	3.5/ea
Mashed avocado	370/cup

Nuts

Dried almonds	167/oz
Roasted peanuts	163/oz
Peanut butter	94/tbsp

Background material on calorimetry can be found in CALORIE; FITNESS; KILOCALORIE; *and* NUTRITION. *Further information is contained in* DIET AND DISEASE *and* ENERGY. *Subjects related to calorimetry include* FOOD *and* NUTRITIONAL DISORDERS.

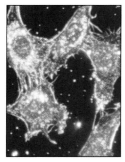

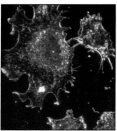

Cancer Cells.
Cancer cells multiply in an uncontrolled way, resulting in malignant growths. Above, top, culture of normal cells in human connective tissue. This image can be contrasted with the cancerous connective tissue cells pictured (bottom). Right, cancerous breast tissue. The pink spots are normal connective tissue and the blue areas are cancer cells. Below, a diagram of normal and cancer cells.

Cancer

A disease in which there is a dangerous, unrestrained growth of cells in a body tissue or organ.

The billions of cells in the human body are in a constant cycle of activity, death and replacement. A cell is created by the division of a parent—or precursor—cell. It matures, divides, and dies, to be replaced by another cell.

Signals within the cell and those sent to neighboring cells keep this process under control. This regulated rhythm of cell creation, reproduction, and death varies from organ to organ and tissue to tissue.

But sometimes a cell regenerates out of control. It begins to multiply in an uncontrolled way, passing its loss of control to its created—or daughter—cell, which repeats the disorderly cycle of uncontrolled growth and failure to die. The result is a tumor, also known as a growth. Some tumors are benign, with their overgrowth limited. Warts are an example of growths that are benign. Malignant tumors are dangerous because their growth is unrestrained.

Cancer, the Greek word for "crab," has been used since ancient times to describe the appearance of a tumor. As a cancer grows, it pushes into surrounding tissue. It may damage nerves, bones, and other tissues and block passageways in the body. Some abnormal cells can split off the parent cancer and travel through the bloodstream or the lymph system to other parts

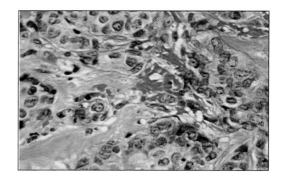

of the body, establishing colonies called metastases. Eventually, this uncontrolled growth interferes with bodily functions enough to cause death.

CAUSES

The underlying cause of all cancers lies in the genetic material in the nucleus of cells that controls all their replication processes. This genetic material is deoxyribonucleic acid, or DNA, a molecular chain made up of two intertwined strands of nucleic acids.

DNA is arranged in sequences, or segments, called genes, which together form chromosomes. There are 23 sets of chromosomes in a normal cell. Genes govern the production of proteins that do the business of the body.

Genes and chromosomes are subject to change, or mutation. A cell has genes that keep division and growth under control. If a mutation occurs in these tumor suppressor genes, as they are called, growth becomes uncontrolled.

Cells also contain oncogenes, which can initiate cancerous growth. They are normally inactive, but can be activated by mutation. The possibility of mutation increases with age, and so the incidence of cancer rises accordingly.

Mutations can also be caused by environmental factors, ranging from the ultraviolet rays of sunlight to viruses to the carcinogens—cancer-causing substances—in tobacco and industrial chemicals.

In addition, research has shown that every time a cell divides, some DNA is clipped off the ends of the chromosomes in the daughter cells. When enough of the chromosomes is lost, the cell dies. How-

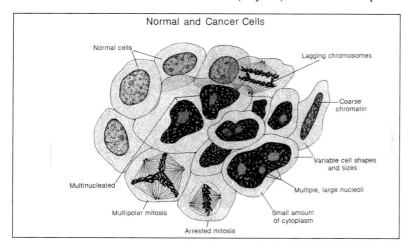

Normal and Cancer Cells

Normal cells

Lagging chromosomes

Coarse chromatin

Variable cell shapes and sizes

Multiple, large nucleoli

Multinucleated

Multipolar mitosis

Small amount of cytoplasm

Arrested mitosis

ever, cancer cells produce a substance called telomerase, which replaces the lost DNA, so that the cells do not die but multiply and reproduce endlessly.

PROGRESSION

The growth of a cancer begins with a mutation that alters a cell's genetic controls. In some cases, a single mutation is enough; in others, several mutations must take place. In this initiation stage, it may take several cycles of reproduction for a cell to become cancerous, as the necessary mutations accumulate. As that cell divides, it creates a growing group of abnormal cells, with unusual characteristics. They tend to divide more often than normal cells, and they usually lose the ability to perform the specialized tasks of normal cells.

It may take years for any symptoms of a small cancer to appear. During that time, the growth of the cancer can be accelerated by factors called promoters.

A promoter is anything that accelerates the tendency of cells to grow; some carcinogens also act as promoters. In this silent phase of a cancer, cells can drift away to form metastases in different parts of the body. This process of metastasis makes treatment of cancer more difficult.

TYPES

Cancers can be classified by the tissues in which they arise. The major classes of cancer are:

Carcinomas, which arise in the epithelial tissue that forms the lining of organs and internal tracts, such as the gastrointestinal system. More than 80 percent of all cancers are carcinomas. They are most common in organs that have a secretory function, such as the breasts. Carcinomas are subdivided into adenocarcinomas, which develop in an organ or gland, and squamous cell carcinomas, which develop in the skin or lining of the upper airways or other membranes.

Sarcomas, which arise in connective tissue, a class that includes bone, tendon, cartilage, muscle and fat.

Leukemias are cancers of forming tissues of the bone marrow, and the lymph system.

Myelomas, which arise in the plasma cells of the bone marrow.

Lymphomas, which arise in the lymphatic system, a network that runs all through the body and includes lymph nodes, the spleen, the tonsils, and the thymus gland.

Nerve Tissue Cancers, which are named for the specific cells in which they arise. A glioma is a cancer of a glial cell of the brain; a meningioma is a tumor in the meninges, the tissue covering the brain.

GRADE AND STAGE

Another way of classifying cancers is based on the extent to which their cells have become abnormal. As mentioned, cancer cells tend to lose the ability to perform the specialized tasks of normal cells. In formal language, they are less differentiated. One of the earliest stages of cancer is carcinoma in situ, in which cells have just begun to appear abnormal.

As the cells become less differentiated, they are classified by grade. A Grade I cancer is one in which fewer than 25 percent of cells are undifferentiated; in Grade II tumors, 25 to 50 percent of cells are undifferentiated; in Grade III tumors, 50 to 75 percent of cells are undifferentiated; and in Grade IV tumors, more than 75 percent of cells are undifferentiated.

Stage refers to the size of the tumor and the extent to which it has spread to adjacent tissue, lymph nodes, and distant sites (metasteses). Most tumors range from stage I (small and local) to stage IV (large and spread).

RISK FACTORS

Some persons run a higher-than-average risk of developing cancer. One major risk factor is exposure to known carcinogens, cancer-causing agents. One of the clearest associations between exposure to carcinogens and cancer is seen in lung cancer, which is directly related to smoking—a fact that somehow does not prevent more than 25 percent of Americans from smoking cigarettes. Occupational exposure to substan-

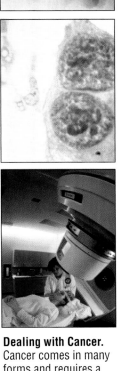

Dealing with Cancer. Cancer comes in many forms and requires a variety of therapeutic approaches. Treatment for lung cancer, shown in the x-ray, top, may not apply to the osteosarcoma (bone cancer), middle. Some cancers respond best to radiation treatments, bottom, while others respond best to chemotherapy.

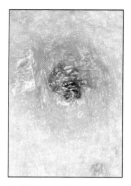

Is it Cancer?
Lumps and bruises of the skin come in many shapes and forms. It often requires a physician to tell whether the crusty lump, above, is cancerous or not—and even then, only microscopic analysis in the laboratory can determine the true nature of the suspect cells.

ces such as asbestos and environmental exposure to air pollutants (i.e., secondary smoke) and the ultraviolet radiation in sunlight are also risk factors. Screening to detect cancer at an early, treatable stage is advised in such cases. Other persons at higher risk of cancer include:

- People with a family history of a specific cancer, meaning that one or more close relatives—brother, sister, parent, grandparent—have been diagnosed with that cancer. Colorectal cancer and breast cancer are among those known to be related to family history.
- Persons with certain other disorders that can lead to specific cancers, such as those infected with HIV.
- Persons who have had one cancer. For example, cancer in one breast indicates a higher risk not only of cancer in the other breast, but also of cancer of the colon and the endometrium, the lining of the uterus.

OUTLOOK

"Cancer" is perhaps the most dreaded word in the language, but a large percentage of cancers are curable. Statistics show that more than half of the patients now diagnosed with cancer will be cured, and many others will achieve long-term survival and live complete lives.

Traditional treatments such as surgery, radiation therapy, and chemotherapy are continually being refined, and new treatments in the form of more effective medications and biological agents derived from the body's own defense system are coming into play.

Cancerous growths can be frozen, blasted with laser light, scraped away, or eliminated in several other ways. The gains against some cancers are impressive.

In the early 1960s, for example, only four percent of young children diagnosed with acute lymphocytic leukemia survived for five years; by 1991, the five-year survival rate reached 77 percent.

Improvements in cancer treatment have helped, while better methods of early detection, combined with improved knowledge of risk factors to be avoided, have

contributed to continued progress.

> *Background material on cancer can be found in* CELLS; MALIGNANCY; *and* TUMOR. *Additional material is contained in* GROWTH; LESION; LYMPHOMA; *and* METASTESES. *Details on treatment and diagnosis is available in* BIOPSY; CHEMOTHERAPY; *and* RADIATION THERAPY.

Cancer, Diet Therapy for

An approach to preventing and treating cancer that is based on diet.

Some evidence indicates that at least one third of cancers are influenced by diet. Thus, the foods a person eats may affect the likelihood of developing cancer and may help restore physical health after treatment with conventional medical therapy.

However, dietary approaches to preventing and treating cancer are often controversial and are rarely supported by solid clinical evidence.

Cancer Prevention. It is commonly accepted that a diet high in fiber, low in fat, and rich in vegetables, fruits, and whole grains can decrease the risk of cancer.

Recent research has investigated the role that antioxidants play in preventing cancer. Antioxidants are found primarily in vitamins A, C, and E and are plentiful in a diet that includes a high intake of vegetables. These substances limit the effects of free radicals—charged particles produced as a byproduct of metabolism that can damage cells and have been linked to cancer and age-related degeneration.

Cancer Treatment. Medical techniques to treat cancer include surgery, chemotherapy, and radiation therapy. When cancer is caught early enough, these techniques are highly effective. However, if a cancer has spread throughout the body, conventional treatments are less effective.

Many alternative treatments claim to be effective against even advanced cancer. These often entail a strict diet and may include additional supplements, treatment measures, and lifestyle changes.

Macrobiotics is probably the most popular alternative diet today. Based on a combination of ancient and modern philosophies, it claims that many modern ailments arise from people being out of balance with the natural environment. The diet it proposes is based on organic, unprocessed foods, primarily whole grains supplemented with vegetables and some sea vegetables, beans, and soups. Substances such as alcohol, coffee, and refined sugars are strictly avoided.

Other diet therapies include:

• **The Gerson Diet**—a highly involved regime that includes high doses of fresh, organic vegetable and fruit juices, a vegetarian diet, numerous supplements, and frequent coffee enemas.

• **The Wheatgrass Diet**—a diet consisting entirely of raw foods, including seeds, nuts, vegetables, and sprouts, supplemented by wheatgrass juice and accompanied by detoxification with enemas and high colonics.

• **Megadoses of Vitamin C**—consuming upwards of 10,000 milligrams of vitamin C each day.

In general, alternative diet treatments are almost entirely vegetarian and thus tend to be quite high in fiber and low in fat.

PRECAUTIONS

Some diet therapies may include the use of toxic substances or may not be nutritionally complete; some may be quite expensive. Also, some diet therapies rely on antictodal evidence, rather than on clinical testing. A more serious problem with these therapies is that many of them call for stopping conventional treatments.

> *See* ALTERNATIVE MEDICINE; NUTRITION AND DIET, *and* ALTERNATIVE THERAPIES *for a discussion of the foundations of diet theray for cancer. Further material is contained in* VITAMIN C. *Related information is found in* CANCER.

Cancer Screening

Tests that detect the possibility of cancer being present in a person's body.

Cancer screening starts with a cancer related checkup that is recommended periodically for all adults but is especially important for persons in high-risk groups. These include persons in a family with a history of specific cancers; those who have a disorder that predisposes them to cancers; those exposed to carcinogens, such as cigarette smokers or workers in some industries; and those who have already had one cancer that might recur or might increase the risk of other cancers.

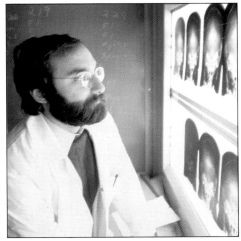

Cancer Screening. Above, examining a series of x-rays of the head in search of cancerous growths.

The ultimate goal of cancer screening is to accurately detect cancerous development at an early, treatable stage. Physicians strive for infallibility in screening because a misdiagnosis could result in delayed treatment or treatment that leads to undue risk for a healthy person. Physicians also seek to create procedures that are safe and cause a minimum of discomfort.

The American Cancer Society guidelines recommend a checkup every three years for men and women over the age of 20, with annual checkups for those 40 and older. Tests to screen for specific cancers recommended by the society include:

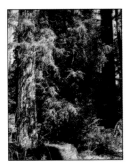

Yew Tree. The yew tree of the Pacific Northwest is the source for the cancer drug Taxol (a brand name for paclitaxel).

• Sigmoidoscopy to screen for colon cancer, every three to five years for men and women 50 and older.

• Fecal occult blood test to screen for colon cancer every year for men and women 50 and older.

• Digital rectal examination to screen for intestinal cancer every year for men and women 40 and older.

• Prostate examination to screen for prostate cancer every year for men 50 and older. The test looks for abnormally high levels of prostate-specific antigen (PSA), a substance produced by the prostate.

• Pap smear test and pelvic examination to screen for cervical cancer for women 18 or older or those who are sexually active every year. After three

Cancer Diagnostics.
Mammography, right, is among the most effective ways of detecting breast cancer early. Cancers are also detectable through the use of magnetic resonance imaging, or MRI. Bottom, frozen breast tissue is analyzed in the estrogen receptor assay test, used to diagnose breast cancer.

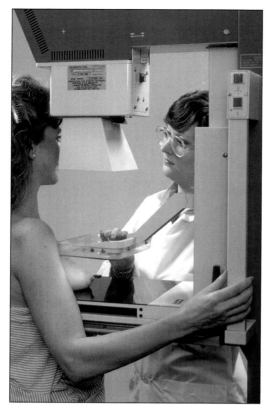

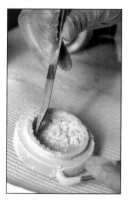

negative tests, the screening can be done less frequently at the discretion of the physician.

- Mammography to screen for breast cancer every one to two years for women ages 20 to 40 and every year for women over 40. Breast self-examination is recommended every month for women 20 and older.
- Endometrial tissue sample is used to screen for endometrial cancer at menopause for women at high risk because of failure to ovulate, abnormal uterine bleeding, estrogen therapy, or other indications.

Other tests may be recommended for persons whose family history or environmental exposure indicates a higher than normal risk of certain cancers.

Background material may be found in CANCER; IMAGING TECHNIQUES; MEDICAL TESTS; *and* RADIATION. *Further information regarding cancer screening techniques may be found in* BIOPSY; BLOOD TESTS; MAMMOGRAM; PAP SMEAR; SIGMOIDOSCOPY; *and* X-RAY. *Related material is contained in* ABSCESS; LYMPHOMA; METASTESES; *and* TUMOR.

Candidiasis

A fungal infection of the mucous membranes that affects the mouth or the genitals.

This infection occurs in people with a normally functioning immune system, but is more common or persistent in pregnant women and people with diabetes or AIDS. An individual with an impaired immune system can develop candidiasis that spreads throughout the whole body.

When the infection is present in the bloodstream, it is called candidemia and occurs most often in people with a low level of white blood cells (i.e., those with leukemia). It also occurs frequently in persons who are undergoing cancer treatment or have a catheter present in a blood vessel. The heart valves may become infected after surgery or another invasive procedure involving the heart or blood vessels.

Genital candidiasis involves an infection of the vagina or penis. The fungus is normally present in the skin or intestines and spreads to the genitals. Candidiasis is a common cause of vaginitis and is becoming more common due to the increasing use of antibiotics, oral contraceptives, and other drugs that affect vaginal acidity.

Symptoms. Women may experience itching and irritation and possible vaginal discharge, including a white, cheesy coating. The vulva will be reddish and swollen. Men often have no symptoms, but the tip of the penis may be sore after sexual intercourse. The penis may also have blisters or sores or a white, cheesy coating.

Treatment. In cases of candidiasis that affects the genitals or the mouth, antifungal drugs can be applied directly to the area. Antifungal medications such as fluconazole can also be taken orally. If the infection has spread throughout the body, it must be treated with antifungal drugs given intravenously. Diabetes can make the condition worse and must be brought under control prior to treatment. Women may need to discontinue taking oral contraceptives for a few months. *See also* AIDS; ANTI-FUNFAL DRUGS; DIABETES; *and* FUNGUS.

Canker Sore

Also known as aphthous ulcer

An open sore in the mouth that, though painful, is benign; it is characterized by a white or yellow sore surrounded by a bright red area.

Canker sores are a common type of mouth ulcer. They usually appear on the inner surface of the cheeks, lips, palate, and gums.

Cause. The cause of canker sores is unknown. Heredity may play a role in their development; there may also be a link to the immune system. Canker sores may result from mouth injury or excessive tooth cleaning; they may also be associated with stress, dietary insufficiencies, the menstrual cycle, changes in hormone levels, and food allergies.

Symptoms. These include a tingling sensation in the mouth, a skin lesion or red bump in the mouth, single or cluster-like sores, and mouth pain. Occasionally fever, a generalized feeling of sickness (malaise), swollen lymph nodes, and lethargy also occur.

Treatment. Usually no treatment for canker sores is necessary, as they tend to heal on their own. Severe cases may need to be treated with tetracycline, although this medication is not given to children unless all of their permanent teeth have come in, because otherwise the teeth can become discolored. Corticosteroids, such as dexamethasone and prednisone, are also sometimes used to treat canker sores. *See also* GUM; MOUTH; *and* TEETH.

Cannula

Hollow tube that allows passage of air or fluid during aspiration or artificial respiration.

A cannula is generally used with a sharp object known as a trocar for the aspiration of fluid from the body. The cannula encloses the trocar, which punctures the area from which fluid is to be removed. The trocar is then withdrawn while the cannula remains, and fluid flows out through the cannula.

Another type of cannula, known as a nasal cannula, is used for introducing oxygen through flexible tubing into each opening in the nose (naris). The nasal cannula is commonly used in treatment of cardiac disease, where a low air flow with small oxygen concentration is required. The percentage of oxygen delivered by this method varies, depending on patient respiration. *See also* ASPIRATION.

Capillary

A tiny blood vessel, the smallest in the circulatory system.

Capillaries are tiny blood vessels arranged in vast networks. The heart pumps blood into the arteries, which narrow into arterioles and then further into capillaries. In the capillaries the blood feeds tissues with oxygen and nutrients and takes in waste products, all through diffusion. Blood leaving the capillaries is a dark red color. It enters the venules, the venous system's equivalent of the arterioles, and then the veins, which take the blood back to the heart and lungs to be nourished again. *See also* ARTERIES; BLOOD; HEART; *and* VEINS.

Carbamazepine

An anticonvulsant used to treat certain kinds of seizures; also used to relieve the symptoms of facial nerve inflammation (tic douloureaux).

One of many of antiseizure drugs, carbamazepine is also used to relieve the pain of some types of neuralgia, including tic douloureaux, a facial nerve disease. Carbamazeine is often a first-choice anticonvulsant; as there are relatively few side effects; it is also useful in treating bipolar depression. Concentrations of the drug in the bloodstream must be balanced to produce a maximum effect while minimizing side effects. It should not be taken with other drugs unless approved by a doctor; drug interactions are common. Side effects include dizziness, drowsiness, confusion, mood changes, nausea, fever, and chills. There is also a danger of life-threatening toxicity of the blood, indicated by blurred or double vision and rapid, involuntary eye movement.

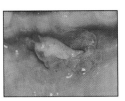

Canker Sore. An open sore or ulcer, that grows on the inside of the mouth. Most canker sores will heal themselves.

Carbohydrates

Any one of a number of organic compounds that, when metabolized, supply the body with energy.

Carbohydrates are made up of molecules that are the components of dietary sugar. Their main function is to provide the body with energy, but they also serve other important functions. The two types of carbohydrates are simple and complex.

Simple Carbohydrates. Simple carbohydrates, commonly known as sugars, are generally either monosaccharides or disaccharides. Fructose and glucose are examples of monosaccharides, while sucrose and lactose are examples of disaccharides.

Complex Carbohydrates. These are commonly known as starches; they are made up of many sugar molecules and are called polysaccharides. One starch molecule can contain hundreds of sugar molecules. Starches are broken down by enzymes in the mouth and the intestines into single sugar molecules, which are then absorbed by the intestines and stored in the liver and muscles as glycogen. When needed, glycogen is broken down into monosaccharides and distributed throughout the body via the liver as blood sugar. Carbohydrates are critical to the body's regulation of blood sugar levels.

Complex carbohydrates are usually an excellent source of dietary fiber, primarily from cellulose, the chief component in plant cell walls. Cellulose is constructed with bonds that cannot be broken apart by the human body; it thus passes through the digestive tract virtually undigested. The dietary fiber provided by cellulose and other indigestible complex carbohydrates, such as pectin and hemicellulose, is essential to the maintenance of the digestive tract. By bringing water into the digestive tract, fiber softens the stools and prevents constipation. Fiber also sustains the muscle tone of the digestive tract. It expedites the passage of food, reducing the amount of time carcinogenic (cancer-producing) substances are in contact with the intestines. Dietary fiber binds to fats such as cholesterol,

Resources on Carbohydrates

Groff, James L, and Sareen S. Gropper, *Advanced Nutrition and Human Metabolism* (1999); Heimburger, Douglas C. and Roland L. Weinsier, *Handbook of Clinical Nutrition* (1997); Mahan, Kathleen L. and Sylvia Escott-Stump, *Krause's Food, Nutrition, and Diet Therapy* (2000); Shils, Maurice E., et al., *Modern Nutrition in Health and Disease* (1999); American Dietetic Association, Tel. (800) 366-1655, Online: www.eatright.org; Center for Nutrition Policy and Promotion, Tel. (202) 418-2312, Online: www.usda.gov/cnpp; Food and Drug Administration, Tel. (888) INFOFDA, Online: www.fda.gov; www.ny-cornell.org/medicine/nutrition/index.html.

Carbohydrates in the Diet

Carbohydrates should provide more than half of the energy in the human diet—between 55 and 60 percent of total calories consumed—and should primarily be complex carbohydrates such as grains, beans and peas, bread, and pasta. Simple sugars contribute calories to the diet but contain few nutrients. In addition, foods containing large amounts of refined sugar tend to be low in dietary fiber, vitamins, and minerals, and high in fat. Each gram of carbohydrate yields four calories. Complex carbohydrates tend to have fewer calories per serving because of the bulk provided by cellulose and other dietary fibers.

which are then excreted in the feces, thus aiding in the maintenance of low blood levels of cholesterol. *See also* DIETARY FIBER; GLUCOSE; GLYCOGEN; KETOSSI; *and* LACTOSE.

Carbon Dioxide

A colorless, incombustible gas found in the atmosphere and used during respiration.

Under compression, carbon dioxide liquefies; its solid form is known as dry ice. It is released into the air by combustion, animal respiration, fermentation, and volcanic activity. In the gas-exchange function of respiration, oxygen is inhaled and enters the bloodstream, while the carbon dioxide is removed from the bloodstream and exhaled as a waste product.

Carbon dioxide is widely used in industry. It serves as a refrigerant and is used in carbonated beverages, fire extinguishers, and greenhouses.

When the concentration of carbon dioxide in the air reaches a certain level, it displaces oxygen and becomes an asphyxiant (causing suffocation). Some respiratory diseases cause a buildup of carbon dioxide in the blood. Symptoms of exposure to low levels of carbon dioxide include headache and shortness of breath. Higher levels can cause ringing in the ears, tremor, visual disturbances, and unconsciousness.

Carbon dioxide also presents an environmental concern: atmospheric levels are increasing steadily due to deforestation and the use of fossil fuels. Like other greenhouse gases, carbon dioxide traps some of the sun's heat, raising global temperatures. *See also* AIR *and* ENVIRONMENTAL MEDICINE.

Carbon Monoxide

A colorless, odorless, highly toxic gas.

Carbon monoxide is one of the leading causes of death in the United States. All combustion devices, including car engines, heaters, stoves, and furnaces, emit carbon monoxide. Tobacco smoke is another source. Methylene chloride, a paint stripper, is metabolized into carbon monoxide, posing an occupational risk.

ALERT
Exposure to Carbon Monoxide

Indications of exposure to carbon monoxide may appear slowly and resemble flu symptoms. A person may also experience headache, shortness of breath, chest pain, nausea, confusion, and fainting. Exposure to higher concentrations may cause drowsiness, unconsciousness, and even death. In chronic cases, it can cause bizarre and hyperactive behavior, and convulsions may occur. Chronic exposure at low levels has been correlated with mental deterioration and hearing loss. Treatment for acute carbon monoxide poisoning involves oxygen therapy.

Prevention. To prevent exposure to toxic levels of carbon monoxide, heating appliances should be properly vented, with vents and chimneys kept clean and unobstructed. Car engines and exhaust systems should be properly maintained. Cars and other power equipment should never idle in an attached garage. Homes should be equipped with carbon monoxide detectors. *See also* RESPIRATION.

Carbon Tetrachloride

A highly toxic liquid solvent with a distinctive odor.

Carbon tetrachloride is a clear, colorless liquid used as a solvent. It is thought to be carcinogenic and is banned by the Food and Drug Administration in most applications, is being replaced by less toxic sol-

vents. Exposure may occur from ingestion, skin absorption, or inhalation.

Initial symptoms may include nausea, stomach pain, headache, dizziness, eye, nose and throat irritation, blurred vision, loss of coordination, confusion, and unconsciousness. Following exposure, symptoms may subside in a period of time ranging from one day to two weeks.

Further symptoms may indicate liver or kidney damage; these include jaundice, nausea and vomiting, decreased urine output, swelling, and fluid retention. In extreme cases, death may even result. *See also* LIVER *and* TOXICITY.

Carbuncle

A cluster of deep boils that form connections inside the skin as well as on the skin's surface.

Carbuncles are usually very painful. They can develop anywhere but are most common on the back and neck. When the boils break open and drain, the pain subsides.

Carbuncles are caused by a contagious staphylococcal (bacterial) infection. Poor hygiene or physical condition and friction from razors or clothing may increase the likelihood of infection. People with diabetes and with suppressed immune systems are at greater risk.

Symptoms. These include painful pink or white skin lesions, ranging from pea-sized to golf ball-sized, that may ooze or contain pus. There may be redness and inflammation around the boils. Fever and fatigue may also occur.

Treatment. Carbuncles usually must drain before they can heal. The boils generally drain within two weeks. If the condition lasts for more than two weeks, is accompanied by a fever, is located on the spine or the face, or recurs, a physician should be consulted. Antibiotics may help control the infection. Warm, moist compresses help carbuncles drain more quickly. Lancing the boils at home is not recommended, as this may actually spread the infection. *See also* ANEMIA; DERMATITIS; *and* DIABETES.

Carcinogen

Any substance that can cause cells to become cancerous.

Carcinogens are substances, either in the body or introduced from the environment, that can damage cells and their DNA. Carcinogens interfere with cells' ability to receive information from hormones and the brain, corrupting the cells' built in mechanism for regulating growth and death.

CARCINOGENISIS

Normally, cells have built-in reproductive life spans. Some reproduce throughout the life of the body, such as hair and skin cells. Others, notably in the liver and kidney, have a more limited ability to reproduce, and reproduction is triggered only when repair is needed. Still other cells, such as those in the muscles and bones, have no ability to regenerate at all once they have passed the initial growth stages.

A cell receives instructions from its DNA that determine growth, function, reproduction, and life span. However, cells are exposed constantly to carcinogens that have the potential to alter their genetic material. After significant exposure to a carcinogen, the genetic material that controls a cell's life and behavior can become altered. Normally, this genetic damage is repaired, but if it is not, the cell's offspring inherit the abnormal DNA and, with it, abnormal growth and reproduction patterns. A cell whose controlling mechanisms have mutated is considered cancerous; the process by which a cell becomes cancerous is known as carcinogenesis. Cancerous tissue characteristically grows unchecked. It invades nearby tissue, and, over time, it may enter the bloodstream and invade other areas of the body (metastasis).

TYPES OF CARCINOGENS

Tobacco. This is the leading cause of cancer, responsible for 85 percent of deaths caused by lung cancer. Tobacco is also implicated in cancer of the digestive tract, bladder, pancreas, and cervix. Though chewing tobacco and snuff are harmful, smoking is the most hazardous use. Although it may be difficult to avoid secondhand smoke, not smoking is the easiest way to avoid exposure to tobacco.

Chemicals. Most chemical carcinogens are encountered through industrial exposure. The incidence of cancer among those who work with asbestos, benzene, vinyl chloride, chromate, industrial dyes, and nickel is uncommonly high. Workers in industries that involve rubber, tar, and pitch are frequently exposed to carcinogens. Protective clothing and face masks are available for people who work with dangerous materials.

Ionizing Radiation. This carcinogen is named for its ability to disturb the electrons of atoms, including those in DNA. Ionizing radiation sources can be found in healthcare facilities, research institutions, nuclear reactors, and various manufacturing facilities. If not properly monitored and safeguarded, these sources can pose health risk to workers. A number of technical and regulatory sources offer information about the recognition, evaluation, and control of occupational health hazards associated with ionizing radiation, including the Nuclear Regulatory Commission

---

Diet and Cancer

The role of diet in preventing cancer is a controversial subject. Until recently, a diet rich in fiber from fruits and vegetables has been recommended to help prevent cancer of the gastrointestinal tract. But several large-scale, long-term studies have found no reduction in cancer risk associated with such a diet. The recommendation for such a diet still stands, but for its beneficial effects on cardiovascular disease rather than its role in preventing cancer.

One significant contributor to carcinogenesis is obesity, because an estimated 60 percent of Americans over the age of 20 are overweight or clinically obese. Fat cells convert estrogen to estriadol, a more active form of the hormone that can promote tumor growth.

Abdominal fat can cause increased production of insulin-like growth factor, a body chemical related to cancer promoters. Obesity is also related to an increased risk of cancer of the breast, colon, and prostate, among other malignancies.

(NRC) and the Occupational Safety and Health Administration (OSHA).

Sunlight. Although ultraviolet radiation from sunlight is not ionizing, prolonged exposure can cause skin cancer, particularly in people with fair skin. The incidence of skin cancer has been increasing in the United States in recent years. This is attributed to two main factors. First, Americans are spending more time outdoors without appropriate protection, such as a hat or sunscreen. Second, the earth's ozone layer, which absorbs ultraviolet radiation, is deteriorating, resulting in a higher percentage of the sun's ultraviolet rays penetrating the atmosphere.

Viruses. The viruses responsible for genital herpes and warts lead to a higher risk for cervical cancer. Hepatitis viruses B and C lead to higher ocurence of liver cancer. Human immunodeficiency virus (HIV) can cause acquired immunodeficiency syndrome (AIDS), which can result in the development of cancer, especially of lymphoid tissue (lymphoma). AIDS is also associated with tumors of the skin and mucous membranes, called Kaposi's sarcoma.

PROMOTERS AND ENHANCERS

The process of carcinogenesis, in which a normal cell becomes cancerous, is not a simple one. A number of agents can play a role in the transformation. While carcinogens cause mutations in DNA, some carcinogens damage other parts of the cell.

In addition to carcinogens, there are substances known as promoters that accelerate the process of malignant transformation. Promoters can be synthetic chemicals, such as polychlorinated biphenyls (PCBs), or they can be substances normally found in the body, such as estrogen, a hormone that promotes the growth of breast cancer.

Another class of agents involved in carcinogenesis, known as enhancers, acts indirectly in the development of cancer. For example, nitrites, a group of compounds used as food preservatives, are not directly carcinogenic, but they can be transformed in the digestive tract into nitrosamines, which are carcinogens.

Known and Suspected Carcinogens

The following known and suspected carcinogens are among the over 200 listed in the Ninth Annual Report on Carcinogens published by the Environmental Health Information Service of the U.S. Department of Health and Human Services. The full report is available online at:

http://ehis.niehs.nih.gov/roc/tos9.html

The following carcinogens may cause cancer after prolonged exposure or contact.

KNOWN CARCINOGENS

- nuclear radiation and x-rays (leukemia, skin)
- radon (lung)
- solar radiation, sunlamps and sunbeds (skin)
- polycyclic aromatic hydrocarbons (PAHs) :
    tobacco smoke, pitch, and tar fumes (lung)
    solid pitch and tar (skin)
    soot (scrotum)
- smokeless chewing tobacco (mouth, stomach)
- alcoholic beverages (liver)
- insulation materials :
    white asbestos (lung)
    brown asbestos
        (organ and body cavity membranes)
    blue asbestos, short-term exposure
        (organ and body cavity membranes)
- aromatic amines, ammonia derivitives in the chemical and rubber industries (urinary bladder)
- aflatoxins, in molds that contaminate stored grains, cassava, peanuts (liver)
- arsenic, a poisonous component of pesticides (various)
- creosote, a wood preservative (various)

SUSPECTED CARCINOGENS

- ceramic fibers
- chloroform
- DDT, an insecticide
- glasswool
- lead acetate
- lead phosphate
- progesterone
- diesel exhaust particulates
- trichloroethylene, found in adhesives, paint removers, and spot removers

---

For background information on carcinogen, see CACNER; MUTAGEN; *and* MUTATION. *Related material can be found in* AIDS; GENE; GENETICS; GROWTH HORMONE; LYMPHOMA; KAPOSI'S SARCOMA; METASTASIS; OCCUPATIONAL MEDICINE; RADIATION; TOBACCO SMOKING; *and* VIRUSES.

Resources on Carcinogens

Renneker, Mark, ed., *Understanding Cancer* (1988); Steen, R. Grant, *A Conspiracy of Cells: The Basic Science of Cancer* (1993); Steward, Clifford T., ed., *Cancer: Prevention, Detection, Causes, Treatment* (1988); American Cancer Society, Tel. (800) ACS-2345, Online: www.cancer.org; National Cancer Institue, Tel. (800) 4-CANCER, Online: www.nci.nih.gov; Nat. Alliance of Breast Cancer Organizations, Tel. (888) 80-NABCO, Online: www.nabco.org; www.nycornell.org/medicine/hematology/.html

Carcinoid Syndrome

Symptoms resulting from the excess production of hormones by a tumor.

A carcinoid is an abnormal growth within the lungs or the intestine that can cause overproduction of serotonin. Most carcinoids that produce serotonin are malignant tumors in the intestine. Serotonin is a neurotransmitter—a chemical that helps transmit nerve signals. In the brain, serotonin plays a role in mood. In the body, it causes blood vessels to constrict.

The most common symptom of carcinoid syndrome is an uncomfortable episode of flushing of the head and neck, often triggered by an emotional experience or ingestion of food or alcohol. Other symptoms include recurrent diarrhea, abdominal cramps, and wheezing.

The diagnosis can be confirmed by testing urine for 5-hydroxyindoleacetic acid, a breakdown product of serotonin. When surgical removal is not possible, drugs that prevent the formation or block the action of serotonin can provide some relief. *See* Blood *and* Lungs.

Carcinoma

Cancer originating in organ-lining tissue.

Carcinoma is the most common cancer, accounting for 80 to 90 percent of cases. It arises in epithelium, the tissue that forms the surface layer of organs, such as skin, the surface of glands, and the lining of the digestive tract. Most carcinomas arise in organs whose function is secretion, including the breast, whose glands produce milk, and in the lungs, whose epithelium secretes mucus. There are two subtypes of carcinoma: adenocarcinoma, which develops from a gland; and squamous cell carcinoma, which originates in the skin or lining of some body organs. Carcinoma is distinguished from sarcoma—cancer of connective tissue such as bones, tendons, and cartilage. *See also* Cancer; Digestive System; Epithelium; Sarcoma; *and* Skin.

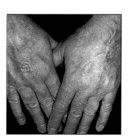
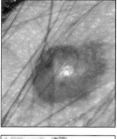
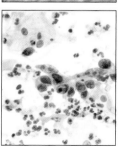

Carcinoma. Above top and middle, skin cancer can appear as a firm, red lump. Bottom, histological section showing cervical cancer specifically squamous cell carcinoma in the cervix. Tissue is stained with pap stain and magnified 200 times.

Carcinomatosis

Spread of carcinoma throughout the body.

Carcinomatosis is the result of metastasis, the process by which malignant cells spread from a tumor. It can occur with many kinds of carcinoma, with symptoms depending on the site or sites to which the cancer has spread. Cancer that spreads to the lungs can cause breathing difficulty and a persistent cough; cancer that spreads to the abdomen can result in jaundice and bloating. Weight loss and weakness are common.

Treatment. Removal of the original tumor generally will not affect the spread of cancer, unless that tumor produces a hormone that stimulates the growth of the metastases. Drug, radiation, or hormone therapy are often effective against secondary cancer that originates from the prostate, thyroid, or testis. Secondary cancers that originate from malignancies of the lung or intestines are more difficult to treat. The prognosis for carcinomatosis depends on the extent and location of the metastases. *See also* Cancer.

Cardiac Arrest

The sudden failure of the heart to pump blood.

Cardiac arrest is frequently caused by ventricular fibrillation, a severely irregular rhythm of the heart. Ventricular fibrillation is ousually brought on by a heart attack (myocardial infarction). Cardiac arrest can also be caused by asystole, which means the heart has ceased to beat. Cardiac arrest can be related to an underlying cardiovascular condition, such as cardiomyopathy, heart failure, or hypertension. It can also occur in people with severe burns, major injuries that result in the massive loss of blood, severe allergic reactions, drug overdoses, or electric shock. *See* Cardiovascular Disorders.

Symptoms. These are swift and devastating and include: failure to breathe, loss of consciousness, physical collapse, and absence of the normal pulse. Symptoms usually occur without warning, although the patient may have felt chest pain, shortness of breath, or severe fatigue in the days before cardiac arrest takes place.

Treatment. Emergency teams are trained in defibrillation—the delivery of a shock to the heart or administration of medication intended to start it beating properly again. In a hospital, more advanced techniques can be used, and drugs such as lidocaine can be given intravenously to stabilize the heartbeat.

Prognosis. When the heart stops beating quick treatment is necessary to prevent major damage to the brain can occur from lack of oxygen. Permanent damage can take place in as little as three minutes. Even with treatment, the outcome may not be favorable. About two-thirds of cardiac arrest patients die immediately, and the death rate for survivors in the year following the arrest is high. People at high risk of cardiac arrest should be on the alert for warning signs. For patients with serious arrhythmia affecting the ventricles, implantation of a defibrillator can reduce the risk of cardiac arrest. *See also* DEFIBRILLATION *and* MYOCARDIAL INFARCTION.

ALERT
In Case of Cardiac Arrest

If cardiac arrest occurs in a home or public place, emergency cardiopulmonary resuscitation must be administered to restore heart function or to maintain viability until more sophisticated measures and rescue personnel arrive. In CPR, the patient's airway is opened, and the person administering CPR breathes into the mouth while compressing the chest at regular intervals. Emergency medical help should be called while CPR is being performed.

Cardiac Output

The amount of blood pumped by the left ventricle, the chamber that pumps blood to most of the body.

Cardiac output is determined by measuring the heart rate and the amount of blood emitted with each beat. For healthy adults, cardiac output is about 5 quarts per minute at rest and as much as 32 quarts during exercise. Low output can indicate heart muscle damage or another condition requiring preventive measures or treatment. *See also* HEART *and* VENTRICLE.

Cardiac Stress Test

An exercise test carried out while the patient's heart is monitored.

The cardiac stress test is used to determine overall cardiovascular fitness and to diagnose and assess heart disorders. It can reveal cardiovascular ailments that may not be apparent while the patient is at rest.

During the test, the subject walks on a treadmill or rides a stationary bicycle. An electrocardiogram, or ECG, continuously monitors the heart rate, and blood pressure is recorded at even intervals. The pace of the exercise is increased until the patient's heart rate reaches 80 to 90 percent of maximum, or until acute shortness of breath or chest pain stops the test. A simultaneous nuclear scan and echocardiogram may be done.

In addition to diagnosing cardiac or lung ailments, a stress test may be given to establish a baseline for an exercise program or insurance purposes. *See also* ECG; FITNESS; HEART*; and* INSURANCE .

Cardiology

The study of the function of the heart and its related blood vessels, and the diagnosis and treatment of disorders affecting them.

Because cardiovascular disorders, including stroke, are the leading causes of death in the United States, family physicians are familiar with basic cardiology and conditions affecting the heart, such as atherosclerosis and hypertension. Many patients with serious conditions, however, such as arrhythmia, congestive heart failure, cardiomyopathy, and heart valve abnormalities, must be referred to a cardiologist or to a cardiovascular surgeon for corrective treatment. *See also* CARDIOVASCULAR DISORDERS; CIRCULATORY SYSTEM; *and* HEART,

Resources on Cardiology
Berne, Robert M., et al., *Cardiovascular Physiology* (2001); Debakey, Michael E. and Antonio M. Gotto, *The New Living Heart* (1997); Gould, Lance K., *Heal Your Heart: How You Can Prevent or Reverse Heart Disease* (2000); Neill, Catherine A., *The Heart of a Child: What Families Need to Know About Heart Disorders in Children* (1992); American Heart Association, Tel. (800) 242-8721, Online: www.amhrt.org; Heart Information Network, Tel. (973) 701-6035, Online: www.heart-info.org; National Heart, Lung, and Blood Institute, Tel. (301) 496-4236, Online: www.nhlbi.nih. gov; www.nycornell.org/ cardiothoracic.surgery/ www.nycornell.org/medi-cine/cardiology/html

Cardiomegaly

Also known as an enlarged heart

Abnormal enlargement of the heart.

Cardiomegaly can take the form of hypertrophy, thickening of the heart muscle, or dilation, in which one or more chambers of the heart widen as their tissue is weakened. Hypertrophy occurs when the heart must regularly work harder than normal. This may be caused by a condition such as high blood pressure (hypertension), in which more pressure is needed to push blood out to the body. Hypertrophy can affect the left ventricle, which pumps blood to most of the body, or, if there is high blood pressure in the lungs (pulmonary hypertension) or the right ventricle, which pumps blood to the lung. Dilation can be caused by an abnormality of a heart valve that reduces the efficiency with which blood is pumped.

Symptoms. Cardiomegaly often causes few symptoms until the activity of the heart is seriously impaired. Symptoms include breathlessness and swelling of the feet.

Diagnosis. Cardiomegaly is diagnosed by a physical examination and tests such as a chest x-ray, electrocardiogram and echocardiogram.

Treatment. Cardiomegaly is usually treated by drugs to manage the underlying condition that causes it. Surgery may be needed to repair a valve abnormality. *See also* BLOOD; HEART; *and* HYPERTENSION.

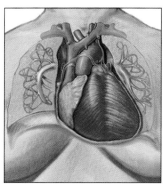

Cardiomegaly. The left ventricle is enlarged due to high blood pressure, This condition makes blood out of the heart more difficult.

Cardiomyopathy

Any degenerative disease of the heart muscle (myocardium).

There are three major types of cardiomyopathy: dilated, hypertrophic, and restrictive. The causes of most cases of cardiomyopathy is unknown.

Dilated Cardiomyopathy. This is the most common form. The walls of the heart balloon out, and the heart muscle cannot pump blood adequately. The result can be inability to meet the body's need for oxygen-carrying blood (congestive heart failure); disturbance of the normal pace of the heartbeat (arrhythmia); or inability of the heart valves to close properly, causing a heart murmur. The risk of a blood clot that can block an artery and cause a heart attack

---

The Options Available

Patients with cardiomyopathy are often told to limit stressful activities. Drug treatment of dilated cardiomyopathy is aimed at improving heart function, with medications such as digitalis, lanoxin, diuretics, or ACE inhibitors. Some patients may require an implanted pacemaker or defibrillator. Hypertrophic cardiomegaly is treated with beta-blockers, calcium channel blockers or, if necessary, antiarrhythmic drugs. Surgery may be performed to remove excess heart tissue that obstructs the flow of blood within the heart. Restrictive cardiomyopathy is treated with diuretics to relieve symptoms. In severe cases, a heart transplant may be necessary.

---

or stroke is increased. Some patients may develop rapid or slow heartbeats. Symptoms can include palpitations, fatigue, fainting, and sudden death.

Hypertrophic Cardiomyopathy. This the second most common form; it is an abnormal enlargement of the heart. It often affects the left ventricle, which pumps blood to most of the body. A heart valve may become damaged or an arrhythmia may develop. Symptoms include chest pain, dizziness, and shortness of breath, or even fainting during physical exertion.

Restrictive Cardiomyopathy. This causes the heart muscle to become rigid and lose the ability to pump blood. The most common cause is amyloidosis, a condition in which an abnormal protein material is deposited in heart tissue. Symptoms include fatigue, difficulty breathing during physical activity, and swelling of the arms and legs.

Background information on cardiomyopathy can be found in CIRCULATORY SYSTEM *and* HEART. *For further material, see* ARRHYTHMIA; HEART FAILURE; THROMBOSIS; *and* VENTRICLE. *See also* ACE INHIBITOR DRUGS; BETA BLOCKER DRUGS; CALCIUM CHANNEL BLOCKERS; DEFIBRILLATION; DIGITALIS; *and* PACEMAKER *for more on treatment options.*

Cardiopulmonary Resuscitation (CPR)

An emergency method used to restart the heart and initiate breathing when a person's pulse has stopped (cardiac arrest).

Cardiopulmonary resuscitation combines cardiac compression to restart or maintain the heartbeat and if possible mouth to mouth resuscitation to supplement or enhance ventilation and oxygen delivery to the lungs. When the heart stops beating its pumping action ceases and, oxygen-rich blood fails to reach the brain. This can result in permanent brain damage after only three or four minutes and death after eight to ten minutes. It is therefore crucial to begin CPR as quickly as possible.

Ideally, a person performing cardiopulmonary resuscitation should be formally trained. You can locate the nearest CPR class in your area by contacting your local chapter of the American Heart Association or the American Red Cross. Mouth-to-mouth resuscitation can be successfully administered by an untrained individual, but the most effective method of restoring circulation is cardiac compression massage performed by a trained individual. The instructions included here are **not** a substitute for classroom training.

How to Perform CPR

First, it is important to verify that the victim has indeed suffered cardiac arrest and is not merely unconscious. Look in the victim's mouth to make sure that no food or foreign material is obstructing the airway, then with your ear over the victims mouth and nostrils listen for signs of breathing. If a spinal injury is suspected, do not move the head or neck, as that may worsen the injury.

Immediately call for emergency medical help. Have a person not performing CPR make the call. If you are alone, call before starting CPR.

Remember to be gentle when applying pressure to the chest, particularly with children. Be sure to press straight down; do not

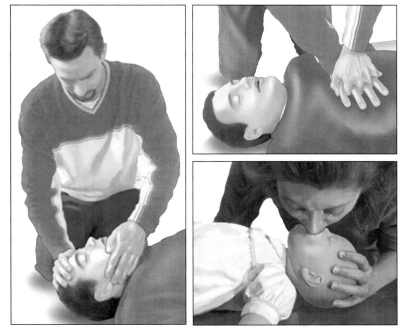

rock. Count the compressions so that they are evenly spaced.If the victim vomits while CPR is being administered, roll him over to his left side until he is finished. Clear the air passages, and resume CPR if there is still no heartbeat or breathing.

Adults

- Place the person on his back, tilt the head back, and lift the chin.
- Pinch the nose and make an airtight mouth to mouth seal. Give two full breaths. The victim's chest will rise if he is getting enough air.
- If there is no response or pulse, begin chest compressions at about 100 per minute, with two breaths given after every 15 compressions. Place one hand on top of the other and position the hands about two finger-widths above the lowest part of the person's breast bone. Press straight down, about one and one-half to two inches. and release.
- Continue until help arrives, or breathing and pulse begin again, or your fatigue becomes overwhelming.

Children Ages One to Eight

- Place the child on his back, tilt the head back, and lift the chin.

Performing CPR.
Above left, first check for breathing. Right, top, apply chest compressions. Bottom, apply mouth to mouth resuscitation.

- Pinch the nose and make an airtight mouth to mouth seal. Give two full breaths. The victim's chest will rise if he is getting enough air.
- If there is no pulse, begin chest compressions at a rate of 100 per minute. Place the heel of the hand about two finger-widths above the lowest part of the child's breastbone. Press gently straight down about one to one and one-half inches and then release. After every five compressions, give one breath.
- Continue until help arrives, breathing and pulse begin again, or your fatigue becomes overwhelming.

INFANTS

- Place the infant on his back across your knees, tilt the head back, and lift the chin.
- Create a seal over the mouth and nose of the victim. Give two small puffs. The child's chest will rise if he is getting enough air.
- If there is no pulse, begin quick chest compressions at a rate of 100-120 per minute; after every five compressions give one puff of breath. Place two fin gers in the middle of the breastbone, between the nipples. Press gently straight down about a one-half inch to one inch and release.
- Continue until help arrives, breathing and pulse begin again, or your fatigue becomes overwhelming.

Performing CPR on an Infant. First, check the breathing of the infant. Then create a seal over the mouth and nose and give two small puffs (right) . Afterwards, begin quick chest compressions.

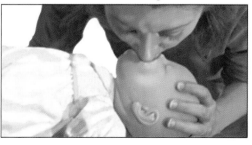

For background material on cardiopulmonary resuscitation, see ANOXIA; ARTIFICIAL RESPIRATION; CHOKING; HEART RATE; and HEIMLICH MANEUVER. Further information can be found in EMERGENCY FIRST STEPS and FIRST AID. See also HEART ATTACK.

Cardiovascular Disorders

Disorders of the heart and blood vessels.

Heart disorders are the most common cause of death in the United States and in other industrialized nations.

Disorders that impair blood flow include the major causes of death, such as heart attacks (myocardial infarction). Underlying most of these conditions is deterioration of blood flow through the coronary arteries, which supply blood to the heart muscle. Over time, the coronary arteries can become narrowed and less flexible because of a buildup of fatty deposits in the artery walls (atherosclerosis). As all or part of the heart muscle is deprived of its normal blood supply, it must work harder to maintain blood flow to the rest of the body.

One result can be congestive heart failure, in which the heart cannot supply enough blood to the body. Another can be angina pectoris, pain that occurs at first during exertion and later even at rest. The heart can experience a disturbance of its normal rhythm (arrhythmia), which in extreme cases can lead to a complete loss of rhythm (fibrillation). Also, an artery can become blocked, causing myocardial infarction, the death of part of the heart tissue, which can result in sudden death.

Congenital Disorders. These consist of abnormalities in the structure of the heart or its major blood vessels that are present from birth. They include septal defects, "holes in the heart," and malformations of the heart valves such as stenosis or prolapse.

Infection. A bacterial, fungal, or viral infection can cause inflammation of the tissue lining the inside of the heart muscle (endocarditis) and often damage the heart valves. The result can be conditions including mitral insufficiency, in which the mitral valve does not close properly, and mitral stenosis, narrowing of the valve opening .

Muscle Disorders. Cardiomyopathies result in a weakening of the heart muscle and reduced blood flow. They can be due to a congenital condition, a vitamin deficiency, overconsumption of alcohol, or an infection. Myocarditis is inflammation of the heart muscle as a result of infection, certain drugs, or radiation therapy.

Injuries. Many highway fatalities are caused by blunt injuries to the heart, as in auto accidents. Mild compression can bruise the heart, but a severe impact may result in fatal rupture of the heart muscle. Seat belts and air bags have reduced the incidence of these injuries. There is no similar protection against a stab or bullet wound to the heart, which can be fatal unless treatment is given within minutes.

Nutritional Disorders. The most common nutritional disorder affecting the heart is obesity, which leads to high blood pressure, atherosclerosis, and an excessive demand on the heart's pumping ability. A diet low in fat and cholesterol and high in fibers, fruit, and vegetables can slow the progression of atherosclerosis.

Beriberi is a deficiency of vitamin B_1 leading to heart failure. While most Americans get enough vitamin B_1 in their diets, it still is a major problem for alcoholics.

Alcohol. Alcoholism can cause cardiomyopathy, which is reversible if the intake of alcohol is ended. Drinking heavily at a single sitting can cause the heart to swell, weaken, and ultimately fail.

Drugs. Some anticancer and heart disease drugs, as well as tricyclic antidepressants, can potentially permanently damage the heart.

DISORDERS OF VEINS

Thrombosis. The most common disorder of the veins is venous thrombosis, formation of blood clots in the veins. A blood clot (thrombus) that forms in the deep veins of the legs or the abdomen can break away and float to the lungs, where the blockage it causes can be life-threatening. Thrombosis can also lead to chronic venous insufficiency, in which a blood clot blocks a vessel in a leg and causes swelling and discoloration.

Phlebitis. This is a painful inflammation of the veins close to the surface of the legs, which can be caused by infection or injury and increases the risk of thrombosis.

Raynaud's Phenomenon

Raynaud's phenomenon is an excessive constriction of the small arteries of the fingers and toes that is triggered by exposure to cold weather or a number of other factors, such as smoking or emotional stress. It is caused by a number of primary diseases: arterial diseases (Buerger's disease, atherosclerosis, embolism, and thrombosis), connective tissue diseases (rheumatoid arthritis, scleroderma, and lupus erythematosus), the drugs ergotamine and methysergide, and beta-blockers. It is also found among people who use pneumatic drills, chain saws, or other vibrating machinery, and among pianists, typists, and others who subject their fingers to heavy, repetitive use.

Varicose Veins. These result in swelling and distortion of the blood vessels. Varicosity usually occurs in veins just below the skin of the leg, but they can also affect veins of the anus, esophagus, and scrotum.

DISORDERS OF ARTERIES

Arteriosclerosis. This thickening and loss of elasticity of the artery walls is most often caused by atherosclerosis. The buildup of plaque or the formation of blood clots can reduce blood flow. In the legs this can produce pain called intermittent claudication. Complete blockage of a heart artery can cause a heart attack. Blockage of a brain artery can result in a stroke.

Atherosclerosis. This is a buildup of fat deposits that cause artery walls to thicken. It is the most common artery disease and can occur in the legs (peripheral vascular disease), heart (coronary heart disease), and brain (cerebrovascular disease). Severely restricted blood flow in the arteries to the heart muscle leads to symptoms such as chest pain.

Arteritis. An inflammation of the arterial wall can block blood flow. It can occur in the scalp (temporal arteritis) or in the limbs (Buerger's disease, which occurs mostly in male cigarette smokers).

Aneurysm. Congenital defects or atherosclerosis may cause artery walls to thin and swell, forming an aneurysm.

Hypertension. High blood pressure can cause arteries to thicken and narrow, increasing a person's susceptibility to heart disease, stroke, and kidney failure.

Thrombosis. Arteries, like veins, may also be susceptible to clotting. *See also* ALCOHOLISM; BLOOD; *and* HEART.

Resources on Cardiovascular Disorders
Debakey, Michael E. and Antonio M. Gotto, *The New Living Heart* (1997); Gotto, Antonio, *A Patient's Handbook of Cholesterol Disorders* (2000); Gould, Lance K., *Heal Your Heart: How You Can Prevent or Reverse Heart Disease* (2000); Neill, Catherine A., *The Heart of a Child: What Families Need to Know About Heart Disorders in Children* (1992); American Heart Association, Tel. (800) 242-8721, Online: www.amhrt.org; Heart Information Network, Tel. (973) 701-6035, Online: www.heart-info.org; www.nycornell.org/cardiothoracic.surgery/ www.nycornell.org/medicine/cardiology/html.

Carditis

Inflammation of any part of the heart muscle or the tissue that lines it.

Inflammation of the heart muscle (myocarditis) usually results from infection by a virus. Inflammation of the lining of the chambers of the heart and the heart valves, called endocarditis, usually results from a bacterial infection.

Inflammation of the outer lining of the heart is called pericarditis and can result from a bacterial infection; a viral infection, or a heart attack (myocardial infarction); or other systemic illnesses like lupus. Pericarditis is sometimes caused by an autoimmune disease, such as systemic lupus erythematosus or rheumatoid arthritis. Carditis often occurs very transiently in patients with Lyme disease, an infection caused by a spirochete, a microbe transmitted by the bite of ticks.

Symptoms of carditis include shortness of breath, fatigue, fever, chills, and chest pain that may mimic that of a heart attack; and a number of other discomforts, including fever, chills, and breathlessness.

Treatment of endocarditis starts with antibiotic medication to attack the underlying infection. Pericarditis is treated with anti-inflammatory drugs and occasionally antimicrobial agents as well. Severe cases may require other medications to stabilize the function of the heart and prevent major complications. *See also* HEART ATTACK *and* LYME DISEASE.

Caries, Dental

Medical term for tooth decay.

Dental caries begin when bacteria in plaque eat away at the outer layer (enamel or cementum) of a tooth. Normally, these layers are strong enough to withstand invasion, but when the residue of built up food (plaque) remains on the teeth, it gives the bacteria a chance to work more steadily.

Tooth decay may start as a small spot on a tooth. Left untreated, it can destroy teeth, gums, and even the bone around the teeth. The bacteria work their way into the tooth and into the pulp. The further the bacteria go, the more damage is done.

Early stage caries often go unnoticed. As the tooth deteriorates, it becomes increasingly sensitive to sweet, hot, or cold food. Removing the decayed area and filling the cavity is the usual form of treatment. For severe cases, removal of the tooth pulp (root-canal treatment) or the tooth itself (dental extraction) is necessary.

People can prevent caries by reducing the amount of sugar and other refined carbohydrates in their diet. The next step is proper oral hygiene. The fluoride in toothpaste and flouridated water strengthens enamel. *See also* EXTRACTION, DENTAL; FILLING, DENTAL; ORAL HYGIENE; PLAQUE; *and* ROOT-CANAL TREATMENT.

Carotene

Any of a number of organic compounds some of which are converted in the liver into vitamin A.

Carotene is a family of plant pigments, of which beta carotene is one of about 500. Approximately 10 percent of carotenoids (retinoids) are converted into vitamin A by the body. Beta carotene is one of these, and is found in foods such as carrots, apricots, squash, sweet potatoes, and leafy green vegetables. Increased consumption of these foods has been linked to the prevention of cancer and other illnesses through their antioxidant effects. As antioxidants, carotenes prevent cell damage from oxidation, a process that make cells more sensitive to cancer-producing agents. Phytochemicals in the plant sources are also thought to have disease-fighting properties.

It is possible to overdose on vitamin A supplements if the amounts are too high. While not toxic in excessive quantities as is vitamin A, carotenes if eaten in abundance will result in temporary yellowing of the skin. There is some concern that carotenes consumed in large amounts in supplements by heavy smokers may increase the risk of lung cancer. *See also* VITAMIN A.

Carotid Arteries

The two main arteries that carry blood to the neck and head.

There are two common carotid arteries, right and left, which originate from or near the aorta, the main artery leading from the heart. Each of the common carotid arteries divides into two branches, one internal and one external. *See* AORTA *and* NECK.

The left common carotid artery runs from the aorta, above the heart, up the neck on the left of the windpipe (trachea),

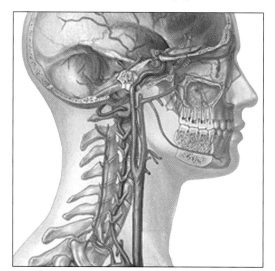

then divides into the left internal and external carotid arteries just above the larynx.

The right common carotid artery originates at the subclavian artery, which branches from the aorta soon after it leaves the heart, and divides into the right internal and left external carotid arteries on the level with the left common carotid artery.

The internal and external carotids supply different parts of the head and neck. The internal carotids carry blood to the brain and eye through a series of progressively smaller branches. The external carotids carry blood to the scalp, face, mouth, and jaws. Two sensory regions in the neck, the carotid sinus and the carotid body, monitor the pressure and oxygen content of the blood vessels to ensure an adequate supply of oxygen to the neck and head.

Carpal Tunnel Syndrome

Numbness or tingling in the thumb, index, and middle fingers, often accompanied by pain of the hand, wrist, and arm.

Carpal tunnel syndrome is a condition in which the median nerve, the main nerve that supplies sensation to the thumb and adjacent two fingers, is compressed where it passes through the wrist. As a result, the area supplied by the nerve becomes numb and at times painful. Carpal tunnel syndrome can affect one or both hands.

Causes. The median nerve and the flexor tendons, which are vital for fine movement of the fingers, enter the hand through a gap in the wrist known as the carpal tunnel. If the flexor tendons become inflamed, the substance covering the tendon (tenosynovium) swells. This put pressure on surrounding issues. The bones and ligaments cannot stretch, due to a lack of space, and the median nerve is pressed against the carpal ligament. The nerve can no longer function, and the hand becomes painful and numb.

Swelling of the flexor tendons occurs most commonly as a result of repeated stress on the hands and wrist, such as occurs in typing or operating hand-held power machinery (which causes the hands to vibrate).

Treatment. A brace may be worn at night to keep the wrist in a neutral position and alleviate the discomfort. Anti-inflammatory drugs such as ibuprofen and aspirin may control the swelling. If the condition is more serious, a physician may prescribe injections of corticosteroids. In extreme cases, the carpal ligament may be surgically disconnected in order to reduce pressure on the nerve.

Prevention. The likelihood of developing carpal tunnel syndrome is reduced when repetitive stress on the hands and wrists are minimized. For example, wrist supports should be used when typing, and vibration-absorbing gloves should be worn for operating power machinery. *See also* BRACE; MEDIAN NERVE; *and* OVERUSE INJURY.

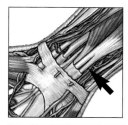

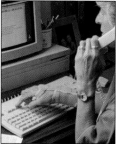

Carotid artery. Left, the artery that carries blood from the aorta to the brain.
Carpal Tunnel Syndrome. Above, if the flexor tendons become inflamed, the substance covering the tendon swells and carpal tunnel syndrome occurs, causing numbness in the hand, wrist, and arm. Many computer users use a brace on their wrists to offset the effects of carpal tunnel syndrome.

Carrier

A person or animal infected with a disease, who transmits it to others but exhibits no symptoms.

A carrier may have no or very mild symptoms of disease. The most famous case of a carrier was Typhoid Mary, a woman who lived shortly after the turn of the twentieth century and who was discovered to have infected with typhoid a number of families with whom she worked as a cook. Today about three percent of people infected with *Salmonella typhi*, the bacteria that causes typhoid fever, have no symptoms of typhoid but continue to eliminate the bacteria in their stools for a year or more. *See also* BACTERIOLOGY *and* TYPHOID FEVER.

Cast

Casing designed to hold a body part in place so that a broken bone or dislocated joint will heal in the correct position.

Casts are rigid, usually made of plaster of Paris, though some are now made of lighter materials such as fiberglass. *See also* DISLOCATION *and* FRACTURE.

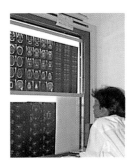

Cast. Above this plaster cast is holding an ankle in place for proper healing.

CAT Scan

Acronym for computerized axial tomography, also known as CT (computed tomography) scan

An x-ray imaging technique that uses computers to compose a detailed cross-sectional view of part of the body.

CAT scanning is a high-resolution imaging technique that, along with Magnetic Resonance Imaging (MRI) and ultrasound, has revolutionized noninvasive visualization of the body. CAT is a rapid and painless procedure during which a bodily area is scanned by a computerized x-ray device, resulting in a detailed, three-dimensional (3-D) image.

CAT scans are often used to study the brain, chest, and abdomen. Treatment for a range of disorders may also be monitored using this technique.

The CAT scan works on the same basic principle as conventional x-ray the differ-

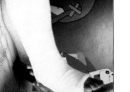

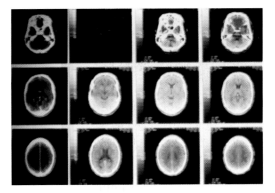

CAT scan. Above and above right, CAT scans are often used to study the brain, chest, and abdomen.

ential absorption of x-rays resulting from the varying density of body tissue. The impressive sensitivity and detail of the CAT scan however, far outweigh conventional x-ray, providing a thousandfold increase in resolution, and identifying lesions less than two millimeters in diameter.

The Technique. The CAT-scanning machine consists of a donut shaped x-ray apparatus and a moveable table on which the patient lies. Transverse sections of tissue are swept with a very fine radiographic beam. Opposite the beam is a detector that records unabsorbed x-rays passing through the body. The entire apparatus rotates about the area being imaged, collecting x-ray data. Unlike conventional x-ray film, which acquires a flat image from a single scan, CAT scan acquires many projections around the body to compose a 3-D representation of the body's anatomy, which most often is viewed as individual "slices," or tomograms.

The table slides the patient under the scanning apparatus for 10 to 15 minutes (though a 3-D image can be created in under a minute). Often, a contrast "dye" will be injected prior to the CAT scan to clarify or enhance the image. Fasting for several hours is required should a "dye" be used, and some nausea may be experienced as a result.

For background information on CAT scan, see IMAGING TECHNIQUES. Further material can be found in DIAGNOSTICS; MRI; PET SCAN; RADIONUCLIDE SCAN; RADIOPAQUE; *and* X-RAY. See also ABDOMEN; BRAIN; *and* CHEST X-RAY for more on areas of the body that might be subjected to a CAT scan.

Catalepsy

A condition usually associated with schizophrenia in which the muscles of the face, arms, and legs become rigid.

Catalepsy is a condition in which an individual maintains a facial expression or a bodily position for a prolonged interval. It is characterized by a loss of consciousness, paralysis of parts of the body, and a lack of response to external stimuli. The person's expression or body position will not change no matter how uncomfortable the position may appear to be. Breathing slows to an abnormally low rate. Efforts to alter the individual's pose are met with resistance. A cataleptic person can remain in a trance-like state for as long as several hours or even days.

Catalepsy is most often seen in people with schizophrenia, epilepsy, and brain tumors. It may also be a side effect of certain drugs. A cataleptic condition can be induced by hypnosis. *See also* BRAIN TUMORS; EPILEPSY; HYPNOSIS; *and* SCHIZOPHRENIA.

Cataplexy

A loss of muscular power and control without a loss of consciousness.

Cataplexy is an attack in which an individual may become temporarily paralyzed. The episode of muscular limpness may last only a few seconds. It can be triggered by an emotional response, such as fear, anger, joy, or laughter. Often the individual may fall to the ground or drop what is in his or her hand. Speech becomes slurred and eyesight impaired, but hearing and awareness remain intact.

Cataplexy occurs in individuals with sleep disorders such as narcolepsy, in which a person tends to fall asleep suddenly in the course of the day.

The cause of cataplexy is not known. Research has suggested that cataplexy and related disorders may run in families, indicating that there may exist a genetic predisposition to the condition. *See* NARCOLEPSY.

Cataract Surgery

Surgical removal and replacement of a clouded lens (cataract) from the eye, to restore vision.

The lens is the part of the eye that focuses light. To produce a sharp image, the lens must be clear. The changing of proteins in the lens causes the lens to become cloudy, creating a cataract and leading to blurriness, glare, and other vision problems. Often cataracts develop with age, although they may also be present at birth (congenital cataracts) or develop as a result of injury or complications from other health problems.

Cataract surgery may be recommended when impaired vision begins to interfere with quality of life. About seven percent of people ages 45 to 64 have cataracts that require surgery, while 45 percent of people over 75 years old do. About 1.5 million cataract operations are performed in the United States every year.

Cataract surgery is not an emergency procedure; the patient can wait until he or she feels it is necessary. However, the lens may be easier and safer to remove when the cataract is immature. It was previously thought that cataracts had to develop a hard nucleus (ripen) before surgery was possible; with current techniques, however, waiting is not necessary.

PROCEDURE

The specific techniques used by different surgeons can vary greatly, and it is advisable to explore the various options before having the surgery. The basic outline of the procedure is the same for the various techniques currently practiced.

Cataract surgery is almost always done on an outpatient basis. Before surgery, the eye is examined for its length and curvature, to determine the shape of the replacement lens. The patient is then given a local anesthetic, either through injection or eyedrops, and a sedative, in order to make the procedure painless and to keep the patient relaxed. In almost all cases, general anesthesia is not needed. An incision

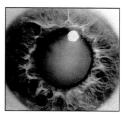

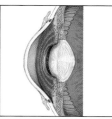

Cataract. Top, a close-up of an eye with cataracts. This condition makes it impossible to focus light. Bottom, a cross section of an eye with cataracts; surgery is the only way to reverse this condition.

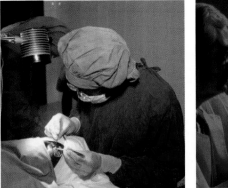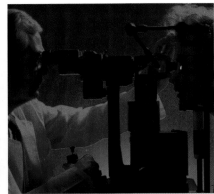

Cataract Surgery. .
Left, the outermembrane of the eye is cut and the defective lens is removed. Right, cataracts are also now being removed with lasers as opposed to more conventional surgical incisions.

Resources on Cataract Surgery
Davson, Hugh, ed., *The Eye* (1984); King, John Harry and Joseph A.C. Wadsworth, eds., *An Atlas of Ophthalmic Surgery* (1970); Vaughan, Daniel, et al., *General Ophthalmology* (1995); Wolf, K.P., *Eyewise: Eye Disorders and Their Treatment* (1982); American Council of the Blind, Tel. (800) 424-8666, Online: www.acb.org; American Foundation for the Blind, Tel. (800) 232-5463, Online: www.afb.org; www.nycornell.org/op/.

is cut in the outer membrane of the eye (the cornea) and the lens is removed. In most cases, an artificial lens is inserted into the eye through the incision and anchored in place. If necessary, the incision is stitched. The procedure takes between 12 minutes and an hour, and the patient can be discharged that day.

TECHNIQUES OF LENS REMOVAL

The two primary ways used to remove a cataract are extracapsular surgery, a more traditional form of surgery, and phacoemulsification, which involves dissolving the lens before removing it.

Extracapsular Surgery. This is the traditional form of cataract surgery. The ophthalmologist makes a semicircular incision, from a third of an inch to half an inch long, around the edge of the upper part of the cornea around.

The lens is removed from its surrounding lens capsule using surgical tools, and remaining soft parts of the lens are sucked out (aspirated). A gel (sodium hyaluronate) is injected to maintain the spacing in the lens capsule until the artificial replacement lens is dropped in. Plastic loops in the lens anchor it in place. The incision is then stitched up.

Phacoemulsification. A more recently developed method, phacoemulsification uses a much smaller incision, usually only an eighth of an inch long, but can remove larger cataracts. The surgeon probes the cataract with a hollow needle that vibrates at 40,000 times per second. This ultrasound vibration causes the lens to dissolve

(emulsify). It is aspirated through the needle while fluid is simultaneously injected to keep the space open. The artificial lens, which can be folded to fit through the tiny incision, is then inserted into the lens capsule. Depending on the size of the incision, no stitches or one stitch may be needed.

RECOVERY

The patient, with a bandage or eye shield, is encouraged to resume normal activities in a few days. Full recovery generally takes four to six weeks. The eye stabilizes fully in six to twelve weeks, after which corrective lenses can be prescribed.

Complications are very rare; cataract surgery is one of the safest surgical procedures. However, as with any surgery, infection or bleeding may occur. Other complications may include drooping eyelid, damage or dislocation of the artificial lens, high pressure in the eye, retinal detachment, swelling or clouding of the cornea, and loss of vision.

PROGNOSIS

In about 98 percent of cases, surgery is successful; in 90 percent of cases vision improves to 20/40 or better, with or without glasses. The artificial lens can correct nearsightedness or farsightedness, as well as astigmatism, which was not previously correctable by this kind of surgery.

Once removed, a cataract cannot return. However, within a year, approximately half of people with cataract surgery develop a recurrence of symptoms because the lens capsule becomes cloudy.

This can be corrected with a procedure known as YAG capsulotomy, in which an ophthalmologist makes a tiny hole in the capsule with a laser beam. This procedure is painless, does not require a hospital stay, and rarely develops complications. However, it is of sufficient risk that it should not be performed as a preventive measure.

Background material on cataract surgery can be found in EYE, DISORDERS OF *and* SURGERY. *For further information, see* BLINDNESS; CORNEA, DISORDERS OF; EYE; EYE, EXAMINATION OF; GLAUCOMA; LENS; *and* VISION, LOSS OF.

Catastrophic Health Insurance

Also known as major medical insurance

A health insurance policy with an extremely high deductible that covers all costs above the deductible.

Catastrophic health insurance is an insurance policy that has a high deductible and covers health care expenditures in excess of a predetermined level, often thousands of dollars or more. Individuals pay all the costs for a medical service up to the level of the deductible. In some cases catastrophic insurance covers only some medical expenses, such as treatment and hospitalization for specific serious illnesses.

Policy holders sometimes supplement basic medical insurance with catastrophic insurance, which are used to cover costs if the policy holder exhausts the basic coverage. *See also* ACCESS TO CARE; ACCIDENTS; EMERGENCY HOSPITALIZATION; *and* HEALTH INSURANCE.

Catheter

A surgical tube, usually flexible, used either to drain fluid from a cavity or organ or to inject fluid into the body.

The most common type of catheter is the Foley catheter, which is inserted through the urethra into the bladder to drain urine. Other types of catheters are used in heart operations (such as in angioplasty and valvuloplasty); in hemodialysis and peritoneal dialysis; to sample blood from the heart; to inject radioactive dye into the blood system during x-ray screening; and to provide intravenous fluids and nutrition. Catheters are also used to perform liver biopsies. *See also* BALLOON CATHETER *and* CATHETERIZATION.

Catheterization

The insertion of a thin, hollow tube into the body to remove or inject fluid.

The two most common types of catheterization are cardiac and urinary catheterization, which, respectively, help diagnose heart disease and allow drainage of urine.

CARDIAC CATHETERIZATION

In cardiac catheterization, a catheter is inserted into the heart to obtain information about its anatomy and function.

The procedure is done under local anesthesia and usually requires an overnight hospital stay. The catheter is inserted into a blood vessel in the leg near the groin or in the arm and threaded through the blood vessel into the heart. The catheter can be used to measure blood pressure in the heart and nearby blood vessels. A contrast dye may be injected to make x-ray images of the heart. Instruments may also be inserted to obtain a sample of heart tissue for diagnosis of specific disorders.

Cardiac catheterization carries a small risk of damaging the blood vessel at the point of insertion, disturbing heart rhythm, or causing a potentially fatal blockage of an artery near the heart. It is performed, however, to diagnose life-threatening disorders and produces invaluable information about the heart's condition.

URINARY CATHETERIZATION

A urinary catheterization involves the insertion of a hollow tube into the bladder to drain urine. This procedure may be done to test bladder function during surgery, to monitor urine production, or for persons who cannot empty their bladder normally. It does not require anesthesia and can be done in minutes. The end of the urethra is cleaned with an antiseptic solution and the catheter is passed up the urethra to the bladder. If the catheter cannot reach the bladder through the urethra, it can be inserted through the abdominal wall. Some patients with chronic urinary problems may require permanent catheterization.

For background information on catheterization, *see* DIAGNOSIS *and* SURGERY. *Related material can be found in* ANESTHESIA, LOCAL; ARRHYTHMIA; BLOOD PRESSURE; HEART ATTACK; HEART, DISORDERS OF; HEART FAILURE; INCONTINENCE, URINARY; *and* X-RAY.

Cats, Diseases from

Diseases contracted from contact with a cat.

Although many feline diseases cannot be transmitted to humans, there are health risks posed by interaction with cats. Cats can transmit certain parasites, viruses, and bacteria to humans and may trigger an allergic response in some individuals.

MODES OF TRANSMISSION

Transmission of disease can occur through the air, from physical contact, and from injuries as a result of contact with the cat.

Through the Air. The most common health risk from cats is an allergic response to cat dander. Studies show that nearly 20 percent of people who are exposed to animals develop an allergy; fewer than half of those allergies involve asthma. Fleas and other parasites may pass from a cat to a human being. Cats are also susceptible to the fungus that causes ringworm, an infection of the skin that is highly contagious to humans but may produce no symptoms in cats. Some studies estimate that almost 40 percent of cats are infected with ringworm.

Physical Contact. Contact with feline waste products also carries certain health risks. Toxoplasmosis, a parasitic disease picked up from the feces of infected cats, causes cold-like symptoms in most people; but it can produce severe complications in pregnant women and people with compromised immune systems. Salmonella, which can cause illness in humans, may be present in cat feces.

Scratches and Bites. Deep lacerations allow dirt and bacteria to penetrate below the skin. Tetanus, rabies, and even strep throat may result from injuries inflicted by cats. In addition, nearly 60 percent of cats have the bacteria *Pasteurella* in their mouths, which may infect bite wounds.

Cat-Scratch Fever. This is a bacterial infection (*Bartonella henselae*) that develops from a scratch or bite of a cat or dog and occasionally from fleas. It forms a crusted blister on the skin and causes swelling and tenderness of nearby lymph nodes. The victim may have a low-grade fever and experience flu-like symptoms. In extreme cases the victim may develop high fever, pneumonia, tonsillitis, encephalitis, or hepatitis, but this usually only occurs in people with compromised immune systems. Usually cat-scratch fever is self-limiting and mild. It is treated with pain relievers and hot compresses; antibiotics may be prescribed to destroy the bacteria.

PREVENTION

Both cats and humans should receive all routine vaccinations, and humans should receive vaccinations for diseases such as tetanus and rabies . Owners should try to avoid serious scratches or bites. After handling a cat, hands should be washed with soap and water. In case of a bite or a scratch, the wound should also be carefully cleaned. If the wound is serious or if the person is at risk for infection, a doctor should be consulted. Individuals, especially those at high risk for toxoplasmosis, should avoid contact with cat feces. Most bacterial infections that result from contact with a cat can be treated with antibiotics.

Factors That Increase Risk

Pregnant women who contract certain diseases transmitted by cats, such as toxoplasmosis, can suffer a miscarriage; or the fetus can develop serious disorders of the brain, heart, lungs, eyes, or liver. Individuals with diabetes or arteriosclerosis must monitor wounds from scratches or bites carefully, as there is a risk of serious infection. The individuals at greatest risk, however, are those with compromised immune systems, such as those infected with HIV or who are undergoing chemotherapy. Cats can infect immunodeficient individuals with cryptosporidiosis, toxoplasmosis, *Mycobacterium avium* complex, and other diseases. People with normal immune systems may resist infection or develop only mild symptoms from these diseases, but immunodeficient individuals may develop severe diarrhea, brain infections, and skin lesions.

For background information, see ALLERGY *and* RINGWORM. *Further material can be found in* ANTIBIOTIC DRUGS; BACTERIA; DOGS, DISEASES FROM; PARASITE; RABIES; SALMONELLA; TETANUS; *and* TOXOPLASMOSIS.

Caudal Block

Regional anesthesia used for pain relief during childbirth.

A caudal block is a type of regional anesthesia. In regional anesthesia, a local anesthetic is injected into an area where it will affect a nerve root, a nerve that branches out into a number of smaller nerves that supply various body parts. The anesthetic then provides pain relief for body parts, the nerves of which branch off the affected root.

In a caudal block, an anesthetic is injected into a space in the tailbone (caudal area), blocking the lower back and pelvis.

During childbirth, a needle is inserted into the caudal area and a local anesthetic is slowly and continuously applied. This numbs the cervix, vagina, and perineum. Because there is risk of accidentally injecting the anesthetic into the bloodstream or the fetus, other, safer methods of regional anesthesia are preferred.

Caudal anesthesia is sometimes used to relieve postoperative pain for children. It can provide pain relief when given continuously for up to ten hours. *See* ANESTHESIA; CHILDBIRTH; EPIDURAL; *and* TAILBONE.

Cauliflower Ear

Also known as auricular hematoma

A condition in which the shape of the ear becomes distorted due to an accumulation of blood in the cartilage of the outer ear.

Cauliflower ear is caused by trauma, friction, or infection of the ear. It may result from a single injury but is more common among those whose ears are repeatedly subjected to trauma, such as boxers and other athletes. Cauliflower ear causes swelling and extreme sensitivity to touch.

Prompt treatment can prevent or limit deformity of the ear. The ear is usually drained of excess fluid. Antibiotics may be prescribed to cure an underlying infection. If the condition is left untreated, the ear can become permanently disfigured. *See also* ANTIBIOTICS; EARS; *and* HEMATOMA.

Causalgia

Intense burning pain caused by damage to nerves.

Causalgia is an intense, continuous pain that may follow an injury or disease in a major nerve pathway. It is accompanied by changes in blood flow. Other symptoms include swelling, sweating, and red and tender skin around the affected area. It is often a result of a gunshot wound in the leg, a fracture, or a deep cut severing a nerve. Physicians may treat patients with a sympathetic nerve block. In extreme cases, a surgical procedure severing the affected nerves (sympathectomy) is performed. *See also* NERVES.

Cauterization

Also known as diathermy

The use of a heated instrument or caustic chemical, such as silver nitrate, to destroy abnormal cells, stop bleeding, or promote healing.

Heat cauterization may be used to stop bleeding during operations and to treat cervical erosion and inflammation of the cervix. Chemicals such as silver nitrate have been used to cauterize nosebleeds and remove warts. Heat was also commonly used to destroy hemorrhoids, but the use of high-frequency electric current (electrocoagulation), which is easier and more efficient to use, is now the preferred method of cauterization. *See also* ABLATION *and* ELECTROCOAGULATION.

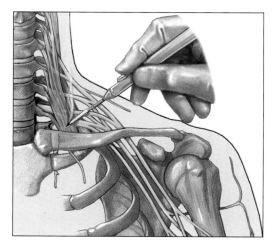

Cauterization. Heat is often used to stop bleeding during operations.

Cavernous Sinus Thrombosis

Blockage of a large group of veins in the brain.

Cavernous sinus thrombosis is a blood clot in a major vein located at the base of the brain just behind the eye socket. The clot is usually a complication of a bacterial infection of the sinuses or the eye or nose region. It results in headaches, seizures, bulging eyes, and high fever, and if untreated, may be life-threatening. Cavernous sinus thrombosis is rare today because of the routine use of antibiotics.

Causes. Infections that may result in thrombosis include: skin infection occurring on the face (cellulitis); infection and inflammation in the nose (sinusitis); infection in the bloodstream (septicemia); infection in the middle ear, eye, or mouth; a tumor crushing the veins; and excess red blood cells in the blood (polycythemia).

Symptoms include high fever, persistent headache, loss of sensation in the cornea, protrusion of the eye as a result of swelling (exophthalmos), and blurred vision from pressure on the optic nerve.

Treatment involves intravenous administration of antibiotics and anticoagulants to heal the infection and break up the clot. If the condition does not improve within 24 hours, surgery may be performed to drain the sinus. If the clot is not treated, blindness may result, and the infection may prove fatal. *See also* BACTERIAL INFECTIONS.

Celebrex

Brand name for celecoxib

Anti-inflammatory drug used to treat arthritis.

Celebrex is a recently developed anti-inflammatory and pain relief (analgesic) drug known as a COX-2 inhibitor. It limits the action of an enzyme, COX-2, that plays a role in pain and inflammation. Celebrex is similar to older nonsteroidal anti-inflammatory drugs (NSAIDs), but it may not be as damaging to the gastrointestinal tract.

Celebrex may also be used to reduce the number of polyps in familial adenomatous polyposis, an inherited disease in which numerous precancerous polyps develop in the colon and rectum.

People who have had an allergic reaction to sulfa drugs or NSAIDs should not take Celebrex. Side effects may include stomach pain, ulcers, internal bleeding, and fluid retention. There may be an increased risk of cardiovascular disease associated with using Celebrex. *See also* ANALGESIC DRUGS; ARTHRITIS; FAMILIAL ADENOMATOUS POLYPOSIS; *and* NSAIDs,

Celiac Sprue

Damage to the small intestine as a result of an inability to digest gluten.

Celiac sprue is one of several malabsorption problems that arise from the body's inability to digest a certain type of food, in this case, gluten, a protein found in several grains including wheat, rye, oats, and barley. Exposure to gluten causes the villi, small folds in the intestine through which nutrients are absorbed, to disappear, and causes the intestinal lining to produce large amounts of digestive enzymes.

Symptoms. The common symptoms of sprue are foul-smelling diarrhea, bloated abdomen, anemia, weight loss, abdominal cramps, gas, and a general feeling of weakness (malaise).

Celiac sprue is most commonly seen in young children, who fail to grow. Lack of absorption of nutrients may cause a vitamin D deficiency, resulting in a softening of the bones (rickets or osteomalacia).

Diagnosis. Celiac sprue is diagnosed through barium x-rays of the small intestine, as well as a biopsy of the lining; an accurate blood test has also recently been developed.

Treatment. Foods containing gluten are permanently eliminated from the diet. Vitamin and mineral supplements may be administered. A gluten-free diet over time results in the reversal of the changes seen in the small intestine. *See* DIGESTIVE SYSTEM.

Cell

The fundamental unit of a living organism.

Cells were first described in the 17th century. In the 19th century, the cell was established as the basic unit of all living organisms and cell division as its means of multiplication. Further research found that the cell nucleus contained hereditary information. In the 1940s, DNA was suspected to be the molecule that controls heredity; its structure was discovered in 1953.

A human cell is made of two main components: the nucleus and cytoplasm. The nucleus contains DNA and is responsible for giving the cell instructions and passing on hereditary information. Cytoplasm contains the nucleus and makes up the body of the cell. It is responsible for movement, protein production, and converting substances into chemical energy.

Nucleus

The nucleus is separated from the cytoplasm by two membranes known as the nuclear envelope. The nucleus contains molecules of deoxyribonucleic acid (DNA), which store the hereditary information responsible for cell growth and reproduction. This information is divided into 46 chromosomes. Enzymes in the nucleus copy parts of the DNA into strands of ribonucleic acid (RNA). Each segment of a chromosome used to produce a strand of RNA is known as a gene. Some types of RNA (messenger) are used to produce new copies of DNA. Other types (ribosomal) enter the cytoplasm through the nucleic membrane. There they form protein-RNA structures known as ribosomes, used as blueprints for producing molecules that fuel and organize cell activity.

Cytoplasm

The cytoplasm is contained inside the plasma membrane. Nutrients and waste materials pass through this membrane by slowly dissolving through or by way of channels formed out of proteins. Similar internal membranes distinguish or-

ganelles, compartments in the cell that specialize in a particular function, from the cytoplasm. Ribosomes and organelles inhabit the cytoplasm as separate membrane-bordered chemical and molecular environments.

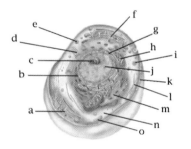

Ribosomes. Free-floating ribosomes use proteins to make enzymes, structural supports, and elements used for movement. Other ribosomes attached to a cluster of flattened, membranous sacs (endoplasmic reticulum) build proteins that are stored, used in membranes, or released from the cell altogether. The Golgi complex, another system of sacs, modifies proteins made in the endoplasmic reticulum.

Some Types of Organelles. The mitochondrion produces most of the chemical energy needed by the cell. Carbohydrates, fats, proteins, and nucleic acids provide fuel for reactions inside the mitochondria that release energy to spur cell growth and development.

The lysosome contains the cell's digestive enzymes. Substances engulfed by the cell may be directed to a lysosome for digestion. In case of disease or as part of cell division, lysosomes may release their enzymes into the cytoplasm, killing the cell.

Microtubules and microfilaments are used for cell locomotion. They also form the cytoskeleton, an internal structure that supports the cell.

Background information on cell can be found in DNA *and* RNA. *For related material, see* Bacteria; Chromosome; Familial; Gene; Genetics; Heredity; Metabolism; Parasite; *and* Viruses. *See also* Cancer; Carcinogen; Mutagen; *and* Mutation *for more on diseases caused by abnormalities of cell DNA.*

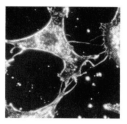

Cells. Above, cells can be said to lead lives: they move as if driven to perform certain functions, and they can suddenly destroy themselves. Left, there is much variation from cell to cell, even within a family of cells with the same function. But a eukaryotic cell will generally have the following complement of organelles: (a) the smooth endoplasmic reticulum; (b) the nucleus; (c) the nucleolus; (d) a centriole; (e) a secretion granule; (f) a Golgi apparatus; (g) the nuclear envelope; (h) a mitcochondrion; (i) a lysosome; (j) chromatin; (k) the cell membrane; (l) a microtuble; (m) the rough endoplasmic reticulum; (n) cytoplasm; and (o) a ribsome.

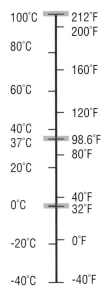

Celsius. Above, the Celsius and Fahrenheit scales. Highlighted are the freezing and boiling points of water (0°C and 100°C), and 37°C approximately body temperature.

Central Nervous System. Right, the basic elements of a human nervous system: (a) the brain; (b) the cervical spinal nerves; (c) the lumbar spinal nerves; (d) the spinal chord; (e) the thoracic spinal nerves; (f) the sacral spinal nerves.

Celsius Scale

Also known as the centigrade scale

A scale of temperature.

The Celsius scale is named for Swedish astronomer Anders Celsius (1701-1744). The scale is based upon the boiling and freezing points of water, which are assigned 100° and 0° respectively. Other common temperature systems include the Kelvin and Fahrenheit scales. *See also* FAHRENHEIT SCALE *and* THERMOMETER.

Centers for Disease Control

The agency that heads the federal government's efforts to prevent the spread of disease.

The Centers for Disease Control (CDC), headquartered in Atlanta, Georgia, is part of the Department of Health and Human Services. It works to control the spread of disease, improve the nation's environmental health, and educate the public about disease prevention,

The CDC has more than 2000 employees who work in its US offices and more than 100 overseas. The CDC's activities range from analyzing the epidemiology of infectious diseases to training people in HIV prevention and traveling to foreign locales to help stop outbreaks of infectious diseases. *See also* DISEASE; INFECTION; *and* PUBLIC HEALTH.

Central Nervous System

The brain and spinal cord.

The central nervous system (CNS) processes and responds to messages from the rest of the body. Organs such as the skin, eyes, ears, nose, and glands communicate with the CNS via the peripheral nervous system (PNS), made up of nerves throughout the body that connect to the spine or brain. The CNS receives sensory information, analyzes and interprets it, and then responds

in some way—for instance, by scratching an itch. Some messages, such as those that prompt reflexes, do not require in-depth analysis and thus need not climb all the way to the brain, but are handled by the spinal cord. Complex information requires a trip to the brain for conscious, prolonged analysis. Neurons and nerve cells supported by tissue comprise the CNS and extend into nerve fibers that form the PNS. The skull and spine protect the CNS.

Damage to the CNS may be caused by injury or illness. In some cases, as in the

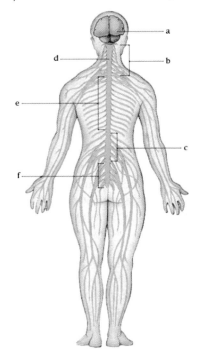

case of a tumor in the brain, damage may be minimized or repaired through surgical intervention. In other cases, as after a stroke or some other form of head injury, varying degrees of spontaneous recovery may occur over time. In still other cases, as in progressive disease or serious injury, damage may be permanent or fatal.

For background material on central nervous system, see BRAIN; NERVOUS SYSTEM; *and* SPINAL CORD. *Further information can be found in* BRAIN, DISORDERS OF; BRAIN TUMOR; EAR; EPIDURAL ANESTHESIA; EYE; GLAND; HEAD INJURY; NERVE; NERVE BLOCK; NERVE INJURY; NERVE, TRAPPED; NOSE; PARALYSIS; SKIN; *and* STROKE

Centrifuge

A machine for spinning fluids in test tubes at high speed to separate their contents.

A centrifuge is a device used to separate fluids, especially blood, into component parts. When the centrifuge is spinning, centrifugal force causes the heavier particles in the solution to sink and the lighter ones to float to the surface. When, for example, whole blood is centrifuged, heavier red blood cells sink to the bottom of the test tube while plasma rises to the surface. White blood cells (leukocytes), which are lighter than red blood cells but heavier than plasma, form a thin layer in the middle. *See also* BLOOD TESTS.

Cephalhematoma

A firm swollen mass on a baby's head caused by pressure exerted during labor.

A cephalhematoma is caused by the accumulation of blood under the outside covering of the skull. It is sometimes accompanied by a minor skull fracture. A cephalhematoma may also occur during forceps or vacuum-assisted delivery. Treatment is rarely necessary, as the blood usually disappears within 2 to 12 weeks. A cephalhematoma is not associated with long-term problems, although infants with a cephalhematoma may be at risk for elevated bilirubin levels, which should be monitored, since this can result in brain damage or jaundice. *See also* BIRTH INJURY.

Cephalosporins

A family of antibiotic drugs that are effective against a number of bacteria, including staphylococci and streptococci.

Originally used as an alternative to penicillin, cephalosporins have over time been developed for wider use. They attack a wide range of bacteria and seem to induce fewer instances of allergic reactions. Early cephalosporins were used against penicillin-re-sistant strains of staphylococci, streptococci, proteus, and *E. coli.* They are now also used in treating infections of the skin, urinary tract, blood, bones, lungs, and heart. Side effects may include gastrointestinal upset, diarrhea, yeast infection, nausea, and allergic reactions. They should not be taken with alcohol. *See also* ANTIBIOTIC DRUGS; PENICILLIN; STAPHYLOCOCCAL INFECTIONS, *and* STREPTOCOCCAL INFECTIONS.

Cerebellum

Portion of the brain that controls coordination.

The cerebellum is located below the cerebrum (the main portion of the brain responsible for complex, conscious functions such as movement, speech, and thought) and behind the brain stem (the portion of the brain responsible for involuntary functions such as heartbeat and reaction to stress). The cerebellum is connected through the brain stem to the motor area of the cerebrum (responsible for directing the muscles), the spinal cord, and the semicircular canals in the inner ear (key in maintaining balance).

The main function of the cerebellum is to aid in coordination, balance, and fine motor control. While the motor area in the cerebrum is responsible for directing conscious movements of the muscles—for example, directing the legs to walk—the cerebellum is responsible for interpreting that direction into the many fine muscle variations that allow movement to be smooth and coordinated.

Disorders of the Cerebellum. Damage to the cerebellum may occur as a result of head injury, internal bleeding (hemorrhage), stroke, benign or malignant tumors, or congenital nervous system disorders. Disorders that affect the cerebellum may include:

• **Astrocytomas**, one of the most common types of brain tumors; astrocytes in the cerebellum more commonly occur in children than in adults.

• **Medulloblastomas**, tumors that arise

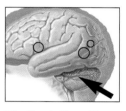

The Cerebellum. The part of the brain (arrow) that controls coordination, balance and fine motor control.

in the cerebellum from primitive nerve cells; medulloblastomas occur most often in children.

- **Friedrich's Ataxia**, a congenital disease of the nervous system that results in progressive damage to the cerebellum, spinal cord, and peripheral nerves.

Impairment of the cerebellum generally results in uncoordinated movement (ataxia). A person may stagger while walking; movements may be uncontrolled and jerky. The eyes may jerk back and forth (nystagmus). Posture may be abnormal. If only one side of the cerebellum is damaged, symptoms occur on the same side.

Some types of damage to the cerebellum can be treated. A tumor may removed surgically or through radiation therapy. An abscess or blood clot from injury or infection may be surgically removed. In other cases, such as stroke, some amount of recovery may occur spontaneously. *See* BRAIN; BRAIN TUMORS; BALANCE ATAXIA; *and* FREIDRICH'S ATAXIA.

Cerebral Palsy

A nonspecific term for chronic, nonprogressive disorders impairing muscle alignment and movement.

Cerebral palsy usually occurs as a result of brain injury before, during, or shortly after birth. It is characterized by weakness, rigidity, or tremors in the arms and legs.

Causes. A number of different types of injury can cause cerebral palsy, but in any specific case, the cause is usually not known. It can be caused by lack of oxygen to the brain prior to, during, or just after birth. Other causes include infection by German measles (rubella) during pregnancy; extreme jaundice in newborns, leading to a condition known as kernicterus; and trauma, meningitis, or dehydration after birth. As a result of these injuries, the areas of the brain that control coordination and movement are damaged and do not develop properly.

TYPES

There are four types of cerebral palsy:

Resources on Cerebral Palsy

Geralis, Elaine, *Children With Cerebral Palsy : A Parents' Guide* (1998); Kandel, Eric R., et al., *Principles of Neural Science* (1991); Miller, Freeman, and Steven J. Bachrach, *Cerebral Palsy: A Complete Guide for Caregiving* (1998); Sanes, Dan Harvey, et al., *Development of the Nervous System* (2000); United Cerebral Palsy, Tel. (800) USA-5-UCP; Online: www.ucp.org; American Academy of Neurology, Tel. (651) 695-1940, Online: www.aan.com; www.med.cornell.edu/neuro/html.

Early Signs of Cerebral Palsy

Doctors begin to suspect cerebral palsy if an infant is consistently slow to reach first year developmental stages such as smiling, rolling over, and crawling. The infant may also have trouble sucking and swallowing. Muscle floppiness and poor coordination may prevent a child from exploring the world to a full extent, thus delaying many forms of learning. Early diagnosis and treatment is essential in helping an affected child reach his or her full potential.

- **Spastic**—muscles are rigid and weak; this occurs in 70 percent of cases.
- **Dyskinetic**— in which muscles move haphazardly without control.
- **Ataxic**— in which coordination is impaired and movement is shaky.
- **Mixed**— in which a combination of symptoms is seen.

Symptoms. These vary greatly from one person to the next. Some people may have only mild impairment to coordination, while others may have near complete paralysis of all four limbs. The disease is not progressive, but symptoms may modify over time—often for the better.

An infant with cerebral palsy may exhibit a lack of muscle tone (hypotony), posture abnormalities such as crossed legs, and delays in walking and speaking. In older children, balance and fine motor skills may be impaired, and speech may be hard to comprehend. Some children with cerebral palsy experience other disorders such as seizures or mental impairment.

Treatment. There is no cure for cerebral palsy. The objective of treatment is to enable the child to live as full and independent a life as possible. Physical, occupational, and speech therapy can help a child develop muscle control and coping skills. Depending on the degree of impairment and whether mental impairment is also involved, a child may need assistance in school or may need to attend a school geared toward children with disabilities.

Background information on cerebral palsy can be found in CENTRAL NERVOUS SYSTEM; MUSCLE; *and* NERVOUS SYSTEM. *For further information, see* BIRTH INJURY; DEHYDRATION; HYPOTONIA; JAUNDICE; MENINGITIS; *and* RUBELLA.

Cerebrovascular Accident

Sudden interruption of blood flow in the brain caused by blockage or rupture of a blood vessel.

In a cerebrovascular accident, blood flow to the brain is interrupted by a blood clot (thrombosis) or the rupture of a blood vessel, classified either as an intracerebral hemorrhage (within the brain) or a subarachnoid hem orrhage (between the brain and its lining).

Interruption of blood flow can kill a significant number of brain cells within minutes. It can also lead to a stroke, resulting in paralysis, loss of mental function, or death. *See also* STROKE.

Cerebrovascular Disease

Any condition that affects the normal function of an artery supplying blood to the brain.

Cerebrovascular disease includes atherosclerosis (narrowing of an artery caused by the buildup of deposits in its walls) and aneurysm (ballooning out of an artery wall resulting from defect, injury, or high blood pressure). These conditions may result in cerebrovascular problems or stroke—the death of brain cells. Excessive narrowing of arteries can lead to progressive loss of mental function (dementia). *See also* BRAIN.

Cerebrum

Main portion of the brain; receives and interprets sensory information, and is the seat of conscious thought.

The cerebrum, the uppermost portion of the brain, is responsible for a great number of functions, including interpretation of sensory input; recognition of familiar objects; and control of movement, speech, memory, thoughts, and feelings.

The cerebrum is dividied into the left and right hemispheres, which are connected by a structure known as the corpus callosum. The left hemisphere is associated with language and speech, and the right hemisphere is associated with visual and spatial interpretation. Each hemisphere is responsible for controlling functions on the opposite side of the body. For example, a signal from the right hemisphere causes the left arm to move.

Cerebral Cortex. The outer layer of the cerebrum is known as the cerebral cortex. It is grayish brown and thus is said to be made up of gray matter. The inner core of the cerebrum is white.

The cerebral cortex is responsible for the bulk of the cerebrum's functioning. It is highly convoluted and contains a great number of grooves and bulges. Several of the largest of the grooves divide the cerebrum into lobes. Each lobe contains areas that control specific functions. The lobes and some of their functions are:

- **Frontal lobe**—movement, language, associative thought, intelligence, feelings, personality.
- **Temporal lobe**—memory, interpretation of sounds, speech and language.
- **Parietal lobe**—interpretation of multiple sensory inputs used to recognize objects.
- **Occipital lobe**—interpretation of visual images.

Damage to the cerebrum may occur as a result of trauma, injury or infection during or shortly after birth (cerebral palsy), stroke, or tumors. Cerebral damage may result in a range of impairments, from impaired movement to difficulty speaking to memory loss to inability to interpret sensory information.

Damage that affects only one side of the brain affects the opposite side of the body. Some disorders, such as tumors and blood clots, may be removed surgically. Other disorders, such as from injury and stroke, may improve over time. The prognosis is highly variable, depending on the extent and location of damage.

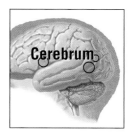

The Cerebrum. The main portion of the brain responsible for complex, conscious functions such as movement, speech and thought

For background information on cerebrum, see BRAIN; CENTRAL NERVOUS SYSTEM; *and* NERVOUS SYSTEM. *Related material can be found in* GRAY MATTER; MEMORY; *and* SPEECH. *See also* BRAIN TUMOR; CEREBRAL PALSY; HEAD INJURY; *and* STROKE.

Certificate of Need

Legal document that a health institution must receive to offer a new service or expand facilities.

A certificate of need is a legal document that a health facility, such as a hospital, must receive to install or modify some facilities or major new equipment, or offer some new service. In most cases, the facility applies to a state review board for the certificate. Most states have certificate-of-need laws, as a result of the Public Health Services Act of 1974, which provides incentives for states to create these laws. Facilities that require certificates of need include hospitals, ambulatory surgical facilities, nursing homes, and rehabilitation centers. *See also* CAT SCAN *and* HOSPITALS.

Certification

Process by which an individual or an institution demonstrates that it meets requirements to engage in certain health care activities.

In the interest of public health, institutions and individuals undergo a certification process before engaging in specialized activities. National licensing and certification programs that measure competency exist for nurses, physicians, health educators, laboratory technicians, environmental health specialists, and many allied health professionals.

Practitioners must be trained at institutions that have themselves received certification. The certification process for medical schools, hospitals, residency programs, and other health institutions is called accreditation. In this process, a national review board certifies that the institution meets predefined standards. *See also* ACCREDITATION *and* BOARD CERTIFICATION.

Cervical Erosion

Scraping of or damage to the cervix.

Cervical erosion occurs when the cervix has been scraped or damaged, possibly during sexual intercourse or from an intrauterine device (IUD).

Symptoms may include a whitish or slightly bloody discharge, and bleeding during or following intercourse. A reddish patch may be visible on the cervix. If an abrasion is visible, a pap smear should be done to ensure that it is not cancer. A biopsy may be performed as well.

Treatment usually consists of cauterizing the area with heat or cryosurgery to speed healing.

A related disorder is cervical eversion, which occurs when cells that normally line the inside of the cervical canal grow on its outside. *See also* CERVIX.

Cervical Incompetence

Weakness of the cervix.

The cervix is the neck of the uterus; during pregnancy, it usually stays closed until the onset of labor. With cervical incompetence, the weight of a growing fetus forces the cervix open during pregnancy, in the absence of contractions resulting in a miscarriage or premature birth. The problem can be solved with a cerclage procedure, in which the cervix is literally stitched closed. At the beginning of the ninth month, the stitches are cut so childbirth can occur. *See also* MISCARRIAGE *and* PREMATURE LABOR .

Cervical Osteoarthritis

Also known as cervical spondylosis

Neck stiffness as a result of abnormal bone growth, as well as degeneration and calcification between the cervical disks.

Cervical osteoarthritis is caused by the deterioration of the disks that rest between the vertebrae of the neck. Further loss of mobility may be caused by mineral deposits known as calcification, or bone growths (spurs) on the vertebrae. This disorder usually occurs in older people as a normal part of aging but may occur earlier in those who have suffered a neck injury.

Symptoms include neck pain and stiffness that may worsen over time, and a loss of sensation or abnormal sensation in the arms, shoulders, and occasionally legs. Other symptoms include headaches in the back of the head, loss of balance, and muscle weakness. Loss of or exaggerated sensations may be the result of nerves in the spinal cord being compressed by the vertebrae.

Diagnosis is confirmed by spine or neck x-rays, CT scans, or MRIs. Myelograms can further explore the depth of the condition.

Treatment concentrates on the relief of pain and prevention of further damage. For mild cases, exercises to strengthen the neck may be recommended. For others, a cervical collar may be worn to reduce movement that causes pain. Surgical decompression may be performed if the neck is not responding to treatment, or if there is a significant loss of ability. Nerve damage prior to surgery is usually permanent. *See* ARTHRITIS; NECK; *and* SPINAL CORD.

Cervical Rib

Disorder in which the lowest of the neck bones (cervical vertebrae) overdevelops and forms a rib.

The growth of a cervical rib appears to be a congenital disorder with no external cause. The rib, which rests parallel to the rib of the first thoracic vertebra, usually develops in early adulthood.

Symptoms may include pain, stiffness, numbness, and tingling in the forearm and hand. These symptoms occur when the newly developed rib presses against the nerves that pass from the spinal cord into the arm. Compression of the nerves or veins in the region may cause thoracic outlet syndrome, characterized by numbness in the hand and a weakening of the grip. As these sensations can indicate a variety of disorders, the only certain way to diagnose a cervical rib is with an x-ray.

Treatment may include exercises to strengthen and improve posture so that the extra rib does not press on the nerves. In extreme cases, surgery may alleviate the symptoms. *See also* NECK; SPINE; *and* THORACIC OUTLET SYNDROME.

Cervicitis

Inflammation of the cervix.

Cervicitis can be caused by a local infection, particularly after giving birth if any damage was sustained at that time. It can also be a symptom of vaginal infection, pelvic inflammatory disease (PID), or various sexually transmitted diseases.

While acute cervicitis often produces no symptoms, chronic cervicitis may be accompanied by pain, bleeding, and vaginal discharge. Cervicitis is diagnosed by means of a biopsy. A pap test is also usually performed at the same time to rule out cervical cancer.

Treatment. An antibiotic, geared to the particular organism causing the infection, is administered. Severe cases of cervicitis are treated by cauterizing the cervix either with heat or freezing (cryosurgery). Cauterization and cryosurgery destroy problematic tissue and stop bleeding. Both procedures can be performed in a doctor's office. *See* CERVIX, PAP SMEAR; *and* REPRODUCTIVE SYSTEM, FEMALE.

Cervix

The neck of the uterus, the lower portion of which protrudes into the vagina.

The cervix is the lowest part of the uterus. The cervical canal, is the opening into the uterus that passes through the cervix. Menstrual fluids are expelled from the uterus and sperm enters the uterus through the cervical canal. During birth, the cervix dilates to allow the infant to pass into the birth canal.

It is important for women to regularly receive a pap smear, a safe diagnostic test in which a small sample of cells is scraped off the cervix and examined under a microscope. This test can reveal changes that might indicate a precancerous or cancerous condition. Early detection is key in preventing and limiting cervical cancer. *See also* BIRTH; CERVIX, CANCER OF; PAP SMEAR; *and* REPRODUCTIVE SYSTEM, FEMALE.

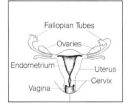

The Female Reproductive system. The cervix is the lowest portion of the uterus. It is scraped when women have a Pap smear test taken, to detect cancer.

Cervix, Cancer of the

Malignant tumor of the cervix, the lower part of the uterus that protrudes into the vagina.

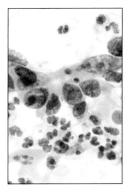

Cancer of the Cervix. The great majority of cervical cancers are squamous cell carcinomas, which arise in the surface layer of cells.

Resources on Brain Tumors

Dahm, Nancy Hassett, *Mind, Body, and Soul: A Guide to Living with Cancer* (2001); Murphy, G., et al., *Informed Deci-sions: The Complete Book of Cancer Diagnosis, Treatment, and Recovery* (1997); Renneker, Mark, ed., *Understanding Cancer* (1988); Steen, R. Grant, *A Conspiracy of Cells: The Basic Science of Cancer* (1993); Steward, Clifford T., ed., *Cancer: Prevention, Detection, Causes, Treatment* (1988); American Cancer Society, Tel. (800) ACS-2345, Online: www.cancer.org; National Cancer Institue, Tel. (800) 4-CANCER, Online: www.nci.nih.gov.

Cancer of the cervix is one of the most common cancers among women. The incidence is highest among women in their 40s. It appears to be associated with human papilloma virus (HPV), which is primarily transmitted through sexual contact. Ninety percent of all cervical tumors contain genetic material from HPV. The herpes virus is also suspected to be a risk factor. Daughters of women who took the synthetic estrogen diethylstilbestrol during pregnancy are at increased risk, as are smokers and women who have had more than five pregnancies.

The great majority of cervical cancers are squamous cell carcinomas, which arise in the surface layer of cells. A small percentage are adenocarcinomas, which arise in deeper layers of tissue.

SYMPTOMS

Early stages of cervical cancer usually causes no symptoms. Symptoms that may appear include painful intercourse, bleeding during intercourse or between menstrual periods, heavy menstrual flow, and foul-smelling discharge.

A cervical test called the pap smear is recommended by the American Cancer Society annually for women, starting at age 18 or the beginning of sexual activity. In a pap test, a sample of cells is taken from the cervix and examined for the presence of abnormal cells that may be precursors to a malignant tumor.

STAGES OF CERVICAL CANCER

The first sign of potential cervical cancer is dysplasia, the appearance and growth of abnormal cells. Dysplasia does not always progress to cancer, but the cells can proliferate until they cover the whole surface of the cervix. Dysplasia is treated by removal of the abnormal cells with cryosurgery, which freezes the cells, or laser therapy.

The extent and severity of cervical can-

Cervical Cancer and HPV

Several strains of the sexually transmitted human papilloma virus (HPV) are associated with an increased risk for cervical cancer. HPV is the most common sexually transmitted disease (STD) in the United States. A number of factors, such as pregnancy and smoking, are associated with HPV, but the greatest indicator for HPV infection is the number of sexual partners a person has had.

In the majority of cases, HPV does not result in any symptoms, although some strains cause the growth of warts in the genital area. Warts can be removed surgically or by use of a drug, but they may recur. Also, removing the warts may reduce but does not eliminate the risk of transmission. Condoms, which are highly effective in the prevention of many STDs, have not been shown to reduce transmission of HPV. The spermicide nonoxynol-9 has also not been shown to limit the spread of the virus.

Aside from abstinence, the most effective means of reducing risk for HPV is to limit the number of sexual partners. However, even a monogamous partner may have already been infected with HPV.

cer is classified according to numbered stages, with a lower number indicating a more localized and easily treatable cancer. Stage 0 cervical cancer is known as *carcinoma in situ*. In this case, the cancerous tissue is confined to an area on the surface of the cervix. Cryosurgery may be performed to remove the cancerous cells, or a technique called cone biopsy to remove the cells and some of the nearby tissue. A hysterectomy may be recommended for a woman who has completed childbearing or who has other conditions that might benefit from removal of the uterus.

In stage 1 cancer, the tumor has spread to the interior of the cervix or to the

ALERT

Cervical Cancer and Pregnancy

If cancer of the cervix is detected during pregnancy, the health of the fetus as well as of the mother is a consideration in treatment. Therapy may be delayed until after delivery for carcinoma in situ—if tests show that the cancerous cells have not spread. If the cancer has spread, the stage of pregnancy, the extent of spread and the wishes of the parents are issues to be considered, since most treatments may cause the death of the fetus.

uterus. It can be treated by cone biopsy or by surgery. The extent of surgery depends on the extent of the cancer and may involve a hysterectomy. Radiation therapy is often performed to prevent further spread.

At later stages, in which the cancer has spread to the lower part of the vagina and nearby lymph nodes (stage 2) or the wall of the pelvis (stage 3), it can be treated by hysterectomy, removal of the lymph nodes, and radiation therapy. If the cancer is even more widespread (stage 4), radiation therapy is considered, usually with the addition of chemotherapy.

PROGNOSIS

The results of treatment depend largely on the stage at which the cancer is detected. The five-year survival rate for carcinoma in situ is almost 100 percent. For stage 2 cancer, the five-year survival rate is about 60 percent for squamous cell carcinoma, and up to 40 percent for adenocarcinoma. The risk of recurrence is highest in the three years after treatment, so periodic follow-up visits for pelvic examinations, pap smears, x-rays and CT scans are recommended. *See also* CANCER; CANCER SCREENING; CERVIX DISORDERS OF THE; CERVICAL EROSION, CERVICITIS; HYSTERECTOMY; *and* UTERUS.

Cervix, Disorders of the

Pain, disease, or injury related to the cervix.

The cervix is the connection between the uterus and the vagina. Common disorders of the cervix include cervical erosion, cervicitis, polyps, Nabothian cysts, dysplasia, and cancer. *See* CERVIX, CANCER OF THE.

Cervical polyps are harmless growths that protrude from the mouth of the cervix. They may occur singly or in clusters. They often appear after pregnancy, due to hormonal changes, or any time after the cervix has been injured. They are rarely cancerous. Polyps may cause no symptoms or may result in bleeding after intercourse, in the middle of the menstrual cycle, or after menopause, or very heavy periods accompanied by cramps. These symptoms

may also be indicative of cervical cancer, so it is important to determine the cause.

Surgical removal of polyps is performed in the doctor's office with local anesthesia. If the polyps are numerous or unusually large, the procedure is done in the hospital. If the polyps recur, the uterus may need to be dilated and the inside lining scraped with a curette.

Nabothian Cysts. These are fluid-filled lumps found on the cervix. They occur when a mucus gland on the surface of the cervix becomes obstructed. This sometimes happens after childbirth or after menopause. Nabothian cysts rarely require treatment. In some cases, destruction of the area of tissue (cauterization) is necessary, either with heat or cryosurgery.

Cervical Dysplasia. This term refers to the presence of abnormal cervical cells, often found during a pap test. These cells are considered to be precancerous and, if untreated, may progress to cervical cancer. Dysplasia is found most often between the ages of 25 and 35 and occurs more often in women who have multiple sex partners or who became sexually active at a young age. Dysplasia has been linked to various viruses that cause sexually transmitted diseases.

A mild case may be resolved without treatment or may require cauterization, either by cryosurgery or laser.

Advanced dysplasia requires a cone biopsy, a major surgical procedure in which a cone-shaped section of the cervix is removed. A severe case may require the removal of the reproductive system (hysterectomy).

A woman who has had advanced dysplasia and has a had a hysterectomy will not be able to become pregnant. A woman who has been treated for dysplasia should have a pap test performed twice a year for two years and then annually to make sure the condition does not recur.

> *For background information on disorders of the cervix, see* CERVIX *and* REPRODUCTIVE SYSTEM, FEMALE. *Further information can be found in* CANCER; CERVICAL EROSION; CERVICAL INCOMPETENCE; CERVICAL OSTEOARTHRITIS; CERVICITIS; *and* CERVIX, CANCER OF.

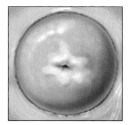
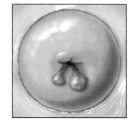
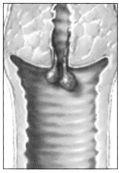

Disorders of the cervix. Top, cervical neoplasia a precancerous change of the cervix. Middle and bottom, fingerlike growths originating from the mucosal surface of the cervix or endocervical canal. Small fragile growths hang from a stalk and protrude through the cervical opening.

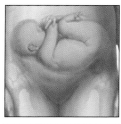

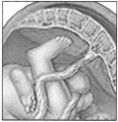

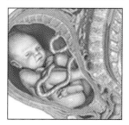

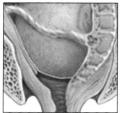

Cesarean Section.
Right, the surgeon reaches into the abdomen with both hands and lifts the baby as an assistant pushes down on the uterus. Above, causes for a C-section include—from the top—transverse position; placenta abruptio; breech presentation and placenta previa.

Resources on Cesarean Section
Chervenal, Frank A., *Fetal Medicine* (1999); Creasy, Robert K., and Robert Resnik, eds., *Maternal-Fetal Medicine: Principles and Practice* (1994); Gonik, Bernard and Renee A. Bobrowski.

Cesarean Section

Also known as a C-section or surgical delivery

An operation to remove a baby from the uterus. Incisions are made in the mother's abdomen and uterine wall, and the baby is lifted out.

A Cesarean section is often performed under the following conditions:

- The baby is in the breech position.
- The infant is unusually large or the birth canal is unusually small.
- There are uterine or vaginal abnormalities or obstruction.
- Placenta previa, or premature separation of the placenta from the uterine wall, occurs.
- The mother has preeclampsia, diabetes, genital herpes, or hypertension.
- There is fetal distress.
- Labor is prolonged with insufficient uterine contractions.

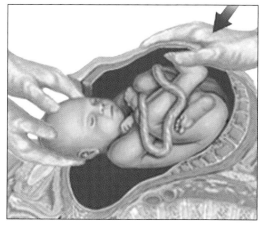

In recent years the number of Cesarean sections has increased greatly. This may be partially due to physicians' tendency to opt for surgical delivery whenever there is a possibility of a difficult birth. As fetal monitoring has improved, problems are more likely to be spotted, and doctors perform a Cesarean section to safeguard the baby's health. Additionally, women are increasingly waiting to have children at a later age and are consequently at a higher risk of complications in labor and delivery.

PROCEDURE

In the case of an emergency Cesarean section, general anesthesia may be necessary. Otherwise, a local anesthetic such as an epidural is usually given, allowing the mother to remain awake. The operation takes approximately one hour. The abdominal incision is either vertical or horizontal (the "bikini cut" near the pubic bone). The uterine incision may be horizontal across the lower part of the uterus or vertical. The lower uterine incision heals more readily and lessens the chance of uterine rupture. The vertical incision, on the other hand, allows more access inside the uterus. Once the baby and placenta are removed, the incisions are closed.

RECOVERY AND COMPLICATIONS

Most women experience few problems in recovery from a Cesarean section. However, as with any form of major surgery, there is a chance of postoperative infection. Heavy bleeding is rare but may be severe when it does occur. Cesarean section is associated with a death rate up to four times higher than a vaginal delivery. However, this operation is performed on women whose pregnancies are in the high-risk category; the numbers may reflect preexisting conditions and not the surgery itself.

Recovery after a Cesarean section is longer than after a vaginal birth. The average hospital stay is five or six days, compared to one to two days for a nonsurgical delivery. Afterwards, the mother must continue to rest for a few weeks and avoid heavy lifting.

In previous years, once a woman had a Cesarean section, future deliveries would have to be done surgically as well, because of the risk of uterine rupture during labor. However, today more than half of women with a history of Cesarean section can have vaginal deliveries. Whether a woman can undergo a vaginal birth after Cesarean depends on two factors: if the condition that necessitated the earlier Cesarean is absent, and what type of uterine incision was made. Women who had a lower transverse incision are more likely to be able to sustain a vaginal delivery. *See also* CHILDBIRTH *and* VAGINA.

Chagas' Disease

Parasitic disease common in Central and South America.

Chagas' disease is caused by a parasitic one-celled organism, *Trypanosoma cruzi*, transmitted through the bite of several blood sucking insects.

Immediately following infection, redness and swelling may develop around the bite, and nearby lymph nodes and one eye may swell and become tender. The infected person may then develop a fever and swollen lymph nodes, and the heart may beat rapidly and irregularly. Although some people may experience no or only mild symptoms, about 10 percent of infected people die during this phase of the disease.

Over time, about 20 percent of infected people develop chronic Chagas' disease, which leads to progressive and potentially fatal heart disease and digestive problems.

Treatment

The drugs benznidazole and nifurtimox may be used to kill the parasite that causes Chagas' disease; these drugs are not available in the United States. The disease may be prevented by using insecticides, wearing protective clothing, and avoiding areas where Chagas' disease is endemic. *See also* INSECT BITES *and* PROTOZOA.

Chalazion

A cyst-like lump on the eyelid.

A chalazion develops when a gland that provides part of the eye's lubricating layer becomes blocked. The swelling is preceded by pain, inflammation, and possibly increased tearing. Usually a chalazion disappears on its own in a month or so, but it may recur. Warm compresses applied several times a day may help a chalazion heal faster; this is most effective before the cyst has fully developed. A large chalazion may be surgically removed. If a chalazion continually recurs, it should be biopsied to rule out the possibility of a malignancy. In people prone to developing chalazions, regular cleansing of the eyelid may limit incidence. *See also* CYST *and* EYE.

Chancre, Hard

A sore or ulcer associated with various sexually transmitted diseases (STDs), particularly syphilis.

A chancre is a hard, open sore that is most often painless. It does not bleed, although it may leak fluid, particularly pus, which is highly infectious. A hard chancre is usually found at the site where infection occurred: in men the penis, and in women the vulva or vagina. In both sexes it may also be found on the anus, rectum, lips, throat, and tongue. Nearby lymph nodes may become enlarged. The sore usually heals without treatment in 3 to 12 weeks.

Diagnosis of the cause of the chancre is made by a physician or a blood test. Abstinence and monogamy are effective means of preventing infection. Using a condom reduces the risk of contracting many STDs, but it is not 100 percent effective. *See* SEXUALLY TRANSMITTED DISEASES; *and* SYPHILIS.

Chancroid

Also known as soft chancre

A sexually transmitted disease caused by the bacteria *Hemophilus ducreyi*.

Chancroid often causes no symptoms; therefore it can be spread unwittingly. The disease is more commonly found in tropical climates but is becoming increasingly common in North America. It is spread by either sexual or skin contact. There is some evidence that the presence of chancroid may cause an individual to become more susceptible to HIV infection.

Symptoms. Some people develop small, raised painless or slightly tender sores with reddish borders. In women these sores are found on the vulva, vagina, urethra, cervix, or inner thighs; in men, on the penis or urethra. The sores develop anywhere from three to seven days after the initial infection and may fill with pus and rupture, causing an open sore that resembles a herpes lesion. Many sores often run together to form one large ulcer. The sores occasionally heal spontaneously, but the bacteria can infect nearby lymph glands, which become hard and swollen and sometimes form an abscess, called a bubo, that can rupture if left untreated.

Diagnosis is based on the appearance of the sores after other sexually transmitted diseases that may cause similar symptoms are ruled out. Chancroid is difficult to diagnose in most women.

Treatment. Chancroid can be treated with several types of antibiotics, including sulfa drugs, streptomycin, and erythromycin. Any buboes present are lanced.

Prevention. Like other sexually transmitted diseases, the spread of chancroid can be limited by means of safe sex practices. *See also* Barrier Methods; Safe Sex; *and* Sexually Transmitted Diseases.

Chapped Skin

Roughening of the skin caused by exposure to wind or cold temperatures.

Chapped skin is most common during the winter months. People who have less protein and lipids in their skin have less defense against chapped skin. These oils help keep skin soft and repel water.

Dry skin should be treated with moisturizer several times a day, especially after bathing. Vaseline is a good moisturizer. Products with perfumes and other additives can be irritants and should be avoided. Tepid, not hot, water should be used for bathing. Wet skin should be patted, rather than rubbed dry. Scratching and scrubbing skin can irritate it.

Chapped and inflamed lips may occur as a result of infection, allergy, sunburn, or vitamin B_2 deficiency. Skin creams can soothe the lips, and if necessary, the underlying cause should be treated.

If the skin is extremely itchy and includes red patches, especially behind the knees and on the arms, neck, and face, it may indicate eczema, a more serious skin condition. Eczema, which is often an inherited condition, can be treated with a topical corticosteroid ointment. *See also* Eczema; Ointment; *and* Skin.

Charcot's Joint

Also known as neuropathic joint

Loss of sensation in a joint.

Causes of Charcot's joint may include diabetes and untreated syphilis. The affected joint does not react to stress or damage with the usual signals of pain. Repeated, incorrect movement without pain to deter it can cause severe, long-term damage. Joint degeneration and damage from repeated injury may be detected on x-rays. Treatment may include a brace or splint to restrict movement, or joint fusion may be performed. Nerve damage cannot be reversed. *See also* Diabetes *and* Joints.

Chelating Agents

Chemicals used to treat heavy metal poisoning.

Chelating agents are compounds that form bonds to metal ions. They are used as antidotes for poisoning from substances such as mercury, lead, cadmium, arsenic, and iron. Chelating agents draw the metal from the blood and tissues into the bloodstream, a process known as chelation. The patient is then saturated with fluids so that both the chelating agents and the toxic buildup are excreted through urine and the bile in feces. Sometimes drugs chelate beneficial metals, such as zinc, and can result in significant depletion. *See also* Poison.

Chelation Therapy

A controversial therapy involving the use of chelating agents, which are chemicals used to treat heavy metal poisoning, to treat other disorders.

Chelation therapy grew out of the standard medical treatment for removing toxic metals, like lead, from the bloodstream. The chemicals most frequently used are EDTA, ethylenediaminetetraacetic acid, BAL 9dimercaprol), penicillomine, and desferrioxamine (for iron poisoning).

In addition, chelation therapy has been administered as part of a comprehensive program involving diet, exercise, and the cessation of smoking or other drugs. A chelation session may take several hours and will often be accompanied by the introduction of vitamins and nutritional supplements.

Chelation therapy has been used in treating atherosclerosis; circulatory disorders that result in leg cramps; and degenerative disorders such as arthritis, scleroderma, gangrene and lupus. It is not approved by the FDA. *See also* GANGRENE; POISONING; *and* SCLERODERMA.

Chemonucleoysis

The injection of the enzyme chymopapin into a prolapsed disk to dissolve the center of the disk and relieve pressure.

Chemonucleolysis is performed to relieve sciatica, a painful condition resulting from a prolapsed disk pressing against the spinal nerve root. In chemonucleolysis, the enzyme chymopapin is injected into the prolapsed disk. This enzyme dissolves the soft center of the disk (nucleus pulposis), thus relieving pressure. It does not affect healthy surrounding tissue.

Chemonucleolysis may be used when treatments such as bed rest and traction prove ineffective. It is less invasive than surgical removal of the disk or decompression of the spinal nerve root. Usually the procedure results in relief. There is a postoperative period of recuperation of lower back pain that can range from a few days to two weeks. *See* PROLAPSED DISK *and* SCIATICA.

Chemotherapy

A general term used to describe a course of medication to combat cancer.

There are two main avenues to attack cancer. Local therapies, such as radiation and surgery, treat cancer where it is located. Systemic therapies, such as chemotherapy, affect the entire body. In chemotherapy, drugs circulate in the bloodstream and attack tumors that are unreachable by local means. They may have begun to spread throughout the body (metastasized), or have been partially removed by surgery or radiation but still have the potential to return.

Major types of chemotherapy include:
- **Alkylating agents**, such as cyclophosphamide and Cis-platin, attack the cancer DNA directly so cancer cells cannot grow. Side effects include nausea, vomiting, hair loss, blood in the urine, low blood cell counts, low sperm counts in men, and a long-term risk of leukemia.
- **Asparaginase** removes an enzyme from the blood that leukemia needs to support growth. In addition to nausea and vomiting, asparaginase can cause fever and high blood sugar levels.
- **Hormone therapies** raise or lower hormone content in the blood. These limit some tumors that need hormones for growth. Examples include flutamide for prostate cancer and tamoxifen for breast cancer.
- **Anti-metabolites**, such as 5-fluorouracil and methotrexate, prevent DNA replication by interfering with the building blocks of DNA, purines and pyrimidines.
- **Antibiotics**, such as doxorubicin (adriamycin), and bleomycin, attack cancer DNA, with side effects similar to those of alkylating agents. In addition, they may darken the skin and may cause kidney failure, heart failure, and lung disease.
- **Antimitotic Agents**, such as taxol, vincristine, and vinblastine, bind to microtubles in cells and prevent cell division.
- **Interferon** is used to combat multiple myeloma and Kaposi's sarcoma. It works by stimulating the body's own immune system to fight the cancer.

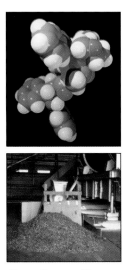

Chemotherapy. Top, an illustration of a taxol molecule; Monroe E. Wall and Mansukh C. Wani isolated taxol in 1967. Since then it has been used as a paradigm for new chemotherapy treatment. Above, the Pacific yew tree (Taxux brevifolia) is used in the synthesis of anticancer drugs including Paclitaxel. The National Cancer Institute, in cooperation with private research institutions, continue to work to make this treatment—as well as synthetically similar treatments that come from the Himalayan yew—more readily available. Below, an image of cisplatin crystals; this is a type of chemotherapy that is given as an infusion into a vein or under the skin.

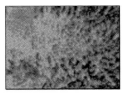

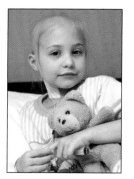

Cancer Treatment.
While chemotherapy is a useful tool in the battle against cancer, one of the most notable side effects is rapid hair loss; the hair usually grows back when the treatment is over. Below, this mouse has been engineered so that its bone marrow is protected from the effects of chemotherapy.

Side Effects and their Treatment

• *NAUSEA AND VOMITING* are controllable with anti-emetics. Nausea in particular can be controlled by eating small, frequent meals. Marijuana has proven to reduce the discomfort of nausea and vomiting and is slowly becoming recognized by state governments as a legitimate means of countering these side effects of chemotherapy.

• *HAIR LOSS* results from many of the chemotherapies. The hair will grow back after the course of treatment has ended. If scarves or hats seem inappropriate, a person may wish to buy a wig.

• *LOW BLOOD CELL COUNTS* usually do not need to be treated, but if low red cell count (anemia) is severe, it can be treated with transfusions. Low white cell count increases risk of infection, which may require antibiotics. Platelets can also be added to the blood by transfusion if there is risk of bleeding.

• *STERILITY* or induction of menopause is sometimes a side effect of chemotherapy.

• **Retinoic acid** is used to treat acute myelocytic leukemia.
• **STI-157** is used to treat chronic myelogenous leukemia.

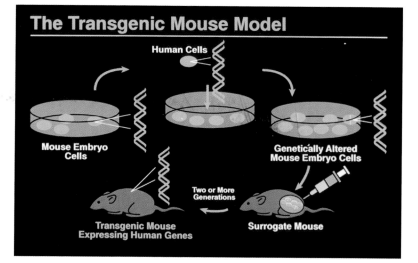

The Transgenic Mouse Model

Human Cells

Mouse Embryo Cells

Genetically Altered Mouse Embryo Cells

Two or More Generations

Transgenic Mouse Expressing Human Genes

Surrogate Mouse

For many cancers, the therapy of choice is a combination of surgery, radiation, and several of the drugs mentioned above.

The problem with all chemotherapies is that these chemicals attack all cells whether they are cancerous or not. Thus, drugs and their dosages must be carefully chosen to be effective against the cancer but minimize side effects. Many drugs are given together to cancer patients to prevent the tumor cells from becoming resistant to the chemotherapy. Some patients tolerate chemotherapy with few side effects. Others may need additional medications, such as anti-nausea medication, to counteract undesirable side effects.

> *Background material on chemotherapy can be found in* ANTICANCER DRUGS *and* CANCER. *For further information, see* RADIATION THERAPY *and* TUMOR. *See also* BREAST CANCER; COLON CANCER; *and* LUNG CANCER *for more on common types of cancer.*

Chenodiol

Medication used in the treatment of gallstones, taken orally to dissolve the stones.

Chenodiol (chenodeoxycholic acid) is a prescription medication taken to dissolve gallstones. It only works in patients who have a functional gallbladder and whose gallstones are made of cholesterol. Chenodiol is most effective when the stones are small and of the floating kind. A high-fiber diet may also be recommended to help dissolve the stones and to prevent new ones from forming.

Chenodiol should not be taken with antacids that contain aluminum, since this may diminish its effectiveness. Side effects may include diarrhea, constipation, nausea or vomiting, and stomach pain. *See also* GALLSTONES *and* FIBER.

Cherry Angioma

A benign skin growth that looks like a smooth, cherry-colored bump.

Cherry angiomas can occur anywhere on the body, although they usually appear on the trunk. They are usually painless but may bleed if injured.

Cherry angiomas occur commonly after the age of 40. Their cause is unknown. Cherry angiomas are not serious. If the angioma is unwanted, it can be removed using surgery, cryotherapy, or electrosurgery. Removal usually does not cause scarring. *See also* BENIGN *and* SKIN.

Chest Pain

Discomfort in the chest region that may vary in severity, type of sensation, and location.

Chest pain comes in many forms, can have many different causes, and can be nothing more than a minor annoyance. But it can also be an urgent signal of a life-threatening condition—it is the second most common symptom of heart disease, ranking just behind shortness of breath.

NONCARDIAC CAUSES

Chest pain that is not caused by a heart disorder may stem from a condition such as a muscle strain or a broken or bruised rib. An infection such as bronchitis or pneumonia can cause chest pain by inflaming the tissue that lines the lungs. Bronchitis in the airways of the lung can cause pain in the upper chest that becomes worse when the patient coughs. Acid indigestion can cause the discomfort behind the breastbone called heartburn, and the viral infection called shingles can cause severe pain in the chest, accompanied by skin blisters.

CARDIAC CAUSES

Angina Pectoris. The most common chest pain related to heart disease is angina pectoris. It occurs when the heart muscle does not receive enough oxygen because the arteries that carry blood to it become narrowed, usually from a buildup of deposits containing cholesterol. Angina pectoris resembles the pain of a severe bout of indigestion. It is often felt as a heavy pressure in the center of the chest, often spreading out to the jaw, throat, or arms. Angina is usually brought on by physical exertion; even a brisk walk can increase the heart's demand for oxygen beyond the ability of narrowed arteries to meet. Emotional stress can also increase the burden on the heart, as can a heavy meal, which requires extra oxygen for digestion.

Pericarditis. This is another common chest pain, and it may sometimes cause pain severe enough to mimic a heart attack. The pain is caused by friction when

the two membranes that cover the lung and heart become inflamed and rub against each other. Diagnosis of pericarditis can be made by a physician, who listens for the sound through a stethoscope.

Mitral valve prolapse. This is deformation of the valve between chambers of the heart; it can cause sharp pain on the left side of the chest that does not require emergency treatment. It can be diagnosed by the sound, or murmur, caused by backflow of blood through the valve.

Aortic Valve Regurgitation. Chest pain resembling that of angina can be caused by another valve problem, aortic valve regurgitation, due to malformation of or damage to the main valve through which blood flows out of the heart.

Arrhythmia. This is abnormal heartbeat; it can also cause chest pain or pressure that can be mistaken for angina.

Dissection of the Aorta. One cause of chest pain requiring emergency treatment is dissection of the aorta, a disruption of the inner lining of the main artery from the heart. Dissection produces pain that radiates out from the front to the back of the chest, or from between the shoulder blades. This disorder is most common in older people with high blood pressure that has produced an aneurysm, a ballooning out of the wall of the aorta. *See also* CONGESTIVE HEART FAILURE; CORONARY HEART DISEASE; HEART; HEART ATTACK; *and* STRESS.

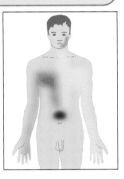

Angina. Above, an image of angina. This is a form of recurring chest pain that affects certain sections of the chest whenever part of the heart is not receiving enough oxygen. It often feels as though another person is pressing on the body or squeezing tightly just below the ribs or breast bone. Angina can usually be treated with some simple lifestyle changes that reduce a person's risk of suffering such pains.

Chest X-Ray

Use of x-rays to create an image of the chest region for diagnosis.

X-rays are useful in medicine because they can penetrate soft tissue but are absorbed by bone and other dense structures. This property allows a physician to produce an image of the body's interior, which can be a vital diagnostic aid. Chest x-rays are most useful for diagnosis when they can be compared with an earlier chest image of the same patient. The doctor can then identify changes and irregularities over time.

Examination of the lungs with chest x-rays allows the physician to detect unhealthy tissue, which appears whiter than normal lung tissue. The technique is helpful in the diagnosis of pneumonia, collapsed lung (atelectasis), lung cancer, emphysema, or fluid around the lung (pleural effusion).

Suspicion of heart disease usually requires a chest x-ray, taken from the side and from the back. The doctor will note the size and shape of the heart and will use the image to visualize the blood vessels of the chest.

Abnormal shape or size of the heart will be apparent, as will calcium deposits in heart tissue and other irregularities of the heart muscle.

The condition of the lung's blood vessels, also readily detected, is sometimes a key diagnostic indicator for certain heart diseases, such as constrictive pericarditis, in which the heart undergoes scarring but remains the same size and as in heart failure.

Standard chest x-ray may be supplemented with a battery of noninvasive imaging procedures, including CT and MRI. The field of radiological diagnostics is growing continuously as new technologies are applied to medical situations.

> *For background information on chest x-ray, see* LUNG IMAGING *and* X-RAY. *Related material can be found in* BRONCHITIS; DIAGNOSIS; LUNG CANCER; PNEUMONIA; *and* RESPIRATORY SYSTEM. *See also* CAT SCAN; MRI; *and* PET SCAN *for more on other imaging techniques.*

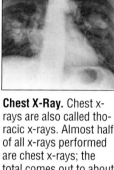

Chest X-Ray. Chest x-rays are also called thoracic x-rays. Almost half of all x-rays performed are chest x-rays; the total comes out to about 145 million images per year in the United States.
Above, an x-ray of the chest. If possible, have a thoracic imaging specialist or a certified radiologist interpret any findings. As important as chest x-rays are, they sometimes produce poor-quality images.

Resources on Chicken Pox

Behrman, Richard E., *Nelson's Textbook of Pediatrics* (1996); Burg, Fredric D., ed., *The Treatment of Infants, Children, and Adolescents* (1990); Fettner, Ann Guidici, *The Science of Viruses* (1990); Grist, Norman R., et al.

Cheyne-Stokes Respiration

Abnormal variation in rate and depth of breathing.

Cheyne-stokes respiration is characterized by progressively slower and shallower breaths that eventually result in a temporary stop in breathing, which may last for 20 seconds before breathing is resumed. Resumed breathing is deep and rapid, and the pattern is begun again.

Cheyne-stokes respiration can be caused by a disease, stroke, or head injury that affects the part of the brain that controls breathing, by a drug overdose, or by heart failure—which slows blood circulation enough to affect respiration. It can also occur in healthy people unaccustomed to high altitudes. Treatment is directed at any underlying condition. *See also* ALTITUDE SICKNESS; HEAD INJURY; *and* RESPIRATION; STROKE;

Chickenpox

An extremely contagious viral disease spread by contact or through airborne droplets of water.

The virus that causes chickenpox is called *Varicella zoster*; the disease is technically called varicella. A person with chickenpox remains contagious from the first symptoms until the last blisters have formed hard crusts. It is frequently considered a disease of childhood, since once a person has had it, he or she will be immune for the rest of his or her life.

SYMPTOMS

Symptoms of chickenpox begin two to three weeks after exposure. Low-grade fever, mild headache, and general malaise are common among adult sufferers. Children may have none of these early symptoms. Within a day or two, a rash of small red spots appear, which soon turn into raised bumps that blister and itch. The blisters then open, drain, and crust over. The spots originate on the face, head, and neck, and quickly spread to the body and arms. Spots in the mouth and throat open into ulcers that may make swallowing painful. Spots in the voice box and chest may make breathing difficult. Lymph nodes on the sides of the neck may become swollen and tender. In a week or two the full course of the disease is completed, with all spots crusted over and healing.

Reye's Syndrome

Children or teenagers with chickenpox or other viral diseases should not be given aspirin. For reasons that are not understood, salicylate (the active ingredient in aspirin) in the presence of a virus increases the incidence of Reye's syndrome by more than 30 times. Reye's syndrome is a rare but life-threatening disease that causes the brain to swell and fat to accumulate in the liver. Four or five days after the onset of chickenpox, a child with Reye's syndrome may develop severe nausea and vomiting, followed after a day or so by confusion, agitation, seizures, and coma. The child may die soon afterwards.

Treatment for chickenpox is bed rest and clear fluids to avoid dehydration. Aspirin should not be given to children, because of the risk of Reye's syndrome. Wet compresses on the skin and showers with a mild antibacterial soap reduce the possibility of bacterial infection. Antiviral agents (Acyclovir) can be used in severe cases. Scratching can promote infection and may lead to scarring.

A chickenpox vaccine is available; it is not recommended for people with compromised immune systems. Children recover from chickenpox easily with few complications. Adults run the risk of contracting pneumonia, which can be fatal. Enlarged heart, heart murmur, enlarged liver, and inflamed joints are also associated with chickenpox and can cause pain. Infection of the skin sores by bacteria is possible, and brain infections have been reported, causing headache, convulsions, and vomiting.

Background material on chickenpox can be found in Viruses. *For further informaiton, see* Antiviral Drugs; Bacteria; Fever; Lymphatic System; Pneumonia; Reye's Syndrome; Seizure; Vaccine; *and* Vomiting.

Chigger Bite

Irritating bite of the blood-sucking larva of the harvest mite.

Chiggers are six-legged reddish larval parasites that inhabit grass and weeds in warm months and exist worldwide.

The larvae attach themselves to human skin if contact is made, generally to the areas of the feet, legs, waist, armpits, and groin. They attach themselves with specialized mouth parts and inject a saliva beneath the skin that destroys skin cells and produces intense irritation known as redbug dermatitis. Infested areas become swollen and may develop a blister. The Asian species of chigger carries tiny organisms (rickettsia) that produce scrub typhus in humans. Chigger bites, in general, are entries for dirt and may result in tetanus.

Insect repellents offer significant protection against chiggers. Checking clothing and target areas of the body after traveling in wooded areas is also advisable. The bites are treated by lancing the blister with a sterilized needle and removing the chigger with sterilized tweezers. Antiseptic cream and a bandage are then applied to the wound. *See also* Insect bites; Parasite; Rickettsia; Tetanus; *and* Typhus.

Chigoe

Also known as a sand flea

Parasitic flea, *Tunga penetrans*, found in tropical and subtropical regions of the Americas and Africa.

In a chigoe infestation, the pregnant female burrows into the skin, most often on the feet or legs. The skin around the flea swells, becomes itchy, and ulcerates, forming an open sore. Severe chigoe infestation may make walking painful and difficult, and the ulcers may develop secondary infections. Chigoes can be removed surgically. Since most chigoes are picked up through direct contact with infested soil, prevention includes eradicating chigoe populations and wearing protective clothing in infested areas. *See* Parasite *and* Skin.

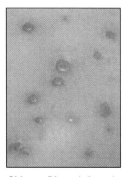

Chigger Bites. Infested chigger bite ares become swollen and may develop blisters. This inflammation is sometimes referred to as chigger dermatitis. It is quite common in tropical areas and forested areas around the United States. Hikers, campers, mountain climbers and naturalists should be especially aware of the effects and incidence of chigger bites before going into a new environment.

Child Abuse

Physical or emotional mistreatment of a child.

Child abuse is the willful infliction of injury, pain, or suffering on a child by an adult. It includes physical, emotional, or sexual mistreatment or neglect of a child by a parent, caregiver, or other adult. Child abuse not only may result in physical harm, but can cause lasting emotional and psychological damage. Children from infancy to late adolescence, are vulnerable to abuse. The definition of what constitutes child abuse varies from culture to culture.

Physical abuse is the deliberate use of force on a child, which may result in injury.

Emotional abuse refers to attacks on a child's sense of self. Humiliation, isolation, rejection, intimidation, and name-calling are all forms of emotional abuse.

Sexual abuse involves any type of sexual behavior directed at a child under any circumstances; any sexual activity is considered abusive, even if the child appears to consent.

Neglect consists of deliberate failure by a parent or caregiver to provide basic necessities such as food, clothing, shelter, medical care, or supervision.

INCIDENCE
It is difficult to determine the actual incidence of child abuse, as many cases go unreported. Over the last decade, there has been an increase in the cases of abuse reported. At least 500,000 children are physically abused in the United States each year, and many more are emotionally abused, sexually abused, or neglected.

CAUSES
Child abuse and neglect occur in all socioeconomic, religious, and ethnic groups. While abuse may have a number of different causes, some factors are common to nearly all cases of abuse.

Abusive behavior is often a maladaptive response to stress and feelings of powerlessness. Abusive parents were often abused as children; they may repeat the same patterns they suffered in childhood, often mistaking that they are exercising legitimate parental rights.

Marital conflict, domestic violence, employment problems, and social isolation tend to create an environment conducive to abuse. Infants who are constantly ill or who were born prematurely may be more vulnerable. Children who are perceived as different, including disabled children, are also at greater risk.

SYMPTOMS
Multiple injuries in various stages of healing are an indication of possible physical abuse. Other signs include: bruises or abrasions; burns; fractures and dislocations, particularly in children under two; and delays in seeking medical attention.

Sleep disturbances, physical complaints with no medical basis, low self-esteem, and depression are all signs of emotional abuse.

The genitals, anus, and mouth are the main areas that show signs of sexual abuse. Indications may include bruises, sores, and other injuries in these areas.

Hunger, inadequate attire for the weather, and extremely irregular attendance at school may all be signs of neglect.

Symptoms that appear to indicate the presence of abuse may actually reflect other emotional or physical problems in a child's life.

Individuals who suspect abuse should report their concerns to a school official, child welfare agency, social service department, or local police department. In many states, physicians are required by law to report suspected child abuse.

PREVENTION
Increasing the perceived value of children and the economic self-sufficiency of families, discouraging corporal punishment, and expanding the effectiveness of social services organizations are some steps toward prevention. Programs to help parents provide for their children and educate parents about child behavior are effective ways of preventing abuse within the family. *See also* DISABILITY; INCEST; *and* SEXUAL ABUSE.

Resources on Child Abuse
Barnett, Ola W., Cindy-Lou Miller-Perrin, and Robert D. Perrin, *Family Violence Across the Lifespan: An Introduction* (1997); Levine, Murray, *Helping Children: A Social History* (1992); Pagelow, Mildred, *Family Violence* (1984); American Academy of Family Physicians, Tel. (800) 274-2237, Online: www. aafp.org; Child Abuse Prevention Network, Online: Http://child-abuse.com.

Child Development

Physical, mental, and social growth of a child.

From birth until adolescence, children develop fundamental skills: motor control, self-care, intellectual accomplishments, and social interaction. Generally, a child's development is predictable and conforms to a certain order. Rates of development, however, can differ drastically from one child to the next; children may learn some skills easily and take more time to learn other skills. Only extremes of development—whether advanced or delayed—warrant consultation with a pediatrician.

Genetics, factors while in the uterus, and postbirth environments all influence a child's development. A child's capacity to learn depends on the normal growth of the nervous system. Any intellectual or sensory defect can lead to a delay in normal physical or mental development. For example, a baby born near its due date benefits from time in the uterus that a premature baby loses; the latter's growth should be tracked from the due date and not the birth date.

The role played by a healthy home environment is paramount to a child's health and quality and rate of development. Factors ranging from nutrition to interactions with others can affect a child's development on many levels. For example, a child of two or three who does not interact with other children will not receive sufficient stimulation to facilitate learning social, language, intellectual, and physical skills.

BEFORE THE AGE OF ONE
An infant develops the ability to control movement slowly. The jerky reflexes of a newborn are gradually replaced by conscious movement. This usually works from the top down: first comes a mastery of the head, followed by improved coordination of the arms, trunk, and legs. The baby gains strength by efforts to lift the head, sit up, and maintain balance while sitting.

Immediately after birth, a baby's eyes cannot focus on faraway objects or stay settled on an object unless it is extremely close to the face. Soon, the baby notices its hands and uses them to practice hand-eye coordination, moving the hands and trying to follow them with the eyes. In this way the baby learns how to focus and judge distances.

Crying is an infant's sole means of communication. A three-week-old infant will cry when hungry every two to three hours. Up to twelve weeks of age, some crying will have a mysterious cause and the child may remain inconsolable. Once able to connect hearing and vision, a baby pays attention to parents' mouths, progressing from smiling to uttering sounds. An infant knows a parent's face and voice and is comforted by hearing voices and singing. Finger or thumb-sucking is normal and comforting and should not be discouraged.

A six- to eight-week-old infant eats every three to four hours and becomes irritable at the end of the day. At four months, the infant may be able to eat solid food, but learning how to swallow requires a lot of practice and parental patience. The infant sleeps six to twelve hours each night and becomes visibly and audibly frustrated when unable to turn over.

At seven months, eating becomes a way of practicing motor skills; small bite-sized foods are best. Objects will be dropped again and again in an ongoing exploration of cause and effect. Everything becomes a toy, and many objects find their way to the child's mouth. Harmful objects should be placed out of reach, and the baby should be carefully monitored to prevent choking.

At nine months the child may become irritable and demand to feed himself; he may be successfully preoccupied by having something else to hold on to and examine while being fed. The child will better learn how to go to sleep if the parent refrains from picking him up every time he cries.

FROM AGE ONE TO THREE
A one-year-old begins to develop a sense of independence. One way this may appear is in food-fights; food may be rationed and doled out in increments to prevent messes and reward civil eating habits. Speech and body language blossoms; parents should

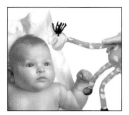

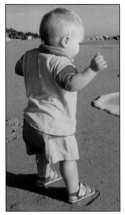

The Early States. Above, images of the early stages of human development. A small child will develop hand-eye coordination by playing with toys in the crib; this can be an important skill at any age. Bottom, by their first birthday some children are beginning to walk.

Milestones in Child Development

Between six and seven months of age most children can:
- Sit without support and hold the head steady when in a sitting position
- Bear some weight on the legs when held as if to stand
- Control head and arm movements, grasp items, and transfer objects from one hand to the other; babies of this age are not yet clearly right or left handed
- Investigate cause and effect—for example, what happens when a toy falls from the baby's hands to the floor
- Recognize the parents and distinguish between familiar and unfamiliar people
- Expect to be fed, dressed, and bathed
- Enjoy being cuddled
- Babble vowel sounds and about half of the consonants

At nine months, most children can:
- Crawl and sit up unassisted, and possibly pull themselves up to stand and walk a bit, supported by furniture or a caregiver
- Be aware when a favorite toy has been taken away and demand it back
- Try to get objects that are out of reach
- Play games such as peekaboo
- Babble words such as "mama" and "dada"
- Begin to understand what the word "no" means
- Exhibit specific emotional attachment to the primary caregiver and protest being left with another caregiver

By age one, most children can:
- Begin trying to walk
- Play interactive games such as pattycake
- Pick up small objects with thumb and forefinger
- Drink from a cup and feed themselves
- Possibly say "mama" and "dada," and perhaps one other word
- Respond to simple commands and their own name
- Express anger, affection, fear of strangers, and curiosity

At eighteen months, most children can:
- Eat, if sloppily, with a knife and fork
- Run, kick a ball, and draw with crayons
- Possibly act dependent on their parents, have temper tantrums, and do the opposite of what they are told

At ages two to three, most children can:
- Jump off a step, ride a tricycle, color with crayons, and build a tower of blocks
- Copy their parents' actions
- Enjoy playing alongside another child, though they are extremely possessive
- Try to give orders and ignore their parents' commands

Most children between the ages of three and four can:
- Stand on one leg, jump up and down, and draw a circle and a cross
- Share and cooperate with other children
- Be afraid of the dark
- Act affectionately toward their parents
- Develop ideas about sex roles; they may identify with the same sex parent and develop a romantic attachment toward the opposite sex parent
- Take pleasure in their genital development and exhibit curiosity about other children's bodies

By four or five years of age, most children can:
- Exhibit mature motor control: skip, broad-jump, dress themselves, and copy a square and a triangle
- Speak clearly
- Use adult speech patterns and know basic grammar
- Relate a story and use over 2,000 words

listen closely and echo words. Separation fears surface, as the child learns the difference between friends, family, and strangers. The child begins to learn to walk. Creating a safe, closed environment can both reassure and contain the child.

At 15 months, the child will imitate the parent's speech and become frustrated by his shortcomings; pushing the child to speak may actually slow progress. Sounds become signals; for example, the slam of a car door can mean a parent is home. Rhythms in games are sensed.

An 18-month-old begins to learn from observing and interacting with other children; having playmates becomes important to development. Parents should keep an eye on the child always, as he may run away or act rashly. Some children of this age have a vocabulary of close to 200 words.

A child of between two and three years old may start to speak in short sentences, control and explore the world using language, and develop a brief stutter. Emotionally, the child will still display a fear of separation from parents. The child may also display violent emotions, anger, a sense of humor, and negativity.

In Later Childhood

Children of four or five take pride in their accomplishments and enjoy responsibilities. They prefer to play with other children and usually engage in stereotypical sex-appropriate activities. Four to five-year-olds want to fit in with the crowd and usually try to conform to others their age.

In late childhood, before the start of adolescence, children try to meet the expectations of family, classmates, and school successfully. It is important during this stage that children learn how to deal with frustration without developing low self-esteem or feelings of inferiority.

For background information on child development, see DNA *and* Gene. *Related material can be found in* Chromosome; Crying in Infants; Genetics; Infant; Learning Disabilities; Nutrition; Pediatrics; Puberty; Prematurity; Reflex; School Phobia; Separation Anxiety; Speech; Speech Disorders; *and* Stuttering.

Childbirth

The process of giving birth.

Giving birth, which consists of labor and delivery, is the culmination of nine months of pregnancy. A vaginal delivery, in which the baby emerges from the birth canal, propelled by contractions, is the most common. However, some births, for reasons ranging from fetal distress to the baby being too large to pass easily through the birth canal, require surgical intervention in the form of a Cesarean section.

Few women deliver exactly on their expected due date. Delivery can occur anywhere from two weeks before to two weeks after the projected date. A baby is considered premature if it is born before the 37th week of pregnancy. Postmaturity is when the baby is born after 42 weeks. Both types of labor carry their own risks.

WHEN LABOR BEGINS

First time mothers, and even those who have given birth before, may have trouble distinguishing real labor from false. Real labor is characterized by regular contractions that are from 10 to 20 minutes apart at first and last 45 seconds to one minute. Within an hour or two they become more frequent. True contractions begin in the lower back and travel across the front of the abdomen, which hardens in response.

Another sign of real labor that is usually seen is a blood-tinged clump of mucus known as the "show." This is the mucus plug that sealed the neck of the uterus during pregnancy. The show may appear up to a few days before labor actually begins.

Rupture of the membranes, or "breaking the waters," is a sudden flow of liquid, in a gush or slow leak. During pregnancy, the baby is surrounded by amniotic fluid that acts as a protective cushion. Rupture of the membrane may occur from shortly before labor to well into labor.

False labor is often associated with Braxton-Hicks contractions, which appear from the fourth month of pregnancy on and intensify toward the end of pregnancy. Some women may also mistake "lightening," the sensation when the baby settles further down in the pelvis in preparation for birth, for the onset of labor.

LABOR

Once labor has begun, it is important that the mother not eat any solid food. If anesthesia is administered, a full stomach can result in severe nausea and complicate delivery. The mother should also try to empty her bladder frequently.

Labor and delivery consist of three stages. The first stage, which lasts the longest (18 hours or more in first births is not unusual), consists of gradually strengthening contractions at increasingly closer intervals. These contractions cause the cervix to start to open (dilate) and thin out (efface). In women who have previously given birth, it is not unusual for the cervix to begin dilating and effacing somewhat during the last month of pregnancy. This stage is completed when the cervix is at 10 cm dilation and is completely effaced.

During this stage, the mother may move around. Walking can in fact help advance labor. The contractions gradually intensify and occur at closer intervals. The woman should notify her doctor that labor has begun. For first babies, unless the mother lives far from the hospital or there are other concerns, it is usually recommended

Procedures Encountered During Labor

- *Episiotomy*—a small incision made between the vagina and anus to prevent any rips from occurring when the skin is stretched by delivery. A cut is easier to repair than a tear. These are the "stitches" many women have after giving birth.
- *Fetal monitoring*—belt monitors placed over the mother's abdomen during labor keep track of the baby's heart rate. The heart rate increases in response to a contraction. Sometimes, a monitor is attached to the fetus' scalp, or a small sample of blood is withdrawn to test oxygen and acidity levels.
- *Induction*—in case of postmaturity or failure of labor to progress, various drugs are administered to the mother to induce or strengthen contractions. The most common drug is pitocin, which is very similar to the body's natural labor hormone, oxytocin.

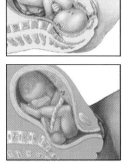
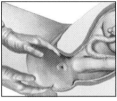
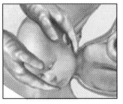
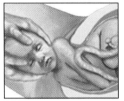

Birth. Doctors must first evaluate the delivery presentation, that is, the position the fetus is in as it comes down the birthing canal. If the fetus is in Cephalic presentation (top) normal childbirth procedures are used (as illustrated by the bottom three images) But if the fetus is in breech position, second from the top, a Cesarean section may be necessary.

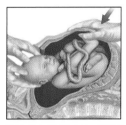

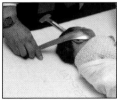

Cesarean Section. Top, with both hands the surgeon reaches into the abdominal incision and lifts the baby's head as an assistant pushed down on the upper uterus. Bottom, forceps may be used to assist the surgeon in removing the baby from the abdomen.

Resources on Childbirth

Gonik, Bernard and Renee A. Bobrowski, *Medical Complications in Labor and Delivery* (1996); Karte, Diana and Roberta M. Scaer, *A Good Birth, A Safe Birth* (1991); New, Maria I., *Diagnosis and Treatment of the Unborn Child* (1999); Sears, William, et al., *The Pregnancy Book: Month-by-Month, Everything You Need to Know From America's Baby Experts* (1997); International Childbirth Education Association, Inc., Tel. (612) 854-8660, Online: www.icea.org; Maternity Center Asso-ciation, Tel. (212) 777-5000, Online: www.ma-ternity.org; Universe of Women's Health, Tel. (512) 418-2922, Online: www.obgyn.net; www.ny-cornell.org/obgyn/.

that she go to the hospital when the contractions are about five minutes apart. For women who have given birth before, the recommended time is when contractions are 10 minutes apart, as subsequent labors generally progress faster.

It is important that the mother remain relaxed, as tensing up or trying to fight the contractions just makes them worse. Many women find Lamaze techniques of controlled breathing to be useful. Various medications are available if the mother so desires. Other women prefer to try alternative means of pain management such as hypnosis or acupuncture.

DELIVERY

The second stage, which lasts about 50 minutes in first mothers and 20 minutes in later prognancies, consists of pushing the baby out. This stage begins when the cervix is fully dilated. The mother starts feeling an uncontrollable urge to push, and is encouraged to bear down and push with each contraction, which helps propel the baby down the birth canal.

Pain Management in Labor

Natural childbirth refers to giving birth without the use of drugs or anesthesia. Often women who choose natural childbirth seek alternative ways of managing pain, such as Lamaze breathing techniques, hypnosis, or acupuncture.

Analgesics can relieve pain and help the mother relax between contractions. Common medications include narcotics, tranquilizers, and barbiturates. All of these cross the placenta and can affect the baby. If administered too early, they can slow labor.

General anesthesia is rarely used during childbirth, except in cases of emergency Cesarean sections. Regional anesthesia such as epidurals are more common. In an epidural, a local anesthetic is inserted into the space below the spinal column, resulting in a loss of sensation in the lower body. This may or may not interfere with the urge to push. If administered too early, an epidural can slow labor. It can also cause a headache or a sudden drop in blood pressure. A less common regional anesthetic is the spinal block, in which a local anesthetic is injected into the membrane surrounding the spinal cord. Its benefits and disadvantages are roughly similar to those of an epidural.

Most babies are born head first, with the face downward. The baby is said to have crowned when the head is visible from the vaginal opening. The doctor helps to maneuver each shoulder out of the birth canal. Once the shoulders are free, the rest of the body follows quickly.

Once the baby has emerged, labor and delivery are still not over. The third stage involves the delivery of the placenta, or afterbirth. The placenta has usually already separated from the uterine wall in response to contractions; the doctor may tug gently on the umbilical cord, taking care not to damage it. In rare circumstances the placenta may have to be surgically removed. Once the placenta has emerged, it is examined to make sure that no pieces have broken off and been left behind. Any retained portions of the placenta can contribute to postpartum hemorrhage.

Many women breast-feed on the delivery table, which, in addition to being a way of bonding with the baby, stimulates contractions that can assist with pushing out the afterbirth. *See* EMERGENCY CHILDBIRTH.

Childbirth Complications

Difficulties or abnormal situations that arise during the process of giving birth.

In most cases, an uneventful pregnancy is followed by a smooth labor and delivery of a healthy child. However, various complications can arise in childbirth. These may stem from due to preexisting health problems, the mother's age, or previous problems with childbirth. Sometimes complications arise or are diagnosed during pregnancy. Other times, however, complications appear without warning during the birth process itself.

Problems During Pregnancy. Maternal health problems, such as high blood pressure, uncontrolled diabetes, preeclampsia, and, eclampsia can all cause problems during pregnancy. If the threat to the mother's health becomes severe, it may be necessary to deliver the infant prematurely by Cesarean section.

Excessive Vaginal Bleeding. During early pregnancy this is usually indication of a possible miscarriage. Bleeding during the second half of pregnancy may be due to a damaged cervix or a problem with the placenta, such as placenta previa, in which the placenta is blocking the cervix, or placenta abruptio, in which the placenta prematurely separates from the uterine wall.

Preterm Labor. This occurs when labor begins before the 37th week of pregnancy. The baby may be born before it is capable of surviving outside the uterus. The lungs are the last organs to develop, and many premature infants have difficulty breathing. There is also an increased chance of neurological disorders. The earliest a baby can be born and have a 50 percent chance of survival is approximately 24 weeks.

If preterm labor is likely, an attempt is made to slow or stop labor. The mother may be placed on bedrest. If that does not help, she will be hospitalized. Drugs such as magnesium phosphate may be administered in an attempt to stop labor.

Post-Term Pregnancy. Postmaturity, or failure to go into labor after 42 weeks, carries its own risks. The baby depends on the placenta to provide it with oxygen and nutrients from the mother's bloodstream, and to eliminate wastes. If pregnancy has gone on too long, however, the placenta becomes "senile" and is no longer capable of fulfilling its functions. If pregnancy is very late, labor is induced with drugs.

Failure to Progress. Sometimes a woman remains in labor for several hours but does not progress to delivery. The contractions do not cause the cervix to dilate and efface. A drug such as pitocin may be administered to strengthen the contractions. If a woman has been in labor for over 24 hours without progressing, a Cesarean section may be performed.

Premature Rupture. Rupture of the membrane usually occurs at the beginning of or during labor. In premature rupture, labor does not begin shortly afterwards. Once the membranes have ruptured, there is an increased chance of infection; the mother may be hospitalized.

Abnormal Presentation. Most babies are born head first, with the face toward the mother's back. A breech baby lies in the uterus so that its feet or buttocks are located near the cervix. As a result, these are the first body parts to emerge from the birth canal. Breech presentation may interfere with the newborn's first attempts to breathe. Doctors can usually tell in advance that a baby is in a breech position and may attempt to turn the baby around.

Other abnormal presentations include occiput posterior, in which the baby is head down but turned toward the mother's front. Transverse presentation is when the baby is sideways in the uterus. The shoulder is usually blocking the birth canal, making vaginal delivery impossible. Of more immediate concern is the possibility that the umbilical cord will become obstructed, interfering with the baby's oxygen supply.

Shoulder Dystocia. This term refers to an uncommon situation during delivery in which the baby's shoulder gets jammed against mother's pubic bone.

Prolapsed Umbilical Cord. A prolapsed umbilical cord occurs when the umbilical cord emerges from the birth canal before the baby. The cord may become compressed, cutting off the baby's oxygen supply. Other problems with the umbilical cord can arise when the cord becomes entangled with the fetus.

Fetal Distress. The fetus is carefully monitored during labor. The fetal heart rate usually rises in response to a contraction. If fetal heart rate abnormalities occur, this may be an indication of fetal distress and may necessitate an emergency Cesarean section.

Retained Placenta. Usually, the placenta emerges after the baby is born. A retained placenta, in which part or all of the placenta remains in the uterus, can be a source of postpartum hemorrhage.

Background information on childbirth complications can be found in CHILDBIRTH; DELIVERY; *and* PREGNANCY. *For further information, see* BIRTH INJURY; BREECH DELIVERY; ECLAMPSIA; NATERNAL MORTALITY; PLACENTA PREVIA; POSTPARTUM HEMORRHAGE; PREECLAMPSIA; *and* PREMATURITY.

Chill

A sensation of cold, accompanied by goose bumps and shivering, that occurs when the body temperature rises, making the environment seem colder.

Normal body temperature is lowest in the early morning hours (as low as 97°F), but it rises during the day to a level as high as 99.3°F in the afternoon. A fever occurs when the body reacts to infection. When the body detects invading pathogens (disease-causing organism), the hypothalamus, a structure in the brain responsible for regulating body temperature, raises the temperature above normal. This makes it more difficult for the pathogens to survive and enhances the body's immune response to be more effective.

Often a fever rises and falls cyclically, resulting in chills alternating with a sensation of heat.

Treatment for chills includes drinking fluids and getting plenty of rest. A persistent chill, a very high fever, or a low-grade fever that persists for several days may require medical attention. *See also* FEVER *and* HYPOTHALAMUS .

Chinese Medicine

A preventive approach using a combination of medicinal plants, diet, acupuncture, massage, and exercise to diagnose and treat individuals.

Traditional Chinese Medicine (TCM) is an ancient system of medicine that is endorsed by the World Health Organization and presently used by more than a quarter of the world's inhabitants. TCM differs in approach from traditional Western medicine in that, instead of emphasizing the illness, TCM is concerned with how an illness manifests itself in the patient. Thus, treatment, through a combination of herbs and other therapies, is tailored to treat the specific bodily imbalances of the client.

Central to TCM is the idea of yin and yang, which describes the oppositional and complementary forces at work in every body. For instance, a practitioner of Chinese medicine might describe the patient's body condition in naturalistic terms (i.e. hot or cold, dry or wet), stressing the way these yin and yang characteristics must work in harmony with each other.

TCM also integrates the idea of *"ch'i"* (pronounced chee) into its understanding of physical wellness. *Ch'i* is understood as the vital flow of energy through the body. When a person's *ch'i* is blocked, illness and disease can result. Acupuncture is often prescribed to help "unclog" blocked pathways and restore the natural flow of *ch'i* through the body.

METHOD OF DIAGNOSIS

To ascertain a person's physical state, a practitioner of Chinese medicine will observe the following:

- Complexion, body and disposition
- Patient's response to questions about symptoms, medical history, and lifestyle
- Tone and quality of voice
- Bodily odor and excretions
- Rate of pulse where *ch'i* flows through the body.

The pulse determines the strength of *ch'i* throughout the body and the condition of the person's internal organs. After a careful evaluation using these tools, the doctor will make a diagnosis.

METHOD OF TREATMENT

Herbal medicine has long been a cornerstone in TCM. Most Chinese herbal remedies consist of six to 19 raw ingredients (mostly of plant origin) that have been dried and then boiled into soups or teas. Sometimes these can also be processed into pills, powders, and topical ointments.

TCM encourages a patient to combine medicinal herbs, acupuncture, massage, and a well-balanced diet and exercise to promote overall wellness.

Background material on Chinese medicine can be found in ALTERNATIVE MEDICINE. *For further information, see* ACUPRESSURE *and* ACUPUNCTURE. *See also* AYURVEDIC MEDICINE *and* HOLISTIC MEDICINE *for more on other types of alternative medicine.*

Chinese Restaurant Syndrome

Adverse physical reaction to monosodium glutamate.

Chinese restaurant syndrome refers to the brief physical illness some sensitive individuals experience after ingesting monosodium glutamate (MSG), a seasoning and flavor enhancer often used in Chinese food. Since first reported in the 1960s, hundreds of studies have been carried out to determine whether the symptoms are actually caused by MSG. The results are not conclusive. While some tests suggest that MSG in high doses does cause the syndrome, the same symptoms have also been linked to consumption of other foods, such as coffee, chocolate, and alcohol.

Symptoms. Sensitivity to MSG include severe headaches, warmth and facial flushing, numbness, and tingling (mainly in the shoulders, neck, and face), and chest pain and pressure. These symptoms are temporary, and cause no lasting harm. In some asthmatics, MSG can induce an attack.

Prevention. People who experience symptoms of Chinese restaurant syndrome, should avoid foods containing MSG and read the ingredients of prepared foods and seasonings carefully. Both the Food and Drug Administration and the World Health Organization have deemed MSG safe for most people, even though its safety is being reexamined. Since MSG is high in sodium, those on a low sodium diet should avoid it or limit their consumption. *See* SODIUM.

Chiropractic

A form of therapy using adjustment and manipulation of the joints to alleviate conditions related to the nerves, muscles, bones, and joints.

Many of the principles on which contemporary chiropractic therapy is based were developed as part of the Chinese healing arts in the third century BC. Recent evidence suggests that the idea of soft-tissue manipulation, for instance, was introduced to the West through Chinese Confucian writings brought over by missionaries. In fact, many cultures have documents attesting to the use of similar techniques, such as massage, adjustment, and back-walking, as part of traditional healing therapies.

In the late 19th century, Daniel David Palmer, a teacher and magnetic healer (someone who performs hands-on healing therapy) discovered that he was able to restore a man's hearing by adjusting one of the vertebrae in his spine. Following this episode, Palmer went on to develop the foundational principles of modern chiropractic medicine. His technique is based on the premise that the health of the nervous system, and therefore the entire body, is contingent on the proper alignment of the spine.

By manipulating or adjusting these joints, Palmer believed that he was able to reduce undue pressure on the nerves; and thereby lessen tension, stiffness, and pain.

DIAGNOSIS

Today, chiropractors use two primary methods for diagnosing disorders. X-rays of the spine are taken in order to rule out any deformity or disease and to reveal the client's bone structure, providing a detailed view of the area of concern. Chiropractors also measure the range of motion in each of the joints to determine which regions are under the most stress.

TREATMENT

Before administering treatment, the chiropractor will take into consideration the client's age, shape, overall health, and the degree of pain that is suffered. Treatment involves a combination of two techniques, which employ mobilization and manipulation. Mobilization stretches the joint to its maximum range of mobility.

Manipulation consists of the adjustment of segments of the spine using a number of techniques to alleviate tension, swelling, and pain. Often the practitioner will apply short and rapid, twisting movements (high velocity, low amplitude) into the spinal cord in order to realign the vertebrae. Un-

Resources on Chiropractic

Pizzorno, Joseph E., et al., *Clinician's Handbook of Natural Medicine* (2001); Swenson, David, *Ashtanga Yoga* (1999); Tousley, Dirk, *The Chiropractic Hand-book for Patients* (1985); National Center for Complementary and Alternative Medicine, Tel. (888)644-6226, Online: nccam.nih.gov; American Chiropractic Association, Tel. (703) 276-8800, Online: www.amerchiro.org; Association for Applied Psychophysiology and Biofeedback, Tel. (303) 442-8892, Online: www.aapb.org; http://www.nycornell.org/medicine/gim/index.html.

like other forms of bodywork, the chiropractor will generally concentrate on specific areas of concern rather than on the entire body. The chiropractor may also suggest certain stretching exercises to be done in conjunction with regular therapy sessions. *See also* BACK PAIN *and* BODYWORK.

Chlamydia

A sexually transmitted disease caused by the parasitic organism *Chlamydia trachomatis*.

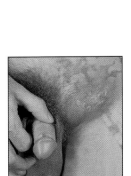

Chlamydia. Above, genital lesions on a man; these are caused by infection with the bacteria *Chlamydia trachomatis*. Chalamydia is a serious infection; it affects both men and women. In the United States, about 3 out of every 1,000 people are infected.

Chlamydia is usually transmitted by sexual activity. The bacteria are found in semen, vaginal fluid, and blood, so any exchange of these fluids can transmit the disease. It is the most widespread of venereal diseases. Since chlamydia can be asymptomatic, an accurate count of infected people is impossible; it is estimated, however, that 45 percent of sexually active teenagers have been exposed to the disease.

SYMPTOMS

Half of infected men and three-quarters of women have no symptoms. The major symptoms for men include a white, pus-like discharge from the penis, swollen testicles, and painful urination. For women there may be a yellow vaginal discharge, pain during urination, pain in the lower abdomen, pain during intercourse, nausea, and fever. Women may experience bleeding during intercourse or between periods. Some women with chlamydia also get cervicitis, an inflammation of the cervix.

DIAGNOSIS

A diagnosis may be based on the symptoms; if the disease is asymptomatic, it may not be diagnosed until complications appear. A new test for chlamydia has recently been made available, called the amplicor chlamydia trachomatis test. It is done with a sample of a man's urine or a swab from the woman's cervix or urethra. Results are available in four hours.

COMPLICATIONS

If the disease is left untreated, men may de-velop inflammation of the epididymis or testicles, which may lead to infertility. Women risk developing pelvic inflammatory disease (PID), which produces severe inflammation or scarring of the fallopian tubes and the lining of the uterus. This may lead to infertility, or the inflammation may cause a fertilized egg to become lodged in the fallopian tubes (ectopic pregnancy). If a pregnancy is normal, the bacteria can pass to the child, who may be born blind or may develop a severe case of pneumonia. Women who have chlamydia also have a much increased risk of acquiring HIV if exposed to the virus.

PREVENTION AND TREATMENT

Abstinence or a monogamous relationship with a partner known to be healthy are ways to prevent transmission. The use of condoms limits but does not completely eliminate transmission of the organism.

Infection must be treated with antibiotics, such as tetracycline and azithromycin. Sexual partners of people infected with chlamydia should also be tested for the disease and treated. Many people who have chlamydia also have gonorrhea. *See also* ANTIBIOTIC DRUGS; HIV; *and* SEXUALLY TRANSMITTED DISEASES.

Chloasma

Also known as melasma and mask of pregnancy

A discoloration of the skin of the face.

Chloasma refers to the darkening of patches of skin due to an increase in skin pigment. The condition is usually associated with pregnancy, although it can also be associated with other situations that increase the amount of female hormones in the body, such as taking birth control pills and hormone replacement therapy. Chloasma is not dangerous and does not need to be treated. Darkening may be lessened by avoiding sun exposure and female hormone intake. Bleaching preparations and, sometimes, chemical peels are used. *See also* CHILDBIRTH; ESTROGEN; HORMONES; PREGNANCY; *and* SKIN.

Chlorate Poisoning

The ingestion of toxic chlorates, which can result in kidney and liver damage.

Symptoms of chlorate poisoning include diarrhea, abdominal pain, and ulceration of the mouth.

TREATMENT

Skin that has come in contact with chlorates should immediately be washed with soap and water. Eyes should be flushed out with liberal amounts of water. In case of ingestion, medical help should be contacted immediately. Depending on the severity of symptoms and the amount of time elapsed since poisoning, treatment may involve administering oxygen or intravenous fluids, washing the stomach with activated charcoal, or even hemodialysis.

ALERT

Highly Toxic

Chlorates are highly toxic substance present in defoliant weed killers and fertilizers. Ingestion of chlorates can result in kidney and liver damage, corrosion of the intestine, a chemical change in hemoglobin (methemoglobinerria), and depression of the central nervous system. In some cases, ingestion can be fatal.

PREVENTION

Pesticides and fertilizers should be kept out of the reach of small children. When assisting a victim of chlorate poisoning, avoid direct contact with clothing that may be contaminated, and use rubber gloves while cleaning the toxins from hair and skin. *See also* ANTIFREEZE POISONING *and* POISONING .

Chloroform

A colorless, heavy, volatile liquid that produces a vapor that, if inhaled, acts as a general anesthetic.

Once widely used during surgical operations, chloroform was found to cause a high incidence of liver and heart problems. Its main uses today are as a solvent, fumigant, and insecticide, or as a flavoring and preservative for other medicines. Chloroform is rarely used as an emergency anesthetic for first aid or armed-service field surgery. *See also* ANESTHESIA, GENERAL; *and* SURGERY.

Chlorosis

A form of anemia resulting from iron deficiency.

A fairly rare disease that has all but disappeared, chlorosis was common during the 19th century and before the First World War in malnourished adolescent girls. Chlorosis is characterized by a greenish-yellow tinge to the skin. Other symptoms of anemia caused by this sort of iron deficiency include fatigue, pallor, breathlessness, and rarely, pica, a condition in which a person craves nonfood items. Iron deficiency anemia can be treated and often quickly reversed with the use of iron rich foods and supplements. It is most important to determine and treat the underlying cause of the iron deficiency. *See also* ANEMIA; IRON DEFICIENCY ANEMIA; IRON; NUTRITION; PICA; SKIN; *and* VITAMIN SUPPLEMENTS.

Chlorthalidone

Diuretic drug used primarily to treat hypertension.

Chlorthalidone is a thiazide diuretic, a drug that removes excess water and sodium from the body by acting on the area of the kidney known as the tubules, the structures that filter the blood to determine content of urine. It can be prescribed for conditions including congestive heart failure and liver disease, but its main use is in the treatment of high blood pressure .

While chlorthalidone generally causes few problems for patients, it can produce side effects such as lethargy, cramps, or impotence. Because some of these side effects are due to excess loss of potassium, patients taking the drug may also be told to take a potassium supplement. Pregnant women should consult their physician before taking this drug. *See also* ANTIHYPERTENSIVE DRUGS; DIURETIC DRUGS; *and* SODIUM.

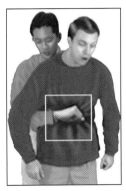

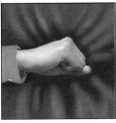

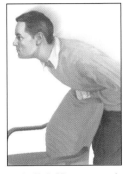

Heimlich Maneuver. A choking victim can be helped by using the Heimlich maneuver. Top, the person helping the victim should go behind the person, wrap their arms around the victims upper abdomen and thrust inward near the bottom of the rib cage (middle). Choking victims who are alone may use the back of a chair (bottom) to simulate the thrust another person would give them.

Choking

Partial or complete obstruction of the airway, resulting in coughing, gagging, or wheezing.

SYMPTOMS

A choking victim will not be able to speak. The person who is choking may, occasionally, place both hands around the neck or lean forward in an attempt to dislodge the obstruction. The victim is likely to make wheezing or snorting sounds and may become pale or blue in the face. Sometimes choking victims will faint.

If a person appears to be choking but there is no obstruction, he or she may actually be suffering from anaphylactic shock. This is a severe allergic reaction to food, medication, or an insect bite that results in shock and can be fatal in as little as 15 minutes. Accompanying symptoms may include hives, swelling, and redness or blueness of the skin (cyanosis).

TREATMENT

An object caught in the air passages may be removed by using the Heimlich maneuver (see picture). The Heimlich maneuver should only be preformed on a conscious person. Once normal breathing resumes, it is important to determine if any part of the object was inhaled into the lungs, since this can cause subsequent medical problems (pneumonia).

In all cases of blockage, emergency

ALERT

Preventing Choking in Children

- Keep chunks of meat or cheese, grapes, hard candy, and other foods that children may choke on, out of their reach. Nuts should not be given to any child under the age of seven.
- Teach older children not to offer foods that may cause choking to younger siblings.
- Cut firmer foods into small pieces before feeding to a small child.
- Teach children to chew well before swallowing.
- Children should never be allowed to run or play with food or drinking straws in their mouths.
- Always keep small toy parts and other household objects out of the reach of small children.

medical help should be sought immediately. If the Heimlich maneuver does not remove a blockage, or if there is no object in the air passages, medical technicians will decide if a surgical procedure on the airway should be used and whether or not the victim should be taken to the hospital. Oxygen deprivation for more than five or six minutes may cause brain damage.

CHOKING IN CHILDREN

Children beginning solid food for the first time and children under the age of four who do not chew their food well are at high risk for choking. Nuts, chunks of meat such as hot dogs and cheese, grapes, hard candy, and popcorn are the most dangerous foods for small children. Common household items may also pose a potential hazard to a young child's air passages. Rubber or latex balloons, coins, marbles, small parts of toys, pen caps, and button-type batteries are also frequent causes of airway obstructions. *See* ANAPHYLAXIS; ARTIFICIAL RESUSCITATION; CARDIOPULMONARY RESUSCITATION (CPR); *and* HEIMLICH MANEUVER; ANOXIA.

Cholangiocarcinoma

Cancer of the tissue lining the bile ducts of the liver and the gall bladder.

Cholangiocarcinoma is a malignancy of the epithelium lining the channels that transport bile from the liver and gallbladder to the small intestine. It is rare in Western countries, with only 1 case per 100,000 in the United States every year. The incidence is much higher in the eastern Hemisphere, where an underlying infestation with liver flukes is believed to be at least partially responsible. Symptoms are caused by blockage of the bile-ducts; they may include jaundice clay-colored stools, pain in the upper right abdomen, unexplained weight loss and loss of appetite, and fever or chills. Patients with chronic ulcerative colitis or sclerosing cholangitis are at higher risk for developing cholangiocarcinoma. *See also* BILE DUCT; CHOLANGITIS; GALL BLADDER; SMALL INTESTINE *and* ULCERATIVE COLITIS .

Cholangiography

Examination of the bile ducts by radiography.

Cholangiography is performed to examine the biliary ducts, which carry bile from the liver and gallbladder to the intestines. It is often used to assist a doctor in finding the exact location of a biliary obstruction after its discovery by computerized tomography (CT) scanning or ultrasound. Through this technique, a detailed view of the obstruction is possible.

Types. There are two types of cholangiography. In endotropic retrograde choiangiography (ERCP), the bile duct is evaluated via an endoscope and a contrast "dye" is injected into the bile duct through its opening into the intestines. X-ray images are then taken to outline the duct, assess its size, and detect any internal or external obstruction, such as gallstones or a tumor.

In percutaneous hepatic cholangiography (PCT), the contrast medium is injected directly into the liver. This technique gives a detailed picture of the bile duct. It is invasive, however, and carries the potential risk of side effects. The procedure may be performed under local or general anesthesia. A needle is inserted into the liver with the aid of a viewing instrument known as a fluoroscope. Contrast medium is injected while liver bile is aspirated by the needle. The liver is x-rayed at intervals to provide an ongoing record of activity. More recently, MRI has been used to make non-invasive cholangiography, and it may be suitable for some individuals.

Side Effects. Both types of cholangiography may result in nausea or hives. ERCP may cause pancreatitis, perforation, and bleeding. Complications of PTC include internal bleeding, bacterial infection of the blood (septicemia), and peritonitis caused by leakage of bile into the bloodstream.

Results. Irregular results of cholangiography may indicate any of the following abnormalities, possibly requiring prompt medical attention: jaundice caused by an obstruction of the biliary tract; gallstones; or cancer of the biliary system. *See also* BILIARY SYSTEM; CHOLANGIOCARCINOMA; GALLSTONES; JAUNDICE; PERITONITIS; AND SEPTICEMIA.

Cholangitis

Inflammation of the bile ducts.

Cholangitis is a disease of the bile ducts, usually bacterial in origin, that results in inflammation, scarring, and blockage of the bile-ducts. The bile-ducts conduct bile from the gallbladder to the small intestine to assist in the digestive process; cholangitis may prevent bile from reaching the small intestine, thus interfering with digestion.

Causes. Most often, cholangitis is caused by bacterial infection, often by *Escherichia coli* bacteria, in a bile-duct that is already blocked, as may occur with a gallstone, tumor, or parasite, such as a liver fluke. In this case it is called ascending cholangitis. Primary sclerosing cholangitis is a type of cholangitis of unknown cause, characterized by a scarring of the bile ducts. The disease is more common among men than women. As many as 80 percent of people who have primary sclerosing cholangitis also have ulcerative colitis.

Symptoms of cholangitis may include pain in the upper right abdomen, possibly spreading to the back, jaundice, fever, and chills. Feces may be clay-colored, due to a lack of bile.

Treatment for ascending cholangitis involves the administration of antibiotics. Since an obstruction of the bile-duct is usually involved as well, the underlying cause of the obstruction should be treated. In primary sclerosing cholangitis, clogged ducts are opened surgically, or a drain may be placed in the ducts. In some cases, a liver transplant may be possible.

Prognosis for ascending cholangitis is good with treatment. With primary sclerosing cholangitis, outlook is poor; often the disease is fatal a few years after symptoms appear. *See also* BILE DUCT OBSTRUCTION *and* GALLBLADDER, DISORDERS OF.

Cholecalciferol

Another name for vitamin D$_3$.

Cholecalciferol may be taken as a dietary supplement for the prevention and treatment of vitamin D deficiency when dietary intake or exposure to sunlight (which stimulates the skin to produce vitamin D) is inadequate. As with calciferol, or vitamin D$_2$, cholecalciferol should not be taken without medical supervision by anyone whose levels of either calcium or vitamin D are already high, since excessive amounts of the vitamin will cause calcium to be deposited in tissues other than bone. Cholecalciferol supplements may be necessary to prevent bone loss in individuals who have a deficiency of either calcium or vitamin D, a severe malabsorption problem, or other disorders. *See also* CALCIUM *and* VITAMIN D.

Cholecystectomy

Surgical removal of the gallbladder.

Cholecystectomy is usually performed in response to the presence of gallstones that cause recurrent attacks of abdominal pain (biliary colic) and nausea, or to treat acute infection of the gallbladder (cholecystitis). An emergency cholecystectomy is occasionally required for perforation of the gallbladder or for pus formation (empyema) in the gallbladder.

About 500,000 gallbladders are removed every year in the United States, making it the most commonly performed abdominal surgery in medicine.

Open Cholecystectomy. Before 1988, this procedure was performed by cutting a large incision in the abdomen and cutting through layers of skin, fat, and muscle to reach and remove the gallbladder. The incision made was five to eight inches long, and could be vertical, horizontal, or oblique, from below the ribs on the right side to just below the waist. An uncomplicated operation could take an hour, but exploration of the bile-ducts could prolong the procedure. The patient would have to remain in the hospital for five to seven days, with recovery taking several weeks.

Laparoscopic cholecystectomy, in which flexible tubes are passed through tiny incisions to access and remove the gallbladder, is now used in 90 percent of gallbladder re-

---

Robotic Surgery

The first operation performed by a robot was a cholecystectomy, preformed by the newly FDA-approved da Vinci Surgical System in July 2000. Surgeons operated by the use of joysticks, a computer terminal, and 3-D perspectives of the site on a TV screen. Once fully developed, robotic surgery could reduce the cost of surgery, enable surgeons to operate from a distance, and increase the precision and steadiness of surgery, thus reducing trauma to the patient.

---

movals. The surgeon uses a laparoscope, a thin, tubular instrument with a light and video camera, to probe the gallbladder, and then makes three small incisions through which instruments can be inserted. The gallbladder is removed through one of these incisions. No abdominal muscles have to be cut. The operation occurs under under general anesthesia and takes about an hour. Approximately one in twenty laparoscopic cholecystectomies require a subsequent open cholecystectomy because of complications in diagnosis or removal.

After laparoscopic cholecystectomy, most patients can leave the hospital within a day and return to work soon thereafter, with little postoperative pain.

Risks. Although the gallbladder can be removed with little ill effect, the common bile-duct, which carries bile from the liver to the small intestine, is essential to digestion. The chief risk of cholecystectomy is inadvertent damage to the common bile-duct. Other complications, which are rare, may include bleeding, infection, or damage to the intestines.

Prognosis. The vast majority of cholecystectomies result in cessation of pain and nausea. About 10 percent of patients have continued symptoms, indicating possible stones in the bile-duct. *See* ABDOMEN, PAIN IN THE; GALLBLADDER; *and* GALLSTONES.

Cholecystitis

Inflammation of the gallbladder.

Cholecystitis may be acute, usually resulting from a gallstone in the cystic duct, or it may be a chronic condition. Acute cholecystitis is only rarely due to a bacterial infection. In the absence of gallstones, the condition usually occurs after severe injury or illness in a patient in an intensive care unit, and can lead to gangrene or perforation of the gallbladder. Chronic cholecystitis is a result of scarring and other accumulated damage from previous episodes of acute inflammation.

SYMPTOMS

The most prominent symptom is severe, sharp pain in the right upper part of the abdomen. The pain increases when the patient breathes deeply and may extend to the lower portion of the right shoulder blade. The pain may worsen after eating food, especially if it is high in fat. There may be a feeling of severe pressure or gaseousness in the abdomen, yellowing of the skin (jaundice), nausea, vomiting, and fever.

In the absence of complications, the pain usually subsides within a few days. Chills and high fever, an increase in the white cell count, and cessation of normal intestinal movements may indicate an abscess, a perforation, or gangrene of the gallbladder, requiring emergency surgery.

Chronic cholecystitis is indicated by repeated attacks of acute cholecystitis. Eventually, chronic abdominal pain and indigestion develop.

TREATMENT

A patient with severe acute cholecystitis is hospitalized and receives only intravenous fluids. A nasal-gastric tube may be inserted into the stomach to reduce abdominal pressure. Most cases pass on their own. In the case of complications, the gallbladder may be removed surgically. Chronic cholecystitis is treated with surgical removal of the gallbladder. If surgery is inadvisable, a low-fat diet and the use of antacids may help limit symptoms. *See* GALLBLADDER.

Cholecystography

Procedure for studying the gallbladder with x-rays.

Cholecystography, also known as a gallbladder series, examines the gallbladder following the ingestion of a contrast medium, a solution that fills the gallbladder and blocks the passage of x-rays and thus makes the gallbladder clearly visible under x-ray. The test typically requires the patient to eat a fatty meal beforehand, so that the emptying of the contrast medium into the gallbladder may be observed.

Noninvasive techniques, particularly gallbladder ultrasonography, have largely replaced cholecystography as a diagnostic tool. *See also* GALLBLADDER.

Cholera

An infectious disease characterized by severe diarrhea and danger of dehydration.

Cholera is caused by the bacterium *Vibrio cholerae*, which produces a toxin that causes the small intestine to secrete large amounts of fluids, salts, and minerals. This produces severe diarrhea, which can rapidly lead to dehydration.

Cholera is contracted by ingesting water or foods contaminated with the stools of infected individuals. It is found mostly in parts of Asia, the Middle East, Africa, and Latin America. Outbreaks usually occur during the summer months. The incidence is highest among young children.

Individuals deficient in stomach acids are more susceptible to the disease. People living in cholera-endemic areas gradually develop a limited natural immunity.

SYMPTOMS

Cholera symptoms usually begin one to three days after infection and include sudden, painless, watery diarrhea, and vomiting. Within hours, severe dehydration sets in, as a loss of more than one quart of fluid per hour may occur. The patient experiences intense thirst, muscle cramps, and weakness. Symptoms last from three to six days. If left untreated, the electrolyte imbalance and water loss may lead to kidney failure, shock, coma, and death.

TREATMENT

Prompt replacement of lost fluids, salts, and minerals, either by mouth or intravenously, is essential. Early treatment with tetracycline or other antibiotics kills the bacteria and halts the diarrhea within 48 hours. Full recovery usually follows.

PREVENTION

Uncontaminated sources of water and proper disposal of wastes are essential for controlling outbreaks of the disease. During an outbreak, all water should be boiled and raw vegetables should be avoided, as should any fish or shellfish that has not been cooked thoroughly.

For background information on cholera, see BACTERIA *and* INFECTIOUS DISEASE. *Related material can be found in* ANTIBIOTIC DRUGS; COMA; DEHYDRATION; DIARRHEA; KIDNEY FAILURE; SHOCK; WATER SAFETY; *and* VOMITING.

Cholestasis

Reduction or cessation in the flow of bile from the liver to the small intestine.

Cholestasis occurs when the bile-ducts become blocked because of inflammation or obstruction. It is divided into two categories, depending on whether the problem affects the bile-ducts in the liver or outside it. If the problem is within the liver, it may be due to hepatitis, alcohol-related liver disease, chronic inflammation of the bile-

Resources on Cholera
Barua, Dhiman, and William B. Greenough, eds, *Cholera* (1992); McNeill, William H. *Plagues and People* (1972); Grist, Norman R., et al., *Diseases of Infection: An Illustrated Textbook* (1992); Shaw, Michael, ed., *Everything You Need to Know About Diseases* (1996); Centers for Disease Contol and Prevention, Tel. (800) 311-3435, Online: www.cdc.gov; Infectious Disease Society of America, Tel. (703) 299-0200, Online: www.idsociety.org; National Institute of Allergy and Infectious Disease, Tel. (301) 496-5717, Online: www.niaid.nih.org; www.nycornell.org/medicine/infectious/index.html.

ducts, or a side effect of some drugs. Causes outside the liver include a bile-duct obstruction due to gallstones or tumor, inflammation, or cancer of the pancreas.

Symptoms include itching jaundice, dark urine, and pale stools. The stool may contain fat, because the reduced amount of bile interferes with fat digestion. Bone loss and a tendency to bleed easily may also occur due to the impaired absorption of several important fat-soluble vitamins, such as vitamins D and K. Abdominal pain, loss of appetite, vomiting, and fever may also be present.

Treatment depends on what is impeding the flow of bile. It may be treated surgically or with medication. *See also* BILE DUCT OBSTRUCTION; BILIARY CIRRHOSIS; CHOLECYSTITIS; *and* PANCREAS, CANCER OF.

Cholesteatoma

Accumulation of skin debris in the middle ear.

A chronic or persistent middle-ear infection may cause a rupture in the eardrum. When the eardrum breaks, it usually heals on its own; in some cases, however, a pocket of new skin may grow into the middle ear and form a cyst-like lump. If left on its own, it will continue to grow, and may damage the bones of the middle ear, as well as the surrounding bony structure, resulting in hearing loss in the affected ear, chronic draining of fluid from the ear, or dizziness.

Treatment. Cholesteatoma usually needs to be removed surgically. The middle ear may be accessed through the eardrum or by removing the bone behind the ear (the mastoid). The cholesteatoma has a tendency to recur and may need to be removed periodically.

Prevention. Prompt treatment of ear infections can prevent rupture of the eardrum and resulting complications.

Background material on cholesteatoma can be found in EAR *and* OTITIS MEDIA. *For further information, see* EAR ACHE; EAR, DISCHARGE FROM; EAR, DISORDERS OF; HEARING; *and* HEARING LOSS. *See also* SURGERY *for more on treatment options.*

Cholesterol

An organic compound present in animal fats and manufactured by the human body.

About twenty percent of blood cholesterol is normally derived from food; the rest is produced by the body, primarily by the liver and intestines. Cholesterol is essential to the function of every cell in the body: for structural support in cell membranes; as a component of the brain and of nerve cells; and in the makeup of hormones such as estrogen, progesterone, testosterone, cortisol, and aldosterone. Since cholesterol is a fat, it is not water soluble and therefore requires a carrier to be transported in fluids. Lipoproteins are particles containing, among other substances, cholesterol and "carrier proteins" that transport cholesterol throughout the body.

Types. Several types of lipoproteins are usually referred to when discussing health and cholesterol: high-density, low-density, and very-low-density lipoproteins. High-density lipoprotein (HDL) is considered the "good" cholesterol, as it is high in protein and low in cholesterol. Low-density lipoprotein (LDL), is considered the "bad" cholesterol, as it is low in protein and high in cholesterol. Very-low-density lipoprotein (VLDL) contains mainly triglycerides, which are fat molecules.

High blood levels of HDL cholesterol are desirable, since the HDL carries cholesterol away from the arterial wall to the liver for recycling or removal from the body. LDL transports cholesterol throughout the body for hormone production and cell membrane repairs, but in large quantities it often leaves cholesterol deposits on walls of blood vessels, increasing the risk of heart disease, heart attacks, peripheral vascular disease, and stroke. High levels of triglycerides also increase the risk of heart disease.

Risk Factors. High cholesterol is a risk factor for coronary heart disease. Individual cholesterol levels are determined by a combination of genetic makeup and the amount of saturated fat and cholesterol in the diet, as well as lifestyle factors, such as

---

Cholesterol and Heart Disease

Lowering blood cholesterol levels can significantly decrease the risk of heart disease. You can modify your diet by limiting intake of saturated fats to no more than 10 percent of caloric intake, limiting consumption of cholesterol to less than 300 milligrams per day, and increasing dietary fiber. Cholesterol-lowering medications are available, but modifying diet and exercise should be the first line of action.

---

amount of exercise and alcohol consumption. Preventive and risk-reducing measures include avoiding or limiting consumption of highly saturated fats, since they hinder the removal of cholesterol from the blood. Risk factors include cigarette smoking, high blood pressure, low HDL cholesterol (less than 35 mg/dL), diabetes, sedentary lifestyle, and a family history of coronary heart disease. Conversely, high HDL cholesterol (60 mg/dL) is a protective factor.

For background information on cholesterol, see FATS AND LIPIDS. *Further information can be found in* ANGIOPLASTY, BALLOON; ARTERIOSCLEROSIS; ATHEROSCLEROSIS; ESTROGEN; HEART DISORDERS; HORMONES; PLAQUE; PROGESTERONE; *and* TESTOSTERONE.

Chondritis

Inflammation of cartilage, caused by unusual pressure or stress.

Chondritis is a condition in which the cartilage has become irritated. A good example is costal chondritis, in which the cartilage between the ribs and breastbone becomes inflamed because of excessive and repeated coughing or lifting something that is unusually heavy. The cartilage is overstretched because of the strain and it becomes tender and painful. Cartilage in other areas, such as the hip or knee, can also suffer this kind of inflammation.

Treatment should consist of about two to three days of rest, a daily application of ice, and over-the-counter medicines for pain. A physician should be contacted if pain and swelling persists or increases. *See also* KNEES.

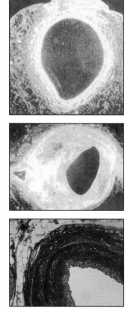

The effects of cholesterol. Top, a normal arterial cross-section, unobstructed by atherosclerotic plaque, as it is in the middle image. Bottom, a cross section micrograph of a blood vessel, shows a large artheroma that can decrease blood flow.

Resources on Cholesterol

Berne, Robert M., et al., *Cardiovascular Physiology* (2001); Debakey, Michael E. and Antonio M. Gotto, *The New Living Heart* (1997); Neill, Catherine A., *The Heart of a Child : What Families Need to Know About Heart Disor-ders in Children* (1992); American Heart Association, Tel. (800) 242-8721, Online: www.amhrt.org; Heart Information Network, Tel. (973) 701-6035, Online: www.heartinfo.org; Nat. Heart, Lung, and Blood Inst., Tel. (301) 496-4236, Online: www. nhlbi.nih. gov; www.nycornell.org/ cardiothora-cic.surgery/; www.nycornell.org/medi-cine/cardiology/index.htl.

Chondromalacia Patellae

Damage to the cartilage of the knee, due to mis-alignment of the kneecap.

Overuse or trauma of the knee may throw the kneecap out of alignment, leading to a wearing-down of the cartilage. The kneecap normally glides across the lower end of the thigh bone. Instead, the misplaced kneecap tilts against the cartilage when straightened, causing wear and tear on the smooth surface.

Chondromalacia is most common in adolescents, especially girls and young women. Participation in sports where the knee is bent most of the time, such as biking or horseback riding, may increase the tendency towards this condition.

Symptoms include pain, tenderness, and a grating sensation when the knee is bent. The pain worsens when climbing, notably stairs. X-rays confirm the condition.

Treatment. The usual treatment consists of rest, painkillers such as analgesics, and, most importantly, strengthening the quadriceps to help keep the kneecap correctly aligned. *See also* KNEE.

Chondromatosis

Multiple benign tumors within bones.

Chondromatosis generally occurs in younger people, usually between the ages of 10 and 30. The tumors, known as chondromas, are made up of cartilage cells and may occur inside the bones or on the surface. They most often occur in bones of the hand, although they can also affect the pelvis. These tumors are not malignant and often cause no symptoms; they are generally detected when x-rays are taken for other reasons. They can sometimes cause pain, but the most common problem is an increased risk of fractures, since the tumors increase the brittleness of bones by thinning their lining.

In synovial chondromatosis, cartilage tumors form in the membranes that line the joints. Sometimes the tumors break free, forming loose bodies in the joints. *See also* BONES *and* BENIGN.

Chondrosarcoma

A cancerous growth arising from cartilage.

Chondrosarcoma is the second most common form of bone cancer, behind osteosarcoma. It most often develops during middle age. It begins in cartilage, either within the cartilage or on its surface, and usually occurs in the pelvis, upper leg, or shoulder. Chondrosarcomas generally grow slowly and do not spread during their early stages.

Causes. Chondrosarcoma often originates from a benign tumor that becomes malignant. While some of these sarcomas can be linked to exposure to radiation or carcinogenic chemicals, the cause of most of them is unknown.

Symptoms. As the chondrosarcoma grows, it causes swelling, pain, and sometimes tenderness in the affected area.

Diagnosis. Chondrosarcomas can be diagnosed by x-ray, which will show the abnormal region of the bone, as well as by computerized tomography (CT) or magnetic resonance imaging (MRI) scans. A biopsy is done to confirm the diagnosis.

Treatment. The usual treatment is surgery to remove the affected area of the bone, by amputation if the cancer is in a bone of an arm or leg. Chemotherapy may be done after surgery. Radiation therapy after surgery is generally not helpful. *See also* CANCER *and* CARTILAGE.

Chordee

Birth defect causing abnormal curvature of the penis.

Chordee is usually seen in male infants with hypospadias, a birth defect in which the urethra has an opening along the shaft of the penis rather than at the tip. Due to this abnormality, the penis bends downward. If uncorrected, chordee can cause later difficulties with sexual intercourse.

Surgery is usually performed to correct

the abnormality; it can be done in the first years of life with great success. Hypospadias can also be corrected by surgery, which is performed as soon as the sixth month after birth. The repair is done using tissue from the foreskin (or the lining of the bladder) to create a new urethra that properly extends to the tip of the penis. *See also* Hypospadias; Penis; *and* Urethra.

Chorea

An involuntary and random twitching of the muscles of the face and limbs.

Chorea is a nervous system disorder characterized by sudden, unintentional movements. It predominantly affects the muscles of the face, arms, and legs, and it may abruptly move from one part of the body to another. It initially appears as grimacing or as randomly moving fingers, and it advances to the lower body. It often appears in conjunction with slower involuntary writhing movements, known as athetosis.

Causes. Chorea is caused by damage to the basal ganglia, a part of the brain that is responsible for controlling movement. This results in an excess of dopamine, a chemical that helps signals pass between nerve cells (neurotransmitter), which leads to the characteristic movements.

Huntington's chorea is the disease perhaps most commonly associated with chorea. Huntington's chorea generally appears between the ages of 35 and 50 and is characterized by progressive involuntary movement, slow eye movement, rigidity, dementia, and depression.

A second disease associated with chorea is an acute childhood disorder, Sydenham's chorea, or St. Vitus' dance. This disease is characterized by slurred speech, muscle weakness, and purposeless arm and leg movements. It appears among four to seven-year-olds after the onset of rheumatic fever and generally clears up several months following treatment of that disease.

Chorea that occurs during pregnancy is called chorea gravidarum. Chorea may also

be a side effect of certain drugs, particularly after long-term use of antipsychotic drugs used to treat schizophrenia.

Treatment. If the chorea is a result of a drug side effect, it should improve with the removal of the drug. If it is caused by an underlying disease, drugs that block the effect of dopamine or limit the nervous system pathways involving movement can help control the movements. *See also* Tourette's Syndrome.

> *Background material on chorea can be found in* Athetosis *and* Basal Ganglia. *For related informaiton, see* Antipsychotic Drugs; Brain; Brain Disorders; Central Nervous System; Dopamine; Muscle Spasm; Nervous System; Pregnancy; Schizophrenia; Sydenham's Disease; *and* Tourette's Syndrome.

Choriocarcinoma

A malignant tumor of the placenta.

Choriocarcinoma is an uncommon cancer, occurring in about 1 out of every 20,000 pregnancies. It usually originates from a hydatidiform mole, a type of abnormal pregnancy in which the tissue around the fertilized egg, which usually attaches to the uterine wall and develops into the placenta, instead develops into a nonmalignant tumor of abnormal cells. Choriocarcinoma occasionally occurs after an abortion. In some cases, the tumor can develop months or years after a molar pregnancy; a woman who has had a hydatidiform mole must be examined regularly for at least a year to detect a possible cancer.

Symptoms. The tumor often causes no symptoms, but it can cause persistent vaginal bleeding. Untreated, the cancer can spread to the lungs or brain.

Diagnosis. Tests done to detect choriocarcinoma include ultrasound scans and assays of the blood and urine to measure for abnormally high levels of human chorionic gonadotropin, a hormone produced during pregnancy by the placenta that is also produced by a hydatidiform mole.

Treatment. Chemotherapy is a first line

of treatment, but a hysterectomy may be performed to remove the uterus if drug treatment is not effective. The prognosis after treatment is good; patients have a 70 percent chance of survival.

Chorionic Villus Sampling

A form of fetal biopsy that tests for prenatal chromosome irregularities and other disease.

In chorionic villus sampling (CVS), a sample of placental tissue is removed from the uterus and tested for genetic abnormalities. Chorionic villi, from which the sample is obtained, are tiny finger-like projections on the far side of the placenta from the fetus; they are genetically identical to the fetus.

CVS can be performed in the first trimester, earlier than amniocentesis, which cannot be performed until the 15th to 18th week of pregnancy. As it is slightly more dangerous than amniocentesis, CVS is usually performed only if the fetus is at risk of genetic defect. As the test may be performed within the first trimester, a report of abnormalities may, if the parents so decide, allow for safer termination of pregnancy, with less physical and emotional trauma, and with faster recovery, than results received later. Furthermore, early detection of some fetal abnormalities can greatly improve the baby's prognosis.

PROCEDURE

There are two ways of performing CVS, depending on the location of the placenta in the uterus. Transabdominal sampling is performed if the placenta lies on top of or in front of the uterine wall. In this case it can be reached directly through the abdomen; a needle is inserted through the abdomen and a sample of tissue removed from the placenta.

Transcervical sampling is done when the placenta is not as easily accessible. A catheter is inserted through the cervix and into the uterus and guided to the placenta using ultrasound. The transcervical method carries a somewhat higher risk of infection and fetal loss than the transabdominal

method; also, the catheter cannot be guided as accurately as the needle.

RESULTS

The tissue sample is sent to a laboratory for chromosome analysis. Analysis can diagnose a range of genetic disorders, including Down's syndrome, thalassemia, and hemophilia.

The information obtained with CVS is the same as that obtained by amniocentesis, and the accuracy rates of the tests are comparable, though neural tube defects are not detected by chorionic villus sampling. For this reason, the test is usually followed by further testing several weeks later. The sampling of chorionic villi, though generally safe, carries a somewhat higher risk of miscarriage or defect than amniocentesis, though refining of techniques has further reduced this hazard.

For background information on chorionic villus sampling, see BIOPSY *and* AMNIOCENTESIS. *Further information can be found in* BIRTH DEFECT; CATHETER; CERVIX; DOWN'S SYNDROME; GENE; GENETIC DISORDERS; HEMOPHILIA; PLACENTA; PREGNANCY; THALASSEMIA; *and* UTERUS.

Choroiditis

Inflammation of the choroid, the blood vessels and connective tissue between the white of the eye and the retina.

Choroiditis can be caused by injury; an underlying infection such as tuberculosis, cytomegalovirus, or toxoplasmosis; an underlying condition that causes inflammation such as sarcoidosis or ulcerative colitis; or it may have no definable cause. The inflammation can lead to the development of patches of scar tissue, which may cause corresponding patches of vision loss. Symptoms include pain; redness; sensitivity to light; blurred vision; and dark spots in the field of view. Treatment involves identifying and treating the underlying cause, if possible. Corticosteroids may be given to reduce inflammation. *See also* CORTICOSTEROIDS; CYTOMEGALOVIRUS; EYE; SARCOIDOSIS; TOXOPLAMOSIS; *and* TUBERCULOSIS.

Christmas Disease

Also known as hemophilia B

One of two types of hemophilia.

Hemophilia is a disease in which the blood clotting function is impaired. In Christmas disease, one of the many substances necessary for blood clotting, factor IX, is missing. As a result, even minor bleeding may become life-threatening. Sufferers must be extremely careful to avoid situations in which bleeding can occur, such as accidental cuts or bruises, minor surgery, or dentistry.

The disease is X-linked, meaning that 50 percent of male children of mothers who are carriers will have the disease. Females can only get the disease if the father is a hemophiliac and the mother is a carrier; thus the disease is very rare in females.

Typically, bleeding occurs in the joints, skin, and muscles; and patients with this disease often develop severe arthritis, requiring joint replacement. The disease can be treated by administering a pure form of factor IX intravenously. *See also* BLOOD; BLOOD CLOTTING; *and* HEMOPHILIA.

Chromium

Natural substance that regulates the body's use of sugar and metabolizes fatty-acid.

Chromium is a mineral essential to normal absorption of glucose. The adult requirement is between 50 and 200 micrograms per day, supplied by such foods as brewer's yeast (the richest source of chromium), whole grains, cheeses, and meats. Chromium allows insulin to function by facilitating blood glucose absorption by the body's cells. Chromium deficiency can lead to diminished insulin function and symptoms similar to diabetes. Supplemental chromium can improve the ability to absorb glucose in people who either have adult-onset diabetes or who are elderly and have difficulty in absorbing chromium. Because chromium is not well absorbed and is easily excreted, overdose is rare. *See also* DIABETES; GLUCOSE; *and* METABOLISM.

Chromosomal Abnormalities

Defects of the chromosomes that may lead to irreversible birth defects.

Chromosomal abnormalities are irreversible and are one of the leading causes of birth defects. Normally, there are 23 pairs of chromosomes—22 pairs of regular (autosomal) chromosomes and one pair of sex chromosomes, XX for females and XY for males. A chromosomal abnormality can be due to the presence of an extra chromosome (trisomy) or the lack of all or part of a chromosome (deletion syndrome).

Autosomal trisomies, the presence of an extra non-sex chromosome, are usually fatal. An exception is Down's syndrome, which is caused by an extra copy of chromosome 21. The characteristics of Down's syndrome include delayed physical and mental development, a broad face with slanting eyes, and a single crease across the palm. Thirty-five percent of children with Down's syndrome have heart defects. Most individuals with Down's syndrome can be well integrated into society and can live until their 30s or 40s.

Trisomy 18, known as Edward's syndrome, is due to the presence of an extra copy of chromosome 18. Children with this syndrome have facial abnormalities as well as severe retardation and usually only survive for a few months. Trisomy 13, known as Patau's syndrome, involves the presence of an extra chromosome 13. Infants born with this syndrome have severe brain and eye defects and rarely survive past one year.

Sex chromosome trisomies are not fatal but can have a wide range of effects. Triple X syndrome, which occurs once in 1000 female births, can result in mental retarda-

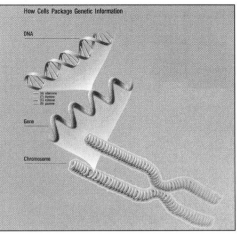

How Cells Package Genetic Information

DNA

(A) adenine
(T) thymine
(C) cytosine
(G) guanine

Gene

Chromosome

Chromosomes. Genetic information is contained in DNA molecules that are, in turn, contained in the chromosomes.

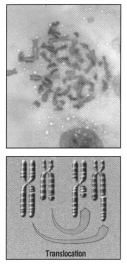

Chromosome. Top, the chromosomes of a human cell undergoing mitosis.Bottom, translocation, which causes some types of cancers.

Resources on Chromosomal Abnormalities

Davies, Kevin, *Cracking the Genome: Inside the Race to Unlock Human DNA* (2001); Moore, Keith L., *Before We Are Born : Essentials of Embryology and Birth Defects* (1998); Nussbaum, Robert L., et al., *Thompson & Thompson Genetics in Medicine* (2001); Pollack, Robert, *Signs of Life: The Languages and Meanings of DNA* (1994); Ridley, Matt, *Genome* (2000); Alliance of Genetic Support Groups, Tel. (800) 336-GENE, Online: www.medhelp.org/geneticalliance; Easter Seals, Tel. (800) 221-6827, Online: www.seals.org; National Center for Biotechnology Information, Tel. (301) 496-2475, Online: www.ncbi.nih.gov; Office of Rare Diseases, Tel. (301) 402-4336, Online: rarediseases.info.nih.gov/org; http://www.med.cornell.edu/research/cores/genetherapy/index.html.

tion. Females with this syndrome may be sterile, although some are not. "Triple" X is a misnomer, as there can be more than one additional chromosome. As the number of addition chromosomes increases, so does the chance of mental retardation and physical abnormalities.

Boys born with Klinefelter's syndrome have an extra X chromosome, resulting in a pattern of XXY. This occurs in approximately 1 in 700 male births. These males are tall, with somewhat feminized bodies, including breast development. Their testes are small and are usually sterile. Boys with this syndrome have normal intelligence but exhibit speech and reading disabilities.

Sometimes a male has an extra Y chromosome, resulting in a pattern of XYY. These males are usually tall and experience language difficulties.

Deletion syndromes are those in which an individual is missing either a partial or entire chromosome. Cri du chat ("cry of a cat") syndrome, caused by 5p- deletion, involves physical abnormalities and mental retardation. Affected babies have a high-pitched cry like that of a kitten and rarely survive to adulthood. 4p- deletion is extremely rare and results in extreme mental and physical defects. Most children with this syndrome die in infancy. If they do survive, they are severely handicapped.

Deletion Syndromes of the Sex Chromosome. In fragile X syndrome, the presence of an abnormal X chromosome can result in mental retardation. Effects of this syndrome, however, can vary widely. For example, some boys with the syndrome have normal intelligence, whereas some girls who have one normal X as well as one abnormal X may be mentally retarded.

In Turner's syndrome, which occurs in 1 in 3000 births, a girl has only a single X chromosome. This results in short stature and limbs, a wide chest with broad-spaced nipples, and undeveloped breasts and genitals. The ovaries do not produce eggs, and menstruation does not occur. Mental retardation is rare, although girls with Turner's syndrome may experience difficulty with spatial relationships and mathematics.

Chromosome

The body that is the bearer of genes in cells.

Chromosomes are lengths of genetic material that determine the growth and function of every living cell and thus of every living organism. Each chromosome is made of several thousand genes, and each gene is a chain of deoxyribonucleic acid (DNA). The links in the DNA chain are known as base pairs, which, through the order in which they are arranged, code for a cell's operating instructions.

A cell's nucleus contains chemicals that can read, distribute, and follow through on genetic instructions. Because of the aggregate effect of the many genes, physical traits such as height, hair color, and facial features, as well as some mental ones, owe their qualities to chromosomes.

HUMAN CELLS. Most human cells contain 23 pairs of chromosomes and are called diploid cells. Each pair of chromosomes is attached mid-segment by a constriction called a centromere; larms on either side form a narrow, gangly "X."

Egg and sperm cells are called haploid cells, because they contain only half the normal number of chromosomes—one from each pair.

When an egg is fertilized, the egg and sperm cells' genetic material combines to form a diploid cell. Copied again and again in the process of growth called cell division, these cells eventually grow into a full human being, with identical genetic material in each cell. Mosaicism, an abnormality in which some cells contain a slightly different set of chromosomes, is rare.

Identical twins are the only genetically identical humans. The rest differ from one another because of slight differences in chromosomal material.

For background information on chromosome, see DNA; GENE; *and* RNA. *Related material can be found in* CELL; CONCEPTION; CYSTIC FIBROSIS; DOWN'S SYNDROME; GENETIC DISORDERS; HEMOPHILIA; HEREDITARY; *and* THALASSEMIA. *See also* CLONE *and* TWINS *for more information on individuals with identical DNA.*

Chromosome Analysis

Also known as karyotyping

An analysis of the genetic material in cells to detect any abnormalities in the number or structure of the chromosomes.

Chromosome analysis is most often performed on fetal tissue to detect any genetic irregularities before birth. Tissue to be tested is obtained from amniotic fluid (amniocentesis), or by extracting a sample from the placenta (chorionic villus sampling). It can be used to identify a predisposition to genetic disease, assess the genetic health of a fetus, or identify chromosome irregularities that may be associated with birth defects. In addition, chromosome analysis may be performed after birth and into adulthood. There are an increasing number of genetic counseling facilities in the United States that perform chromosome analysis.

Chromosomes form a linear thread within the nucleus of all cells. They are made up of genes, which in turn are made up of deoxyribonucleic acid (DNA), the basic genetic building block of all living organisms.

Most human cells have 46 chromosomes; with the exception of the sex cells, sperm and ova, each of which contain 23 chromosomes. Each fetus receives half of its chromosomes from its mother and half from its father. The chromosomes are divided into 23 pairs, called homologues, which are similar in size, shape, and function. The one exception to this is the sex chromosomes, known as X and Y, which determine an individual's sex. Y chromosomes are significantly smaller than X chromosomes. An individual with two X chromosomes is female, while an individual with one X and one Y chromosome is male. Each homologue contains one member from the mother and one member from the father.

TESTING

Chromosome analysis allows the analyst to visually identify and classify chromosomal defects according to type. Common defects include breakage, inversion, duplication, and loss of chromosomes.

To view the chromosomes, the analyst treats the sample cells in a process that makes the chromosomes easily visible. Using a high-power microscope, the analyst chooses the cell or cells with the clearest chromosomes and photographs them. The resulting picture is enlarged, and the chromosomes are cut out and arranged according to size on a chart known as a karyotype. A standard karyotype orders the 22 "standard" chromosome pairs from largest to smallest, with the X and Y chromosomes appearing separately at the end of the karyotype. In the case of chromosomes that appear close in size and shape, the researcher identifies specific chromosomes by a characteristic sequence of banding, which resembles a bar code.

TYPES OF CHROMOSOMAL ABNORMALITY

Nondisjunction. Occasionally, paired chromosomes fail to properly separate during cell division. This is known as nondisjunction. If nondisjunction occurs during the formation of sperm or ova, these cells have one too many or too few chromosomes. The most well-known case of nondisjunction is Down's syndrome, in which an individual has an extra copy of the 21st chromosome. Down's syndrome is characterized by certain facial features and body type, mental retardation, and a variety of other abnormalities ranging in severity.

ALERT

When Analysis Is Recommended

Chromosome analysis is used to detect a variety of abnormalities that may produce severe symptoms and deformities, including birth defects and mental retardation. Samples of chromosomes in a developing fetus may be obtained through chorionic villus sampling or amniocentesis. Chromosome analysis is recommended in the following instances:

- Pregnancy in women over the age of 35.
- Anatomical irregularity of the fetus discovered by ultrasound.
- The birth of a newborn displaying obvious or suspected birth defects.

Most often, nondusjunction prevents the development of a viable embryo or, rarely, results in an infant with widespread abnormality. Such an individual will be still-born or survive at most a few months.

Nondisjunction of the sex chromosomes is more common and less severe than nondisjunction of the 44 regular chromosomes. In Turner's syndrome, a girl is born with only one X chromosome, resulting in short stature, infertility, and associated health problems. In Kleinfelter's syndrome, a boy has one or more extra X chromosomes, resulting in a lack of sexual development, infertility, and possible delays in language development.

Translocation. In this condition, a deleted portion of one chromosome is attached onto another chromosome in a different pair. This person generally will be normal, but may pass on an abnormality to his or her children. Some diseases are suspected to be related to this abnormality.

For background informaiton on chromosome analysis, see CHROMOSOME; DNA; GENE; *and* RNA. *Further information can be found in* AMNIOCENTESIS; CHORIONIC VILLUS SAMPLING; DOWN'S SYNDROME; FRAGILE X SYNDROME; GENETIC DISORDERS; HEMOPHILIA; KLEINFELTER'S SYNDROME; PLACENTA; *and* TURNER'S SYNDROME.

Chronic Fatigue Syndrome

A disorder characterized by feelings of debilitation and lack of energy.

Chronic fatigue syndrome is a disorder that affects the body's immune system. It occurs mainly among young adults and twice as often in women than men. It is often misdiagnosed, because its symptoms resemble those of mononucleosis, multiple sclerosis, fibromyalgia, and Lyme disease.

CAUSE

The cause of chronic fatigue syndrome remains unknown. The Epstein-Barr virus was once thought to be the cause, but more recent research points to an immune system dysfunction originating in the central nervous system. Chronic fatigue syndrome is not thought to be contagious.

SYMPTOMS

Symptoms of chronic fatigue syndrome include an unexplained, lingering fatigue that is not alleviated by bed rest. The ability to function on a personal or occupational level is curtailed due to a lack of stamina. Short-term memory and concentration may be impaired, and an affected person may experience a sore throat, tender lymph nodes, muscle pain, headaches, and exhaustion after any exertion.

Some people may experience speech impairment, visual difficulties, shortness of breath, low-grade fever, or a low body temperature, as well as psychological problems such as anxiety or depression. Physical or mental stress may aggravate the symptoms. Symptoms must persist for at least six months for the patient to be diagnosed with chronic fatigue syndrome. Diagnosis generally occurs after an extensive process in which all other possible causes for the symptoms are ruled out.

TREATMENT

Lifestyle changes, including increased rest and coping strategies to minimize stress and pace activities, can help manage the disease in the long term. Over-the-counter drugs, such as aspirin and ibuprofen, may help to relieve muscle aches. Some prescription medications, such as antidepressants or drugs that boost the immune system, can also help to manage symptoms. The condition has also encouraged investigation of alternative medical techniques.

PROGNOSIS

Prognosis is variable, but some people with chronic fatigue syndrome recover in time, while others learn to effectively manage their condition.

Background information on chronic fatigue syndrome can be found in CENTRAL NERVOUS SYSTEM *and* IMMUNE SYSTEM. *For related material, see* ANXIETY; DEPRESSION; EPSTEIN-BARR VIRUS; FIBROMYALGIA; LYME DISEASE; MEMORY; MONONUCLEOSIS; *and* MULTIPLE SCLEROSIS.

Resources on Chronic Fatigue Syndrome
Collinge, William, *Recovering from Chronic Fatigue Syndrome: A Guide for Self-Empowerment* (1993); Ravicz, Simone, *Thriving With Your Autoimmune Disorder: A Woman's Mind-Body Guide* (2000); Yehuda, Shlomo, and David Mostofsky, eds., *Chronic Fatigue Syndrome* (1997); American Acade-my of Allergy, Asthma & Immunology, Tel. (800) 822-2762, Online: www.aaaai.org; American Autoimmune Related Diseases Association, Tel. (800) 598-4668, Online: www.aarda.org.

Circulatory System

Also known as the cardiovascular system

The organs and conduits that transport blood, carrying oxygen, nutrients, waste, and enzymes through the body.

The circulatory system is the name given to the complex system of organs, conduits, and fluids that move gases, nutrients, waste, and other substances through the body. The system ensures the uninterrupted flow of oxygenated blood and nutrients to all tissues and the expulsion of waste and carbon dioxide from the body.

There are three main types of circulation: systemic circulation is the movement of blood through arteries and other vessels; pulmonary circulation is the movement of blood from the heart to the lungs and back to the heart again; coronary circulation is the movement of blood through the tissues of the heart.

Systemic Circulation. As the engine of systemic circulation, the heart's left side pumps oxygenated blood into the aorta for distribution to all areas of the body. Even in the distant arteries and the smaller arterioles, blood flows owing solely to the heart's beat. Blood slows as it exits the arterioles and enters vast networks of capillaries. These tiny vessels eventually widen into veins, the blood vessels of the venous system, which carry blood back to the heart. While arteries are thick-walled and elastic to withstand the pressure of blood surging from the heart, veins have thinner walls and are less resistant, allowing the contraction of surrounding muscles to propel blood back to the heart. Deep veins run parallel to arteries, while superficial veins are found closer to the skin.

The venous system does not have a heartbeat to move blood, so veins expend more energy in returning blood to the heart than arteries do in carrying it away from the heart. The venous system uses three tools, collectively called the venous pump, to make blood flow. First, the surrounding muscles, from those that generate breathing to those used in strenuous exercise, exert pressure on veins, forcing blood to move. Second, pressure in the abdomen, dictated by changes in respiration, draws blood in the same way that atmospheric pressure encourages the siphoning of a liquid from one chamber into another. Third, venous valves, funnel-shaped structures that converge in the ends of veins in the pelvis and extremities, make it difficult for blood to flow in the opposite direction. The veins are responsible for returning the blood to the heart for pulmonary circulation, which results in the exchange of gases in the lungs.

Blood also passes through the kidneys, in a phase of systemic circulation known as renal circulation. During this phase, the kidneys filter much of the waste from the blood. During another phase called portal circulation, blood passes through the small intestine, stomach, and other digestive organs, and collects in the portal vein, which

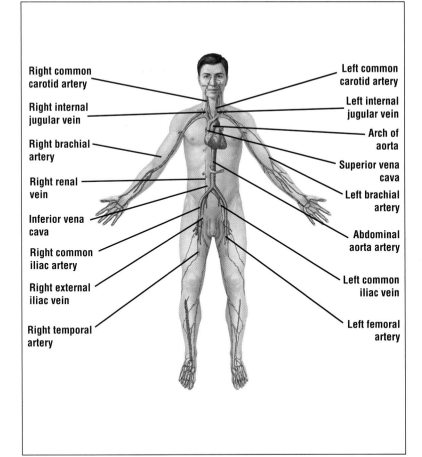

Right common carotid artery

Right internal jugular vein

Right brachial artery

Right renal vein

Inferior vena cava

Right common iliac artery

Right external iliac vein

Right temporal artery

Left common carotid artery

Left internal jugular vein

Arch of aorta

Superior vena cava

Left brachial artery

Abdominal aorta artery

Left common iliac vein

Left femoral artery

Circulatory System.
The circulatory system, above, consists of all the vessels and organs that transport nutrients and wastes throughout the body. The three types of circulation are systemic (the movement of blood through the blood vessels), pulmonary (the movement of blood to and from the lungs), and coronary (the movement of blood within the heart).

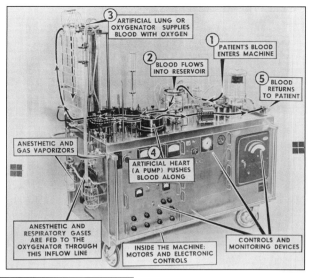

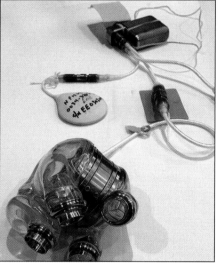

Circulatory System. Throughout the past fifty years, many artificial devices have been invented to assist in circulation for patients with circulatory disease. Top, an artificial heart/lung machine from 1955. Bottom, the type of artificial heart that was surgically implanted in the chest of Robert Tools, a 59-year-old man with end-stage heart disease, in July 2001.

passes through the liver. The liver filters sugars and other nutrients from the blood, storing them for later use, and routes blood through the inferior vena cava and back into systemic circulation.

Pulmonary Circulation. Between contractions, the heart rests. At this point, the right atrium receives oxygen-poor blood from the venous system via the caval veins (the body's two primary veins), and pulmonary circulation begins. This blood is dark red due to its depleted oxygen content. The next contraction pushes the blood through a one-way valve into the right ventricle. The right ventricle then contracts, pushing the blood into the pulmonary artery leading to the lungs. There the blood flows into lung capillaries that infuse it with oxygen and drain carbon dioxide and waste; both processes are accomplished by diffusion. The blood turns bright red and returns to the heart through the pulmonary veins, then flows in and out of the left atrium and into the left ventricle. The strongest of the heart's four chambers, the left ventricle pumps blood into the aorta and beyond.

The valves in the heart are part of the circulatory system's network of one-way streets. If blood started flowing the wrong way, oxygen and carbon dioxide could mix and cause serious harm to the body. Arteries branch into the arterioles, which in turn split into capillaries, where organ tissue absorbs the oxygen in the bloodstream and unloads waste and carbon dioxide by diffusion, turning the blood from bright red to dark red again. Leaving the capillaries, it enters the venules and the wider veins.

Coronary Circulation. While the circulatory system provides oxygen and nourishment to every cell of the body, the heart also needs nourishment. Serious heart damage may occur if the heart does not receive a normal supply of food and oxygen. Coronary circulation delivers nourishment through arteries in the heart.

Blood pressure measures the strength of blood flow at the moment the heart contracts (systolic pressure) and when it is at rest (diastolic pressure). Someone testing blood pressure expresses it as, for example, 110 over 90. Pulmonary circulation is audible through a stethoscope. The two sounds, "lub" and "dub," are the ventricles contracting and the valves closing.

A total of five liters of blood circulate in the average human body. In the average person's lifetime, the heart beats approximately three billion times. In the body, about eight million blood cells die and another eight million are born every second. Within a tiny droplet of blood, there are five million red blood cells, and it takes about 20 seconds for one of them to circle the whole body. From the time of their birth in the bone marrow, red blood cells make approximately 250,000 round trips of the body before returning to the bone marrow to die. Red blood cells may live for four months circulating throughout the body, feeding the body's 60 trillion cells.

For background information on circulatory system, see CARDIOLOGY. *Further information can be found in* CARDIAC OUTPUT; HEART; HEART ATTACK; HEART FAILURE; *and* HEART SOUNDS. *See also* ARTERIES, DISORDERS OF *and* HEART DISORDERS *for more on circulatory system disorders.*

Circumcision, Female

The ritualistic surgical removal of all or parts of a female's clitoris (clitoridectomy) and inner and outer labia, sometimes combined with narrowing of the entrance to the vagina.

Female circumcision is common in parts of Africa (including Ethiopia, Egypt, Sudan, Somalia, and Nigeria), New Guinea, the Middle East, Mexico, Brazil, Peru, India, and over a dozen other countries. The ritual has its origins in social and religious practices aimed at protecting virginity and reducing sexual desire.

All evidence indicates that the procedure has no benefits and no valid medical purpose. In fact, female circumcision may cause severe bleeding, tetanus, painful urination, painful sexual intercourse, sexual dysfunction, menstrual problems, and birth complications. Women's groups and medical organizations have attempted to end the practice throughout the world, but progress toward that end has been slow. *See also* SEXUAL DYSFUNCTION *and* TETANUS.

Circumcision, Male

The surgical removal of the foreskin (prepuce) from the tip (glans) of the penis.

Circumcision, a procedure in which the foreskin is cut from the tip of the penis, is routinely performed on newborn male babies in the United States. It was originally performed for religious reasons but in the late nineteenth century began to be performed as a sanitary measure. Occasionally, circumcision is performed on older males.

Circumcision is also part of a religious ritual that has been practiced for thousands of years by Jewish and Muslim individuals. Among Jewish people, it is performed on the eighth day after birth; among Muslim people, it is done either before or at puberty, or sometimes immediately before marriage.

In some countries circumcision is routinely carried out for reasons of hygiene, in the belief that it prevents the accumulation of secretions under the foreskin and therefore minimizes the probability of infection or cancer in the genital region. The medical benefits of circumcision are controversial, however, and reasonable hygiene measures can also prevent the accumulation of secretions under the foreskin. For this reason, rates of circumcision have declined since the 1970s. However, it is unlikely that circumcision will cease to be performed altogether.

> ### Circumcision as Prevention
> In the early twentieth century, it was believed that circumcision reduced the risk of infection and penile cancer. In recent years, however, the medical benefits of circumcision have been called into question, and most physicians now believe that the procedure serves no medical purpose. It has been suggested that circumcision reduces the risk of sexually transmitted diseases, but studies have produced conflicting results. Today, the decision whether or not to circumcise a child is generally made for religious or cultural reasons.

Reasons. The most common medical reasons for circumcision in older males include ballooning of the foreskin during urination, pain during sexual intercourse, or recurring painful compression of the shaft of the penis, caused by retraction of the foreskin (paraphimosis).

Procedure. Circumcision takes only a few minutes for babies or young children, and the procedure is increasingly performed with some type of local anesthetic. In adolescent and adult males, a general anesthetic is used.

The foreskin does not retract easily until a boy reaches three or four years of age. Prior to that time, attempting to pull the foreskin back from the glans can cause pain or injury. When washing an uncircumcised infant, only the visible parts of the glans should be washed.

> *Background information on male circumcision can be found in* REPRODUCTIVE SYSTEM, MALE. *For further information, see* PENIS; PENIS, CANCER OF; *and* SURGERY. *See also* CHILD DEVELOPMENT *and* HYGIENE *for more on hygiene in the genital region after birth.*

Circumcision.
The three images above illustrate the procedure of male circumcision. In the procedure, the foreskin is forcibly retracted and surgically removed. The remaining skin is then stitched together and the penis is left to heal.

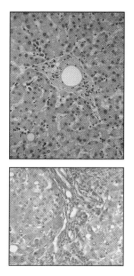

Cirrhosis.
Patients with cirrhosis suffer scarring of the liver tissue, which is visible under a microscope. Above, top, normal liver cells viewed through a microscope. Above, bottom, cirrhotic liver cells, with prominent and extensive scarring .

Resources on Cirrhosis of the Liver

Knapp, Caroline, *Drinking: A Love Story* (1997); Ketcham, Katherine, *Beyond the Influence: Understanding and Defeating Alcoholism* (2000); Knott, David H., *Alcohol Problems: Diagnosis and Treatment* (1989); Alcoholics Anonymous (local chapters in the phone book); Al-Anon: (800) 356-9996, On-line: www.alanon.alateen.org; Mothers Against Drunk Driving: (800) 438-MADD, National Council on Alcoholism and Drug Dependence, (800) 622-2255, www.ncadd. org/problems.html; www.nycornell.org /psychiatry/.

Cirrhosis

A liver disease characterized by progressive and irreversible scarring of the liver tissue.

Liver damage may occur as a result of various diseases or chronic consumption of alcohol. As liver cells die, they are replaced by scar tissue. In time, fewer and fewer healthy cells remain available to remove toxins from the blood, manufacture critical bodily proteins, or process other compounds. The liver may initially become enlarged in an attempt to compensate, but it will shrink with additional scarring.

TYPES AND CAUSES

There are various causes of cirrhosis, including alcohol abuse, chronic infection with hepatitis B or C viruses, certain genetic liver diseases, immune-mediated liver disease, or fatty deposition.

Alcohol-induced cirrhosis usually occurs after many years of heavy drinking and may affect up to 15 percent of all alcoholics. It is believed that just 45 grams of alcohol per day for several years may be enough to damage the liver.

Cryptogenic cirrhosis is a term used to describe cirrhosis of unknown origin.

Primary biliary cirrhosis occurs due to inflammation of the small bile ducts inside the liver, leading to eventual scarring and obstruction. It has been linked to autoimmune disorders. The majority of primary biliary cirrhosis cases occur in women between the ages of 35 and 60.

Hemochromatosis is a disease in which excessive amounts of iron accumulate in the liver, leading to scarring and damage. Wilson's disease is similar, except copper is the material that accumulates. Both conditions, if left untreated, can lead to cirrhosis.

SYMPTOMS

The symptoms of the various types of cirrhosis are similar, and may develop slowly over time. They include an enlarged liver or spleen, water retention, the appearance of spider-like blood vessels on the skin, jaundice, a lack of appetite, weight loss, weakness, fatigue, easy bruising, and esophageal bleeding.

COMPLICATIONS

In individuals suffering from cirrhosis, blood flow to the liver becomes increasingly compromised, resulting in increased pressure in the veins supplying the liver (portal hypertension), enlargement of the spleen, and collapsed blood vessels in the esophagus. One of the liver's primary functions is to process toxic materials in the blood; with increasing liver impairment, these substances accumulate in the blood and can affect other organs, including the brain. This will eventually lead to mental confusion and then coma. Blood clots may form either in the portal or hepatic veins, the latter resulting in accumulation of fluid in the abdominal region (ascites).

TREATMENT

Treatment is aimed at alleviating the complications of cirrhosis, as the damage itself is irreversible. Giving up alcohol can reduce further liver damage and increase life expectancy. In severe cases, a liver transplant is the best option.

For background information on cirrhosis, see LIVER. *Further information can be found in* LIVER DISEASE, ALCOHOLIC. *See also* ADDICTION; ALCOHOL DEPENDENCE; AUTOIMMUNE DISORDERS; *and* HEPATITIS, VIRAL *for more on possible causes of cirrhosis.*

Claustrophobia

Intense fear and avoidance of closed spaces, such as elevators and small rooms.

A person with claustrophobia often realizes that the fear is irrational. Nevertheless, the fear is such that the person will either avoid closed spaces or experience substantial anxiety when in such places.

Various approaches, including psychotherapy, cognitive-behavior therapy, behavioral therapy, and anti-anxiety medications, may be used in combination to treat claustrophobia. *See also* BEHAVIOR THERAPY; PANIC ATTACK; *and* PHOBIA.

Claw Foot and Hand

Deformities causing a claw-like appearance of the hand and/or foot.

In claw foot, the toes are permanently pointed down and the arch is high, giving the foot a claw-like appearance. Claw foot is usually a congenital deformity, but it can also be acquired as a consequence of other disorders, such as muscular dystrophy.

Claw toe, or hammer toe, is a similar deformity of a single toe, in which the joint nearest to the foot is bent upward and the other joints bend downward. It generally occurs as a result of nerve damage.

Claw hand is a deformity in which the digits remain permanently flexed. The curved or bent fingers give the hand a claw-like appearance. Claw hand usually results from a congenital deformity but can also result from other disorders such as muscular dystrophy. Partial claw hand occurs when the ulnar nerve is damaged, and this will generally affect only the ring and little fingers. When the median nerve is also affected, the condition is known as complete claw hand.

Treatment for mild cases of these conditions may include splinting or manipulation of the affected area, along with exercises to strengthen the muscles in the region. More severe cases may require surgery to straighten the joints. *See also* CONGENITAL; MUSCULAR DYSTROPHY; NERVE; NERVE BLOCK; NERVE INJURY; PHYSICAL THERAPY; *and* SPLINT.

Cleft Lip and Palate

Incomplete formation of the upper lip and/or the roof of the mouth.

Cleft lip and cleft palate are the most common birth defects involving the skull and face. A cleft lip, sometimes referred to as a harelip, is an incomplete joining of the upper lip, ranging from a small notch to a split that extends up to just below the nose. A cleft palate refers to incomplete closure of the roof of the mouth, which results in an abnormal passageway through the roof of the mouth into the nose.

Incidence. Cleft lip occurs in approximately one in every 1000 births. Cleft palate occurs in about one in every 1800 births. Either one or the other defect occurs once in 600 to 700 births.

Symptoms. The presence of a cleft lip prevents an infant from completely closing his or her mouth and lips and may affect the ability to suck properly. A cleft palate may interfere with both speech and eating.

Treatment. A dental device can be used to temporarily seal the roof of the mouth of a baby with cleft lip or palate so the baby can suck. Both cleft lip and cleft palate can be permanently corrected with surgery.

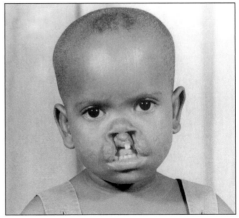

Cleft Lip and Palate. Cleft lip and palate is marked by incomplete development of the upper lip or the roof of the mouth.

> *Background information on cleft lip and palate can be found in* BIRTH DEFECTS. *For further information, see* CONGENITAL; COSMETIC SURGERY; DENTISTRY; DIGESTIVE SYSTEM; *and* SURGERY. *See also* FAILURE TO THRIVE *for possible consequences of severe cases in infants.*

Clitoris

The erectile organ of the vagina.

Located below the pubic bone, above the opening of the urethra, and slightly covered by the lip-like labia, the clitoris is a small, round erectile organ that contains many touch receptors. When stimulated, the clitoris swells, lengthens, and becomes highly sensitive. Together, the clitoris, labia, and vaginal and urethral openings comprise the vulva, the externally visible part of the highly complex female genitalia. Normally, only the head of the clitoris is exposed. Underneath the labia major, or outer lips of the vagina, lie the labia minor, which provide skin cover, called a prepuce, for the clitoris. This corresponds to the male prepuce at the head of the penis. *See also* CIRCUMCISION, FEMALE *and* ORGASM.

Resources on Birth Defects

Clifford, Edward, *The Cleft Palate Experience* (1987); Moore, Harold, and Barry O'Donnel, *The Developing Human* (1992); American Academy of Pediatrics, Tel. (847) 228-5005, Online: www.aap.org; Fed. for Children with Special Needs, Tel. (800) 331-0688, Online: www.fcsn.org; Birth Defects Reseach for Children, Tel. (407) 895-0802, Online: www.birthdefects.org; Spina Bifida Association of America, Tel. (800) 621-3141, On line: http://sbaa@sbaa.org; www.ny-cornell.org/pediatrics/.

Clomiphene

Medication used to treat infertility.

Clomiphene is used in the treatment of infertility caused by lack of ovulation in women and decreased sperm production in men. *See also* CONCEPTION.

In women, ovulation is stimulated by hormones (gonadotropins) released by the by the pituitary gland, which is stimulated by hormones produced by the hypothalamus in the brain. Since a common cause of infertility is the failure to ovulate, clomiphene works by increasing the hypothalamus' stimulation of gonadotropin production, which can result in ovulation.

In men, clomiphene can increase sperm production through stimulation of gonadotropins. A sperm count is taken at regular intervals to check for the effectiveness of the drug, which is normally administered for a period of six to twelve months.

Side effects of clomiphene include nausea, blurred vision, headache, and hot flashes. There is also a small chance that women who take the drug can develop ovarian cysts, which then decrease in size when the dosage of the medication is reduced. A very rare side effect is alopecia (hair loss). Multiple pregnancies may also result from the use of clomiphene. *See also* INFERTILITY *and* OVULATION.

Clone

A copy of a cell or organism.

A clone is a cell or organism that is an exact genetic duplicate of another cell or organism. Recent scientific advances have resulted in the cloning of animals, which may eventually be used in medical testing. The ethical implications of cloning humans are complex, and research is ongoing.

When a gene is cloned, it is inserted into the DNA of a bacterium. Every time the bacterium reproduces, the new bacteria contain exact copies of the DNA of the original bacterium, including the inserted gene. *See also* GENETICS.

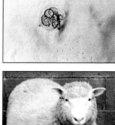
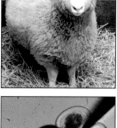
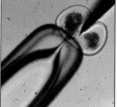

Clone.
A clone is an identical copy of a cell or organism. Above, top, a cloned embryo in an early stage of development. Above, middle, Dolly the sheep, the most famous successfully cloned animal. Above, bottom, an egg that is being fertilized outside of the womb (in vitro), in a process similar to that which is used in cloning.

Clubbing

Also known as osteoarthropathy

A broadening and thickening of the fingers or toes, with increased curvature of the nails.

Clubbing is associated with a number of diseases, most often involving the heart and lungs. These diseases include congenital heart disease, cystic fibrosis, emphysema, tuberculosis, atrial myxoma, celiac disease, cirrhosis, lymphoma, chronic active hepatitis, and Crohn's disease. Clubbing results from an accumulation of body fluids. It is associated with decreased blood oxygen and causes cyanosis (blueness) in the fingers and toes. Clubbing is also associated with malabsorption of nutrients and diseases of the liver and intestines.

If clubbing occurs, a healthcare provider should be contacted. A doctor may perform a chest x-ray, an echocardiogram, an electrocardiogram, and arterial blood gas and pulmonary function tests to determine the cause. If the underlying cause is treated, the clubbing will lessen and may totally disappear. *See also* CELIAC DISEASE; CONGENITAL HEART DISEASE; CROHN'S DISEASE; CYANOSIS; CYSTIC FIBROSIS; EMPHYSEMA; HEPATITIS; *and* TUBERCULOSIS.

Coarctation of the Aorta

A congenital condition in which the aorta is abnormally narrowed.

Coarctation of the aorta reduces blood flow to the lower half of the body. The heart works harder to compensate, resulting in higher than normal blood pressure in the upper part of the body, while the legs may exhibit normal or low blood pressure. The narrowing (coarctation) usually occurs at the point where the ductus arteriosus, a heart valve that bypasses the lungs and closes shortly after birth, is joined to the aorta. Coarctation is usually accompanied by an abnormal aortic valve. The condition may also occur together with aortic stenosis, an abnormal mitral valve, or a ventricular septal defect, all of which require medical attention and treatment.

SYMPTOMS

In most cases, coarctation of the aorta does not cause any symptoms and is discovered during a routine physical exam because of changes in pulse and blood pressure. Some children may experience headaches or leg pains, but most have no symptoms.

Some infants with coarctation of the aorta experience heart failure before the age of two weeks or may develop respiratory distress. These are life-threatening emergencies.

TREATMENT

Treatment consists of giving prostaglandins to reopen the ductus arteriosus (a valve in the heart that closes shortly after birth) and to administer various other drugs to support the heart. Surgery is recommended to repair the aorta; otherwise the heart will have to work abnormally hard to pump blood into the narrowed aorta, causing high blood pressure. Corrective surgery is usually performed when a child is between the ages of three and five. *See also* AORTIC STENOSIS; EXAMINATION, PHYSICAL; *and* VENTRICULAR ECTOPIC BEAT.

Cocaine

An illegal, extremely addictive stimulant.

Cocaine is a stimulant, the effect of which is like an amphetamine—it produces euphoria and a sense of alertness by increasing blood pressure and heart rate. It can also cause severe constipation, delusions, hallucinations, paranoia, and violent reactions. A person under the influence of cocaine can be dangerous to self or others.

Cocaine is highly addictive. Tolerance to the drug builds up rapidly, and larger and larger doses are needed to produce the desired effect. Withdrawal from cocaine addiction is extremely painful, with symptoms including severe depression and suicidal tendencies. *See also* ADDICTION; AMPHETAMINE DRUGS; DRUG DEPENDENCE; *and* SUBSTANCE ABUSE.

Coccygodynia

A pain in the tailbone (coccyx), located at the base of the spine.

Coccygodynia, or coccygeal pain, refers to a back pain originating at the base of the spinal column in the coccyx region. It usually appears after a bad fall or injury to the buttocks. Women may experience coccygodynia after childbirth as a result of excess pressure to the coccyx area.

Classic treatment for back pain is helpful for individuals with coccygodynia, such as the use of a heating pad, massage, or manipulation. A specifically designed cushion can ease the pressure on the coccyx bone and diminish pain. Coccygeal pain usually disappears over time. *See also* CHILDBIRTH; CHILDBIRTH, COMPLICATIONS; COCCYX; MASSAGE; *and* PREGNANCY.

Coccyx

The tailbone.

Four small bones fused in the shape of a triangle form the coccyx, the lower tip of the spine. The equivalent of the tail in mammals, the coccyx is a vestige of the human evolutionary ancestors' tailbone. Its main function is to serve as a site of insertion for pelvic floor muscle. It joins a much larger bone, the sacrum, to form the bowl-shaped back of the pelvis, which protects the uterus and bladder and supports the upper body. It can be felt above the hollow between the buttocks.

Even prior to fusing together in middle age, the coccyx and sacrum hardly move, except during childbirth, which can cause coccyx pain after delivery. Tenderness, swelling, or bruising are symptoms of a fracture. Treatment may include manipulation or surgical removal of the broken coccyx, physical therapy, and rehabilitation, and specific doctor-prescribed exercises. Obesity, calcium deficiency, and a history of osteoporosis increase the risk of fracture. *See also* BACK PAIN; CHILDBIRTH, COMPLICATIONS; *and* COCCYGODYNIA.

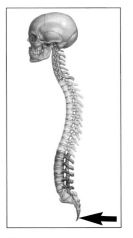

Coccyx.
Above, the coccyx is the lower tip of the spine, located at the bottom of the spinal column. The coccyx is the remnant of the tailbone that was present in the evolutionary ancestors of humans.

Cochlear Implant

An electronic device that can restore partial hearing to a severely or completely deaf person.

The cochlea is a coiled structure in the inner ear that transforms sound vibrations into nerve impulses, which are then sent to the brain. When the cochlea is damaged (through birth defect, disease, injury, or poisoning) to the point that not even powerful hearing aids work, a cochlear implant can substitute for the cochlea, sending electrical impulses to the auditory nerves in response to sound. For this to be effective, at least some healthy nerve fibers must be present.

How It Works

A cochlear implant consists of electrodes surgically implanted in the cochlea and an external portion consisting of a microphone, a speech processor, and a transmitter. The microphone and the transmitter are worn behind the ear. A thin cord connects the microphone to the speech processor and transmitter. Magnets hold the transmitter over the surgically implanted electrodes.

The microphone receives sound and transmits it to the speech processor, which translates the sounds into corresponding electrical signals. The signals are then sent through the transmitter, which touches the skin, to the internal electrodes. The electrodes then send signals to the auditory nerve fibers, which carry them to the brain.

Early implants used only a single electrode, but more recent implants use multielectrode arrays that provide several independent channels of stimulation. The multielectrode implants, with at least four to six channels, provide more information about the acoustic signal and improve speech recognition.

Implant Surgery

Electrodes are implanted in the cochlea through an incision in the bone leading to the inner ear. The procedure takes place under general anesthesia and can last up to five hours, depending on the type of implant and the anatomy of the patient's inner ear. Recovery generally requires at least one night in the hospital.

Prognosis

Cochlear implants do not restore hearing to normal, but rather transmit sounds that the patient must learn to interpret. The effectiveness of the implant depends on a person's existing language skills and motivation to learn, and on the number of working nerve fibers. A majority of patients are able to detect speech at comfortable listening levels. Many patients are able to combine lip-reading with cues from the sounds and rhythms of speech, while a smaller number are able to learn to understand words or sentences without the use of lip-reading.

For background information on cochlear implant, see HEARING. *Further information can be found in* BIRTH DEFECTS; CONGENITAL; DEAFNESS; GENE; GENETICS; HEARING AID; *and* HEARING TEST. *See also* ANESTHESIA, GENERAL *and* SURGERY *for more about what will happen during the implant procedure.*

Cod Liver Oil

Oil from the liver of codfish, used as a nutritional supplement and as a laxative.

Cod liver oil has been used as a laxative and nutritional supplement for many generations. Fish oils such as cod liver oil are also a supplemental source of omega-3 fatty acids, which can lower blood fat. However, cod liver and some other fish oils may contain large amounts of vitamin D and vitamin A, which are toxic in great quantities. In order to safely obtain the benefits of omega-3 fatty acids, the American Heart Association recommends consumption of fish and not of fish oil supplements. There are also vegetable sources of omega-3 fatty acids, which are fairly similar to fish oils. Some plant sources include walnuts and walnut oil, wheat germ oil, rapeseed oil, butternuts, beans, seaweed, and flaxseed oil. *See also* CONSTIPATION *and* NUTRITION.

Codeine

A pain-relieving (analgesic) medication often used in conjunction with cough medicines as a cough suppressant.

Codeine mildly sedates the brain and nervous system and suppresses the cough reflex. It is an opioid analgesic and, while less addictive than most of these types of drugs, is available only through prescription. People who have diarrhea, heart disease, kidney disease, liver disease, seizures, or allergies, or who are pregnant or trying to get pregnant should speak with their doctor before taking codeine. It interacts with alcohol, medications used for seizures, and antidepressants. Side effects may include cold, clammy skin; seizures; changed heart rate; breathlessness; wheezing; and rash. Milder side effects include constipation, vision problems, dizziness, drowsiness, headache, nausea, vomiting, and sweating. *See also* ADDICTION; ANALGESIC DRUGS; CONSTIPATION; COUGH; COUGH REMEDIES; NAUSEA; *and* VOMITING.

Cognitive-Behavior Therapy

Psychological treatment that addresses the thought processes, rather than the underlying motivation, of a person suffering from a mental disorder.

Cognitive-behavior therapy was developed in the 1960s by Dr. Aaron Beck and Dr. David Barlow for the treatment of anxiety disorders, especially panic disorder. Based on the idea that thoughts and beliefs affect emotions and behavior, this treatment attempts to help the patient pay attention to the self-defeating thoughts that cause anxiety or depression. Cognitive theory suggests that a depressed person who makes a mistake is more likely to have thoughts such as "I am a failure" or "I never do anything right," rather than to recognize that everyone makes mistakes.

Cognitive-behavior therapy aims to help the patient pay attention to this thought pattern and replace such thoughts with a more realistic assessment of the situation. An individual who suffers from panic attacks and starts to notice his or her heart beating faster is taught to understand that fear, rather than a heart attack, is causing the heart to beat faster.

STAGES

Cognitive-behavior therapy is usually brief, lasting no longer than a few months. The first stage is education, when a patient is taught about how the mood or anxiety disorder results from overwhelming negative thoughts and beliefs. Because patients suffering from anxiety disorders and depression tend to interpret situations as catastrophic, in cognitive restructuring the goal is to train patients to monitor dysfunctional thoughts and replace them with more rational and helpful thoughts. This form of therapy requires a good deal of practice and effort by the patient and is tailored specifically to the individual's unique thought patterns.

PANIC ATTACKS

When used for treating panic attacks, cognitive-behavior therapy teaches patients breathing exercises and relaxation techniques. This type of therapy helps the individual to slow and regulate breathing and to avoid hyperventilation, which often initiates a panic attack. He or she will be gradually exposed to panic-inducing situations, in the presence of a supportive therapist, while learning strategies to cope with accompanying anxiety.

The patient-therapist relationship in this form of therapy is collaborative. Cognitive-behavior therapy does not delve into the underlying meaning of the symptom but attempts to retrain the mind in order to deal with the difficult, painful, and limiting emotions that plague those who suffer from depression and panic.

> *Background information on cognitive-behavior therapy can be found in* PSYCHIATRY. *For further information, see* BEHAVIOR THERAPY *and* PSYCHOTHERAPY. *See also* ANXIETY DISORDERS *and* PANIC DISORDER *for more on disorders for which cognitive-behavior therapy might be used.*

Cold Injury

Tissue injury due to freezing temperatures and outdoor exposure.

The three stages of cold injury are chilling, frostnip, and frostbite. The first stage, chilling, involves a rapid lowering of body temperature. The skin then becomes numb and loses color, marking the second stage, frostnip. At this stage, tissue damage is still reversible. In the last stage, frostbite, normally red skin becomes pale or white, and ice crystals form on the skin's surface. As the skin warms, it will appear blue or purple. Burning, swelling, and chilblains (burning or chilling sensations) may also occur. Chilblains (also known as pernio) are usually experienced in areas of the body that were previously frostbitten.

Warning signs to look for if cold injury is suspected include shivering, a change in skin color (to pale or blue), and numbness. Affected children who have been complaining about the cold may suddenly stop complaining.

Compared to adults, children have a higher ratio of body surface to weight, and thus are more likely to suffer cold injury. Factors that may cause cold injury include low temperature, moist skin subjected to low temperature, wind, and high altitude. Cold injury is treated by warming the affected area (in the case of frostbite, the area must be warmed slowly and carefully). Chilblains usually resist attempts at treatment and can persist for months or even years. *See also* Frostbite; Hypothermia; *and* Pernio.

Cold Sore

A viral infection that produces small blisters, usually on the lips and gums, but also on the nose, chin, and cheeks.

Cold sores are painful sores caused by the type I herpes simplex virus. Symptoms are usually visible from one to two weeks after the infection, but the virus remains dormant in the body and will recur when triggered by stress, fatigue, or another infection. The disease is extremely contagious and is transmitted by direct contact. It remains contagious until the blisters crust over and begin to heal.

There is no cure for the virus that causes cold sores, but acyclovir tablets and ointment applied over a period of ten days may reduce blistering and promote healing. Common side effects of acyclovir may include a rash, hives, mild burning or stinging at the application site, headache, and lightheadedness.

The herpes simplex virus can never be entirely eliminated from the body. People with immune deficiency or diseases, such as AIDS, those who are recovering from transplant surgery, and those being treated with chemotherapy for cancer, are at increased risk, because the virus can spread to the brain. *See also* AIDS; Antiviral Drugs; Cancer; Chemotherapy; Fever Blisters; *and* Herpes Zoster.

Cold, Common

A viral infection of the upper respiratory tract.

Any one of over a hundred different viruses can cause a cold. The virus is transmitted in droplets that are coughed or sneezed into the air, but it is also transmitted when one person touches an infected person, handles an object that has been touched by an

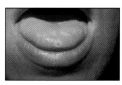

Cold Sore.
Cold sores are caused by an infection with type I of the herpes simplex virus. Above, a cold sore located on the tongue.

Cold Remedies

Hundreds of different viruses may produce symptoms typical of the common cold—runny nose, sneezing, coughing, sore throat, fatigue, muscle aches, and headache. Unless the infection moves to other parts of the body, colds are self-limiting—the symptoms will subside on their own. No cure exists for the common cold. Instead, cold remedies are used to control symptoms. These remedies include decongestants, cough suppressants, and acetaminophen. There is some anecdotal evidence that zinc tablets may shorten the duration of a cold.

The best treatment for colds is prevention, which can be no more complicated than washing hands frequently and avoiding physical contact with someone who has a cold.

infected person, or eats food prepared by an infected person. People who are fatigued or have allergies are more susceptible to colds.

Symptoms of the common cold include watery discharge from the nose, sneezing, nasal congestion, sore throat, watery and itchy eyes, fatigue, muscle aches and pains, a headache, and low-grade fever. The common cold is self-limiting; the course of an infection is usually seven to ten days.

TREATMENT

There is no cure for the common cold, but the symptoms can be treated. The infected person should stay warm and drink plenty of fluids to keep secretions loose and easier to remove. Dozens of cold remedies are sold over the counter. Nasal decongestants may provide temporary relief, and antihistamines may dry up a runny nose. Inhaling the mist from a vaporizer may relieve some congestion. These drugs are not without side effects, however. They may cause drowsiness, particularly in the elderly. Coughing is how the body brings up secretions from the lungs, so cough suppressants should be avoided unless the cough interferes with sleep or is very painful. Antibiotics should not be used unless there is also a bacterial infection, since the common cold is caused by a virus.

For background information on common cold, see INFECTIOUS DISEASE. *Further information can be found in* ALLERGY; BACTERIA; BREATHING DIFFICULTIES; COUGH; COUGH REMEDIES; EXPECTORANT; FEVER; HYGIENE; MICROORGANISM; RESPIRATORY TRACT INFECTION; *and* VIRUSES. *See also* ANTIBIOTIC DRUGS; ANTIHISTAMINE DRUGS; ANTIVIRAL DRUGS; *and* ZINC *for more on treatment.*

Colectomy

The surgical removal of the large intestine (colon) or part of the colon (partial or hemi-colectomy).

A colectomy is recommended for serious diseases of the colon that cannot be controlled nonsurgically.

A partial colectomy is performed when disease or damage is confined to a portion of the colon, as in the case of a specific malignant tumor or an obstruction. The diseased or damaged portion of the colon is removed and the remaining healthy sections are rejoined. Occasionally, a temporary colostomy, in which the colon is connected to an artificial opening (stoma) in the abdominal wall, is performed so that the rejoined section has time to heal.

A total colectomy is performed in cases where disease or damage affects the entire colon. These may include some cases of ulcerative colitis and familial adenomatous polyposis. A total colectomy may involve both removal of the rectum and a permanent ileostomy.

In a laparoscopic colectomy, a tube with a light and camera at the end is inserted into the abdomen through a small incision and is used to guide instruments also inserted through small incisions. This type of colectomy is being performed with increased frequency and with promising results. It reduces abdominal wall damage and shortens the recovery period, which is usually eight to twelve days.

Prognosis. Generally, the colon functions normally after a partial colectomy. If a large section or all of the colon is removed, it greatly reduces the ability of the intestines to absorb water from the feces and can cause diarrhea; this requires ongoing drug treatment. A patient who is about to have a colostomy will need training for proper aftercare.

Background material on colectomy can be found in COLON *and* DIGESTIVE SYSTEM. *For further information, see* COLOSTOMY; DIARRHEA; LAPAROSCOPY; *and* POLYPS. *See also* COLON CANCER *and* ULCERATIVE COLITIS *for more on diseases that may necessitate a colectomy.*

Resources on the Common Cold

Kolata, Gina, *Flu: The Story of an Epidemic* (1999); Grist, Norman R., et al., *Diseases of Infection: An Illustrated Textbook* (1992); Shaw, Michael, ed., *Everything You Need to Know About Diseases* (1996); Fettner, Ann Guidici, *The Science of Viruses: What They Are, Why They Make Us Sick, How They Will Change the Future* (1990); Centers for Disease Contol and Prevention, Tel. (800) 311-3435, Online: www.cdc.gov; Infectious Disease Society of America, Tel. (703) 299-0200, Online: www.idsociety.org; National Institute of Allergy and Infectious Disease, Tel. (301) 496-5717, Online: www.niaid.nih.org.

Colic

A term used to refer to digestive disorders or illnesses related to the gastrointestinal tract.

Biliary colic is pain that is caused by obstruction of the flow of bile from the gallbladder. This condition is most often caused by gallstones.

Renal colic is caused by obstruction of the ureter by kidney stones. The pain is intermittent and felt in the left or right flank, later spreading to the abdomen, the inner thigh, and genital areas. It is accompanied by nausea, vomiting, abdominal distention, and fever.

Colic in infants refers to attacks of abdominal pain that are thought to originate in the intestines. A baby with colic usually begins to cry after a feeding. The severity and frequency of attacks may vary. The cause is unknown, but may be associated with swallowed air that has entered the intestines. Some babies seem to be more susceptible to colic than others. *See also* BILIARY COLIC; CALCULUS, URINARY TRACT; *and* COLIC, INFANTILE.

Colic, Infantile

Severe crying in infants for which there is no discernible cause.

A baby who suffers from colic is usually not hungry, wet, or dirty, but is clearly experiencing discomfort. The precise cause is unknown. Colic is currently thought to be due to bouts of intense abdominal pain, originating in the intestines. This theory is bolstered by the fact that often the baby stops crying after having a bowel movement or passing gas.

Symptoms. A baby responds to colic, as to any discomfort, with crying. Attacks may last for several hours at any time of day; they do not necessarily occur more frequently at night, although it may certainly seem that way to tired parents. Crying from colic is distinguished from cries of hunger by the timing—crying often begins after a feeding instead of before. Some infants never seem to experience colic, others have only occasional episodes, and others experience colic daily.

Babies often quiet down, or at least are slightly soothed, when held. It is thought that pressure on the abdomen and warmth from the parent's body eases gastrointestinal discomfort. Colicky babies also benefit from being held on a lap. Walking or other motion serves as a distraction.

It is particularly important to burp the baby after each feeding. Sometimes a change in formula may help as well. Colic generally disappears after a few months. *See also* CRYING IN INFANTS.

Colitis

Inflammation of the large intestine.

Colitis can be caused by a number of factors, including viral or bacterial infection, parasitic infestation, and autoimmune disorders. It may be acute or chronic. Both acute and chronic colitis are marked by diarrhea, abdominal pain, and fever.

Antibiotic-Related Colitis. Colitis can be caused by taking antibiotics for a prolonged period of time. Antibiotics can kill beneficial bacteria in the intestines, which may allow for the growth of harmful bacteria, such as *Clostridium difficile*. Inflammation may be mild or severe, and ulcers may also develop.

Symptoms of antibiotic-related colitis include fever, diarrhea, and abdominal pain. Severe dehydration, which can be life-threatening, may occur. Treatment involves stopping the use of the antibiotics causing the condition.

Ischemic Colitis. This is an uncommon condition, affecting mainly the elderly, in which there is less blood supplied to the colon. The major arteries are not affected.

The symptoms of ischemic colitis include pain in the lower abdomen and rectal bleeding. A narrowing of the colon may develop at the site of the ischemia. The problem may resolve on its own, but surgery is usually performed in severe cases.

Hemorrhagic Colitis. Hemorrhagic colitis is a type of gastroenteritis caused by certain strains of *Escherichia coli* bacteria. The bacteria produce a toxin that causes sudden bloody diarrhea. Outbreaks can be caused by eating undercooked beef or drinking unpasteurized milk. *E. coli* can be spread by contact from one person to another. If absorbed into the bloodstream, the toxin can damage other organs, such as the kidneys.

The primary symptom of hemorrhagic colitis is bloody diarrhea. Prevention of dehydration is crucial. Antibiotics will not kill the bacteria or relieve the symptoms. Hospitalization is necessary.

Other Types. Ulcerative colitis and Crohn's disease are two chronic, potentially serious causes of colitis. The cause of these conditions is unknown. They usually appear in early adulthood and are characterized by chronic inflammation and the formation of sores (ulcers) in the colon. Treatment of these conditions aims to control the symptoms and replace lost fluids and nutrients. *See also* CROHN'S DISEASE.

Collagen

> The main structural protein in the body, found in connective tissues such as skin, bone, ligaments, and cartilage.

Collagen is a major protein in the body, responsible for structure. Collagen diseases affect skin, bone, ligaments, and cartilage. They include Ehlers-Danlos syndrome, keloids, mucopolysaccharidosis, and osteogenesis imperfecta.

Ehlers-Danlos syndrome consists of a group of inherited disorders characterized by fragile skin that bruises easily, excessive looseness of the joints, and easily damaged blood vessels. The disease is associated with abnormal formation of connective tissue.

Keloids. The term keloids refers to excessively large patches of scar tissue at the site of a skin injury. Surgical incisions, vaccination sites, burns, acne, and even scratches can cause such scarring. Keloids occur primarily in young women and people of color. Most keloids tend to become less noticeable over time.

Mucopolysaccharidosis (MPS) is a severe genetic disease found in children and adults. In individuals with MPS, the body has too much of a sugar called mucopolysaccharide, caused by the absence of an enzyme. The body is unable to break down mucopolysaccharides completely. MPS causes bone, spleen, eye, and liver abnormalities, and mental retardation in some cases.

Osteogenesis imperfecta is a condition involving abnormally fragile bones. It is an inherited disorder that is usually present from birth. Infants with this condition can suffer multiple fractures of the arms and legs, causing shortening of the limbs. The skull may also be affected, and trauma to the skull of the baby during labor may result in stillbirth. *See also* EHLERS-DANLOS SYNDROME; KELOID; MUCOPOLYSACCHARIDOSIS; *and* OSTEOGENESIS IMPERFECTA.

Collar, Orthopedic

> Collar worn to stabilize the neck.

After a neck injury or repeated stress on bones, nerves, or cartilage, an orthopedic collar can aid healing by preventing excess movement. Soft collars, made from foam, stabilize the neck and lessen movement. Stiff collars, made from foam and plastic, may be used to stabilize a fractured neck that is partially healed or to stabilize vertebrae in the neck. *See also* NECK.

Colles' Fracture

> Break at the end of the lower arm bone, which bends the hand backward from the wrist.

Colles' fractures often occur in people who try to break a fall with their hands. They are more prevalent among the elderly. The bones of a younger person may not break, but an older adult or an individual with osteoarthritis may have fragile bones. Young people tend to suffer Colles' fractures from violent trauma, such as that encountered in skateboarding or in-line skating accidents. *See also* FRACTURE.

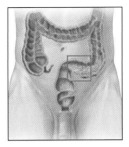

Colon.
Above, the colon forms the main portion of the large intestine. The four sections of the colon are, in order from the junction with the small intestine, ascending, transverse, descending, and sigmoid.

Resources on Colon Cancer
Murphy, G., et al., *Informed Decisions: The Complete Book of Cancer Diagnosis, Treatment, and Recovery* (1997); Renneker, Mark, ed., *Understanding Cancer* (1988); Steen, R. Grant, *A Conspiracy of Cells: The Basic Science of Cancer* (1993); Steward, Clifford T., ed., *Cancer: Prevention, Detection, Causes, Treatment* (1988); American Cancer Society, Tel. (800) ACS-2345, Online: www.cancer.org; Nat. Cancer Institue, Tel. (800) 4-CANCER, Online: www.nci.nih.gov; www.nycornell.org/medicine/hematology/html.

Colon

The primary section of the large intestine.

Four and a half feet long and two and a half inches wide, the colon is a segmented tube draped over and around the small intestine. The serous coat, the colon's fibrous outer layer, is a smooth protective membrane. Consecutive, uniform bulging segments called haustrations give the colon the outline of a thick chain.

The colon has four sections. From the lower right abdomen, the ascending colon stretches straight up to the liver and bends ninety degrees to form the hepatic flexure. Here the second section, the transverse colon, begins, drooping above the small intestine before climbing slightly under the stomach to the splenic flexure, an acute downward bend near the spleen. The descending colon drops straight down along the left side of the abdomen to the top of the pelvis. The subsequent S-turn in the bowel is the sigmoid colon, which leads to the rectum. *See also* COLON CANCER; COLONOSCOPY; *and* COLOSTOMY.

Colon Cancer

Also known as colorectal cancer

An abnormal growth of cells in the large intestine.

Over 100,000 people in the United States are diagnosed with colon cancer every year. Contrary to popular conception, colon cancer is common in both men and women, and is actually slightly more prevalent in women.

INCIDENCE
Colon cancer is the second most common form of cancer in the United States (lung cancer is the first) and causes the second highest number of deaths from cancer, accounting for over 15 percent of cancer deaths. About 2 out of every 1000 people will suffer from colon cancer at some point in their lives. The incidence of colon cancer grows with age, starting to rise at age 40 and peaking between the ages of 60 and 75.

TYPES
Carcinoma is the most common type of colon cancer. Carcinoid tumors, which slowly increase in size, can also develop in the colon, as can lymphomas, which can damage the intestinal wall.

CAUSES
There is no single identifiable cause of colon cancer. Instead, there are a number of factors that increase a person's risk of developing the disease. The high occurrence of colon cancer in Western countries points to factors such as a high fat, meat-rich, and low-fiber diet. A family history of colon cancer is also a contributory factor. Colon cancer more commonly occurs in people who have other disorders of the colon, such as colon polyps, ulcerative colitis, and granulomatous colitis.

SYMPTOMS
Most patients with colon cancer are asymptomatic (without noticeable symptoms). The first symptom of colon cancer can be a distinct change in bowel habits (either diarrhea or constipation) lasting longer than ten days. Other symptoms of the disease may include blood in the feces, abdominal pain and tenderness, unexplained weight loss, and a feeling of fullness or gaseousness. Patients may also feel weak, owing to anemia (low red blood cell count).

DIAGNOSIS
Colon cancer is detected by tests on feces and on the colon. These may include a manual rectal examination, a fecal blood test, a colonoscopy, or a sigmoidoscopy.

In a manual or digital rectal examination, the doctor examines the rectum with a lubricated finger to check for abnormalities. In a fecal blood test, a laboratory tests the feces of the patient for the presence of blood. The patient must follow a special diet and submit fecal samples to a doctor for three consecutive days.

In a colonoscopy, the intestine is emptied with enemas or laxatives. A flexible tube with a light at one end is inserted into the rectum. The doctor then inspects the colon for polyps or growths. Any growth is removed and sent to a laboratory to be examined and tested. Since a colonoscopy can be uncomfortable, some patients will receive a mild sedative before the procedure. A sigmoidoscopy is similar to a colonoscopy, except that the tube inserted into the rectum is smaller and only the sigmoid colon is examined.

TREATMENT

Treatment varies depending on the stage of development of the cancer. Surgery to remove the affected part of the colon is the primary treatment, however, nonsurgical treatments may be successful in treating rectal cancer.

In a procedure called a partial colectomy, the tumor is removed along with a small amount of surrounding normal tissue. If the cancer has spread through the wall of the intestine or invaded the body's lymph system, chemotherapy or radiation treatment may be necessary.

In an operation called an abdominoperineal resection (or APN), the rectum and anus are removed and a permanent colostomy is necessary, in which an artificial opening (stoma) is created so that feces can empty into a bag outside the body. This operation is usually necessary only with tumors of the lower portion of the rectum.

OUTLOOK

The outlook for colon cancer patients depends on how long the cancer has gone undetected. If colon cancer is caught in its earliest stages, the cure rate is very high, up to 80 to 90 percent. If surgery must be followed by chemotherapy or radiation treatment, the survival rate after five years is 50 percent. If the cancer spreads to the lymph nodes, the five-year survival rate drops to 30 percent. Since the survival rate increases the sooner colon cancer is detected, it is important to see a doctor at the onset of any changes in bowel habits.

PREVENTION

Colon cancer can be easily cured if it is caught early enough, but it is even easier to

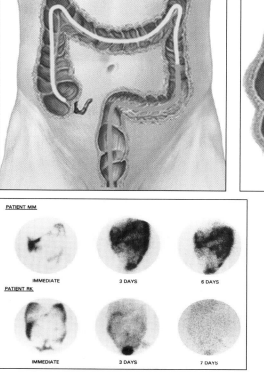

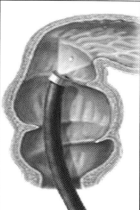

Colon Cancer.
Colon cancer is the uncontrolled growth of cells in the large intestine. This type of cancer is often diagnosed with a colonoscopy or sigmoidoscopy. Above, left, a sigmoidoscopy examines only the lower third, or sigmoid, portion of the colon. The area examined is shaded in green. Above, right, in both a sigmoidoscopy and a colonoscopy, a thin tube with a light on the end is passed into the colon, which is examined for any signs of abnormal growth. Left, camera scans of two patients who were injected with a monoclonal antibody, a substance that recognizes colon cancer.

prevent. After lung cancer, colon cancer is the second most preventable type of cancer. To prevent colon cancer, it has long been thought that individuals should be screened regularly using tests such as fecal blood tests, manual rectal examinations, and sigmoidoscopy. Any colon polyps, although they may not be cancerous, should be removed. Recently, there has been a pronounced trend toward the periodic performance of full colonoscopy. It is important that individuals at risk for colon cancer eat a diet low in fat and high in fiber, drink alcohol in moderation, refrain from using tobacco or tobacco products, and stick to a regular program of moderate exercise, such as walking. As many as 40 percent of colon cancer cases could be prevented by these simple precautions.

For background information on colon cancer, see COLON *and* DIGESTIVE SYSTEM. *Further information can be found in* COLECTOMY; COLOSTOMY; *and* POLYPS. *See also* DIET AND DISEASE *and* OBESITY *for more on possible risk factors for colon cancer.*

Colonoscopy

A procedure for directly viewing and performing minor surgery on the large intestine, using a fiberoptic endoscope.

Colonoscopy is used to examine the large intestine as a means of diagnosing disorders such as bleeding, benign or malignant tumors, polyps, stricture, diverticulosis (the presence of inflamed sacs in the inner lining of the intestine), and inflammatory bowel disease (also known as Crohn's disease or ulcerative colitis).

PROCEDURE

A patient is generally given a sedative and pain reliever immediately prior to a colonoscopy, since the procedure can be uncomfortable. A fiberoptic device known as a colonoscope is guided through the colon. Air is injected through the colonoscope into the bowel, distending the colon and providing better visualization through the endoscope. The bowel lining can be seen and photographed through a lens at the tip of the colonoscope. Should the doctor suspect a lesion, he or she may remove a biopsy sample through a chamber of the endoscope. In addition, any polyps can be removed and laser surgery can be performed during the procedure if necessary.

RISKS

Use of a colonoscope carries a very slight risk of intestinal perforation. If a polyp removal is performed, there is also a risk of bleeding. After age 50, it is recommended that the colon be examined regularly every five years. For those whose family history includes colon cancer, screening should begin at age 40 or at least 15 years before the age at which the relative was diagnosed. Regular screening is considered among the best means of lowering the risk of diseases of the digestive system.

Background information on colonoscopy can be found in COLON; DIAGNOSIS; *and* DIGESTIVE SYSTEM. *For further information, see* COLON CANCER; GASTROINTESTINAL TRACT; INTESTINE; LAXATIVE DRUGS; *and* POLYPS.

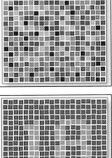
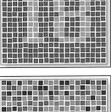
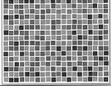
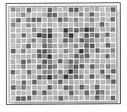

Color Vision.
Above, four tests of color vision. The number 58 should be visible in the top test, the number 18 in the second test from the top, the capital letter E in the third test from the top, and the number 17 in the bottom test.

Color Vision

The ability to differentiate colors.

Light consists of radiation of different wavelengths. Each wavelength produces a different color in the color spectrum, which consists of red, orange, yellow, green, blue, indigo, and violet. When the wavelengths affect the light-sensitive cells in the retina of the eye, nerve impulses are stimulated, which then are sent to the occipital lobe in the rear of the brain to be processed. Most light consists of many different wavelengths mixed together, which is interpreted as a single color by the retina and the brain.

The retina contains two types of light-sensitive cells: rods and cones. The rods do not respond differently to different wavelengths, and thus do not affect color vision. Because the cones are concentrated in the center of the retina, color vision is not as accurate for objects at the periphery of the viewed area. Since cones need a certain amount of total light to function, if it is too dark, only the rods will respond, and everything will appear gray.

When a cone receives light, the visual pigments it contains are changed structurally and send electrical signals to the brain. Each cone sends electrical impulses more frequently when stimulated by specific wavelengths. Thus a single cone responds more positively to light with a wavelength of 570 nanometers, enabling the brain to process this information and distinguish the presence of colors in this wavelength (i.e., blue color). *See also* EYE, DISORDERS OF *and* VISION, DISORDERS OF.

Colostomy

An operation to create an artificial opening (stoma) from part of the large intestine (colon) to the outside of the abdomen.

A colostomy is performed to temporarily bypass a blocked or healing intestinal tract or to permanently replace colonic or rectal function. The colon may be removed or may not function as a result of injury, cancer, or certain chronic diseases, such as ulcerative colitis, in which the bowel becomes inflamed and develops numerous sores, and familial adenomatous polyposis, in which hundreds of potentially cancerous growths develop in the colon.

TYPES

A temporary colostomy is often performed in conjunction with the removal of all or part of the colon (colectomy). The remaining healthy portions of the colon, or the small intestine and the rectum, are joined together, and a colostomy is performed above the junction. This allows the colon to heal without passing feces. A temporary colostomy is closed when the rejoined colon has healed. A permanent colostomy is performed when it is not possible to rejoin any portion of a functioning colon; this is most often as a result of rectal or colon cancer.

PROCEDURE

Colostomy is performed under general anesthesia. After making an incision in the abdomen, the surgeon separates the abdominal muscles, exposing the intestines. The diseased section is clamped and excised. The top end of the colon is brought to the surface of the abdomen and stitched to the skin, and the bottom end is sealed.

Complications. A colostomy can sometimes slip forward (prolapse) and protrude out of the abdomen. The opening or path can also narrow, blocking the passage of feces. Additional surgery may be required.

RECOVERY

After the operation, the patient is fed intravenously for several days and then given a light diet. The average hospital stay is seven to ten days, and full recovery is usually achieved in six weeks.

After a colostomy, feces pass through the intestines normally and are emptied through the stoma into a lightweight plastic bag attached to the body. The patient must be trained to properly care for the colostomy and often receives therapy to help adjust to the day-to-day implications of living with a colostomy.

For background information on colostomy, see COLECTOMY. *Further information can be found in* COLON; DIGESTIVE SYSTEM; *and* SURGERY. *See also* COLON CANCER *and* INTESTINE, OBSTRUCTION OF *for more on conditions that may require a colostomy as treatment.*

Colostrum

A thin, yellowish, sticky liquid secreted by the breasts before milk production begins.

Colostrum may begin to leak from the breasts from about the fourth month of pregnancy on. During the first 12 to 24 hours after delivery, the amount of fluid produced increases greatly.

Colostrum is a valuable fluid; it has a higher protein content than milk, and is rich in calories yet low in fat. It acts as a laxative, helping to clear the baby's intestines of mucus and meconium, dark greenish fecal matter that accumulates during pregnancy. Colostrum also contains antibodies that protect the newborn against disease. Above all, colostrum provides an opportunity for mother and baby to become proficient at breast-feeding before true milk production begins, on the third or fourth day after delivery. *See also* BREAST FEEDING.

Colposcopy

Process of evaluating tissue of the cervix or upper vagina, and, in case of abnormal pap smear results, performing a biopsy.

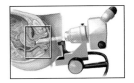

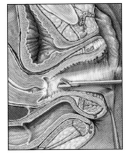

Colposcopy.
A colposcopy is used to further evaluate tissue of the cervix when the results of a pap smear are abnormal. Above, top, an instrument called a colposcope illuminates the cervix for examination. Above, bottom, forceps are then used to sample a small portion of tissue from the cervix.

A colposcope is a specialized microscope used to examine the lining of the cervix and upper vagina. Generally, abnormal tissue is first identified by a pap smear, a technique for diagnosing cancer by removing cells from the cervix and vagina.

Colposcopy is particularly useful for defining the extent of tumors and evaluating benign lesions. Further, it is a recommended technique for vaginal examination in prepubescent youth at risk for DES syndrome—a disorder caused by prenatal exposure to diethylstilbestrol, a synthetic form of the hormone estrogen, once thought to prevent miscarriage.

A painless procedure, colposcopy requires only a few minutes to complete. A gynecologist can use colposcopy to identify cervical warts, tumors, and precancerous or cancerous tissue changes.

If a biopsy is required, the doctor may remove a tiny piece of cervix observed by the colposcope (punch biopsy) or perform endocervical curettage, in which tissue is scraped from the cervical canal. These techniques are often used in combination for a thorough diagnosis.

Yearly pap smears are strongly recommended, as they provide early warning for cervical irregularities, particularly cervical cancer. *See also* CERVIX; CERVIX, CANCER OF; EXAMINATION, PHYSICAL; GYNECOLOGY; *and* PAP SMEAR.

Coma

A state of deep unconsciousness caused by disease or injury.

Coma is a state similar to deep sleep, but a person cannot be roused from it. A person in a coma does not respond to external stimuli, such as light, touch, sound, or pain. The patient is also unaware of internal sensations, such as an urgency to empty

a full bladder. Patients in comas thus need urinary catheters, intravenous feeding, and sometimes even artificial respiration. In a mild coma, the patient may be able to move the limbs in response to pain. In a deep coma, there is no such response.

CAUSES

Coma results from damage or injury to the cerebrum, brain stem, or other parts of the brain. Coma may be caused by:

- head injury, such as a concussion or bleeding around the brain;
- infections, such as meningitis and encephalitis, that produce high fever;
- oxygen deprivation resulting from cardiac arrest;
- carbon monoxide inhalation;
- extreme high/low body temperature;
- low blood sugar (hypoglycemia); and
- drug and alcohol abuse.

DIAGNOSIS

The severity of a coma can give important information about prognosis and the best choice of treatment, so a physician will test the patient's level of response and functioning of vital signs. To determine the cause of the coma, blood tests check for anemia, infection, and abnormal levels of alcohol, oxygen, or carbon dioxide. Computed tomography (CAT) or magnetic resonance imaging (MRI) can be used to detect possible brain damage.

TREATMENT

In some instances, the coma can be treated by treating the underlying cause. Otherwise, the patient can only be made as comfortable as possible. A deep coma may last for years, or a person may recover after a shorter period of time. The outlook is better in cases of injury than in cases where the coma is caused by tissue death due to a lack of oxygen.

Background information on coma can be found in BRAIN DISORDERS *and* NERVOUS SYSTEM. *For further information, see* CAT SCAN; INVOLUNTARY MOVEMENTS; MRI; *and* PARALYSIS. *See also* ACCIDENTS *and* HEAD INJURY *for possible causes of a coma.*

Resources on Coma
Calvin, William, *Inside the Brain* (2001); Le-Doux, Joseph, *The Emoional Brain* (1998); Pierce, Howard, *Owner's Manual for the Brain* (2000); Restak, Richard, *The Secret Life of the Brain* (2001); Restak, R., *The Brain Has a Mind of Its Own* (1993); Sacks, Oliver W, *Awakenings* (1989); www.med.cornell.edu/neuro/html.

Commensal

A term used to refer to microorganisms that live on the skin or in the intestinal tract and that do not harm (and may indeed benefit) the body.

Within the body, there are billions of microorganisms that do not harm the body; many of these organisms actually benefit the body by breaking down dying skin cells and cleaning up other debris. For example, there are commensal bacteria in the intestinal tract that help in the digestive process. If antibiotics are administered in an effort to destroy disease-causing bacteria, some commensal bacteria will also be destroyed and may be replaced by less benign organisms that can cause a disease different from that which was the original target of the drug. *See also* ANTIBIOTIC DRUGS *and* ANTIBIOTIC RESISTANCE.

Compliance

Adherence to health regulations or medical advice.

Many federal, state, and local laws govern the ways in which institutions, individuals, health practitioners, and businesses can engage in certain activities that affect the health of the community. For example, manufacturing facilities must keep their emissions to a prescribed level and toxic waste handlers must dispose of waste in a federally regulated manner. Employers and local governments must create a work environment that adheres to federal regulations governing occupational safety and the treatment of people with disabilities.

In medicine, compliance refers to both how well medical institutions meet these standards and how adequate the documentation is for levels of billing and for payment from insurance providers or government agencies. The penalties for failing to comply with regulations include fines, civil lawsuits, and criminal prosecution.

Compliance also refers to the degree to which patients adhere to a treatment plan, often a critical element in recovery. *See also* PUBLIC HEALTH.

Complication

Negative reaction to or undesirable side effect of an illness or surgical procedure.

Complication is a general term covering the full scope of side effects and undesired consequences. A complication can be further damage brought on by an existing condition, or can be caused by the treatment itself. A patient might have a negative reaction to a procedure or to a medication or anesthesia.

Even the most common surgeries have potential complications. A tonsillectomy (a removal of the tonsils) can cause severe bleeding that may be fatal if left untreated. Oral surgery to remove wisdom teeth can lead to facial paralysis. One of the most common sources of surgical complications is the use of general anesthesia. Complications from anesthesia include heart attack, stroke, sore throat, damage to the teeth, blood clots, and allergic reaction. *See also* ANESTHESIA, DENTAL; ANESTHESIA, GENERAL; *and* SURGERY.

Compress

Padded material used either to apply heat, cold, or medication to a part of the body or to stop bleeding from a wound.

A compress is usually applied under pressure to an injury or wound and held in place by a bandage. Compresses can be made of gauze, linen, or plastic envelopes filled with heat- or cold-retaining jelly or ointment. Hot-packs are commonly heated up in warm water, while cold packs are usually chilled in a refrigerator. Fabric compresses are cooled by ice or cold water, or heated by warm water.

USAGE

A cold compress can reduce pain, swelling, and bleeding under the skin (bruising) after an injury. A dry compress can stop bleeding or can be used to apply medicated cream to infected skin. *See also* BANDAGE; EMERGENCY FIRST STEPS; FIRST AID; *and* ICE PACKS.

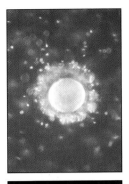

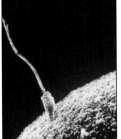

Conception.
When a sperm fertilizes an egg, conception occurs and a zygote is formed. Above, bottom, only a single sperm is needed to fertilize an egg and create a zygote. Above, top, the zygote in the first days after conception.

Conception

Another name for fertilization; the union of sperm and egg, creating a zygote.

Conception takes place in the upper third of the fallopian tube. When ejaculation occurs, hundreds of millions of sperm are released, of which a small fraction travel through the uterus up one of the fallopian tubes to the egg. Some sperm die along the way. Those that survive swarm over the egg's surface, but only one succeeds in entering. The sperm penetrates the egg by releasing an enzyme that dissolves the egg's firm outer layer, the zona pellucida. Upon entry, the sperm sheds its tail. A chemical change then occurs in the egg's outer membrane, keeping all other sperm out. The chromosomes of the successful sperm unite with those of the egg. A fertilized egg is known as a zygote. It is first a single cell and then divides multiple times.

The day of ovulation, when a mature egg is released from the ovary, is the time when conception is most likely to occur. An egg may be fertilized for 24 to 36 hours after its release. Sperm remain alive in the uterus from two to five days after ejaculation. It is possible to pinpoint the exact day of ovulation with frequent blood or urine tests; it usually occurs 13 or 14 days before the next menstrual period.

For background information on conception, see REPRODUCTION, SEXUAL. *Further information can be found in* EMBRYO; FERTILIZATION; OVULATION; REPRODUCTIVE SYSTEM, FEMALE; REPRODUCTIVE SYSTEM, MALE; *and* ZYGOTE. *See also* INFERTILITY *and* IN VITRO FERTILIZATION *for more on problems with conception.*

Concussion

Mild injury to the brain as a result of a blow to or violent motion of the head.

Any blow to the head may force the brain against the bony structure of the skull. Concussion is a form of injury to the brain that is sometimes associated with a brief loss of consciousness.

Symptoms. Beyond a loss of consciousness, symptoms can include loss of memory, dizziness, vomiting, nausea, and headache. Head injury causing unconsciousness should be investigated by a doctor. Recovery generally occurs without treatment and is complete within 24 to 48 hours.

ALERT

Children and Head Injury
Children are at particular risk for brain injury because they are more prone to accidental falls. Also, infants and toddlers are, accidentally or intentionally, easily shaken by adults and can suffer severe brain injury. Any vomiting, paleness, drowsiness, or even a very brief period of unconsciousness following a blow to the head is evidence of brain injury, and the child should be checked by a physician as soon as possible.

Serious symptoms may develop after a period of time, including persistent headaches, amnesia, confusion, and increasing sleepiness and lethargy. Emergency symptoms include persistent unconsciousness, seizures, drowsiness, repeated vomiting, unequal pupil size, confusion, and difficulty walking.

Children and Concussion. Children are particularly at risk for brain injury, because they are more prone to falls. Any fall or blow to the head of a child that results in a loss of consciousness warrants an immediate evaluation by a medical pofessional.

Background information on concussion can be found in BRAIN *and* HEAD INJURY. *For further information, see* ANXIETY; CENTRAL NERVOUS SYSTEM; CONFUSION; DEPRESSION; NAUSEA; NERVOUS SYSTEM; SEIZURE; *and* VOMITING. *See also* SPORTS INJURIES *and* SPORTS MEDICINE *for more on sports-related concussions.*

Condom

A barrier placed on the penis to prevent semen from entering the vagina during intercourse.

Condoms are made of latex or rubber, and usually contain a spermicide. They are rolled over the erect penis and contain a reservoir or space in the tip to hold the semen. Condoms can also be made of materials such as lamb intestine, but those have microscopic holes and therefore are not as effective as their latex counterparts. If used correctly, condoms are 99 percent effective in preventing pregnancy. They also provide very good protection against sexually transmitted diseases, but must be put on before any contact with the partner's genitals in order to be fully effective.

Condoms can be used with or without additional lubricant, but only water-based substances should be used, as petroleum-based materials may weaken the condom and lead to breakage. A fresh condom must be put on prior to each incident of intercourse.

Condoms are recommended for use during oral sex as well to prevent any sexually transmitted disease.

Manufacturers are responding to society's demand for healthier lifestyles and are creating a wide variety of condoms. Various condom sizes and thicknesses are available for comfort. In attempts to intensify sensitivity and pleasure for both partners, small ridges and nodules are manufactured into the material of certain types of condoms.

The female condom, which lines the vagina, has a similar construction to the male version. It is larger and is held in place with a ring. The failure rate of the female condom is higher than for the male condom. *See also* BARRIER METHOD; CONTRACEPTION; SAFE SEX; SEXUAL INTERCOURSE; *and* SEXUALLY TRANSMITTED DISEASES.

Cone Biopsy

Also known as conization

A specialized biopsy used to remove a cone-shaped section of the uterine cervix.

A cone biopsy entails removing a cone or doughnut-shaped segment that contains both the inner and the outer portions of the cervix.

If a pap smear or cervical biopsy indicates a tumor on the cervix (cervical intraepithelial neoplasia, or CIN), this technique may be used to remove the tumor. A cone biopsy may also be used to diagnose squamous cell cancer, human papilloma virus (HPV), and various lesions.

Procedure. A cone biopsy is performed under general anesthetic. A one-half- to one-inch long and three-quarter-inch wide section of tissue is removed using a carbon dioxide laser, heat (electrocautery), or a knife. Once a lesion has been removed, it is sent to a pathologist for analysis under a microscope.

Cone biopsy is generally reserved for CIN, severe abnormal tissue growth (dysplasia), or cancerous tissue. Side effects of cone biopsy may include bleeding, infection, cervical stenosis, or incompetence. *See also* BIOPSY; CERVIX; CERVIX, CANCER OF; *and* CERVIX, DISORDERS OF.

Confabulation

The act of devising a story to cover up unexplained memory lapses.

People who confabulate are creating a fiction to make sense of their experience, not to deliberately deceive the listener. Confabulation is seen in patients with brain injuries, amnesia, and Wernicke-Korsakoff syndrome—a disease associated with chronic alcoholism. *See also* AMNESIA; BRAIN DISORDERS; BRAIN TUMORS; *and* WERNICKE-KORSAKOFF SYNDROME.

Confusion

An abnormal mental state in which a person is unsure of time or place.

Confusion, also known as mental dysfunction, is an altered mental state in which a person experiences uncertainty about time, place, identity, or situational context. While even a healthy individual can become confused for isolated periods of time, serious or prolonged mental confusion can be cause for alarm.

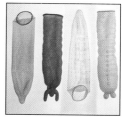

Condom. Condoms are used to prevent sperm or semen from coming into contact with the vagina during sexual activities, as well as to prevent the transmission of sexually transmitted diseases. Above, condoms come in many colors, shapes, and sizes.

INCIDENCE

Confusion may come on suddenly, or it may appear gradually over time. In some cases it is temporary, in others it is permanent and irreversible. Confusion is more common in the elderly than it is in the general population.

CAUSES

Confusion has numerous causes. Among the most common is alcohol intoxication. Low blood sugar, head injury or trauma, a fluid imbalance, a sudden drop in body temperature, heat-related disorders, nutritional deficiencies, hypothermia, stroke, high fever, and certain types of medications may also cause confusion. Confusion is often exacerbated by stress.

SYMPTOMS

Affected individuals may show seriously impaired judgment, a diminished ability to communicate with others, physical disorientation, a general sense of bewilderment or an inability to make decisions. In extreme cases, the individual may experience perceptual delusions, extreme insomnia, agitation, and paranoia.

TREATMENT

In some cases, confusion disappears on its own. Patients should consult their doctors if confusion is severe or persistent, or if it is accompanied by excessive thirst, frequent urination, unexplained weight loss, numbness, or tingling of the hands and feet. If confusion is a side effect of medication, it can be treated by discontinuing or adjusting the dosage.

Severely confused patients should never be left alone. A calm and peaceful setting helps confused people orient themselves to their environment. Placing a clock and calendar near the patient can help reduce time-related confusion.

> *For background information on confusion, see* GERONTOLOGY *and* PSYCHIATRY. *Further information can be found in* ALZHEIMER'S DISEASE; CONCUSSION; HEAD INJURY; *and* MENTAL ILLNESS. *See also* DEMENTIA *for more on severe cases of confusion.*

Congenital

Present from birth.

The term congenital refers to a physical defect or disease present from the time of birth. A congenital disorder can often be traced to genetic or chromosomal cause, or an infection or other environmental abnormality that occurs during pregnancy. *See also* GENETIC CODE; GENETIC ENGINEERING; *and* GENETICS.

Congenital Sexually Transmitted Diseases (STDs)

Sexually transmitted diseases passed by a mother to her child and present in the child at birth.

Congenital sexually transmitted diseases (STDs) are present in an individual at birth. If a pregnant mother is infected with an STD, such as AIDS, syphilis, or gonorrhea, it can be passed to the fetus in the uterus or during delivery. *See also* SEXUALLY TRANSMITTED DISEASES.

Congestion

A condition in which mucous collects in the lungs and nasal passages, or the passages themselves swell, interfering with breathing.

The nasal passages run from the nostrils to the back of the throat. They are lined with mucous membranes that lubricate the area and help to filter the air. When there is an infection, the mucous membranes may become inflamed, blocking the passage of air and causing fluid to build up.

Chest or pulmonary congestion frequently occurs when a person suffers from upper respiratory infections like a cold or the flu. Allergic reactions can also trigger congestion when the nasal passages and sinuses swell.

Symptoms include runny nose, itchy and watery eyes, headache, and difficulty breathing through the nose.

Treatment. Recommended treatments for congestion include over-the-counter expectorants, the ingestion of large amounts of liquid, and inhalation of steam. If a fever or cough persists, or if there is chest pain or blood in the sputum, a medical professional should be consulted. *See also* ALLERGY; COLD, COMMON; NASAL DISCHARGE NOSE; *and* SINUSITIS.

Congestive Heart Failure

A condition in which the heart is unable to pump blood efficiently.

Congestive heart failure can affect the left side of the heart, the right side, or both sides. Left-sided heart failure can be caused by hypertension (high blood pressure), a congenital heart defect, a heart valve disorder such as aortic stenosis, hyperthyroidism (an overactive thyroid), or anemia. If the left side of the heart cannot pump out blood completely, blood will back up into the lungs. Right-sided heart failure can also result from a congenital heart problem or a valve defect, but is most often caused by pulmonary hypertension (increased blood pressure with a resistance to blood flow through the lungs). Right-sided failure is characterized by an inability of the right side of the heart to accept enough blood from the rest of the body. The result is that blood backs up into the veins, enlarging them as well as the organs.

Treatment. The goals of treatment for congestive heart failure are to reduce the work load of the heart. Vasodilator drugs may be used to open the blood vessels, reducing the work load of the heart. Diuretic drugs may be administered to rid the body of excess fluid. ACE inhibitor drugs have also proven effective. If the condition cannot be stabilized with medication, surgery or a heart transplant may be needed.

> **Background information on congestive heart failure can be found in CIRCULATORY SYSTEM and HEART DISORDERS. For further information, see ARTERIOSCLEROSIS; ATHEROSCLEROSIS; HEART; HEART ATTACK; HEART FAILURE; HEART IMAGING; and HEART SOUNDS.**

Conjunctivitis

Also known as pink-eye

Inflammation of the conjunctiva, the membrane that covers the white of the eye.

Conjunctivitis can be infective or allergic. Infective conjunctivitis is most often caused by bacteria, such as staphylococci, or viruses, such as those that cause colds. Viral conjunctivitis may occur in epidemics in schools or day-care centers. Allergic conjunctivitis is an allergic response of the conjunctiva to cosmetic products, contact lenses, or pollen.

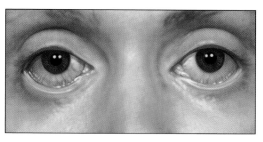

Symptoms. All types of conjunctivitis can cause redness, discomfort, and discharge from the eye. In infective bacterial conjunctivitis, the discharge contains pus.

Other symptoms may include increased tearing, eye pain, itching, and blurred vision. Diagnosis is made through a swab of the conjunctiva, which is taken for laboratory analysis.

Treatment. Infective conjunctivitis can be treated with antibiotic drugs if the cause is bacterial. Viral conjunctivitis disappears on its own without treatment, but may result in scarring if left untreated. Allergic conjunctivitis may disappear if the allergen (allergy-causing agent) is removed.

> **For background information on conjunctivitis, see EYE, DISORDERS OF. Further information can be found in ALLERGY; BACTERIA; EYE; INFECTIOUS DISEASE; INFLAMMATION; VISION; and VIRUSES. See also ANTIBIOTIC DRUGS and EYE DROPS for more on treatment.**

Conjunctivitis. Conjunctivitis may be caused by a bacterial infection or an allergic reaction. Left, the eyes of an individual with conjunctivitis appear red; there may be discomfort and a discharge. Below, the conjunctiva, the membrane that surrounds the white of the eye, is inflamed in patients with conjunctivitis.

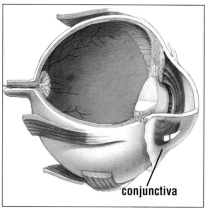

conjunctiva

Conn's Syndrome

Excess secretion of aldosterone.

The hormone aldosterone helps to control the balance of sodium and potassium levels in the blood. When a tumor of the adrenal gland causes overproduction of aldosterone, the result is a condition known as Conn's syndrome, in which sodium levels in the blood are increased and potassium levels are decreased. The increase in sodium in the blood causes hypertension and symptoms of hypokalemia or low potassium, including tiredness, weakness, and increased urination. Decrease in potassium causes weakness of the muscles. Usually, aldosterone levels will return to normal if the growth (not the adrenal gland itself) is removed. *See also* ALDOSTERONE.

Consent

A patient's permission to receive a treatment or to allow a doctor to disclose information.

In health care, there are two main ways a patient can give consent. First, the patient, unless deemed mentally unfit to make decisions, must agree to receive a specific medical treatment. Second, the patient must give consent to allow a doctor to disclose his or her medical history, as, in most countries, laws of confidentially protect medical records and information from release without patient consent.

Informed Consent. The right of patients to consent to medical treatment has led in the United States to the principle of informed consent. This doctrine requires physicians to share certain information with patients before asking for their consent to treatment. Physicians must describe the procedure and list its major risks, benefits, and alternatives. This is based on the principle that patients have a right to self-determination. Since they have the most at stake in treatment, they have the right to make an informed choice.

Physicians and health care institutions have the responsibility to maintain confidentiality of patient information. Consent is required before this type of information is released. Institutional review boards must approve any research requiring patient information and the researchers must maintain the confidentiality of patients and guarantee the safety of such data before a study may be approved.

> *Background material on consent can be found in* PUBLIC HEALTH. *For further information, see* ACCREDITATION; BOARD CERTIFICATION; CERTIFICATION; COMPLIANCE; CONFIDENTIALITY; *and* LIABILITY INSURANCE, PROFESSIONAL. *See also* MENTAL ILLNESS *for cases in which a patient may be deemed unfit to give consent.*

Constipation

Uncomfortable or infrequent bowel movements.

Bowel habits are subject to change by factors as varied as diet, stress, medication, and disease. Constipation is defined as the passing of hard stools less than three times a week. Constipation may be accompanied by other symptoms, such as abdominal cramps, bloating, and a sensation that the rectum has not been fully emptied.

The large intestine removes water from waste products, compacting the feces into a form that is eliminated. The feces are moved along by muscular contractions of the large intestine. Alterations in the speed at which fecal matter moves affect how much water is reabsorbed. Removal of too much water results in hard, dry stools; if insufficient water is removed, the result is diarrhea. Frequently, one condition changes abruptly to the opposite extreme.

Types. Acute constipation refers to the abrupt and sudden onset of the condition. Chronic constipation begins slowly and gradually, and may continue for extended periods of time. In spastic constipation, the feces are passed as a series of small hard balls or ribbons.

Chronic constipation may result in fecal impaction, in which the last part of the large intestine and the rectum contain a hardened mass of feces, which acts as a plug. Fecal impaction is accompanied by cramps, rectal pain, and the frequent though unsuccessful urge to have a bowel movement. Often watery mucus seeps out around the blockage. Fecal impaction requires an enema to remove the hardened material, as well a stool softener regimen to prevent it from recurring.

If hemorrhoids are present, constipation can make the condition more severe or cause the formation of new ones.

CAUSES

The causes of constipation include a low-fiber diet, certain types of medication, change in the diet, change in exercise pattern, irritable bowel syndrome, intestinal obstruction, and Parkinson's disease.

DIAGNOSIS

Diagnosis can be facilitated with either a flexible proctosigmoidoscopic exam or a barium x-ray, which rule out serious factors that may be causing constipation.

TREATMENT

Before resorting to laxatives, the following measures are recommended:

- Increase water intake to six to eight glasses daily.
- Increase fiber in the diet through increased consumption of fruits and vegetables.
- Take a fiber or bran supplement or a bulk former like psyllium, a vegetable fiber.
- Try to make bowel habits regular, i.e., at the same time each day.
- Don't resist the urge to have a bowel movement.
- Increase the amount of daily exercise.
- Avoid overuse or dependence on enemas and laxatives.

Laxatives. The use of laxatives to alleviate constipation should be a short-term measure only and should not be used to prevent *possible* constipation. Laxatives can have long-lasting effects on the body, causing nutrients to be flushed out before they are able to be properly absorbed. Laxatives can also result in excessive excretion of water, sodium, and potassium. Prolonged use can weaken the muscles in the intestine to the point where a person may find it impossible to have an unaided bowel movement. Excessive use of laxatives can also cause diarrhea.

> *For background information on constipation, see* DIGESTIVE SYSTEM *and* GASTROINTESTINAL TRACT. *Further information can be found in* AGING; COLON; COLON CANCER; DIARRHEA; INTESTINE; IRRITABLE BOWEL SYNDROME; *and* POLYPS. *See also* ENEMA *and* LAXATIVE DRUGS *for more on treatment options.*

Contact Lenses

Thin optical disks placed on the cornea of the eye to correct vision.

Contact lenses are placed on the outer surface of the eye to correct vision. They are most often used for convenience and cosmetic reasons but can also be useful for hiding scars or corneal abnormalities.

The three main types of contact lenses are hard plastic lenses, hard gas-permeable lenses, and soft lenses. Hard plastic lenses are long-lasting, inexpensive, and durable. They may be difficult to tolerate, however. The wearer may also suffer pain if dust or dirt gets between the eye and the lens.

Rigid gas-permeable lenses are similar to hard plastic lenses, but they allow air to get between the lens and the eye and are therefore more comfortable. They are not as durable and are more expensive than hard plastic lenses.

Soft lenses are the most comfortable and can be worn for long periods of time. They do not last as long as hard lenses, however, and they require complicated maintenance procedures. Soft lenses with a high water content can be designed for extended wear, and they can be thrown away after use. These lenses, called disposable lenses, may increase the risk of infection if they are worn for long periods.

Problems that can develop from wearing contact lenses include eye irritation and sensitivity. Hard-lens wearers may suffer abrasion of the cornea, which is treated with antibiotics. *See also* CORNEAL ABRASION.

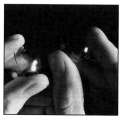

Contact Lenses. Contact lenses are often worn instead of glasses by individuals with vision problems. They are placed directly on the surface of the eye. Above, a pair of soft contact lenses, the most commonly worn type of contact lens.

Contact Tracing

The process of contacting the sexual partners of an individual with a sexually transmitted disease.

To help control the spread of sexually transmitted disease, partners of infected individuals must be notified that they have been exposed to infection and encouraged to seek testing, and, if necessary, treatment. The objectives of contact tracing are to interrupt the transmission of the disease, prevent or decrease complications arising from infection, and encourage individuals to change their behavior and thereby avoid infecting others.

While contact tracing is a standard weapon in public-health efforts against sexually transmitted diseases, the method's use for HIV infection has been the subject of debate since the epidemic began. With the advent of new treatments to hinder disease progression and prevent viral transmission, health officials are pushing to expand contact-tracing efforts, to reach the approximately 250,000 people in the United States who do not know they are infected. In confidential contact tracing, health workers notify people that they have been exposed to the disease but do not identify the person who exposed them.

Half of all states require confidential reporting of HIV-infected persons by name to state or local health departments, and all 50 states require reporting of AIDS patients. *See also* AIDS; CONSENT; *and* SEXUALLY TRANSMITTED DISEASES.

Contraception

Also known as birth control or family planning

Various methods used to prevent conception.

Barrier methods are designed to prevent sperm from entering the uterus. These include condoms, diaphragms, cervical caps, sponges and contraceptive creams, foams and jellies. They have varying success rates.

The male condom is used to prevent semen from entering the vagina. Made of latex or rubber, it is rolled over the erect penis and contains a reservoir—space in the tip—to hold sperm upon ejaculation. Most condoms also contain spermicide. Condoms are 99 percent effective in preventing pregnancy. A fresh condom must be used for each incident of intercourse.

The female condom, which lines the vagina, is similar in construction to its male counterpart. It is larger than the male condom and is held in place with a ring. The failure rate of the female condom is higher than that of the male condom.

The diaphragm is a dome-shaped rubber cup that fits over the cervix and prevents sperm from entering the uterus. It is filled with a contraceptive cream or jelly that contains a spermicide. The diaphragm, which must be fitted by a medical practitioner, should cover the entire cervix without causing discomfort when positioned properly. The diaphragm must be inserted prior to intercourse and should remain in place for at least 8 hours afterwards but not for more than 24 hours.

The diaphragm must be refitted after a woman gives birth, undergoes an abortion or miscarriage, or gains or loses more than 10 pounds. Some doctors recommend refitting after a year, whether or not any of these events have actually taken place. The diaphragm is 80 percent to 90 percent effective in preventing pregnancy.

The cervical cap is a smaller and more rigid version of the diaphragm. It fits directly over the cervix. It also must be fitted by a healthcare professional. A contraceptive cream or jelly must be used as well. The cap should be inserted before intercourse and left in place for at least 8 hours afterwards, but not for longer than 48 hours. Cervical caps are approximately as effective as diaphragms.

Contraceptive creams, foams, and jellies contain spermicide. Usually used in conjunction with diaphragms or cervical caps, they can also be used alone. When placed in the vagina, these products block sperm from entering the reproductive tract as well as kill any sperm with which they come in contact. Creams, foams, and jellies are 60 percent effective.

Hormonal methods involve the use of progesterone and estrogen, naturally occurring female hormones. They prevent pregnancy by inhibiting ovulation and keeping the cervical mucus thick enough to complicate the easy passage of sperm.

Oral contraceptives are pills containing the hormones estrogen or progesterone. They are taken daily for 3 weeks, then stopped for 7 days to allow menstruation to occur. Pills containing only progesterone are taken daily throughout the entire month. Skipping a day for either type of pill may result in pregnancy. Oral contraceptives have a success rate of 97 percent or higher. Certain drugs, such as antibiotics, can decrease the effectiveness of birth control pills.

Hormone injections, or implants such as Norplant, release estrogen and progesterone into the body over a period of time. Although the delivery method is different, their function, effectiveness, and side effects are the same as contraceptive pills.

Periodic abstinence is another name for the rhythm method. In this method, a couple abstains from intercourse during the time of month deemed the fertile period—when the woman is most likely to conceive. This is not always effective, since fertilization can occur several days after intercourse, not only during ovulation.

The intrauterine device (IUD) is inserted into the uterus to prevent the implantation of a fertilized egg. One type of IUD releases copper, another type releases progesterone. This causes inflammation and the release of white blood cells into the uterus. The white blood cells produce a substance that is poisonous to sperm, thus preventing contraception. The progesterone type must be replaced annually, whereas the copper type is effective for approximately 10 years. The IUD is close to 100 percent effective, but has been associated with uterine and tubal infections.

Sterilization is a more or less permanent form of contraception. A vasectomy is the male operation, involving severing the sperm pathway (vas deferens) and thereby preventing sperm from being released in the semen. This operation is close to 100 percent effective and is only rarely, and with great difficulty, reversible. Even after surgery, there may still be sperm present in the seminal vesicles and thus in the semen for a few weeks; during that time another method of contraception should be used.

A tubal ligation involves surgically cutting and tying off a woman's fallopian tubes in order to prevent the sperm from having access to the egg. Tubal ligation is close to 100 percent effective. Possible side effects include scarring and increased chance of a fertilized egg developing in the fallopian tubes or cervix (ectopic pregnancy). Tubal ligation is only rarely irreversible; about one quarter of women who undergo the reversal procedure fail to regain fertility.

Morning-after pills, or high doses of oral contraceptives, are sometimes used to prevent pregnancy after a single act of unprotected sex. This must be taken within 72 hours of intercourse to be effective.

Douching (artificial flushing of the vagina) immediately after intercourse is an attempt to remove semen and prevent the sperm from reaching the uterus. This may be too late, as sperm may have already traveled beyond the point where douching can reach. In some cases, douching may actually help propel sperm farther up the reproductive tract.

Abortion should not be viewed as a method of birth control, but rather a means to terminate an unwanted pregnancy for medical or other reasons.

Aside from a conventional surgical abortion, there exist chemical means of ending a pregnancy in the early stages. Mifepristone, known widely as RU-486, can be taken in combination with contraction-inducing chemicals known as prostaglandins. This has been an effective method of terminating a pregnancy before the ninth week.

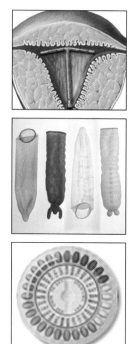

Contraception.
There are many different forms of contraception, all of which prevent pregnancy but not necessarily the transmission of sexually transmitted diseases. Above, top, an intrauterine device (IUD) in place. Second from the top, a variety of condoms. At bottom, oral contraceptives (birth control pills).

Background information on contraception can be found in REPRODUCTION, SEXUAL. *For further information, see* CONTRACEPTIVE. *See also* CONDOM; DIAPHRAGM; INTRAUTERINE DEVICE (IUD); *and* NATURAL FAMILY PLANNING *for more on specific methods of contraception.*

Contractions

The muscular movements of the uterus and vaginal canal during labor.

Contractions are experienced as a pain beginning in the lower back and moving across the abdomen, which tightens in response to the movements. They may start out feeling like menstrual cramps. Each contraction intensifies to a peak and then slowly subsides. In the early stages of labor, contractions cause the cervix to dilate and thin out (efface). Once the cervix is fully dilated, the contractions serve to expel the baby from the mother's body. As labor progresses, the contractions become more intense and occur closer together. *See also* CHILDBIRTH; CHILDBIRTH, COMPLICATIONS; *and* PREGNANCY.

Contracture

Deformity caused by a tightening of muscle, skin, tendons, ligaments, or skin.

When an injury heals or after a surgical procedure, the affected area may shrink and impair movement or alter in appearance. A good example is the way skin can shrink after a burn; in a severe case shrinkage can prevent virtually all movement. Reduced usage of a body part can also lead to contracture, as can nerve damage. Disorders such as muscular dystrophy sometimes cause contracture.

Decreased mobility in a joint is an indication of contracture. Physical therapy, orthopedic appliances, or surgery may be used to resolve the problem. *See also* BURNS *and* MUSCULAR DYSTROPHY.

Controlled Trial

An experimental study that eliminates the effects of outside variables on the outcome.

Medical experiments often test the effect of one or more variables on human populations. A controlled trial is designed so that only the variables under study affect the results. In other words, the design eliminates the effect of a systematic bias on the study's data.

A study on fat intake, for example, might examine the difference in lifespan between two groups, one with high fat consumption and the other with low fat consumption. Fat intake, however, might not be the only variable that differs from subject to subject in a dietary study. Exercise, total food consumption, and stress levels, among other factors, may also vary. For example, the low-fat intake group may exercise more than the other group. To avoid the effects of exercise or stress, a controlled trial would be designed so that these other variables did not vary systematically from one group to the other; i.e., the study would control for the effects of possible outside variables.

Polling experiments, on the other hand, must prevent a systematic bias in the population sample surveyed. If a survey on presidential candidates polls only people with a certain income or education level, it may skew the results of the survey. The poll would fail to reflect the preferences of the larger population under study (i.e., all voting Americans). To eliminate the effect of a systematic bias, the study will use a random selection process that ensures a even mix of many different demographics. *See also* STATISTICS, MEDICAL.

Contusion

A bruise.

Blunt trauma causes contusions. For example, a fall can result in a contusion to the brain. Tissue damage usually results from the movement of the brain in the skull during a head trauma.

Once a contusion occurs, discoloration appears just underneath the skin. The contusion first appears black or blue due to the accumulation of blood. When hemoglobin, one component of the blood, begins to break down, the contusion starts to appear greenish or yellow. *See also* BLOOD CLOT *and* BRUISE.

Convalescence

The period of recovery following an illness, injury, or surgical operation.

During convalescence, the patient regains strength before resuming regular activities. The convalescent period varies, depending on the nature of the injury or illness. For example, recovery from an illness such as tonsillitis or influenza can require only a few days, while recovery from a major operation or a bad heart attack may take several weeks to more than a month. Older people take longer to convalesce, and are sometimes encouraged to enter a nursing or convalescent home for better care and to minimize the risk of complications. *See also* HEART ATTACK; INFLUENZA; STROKE; *and* TONSILLITIS.

Copper

Metallic element essential for the formation of hemoglobin in the blood and the maintenance of other bodily functions.

Copper is a metal found in the earth's crust and as a trace mineral in the body. Copper enables red blood cells to carry oxygen to tissues, and assists in the formation of hemoglobin. Copper is also necessary for production of energy, proper hormone balance, and as part of many important chemical reactions. For most people, a balanced diet will supply the body with the recommended allowances of copper. Foods rich in copper include seafood, organ meats, nuts, and green vegetables.

Although copper poisoning is rare, exposure to toxic levels can occur through inhalation of dust, fumes, or sprays, or absorption through the skin. Copper may also contaminate food and water. Symptoms of copper poisoning include a burning mouth and throat, nausea, diarrhea, greenish-blue vomit, eye irritation, cough, and sinus irritation. In addition, an increased incidence of lung cancer has been linked to workers exposed to sprays containing copper. *See also* POISONING.

Cordotomy

A surgical incision, performed to alleviate pain, in which the bundles of nerve fibers in the spinal cord are divided.

Cordotomy is a procedure to alleviate pain of the back or lower body by decreasing the perception of pain. Cordotomy is performed only after painkillers (analgesics), muscle relaxants, corticosteroid injections, and physical therapy have failed. It is often performed on people with cancer. Most cordotomy procedures are carried out with a local anesthetic. *See also* ANALGESIC DRUGS; ANESTHESIA, LOCAL; BACK PAIN; CANCER; *and* PHYSICAL THERAPY.

Cor Pulmonale

Abnormal thickening of the pulmonary arteries caused by chronic lung disease.

Damage to the lungs can increase resistance to the flow of blood from the heart to the lungs through the pulmonary arteries, causing them to become thicker and narrower. The heart must work harder, so its right side becomes enlarged. The end result may be right-sided heart failure. Shortness of breath and swollen ankles are common symptoms; patients may also experience chest pain and drowsiness. Cor pulmonale often occurs in heavy smokers. Home treatment with oxygen and bed rest can ease the symptoms. *See also* HEART FAILURE *and* TOBACCO SMOKING.

Corn

A small area of thickened skin that occurs on a toe.

Corns are hardened areas on the toe, similar to calluses. For example, pressure or friction on the foot from poorly fitting shoes causes corns. *See also* CALLUS.

If the cause of the pressure or friction is removed, corns will disappear. Corns can be dissolved with medications containing acid, but care should be taken to prevent the acid from harming normal tissue.

Cornea

A lens and the protective front cover of the eyeball.

The cornea is transparent and dome-shaped to focus light rays onto the retina. It covers the pupil and iris and joins the white of the eyeball, or sclera, just outside the border of the iris. To remain healthy, the cornea must be moist; the lacrimal gland produces tears, while the lining of the eye and the inside of the eyelids, the conjunc-

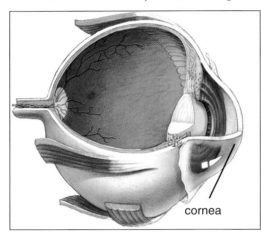

Cornea.
The cornea, right, covers the eyeball and protects the eye from irritants. Disorders that may affect the cornea include abrasions, infections, and ulcers.

cornea

tiva, secrete mucus and fluid. Scratches and foreign debris can cause extreme pain, as the cornea is very sensitive. Endothelial cells in the inner layer remove excess water from the cornea to maintain transparency. *See also* CORNEA, DISORDERS OF; CORNEAL ABRASION; *and* CORNEAL ULCER.

Cornea, Disorders of

Conditions that affect the cornea of the eye

The cornea is prone to various disorders. These disorders include congenital defects, injury, inflammation, infection, degeneration, and nutritional conditions. Most corneal disorders are diagnosed by microscopic examination.

Congenital defects of the cornea are present at birth, and are not common. Small cornea (microcornea) or large cornea (megalocornea) can occur in either eye or in both eyes.

Injury. Trauma to the cornea is fairly common and usually minor. Corneal abrasion is a scratch to the cornea that can be caused by overuse of contact lenses or by a foreign particle in the eye. If the abrasion becomes infected, it can worsen and become a corneal ulcer, a condition that may eventually lead to loss of vision. Chemical injuries to the eye can also result in visual loss and can be caused by acids or by alkalis. In the case of a chemical injury, the eye should immediately be flushed with large amounts of water.

Infection. The cornea can be infected by viruses, fungi, or bacteria. Corneal infection with the herpes simplex virus is very serious, and may cause ulceration and vision loss.

Vitamin A deficiency causes keratomalacia, a disorder in which the cornea softens and easily perforates, resulting in blindness. Keratomalacia, common in children who are malnourished, is a major cause of blindness in developing countries. *See also* CORNEA *and* CORNEAL ABRASION.

Corneal Abrasion

A scratch in the cornea.

A corneal abrasion is a scratch or abnormality in the outer layer of the cornea. It can be caused by a foreign particle in the eye or by an injury to the cornea. Corneal abrasions can be painful, cause sensitivity to bright lights (photophobia), and increase tear production. Keeping the eye closed or covered will relieve some of these symptoms. Pain killers (analgesics) can be prescribed to relieve the pain associated with the condition, and antibiotics will prevent infection of the area, which could otherwise cause ulceration and loss of vision.

Corneal abrasions usually heal within a few days, unless there is an infection. Occasionally, an abrasion can recur, particularly if the outer layer of the cornea does not heal properly. In this case, patching or ointments may help, as may the application of a specially designed contact lens to hold the cornea in place. *See also* CORNEA.

Corneal Graft

Also known as keratoplasty

The surgical replacement of diseased corneal tissue with healthy tissue from a donor eye.

A corneal graft or transplant may be appropriate when the eye functions well but the outer covering of the eye (cornea) is clouded or otherwise obscured. The cornea may become clouded from injury; scarring; bacterial, viral, or fungal infection; inflammation; a congenital defect; fluid collection; degeneration; and aging.

Transplanted corneas are most often taken from another human (heterograft), but a few may come from the patient's own cornea (autograft), if enough healthy tissue is available from a peripheral part of the eye. Most donated corneas come from recently deceased people. Donated corneas can be frozen and later stored for several days.

PROCEDURE

Corneal transplants are usually performed with a local anesthetic; the patient may also receive a sedative to further relax him or her. The ophthalmologist removes the defective part of the cornea with scissors and a trephine, an instrument used to cut a circular section (button). The donor corneal button, slightly larger than the recipient's, is then sutured in place.

The sutures are removed from the eye three to four weeks later; topical corticosteroids are used for several months to reduce inflammation. Full recovery may take up to a year.

PROGNOSIS

The success rate for corneal grafts is high. Usually there is a significant risk of rejection with a transplant, but the cornea is free of blood vessels; so white blood cells, which are responsible for fighting off foreign tissue, do not typically reach the cornea. It does help, however, to have the tissue type of the donor and recipient matched as closely as possible. *See also* ANESTHESIA, LOCAL *and* CORNEA, DISORDERS OF.

Corneal Ulcer

A sore in the outer layer of the cornea, which may penetrate the tissue underneath.

A corneal ulcer is an infection of the cornea. It is usually caused by a bacterial, viral, or fungal infection. Corneal ulcers may also be caused by scratches (abrasions), foreign particles in the eye, severe allergic eye disease, dry eyes, and some inflammatory disorders. Symptoms of a corneal ulcer include eye pain and redness, increased tearing, impaired vision, sensitivity to bright lights (photophobia), and a white patch on the cornea. There may also be eye itching, burning, and a discharge.

Diagnosis. Corneal ulcers are normally diagnosed by a laboratory analysis of a small tissue sample that is taken from the cornea. They are treated based on the cause, preferably as soon as possible to prevent loss of vision. Infections causing corneal ulcers are treated with antibiotic, antiviral, or antifungal eye drops, depending on the organism causing the infection. Corticosteroids are sometimes prescribed to reduce associated inflammation.

For background information on corneal ulcer, see CORNEA, DISORDERS OF *and* EYE, DISORDERS OF. *Further information can be found in* CORNEA; CORNEAL ABRASION; EYE; VISION; *and* VISION, LOSS OF. *See also* ANTIBIOTIC DRUGS; ANTIFUNGAL DRUGS; ANTIVIRAL DRUGS; *and* CORTICOSTEROID DRUGS *for more on treatment options.*

Resources on Corneal Disorders

Brightbill, F.S., *Corneal Surgery* (1993); King, John Harry and Joseph A.C. Wadsworth, eds., *An Atlas of Ophthalmic Surgery* (1970); Weihenmayer, Erik, *Touch the Top of the World: A Blind Man's Journey to Climb Farther Than the Eye Can See* (2001); Wolf, K.P., *Eyewise: Eye Disorders and Their Treatment* (1982); American Council of the Blind, Tel. (800) 424-8666, Online: www.acb.org; American Foundation for the Blind, Tel. (800) 232-5463, Online: www.afb.org; Glaucoma Research Foundation, Tel. (800) 826-6693, Online: www.glaucoma.orgw.nycornell.edu/op/.

Coronary

Referring to the heart and the arteries that supply the heart.

Coronary is a word derived from *corona*, the Latin word for crown. It is used to refer to the arteries that supply the heart, because they encircle the heart like a crown. The word "coronary" is commonly used to describe a heart attack, which is often a result of arterial problems.

Coronary artery disease is a condition affecting the arteries that carry blood to the heart. *See also* HEART ATTACK.

Coronary Artery Bypass

Surgery that improves the flow of blood to the heart by grafting blood vessels to loop around narrowed or blocked coronary arteries.

Bypass surgery is performed when other treatments for coronary heart disease, such as medication, angioplasty, or lifestyle changes, do not prevent progression of the disease. A vein removed from a leg or arm of the patient is used to construct new paths for blood flow around one or more affected arteries.

Bypass surgery is done under general anesthesia and requires a hospital stay of several days; it allows most patients to resume normal lives. *See also* BYPASS.

Coronary Care Unit

A hospital ward devoted to monitoring and treating patients who have suffered or are believed to have suffered heart attacks.

Coronary care units are staffed by specially trained cardiologists and nurses. These units are equipped with specialized devices, such as computerized electrocardiographs, that give detailed information about the status of the heart from minute to minute, and with defibrillators and other lifesaving equipment used to treat emergencies such as cardiac arrest or life-threatening arrhythmia. The patient is transferred from the coronary care unit to an ordinary hospital ward when his or her condition stabilizes. *See also* HEART ATTACK.

Coronary Heart Disease

Also known as coronary artery disease

A chronic, progressive condition in which the arteries supplying the heart become narrower and harder, impeding the flow of blood to the heart muscle.

Coronary heart disease is the leading cause of death in the United States, resulting in almost half of deaths.

CAUSES
While some degree of coronary heart disease occurs in many individuals with age, the risk is raised significantly by lifestyle practices, such as smoking, obesity, lack of exercise, and a diet rich in fat and cholesterol. Medical conditions, such as high blood pressure and diabetes, are also associated with coronary heart disease. Certain personality traits, such as a tendency to be easily upset or to feel constant time pressure or stress, are also believed to be associated with an increased risk of coronary heart disease.

Coronary heart disease generally begins in the early adult years. In childhood, the arteries are wide, with a smooth lining that permits the easy flow of blood. In individuals with coronary heart disease, however, blood flow is gradually impeded by atherosclerosis, in which the walls of the arteries gradually become thicker and less flexible because of the accumulation of plaque—deposits consisting of cholesterol, fat, and cells. In most people with coronary artery disease, the effects of the condition are felt in the middle and later years, generally after the age of 50.

SYMPTOMS
Angina. The first symptom of coronary heart disease is often angina. Angina can occur in men as early as their 30s; in women, it generally does not occur until after menopause.

Angina can be felt as a dull pain or pressure in the the chest that extends up the neck or down an arm (most often the left arm). The pain or pressure often occurs after physical exertion, even something as moderate as walking up a hill or a flight of stairs, or after some emotional stress. A variant form of the condition, called vasospasm or Prinzmetal's angina, can progress quickly, when a spasm in an artery blocks blood flow to the heart. Vasospasm is uncommon and usually occurs when a person is at rest, but like the common kind of angina, it indicates the presence of severe coronary heart disease.

DIAGNOSIS
Symptoms of coronary heart disease may be so obvious that diagnostic tests are not

Angina

Any kind of chest pain, discomfort, or pressure (angina) is a warning sign of a high risk of myocardial infarction (heart attack), in which blood flow through a coronary artery is blocked completely. Angina is most commonly experienced after strenuous exercise. While anyone experiencing angina should see a doctor regularly, this is even more important when angina occurs frequently and without any external cause.

needed; instead, treatment is given immediately. If the diagnosis is not clear, a battery of tests may be done. A basic test is the electrocardiogram, which gives a printed record of the heartbeat through electrodes placed on the chest, arms, and legs. Damage to the heart alters the electrocardiogram pattern.

Other diagnostic tests are echocardiography, which uses ultrasound to obtain images of the beating heart; a coronary angiogram, in which dye is injected so that x-ray images of the circulatory system in and around the heart can be obtained; a nuclear scanning test, which uses a short-lived radioactive substance injected into a vein to generate a computer image of the heart; and a Holter monitor examination, which requires the patient to wear a portable electrocardiogram device in a sling for as long as 24 hours, to provide a continuing record of the electrical activity of the heart.

TREATMENT

If lifestyle changes cannot stop the progression of coronary heart disease, drug treatment can help to slow the process or control the symptoms. Medications are chosen on the basis of the degree to which the condition has progressed and the symptoms the patient feels.

Medication. Vasodilators, drugs that cause arteries to relax and widen, may be prescribed for angina pectoris. In angina pectoris, the chest pain or discomfort results when the myocardium, the heart muscle, is no longer receiving an adequate supply of oxygen because of reduced blood

flow through the arteries. One of the oldest and most commonly used vasodilators is nitroglycerine, which can have a beneficial effect in a matter of minutes after a pill is dissolved under the tongue or a dose is sprayed into the mouth.

Another class of drugs prescribed for angina are calcium channel blockers, which slow the absorption by heart muscle cells of calcium, a blood element that causes arteries to contract.

Beta blockers are drugs that lower heart rate and blood pressure, reducing the load on the heart muscle by decreasing the activity of the hormone adrenaline (epinephrine). Beta blockers are often prescribed for hypertension.

Angiotensin-converting enzyme (ACE) inhibitors widen arteries and reduce blood pressure by preventing the conversion of an inactive form of the chemical enzyme to the active form. ACE inhibitors can also prevent inflammation of the arteries. However, these treatments often do not prevent coronary heart disease from progressing to the point where it causes symptoms.

Surgery. If coronary heart disease progresses to the point where blockage of one or more arteries is imminent, one of several techniques can be used to keep the arteries open and blood flowing adequately. A narrowed region of an artery can be widened by balloon angioplasty. In balloon angioplasty, a catheter is inserted to the point of blockage, with a balloon at its end, which is inflated to open the artery. Balloon angioplasty may be followed by implantation of a stent, a metal tube that keeps the artery open. If there is excessive blockage or multiple blockages, coronary

ALERT

In Case of a Heart Attack

Severe chest pain, fainting, and pain in the middle of the chest spreading to the back or left arm is a medical emergency. Half of all heart attack deaths occur in the first few hours after the onset of symptoms. The sooner the person is treated, the greater the chance of survival. Medical help should be sought immediately by dialing 911.

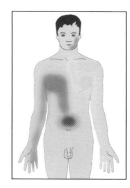

Angina. Angina pectoris is often the first symptom of coronary heart disease. The illustration above shows the areas of the body that are most often affected by angina.

Resources on Coronary Heart Disease
Berne, Robert M., et al., *Cardiovascular Physiology* (2001); Debakey, Michael E. and Antonio M. Gotto, *The New Living Heart* (1997); Gould, Lance K., *Heal Your Heart: How You Can Prevent or Reverse Heart Disease* (2000); American Heart Association, Tel. (800) 242-8721, Online: www.amhrt.org; Heart Information Network, Tel. (973) 701-6035, Online: www.heartinfo.org; National Heart, Lung, and Blood Institute, Tel. (301) 496-4236, Online: www. nhlbi.nih.gov;www.nycornell.org/cardiothoracic.surgery/; www.nycornell. org/medicine/cardiology/index.html.

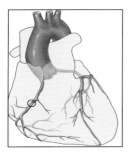

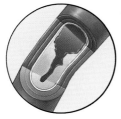

Coronary Heart Disease. The arteries supplying the hearts of patients with coronary heart disease become narrowed and blocked due to the accumulation of deposits of plaque. Above, top, the coronary arteries are shown in red. It is these arteries that are often blocked. Above, bottom, the inside of an artery affected by the buildup of plaque (circled in the top image). The space through which the blood can flow is smaller.

Psychological Risk Factors

Some cardiologists have identified what they call a type A personality, which describes a person who is constantly in a hurry, angry, impatient, hostile, and easily irritated, as an important factor in development of coronary artery disease. Studies have found that type A individuals have higher than normal levels of stress hormones. While some studies have found an increased risk of coronary heart disease in type A individuals, the exact relationship between personality and heart disease remains uncertain.

artery bypass graft surgery may be done. A section of a vein can be taken from another part of the body and sewn into place so that blood is routed around the severely narrowed coronary arteries.

Hundreds of thousands of bypass operations are performed in the United States each year. An alternative technique, still under development, is atherectomy, in which a cutting device carried by a catheter is used to shave away the artery-blocking plaque deposits. But in spite of all these techniques, myocardial infarctions (heart attacks) still strike many people with severe coronary heart disease.

PREVENTION

Measures to prevent coronary heart disease include weight loss; a diet rich in fruits and vegetables and low in fat, cholesterol, and salt; a program of exercise that includes at least 30 minutes of moderate activity at least five days a week; avoidance of smoking; alcohol intake that is low to moderate (no more than a drink or two a day); and stress-reduction techniques, especially for those individuals in the type A personality category, who are usually impatient, angry, and easily annoyed. Regular monitoring of risk factors for coronary heart disease, recommended for all adults, is even more important for type A individuals.

Background information on coronary heart disease can be found in CIRCULATORY SYSTEM *and* HEART DISORDERS. *For further information, see* ARTERIOSCLEROSIS; ATHEROSCLEROSIS; HEART; *and* HEART ATTACK. *See also* ANGIOPLASTY, BALLOON; HEART SURGERY; *and* SURGERY *for more on treatment.*

Coronary Thrombosis

The narrowing or blockage of an artery of the heart by a clot or thrombus.

Complete blockage of a coronary artery causes myocardial infarction, also known as a heart attack. Coronary thrombosis is generally the culmination of a long-term buildup of arterial plaque, deposits consisting of cholesterol, fat, and cells. This buildup, called atherosclerosis, causes the walls of the artery to become thicker and less flexible. The result is ischemia, a reduction in the flow of oxygen-carrying blood that can cause symptoms including angina (chest pain).

As plaque accumulates, some may break off to form a thrombus, a clot that can travel to a narrowed place in the artery, blocking it and causing a myocardial infarction. Sometimes coronary thrombosis is caused by plaque that does not break away, but has grown enough at its original site to form what is called a coronary thrombus. *See also* ANGINA; ARTERIOSCLEROSIS; *and* ATHEROSCLEROSIS.

Corset

Support device for the back.

A corset is generally used to help relieve lower back pain and strain, or to treat abnormalities or injuries of the spine. Corsets are worn around the trunk. They work by applying extra pressure on the abdomen, which helps to take the weight of the trunk off the lower back. Corsets restrict movement and provide an extra layer of warmth for healing.

Soft corsets are made of cotton reinforced with plastic or metal. They have straps that can be used for tightening. Hard corsets are made of plaster or light plastic and must be molded to fit the individual's body. This type of corset restricts movement and is generally used to support unstable spines or to correct curvature of the spine, in cases such as scoliosis. *See also* SCOLIOSIS *and* SPINAL INJURY.

Corticosteroid Drugs

A family of drugs used to mimic the hormone cortisol, produced in the adrenal glands.

Corticosteroid drugs are a family of drugs that are used to treat allergies, asthma, and other diseases that cause inflammation in the body. Available as nasal sprays, pills, liquids, and shots, corticosteroid drugs are prescribed for chronic respiratory diseases, nasal allergies, and inflammatory conditions, particularly those affecting the joints and muscles. Occasionally, the drugs may be injected directly into the joints to relieve inflammation. However, because of undesirable side effects, these medications are generally used only when other drugs have been ineffective. *See also* ANTI-INFLAMMATORY DRUGS; ARTHRITIS; ASTHMA; CORTICOSTEROID HORMONES; INFLAMMATION; *and* JOINT.

Corticosteroid Hormones

Hormones produced by the adrenal glands.

The adrenal cortex, which is the outer region of the adrenal gland, produces the corticosteroid hormones. These hormones —hydrocortisone (also known as cortisol) and corticosterone—help the body use and store fats, proteins, and carbohydrates. They also can help to suppress inflammation. The corticosteroids are secreted directly into the bloodstream and are regulated by the release of hormones from the pituitary gland. *See also* ADRENAL GLANDS; CORTICOSTEROID DRUGS; HORMONES; *and* PITUITARY GLAND.

Cosmetic Dentistry

Field of dentistry that seeks to improve the appearance of teeth and the face around the mouth.

While basic dentistry focuses on the health and efficiency of teeth and gums, cosmetic dentistry combines this objective with an aesthetic goal.

Incorrectly aligned teeth are not merely sources of gathered plaque, but can be a source of embarrassment. Braces (orthodontic appliances) fixed onto the teeth can help to properly position them within a few months. Braces are now readily available to children, teenagers, and adults.

Chipped, malformed, or stained teeth, as well as decayed or broken teeth, can also be repaired cosmetically. Dentists bleach teeth, bond a tooth-colored material onto natural teeth, bond a complete veneer or facing over a tooth, or, if appropriate, completely cover a tooth or teeth with crowns. The dentist takes into account the color, shape, and size of the teeth, and the shape of the smile and face, when treating a patient cosmetically. *See also* BRACES, DENTAL *and* ORTHODONTIC APPLIANCES.

Cosmetic Surgery

An operation performed primarily to improve the appearance of an individual, rather than to correct functions of tissues and organs.

Cosmetic surgery can improve a person's appearance in many ways. A cosmetic surgery procedure may be as simple as removing a mole (nevus) or skin blemish from the face, or as complex as a comprehensive facelift and liposuction. Cosmetic surgery can enlarge the breasts or remove excess and unwanted fat from the hips and thighs. Yet cosmetic surgery cannot cause drastic physical change, nor can it cure depression or self-esteem problems. It is important to have realistic expectations of what the surgery can and cannot accomplish. It is also important to understand that with all surgical procedures comes the possibility of complications.

TYPES
There are many types of cosmetic surgery. Some common procedures include facelifts, performed to correct sagging of the skin on the face and neck; eyelid surgery (blepharoplasty), to remove bags from under the eyes; nose surgery (rhinoplasty), to correct the nose; liposuction, to remove unwanted fat; dermabrasion, a type of laser

Cosmetic/Reconstructive Procedures in the United States—1999

PROCEDURE	# PERFORMED
Tumor removal	521,678
Liposuction	230,865
Hand surgery	171,510
Breast augmentation	167,318
Eyelid surgery	142,033
Breast reconstruction	82,975
Breast reduction	78,169
Facelift (rhytidectomy)	72,793
Laceration repair	69,729
Tummy tuck	54,977
Collagen injections	53,197
Chemical peel	51,589
Laser skin resurfacing	50,505
Nose reshaping	46,596
Scar revision	46,242
Forehead lift	40,969
Breast lift (mastopexy)	38,276
Birth defect reconstr.	30,702
Microsurgery	23,200
Burn care	22,202
Fat injections	20,503
Maxillofacial surgery	20,347
Breast implant removals	13,009
Animal bite repair	11,600
Dermabrasion	11,550
Breast reduction in men	9,152
Ear surgery (otoplasty)	8,716
Chin augmentation	6,059
Cheek implants	3,042
Endoscopic procedures	2,707
Subcutaneous mastectomy	1,798

surgery used to rid the skin of wrinkle lines, stretch marks, or scars; and tummy tucks (abdominoplasty), to diminish the size of the abdomen.

RECOVERY

All cosmetic surgery carries risks and requires substantial recovery time. Pain felt after cosmetic surgery can generally be treated with analgesic drugs (painkillers).

For background material on cosmetic surgery, see BIRTH DEFECTS and SURGERY. Related information can be found in ACCIDENTS; BLEPHAROPLASTY; BREAST CANCER; BURNS; CLEFT LIP AND PALATE; FACE-LIFT; HEAD INJURY; KELOID; MASTECTOMY; and SCAR.

Resources on Cosmetic Surgery

Converse, J.M., *Reconstructive Plastic Surgery* (1977); Engler, Alan, *Body Sculpture: Plastic Surgery of the Body for Men and Women* (2000); Grazer, F.M. and J.R. Klingbeil, *Body Image: A Surgical Perspective* (1980); Henry, Kimberly A., et al., *The Plastic Surgery Sourcebook: Everything You Need to Know* (1999); Rudolph, Ross, et al., *Skin Grafting* (1979); American Society of Plastic Surgeons, Tel. (888) 475-2784, Online: www.plasticsurgery.org; American Society for Aesthetic Plastic Surgery, Tel. (800) 364-2147, Online: surgery.org; www.nycornell.org/ent/.

Costalgia

Discomfort in the chest cavity due to an injury to a rib or to one of the nerves beneath the rib cage (intercostal nerves).

Costalgia is a condition marked by deep chest pain. It is a result of a broken rib or damage to a nerve located beneath the rib cage. Deep breathing aggravates costalgia, and severe pain may persist for as long as a few weeks.

Rib fracture can result from a fall or a blow. It can also result from repeated stress on the rib cage, such as that produced by repeated and severe coughing. The most common cause of damage to the nerves underneath the ribs is infection by the herpes zoster virus (shingles). Research suggests that the herpes zoster virus enters the ganglia of the spine, where it remains latent. The virus later reactivates when the immune system is damaged by AIDS, Hodgkin's disease, or drugs. When the virus is reactivated, it multiplies quickly and causes excruciating pain.

Rib fractures usually heal without treatment. If costalgia is caused by shingles, there is no cure, but antiviral drugs can lessen the severity of the symptoms. Aspirin, ibuprofen, acetaminophen, or codeine can also reduce the pain. *See also* AIDS; ANTIVIRAL DRUGS; *and* HERPES ZOSTER.

Cough

A sudden explosive reflex action that tends to clear material from the airway.

A cough is usually a natural reflex that protects the respiratory system from irritants such as dust or smoke. Receptors in the nose, throat, and chest detect irritants and stimulate a cough center in the brain. Muscular portions (such as the vocal cords) of the windpipe tighten, trapping air in the lungs. The muscles of the abdomen and chest tighten forcefully, pushing against the diaphragm. Then the vocal cords and epiglottis open suddenly, and the trapped air leaves explosively.

CAUSES

A persistent or unusually forceful cough can be a symptom of a medical problem, ranging from the common cold to influenza to lung cancer. Some causes of coughing are:

- environmental pollutants, such as cigarette smoke, dust, smog, and aerosol sprays;
- unusually cold or dry air;
- gastrointestinal reflex, or the backup of stomach acid into the esophagus or lungs while lying down;
- the inflammation and constriction of air passages (bronchi) in the lung, owing to asthma;
- bronchitis, or inflammation of the air passages in the lung;
- postnasal drip, or overproduction of mucus that trickles from the back of the nose into the throat;
- drugs, such as inhaled steroids or medications for hypertension and heart disease; and
- bronchospasm, or temporary narrowing of the bronchi resulting from asthma, an allergic reaction, or an infection.

A Coughing Child

Children between the ages of one and three often develop a hoarse, barking cough accompanied by wheezing. This condition, called croup, results from infection by a respiratory virus. The cough is usually worse at night. Croup can often be relieved by turning on the hot water in the bathroom and having the child sit in the enclosed room. If this measure is not effective, a doctor should be called, because the cough may be due to a more serious infection.

TYPES

A cough is described as nonproductive (dry) when it does not bring up mucus (phlegm) and productive when it does. A cough that brings up mucus helps to remove irritants from the lungs and airways. A cough can be made more productive by drinking a great deal of water or using a humidifier to loosen mucus.

Observing Different Types of Phlegm. The type of phlegm produced by a cough is significant for diagnosis. Lung cancer, for example, is associated with blood-stained phlegm. The inflammation of the lungs in pneumonia can also result in blood-containing mucus. Yellowish, green, or brownish phlegm indicates a respiratory infection. Any cough that lasts for several days, is accompanied by symptoms such as chest pain, or brings up discolored phlegm should prompt a visit to a physician for diagnosis and treatment.

TREATMENT

While many over-the-counter cough medications are available, they fall into two general classes, based on the active ingredient they contain. It is important to read the label of a combination cold medicine carefully to determine if the active ingredients it contains are appropriate for a specific type of cough.

One class of cough remedies is intended for productive coughs. These drugs contain an expectorant, which stimulates the body to expel phlegm. Expectorant remedies may also contain an ingredient to enhance expulsion by reducing the stickiness of the phlegm.

A second class of remedies is intended for nonproductive or dry coughs. These drugs contain suppressants, ingredients that depress the part of the brain that controls coughing.

Choosing the correct cough remedy for the kind of cold being treated is important, since a nonproductive cough remedy may not help the body to clear the amount of sputum produced by a productive cough. Cough remedies should be used with care, because many of them can cause drowsiness. A cough that persists despite the use of over-the-counter remedies could indicate a serious condition requiring attention from a doctor.

Background information on cough can be found in RESPIRATORY SYSTEM. *For further information, see* ALLERGY; ASTHMA; BRONCHITIS; BRONCHOSPASM; COLD, COMMON; COUGH, SMOKERS'; COUGHING UP BLOOD; CROUP; RESPIRATORY TRACT INFECTION; WHOOPING COUGH; *and* VIRUSES. *See also* EXPECTORANTS *for more on treatment.*

Resources on Coughing and Respiration
Crystal, Ronald G., *The Lung: Scientific Foundations* (1997);Haas, Francois, and Shela Sperber Haas, *The Chronic Bronchitis and Emphysema Handbook* (2000); Parker, Steve, *The Lungs and Breathing* (1989); Perry, Angela R., *Essential Guide to Asthma* (1998); Scott, Walter J., *Lung Cancer: A Guide to Diagnosis and Treatment* (1999); American Lung Association, Tel. (800) LUNG-USA, Online: www.lungusa.org; Lung Line Information Service, Tel. (800) 222-5864, Online: www.nationaljewish.org; www.nycornell.org/medicine/pulmonary/index.html

Cough, Smokers'

A recurrent cough caused by prolonged smoking.

Smokers' cough is a repeated effort to clear away phlegm from the airways. It cannot succeed, since the irritation that causes the buildup of phlegm is aggravated with each cigarette or cigar that is smoked.

Smokers' cough is the result of the irritation caused by long-term tobacco use. Irritation causes inflammation, to which the respiratory tract responds by producing unusually large amounts of mucus, which blocks the airways.

Smokers' cough is common in anyone who smokes heavily or for a long period of time. Smokers' cough is associated with increased risk of lung cancer, heart attack, and other life-threatening conditions.

Cough remedies may provide some temporary relief, but they cannot succeed as long as smoking continues. The only effective treatment for smokers' cough is to quit smoking. Even though smokers may become accustomed to their cough, they should consult a doctor, especially if the frequency or character of the cough changes, as this could indicate a serious disease. *See also* BRONCHITIS; COUGH; HEART ATTACK; LUNG CANCER; SUBSTANCE ABUSE; *and* TOBACCO SMOKING.

Coughing Up Blood

Also known as hemoptysis

Blood in the sputum.

Any number of medical conditions can result in the presence of blood in the sputum (hemoptysis), including bacterial infections, lung cancer, bleeding disorders such as hemophilia, inflammation of the trachea, heart failure, mitral stenosis, and congestive heart failure. Any of these conditions can result in broken blood vessels in the airways, nose, throat, or another part of the respiratory system. While a simple persistent cough can cause blood in the sputum, such blood is usually a sign of a serious underlying condition that requires medical attention.

CAUSES

Most often, coughing up blood is the result of a respiratory tract infection such as tuberculosis, bronchitis, or pneumonia. Such an infection can inflame the airways (bronchi) of the lung or the small sacs (alveoli) where air is exchanged in the lung. An infection may also damage a blood vessel of the respiratory tract enough to cause it to rupture.

When the bronchi become enlarged and distorted (bronchiectasis), one of the blood vessels within the bronchi may break open. This can also happen with tracheitis, or inflammation of the windpipe. Within the lung itself, congestion can put enough pressure on blood vessels to cause them to rupture. Congestion can be due to a narrowing of the valve between the upper and lower chambers of the heart (mitral stenosis), or blockage of a lung artery by a clot (pulmonary embolism). Lung cancer can also weaken and eventually rupture a blood vessel, causing hemoptysis.

DIAGNOSIS

The appearance of the blood coughed up can give clues to the underlying disorder. Only rarely is the blood bright red and unmixed with other secretions. It may have a pink, foamy, or streaked appearance, or take the form of clots.

A cough that persists for months, worsens dramatically, and produces blood may be an indication of lung cancer. A high fever and shortness of breath may suggest pneumonia. A chest x-ray can be done to detect abnormalities in the lungs and respiratory tract. In some cases, visual examination of the respiratory tract with a bronchoscope may be performed.

TREATMENT

Treatment may include antibiotic drugs for bacterial infections, diuretics to reduce fluid retention, and anticoagulant drugs to prevent abnormal blood clotting. *See also* ANTIBIOTIC DRUGS; ANTICOAGULANT DRUGS; BRONCHOSCOPY; CONGESTIVE HEART FAILURE; HEART FAILURE; HEMOPHILIA; MITRAL STENOSIS; *and* RESPIRATORY TRACT INFECTION.

Counseling

Care and psychological support given by a medical professional to help a patient deal with a health problem.

Counseling is helpful for a number of individuals. It can be given to those with drug or alcohol addictions; people with problems at school, at work, or in the home; individuals who need information about family planning; and those who are experiencing crises.

During a counseling session, the patient or client is given information by a healthcare professional, usually in a one-on-one setting but sometimes in small groups with other clients. The client is then given the chance to ask questions or to discuss concerns he or she may have.

Counseling is offered to clients by a number of organizations, including nonprofit volunteer organizations, hospital crisis-intervention centers, or social services departments. These organizations specialize in providing short-term care. Psychotherapists provide longer-term counseling. *See also* ALCOHOL DEPENDENCE *and* CRISIS INTERVENTION.

Cowpox

A very rare disease caused by a virus called variola, which is similar to the virus that causes smallpox in humans.

Cows infected with cowpox have pus-filled lesions on the teats and udders. Today the disease is transmitted to humans by small animals, mostly cats, though it has never been reported in the United States and is only rarely found in Europe.

Cowpox produces a mild, self-limiting infection in humans. Edward Jenner based his smallpox vaccine on the less dangerous cowpox virus to demonstrate the efficacy of vaccination as a means of building immunity to diseases in humans. As a result of this vaccine, smallpox has been virtually eradicated throughout the world. *See also* SMALLPOX *and* VACCINATION.

Coxa Vara

Deformity of the hip, causing shortening of the leg.

When the angle between the neck and head and the shaft of the femur is reduced, the leg is shortened, which may lead to a limp. This is most likely to occur with injury. In adolescents, coxa vara may be the result of injury to the still-developing head of the bone. Bone softening, due to such conditions as rickets or Paget's disease, may also be the cause.

Pain, stiffness, and difficulty walking are symptoms of coxa vara; the diagnosis is usually confirmed with x-rays. Treatment can harden bones that have become soft through a bone disorder. An osteotomy, in which the neck of the bone is cut to reposition it, may be performed to relieve pain and stiffness. *See also* FEMUR; PAGET'S DISEASE; *and* RICKETS.

Cradle Cap

Also known as seborrheic dermatitis

A scaly, yellowish rash on the head, face, and ears of infants, caused by overactive oil glands stimulated by maternal hormones in breast milk.

Cradle cap, the common name for seborrheic dermatitis, is an inflammation that occurs on the oily parts of the body. It is yellowish and crusted in appearance, usually a collection of shedding skin caught around an infant's growing hair.

The cause of cradle cap is overactive oil glands in the infant's scalp, which are stimulated by the mother's hormones. A contributing factor is not washing the infant's scalp thoroughly.

Treatment. Cradle cap is treated with a mild dandruff shampoo two or three times a week. The shampoo should be left on the baby's scalp for five minutes, then rubbed off with a wet washcloth. If cradle cap is severe, mineral oil should be applied to the scalp one hour before bathing the infant. Dandruff shampoo should be used until the condition clears. *See also* DANDRUFF; DERMATITIS; *and* SEBUM.

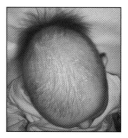

Cradle Cap.
Cradle cap, also known as seborrheic dermatitis, is found on the heads, faces, and ears of infants with overactive oil glands. Above, the scaly, yellowish rash characteristic of cradle cap can clearly be seen on the head of this infant.

Cramp

A sudden, painful contracting of the muscles.

Painful muscle spasms or cramps are common in healthy people and usually last only a few minutes. Cramps may result from vigorous activity or remaining in the same position for an extended period.

CAUSES

Cramps that occur during or just after strenuous exercise are caused by a buildup of lactic acid in the muscles. A muscle cramp may also indicate a minor injury to muscle fiber. Prolonged exercise accompanied by excessive sweating can lead to a loss of electrolytes and cause cramps in resting muscles. Some individuals experience leg cramps at night while sleeping; this may be caused by poor blood circulation to the leg muscles.

SYMPTOMS

Attempting to move a cramped muscle causes the muscle to vigorously contract. If pressure is placed on the cramped muscle, the pain is temporarily eased.

TREATMENT

A cramp usually lasts only a few minutes and will improve by itself. Gently massaging and stretching the muscle can help to ease the cramp. To prevent cramping, it is important to drink plenty of water and stretch properly before exercising. Adding calcium to the diet and raising the legs may relieve leg cramps.

WRITERS' CRAMP

Writers' cramp is a series of muscle spasms that makes writing painful. Half of people with writers' cramp develop a tremor in the arms. It may be a form of dystonia (an involuntary muscle spasm), or it may be psychological in origin, as often writing is the only affected movement. However, the cramp does not generally respond to psychotherapy. The main treatment is rest; muscle relaxants are usually ineffective. *See also* DYSTONIA *and* MUSCLE SPASM.

Craniopharyngioma

A rare tumor of the pituitary gland.

A craniopharyngioma is a tumor of the pituitary gland. It can cause dwarfism by interfering with the activity of the growth hormone produced by this gland. It is a rare condition, occurring in about one of every million births in the United States. In addition to growth retardation, other symptoms of the condition are headaches, vomiting, vision problems, and incomplete sexual development. The condition can be diagnosed by brain scans and treated effectively in most cases by surgical removal of the tumor. *See also* BRAIN IMAGING; DWARFISM; *and* PITUITARY GLAND.

Craniosynostosis

A condition in which an infant's skull bones fuse together prematurely, resulting in an abnormally shaped head.

A newborn's head contains two "soft spots" where the bones of the skull have not yet grown together. These areas, known as fontanels, are a necessity dictated by the birth process, as a completely formed skull would have difficulty negotiating the narrow birth canal. Additionally, they ensure sufficient room in the skull to accommodate the growing brain. Closure of the fontanels usually occurs 12 to 18 months after delivery.

In craniosynostosis, the skull bones close prematurely, causing an abnormally shaped head. It may be due to a genetic anomaly, or there may be an unknown cause. Some cases of craniosynostosis are associated with other disorders such as microcephaly (small head) and hydrocephalus (excessive fluid in the brain). The first sign of craniosynostosis is an abnormal head shape. Other symptoms, possibly caused by constriction of the growing brain, are developmental delay and mental retardation. Surgery is required to increase skull capacity. *See also* CHILD DEVELOPMENT; HYDROCEPHALUS; *and* MICROCEPHALY.

Craniotomy

The surgical removal of part of the skull (cranium) to give access to the brain.

A craniotomy exposes enough of the brain for a neurosurgeon to perform an operation such as the removal of tumors, aneurysms, or blood clots; tissue sampling for biopsy; repair of tears in the brain's membrane; or drainage of a brain abscess.

In a craniotomy, a portion of the patient's head is shaved; incisions are made through the skin, muscle, and membranes of the scalp; and a segment of bone is cut away; then the operation is performed. After the operation, the cranial segment is replaced, and the membranes, muscle, and skin are sewn back into position. The scalp is closed with sutures or clips. *See also* ABSCESS; ANEURYSM; BIOPSY; BRAIN; BRAIN TUMOR; *and* SUTURING.

Crepitus

Grating sound that occurs when two rough surfaces rub together.

Crepitus occurs when bone is left without any kind of cushioning or padding, for example, when the two ends of a broken bone rub against each other, or in osteoarthritis, where the protective cartilage has worn away, leaving the joints to grind together. The sound is loud enough to be heard with the ear alone, but a stethoscope can pick it up more clearly. Crepitus also occurs when air under the skin, or the gas in infected tissue, is pressed. *See also* ARTHRITIS *and* FRACTURE.

Creutzfeldt-Jakob Disease (CJD)

A disease thought to be caused by a virus-like organism called a prion.

Creutzfeldt-Jakob disease is related to mad cow disease (bovine spongiform encephalopathy—BSE), and it may be transmitted by eating the flesh of infected animals. It is characterized by a number of tiny, almost invisible holes in the brain that produce a form of dementia. Sufferers may go without symptoms for months or even years after exposure, but once the symptoms begin, the disease progresses rapidly, much more so than Alzheimer's disease.

Symptoms. Early on, the victim exhibits muscle twitching and poor coordination, soon followed by a loss of intellectual capacity. Other symptoms include irritability, apathy, indifference to hygiene, and confusion. Sleep disorders are common in the later stages of Creutzfeldt-Jakob disease, and patients' vision is blurred. Death usually follows within six to twelve months of the first symptoms, with pneumonia usually as the final cause of death. A tiny percentage of sufferers may live two to five years after being infected.

Treatment. Treatment of Creutzfeldt-Jakob disease consists of making the sufferer as comfortable as possible with medications to control more aggressive behavior and sedatives for the twitching. There is no cure for this disease. *See also* ALZHEIMER'S DISEASE; BRAIN DISORDERS; CONFUSION; DEMENTIA; ENCEPHALOPATHY; PNEUMONIA; *and* PRION.

Cri du Chat Syndrome

A rare condition caused by a chromosomal deficiency.

Cri du chat syndrome is a chromosomal abnormality. The name literally means "cat's cry," as newborns with this condition have a high-pitched cry closely resembling that of a kitten. The cry persists for several weeks.

Other symptoms include low birth weight, a mouth that does not close properly, a round or asymmetrical face, wide-set eyes, a wide nose, low ears with an abnormal shape, webbed fingers, heart defects, and severe mental retardation.

Children with cri du chat syndrome often survive to adulthood; they need care throughout life. *See also* CHROMOSOMAL ABNORMALITIES; CRYING IN INFANTS; *and* MENTAL RETARDATION.

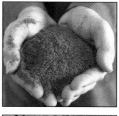

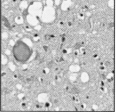

Creutzfeldt-Jakob Disease. Creutzfeldt-Jakob disease is a serious degenerative brain disease that is related to mad cow disease. Above, top, mad cow disease originally may have spread among cattle because of the presences of parts of infected cows in the cattle's feed. Above, bottom, this type of infection produces tiny holes in the brain cells of affected individuals, resulting in progressive dementia and related symptoms.

Crisis Intervention

Emergency counseling given to people with serious social or medical problems.

Crisis intervention is provided for people who are experiencing severe distress or emotional difficulty. There are many organizations that help people in crisis, including nonprofit volunteer organizations, social services departments, and hospital walk-in centers.

Crisis centers offer counseling sessions, during which clients are given advice or information about their particular problem and about ways to deal with it. The client is then given the opportunity to raise questions or to discuss any additional questions or doubts he or she may have.

Crisis centers are set up to provide emergency care on a short-term basis. For longer-term help, these centers may refer clients to psychotherapists or other health professionals. *See also* COUNSELING; PSYCHOTHERAPY; *and* THERAPY.

Crohn's Disease

Also known as ileitis or regional enteritis

A disease of unknown origin, characterized by chronic inflammation and ulceration of the intestines.

Crohn's disease is a chronic and progressive inflammation of the intestine, involving the lower part of the small intestine (ileum) and, in some cases, the colon. However, Crohn's disease may also affect any portion of the digestive tract from mouth to anus.

INCIDENCE AND CAUSE

Crohn's disease occurs in 1 in every 50,000 people. In recent years, the disease has become more prevalent in the United States and other Western countries. The typical patient suffering from Crohn's disease is Caucasian and between the ages of 15 and 35. The disease may be inherited, and it is suspected that it may result from an abnormal reaction of the immune system to a substance in the digestive tract.

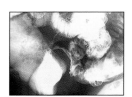

Crohn's Disease. Crohn's disease is marked by chronic inflammation of the intestines. Above, this inflammation can clearly be seen on an abdominal x-ray.

SYMPTOMS

Symptoms of Crohn's disease include periodic pain and cramping on the right side of the abdomen or around the navel, abdominal swelling or tenderness, chronic diarrhea, nausea, a low-grade fever, fatigue, malaise (a generalized feeling of illness), weight loss, and lesions, especially in the intestine and around the mouth. Crohn's disease is thought to be hereditary; if an individual has a family history of symptoms, there is a greater chance of that individual developing the disease.

DIAGNOSIS

Crohn's disease is diagnosed with barium x-rays, which reveal abnormal areas of the intestine. Parts of the intestine may appear narrower and more rigid than normal. Colonoscopy, also used, may reveal a cobblestone-like texture of ulcerations in the lining of the intestines.

COMPLICATIONS

The diarrhea that characterizes Crohn's disease can be quite debilitating and can result in severe malnutrition, as nutrients are not properly absorbed by the intestines. Abdominal pain helps suppress the appetite, resulting in further weight loss. Other complications include progressive obstruction of the small intestine, development of abnormal connections (fistulas) and fissures in the rectal and anal areas, bleeding, and development of abscesses.

TREATMENT

There is no single cure for Crohn's disease. Supplements of certain vitamins and minerals, such as vitamin B_{12}, are often needed to counter reduced absorption of nutrients. A special diet may be required. Generally, foods that are difficult to digest, such as high-fat or high-fiber foods, as well as irritants, such as caffeine and spicy foods, should be avoided. Some physicians recommend liquid diets or intravenous feeding during severe attacks, to give the intestine a chance to rest.

No specific treatment is required if the patient does not exhibit symptoms. Mild

When Crohn's Disease Results in Dehydration

Dehydration may not seem very threatening to overall health, but it can cause serious damage. Young children can dehydrate rapidly, causing serious damage to the digestive tract and even death. Adults, too, should pay attention to frequent spells of diarrhea. Oral rehydration therapy is simple and effective: replace what diarrhea takes out of the body by drinking glasses of water mixed with a half-teaspoon of salt or baking soda. Dementia in the elderly may be a sign of dehydration.

symptoms can be helped by antidiarrheal medications and adequate intake of fluid.

More severe cases can be helped by anti-inflammatory medications such as s-amino-saliylate drugs and corticosteroids. If only the rectum is affected, corticosteroid enemas may suppress inflammation. Immuno-suppressive therapy may also be effective, including a recently introduced drug called infliximab. All of these treatments provide relief from symptoms of the disease, but they cannot cure the disease itself.

Surgery is performed for complications such as obstruction, abscesses, and perforation. The large intestine may be removed if the disease is limited to one area and medications have proven ineffective. When the disease is found only in the small intestine, the diseased segment is removed and the healthy portions joined together.

Approximately 70 percent of patients with Crohn's disease require surgery at some point. Surgery is not a permanent cure; recurrence of the disease in other areas of the intestinal tract is common.

PREVENTION

Since Crohn's disease is most likely caused by genetic factors, there is no way to prevent this condition. Individuals with the disease should get plenty of rest.

For background information on Crohn's disease, see COLON *and* DIGESTIVE SYSTEM. *Further information can be found in* ABDOMINAL PAIN; DIET AND DISEASE; DIARRHEA; INTESTINE; IRRITABLE BOWEL SYNDROME; *and* ULCERATIVE COLITIS.

Cromolyn Sodium

A prescription medication used on a long-term basis to prevent asthma attacks, as an alternative to inhaled corticosteroids.

As a treatment for chronic asthma, cromolyn sodium is a slow-acting drug intended for long-term control of the symptoms and a preventive measure if a crisis is anticipated. However, it is not effective during a severe asthma attack. It is also used for the treatment of mastocytosis, a rare disease marked by excess mast cells in the body.

Side effects of cromolyn sodium that should be reported to a physician include skin rash and itching, swelling of the face or lips, coughing, or wheezing. Individuals may also experience sneezing, dry mouth, nasal congestion, and watery eyes. *See also* ASTHMA *and* MASTOCYTOSIS.

Crossmatching

A test to establish the compatibility of blood before transfusion.

Blood transfusion is necessary during a variety of medical emergencies and surgical procedures. The blood is generally needed to replace blood lost through injury or during surgery, or to treat certain blood disorders, such as hemophilia. While it is always best to use the patient's own blood, blood banks can crossmatch blood of the recipient with a donor to ensure that they are compatible. Crossmatching involves testing the blood for the presence of ABO blood type and Rh antigens.

Testing for A, B, and Rh antigens is crucial. If patients without one of these antigens receive blood containing that antigen, they will develop an immune response to the transfused blood. Their bodies will treat the blood as a foreign invader and produce antibodies to rapidly destroy the transfused cells. This process is known as hemolysis. *See also* AUTOIMMUNE DISORDERS; BLOOD GROUPS; HEMOPHILIA; IMMUNE SYSTEM; THALASSEMIA; *and* TRANSFUSION.

Resources on Crohn's Disease

Sapolsky, Robert M., *Why Zebras Don't Get Ulcers: An Updated Guide to Stress, Stress-Related Diseases, and Coping* (1998); Sachar, David B., et al., *Pocket Guide to Gastroenterology* (1991); Thompson, W. Grant, *The Angry Gut: Coping with Colitis and Crohn's Disease* (1993); Crohn's and Colitis Foundation of America, Inc., Tel: (800) 932-2423, Online: www.ccfa.org; Digestive Disease National Coalition, Tel. (202) 544-7497, Online: www.ddnc.org; National Institute of Diabetes and Digestive and Kidney Diseases, Tel. (301) 496-3583, Online: www.niddk.nih.gov; www.nycornell.org/medicine/digestive/index.html

Cross-Eye

Also known as strabismus

Misalignment of the eyes.

Cross-eye, or strabismus, is a type of eye defect in which one eye looks in a different direction than the other. The condition can cause double vision. It can be corrected by glasses in some cases, but may be surgically corrected for visual and cosmetic reasons. Most types of cross-eye can be repaired. *See also* EYE, DISORDERS OF.

Croup

A respiratory condition marked by a cough and stridor (a harsh barking sound caused by obstructed airways).

There are many different kinds of croup; all include a swelling of the membranes lining the larynx, trachea, or bronchi.

Viral croup is most commonly seen in children between six months and three years of age. This type of croup is usually mild. Along with noisy breathing there may be a low-grade fever. If the child is having trouble breathing, a humidifier and generous intake of liquids may help.

If a child with viral croup has labored breathing, he or she may require hospitalization. The parent or caregiver should watch a child with viral croup for signs of labored breathing or blue lips or fingertips. If any part of the child appears blue, this signifies a medical emergency, and emergency care (911) should be called immediately. In the hospital, the child will receive humidified air to breathe and might recline in a croup tent. The child may be given medications to shrink the swollen membranes and open the airways.

Acute epiglottitis is another type of croup that most often affects children older than three. Children with this serious infection tend to drool, because it hurts to swallow. It can progress from stridor to complete obstruction in four to twelve hours, so prompt treatment is necessary. Frequently, a tube is placed in the trachea, and the child is kept in the intensive care

---

In the Middle of the Night

A parent awakened in the middle of the night and hearing a child having a croup attack should remain calm. Hold the child and help him or her relax, which may help stop the windpipe from restricting. Go into the bathroom, close the door, and turn on the hot water in the tub and sink. Have the child sit on the toilet while you read aloud to pass the time. Opening the window will create more steam. Allow 15 minutes in the bathroom, and if the symptoms persist, call the doctor or hospital.

---

unit. The child will also be given antibiotics and oxygen. Sometimes a tracheotomy must be performed. If acute epiglottitis is treated quickly, it is not fatal.

Spasmodic croup occurs frequently, usually at night, and involves severe obstruction that lasts for only a few hours. For relief, the child should be placed in a warm bath to breathe the steam. Using an inhaler to open the swollen passageways may also help. In more serious cases, the child should be taken to the emergency room.

Diphtheritic croup is a rare form of croup, due to an increase in the number of immunizations for diphtheria. It is considered a possibility only when the child is very ill and has not yet been immunized against diphtheria. A child with this type of croup appears quite ill. Diphtheritic croup is treated with a diphtheria antitoxin as well as antibiotics.

Background material on croup can be found in INFECTIOUS DISEASE *and* PEDIATRICS. *For further information, see* COUGH; INFLAMMATION; RESPIRATORY SYSTEM; RESPIRATORY TRACT INFECTION; STRIDOR; *and* VIRUSES. *See also* EXPECTORANTS *for more on treatment options.*

Crowding, Dental

Insufficient room along the jawbone to allow correct alignment of teeth.

Sometimes the mouth is too small to accommodate the human body's 32 teeth. Other times the mouth is not small but the teeth are too large. In either case, the teeth can become crowded, which causes them to grow irregularly. Crowding can cause pain and discomfort.

The common procedure for dealing with dental crowding is to better align the teeth with orthodontic treatment. Occasionally, it is necessary to reduce the width of some teeth or remove one or more teeth to create more space for the remaining teeth. *See also* ORTHODONTIC APPLIANCES *and* ORTHODONTICS.

Crush Syndrome

Also known as compression syndrome

Failure of the kidneys, resulting from violent compression of muscle tissue.

Victims of collapsed buildings or auto accidents often suffer crush syndrome. The damaged muscle tissue releases large amounts of protein into the bloodstream. This sudden deluge interferes with the ability of the kidneys and liver to remove toxins from the blood. Crush syndrome is a life-threatening condition, since toxic substances build up to high levels in the blood instead of being excreted in the urine.

Crush syndrome is almost always complicated by shock. Hospitalization with artificial cleansing of the blood (kidney dialysis) removes high levels of toxins in the blood, while allowing the kidneys to recover. *See also* ACCIDENTS; DIALYSIS; KIDNEY; LIVER FAILURE; RENAL FAILURE; *and* SHOCK.

Crutch Palsy

Muscle weakness in the wrist, fingers, and thumb due to pressure from a crutch.

If a crutch is too long for an individual, excess pressure will be exerted under the arm, which will affect the nerves that operate the muscles in the wrist, fingers, and thumb. The condition occurs in other situations in which these nerves are pressured, such as falling asleep with an arm over the back of a chair.

Crutch palsy usually does not require treatment, as it will resolve itself once the pressure on the nerves is relieved. *See also* FRACTURE.

Crying in Infants

Crying is a baby's primary means of communication. Babies cry when they are hungry, wet, tired, overstimulated, or in pain. It is often overwhelming for a new parent to determine what is causing a baby to cry and how to correct the situation.

With time and experience, parents can learn to distinguish between their baby's different cries. Until then, the process of elimination can be quite helpful.

If it has been more than an hour or two since a baby has been fed, the baby may simply be hungry. If it has been less than an hour since the last feeding, chances are the baby is not hungry. In that case, crying may due to an irritating air bubble in the stomach, which can be alleviated by burping.

Some babies do not seem to mind being wet or dirty, whereas others do. A baby with sensitive skin or with a propensity for developing diaper rash may cry when he or she needs to be changed.

A baby who has been up for a relatively long time may be overtired and need to sleep. Some babies settle down on their own; others may be overstimulated and need to be rocked or sung to.

Some babies seem to prefer being swaddled or wrapped up tightly with a blanket and will cry if they are unwrapped.

Babies may also cry because of illness or pain. A doctor should be notified of any excessive or inconsolable crying, as this may indicate an illness or other medical condition that requires treatment.

COLIC

Sometimes no discernible cause for crying can be found, in which case the baby is said to be suffering from colic. Babies with colic tend to cry for prolonged periods of time, often at the same time of day or night. This crying may be the result of gastrointestinal discomfort. Being held and walked tends to quiet colicky babies, either from the warmth and pressure on the abdomen or simply from the distraction of the motion. *See also* ABDOMINAL PAIN; COLIC, INFANTILE; CONSTIPATION; *and* DIAPER RASH.

Cryopreservation

The preservation of tissue, sperm, fluid, blood, or plasma at extremely low temperatures.

Cryopreservation stabilizes human fluid and tissue for later use, often for use in a different recipient. Long-term preservation of biological material may be accomplished by deep-freezing and freeze-drying at low temperatures. Cryopreservation employs liquid nitrogen, preserving samples at $-196°C$. At such extremely low temperatures, biological material will keep its structure and its viability (capacity to function and grow) indefinitely.

Cryopreservation technology has been a stimulus to both agriculture and medicine alike, particularly as an aid to the development of technologies that aid in reproduction. Bovine sperm cells, for example, have been stored for more than 50 years without any noticeable reduction in fertility or increase in abnormalities.

The most important factor in cryopreservation is the temperature of cryogenic freezing. If human fluid or tissue is not kept below $-135°C$, its viability decreases over the course of long-term storage. Warmer temperatures may be suitable in tissue where some loss of viability does not pose a problem, but cryopreservation of eggs and embryos (used for implantation), now a common practice in infertility treatment, requires lower temperatures. *See also* BLOOD TRANSFUSION; EGG; EMBRYO; IMPLANTATION; *and* IN VITRO FERTILIZATION.

Cryosurgery

Surgical technique using localized freezing, usually with liquid nitrogen, to remove or destroy diseased tissue.

Cryosurgery works by rapidly cooling body tissues to below-freezing temperatures, causing ice crystals to form, which disrupts cell structure and kills the cell. Cryosurgery is also used to withdraw tissue with a probe, as the low temperatures cause the tissue to stick to the probe.

Cryosurgery is primarily used in the removal of skin lesions and cancers, control of tumors in the reproductive and urinary systems, removal of cataracts, treatment of retinal detachments, elimination of hemorrhoids, and treatment of pancreatic and prostate cancer. Since it involves minimal scarring, cryosurgery is favored for surgery on the cervix, liver, and bowel; organs in which scarring can cause blockages.

Skin problems, external disfigurements such as birthmarks, and hemorrhoids are usually treated on an outpatient basis. A metal probe is cooled to the temperature of liquid nitrogen (about $-256°F$ or $-160°C$) and is used to freeze the affected area. The extreme cold paralyzes the nerves in the skin and is thus painless. After treatment, a blister develops and then heals after a few days. Scarring is minimal, though the skin may appear slightly paler than surrounding skin.

Treatment of an internal tumor with cryosurgery is major surgery, requiring general anesthetic. The tumor is destroyed by applying a metal probe cooled to the temperature of liquid nitrogen or by spraying the tumor with liquid nitrogen. *See also* CATARACT SURGERY *and* HEMORRHOIDS.

Cryptococcosis

A fungal infection usually acquired by breathing dust particles contaminated with bird feces.

Although cryptococcosis infects many people, symptoms will only appear in people who have compromised immune systems, such as those with AIDS, people with autoimmune diseases, people who are being treated with chemotherapy, or those who have had an organ transplant.

Symptoms. Symptoms of cryptococcosis include weight loss, night sweats, shortness of breath, a red rash on the face, and pain in the bones and joints. If the central nervous system is attacked, there may be blurred vision, dizziness, aphasia, or vomiting. Symptoms appear when the infection spreads from the lungs to other organs, such as the brain, the prostate, the liver, or the kidneys.

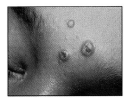

Cryptococcosis Lesion.
Cryptococcosis is a fungal infection that only produces symptoms in people with compromised immune systems. One of these symptoms may be a red rash on the face, as seen above.

Treatment. Cryptococcosis is treated with intravenous amphotericin B or fluconazole, which are antifungal medications. If the disease spreads to the brain, it may be fatal. *See also* AIDS; ANTIFUNGAL DRUGS; *and* IMMUNE SYSTEM.

Culture

The growth of bacteria, viruses, or tissue cells in a specialized medium.

Cells and organisms are generally cultured for identification and study. There are many types of cultures used for diagnostic purposes.

Perhaps the most familiar culture is for strep throat. Cells are scraped from the throat with a cotton swab, and the material is sent to a microbiology lab for culturing. Once the cells are cultured, the researcher will attempt to identify beta-streptococcus, the bacterium that causes strep throat.

Blood and other body fluids are also subject to culture. Urine cultures are used to identify bacteria associated with urinary tract infections.

Infectious diseases are often studied through blood culture. Bacteriological methods may then be used to identify these organisms. Once infectious microorganisms are identified, culturing may be applied to establish effective antibiotic treatment. Specific microorganisms are isolated in culture, and then their rate of growth following exposure to various antibiotics is studied.

PCR. Culturing takes from 2 to 15 days, though new techniques such as polymerase chain reaction (PCR) have reduced the time necessary for results and improved the identification of bacteria and viruses. Generally, PCR culture tests for bacteria take only 12 to 48 hours, whereas viral cultures may require up to 2 weeks. However, a new strategy, known as shell vial assay, may cut the time needed for a viral culture to a day. Tuberculosis is the most time-consuming culture to produce for diagnosis and analysis, requiring up to six weeks. *See also* STREP THROAT *and* TUBERCULOSIS.

Curettage

The removal of tissue with a curet, a sharp-edged, spoon-shaped surgical instrument.

In curettage, abnormal tissue or tissue for lab analysis is taken from the lining of a body cavity or from the skin. Curettage is often used to scrape tissue from the lining of the uterus as part of a dilatation and curettage (D & C) operation, to remove infected material from an abscess, and to remove small growths from the skin.

Dental curettage is used to clean the tooth root and the gums. When calculus forms beneath the gums, the gums become inflamed. Calculus and inflamed tissue can be cleaned and removed by scaling and curetting the teeth and gums. Dental curettage is part of the treatment for inflammation of the tissues that support the teeth, a condition also known as periodontitis. *See also* ABSCESS; D AND C; DILATATION; PERIODONTAL DISEASE; PERIODONTICS; PERIODONTITIS; *and* SKIN CANCER.

Curling's Ulcer

A type of ulcer that develops in people who have suffered extensive burns.

Stress ulcers form in the lining of the stomach or duodenum following severe physical or mental stress. Curling's ulcer is a specific type of stress ulcer that occurs in people who have suffered extensive skin burns. Multiple small ulcers develop 24 hours after the burns are sustained.

Symptoms. Initially, there may be mild discomfort in the upper abdomen. As the ulcers enlarge and begin to bleed, the stools may turn a tarry black. In severe cases, bleeding can be massive and cause blood pressure to drop precipitously. Diagnosis is performed through gastroscopy.

Treatment. Treatment for Curling's ulcers is the same as for other types of stress ulcer; once the condition that has caused the ulcers is treated, they begin to heal. *See also* BURNS; EMERGENCY FIRST STEPS; SHOCK; *and* STRESS ULCER.

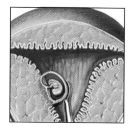

Curettage.
In curettage, a sharp, spoon-shaped surgical instrument called a curet is used to remove tissue from body cavities, including the uterus, as seen above.

Cushing's Syndrome

Disorder caused by overproduction of hydrocortisone by the adrenal glands.

Resources on Cushing's Syndrome

Greenspan, Francis S., et al., *Basic and Clinical Endocrinology* (2000); Krimsky, Sheldon, and Lynn Goldman, *Hormonal Chaos: The Scientific and Social Origins of the Environmental Endocrine Hypothesis* (1999); Shin, Linda M., et al., *Endocrine and Metabolic Disorders Sourcebook* (1998); Nat. Institute of Diabetes and Digestive and Kidney Diseases, Tel. (301) 496-3583, Online: www.niddk. nih.gov; Thyroid Foundation of America, Tel. (800) 832-8321, Online: www. tsh.org; www.nycornell .org/medicine/edm /index.html.

Hydrocortisone, a hormone secreted by the adrenal glands, controls the use and distribution of nutrients. Reduced production of hydrocortisone is called hypoadrenalism. Overproduction of the hormone is known as Cushing's syndrome.

CAUSES

Conditions that can lead to Cushing's syndrome include:

Pituitary Gland Disorders. The rate and amount of release of hydrocortisone are regulated by a hormone secreted by the pituitary gland, called ACTH. Therefore, diseases that attack the pituitary gland influence the production of hydrocortisone. Some tumors can cause the pituitary gland to overproduce ACTH, and hence cortisol by the adrenal gland.

Adrenal Gland Disorders. A benign or cancerous tumor can lead to overproduction of hydrocortisone.

Exogenous Cushing's Syndrome. The symptoms of Cushing's syndrome may be caused by overmedication with corticosteroids. These synthetic hormones are commonly prescribed to reduce inflammation caused by diseases such as rheumatoid arthritis and asthma, or injuries that need urgent treatment of inflammation.

Ectopic Cushing's Syndrome. Occasionally, tumors in parts of the body far from the pituitary gland secrete extra ACTH, resulting in excess hydrocortisone production by the adrenal glands. These tumors are most commonly lung cancers, although other types of cancer, such as tumors of the thyroid and pancreas, may be involved.

SYMPTOMS

Cushing's syndrome is usually characterized by moon face (puffiness and redness in the face), weight gain only in the abdomen, a hump of fat in the upper back, acne or stretch marks, bone weakening, depression, and susceptibility to infections.

DIAGNOSIS

Cushing's syndrome can be difficult to diagnose, as its symptoms may easily be confused with those of other diseases. Any of the above symptoms warrant investigation. Tests can measure the levels of ACTH and cortisol in the blood or urine, and computed tomography (CT) scans can be used to search the glands for tumors.

TREATMENT

Finding the cause of Cushing's syndrome will help physicians to determine the appropriate treatment. If the disorder is caused by overmedication with corticosteroids, then decreasing the drug will relieve the symptoms of Cushing's syndrome. If a tumor is the problem, early discovery and removal is generally successful. If an adrenal gland itself needs to be removed, then long-term cortisol replacement may be necessary until the other adrenal gland begins to function.

For background material on Cushing's syndrome, see ACTH *and* ENDOCRINOLOGY. *Related information can be found in* ADRENAL GLANDS; PANCREAS; PITUITARY GLAND; *and* THYROID GLAND. *See also* ATROPHY; HEADACHE; OBESITY; *and* WEIGHT GAIN *for more on possible symptoms of Cushing's syndrome.*

Cusp, Dental

A point on the grinding surface of a tooth.

Although the teeth are usually believed to be smooth, their chewing and cutting surfaces are actually rough. The chewing surface of the back teeth contains points and indentations; the points are known as dental cusps. Their irregular shape better equips teeth to do their job, including holding food and grinding it so that it can be swallowed.

When an artificial tooth (or crown) is being made for a patient, the dentist is careful to make irregular curves, indentations, and points that meld with the shape of the opposing tooth, so that the patient is easy able to chew food. *See also* DENTAL EXAMINATION *and* DIGESTIVE SYSTEM.

Cutdown

Surgical incision of the skin to expose a vein and permit the insertion of a catheter or needle for administration of medication, withdrawal of blood, or diagnostic or therapeutic catheterization.

A cutdown is usually performed when it is not feasible to insert a needle through unbroken skin into a vein. This may occur if veins cannot be clearly located through the skin or if they have become damaged as a result of repeated intravenous infusions. After the vein is exposed, a catheter is inserted and held in place with sutures. The preferred sites for a venous cutdown are at the wrist, elbow, and shoulder (the cephalic vein), and at the ankle (the saphenous vein). *See also* INTRAVENOUS INFUSION.

Cyanide

One of a group of lethal compounds that exist in liquid and solid form.

Cyanides are a group of highly toxic compounds used in chemical processes, such as the production of rubber or plastics, fumigation, and electroplating.

The ingestion or inhalation of large doses of cyanide or its compounds may result in convulsions, unconsciousness, and death within fifteen minutes. Smaller doses may cause weakness, dizziness and drowsiness, headache, rapid breathing and pulse, diarrhea, vomiting, headache, flushed skin, unconsciousness, and possibly death.

Immediate treatment for cyanide poisoning is essential to avoid serious complications. A patient who has inhaled cyanide will be given 100 percent oxygen to

ALERT
Deadly Seeds

Fruits such as apples, apricots, and pears contain natural cyanide compounds in their seeds; other plants contain cyanide compounds in bark, leaves, or roots. Small children may be poisoned by nibbling on deadly plant parts, and thus their eating habits should be monitored closely.

breathe. In the case of cyanide ingestion or inhalation, an antidote is available but is not always reliable. *See also* EMERGENCY HOSPITALIZATION *and* POISONING.

Cyanosis

Blue coloring of the skin caused by a lack of oxygen in the blood.

Oxygenated blood coming from the lungs is bright red, but as the oxygen is taken up by the tissues of the body, the hemoglobin turns dark red and appears blue through the skin. If the blood supplied by the heart to the arteries does not have a sufficient supply of oxygen, it will be dark red and unable to meet the needs of the body's tissue.

CAUSES
Cyanosis may be a relatively normal occurrence in certain situations, as is frequently seen in newborn infants who are just beginning to breathe. Cyanosis can be caused by asphyxiation, by certain chemical compounds, or by drugs that interfere with hemoglobin's ability to acquire oxygen. Carbon monoxide is such a compound; a person who inhales a sufficient quantity of carbon monoxide will have blue lips and fingernails. Cyanosis can also be a symptom of a number of severe heart and lung ailments that starve the blood of oxygen.

TREATMENT
Treatment for cyanosis depends on the underlying cause of the condition. Newborn infants who are cyanotic generally do not require treatment. Pure oxygen is usually administered to cyanotic patients, but it must be monitored carefully, since oxygen is an extremely reactive and flammable compound and has the potential to be dangerous for both the patient and his or her immediate environment.

Background information on cyanosis can be found in BREATHING DIFFICULTIES *and* RESPIRATORY SYSTEM. *For related material, see* ANOXIA; CHILDBIRTH, COMPLICATIONS; EMERGENCY FIRST STEPS; FIRST AID; HYPOXIA; *and* RESPIRATORY DISTRESS SYNDROME.

Cyclophosphamide

A drug often used in chemotherapy for several types of cancer.

Cyclophosphamide works by interfering with a cancer cell's ability to grow and reproduce. As an alkylating agent, it attaches to and modifies the DNA of tumors. Cyclophosphamide is used to treat many different types of cancer, including cancer of the ovaries, breast, blood, lymph system, eyes, bone marrow, and skin.

Cyclophosphamide's ability to suppress the immune system makes it useful in bone marrow and other types of organ transplantation to prevent rejection. Since cyclophosphamide suppresses the immune system, a person taking the drug will be more susceptible to infection. Common, less serious side effects of cyclophosphamide include sore throat, fever, hair loss, darkened skin, and nausea. More serious side effects include missed menstrual periods, painful urination, blood in the urine, dizziness, increased heart beat, and joint pain. *See also* CHEMOTHERAPY.

Cyst

A closed pocket of tissue, which can be filled with air, fluid, pus, or other material.

Cysts are closed pockets of tissue that can form inside any tissue in the body. Cysts within the lungs are ordinarily filled with air, while cysts involving the lymph system, skin, or kidneys are usually filled with fluid.

CAUSES

Parasites, such as trichinosis, dog tapeworm, and echinococcus, cause cysts to form within muscle, the liver, brain tissue, the lungs, and the eye. They may also develop as a result of developmental abnormalities. Cysts are also common on the skin, developing as a result of infection or clogging of sebaceous glands.

Sebaceous cysts are caused by the accumulation of oily material (sebum) and dead cells, resulting from clogged pores.

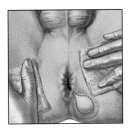

Anal Abscess.
An abscess is a cyst-like collection of pus resulting from an infection by bacteria. Abscesses may be painful and may have to be drained to relieve the pain. An anal abscess is pictured above.

They are common and benign, and most often occur on the back of the neck, the upper chest, the back, the vulva, or the labia. Cysts on or inside the vulva normally grow slowly and are small. Although cysts may swell, most are not painful.

TREATMENT

Cysts can be ignored unless they become infected. An infected cyst can form a painful abscess. If this occurs, antibiotics may be given, but usually surgical drainage of the abscess is necessary to relieve the pain. Cysts typically recur, unless the cyst lining is removed. There is no known prevention for cysts. *See also* TRICHINOSIS.

Cystectomy

The surgical removal of the bladder, usually as a treatment for cancer.

A cystectomy is sometimes performed as an alternative to radiation therapy, cobalt irradiation, and chemotherapy if bladder cancer is invasive. A radical cystectomy requires the additional removal of adjacent tissue. In men, the prostate is removed in addition to the bladder; in women, the uterus, ovaries, fallopian tubes, and part of the vaginal wall located adjacent to the bladder are removed.

After the bladder is removed, a portion of the small intestine is used to create an artificial bladder that empties through an opening (stoma) on the lower abdomen and collects in an external plastic bag. A ureter can also be implanted into the large intestine (in a ureterosigmoidostomy) and urine passed via the rectum.

Alternative methods, known as orthotopic neobladder and continent cutaneous diversion, are becoming increasingly common. An internal reservoir (neobladder) is constructed from the intestine and connected to the urethra or a continent abdominal stoma.

A radical cystectomy may cause impotence in males because of pelvic nerve damage; it causes infertility in women. *See also* BLADDER *and* INFERTILITY.

Cystic Fibrosis

An inherited condition characterized by the production of abnormal secretions from the glands.

Symptoms of cystic fibrosis can be present at birth (congenital), or they can develop at any time afterwards. In cystic fibrosis, certain glands produce abnormal secretions. Pancreatic and intestinal secretions tend to be solid and thick and may clog the pancreas completely. Glands in the respiratory system produce thick, dry mucus that clogs the lungs and creates a breeding ground for bacteria. Sweat and salivary glands produce fluids with a higher than normal salt content.

CAUSE

Cystic fibrosis is caused by a defective gene. It is an autosomal recessive condition; it requires the combination of faulty genes from both parents. If a person has one normal gene and one gene for cystic fibrosis, he or she will be a carrier and thus may pass the gene on to children. If both parents are carriers (one normal gene and one defective), each child has a 25 percent chance of having the disease. One in 2,500 Caucasians and 1 in 17,000 African Americans have cystic fibrosis; the disease is rare among Asians.

SYMPTOMS

Symptoms arise from complications related to thickened or otherwise abnormal secretions. One of the first signs of the disease may be meconium ileus, an intestinal blockage in newborns due to abnormally thick fecal matter (meconium). If it is left untreated, this condition can lead to a perforated or twisted intestine. Babies with meconium ileus almost always develop other symptoms of cystic fibrosis later on.

Another early symptom of cystic fibrosis is poor weight gain. This is due to insufficient pancreatic secretions, which contain enzymes for proper digestion and absorption of nutrients. The babies will have frequent, foul-smelling, and oily feces; they may also have protruding abdomens. De-

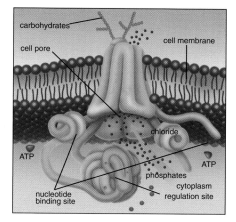

Cystic Fibrosis.
A normal cell, above, contains a substance called cystic fibrosis transmembrane conductance regulator (CFTR), which forms a choloride-permeable channel in the cell membrane. Chlorides cleave onto ATP and cross the membrane with ATP. In people with cystic fibrosis, a lack of CFTR confuses the regulatory mechanism of the cell, and thus the transferance of chloride never takes place.

spite a good appetite, these children will also exhibit signs of malnutrition and vitamin deficiency, rectal prolapse (in which the rectum protrudes through the anus), and anemia from lack of protein.

The lungs are normal at birth but breathing problems soon develop. Thick bronchial secretions begin blocking small airways in the lungs, reducing the lungs' ability to transfer oxygen to the blood.

Other early signs of cystic fibrosis are chronic respiratory tract infections accompanied by excessive coughing, gagging, and vomiting. Parents may also notice that the baby's skin tastes salty when kissed, as sweat secretions of people with cystic fibrosis have an unusually high salt content. Teenagers with cystic fibrosis experience slow growth and delayed puberty.

COMPLICATIONS

Complications of cystic fibrosis include collapsed lungs and heart failure. Recurrent infections such as bronchitis and pneumonia gradually destroy the lung tissue. Two to three percent of patients develop insulin-dependent diabetes owing to scarring of the pancreas. Blockage of bile ducts may lead to liver damage and cirrhosis.

Reproductive function is impaired as well, with 98 percent of adult male patients having low sperm counts or producing no sperm at all. Women exhibit decreased fertility and abnormally thick cervical secretions, and they have a higher likelihood of complications during pregnancy.

TREATMENT

Treatment is geared toward prevention of organ damage through a comprehensive program of physical and respiratory therapy. Children must have a diet that includes sufficient calories and protein for proper growth. All patients must ingest higher than normal amounts of fat, because it is not absorbed well, as well as additional vitamins. A patient with an affected pancreas must also take enzyme replacements throughout life.

Airway blockages and subsequent infection can be prevented or reduced with percussion therapy and assisted coughing. Any respiratory infection must be treated immediately to prevent damage. Surgery may be needed in more severe cases. Heart-lung transplants have proven effective when there is extensive damage.

PROGNOSIS

While cystic fibrosis cannot be cured, improving technology in treating the symptoms has led to an improved outlook for those born with the disease. The prognosis depends on the severity of the disease and the degree to which the lungs are affected and damaged. The outlook has been improving in recent years with the development of new treatments that postpone lung damage. Fully half of all people with the disease live past age 28. Long-term survival is better in males, as well as in those who do not experience problems related to the pancreas and whose initial symptoms do not involve the respiratory system.

> For background material on cystic fibrosis, see GENETIC DISORDERS. Further information can be found in GENE; GENETICS; INHERITANCE; MECONIUM; and RESPIRATORY TRACT INFECTION. See also GENETIC ENGINEERING for more on ongoing genetic research.

Resources on Cystic Fibrosis

Harris, Ann, and Maurice Super, *Cystic Fibrosis: The Facts* (1991); Moore, Keith L., *Before We Are Born: Essentials of Embryology and Birth Defects* (1998); Nussbaum, Robert L., et al., *Thompson & Thompson Genetics in Medicine* (2001); Cystic Fibrosis Foundation, Tel. (800) FIGHT-CF, Online: www.cff,org; Alliance of Genetic Support Groups, Tel. (800) 336-GENE, Online: www.medhelp.org/geneticalliance; Easter Seals, Tel. (800) 221-6827, Online: www.seals.org; www.ny-cornell.org/medicine/infectious/index.html.

Cystitis

Inflammation of the bladder resulting from an infection.

Cystitis is more common in women than men. At least one in every five women will experience cystitis at some time, most often from a bacterial infection. In sexually active women, the infectious agent is often *Escherichia coli (E. coli)*, which may be introduced during intercourse. An obstruction of the flow of urine due to a bladder stone or other cause also increases the risk of infection. In men, cystitis can result from obstruction owing to an enlarged prostate gland pressing on the urethra. In children, cystitis can result from a congenital malformation of the ureters, which carry urine from the kidney to the bladder.

SYMPTOMS

A major symptom of cystitis is an urgent need to urinate, with pain felt during and after urination. A patient may also experience fever, chills, and abdominal discomfort. Children with cystitis may only experience a slight fever and pain; a child who cries during urination should be examined by a physician for signs of infection or malformation.

DIAGNOSIS

Cystitis is diagnosed by microscopic examination of the urine to detect bacteria, blood, and pus. Tests can then be done to identify the infectious agent. If no bacteria are found, the cystitis may be caused by inflammation of the urethra or by trauma to the urethra.

TREATMENT

With proper treatment, cystitis is often resolved within days. One basic treatment is to increase the intake of water and other fluids such as cranberry juice, which makes the urine less friendly to bacteria. If bacteria are identified, antibiotics will be prescribed. In many cases, antibiotic therapy will be started before a specific infectious agent is identified. If cystitis recurs on a regular basis, a long-term course of low-dose antibiotics may be prescribed. In some cases, patients will be told to take an antibiotic before sexual intercourse. As a preventive measure, some patients may be told to avoid sexual intercourse until the infection has cleared to avoid exacerbating their condition.

For background information on cystoscopy, see BLADDER. *Related material can be found in* ANTIBIOTIC DRUGS *and* PROSTATE, ENLARGED.

Cystocele

Also known as dropped bladder or fallen bladder

A pushing through (herniation) of the bladder into the vagina.

Cystocele results in the bladder bulging into the front of the vagina. It is generally caused by the stretching and weakening of the pelvic muscles resulting from multiple instances of pregnancy, large babies, or long, difficult labors. Decreased estrogen levels after menopause can also cause cystocele. Women suffering from cystocele may experience uncontrollable release of urine (urinary incontinence) and may be more prone to urinary tract infections.

SYMPTOMS

Symptoms of cystocele include pressure or aching in the vagina, difficulty urinating, incontinence, and difficulty with penetration during intercourse. Weakened pelvic muscles can also cause the tube that carries urine from the bladder (the urethra) to bulge into the vagina, a condition known as urethrocele, which commonly occurs together with cystocele.

TREATMENT

Kegel exercises, in which a woman practices alternately contracting and relaxing the pelvic floor muscles, are recommended as treatment for cystocele. Cystocele can be corrected surgically if a woman is suffering from severe discomfort or incontinence. The recovery period varies. *See also* INCONTINENCE; MENOPAUSE; PREGNANCY; *and* URINARY TRACT INFECTION.

Cystometry

Also known as cystometrography

A test used to measure the function of muscles controlling the bladder.

Cystometry is used to diagnose bladder dysfunction by measuring the performance of bladder control muscles. This information is used to determine bladder capacity, its compliance (elasticity when full), and the efficiency of the voluntary and involuntary detrusor muscle.

Using a catheter, the extent to which the bladder empties is measured and a record of the bladder filling at various stages is made. Cystometry involves the introduction of saline solution into the bladder. The patient is asked to report any discomfort or unusual sensations. The saline is then drained and the process is repeated with saline or carbon dioxide, which may be introduced through a cystometer, a device that can measure pressure and volume within the bladder. The procedure should not be performed in patients with urinary tract infections. *See also* CATHETER; CARBON DIOXIDE; INCONTINENCE; URINARY SYSTEM; *and* URINARY TRACT INFECTION.

Cystoscopy

Also known as cystourethroscopy

Examination of the urethra and bladder by means of a fiberoptic endoscope for the purpose of diagnosing urinary tract diseases.

Cystoscopy employs a special type of endoscope known as a cystoscope or urethroscope. With it, a doctor can examine the urethra and bladder for indications of urinary tract disease. Fiberoptic light is used to guide the instrument through the urethra and into the bladder. The cystoscope also allows the doctor to perform biopsies or remove small stones by passing instruments through a specialized hollow channel in the cystoscope. Small areas of abnormal tissue lining the walls of the bladder may be burned away during the procedure. The urethra and bladder may also be visually examined or they may be photo-graphed

graphed through the cystoscope.

Cystoscopy, which allows for diagnosis of abnormalities such as tumors, inflammation, or prostatic enlargement, is sometimes supplemented with cultured urine analysis. The procedure is generally carried out under local anesthesia, although children may require general anesthesia. Diagnostic viewing alone should cause only mild discomfort. Some irritation may accompany biopsy because of blood in the urine following the procedure. *See also* PROSTATE, ENLARGED.

Cystostomy

The surgical creation of an opening (stoma) in the bladder, usually performed to siphon off urine when the introduction of a catheter into the bladder through the urethra is not possible.

Drainage of urine over the pubic area (suprapubic cystostomy) is an option after urethral trauma. A cystostomy is often the first stage of a two-stage prostate operation in which a rubber tube is placed into the bladder through an abdominal incision. A permanent suprapubic cystostomy can provide adequate drainage for a weak or spastic bladder; but this is undesirable as it predisposes patients to infection, formation of stones, and, more rarely, cancer. *See also* BLADDER TUMORS *and* INCONTINENCE.

Cytology

Field that investigates the formation, structure, and function of cells.

Cytology is concerned with how cells relate to disease and how they can be studied to diagnose abnormalities. Cytological specimens may be obtained from urine, cerebrospinal fluid, blood, sputum, irregular discharge, or other fluid, or they may be examined in the context of masses of cells making up tissues and organs. The pap smear is one example of a cytological specimen used for diagnostic purposes.

The purpose of clinical cytology is to detect and identify abnormal cells, particularly those that are cancerous, as well as viral, fungal, and other types of infection. Cytological studies may identify, through varying techniques, irregularities in cell size, shape, number, and type; the malfunction of component parts (organelles) of the cell; genetic irregularities; malignancy; and infection. *See also* CANCER.

Cytomegalovirus

Also known as CMV

A type of herpes virus that usually remains dormant and causes no symptoms in healthy people.

Cytomegalovirus (CMV) is a common virus of the herpes family. It is especially prevalent among individuals living in the developing world, and among people infected with HIV. CMV is transmitted by bodily fluid (especially blood), but a sufficiently strong immune system limits the activity of the virus.

Symptoms. When an impaired immune system allows CMV to become active, the virus first attacks the eyes. Visual problems like blind spots, distorted vision, and noticeable blurring are symptoms that signal the onset of CMV. Retinitis follows, and other organs of the body are later attacked.

Diagnosis. The physician will diagnose the disease after seeing yellow-white lesions in the retina, a sign characteristic of CMV.

Treatment. A number of new antiviral drugs to treat CMV have been approved by the Food and Drug Administration (FDA). They can be taken orally, injected into the eye, or implanted. Side effects, however, can be serious and include seizures and damage to the bone marrow or kidneys. If possible, bolstering the immune system may be a better approach, since the immune system can control the disease.

Prognosis. Prognosis for healthy people with CMV is excellent, as these people do not exhibit symptoms. Prognosis for individuals with depressed immune systems depends on when the CMV infection was discovered. If CMV is caught early, it can be treated with antiviral drugs. If it is caught only after the virus has damaged body tissues, it may be too late for treatment. *See also* AIDS *and* AUTOIMMUNE DISORDERS.

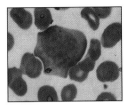

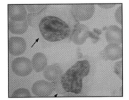

Cytomegalovirus. Downy cells are white blood cells infected by cytomegalovirus. Downy cells are characterized as type I, II, or III. Above, a type III Downy cell. Below, a type I Downy cell.

Resources on Cytomegalovirus (CMV)
Fettner, Ann Guidici, *The Science of Viruses* (1990); Fields, Bernard, et al., *Fields'Virology* (1996); Radetsky, Peter, *The Invisible Invaders* (1991); Centers for Disease Contol and Prevention, Tel. (800) 311-3435, Online: www. cdc.gov; Infectious Disease Society of America, Tel. (703) 299-0200, Online: www.idsociety.org; National Institute of Allergy and Infectious Disease, Tel. (301) 496-5717, Online: www.niaid.nih.org; Office of Rare Diseases, Tel. (301) 402-4336, Online: rarediseases.info. nih.gov/org; www.nycornell.org/medicine/infectious/index.html.

Dacryocystitis

Also called tear sac infection

An inflammation of the tear sac that occurs when the nasolacrimal duct is obstructed.

The nasolacrimal duct runs between the nose and the tear sac. When it is obstructed, it may result in an infection that is called dacryocystitis.

Dacryocystitis is marked by the discharge of mucus or pus from the eyelid whenever light pressure is applied. It may also cause redness, some pain, and swelling on the inside corner of the infected eye.

Dacryocystitis will regularly cause tearing to occur. In more serious cases there may be an abscess in the tear sac, where tears are stored before exiting the body when the eyes water or when an individual is crying. *See also* ABSCESS.

Causes. Dacryocystitis can be caused by an infection, nasal polyps, or trauma. Dacryocystitis often appears after serious facial traumas, particularly those involving the nose; this may explain the increased incidence in children.

Treatment. A warm compress applied to the affected region of the face may help treat some of the pain and redness. A health care professional should be consulted as soon as possible in order to ensure that the infection is not serious.

Antibiotics may be prescribed to combat any infection related to the dacryocystitis. Although medication completely heals dacryocystitis most of the time, in the most severe cases surgery may be necessary. *See also* ANTIBIOTIC DRUGS; EYES; INFECTION; SINUS; SURGERY; *and* TRAUMA.

D and C

Generally written as D&C

Procedure for expanding the cervical canal of the uterus, allowing the surface lining of the uterine wall to be scraped.

Dilation and curettage (D&C) is a procedure in which tissue is scraped from the lining of the uterine wall. A gynecological surgeon will dilate the cervix with metal rods and insert a spoon-shaped curette into the uterine lining. The surgeon can obtain a sample of the uterine lining with the curette for diagnostic purposes (endometrial biopsy) or to clear the lining of any excess tissue. *See also* BIOPSY.

Procedure. The first phase of a D&C involves relaxing and enlarging (dilating) the cervical opening to allow the passage of tools into the uterine canal. Often the procedure is carried out in a doctor's office under local anesthesia. Mild discomfort may accompany the widening of the cervix. Should greater dilation be required for an adequate endometrial biopsy, the procedure will be performed under general anesthesia in a hospital setting.

Endometrial biopsy is often performed when a condition known as endometrial hyperplasia is suspected. This disorder involves a thickening of the uterine lining, which may cause midcycle bleeding or excessive menstrual flow. The condition often affects women in their teens and those approaching menopause. D&C is especially important in older women as a means of determining whether or not the condition is benign. The D&C technique may also be applied in cases of incomplete miscarriage or as part of an early elective abortion. *See also* ABORTION; GYNECOLOGY; *and* UTERUS.

Danazol

A synthetic male hormone (androgen) used to treat endometriosis.

Endometriosis is a condition in which the uterine tissue grows outside of the uterus. Danazol, a male hormone, alleviates the symptoms of endometriosis by inhibiting menstruation. It is also used to relieve the pain of fibrocystic disease, in which lumps form in the breast. Like all steroids, danazol has a number of side effects that need to be monitored carefully, including: unnatural hair growth in women; nosebleeds; dizziness; reddened skin tones; muscle cramps; headache; weight gain; acne; lowered voice; mood swings; carpal tunnel syn-

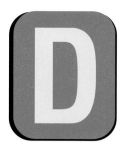

drome; and vaginal itching or dryness. *See also* ENDOMETRIOSIS; FIBROCYSTIC DISEASE; MENSTRUATION; STEROID DRUGS; UTERUS; VAGINA; *and* VAGINAL ITCHING.

Dandruff

Also known as seborrheic dermatitis and cradle cap

A skin condition, generally of the scalp, characterized by dry or greasy white scales, with or without reddening of the skin.

Besides the scalp (the primary site), dandruff can also affect the face, the nose, the eyebrows, behind the ears, and the skin that covers the body's trunk.

Symptoms. Skin lesions, flaky white or, less often, yellow skin, patches of dry skin on the nose or forehead, and mild redness, which may or may not itch, are typical symptoms of this condition.

Treatment. Controlling risk factors and practicing good skin care may reduce the severity of dandruff, although the tendency to develop the condition is inherited. Dandruff shampoos, which contain salicylic acid, coal tar, zinc, or selenium, may reduce flaking and dryness of the scalp.

Prescription shampoos that contain selenium, ketaconazole, or corticosteroids are used in severe cases. However, the condition has a tendency to recur.

Risk Factors. Fatigue, stress, weather extremes, oily skin, and improper hygiene may increase the risk of the development of dandruff. There are also certain conditions, such as AIDS and Parkinson's disease, that are associated with an increased incidence of dandruff. *See also* AIDS; CHAPPED SKIN; CRADLE CAP; DERMATOLOGY; DRY SKIN; *and* PARKINSON'S DISEASE.

Deafness

A complete or partial inability to hear.

Impaired hearing is the single most common physical disability in the United States. It can vary in severity, cause and prognosis and can be the result of disease, injury, or old age.

TYPES

Deafness can be classified as either conductive, sensorineural, or a combination.

Conductive hearing loss refers to a mechanical problem that blocks the transmission of sound through the outer or middle-ear. It is frequently a result of damage to the eardrum or the middle-ear bones. In a healthy ear, sound enters the outer ear and passes down the ear canal to the eardrum (tympanum). The sound causes the eardrum to vibrate, activating the middle-ear bones, which then carry the vibrations to the inner ear.

Conductive hearing loss has a number of possible causes. Earwax blocking the outer ear canal is the most common cause in adults, while middle-ear infection (otitis media) is the most common cause in children. The eardrum may become perforated due to middle-ear infection or ear surgery, or the eardrum or middle-ear may be damaged by abrupt pressure changes (barotrauma).

Sensorineural Hearing Loss. This is the result of damage to the inner ear, auditory nerve, or nerve pathways. Vibrations reach the inner ear but are not transmitted to the brain. Common causes include:

- genetics;
- injury to developing fetus because of exposure to German measles (rubella);
- repeated exposure to loud noise; and
- fluid in the labyrinth of the inner ear.

The quality of an individual's hearing also gradually declines with age. One-third of people over 65 experience some form of hearing impairment.

SYMPTOMS

A child who is born deaf will not react to startling sounds or to his or her parents' voices. As the child approaches one year of age, he or she will not babble or mimic other people's voices. In general, a child's failure to meet any of the developmental milestones in relation to sound or developing speech is cause for a hearing test.

In adults, hearing loss may be gradual and difficult to notice. Generally, hearing high-frequency noises is first to be impaired, and the hearing loss progresses until it is difficult to understand normal conversation. Sounds are not only softer but also become indistinct. Consonants, such as "f," "s," and "z," may sound alike or may be inaudible. If hearing loss is in one ear only, it may not become apparent until a person uses a telephone with the impaired ear.

DIAGNOSIS

Several hearing tests are used to determine the type and severity of hearing loss. A person's responses to different sounds in each ear, both heard through the ear and transmitted through the bone at the back of the ear, can help a physician determine whether the middle- or inner-ear is impaired and what the underlying causes are.

TREATMENT

Proper diagnosis is crucial for the treatment of hearing loss. A simple accumulation of fluid or wax can be drained or removed, and hearing will be restored. Children who have continuous otitis media causing hearing loss can be treated with antibiotics and, if necessary, surgery can drain accumulated fluid (myringotomy). A perforated eardrum that fails to heal naturally can be surgically rebuilt (typanoplasty).

In cases in which there is no cure for deafness, a hearing aid is recommended. Basically, hearing aids consist of a microphone, an amplifier that makes sounds louder and clearer, and a speaker. Different hearing aids meet different individuals' needs; there are many types that vary in clarity, ease of adjustment, and visibility. Presently, hearing aids have been developed that are controlled by computer to adjust for different environment, such as a crowded restaurants or a quiet room. Those with hearing impairments can also purchase amplifiers that attach to telephones and doorbells.

Cochlear Implant. If a hearing aid is not effective, a cochlear implant may be surgically embedded in the ear. The implant consists of internal and external coils, electrodes, a speech processor and a micro-

phone. The microphone accumulates sound waves that the processor then transforms into electrical impulses. These impulses are transmitted from the external coil through the skin to the internal coil and then to the electrodes, which activate the auditory nerve. Since it is a surgical procedure, the cochlear implant is used as a last resort; the person must work with a speech therapist to learn how to interpret the sounds produced by the implant. *See also* ACOUSTIC NERVE; COCHLEAR IMPLANT; EAR; EAR, DISORDERS OF THE; *and* TINNITIS.

Death

The cessation of life.

The certification of death is usually issued with the cessation of either heart or lung function. In the 1970's legislation was passed in many states that allowed for the pronouncement of brain death, which is the cessation of the brain's vital activities, to be considered another criteria for death. Thus, when any one of these three organs irreversibly ceases to function, a person may be considered legally dead.

Diagnosis of Death. The specific criteria for making such a determination, in the absence of a breathing machine, include: the absence of spontaneous breathing; a lack of a heartbeat; and dilated pupils that do not respond to light.

The pronouncement of brain death is made when it can be ascertained that the brain is irreversibly damaged or when the person remains in a comatose state for a prolonged duration of time, and there appears an absence of "brain stem function" indicated by the pupils' lack of response to light or pain or the eyes' failure to blink. An electroencephalogram may confirm a absence of electrical activity in the brain.

Sudden Death. Sudden death may occur under certain circumstances to both infants and adults. Sudden infant death syndrome (SIDS), or crib death, can occur unexpectedly to infants in their first year. There are still no known causes for this occurrence, only conjecture. Among adults,

Resources on Deafness

Davis, Hallowell, and S.R. Silverman, *Hearing and Deafness* (19078); Jerger, James, *Hearing Disorders in Adults* (1984); Pender, Daniel J., *Practical Otology* (1992); Stevens, S., and H. Davis, *Hearing: Its Psychology and Physiology* (1983); Strong, W.J., *Music, Speech, Audio* (1992); National Association of the Deaf, Tel. (301) 587-1788 (voice), -1789 (TTY), Online: www.nad.org; American Academy of Neurology, Tel. (651) 695-1940, Online: www.aan.com; American Board of Neurological Surgery, Tel. (713) 790-6015, Online: www.abns. org; www.med.cornell.edu/neuro/.

unexpected death may result from fatal injury, a heart attack, or brain hemorrhaging. A medical examiner will decide if an autopsy is required.

Preparation for Death. While statistics have shown that most Americans will live into their seventies and eighties, anticipating death evokes a great deal of uncertainty and fear. Caring for someone who is dying can take a heavy emotional toll on the caregiver and can raise a number of questions for all of those involved. While medical professionals may offer some assistance in responding to these concerns, every person ultimately confronts impending death in different and intensely personal ways. For some, the period im- mediately preceding death may offer a unique opportunity to comfort the dying, relieve their pain, and to gain a sense of closure.

After Death. Grief is an important part of processing and dealing with death. Most people experience different stages of grief. Initially there may be shock, denial, or disbelief. Some may immerse themselves in the affairs surrounding the death (the funeral or memorial service), while others may withdraw entirely. Guilt and anger are common reactions following the death of a loved one. In many instances, the bereaved experience physical symptoms such as irregular sleeping and eating habits; a weakened immune system; and an overly sensitive digestive system.

In such cases, a regular daily routine is advisable. For some, therapy is an effective means of coping with extreme feelings of grief and despair. Eventually, it is important that the grieving person find the strength to resume activities of personal meaning and purpose. For many, interaction with friends and family is a vital part of the recovery process.

For an in depth discussion of Death see BRAIN DEATH; SUDDEN DEATH; *and* SUDDEN INFANT DEATH SYNDROME. *Regarding the emotional and psychological effects of Death see* ANXIETY; ANXIETY DISORDERS; BEREAVEMENT; *and* DEPRESSION. *See also* HOSPICE CARE.

Debridement

Surgical removal of dead, damaged, or infected tissue, or foreign material from a wound or a burn.

Debridement exposes healthy tissue and promotes healing of damaged skin, muscle, bone, and other tissue. It may be performed on bedridden patients who have developed ulcers, or used in the treatment of tetanus, especially in deep-puncture wounds. *See also* TETANUS.

Debridement is also used to treat diabetic foot ulcers, and on victims of snakebites to remove blisters or pustules, bloody vesicles, or dead tissue. *See* SNAKEBITES.

A scalpel and tweezers are the traditional tools. Lasers and a new fluid-jet removal system are now used in treating burn and accident victims. *See also* LASER TREATMENT; MUSCLE; SKIN; *and* ULCER.

Decalcification, Dental

A deficiency or an erosion of calcium in the enamel of one or several teeth.

When calcium erodes in the enamel of teeth, they grow weak. This is usually a result of poor dental hygiene and will lead to cavities and tooth deformities, as well as other infections throughout the body. Dental decalcification is also found in individuals with eating disorders as a result of severe and repeated vomiting. The only treatment for dental decalcification is proper preventative hygienic habits. *See also* EATING DISORDERS *and* TOOTH CARE.

The Hospice Program

For people expected to die within six months, hospice programs offer a team of professionals, including doctors, nurses, physical therapists, and dietitians, to assist families through a loved one's final months, either at home or in nursing facilities.

Your doctor or hospital will be able to recommend a hospice chapter in your area; there is also a national referral service:

The National Hospice and Palliative Care Organization
1700 Diagonal Road, Ste. 300
Alexandria, VA 22314
703-243-5900 or www.NHPCO.org

Decerebrate

Lacking a functioning cerebrum.

A person becomes decerebrate if the brain stem is severed, cutting off the cerebrum from the spinal cord. Characteristics of a decerebrate condition, known as decerebrate posture, include rigidity in the arms, legs, and back, with the limbs rotated inward. A person exhibiting decerebrate posture must be immediately hospitalized to stabilize the condition and assess and treat the underlying cause.

Decerebrate posture, which may be accompanied by reduced consciousness and may occur on one or both sides of the body can indicate an injury of the central nervous system. This may be caused by a stroke, hemorrhage, brain tumor, or encephalopathy. *See also* BRAIN; BRAIN HEMORRHAGE; BRAIN STEM; BRAIN TUMOR, ENCEPHALOPATHY; HEAD INJURY; *and* STROKE.

Decompression Sickness

Also known as the bends

Physical problems caused by an overly rapid ascent from deep under water.

When decompression sickness was an occupational disease of workers in high-pressure conditions, such as underwater construction and marine bioengineering, it was called caisson disease. Now it is largely a hazard for scuba divers.

In high-pressure environments, such as deep water, gases build up in the tissues of the body. If pressure drops suddenly when a diver rises to the surface too quickly, those gases will expand and form bubbles that block blood vessels.

Symptoms can occur within 24 hours after the event. They include severe pains of the larger joints, itching, chest tightening, and mottling of the skin. Decompression sickness can cause neurological problems such as visual disturbances or difficulty with balance. If the blood vessels blocked by the bubbles are in the heart or lungs, the condition can be fatal.

Decompression sickness is treated by putting the person in a decompression chamber, where high pressure dissolves the bubbles; the pressure is then reduced gradually so that excess gas can be breathed out. A carefully timed, slow ascent from a deep dive is necessary to prevent decompression sickness. *See also* BAROTRAUMA.

Decompression, Spinal Canal or Cord

Also known as decompression laminectomy

A surgical procedure used to decompress the spine after severe trauma.

In many cases of spinal injury, the spinal cord is compressed rather than cut, which may be remedied by decompressing the spinal canal. Spinal canal decompression is often performed in conjunction with spinal stabilization or fusion. This surgery is fairly new and is still quite controversial; presently there are no guidelines for when neurosurgeons should perform this procedure. *See also* SPINAL INJURY *and* SPINE.

Decongestant Drugs

Drugs used to alleviate nasal congestion.

Decongestant drugs help nasal passages to drain when fluids accumulate. Conditions that may call for the use of decongestants include upper respiratory tract infections such as colds, inflammation of the tonsils (tonsillitis), and croup (inflammation and narrowing of the air passages). Decongestants are usually available in tablet form or as nose drops. Some common decongestants are ephedrine, oxymetazoline, phenylephrine, pseudoephedrine and xylometazoline. *See also* INFECTION.

Decongestants act on the blood vessels in the membrane of the nose. When an infection or irritation is present, blood vessels enlarge and more fluid passes into the membranes, which become swollen, generating more mucous. The swelling prevents drainage of fluids, which creates the feeling of a stuffy nose. *See* ANTIVIRAL DRUGS.

Decongestants work by helping the blood vessels in the area constrict; this reduces the swelling and fluid production, and allows fluids to pass through.

Risk Factors. Decongestant tablets are not recommended for those with heart conditions, as they may increase heart rate, resulting in tremors and palpitations. Nose drops do not have this effect, but if taken for too long, the system may become dependent on them and a worse form of the congestion may occur. *See also* CONGESTION, NASAL; OTIS MEDIA; RESPIRATORY TRACT INFECTION; *and* SINUSITIS.

Defibrillation

The technique of giving the heart a brief electric shock to terminate a rapid, irregular and ineffective heartbeat and restore normal heart rhythm.

In an emergency situation where an abnormal heartbeat such as ventricular fibrillation or ventricular tachycardia is life-threatening, paddles are placed over the heart and a shock is given to restore normal electrical activity.

Experience Not Mandatory

Automatic defibrillators are available in many public places, such as airports and stadiums, so that persons with even minimal training can use them in the short period, only a few minutes long, when restarting the heart can save a life. Defibrillation using advanced devices does not require extensive training.

Defibrillation is also used routinely to restart the heart after open-heart surgery. Defibrillators are standard equipment in ambulances and are carried by emergency medical teams. Persons with conditions that place them at high risk of life-threatening arrhythmias now often have implanted defibrillators that are programmed to detect an arrhythmia and administer a shock automatically.

For anatomical information related to Defibrillation see HEART; HEART VALVE; ECTOPIC HEART BEAT; *and* FETAL HEART MONITORING. *Disorders related to Defibrillation are related in* HEART ATTACK; *and* CONGESTIVE HEART FAILURE.

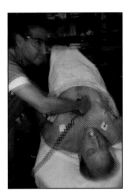

Defibrillation. Above, a physician is using a defibrillator to restart a man's heart. All physicians and emergency medical technicians, as well as others, are trained in defibrillator use. Early defibrillation is essential to effective emergency heart treatment.

Defoliant Poisoning

Poisoning from a substance intended for killing plants.

A defoliant is a substance used to kill or accelerate the drying of plant tissues, usually causing the leaves or flowers to fall off. Usually sprayed or dusted onto crops, defoliant insecticides can be hazardous to human health. During the Vietnam War, a controversy arose after the United States sprayed the defoliant Agent Orange on the jungle growth in Vietnam. Agent Orange is an herbicide containing trace amounts of the toxic contaminant dioxin. Victims of Agent Orange poisoning have reported symptoms that include cancer, adult-onset diabetes, birth defects, cardiovascular disease, and many others. *See also* AGENT ORANGE; PLANTS, POISONOUS; *and* POISON.

Deformity

An abnormality involving an organ or limb.

When a deformity occurs, it is usually present at birth or develops shortly afterwards. Deformities may be caused by either genetic or environmental factors. The most commonly affected systems are the cardiovascular, skeletal, gastrointestinal, urogenital, and central nervous system. Depending on the type and location, the severity ranges from relatively minor to quite serious. Severe deformities may result in a baby being stillborn or dying within a few days of birth. Many less serious conditions can be corrected surgically. *See also* BIRTH; BIRTH DEFECTS; *and* ENVIRONMENTAL MEDICINE.

Degeneration

A progressive deterioration of the organs and tissues of the body.

As the body ages, certain physical and chemical changes occur in the tissues that slow the process of regeneration. In conjunction with this, many organs begin to work less efficiently. The reduction of elasticity causes the skin to appear thinner, more wrinkled, and drier. Typically, bones become less dense and are consequently more fragile, as is the connective tissue, like the ligaments. While degeneration is a natural part of the process of aging, certain degenerative disorders may result from other causes such as injury, reduced blood supply, poisoning, or vitamin deficiencies. *See also* AGING; DEATH; DEGENERATIVE DISORDERS; GERONTOLOGY; *and* SKIN.

Degenerative Disorders

A number of diseases associated with the progressive deterioration of the body's organs and tissues.

"Degenerative disorders" is an umbrella term to describe conditions in which degenerative changes appear prematurely. The term does not include diseases that cause degeneration as the result of infection, inflammation or physical damage.

Degenerative diseases are diagnosed through microscopic examination of the organ or tissue. Such an examination would reveal scar tissue where there should otherwise be normal regenerative replacements. Degenerative disorders can affect the nervous system, eyes, joints, arteries, and muscles.

Alzheimer's disease is the most common degenerative disorder of the nervous system. Persons suffering from Alzheimer's are afflicted with early dementia. Huntington's chorea and Parkinson's disease are also examples of degenerative disorders that result in abnormalities of movement and functioning. Recent research also traced the onset of Parkinson's disease to certain poisons such as MPTP, commonly found in some designer drugs.

Other degenerative disorders affecting the eyes, joints, muscles, and arteries include: early blindness (Leber's optic atrophy); retinal degeneration (retinal pigmentosa); degenerative joint disease (osteoarthritis); the form of arteriosclerosis known as Monckeberg's sclerosis; and various forms of muscular dystrophies that cause severe muscular weakness.

Related Degenerative Disorders are discussed in ALZHEIMER'S DISEASE; ARTERIOSCLEROSIS; HUNTINGTON'S CHOREA; MUSCULAR DYSTROPHY; OSTEOARTHRITIS; PARKINSON'S DISEASE; *and* RETINITIS PIGMENTOSA. *Also see* AGING; ELDERLY, CARE OF THE; *and* GERONTOLOGY.

Dehiscence

The splitting open of an unhealed wound along natural or surgical suture lines.

Risk factors for dehiscence include diseases that impair the body's ability to heal itself, such as diabetes, malnutrition or a depressed immune system; advanced age; excessive movement or trauma to the partially healed wound, as may occur with excessive coughing, seizures, or too much activity occurring too soon; abdominal distention and accumulation of fluid; infection of the wound; extensive trauma; and any other factors that hamper the healing process of the wound or expose it to undue stress. *See also* DIABETES; SURGERY; *and* TRAUMA.

Dehydration

A loss of water through vomiting, diarrhea, inadequate fluid intake or perspiration.

If not restored by fluid intake, dehydration can have many serious consequences, including low blood pressure, loss of consciousness, heart failure, and, in the most extreme cases, even death. Water enters the body through the ingestion of food and liquids. Water leaves the body in the form of urine, perspiration, vomiting, in the stool, and as air that is exhaled. Most of the water retained in the body is in the cells themselves or in the spaces surrounding the cells. *See also* DEHYDRATION IN INFANTS.

Only about eight pounds, or four to five quarts, of water is needed in the bloodstream, so there is always a large reserve available in the rest of the body when the water in the blood is depleted. The water in the bloodstream acts as the vehicle for the various types of blood cells, and it also carries dissolved mineral salts necessary for bodily functions.

The percentages of sodium and potassium in the bloodstream are carefully monitored by the body. If the percentage rises, the body attempts to reduce loss of water through the kidneys. Thirst increases causing greater water intake and retention. When the body's sodium percentage lowers, the body excretes more water through the kidneys. This mechanism is controlled in part by the pituitary gland in the lower part of the brain, which senses the need to retain water and secretes an antidiuretic hormone. *See also* HORMONES.

When this hormone is present in the bloodstream, the kidneys drain less water from the blood, and other cells of the body give up their retained water. When blood volume and pressure is at healthy levels, the pituitary gland ceases to release the antidiuretic hormone, and the kidneys resume their normal draining function.

Over 60 and Under 6

Dehydration is particularly dangerous to small children and the elderly. Over two million infants die of dehydration every year often because of diarrhea.

An elderly person does not respond as quickly to the signals of low water content and may be slow to replenish the depleted water supply. In addition, older people have underlying conditions that predispose them to dehydration. They are more likely to suffer from diarrhea due to diseases that are more common among the elderly (such as diabetes) and from medications, including some antibiotics. The elderly are also at risk of kidney failure caused by the reduced blood flow to the kidneys when dehydrated.

CAUSES

Dehydration occurs when there is an imbalance between intake and outflow of bodily fluids—when the body loses more water than it takes in. This can happen during strenuous exercise with heavy perspiration or when the person is in hot dry environments. Fluid loss can be the result of diarrhea and vomiting. Sometimes inadequate ingestion of water or foods with high water content is caused by simple forgetfulness, particularly among the elderly, whose thirst and hunger signaling mechanisms may be impaired. Dehydration is also a consequence of many diseases, such as diabetes or viral infections like *Escherichia coli*. In the case of children too young to feed themselves, dehydration may be caused by parental neglect.

SYMPTOMS

In the early stages, a person with dehydration becomes very thirsty. An infant may cry without tears. Symptoms include dry mouth and nasal passages; an individual may have a flushed face; dry, warm skin; feel dizzy and weak; experience cramped limbs; he or she will become confused and have headaches of varying degrees of intensity; and urinary output may decrease. Severe dehydration can produce low blood pressure leading to a loss of consciousness; this is a medical emergency.

TREATMENT

Mild dehydration is easily treated by drinking water. There are a number of commercial drinks specially fortified with potassium and sodium that can be used to treat dehydration. Before, during, and after strenuous exercise, a person should drink plenty of fluids and increase salt intake somewhat. People with heart or kidney problems should be especially careful and consult a physician before starting heavy exercise; they should also be extremely cautious in utilizing any supplemental salt or potassium preparations.

In emergencies involving excessive blood loss, severe dehydration or the onset of shock, medical personnel will rapidly apply intravenous solutions of salt water.

If the kidneys excrete too much water (leading to dehydration), a doctor may perscribe medication. If the dehydration is caused by diarrhea, the cause of diarrhea must be addressed by whatever means necessary, or else the rehydration process will be thoroughly ineffective.

Further discussion of Dehydration can be found in ANTIDIARRHEAL DRUGS; SALT; *and* WATER. *Disorders related to Dehydration can be found in* DIARRHEA; KIDNEY FAILURE; SHOCK; *and* VOMITING. *See also* KIDNEY; POTASSIUM; SODIUM; TISSUE FLUID; *and* URINARY SYSTEM.

Dehydration in Infants

Water and salt (electrolytes) loss as it pertains to infants.

Dehydration in infants is most often caused by vomiting, diarrhea, or inadequate fluid intake. Gastroenteritis, an infection of the digestive tract, often causes the condition. Diarrhea is most often caused by viral or bacterial gastroenteritis.

Other possible causes of acute diarrhea include: contaminated foods; consuming poisons, such as iron, arsenic, or pesticides; ingestion of too many laxatives; food intolerance; emotional stress; and constipation with fecal soiling. Diarrhea can also be caused by a reaction to antibiotics, acquired sugar intolerance, Hirschsprung's disease (a condition in which the large intestine is obstructed due to inadequate muscular motion), milk protein allergy, upper respiratory infection, and urinary tract infection.

SYMPTOMS

In addition to diarrhea, fever, abdominal pain, and upper respiratory infection may be present when an infant is dehydrated. There is also the possibility of parasitic infection. Vomiting, which will often cause dehydration in an infant, is usually due to upper respiratory infection, flu-like infection, or gastroenteritis.

Infants who are five percent dehydrated will probably show signs of a poor appetite, fever, dry mucous membranes, concentrated urine output (that is, very dark urination), dry and sunken eyes, drowsiness, and a slightly increased heart rate.

Rotavirus and Diarrhea

Rotavirus, which kills about 600,000 children a year worldwide, causes an acute form of diarrhea that leads to life-threatening dehydration. But, in the past, how the disease worked was a mystery. It now appears that the rotavirus attacks nerves in the wall of the gut, stimulating the secretion of water and salt. This discovery has led to new treatments for viral gastroenteritis in children.

An infant or child who is 10 percent dehydrated will usually have a depressed fontanel, or soft spot, as well as the symptoms listed above.

The most severely dehydrated infants—those who are more than 15 percent dehydrated—experience decreased blood pressure or shock.

ALERT
When to Call a Doctor

Infants and children dehydrate more rapidly than adults. Parents need to know the warning signs of dehydration and be aware of certain other factors and situations that may exacerbate or increase a child's susceptibility to dehydration. A child's chronic medical condition, especially if he or she is less than two months old, may contribute to a dehydration. Parents should call a doctor if they observe any of these conditions:

- the soft top of the infant's head has shrunken;
- the infant has gone 8 to 12 hours without wetting a diaper;
- bloody, particularly pungent, or increased frequency or amount of bowel movements;
- crying brings no tears;
- a weak, raspy cry or decreased activity;
- mouth, eyes, or skin are dry;
- the child shows signs of malnutrition; or
- frequent vomiting.

TREATMENT AND PREVENTION

The best way to prevent dehydration in an infant is to maintain sufficient electrolyte balance and to replace fluids lost through diarrhea or vomiting. Since dehydration can be serious in an infant, it is important for a doctor to examine a sick child and evaluate severity on a case-by-case basis.

Treatment regularly includes intravenous fluids and electrolytes. For treatment of slight dehydration, a nonprescription drink, such as Pedialyte, may be used to balance the infant's electrolytes, unless the child's pediatrician recommends otherwise.

For more information about Dehydration in Infants see CRYING IN INFANTS; FEEDING, INFANT; SALT; *and* WATER. *In depth discussions of related diseases and disorders can be found in* DIARRHEA; *and* HIRSCHSPRUNG'S DISEASE.

Delirium

Acute and sudden onset of abnormal mental symptoms resulting from physical illness.

Delirium is characterized by extreme confusion, often accompanied by agitation. The individual often appears disoriented, frightened, and confused. Symptoms may also include disorganized speech, screaming, threatening, visual and auditory hallucinations, and mood swings. The person's mood, memory, and awareness fluctuate significantly, so he or she may be calm and lucid at times and extremely agitated and incoherent at others. Delirium usually disappears as abruptly as it arrives, often after a few days. It may, however, be an early sign of chronic dementia and it may even be life-threatening. *See also* CONFUSION.

There are many physical causes for delirium, including brain injury or disease, metabolic disorders, low blood sugar, vitamin deficiency, infection, and anesthesia. Diagnosis is urgent so that the underlying illness may be treated. *See also* DEMENTIA.

Delivery

The last stage of pregnancy, when the baby leaves the uterus.

Delivery refers to the actual birth of a baby—the moment it leaves its mother's uterus. The mother will feel a strong urge to push when the uterus contracts; this will help the baby along.

Pushing is hard work for the mother. She will often be red in the face and perspire heavily; it is normal for some stool to escape during delivery. At this point, she may feel frightened and hold back her pushing. The mother may also experience burning and stinging sensations and a feeling as though her body will tear apart—it will not, but if these sensations are intense, an episiotomy may be recommended.

Delivery may be performed in a number of positions, which can be adjusted to accommodate the mother's comfort. *See also* CESAREAN SECTION *and* PREGNANCY.

Dementia

The loss of mental agility.

Dementia describes the mind after disorders in which brain cells die. Usually caused by brain disease, such as Alzheimer's or cerebrovascular disease, dementia can affect a person's memory, intellect, emotional stability, sense of direction, and attention to personal health and hygiene. The onset of symptoms may go unnoticed at first. People may get lost in their own neighborhood or become confused in what should be familiar situations—many people try to cover up what they can not do. *See* CONFUSION.

Demyelination

The destruction or removal of the myelin fatty sheaths that surround the nerve fibers.

Myelin sheaths insulate the nerve fibers (axons) in the brain and spinal cord. Myelin sheaths increase the velocity and improve the nerve impulses' precision and movement. Demyelination occurs when the myelin sheath becomes irritated, inflamed, or distended by a disease. Demyelination can be the result of a stroke, immune disease, or toxins—such as alcohol when it is abused. The greater the degree of demyelination, the more extensive the nerve destruction and the less likely the prospects for repair and recovery.

Demyelinating Diseases. Multiple sclerosis is a demyelinating disorder without a known cause. This disease results in blurred vision, muscle weakness, and loss of coordination. Encephalomyelitis (often called disseminated encephalomyelitis) is a less common form of demyelination. It may be caused an infection. Adrenoleukodystrophy and adrenomyeloneuropathy are metabolic disorders that affect young boys. In addition to demyelination, affected individuals become blind, have deteriorated mental health, and suffer from seizure-like movements. *See also* BRAIN; BRAIN STEM; LEUKODYSTROPHY; MULTIPLE SCLEROSIS; NERVE; *and* NERVOUS SYSTEM.

Dengue

Also known as breakbone fever or dandy fever

An illness caused by any of the numerous dengue viruses.

There are many viruses that cause dengue fever and dengue hemorrhagic fever. This class of viruses includes West Nile and O'nyong-nyong fever. Dengue hemorrhagic fever sets in when multiple viruses infect the victim at the same time or when another dengue virus infects an individual who previously suffered from dengue fever.

SYMPTOMS

Victims of dengue will experience the sudden onset of a very high fever, often above 104° Fahrenheit. That usually coincides with the onset of a severe headache; muscle and joint pains will come later in dengue hemorrhagic fever than in dengue fever. Appetite virtually disappears and vomiting may also occur.

After a few days, in the later phase of dengue hemorrhagic fever (the most severe form of dengue), the victim will experience shock-like symptoms, including perspiration, clammy skin, and restlessness. This will be accompanied by a rash all over the body and petechiae, which looks like a bruise bleeding under the skin.

DIAGNOSIS

An examination will find the pulse has quickened and blood pressure is below normal levels; an external examination of the liver will find it enlarged—a condition known as hepatomegaly—so that it can be felt with the fingertips below the edge of the ribcage on the right side. A "tourniquet" test will reveal petechiae just below where it is applied and chest x-rays will show that the lungs are filled with fluid, a condition known as pleural effusion. Blood tests will show antibodies to dengue viruses.

PREVENTION

The virus is transmitted by mosquitoes (*Aedes aegypti*), so repellent and wearing long sleeves in areas where it is known to occur may help. At night, beds and mattresses should be covered by mosquito netting. It may also be beneficial to research the "mosquito season" if a destination is known to harbor infected insects.

> ### Dengue Warnings for Travelers
>
> Dengue is a particular concern among many people going overseas. Dengue is particularly virulent in the Caribbean islands, however, it also shows up in places such as the tropical regions of Asia, Africa Central, and South America. Infected mosquitoes have also been found in the Northeastern U.S.

TREATMENT

The only course of action involves treating the the symptoms. An intravenous unit is used to rehydrate the patent and normalize electrolyte levels. The fever should be treated with acetaminophen.

Transfusions and injections of platelets to treat bleeding problems are common as is oxygen therapy. If dengue is treated before shock sets in, the prognosis is good; if shock sets in, there is about a 50 percent mortality rate. There is not yet a vaccination for dengue so preventative measures are the best steps to take.

> *For background material on Dengue see* BRUISE; FEVER; LIVER; MOSQUITO BITES; PETECHIAE; RASH; SHOCK; *and* VIRUS. *A further discussion of topics related to Dengue can be found in* BLOOD TESTS; FEVER; *and* TROPICAL MEDICINE.

Resources on Dengue
Fettner, Ann Guidici, *The Science of Viruses* (1990); Garrett, Laurie, *The Coming Plague: Newly Emerging Diseases in a World Out of Balance* (1994); Gubler, D.J., and G. Kuno, *Dengue and Dengue Hemorrahgic Fever* (1997); Radetsky, Peter, *The Invisible Invaders: The Story of the Emerging Age of Viruses* (1991); Centers for Disease Contol and Prevention, Tel. (800) 311-3435, Online: www.cdc.gov; Infectious Disease Soc. of America, Tel. (703) 299-0200, Online: www.idsociety.org; National Inst. of Allergy and Infectious Disease, Tel. (301) 496-5717, Online: www.niaid.nih.org; Office of Rare Diseases, Tel. (301) 402-4336, Online: rarediseases.info.nih.gov/org.

Dental Emergencies

Situations of injury to or severe pain in the teeth.

Dental emergencies require immediate medical attention either because the pain is debilitating or because a slow response might result in infection, deformity or other complications.

Tooth Avulsion. A tooth that has been knocked out or badly loosened (avulsed) in an accident is treatable. The more immediately tended to, the better the chances are that the tooth or teeth will be reimplanted. The procedure involves attaching the tooth or teeth to surrounding teeth, or dental splinting, a process similar to placing a cast on a broken bone.

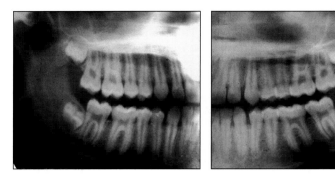

Dental X-Rays . Above, an x-ray of the mouth; dental x-rays are often used to diagnose tooth and mouth disorders. This image shows a good bite and excellent dentition. Dentition refers to the type, number, and growth of the teeth.

Resources on Dentistry

Breiner, Mark A., *Whole-Body Dentistry: Discover The Missing Piece To Better Health* (1999); Cutler, Andrew Hall, *Amalgam Illness, Diagnosis and Treatment : What You Can Do to Get Better, How Your Doctor Can Help* (1999); Malamed, Stanley F., *Handbook of Local Anesthesia* (1996); Moss, Stephen, *Growing Up Cavity Free: A Parent's Guide to Prevention* (1994); Wynn, Richard L., *Drug Information Handbook for Dentistry, 2001-2002* (2001); Academy of General Dentistry, Tel. (312) 440-4000, Online: www.agd.org; American Academy of Pediatric Dentistry, Tel. (312) 337-2169, Online: www.aapd. org; American Dentistry Association, Tel. (312) 440-2500, Online: www. ada.org; National Inst. of Dental & Craniofacial Research, Tel. (301) 496-4261, Online: www.nidr. nih.gov.

Fractured Tooth. Another dental emergency is a fractured tooth. Treatment varies, depending on the size and location of the break. Fractures in the upper part of the tooth (crown) receive fillings that prevent pain and infection. A fracture that affects the inner nerve and blood vessels of the tooth requires a root canal and rebuilding. A fracture in the lower portion of a tooth (root) is often not repairable, requiring that the tooth must be removed.

Broken Jaw. If the jaw breaks, the parts are wired together, immobilizing them in order to heal. *See also* CAST.

Swelling, inflammation, and general pain in the mouth can be caused by toothache, dental abscesses, or gingivitis. Sometimes pain can be relieved simply by brushing and flossing. If these measures are insufficient, a visit to the dentist is usually necessary. *See also* DENTAL EXAMINATION; DENTAL X-RAY; RESTORATION, DENTAL; *and* SPLINTING, DENTAL.

Dental Examination

An examination of the teeth that should be performed biannually.

Everyone should have dental examinations twice a year. This ensures that the teeth are cleaned professionally on a regular basis; it also provides the dentist with a chance to spot problems while they are still minor.

Typically, the dental examination begins with the dentist making a visual inspection of the teeth, gums, and mouth aided by a small mirror and a tool known as a probe. The dentist may take x-rays of the teeth to check for decay and periodontal problems. Sometimes, a cavity can be so small, or decay so well hidden, that x-rays provide the only meagre clue.

If the dentist finds a cavity, the decay will be drilled out, the area will be cleaned, and a filling will be inserted. If the x-rays reveal healthy teeth, the dentist or the dental hygienist will clean the teeth with special tools designed for that purpose. Both the hygienist and the dentist look for potential trouble spots.

Often the dentist will inspect previous work to make sure that it is still functioning. The dentist also examines the soft tissues of the mouth (the tongue, floor of the mouth, gums, and lips) for ulcers or other lesions, including oral cancer. *See also* DENTAL X- RAYS; DENTURE; *and* TEETH.

Dental X-Ray

X-ray of the teeth and surrounding tissue.

X-rays are of particular importance to dental hygiene. Often, the early stages of tooth decay are invisible to the naked eye. An x-ray can show whether decay is present and how far into the tooth it has penetrated. X-rays also show how healthy the supporting bone is and can show growth.

Typically, the dentist will take a series of x-rays that include the bitewing (which checks the tooth enamel) and the occlusal (which is taken while the patient is biting down). X-rays show whether decay is present, whether a tooth is growing in improperly and whether there are other infections in the tooth, such as abscesses. X-rays are not harmful, but dentists routinely place lead aprons on patients to protect them from the minuscule amount of radiation released in the process.

A patient visiting a dentist for the first time, or seeing a new dentist, should expect to have a set of dental x-rays taken. If dental work is done, the dentist will take x-rays to make sure it is healing properly and to see whether infection has set in. Thereafter, dentists periodically x-ray the teeth during routine exams. *See also* DENTAL EXAMINATION; TEETH; *and* X-RAY.

Denture

An artificial replacement for one or more teeth.

Most people think of false teeth, or dentures, as one of the inevitable aspects of aging. In fact, properly cared for, a single set of teeth can last a lifetime. In the course of an individual's life, however, disease and injury can cause teeth to decay and fall out. Rarely do all of a person's teeth fall out, but when a full denture is called for, the dentist may remove whatever teeth still remain.

The goal of the dentist, in fact, is to save as many of the patient's real teeth as possible. The reason is that nothing can take the place of real teeth. Even the best dentures will never provide the same sensation while eating that natural teeth offer. Dentists will therefore do everything possible to save a tooth before they extract it. But sometimes saving teeth is impossible.

PARTIAL DENTURE

A partial denture is used to replace several teeth when a permanent bridge is not a feasible option. The partial denture is anchored by healthy teeth. An overdenture fits over a much smaller number of teeth, which are nonetheless strong enough to anchor false teeth.

FULL DENTURE

A full denture is called for when the remaining teeth are not strong enough to anchor an overdenture, or when the teeth or gums have been ravaged by disease. Typically, the mouth takes several months to heal, so a set of conventional dentures cannot be fitted. Instead, the dentist will make a set of temporary dentures to allow an individual to function fairly normally while the gums have a chance to heal. As the gums heal, they will shrink. The temporary dentures may need to be reshaped to fit the mouth. In some cases, the patient's mouth is too sore to accommodate dentures, in which case no teeth can be fitted until the gums have healed somewhat.

Once the mouth is ready for conventional dentures, the dentist will measure the mouth and the gums before making a set of teeth. The dentures resemble real teeth. Although they are straighter and more uniform than real teeth, they are purposely not made to look perfect; otherwise they would hardly look real.

Getting Accustomed. On average, it may take several weeks to get accustomed to dentures. Eating and talking may be affected slightly. Typically, it will take several weeks for a person to adjust to the feeling of dentures. A person wearing dentures for the first time may be self-conscious and eat very carefully at first. Some people unconsciously make faces as they try to adjust to the new feeling in their mouth.

Dentists recommend that people eat small bites of soft food at first until they get used to chewing with dentures. Extremely hot foods should be avoided, as should hard foods like candy or apples.

Poor Fit. Properly fitted dentures usually do not require adhesives (despite the prevalence of these products in television commercials). If dentures feel loose or if they cause sores, the problem is that the dentures do not fit properly and must be readjusted; adhesive is not the answer. Denture adhesive can be helpful as a temporary measure, but otherwise is rarely a necessity.

Eventually, dentures wear out or else the mouth changes shape gradually. Dentures can be refitted, or new teeth may have to be made. As with any foreign object placed in the body, care must be taken to keep dentures clean and hygienic.

Titanium Implants. A new procedure known as osseointegration is helpful for people who have difficulty with traditional dentures. Artificial teeth are prepared like dentures, except that these teeth are permanently attached to the jaw with small titanium screws. These teeth, anchored in the mouth, make chewing easier than traditional dentures since they can withstand more pressure.

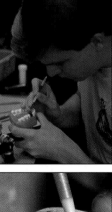

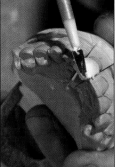

Denture Molding. Top, a man is fashioning a set of false teeth. A full set is only built after all of the teeth are gone. Teeth may fall out due to decay or trauma. Below, a porcelain crown is shaped to fit the model of a person's teeth. Platinum is often used to fashion the model.

> ***Background information about Dentures can be found in*** CARRIES, DENTAL; COSMETIC DENTISTRY; *and* EROSION, DENTAL. ***Related topics include*** PUBLIC HEALTH DENTISTRY; PREVENTIVE DENTISTRY; FRACTURE, DENTAL; *and* IMPRESSION, DENTAL.

Dependent Personality Disorder

A personality disorder characterized by extreme neediness for others—a tendency to be submissive, exhibiting a persistent fear of separation.

Throughout life, people experience neediness and dependence at various times and to varying degrees. People with dependent personality disorder, however, constantly seek the direction and acceptance of others because of a pervasive sense of inferiority. Lacking in self-confidence, they have an intense insecurity about their own ability to care for themselves. As a result of these traits, they rely on others to make decisions for them and look to others to take responsibility for their needs. Such individuals are highly suggestible, and may fall victim to cults; their behavior is easily influenced and informed by stronger personalities.

Cause. Like other personality disorders, dependent personality disorder probably arises out of a combination of inborn tendencies and environmental factors. People with dependent personality disorder are likely to have parents who were overly intrusive and excessively critical of the child's attempts to establish independence.

Treatment. While medication is of little use in treating dependent personality disorder, the individual's willingness to please can be of benefit in a therapeutic situation. A therapist may provide the person with the opportunity to develop the necessary behaviors of assertiveness and independence to counteract his or her own tendency to rely on others. *See also* ANTIANXIETY DRUGS; BEHAVIOR THERAPY; BONDING; EGO; *and* PSYCHIATRY.

Depersonalization

A feeling of being unreal and insubstantial.

Depersonalization is a loss of personal identity that often occurs without warning and makes a person feel illusory, and ephemeral. It can happen to perfectly healthy people walking down the street—they suddenly feel like a robot controlled by some unknown force, or see themselves as though from a distance, or as though they were watching someone else.

While rarely dangerous, depersonalization may occur in those susceptible to panic attacks, migraines or epilepsy, or owing to the effects of antidepressant medication or LSD. *See also* DEPRESSION; EPILEPSY; MIGRAINE; *and* MEMORY.

Depilatory

A chemical cream or paste used for hair removal.

Depilatories are generally used for cosmetic reasons, although they may be prescribed for such conditions as excess hairiness (hirsutism). Depilatories do not remove the hair completely, but instead dissolve it at the skin's surface. The hair will grow back in a few days.

Before using a depilatory, allergic reactions should be tested for and ruled out, as such reactions may cause painful swelling of the skin. To test for an allergic reaction, the depilatory should first be used on a small patch of skin. Depilatories should not be used after exposure to heat, such as in a hot shower or sauna, as heat opens the skin's pores and increases absorption of chemicals. *See also* HIRSUTISM.

Depot Injection

A medicating technique in which a drug is released over a period of two to four weeks.

When a medication level must be maintained in the body over long periods, it can be injected in a slow release form. Antipsychotic medications, in particular, benefit from this mode of delivery since the patient does not have to take pills on a daily schedule, but can receive an injection once every two to four weeks. Depending on the medication, side effects may include some discomfort at the site and drowsiness, especially when combined with alcohol. *See also* DPT VACCINATION *and* VACCINATIONS.

Depression

A disorder characterized by pervasive depressed mood, pessimistic, thoughts and feelings of despair and hopelessness, accompanied by a loss of interest in otherwise pleasurable activities and changes in eating and sleeping habits.

Depression is one of the most common of all mental disorders and is seen twice as often in women than in men. It is also one of the most treatable illnesses, but often goes untreated because it tends to be tolerated or denied by those suffering with it.

Situational Depression (Grief). Feelings of sadness and depression are normal reaction to certain situations, such as losing a loved one due to a breakup, divorce, or death; relinquishing an important goal; retirement; or experiencing a long-term frustration. Anyone may suffer from transient feelings of hopelessness or despair.

Often, this sort of depression will eventually lift without intervention. When dark thoughts and depressed mood persist longer than several weeks and making it difficult to get up in the morning, experience happiness or function normally; it may be useful to seek treatment, particularly if there are prominent feelings of guilt or thoughts about suicide.

Major Depressive Disorder. Major depression overwhelms a person with feelings of sadness and hopelessness that do not seem to have a specific cause or are out of proportion to a troubling situation. Depressed patients lose the zest for life and may become suicidal. These feelings are accompanied by physical symptoms, including exhaustion, decreased concentration, sleep disturbances, and appetite problems.

Major depressive disorder is often (although not always) a recurring disorder. Once a person has experienced this problem, the likelihood of a relapse is higher and increases with each occurrence. For this illness to be diagnosed, at least five criteria must be continuously present for at least two continuous weeks.

Dysthymic Disorder. Dysthymic disorder is a chronic form of depression with similar but less severe symptoms than

Signs of Major Depressive Disorders

Sufferers of major depressive disorders feel *sad all the time*; they are down, often tearful, guilt-ridden, and hopeless. They no longer enjoy doing things that previously gave them pleasure.

There are significant *changes in appetite*: either the sufferer loses all interest in food or else he or she feels the need to overeat.

Sleeping habits are also altered so that an individual with major depressive disorders sleeps significantly more or less than usual. He or she may experience major sleep disturbances, often in the middle of the night.

Sufferers have *a diminished ability to concentrate*, to think clearly, and to make decisions. Anxiety and agitation are common in individuals with major depressive disorder.

Thoughts of suicide—or the wish no longer to be alive—are common in a depressed person, who may express these feelings to others.

If these signs should appear in an individual, persuade him or her to seek the care of a trained professional—a psychiatrist or psychologist.

major depressive disorder.

It usually starts at an early age and continues throughout life. A general feeling of melancholy envelops a person with this disorder. Those affected suffer from low self-esteem and tend to view life with a sense of regret and dissatisfaction.

While those with this disorder function on a higher level in common social situations than those with major depressive disorder, their symptoms limit their enjoyment of life. People with dysthymic disorder may be difficult to be around and may have a limited social circle, which exacerbates their sense of isolation. Consequently sources of emotional support in times of need are limited.

CAUSES

The tendency to be depressed may be inherited, or based on the biology of the brain, or it may be associated with adult or childhood trauma. Some medications, including antihypertensives and sleeping pills, may trigger depressive episodes. Certain diseases, such as stroke or hypothyroidism, are also associated with depression. The risk of depression increases after surgery, particularly heart surgery, or childbirth (postpartum depression). People who suffer from seasonal affective disorder experience bouts of depression in the winter that are related to lack of daylight.

Depression in the Elderly

The incidence of depression increases with age. Several factors that may be part of the aging process contribute to this. Loneliness, physical illness, reactions to medications, weakened physical and mental powers, and chronic pain are all factors that tend to increase the chances of depression. At the same time, depression is not diagnosed as easily at this stage in life. Patients may believe it is an inevitable part of aging and not report it as a problem. Any one of the symptoms may be indicative of another illness or normal aging, but the constellation of symptoms seen together indicates depression and calls for treatment.

TREATMENT

Depression is a highly treatable disorder. A number of therapies address the physiological, biochemical, emotional, and cognitive aspects of depression.

Antidepressant Medication. Antidepressants have become safer and more tolerable recently because the number of side effects has been dramatically reduced. These new medications may require three or four weeks to take effect and can take up to two months to reach full potency. The likelihood that these medications will work is high, although one may need to try several different drugs to find one that is effective in a particular case.

If an antidepressant medication is effective, it can be taken safely for a long period of time; these drugs are not addictive and will not produce an unnatural high. The most widely prescribed antidepressant medications are fluoxetine (Prozac), sertraline (Zoloft), and paroxetine (Paxil). Although side effects are usually minimal, some people may experience nausea, upset stomach, headaches, or sexual side effects.

Electroconvulsive Therapy. ECT is safe, effective, and appropriate treatment for individuals with depression that does not respond well to medication. The electrical current that passes through the brain may improve chemical imbalances associated with depression. Negative attitudes towards ECT have been fostered by fictional depictions of inappropriate use.

Cognitive Interpersonal Therapy. Because many depressed people feel hopeless, helpless, and worthless, cognitive therapy can be helpful in addressing the negative thinking patterns that perpetuate a depressed individual's downward spiral in mood. Interpersonal therapy deals with the patients current interactions.

Other Treatments. Insight psychotherapy helps a patient define the unconscious psychological conflicts that may have con-

Women and Depression

Why is major depression far more common in women than in men? Several studies posit theories to explain the difference. One suggests that it is a result of the fact that women are more likely to report and seek help for depression than men because of either a cultural bias, a biological predisposition to therapy, or both. Another theory recognizes that depression may have a biological basis; that there are differences in brain structure, including factors like neurotransmitters, circadian rhythms, and hormonal makeup. Women, more likely to experience depression during the premenstrual period, during and after pregnancy, and during menopause, are subject to hormonal changes that affect neurotransmitters, thereby increasing their susceptibility to depression. Women are more likely to attempt suicide, but men are more likely to succeed when attempting it. This may be a function of the methods used: women are more likely to use pills, and men tend to use guns or rope—which have a very high comparative mortality rate.

tributed to depression. Behavior therapy attempts to affect mood by changing behavior first.

In light therapy, which is appropriate for those affected by seasonal affective disorder, a person suffering from seasonal affective disorder is exposed to a source of bright light at work or at home during the winter months.

Background information about Depression can be found in BIPOLAR DISORDER; POSTPARTUM DEPRESSION; *and* PSYCHIATRY. *Other related articles include* ANTIANXIETY DRUGS; ANTIDEPRESSION DRUGS; *and* INSIGHT PSYCHOTHERAPY.

Resources on Depression
Greist, John H. and James W. Jefferson, *Depression and Its Treatment* (1992); Hardman, Joel G., and Lee E. Limbird, *Goodman and Gilman's The Pharmacological Basis of Therapeutics* (1996); Wender, P.H., and D.F. Klein, *Mind, Mood, and Medicine: A Guide to the New Biopsychiatry* (1981); National Alliance for the Mentally Ill, Tel. (800) 950-6264, Online: www. nami.org; Nat. Depressive & Manic-Depressive Association, Tel. (800) 82-NDMDA, Online: www. ndmda.org; National Mental Health Association, Tel. (800) 969-NMHA, Online: www.nmha.org; www.ny-cornell.org/psychiatry/.

Dermabrasion

Also known as skin-smoothing surgery

The surgical removal of the top layers of severely scarred skin.

Dermabrasion is given to patients who have had disfiguring acne, accidents, surgery, facial wrinkles, or precancerous growths (kera- toses). A surgical instrument is used to "sand away" the upper portion of the skin, which then heals improving skin appearance. After the procedure, the affected skin is treated with ointment, a wet or waxy dressing or a dry treatment. Aching, tingling, and a burning sensation usually occurs for a while after surgery. For three to four weeks after the surgery, alcohol consumption may cause the recovering person's skin to flush. *See also* KERATOSIS.

Dermatitis

An inflammation of the skin.

Dermatitis affects one in five people at some point in their lives. It results from numerous causes and it has many different patterns.

Causes. Causes of dermatitis are varied and may include contact with irritants (including detergents, solvents, and harsh chemicals); friction; contact with allergens (such as nickel, perfume, or rubber); inherited factors (such as a family history of dermatitis or asthma); dry skin; injury to the skin; infection as a result of bacteria; yeast; or fungus; psychological stress; and unknown factors.

Dermatitis Artefacta

Any self-induced skin condition is called dermatitis artefacta. It may range from a small self-inflicted scratch by a person under stress to extensive self-mutilation by a psychologically disturbed individual. Dermatitis artefacta may take the form of ulcers, blisters, or scratches. Self-induced wounds may appear symmetrical or in a bizarre pattern. The wounds are never consistent with any skin disease, as they are self-inflicted.

Skin-Writing

Dermographia, also called dermatographism, is a form of urticaria, better known as hives. The word dermographia means "skin-writing." It is marked by an exaggerated tendency to produce trace marks when the skin is scratched.

Dermographia is caused by histamine released from a mast cell in the skin, but other chemicals may be involved as well. Individuals with a severe form of the disorder may have an antibody in their blood directed against mast cells. Occasionally, dermographia is triggered by an allergy to an external agent, such as a reaction to penicillin, scabies, or worm infestation. In unaffected people, firm stroking of the skin produces a white line, a red line, a slight swelling down the line of the stroke, and finally a mild red flare in the skin surrounding the line. Individuals with dermographia have an intense reaction to "skin tracing." Those with this allergy can, very literally, write on themselves.

Dermographia can occur at any age but is most common in young adults. The symptoms usually worsen in hot weather or after a hot shower or bath. Antihistamines often give relief to patients with dermographia. Hot baths, rigorous towel drying, and rough clothing should be avoided by those who suffer from the condition.

Types. Dermatitis can be acute, chronic, or both. Acute dermatitis, which is also called acute eczema, refers to a rapidly changing, red (or pink), swollen, blistered rash. Chronic dermatitis refers to an area of the skin that has been periodically irritated for a great deal of time. This area is usually darker and thicker than the surrounding skin.

Treatment. A doctor may prescribe topical corticosteroids, antibiotics, or antihistamines for dermatitis. Oral corticosteroids (including prednisone and prednisolone) and phototherapy—UV light treatment—may be prescribed in severe cases. At home, patients should reduce the number of baths they take and use a doctor-recommended soap. They should protect themselves from dust, water, solvents, detergents, and injury. An emollient should be applied often, especially after baths.

*Background information about **Dermatitis** can be found in DERMATOLOGY; DERMATITIS HERPETIFORMIS; DERMATOMYOSITIS; and SKIN. Also see INFLAMMATION and RASH.*

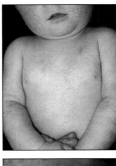
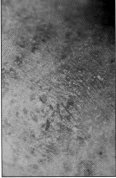

Infant Atopic Dermatitis. Top, infants regularly show signs of atopic dermatitis and the condition also tends to run in families. The word atopic refers to conditions that are frequently found together in individuals or families. It is derived form the Greek word atopia, which means uncommonness. Below, a skin reaction caused by hair dye (allergic dermatitis). Both conditions show signs of erythematous (redness) but only the allergic dermatitis has thickened (lichenified).

Dermatitis Herpetiformis

An uncommon skin disease, caused by a gluten or wheat allergy.

Dermatitis. Top, dermatitis herpetiformis is a chronic inflammatory disease that produces raised blisters that may burn. Middle, seborrheic dermatitis is marked by redness and mild scaling. Individuals living with AIDS have an especially high incidence of seborrheic dermatitis. Bottom, this skin disorder on the leg is known as stasis. It exhibits a brownish discoloration that is the result of decreased blood flow and puts a person at risk for a deep skin infection known as cellulitis. All three conditions are treated by dermatologists.

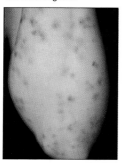

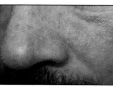

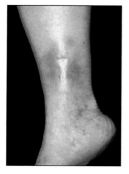

Dermatitis herpetiformis is characterized by plaques and blisters on the skin of the elbows, buttocks, knees, hands, forearms, thumbs, cheeks, and other areas. Clusters of itchy bumps and small blisters may appear on the legs and back. The affected skin is red, thickened, and bumpy. It burns and itches quite severely.

Only about 1 person in 10,000 develops dermatitis herpetiformis. Only 10 to 25 percent of patients with the disorder have spontaneous remission within 25 years after the first symptoms appear. Wheat gluten is responsible for triggering the attacks. If wheat is eliminated from the diet, dermatitis herpetiformis will clear up.

The drugs dapsone, sulphapyridine, and sulfamethoxypyridazine are often used to suppress an outbreak. *See also* ALLERGY; BLISTER; DERMATOLOGY; SKIN; SKIN ALLERGY; SKIN TESTS; *and* SKIN TUMORS.

Dermatology

The study of the skin, hair, and nails, and their associated disorders.

The skin consists of three layers, and each is affected by different disorders. The top layer is the epidermis. The middle layer layer is the dermis, which contains lubricating (sebaceous) glands. The deepest layer of the skin is made up of fat and contains sweat glands. Dermatologists must determine if symptoms or lesions are caused by a certain disorder or if they are secondary to that disorder (not directly caused by it). If a visual diagnosis can not be made, a skin biopsy is often performed. This involves the removal of a small portion of the affected area for analysis and diagnosis.

TYPES OF SKIN DISORDERS

The four most common diseases found in the dermatological study are acne, eczema, skin cancer, and psoriasis. Acne is a condition characterized by skin eruptions, on the face and other body parts, caused by clogged pores. Eczema, also called dermatitis, is a group of skin conditions that cause red, itchy skin. Melanoma is a form of skin cancer, a malignant tumor of the pigment cells of skin. Psoriasis is an inflammatory skin condition that causes episodes of itching, redness, and thick, dry, silvery scales on the skin.

Acne. Acne, a common skin disorder in people of all ages, is most common in teenagers, especially teenage boys. Acne is caused when the sebaceous glands within the skin pores become clogged, because dead skin cells and oil occlude the opening of the pores. The clog causes the pores to bulge (causing whiteheads) or darken (causing blackheads). If the clogged pores rupture, inflamed bumps containing pus, called pustules, will break on the surface of the skin.

Eczema. Eczema is a skin condition that affects one in five children, and 1 in 12 adults. Mild eczema causes dry, itchy skin, while severe eczema may cause the skin to become broken and raw, and to bleed. There are numerous forms of eczema.

Atopic eczema, which is thought to be hereditary, affects people who are sensitive to allergens in the environment; these allergens may cause inflamed, irritated, sore skin. Atopic eczema is the most common type of eczema. Asthma and hay fever are also associated with this form of eczema. Constant scratching of the itchy skin can cause the skin to break, leaving it prone to infection. Treatments for eczema regularly include emollients to maintain skin hydration and corticosteroids to reduce inflammation. Other forms of eczema include irritant contact dermatitis, infantile seborrheic eczema (cradle cap), adult seborrheic eczema (dandruff), varicose eczema, and discoid eczema.

Psoriasis. Psoriasis, a common condition that causes redness, itching, and scaly skin, may be an inherited disorder. It is most common in Caucasian individuals between 15 and 35 years of age. This skin disorder is characterized by frequent episodes of recurrences and remissions. It is most often seen on the body trunk, elbows, knees, scalp, skin folds, and fingernails. Skin normally takes about one month to regenerate cells. In psoriasis, this process takes only a few days, causing a build-up of dead skin cells.

Psoriasis can be aggravated by injury, irritation, and insect bites. Flare-ups may be triggered by medications, viral or bacterial infections, excessive alcohol consumption, obesity, and stress. People with compromised immune systems, such as those with AIDS, cancer, and autoimmune disorders such as rheumatoid arthritis, may have more severe cases of psoriasis than others.

TYPES OF SKIN CANCER

Melanoma is a malignant skin tumor derived from skin cells that produce pigment (melanin). It is an aggressive type of cancer that can spread quickly. Risk factors for developing melanoma include a family history of melanoma, red or blond hair, development of precancerous actinic keratoses, obvious freckling on the upper back, and three or more episodes of blistering sunburn before age 20. Melanoma is most common among young women. Although malignant melanoma is the most deadly form of skin cancer, it is also the least common. However, its incidence has doubled in the United States since 1975.

Melanoma is marked by cancerous changes to the skin cells that produce melanin. About 70 percent of melanomas appear on normal skin, while 30 percent occur in moles or other lesions that have changed appearance. The tumor spreads to the adjacent skin rapidly. In this stage, the cancer is highly curable. If melanoma is not detected early, it can spread to the internal organs (metastasize). Once this has occurred, melanoma has a much lower survival rate.

Squamous Cell Carcinoma is a malignant skin tumor. It originates in the layer of tissue just below the epidermis, the outermost layer of the skin. Squamous cell carcinoma first appears as a small patch or lump that usually resembles a wart, is pain-

less and grows slowly. This form of skin cancer must be completely destroyed by surgery, by freezing (cryotherapy), and sometimes by curettage (scraping). Radiation may be used if surgery will be disfiguring, such as when the face or nose needs treated. Sites treated with radiation may develop unwanted changes years later (radiation dermatitis) so it is usually reserved for older individuals.

Basal Cell Carcinoma. This type of skin cancer begins in the basal cells at the innermost layer of the skin. About half of all cases are nodular cancers, which are flesh-colored, translucent nodes. Less common are superficial lesions—red and scaly patches. A smaller percentage of cases are morpheaform lesions, which are off-white or yellow areas that resemble scar tissue. Least common are pigmented lesions, which are darker than the skin surrounding them. Those over the age of 50 with fair skin who live in regions that get a lot of sunlight are at highest risk.

About 80 percent of basal cell carcinomas occur on the head and neck, although they also can occur elsewhere. Basal cell carcinomas can be removed surgically or by radiation therapy, freezing or cutterage and electrocauterizing (burning) and a complete cure is common.

TREATMENTS

The most frequently prescribed treatments by dermatologists are topical medications, which are placed directly on the affected area. A variety of topical medications are used for different diseases and conditions.

Surgery may also be performed, especially in cases of different forms of skin cancer. The most prevalent types of skin can- cer are basal cell epithelioma, basal cell carcinoma, and, less frequently, squamous cell carcinoma. Melanoma is the most dangerous form of skin cancer, as it tends to spread to other parts of the body.

> *Specific aspects of Dermatology can be found in* SKIN CANCER; SMALL-CELL CARCINOMA; *and* SQUAMOUS CELL CARCINOMA. *Articles about other disorders include* ACNE; ECZEMA; *and* DERMATITIS HERPETIFORMIS. *See* DERMABRASION.

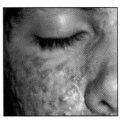

Acne. Above, a severe case of acne covering a man's face. A dermatologist will have to treat such a condition so as to minimize scarring in such a visible and sensitive place.

Lentigo Melanoma. Below, lentigo melanoma appears only in about five percent of cases, but the incidence of this dark brownish skin marking is on the rise. This condition tends to occur in the elderly; it is caused by exposure to sunlight.

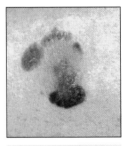

Resources on Dermatology

Kenet, Barney J., *Saving Your Skin: Prevention, Early Detection, and Treatment of Melanoma and Other Skin Cancers* (1998); Turkington, Carol A. and Jeffrey S. Dover, *Skin Deep* (1998); American Academy of Dermatology, Tel. (888) 462-DERM, Online: www.aad.org; American Board of Der-matology, Tel. (313) 874-1088, Online: www.ab derm.org; Nat. Psoriasis Foundation, Tel. (800) 723-9166, Online: www.psoriasis.org; www.nycornell.org /dermatology.

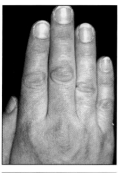

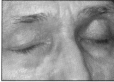

Dermatomyositis on the Right Hand. Top, an individual affected by dermatomyositis may exhibit Grotton's papules on the hands. This is an inflammatory disease of the muscles and skin that causes a violet color on the skin. Grotton's papules are important in the diagnosis of dermatomyositis. Bottom, some people affected by dermatomyositis are also affected by heliotrope eyelids. The eyelids will develop a brownish color, rather than a reddish hue, such as is common in other dermatological disorders.

Dermatomyositis

A chronic disease of the connective tissue, characterized by inflammation and degradation of the muscles, as well as inflammation of the skin.

Dermatomyositis usually occurs in children between the ages of 5 and 15, or in adults between the ages of 40 and 60. Women about are twice as likely to develop the condition as men.

CAUSE

The cause of dermatomyositis is still unknown; however, viruses and autoimmune reactions are thought to play a role. Often an immune reaction to cancer results in an attack on the muscles as well. Dermatomyositis usually affects the shoulders and hips, but other muscles of the body may also be infected.

Symptoms of the condition include muscle weakness, pain in muscles and joints, a rash, difficulty in swallowing, fever, fatigue, and weight loss. In addition to the rash, which appears at the same time as the onset of muscle weakness, there will be a reddish-purple swelling around the eyes. The rash may be scaly, smooth, or red. It can appear anywhere on the body but is especially prominent on the knuckles. The fingernail beds may also be affected. After the rash fades, there may be areas affected by pigmentation. The internal organs are usually not affected, although dermatomyositis may affect the lungs.

TREATMENT

Corticosteroids such as prednisone usually help to control the symptoms of dermatomyositis. The medications are given orally in high doses for four to six weeks until the symptoms begin to subside. The dose is then gradually decreased, but most adults must continue taking prednisone for years to prevent a relapse. Children may be able to discontinue the drug after a year. Occasionally prednisone is ineffective or makes the condition worse; in these cases immunosuppressive drugs are given instead. *See* IMMUNE SYSTEM; SKIN; *and* SKIN TESTS.

Dermatophyte Infections

Infections of the skin due to dermatophyte (ringworm) fungi.

Dermatophytes are fungi that infect the skin and are typically transmitted from person to person, though they may be acquired from animals or through exposure to contaminated soil.

The fungi attach themselves to the superficial outer layers of the skin, where they proliferate, sometimes living in the fingernails and hair. Poor nutrition, improper hygiene, warm climate, and contact with infected individuals, animals (wild and domestic), or clothing (fomites) contribute to the proliferation of dermatophyte fungi.

Common dermatophyte infections include *Tinea capitis* (scalp ringworm); *Tinea manum* (hands); *Tinea barbae* (infection of beard or mustache); *Tinea pedis* (feet); *Tinea corporis* (infection of non-hairy skin); *Tinea unguium* (nails, also known as onychomycosis); and *Tinea cruris* ("jock itch").

Dermatophyte infections are prevented by avoiding heat and moisture and implement proper hygiene. Topical antifungal medications are used to treat theses sorts of infections. *See also* FUNGAL INFECTIONS.

Dermoid Cyst

A benign tumor that has the cell structure of skin.

Cysts are usually fluid-filled lumps or swellings. Dermoid cysts have a cell structure that resembles skin, and may contain hair, sweat glands, and sebaceous glands. There may even be bone fragments, pieces of cartilage, or sometimes tooth material in dermoid cysts. Most of these cysts are removed surgically. Dermoid cysts account for approximately 10 percent of all ovarian cysts. These cysts occur in the ovaries when the follicle—or tissue around the egg—does not burst as the egg matures. Instead, the follicle fills with fluid deposits of precursor cells, cells that allow for the development of nails, hair, skin, and teeth.

These cysts may grow to about three inches and occasionally will occur in both ovaries at the same time. They are rarely cancerous. Dermoid cysts can cause severe abdominal pain, because of their size. Dermoid cysts often occur in young womens' ovaries, they must be surgically removed. *See also* CYSTS *and* OVARIES.

Desmoid Tumor

Also known as aggressive fibromatosis

A benign soft-tissue tumor that rarely metastasizes (spreads through the body).

Desmoid tumors tend to show up most often in young adults. They do not metastasize but instead interweave with the surrounding tissue, usually muscle tissue, which complicates treatment.

Desmoid tumors are sometimes surgically removed, but they can recur. The combination of surgery and radiation therapy is also used, but such an aggressive procedure exposes the patient to high levels of radiation, and therefore the possibility of a secondary malignancy; this is not necessitated by a benign condition. Low-dose chemotherapy is preferred. *See also* BENIGN; CANCER; *and* RADIATION THERAPY.

Detergent Poisoning

Poisoning brought about by the intake of any product containing cleaning agents.

The chemical ingredients of many household products, including shampoos, laundry detergents, and cleaning fluids, are very dangerous when ingested. In some cases the Ph is very high and creates a caustic hazard to the gastrointestinal (GI) tract. Accidental detergent poisoning is particularly common in small children, who are drawn to these products because of their pleasant scent or attractive color. Symptoms of detergent poisoning may include nausea, difficulty in swallowing or breathing, and unconsciousness. If a child ingests detergents, first contact the poison control center, then the label of the household product should be checked for emergency instructions. The victim should drink lots of water to dilute the poison.

Developmental Delay

A condition in which a child is significantly behind typical growth patterns for his or her age group.

Maternal, fetal, and environmental factors can affect the size and growth of a newborn. Infections such as rubella, toxoplasmosis, and syphilis can affect the size of a newborn. A woman carrying multiple births sometimes does not have enough room or adequate nutrition for all the babies to grow normally. The age of the mother also plays a role—adolescent mothers often have undersized babies.

Serious environmental factors that can cause delayed growth in a fetus include the use of drugs such as crack, cocaine, and heroin, as well as prescription medications like Dilantin. Alcoholic mothers can give birth to infants with fetal alcohol syndrome (FAS), which stunts normal growth in a baby. There is evidence that even moderate drinking during pregnancy can affect the baby. Cigarette smoking contributes greatly to undersize babies at birth.

Physical Growth. Hormonal growth disorders prevent the bones from developing. Growth is stunted when the pituitary gland does not make enough hormones. The cause may be a pituitary tumor, disease, malnutrition, or it may be of unknown origin. Growth problems in children usually become apparent between the ages of two and four. Sometimes the sex glands are affected too, stunting a child's sexual growth as well as his or her height and weight. If there is a growth hormone deficiency, the child is treated with replacement therapy.

IGR. Some children have growth problems due to intrauterine growth retardation, which involves a problem during pregnancy that slows fetal growth. This condition causes a baby to be born significantly smaller than normal. In about 90 percent of cases, the cause of intrauterine growth retardation is unknown.

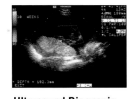

Ultrasound Diagnosis. A normal ultrasound is shown above. Ultrasound examinations are often given in order to determine weather or not a fetus is predisposed to a developmental delay after it is born. In the above image, the umbilical cord is shown in color.

There may also be problems within the fetus that can cause retarded fetal growth. If a fetus displays chromosomal abnormalities, such as Down's syndrome or Turner's syndrome, inadequate growth is typical. Children with Down's syndrome, which occurs in about 1 of every 600 to 800 births, have an extra copy of chromosome 21. Down's syndrome affects both physical and mental development; many children with Down's syndrome also have heart defects.

Turner's syndrome is a chromosomal defect that only affects girls. Girls with this disorder are missing one of the two X chromosomes. Their ovaries fail to develop properly and they are often shorter than other individuals in the same age group; growth hormones can improve height. Since the ovaries are deficient at puberty, girls afflicted with Turner's syndrome are infertile owing to the failure to ovulate.

Chondrodystrophy is characterized by abnormal cartilage in the bones, causing shortness. X-rays of the bone can usually show what is causing the underlying problem. Sometimes chondrodystrophy is inherited. Achondroplasia is a type of chondrodystrophy that causes a child's trunk and head to develop normally, while their arms and legs are stunted. However, these individuals may grow up to produce normal-sized children.

Resources on Developmental Delay

Apgar, Virginia and Joan Beck, *Is My Baby All Right?* (1972); Moore, Harold, & Barry O'Donnel, *The Developing Human* (1992); New, Maria, *Growth Disorders: State of the Art* (1992); American Academy of Pediatrics, Tel. (847) 228-5005, Online: www.aap. org; Fed. for Children with Special Needs, Tel. (800) 331-0688, Online: www. fcsn.org; Birth Defects Research for Children, Tel. (407) 895-0802, Online: www.birth-defects.org; Spina Bifida Association of America, Tel. (800) 621-3141, On line: http:// sbaa@sbaa. org; www.nycornell.org/pediatrics/.

Fetal Alcohol Syndrome

Fetal Alcohol Syndrome (FAS) is the manifestation of growth, mental, and physical birth defects that are associated with a mother's use of alcoholic beverages during pregnancy. The incidence of this disorder varies: 1 out of 1500 to 1 out of 600 newborns may be affected. Heavy alcohol use during the first trimester is especially harmful to a growing fetus. Development problems the baby may face include growth retardation, delayed or decreased mental functioning, facial abnormalities, heart defects, and limb abnormalities.

INTELLECTUAL DEVELOPMENT PROBLEMS

A number of factors can influence intellectual developmental disorders. Some studies are trying to trace genetic patterns to find a link with autism, while others attribute prebirth environmental factors to conditions such as dyslexia. There is still no conclusive evidence as to the causes of these problems. The following are the more common intellectual development disorders:

Autism. This is a serious cognitive disorder in which children cannot relate socially to others. Autistic children often perform ritualistic tasks repeatedly, have problems with speech development, and have difficulty conceptualizing. In addition, many autistic children are mentally retarded. The cause of autism is unknown, although it may be caused by a structural abnormality in the brain. Treatment of autistic children is very difficult, although there is some evidence that intense one-on-one counseling may improve the symptoms.

Cerebral palsy affects about 1 in 500 newborns. Cerebral palsy is caused by an abnormality in the central nervous system or damage to the immature, prebirth brain. It affects movement and posture. Its symptoms can manifest in something as mild as awkward running or as intense as major muscle spasticity.

Developmental Aphasia. This is the inability to acquire language skills. Children with developmental aphasia have trouble listening, and some have trouble both listening and speaking. It is caused by an abnormality in the part of the brain that deals with auditory learning.

Dyslexia. Dyslexics have difficulty recognizing certain letters and numbers and reading certain words. A dyslexic child with normal intelligence will often lag behind in reading while doing well in other areas. A dyslexic child may have trouble reading out loud. Changing teaching techniques often helps dyslexic children. Most people with dyslexia eventually learn to read, although they may still prefer the spoken word to the written word.

Background material on Developmental Delays can be found in GROWTH, CHILDHOOD; ENVIRONMENTAL MEDICINE; GROWTH HORMONE; *and* HORMONES. *Specific topics include* APHASIA; AUTISM; CEREBRAL PALSY; DOWN'S SYNDROME; DYSLEXIA; *and* TURNER'S SYNDROME. *See also* FETUS.

Dextrocardia

A rare congenital condition in which the heart is located on the right side of the chest, as opposed to the left.

Dextrocardia may occur in combination with many other inherited forms of heart disease. It may be just one aspect of a disorder known as situs inversus, where the abdominal organs are also transposed. If the heart is structurally normal, no health hazard exists. However, when dextrocardia occurs with other forms of congenital heart disease, prognosis is contingent upon the severity of the additional defects. *See also* HEART *and* SITUS INVERSUS.

Dextrose

A monosaccharide sugar.

Dextrose is one of the many simple sugars that is stored and used by the body to provide energy. Dextrose comes from digested carbohydrates, and is absorbed into the bloodstream through the wall of the intestines.

Hormones such as insulin, epinephrine, corticosteroids, and growth hormone all play a part in maintaining normal blood sugar levels in the body. If the blood sugar level is too high, it is called hyperglycemia; when it is too low, it is known as hypoglycemia.

> *For further information about sugar levels see* EPINEPHRINE; GLUCAGON; GLUCOSE; GROWTH HORMONE; HYPOGLYCEMIA; HYPERGLYCEMIA; *and* INSULIN. *See also* CORTICOSTEROIDS; HORMONES; *and* METABOLISM.

Diabetes Insipidus

Lack of antidiuretic hormone, which causes excessive urination.

Diabetes insipidus is very different from the much more common diabetes mellitus, although both conditions have frequent urination as a symptom. A person with diabetes insipidus will pass as much fluid as he or she drinks, as there is no hormone released to stop the output. If more water leaves the body than can be replaced, dehydration will set in.

ADH (antidiuretic hormone) is responsible for helping the body maintain a healthy balance of water. When the body has too little water, the hypothalamus signals the pituitary gland to release ADH, which stops water loss through urination. When there is too much water, ADH is not released, allowing water to flow out of the body. A disease of the pituitary hypothalamus, such as a tumor, injury, or inflammatory lesions, can interfere with the production of ADH, causing diabetes insipidus.

Treatment. Diabetes insipidus is usually treated with synthetic ADH, although in the congenital form, it will be relatively ineffective. For those people, a low-sodium diet is recommended and treatment will include a drug that inhibits development of the symptoms.

> *Information related to this topic can be found in* DIABETES MELLITUS; HORMONES; KIDNEYS; UREA; URIC ACID; URINALYSIS; URINARY SYSTEM; *and* URINE. *Related source information can be found in* CONGENITAL; URINARY SYSTEM; *and* WATER.

Diabetes Mellitus

Often referred to simply as diabetes

A disease, based in the pancreas, that results in abnormally high blood sugar levels.

The pancreas, a gland located behind the stomach and next to the small intestine, helps the body absorb and digest food so that it can provide the nutrients needed by the body. The hormones produced by the pancreas—including glucagon, insulin, and somatostatin—regulate nutrients and the energy used by the body. The food taken in helps regulate the energy that is put out, while some calories are stored. Insulin is a hormone that is essential in the regulation of sugars in the body and in energy production. An individual with diabetes mellitus may not produce insulin, causing problems with the body's regulation of nutrients and energy, or may have insulin resistance.

Resources on Diabetes

Groff, James L. et al., *Advanced Nutrition and Human Metabolism* (1999); New, Maria, *Genetics of Endocrine Disorders* (2001); Walker, Elizabeth A., et al., *American Diabetes Association Complete Guide to Diabetes: The Ultimate Home Diabetes Reference* (2000); American Diabetes Association, Tel. (800) 342-2383, Online: www.diabetes. org; The Juvenile Diabetes Foundation International, Tel. (800) JDF-CURE, Online: www.jdf-cure.org; National Inst. of Diabetes and Digestive and Kidney Diseases, Tel. (301) 496-3583, Online: www.niddk.nih.gov.

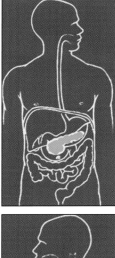

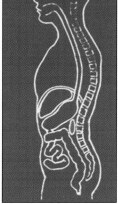

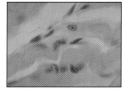

The Pancreas and its Composition. The position of the pancreas in relation to the other abdominal organs is outlined in the top 2 images. At bottom are the islets of Langerhans. This sample is taken from a monkey but they are otherwise the same as those found in a human pancreas. These islets make up barely one percent of the total pancreatic mass but provide vital hormones to regulate sugar levels.

HOW DOES INSULIN WORK?

After eating, the various digestive enzymes break down food into amino acids, sugars, or fatty acids. As the body begins to absorb these, the amount of glucose in the blood rises. The increased level of glucose acts to release insulin, which helps send nutrients into the body where they are needed. The release of insulin stops the production of glucose by the liver, with serum glucose levels then returning to normal.

However, without any or enough insulin, diabetes mellitus results. The two types of diabetes include type 1 diabetes and type 2 diabetes. The terms "insulin-dependent" and "juvenile" diabetes have gone out of use as they are no longer accurate descriptions.

TYPE 1 DIABETES

This form of diabetes occurs when there is no insulin production. When the body does not produce any insulin, glucose production continues unchecked, causing problems with the body's ability to balance the intake and use of nutrients. Glucose flows into the kidneys, escaping through increased urination, while the body continues to use its store of fats, rather than the new nutrients that the body has consumed. Weight loss and dehydration follow. Without insulin, the body can in effect starve itself despite the intake of nutrients because it cannot use them properly.

CAUSES OF TYPE 1 DIABETES

Type 1 diabetes usually occurs in individuals under the age of 30. It is the result of an autoimmune disorder, in which a toxin or virus may cause the body's own immune system to attack the pancreas. This results in the destruction of the cells that produce insulin. Although it does seem to run in families, the exact cause for a familial link is not known.

SYMPTOMS OF TYPE I DIABETES

The symptoms of type 1 diabetes may include: excessive thirst and hunger; significant weight loss; regular feelings of fatigue; blurred vision; a slowing of mental reactions; nausea; and frequent infections.

COMPLICATIONS OF TYPE 1 DIABETES

If no insulin is sent in to stop the production of glucose, a variety of complications may develop.

Diabetic Ketoacidosis. With a lack of sufficient insulin plus an excess of fat breakdown, the body may be unable to eliminate the resulting waste products (ketoacids). These acids provide fuel for the muscles and heart, however, when ketones are produced faster than they are evacuated, these acids can overwhelm the body. High blood acidity can be fatal in some cases.

Retinopathy. Long-term diabetes may, despite treatment, cause organ breakdown The eyes are especially susceptible. Retinopathy occurs when the arteries in the retina weaken and rupture, causing hemorrhages that can kill parts of the retina. Scar tissue builds up in the area and attempts to create new blood vessels that can cause the retina to detach, leading to blindness. Though this condition may occur to some degree in many individuals with type 1 diabetes, only a small percentage of these people suffer serious loss of vision.

Kidney Damage. Although under 50 percent of people with type 1 diabetes are likely to develop kidney damage, the failure of this organ is a very real danger for those individuals who do develop such damage. Controlling diabetes by maintaining normal blood pressure and glucose levels is the best defense against diabetes-related kidney disease.

Numbness and Poor Circulation. Diabetes impedes the flow of blood to the body's extremities, leading to poor circulation in the hands and feet. This means that otherwise minor foot problems, such as tight shoes, blisters, or poor nail care can be dangerous. Impaired healing ability can lead to gangrene, and possibly amputation. Proper foot care is a must for people with diabetes.

Neuropathy. Poor blood flow and increased levels of glucose and can lead to nerve damage. Correct maintenance and control of blood glucose levels can help to avoid this complication.

TREATMENT FOR TYPE 1 DIABETES

Type 1 diabetes is a lifelong disease, so treatment is aimed at replacing insulin. This may involve regular insulin injections, and learning to recognize, or self-test, for abnormal glucose levels. Drops in glucose, usually due to lack of food or overexertion, can be treated with glucose pills, or, in an emergency, candy or juices.

An exercise plan is an effective way to control glucose production; a doctor can design an appropriate mix of aerobics and strength-training for each case. Eating regular meals at consistent times helps to maintain the correct levels of insulin, and a diet low in simple sugars and high in proteins, fruits, and vegetables is recommended. A healthy diet and the right exercise cannot cure type 1 diabetes but they can help to limit the amount of medication necessary to control glucose levels.

TYPE 2 DIABETES

With this form of diabetes, some insulin is produced, but the body is unable to use it properly. Type 2 diabetes is very often linked to obesity, which itself is linked to insulin resistance. This occurs when the body's response to the insulin produced by the pancreas is impaired, thus urging the pancreas to produce more in an attempt to maintain blood glucose levels.

When the insulin level rises, the kidneys begin to reserve sodium, causing fluid retention. The muscle layers of the arteries thicken and tighten, and blood pressure rises. The liver puts out an excess amount of triglycerides, the molecules that help the body store fat. The body is ignoring the signals from the insulin, and therefore the pancreas becomes overworked while trying to keep up with the amount of glucose put out by the liver.

CAUSES OF TYPE 2 DIABETES

While the exact cause of type 2 diabetes is unknown, however, obesity is common to many individuals with this kind of diabetes. Excess fat in the abdominal area especially seems to trigger insulin resistance. Up to 90 percent of all diabetes cases are type 2, and 75 percent of those are found in people who are overweight.

As the U.S. population is steadily becoming more obese, the incidence of type 2 increases as well. Family history can play a part, and incidence seems to be particularly high among African Americans, Native Americans, and Hispanics. Most people develop the disease after age 40.

SYMPTOMS OF TYPE 2 DIABETES

The symptoms of type 2 diabetes are similar to type 1. There may be increased urination; excessive thirst; unexplained weight loss; susceptibility to infections, such as bladder, vaginal, or yeast infections; loss of sensation, or numbness in the feet and hands; and blurred vision.

COMPLICATIONS OF TYPE 2 DIABETES

Many of the complications of type 2 diabetes are similar to those associated with type 1 diabetes. Eventually the overstressed pancreas fails in type 2 diabetes. Insulin will no longer be produced. Additionally, in obese individuals, there are also effects such as heart disease and arthritis.

TREATMENT FOR TYPE 2 DIABETES

Type 2 diabetes often requires medication; for most people, however, the disease can be managed by achieving a healthy weight, exercising, and avoiding foods that can exacerbate blood-glucose levels.

As with type 1 diabetes, a diet that limits simple sugars and overprocessed carbohydrates, but is high in lean proteins, vegetables, fruits, and grains, will help with weight loss and glucose management.

If both forms of diabetes are treated carefully, through attention to diet, exercise, and monitoring of insulin and glucose levels, the disease can have minimal impact on daily life. Early diagnosis and understanding the responsibilities of self-treatment make for an excellent prognosis.

> *Related topics include* BLOOD TESTS; GLUCAGON; GLUCOSE; *and* INSULIN. *Anatomical aspects of this disorder can be found in* CIRCULATORY SYSTEM; ENDOCRINE SYSTEM; HORMONES; LIVER; KIDNEY; *and* PANCREAS. *See also* RETINOPATHY.

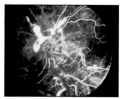
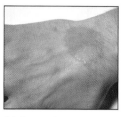

Diabetes. Insulin self-injections are required regularly by people living with diabetes in order to maintain a healthy and safe blood sugar level. Levels are monitored regularly and adjusted as necessary. Top, diabetic retinopathy is a complication of diabetes that affects the retina; nearly half of all individuals in the United States who live with diabetes are affected by diabetic retinopathy. Bottom, diabetes-associated granuloma annulare affects women about twice as often as it affects men. This is a harmless condition that causes a reddish skin discoloration. It resolves itself in about half of all cases.

Diagnosis

An evaluation of the nature and cause of an illness, which leads to a general outlook for the disease, and suggested treatment.

A proper diagnosis is essential to an effective treatment plan. It is the first stage in any battle with disease. In many cases, diagnosis requires only a brief consultation with a general practitioner. This is true when the symptoms are clear, familiar to the doctor, and produced by a common underlying cause.

At the other extreme, proper diagnosis can be enormously involved. A range of sophisticated tests, examinations, and procedures have been developed to aid physicians in diagnosis. Often one or more specialists may be consulted when a diagnosis is in question.

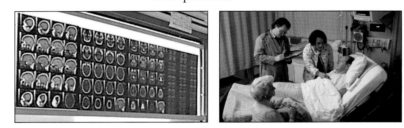

Diagnostic Techniques. Above, left, CAT scan images are regularly used in radiographic diagnosis. They provide highly accurate images that enable physicians to diagnose disorders with the utmost accuracy. Above, right, the simplest test of all—just looking at someone—often tells a doctor more than one might imagine. A physical examination and medical interview (history), are usually the first steps in the diagnosis of any disease or disorder.

The misdiagnosis of disease will often lead to an ineffective or harmful treatment, and, in the most severe cases, it can be fatal. Thus, the use of careful and thorough diagnostic strategy and an awareness of the range of possible causes are among the most important factors in the successful treatment of illness.

The Importance of Testing

Proper diagnosis almost always requires some form of testing. Testing may be as simple as listening to the sounds of the heart and lungs with a stethoscope (auscultation) during a routine checkup, or it may involve studies of blood cells, advanced imaging to identify internal disorders, or exploratory surgery. Often, a combination of tests is used to narrow down possible causes and firm up a diagnosis so that effective treatment may begin.

If treatment is ineffective, the doctor may reassess the diagnosis, often through further tests and tracking the patient's response to current treatment.

ALERT

Paying Attention to the Body

Symptoms that seem frightening may have a benign origin and require little or no treatment. On the other hand, persistent unusual conditions, even if they are not particularly bothersome, could indicate a serious underlying disorder requiring prompt medical intervention. Symptoms that should be brought to a physician's attention include:

- Irregularities of heart and lungs;
- Irregular gastrointestinal conditions;
- Shortness of breath or cough;
- Sleep disorders;
- Persistent infections;
- Prolonged weakness; and
- Abnormal bleeding.

A physician can establish proper diagnosis and, when needed, appropriate treatment. Careful testing by a physician is advised in all such cases, and self-diagnosis should always be avoided.

TYPES OF DIAGNOSIS

Diagnostic procedures differ in their sensitivity and specificity. A highly sensitive test is more likely to detect an existing disease, while a highly specific test is often used to rule out a given illness. All diagnostic tests are subject to some degree of error. When diagnosis is tricky, the combined information of several tests greatly improves the reliability of diagnosis.

Physical diagnosis, or a physical examination, is the simplest form of diagnosis. It is carried out as an external examination.

Clinical diagnosis combines patient disease history, laboratory studies, and symptoms. It is common for a number of diseases to share symptoms. A variety of tests may be required to pinpoint the precise cause of an ailment.

Diagnosis by exclusion, as the name implies, narrows down the potential causes of a particular malady by eliminating other possibilities. A skin sensitivity test to a number of possible allergic irritants is a simple example of this process.

Pathologic diagnosis is carried out through the microscopic examination of cells in tissue or body fluids. The size, shape, number, composition, and reproduction of these cells may suggest a range of possible diseases.

Differential diagnosis is carried out by comparing the symptoms of two similar diseases or disorders in order to arrive at a specific cause.

Radiographic diagnosis involves the interpretation of radiographic images, such as x-rays, computed tomography (CT) scans, MRIs, and other means of medical imaging. Radiographic studies may be used to diagnose abnormalities ranging from simple bone fractures to gastrointestinal lesions, tumors, and cerebral aneurysms.

Prenatal Diagnosis. Fetal health problems may be diagnosed through any of several technologies, including amniocentesis, cell culture, biochemical methods, amnioscopy, amniography, ultrasound, and chorionic villi biopsy. Prenatal tests can be some of the most important diagnoses in a person's lifetime.

> *For background information about methods of* DIAGNOSIS *see* BIOPSY; BONE IMAGING; BRAIN IMAGING; CAT SCAN; HEART SOUNDS; IMAGING TECHNIQUES; *and* MRI. *Other aspects of this subject are discussed in* DOCTOR, CHOOSING A; HOSPITAL; INOPERABLE; LAPAROSCOPY; SYSTEMIC; *and* TESTS, MEDICAL.

Diagnosis-Related Group

Also known as DRG

A classification system that groups patients with have similar illnesses and treatments.

DRGs form a patient classification system that defines different types of hospital patients. This system groups patients who have a similar clinical history according to their diagnosis and treatment. The system is used as an analytical tool by federal policy-makers to compare the consumption of resources at hospitals in different regions, even though different hospitals may not have the same mix of patient types.

Ever since the idea was developed at Yale University, diagnosis-related groups have been used by Medicare since 1983 as part of the Prospective Payment System for funding hospitals, because they provide an easy and convenient means of standardizing the system of reimbursement. *See also* HOSPITALS; MEDICAID; *and* MEDICARE.

Diagnostics in Women's Health

Methods to identify illness or injury in women.

Diagnostics in women's health begins with a doctor whose professional and personal qualities suit the patient's needs, preferences, and comfort level. A woman and her doctor discuss the purpose of the visit. The doctor may ask about menstrual history; birth control methods; number and descriptions of pregnancies; whether self-examinations are performed or instruction is needed; prescription, over-the-counter, or illicit drug use; alcohol consumption; smoking, or whether physical or sexual abuse has ever occurred.

The doctor may have or request access to a woman's full medical records in order to review her nongynecologic medical history. There has been less research performed on nongynecologic illness owing to an emphasis on the reproductive system and breast cancer. Diseases such as osteoporosis, thyroid disorders, systemic lupus erythematosus, rheumatoid arthritis, and multiple sclerosis affect women more often than men, while heart disease develops in women differently than it does in men.

Diagnostic tests for women include: bone densitometry; endometrial or uterus lining biopsy; follicle-stimulating hormone and luteinizing hormone (LH) measurements to determine causes of abnormal menstrual cycles, lack of ovulation, and confirmation of the onset of menopause; hysteroscopy, which entails the insertion of a thin wand into the vagina and cervical canal to examine the uterus; a mammogram, or breast x-ray; pap smear—scraping of cells from the cervix for microscopic examination, a test for cancer; pelvic, vaginal, and breast examinations; and ultrasounds. Women should also be screened for colon cancer and heart disease after the age of 50.

> *Diagnostics in Women's Health is also discussed in* BREAST CANCER; BREAST DISORDERS; COLONOSCOPY; *and* PAP SMEAR. *Related topics include* FAMILY PLANNING; INCOMPETENT CERVIX; GYNECOLOGY; *and* MENSTRUATION, DISORDERS OF.

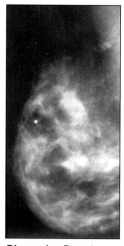

Diagnosing Breast Cancer. The diagnostic procedures involved in diagnosing breast cancer usually involve mammography. Mammography is a imaging technique that is meant to discover breast cancer at the earliest stage possible so that the most effective treatments can be applied. Mammography is, however, only one of a number of diagnostic tests that women should take regularly.

Resources on Diagnostics

Cullinan, John Edward, *Illustrated Guide to X-Ray Techniques* (1980); Kee, Joyce LeFever, *Handbook of Laboratory and Diagnostic Tests with Nursing Implications* (1994); Ravin, Carl E., ed., *Ima-ging and Invasive Radio-logy in the Intensive Care Unit* (1993); Segen, Joseph C., and Joseph Stauffer, *The Patient's Guide to Medical Tests* (1998); American Hospi-tal Association, Tel. (800) 242-2626, Online: www. aha.org; The American Board of Radiology, Tel. (520) 790-2900, Online: www.theabr.org; Ameri-can Healthcare Radiology Administrators, Online: www.ahra.org; www.ny-cornell.org/radiology/.

Dialysis

A treatment to remove waste compounds from the blood and excess fluid from the body in cases of kidney failure.

More than 150 quarts of blood pass through the two kidneys of an adult every day. As the blood passes through, the kidneys absorb essential substances such as glucose, sodium, potassium, and amino acids (the building blocks of protein).

The kidney also filters out waste products such as urea and toxins, which are excreted in the urine. If the kidneys fail to work properly, toxic compounds accumulate in the blood and excess fluid accumulates in the body, causing progressive damage that can be fatal.

Until about 40 years ago, kidney failure inevitably resulted in death. Now many patients can be saved by dialysis or a kidney transplant. A single transplanted kidney is enough to maintain life and health. But the supply of donor kidneys is limited, and any donated kidney must be matched closely to the immune system of the recipient to avoid rejection of the transplant.

Dialysis keeps patients alive until a donor kidney becomes available. It can also be used to keep patients with kidney failure alive indefinitely.

TIMING

Because dialysis carries risks, such as infection and abnormally low blood pressure, the decision to start the treatment is based on an analysis of the patient's needs.

One basis for the decision is the extent to which the kidneys, with the help of diuretic medications, are able to excrete enough urine to maintain the body's fluid balance. Another factor that determines whether dialysis is necessary is the extent to which the kidneys are able to remove enough of the body's waste products, such as acid and magnesium.

Sometimes problems such as seizures, loss of consciousness, inflammation of the membrane lining the heart (pericarditis), or symptoms including persistent nausea and vomiting indicate the need for dialysis. Two blood tests often help decide the issue: the test for blood creatine and the test for blood urea nitrogen (BUN), both indicators of kidney function. If levels of these substances in the blood rise above given points, the benefits of dialysis generally are greater than the risks. Usually dialysis is indicated when kidney function falls to less than 10 percent in most people, or when it falls to 15 percent for people with diabetes.

There are two methods of dialysis that are regularly used: hemodialysis, which uses an artificial kidney machine, or peritoneal dialysis, in which the abdominal cavity of the patient is the site where treatment takes place.

Diet and Dialysis

The need for dialysis can be delayed in many cases by a treatment regimen that includes dietary changes. Patients will be told to measure their protein intake carefully, getting enough protein in the diet to maintain normal function but not enough to overburden the kidneys. Intake of both salt and water may be restricted for persons with hypertension or a buildup of fluid in the lower part of the body. Limiting intake of food high in potassium, phosphorus and magnesium can delay the need for dialysis and limit damage to the bones.

TYPES

Hemodialysis. A patient's bloodstream can be connected to an artificial kidney machine through blood vessels in the arm, with a shunt or fistula connecting to an artery and a vein. In some cases, a hemodialysis catheter, a large tube, will be inserted in a vein in the neck for temporary use until a shunt or fistula can be created.

Blood flows into the dialysis machine, where artificial membranes carry out the functions of the kidneys, clearing toxic wastes from the blood, which then is returned to the body. Carefully prepared fluids in the machine maintain the proper water level and chemical content in a person's body.

A dialysis session usually takes three to four hours. Most patients with progressive kidney failure undergo three sessions a week. These sessions usually take place in specialized dialysis centers or at hospitals. A select few patients are able to perform hemodialysis at home.

Peritoneal Dialysis. For peritoneal dialysis, a small incision is made in the abdomen and a catheter—a little hollow tube—is inserted into the abdominal cavity. Peritoneal dialysis takes advantage of the fact that fluids can easily pass through the walls of the small blood vessels lining the abdominal cavity.

A patient can conduct home self-treatment, putting a set amount of dialysis fluid into the abdominal cavity through the catheter. The fluid is left in place long enough for toxic wastes to be filtered from the blood, after which the fluid is then drained from the body.

This one-hour session generally is done four times a day in what is called continuous ambulatory peritoneal dialysis. Some patients undergo continuous cycler-assisted peritoneal dialysis, in which a machine automatically performs the exchange of fluids at night, while the person undergoing treatment sleeps.

The major risk of peritoneal dialysis is infection of the peritoneal tissue through the catheter in the abdominal cavity. Its main advantage is that it can be done at home, so that patients do not have to make repeated trips to a dialysis center.

Special topics related to Dialysis *include* Biomechanical Engineering; Diet and Disease; Donor; Hemodialysis; Seizure; *and* Toxin. *Related anatomical issues include* Kidney; Kidney Transplant; Circulatory System; Blood; *and* Blood Tests. *Also see* Catheter; *and* Infection.

Diaper Rash

A condition that irritates the baby's diaper area, causing red, chafed skin, and possibly blisters.

Diaper rash is the most common form of irritant dermatitis. Chemicals formed inside the soiled diaper irritate the baby's skin, making it easily infected. If left untreated, diaper rash can progress from simple redness to oozing sores. The buttocks, anal area, genitals, lower abdomen, and thighs are the areas most commonly affected.

Cause. Leaving the baby in a wet or soiled diaper for too long is the most common cause of diaper rash. Babies who have frequent bowel movements usually have diaper rash more often than babies who have less frequent bowel movements. Sometimes babies treated with antibiotics develop diaper rash as a result of excess yeast on the skin. Strong detergents used on the baby clothes may also contribute to the problem, as may certain fabric softeners, baby oils, and plastic or rubber diaper covers. Diaper rash is most common in the baby's third or fourth week of life.

Treatment. If treated, diaper rash will usually go away in three or four days. A pediatrician should be contacted if there is no improvement after three days. Treatment for this condition includes frequent diaper changing—as soon as it becomes wet or soiled. Wash the skin with mild soap and dry it thoroughly. Ointment, petroleum jelly, cornstarch powder, or baby powder may also help to keep the area dry. A mild laundry soap, one without fragrances or dyes, should be used on all of the baby's clothes and blankets—never use bleach. Heavy rubber or plastic diaper covers that prevent moisture from evaporating should be avoided. The baby should also be allowed time each day to go without the diaper, as this will promote healing.

Details about Diaper Rash can be found in Crying in Infants; Dry Skin; Rash; *and* Skin. *Articles about related fields include* Dermatology; *and* Pediatrics; *and* Postnatal Care. *Important information is also included in* Dehydration; Dehydration in Infants; Diarrhea; *and* Water.

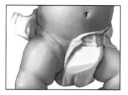

Chemical Diaper Rash. Diaper rash is often caused by a baby's reaction to chemicals in the diaper—such as ammonia—that are produced by the break down of urine and other wastes and chemical residues that may be left on a cloth diaper after laundering.

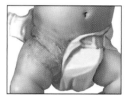

Bacterial Diaper Rash. Diaper rash can also be caused by bacteria and the *Candida* organism, which is a type of yeast microorganism. This organism shows up as a bright red patch or a set of bright red stripes that look like sores along a baby's diaper area.

Diaphragm

A semi-circular muscle that separates the abdomen from the chest.

Attached to the sternum, ribcage, and spine, the diaphragm draws air into the lungs by contracting. The phrenic nerve controls contractions, which pull downward on the central tendon of the diaphragm, expanding the chest; inflated lungs take up additional space. *See* Lungs.

Diarrhea

An increase in the volume, wateriness, or frequency of bowel movements.

As waste products pass through the intestines, water is removed and wastes are compacted into a solid form that is eliminated. If too much water is removed, stools will become hard and dry; if insufficient water is removed, the result is diarrhea.

Causes

The most common causes of diarrhea include:
- bacterial, viral, fungal, and parasitic infection;
- inflammation of the intestinal lining;
- altered intestinal transit; and
- antibiotics.

The most common cause of diarrhea is infection. Viral infections that affect children are quite common; a minor epidemic of "stomach flu," which is usually a viral infection causing both diarrhea and vomiting, will occur in a school from time to time. Most infectious causes of diarrhea are self-limiting or easily treated. Common infectious causes of diarrhea include:

Rotavirus affects mostly children under two, but is also implicated in epidemics in nursing homes.

Norwalk virus is similar to rotavirus and it is often contracted through exposure to contaminated water or eating contaminated shellfish.

Cytomegalovirus occurs in people with compromised immune systems.

Campylobacter is the most common bacterial cause of infectious diarrhea in young adults; it is caused by the consumption of contaminated foods such as raw milk and poultry.

Salmonella causes a third of all cases of diarrhea. It comes from contaminated food.

Parasitic infestations include *Giardia lamblia, Entamoeba histolytica* and *Cryptosporidium.* All of these parasites cause diarrhea.

Malabsorption can be caused by a malabsorption syndrome, in which the body is unable to digest certain foods, or by laxative drugs, which contain soluble substances (such as magnesium) that are poorly absorbed by the intestines. Poorly absorbed soluble substances cause the intestines to retain extra water. Malabsorption of fats, which do not dissolve in water, results in water retention, but may cause the intestines to excrete more salts and water than they are able to reabsorb (secretory diarrhea).

Malabsorption syndromes include an inability to process milk sugar, (general malabsorption disorders) and an inability to process gluten. Other related to malabsorption include problems of the pancreas, surgical removal of part of the intestine, lack of sufficient enzymes in the small intestines, and liver disease.

Inflammation can also cause diarrhea. When the lining of large intestine is inflamed, ulcerated, or engorged, proteins, blood, and mucus are excreted. The colon or rectum may also be more sensitive to distention, leading to increased urgency and frequency of bowel movements. The intestinal lining can become inflamed as a result of diseases such as ulcerative colitis, Crohn's disease, tuberculosis, lymphoma, and cancer.

Altered intestinal transit occurs when feces are moved too quickly through the large intestine. As a result, the intestine does not have time to absorb enough water. This may be caused by hyperthyroidism, surgical removal of part of the small or large intestine or stomach, damage to the vagus nerve, antacids, caffeine, and laxatives that contain magnesium.

Bacterial overgrowth refers to the abnormal growth of bacteria that are normally found in the intestinal tract.

Antibiotics such as clindamycin, ampicillin, and cephalosporins can alter the normal intestinal environment, killing necessary intestinal bacteria and allowing harmful bacteria to flourish—most commonly *Clostridium difficile.*

COMPLICATIONS

Severe diarrhea carries the risk of dehydration as well as malnutrition. Dehydration can result in a precipitous fall in blood pressure, leading to shock. Electrolyte levels can be disrupted, leading to abnormal blood acidity (metabolic acidosis).

ALERT

Complications Arising from Diarrhea

Diarrhea may lead to serious complications or indicate a serious underlying disorder if it is accompanied by high fever, severe abdominal pain, painful passing of stools, or bloody or black diarrhea. In these cases, or if diarrhea persists for more than a few days, a physician should be consulted.

The most common complication of diarrhea is dehydration. Symptoms of dehydration include weakness, rapid heartbeat, confusion, and a loss of skin elasticity. In infants, the soft spots (fontanelles) may appear sunken. If any of these symptoms occur, seek medical treatment immediately.

DIAGNOSIS AND TREATMENT

Diagnosis of the cause of diarrhea often requires an examination of a stool sample as well as a description of the symptoms and when the condition began.

Treatment ultimately depends on the cause. For minor cases of diarrhea, this simply involves making sure fluids are replaced; if the diarrhea is accompanied by vomiting, small amounts of fluid should be taken frequently. High fiber foods and bulking agents such as psyllium, found in commercial fiber supplements, may absorb water and add some solidity to the stools. Over the counter medications such as attapulgite and loperamide hydrochloride also add bulk and reduce the frequency of bowel movements.

In cases of more severe diarrhea, prescription drugs including diphenoxylate, codeine, and loperamide can be administered to halt the diarrhea. These should be used only after consulting a physician. Antiemetic drugs may be prescribed to control associated vomiting.

PREVENTION

The easiest way to prevent infectious diarrhea is to observe proper hygiene. Wash hands before and after using the bathroom and before handling or eating food, and make sure utensils and plates are clean. Children should be taught not to put objects in their mouths.

Further information about Diarrhea can be found in ANTIBIOTIC DRUGS; DEHYDRATION; DIURETIC DRUGS; INFLAMMATION; MALABSORPTION; *and* MALNUTRITION. *Related topics include* BACTERIA; HYGIENE; INTESTINE; *and* PARASITE.

Diastole

The resting phase of the rhythmic expansion and contraction of the heart.

Diastole alternates with systole; it is the period when the heart pumps blood. It is the longer period of the heart's rhythmic cycle. During diastole, the heart generates an electric pulse that impels the two atria, the lower chambers of the heart, to contract. Diastole ends when the electric pulse reaches the ventricles and they contract, expelling blood to the lungs and the rest of the body. *See* BLOOD PRESSURE *and* SYSTOLE.

Diathermy

The use of high-frequency current to generate heat in a part of the body, for therapeutic purposes.

The application of heat through high-frequency current is sometimes beneficial because the current may be used to increase blood flow to specific areas or warm tissues without damaging them. Diathermy may also be applied in surgical procedures to stop bleeding through electrocoagulation and wound cauterization. *See* BLEEDING.

Resources on Diarrhea

Levine, Joel S., ed., *Decision Making in Gastroenterology* (1992); Miskovitz, Paul F., and Arnold M. Rochwarger, *The Evaluation and Treatment of the Patient With Diarrhea* (1993); Sapolsky, Robert M., *Why Zebras Don't Get Ulcers: An Up-dated Guide to Stress, Stress-Related Diseases, and Coping* (1998); Sa-char, David B., et al., *Poc-ket Guide to Gastroentero-logy (*1991); Thompson, W. Grant, *The Ulcer Story: The Authoritative Guide to Ulcers, Dyspepsia, and Heartburn* (1996); Crohn's and Colitis Foundation of America, Inc., Tel: (800) 932-2423, Online: www. ccfa.org; Digestive Disease Nat. Coalition, Tel. (202) 544-7497, Online: www.ddnc.org; Gastro-Intestinal Research Found., Tel. (312) 332-1350, Online: www.girf.org; National Institute of Dia-betes and Digestive and Kidney Diseases, Tel. (301) 496-3583, Online: www.niddk.nih.gov; www. nycornell.org/medicine/digestive/index.html.

Diet and Disease

While disease is generally precipitated by a variety of factors, including heredity, environment, activity level, alcohol consumption, cigarette smoking, and illnesses, diet plays an important role both in preventing and in causing disease.

Malnutrition weakens the body and makes it susceptible to a range of diseases. Specific nutritional deficiency diseases include kwashiorkor, beriberi, marasmus, pellagra, scurvy, rickets, and osteoporosis.

Diet and Type 2 Diabetes

Diabetes is a disease in which treatment nutrition plays a significant role, and in Type II diabetes, obesity often is a determining factor. Type I, or insulin-dependent diabetes, generally occurs early in life and is thought to be of autoimmune origin. Adult-onset or Type II diabetes, however, occurs mainly in overweight or obese adults—over 90 percent are significantly overweight—though it can also be brought on by illness. Often by getting weight under control and making dietary changes people can manage Type II diabetes without insulin. In fact, drug therapy is often used for such patients only if, after six to eight weeks on a low-calorie diet, blood sugar (glucose) levels have not returned to normal. People who have a family history of diabetes should carefully monitor their weight.

DIET AND PROSPERITY IN THE WEST

Until the mid-20th century, most cultures consumed a diet low in fat and protein. However, the advent of industrialization and wealth has led to a concentration in the consumption of foods that were eaten sparingly in the past.

Wealthy lifestyles have brought with them serious illnesses. Obesity, heart disease, diabetes, and cancer are some examples. One type of hardening of the arteries (atherosclerosis) and high blood pressure are diet-related. They are also the most common forms of cardiovascular disease, the main cause of death in America today.

Heart disease is directly affected by diet and is vastly more prevalent in industrialized cultures like the United States. In cases of heart disease, an individual's diet should be carefully scrutinized before med-

ication is prescribed. Even when cholesterol-lowering drugs are prescribed, dietary modifications must be adhered to.

HIGH-CALORIE DIETS AND CANCER

The links between diet and cancer incidence are being researched, and it appears that a high-calorie diet raises the likelihood of developing certain types of cancer. Studies indicate that a high-fat diet, a sedentary lifestyle, obesity, cigarette smoking, and alcohol consumption increase the risk of breast cancer, while the risk is decreased in individuals who exercise regularly and follow a low-fat, low-calorie diet.

Comparisons of breast cancer rates in American and Japanese women have found that the disease is rare in Japan, where a low-fat diet is the norm. Among Japanese women moving to the United States and eating an American diet, breast cancer rates tend to approach those of Americans.

FAD DIETS

Fad diets can also have a profound effect on health. Any diet that stresses the exclusion of a variety of foods, or any diet that emphasizes one type of food, can lead to nutritional imbalances and can cause serious health problems. "Crash diets" are essentially short-term periods of starvation that cause the body to turn on itself and literally consume lean muscle for sustenance.

A balanced diet is an important component of a healthy lifestyle. While diets lacking nutritional balance cause diseases of deficiency; the illnesses of overconsumption cause a different set of diseases. This is particularly true of diets high in saturated fat and processed foods, which contain large amounts of fat. These types of diets often contain little fiber and few nutrients—contributing to the epidemic of obesity and related diseases so prevalent in the United States today.

For more information about Diet and Disease see FATS AND OILS; *and* CHOLESTEROL. *Information about related disorders can be found in* BERIBERI; DIABETES; KETOSIS; MARASMUS; OSTEOPOROSIS; RICKETS; *and* SCURVY. *See also* DIET, ATKINS; DIETARY FIBER; *and* NUTRITION.

Resources on Diet and Disease

Debakey, Michael E. and Antonio M. Gotto, *The New Living Heart* (1997); Heimburger, Douglas C. and Roland L. Weinsier, *Handbook of Clinical Nutrition* (1997); Mahan, Kathleen L. and Sylvia Escott-Stump, eds., *Krause's Food, Nutrition, & Diet Therapy* (2000); National Academy Press Food and Nutrition Board, Recommended Dietary Allowances (1989); Shils, Maurice E., et al., *Modern Nutrition in Health and Disease* (1999); American Dietetic Association, Tel. (800) 366-1655, Online: www.eatright.org; Center for Nutrition Policy and Promotion, Tel. (202) 418-2312, Online: www. usda. gov/cnpp; Food and Drug Administration, Tel. (888) INFOFDA, Online: www. fda.gov; www.nycornell.org/medicine/nutrition.html

Diet, Atkins

A diet introduced in the 1970s by Robert C. Atkins.

The Atkins Diet is a weight-loss program based on decreased consumption of carbohydrates and increased consumption of fat and protein. According to Atkins, foods high in sugar and carbohydrates, such as pasta, bread and cereal, increase the body's production of insulin, which breaks down carbohydrates into fat according to his theory. If an individual consumes carbohydrates regularly, insulin will always be in the blood converting carbohydrates into fat. Meats, cheeses, and eggs form the cornerstone of the Atkins Diet; sugars, grains, cereals, and carbohydrates of every kind are minimized; and fruits and vegetables are not particularly encouraged. This may make the body burn fat for energy. The dietary regimen has come under attack as unhealthy, increasing the chance of heart and liver disease, high blood pressure, and malnutrition. *See also* DIET AND DISEASE.

Dietary Fiber

The essential component of many carbohydrates, comprised of the structural materials of plants. It is not directly digestible by humans.

Fiber is classified in one of two ways; it is either soluble and fermentable, or insoluble and nonfermentable.

Soluble fibers form a gel when mixed with water, and include guar, pectin, mucilages, and the fiber in barley, oat bran, beans, and other legumes. The more soluble the fiber, the more fermentable. This means that it is broken down (fermented) in the lower small and upper large bowel by bacteria into short-chain fatty acids. These acids aid in chemical processes and provide energy after they are absorbed. Soluble fibers lower blood cholesterol but do not have a large influence on stool bulk.

Insoluble fiber passes largely unchanged through the digestive tract, absorbing as much as fifteen times its weight in water, softening and increasing the size of the

ALERT

The Dangers of Excessive Fiber
Too much fiber can be dangerous, especially if obtained through supplements in excessive dosages. They can cause bowel obstructions, requiring surgical removal in some cases. An excess of fiber can also impede the absorption of nutrients, and may result in deficiencies of calcium, zinc, and iron, which bind to fiber and are excreted. Consult a specialist about a diet with the right amount of fiber before making any major changes in dietary supplements.

stool. This added bulk promotes peristalsis, the contractions of the bowel, preventing constipation by moving stool through the body more quickly. Thus insoluble fiber decreases the amount of intestinal muscle pressure necessary to move the stool through the bowel; it also reduces the amount of pressure inside the intestine. Insoluble fiber aids the treatment of diverticular disease by lowering the likelihood that fecal matter will fill the pouches in the intestinal wall and by reducing the pressure that stimulates the formation of these pouches (diverticulae). A diet high in insoluble fiber is sometimes helpful in treating irritable bowel syndrome. Insoluble fiber does not significantly influence blood sugar levels or the body's cholesterol level.

High-fiber foods play an important role in weight-loss programs, since they are often low in calories and their bulk can enhance the feeling of satiety after eating a reasonable meal. High-fiber foods, in extremely large amounts, seem to reduce the absorption of some nutrients, perhaps because they cause food to move through the digestive tract quickly or bind to the nutrients.

The daily fiber consumption for an adult should be no less than 20 grams and generally no more than 35 grams. Increasing the amount of dietary fiber consumed should be done gradually, particularly when making the switch from a diet low in fiber to one high in fiber. The sudden addition of large amounts of fiber to the diet can cause gastrointestinal problems, ranging from gas and bloating to cramps and diarrhea. *See also* CARBOHYDRATES; DISEASE; DIVERTICULAR DISEASE; *and* NUTRIENTS.

Diethylstilbestrol

Also known as DES

A synthetic form of estrogen that causes vaginal cancer in women with mothers who took it during pregnancy.

In the 1930s researchers created a synthetic estrogen called diethylstilbestrol, or DES. At the time, they thought it would be an effective preventative for women with a high risk of miscarriage. It later proved not only ineffective but dangerous, even though it was prescribed to millions of women between 1938 and 1971.

Studies have found that DES causes vaginal cancer in women whose mothers took the medication during pregnancy. Women exposed to DES should seek a practitioner with special experience in diagnosing and treating DES-daughters, especially those who are pregnant and those who are planning on becoming pregnant, because they may wish to inquire about high-risk obstetric care. Men who were exposed to DES have a greater incidence of testicular abnormalities, testicular cancer and reduced fertility. Men should also consult a specialist about options or need for treatment. *See also* ESTROGEN HORMONES.

Differentiation

A process whereby cells of a fertilized egg develop into different cells for different body parts.

The embryo starts out as a single cell that undergoes several rounds of rapid divisions. As the number of cells increases, they become different from each other, both in structure and function; this process is known as differentiation.

A cell is completely differentiated when it possesses all the features characteristic of a specific cell type. In prenatal development process, the cells continue to differentiate in the period of the zygote, the period of the embryo, and the period of the fetus. As the process proceeds, a variety of shaping and patterning processes organize the cells into tissues and organs. *See also* BIRTH; DELIVERY; *and* PREGNANCY.

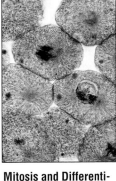

Mitosis and Differentiation. Above, fertilized human cells after only two divisions. These cells will continue to divide. Mitosis is the process of cell division. How divided cells know what body parts they will develop into is still a mystery.

Digestive System

A group of organs that delivers nutrients to the bloodstream and turns food into energy, cells and tissue, and waste.

Digestion, and thus the digestive system, can be thought of as a process that holistically operates in three primary stages: consumption, absorption, and secretion. The most important of these is the second stage because that is how the body supports all of its daily operations.

The Mouth. This complex system begins with consumption so it also starts in the mouth. Saliva softens food and starts the process of chemically breaking down carbohydrates, sometimes called intraluminal digestion. Taste buds on the tongue sense flavor, while the tongue pushes food into the line of teeth that grind and tear food into pieces small enough to move to the back of the throat, or the pharynx.

Swallowing is achieved by peristalsis—muscle contractions strong enough to squeeze food through the esophagus to the stomach even if the person stands on his or her head; peristalsis continues throughout the digestive system, from throat to rectum.

The Stomach continues the physical operation of digestion by twisting and churning, of partially liquefying the food. The stomach also begins the process of chemical digestion by secreting digestive acids and gastric juices, including the enzyme pepsin and hydrochloric acid, from its lining. These secretions break down proteins before they move along through to other parts of the digestive tract.

The Small Intestine. Once the food is reduced to a chunky liquid that is often called chyme, it moves into the first tract of intestine, the duodenum. This is where two hormones, secretin and cholecystokinin, are released. This signals the gallbladder to release its contents into the bile-duct that connects to the duodenum: bile salts and acids, produced by the liver and stored in the gallbladder, enter the duodenum to break down fats. Pancreatic enzymes, most notably trypsinogen and chymotypsinogen, also arrive in the duodenum to help break down proteins, fats, and carbohydrates into substances that body can easily absorb.

The food then moves through the next sections of the small intestine, the jejunum and ileum, where most of the body's vitamin and mineral absorption takes place. The rest of the small intestine releases more enzymes and completes the process of chemical breakdown.

The thin intestinal walls, lined with tiny finger-like organs called villi, absorb nutrients and pass them into the bloodstream or into the lymphatic system. Villi also line the walls of the duodenum, jejunum, and ileum, but they are largest in the small intestine.

The Large Intestine. Moving into the large intestine (comprised of the cecum, colon, and rectum), undigested materials, waste products, and intestinal lining cells cast off in the digestive process coalesce and are excreted through the rectum and anus as feces.

Absorbing the Food. Food spends about four minutes in the mouth and throat, two to four hours in the stomach, one to four hours in the small intestine, and somewhere between ten hours to several days in the large intestine. Most vitamins and minerals do not need to be digested to pass into the bloodstream. The body's primary source of energy comes from sugary or starchy foods; the digestive system reduces their carbohydrate content into the sugars fructose, galactose, and glucose.

The proteins in meat, fish, cheese, eggs, and beans are converted into amino acids, peptides, and polypeptides, which repair and replace the body's cells. The pancreatic and intestinal enzymes that break down fats into fatty acids, glycerides, and glycerol are called lipases. Fats provide the body with the fat-soluble vitamins A, D, E, and K, energy, and materials that repair and produce cells.

Aspects of the Digestive System are discussed further in EXCRETORY SYSTEM; INTESTINE; STOMACH; and TEETH. the ENZYME. Related topics include DIET AND DISEASE; NUTRITION; and NUTRITION AND DIET, ALTERNATIVE THERAPIES.

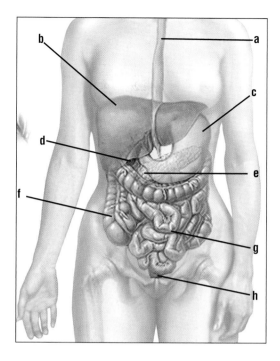

The Digestive System. The digestive system is basically a very long tube that passes through the human body. At various stages this tube takes in (consumes) and absorbs nutrients, and removes food from the body. This diagram of the digestive system shows the order and comparative positions of the esophagus (a); liver (b); stomach (c); gallbladder (d); pancreas(e); large intestine (f); small intestine (g); and rectum (h).

Digitalis Drugs

The oldest group of medications prescribed for cardiovascular conditions.

Digitalis drugs come from the leaves of the foxglove plant (*digitalis purpurea*) and are prescribed for heart failure cases. They can also be used against some forms of arrhythmia (abnormal heart rhythms). Digitalis drugs vary in potency and activation time. The two most commonly used digitalis medications are digoxin and digitoxin.

Digitalis drugs cause the heart to beat more slowly and with greater force, so that it pumps blood more efficiently. Digitalis drugs can also slow abnormally rapid electric signals that cause rapid, irregular heartbeats. The main side effects are stomach upset and loss of appetite, and the drugs may also cause an abnormally slow heartbeat in some patients.

Even though digitalis drugs are the fourth most prescribed medicine in America, they are highly potent drugs. Dosages must never be doubled and they should always be carefully measured because, when taken in excess, they can be highly toxic. *See also* HEART *and* HEART DISORDERS.

Resources on the Digestive System

DLevine, Joel S., ed., *Decision Making in Gastroenterology* (1992); Berkson, D. Lindsey, et al., *Healthy Digestion the Natural Way* (2000); Sapolsky, Robert M., *Why Zebras Don't Get Ulcers: An Updated Guide to Stress, StressRelated Diseases, and Coping* (1998); Sachar, David B., et al., *Pocket Guide to Gastroenterology* (1991); Thompson, W. Grant, *The Ulcer Story: The Authoritative Guide to Ulcers, Dyspepsia, and Heartburn* (1996); Crohn's and Colitis Found. of America, Inc., Tel: (800) 932-2423, Online: www. ccfa.org; Digestive Disease National Coalition, Tel. (202) 544-7497, Online: www.ddnc. org; Gastro-Intestinal Research Found., Tel. (312) 332-1350, Online: www. girf.org; National Institute of Dia-betes and Digestive and Kidney Diseases, Tel. (301) 496-3583, Online: www.niddk. nih.gov; www. nycornell.org/medicine/digestive/index.html.

Digoxin

A medication used to strengthen the heart and slow the heartbeat.

Digoxin is one of a family of drugs, known as digitalis drugs, that has been used for over 200 years to treat congestive heart failure, in which the heart muscles are too weak to sufficiently circulate blood throughout the body.

Digoxin stimulates the heart to pump more powerfully with each beat, so that the heart rate slows and blood more effectively reaches the extremities. Digoxin is a long-term medication. It may take weeks or even months for the full effect to be felt.

Drug Interactions. Digoxin interacts with many other drugs that may result in serious side effects. Therefore, a person taking digoxin should consult a physician about taking any other drugs. For example the combination of quinidine (a derivative of quinine that is often prescribed for heart rate disturbances) and digoxin exaggerates the effect of digoxin leading to an overdose that can be life-threatening. Digoxin can also interact with amiodarone to stop the heart from beating entirely.

Some nutritional supplements and over the counter medications that interact with digoxin include liquid antacids, antidiarrheal medications like attapulgite, bulking laxatives like psyllium or methylcellulose, high fiber supplements and nutritional supplements such as Ensure. These foods may result in too little of the digoxin finding its way into the blood stream.

Side Effects. The exact dosage of digoxin is critical. Too much digoxin can be very dangerous, producing nausea, vom-

---

Mistaken Side Effects

In an elderly patient, if there is too much digoxin in the blood, as a result of too high a dosage or interaction with other drugs, side effects may include confusion, weakness, and disorientation. It is not entirely uncommon for a physician to attribute these symptoms to Alzheimer's disease rather than to this simpler, more treatable cause.

---

iting, drowsiness, vision abnormalities, headache, confusion, depression, hallucinations, and seizures. *See also* CONGESTIVE HEART FAILURE; DIGITALIS DRUGS; HEART ATTACK; HEART DISEASE; *and* KIDNEY.

Diminished Ovarian Reserve

Also known as diminished fertility

A decrease in the number and quality of eggs in a woman's ovaries.

As a woman ages and approaches menopause, the number and quality of her eggs decreases, with the sharpest decrease generally coming after the age of 37, but still well before the onset of menopause. This figure varies from woman to woman, but since women do not produce any new eggs, the fertility of existing eggs will decline with age. Due to the decreasing quality of the eggs, the likelihood of pregnancy decreases and the possibility of miscarriage sharply increases.

Diminished ovarian reserve is not always associated with age and the approach of menopause. It may also affect the fertility of a young woman, complicating her ability to conceive a child.

Diagnosis. An accurate estimate of ovarian reserve is problematic, since there are no perfect tests. However, there are related tests for follicle stimulating hormone level, or FSH, which is the hormone that controls the ripening of eggs in the ovaries. The baseline FSH levels are measured on the third day of the menstrual cycle, so the test is usually called a Day-3 FSH test. This test can provide an indication of diminished ovarian reserve when the results are abnormal. However, normal results do not always indicate a high level of fertility or a normal ovarian reserve.

Elevated FSH levels are often found in perimenopausal (women in the years immediately preceding menopause) women who are experiencing diminished ovarian reserve due to age. When this type of disorder is found in younger women, it may be an indication of diminished fertility.

Treatment. Individuals with infertility problems due to diminished ovarian reserve can sometimes be treated with controlled hyperstimulation of the ovaries, which is a procedure that may induce ovulation. There are also a number of different forms of injectable FSH, including menotrophin, urofollitropin and human chorionic gonadotropin or hCG; these are usually taken for about nine days. All of these medications should be closely monitored by fertility specialists. Gonadotropin is not effective with elevated FSH levels.

Diminished ovarian reserve is sometimes treated with hyperstimulation in conjunction with in vitro fertilization and intrauterine insemination in order to produce pregnancy. Pregnancy rates in women with diminished ovarian reserve are sill lower than in others. *See also* IN VITRO FERTILIZATION; MENOPAUSE; *and* PERIMENOPAUSE.

Diphtheria

A bacterial disease caused by the *Corynebacterium diphteriae* bacterium, and spread by breathing droplets of moisture coughed into the atmosphere.

The bacteria that cause diphtheria die quickly if they do not find a host, so the disease is rarely spread by contact with utensils, tools, or clothing.

Symptoms. In the early stages of diphtheria, the sufferer experiences a sore throat and painful swallowing. There is also a low-grade fever, nausea, vomiting, a rapid pulse rate, chills, and a headache. The lymph nodes swell, causing breathing difficulties. The bacteria build a gray membrane in the throat that may further narrow the air passages. Some strains of the bacteria release a toxin that travels in the bloodstream to the heart and nerves. This toxin can be fatal.

Diagnosis. Diphtheria is diagnosed by growing a culture in the laboratory and identifying the bacteria as *Corynebacterium diphtheriae*. If diphtheria is diagnosed, the individual must be taken to the hospital for intensive care. In the hospital, an antitoxin will be administered, first in small quantities to be sure the sufferer is not allergic to it and then in progressively larger quantities. The patient will be monitored closely for breathing difficulties, and an antibiotic will be administered to destroy the bacteria. Diphtheria is a long-term disease, and full recovery takes weeks.

If You Have Been Exposed

If you have had contact with someone with diphtheria, have a physician examine you and have a throat swab sent to a laboratory for culturing. Antibiotics will be given for a seven-day course, and you should be monitored closely for evidence of the disease. A vaccine booster shot is advisable if you have not had one within the last five years. Some people may be carriers of diphtheria and not experience any symptoms. These carriers will be revealed by the throat culture and should be given the full sequence of antibiotics to destroy the bacteria so that they do not spread the infection to others.

Prevention of diphtheria is much preferred to treatment for the disease. Routine immunization shots given to children for diphtheria, whooping cough, and tetanus have essentially eliminated these disease in developed countries. The shots are given in a five-part series that should be administered over the first five years of a child's life. Booster shots should be given every ten years thereafter to maintain the body's immunity. *See also* ANTIBIOTIC DRUGS; BACTERIA; DPT VACCINATION; HEART; NERVE; SORE THROAT; TOXIN; *and* VACCINATION.

Dipyridamole

A drug that increases the blood supply to the heart tissue and blocks platelet function.

Dipyridamole is used to ease the pain of angina pectoris and to prevent the formation of blood clots. It dilates the blood vessels, increasing the flow of oxygenated blood to the heart. It also reduces the stickiness of platelets, protecting against blood clots, particularly those forming in the body after heart surgery. It may be used in conjunction with warfarin and aspirin without side-effects. *See* ANGINA PECTORIS.

Disability

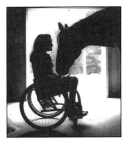

Living With a Disability. There are very few activities that an individual with a disability can not participate in, including horseback riding. According to American law, people with disabilities cannot be discriminated against when they try to participate. Enacted in 1990, the Americans with Disabilities act legally defines and describes the nature of discrimination against individuals who live with disabilities. This law makes any sort of discrimination illegal, and carries severe fines. The law protects some 43 million Americans.

A physical or mental impairment that affects an individual's ability to carry out some normal everyday activities.

A disability is any physical, mental, or sensory impairment that substantially limits an individual's ability to engage in one or more major life activities, such as walking, talking, seeing, or reading. Disabilities commonly affect mobility, manual dexterity, physical coordination, continence, or vision and hearing.

In the United States, federal law prohibits private employers, states, and local governments from discriminating against disabled individuals in a work setting. Employers must design work facilities and job schedules to accommodate disabled employees capable of performing their jobs competently.

Incidence. In the United States, more than 49 million people have physical and mental disabilities, according to a study in 1998 by the Pan American Health Organization (PAHO). For these individuals, disability affects all aspects of their well-being, and has emotional, social, and financial consequences. A 1994–95 survey by the National Center for Health Statistics (NCHS) revealed that the prevalence of disabilities is disproportionately high among people in minority, elderly, poor, and rural populations. The Department of Health and Human Services devotes tens of millions of dollars a year to programs for people with disabilities. *See also* BLINDNESS; DISABLED, AIDS FOR THE; *and* PARAPLEGIA.

Disabled, Aids for the

Devices that help the disabled carry out everyday tasks.

Aids for the disabled include a wide variety of appliances that have been created over the years to help those with disabilities lead unassisted (or minimally assisted) lives. As people with disabilities have been integrated into society and have gained more

In the Home and at Work

Households and workplaces can be outfitted with devices to make it easier for a person with a disability to function. For example, appliances may be lowered or automated for a person in a wheelchair; flashing lights may take the place of phone rings and doorbells for the deaf; tools, such as cutlery, knobs and faucets, can be made so that a person with limited mobility can use them; and computers can be voice-activated for the blind or for those who are unable to use a keyboard.

independence, devices have been designed to allow them to participate in sports, drive, and live on their own, whereas in the past they may have been institutionalized.

Aids for the disabled include such correctives as glasses, hearing aids, wheelchairs, leg and back braces, and artificial limbs. The trend towards using animals to assist the disabled is one of the more interesting aids. Sparked by the use of guide dogs for the blind, a movement is now underway to train dogs (and other animals) to live with disabled individuals. These animals will be able to open doors, operate some specially equipped appliances, help fetch and carry, and most importantly, provide companionship.

Background information about Aids for the Disabled can be found in BIOMECHANICAL ENGINEERING; BRAILLE; DISABILITY; EYE INJURIES; WALKING AIDS; *and* WHEELCHAIR. *Regarding special subjects in this area, see* BLINDNESS; PARAPLEGIA; *and* SIGHT, PARTIAL. *Also see* DEAFNESS; *and* HEARING AIDS.

Discharge

Secretion or excretion of pus, feces, urine or other material from the body. Also the material itself.

Abnormal discharges from the body usually indicate an underlying disorder that needs treatment. Often, the the discharge may be used diagnostically in order to identify the nature of a disease or ailment.

Discharge from the Eye. There are several types of irregular discharge that issue from the eyes because of illness or inflammation. Conjunctivitis results from an inflammation of the tissues protecting the eye surface and inner eyelid, producing a clear or yellowish crusting discharge that may be viral or bacterial in nature. Both are highly contagious and may be transmitted through the discharge. Other eye disorders producing discharge include corneal ulcer and dacryocystitis.

Pus. A variety of bacterial and viral wound infections are accompanied by the discharge of pus, a by product of inflammation composed of white blood cells, albuminous substances and thin fluid. The color, texture and occasionally the smell of this pus can indicate the particular form of infection. Pus is generally yellow. Blue or green pus indicates the presence of *Pseudomonas aeruginosa*, a species of bacteria. Discharges of pus may also occur in the urine, and may indicate any of the following: cystitis, pyelitis, urethritis, tuberculosis of the kidney, infection of the genitourinary tract or trauma.

Blood. Abnormal discharges of blood from any of the bodily orifices are of particular concern. Such discharges, particularly vaginal, are not uncommon and may indicate a range of disorders. Any atypical discharges should be reported to a health care professional for diagnostic analysis and, when needed, treatment.

For further reading about DISCHARGE *see* BLOOD; CONJUNCTIVITIS; DACROCYSTITIS; INFECTION; INFLAMMATION; *and* PUS. *Related articles about specific kinds of* DISCHARGE *can be found in* ANAL DISCHARGE; EAR, DISCHARGE FROM; NASAL DISCHARGE; *and* VAGINAL DISCHARGE; *Also see* TUBERCULOSIS.

Disclosing Agents

Temporary dyes applied to the teeth to locate plaque.

Plaque is often invisible to the naked eye. It may remain on the teeth after they have been brushed and flossed, causing damage to teeth and gums. To ensure that all plaque has been removed, some dentists recommend the use of disclosing agents. Essentially, disclosing agents act as a dye. Chewing a tablet containing the agent causes the plaque on the teeth to acquire the color of the tablet, pinpointing the areas that need more attention and brushing until the coloring is gone. *See also* ABRASION, DENTAL; CARIES, DENTAL; DISCOLORED TEETH; GINGIVITIS; PLAQUE, DENTAL; *and* PREVENTIVE DENTISTRY.

Discolored Teeth

Teeth, like other parts of the body, are affected adversely by age and environment. Sometimes this results in enamel discoloration. Discoloration may be caused by certain medicines or when certain foods are eaten. These can affect the enamel over a long period of time. Smoking also causes discolored teeth.

Teeth are not "true white"; they vary in shade. Whitening toothpaste can remove some undesirable color from the teeth, either through bleaching or abrasion. But their effect is somewhat limited.

Dentists can whiten or brighten discolored teeth by applying a bleaching substance that gradually whitens the teeth. Sometimes they will do this when a person is having a crown or a bridge placed where the new artificial teeth will show. The surrounding front teeth may be whitened so that the artificial teeth do not stand out. Teeth can also be whitened for cosmetic reasons. Again, the natural color of teeth can vary and dentists will try to create and match the color and shade to each individual patient. *See also* BLEACHING, DENTAL; FLOSSING, DENTAL; *and* PERIODONTICS.

Disk Imaging

Imaging techniques used to assess disease or injury to the disks of the spine.

The disks are located between the vertebrae of the spine. They are composed of cartilage filled with a gel-like tissue. Being compressible, they give the back flexibility. Age and disease may impair the resiliency and general condition of disks, causing pain and impaired movement. The spinal cord, which houses the nerve cord within

The Shape of the Spine. As the spine moves downward, it changes shape, reflecting the varying function of various parts of the back. The disks between the vertebrae that cushion the space between theses bones also must change shape, but to a lesser degree—especially as they are malleable gel-like tissue.

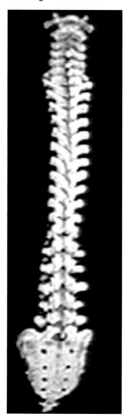

the spinal column, may become damaged as a result of a disk disorder.

A range of imaging techniques can be used to evaluate the condition of the vertebral disks and assess possible treatment for back injury, disease, or age-related degeneration. In the past, disks were examined by x-ray through myelography or diskography, in which a dye opaque to radiation had to be injected into the spinal canal or when dye was injected directly tin a disk. Now, however, the more accurate and less invasive techniques of computed tomography (CT) and magnetic resonance imaging (MRI) are usually preferred.

Disk ruptures are a relatively common affliction; age or excessive strain weakens the fibrous shell and allows the gel within the disk to bulge or rupture (herniate). The severity of disk impairments often depends on the location. Most herniated disks occur in the lower back (lumbar) region. Damage to lumbar disks often causes pain, not only to the lower back but along the sciatic nerve, which runs from the spinal column to the leg and heel. Rupturing more centrally located disks may cause more severe symptoms and, in some cases, disability. *See also* SPINE.

Rest, medication (muscle relaxants), and sometimes physical therapy, are prescribed to treat ruptured disks. In severe cases, a physician may recommend back surgery. This, however, is generally the last choice of treatment, as it carries a risk and varying degrees of success in alleviating pain or disability. *See also* BACK PAIN; CAT SCAN; MRI; MUSCLE; *and* PHYSICAL THERAPY;.

Disk Prolapse

The rupturing of a disk between the vertebrae of the spine, which pushes the disk out, putting pressure on a nerve.

The disks between the vertebrae provide cushioning and the flexibility that allows the spine to bend, lean, and bear weight. The disks—gel cores surrounded by tough, fibrous material—are susceptible to the wear and tear of age, as well as to damage

The Aging of the Spine. As the spine ages, it weakens. This weakening may cause bending, especially towards the lumbar region and near the shoulders. The bones of the spine also become significantly more fragile. Those who have had a previous spinal cord injury (SCI) are more likely to develop bending and weakness sooner than those who have not.

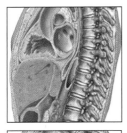

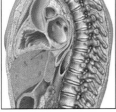

from excessive strain. Sudden strenuous activity, such as heavy lifting, may rupture a disk, but the condition is more likely to occur as a result of repeated activity or degeneration from age. The ruptured disk may protrude, compressing nerves in the spinal cord, and causing pain in the areas controlled by those nerves. Disk prolapse may occur in any part of the spine, but is most common in the lower back.

SYMPTOMS

Indications of a disk prolapse include sharp, shooting pains that run down the buttock and leg; these may worsen while coughing or sneezing. Tenderness, lack of mobility, and occasional numbness or tingling may also signify a disk prolapse.

Physicians may diagnose disk prolapse with examination and movement tests, or may take x-rays or MRI scans.

> **The Age Range for Disk Prolapse**
>
> Disk prolapse is most common in those between the ages of 30 and 40. During this time, the disks begin to wear out, but after age 40, they develop an extra fibrous coating that adds an extra layer of protection and stability. Disk prolapse is a little more common in men than women. Spending long periods of time sitting in one position increases the risk.

TREATMENT

Bed rest and pain relievers may reduce the inflammation, and special exercises may help to alleviate the condition. In cases where nerve roots are compressed, surgery may be required. This may involve full or partial removal of the problem disk in order to prevent long-term nerve damage. Surgery has its risks, but in cases where there is a risk of severe nerve damage, it may be the best option. New procedures, in which the surgery is performed with lasers, may prove to be safer and more effective, but no definitive comparisons have been made as of yet.

> *Additional relevant information related to Disk Prolapse is in* BACK PAIN; DECOMPRESSION, SPINAL CANAL OR CORD; MRI; SPINAL INJURY; SPINAL NERVES; *and* SPINE. *Important related material also includes* PAIN RELIEF.

Dislocation, Joint

The displacement of two bones in a joint, so that they no longer touch each other.

Joint dislocation often occurs with an injury, usually a car accident, sports injury, or a fall. Tearing of ligaments and additional injury to the joint capsule may occur; one of the bones involved may fracture as well.

ALERT
Not For Beginners

Nonprofessionals should not try to pop the dislocated joints back into place. Unqualified people may not know how to avoid additional nerve damage and may not be able to tell if fractures are present. A splint or sling may be worn to restrict movement until a doctor is available to correctly reset the bones. In most cases, a physician will test to see if there are any additional fractures, then may simply manipulate the bones back into place. In extreme cases, surgery may be necessary to reposition the bones. Afterwards, a splint or cast may be fitted to restrict movement as the affected area heals.

Symptoms of joint dislocation include severe pain, lack of mobility, and swelling. Dislocation of one of the vertebrae can lead to paralysis. A shoulder or hip dislocation that injures surrounding nerves can also result in paralysis of the limb. *See also* NERVE INJURY; PARALYSIS; SLING; *and* SPLINT.

Diuretic Drugs

Medications that help the kidneys remove excess fluids and sodium.

By decreasing the blood's volume, diuretic drugs ease the workload of the heart and swelling caused by excess fluid throughout the body. Diuretic medications are used to treat high blood pressure, heart failure, kidney failure, and other conditions involving excess fluid accumulation. Diuretics were the first drugs to show that treatment of high blood pressure could reduce the risk of myocardial infarction and stroke.

Types. Thiazide diuretics act in the channels through which urine travels in the

Nutrition and Diuretics

A patient who is told to take a diuretic drug may also be told to change eating habits to reduce the severity of the side effects. Adding certain fruits and vegetables to the diet can help replace the potassium lost by diuretic action. A mineral supplement may be advised to help prevent other side effects.

kidneys (tubules). There are several thiazide diuretics, including chlorothiazide and hydrochlorothiazide. Thiazide diuretics are often the first prescribed.

There are also loop diuretics. These affect the loop of Henle, a structure within the kidneys. They may be prescribed when a patient does not respond well to a thiazide diuretic or when kidney function is inadequate. Loop diuretics include bumetanide and furosemide.

Potassium-sparing diuretics reduce the loss of potassium that can accompany diuretic action. They are prescribed along with a thiazide diuretic or a loop diuretic to minimize this side effect.

Carbonic anhydrase inhibitor diuretics block an enzyme that helps to control the amount of bicarbonate ions in the blood. Their use is limited because they are active only for short periods. In contrast, osmotic diuretics are highly active. They are generally prescribed to maintain an adequate level of urine production after surgery or during recovery from an injury.

Risk Factors. Prolonged use of diuretic drugs will increase the risk for, or aggravate the effects of, some diseases. Because they increase the blood level of the waste product uric acid, some diuretics are associated with an increased risk of gout. Other drugs in this family can lead to higher levels of blood sugar, which has ill effects on those with diabetes.

Some men taking diuretics may experience impotence or gynecomastia (enlargement of the breasts). Excess loss of both potassium and magnesium resulting from diuretic treatment can cause muscle cramps, dizziness, and fatigue. As with all drug treatment, careful monitoring prevents such adverse side effects. *See also* BLOOD PRESSURE; KIDNEY; *and* STROKE.

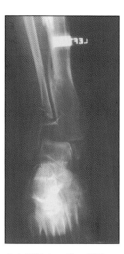

Joint Dislocation X Ray Imagery. Dislocations can be seen most clearly under the scrutiny that x-ray images offer. Due to the nature of dislocations, any more complex imaging techniques, such as MRIs or CAT scans, are usually excessive. Dislocations can be seen with or without contrast agents (radiopaque dyes that cause disorders to show up more clearly).

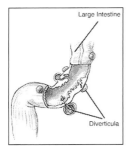

Diverticulosis. The sacks that form off of the side of the large intestine are of varying sizes. Even though this condition rarely cause any serious symptoms, it should always be diagnosed by a physician and treated.

Diverticular Disease

A disease resulting from formation of diverticula, small pouches in the inner lining of the intestine.

The occurrence of diverticula is directly associated with aging. For an 80-year-old American, there is roughly a 50 percent chance that diverticula are present in the intestinal tract, most likely in the lower part of the intestines. They form when parts of the intestines lose their ability to withstand the pressures of digestion, as contraction of the muscles around the colon causes slowed movement of the contents of the intestine. *See* Diverticulitis *and* Intestine.

Symptoms. Most people will not experience symptoms from diverticula. This symptom-free condition is called diverticulosis. In some cases, rectal bleeding will occur; if the bleeding is frequent, treatment such as the injection of an artery-constricting drug may be necessary. When there is rectal bleeding, tests are done to rule out the possibility of cancer.

In case of infection, one or more diverticula may become inflamed, causing a fever, pain, tenderness, and rigidity in part of the abdomen. In severe cases, an abscess or hole will form in the intestine. Material from the intestine can spill into the abdominal cavity, causing peritonitis, an inflammation that is a medical emergency. Sometimes diverticulitis results in the formation of a stricture, narrowing of the intestine, or a fistula, an abnormal channel between parts of the intestine.

Diagnosis. Diverticulosis can be diagnosed by views of the intestine obtained though barium x-ray examinations or from

---

Preventing Diverticular Disease

The risk of diverticular disease may be linked to a diet that is low in fiber. Eating fiber-rich foods such as whole grains, beans, fruits, and vegetables is advisable for older persons, not only for intestinal health but also for its beneficial effects against heart disease. Avoiding popcorn, nuts, and seeds, which can become lodged in the diverticula, is another preventive measure.

---

a fiberoptic instrument that lets a health care professional view the interior of the intestine (colonoscopy). *See* Barium X Ray.

Treatment. The first recommended treatment is usually bed rest, accompanied by antibiotic medication. If symptoms are severe, the patient will stop eating, with nutritional needs met by a liquid diet or intravenous fluids. This regimen can be continued for a few days or several weeks. If the symptoms do not go away, or if tests detect an abscess (fistula), surgery may be performed. *See also* Anal Fistula.

In many cases, it will be a two-part procedure. First, a temporary colostomy is performed, an operation to open the intestine through the abdominal wall. The diseased part of the intestine is then removed. Weeks or months later, the colostomy will be closed and the remaining sections of the colon will be connected. *See* Peritonitis.

Diverticulitis

The presence of multiple small pouches in the large intestine that are infected and inflamed.

Diverticulosis is a common condition in which small pouches develop in the lining of the large intestine. The cause is unknown, but is thought to be related to a low fiber diet. Diverticulitis results when one or more of these pouches become infected, usually from food or bacteria lodged in the pouches. The infection in turn may lead to the development of a small abscess or perforation in the colon. Symptoms include cramp-like pains on the left side of the abdomen, fever, and nausea. Attacks may recur. *See also* Diverticulosis.

Complications include the rupture of an inflamed diverticulum, causing the contents of the intestine to enter the abdominal cavity; this may result in peritonitis, which is an emergency situation. Internal bleeding may also occur.

Treatment for a mild case includes bed rest, stool softeners, a liquid diet, and antibiotics. In cases with complications, hospitalization is required for the administration of intravenous antibiotics. In severe, recurrent cases, surgical removal of the affected segment of the intestine (ileostomy or colostomy) may be required.

Diverticulosis

The development of multiple small pouches, called diverticula, in the wall of the large intestine. Alternatively, a single giant diverticulum.

Diverticulosis usually affects the lower portion of the large intestine when pouches form. When these pouches become inflamed, a condition known as diverticulitis results. The cause of diverticulosis is unknown, although it may be related to a low-fiber diet. The risk of developing diverticulosis increases with age. Most patients are over the age of 50, about half of people over age 80 have some of diverticulosis.

In the absence of inflammation there are usually no symptoms, so diverticulosis may go undetected. In some cases, gastrointestinal bleeding may occur. Barium enemas are often used to diagnosis this disorder; it may also be found during a colonscopy. In the absence of symptoms, treatment is unnecessary. Bleeding usually ceases on its own. Some physicians recommend a high-fiber diet to prevent diverticulosis and diverticulitis. *See also* INTESTINE.

Dizziness

A condition in which an individual feels a general sense of lightheadedness or that the surroundings are spinning around.

Dizziness is a symptom of a malfunction in the ear, along the nerve pathways, or in the brain itself. Dizziness can refer to either fainting or vertigo. Fainting is a classification of dizziness characterized by a sensation of grogginess, lightheadedness, queasiness, and nausea. Vertigo is a form of dizziness in which a person may feel as though the room is whirling about or that he or she is falling down. Vertigo may last for a few minutes or continue for a period of days. The condition may be improved by lying down flat. *See also* BALANCE.

Balance and Age

The sense of balance becomes less exact as we age. The greater incidence of falls among the elderly and an increase in brittleness in older bones can lead to serious injury. In addition, many prescribed drugs, such as sleeping pills and tranquilizers, actually increase the chances of the elderly losing their balance. Falls are responsible for more than half of accidental deaths among the elderly.

CAUSES

Most episodes of dizziness are innocuous. They can be caused by either a temporary reduction of the blood pressure to the brain or a change in the pressure of the fluid in the inner ear. This can be manifested when abruptly leaping out of bed or bending to pick up an item from the floor. Dizziness is also a side effect of anemia, epilepsy, heart trouble, blockage in the arteries that supply the brain, and inner ear disorder. Dizziness may be caused by malfunctioning balance-controlling organs located in the inner ear or along the nerve impulses traveling to the brain. Common causes for vertigo include:

- Bacterial infections;
- Viral infections;
- Brain tumors;
- Abnormal pressure;
- Nerve inflammation;
- Labyrinthitis (infection in the labyrinth, which controls balance in the ear);
- Ménière's disease (fluid in the labyrinth, increasing pressure);
- Motion sickness;
- Drugs, such as alcohol or tranquilizers;
- Multiple sclerosis.

TREATMENT

Episodes of dizziness usually pass by themselves; lying down may make a person less disoriented. Prolonged and repeated attacks of dizziness should be brought to the attention of a physician. Treatment then depends on diagnosing and treating the underlying cause. Drugs that may be effective in treating vertigo include meclizine, dimenhydrinate, and scopolamine. *See also* EAR; INFECTION; NERVE; *and* VERTIGO.

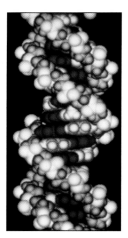

The Double Helix. First modeled by James Watson, Francis Crick, and the lesser known Maurice Wilkins, who won the Nobel Prize in 1962 for their work, DNA (as seen above) is now modeled with computer graphics that can clearly render the most basic component of all life on Earth.

Resources on DNA

Davies, Kevin, *Cracking the Genome: Inside the Race to Unlock Human DNA* (2001); Moore, Keith L., *Before We Are Born: Essentials of Embryology and Birth Defects* (1998); Alliance of Genetic Support Groups, Tel. (800) 336-GENE, Online: www.medhelp.org/geneticalliance; Easter Seals, Tel. (800) 221-6827, Online: www.seals.org; National Center for Biotechnology Information, Tel. (301) 496-2475, Online: www.ncbi.nih.gov; Office of Rare Diseases, Tel. (301) 402-4336, Online: rarediseases.info.nih.gov/org; http://www. med.cornell.edu/research/cores/genetherapy/index.html.

DNA

The abbreviation for deoxyribonucleic acid, the hereditary blueprint for the development and functioning of a living organism.

Shaped like a twisted rope ladder, or a double helix, DNA is found in the chromosomes in cell nuclei. It is one of two nucleic acids; the other one, ribonucleic acid, or RNA, helps transport, interpret, and carry out the genetic instructions provided by the DNA.

Sugar and phosphates form the two sides of DNA's double helix. Each "rung" of the double helix consists of a pair of the following chemicals: adenine, cytosine, guanine, and thymine. Called bases, these chemicals can be arranged in any sequence. The sequences are millions of bases in length and amount to the chemical code of operation for each and every one of a cell's numerous activities, from reproduction to cell repair. DNA is to life what letters are to written language.

The bases that form the rungs conform to strict pairing rules: adenine always pairs with thymine, and cytosine pairs with guanine. Thus one need only know one of the bases on the rung to know the identity of the other one. Different sections of DNA are called genes.

DNA pinpoints and directs the production of enzymes that control cell activity. Different genes determine which proteins are produced and how. RNA acts as a messenger that copies DNA; it migrates outside of the nucleus, and combines strings of amino acids to form a protein molecule. The type, amount, and rate of production of a protein is determined by the DNA blueprint.

Growth by cell division means that the DNA of the parent cell is copied into each of the resulting cells. This is achieved by the unzipping of DNA: the two sides of the rope ladder peel apart and each side is mated to a new side comprised of free-floating nucleotides in the cells. Two separate chains are born, identical to the original due to the conformity of parings.

The process goes on, with the DNA in the first and latest cell, and all those in between, remaining identical.

Sources for related information include HEREDITY; HERITABILITY; *and* INHERITANCE. *Closely related and highly relevant information can also be found in* GENE; GENETIC COUNSELING; GENETIC PROBE; GENETICS; *and* ONCOGENE.

DNR

Abbreviation for: do not resuscitate

The order that cardiopulmonary resuscitation should not be performed on a person should his or her heart or breathing stop.

Some patients in the advanced stages of illness complete a do-not-resuscitate order. DNR orders are advance directives that individuals provide their physicians to direct them through emergency situations. Usually appearing in the patient's chart, the DNR instructs nurses, emergency medical personnel, and hospital medical staff not to revive the patient in the event of cardiopulmonary arrest. The DNR applies to situations in which the patient experiences an acute problem of the heart or lungs that poses a threat to the person's life. To honor a DNR, medical personnel refrain from inserting tubes into the patient, from strong chest massage, or from any means to aid a patient who has stopped breathing. Medical workers also avoid using a defibrillation machine or chest compressions to reverse cardiac arrest. *See also* DEATH.

Legal Responsibilities and DNR

Choosing to sign a DNR order can be one of the hardest decisions an individual will ever have to make with the family. In order to ensure that last wishes and arrangements are fulfilled, it may be best to sign over the rights and power of attorney of a health care proxy to a trusted loved one. This is someone who will relay the dying individual's final wishes to health care professionals in the event that the patient should lose consciousness.

Further information about Do Not Resuscitate orders can be obtained from:

Partnership for Caring
475 Riverside Drive
New York, NY 10115 or partnershipforcaring.org

Doctor, Choosing a

The evaluation of and the selection of a physician.

There is more information available to the public than ever before on any given physician's background, specialties, and consultation style. Individuals and families should use this information to choose a physician based on their particular needs. The first step is to identify an appropriate health insurance plan and the healthcare providers whose costs are covered by that plan.

The American Medical Association (AMA) maintains a web site (www.ama-assn.org/aps) that lists doctors and the medical schools they attended. The web site also provides a Physician Select Service at no cost, availing users of any doctor's location, gender, medical school, graduation date, residency site and completion date, specialty, and board certification.

Board certification is recognition of a physician's competence in a particular field by a group of medical authorities called the American Board of Medical Specialties. ABMS certifies doctors in 24 specialties by offering exams to those who have completed a residency program. These "board-eligible" doctors become "board-certified" upon passing the exam. Those who have practiced for a long time but remain merely board-eligible may have failed the exam. There are also outstanding physicians who choose not to take the exam. To learn whether a particular doctor is board-certified, a prospective patient can call ABMS (1-800-776-CERT) or consult the ABMS Public Education web site (www.certifieddoctor.org/verify).

National medical education certification boards establish standard courses of study for all medical schools. Thus, doctors who attended medical school in the United States may receive a higher and more consistent education, owing to a high degree of curriculum monitoring, than those in other countries. However, it is not guaranteed that each individual doctor performed well in medical school; a more reliable measure of academic performance is whether a doctor trained in residency, which is typically selective and intensive.

Most malpractice suits are either thrown out of court as frivolous or defeated. However, doctors with a history of finding themselves in court should be thoroughly researched and evaluated. State insurance departments, licensing boards, and a web site (www.docboard.org) can provide relevant information about malpractice.

Physicians affiliated with reputable hospitals are often exemplary, since hospitals select doctors who are the best in their field. By choosing such a physician, a person will have access to the same hospital should the need for hospitalization arise.

A doctor on staff at a hospital is exposed to the experiences and ideas of highly qualified colleagues, medical teams, and state-of-the-art equipment, all of which make him a better doctor. A doctor's personal attributes may be important to prospective patients; others may place a higher priority on a doctor's skills.

> *Background information about Choosing a Doctor can be found in* AMERICAN MEDICAL ASSOCIATION; HOSPITAL; MEDICARE; MEDICAID; NIH; *and* PUBLIC HEALTH. *Related materials can be found in* ETHICS *and* MEDICAL TESTS. *Also refer to* NURSE; *and* NURSE, HOME CARE.

Dogs, Diseases from

Human diseases contracted from contact with a dog.

There are many canine diseases that are transmittable to humans through airborne contagions, from physical contact with the animal, or from injuries that result from contact with the animal. Dogs can transmit certain parasites, fungi, viruses, bacteria, and other airborne contagions.

How Diseases are Transmitted. Several diseases are transmitted from dogs to humans. Dog dander inflames allergies in some people and asthmatic individuals may have a severe reaction to it. Numerous parasites from dogs can infect people, and children are especially prone to such infections. *See also* PARASITE.

The most common, and perhaps most dangerous, parasite that can be transmitted from dogs to people is a type of tapeworm that creates cysts in the human body. Roundworms are another transmittable parasite that comes from dogs. Scabies, a mite infestation that causes redness and itching, can also be passed along to people.

Contact with a dog or waste products presents a risk of infection or disease. Weil's disease can infect humans who come into contact with dog urine. The bacteria enters the human body through the mucous membranes and cause soreness, redness, and bruises. Weil's disease is fatal in 10 percent of cases.

The most common serious illness transmitted from dogs to humans is rabies. Rabies is a viral disease that can affect all warm-blooded animals. It is transmitted through the saliva of affected animals, and thus it can pass from dogs to human beings through a bite or scratch. Though there is a vaccine for rabies, there is no cure once the disease is contracted.

PREVENTION

To prevent the transmission of diseases from dogs to humans, both dog and owner should have all the appropriate vaccinations. After handling dog feces or urine, hands should be washed thoroughly with soap and water. At-risk individuals (such as pregnant women or individuals who are HIV-positive) should always wash their hands carefully after contact with dogs. At-risk owners should take extra measures to ensure that their dog is clean and healthy.

TREATMENT

The site of any wound inflicted by a dog should be cleaned carefully, and the affected individual should receive any needed vaccinations. If bacterial infection is suspected, a doctor may prescribe an antibiotic medication.

Essential topics discussed elsewhere related to Diseases From Dogs include ALLERGY; RABIES; SNAKEBITES; SPIDER BITES; STINGS; *and* VENOMOUS BITES AND STINGS. *See also* BLEEDING, TREATMENT OF; TRAUMA; *and* WOUND.

Donor

An individual who donates a body organ or substance to help treat others.

A donor is any individual who donates an organ, body fluid, or other bodily substance to treat a sick person who may be someone the donor knows personally or an anonymous patient in another part of the country. Donors often contribute blood, bone marrow, or a body organ. All a person needs to do in order to become an organ-donor is to designate it on a driver's license or carry an organ-donor card. Every day 60 people receive organ transplants that either save or extend their lives and 17 die on waiting lists because there are not enough organs, blood, or tissue available.

The term donor usually refers to organ-donors. There are three types of donors: living donors (living people who donate organs or tissue such as bone marrow, kidney, liver, or lung), brain-dead donors, and non-heartbeating donors; the last are cases of circulatory death. Each type has to fulfill specific medical criteria in order to be eligible to donate. Donors may specify which organs they wish to donate. Tens of thousands of people benefit from organ-donations every year. *See also* ORGAN DONATION.

Dose

Amount of a medication taken at any one time.

When a person takes a medication, its effectiveness and the severity of its side effects depend on the drug's concentration in the bloodstream. This is why prescriptions are held to exacting standards.

Sometimes, the medication works for a limited period of time and then is absorbed or eliminated by normal body processes. Alternatively, the medication's concentration may need to be maintained for a long period of time or even indefinitely. Generally, a balance must be maintained, so that there is enough of a drug for it to be effective, but not so much that the side effects outweigh the benefits.

Determining dosage can sometimes be difficult, as humans come in all sizes and weights, from a few ounces for a premature infant to several hundred pounds for a large adult. Further, different metabolism rates in different people lead to different dosage levels. It is critically important that a patient make his or her feelings and physical responses known to the prescribing physician, so that proper dosage may be determined. *See also* ANTIBIOTIC DRUGS; METABOLISM; *and* PREMEIDCATION.

Double Vision

Also known as diplopia

The sensation of seeing two images of everything in the visual field.

When the eyes are working properly, an individual sees a single 3-dimentional image of the world; this is called stereovision. The brain filters and interprets information about the visual field from both eyes to make one image. This also allows an individual to perceive depth. However, when there is a disorder in either eye, in the pathways that transport information about the visual field from the eyes to the brain, or in the image processing function of the brain, then double vision may be the result.

Types. There are two principal types of double vision: monocular and binocular. Monocular double vision is often due to a disorder in one eye. If one eye is covered and the visual field is double, then the disorder is probably within the eye itself. The person could be suffering symptoms associated with astigmatism from an abnormality in the lens, retna, cornea, or a cataract.

Binocular double vision usually has a neurological basis or is associated with defects related to a misalignment of the eyes—this is similar to symptoms associated with crossed eyes. If one eye is covered and the double vision is relieved then the particular case of double vision is binocular.

Treatment. Usually, double vision is not a disorder in itself, so it can be alleviated by treating underlying ailments. Trauma to the head, myasthenia gravis, multiple sclerosis, nerve palsy, or a brain tumor may need to be treated before double vision disappears. Glasses with the proper corrective prism may treat some cases, while surgery on the muscles that control the eyes may correct vision in others. *See also* BLURRED VISION; TUNNEL VISION; *and* VISION.

Douche

A method used to rinse out the vaginal canal, either for cleanliness or as an extremely ineffective means of birth control.

Douching is not necessary for either health or normal cleanliness. The body's own secretions are sufficient when coupled with regular bathing. In terms of health, douching may actually be harmful, as it can result in forcing bacteria farther up the vagina, promoting infection.

As a method of birth control, douching immediately after intercourse is an attempt to flush semen out of the vagina. This may be too late, as sperm may have already traveled beyond the point where douching can reach. In some cases, douching may actually help propel the sperm easily travels up the reproductive tract. Douching is not an effective preventive measure against sexually transmitted disease.

If an individual feels that it is necessary to douche, use either plain water or a very diluted vinegar solution. Commercial hygiene products may contain chemicals that act as irritants. In some cases, these products may cause inflammation, various degrees of allergic reactions, or even excessive dryness. *See also* D AND C.

It is recommended that women not douche under the following four circumstances:
- during pregnancy;
- within six weeks of giving birth;
- within two weeks of a D&C, an abortion, or an IVF retrieval; and
- 24 hours before a pelvic exam.

The rationale for not douching under the first three circumstances is to guard against infection, and in the last it is so as to not wash away any secretions that are vital to make an accurate diagnosis. *See* VAGINA.

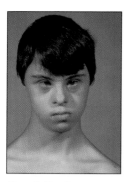

Down's Syndrome.
Down's Syndrome is named for John Langdon Down, the British doctor who first identified the condition in the middle of the 19th century. The chromosomal abnormalities were not discovered until 1959, when they were identified by Dr. Jerome Lejeune and Dr. Patricia Jacobs. There are three different types of Down's syndrome; the most prevalent being trisomy 21 (three copies of the 21st chromosome); translocation Down's syndrome is much rarer—it causes a part of the 21st chromosome to attach to another chromosome. About half of all cases of Down's syndrome show signs of mosaicism—a condition in which some, but not all, cells have an extra copy of chromosome 21.

Down's Syndrome

Also known as trisomy 21

A chromosomal disorder resulting in varying levels of mental retardation and characteristic physical features.

Down's syndrome is caused by an extra copy of chromosome number 21. In most cases, the presence of an extra non-sex chromosome (trisomy) is fatal within the first year. Children born with Down's syndrome, however, usually live into their 30s or 40s.

Down's syndrome occurs approximately once in every 600 to 800 births. The chance of giving birth to a child with this condition rises with age. For a 25-year-old woman, the chances are about 1 in 1205, but for a woman who is 35 years old, the probability rises to about 1 in 365.

Some of the characteristics of Down's syndrome include:

- delayed physical and mental development;
- mental retardation;
- small head;
- broad face with slanting eyes;
- large, prominent tongue; and
- a single crease across the palm of the hand.

Thirty five percent of individuals with this syndrome have heart defects as well. These can be surgically repaired.

Down's Syndrome in the Family. Children with Down's syndrome tend to be extremely good-natured and loving. There are different degrees of Down's syndrome, depending on whether there is an entire extra copy of the chromosome present or just a segment. Many individuals with Down's syndrome may function relatively well. *See also* CHROMOSOME *and* DNA.

DPT Vaccination

A combined immunization against the diseases diphtheria, pertussis (whooping cough), and tetanus.

The DPT vaccination is administered as a series of five shots, beginning when a child is two months old and ending prior to the his or her entrance into school. Some children may have a reaction to the shot, in which case no further injections should be given. The vaccine is usually not administered to children past the age of six.

This series of shots prevents three serious diseases in the vaccinated individual:

Diphtheria. Diphtheria is now an extremely rare disease in the United States, owing to the intensive vaccination program. This disease is caused by the bacterium *Corynebacterium diphtheriae* and easily treated with antibiotics; however, if complications develop, it can be a serious disease. A booster shot, usually in combination with one for tetanus, should be given every ten years. *See also* ANTIBIOTIC DRUGS.

Pertussis. Pertussis can be mistaken for a common cold in its early stages, prior to the development of the characteristic cough, the whooping cough. Breathing difficulties may occur; if they are severe this can deprive the brain of oxygen. If a child's lips turn blue, emergency medical help should be sought, because pertussis is highly contagious.

Tetanus. Tetanus, also known as lockjaw, can cause muscle spasms and eventually affect breathing. It is a disease that is often fatal. Once the initial immunization series is completed, a booster shot should be given every ten years.

In recent years, the DPT vaccination has been replaced by what is known as the tetramune shot, consisting of the vaccinations for diphtheria, pertussis, and tetanus, as well as a fourth agent against bacterial meningitis, which is caused by a bacteria called *Haemophilus influenzae* Type B. The HiB immunization, which prevents bacterial meningitis, and which used to be administered as a single shot at the age of 18 months or two years, is now included in the DPT vaccination.

Articles related to DPT Vaccination include IMMUNITY; PUBLIC HEALTH; *and* VACCINATIONS. *Entries about the diseases that this vaccination prevents are included in* DIPHTHERIA; PERTUSSIS; *and* TETANUS. *Other related information is included in* BACTERIA; MENINGITIS; *and* MUSCLE.

Drain, Surgical

A tubular apparatus inserted into a wound or body cavity to permit drainage of secretions.

The three main types of surgical drains are the Penrose drain, the Jackson-Pratt drain, and the Hemovac drain.

The Penrose drain is the simplest and is used for small quantities of drainage. It usually consists of a somewhat flattened, thin rubber tube passed from a body cavity into a dressing. The Penrose drain has no collection device, so the dressing has to be changed periodically.

The Jackson-Pratt drain is an airtight, closed-drainage system with tubing attached to a plastic suction bulb for an above-average amount of drainage. The end inserted into the wound has small holes along the sides to facilitate drainage from the site.

The Hemovac is similar to the Jackson-Pratt drain except that its tubing is attached to a large cylindrical collection device that can hold a larger amount of drainage.

Another type of drain is T-shaped and is used to remove bile from the biliary system (gallbladder and ducts) after surgery. The T-shape holds it in place. Drainage fluid that is odorous and yellow or blue-green is usually a sign of infection and requires treatment. *See also* BILE; BILIARY SYSTEM; *and* GALLBLADDER.

Dreaming

The imagining of sensory stimuli during sleep.

Dreaming is a mental activity in which a sleeping person imagines sights, sounds, events, and other stimuli. Dreams often seem to be real when they are taking place. They are usually based on the dreamer's daily experiences, although time, logic, and objects are distorted.

REM Sleep. Scientific research indicates that dreaming occurs during REM (rapid eye movement) sleep. Brain waves as measured on an electronencephalograph are usually large and slow throughout the night. During REM sleep, brain waves are much more active and the eyes move rapidly. The body, however, does not move during a period of REM sleep because the pathways that carry nerve impulses from the brain to the muscles are blocked. In adults, REM sleep usually occurs for about 20 minutes three to five times a night; children dream more frequently. If a person is awakened during REM sleep, he or she usually remembers the particulars of the interrupted dream.

Why we dream remains a matter of debate. For psychoanalysts, dreams "speak" in the symbolic language of the unconscious mind. They may not make logical sense and cannot be taken as literal messages. In a dream, for example, an animal may represent a person, or a person may represent several people with a similar characteristic in the mind of the dreamer.

What the symbols and images in a dream mean depend on an individual's life associations. Psychiatrists and psychoanalysts often use dream analysis as a means of understanding the unconscious. By listening attentively to a dream and by helping the dreamer make the associations, it is possible to unearth meanings embedded beneath the dream's surface.

Most psychiatrists maintain that dreams are meaningful and even necessary for healthy psychological functioning. Similarly, the neurological and physiological activities that occur during REM sleep seem to indicate that this is a period when the brain and body are being refreshed for further activity.

Nightmares are peculiar, often frightening dreams that appear more often during periods of stress, alcohol consumption, and fever. A child who experiences a nightmare may awaken with exact details of the dream. Nightmares are common in three- to four-year-olds who are still learning to differentiate between fantasy and reality.

> *See* PSYCHIATRY *and* SLEEP *for fundamental material on dreaming. For additional information, see* NIGHTMARE *and* NIGHT TERROR. *Related material is available in* ELECTROENCEPHALOGRAM; PSYCHOTHERAPY; *and* SLEEP WALKING.

Resources on Sleep and Dreaming

Borbely, Alexander, Secrets of Sleep (1986); Carskadon, Mary A., ed., Encyclopedia of Sleep (1993); Gackenbach, Jayne, Sleep and Dreams (1986); Hobson, J. A., Sleep (1995); National Sleep Foundation, Tel. (202) 347-3471, Online: www.sleepfoundation.org; American Academy of Sleep Medicine, Tel. (507) 287-6006, Online: www.aasmnet.org; www.nycornell.org/psychiatry/.

Dressing

Protective coverings placed on wounds.

Dressings are used to control bleeding and aid the healing process by absorbing secretions and preventing contamination by bacteria. Sterile, absorbent dressings are placed directly over wounds to promote dryness and thereby discourage growth of microorganisms. The dressing should be left undisturbed unless the wound needs to be cleaned.

TYPES

Types of dressings include adhesive and elastic bandages, gauze, butterfly bandages, roller gauze bandages, and circular bandages. In emergency situations, clean, absorbent materials such as clean handkerchiefs and sheets can be used as substitute dressings.

Gauze can be placed directly on a wound and is made either of cotton (woven or nonwoven) or a synthetic material. It is held in place by a bandage, by adhesive strips or by first-aid tape. The commonly used Band-Aid® is a smaller, name-brand variation of this gauze-and-adhesive strip configuration. Gauze is usually applied dry, but sometimes contains a substance to promote regrowth of tissue in a deep wound.

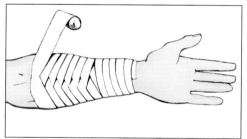

Dressings.
Dressings are used to protect wounds from infection and to stop bleeding. Above, an injured arm is wrapped in a bandage.

Alginate dressings, derived from brown seaweed, are a relatively new form of dressing used mostly for moderate to high exuding wounds. They form a gel capable of absorbing up to 20 times its weight in fluid. An innovative blood-clotting fibrin bandage, made of natural proteins, is currently being tested by the American Red Cross and the U.S. Army.

Background material on dressing may be found in FIRST AID *and* WOUND. *Addition information is contained in* BANDAGE; GAUZE; *and* SURGERY. *Related material is available in* BACTERIA; BLEEDING, TREATMENT OF; EMERGENCY, FIRST STEPS; *and* MICROORGANISM.

Drooling

The slow seepage of saliva from the mouth.

All babies drool to some degree, and drooling may become particularly heavy during bouts of intense teething. If copious amounts are produced and allowed prolonged contact with the skin, a rash may result around the mouth and chin. This will disappear on its own if the skin is kept as dry as possible. Some parents find bibs useful in protecting clothing.

Drooling eventually ends, usually by the child's second year. Any concern about seemingly excessive or prolonged drooling should be reported to the doctor, as drooling in older children and adults can be a symptom of neurological problems.

Drooling during sleep is, however, quite normal, especially if the person is very tired and prone to sleeping deeply. *See* SALIVA.

Dropsy

Accumulation of fluid in the ligaments or tissues of the body, currently called edema.

The term dropsy was first used in the Middle Ages to describe a number of different diseases characterized by swelling of the abdomen or ankles. Now, researchers attribute any abnormal swelling in the body's tissues to a buildup of a clear watery fluid referred to as edema. This fluid may accumulate in many parts of the body, particularly in the legs, abdomen or chest, face, eyes, or fingers. The term dropsy is now generally considered outdated.

Causes. Edema can be caused by heart failure, high blood pressure, medication, malnutrition, kidney and liver disease, and many other diseases. For example, Cushing's syndrome is a disorder of the adrenal glands that causes fluid retention in many parts of the body, especially the legs, and abdomen. Many liver diseases, like cirrhosis, fatty liver, and hepatitis, exhibit abdominal or leg swelling as a primary symptom. *See also* CIRRHOSIS; CUSHING'S SYNDROME; HEART FAILURE; HEPATITIS; *and* SWELLING.

Drowning

Death by suffocation in water or some other fluid.

When a person is subjected to prolonged immersion in water, death can be caused by suffocation and a lack of oxygen (hypoxia). Drowning can occur in two ways. In one instance, a person inhales liquid into the lungs. In the other, no liquid enters lungs, as the water is instead diverted into the stomach. In these cases, the drowning death is completely caused by oxygen deprivation; this is referred to as dry drowning. Near-drowning describes an event in which a drowning victim is resuscitated back to life. Drowning is the third leading cause of accidental death in the United States, following auto accidents and falls.

A large majority of drowning victims are capable swimmers who underestimate the dangers of undertow, fatigue, and panic. In contrast, nonswimmers tend to act with caution and comprise a small number of drowning victims. Other drowning cases occur due to very specific conditions, such as floods, capsizing, falling through ice, or infant drownings.

More than a third of all drowning accidents involve alcohol consumption. There are many physiological reactions to alcohol consumption that may be problematic in drowning incidents. The major problem, however, is that alcohol impairs both judgement and physical coordination, thereby greatly increasing the likelihood of a drowning death.

PROCESS
In the first moments of drowning, an automatic protective reflex is triggered and a muscle at the entrance of the windpipe tightens to direct water to the stomach, rather than the lungs. But this esophageal reflex also interferes with normal breathing, which can lead to a lack of oxygen in the blood that causes loss of consciousness. Dry drowning occurs when a person has a particularly strong esophageal reflex that cuts off their oxygen supply. In this instance, the person drowns from lack of oxy-

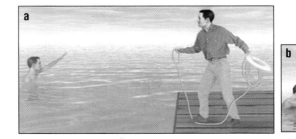

gen, even if only little or no water has entered the lungs.

RESCUE
The best help for a drowning person comes from a trained lifeguard, since a panicking swimmer can pull an untrained rescuer down. The person in danger should be given something—a rope, a large floating object, the end of an oar—to hold onto while the rescuer gets him or her ashore or into a boat.

Once the victim is on a firm surface, the rescuer should immediately check for the presence of breathing and a pulse. It is important to remember that even a swimmer who has suffered cardiac arrest can sometimes be revived. Artificial ventilation or cardiopulmonary resuscitation (CPR) should be provided as needed. If a phone is available, 911 should be called and emergency services contacted. It is essential that all victims of drowning or near-drowning be transported to an emergency department for further evaluation.

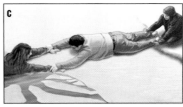

Drowning Assistance. There are several methods one can use when trying to rescue a drowning victim. (a) if available, toss a floating object to the drowning victim to keep him or her afloat until help arrives. Otherwise, try to offer an object such as a board, pole, or stick (b) to the victim and attempt to pull him or her out of the water. One should not place oneself at risk when rescuing a drowning victim, but as a last resort the human chain method (c) may be attempted.

Spinal Cord Damage
Divers rescued from drowning in shallow water or surf might also be victims of spinal cord damage if they slipped and hit their head on a hard surface, or if the strength of the surf tossed them onto the floor of the ocean, resulting in head or neck injury. If a spinal cord injury is suspected, the swimmer should be moved as little as is necessary to restore breathing and should be kept still until medical assistance arrives.

Background material on DROWNING *may be found in* ACCIDENTS *and* SUFFOCATION. *For further information see* CARDIOPULMONARY RESUSCITATOIN; EMERGENCY, FIRST STEPS OF; *and* OXYGEN. *Related material is available in* ALCOHOL INTOXICATION *and* SPINAL CORD.

Drowsiness

The state between wakefulness and sleep.

Drowsiness occurs normally when a person is tired, but excessive or otherwise abnormal drowsiness indicates an underlying health problem that requires the attention of a physician.

The main causes for drowsiness are self-induced sleep deprivation, medication, and sleep disorders. Drowsiness may also be attributed to:

- a head injury;
- high fever;
- narcolepsy (a tendency to fall asleep during normal waking activities);
- meningitis (inflammation of the membranes of the brain and spinal cord);
- liver failure;
- kidney failure (uremia);
- encephalitis (viral inflammation of the brain).

If a person is persistently drowsy and will not become alert in response to strong stimuli, such as loud noises or pinching, the situation should be treated as a medical emergency. *See also* SLEEP APNEA.

Drug

Any substance introduced into the body that changes the way it functions.

Throughout history, humans have used plant and animal products to change their thought processes, heal sickness, and relieve pain. Today drugs play so much a part of people's everyday lives that it is difficult to conceive of a time when they were not as readily available. Their functions vary widely. A drug may be used to relieve pain or swelling, unclog an artery obstructed with a blood clot, control the effects of schizophrenia, or kill cells carrying viruses.

TYPES OF DRUGS

Drugs may be divided into three categories: over-the counter; prescription; and illegal.

Over-the-counter drugs are considered safe for general use and are available without a prescription. They are used mainly to treat minor pain and illnesses. Over-the-counter drugs include drugs like aspirin, antacids, antihistamines, and ibuprofen.

Prescription drugs require the supervision of a physician to be used safely. They are generally more potent and can treat more serious diseases. They include such drugs as antibiotics, anticoagulants, and chemotherapy drugs.

Illegal drugs are not approved for clinical use and are generally used for nonmedical purposes. They include LSD, cocaine, heroin, and marijuana (although some states have begun to approve of the prescribed use of marijuana to control the side effects of chemotherapy, glaucoma, and AIDS treatment). Possessing or selling illegal drugs is against the law and may result in fines or a jail sentence.

Most legitimate drugs have at least three names, and some have more. The chemical name describes the drug's chemical make-up in detail, but it is usually so long and complex that only a specialist can remember it. The generic name is given by the United States Adopted Name Council and is generally used to identify the drug. Acetominophen is an example of a generic name. Proprietary names are given by drug manufacturers. They are intended to be memorable and link the drug with the company that manufactures it. Tylenol®, for example, is the proprietary name for acetominophen.

NEW DRUGS

Drug manufacturers submit new formulations to the Food and Drug Administration for approval. This is a lengthy and expensive process, involving many tests to prove the safety and efficacy of the drug. If approved, the drug manufacturer receives a patent, giving it the exclusive right to manufacture and sell the drug for a specific purpose for a period of 17 years. After the patent has expired, the drug can be manufactured by other drug companies. These generic versions are generally less expensive than the original but are of exactly the same chemical structure.

HOW A DRUG WORKS

Generally, drugs work by stimulating the natural processes of the body either to speed them up or to slow them down. For example, dilantin is administered to control seizures. It works by slowing the production of certain brain chemicals that cause seizures. The drug itself does not stop them; rather, it alters the body's chemical processes, so that the brain does not produce a condition that triggers seizures.

SIDE EFFECTS

When a drug enters the bloodstream, it is carried throughout the body, not just to the site of the problem. This means that the drug may cause effects other than those intended. Side effects generally are unpleasant and unwanted, although the benefits of certain drugs tend to outweigh the resulting discomfort. In chemotherapy, anticancer drugs work to kill cancer cells, but, they upset the stomach, producing nausea and vomiting. Many people are willing to endure the effects of anticancer drugs in the hope that they may rid their body of cancer cells. Other patients may instead seek unconventional therapies to avoid the intolerable discomforts.

Certain drugs may cause allergic reactions ranging from a mild rash to severe anaphylactic shock, a potentially life-threatening reaction in which breathing is impaired and a person may lose consciousness. In the case of severe allergies, drugs should not be administered.

DRUG INTERACTIONS

Each drug may, by itself, be entirely benign and produce the desired result, but when mixed with other drugs, the combination is capable of producing an entirely different response. Sometimes the interaction may be dangerous and even life threatening. Some drug interactions may actually help achieve a desired result. To avoid potentially dangerous interactions, a person should inform a physician of all the drugs he or she is taking—over-the-counter, prescribed, and illegal—before a new prescription is issued.

COMPLIANCE

An interesting and often neglected aspect of drug prescription is that as many as 50 percent of all people who are prescribed drugs do not take them as directed. This is referred to as the compliance problem, and it may be attributed to a number of different causes. Some people are forgetful, particularly when the drug has proven ineffective. Others consider it unnecessary to take the drug once they begin feeling better, believing that the drug has repaired their problem. Discontinuing use of a drug may be harmful, however, and often results in a relapse.

Many patients are concerned that they will become addicted to their medication, although studies have shown that even the most addictive drugs, like morphine, have relatively mild withdrawal effects if a person uses them as prescribed and is motivated to stop using the drugs when finished with the prescription. For a drug to work effectively, it must be taken only as prescribed and for the recommended duration.

Liver Function and Aging

Liver function declines with age, and because the liver does most of the metabolizing and modifying of the chemicals and nutrients that move through the digestive system, sensitivity to drugs increases with age. Any compromise of liver function means a drug will remain longer and in higher concentrations in the bloodstream. Also, there are proteins in the blood—which also become fewer with age—that bind to drugs and thus prevent them from affecting the body. Thus, as people age, the concentration of a drug in the bloodstream increases, as does the percentage of unbound drug. Thus, those over fifty are likely to be more sensitive and react more strongly to drugs than younger people. Given the slower elimination of drugs from the system, the chemicals will remain in the body longer.

See DRUG DEPENDENCE; DRUG OVERDOSE; DRUG POISONING; NARCOTICS; *and* PRESCRIPTION *for information directly relating to drugs. Additional information is contained in* BARBITURATE DRUGS; MARIJUANA; NICOTINE; OPIATE; *and* STIMULANT DRUGS. *Related information is contained in* FOOD AND DRUG ADMINISTRATION.

Resources on Drugs
Hardman, Joel G. and Lee E. Limbird, eds., *Goodman and Gilman's The Pharmacological Basis of Therapeutics* (1996); Hobson, J. Allan, *The Dream Drugstore: Chemically Altered States of Consciousness* (2001); Griffith, H. Winter, *Complete Guide to Prescription and Non-Prescription Drugs* (1992); Temin, Peter, *Taking Your Medicine* (1980); Winter, Ruth, *A Consumer's Dictionary of Household, Yard, and Office Chemicals* (1992); American Pharmaceutical Association, Tel. (202) 628-4410, Online: www. aphanet.org; American Association of Colleges of Pharmacy, Tel. (703) 739-2330, Online: www. aacp.org; American Association of Pharmaceutical Scientists, Tel. (703) 243-2800, Online: www.aapspharmaceutica.com;www w.nycornell.org/medicine /pharmacology/index.html

Drug Dependence

The craving of a drug to produce a desired effect or to prevent the uncomfortable effects of withdrawal.

Drug dependence is the compulsion to use a drug, particularly to produce certain desired effects, despite the presence of any number of social, medical, or psychological risks accompanying its usage. Dependence reflects an unhealthy psychological or, in some cases, a physical need to continue using a drug despite its harmful effects.

CAUSES

A number of factors contribute to the likelihood of an individual becoming drug dependent: genetic predisposition; peer pressure; the need to relieve stress or discomfort; mood-enhancing pleasure. In some cases, use of a drug may be a form of self-medication; for example, a person with an undiagnosed and untreated anxiety disorder may use marijuana regularly for its calming effect.

Continued use or abuse of drugs often leads to dependence. In the case of physically addictive drugs, an individual begins to require increasingly greater amounts of the substance to achieve the same effect (referred to as tolerance). Eventually the person's body becomes so accustomed to the drug that ceasing use causes symptoms of withdrawal. An addict will continue to use the drug to avoid this physical discomfort. In the case of less physically addictive drugs (such as marijuana), emotional dependence—a reliance on the feeling the drug produces—may be the primary motivator for continued use, despite social, psychological, and financial burdens.

TREATMENT

The first step in treating any type of substance abuse is recognition and admission of the problem. In cases where an individual has developed tolerance and will experience withdrawal symptoms, intake of the drug should be stopped, and it is necessary for that person to go through a period of detoxification. Sudden withdrawal from a physically addictive drug, such as alcohol or opioids, can produce life-threatening symptoms, such as: severe vomiting; drop in blood pressure; tremors; headaches; and hallucinations. During a detoxification treatment program, intake of a drug will be systematically decreased, often in a super-

Drug Dependence

Drug Type	Effects	Indications of Use	Long-Term Effects
Opiates (heroin, opium, morphine, methadone, codeine)	Eases physical and mental pain; produces feeling of euphoria.	Constricted and dilated pupils; weight loss; slurred speech; mood swings; needle needle marks; anxiety.	Absence of menses; respiratory failure; Risk of HIV or hepatitis from an infected needle; coma.
Stimulants (amphetamines, crack cocaine, ecstasy)	Accelerated physical and mental states; rapid heartbeat; physical dependence (cocaine).	Dilated pupils; trembling; sweating; fever; high blood pressure; insomnia.	Weight loss; hallucinations; paranoia; psychosis; heart attack; stroke; hemorrhage; coma.
Depressants (tranquilizers, inhalants)	Sedative; lethargy; drowsiness; mood swings; physical dependence.	Lack of alertness; coordination problems; suicidal behavior.	Anxiety; insomnia; weakness; memory impairment; paranoia; respiratory arrest; coma; death.
Hallucinogens (LSD, PCP, mescaline)	Hallucinations (positive or or negative); anxiety; paranoia.	Dilated pupils; trembling; sweating; chills; fever.	Psychosis; panic attacks; schizophrenia; hallucinations.
Marijuana (hashish)	Lack of motivation; heightened perception; relaxation.	Bloodshot eyes; dilated pupils; lack of energy; memory problems.	Impaired immune response; respiratory disease; lung cancer.

vised, hospital setting. Most treatment centers aim to provide a supportive and open environment to help patients come to terms with their addiction.

Cigarettes. To give up cigarette smoking, a nicotine patch may be used. This allows for a step-by-step reduction in the level of nicotine absorption into the bloodstream, while the individual breaks the habit of smoking itself. Nicotine gum and nasal spray work similarly. Non-nicotine treatments, namely hypnosis and anti-depressants, may also be beneficial.

A variety of other treatments are available to help a person recover from drug dependence; these include psychotherapy, group and behavior therapy, and a number of alternative medicine treatments. The goal of these therapies is to provide healthier environments and habits to replace the settings and activities that lead to addictive behavior.

> *See* DRUG *and* SUBSTANCE ABUSE *for basic information on drug dependence. For information on treatment, see* DRUG OVERDOSE; GROUP THERAPY; REHABILITATION; *and* WITHDRAWAL. *Related material is available in* MARIJUANA; NARCOTIC DRUGS; NICOTINE; OPIATE; *and* STIMULANT DRUGS.

Drug Overdose

> The accidental or deliberate ingestion of an excessive amount of a drug.

Deliberate and unintentional drug overdoses are leading causes of poisoning and death in the United States. The Food and Drug Administration decides which drugs are safe to be sold over the counter, which require a doctor's prescription, and which are illegal. Considerations for a given drug's safety include whether the drug can be harmful when taken by itself and whether it is habit-forming.

Legal drugs are usually safe when a recommended dosage is taken, but they can be dangerous if too much is consumed at once or if they are combined with other drugs. Some accidental medication overdoses occur because a patient believes that increasing the dosage will speed up or en-

hance the drug's effect. For patients prone to forgetfulness, the dosage should be written and highlighted on the label, so they can check it every time the medication is taken. Sometimes overdose occurs as a complication of kidney or liver malfunction, in which case the medication is not effectively processed and builds up in the bloodstream.

Illegal Drugs. The effects of illegal drugs vary; an overdose can often cause unpredictable reactions. Because such drugs do not have to pass any regulations before they are sold, users may expose themselves to illegal drugs that have been mixed together or diluted with potentially harmful substances.

Accidents. Children are at high risk for accidental drug overdose, because they may not realize what they are consuming. It is important to keep drugs out of childrens' reach and in childproof containers, as well as to educate older children about drug safety.

SIGNS OF A DRUG OVERDOSE

Indications of a drug overdose vary depending on the drug and the dosage. Symptoms include: abnormal breathing; slurred speech; lack of coordination; abnormal pulse rate; abnormal body temperature; enlarged or constricted pupils; sweating; drowsiness; convulsions; and hallucinations.

> ## Drugs and Age
> The elderly are particularly sensitive to drugs like barbiturates and benzodiazepines. Psychoactives and alcohol can lower the body temperature, and nonsteroidal anti-inflammatory drugs can cause gastrointestinal bleeding and kidney malfunction.

IN CASE OF AN EMERGENCY

If the victim is a child, his or her mouth should be checked for pills or other medication, which must be removed at once. If the victim is an adult and unconscious, make sure he or she is breathing. Act immediately if there is any sign of bluish coloring. The air passages should be checked

Resources on Barbiturate Drugs
Barchas, Jack D., *Biological Basis for Substance Abuse* (1993); Dupont, Robert L., *The Selfish Brain: Learning from Addiction* (1997); National Mental Health Association, Tel. (800) 969-NMHA, Online: www.nmha.org; www.ny-cornell.org/psychiatry/.

for obstructions. Opening the air passageways to allow the person to breathe is essential. This is done by pushing on the forehead while pulling the jaw upward. This is also good preparation in case the victim is still not breathing and needs mouth-to-mouth resuscitation (artificial respiration). In addition to the air passages, it is important to check breathing, temperature, and pulse. Cardiopulmonary resuscitation (CPR) should be administered if necessary.

A poison control center should be called immediately. Information about the specific drug ingested is vital to determining proper treatment. Vomiting should not be induced unless it is specifically advised by the poison control center or a qualified health professional.

If a victim is conscious and hallucinating, convulsing, or breathing slowly and shallowly, emergency medical help should be called. Do not administer anything by mouth. *See also* ACCIDENTS; DRUG; DRUG DEPENDENCE DRUG POISONING; EMERGENCY, FIRST STEPS *and* POISONING.

Drug Poisoning

The accidental or intentional overdose of over-the-counter, prescription, or illegal drugs.

Drug poisoning can occur in a variety of ways. Many medications can be deadly if taken in amounts greater than prescribed, or if combined with alcohol or other medications. Patients should inform a doctor of all chronic and short-term conditions and all prescription and over-the-counter medications being taken, including vitamins and supplements, herbs, laxatives, antibiotics, pain relievers, cold and allergy medicines, oral contraceptives, and antibiotics. Filling prescriptions at the same pharmacy reduces the possibility of dangerous medicinal reactions, as the pharmacist can identify negative drug interactions.

If drug poisoning is suspected, a poison control center should be called, even if no symptoms have appeared yet. The drug container should be on hand in order to read the ingredients to the poison control

ALERT

Precaution for Children

Children are extremely curious. All drugs should be kept out of their reach, as they are potential sources for poisoning. Vitamins and other supplements behave as drugs and can be dangerous, especially to children. Medications and vitamins should be kept in their original packaging and also put out of reach. The strengths of most medicines are calibrated for adults, and even a small amount can be toxic to a child. All medicine containers need to be childproof. Also, taking medication in front of children is not advised, as they like to mimic adult behavior.

center operator. It is thus recommended that medications be kept in their original packaging.

The operator will ask for a description of what was taken, the quantity, and how recently, and will also want to know the person's age and whether he or she is conscious or not, drowsy, vomiting, convulsing, or experiencing changes in body temperature or skin color.

Vomiting should not be induced unless directed by medical personnel. For such situations, it is wise to keep a bottle of ipecac syrup in the medicine cabinet, as well as activated charcoal, which is indicated for certain cases of poisoning, and which may be purchased at most pharmacies. Activated charcoal should be used only when advised by a physician.

If the victim loses consciousness, stops breathing, or is having convulsions, an ambulance should be called immediately.

See DRUG *and* POISONING *for basic information on drug poisoning. For further information see* ACCIDENTS; DRUG OVERDOSE; *and* EMERGENCY, FIRST STEPS. *Related material is available in* IPECAC; *and* VOMITING.

Dry Ice

Solid carbon dioxide used to destroy warts.

Carbon dioxide changes from a gas to a solid without going through a liquid phase. Dry ice is produced when carbon dioxide gas is kept under pressure and allowed to escape through a small nozzle. This cools the carbon dioxide to –95° F (–70° C). The dry ice is formed as a powder, then made into cakes when it is needed for use.

Dry ice is effective in the treatment of warts, plantar warts, and certain other benign growths. *See also* CRYOSURGERY.

Dry Skin

A skin irritation caused by a lack of moisture.

Dry skin is very common, especially in the elderly. It occurs most often in winter.

Symptoms of dry skin include cracked skin, which may have a scaly appearance, and round patches of irritated skin, most commonly found on the lower legs, arms, and thighs. The skin may also become irritated and inflamed.

Using a forced-air furnace increases the risk of dry skin because of the decrease in humidity it may produce in the home. To prevent dry skin, it is important to maintain moisture. Dry skin can be helped through the use of a humidifier. Changing bathing habits may also help. Short baths in lukewarm water are preferable, with minimal use of soap to the armpits, face, and genitals. The frequency of bathing should be reduced and a bath oil or moisturizer should be used. Moisturizers are best applied while the skin is still damp. If symptoms persist, a doctor should be consulted. *See also* DERMATITIS *and* ECZEMA.

Dry Socket

Severe pain at the site of a tooth extraction.

When a tooth is removed (extracted), the socket remains exposed. Usually the socket heals without incident, but in rare instances it can become very painful when proper healing does not occur, leaving the bone exposed. This is called a dry socket and is treated with a sedative, dressing or packing, plus pain medication, until the socket heals.

If infection of the socket is suspected, antibiotics may also be prescribed. *See also* BLOOD CLOTTING *and* EXTRACTION, DENTAL.

DSM IV

Abbreviation for Diagnostic and Statistical Manual of Mental Disorders, fourth edition

A publication that establishes definitions that set the standards for psychiatric diagnosis.

Published in 1994, by the American Psychiatric Association, the DSM IV describes the criteria for each currently recognized psychiatric disorder. In addition to listing symptoms and associated features of each disorder, the DSM describes how serious or extensive certain behaviors or symptoms must be to be considered an illness.

By defining disorders and setting standards for diagnosis, clinicians can use the DSM to classify illnesses and to begin selecting treatment options.

Background material on DSMIV may be found in DIAGNOSIS *and* PSYCHIATRY. *For further information, see* MENTAL ILLNESS; NEUROSIS; *and* PSYCHOSIS. *Related material is available in* PSYCHOANALYSIS *and* PSYCHOTHERAPY.

Duct Disease

Disease of a tubular body canal, often in the digestive system.

Duct disease is an inflammation, obstruction, infection, or other disorder relating to a duct. A duct is a tubular canal that often carries a glandular secretion (e.g., tears). Examples include bile-ducts in the digestive system, lacrimal (tear) ducts, or mammary (breast) ducts. There are a number of ducts found throughout the body.

Types. Duct disease often affects the bile-releasing ducts of the digestive system. Bile-duct disease is commonly an obstruction or inflammation of the bile-ducts, usually caused by gallstones (stones that form in the gallbladder). Tear ducts may also become obstructed, as can the mammary ducts, which are susceptible to multiple diseases, including breast cancer.

See BILIARY SYSTEM *and* DIGESTIVE SYSTEM *for basic information on duct disease. For additional information, see* BILE; GALLSTONE; *and* TEARS. *Related material is available in* BREAST CANCER; INFECTION; *and* INFLAMMATION.

Dumping Syndrome

A combination of gastrointestinal symptoms that result from partial or complete removal of the stomach.

In dumping syndrome, due to the reduced capacity of the stomach, food is passed through the stomach too rapidly and "dumped" into the small intestine. This results in a decrease in blood pressure shortly after eating (early dumping syndrome) or a drop in blood sugar two to three hours after eating (late dumping syndrome).

Symptoms. Symptoms include lightheadedness, sweating, abdominal discomfort, vomiting, and diarrhea after meals.

Treatment. Eating frequent small meals throughout the day and eliminating liquids at mealtime will lessen the severity of the symptoms. Recovery is usually spontaneous in a few months to a year, but symptoms may persist indefinitely. *See* STOMACH.

Duodenal Ulcer

A sore in the lining of the opening of the small intestine.

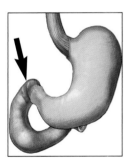

Duodenum.
Above, bacteria in the lining of the duodenum may result in a peptic ulcer.

Duodenal ulcers, which occur in the opening of the small intestine (duodenum), are the most common form of peptic ulcer. An ulcer is a round or oval sore in the lining of the stomach or duodenum. Frequently, ulcers are caused by the bacterium *Helicobacter pylori* (*H. pylori*) which, unlike most bacteria, thrives in the warm and highly acidic environment of the human stomach.

Most duodenal ulcers appear in people between the ages of 30 and 50; they are more common in men. Symptoms include belching, a feeling of being bloated, vomiting, and loss of appetite. Risk factors for peptic ulcers include the presence of *H. pylori* bacteria, smoking, and a family history of ulcers. Diagnosis usually involves a blood test that measures the antibodies of the bacterium in the blood, and possibly an endoscopy. A regimen of antibiotics and other medications will often eradicate the bacteria. *See* PEPTIC ULCER.

Duodenitis

An inflammation from unknown cause that affects the duodenum, the first part of the small intestine.

Patients with duodenitis exhibit only vague symptoms. Diagnosis is made with a fiber-optic viewing scope (gastroscopy), which is inserted in the mouth and fed through the esophagus and stomach. Instead of a well-defined ulcer, there is a diffuse area of inflammation, accompanied by redness and swelling of the lining. Contact of this area with the tip of the gastroscope often causes bleeding.

Treatment for duodenitis is similar to treatment for a duodenal ulcer. However, due to the lack of clear physical signs of the condition, it is still not certain if such treatment is truly effective. *See also* DUODENAL ULCER *and* INTESTINE.

Dupuytren's Contracture

A thickening and tightening of tissue beneath skin on the palm of hand.

Most common in the area of the ring fingers and little fingers, Dupuytren's contracture begins as a nodule in the connective tissue in the hand, which then spreads and forms a hard cord. First this reduces the movement of the fingers, then it causes them to curl inward. No single cause has been identified for Dupuytren's contracture; it may be more common in people who spend long periods of time tightly gripping tools, yet it also occurs in people with cirrhosis of the liver. It tends to run in families, but does not seem to be a hereditary disorder. The condition is most common in men over 40.

TREATMENT

Warm baths, exercise and splints may help, but as the condition worsens, surgery may be recommended. In this procedure, the bands that are constricting the hands are cut to free the tendons. Afterwards, physical therapy is recommended to help to restore movement to the hands.

Dust Disease

Also known as pneumoconiosis

An illness or injury resulting from the inhalation of dust particles.

Several types of lung disease are caused by persistent or severe inhalation of dust particles, particularly mineral or metallic dust. The names of dust diseases derive from the substances that produce them. The best known of these disorders are silicosis and asbestosis.

Silicosis results from breathing silica, or quartz dust, and causes severe coughing, fatigue, chest pains, and other symptoms. Asbestosis is a result of exposure to particles of asbestos, a fibrous material used for insulation. Exposure to asbestosis can cause shortness of breath, coughing, weight loss, and eventually lung cancer.

Prevention. Adequate ventilation, a constant supply of fresh air, and facial masks can help reduce the threat of airborne dust. People should not be regularly exposed to such hazards and those that are should have frequent medical examinations in order to detect dust-related illness early and prevent severe damage. *See also* ASBESTOSIS *and* SILICONE.

Dysarthria

Loss of speech due to nerve or muscle damage.

Dysarthria is the term that describes a loss of speech caused by a defect or injury to the actual muscles that convert sound into words. It may also refer to impaired functioning of the muscles and nerves that control the tongue and mouth.

A person suffering from dysarthria does not have any brain injury that has disrupted the speech center, nor is there any damage to the voice box (larynx) that would affect the ability to actually create sound. At times speech may be slow and slurred; for those who have suffered a stroke, one side of the face may sag owing to muscle paralysis on that particular side of the body. Drooling is also common in patients with dysarthria.

CAUSE

As its relationship to the actual mechanics of speech may suggest, dysarthria is often found in those suffering from degenerative diseases that affect the nerves. Parkinson's disease, Huntington's chorea, and multiple sclerosis can all cause dysarthria. Conditions that attack the nervous system in the brain, such as strokes or tumors, may also cause dysarthria, as may injuries to specific nerves, such as the hypoglossal nerve (the nerve that controls tongue movements). Mouth defects or injuries, such as a cleft palate, may also disrupt speaking ability. Children with cerebral palsy or other movement disorders, may be affected.

TREATMENT

There is no cure for dysarthria, unless surgery can correct any mechanical defects. In some cases, speech therapy may help. For a stroke victim, ongoing support and encouragement from family and friends is essential in order to assist the patient in the recovery process.

Background material on dysarthia may be found in MUSCLE; NERVE; *and* SPEECH DISORDERS. *For further information, see* CEREBRAL PALSY; DROOLING; HUNTINGTON'S CHOREA; HYPOGLOSSAL NERVE; LARYNX; MOUTH; PARKINSON'S DISEASE; SPEECH; STROKE; *and* TONGUE. *Related material on treatment is available in* SPEECH THERAPY.

Dyschondroplasia

The development of multiple tumors within bones of an infant.

Dyschondroplasia is a rare condition that is present at birth and can cause deformity of an arm or leg. The tumors associated with the condition arise from a congenital defect that interferes with the normal process by which bone develops from cartilage. The condition can be diagnosed with x-rays of the bones. In most cases, only one limb of the infant is affected. Failure of bone to develop properly causes the affected limb to be shorter in size than normal. *See also* BONE; BONE, DISORDERS OF; CONGENITAL; DEFORMITY; *and* TUMORS.

Dysentery

A disease characterized by inflammation of the intestines.

Dysentery refers to painful, often bloody bouts of diarrhea accompanied by abdominal pain. The two major types are amoebic dysentery, caused by a shapeless microscopic organism by the name of *Endamoeba histolytica*, and Sonne dysentery, which is caused by the *Shigella* bacteria.

In amoebic dysentery, the parasite infects the large intestine. Direct transmission occurs through contact with infected feces, usually because of poor sanitation or through sexual contact. Even when the individual does not have an active case of diarrhea, the parasite may form cysts through which it can be spread. Dysentery caused by the *Shigella* bacteria is acquired by the ingestion of contaminated food or water. Most often this occurs in unsanitary environments where food is handled.

Symptoms include constant diarrhea, increased gas, and abdominal cramps. Extreme weight-loss (emaciation) as well as low oxygen level in the blood (anemia) frequently occur. Dehydration can also occur. The dysentery-causing organism may spread through the bloodstream and infect the lungs and brain, as well as the skin and any sustained wounds.

Treatment. Replenishing fluids lost from diarrhea is advised for the treatment of the resulting dehydration. A stool sample is required for accurate diagnosis, after which several different amoebicide drugs, such as iodoquinol, paromomycin, and diloxanide, can be administered to kill the parasite. Metronidazole is usually prescribed in severe cases or when the infection has moved beyond the intestines. Stool samples must be examined at one, three, and six month intervals to ensure that the patient is cured.

See INFLAMMATION *and* INTESTINES *for fundamental material on dysentery. For additional information see* ANEMIA; BACTERIA; DEHYDRATION; DIARRHEA; *and* WEIGHT LOSS. *Related material is available in* PARASITE.

Dyskinesia

Abnormal muscle movements caused by a brain disorder.

In dyskinesia, uncontrolled random movements are caused by an abnormality in the basal ganglia of the brain; it may impair a person's ability to perform willed, controlled movements.

Causes. Dyskinesia may be caused by congenital brain damage. More frequently, it is a side effect of some types of medication, most notably antipsychotic drugs and neuroepileptic tranquilizers.

Symptoms. Dyskinesia can be exhibited in different forms:
- jerky movement (chorea);
- writhing movement (athetosis);
- repetitive fidgeting (tics);
- tremors;
- muscle spasms (myclonus).

Symptoms may involve the arms, legs, head and face. The movements may lead to respiratory difficulty and oral ulcerations.

Treatment. Individualized treatment is preferred because of the lack of a successful standard treatment. If the dyskinesia is drug-induced, the easiest approach is to discontinue the use of the offending drug. However, sometimes discontinuing the drug can worsen the dyskinesia. Drugs that block the effects of dopamine may help lessen the uncontrolled movements. *See also* BASAL GANGLIA.

Dyslexia

A neurological ailment that causes a learning disability specific to difficulty in reading and spelling.

Dyslexia is a disorder in which a child has difficulty learning to read properly. It is caused by a neurological condition that results in problematic processing of sounds and visual input in the language areas of the brain. A person with dyslexia finds it difficult to discern and transcribe the written word without error. A child with dyslexia has average or above average intelligence but, if the dyslexia is not diagnosed and treated, does not excel in school. Dyslexia is seen more often in boys than in girls and tends to run in families.

SYMPTOMS

A child with dyslexia may excel in mathematical or musical ability yet do poorly in spelling and writing. Dyslexic preschoolers may be delayed speakers and have trouble learning the letters of the alphabet. They may use incorrect words in sentences. They often confuse one letter for another similar letter, reverse letters when writing, or transpose letters in a word—for example, writing "b" for "d" or writing "nad" for "and."

TREATMENT

The sooner dyslexia is identified, the greater the chance for the dyslexic child to advance in school. Individualized teaching can help a child learn coping skills to better read, write, and deal with frustration. Tricks and mnemonic devices can counter the tendency to transpose and reverse letters. Perhaps most importantly, parents and educators should be patient with reading and writing activities. They should recognize and praise the areas in which the child excels. This will help the child develop a healthy self-esteem and approach the task of reading and writing without anxiety. *See also* LEARNING DISABILITIES.

Dysmenorrhea

Severely painful menstrual periods that cannot be tolerated without medication.

More than half of all women experience mild cramps during the first few days of a period. Severe cramping, however, occurs in only about 10 percent of women. Secondary dysmenorrhea is suspected when cramps and pain extend past the first three days of a period, occur between periods, or precede a period by a few days, accompanied by vaginal bleeding.

If the pain is not a sign of another gynecological problem, the condition is called primary dysmenorrhea. This is relatively common during adolescence or until a woman gives birth to her first child. Primary dysmenorrhea is caused by excessive levels of prostaglandins, chemicals that are found in menstrual fluids and semen and that trigger uterine contractions. Severe cramps may also be due to internal "gridlock"—a lot of fluid and tissue attempting to exit all at once through a relatively small opening. Pain therefore persists until enough material has been expelled. Once a woman has given birth, the opening has been somewhat stretched.

Secondary dysmenorrhea is caused by an underlying condition such as noncancerous growths (fibroids, endometriosis, or adenomyosis), a sexually transmitted disease, a pelvic inflammatory disease, or an ovarian cyst.

Diagnosis of primary or secondary dysmenorrhea may involve investigation through a fiber optic viewing tube, a pelvic exam, or an ultrasound.

Treatment involves routine medication to alleviate pain in cases of primary dysmenorrhea. Secondary dysmenorrhea is treated by determining and correcting the underlying condition.

See FEMALE REPRODUCTIVE SYSTEM *and* MENSTRUATION *for fundamental material on dysmenorrhea. For further information see* BLEEDING; CRAMPS; *and* MENSTRUATION, DISORDERS OF. *Related material is available in* ENDOMETRIOSIS; FIBROIDS; *and* ULTRASOUND.

Dysphasia

Difficulty understanding or using language.

Dysphasia is an impairment in the ability to understand or choose the words necessary for speech. Caused by an injury to the language areas of the brain, it can affect understanding, speaking, reading, and writing. Over one million Americans suffer from a form of dysphasia. Causes of dysphasia include stroke, head injury, and neurological disease. Speech therapists can help individuals whose speech has been impaired to restore their verbal communication abilities. *See also* APHASIA; DYSARTHRIA; SPEECH THERAPY; *and* STROKE.

Dysphonia

Difficulty vocalizing sounds because of disease to the voice box (larynx) or the nerves that supply it.

Dysphonia is a speech dysfunction that occurs because of impairment of the laryngeal nerves or muscles. Paralysis, nodules on the vocal cords, spasms, or other disorders can cause hoarseness, stuttering or garbled speech.

Speech can also be affected by injury or disease to the muscles or nerve pathways of the auxiliary speech components, such as the tongue and lips (dysarthria), or in the speech-processing areas of the brain itself (aphasia). *See also* APHASIA; DYSARTHRIA; DYSPHASIA; *and* SPEECH.

Dysplasia

An abnormal growth occurring in the tissues of an organ or limb of the body.

Dysplasia is the term used to describe any growth abnormality. An example is hip dysplasia, in which the incorrectly positioned hip of an infant may cause dislocation in the hip socket or instability. Fibrous dysplasia occurs when growing bones replace themselves with fibrous tissue instead of new healthy bone, leading to pain, difficulty walking, and possibly rickets. Cellular dysplasia describes any abnormality in the size, shape, or growth of cells.

Dystonia

An unusual stiffening of the muscles that causes painful spasms.

Dystonia can be either local or general. Neck spasms, or torticollis, are the most common instances of local dystonia. Muscle spasms from a back injury may lead to dystonia in the form of scoliosis (curvature of the spine). General dystonia is usually the result of a neurological disorder, such as a stroke or Parkinson's disease.

Treatment. Although treatment depends on the specific nature of the disorder, heat treatment, ultrasound treatment, and physical therapy may reduce the spasms. A number of alternative therapies can also be beneficial. *See also* ALTERNATIVE MEDICINE; PARKINSON'S DISEASE; SCOLIOSIS; *and* ULTRASOUND TREATMENT.

Dystrophy

The disruption of growth or normal activity of a cell, due to poor nutrition.

The term "dystrophy" refers to a progression of changes that occur to an organ or tissue when cells do not receive an adequate supply of nutrients. This may occur when there is an interruption in the blood supply to a cell, nerve damage that prevents cells from receiving nutrition, or lack of a certain protein or enzyme that is necessary for the cell to function.

TYPES

The most well-known dystrophy is muscular dystrophy, in which the muscle cells do not develop normally, causing weakness and paralysis. In most cases of muscular dystrophy, the arms, legs, and spine become increasingly deformed. By a person's teenage years, most sufferers are confined to a wheelchair. Death may result from pneumonia or some other form of respiratory infection.

Duchenne's muscular dystrophy is the most common form of muscular dystrophy, affecting 20 to 30 in 100,000 males. It occurs only in males. The onset of the disease is usually before age five. One of the first signs is when a toddler exhibits a decrease in mobility. The disease then progresses throughout childhood. Few affected children survive into their 20s.

Less commonly known are leukodystrophies and corneal dystrophies—one destroys the protective covering of nerves, the latter damages the outer lining of the eye.

For background material on dystrophy, see CELLS *and* NUTRITION. *For additional information, see* LEUKODYTROPHIES; MUSCULAR DYSTROPHY; MENIERE'S DISEASE; *and* NERVE. *Related material is available in* NUTRITIONAL DISORDERS.

Ear

The organs of hearing and balance.

The ear is a structure composed of three parts: the outer-ear, the middle-ear, and the inner-ear. The outer-ear is separated from the middle-ear by the eardrum, a membrane that vibrates in response to sound; the middle-ear is a cavity that transports sound across three bones called the ossicles; and the inner-ear is responsible for sending sound to the brain.

A swirl of skin and cartilage forms the outer-ear (also called the pinna or auricle) and leads into the ear canal. The adult ear canal (meatus) is one inch long and is covered by wax-producing skin that keeps dust from penetrating to the eardrum. A tympanic membrane, the eardrum is thin and round; it forms the border between the outer- and middle-ear. Sound causes changes in air pressure that make the ear-drum vibrate.

The middle-ear consists of three tiny bones that straddle the small cavity between the eardrum and the inner-ear. The hammer, anvil, and stirrup connect the eardrum to an oval window that forms the wall between the middle- and the inner-ear.

Deep within the skull, a maze of passages, called the labyrinth, comprise the inner-ear. The cochlea (the primary organ of hearing), is an intricate, hollow tube shaped like a snail's shell. Fluid-bathed hair cells in the cochlea vibrate when sound is transmitted from the middle ear to the inner ear. Different sounds cause various hair cells to respond with nerve impulses to the brain. The auditory nerve transmits these impulses to the brain.

The semicircular canals of the inner-ear control balance. These canals, which are situated at right angles to one another, are filled with fluid. When a person moves his or her head, the fluid in the canal moves, stimulating the nerve endings to send a signal to the brain concerning the direction of movement. The brain then sends the appropriate signals back to the ear to maintain balance. *See also* EAR, DISORDERS OF.

Earache

Pain or pressure in or around the ear.

Earaches, one of the most common pains experienced in childhood, usually take place in the outer-ear or middle-ear, often caused by infections, and on occasion, by earwax or jaw problems. An earache may result in throbbing, tenderness, pressure or splitting pain that occurs inside the ear or in the surrounding areas. Infants and children commonly suffer from infections that cause earaches.

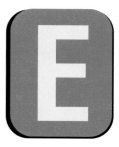

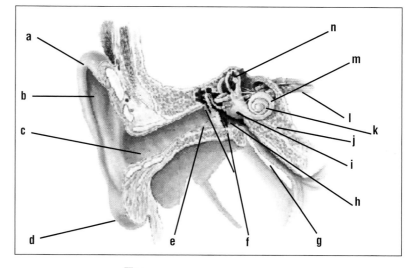

TYPES

Outer-ear infections (otitis externa) are the result of a blockage or buildup of pressure in the outer-ear. Often called swimmer's ear, the most common cause of this type of pain is water buildup in the ear, a recurring problem for frequent swimmers. While the water sits in the ear, bacteria may grow. The ear may itch and the contact with the skin, plus any dirt or residue on it, will cause the bacteria to multiply, resulting in an infection. In addition to pain, symptoms of this type of earache may include itching, a small discharge, and minor hearing loss.

Middle-ear infections (otitis media). The most common earache, otitis media is an accumulation of fluid in the middle ear, causing pressure on the eardrum. The fluid buildup is the result of an obstruction

Structures of the Ear. The ear is divided into three sections: the outer-ear, which consists of (a) helix, (b) auricle, (c) outer ear canal, and (d) earlobe; the middle-ear, which consists of (e) eardrum, and (f) auditory oscicles; (g) auditory tube, (h) tympanic cavity, and the inner ear, which consists of (i) oval window, (j) temporal bone, (k) cochlea, (l) cochlear nerve, (m) vesticular nerve, and (n) semicircular canal.

in the Eustachian tube, the small tube that carries air from the middle ear to the nasal passages. Infections from bacteria or viruses, as well as allergies, may cause the tube to become inflamed or blocked. Fluid from the mucous membranes in the tube build up, causing the pressure resulting in an earache.

Otitis media is characterized by a sharp, stabbing pain. There may also be a rise in temperature and a slight loss of hearing. Children may pull on their ears, or cry and become irritable. If the eardrum ruptures, a discharge of fluid will follow.

Other causes of an earache may not be directly related to the ear itself. Tooth infections, sinus infections, or injuries to the jaw can all cause earaches—as can foreign objects lodged in the ear.

TREATMENT

Care at home for minor outer-ear infections consists of over-the-counter pain-relievers, antihistamines, and nose drops. A vaporizer can help to thin the mucus in cases of inner-ear infections. If symptoms persist for more than a few days, a visit to a doctor is recommended. Doctors usually prescribe antibiotics for middle-ear infections, as well as stronger forms of antihistamines or decongestants that will help open the Eustachian tube. For severe cases, an ear tube may be inserted to drain fluid. *See also* EAR; EAR, DISORDERS OF; OTITIS EXTERNA; *and* OTITIS MEDIA.

Ear, Discharge from

Fluid passing out of the ear.

Ear infections, whether viral or bacterial, usually cause inflammation in the tissues within the ear that prevents fluids from draining. The result is a buildup of fluid that will begin to leak out via the ear canal.

Middle-ear infections (otitis media) allow fluid to gather in the middle-ear cavity, behind the eardrum. The pressure from the fluid may cause the eardrum to rupture, allowing the fluid to drain out of the ear.

Outer-ear infections (otitis externa) form in the ear canal, outside the eardrum, and may extend to the exterior cartilage that shapes the ear (the pinna); in this case, there may be a discharge directly from the ear canal, or there may be pus from a boil. Occasionally, head injuries may cause a leak of cerebrospinal fluid or blood from the ear.

Discharge from an ear should be investigated by a physician. A sample may be taken and analyzed at a lab to determine what, if any, bacteria or virus is present. *See also* EAR; EARACHES; EAR, DISORDERS OF; OTITIS MEDIA; *and* OTITIS, EXTERNA.

Ear, Disorders of

Conditions that affect the ear.

The ear is an organ that is not only responsible for hearing, but also balance. It is composed of three parts: the outer-ear, which takes in sound; the middle-ear; which sends the sound in the form of vibrations to the inner-ear; and the inner-ear, which sends sound to the brain to be processed and understood. The inner ear is also the part of the ear that controls balance. Disorders may affect both hearing and balance.

EARACHES

There are two major kinds of earaches: otitis media and otitis externa. Otitis media is an earache that is caused by a buildup of fluid in the middle-ear, leading to pressure on the eardrum. The accumulation of fluid is usually the result of an infection that causes inflammation in the tissues in the middle ear, preventing draining of fluids. Otitis externa is an earache based in the outer ear. Also known as swimmer's ear, it is caused by a buildup of water or other fluids in the outer-ear, allowing bacteria to grow and infections to develop.

INJURY

Injuries, such as cuts or blows to the ear, usually affect the pinna, or outer-ear. Sharp blows may affect the eardrum, causing it to rupture. Exposure to extremely loud or sudden loud noises, such as explosions, may cause deafness as a result of the eardrum rupturing. Minor damage can sometimes occur from changes in pressure, such as from diving or flying.

LABYRINTHITIS

An infection of the inner-ear, often resulting in vertigo, loss of hearing, or ringing in the ears, labyrinthitis is usually an after effect of a cold or an upper respiratory infection. The symptoms usually disappear after a few weeks, but if they are severe and disruptive, a doctor may prescribe medication to alleviate the nausea or vomiting.

MÉNIÉRE'S DISEASE

An inner ear disorder, Méniére's disease causes periods of severe vertigo and hearing loss, most commonly affecting people between ages 20 and 50. It seems to be related to a problem with the tissues that line the inner ear; if they cannot filter the fluid that is found in the balance and hearing centers in the inner ear, the labyrinth becomes distorted and the brain cannot understand the signals it is receiving from the nerve cells in the area. Medication can help with vertigo, but if it is severe, surgery to cut the balance nerve may be required.

MASTOIDITIS

If untreated, a middle-ear infection may spread to the mastoid, the large bone behind the ear. There will be pain, swelling, and discharge from the ear; fever; and increasing hearing loss. Antibiotics are needed to treat the infection, or the infected area may be surgically removed.

OBSTRUCTIONS

Foreign objects in the ear, such as insects or cotton swabs, are usually the result of accidents in adults. Children may intentionally insert objects in the ear. In both cases, the object should be removed carefully if it can be seen; if it is out of view, then a doctor should be consulted. Do not try to flush it out with water, as that may cause some objects to swell. Insects may be killed with mineral oil, then removed by suction.

A buildup of earwax can occasionally obstruct the ear canal; it may even cause hearing loss. In most cases, it may be flushed out with warm water, but if that does not work, a doctor may have to remove it.

OTOSCLEROSIS

An abnormal bone growth on the stirrup, an inner-ear bone, otosclerosis can cause hearing loss by preventing the reception of sound vibrations in the inner ear. It usually occurs in both ears, and the growth may speed up during pregnancy. The best treatment is surgery to remove the stirrup, replacing it with an artificial part.

RUPTURE OF THE EARDRUM

The eardrum may burst for several reasons: pressure or puncture from an object; force from a stream of water or air; or buildup of fluid due to infection. Symptoms include hearing loss, tinnitus, pain, and bleeding. Small ruptures heal on their own, but if symptoms persist, a doctor may have to surgically repair the rupture.

TINNITUS

A ringing in the ears, tinnitus is often a symptom of another ear disorder. It is the result of the acoustic nerve picking up vibrations that originate within the head or ear. Treatment should focus on the underlying disorder, although sometimes no treatment is available.

TUMORS

Most tumors of the ear are located in the outer, visible part of the ear (the pinna). An acoustic neuroma, or benign tumor in the inner-ear, may cause hearing loss, imbalance, or ringing in the ear (tinnitus). Radiation may prevent further growth, or the tumor may be surgically removed.

For basic anatomical material on disorders of the ear, see EAR. *For additional information, see* ACOUSTIC NEUROMA; EARACHE; LABYRINTHITIS; MASTOIDITIS; MENIERE'S DISEASE; TINITUS *and* TUMOR. *Related material is available in* ACOUSTIC NERVE; BALANCE; *and* HEARING.

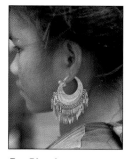

Ear-Piercing.
Though popular, the process of ear piercing is a common cause of injuries to the ear.

Resources on Hearing

Davis, Hallowell, and S.R. Silverman, *Hearing and Deafness* (19078); Jerger, James, *Hearing Disorders in Adults* (1984); Pender, Daniel J., *Practical Otology* (1992); Stevens, S., and H. Davis, *Hearing: Its Psychology and Physiology* (1983); Strong, W.J., *Music, Speech, Audio* (1992); National Association of the Deaf, Tel. (301) 587-1788 (voice), -1789 (TTY), Online: www.nad.org; American Academy of Neurology, Tel. (651) 695-1940, Online: www.aan.com; American Board of Neurological Surgery, Tel. (713) 790-6015, Online: www.abns.org; www.med.cornell.edu/neuro/.

Eardrum, Perforated

A break in the eardrum.

The eardrum is a thin, round fibrous membrane, covered by skin, that separates the middle-ear from the inner-ear. There are several ways this membrane may break: a puncture from a sharp blow or object; a loud noise or explosion; or a change in air pressure, as may happen during flying or diving. The common cause, however, is a middle-ear infection, or otitis media. This is characterized by a buildup of fluid in the middle-ear cavity when inflamed airways prevent the proper drainage of fluid. The pressure may build up to such a level that it ruptures the eardrum, allowing the fluid to burst through and flow out of the ear.

Treatment. A suspected eardrum rupture should be kept clean and dry to avoid infection. A physician will prescribe antibiotics to further reduce the possibility of infection. In most cases, a rupture will heal on its own. If this does not happen within six months, a physician may perform a myringoplasty, a procedure that repairs the break with tissue from another part of the body. *See also* EAR; EAR, DISORDERS OF; *and* OTITIS MEDIA.

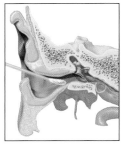

Swab.
A cotton swab can be gently maneuvered into the ear canal to obtain a fluid sample.

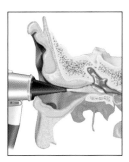

Otoscope.
An otoscope is a lighted viewing device with a tapered end that is inserted into the ear canal. It allows a physician to examine any blockages or inner-ear cysts.

Ear, Examination of

Examination of the ear for diagnostic purposes.

The human ear is an extremely sensitive organ, responsible for hearing and maintaining balance. Its many components may be subject to disease, dysfunction, or abnormality, and various examination procedures exist to diagnose these conditions. The ear is divided into three main regions—the outer, middle, and inner ear. Additionally, the ear chamber is connected to the throat through the Eustachian tube as well as the nose and sinuses, which drain into the throat.

Diagnosis of a range of disorders, including infection, perforation of the eardrum, hearing loss, difficulty with balance, and vertigo, require careful examination of the delicate auditory structures of the inner, middle, and outer ear.

An ear, nose, and throat specialist (otorhynolaryngologist) may perform examinations of the ear when inflammation or infection are present. Hearing loss is often the domain of an audiologist, who will examine the structures of the ear and associated nerves in an effort to diagnose the source of a hearing disability.

Otoscope. Blockage of the ear canal by wax accumulation, foreign objects, or bacterial cysts can be examined directly or by means of an otoscope, a lighted viewing device with a tapered end that is inserted into the ear canal.

Other Techniques. If the physician needs information about the middle or inner ear, x-ray, computerized tomography (CT) scanning, or magnetic resonance imaging (MRI) may be used. Hearing tests, caloric tests, and other tests may be used to diagnose hearing loss or balance disturbance. *See also* AUDIOLOGY; HEARING; HEARING TESTS; *and* OTOSCOPE;.

Ear, Foreign Body in

Matter in the ear that causes an obstruction.

Occasionally objects may become lodged in the outer-ear canal, either accidentally or by intent. Flies or insects may enter and then become trapped in the ear canal. During accidents, an object may be forced into the ear canal. Children frequently insert objects into their ears, such as small toys, beads, buttons, or stones. Small children also often force certain foods, such as peas, into their ears.

Treatment. If an insect has flown or crawled into the ear, a physician may have to remove it. A person should not attempt to remove any type of matter from the ear canal. In these cases, the object should be left alone until a physician can attend to it. Do not attempt to remove foreign objects by flushing the ear with water, as that may cause some objects to swell. A trained physician can safely remove the object with a syringe, tiny forceps, or other specialized suction devices. Occasionally, anesthetic may be required for this procedure. *See also* EAR; EAR, DISORDERS OF; EAR, EXAMINATION OF; *and* OTOSCOPE.

Ear Tube

Tube inserted in ear to allow drainage.

Middle-ear infections (otitis media) cause a buildup of fluid in the middle-ear. In most cases, the fluid will drain on its own as the inflammation from the infection subsides. If the condition persists, or recurs, then a myringotomy—the insertion of a small tube—may help to drain the ear of fluid via the ear canal.

Treatment. A myringotomy is a small slit in the eardrum into which a tiny tube is placed. The tube is usually made of a light plastic, hollow and flared at either end. In adults, the surgery may be performed in a doctors' office with only a local anesthetic; children, however, usually require an operation in a hospital with a general anesthetic. Ear tubes do not need to be removed. As the slit in the eardrum heals, it will push the tube out of its place, and eventually, it will fall out. If the tube has not fallen out within eighteen months, a doctor should remove it.

Risk Factors. Because the tubes create a new passageway for the fluid to drain into the ear canal, precautions should be taken to prevent other fluids from entering the ear. Water containing bacteria, such as may be encountered while swimming or bathing, should not be allowed into the ear. Earplugs should be worn at high-risk times while the tubes remain in place. *See also* EAR; EARACHE; *and* EAR, DISORDERS OF.

Earwax

A secretion from glands in the ear.

The outer-ear canal contains glands that produce a waxy substance that lubricates the skin and captures outside matter that makes its way into the ear. The nature of the wax, known as cerumen, varies from person to person. Some people produce a soft wax, others a stiffer, dryer kind. Most wax easily dissipates with normal cleaning, but some people produce more than the body can dispose of by itself. The wax will build up and form a blockage in the ear canal, called an occlusion. The ear may feel full, and the person may experience some loss of hearing.

Treatment. Most cases of earwax build-up can be taken care of at home. If the wax is soft, it can be flushed out with a stream of room-temperature water delivered via a bulb syringe. There are also over-the-counter earwax removal kits and wax softeners. If there is a large amount of wax, or if it is of the stiff, dry variety, it should be removed by a physician. *See also* EAR; EAR, DISORDERS OF; *and* EAR, EXAMINATION OF.

Eating Disorders

Any disorder that results in long-term, obsessive behavior relating to food or the body.

The number of people affected by eating disorders has significantly increased since the 1970s. Ten to fifteen percent of all adolescent and young women in the United States will develop an eating disorder. While more common in women, weight disorders are also seen in men (especially weight-conscious athletes). The three most common disorders are: anorexia nervosa; bulimia; and binge-eating disorder.

TYPES
Anorexia nervosa is characterized by an obsessive desire to become thin, actualized through methods of self-starvation. Ninety-five percent of all anorectics are women, primarily adolescent girls from middle and upper-class backgrounds. Most anorectics suffer from an extreme fear of becoming "fat." Many have low self-esteem and a distorted perception of their bodies. Feelings of self-loathing are often countered by starvation efforts, obsessive exercise regimes, a preoccupation with detail, and an intense endeavor to excel in school or work.

Many anorectics lose up to 25 percent of

their body weight, and suffer from constipation, abdominal cramping, cold intolerance, weakness, lightheadedness, hyperactivity, depression, and potassium deficiency. Amenorrhea, the complete cessation of menstrual periods, is also common.

Bulimia is characterized by bouts of binge-eating followed by self-induced vomiting. Although most bulimics are of normal weight, many of them suffer from an intense preoccupation with their body and have difficulty with normal food intake. Many may have experienced weight problems or suffered from anorexia at one point in time. A typical binge may last anywhere from one to two hours during which the bulimic may consume as much as 15,000 to 20,000 calories, experience extreme mood swings, and feel as though he or she is out of control. Following such episodes, feelings of shame and guilt cause the person to purge the food from his or her system, using self-induced vomiting, laxatives, or fasting.

Bulimics often suffer from muscle cramping; dental problems, due to frequent exposure to highly acidic gastric juices; electrolyte imbalance; and, in severe cases, cardiac irregularities and seizures.

Binge-eating disorder is characterized by excessive eating of high-caloric foods. It is most prominent in people who are obese and occurs equally in men and women. At least half of all people who binge do so as the result of depression. A combination of psychotherapy and antidepressant drugs has proven relatively effective in reducing binge-eating episodes.

CAUSES

Studies have shown that eating disorders result from a combination of psychological, environmental, and biological factors. Dieting can often trigger the disorder, as can the physical changes that occur with the onset of puberty. Many young women prone to depression and weight gain may also be particularly susceptible. Family problems, low self-esteem, affective disorder, depression, abnormal functioning of the hypothalamus, and social pressure to

be thin may all be factors that lead a person to adopt such extreme behavior toward food and his or her body.

TREATMENT

While treatment varies depending on the disorder and its severity, most therapists recommend a combination of psychotherapy, medication, family and behavioral therapy, as well as nutritional counseling. Some anorectics may require hospitalization (for those who have lost over 30 percent of their bodyweight) to restore lost nutrients and prevent starvation. Through behavior therapy and counseling, doctors attempt to reestablish normal eating habits, and help anorectics reach their ideal weight. Therapy for bulimics aims to end binge and purge cycles of behavior. While therapy and regular eating habits can help return a patient to normal body weight and eating habits, relapses are common, especially during periods of stress and among older individuals. *See also* ANOREXIA NERVOSA; BULIMIA; DEPRESSION; BEHAVIORAL THERAPY; *and* PSYCHOTHERAPY.

Ebola Virus

A highly contagious and usually fatal virus that causes severe hemorrhagic fevers in humans.

Named after the Ebola River in the northern Congo, Africa, the Ebola virus was first identified in 1976 after hundreds of people died in Zaire (the former name of the Congo) and the Sudan. In 1995, another epidemic took the lives of 244 patients (out of 315 reported cases) again in the Congo.

Ebola, similar to the Marburg virus, is classified as a filovirus. It is thought that the virus, once contracted, will produce certain proteins in the body that suppress the immune system and enable the virus to reproduce. It may be transmitted through exposure to bodily fluid, blood, or infected tissue. At first, Ebola victims experience minor symptoms that grow progressively worse. These include fever, appetite loss, headache, muscle aches, diarrhea, and vomiting. Once the virus advances, blood

Resources on Eating Disorders

Brownell, Kelly D., and Christopher G. Fairburn, *Eating Disorders and Obesity: A Comprehensive Handbook* (1995); Bruch, Hilde, *Eating Disorders: Obesity, Anorexia Nervosa, and the Person Within* (1973); Garner, David M., *Handbook of Treatment for Eating Disorders* (1997); Harkaway, Jill Elka, *Eating Disorders* (1987); www. nycornell. org/psychiatry.

clots form (a condition referred to as DIC, disseminated intravascular coagulation) in internal organs, namely the liver, spleen, brain, and their surrounding capillaries. In the final stage, spontaneous hemorrhaging occurs from various body outlets; loss of consciousness, kidney failure, and shock usually results in death in anywhere from eight to seventeen days.

Treatment. As of yet, no treatment has proven successful in treating the virus. The administration of fluids, in addition to blood and plasma transfusions, may produce hemorrhaging. The hospitalization of patients in sanitary, isolated environments helps prevent the spread of the Ebola virus.

Research into the origin and structure of the various strains of Ebola has been slow due to the highly contagious nature of the disease. *See also* EPIDEMIC *and* VIRUS.

Echocardiography

A diagnostic method for examining heart structures by means of high-frequency ultrasound.

Echocardiography is a general term for a family of noninvasive imaging techniques used to evaluate the size, shape, condition, metabolism, and pressures associated with the heart and accompanying blood flow. Echocardiography uses several forms of ultrasonography, in which inaudible, high-frequency sounds are sent into the body. The pattern of echoes that return allows images of internal structures to be constructed. An instrument known as a transducer records the time between the sound transmission to the heart structure and the returning sound echo, displaying this information on a monitor.

The cardiac valves and the dimensions of each ventricle and the left atrium can be visualized and measured through echocardiography. The technique is particularly useful for identifying disease of the lining around the heart (pericardium) and the heart muscle itself, reduced blood supply (ischemia), congenital heart disease, and inflammation of the inner lining of the heart (infectious endocarditis).

Echocardiography is one of the most useful means of examining the heart and diagnosing cardiac diseases. It is noninvasive, does not use ionizing radiation, and is painless.

TYPES

The movement of blood and turbulence of blood flow through the heart and accompanying vessels is accomplished through Doppler ultrasonography, which may be viewed either in color or black and white. In color Doppler ultrasonography, the information obtained can be used to create a detailed color map of the blood vessels around the heart.

M-mode echocardiography uses a single beam of ultrasound directed at the area of the heart under study. Sound waves may also be directed at the heart from varying angles, each sending a distinctive echo back to the transducer. Echoing waves from various depths can be put together to create a two-dimensional image known as an echocardiogram.

Procedure. Echocardiography is a noninvasive, painless procedure. The patient lies flat, and a conducting gel is applied to the chest area to affix the transducer. This converts sound into energy in order to create an image of the heart and surrounding blood vessels. Abnormal results of echocardiology may indicate:

- narrowing of the heart valves (mitral valve or aortic stenosis);
- weakening of the aortic valve (aortic insufficiency);
- collection of fluid in the membrane surrounding the heart (pericardial effusion);
- enlargement of the liver;
- tricuspid valve disease;
- enlargement of the heart (hypertophy).

See DIAGNOSIS *and* IMAGING TECHNIQUES *for fundamental material on* ECHOCARDIOGRAPHY. *For additional information, see* HEART; HEART, DISORDERS OF; *and* ULTRASOUND. *For related material see* AORTIC INSUFFICIENCY; AORTIC STENOSIS; STENOSIS; ENDOCARDITIS; HYPERTROPHY; HEART VALVE; ISCHEMIA; *and* MITRAL STENOSIS.

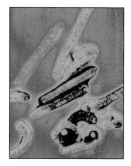

Ebola Virus.
The Ebola virus is a filovirus, characterized by long, curve virions. Research dedicated to the structure of the virus is difficult due to the highly contagious nature of the disease.

Eclampsia

Called the toxemia of pregnancy, a life-threatening condition of late pregnancy characterized by high blood pressure and excessive swelling.

Eclampsia is a serious disease of late pregnancy that occurs when preeclampsia is not brought under control. It can be fatal for both mother and baby. The condition is not as common as it once was, thanks to improved prenatal care and early detection and treatment of preeclampsia. Preeclampsia occurs in five percent of all pregnancies, with eclampsia developing in one in every 1,500 pregnancies.

The cause of eclampsia is largely unknown. It has been thought that it is caused by a toxin in the bloodstream, but no such substance has been identified in either preeclampsia or eclampsia. Women at higher risk of developing these conditions are either very young or older than 40. In addition, the presence of multiple fetuses or a history of high blood pressure predisposes a woman to preeclampsia. *See* HYPERTENSION *and* PREECLAMPSIA.

SYMPTOMS

The earliest symptom of eclampsia is swelling (edema) of the face and hands. Other indications include high blood pressure and protein in the urine. If the condition progresses to an emergency situation, symptoms include pain in the upper right side of the abdomen and visual disturbances, such as flashing lights. At this point, the mother may suffer convulsions, which could lead to a coma.

TREATMENT

For mild preeclampsia, doctors attempt to control blood pressure with diet and medication. Bed rest is prescribed, with the mother lying on her left side so as not to put additional pressure on the blood vessels of the uterus. Hospitalization may be deemed necessary, with the administration of medication to lower blood pressure and remove excess fluid in an attempt to stabilize the condition.

Once eclampsia has set in, it is life threatening and warrants immediate delivery of the baby. In some cases, labor may be induced or a Cesarean section will be performed, after which the eclampsia should abate. Sometimes a decision has to be made weighing the risks and benefits of an early delivery to both mother and child.

The best prevention for eclampsia is consistent prenatal care. If preeclampsia is detected and treated early enough, it is much less likely to progress to a life-threatening stage. *See also* PRENATAL CARE.

Ecstasy

Popular name for methylenedioxymethamphetamine

A recreational drug used as a stimulant in the United States and Europe.

Popular at rave dances and club scenes, ecstasy (or MDMA) is a designer drug that acts as a stimulant, increasing alertness, concentration, and physical performance. It may also cause a sense of euphoria and overall empathy.

Risk factors include heart attacks, stroke, and extreme dehydration, resulting in death in some cases. Over time, MDMA can impair the brain's ability to metabolize serotonin, which can result in depression and, with repeated use, psychotic behavior. *See* DRUG DEPENDENCE *and* DRUG ABUSE.

Ectoparasite

Any of the parasites that live on the skin outside of the body, including lice, fleas, mites, and ticks.

While a large range of organisms fall into the class of ectoparasites, three broad categories are responsible for the most common infestations of humans; fleas, mites, and lice. Such parasites live on the skin outside of the body, feeding on human blood. Though ectoparasites may produce uncomfortable itching in their human hosts, most do not cause disease, and are fairly easily controlled. Some ectoparasites, however, can transmit diseases such as Lyme disease, and therefore constitute a more serious risk to a person's health.

TYPES OF ECTOPARASITES

Fleas are wingless, flat insects, dark brown in color. Their larvae are small, white, and maggot-like, while eggs appear small, white, and spherical. Fleas often prey on cats and dogs. It is not uncommon, however, for fleas to target humans as hosts. In biting the skin and drinking blood, they cause redness, irritation, and itching. Adult fleas remain on the host and eggs are laid in the hair. These eggs may easily fall off onto bedding, where they will hatch into larvae after two to four days.

Fleas are transmitted by direct contact with infected dogs or cats, or from infected bedding. Fleas are visible to the naked eye, and identified on pets by separating the fur with the hands and by closely observing the fur and skin. A spray or powder containing pyrethrin is safe to use on both animals and bedding. Treatment should be carried out weekly for three weeks to ensure all parasites, eggs, and larvae are destroyed.

Mites are tiny arachnids (less than a twentieth of an inch), eight-legged and related to scorpions and spiders. The burrowing mite (*Sarcoptes Scabiei*) is the culprit of human infestation (scabies). Infested persons usually have a violent reaction to the burrowing of the mite, resulting in severe itching (pruritus), which may persist long after the infestation has been eliminated. Topical steroids and other antipruritics are effective in providing relief of itching and irritation. An insecticide lotion treats the infestation.

Lice infestations are also known as pediculosis. Lice are wingless, flat insects with a brownish tinge that may infest the head and hair, or the body or pubic area, depending on the species. Some types of lice are disease carriers; all drink blood from their hosts. Lice are eradicated through pediculocides that kill the lice, larvae, and eggs. This treatment may be applied as a cream or shampoo.

> *For background material on ectoparasite, see* PARASITE *and* SKIN. *For further reading see* LICE; MITES AND DISEASE *and* TICKS AND DISEASE. *For related material see,* INFECTION; LYME DISEASE *and* SCABIES.

ALERT

Ectoparasites and Pets

Ectoparasites often prey on humans as secondary hosts. Primary hosts often include household pets, which should be regularly checked. Proper hygiene, particularly clean clothes and bedding, is critical in controlling many ectoparasites. Additionally, grassy or wooded areas known to harbor such parasites should be approached with caution, with some protection provided for exposed skin.

Ectopic Heartbeat

A heartbeat that originates in an abnormal location of the heart, outside of the normal timed sequence of the heart's muscle contractions.

A normal heartbeat originates in an electric impulse from the sinoatrial node. An ectopic heartbeat originates in a different region, referred to as an ectopic focus. It is usually an irritated area in the heart muscle that somehow starts and sustains a pattern of extra heartbeats. If an ectopic focus is in a ventricle, it affects the beating of the ventricles; a focus in an atrium affects the beating of the atria. The type of abnormal heartbeat induced depends on the time in the cardiac cycle when the focus emits its signal, as well as on the location of the ectopic focus. *See also* HEARTBEAT

Ectopic beats can occur in a normal heart and may be free of symptoms. Factors such as smoking, fatigue, and consumption of coffee or other caffeine-containing beverages can trigger occasional ectopic heartbeats. These can be treated by rest and withdrawal of the stimulants. Persistent ectopic heartbeats caused by damage to the conduction system of the heart from a heart attack are treated by antiarrhythmic drugs. *See* ANTIARRHYTHMIC DRUGS.

Ectopic Pregnancy

The implantation of a fertilized egg in a location other than the uterus.

In 95 percent of ectopic pregnancies, the egg implants in a fallopian tube. This is the

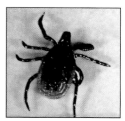

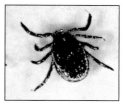

Ectoparasites. Ectoparasites live on the skin of human beings and other animals. Some ectoparasites, such as the Lyme tick (above—top, female; bottom, male—) can transmit Lyme disease and pose a serious threat to a person's health.

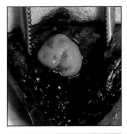

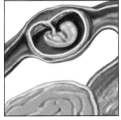

Ectopic Pregnancy.
In an ectopic pregnancy, the fetus (top) grows in a location other than the uterus. This is life-threatening for both the mother and the child. In the most common form of ectopic pregnancy, the egg is implanted in the fallopian tube (bottom) instead of its normal location, the uterus.

Resources on Pregnancy
Creasy, Robert K. and Robert Resnik, eds., *Maternal-Fetal Medicine: Principles and Practice* (1994); Gonik, Bernard and Renee A. Bobrowski, *Medical Complications in Labor and Delivery* (1996); Sears, William, et al., *The Pregnancy Book: Month-by-Month, Everything You Need to Know From America's Baby Experts* (1997); International Childbirth Education Association, Inc., Tel. (612) 854-8660, Online: www.icea.org; Maternity Center Association, Tel. (212) 777-5000, Online: www.maternity.org; Universe of Women's Health, Tel. (512) 418-2922, Online: www.obgyn.net; www.nycornell.org/obgyn

site of fertilization, and the tube is narrow and often convoluted. Rarely, the implantation occurs in the abdominal cavity or on the surface of the ovary. Because it usually occurs in a fallopian tube, ectopic pregnancy is also called tubal pregnancy.

Unlike the uterus, the fallopian tube does not provide adequate room for the growing fetus. Its capacity for expansion is limited. If untreated, an ectopic pregnancy will progress until the embryo has grown too large, resulting in a rupture of the tube. This may result in uncontrolled bleeding and death.

SYMPTOMS

The primary symptoms of an ectopic pregnancy are bleeding, which may range from light staining to heavy spotting, and abdominal pain or cramps. It is sometimes difficult to differentiate between an ectopic pregnancy and a miscarriage.

A woman with an ectopic pregnancy may be unaware she is pregnant at all, as the hormone produced by a growing embryo, human chorionic gonadotropin (hCG), may be at lower levels than in a normal pregnancy. Most pregnancy tests, which test for hCG in the urine, will not detect sufficient levels of the hormone; a test that detects hCG in the bloodstream offers more accurate results.

TREATMENT

The usual treatment for an ectopic pregnancy is surgical removal of the fetus. Depending on the stage of pregnancy, the affected fallopian tube may also have to be removed. Even if the pregnancy is detected early enough for the tube to be saved, it may be too damaged to function normally. Medical treatment with methotrexate may be used to medically abort the fetus.

The incidence of ectopic pregnancy is approximately 1 in 100. The frequency has increased in recent years, possibly because of an increase in pelvic inflammatory disease. Women with damaged or abnormal fallopian tubes, as well as those who have adhesions or endometriosis, are at higher risk for an ectopic pregnancy. Women who

have had an ectopic pregnancy have a one in ten chance of recurrence. Those with a history of two tubal pregnancies have a 50 percent chance.

Women who know they are at risk for an ectopic pregnancy can have an early ultrasound to determine if the egg sac is located in the uterus. The earlier it is discovered, the greater the chances of being able to preserve the fallopian tube.

Long-Term Effects. If the tubes have been damaged or removed, a woman wishing to become pregnant may have to undergo in vitro fertilization. *See also* ABORTION; CHILDBIRTH; ECTOPIC HEARTBEAT; FALLOPIAN TUBE; METHOTREXATE; PREGNANCY; *and* UTERUS.

Ectropion

A condition in which the eyelid is turned inside out (everted).

Usually related to aging, ectropion is caused by muscle weakness. The lower lid is turned outward and its inner surface is exposed. Tears flow out instead of lubricating the eye, which becomes dry and irritated. In some cases, ectropion may be due to an underlying problem, such as atopic dermatitis or lupus erythematosis.

Treatment. Irritation and dryness can be treated with the use of artificial tears and lubricating ointments. A protective eye shield may be used at night to prevent drying. In the condition's early stages, surgery can be performed to reposition the muscles, so that the lid is no longer everted.

Eczema

Also known as dermatitis

A group of skin conditions that cause dry, hot, itchy skin, which occasionally bleeds and becomes raw.

There are numerous types of eczema. Contact dermatitis is caused by exposure to everyday substances, such as detergents. Infantile seborrheic eczema, also called cradle cap, affects babies under one year old. Adult seborrheic eczema, or dandruff, is one of the most common types of eczema.

Varicose eczema affects the lower legs and is caused by poor venous circulation. Discoid eczema causes itchy, coin-shaped areas to develop, usually on the body trunk and lower legs. Atopic dermatitis is an itchy, inflammatory rash associated with individuals and families with asthma, hay fever, and allergies (atopic disorders).

Causes. There are many causes of eczema. Atopic eczema is thought to be hereditary, or genetically linked. Chemicals, detergents, allergens, yeasts, and circulation problems can also cause eczema. Environmental factors and stress have also been linked to cases of eczema.

Symptoms. Itching is one of the most common symptoms of eczema. Other symptoms are redness and inflammation.

Treatment. Treament of eczema includes the use of emollients and topical corticosteroids to reduce inflammation. *See also* ASTHMA; CRADLE CAP; *and* HAY FEVER.

Effusion, Joint

A condition by which a fluid seeps through the walls of blood vessels into a tissue or organ.

The fluids that make up blood can occasionally break out of the capillaries if those blood vessels become congested or inflamed. Any buildup of fluid within a joint can cause swelling, tenderness, and pain. The excess fluid may occur when the lining of the joint (synovium) becomes inflamed or damaged, as in arthritis.

Treatment. The swollen joint should be raised and wrapped with ice packs if possible. Various pain medications, anti-inflammatory drugs, and corticosteroid injections may alleviate some of the pain. In severe cases, the fluid may need to be drawn out with a needle and syringe. *See also* ANTIINFLAMMATORY DRUGS; ARTHRITIS; *and* JOINT.

Ego

A term used to describe a person's sense of self.

According to Freudian theory, ego is the conscious aspect of the human psychologi-

cal makeup that deals with the real world, defending against fears and controlling instinctual drives. The ego also serves to keep these instinctual drives (the id) in check, so the person can behave in accordance with accepted rules of society.

When the ego's mediation between the internal and external self is imbalanced, a person may suffer from a personality disorder resulting in maladaptive behavior and ideas. Colloquially, the term ego is used to refer to one's sense of self-esteem. *See also* PERSONALITY DISORDERS; PSYCHOANALYSIS; *and* PSYCHOTHERAPY.

Ehlers-Danlos Syndrome

Also known as EDS

A connective tissue disorder characterized by excessive joint mobility, skin elasticity, and tissue fragility.

There are six major types of EDS. They include: the classical type; the hypermobility type; the vascular type; the kyphoscoliosis type; the arthrochalasia type; and the dermatosparaxis type. The sensitive skin and unstable joints characteristic of EDS occur as a result of faulty collagen—a protein that acts as a connective "glue" in the body.

Symptoms of EDS include a soft, velvet-like skin surface that bruises easily; increased skin elasticity; severe scarring; slow healing of wounds; lesions; loose joints that are prone to dislocation; joint pain; early onset of osteoarthritis; musculoskeletal pain; scoliosis at birth; poor muscle tone; and gum disease. About one in 5,000 to one in 10,000 people will develop EDS. It affects women and men of all races.

Treatment of EDS includes paying careful attention to gaping skin wounds, which are difficult to repair in EDS patients. Surgery may be necessary to completely rectify the damage. To encourage wound healing, vitamin C may be prescribed, as may bracing, to stabilize weak joints. Since the condition is genetic, genetic counseling should be sought by people with the condition. *See also* COLLAGEN DISEASES; LESION; OSTEOARTHRITIS; SCAR; SCOLIOSIS; SKIN; *and* VITAMIN C.

Eisenmenger Complex

A complication of ventricular septal defect, a congenital condition in which a hole develops between the right and left ventricles, or atria, producing a flow of blood between the two normally separate chambers.

Around ten percent of people with ventricular septal defects develop Eisenmenger complex. The left ventricle, which pumps blood to most of the body, contracts with greater pressure than the right ventricle, which pumps blood to the lungs, so that the hole, or shunt, created by Eisenmenger complex pushes blood into the right ventricle. Pressure in the pulmonary arteries that carry blood to the lungs increases, causing them to become thicker, making the right ventricle work harder and harder.

Symptoms include shortness of breath, a bluish skin (cyanosis), and fainting during physical exertion.

Treatment. Some ventral septal defects close spontaneously in the first years of life. Most others can be closed surgically. Echocardiography is used to determine the size of the defect and its effect on the heart before surgery, which can be done through a small incision on the side of the chest. Most defects are repaired by the operation, and repeat surgery is successful for almost all patients who develop a second shunt. *See also* BIRTH DEFECTS; ECHOCHARDIOGRAPHY; HEART; *and* SEPTAL DEFECT.

Ejaculation

The release of semen from the penis when the climax of sexual arousal is reached.

Ejaculation occurs at the peak of a man's sexual arousal. After sufficient stimulation, nerves stimulate muscle contractions that thrust sperm from the epididymus (the storage duct for sperm) through the vas deferens, which runs from the testes to the beginning of the urethra in the bladder. Further propulsion of the semen is provided by contractions in the muscle structures that surround the urethra from the bladder to the head of the penis.

Sperm are produced in the testes and stored in the seminal vesicles (located behind the prostate gland). The prostate produces a nourishing fluid (semen) that protects the sperm from acid and mucous.

The amount of semen released is usually one or two tablespoons, containing between 300 to 600 million sperm. Once ejaculation occurs, the arteries of the penis constrict and the veins relax. This reduces blood flow and allows the penis to return to its usual, flaccid state.

EJACULATION DISORDERS

Premature ejaculation is defined as ejaculation that occurs too early, either before penetration or very shortly afterwards. There is rarely a physical cause for this occurrence; however, in some instances it may be due to mild inflammation of the prostate or a problem with the nerves in the groin area.

Treatment involves using the "stop-and-start" technique to "train" the person to hold off for longer periods before ejaculating. Drugs that inhibit serotonin reuptake can be prescribed, although this approach is rare.

Retarded ejaculation is when an erection is maintained, but ejaculation is delayed for longer than desired. This is relatively rare. However, as men get older it usually takes longer to achieve orgasm. Certain medications, like those used to treat high blood pressure, have been found to impair ejaculation. Treatment involves behavioral therapy.

Retrograde ejaculation occurs when semen is released into the bladder rather than out of the penis. This can be prevented by constricting the bladder opening. Retrograde ejaculation is more common in men who have had pelvic surgery, including removal of the prostate, and in diabetics. Retrograde ejaculation can also result from abnormal nerve function. There is no current treatment for this disorder. *See also* BEHAVIORAL THERAPY; ORGASM; PENIS; SENSATE FOCUS TECHNIQUE; SEXUAL DYSFUNCTION; SEXUAL INTERCOURSE; *and* SPERM.

Elbow

Joint between the forearm and upper arm bones.

The elbow is the hinge that enables the bicep to bend the arm and the forearm to rotate nearly 180 degrees. Ligaments surround and stabilize the joint. Arthritis and muscle, tendon, and ligament damage are the most common disorders of the elbow. *See also* BASEBALL ELBOW *and* TENNIS ELBOW.

Elderly, Care of

The process of attending to the physical, psychological, spiritual, and emotional needs of the elderly.

The term geriatrics describes the medical science dealing with the diseases and care of the elderly. Most elderly people are completely self-sufficient and need no special assistance. Nearly 30 percent of people over 65 live alone, and while they may be phoned and visited by family members regularly, they are independent and prefer to remain so.

As a person ages, more assistance may be required in the basic tasks of living, especially as the person becomes more vulnerable to certain diseases. But even the so-called geriatric diseases can be controlled and managed today as never before. Conditions that occur in the elderly, such as heart attacks, pneumonia, and hip fractures, are not as likely to result in death with modern medical care. Thus, the elderly tend to live longer and may require more care.

Needs. Typical problems of the elderly include the provision of nutritious meals, clean clothing, personal hygiene, transportation, and legal and professional advice. Depending on their physical condition, they may require special housing facilities and specialized medical care. Depending on the needs of the individual, home care, a nursing home, or a hospital may be best able to provide the services required.

Home. Most of the frail elderly today are cared for at home by family members. In many cases, these family members are women who choose not to work or to curtail work in order to care for an elderly relative. They are responsible for shopping, meals, transporting the elderly person to doctors' appointments, assisting in personal hygiene, and administering medications. This can place great stress on the caregiver. Studies have shown that home care does not necessarily improve the health or life expectancy of an elder person and it may not improve physical or mental functioning, but it may improve the quality of life.

Home-care services are an available option. Trained professionals assist in household tasks like meals, cleaning and laundry, transportation, bathing, physical therapy, and the administering of medications. At present, most of these services have time limitations under Medicare coverage.

Assisted living is a compromise between living at home and in the nursing home. Assisted living facilities offer some of the independence and privacy of living at home, while dining and recreational facilities are offered on a community basis. Most residents have their own rooms or apartments, and they may have the option of cooking for themselves. In each apartment, the resident may ring emergency services for help directly in case of a fall or any other circumstance requiring immediate medical assistance.

Retirement communities offer a lifestyle that is closer to living at home. These residential communities usually provide social, cultural, and recreational facilities to residents as well as access to medical assistance when necessary.

Nursing homes are most suitable for people with serious physical and cognitive disabilities who may wander off and get lost if they are living with relatives, or for those who require 24-hour supervision due to other ailments. Only one percent of all people over the age of 65 live in nursing homes. However, close to 22 percent of all people over the age of 85 reside in nursing facilities. Deciding to place a loved one in a nursing home is always a difficult and complex decision. While nursing homes are

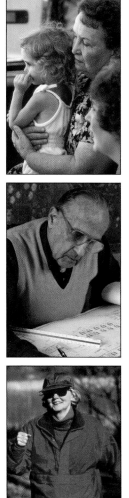

Care of the Elderly.
As a person ages, more assistance may be required in their everyday lives. Some people may choose to receive this assistance at facilities such as nursing homes or retirement communities. Others may seek help from their families (top). In any situation it is important to remain active by participating in activities such as reading (middle) and exercising (bottom).

Choosing a Nursing Home

Making arrangements for a nursing home can be a difficult task. Questions to ask:

- Is the facility licensed by the state and by Medicaid?
- How long has it been in operation?
- Is it clean, odor-free, and well maintained?
- Is the food nutritious and well prepared?
- Do the residents look clean and cared for?
- Are the rooms cheerful and of adequate size?
- Are there social and semi-physical activities available for the residents?
- Are there standard safety features like grab bars in the bathrooms?
- Is the facility fully wheelchair accessible?
- What is the ratio of staff to residents?
- Are professionals and staff and administrators on call at all times? What is the turnover rate?
- Are the professionals trained in geriatrics and other health-related fields?
- How much does it cost and what part of the expense is covered by insurance?

---

patterned somewhat after hospitals, only the senior physicians and administrators are trained medical professionals.

In many cases, nursing homes are the best option for elderly with severe disabilities or advanced dementia whose families are unable to care for them. However, nursing homes have also met with criticism for varying degrees of negligence. The Nursing Home Reform Act, passed in 1987, established basic standards for all nursing homes with respect to nutrition, health codes, and patient care. Ultimately, it is the responsibility of the fa-mily to oversee their loved one's long-term care and to advocate on his or her behalf.

While most private insurance and the Medicare public health care plan do not cover the cost of nursing home facilities, Medicaid recipients are eligible for these services. In fact, according to The Family Caregiver Aliance, Medicaid currently pays more than half of the U.S. total nursing home bill.

See AGING *for fundamental material on care of the elderly. For additional information, see* GERONTOLOGY; MEDICARE; MEDICAID; *and* NURSE, HOME CARE. *For related material see* ACCIDENTS; DEPRESSION *and* HYGIENE.

Resources on Aging and Care of the Elderly
Cassel, Christine, *Geriatric Medicine* (1990), Fries, James F., *Aging Well* (1989); Rossman, Isadore, *Looking Forward: The Complete Medical Guide to Successful Aging* (1989); Schneider, Edward L. and John W. Rowe, *Handbook of the Biology of Aging* (1996); Weiss, Robert, et al., *Complete Guide to Health and Well-Being After Fifty* (1988); American Assoc. of Retired Persons, Tel. (800) 424-3410, Online: www.aarp.org; American Geriatrics Soc., Tel. (212) 308-1414, Online: www.americangeriatrics.org; National Council on Aging, Tel. (800) 424-9046, Online: www.ncoa.org; www.nyc-ornell.org/medicine/geriatrics/index.html; www.cornellaging.org/.

Elective Surgery

Surgery that is performed at the patient's request but is not needed immediately and is not in response to a life-threatening illness or injury.

Common examples of elective surgery include procedures performed on the eyes (laser and LASIK eye operations, as well as cataract removal), back, stomach (hernia), and anus (hemorrhoids). Sclerotherapy is a form of elective surgery used for treating varicose veins in the legs or hemorrhoids. Cryosurgery is another method involving the use of liquid nitrogen or carbon dioxide to freeze off a hemorrhoid. Liposuction is a form of "body contour surgery" used to remove unwanted fat and skin. *See also* BODY CONTOUR SURGERY; COSMETIC SURGERY; CRYOSURGERY; LASER TREATMENT; LIPOSUCTION; *and* SCLEROTHERAPY.

Electrical Injury

Also known as electrical shock

Injury to the skin or internal organs resulting from exposure to an electrical current.

The human body is a good conductor of electricity. Because of this, direct contact with an electric current is potentially fatal. While some resulting burns look minor, the shock is still capable of inflicting serious damage to internal organs.

An electric current can injure the body in three main ways. Cardiac arrest can result from the effect of an electric current on the heart. Massive muscle destruction can be caused from the current passing through the body. Finally, contact with the electrical source can cause thermal burns.

Incidence. In the United States, about 1,000 people die annually of electric shock. Statistically, children under two have a slightly higher risk of electrical injury.

Cause. Electrical injury occurs through exposure to an electric current. Accidental contact with the exposed part of an electrical appliance or wiring; lightning; and contact with high-voltage electric lines are the common sources of electrical injury.

Preventing Electrical Injury in Children

Young children are especially prone to accidental exposure to electricity. They may bite or chew an electric cord or poke a sharp object into an electrical outlet. For that reason, it is important to keep child-safety plugs on all outlets. Children should be taught the dangers of electricity, and parents should take whatever steps possible to minimize electrical hazards in the home. Electrical devices and cords should be kept out of the reach of children, and electrical appliances should be kept out of the bathroom and away from sinks.

SYMPTOMS

Electrical injury causes a diverse range of symptoms. Fatigue, headache, fracture, heart attack, muscle spasms, muscular pain, skin burns, unconsciousness, and loss of vision are some of the signs that exposure to an electric current may have resulted in bodily injury.

TREATMENT

The first step in treatment is to insure that you are not at risk for shock. Having done so, if possible, try to remove the source of the electric current. Often, turning off an appliance will not stop the flow of electric current. The appliance must be unplugged, or the fuse removed from the fuse box. The immediate source of the current should not be touched. If the current cannot be turned off, a non-conducting object, such as a broom or rubber doormat, can be used to push the victim away from the source of the current. Call for medical help. Once the source of the electricity has been stopped, check for signs of breathing and a pulse. If either has stopped, CPR is necessary. Clothing should be removed from burned areas. The victim's head and neck should remain immobile in case internal or spinal injuries have been suffered.

PREVENTION

Simple measures can help to prevent exposure to electric current. Electrical appliances should not be used while showering or while wet. Never touch an electrical ap-

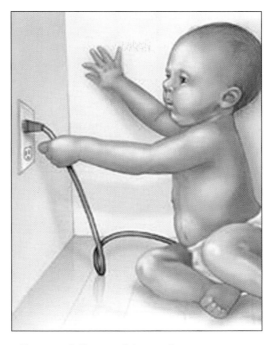

pliance while touching a faucet or water. Frayed or exposed wires should also never be touched and should be replaced to prevent fires.

> *See* ACCIDENTS *for fundamental material on electrical injury. Further reading is contained in* BURNS; CARDIAC ARREST; *and* SHOCK. *For material on treating Electrical Injury, see* EMERGENCY, FIRST STEPS, EMERGENCY HOSPITALIZATION *and* FIRST AID.

Electrocardiogram

Also known as ECG or EKG (after the German)

A diagnostic examination that translates the electrical impulses of the heart into characteristic waves, which can indicate abnormalities of cardiac structure and function.

The electrocardiogram is a noninvasive test that provides information on the functioning of a patient's heart. An ECG records electrical current and maps this information onto a graph; this printout is known as an electrocardiograph. Damage to the heart may be revealed through alterations in the conduction or flow of electrical impulse through the heart.

The electrocardiogram is a painless diagnostic test that may be carried out when the patient is at rest or during exercise, as

Preventing Electrical Injury.
Small children are particularly at risk for electrical injury, because they may be inclined to chew on an electrical wire or stick their fingers or a foreign object into an electrical outlet. Because of this, it is important to teach small children that electricity is dangerous. All electrical cords and devices should be kept out of reach and all accessible outlets should be covered with safety plugs.

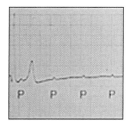

ECG.
An ECG is a diagnostic test that charts electrical impulses from the heart as waves. Above, an ECG from a patient with an arrhythmia.

in a cardiac stress test. In neither case is any specific preparation required. Electrodes (leads) capable of monitoring heart activity are attached to the arms, legs, and chest. These leads are connected to a recording device sensitive to the heart's electrical activity. This recorder will produce the electrocardiograph, which should be interpreted by a cardiologist.

Heart impulses are translated into tracings that allow the cardiologist to indirectly observe the contraction of the small atrial chambers and the larger ventricles, as well as the period of rest and restabilization occurring between heartbeats.

Damage to the heart muscle produces characteristic irregularities in these waves, as do alterations in blood hormones, salts, and various chemicals associated with heart metabolism. Irregularities in these wave forms may indicate the presence and location of a number of disorders including: insufficient blood supply (ischemia); tissue death (cardiac infarction); enlargement of the heart (hypertrophy); abnormal heart beat (arrhythmia); valve disease; congenital heart disease; or defects in electrical conduction.

Prevention. While an electrocardiogram is recommended any time heart irregularities are detected, it is advisable to have such a test before the age of 40. This will establish a baseline of heart function, which may be compared to test results at a later time to assess changes in the condition of the heart.

Resources on Electrocardiogram

Berne, Robert M., et al., *Cardiovascular Physiology* (2001); Conover, Mary B., *Understanding Electrocardiography* (1996); Debakey, Michael E. and Antonio M. Gotto, *The New Living Heart* (1997); (2000); American Heart Association, Tel. (800) 242-8721, Online: www. amhrt.org; Heart Information Network, Tel. (973) 701-6035, Online: www. heartinfo. org; National Heart, Lung, and Blood Institute, Tel. (301) 496-4236, Online: www.nhlbi. nih.gov; www.nycor-nell.org/cardiothoracic.surgery/; www.nycornell.org/ medicine/cardiology/index.html; www.nycornell. org/ medicine/cp/.html.

Risk Factors

Among the preventable risk factors affecting cardiovascular health, particularly those associated with coronary heart disease, are a sedentary lifestyle, obesity, high blood cholesterol, high blood pressure (hypertension), and cigarette smoking. Eliminating or reducing these critical risk factors considerably improves the overall heath of the cardiovascular system. Age, family history, and race are risk factors outside an individual's control, though greater vigilance among those considered at risk (including regular heart checkups after age 50) dramatically improves chances of early detection of cardiac irregularities and effective treatment.

ALERT

Warning Signs

Heart ailments are of critical concern and must always be attended to by a cardiologist. Any of the following warning signs may indicate a potentially life-threatening heart condition or impending heart attack (myocardial infarction). If you experience any of these, seek immediate medical attention!

• Chest pain that travels along the arm, shoulders, neck or jaw;
• Squeezing sensation beneath the breastbone;
• Cold sweat accompanying chest pain;
• Nausea or vomiting accompanying chest pain;
• Chest pain with backache;
• Pale or bluish skin accompanied by chest pain;
• Sensation of irregular heartbeat ;
• Severe anxiety accompanying chest pain.

Cardiac Stress Test. Certain cardiac abnormalities, such as coronary artery disease (atherosclerosis of the heart), may not be readily apparent from a resting ECG trace. By increasing the heart rate through exercise on a treadmill or stationary bicycle, fluctuations in ECG undetectable during rest may be observed and diagnosed. This is commonly known as a cardiac stress test or exercise ECG.

Supplementary Techniques. While ECG is a painless and safe procedure, providing generally reliable information, errors in the ECG can occur, yielding either false positive or false negative results. When conditions warrant, additional supplementary tests may include a stress test, or an echocardiogram, which will improve the reliability of cardiac diagnosis.

Thallium Stress Test. Occasionally, a radioactive dye may be injected to help identify damaged regions of the heart or areas receiving insufficient oxygen supply. This specialized ECG is known as a thallium stress test, since an isotope of the element thallium is used. Areas identified through a thallium stress exam may represent areas more susceptible to future heart attack than their healthier counterparts.

See DIAGNOSIS *and* MEDICAL TESTS *for background on electrocardiogram. For further reading, see* CARDIAC STRESS TEST *and* HEART, DISORDERS OF. *For related material, see* ARRHYTHMIA; HYPERTROPHY *and* ISCHEMIA.

Electrocoagulation

Method of sealing broken blood vessels by applying heat with a high-frequency electric current.

Electrocoagulation is a form of diathermy, which uses high-frequency electric currents, ultrasound, and microwave energy, in medical treatment.

In electrocoagulation, a current is applied to tissue either through a needle or, in surgery, through a knife, allowing the surgeon to make a bloodless incision or close freshly cut blood vessels. In addition to use in surgery, electrocoagulation can be applied to stop nosebleeds or to eliminate abnormal blood vessel formations, such as spider nevi and retinal bleeding. *See also* BLOOD VESSELS; DIATHERMY; NOSEBLEEDS; *and* ULTRASOUND.

Electroconvulsive Therapy

Also known as ECT or shock therapy

Treatment option for major depression in which an electric current is used to induce a seizure, which triggers the release of mood-altering chemicals in the brain.

An individual who receives ECT therapy is first given an anesthetic agent to induce sleep and a muscle relaxant. A small electric shock is then directed through electrodes attached to the head to produce a controlled seizure in the brain. Although the exact nature of how ECT works is not known, the seizure stimulates the brain to restore its overall chemical balance. ECT has often been successful when antidepressant medications have failed. It is administered in a series of six to 12 treatments to induce seizure, two to three times per week, and usually begins to work after only a few treatments

During the 1940s and early 1950s, this treatment form had not been well developed, and anesthetics were not properly administered. As a result of this and a lack of knowledge about advances in administering ECT, it has been portrayed in movies and in popular culture as barbaric and punishing. It is, however, considered one of the safest and most effective treatments for serious mental illness. It is often recommended when other medication has proven ineffective.

The patient must consent before ECT can be administered. The patient must also demonstrate an understanding of his or her illness and the nature of the ECT treatment. Following a comprehensive evaluation (including a blood analysis and electrocardiogram), the patient will be considered for treatment. Side effects of ECT may include headaches and temporary changes in memory.

> *See* DEPRESSION *and* PSYCHOTHERAPY *for background on electroconvulsive therapy. For further reading, see* PSYCHIATRY *and* SEIZURE. *For related material, see* ELECTROCARDIOGRAM *and* MEMORY.

Electrodessication and Curettage

A treatment for skin disorders that dissolves tissue through the use of an electric current.

In this procedure, a surgical instrument called a curette is first used to scrape away some of the tissue. An electrosurgical instrument is then used to stop the bleeding and cauterize the abnormal tissue. This procedure removes the abnormal tissue and minimizes the chance that the skin disorder will recur. *See also* SKIN.

Electroencephalogram

Also known as EEG

A graphic representation of brain wave activity, recorded by scalp electrodes.

Electroencephalography is a painless procedure that allows the physician to evaluate electrical activity of the brain. It is particularly useful for diagnosing major abnormalities, such as epilepsy, inflammation of the brain (encephalitis), and tumors. By means of electrodes attached to the scalp, the activity of masses of brain cells or neurons may be monitored. The record of this brain activity is then traced onto a continuously moving strip of graph paper—the re-

Testing the Brain

Electroencephalogram (EEG) is a painless, noninvasive procedure in which electrodes are attached to the patient's scalp. Recording the activity of the brain, the EEG apparatus converts the data received through scalp electrodes into a visual graph of characteristic brain waves. Analysis of such waves may be used for the diagnosis of various abnormalities caused by tumor, lesion, or stroke. It is of particular use in the diagnosis of epilepsy.

sulting record is known as an electroencephalogram.

Procedures. A typical EEG uses 16 to 30 electrodes, attached to the scalp with an adhesive paste. These electrodes measure the electrical potential flowing between two or more locations. The activity recorded by the electrodes forms recognizable patterns depending on the subject's state of activity. One pattern in normal resting subjects is known as the alpha rhythm. Typical changes in the alpha wave pattern will be noted when the subject falls asleep, opens his or her eyes, or during active mental attention. Other characteristic brain waves recorded in the procedure are known as beta, theta, and delta rhythms, and are defined by different frequencies. An EEG usually takes about 30 minutes.

Uses. While more subtle brain disorders cannot be diagnosed with electroencephalography and require more sensitive procedures, EEG has proven invaluable in the study of epilepsy and other convulsive disorders, as well as in pinpointing cerebral lesions. Changes in brain electrical activity associated with head injury, tumor, stroke, or cerebral infection may be observed in EEG irregularities.

In cases of epilepsy, the physician will often record the brain's normal activity at rest, then expose the patient to various stimuli. These may be visual, auditory or tactile, depending on the form of epilepsy under study. These stimuli produce characteristic jagged wave patterns associated with different kinds of seizures, indicating the nature and severity of the disorder. Such epileptic episodes are more easily

triggered in subjects who are sleep-deprived, and the patient being assessed may be asked to go without sleep for 18 to 24 hours prior to the examination. Once the condition of epilepsy is established through study of the electroencephalogram, further tests are generally required to evaluate the precise cause and possibilities for treatment.

See Diagnosis *and* Medical Tests *for fundamental material on electroenchephalogram. For additional information, see* Brain *and* Brain, Disorders of. *For detailed information on disorders, see* Brain Tumor; Encephalitis; Epilepsy; *and* Seizure.

Electrolysis

A method used to destroy the cells responsible for hair growth as a means of removing unwanted hair.

In electrolysis, a wire that delivers a low electrical current is inserted into the hair follicles destroying both the follicle and the root (papilla). Once the root is destroyed, the hair will not grow back.

There are three different methods of electrolysis. The first method, called galvanic modality, uses direct current to cause a chemical reaction in the hair follicle. This chemical change produces sodium hydroxide, which kills the cells responsible for hair growth. The second method, called thermolysis modality, involves utilizing alternating current to cause heat in the follicle, thereby cauterizing the follicle tissue electrically. Flash thermolysis, the third method, is the application of alternating current at a high intensity and for a short time. Some electrologists use a blend of all three methods. *See also* Hair Removal.

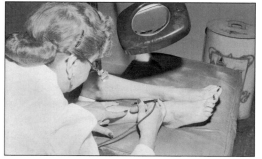

Electrolysis.
Electrolysis is a common method used to remove hair from unwanted areas. Right, a specialist administers an electrical current to a patient's leg in an effort to destroy the hair follicles and prevent regrowth.

Electrolyte

Non-metallic substance vital to energy transference in, and movement of, the body.

Electrolytes are elements (e.g., potassium, sodium, magnesium, and chloride) that, when dissolved in the body's fluids, separate into electrically charged particles, or ions. Electrolytes are essential to the transmission of nerve impulses, muscle contraction, fluid regulation, and maintenance of the acid-base balance of bodily fluids.

Sodium and chloride are mainly found in the fluids surrounding cells. These are the main ions involved in perspiration; they may be lost in large quantities during profuse sweating, although only in extreme situations is salt deficiency an issue. Magnesium and potassium are found largely in fluids inside cells, and are lost through perspiration, but rarely enough to cause deficiency. Excessive or inappropriate use of diuretics may cause severe magnesium or potassium deficiency.

> *Background material on electrolyte can be found in* Cells; Energy; *and* Nutrition. *Additional information is contained in* Acid; Chloride; Energy; Energy Requirements; Magnesium; Perspiration; Potassium *and* Sodium. *Related material is available in* Diet and Disease; Diuretic Drugs; *and* Mineral.

Electronystagmography

A diagnostic technique used to record the speed and direction of involuntary eye movements associated with the disorder nystagmus.

Electronystagmography is sometimes used as a general term referring to tests designed to record the movements of the eyes, sometimes also used for certain ear, nose, and throat examinations. It records electrical signals from the eye muscles as a way to track eye movement. As a diagnostic tool, electronystagmography can help discriminate between inner-ear defects caused by central nervous system damage and defects with other underlying causes.

Nystagmus is a disorder characterized by rapid, involuntary eye movement. When severe enough, it can interfere with vision. The precise nature of the eye movements can indicate the underlying malady. Some forms of nystagmus are congenital and may be recognizable only to a physician. Other forms are occupational, such as those occasionally observed in miners and others working for extended periods in the dark. Opticokinetic nystagmus can result from watching constantly moving objects, such as telephone poles, from a moving train or other vehicle. Still other forms of nystagmus are due to specific neurological disorders. Aural nystagmus causes spasmodic movement of the eye and is the result of a disorder in the labyrinth of the inner ear. *See also* Nystagmus.

Electrophoresis

A technique for separating out tiny particles, such as viruses and proteins, for analysis.

In electrophoresis, substances to be separated are suspended in a gel. Two electrodes are placed on either side of the field of gel, and voltage is applied to the electrodes. Different particles, depending on their charge, size, and shape, are differently affected by the electrical voltage. Particles with positive charges move toward the negative electrode, and particles with negative charges move toward the positive electrode. To improve resolution, a pH gradient can be established in the gel. A protein then moves through the gel until its pH matches that of the gel, at which point it stops and collects, forming a thin band across the gel. *See* Centrifuge *and* Virus.

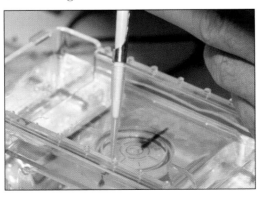

Gel Electrophoresis. Gel electrophoresis (left) is a routine procedure in many life science laboratories. The doubts regarding the reliability of DNA (genetic) fingerprinting, which uses this process, are at odds with the confidence the scientific community has in the procedure.

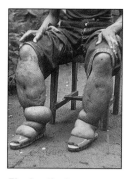

Elephantiasis.
Elephantiasis is a disease in which parasites infest the lymphatic system, resulting in an obstruction. This obstruction causes a hardening, swelling and darkening of the skin (above).

Elephantiasis

Tropical disease produced by filarial parasites, causing enlargement (hypertrophy) of the skin cells, due to lymphatic obstruction.

Elephantiasis, also known as lymphatic filariasis, is caused by several species of parasitic filarial worms, transmitted primarily by mosquitoes. *Wuchereria bancrofti* and *Brugia malayi* are among the more common species responsible for transmitting the disease. Infective larvae infest the lymphatics and lymph nodes. The adult females release larvae (microfilariae) back into the bloodstream, which the mosquitos can then re-ingest, enabling them to transmit the disease to others.

As a consequence of chronic lymphatic obstruction, sufferers experience swelling, darkening, and hardening of the skin, particularly in the legs, arms, and genital area, resulting in skin that resembles the hide of an elephant.

Diagnosis is made by examining the blood for the microscopic presence of the larvae (microfilariae). Treatment with antihelminitic drugs, such as diethylcarbamazine (Hetrazan), invermetin, and albendazole, destroys the parasites, although permanent damage may result from elephantiasis if the disease is well advanced before treatment. *See also* ANTIHELMINITHIC DRUGS; FILARIASIS; INSECT BITES; LYMPHATIC SYSTEM; MOSQUITO BITES; PARASITE; *and* WORM INFESTATION.

ELISA Test

Acronym for enzyme-linked immunoassay

A diagnostic test used to identify the presence and quantity of a variety of antigens and antibodies.

ELISA allows a physician to test for a specific hormone, antibody or antigen in the body, using a sample of the patient's blood. The blood is subjected to a chemical process that attaches the substance being tested for (if it is present) to the surface of a plate or test tube. An enzyme called peroxidase is then introduced to the surface and will stick to the substance. Another chemical is then added; a change in color reveals the substance's presence.

An alternative to traditional immunoassay procedures, ELISA tests are highly specific and have the further advantage of not requiring expensive radioisotopic apparatus and the toxic byproducts of radio-immune assay (RAI). *See also* ANTIBODY; ANTIGEN; ENZYME; IMMUNOASSAY; MEDICAL TESTS; *and* RADIOIMMUNOASSAY.

Embolectomy

Surgical removal of a blood clot (embolus) from a blood vessel.

An embolus is a clot of blood or other material, such as bone marrow (soft, fatty tissue), amniotic fluid, fat, a tumor fragment, or an air bubble, that has traveled in the bloodstream from one blood vessel to a smaller one and become lodged. This can block the supply of blood which poses a threat to life.

Symptoms of an embolus vary depending on the location of the blockage. An embolectomy is often performed with a balloon catheter to dislodge or break up the embolus. Removal of a clot at its original site before it has become dislodged is called a thromboectomy. *See* BALLOON CATHETERIZATION *and* EMBOLISM.

Embolism

A partial or complete blockage of an artery by something traveling in the bloodstream.

A substance that causes a blockage in an artery resulting in an embolism is called an embolus. An embolus can be a piece of tissue, a clump of bacteria, a bit of bone marrow or cholesterol, or a number of other substances (a pregnant woman can suffer an amniotic fluid embolism, in which amniotic fluid escapes from the uterus), but most often it is a blood clot that has broken away from an artery wall and has traveled to a spot where it causes blockage. A moving clot is referred to as a thrombus.

LOCATION

An embolism can occur almost anywhere in the body. The damage that an embolism inflicts is directly related to the site where it occurs.

Leg. An embolism in an artery of a leg or an arm causes pain, numbness, and inflammation in the area that loses its blood supply, sometimes accompanied by cramps and a sensation of cold and pain. If the blood supply is not restored quickly, gangrene can set in, and the tissue of the affected area will die from a lack of oxygen.

Lung. An embolism in an artery supplying the lung can cause chest pain, breathlessness, loss of consciousness, and sudden death if not treated quickly.

Brain. An embolism affecting an artery supplying the brain causes a stroke called a cerebral embolism, which occurs when a thrombus (a small clot that forms in an intact blood vessel) breaks off a blood vessel and travels toward the brain. It is distinguished from a stroke caused by cerebral thrombosis, in which the clot in an artery grows large enough to block the entire diameter of the blood vessel. People at highest risk of cerebral embolism include those with coronary artery disease or a condition affecting the heart valves.

SYMPTOMS

The symptoms of stroke may be mimicked by a transient ischemic attack, TIA, which differs from a stroke in that it does not last long—sometimes only a few minutes, sometimes a few hours. TIAs of longer duration are more likely to be caused by an embolism, while briefer ones are usually due to the narrowing of an artery. A TIA is an important warning signal—as many as half of the persons who suffer a stroke report that it was preceded by one or more TIAs. The risk of TIA or stroke is high in persons with cardiac conditions, such as atrial fibrillation, a disease of a heart valve, congestive heart failure, or endocarditis. An individual with an artificial heart valve or who has suffered a heart attack is also at increased risk, as these increase the chance that an embolus will form.

TREATMENT

Once the diagnosis of an embolism is established, it can be treated either by surgery or by medication. Drug treatment consists of a clot-dissolving (thrombolytic) agent that is injected into the affected artery. Sometimes the thrombolytic agent is administered through a catheter, a thin tube that is inserted in the artery. Thrombolytic agents used to treat embolisms include TPA (tissue plasminogen activator), streptokinase, and urokinase. The process by which the clot dissolves, which can last as long as 48 hours, can be monitored by angiography. Brain damage from a stroke caused by embolism can usually be prevented if TPA is administered within three hours after the onset of symptoms.

Angioplasty. If surgery is required because of an immediate threat of death or major damage, the most common procedure is balloon angioplasty. Alternatively, angioplasty, using a laser, may be performed in facilities equipped for this advanced technique, in which the tip of a catheter inserted into the artery carries a metal probe or a fiberoptic probe that focuses intense laser light on the embolus to dissolve the clot. Laser angioplasty is still being perfected. Angioplasty has replaced embolectomy, the surgical procedure once used for embolism, in which an incision was made in the artery at the site of the blockage, so that the embolus could be sucked out. *See also* BALLOON ANGIOPLASTY; CLOTTING; *and* EMBOLECTOMY.

ALERT

The Need for a Speedy Diagnosis

Quick and accurate diagnosis of an embolism is vital, because arrested blood flow can result in serious, life-threatening death of tissue. If a patient has the symptoms of an embolism, the tests that can be used to make the diagnosis include angiography—an x-ray procedure in which dye is injected to help locate the site of the blockage; an ultrasound examination using computer analysis to detect abnormalities in the flow of blood; and a CT (computerized tomography) scan, which also uses computer processing to produce an image of the blood vessels.

Embryonic Cells.
Right, fertilized human cells after two divisions. Each of these cells will develop into a different part of the embryo.

Embolism, Therapeutic

A surgical procedure performed to obstruct the internal flow of blood to a tumor, blood vessel, or in the event of uncontrollable bleeding.

Therapeutic embolism is often used when an individual is too weak to undergo major corrective surgery. The technique is commonly used for the treatment of tumors. By obstructing the flow of blood to the tumor, therapeutic embolism alleviates pain, prevent tumors from spreading, and, in some cases, can cause some tumors to shrivel, making removal easier. It may also be used to control bleeding in the lining of the intestines. *See* CANCER; *and* EMBOLISM.

Embryo

An unborn baby in the first eight weeks following fertilization. Afterwards, it is referred to as a fetus.

Fertilization occurs within the fallopian tube, which the egg travels through on the way from the ovary to the uterus. Immediately after fertilization, the embryo begins undergoing a series of cellular divisions, known as cleavage.

Embryos.
Right, MRI images of a human embryo at seven weeks. At this point, almost all cell differentiation has taken place. The cells are now in the process of developing into the organs for which they are intended.

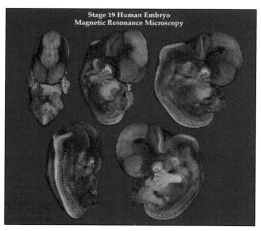

Stage 19 Human Embryo
Magnetic Resonance Microscopy

Sometimes during the early cell stages, cleavage results in the separation of the tissue into two distinct entities. Each entity will develop into a complete individual, or identical twin. Fraternal twins develop from two separate eggs fertilized at around the same time.

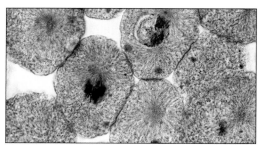

After seven days, the embryo has become a hollow "ball" of cells and has continued to journey through the fallopian tube until it reaches the uterus. It implants onto the uterine wall and is technically known as a blastula.

The blastula is a hollow structure, just one cell layer thick. A portion of its cells make up the embryo, and the rest form the following embryonic membranes:
- Allantois—removes waste;
- Amnion—membranous sac that surrounds the embryo; the cells lining the sac produce the amniotic fluid;
- Yolk sac—a small supply of stored food to be used until the baby "hooks up" to the mother's bloodstream;
- Chorion—supplies the embryo with oxygen and removes carbon dioxide.

These membranes eventually form the placenta. The umbilical cord connects the baby to the placenta.

The blastula subsequently develops into a two layered structure known as the gastrula. These two cell layers are the ectoderm (outer layer) and endoderm (inner layer). A third cell layer, the mesoderm (middle layer) eventually forms between them.

From these three cell layers all of the following body systems develop:
- Ectoderm—central nervous system and skin;
- Mesoderm—skeleton, muscles, reproductive, endocrine and excretory systems;
- Endoderm—digestive system and lungs.

It is not yet clearly understood how the cells "know" which type of tissue and structure they should form; this is known as the problem of cell differentiation. It is be-

Highlights of Embryonic Development

3 weeks: A two-chambered heart begins beating, along with the development of a rudimentary nervous system, called the neural tube. The neural tube will form the brain and spinal cord.

4-6 weeks: Limb buds, which will become the arms and legs, appear. All of the facial features are forming, as well as gonads. The embryo is 1/4 inch long.

8 weeks: The physical structure is complete, although still very tiny. The tail has disappeared, the limbs are becoming jointed, and the fingers and toes have formed. The fetus is between one-half to one inch long and weighs 1 gram.

lieved that there are chemical messengers that "communicate" between the various tissues, encouraging them to develop in certain ways, based upon which other tissues are nearby. This process is known as embryonic induction.

During the embryonic period, a lot of rapid development occurs. All of the major organs form, and the embryo develops from an amorphous ball of cells to a C-shaped creature, complete with gills and tail, to a one-inch-long recognizable hu-

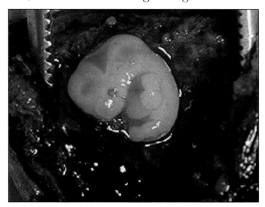

man being. During these first eight weeks, the embryo is highly susceptible to environmental factors, such as drugs or radiation. For this reason, the majority of miscarriages occur during this time.

Background material on embryo can be found in CHILDBIRTH AND ZYGOTE. *Related information is contained in* ABORTION; BIRTH DEFECTS; CHILDBIRTH; CHILDBIRTH, MULTIPLE; EMBRYOLOGY; EMBRYOS; RESEARCH ON; FEMALE REPRODUCTIVE SYSTEM; FETUS; MALE REPRODUCTIVE SYSTEM; *and* PREGNANCY.

Embryology

The branch of biology that deals with the formation, early growth, and development of organisms.

Organisms that reproduce sexually begin as a single fertilized egg cell that undergoes several rapid rounds of cell division. From this collection of cells arise the various cell layers and the many tissues and organ systems which make up the body. The specialization, or differentiation, of the cells into their component layers and structures involves intricate choreography that is not yet completely understood.

Background material on embryology can be found in EMBRYO *and* EMBRYO, RESEARCH ON. *Related information is contained in* CELL; DNA; FETUS; GENETICS; GENETIC CODE; GENETIC DISORDERS; GENETIC ENGINEERING; GENETIC PROBE; PREGNANCY *and* ZYGOTE.

Embryos, Research on

Research that uses a fertilized egg or its cells.

Cells from a fertilized human egg are being used in some types of medical research. Embryonic stem cells, for example, which have the ability to develop into virtually every type of cell in the human body, are used in stem-cell research. This type of research may lead to treatments for serious disorders, including Parkinson's disease, cancer, and diabetes. Research on human embryos also has the potential to help prevent miscarriages and improve scientific understanding of cancer and many types of genetic disorders.

The use of human embryos and fetal tissues is not without controversy, however; opponents of the procedure charge that it is wrong to use a human embryo for the purpose of scientific research. Currently, there is limited federal funding for research involving human embryos.

Background material on research on embryos can be found in EMBRYO AND EMBRYOLOGY. *Related information contained in* BIRTH DEFECTS; CANCER; GENETIC DISORDERS; MISCARRIAGE; PARKINSON'S DISEASE; *and* PUBLIC HEALTH.

Fetus.
During the first eight weeks of a pregnancy, the unborn child is referred to as an embryo. Thereafter it is known as a fetus (left).

Emergency Childbirth

The act of delivering a child without the supervision of a physician or midwife.

NECESSARY ITEMS FOR DELIVERY

- five-inch pieces of clean cloth
- sterilized scissors (boil to make sterile)
- bucket in case of vomiting
- container for afterbirth to be taken to the physician
- towels or sanitary napkins to place over the woman's vagina following the birth.

PREPARATION FOR DELIVERY

- **First.** Call the mother's obstetrician or gynecologist, or the nearest hospital for assistance. Do not, however, delay the birth. It is important to remain calm and to assist the mother in whatever way possible.
- **Second**. Wash your hands and clean underneath the nails. Wash your hands repeatedly during the birth.
- **Third.** Prepare a clean, flat surface with a towel (use newspaper if necessary). If possible, prop up the mother up with pillows so her legs are bent and her feet flat.

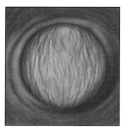

Emergency Childbirth. If the cervix becomes dilated to 10 cm (above), the pregnant woman begins to push out the baby (right) and childbirth is imminent, whether the mother is in the delivery room or not. The mother may experience the urge to have a bowel movement due to the baby's head pushing against the rectum (far right).

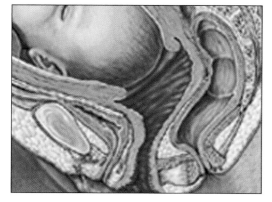

DELIVERY STEPS

- **First.** Encourage the mother to breathe as much as possible. Once the delivery begins, support the baby's head with your hands as it comes into view. Any visible membrane over the face should be torn away and removed. CAUTION: If the umbilical cord is looped around the neck, ease it over the head to prevent breathing problems. DO NOT pull on the baby's head!

- **Second.** Support the shoulders and the head as the baby emerges further. Allow one shoulder to emerge first and the second should follow if you gently raise the baby's head.
- **Third.** Wipe clean any mucus or blood from the baby's mouth so he or she can breathe freely. Continue supporting the body as it emerges.
- **Fourth.** Once the baby is entirely out, check to make sure it is breathing properly. If he or she is unable to breathe, hold the head lower than the body to drain away excess mucus. Blowing onto the chest, or tapping the soles of the feet may also help.

  DO NOT slap the baby's back to initiate breathing! If the infant is still unable to breathe, begin CPR and call 911.
- **Fifth.** Allow the cord to stay connected to the mother. Once it ceases to pulsate, tie the cord four inches from the baby's navel.
- **Sixth.** Wrap the baby and place him or her with the mother.
- **Seventh.** Usually, the afterbirth follows ten minutes after the birth. Gently massaging the mother's abdomen will help control the flow of blood.

Breech Delivery. If the baby's head does

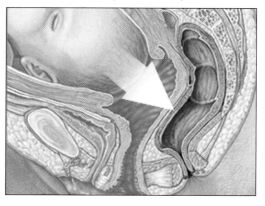

not emerge first, gently press on the mother's abdomen directly above her pubic hair. Support the body of the baby as it emerges, and carefully lift it in the process, exposing the face so as to allow the infant to breathe. DO NOT pull or tug the infant under any circumstances. Clean out the baby's mouth with a towel once the face is outside of the mother. *See also* CHILDBIRTH *and* CHILDBIRTH, COMPLICATIONS.

Emergency, First Steps

Critical situation that requires immediate medical attention.

In the United States, there exists a complete network of emergency services, including medical, fire, police, and psychological departments. Emergency vehicles range from helicopters, to ambulances, to boats. Dialing 911 anywhere in the United States activates a connection between a caller and the nearest emergency service dispatcher. However, in an emergency situation, a bystander must often take the first critical steps before emergency medical assistance is available. In such instances, important considerations include:

Breathing. Are the victim's air passages clear, and is he or she breathing? If there is a foreign object lodged in the throat, use the Heimlich maneuver. If the passages are clear but the victim is not breathing, use artificial ventilation.

Bleeding. Use some form of pressure to control bleeding. If an artery has been injured, a tourniquet may be required as a last resort, but the use of pressure is far more preferable. A cut artery will spurt or pulse; it is far more serious than a cut vein. In contrast, the blood from the latter will have a tendency to ooze. If a ruptured artery is suspected, treat the wound immediately, as a victim can die in minutes.

Heartbeat. Is there a detectable pulse? If not, the patient will require cardiopulmonary resuscitation (CPR) or artificail ventilation.

Protect Yourself. Avoid exposure to the blood or bodily fluids of a victim, as they may be a major source of infection.

Emergency Hospitalization

The treatment and care that an individual receives in a medical emergency.

Emergency departments are designed to deal with unexpected, life-threatening situ-

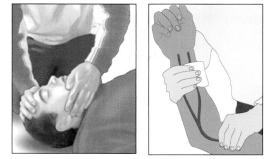

ations that require immediate medical attention, although people often go to the emergency room to treat relatively minor problems.

Triage. Once in the emergency department, patients who are the most severely ill or injured will be treated first. As a result of this need-based system of seeing patients (known as triage), someone with a minor problem may have to wait several hours to be examined. In addition to the wait, the cost of treatment in an emergency department can be as much as three times higher than that of a doctor's office. It can also be difficult to convince some HMOs to reimburse a patient for the costs of a visit to an emergency ward.

WHAT TO EXPECT

Upon arrival at the emergency room, unless you are severely ill or injured and require immediate attention, you will be interviewed by a staff member who will obtain personal and medical insurance information and have you sign treatment consent forms. After you are triaged, you will either be treated and released or admitted into the hospital for extensive care, depending on the nature of your injury.

Even if your life is not in immediate danger, there are still a number of symptoms that may require hospitalization. These include: severe bleeding (especially from an artery); loss of consciousness; pain; high fever; convulsions; difficulty breathing; severe headache; shock; weakness; and numbness in the extremities. All of these symptoms require emergency care, especially if the victim's physician is unavailable. *See also* EMERGENCY CHILDBIRTH; *and* EMERGENCY, FIRST STEPS.

First Steps in Handling an Emergency.
If a victim has lost consciousness, it is important to find out if he or she is breathing by checking for a pulse (above, left). If it appears that the victim is not breathing, open the airways and perform mouth-to-mouth resuscitation or CPR right, if the victim is bleeding, it is important to bandage the wound and apply pressure until help arrives.

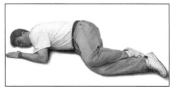

Recovery Position.
An unconscious victim who is still breathing should be placed in the recovery position until help arrives. The person should lie on the stomach with the near arm and top knee bent forward (as pictured).

Emetic

A medicine or substance that induces vomiting.

In certain cases of accidental poisoning (those that do not involve substances that are acidic or alkaline), vomiting is induced. Syrup of ipecac is a commonly used emetic. Soapy water can be used as well. Putting a finger, or other long object, to the back of the throat will induce the gag reflex and will help a person vomit if necessary. *See also* IPECAC; POISON; *and* VOMITING.

EMG

Acronym for electromyogram

A graphic record of muscle contraction following electrical stimulation.

Electromyography is used to measure tiny electrical discharges produced by skeletal muscles. Such activity may be recorded while the muscle is at rest or during muscle contraction. It is a powerful technique in the diagnosis of neuromuscular disease.

Procedure. EMG may be performed with the patient lying down or seated. A physician inserts a fine EMG electrode capable of monitoring the discharge of electricity through the skin. The muscle's electrical output is measured at rest and during muscle contraction, with the results observable on a monitor.

It is possible, through a separate test, to measure nerve conduction properties at the same time the electromyograph is recorded. Nerve conduction studies register the speed at which electrical impulses travel through nerves—often a critical factor in peripheral nerve disorders, such as carpal tunnel syndrome, as well as in central nervous system disorders like Parkinson's disease.

Special Consideration. An electromyogram may produce some discomfort when the needle-like electrode is inserted, although this is generally slight. Smoking should be restricted for several hours before the test, as should cafeinated beverages. Aspirin and related drugs should not be taken a week prior to the test.

Diagnosis. Muscle diseases are diagnosed through specific types of abnormalities that appear in an EMG. Diseases that may be diagnosed through EMG include muscular dystrophy, Lou Gehrig's disease (amyotrophic lateral sclerosis), motor neuron disease, inflammatory muscle disease, muscle degeneration arising from malfunction of the endocrine system (endocrine myopathy), glycogen storage diseases, and other muscular disorders.

See DIAGNOSIS and MEDICAL TESTS *for background on EMG. For further reading, see* AMYOTROPHY; ATROPHY; MUSCLE and MYOPATHY. *For related material, see* NERVE and PARKINSON'S DISEASE.

Emphysema

A respiratory disease that damages the small air sacs (alveoli) of the lungs.

Emphysema, the most common cause of death from respiratory disease in the United States, does its damage by attacking the alveoli, the millions of tiny sacs in the lung where oxygen moves into the blood and carbon dioxide moves into the lungs for exhalation.

Over the years, emphysema can have a harmful effect on a sufferer's heart. The steady decrease in oxygen forces the right side of the heart to work harder as it pumps blood through the lungs. There can be an increase in blood pressure in the pulmonary artery (pulmonary hypertension), which leads to a condition called cor pulmonale, in which the right side of the heart becomes abnormally enlarged because of the strain it experiences. Some people who experience cor pulmonale may experience swelling of the lower legs owing to excess fluid; their skin may take on a bluish tinge because of a lack of oxygen. Because of these symptoms. patients are known as "blue bloaters". Others may retain their normal skin color but will start to breathe more rapidly to get an adequate oxygen supply. These persons are referred to as "pink puffers," due to their reddish coloring from incessant, rapid breathing.

Resources on Emphysema

Haas, Francois and Shela Sperber Haas, The Chronic Bronchitis and Emphyse-ma Handbook (2000); Kittredge, Mary, The Res-piratory System (1989); Parker, Steve, The Lungs and Breathing (1989); Perry, Angela R., Essential Guide to Asthma (1998); Ruck-deschel, John C., Myths & Facts about Lung Cancer (1999); Scott, Wal-ter J., Lung Cancer: A Guide to Diagnosis and Treatment (1999); American Lung Association, Tel. (800) LUNG-USA, Online: www.lungusa.org; Lung Line Information Service, Tel. (800) 222-5864, Online: www.na-tionaljewish.org; Second Wind Lung Transplant Assoc., Tel. (888) 222-2690, Online: www.2ndwind.org; www.nycornell.org/medicine/pulmonary/index.html.

CAUSES

A relatively few cases of emphysema are caused by a genetic mutation that reduces production of alpha-1 antitrypsin (AAT), a protein that protects lung tissue. More than 90 percent of cases are the result of cigarette smoking, with atmospheric pollution sometimes a contributing factor.

The pollutants in tobacco smoke cause the alveoli to rupture or stretch out of their normal shape, as the cells of the lung emit harmful chemicals that cause tissue damage. The amount of damage is directly proportional to the number of cigarettes smoked. Over the years, the lungs lose their elasticity and efficiency, so that breathing becomes more difficult.

The Genetics of AAT

The genetic disorder that reduces production of AAT (or alpha-1 antitrypsin) is generally found in people of northern European descent. Its incidence in the U.S. population is about 1 in 2,500. In these individuals, emphysema can appear as early as their 30s. People from families where AAT deficiency has occurred are advised to be screened for the defect as early as possible and to be especially mindful of the dangers of smoking. They may be prescribed a drug called alpha-1 proteinase inhibitor, which increases lung levels of AAT by blocking activity of a protein that destroys AAT.

SYMPTOMS

Emphysema patients sometimes develop barrel chests, a result of their increasing efforts to supply oxygen to and release carbon dioxide from the body. Most persons with emphysema also develop a chronic cough, with or without a wheeze.

DIAGNOSIS

The disease is monitored by diagnostic tests, such as chest x-rays, pulmonary function tests, and blood tests that measure levels of oxygen and carbon dioxide.

TREATMENT

The damage done to the lungs is irreversible, so treatment is aimed at controlling the disease. For tobacco smokers, the obvious first step is to stop smoking. Bronchodilator drugs can be prescribed to widen the airways (bronchi and bronchioles) of the lung and make breathing more efficient. Corticosteriods sometimes are prescribed to relieve the lung inflammation caused by emphysema. These medications are usually taken through an inhaler, often called a nebulizer, which delivers drugs in an aerosol spray. If a patient retains fluid as the result of lung damage, diuretic drugs may be prescribed to increase the body's excretion of fluid. The doctor will also suggest a diet low in sodium to limit fluid accumulation.

What Accompanies Emphysema

Emphysema is often not the only lung problem that a smoker experiences. The disease is often accompanied by bronchitis—inflammation of the bronchi and bronchioles. The two conditions together are called chronic obstructive pulmonary disease, COPD, the sixth leading cause of death in the United States.

PROGNOSIS

The extent of recovery is dependent on how far the disease has progressed before the patient completely gives up smoking. In addition to smoking cessation, a healthy diet, low in fat and cholesterol and high in fruits, vegetables, and other sources of fiber is recommended. Regular exercise, although it may be difficult at first, can have a beneficial effect on lung function. Patients with emphysema are advised to be immunized against influenza and pneumonia, and to avoid contact with persons who have colds or an infectious lung disease.

Oxygen Therapy. If emphysema progresses enough to cause a dangerous reduction in the oxygen level of the blood, oxygen therapy will be prescribed. Oxygen therapy can be performed at home, using a machine called an oxygen concentrator. This machine extracts oxygen from the air, and pipes oxygen-rich air into a residence. Portable oxygen delivery systems are available for trips outside the home.

Background material on emphysema can be found in LUNGS *and* LUNG DISEASE, CHRONIC OBSTRUCTIVE. *Related information is contained in* AVEOLI; BLOOD PRESSURE; BRONCHITIS, BRONCHI OXYEGEN THERAPY; *and* RESPIRATORY SYSTEM.

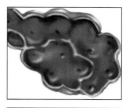
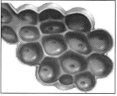

Alveoli.
Emphysema scars and damages the alveoli (air sacs) of the lungs. Above, top, alveoli with emphysema. Bottom, normal alveoli.

Emphysema, Surgical

A condition in which air enters the pleural cavity.

Surgical emphysema is to be distinguished from ordinary emphysema, damage to the airways of the lung caused by cigarette smoking or inhalation of pollutants. Surgical emphysema is usually the result of pneumothorax, a condition in which air enters the pleural cavity, the space between the two membranes that line the lungs and the chest wall. This condition occurs as the result of an injury (chest injury or diving accident) or as a complication from chest surgery; it may also occur unexpectedly for no apparent reason. *See* EMPHYSEMA.

The symptoms include pain in the chest and shortness of breath. Mild surgical emphysema often requires no treatment, but a semisurgical procedure to remove the air through a tube may be necessary. *See* LUNG.

Empyema

The accumulation of pus in a body cavity.

Empyema is associated with the thin membranes (the pleura) that surround the lungs and line the inside of the chest wall. Pus can accumulate when bacterial infections, such as pneumonia, are present in the lungs. Empyema may also result from injuries that cause the puncture of a lung.

Symptoms include chest pain, breathlessness, and fever. X-rays of the chest will confirm the presence of excess pus in the lung cavities. Treatment consists of draining the fluid with a needle and syringe (aspiration), possibly requiring a surgical procedure, and the administration of antibiotics to eradicate infection.

During an episode of gallstone-induced inflammation (cholecystitis), the gallbladder may serve as another site of empyema. As a complication of the inflammation, pus collects in the lining of the gallbladder. This type of empyema is typically treated by the surgical removal of the gallbladder (cholecystectomy). *See also* CHOLECYSTITIS; PLEURA; *and* PUS.

Resources on Encephalitis

Fettner, Ann Guidici, *The Science of Viruses: What They Are, Why They Make Us Sick, How They Will Change the Future* (1990); Fields, Bernard, et al., *Fields' Virology* (1996); Sacks, Oliver, *Awakenings* (1987); Sanes, Dan Harvey, et al., *Development of the Nervous System* (2000); Epilepsy Foundation, Tel. (800) EFA-1000, Online: www.efa.org; American Academy of Neurology, Tel. (651) 695-1940, Online: www.aan.com; American Board of Neurological Surgery, Tel. (713) 790-6015, Online: www.abns.org.

Encephalitis

An inflammation of the brain caused directly by a virus or indirectly by antibodies resulting from an infection of some other part of the body.

Any one of a number of different viruses may cause encephalitis, including the viruses associated with herpes and mumps. The viruses that cause measles, chickenpox, and rubella may not themselves attack the brain but may cause immune reactions that result in an inflammation there.

Symptoms of encephalitis are personality changes, seizures, weakness, confusion, and sleepiness that may lead to coma. Diagnosis is difficult since the symptoms mimic those of a brain tumor, a brain abscess, stroke, or hematoma. A spinal tap can often confirm the presence of a virus.

Treatment. Antiviral drugs (acyclovir) are effective against *herpes simplex* and *varicella zoster* encephalitis. For other forms of the disease, the treatment essentially attempts to control the symptoms. Anticonvulsants may be required to control seizures, analgesics to relieve headaches, and sedatives to encourage sleep. Steroids may be administered to reduce brain inflammation and the accumulation of fluid.

Long-Term Rehabilitation. Encephalitis in infants, small children, and adults over the age of 55 may be fatal. Others will recover slowly, and rehabilitation may be necessary because of brain damage *See also* ANTIVIRAL DRUGS; BRAIN; INFLAMMATION; REHABILITATION; *and* VIRUS.

Encephalitis Lethargica

Also known as "sleeping sickness"

A form of encephalitis that causes extreme lethargy and drowsiness.

Encephalitis lerthargica is caused by a number of different viruses, including herpes, mumps, and, indirectly, by measles, chicken pox, or rubella. There have not been any major outbreaks of encephalitis lethargica since the 1920s.

The initial symptoms of encephalitis lethargica are the same as encephalitis:

fever; extreme lethargy; and paralysis of the eye muscles that produces double vision. The onset of the disease is usually gradual with flu-like symptoms, although these may be preceded by an acute attack of delirium. In severe cases, the delirium may be followed by a coma, and the disease can be fatal. Lethargy, muscular pains, rigidity of the limbs, and convulsions are also symptoms of the disease.

If the patient recovers from the acute stages, tremors and an expressionless face may be exhibited. The posture droops and there is a characteristic shuffling gait. There is no treatment for encephalitis lethargica. Most cases end in chronic invalidism. *See also* ENCEPHALITIS.

Encephalomyelitis

A swelling of both the brain and the spinal cord, usually following a viral infection.

A rare condition that occurs as the result of a complication of measles, and in some instances, other viral infections like chickenpox, rubella, and mononucleosis. Encephalomyelitis is characterized by extreme fatigue after exercise, muscle pain and twitching, and flu-like symptoms, including a sore throat, enlarged lymph glands, and erratic body temperature. The sufferer experiences intellectual and emotional changes as the disease progresses. In severe cases, there will be relapses, but most sufferers recover after a prolonged convalescence.

A physician diagnoses encephalomyelitis based on symptoms, blood tests, and other diagnostic tests such as CT scanning and an EEG (an electroencephalogram). The syndrome may be confused with chronic fatigue syndrome since many of the symptoms are similar, but sufferers of encephalomyelitis exhibit slower recovery of muscle strength and longer lasting fatigue following minimal exercise.

As there is no cure for the disease, treatment involves the use of corticosteroid drugs to reduce inflammation and anticonvulsant drugs to minimize seizures. *See also* CAT SCAN *and* EEG.

Encephalopathy

Diseases of the brain, particularly those that are chronic and degenerative.

Encephalopathy generally refers to one of two diseases, Wernicke's encephalopathy and hepatic encephalopathy.

Wernicke's encephalopathy is a degenerative brain condition caused by a deficiency of vitamin B_1 (thiamine). In developed countries, this occurs most often among alcoholics. Symptoms include weakness, tremors, double vision, memory loss, and mood and behavior changes. One of the marked symptoms of the disease is confabulation, in which an affected person makes up detailed stories to fill in memory gaps. The condition is often complicated by symptoms of alcohol withdrawal or other alcohol-related diseases.

Wernicke's encephalopathy is treated with injections of thiamine, which can improve physical symptoms and slow progression of the disease. Memory and cognition, however, are not usually improved. In the long term, abstention from alcohol and proper nutrition can limit the disease. If untreated, Wernicke's encephalopathy is fatal. *See also* ALCOHOL DEPENDENCE.

Hepatic Encephalopathy, also called portal systemic encephalopathy or hepatic coma, occurs as a result of liver failure or malfunction. Toxic substances that would normally be removed by a properly functioning liver build up in the blood. Ammonia, which is produced when the body breaks down protein, is a common toxin that accumulates.

Symptoms include impaired consciousness, memory loss, personality and behavior changes, tremors, seizures, sluggish speech, and coma. Treatment consists of providing life support, removing toxic substances from the body, and treating the liver, if possible. Prognosis varies. If the underlying cause is treatable, recovery prospects are good; if not, the disease can be progressive and fatal. *See also* BRAIN; BRAIN DISORDERS; CREUTZFELDT-JAKOB SYNDROME; *and* WERNICKE-KORSAKOFF SYNDROME.

Encopresis

Inability to control bowel movements after the age of about four.

Most children are toilet trained, with various levels of encouragement, by the time they are four. Encopresis refers to the condition in which a child passes feces in his or her pants or on the floor after an age when toilet training has been or should have been established.

Encopresis usually occurs when a child holds in stools, causing constipation, then loses control and defecates in a place other than the toilet. It is several times more common in boys than in girls.

Causes. Encopresis is often caused by a physical problem, such as delayed physical development or a gastrointestinal disorder. In the absence of a medical cause, and especially if a child has been successfully toilet trained and later developed encopresis, it is generally a stress-related response. For example, it may be a reaction to the birth of a sibling or moving to a different home.

Treatment. A child who has suffered an uncontrolled bowel movement should not be shamed or berated. Any medical cause should first be identified and treated. Encopresis responds well to behavior modification, using a system of positive reinforcement for using the toilet. It may also be helpful to temporarily use laxatives to help with constipation. *See also* BEHAVIOR THERAPY; CONSTIPATION; *and* ENURESIS.

Endarterectomy

Surgical removal of the lining of a narrowed blood vessel, along with any fatty buildup (atherosclerosis) and blood clots (thrombi).

An endarterectomy is generally performed on major arteries, such as the carotid artery in the neck or the femoral and popliteal arteries in the legs. Carotid endarterectomies are performed to treat victims of minor strokes or transient ischemic attacks who experience narrowing of at least 70 percent of the vessel.

Procedure. The surgeon makes an incision to access the involved artery, puts clamps above and below the obstruction, scrapes out the buildup and lining, and stitches up the artery, using a graft patch. Often, it is necessary for the surgeon to construct a temporary bypass tube to provide circulation around the problem area.

A carotid endarterectomy involves some risk (one to two percent) of causing a stroke or complication; patients with heart problems and high blood pressure are at greater risk. Treating small blockages pharmacologically is generally considered less risky than premature surgical attempts to rectify the problem.

See CLOT *and* SURGERY *for background on endarterectomy. For further reading see* ARTERY; ARTEROSCLEROSIS; CARTOID ARTERY *and* THROMBOSIS. *Related material is contained in* BYPASS; GRAFT; ISCHEMIA; HYPERTENSION; SHUNT *and* STROKE.

Endemic Illness

A disease that is peculiar or native to a locality.

An endemic illness is one that is present in constant levels in a population. Endemic illnesses often occur in low levels in a community, such as a neighborhood or city. An endemic illness is the opposite of an epidemic illness, which affects an unexpectedly large number of people in the population. *See also* CHICKEN POX; EPIDEMIC; LIFE EXPECTANCY; MEASLES; PANDEMIC; PUBLIC HEALTH *and* STREP THROAT;.

Endocarditis

An inflammation of the endocardium (the tissue that lines the interior of the heart and its valves), generally caused by an infection, a congenital heart defect or rheumatic fever.

Damaged or malformed heart valves are especially vulnerable to endocarditis. Nearly 75 percent of cases occur in people with a deformation of a valve or some other part of the heart. People who have had artificial valves implanted are more susceptible to infections also, because these valves tend to attract bacteria. The risk is also high for people who inject illegal drugs, since the needles they use often harbor infectious agents. In the past, endocarditis was almost always due to infection by bacteria such as group A streptococcus. Today, the infectious agents can be any of a variety of bacteria or fungi

SYMPTOMS AND DIAGNOSIS

Symptoms of endocarditis include: fever; weight loss; fatigue; loss of appetite; chills; night sweats; headache; and joint pain. Patients sometimes develop small hemorrhages on the skin of the chest, back, fingers, or toes. Diagnosis starts with a physical examination and a blood test to identify the infectious agent. Doppler echocardiography, nuclear scanning, or magnetic resonance imaging, can provide an image of the damage.

TREATMENT

Aggressive treatment with antibiotics or other therapies can attack the infection once it is identified. While oral or intravenously administered antibiotics taken at home are sometimes prescribed, patients are usually hospitalized for intravenous antibiotic therapy. Antibiotic therapy is continued for at least a month to prevent serious complications, such as heart failure or the formation of blood clots that can cause heart attack or stroke. In some cases, surgery may be performed to cut out the infected area, or repair or replace a damaged valve.

Prevention

Preventive measures are important for individuals at high risk of endocarditis. Many of these measures center on dental care, to prevent the passage of bacteria from the mouth to the heart. Thorough but gentle daily brushing and other oral hygiene measures are recommended, as are frequent visits to the dentist. Antibiotics are prescribed before any visit to the dentist, before dental or medical surgery, and if a significant skin infection occurs. Anyone who has had endocarditis should be monitored for at least a year after the condition is treated, to prevent a relapse or the occurrence of a new infection.

Endocrine Disorders

Any disorder affecting a gland that results in deficient or excessive production of a given hormone.

Benign tumors of the endocrine glands, autoimmune diseases, or disorders of the pituitary or hypothalamus are the most common causes of endocrine disorders. When an excessive or deficient amount of a given hormone is produced, it disturbs the secretion of trophic hormones (stimulating hormones) by the pituitary and hypothalamus, which results in further complications to a person's endocrine system and overall health.

Types. Addison's disease occurs when the adrenal glands do not produce a sufficient amount of corticosterioid hormones to keep the body's sodium, potassium, and sugar levels steady. This condition may occur as the result of cancer, autoimmune disorder, or a severe infection, such as tuberculosis.

Cushing's syndrome results when the adrenal glands overproduce hydrocortisone hormones. A pituitary tumor, for example, may cause the overproduction of corticotropin, the hormone controlling the adrenal glands, leading to Cushing's syndrome.

Thyrotoxicosis occurs when the thyroid secretes excess amounts of hormone (hyperthyroidism). It is also used as another name for Graves' disease.

Diagnosis of an endocrine disorder is based on blood tests that measure the amount of different hormones in the body to determine the exact cause of the disorder. In the case of Addison's disease, because the symptoms start slowly and are minor, this disorder may defy and escape early diagnosis.

Treatment is determined by the underlying cause of the condition.

Background material on endocrine disorders can be found in ADDISON'S DISEASE *and* GLAND *. Related information is contained in* CUSHING'S SYNDROME; GRAVE'S DISEASE; ENDOCRINE SYSTEM; HORMONE; HYDROCORTISONE; TOXOCOLOGY *and* THYROTOXICOSIS.

Resources on Endocrine Disorders

Greenspan, Francis S., et al., Basic & Clinical Endocrinology (2000); Krimsky, Sheldon and Lynn Goldman, *Hormonal Chaos: The Scientific and Social Origins of the Environmental Endocrine Hypothesis* (1999); Shin, Linda M., et al., *Endocrine and Metabolic Disorders Sourcebook* (1998); American Thyroid Association, Tel. (718) 882-6047, Online: www. thyroid.org; www.nycornell.org/medicine/edm/index.html.

Endocrine System

Glands secreting hormones that maintain bodily functions

The endocrine system is composed of glands that help regulate a number of important processes in the body, including: growth and development; metabolism; use and storage of nutrients; sexual development and reproduction; and regulation of fluid and mineral levels. Hormones secreted by the endocrine glands (i.e, pituitary, thyroid, parathyroid, and adrenal glands) flow directly into the bloodstream, as opposed to hormones from exocrine glands (i.e., lacrimal, or tear glands, and sweat glands), which release hormones into ducts (such as tear ducts) that conduct the hormones directly into an organ or to the surface of the body.

The hormones of the endocrine system are released through a series of commands that begin in the hypothalamus, a portion of the brain above the pituitary. The hypothalamus, reacting to signals from the rest of the body and its own monitoring of hormone levels, directs the pituitary gland to decrease or increase production of its hormones. These hormones travel through the bloodstream, sending messages to other glands that tell them how much to produce of their own hormones. These hormones are then released to make their own journey through the bloodstream, searching for the receptors on the organs or tissues that they control. The receptors—highly sensitive areas on the surfaces or in the cells—join with the hormone to send a message into the cells that causes that organ or tissue to commence activity.

With their activities so closely connected, it is easy to see how a disorder in one gland can cause disturbances throughout the whole body. A benign tumor may cause a gland to overproduce its hormone, which will then send the wrong signals to the organs and tissues it controls. Any other glands that are directed by that hormone will then release incorrect amounts of their hormones. Autoimmune diseases that attempt to destroy a gland can lead to underproduction of that gland's hormone, which can result in the same chain reaction throughout the body.

GLANDS AND DISORDERS OF THE ENDOCRINE SYSTEM

Here is a brief overview of the glands of the endocrine system, and the disorders that may affect them:

Pituitary Glands. The pituitary gland consists of anterior and posterior sections. The anterior pituitary gland produces ACTH (adrenocorticotrophic hormone), which directs the adrenal glands; TSH (thyroid-stimulating hormone), which directs the thyroid glands; the growth hormone (GH); and hormones that direct testicular and ovarian function (FSH, LH) and milk production (prolactin) in females.

Disorders may include tumors, which can cause overproduction of one of the pituitary hormones, thereby affecting production of various hormones in other parts of the body. Deficiency of hormones can impair functions and development; for example, low growth hormone production can cause short stature, while overproduction can cause gigantism.

Thyroid. The thyroid gland produces the hormones T_4 and T_3 that help regulate metabolism. Thyroid disorders include:

• **Cretinism.** Too little production of the hormones T_4 and T_3 in infants and children can result in stunted growth; thickened facial features; a large protruding tongue; abnormal bone growth; mental retardation; decreased metabolic rate; and general lethargy. Treatment includes administration of T_4.

• **Graves' Disease.** Also known as hyperthyroidism; an excess production of T_4 and T_3 can cause weight loss; rapid pulse; warm skin; increased metabolism; goiter; tremors; and weakness. Treatments include removal of part of the gland, radioactive iodine therapy, and antithyroid drugs.

• **Myxedema.** Also known as hypothyroidism; insufficient T_4 and T_3 in adults can lead to weight gain; slow pulse; dry skin and brittle hair; decreased metabolism;

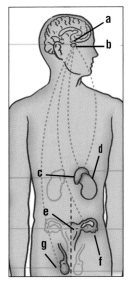

Endocrine System. Above, a diagram of the endocrine system. Pictured (from top to bottom) are the (a) hypothalmus, (b) pituitary gland, (c) adrenal glands, (d) kidney, (e) uterus, (f) ovaries, and (g) testes.

lack of energy; cold intolerance; and diminished perspiration. Treatment consists mainly of the administration of T_4.

• **Goiter.** Insufficient levels of iodine in the body can cause enlargement of the thyroid gland. Treatment requires the administration of iodine, thyroid hormone, or possible surgery.

• **Adrenal Glands.** The adrenal glands are made up of two parts. The adrenal cortex helps regulate metabolism and maintain sodium levels. The adrenal medulla helps speed up the body for greater performance during times of stress. Adrenal gland disorders include:

• **Addison's Disease.** Caused by inadequate production of the corticosteroids, which are secreted by the adrenal cortex, Addison's disease can lead to hypoglycemia; sodium/potassium imbalance; dehydration; hypotension; weight loss; and general weakness. Treatment includes glucocorticoid and a salt-retaining steroid.

• **Cushing's Syndrome.** Oversecretion of the corticosteroids, usually caused by pituitary tumors or overmedication of a corticosteroid (such as prednisone), can cause a puffy face; hyperglycemia; hypertension; recurrent infections; and general weakness. Other causes are glucocorticoid-secreting tumors of the adrenals and tumors elsewhere secreting ACTH. Treatment includes the removal of tumors or the adjustment of medication.

Parathyroid Glands. These glands help regulate levels of calcium in the blood. Disorders include hyperparathyroidism, in which excess production of the parathyroid hormone can disrupt the balance of calcium in the body. Treatment is usually removal of the gland that has the adenoma.

Pancreas. This gland controls the production of insulin, glucagon, and somatostatin in the body, which regulate the amount of glucose, used for energy, in the blood. Disorders include diabetes mellitus, in which there is little or no production of insulin, or even resistance to the glucose-lowering actions of insulin, causing increased glucose levels. Treatment includes artificial insulin injections or glucose-low-

ering pills.

Ovaries and Testes. These glands are responsible for the development of sexual characteristics and reproduction in both sexes. Estrogen and progesterone, the female hormones produced mainly in the ovaries, help with conception and pregnancy. Testosterone, the male hormone produced mainly by the testes, helps with sperm production and male characteristics. Both are controlled by the release of gonadotropins from the pituitary gland.

Disorders of these glands include sexual hormone deficiency, which can result in reproductive problems and underdevelopment of sex characteristics. Overproduction causes early sexual development and exaggerated secondary sexual features.

Endocrinology is the field of medicine that specifically studies disorders relating to the endocrine system. An endocrinologist diagnoses and treats patients suffering from such disorders as diabetes mellitus (disease of the pancreas); hyperthyroidism; goiters; and various adrenal gland disorders, such as Addison's disease and Cushing's syndrome.

Background material on endocrine system can be found in GLANDS *and* HORMONES *Related information is contained in* BRAIN; BRAIN DISORDERS; BRAIN STEM; BRAIN TUMOR; PITUITARY GLAND; SWEAT GALNDS; AND THYROID GLAND.

Endodontics

Branch of dentistry dealing specifically with the pulp (nerves and blood vessels) of teeth.

A dentist who specializes in root canal treatment is an endodontist. Typically, he or she will handle procedures in which the tooth nerve is removed. This is usually performed because the nerve tissue inside the tooth has become infected. A general practice dentist may also do endodontic work. In a root canal, the dentist will remove the pulp from the affected tooth and fill the space with a sedative or protective material. Endodontically treated teeth are often further strengthened and protected with a covering crown. *See also* DENTISTRY.

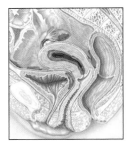

Endometriosis.
In endometriosis, above, the lining of the uterus spreads to other organs resulting in irregular bleeding.

Endometriosis

A condition in which some of the inner lining of the uterus (the endometrium) becomes implanted on other pelvic organs.

Endometriosis may result from menstrual flow that backs up into the fallopian tubes and from there into the abdominal cavity instead of exiting out the uterus and to the vagina. The misdirected cells respond to the changing hormone levels of the menstrual cycle as if they were inside the uterus, first thickening and then bleeding. Because there is nowhere for the blood to go, blood blisters, cysts, scar tissue or adhesions form as a result. If damage occurs on the ovaries or fallopian tubes, it can result in infertility. Women with endometriosis also have an increased risk of a baby developing in the fallopian tube, which is referred to as an ectopic pregnancy.

SYMPTOMS

Symptoms of endometriosis may include:
- Painful menstrual periods that may be unusually heavy;
- Sharp pelvic pain during intercourse;
- Infertility.

It is estimated that 10 to 15 percent of American women of childbearing age experience endometriosis. It is most likely to occur between the ages of 25 and 40 in women who have not yet given birth. For some, it is a progressive and painful disease, and has a tendency to run in families.

TREATMENT

Endometriosis is usually treated with a combination of chemotherapy and surgery. In less severe cases involving smaller endometrial patches, the use of hormone medications (such as estrogen, found in birth control pills) is effective in relieving pain. The hormone progestin may reverse certain symptoms, and reduce endometrial tissue. Surgical removal (laparoscopy) is an option if the endometrial patches are as large as one to two inches in diameter. Laparoscopy is also often used in the case of extreme lower abdominal pain.

PROGNOSIS

Since the invention of laparoscopy in the 1960s and with the use of such techniques as laser surgery and ultrasonography for diagnosis, more women have access to better treatment. Researchers still do not understand, however, what causes endometriosis and how to prevent it; thus, only temporary cures are available. By menopause, endometriosis is usually no longer a problem. *See also* CHEMOTHERAPY; LAPAROSCOPY; *and* MENSTRUATION, DISORDERS OF.

Endometritis

An inflammation of the uterus usually due to an infection, though it may also occur following an abortion, childbirth or the insertion of an intrauterine device (IUD).

Symptoms of endometritis include general discomfort and malaise, fever, lower abdominal or pelvic pain, abnormal vaginal bleeding, and vaginal discharge.

The condition is treated with intravenous antibiotics followed by a course of oral antibiotics. Treatment of sexual partners is also necessary to avoid the possibility of reinfection, and the use of condoms is recommended while undergoing treatment. Repeated endometritis infections can lead to infertility. Sterile techniques during childbirth, abortion, or IUD insertions will reduce the risk of endometritis.

Endorphins

Chemicals that help to inhibit and relieve pain, and which are produced by the central nervous system (the brain and spinal cord).

Endorphins act at specific sites in the body, such as the brain, spinal cord, and possibly other yet-to-be-discovered locations. On the surfaces of these cells are opiate receptors that work to stop pain when joined by substances such as endorphins, or morphine. The full extent of the endorphins' functions are not yet known. They appear to be involved in the body's reaction to stress, and possibly other mood changes. *See also* ENKEPHALINS.

Endoscopy

Use of a fiberoptic device known as an endoscope to examine body organs or cavities for the purposes of diagnosis.

An endoscope is an instrument allowing the diagnostician to directly view organs and cavities in the body. This viewing tool may be inserted into a natural body orifice or through a small incision. There are many types of endoscopy and many kinds of specialized endoscopes, ranging in size from about one to five feet in length and one-quarter to one-eighth of an inch in diameter. Some are flexible and others more rigid, depending on the nature of the diagnostic investigation. In addition to providing a means to view otherwise hidden areas, endoscopes allow small instruments to be passed through hollow channels for the purposes of biopsy and minor surgery.

Risk Factors

Some risk of perforation to the esophagus, stomach, or duodenum exists from upper endoscopy, or of intestinal perforation during colonoscopy. Such injuries are often slight and heal without intervention, though in some cases surgery is required. Further danger is posed by the flow of gastric juices into the lungs—a condition that can develop into pneumonia. Sore throat is common following esophageal endoscopy but rarely involves infection. Both upper and lower endoscopy carry risks of adverse reaction to the sedatives used. The examining physician should be made aware of any existing allergies prior to an endoscopic examination.

How it Works

Endoscopy originally used a fiberoptic system, in which light travels through a plastic tube even when it is bent sharply. This allows unimpeded viewing around corners and in tight areas. Now digital chip technology is used.

As mentioned, many endoscopes are equipped with instruments for removing tissue samples and destroying abnormal tissue. Endoscopy also allows for minor surgery. Tiny tools may be passed through a hollow channel in the endoscope, allowing for the cauterization of wounds, the closing of blood vessels, and the removal of damaged tissue. Bleeding can be arrested; irregular growths, such as polyps, removed; or therapeutic drugs injected through the endoscope to a desired region. Such features make endoscopy an effective means of visualizing and treating irregularities in delicate or hard-to-reach areas of the body.

Types

Endoscopy may be used to directly observe many of the body's internal surfaces. These include: the surfaces of the gastrointestinal tract; the upper respiratory tract; the abdominal cavity; and the knee. Two major types of endoscopy are upper endoscopy and lower endoscopy, which are used to examine the upper and lower gastrointestinal tracts, respectively.

Upper endoscopy, involves passing an endoscope through the mouth in order to study the esophagus, the stomach, and the small intestine (esophagoscopy, gastroscopys and upper gastrointestinal endoscopy, respectively). This may be used to detect gastrointestinal bleeding, tumors, blockages, ulcerations, narrowing (stenosis), and bacterial infections including *Candida esophagitis* or *Heliobacter pylori.*

Lower endoscopy, in which the endoscope is passed through the anus, may involve examination of the large intestine in a procedure known as colon-oscopy. The lining of the bowel can be visualized and photographed through a lens at the tip of the colonoscope. This instrument, like those used in upper endoscopy, is also capable of removing biopsy tissue if a lesion or other abnormality is detected. A different type of endoscope may be inserted into the anus to observe the rectum and lower portion of the large intestine, in a process known as sigmoidoscopy.

Lower endoscopy is used to examine the large intestine in order to diagnose disorders such as bleeding, benign or malignant tumors, polyps, stricture, abnormal sacs in the intestinal lining (diverticulosis), inflammatory bowel disease (Crohn's disease), and others. *See also* ARTHOSCOPY; COLONSCOPY; FIBEROPTICS; *and* SIGMOIDSCOPY.

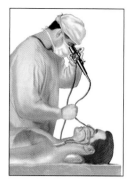

Endoscopy.
Fiberoptic devices that are used to examine internal organs or body cavities are known as endoscopes. In a bronchoscopy (above), a flexible endoscope is inserted through the patient's trachea to view or collect samples from the small airways in the lungs, known as bronchi.

Resources on Endoscopy

Cullinan, John Edward, *Illustrated Guide to X-Ray Technics* (1980); Kee, Joyce LeFever, *Handbook of Laboratory and Diagnostic Tests with Nursing Implications* (1994); Ravin, Carl E., ed., *Imaging and Invasive Radiology in the Intensive Care Unit* (1993); Segen, Joseph C. and Joseph Stauffer, The Patient's Guide to Medical Tests (1998); American Hospital Association, Tel. (800) 242-2626, Online: www.aha. org; The American Board of Radiology, Tel. (520) 790-2900, Online: www. heabr.org; American Healthcare Radiology Administrators, Online: www.ahra.org; www.ny-cornell.org/radiology/

Endothelium

A thin layer of cells that forms the inner lining of blood vessels, the heart, and the lymph system.

The cells of the endothelium are normally thin and flat, allowing for a free flow of blood and lymph fluid. That flow can be impeded by atherosclerosis, the formation of cholesterol deposits that cause the endothelium to become thicker and rougher, increasing the risk of blood clots; the clots may eventually block an artery, causing a heart attack or a stroke. Measures to prevent deterioration of the endothelium include a diet low in fat and cholesterol, and avoidance of cigarette smoking. *See also* ATHEROSCLEROSIS; BLOOD VESSELS; CHOLESTEROL; DIET; *and* LYMPHATIC SYSTEM.

Endotoxin

Term generally referring to poison produced by certain bacteria.

The identifying feature of an endotoxin is that it remains in the cell walls of bacteria until the host bacteria die. This feature is troublesome because endotoxins are usually produced by gram-negative bacteria, which have two cell walls and are adaptable and resistant to bacteria eliminating drugs (antibiotics). Common endotoxin emitting bacteria are *E. coli, Salmonella, Pseudomonas,* and *Staphylococcus aureus.*

Once released, endotoxins have the ability to affect the temperature-regulating part of the brain (hypothalamus), resulting in fever as well as chills. Alternately, endotoxins can also weaken the walls of capillaries. If leakage ensues, there may be a serious drop in blood pressure known as endotoxic shock. Other symptoms include diarrhea and vomiting. *See also* SALMONELLA; *and* STAPHYLOCOCCAL INFECTIONS.

Endotracheal Tube

A tube that delivers oxygen directly to the lungs.

An endotracheal tube is narrow, made of plastic, and has a securing device, called an inflatable cuff, at one end. The purpose of the tube is to provide oxygen for a patient who is not breathing well enough, comatose or anesthetized.

The tube is inserted through the mouth or nose under the direction of an anesthesiologist, then passed through the windpipe or trachea, toward the lungs. The cuff is inflated, securing the tube and creating an airtight seal. Oxygen is delivered through the tube to the lungs. *See also* ANESTHESIA; COMA; ENDOSCOPY; LUNGS; OXYGEN; *and* TRACHEA.

Enema

A fluid injected into the rectum to clear the bowel for the administration of drugs or for diagnosis.

A bowel-clearing enema can be used either to relieve constipation or to prepare the intestinal tract for surgery or an examination, such as a colonoscopy, in which the intestine is examined for polyps, tumors, and cancerous growths. The first fluid used for enemas was ordinary soap and water, which would irritated the intestine enough to cause contractions that expelled feces. Currently, a number of prepared solutions are available.

For treatment, an enema may contain medications such as corticosteroids, administered to treat the inflammation and bleeding caused by ulcerative colitis. For patients with severe dehydration, the enema solution will contain measured amounts of electrolytes—the salts necessary for proper fluid balance.

Barium enemas are given before an x-ray examination of the intestine to aid in diagnosis. These enemas contain barium sulfate, a compound that absorbs x-rays and thus provides an image of the interior of the intestine on an x-ray image. An enema usually is given without anesthetic, since the procedure generally causes only minor discomfort. The solution is introduced into the intestine through a catheter, which is a hollow tube, that is inserted into the rectum of a patient who is lying on one side. *See also* BARIUM X-RAY.

Energy

Fuel produced through the consumption and metabolism of food, which allows for movement and physical change in the body.

The body's energy is produced when cells process, or metabolize, nutrients from food. Carbohydrates, fats, and protein all provide sources of energy, although carbohydrates are the most direct source. Carbohydrates yield blood sugars, which can be used immediately as energy for the central nervous system, brain, and muscles. The central nervous system requires approximately nine tablespoons, or 140 grams, of glucose per day. Carbohydrates continue to provide the body with energy after fat and protein are digested.

Fat also supplies the body with energy, although fat stored in the body is generally broken down for energy only after metabolic needs exceed caloric intake. When an energy deficit exists, fat cells break down stored triglycerides, releasing fatty acids into the bloodstream, where they may be used for energy. Without an adequate supply of glucose, the fat is not broken down completely and ketosis will occur.

Proteins supply the amino acids essential to tissue growth and maintenance. However, when the diet lacks sufficient carbohydrates and fats, protein is converted into glucose for energy.

Carbohydrates and fats are the more efficient energy sources. Carbohydrates and proteins yield four calories per gram, whereas fats yield nine. *See also* AMINO ACIDS; CALORIE; CARBOHYDRATES; ENERGY REQUIREMENTS; FATTY ACIDS; FITNESS; GLUCOSE; GLYCEROL; GLYCOGEN; KILOCALORIE; NUTRITION.

Energy Requirements

An individual's energy needs, usually expressed in calories, and affected by age, gender, height, weight, environmental factors, and activity levels.

Guidelines for consumption of such dietary components as protein, carbohydrates, and fats are general estimates. They will vary somewhat from one individual to another. Body weight is a reflection of one's average caloric intake and average caloric expenditure over time. Therefore, weight gain occurs only when caloric needs are consistently being exceeded.

Caloric requirements vary, but can be roughly calculated. The resting metabolic rate (RMR) is the amount of energy, or calories, necessary for the body to function at rest. To determine caloric requirements, an individual's activity level must also be considered. The RMR for a sedentary individual can be estimated at the rate of 10 calories per pound. Routine daily activity will add about three calories per pound to the individual's caloric requirement; illness and the amount of active exercise that a person experiences also affect the number.

Aging and Energy Requirements

Age is an important factor in determining energy requirements. As people age, their energy requirements gradually diminish. Caloric requirements for those over the age of 30 diminish gradually, by two percent per decade. This occurs primarily as a result of the loss in muscle mass that accompanies the aging process. Nutrient requirements, however, remain constant. Therefore, it is necessary, later in life, to choose nutrient-rich food while eating somewhat less.

Pregnancy and nursing, for example, are times in a person's life when energy requirements, and thus, caloric intake, should rise. In order to give birth to a child of normal weight, and to avoid the health problems and developmental disabilities often associated with low birth weights, pregnant women should increase their caloric intake.

During the first trimester, the pregnant woman should consume approximately 150 extra calories daily, and 350 extra each day in the second and third trimesters. These should not come from sources like candy bars or fast food since these are empty calories that cannot provide the fetus with necessary nutrients, and will simply increase the mother's fat stores.

Energy Requirements for Pregnancy

During pregnancy, a woman can estimate her necessary caloric intake by multiplying her weight by 12 if she is fairly sedentary, 15 if her activity level is moderate, and 20 if she is highly active. To the figure should be added the 150 to 350 calories, depending on the stage of pregnancy. If she is between the ages of 35 and 44, subtract 100 calories from the total. For example, a 32-year-old woman who weighs 120 pounds and is moderately active will require approximately 1800 calories per day, plus 150 calories in the first trimester, and 350 more calories later.

Most fetal growth occurs in the final trimester. Therefore, it is essential that the mother not cut down on calories, even if she thinks that she has gained enough weight by then. Nursing women should add 500 calories per day to their pre-pregnancy energy requirements to balance the nutrient and calorie loss that accompanies lactation. Again, these calories should come from nutrient-rich foods that will serve to nourish both mother and child.

Athletes. An athlete's energy requirements will often be far greater than those of someone who leads a sedentary lifestyle. However, energy costs, or required expenditures, vary from sport to sport, and are also influenced by the athlete's age, weight, height, and sex. While some male athletes may require between 3,500 and 5,500 calories per day, some female athletes such as figure skaters, gymnasts, and dancers stay at their optimal weight on only 1,400 to 2,000 calories per day.

The stress of training and competition can throw off appetite. Often, eating too little is more of a problem in such cases than overeating, so athletes should know the energy requirements for their sport and adjust their diet accordingly. Still, one of the most effective indicators of whether one is meeting (and not exceeding) one's energy requirements is the monitoring of one's body weight.

Background material on energy requirements can be found in CALORIE *and* PREGNANCY. *Related information is contained in* CALORIC TEST; CALORIMETRY; CARBOHYDRATES; EMBRYO; ENERGY; NUTRITION; *and* PRENATAL CARE.

Engagement

A term used to describe the descent of the fetus' head into the mother's pelvis.

Engagement takes place towards the end of the pregnancy, usually by the 37th week. Engagement occurs when the baby's head drops into the pelvis of the mother. It is not uncommon for engagement to not occur until the onset of labor. *See also* CHILDBIRTH *and* DELIVERY.

Enophthalmos

Also known as "sunken eyeball"

The backwards recession of the eyeball in its bony socket.

If the globe of the eye is displaced, it is usually caused either by facial trauma or a cancerous growth. Orbital fat may also atrophy due to age, after radiation therapy or as a disorder related to severe wasting diseases. *See also* CANCER.

When trauma has caused enophthalmos, the bony orbit, the connective ligaments, and the orbital soft tissue have all been either damaged or displaced, thus moving the globe with them.

Treatment of the condition usually involves reconstructive surgery of the bony orbit and a proper repositioning of the globe. *See also* EXOPTHALMOS; EYE; EYE, DISORDERS OF; *and* ORBIT.

Enteritis

An inflammation of the intestines, particularly the small intestine.

Like gastroenteritis, enteritis is a general term for a group of intestinal conditions. They are caused by either bacterial or viral infection, or by eating or drinking something that is already contaminated. Symptoms may include mild to severe diarrhea, abdominal cramps, and discomfort. Dehydration may be a problem if fluid loss is severe, but symptoms will usually disappear within two or three days. *See also* GASTROENTERITIS *and* INTESTINE.

Enterostomy

The artificial formation of an opening, or stoma, from the intestine through the abdominal wall that permits the drainage of fecal matter.

Enterostomy is performed when normal intestinal function is interrupted or because of an intestinal disease that cannot be treated by less drastic means. A portion of the intestine is often removed because of disease and the normal route for eliminating waste is disrupted. A segment of the remaining intestine is positioned so that the feces are eliminated into a pouch worn over the opening in the abdominal wall.

The two main types of enterostomy are ileostomy and colostomy. In a colostomy, the large intestine is drawn to a stoma, a small opening in the abdominal wall that is used for drainage; a colostomy may be either permanent or temporary, depending on the nature of the condition that is being treated. In an ileostomy, the end of the small intestine is brought to the opening; ileostomies may also be either temporary or permanent.

Enterostomies may be temporary treatments for cases of inflamed bowel or penetrating abdominal wounds. They are also useful in the placement of feeding tubes.

Enterostomies are permanent when the removal of diseased sections of the intestine is necessary, as in cases of Crohn's disease, ulcerative colitis, and familial polyposis. *See also* ARTIFICIAL FEEDING; CROHN'S DISEASE; ULCERATIVE COLITIS; FAMILIAL POLYPOSIS; ILEOSTOMY; JEJUNUM; *and* JEJUNAL BIOPSY;

Enterotoxin

A poisonous substance, created by certain species of bacteria, which afflicts the intestinal lining.

The most common producer of enterotoxin is the bacteria *staphylococcus*. It may also be produced by *bacillus, clostridium, escherichia,* and *vibrio*. Bacterial poisons affect the cells of the intestinal mucosa, producing the classic symptoms of food poisoning: diarrhea, vomiting, stomach pain, and cramps. These symptoms are generally violent, but short-lived. However, the very young, the old, and those with compromised immune systems may be very seriously affected.

The bacteria that produce enterotoxins generally infect people via spoiled or contaminated food. Although cooking food thoroughly and cleaning the food preparation area before, during, and after cooking do offer some protection, it should be noted that enterotoxins are extremely resistant to heat and are not always eliminated by cooking. *See also* BACTERIA; ENDOTOXIN; FOOD CONTAMINATION; FOOD POISONING; *and* INTESTINE.

Entropion

A condition in which the eyelids, including the eyelashes, are turned in against the eyeball.

Entropion is most prevalent in babies, the elderly, and those who have suffered an injury to the eye, causing scar formation on the eyelid. In some cases, it is passed on between family members. The condition may cause irritation, tearing, redness, and ophthalmalgia. Common symptoms include strong eye pains, throbbing, burning or aching, and a feeling that there is a foreign body in the eye.

Incidence of entropion has also been linked to the infection trachoma, which, if left untreated, can lead to blindness. Trachoma (granular conjunctivitis) is an infection caused by *Chlamydia trachomatis*.

Entropion poses little harm to babies, as their lashes are soft and will not harm the cornea; in most cases, the disorder will disappear on its own within a few months. A surgical procedure performed on the muscles that control the eyelid can be an effective form of corrective surgery for adults, whose eyes are no longer developing. Eye drops should also be used in order to avoid dryness. *See also* CHLAMYDIA; CONJUNCTIVITIS; CORNEA; ECTROPION; EYE; EYE DROPS; EYELID; SEXUALLY TRANSMITTED DISEASES; *and* TRACHOMA.

Enuresis

Medical term for bed-wetting

Bed-wetting in children after they have been toilet trained or may be expected to be toilet trained; usually, but not always, after age five.

Many children experience periods of bed wetting, but the problem tends to spontaneously stop without any treatment. Bed wetting is about twice as common in young boys than it is in young girls. Because enuresis is embarrassing to children and is not in their control, they should never be punished, chastised, or ridiculed about it.

Enuresis may have physical causes such as diabetes, certain types of spinal cord lesions, infection, or, most likely, the slow development of physical control over waste elimination. There are some disorders of the urinary tract related to a family's medical history that can also cause it.

There may also be emotional causes for bed-wetting, such as separation anxiety or the birth of a new sibling; it may also be caused by the pressure that parents put on children during toilet training; or it may just be a simple form of regression as a reaction to the stress of a new situation. Most children outgrow enuresis, but since it can interfere with a child's self-esteem and ability to be involved in over-night social events, it is best to address the problem.

TREATMENT

To reduce a child's need to void at night, limit the amount of fluids taken before bedtime and have the child urinate immediately before going to bed. Some children may respond to behavior therapy, in which rewards are given after a night without bed-wetting. A doctor may also prescribe drugs, such as imipramine or desmopressin.

Being sensitive to a child's special needs for support at this time may help, particularly if the enuresis is caused by a fear or concern that he or she does not have the ability to verbalize. Patience may prove an effective tool in dealing with the problem. *See also* BEHAVIOR THERAPY; DIABETES; *and* TOILET-TRAINING.

Environmental Medicine

A branch of medicine that studies the medical effects of environmental factors on individuals.

Environmental medicine is the branch of medicine that studies and analyzes the effects of environmental factors on the health of individuals, with a particular focus on the effects of chemicals, water, and air quality. Clinicians estimate that four to five million Americans are affected by illnesses related to their environment, but very few are diagnosed or treated properly. Environmental medicine views each patient as a unique individual exposed to a unique set of circumstances, and therefore in need of individualized evaluation in order to determine the most appropriate forms of therapy.

Physicians who practice environmental medicine focus on the nexus between the patient or a group of people and the environment. They utilize techniques from environmental science to analyze the constituents of the major environmental mediums: air, water, and soil.

Even though environmental medicine looks for alternative reasons for diagnosis, it has less in common with alternative medicine and, as a discipline, environmental medicine is closely allied with occupational medicine, which analyzes potential sources of illness in a patient's work environment.

Some environmental medicine doctors are state-licensed practitioners who combine a conventional allopathic approach with a holistic medical style. They typically have backgrounds in internal medicine, gynecology, psychiatry, or other areas.

CATEGORIES

There are four main categories of environmental factors that can trigger illness:

Chemical factors, which include toxic substances that may be in and around an individual's home or work environment, such as formaldehyde, phenol, solvents, derivatives of gas, oil and coal, pesticides, herbicides, heavy metals, asbestos, chlorine, and sulfur dioxide.

Physical factors affect an individual's well-being; these include factors such as heat, cold, weather cycles, noise, positive and negative ions, electromagnetic radiation, radioactivity from x-ray, atomic explosions, food irradiation, and radon gas.

History of Environmental Medicine

In the 1940s, Theron Randolf, a professor of allergy and immunology at Northwestern University, began writing about food allergies based on tests that he developed with Herbert Rinkel. He testified before the Food and Drug Administration, recommending the labeling of food ingredients. He was the first to describe the concept of chemical sensitivity (abnormal sensitivity to specific constituents of the environment). First called clinical ecology, the field was renamed environmental medicine in 1985. There are now more than 3000 practitioners. Over time, the specialty has evolved from addressing food allergies and chemical sensitivities into a broader discipline that studies all aspects of environmental toxins.

Biological factors, such as bacteria, viruses, molds, parasites, foods, animal dander, dust and pollens from trees, grass, or weeds, affect the quality of life.

Psychological factors, sometimes called stressors, include: prolonged psychological stress in personal relationships, a death in the family, fire, bankruptcy, or job loss.

According to environmental medicine, a patient's health is a result of the interaction of environmental triggers, a patient's genetic tendencies, and the quality of the patient's diet. Inhaled allergies and hypersensitivity to food contaminants are often important factors.

SYMPTOMS

Some chronic illnesses today are the result of poor lifestyle habits or exposure to a variety of substances found in the work or home environment. Patients suffering from environmental disorders often exhibit symptoms in more than one system of the body. The central nervous system is particularly sensitive to toxins.

Some people are abnormally sensitive to environmental toxins. These individuals have sometimes been misdiagnosed or, worse, labeled as malingerers or hypochon-driacs with psychosomatic disorders, while their illnesses have real and identifiable causes. For these people, chronic exposure, even at low levels, can trigger the process. Severe damage to the immune system, organs, or even death can result.

Reactions to low-level exposure to allergins or toxins are especially hard to diagnose because symptoms are not always the same as for higher levels of exposure, which are already considered toxic. Low-levels of exposure often affect target organs, and instead of directly causing disorders, they may cause degenerative affects that may not be diagnosed until later.

Environmental researchers use the term "spreading phenomenon" to refer to two observations: the onset of a reaction to something that was previously tolerated or adapted to, and the spreading of the reaction to that substance from the target organs to other organs or sites in the body. This often happens with chemical exposure; once one affects certain individuals, they suddenly begin reacting to many.

TREATMENT

Among the treatments of environmentally-caused illness are: environmental control (i.e., a change in environment); modified diet; correction of hormonal or metabolic deficiencies; and immunotherapy (enhancement or suppression of the immune system).

DIAGNOSIS

Diagnosis usually relies extensively on an environmentally-oriented medical history (EOMH) to locate a possible source of toxins in the environment. An EOMH relates physical or psychological signs and symptoms to sources of exposure in a patient's home or work environment. Doctors look for possible connections, such as:

- hyperactivity after a school lunch;
- tiredness and sleepiness after a meal;
- muscle pain, bruising, extreme fatigue, or "flu-like symptoms" after exposure to pesticide spraying;
- irritation of the eyes or throat, a breathing problem, or lack of concen-

Resources on Environmental Medicine
Basch, Paul F., *Textbook of International Health* (1999); Moeller, D.W., *Environmental Health,* (1997); National Research Council, Committee on Environ-mental Epidemiology, *Public Health and Hazardous Wastes,* (1991); Turnock, Bernard, *Public Health: What It Is and How It Works* (2000); Mothers and Others for Pesticide Limits, Tel. (212) 727-2700, Online: www. mothers.org; U.S. Public Health Service, Tel. (202) 619-0257, Online: phs.os. dhhs. gov/phs/phs.html; www. med.cornell.edu/ public.health/

How Cancer Spreads.
The process of metastasis (right) involves an enzyme called Type IV collagenase, which allows cancer cells to penetrate the membranes responsible for protecting other parts of the body. Once the cancer cells enter the bloodstream, a secondary tumor may form in another part of the body.

tration after buying new carpets or furniture, etc.; this indicates a heightened sensitivity to chemical exposure;
- recurrent urinary problems;
- recurrent upper respiratory or ear infections.

Environmental physicians also examine the doses in which toxins were absorbed and the exposure timetable (single exposure, intermittent, or chronic). These doctors may employ other, usually noninvasive, tests to diagnosis the illness. Tests may include: EKGs; echocardiograms; cardiac stress testing; organ function tests.

Background material on enviornmental medicine can be found in AIR AND POLLUTION. *Related information is contained in* AIR CONDITIONING; ALLERGY; ANTHRAX; ASBESTOS; CARDIAC STREES TEST; EKG; PUBLIC HEALTH; RADON GAS *and* WATER.

Enzyme

A protein catalyst for chemical change in the body.

Every cell produces enzymes; there are thousands and each one has a unique chemical make-up that determines the reaction that specific enzyme regulates. Enzymes regulate the chemical processes of the body, including such functions as: metabolism; liver activity; and the immune system. Derived from a mineral or vitamin, a coenzyme is a substance necessary to an enzyme's function.

An enzyme acts on a chemical called a substrate by either modifying it, splitting it, or joining it to another substrate. Since its shape determines its function, an enzyme can combine only with a substrate whose molecular make-up complements that of the enzyme. The combination changes the chemical make-up of the substrate, for example, by splitting it in two. This chemical reaction leaves the enzyme unchanged, and it can move on to repeat the process with another substrate.

Drugs can influence enzyme activity by induction. For example, one drug can increase the activity of an enzyme that metabolizes another drug. Enzymes can also be

inhibited in a similar manner, blocking an enzyme that would otherwise continue to spur the growth of cancerous cells.

The measure of enzymes in blood can reveal disease or disorders. A mild heart attack can be confirmed because the damaged muscle releases particular enzymes into the bloodstream. High measures of liver enzymes indicate liver disorders.

Enzymes are also a treatment tool. They can be administered as digestive aids; to loosen phlegm; to reduce blood clots; and to clean wounds. In addition, enzyme therapy, a form of alternative medicine, involves the introduction of plant and pancreatic enzymes into the body for the purpose of improving the absorption of food and the body's immune system. However, research on the effectiveness of these treatments is inconclusive at best.

Background material on enzyme can be found in CELL *and* PROTEIN. *Related information is contained in* ALTERNATIVE MEDICINE; BLOOD CLOTTTING; BLOOD GASSES; HEART ATTACK; IMMUNE SYSTEM; LIVER ACTIVITY; LIVER DISORDERS; METABOLISM; *and* VITAMIN.

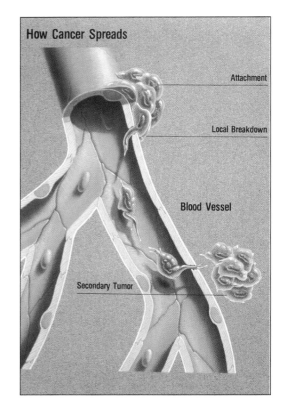

How Cancer Spreads

Attachment

Local Breakdown

Blood Vessel

Secondary Tumor

Ependymoma

Also known as ependymoma

A type of brain cancer that afflicts children.

Ependymoma comprises eight to ten percent of pediatric brain tumors, making it the third most common form of brain cancer. Ependymal tumors begin in the ependyma, cells that line the brain's ventricles. The tumors can obstruct the flow of cerebrospinal fluid and spread to other areas of the brain and spinal cord. Signs include headache, vomiting, and confusion. Treatments include surgery, radiation therapy, and chemotherapy. The overall childhood survival rate is less than 30 percent. Low-grade tumors have a five-year survival rate of 80 percent. *See also* BRAIN TUMORS.

Epidemic

Any disease that spreads rapidly and infects a large percentage of a population.

An epidemic is characterized by the rapid spread of a contagion, generally followed by a leveling off and then a decline of prevalence, as vulnerable subjects die or recover. Influenza is an example of an illness that often becomes an epidemic; new strains of influenza develop every few years, resulting in a rapid increase in the number of people infected with the disease.

An epidemic is often so widespread that it is difficult for individuals to avoid some form of contact with the disease. In some cases, the affected population may be very small, but the sudden rise in the prevalence of the disease in that population marks the infection pattern as an epidemic.

Epidemics occur most often during the warm months of the year. Consequences of epidemics may include the closing of schools, forced shutdown of buildings, and widespread loss of life.

An epidemic that affects multiple geographic regions is known as a pandemic. For example, HIV, which has infected over 54 million people worldwide, is a pandemic. *See also* ENDEMIC *and* PANDEMIC.

Epidemiology

Branch of medicine that studies the causes, distribution, and control of diseases in a population.

Epidemiology analyzes the distribution of disease in human populations and attempts to ascertain the factors responsible for this distribution. The chief tool of epidemiology is statistical analysis. Unlike most other medical disciplines, epidemiology focuses on the presence of disease in groups of people and in populations rather than in individuals. The main goal of epidemiology is to identify populations at high risk for certain diseases and to pinpoint the hidden societal causes of outbreaks. There are two main types of epidemiological analysis—descriptive and analytic.

Descriptive epidemiology uses demographic surveys and information about the characteristics of a population to determine the factors associated with the prevalence of the disease in certain populations. Factors may include age, gender, ethnic group, and occupation, among others. Descriptive studies also chart the progress of a disease over time.

Analytic epidemiology tests the conclusions drawn from descriptive surveys or laboratory observations. A specific factor, such as occupation, is identified as a possible cause of increased incidence of a disease. A sample population is then divided into two groups, based on the presence or absence of this factor. The studies monitor differences in the presence of the disease in the two groups to determine if the factor actually affects the disease's prevalence. *See* ENDEMIC; EPIDEMIC; *and* STATISTICS, MEDICAL.

Epidermolysis Bullosa

Condition in which blisters appear on the skin after minor trauma.

Epidermolysis bullosa is a rare, inherited disorder that can range in severity from mild to fatal. The disease is characterized by large, fluid-filled blisters that appear at the first sign of minor damage to the skin.

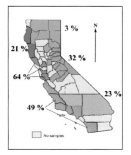

Epidemiology. Epidemiologists use maps like the one above of California to study disease as it affects groups of people using race, sex, age, and geographic location to identify the causes and rate of distribution of disease.

Resources on Epidemiology and Public Health

Basch, Paul F., *Textbook of International Health* (1999); Moeller, D.W., *Environmental Health, revised edition* (1997); National Research Council, Committee on Environmental Epidemiology, *Public Health and Hazardous Wastes* (1991); Timmreck, Thomas C., *Introduction to Epidemiology* (1994); Turnock, Bernard, *Public Health: What It Is and How It Works* (2000); U.S. Public Health Service, Tel. (202) 619-0257, Online: phs.os. dhhs.gov/phs/phs.html; www.med.cornell.edu/public.health/.

Chafing, rubbing, or even change in room temperature can trigger the blisters.

Symptoms include the development of blisters after even mild trauma and blisters around the mouth or in the throat that interfere with eating or swallowing. More severe forms of epidermolysis bullosa can cause deformities, as the skin shrinks from the blisters, causing restricted movement in areas such as the fingers, elbows, and knees. Nutritional problems may occur, as eating can be restricted by the buildup of blisters and scar tissue in the throat and mouth. Secondary infection is a risk in cases where the blisters open up.

Treatment for minor forms of epidermolysis bullosa is based around preventing trauma—the skin is protected as much as possible. In mild cases, children may outgrow the disease. The complications from severe forms of epidermolysis bullosa, such as inability to eat or infections in the blisters, can lead to death. *See also* BLISTER.

Epididymis

Part of the male genital organs, the cord-like structure near the top of the testicles.

The epididymis is a coiled tube that would be nearly 20 feet in length if fully extended. Sperm cells are produced within each testicle and then transported through the epididymis to the seminal vesicles, structures that store the sperm until they are used. *See also* REPRODUCTIVE SYSTEM, MALE.

Epididymoorchitis

Inflammation of a testicle and its sperm-carrying channel, the epididymis.

The usual cause of epididymoorchitis is an infection that originates in the urinary tract and spreads to the testes, causing pain and swelling at the rear of a testicle. In young men, epididymoorchitis is usually caused by the sexually transmitted organism *Chlamydia trachomatis.* Diagnosis is aimed at determining whether the symptoms are caused by inflammation or by a

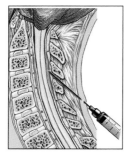

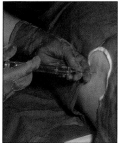

Epidural Anesthesia. Above, a local anesthetic is injected into the lower back to numb the nerves leading to the chest and lower part of the body. The top drawing indicates the anasthetic is injected into the dural, and not beyond. It is commonly used for pain relief during childbirth.

twisting of the spermatic cord (testicular torsion). Epididymoorchitis is treated by identifying the causative organism and administering the appropriate antibiotic; if caused by a sexually transmitted infection, sexual partners should also be treated. In most cases, the swelling in the testicle may take weeks or months to subside after successful treatment. *See also* CHLAMYDIA; TESTIS, SWOLLEN; *and* TESTIS, TORSION OF.

Epidural Anesthesia

A type of regional anesthesia often used for pain relief during labor.

In an epidural anesthesia, a local anesthetic is injected into the durae—the space between two membranes surrounding the spinal cord. The anesthetic affects a major nerve in the lower back, providing pain relief to the lower extremities.

Epidural anesthesia is most commonly used during childbirth and during surgery on the lower limbs. It may also be used as a form of postoperative pain relief and as a way to control some forms of cancer pain.

Generally, the local anesthetic is delivered by a single injection (bolus) or, for longer procedures, continuously through a catheter. The most common anesthetics used in epidural anesthesia are bupivacaine and chloroprocaine. The anesthetics can take 15 to 30 minutes to take effect.

A mobile epidural uses a lower dose of local anesthetic in combination with an opioid such as fentanyl; this permits greater mobility but retains a strong pain-killing ability, which is particularly useful in labor.

Complications. About ten percent of patients experience a drop in blood pressure, which can be controlled through the administration of intravenous fluid. Lowered blood pressure can slow labor, so the hormone oxytocin is often also administered to stimulate uterine contractions. Epidural anesthesia may also cause headaches, but the use of finer needles has reduced the incidence of these to less than one percent. *See also* ANESTHESIA, LOCAL; ANESTHESIA, REGIONAL; CHILDBIRTH; *and* NERVOUS SYSTEM.

Epiglottitis

A bacterial infection causing rapid inflammation of the epiglottis.

The epiglottis is a flap of cartilage that closes while swallowing to keep food and liquid from entering the airways to the lungs. Swelling of the epiglottis can cause a life-threatening blockage of the airways.

INCIDENCE

Epiglottitis is seen most often in children under the age of seven. It is occasionally found in older children and adults; adults with depressed immune systems may be more likely to develop epiglottitis.

CAUSES

Epiglottitis is usually caused by infection with *Hemophilus influenzae* type B bacteria and, more rarely, *Streptococci* bacteria. Because the disease is contagious, family members of a person who has contracted epiglottitis should be tested for the disease and treated if necessary.

SYMPTOMS

The first symptoms are usually sore throat and fever. Swelling usually begins suddenly in the nose and throat and spreads quickly to the epiglottis, where it can block the airway to the lungs. The sufferer develops a high fever and difficulty in breathing, resulting in a buildup of carbon dioxide and a lowered level of oxygen in the blood. Coughing up mucous is difficult if not impossible due to the blocked epiglottis.

TREATMENT

Epiglottitis can be fatal if not treated. A person with epiglottitis should receive emergency medical care as quickly as possible. Antibiotics will be administered to control the infection; breathing difficulties may require an endotracheal tube or surgical opening of a hole in the neck (trachestomy). Once the infection has been controlled, the patient should recover quickly. *See also* ANTIBIOTIC DRUGS; CHOKING; *and* PHARYNGITIS.

Epilepsy

A chronic nervous system disorder characterized by recurring seizures.

Seizures are characterized by a partial or complete loss of consciousness, generally accompanied by convulsions or uncontrolled movements. Seizures result from a breakdown in orderly communication between nerve cells (neurons). Neurons in the brain communicate by sending electrical signals back and forth in an orderly manner. During a seizure, electrical signals from one group of neurons become excessively strong and overwhelm neighboring neurons, resulting in a chaotic pattern.

In epilepsy, seizures are recurrent and are not caused by a nonneurological disorder, such as a fever. About one million people in the United States have epilepsy.

CAUSES

Scientists do not know why the brain sometimes misfires or why certain people are more prone to seizures than others. Two-thirds of people with epilepsy do not have a physical abnormality in the brain that appears to cause the seizures. The remaining third can link the seizures to a brain irregularity, brain damage at birth, head injury, stroke, brain tumor, infection such as meningitis or encephalitis, drug intoxication, or a metabolic imbalance. It is speculated that epilepsy may be genetically related.

SYMPTOMS

The primary symptom of epilepsy is a seizure. There are two different classifications of seizures, generalized and partial. Generalized seizures affect most or all of the brain, influence the entire body, and produce a loss of consciousness. In contrast, partial seizures are caused by a misfiring of a smaller area of the brain and do not necessarily result in loss of consciousness. Many epileptics do not exhibit any symptoms between seizures. Some recognize when a seizure is imminent because of an aura, an often unpleasant feeling or hallucination that precedes an attack.

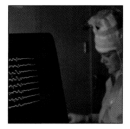

Epilepsy.
Epilepsy is marked by recurrent seizures or temporary alterations in one or more functions of the brain. Above, biofeedback methods are often used to diagnose the condition, as they clearly show the changes in brain activity.

Resources on Epilepsy
Berkow, Robert, and Andrew J. Fletcher, *Living Well with Epilepsy* (1992); Kandel, Eric R., et al., Principles of Neural Science (1991); Sanes, Dan Harvey, et al., Development of the Nervous System (2000); Epilepsy Foundation, Tel. (800) EFA-1000, Online: www.efa.org; Muscular Dystrophy Association of America, Tel. (800) 572-1717, Online: www.md-ausa.org; American Academy of Neurology, Tel. (651) 695-1940, Online: www.aan.com; Epilepsy Foundation, Tel. (800) EFA-1000, Online: www.efa.org; Epilepsy Institute, Tel. (212) 677-8550; American Board of Neurological Surgery, Tel. (713) 790-6015, Online: www.abns.org; www.med.cornell.edu/neuro/.

GENERALIZED SEIZURES

Generalized seizures consist of grand mal and petit mal, or absence, seizures.

Grand mal seizures affect the entire body. The person may cry out and then fall to the ground. The muscles will be rigid for a few moments and will then spasm. Breathing may be irregular or absent; if the seizure lasts for more than one or two minutes, there is danger of brain damage.

Status epilepticus is a type of grand mal seizure in which the convulsions do not cease, producing a medical emergency. It is accompanied by strong muscle contractions, rapid electrical discharge throughout the brain, and difficulty breathing. The patient must get medical help immediately to prevent brain damage or death.

Petit mal seizures are characterized by a

ALERT

First Aid for an Epileptic Seizure

- Do not restrain the person or attempt to put anything in his or her mouth.
- Do not move the person unless he or she is in danger of injuring himself/herself.
- Loosen the clothing around the neck and, if possible, move the head to one side so saliva can drain out of the mouth.
- When the attack has subsided, place the person in the recovery position.
- Remain with the person until he or she regains consciousness, and help reorient him or her.
- If the seizure lasts more than a couple of minutes or if the person does not regain consciousness, seek emergency medical help.

temporary loss of consciousness without any abnormal behavior. They generally occur in children, usually before age five, and disappear after adolescence. A child may appear to be daydreaming but in reality loses awareness for a few seconds. Afterwards, the child continues as if nothing has happened. Petit mal seizures can occur countless times during a day and can impede a child's scholastic performance.

PARTIAL SEIZURES

Partial seizures can be subdivided into simple seizures, in which the victim maintains consciousness, and complex seizures, in which the person loses consciousness.

Triggers

A seizure can appear spontaneously or can be triggered by flashing lights, repetitive sounds, or even by the lights of video games. The most effective triggers are certain drugs and insufficient levels of oxygen or sugar in the blood. These may trigger a seizure in nonepileptics as well.

Simple seizures occur when a chaotic electrical flow in an area of the brain remains confined. The accompanying symptoms are spasm-like movements, tingling of the skin, and hallucinatory sensations. The sufferer remains conscious. In a Jacksonian seizure, movements begin in a hand or foot and slowly travel up the body but remain on one side of the body. The seizure ends after a few minutes.

Complex seizures are characterized by a lack of awareness of surroundings for an interval of a minute or two. The sufferer may perform repeated movements, such as picking at clothes, wandering aimlessly, or babbling unintelligible sounds without conscious intent (automatism).

TREATMENT

Treatment begins with addressing abnormal conditions that are easily correctable, such as high or low blood sugar or sodium levels. At times, this is sufficient to eliminate or reduce seizures. If epileptic attacks persist, anticonvulsant drugs are prescribed to control these attacks; however, these drugs can cause marked drowsiness. A combination of more than one drug may be needed. Fifty percent of patients who successfully respond to anticonvulsant drug therapy can eventually suspend the treatment without relapse. Brain surgery is considered if drug therapy has failed and brain damage in the temporal lobe is the cause of the seizures.

Further information on Epilepsy *can be found in* AUTONOMIC NERVOUS SYSTEM; CENTRAL NERVOUS SYSTEM; NERVOUS SYSTEM; *and* SEIZURE. *Specific topics mentioned in this article are developed in* ANTICONVULSANT DRUGS; BLOOD PRESSURE; BRAIN; *and* FIRST AID.

Epinephrine

A hormone that plays a role in the body's response to stress.

The adrenal glands release epinephrine into the blood in response to exercise, fright, exposure to cold temperatures, and low blood sugar levels. The hormone prepares the body for urgent action—the fight-or-flight response—by raising blood sugar, blood pressure, and heart rate. It is also a neurotransmitter, produced and stored in nerve endings to transport impulses from one nerve cell to another. *See also* ADRENAL GLANDS *and* NOREPINEPHRINE.

Epiphysis

A normal outgrowth of bone or tissue.

Epiphysis commonly refers to the end section of a bone that, at birth and during childhood growth, is separated from the rest of the bone by cartilage. By adulthood, the epiphysis fuses with the bone by the process of ossification. Long bones, such as the thigh bone (femur) and upper arm bone (humerus), have an epiphysis.

The epiphysis is also another name for the pineal body, a small gland that secretes melatonin. It is found in the brains of all vertebrates and is thought to be a vestigial sensory organ. *See also* BONE.

Episcleritis

Swollen blood vessels in the episclera, a tissue that covers the white of the eye (sclera).

Often observed in adults between the ages of 20 and 50, episcleritis may be associated with connective tissue diseases, such as systemic lupus erythematosus and rheumatoid arthritis, but usually the cause is not clear. Symptoms of episcleritis include tearing, mild pain, sudden redness, pink or purple hues to the eyeball, and light sensitivity. They may take up to three days to clear up. If symptoms last longer or seem extreme, consult a physician. *See* SCLERITIS.

Episiotomy

A surgical incision made in the perineum, the soft tissue between the vaginal opening and the anus.

An episiotomy is commonly performed during childbirth. The vagina is extremely elastic and stretches during labor to accommodate the bulk of the baby. However, sometimes the vagina cannot stretch wide enough, and tearing occurs. The purpose of an episiotomy is to prevent the vagina and other nearby tissues from tearing and being damaged. A clean cut, closed with stitches, heals rapidly and with less chance of infection than a comparable tear.

An episiotomy is not made until the baby's head is visible from the vaginal opening (has crowned), signaling that birth is imminent. A local anesthetic is administered immediately prior to the incision, ensuring that it is painless. Between 50 and 90 percent of first-time mothers have an episiotomy, and the procedure is used in 25 to 35 percent of later deliveries.

There are no long-term effects for a woman who has had an episiotomy. The stitches may cause minor discomfort during the first few days after delivery. They do not require removal, and dissolve on their own within a week. *See also* CHILDBIRTH.

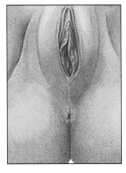

Episiotomy.
An episiotomy, above, is an incision made in the tissue between the vagina and the anus to aid in childbirth.

Epispadias

A rare birth defect in which the urethra opens on the top, or dorsal, surface of the penis, rather than at the tip of the head.

There are three forms of epispadias. The urethra may open at the top of the head of the penis, the whole urethra may be open along the full length of the penis, or the exposed urethra may be accompanied by the bladder opening to the abdomen. Epispadias may be accompanied by other defects of the urinary or reproductive systems.

Epispadias is usually repaired surgically. Incontinence (the leaking of urine) may require further surgery. Repair is usually successful, although incontinence may persist. *See also* HYPOSPADIAS *and* INCONTINENCE.

Epithelium

The cells that make up the top layer of skin.

Epithelial cells also line the internal organs. The three shapes of cells that are found in the epithelium are squamous, cuboidal, and columnar. *See also* SKIN.

Epstein-Barr Virus

The virus that causes mononucleosis.

The Epstein-Barr virus enters the body through the nose and throat and attacks the white blood cells, an important part of the immune system. The virus causes mononucleosis, the symptoms of which are usually mild, and include fever, sore throat, swollen glands, loss of appetite, fatigue, and weakness that may last for several weeks. Treatment for mononucleosis is rest, plenty of fluids, and normal eating habits, even though the sufferer may not be hungry. Nonsteroidal anti-inflammatory drugs can be prescribed to reduce fever and relieve muscle aches. *See also* MONONU-CLEOSIS, INFECTIOUS *and* VIRUS.

Erection

The hardening and lengthening of the penis in response to sexual stimuli.

Erection facilitates the penetration of the penis into the vagina. An erection is the result of a complex interaction between the nervous system and the blood vessels.

When sexual stimuli are transmitted from the brain to the penis, the arteries of the groin supply blood to sponge-like areas in the penis (erectile tissue), that then fill. At the same time, the muscle tissue surrounding the veins tightens, preventing them from removing the excess blood. Under these conditions, the penis can contain up to seven times its original blood volume. Increased blood pressure in the penis causes the increase in length and diameter. *See also* ERECTION, DISORDERS OF; INTER-COURSE; *and* REPRODUCTIVE SYSTEM, MALE.

Erection, Disorders of

Also known as impotence and erectile dysfunction

The inability to achieve or sustain an erection.

Erection disorders may be caused by both physical and emotional problems. Physical causes include circulatory disorders, nervous system problems, and diabetes. Various medications have been known to cause or contribute to the problem as well.

Over half of all cases of erectile dysfunction are caused by nonphysical factors, primarily stress and anxiety. If a man can experience an erection during sleep or while masturbating, then the cause of the problem is psychological rather than physical.

One impotence episode does not indicate a permanent erectile disorder. As men age, they experience more difficulty in achieving or sustaining an erection. Nearly 20 percent of men are impotent at age 60. By age 80, the number is closer to 70 percent.

TREATMENT

Treatment is generally aimed at the underlying cause of the dysfunction.

Drug Treatments. In recent years, pharmaceutical treatments have been developed to treat erectile dysfunctions. The best known of these is the drug Viagra (sildenafil). Certain chemical messengers are responsible for sustaining blood in erectile tissue. Viagra works by inhibiting enzymes that break down these messengers. Viagra has a high success rate, but it will not work for all men. Side effects, experienced by 10 percent of users, include headache, dizziness, indigestion, and visual disturbances. Men with a history of heart disease or with liver or kidney problems are cautioned not to use Viagra.

Surgical implants are available for men who cannot achieve an erection by any other means. One type of implant, a semi-rigid rod, is implanted into the penis so that it permanently remains in a semi-erect state. Another type of implant is an inflatable device that is attached to a pump in the testicles. Neither device should interfere with sensation or ejaculation.

PRIAPISM

Priapism is a painful persistent erection that is unrelated to sexual excitement. Most cases result from drug use or the presence of a blood clot. Sickle cell anemia, leukemia, a tumor in the pelvis or spine, or a genital infection can also cause the condition. In all of these cases, blood may become trapped in the erectile tissue.

Treatment depends on the cause. A shunt may be placed in the penis to restore circulation and drain excess blood. If priapism does not respond to treatment, there is a high probability that sexual function will be permanently impaired. *See also* PRIAPISM.

Ergometer

> **Any device used to measure units of work (ergs) done by a human subject.**

Work refers to a force moving through a distance. Energy is the ability to do work. An erg is a unit measuring work done, and an ergometer is a device to measure and record work. In medicine, various tests allow a physician to measure the amount of work done—by the heart, muscles, etc. A stationary bicycle is often equipped with an ergometer, allowing work by the rider to be measured and compared with other vital data, as in a cardiac stress test. Other types of ergometers can measure muscle contractions. *See also* CARDIAC STRESS TEST.

Ergonomics

> **A branch of science that applies information about the human body to the design of objects, systems, and work-related environments.**

The discipline of ergonomics emerged after World War II, when it became increasingly obvious that certain systems and work environments needed to be better designed to suit the physical needs of the individuals using and working in them. For many years, machines and products had been designed with little or no consideration for the operator. Designs that incorporated ergonomics led to fewer work-related injuries and chronic disorders.

Ergonomists work with designers and engineers to develop better-designed products and machinery, or they evaluate existing products and sites. When evaluating a work site, an ergonomist takes into account several factors, including range of vision, light, ability to hear, excessive noise, motion and vibration, temperature, and the overall workload.

The Occupational Safety and Health Administration of the United States Department of Labor (OSHA) sets ergonomic standards and attempts to enforce these standards in workplaces in order to reduce the number of work-related injuries and disorders. *See also* ACCIDENTS *and* INJURIES.

Erosion, Dental

> **Loss of tooth enamel.**

Caused by chemicals or acids, early dental erosion gives a tooth a frosted appearance. Shallow cavities form as enamel loss continues. Excessive consumption of citrus fruits, fruit juices, or carbonated beverages, or exposure to acids in industry usually causes erosion on the outer surfaces of the front teeth. Tobacco juice or the frequent regurgitation of stomach acid, as can occur with acid reflux or bulimia, tends to decay the inner surfaces of molars. Abrasion and attrition in combination with erosion may cause extensive damage. *See also* ABRASION, TOOTH.

Eruption of Teeth

> **Normal development of teeth out of the jaw and through the gum.**

Normally, baby teeth, or deciduous teeth, begin coming through the gum (erupting) at about the age of six months. These teeth take two to three years to fully grow in. Baby teeth are temporary, and when a child is about six years old, permanent teeth begin to erupt, pushing out the baby teeth over the course of the next three to four years. The wisdom teeth (third molars) may not erupt until young adulthood. *See also* TEETH.

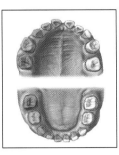

Eruption of Teeth—Deciduous.
Deciduous teeth, begin erupting at six months and continues until 20-24 months. They consist of eight incisors, four canines, and eight molars.

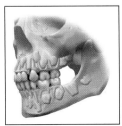

Eruption of Teeth—Permanent.
The full set of permanent teeth (shown set in the skull above the primary teeth) usually start erupting at age six and continue to age 12 Or 13. The third molar (so-called wisdom teeth) erupt (if at all) between the age of 17 and 25. The permanent teeth consist of eight incisors, eight premolars, and twelve molars.

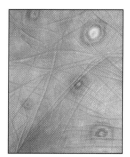

Skin-Related Disorders.
Erythema multiforme lesions, shown above, are often referred to as "target lesions" because of the concentric rings the lesions produce.

Erysipelas

A skin infection caused by streptococci bacteria, which invade the body through a break in the skin.

Erysipelas appears on the face, legs, or arms as a bright red, sharply defined area that tends to spread rapidly. Small blisters may develop and the lymph nodes will swell and become tender. The infection can spread rapidly with fever and chills. Infants, children, and the elderly are most vulnerable to erysipelas, along with people who have had their lymph nodes removed from the groin or underarm.

Erysipelas is treated with penicillin or erythromycin, taken orally if the infection is mild and administered intravenously if the infection is more serious. With treatment, the infection usually clears in about a week. Without treatment, the infection can spread throughout the body and may become life-threatening. *See also* ANTIBIOTIC DRUGS *and* STREPTOCOCCAL INFECTIONS.

Erythema

A bright red or rosy looking rash.

Skin redness, or erythema, is a symptom of many disorders, including dermatitis, rosacea, erythema multiforme, and erythema nodosum. Erythema should be evaluated and treated by a doctor; although the rash is not dangerous, the underlying condition causing it may be. *See also* DERMATITIS.

Erythema Ab Igne

Red skin that may also be dry and itchy, caused by exposure to strong, direct heat.

Erythema ab igne occurs most often in elderly women and is usually found on the shins or the abdomen. In cold weather, sitting too close to a fireplace or hugging a heating pad or hot-water bottle often leaves the skin red and itchy. While the redness will fade, it usually does not disappear completely. The dryness and itching can be relieved with a soothing cream.

Erythema Multiforme

A skin disorder resulting from an allergic reaction.

Erythema multiforme is a type of allergic reaction that occurs in response to certain medications, infections, or illnesses.

CAUSES
The exact cause of the disease is unknown, but damaged blood vessels are suspected to be one cause. About 90 percent of infections are associated with herpes simplex or mycoplasma infections. Allergic reactions to medications such as sulfonamides, penicillin, phenyoin, and barbituates are also associated with the disorder.

SYMPTOMS
Symptoms of erythema multiforme include the appearance of multiple skin lesions of varying kinds, including redness, raised red bumps, and blisters. Other symptoms, such as fever, sometimes, but not always, occur.

TYPES
Stevens-Johnson syndrome is a form of erythema multiforme that causes severe lesions that cover much of the body, especially the mucus membranes.

Toxic epidermal necrolysis (TEN) is the most severe form of erythema multiforme (although it may be a separate disease). In TEN, large blisters form over most or all of the skin and then slough off.

TREATMENT
Treatment of mild erythema multiforme may include moist compresses, antihistamines, medication to reduce fever, and topical anesthetics. Corticosteroids are given to reduce inflammation, and antibiotics are given to control secondary skin infections. For severe forms, hospitalization may be necessary. Mild cases usually resolve in a few weeks. The most severe cases may be fatal.

Issues discussed in this article are further developed in ALLERGY; ARTERIES; ARTERIES, DISORDERS OF; HERPES; HERPES SIMPLEX; *and* SKIN. *Also refer to articles dealing with* ANTIHISTAMINE DRUGS; ANTIBIOTIC DRUGS; *and* FEVER.

Erythema Nodosum

A skin disorder with symptoms that include the formation of painful, reddish skin nodules.

Nodules are large (over half an inch wide) raised bumps on the skin.

CAUSES

The cause of erythema nodosum is unknown, but it appears to be a hypersensitivity, or allergic reaction. Cases have been associated with streptococcal infections, fungal infections, tuberculosis, hepatitis B, syphilis, mononucleosis, and sarcoidosis, as well as other disorders and illnesses. Sensitivity to drugs, especially penicillin, sulfonamides, sulfones, barbiturates, salicylates, and progestin, among others, is also associated with cases of erythema nodosum. Disorders associated with this illness are leukemia, rheumatic fever, and ulcerative colitis. Pregnancy and the use of birth control pills can also be a factor.

SYMPTOMS

Erythema nodosum is characterized by tender nodules, usually on the front of the legs. The nodules may also appear on the buttocks, calves, thighs, and arms. The skin lesions start out as inch-long, elevated, hard lumps. A few days later, they become purple, and they gradually fade to flat, brownish spots. Other symptoms include fever, malaise, joint aches, skin redness and swelling, and swelling of the legs.

TREATMENT

Treatment of erythema nodosum involves diagnosis and treatment of the underlying infection or drug allergy. Nonsteroidal anti-inflammatory drugs or corticosteroids are used to control inflammation. Sometimes, oral potassium iodide (SSKI) is used to treat the nodules. If there is a great deal of pain, analgesics may be given.

For information about disorders that affect the SKIN see DERMABRASION; DERMATOLOGY; DERMATITIS; and DERMATOPHYTE INFECTIONS. Other related issues include ALLERGY; SKIN ALLERGY; and SURFERS' NODULES.

Erythrocyte

Red blood cells.

Red blood cells are one of the many components of blood; their primary function is to carry gases. Erythrocytes are filled with hemoglobin, a molecule that, when enriched with oxygen, gives the red blood cells their scarlet color. They carry oxygen from the lungs to the cells of the body, release it to the tissues, pick up carbon dioxide, and return to the lungs. When the hemoglobin carries carbon dioxide, the blood cells are a much darker red.

Red blood cells also help maintain a balance between the acidity and alkalinity of blood. *See also* ACIDOSIS; ALKALOSIS; BLOOD; CARBON DIOXIDE; HEMOGLOBIN; *and* OXYGEN.

Esmarch Bandage

An elastic bandage used to apply pressure to a wound or muscle.

Esmarch bandages are elastic fabric strips of various widths and lengths, available both sterilized and unsterilized. They are used to wrap around a wound—although gauze is placed to touch the wound itself—or to apply pressure to protect muscles or torn ligaments. *See* BANDAGE *and* DRESSING.

Esophageal Atresia

A congenital condition involving the incomplete development of the esophagus.

In esophageal atresia, instead of connecting to the stomach, the esophagus ends in a blind tube. This condition usually occurs together with an abnormal connection between the esophagus and trachea (tracheoesophageal fistula).

Symptoms accompanying esophageal atresia include excessive saliva, coughing after attempts to swallow, and cyanosis (a bluish cast to the skin). If a tracheoesophageal fistula is present, saliva enters the lungs, putting the infant at risk for aspiration pneumonia.

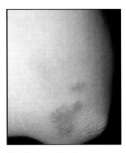

Erythema Nodosum. Red swellings on the shins, thighs, and occasionally the arms, above, are common with erythema nodosum. These swellings, which are shiny and tender, are associated with other diseases, such as streptococcal infections, tuberculosis, and sarcoidosis. Treatment of the underlying condition clears the swellings.

Treatment. Surgery is performed to connect the esophagus to the stomach and to close the fistula. Until then, the infant must be fed intravenously. Continuous suction must also be applied to prevent saliva from entering the lungs. In most cases, surgery is successful, resulting in recovery and healthy development. *See also* ESOPHAGUS.

Esophageal Dilatation

The stretching of a narrowed or blocked esophagus to permit normal eating and drinking.

Narrowing of the esophagus is usually due to inflammation (esophagitis), cancer, or an inability of the muscles in the lower esophagus to relax (achalasia).

Dilatation is performed under sedation. Endoscopy is first performed to locate and identify the cause of the stricture, and then the esophagus is enlarged. A balloon catheter may be inserted down the esophagus and inflated; often a larger balloon follows, so that the esophagus is widened in stages. An older technique is the use of bougies, rounded metal cylinders that are guided down a wire that has been anchored in the intestines, and which push the esophagus open. Gradually increasing diameters of bougies are used until sufficient widening has been accomplished. Depending on the disorder being treated, esophageal dilatation is of varying success and permanence. *See also* ESOPHAGITIS.

Esophageal Diverticulum

A protrusion in the wall of the esophagus.

The two types of esophageal diverticuli are a pharyngeal pouch and a mid-esophageal diverticulum. A pharyngeal pouch typically protrudes backwards at the entrance of the throat from the pharynx. It is caused by a failure of the sphincter muscle to relax during swallowing; when food fails to pass, the throat muscles work harder, forcing the lining of the esophagus to bulge through the esophageal wall, forming a pouch that may trap food. Swallowing becomes a struggle;

bad breath and regurgitation may develop. A pharyngeal pouch can be treated with surgery. A mid-esophageal diverticulum is less serious. It occurs farther down the esophagus, is rarely noticed, and requires no treatment. *See also* SPHINCTER.

Esophageal Spasm

High-pressure, poorly coordinated contractions of the esophagus that occur after swallowing.

Esophageal spasms are contractions of the esophagus that do not send food to the stomach. They affect the smooth muscles in the walls of the lower esophagus. The cause of the spasms is unknown. The symptoms of esophageal spasm include difficulty swallowing and pain that resembles angina. Spasms may be mild and correct on their own, or medication may be prescribed to relax the muscles. *See also* ESOPHAGUS.

Esophageal Stricture

A narrowing of the esophagus, causing difficulty in swallowing.

Types of esophageal constrictions include esophageal webs, which are more prevalent among middle-aged women and may be associated with an iron deficiency, and mucosal rings, which appear near the lower esophageal sphincter. Both of these conditions cause difficulty in swallowing solids.

CAUSES
Acid reflux and the resulting accumulation of scar tissue is a leading cause of esophageal stricture. Scar tissue in the esophagus can also result from previous surgery, bacterial or viral infections, or the ingestion of caustic chemicals.

DIAGNOSIS
It is important to make sure that any difficulty in swallowing is not due to esophageal or stomach cancer. A barium x-ray may be performed, followed by an endoscopic exam, to determine the cause of the difficulty in swallowing.

TREATMENT

Treatment includes esophageal dilation. In this procedure, a topical anesthetic is used on the lining of the throat and a flexible fiber-optic endoscope is inserted into the esophagus. A series of dilators—either balloons or tubes of increasing diameter—are used to widen the esophagus. *See also* ACID REFLUX *and* ESOPHAGEAL DILATATION.

Esophageal Varices

Abnormally expanded veins in the lower esophagus and upper stomach.

Esophageal varices are often an effect of portal hypertension, high blood pressure in the vein carrying blood to the liver (portal vein) as a result of liver disease. The increased pressure diverts blood to veins in the walls of the esophagus and stomach, causing the veins to bulge and possibly rupture.

Symptoms of bleeding esophageal varices include vomiting blood and blood in the feces, which makes them appear black. Treatment may include intravenous injection of blood clotting agents and the insertion into the esophagus and stomach of a balloon catheter, the inflation of which puts pressure on the bleeding veins. Drugs can be used to control recurrent bleeding, and surgery may be performed to relieve pressure in the portal vein. *See also* BLEEDING, INTERNAL; CIRRHOSIS; LIVER DISEASE, ALCOHOLIC; *and* PORTAL HYPERTENSION.

Esophagitis

Inflammation of the esophagus.

Fungal infections and viruses may attack the esophagus and cause esophagitis; but acid reflux is the more common cause, as stomach acids irritate and inflame the lining of the esophagus. Esophagitis is also a frequent side effect of radiation treatment of the chest and neck for cancer.

SYMPTOMS

Symptoms include pain and difficulty upon swallowing and possibly heartburn (if

---

Limiting Symptoms of Esophagitis

A person with esophagitis should avoid nicotine; fried, fatty, or spicy foods; chocolate; coffee; citrus; peppermint; and dairy foods, such as eggs, ice cream, milk, and cream. Foods at room temperature are easier to tolerate than hot foods, and cool liquids may be soothing. Meals should be small and frequent. Antacid medications should be taken 30 to 60 minutes after eating. Food should not be consumed within two hours of bedtime, and the individual should sleep with the head raised eight to ten inches from the bed with pillows. Medications that reduce the secretion of stomach acid may be prescribed.

---

caused by acid reflux) or more systemic symptoms, such as fever or joint pain (if caused by an infection). Correctly diagnosing the root of the discomfort is important, since the symptoms can mimic those of cancer of the esophagus.

TREATMENT

People with acid reflux should take steps to minimize reflux and thus minimize inflammation. If esophagitis is caused by a fungal infection, antifungal oral medications are prescribed. If the causative factor is radiation, the inflammation will usually abate four to six weeks after the cessation of therapy. *See also* ACID REFLUX; ANTACID DRUGS; ANTIFUNGAL DRUGS; ESOPHAGUS; *and* ESOPHAGUS, CANCER OF.

Esophagoscopy

Study of the esophagus by means of a specialized fiberoptic viewing tube or endoscope (esophagoscope), allowing direct observation, tissue biopsy, and photography of the esophagus.

Esophagoscopy is a type of upper endoscopy, which includes the endoscopic examination of the esophagus, stomach, and duodenum by means of specialized fiberoptic viewing instruments. Esophagoscopy can be used to view the esophagus, and instruments can be passed through the hollow endoscope to remove samples or tissue and perform some forms of surgery. Esophagoscopy is useful in diagnosing tumors, erosion, blockage, and narrowing (stenosis) of the esophagus. *See also* ENDOSCOPY; ESOPHAGUS; *and* GASTROSCOPY.

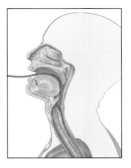

Esophagoscopy.
An esophagoscopy, above, is an examination of the esophagus with an endoscope, a thin, flexible viewing instrument with a light and lens attached.

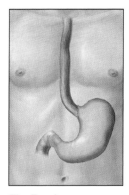

The Esophagus.
The esophagus, above, is a muscular tube through which foods and liquids pass after being swallowed. The esophagus then uses muscle contractions to squeeze the food towards the stomach, where the majority of digestion takes place.

Esophagus

The muscular tube between the throat and the stomach.

The esophagus is a ten-inch-long muscular tube through which foods and liquids pass from the throat to the stomach. Bundles of circular and longitudinal muscles line the esophagus. Sphincter muscles on either end open to let food pass; otherwise they remain closed. Waves of muscle contraction, called peristalsic action, squeeze food toward the stomach; the smooth esophageal lining allows for easier movement of food. Even if a person is upside down, the peristalsic action continues, making it possible to eat and drink. *See also* STOMACH.

Esophagus, Cancer of the

Malignant tumor of the esophagus.

Most cancers of the esophagus develop in the middle or lower section. About 60 percent of esophageal cancers are squamous cell carcinomas, which arise from the surface cells of the esophagus. About 40 percent are adenocarcinomas, which develop in an inner layer. The esophagus lacks the protective lining found in other parts of the gastrointestinal tract. This lining can protect against the spread of cancer cells; without it, esophageal cancer can spread easily to other organs, such as the lungs, liver, brain, bones, and adrenal gland.

INCIDENCE
Cancer of the esophagus occurs mainly in people over the age of 50. It is more common in men, who have three times the incidence as women, and in African-Americans, who are three times more likely to develop esophageal cancer than their Caucasian counterparts. Smoking and heavy drinking are important risk factors.

SYMPTOMS
The first symptom of esophageal cancer usually is difficulty swallowing, noticed first with solids and then with liquids, that is caused by narrowing of the esophagus. Food may be regurgitated. Weight may be rapidly lost. As the cancer progresses, it can cause a chronic cough, pain in the throat, hoarseness, coughing up blood, and an increased incidence of respiratory infections.

DIAGNOSIS
Diagnostic tests can include an x-ray examination in which the patient swallows a drink containing barium; direct visual examination (esophagoscopy); exfoliative cytology, in which cells from the lining of the esophagus are collected and analyzed; computed tomography scanning (CT); and magnetic resonance imaging (MRI).

TREATMENT
Surgery to remove all or part of the esophagus and structures that have been invaded by the cancer can relieve symptoms and prolong survival. Radiation therapy and chemotherapy can accompany surgery or, for patients who cannot withstand the rigors of a major operation, replace it. If swallowing becomes impossible, a tube may be inserted through the cancer so that liquid nourishment can reach the stomach.

PROGNOSIS
Because difficulty swallowing and other symptoms usually do not appear until the cancer is advanced and has begun to spread, the prognosis is often less than a 10 percent survival rate for five years after late-stage treatment.

> ## Diet and Esophageal Cancer
>
> Diet is believed to play a role in the development of esophageal cancer. In parts of Asia, chemicals in certain popular foods are believed to contribute to the risk. In the United States and other Western countries, heavy consumption of foods such as cured ham and bacon are believed to increase the risk, as they contain nitrates and nitrites, which are transformed into nitrosamine, a carcinogen, in the body.

> *Other articles dealing with* CANCER *related issues include* ANTICANCER DRUGS; CANCER SCREENING; *and* PRECANCEROUS. *More information is included in* DIET AND DISEASE; NUTRITION; *and* NUTRITION AND DIET, ALTERNATIVE THERAPIES. *See* AGING; ESOPHAGUS; *and* RADIATION THERAPY.

ESR

Abbreviation for erythrocyte sedimentation rate
Also known as the sed rate

A diagnostic test measuring the rate at which red blood cells settle to the bottom of a test tube.

ESR is generally used to help reveal the presence of a nonspecific inflammatory condition. The test is often part of standard blood testing and is also useful in the ongoing monitoring of patients experiencing a range of rheumatic diseases.

ESR is performed by adding an anticoagulant to whole blood in a long tube; the downward progress of the red blood cells (erythrocytes) is then observed. The distance traveled by gradually settling red blood cells is visually measured over the course of an hour, and the sedimentation rate is recorded.

The test is performed by hand, as opposed to many types of blood tests that today are automated. Normal ESR varies depending on age and sex; it is generally less than 10 mm per hour in adult males and slightly higher in females.

An elevated ESR may indicate anemia, collagen vascular disease, hyperproteinemia, neoplasia, or pregnancy. A low ESR may indicate polycythemia, microcytosis, sickle cell anemia, congenital heart disease, or hypochromic microcytic anemia.

Background information about ERYTHROCYTE SEDIMENTATION RATES *can be found in* ANEMIA; BLOOD TESTS; *and* NEOPLASIA. *More about the treatment of inflammatory conditions can be found in* ANTI-INFLAMMATORY DRUGS *and* NONSTEROIDAL ANTI-INFLAMMATORY DRUGS.

Estrogen Drugs

Natural and synthetic forms of estrogen used to alleviate symptoms of menopause (hormone replacement therapy) and as a form of birth control.

Estrogens, which are produced in the ovaries, are the basic hormones that regulate the female reproductive system. They also influence the role of calcium in the body and so are critical in the prevention of osteoporosis. There is also evidence that they prevent cardiovascular disease.

Estrogen Drug Interactions

Like many drugs, estrogen drugs can interact with other drugs, possibly reducing their effectiveness or causing added side effects. Some drugs that interact with estrogen drugs are:

• *Anticoagulants*	Reduced anticoagulant effect
• *Anticonvulsants*	Reduced estrogen effect
• *Antidepressants*	Increased toxicity and effect of some tranquilizers
• *Antidiabetics*	Unpredictable effect on blood sugar levels
• *Insulin*	Reduced insulin effect
• *Barbiturates*	Reduced estrogen effect
• *Corticosteroids*	Increased corticosteroid effect
• *Tobacco*	Increased blood clot formation

HORMONE REPLACEMENT THERAPY

During menopause, which can start anywhere between the ages of 35 and 55, the amount of estrogen produced gradually declines. Symptoms arising as a result of a lack of estrogen may include hot flashes, urinary frequency, and vaginal dryness. Osteoporosis, cancer, and heart disease are also linked to lower estrogen levels.

To alleviate the symptoms and health risks of menopause, estrogen drugs are often prescribed to replace the body's natural supply. To reduce side effects, such as the risk for uterine cancer, they are often administered with artificial progesterones (progestins). Synthetic forms of estrogen are much more powerful than the natural forms; since the undesirable effects of menopause are ameliorated with very low amounts of estrogen, the natural forms are preferred when used to treat menopause. The lowest effective dose should be used.

BIRTH CONTROL

Estrogens have also been prescribed for birth control, and a high dose of estrogens is sometimes used as a "morning after" contraceptive. However, progestins, either alone or in combination with estrogen, are now preferred for birth control, as they tend to have fewer side effects.

SIDE EFFECTS

Side effects of estrogen drugs may include nausea, vomiting, breast enlargement, swelling of the ankles and legs, loss of appetite, weight changes, water retention, abdominal cramps, headache, and mood changes. They increase libido for women and reduce it for men. If a skin patch has been used, there may be irritation of the skin at the patch site. There may be intolerance to contact lenses.

Long-term use of estrogens increases the risk of endometrial cancer and gallbladder disease in postmenopausal women. Estrogens are also involved in the formation of blood clots and increase the risk of embolism.

SELECTIVE ESTROGEN RECEPTOR MODULATORS

Raloxifene. The drug raloxifene, which is a synthetic estrogen-like drug that modifies the effects of estrogen in the body, can be prescribed to limit some of the health risks of menopause. It is primarily prescribed to prevent osteoporosis, and it may also have beneficial effects in preventing heart disease. Raloxifene limits the effects of estrogen on uterine and breast tissue; because estrogen has been shown to promote the growth of breast cancer, raloxifene is currently under study as a drug to prevent breast cancer. Side effects of raloxifene include hot flashes and an increased risk for blood clots. This medication should not be taken during pregnancy.

Tamoxifen. Another selective estrogen receptor modulator, called tamoxifen, interferes with the activity of estrogen on the breast and is used as a treatment for breast cancer; it is currently being studied as a means of preventing breast cancer. Side effects include symptoms similar to those of menopause (including hot flashes), as well as an increased risk for blood clots, uterine cancer, cataracts, and harmful effects on the liver. The drug should not be taken during pregnancy.

ESTROGEN DRUGS *and other related topics are also discussed in* DIAGNOSTICS IN WOMEN'S HEALTH; HORMONES; MENOPAUSE; PERIMENOPAUS; *and* PREGNANCY. *Disorders related to the use of these drugs are discussed in* BIRTH DEFECTS; CRAMP; EMBOLISM; *and* GALLBLADDER CANCER.

Estrogen Hormones

Hormones responsible for female sexual development and reproduction.

Estrogen is produced primarily by the ovaries and is also produced in small amounts by the adrenal glands of both sexes. It causes the development of female sexual characteristics and reproductive functions, helps prepare the body for pregnancy by thickening the lining of the uterus, and is produced by the placenta as a way of maintaining pregnancy. Estrogen promotes healthy bone density; it also helps prevent cardiovascular disease by lowering levels of LDL cholesterol and raising HDL levels. Production of estrogen diminishes after menopause; at this point, some women may choose to take estrogen in pill form to reduce the symptoms associated with the change in hormone levels. *See also* CALCIUM; CHOLESTEROL; ESTROGEN DRUGS; MENOPAUSE; OVARIES; PREGNANCY; *and* REPRODUCTIVE SYSTEM, FEMALE.

Ethics, Medical

The study of ethical issues in medicine.

Medical ethics is the study of ethical and moral issues in medical treatment and research. It is also used more generally to describe ethical issues in the life sciences and allocation of healthcare resources (healthcare ethics). Medicine, nursing, law, sociology, philosophy, and theology all grapple with ethical problems in medical fields.

HISTORY

Medical ethics traces its roots to ancient Greece. The Hippocratic Oath, which states that physicians should do no harm, is an early example. In the 18th century, the English physician Thomas Percival devised a professional code of ethics for doctors. It served as the model for later codes, such as the one established in 1846 by the founders of the American Medical Association. The Nuremberg Code, written at the close of World War II, laid out guidelines for the

Economic Issues in Medical Ethics

What should society do when the supply of health-care resources cannot meet the demand? That question lies at the heart of the economics of medical ethics. In the 1960s, the development of dialysis machines, which remove wastes from the blood of people with kidney failure, prompted several institutions to create committees in charge of selecting which patients would receive this life-saving treatment. In the 1980s, the United States set up a national system to distribute organs to people in need of transplants, to avoid a free-market crisis in which organs went to those most able to pay for them. In the 1990s, increasing emphasis was placed on minimizing costs in healthcare, with medical ethicists closely examining the fairness of cost-cutting plans.

use of human subjects in medical research. Since 1950, medical ethics has grappled with issues resulting from the advent of new technologies that have brought new complexities to medical treatment.

TOPICS IN MEDICAL ETHICS

Research. There are many areas of long-standing debate in medical ethics. In research, many ethical issues arise surrounding the use of human subjects in medical experiments. In 1966, Henry Beecher, a prominent physician at Harvard Medical School, published a paper detailing abuses suffered by human research subjects at universities and medical centers around the country. For example, some subjects received an experimental treatment without being given the option to choose a standard treatment instead.

Debate intensified when it became widely known that the United States Public Health Service had sponsored a study on syphilis in which researchers withheld diagnostic information and effective treatment from the study's African-American subjects in order to witness the progression of the illness. Eventually, Congress enacted regulations to prevent these ethical abuses.

Artificial Life Support. Technologies developed in the 1960s, such as the mechanical ventilator, allowed physicians to maintain bodily function in the presence of severe brain damage. Many states adop-

ted legislation that defined death in terms of the loss of brain function, to provide patients and their families with the option to end the life of a brain-dead individual. Most other nations define death in a similar way or in terms of the loss of all independent lung and heart function.

Reproductive Technology. During the 1960s and 1970s, new reproductive technologies spurred debate over the rights of human beings to control their bodies and the embryos created from their cells. The debate began with the birth-control pill and culminated in the 1973 Supreme Court decision legalizing abortion. The controversy that followed centered on the definition of personhood, the rights of the pregnant woman, and the role that the state should play in reproductive decisions. Today, the issue is further complicated by the potential to use embryonic cells in important areas of medical research.

Physician-Assisted Suicide. In developed countries, people are less likely to die of infectious diseases and are more likely to die of chronic diseases, such as cancer. People who support physician-assisted suicide believe that terminally ill patients suffering intense pain should have the right to end their own lives, with the help of a physician if necessary. Opponents charge that physician-assisted suicide violates the most basic tenet of medicine: first do no harm. In addition, it could become impossible to draw a meaningful line between patients who can and cannot request help in dying.

New Topics. The distribution of healthcare resources raises questions that draw on concepts of distributive justice, the free market, intrinsic human rights, and the role of the state in allocating resources. Advances in research in genetics, exemplified by progress in mammalian cloning and the mapping of the human genome, have spawned a new set of ethical questions.

Issues related to MEDICAL ETHICS *are discussed in* BLOOD DONATION; DOCTOR, CHOOSING A; DONOR; HOSPITALS, TYPES OF; *and* ORGAN DONATION. *Public organizations and programs that deal with related topics include the* AMERICAN MEDICAL ASSOCIATION; MEDICAID; *and* MEDICARE.

Resources on Medical Ethics
Bauschamp, Tom L., *Principles of Biomedical Ethics* (1989); Basch, Paul F., *Textbook of International Health* (1999); Moeller, D.W., *Environmental Health* (1997); National Research Council, Committee on Environmental Epidemiology, *Public Health and Hazardous Wastes* (1991); Reich, Warren T., *Encyclopedia of Bioethics* (1992); Turnock, Bernard, *Public Health: What It Is and How It Works* (2000); Veatch, Robert M., Case *Studies in Medical Ethics* (1977); U.S. Public Health Service, Tel. (202) 619-0257, Online: phs.os.dhhs.gov/phs/phs.html; www.med.cornell.edu/public.health/.

Etiology

Term referring to the underlying cause of an abnormality or disease, or the study of such causes.

Etiology is a central concept in diagnostic medicine; once the etiology—the underlying cause—of a particular disease or abnormality has been established, the physician may determine appropriate treatment. Often a single underlying cause may be diagnosed for a given symptom or symptoms. In other cases, however, multiple causes produce a variety of symptoms, and the question of etiology becomes more involved. The diagnostician hopes to eliminate incorrect causes and arrive at the correct etiology of a given illness. He or she does so through a combination of experience, the scientific methods at his or her disposal, subjective reports of the patient, and observable symptoms. *See also* DIAGNOSIS *and* EPIDEMIOLOGY.

Euphoria

A positive, glowing sensation of well-being.

Euphoria may arise naturally, as when a person experiences a thrilling life event, such as the birth of a child, a business success, or a new love interest. There are also, however, several pathological causes. Euphoria can be induced by drugs and alcohol, which contributes to the fact that these substances may become addictive. It may also be produced by disorders, such as advanced multiple sclerosis, brain tumors, or dementia, or it may be experienced during the manic phase of manic-depressive illness (bipolar disorder). *See* BIPOLAR DISORDER; MULTIPLE SCLEROSIS; *and* SUBSTANCE ABUSE.

Eustachian Tube

A passage between the back of the nose and the middle-ear.

A Eustachian tube links each ear to the back of the nose. It opens when necessary to maintain hearing and regulate air pressure (relieving stress on the eardrum), and it provides a drainage canal for the middle-ear. An inch and a third long, each tube is lined by a wet mucous membrane and stretches from the inner-ear down toward the middle of the head to the soft palate at the back of the nose. *See also* BAROTRAUMA.

Euthanasia

Also known as physician-assisted suicide

The intentional ending of a person's life to relieve suffering.

Euthanasia is the act of helping a person or animal end his or her life in a painless fashion to relieve unbearable suffering, generally due to the presence of a terminal disease. Voluntary euthanasia is the taking of a person's life at his or her request. Euthanasia is usually performed by inducing rapid unconsciousness, followed by cardiac or respiratory arrest and eventual loss of brain function. The technique attempts to avoid inflicting undue stress on the individual or animal. In the United States, euthanasia is illegal, but many special interests groups continue to lobby to change the law. *See also* DEATH *and* ETHICS, MEDICAL.

Evoked Responses

A diagnostic test that measures the brain's response to certain stimuli.

Evoked responses are a way to detect brain activity too subtle to be detected by electroencephalography (EEG). Stimuli such as touch, sight, sound, and smell stimulate different areas of the brain, and these responses can be measured. If the response is too small to be measured by an EEG, a series of responses can be produced and then analyzed by a computer.

To measure evoked responses, electrodes are fastened to the scalp, and the patient is exposed to a series of stimuli, such as flashing lights or sounds. The electrical impulses picked up by the electrodes are then sent to a computer, which processes them in comparison to a background EEG.

Evoked responses can detect nervous system abnormalities caused by tumor, in-

Eustachian Tube.
The eustachian tube, below, connects the middle ear and the back of the nose. It acts as a drainage passage and maintains hearing by periodically opening to regulate air pressure.

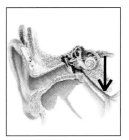

jury, or other changes. Because the test is so sensitive, it can often locate the site of the abnormality. It can also detect small degrees of damage to the optic nerve characteristic in people with multiple sclerosis, as well as electrical discharges characteristic in people with epilepsy. It is also useful in detecting responses in a person who cannot talk, such as testing a baby's ability to hear. *See* BRAIN; CENTRAL NERVOUS SYSTEM; EEG; EPILEPSY; *and* MULTIPLE SCLEROSIS.

Ewing's Sarcoma

A rare cancer of the connective tissue of bone.

Ewing's sarcoma generally occurs in people between the ages of 10 and 15, and it is twice as common in males as in females.

Symptoms include pain and tenderness, sometimes with swelling and an increased incidence of fractures. The cancer is diagnosed by x-ray and a biopsy and is treated by radiation therapy and chemotherapy. Chances of survival are good if the cancer is detected before it has spread to other parts of the body. *See* BONE CANCER *and* CANCER.

Examination, Physical

A general evaluation of health involving a number of standard tests performed by a physician.

A physical exam is a common battery of tests and observations that may be performed for a variety of reasons. A patient may have general feelings of ill health and seek further data regarding his or her condition. A physical may be part of a job requirement or simply part of a periodic monitoring of general health.

Inspection General physical exams involve a painless series of procedures free of attendant medical risk. Usually it is necessary to remove clothing to allow the doctor to fully examine the body. Generally, body weight and height are measured. Vital signs, which include temperature, pulse, respiration, and blood pressure, are recorded. The doctor will note and evaluate any irregularities in these readings.

The patient is inspected by a doctor to assess general health as well as the condition of various physical systems. Physical appearance, body structure, mobility, and behavior are evaluated; and the head and neck, eyes, ears, nose and throat, breasts and underarms, back, chest and abdomen, genitalia, hair, and nails are examined.

Palpation involves applying the sense of touch to inspect the texture of the skin, with attention to any evident swelling, pulsation, or lumps. The position and shape of organs or tissue masses is accompanied by grasping with the fingers. Temperature of the skin may be assessed using the back of the hand, which affords greater sensitivity than the palm. Vibrations may be detected with the base of the fingers. *See* PALPATION.

Percussion requires the physician to tap the skin in short, abrupt strokes to evaluate underlying structures. Information regarding the size, density, and location of underlying organs may be determined through percussion. *See also* PERCUSSION.

Auscultation, or listening to the sounds of the body, generally with a stethoscope, allows the physician to hear and assess the activity of the heart, lungs, blood vessels, and abdomen. *See also* AUSCULTATION.

Tendon reflex test involves tapping a stretched tendon, such as below a bent knee; a normal neurological response is for the muscle to contract. *See* DIAGNOSIS.

Excision

Surgical removal, usually by scalpel, of diseased tissue from surrounding healthy tissue.

Excision is often used to remove benign or cancerous lesions or tumors. Growths removed by excision include polyps, melanomas, moles, carcinomas, hemangiomas, lymphangiomas, fibroids, breast lumps, gangrenous skin, bony outgrowths of the jaw, osteomas, keloid scars, and port-wine stains. Wide excision involves taking additional normal skin or tissue as a defensive measure. Alternatives to excision or follow-up treatments include use of lasers, cryotherapy, and irradiation. *See also* SURGERY.

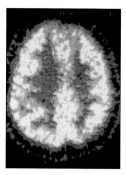
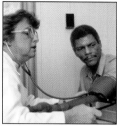
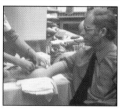

Physical Examination. The photos above highlight certain aspects of a physical examination, an inspection of the various body parts and organs. A physician performs a complete physical examination after a patient's initial visit, which can include a diagnostic image (top); blood pressure test (middle); blood test (bottom); and more. Health experts recommend that physical examinations be done annually.

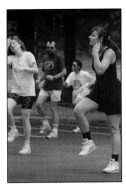

Aerobic Exercise.
Exercise is aerobic when the body is just able to meet the muscles' increased demand for oxygen continuously during increased activity, such as jogging, swimming, or cycling. Aerobic exercise (above), helps the body become more fit and improves the condition of the heart.

Exercise

A physical activity that improves health.

Exercise can increase cardiovascular efficiency, add muscle strength, improve flexibility, and allow for greater endurance. It reduces blood pressure, helps to strengthen the heart, and decreases the likelihood of a heart attack. Increased muscle strength can improve posture, ward off back pain, and help balance, decreasing the possibility of falls. The benefits of exercise can help all people, especially the elderly, to lead independent lives that are both physically and mentally healthier. *See also* AEROBICS *and* FITNESS.

Exocrine Gland

Gland that secretes substances, such as sweat or tears, through ducts or tubes.

Exocrine glands differ from endocrine glands in that they release fluids into ducts or tubes that lead to organs or the skin's surface, while endocrine glands release their chemicals into the bloodstream. Exocrine glands may be triggered by hormones or by signals from nerve endings. Examples of exocrine glands are: lacrimal glands, which secrete tears; salivary glands, which produce saliva; sweat glands, which send sweat to the skin's surface; sebaceous glands, which secrete an oily lubricating substance to the skin's surface; and the pancreas, which secretes digestive enzymes to the small intestine. The pancreas is both an exocrine gland and an endocrine gland. *See also* ENDOCRINE GLANDS.

Exomphalos

Also known as omphalocele

A condition in which the intestines and possibly other abdominal organs are located outside the abdominal wall.

Exomphalos is commonly associated with other abnormalities, particularly those involving the heart. It also has a high association rate with Down's syndrome. As with other abdominal wall defects, exomphalos can be identified by ultrasound scanning as early as the fourteenth week of pregnancy.

Surgery can be performed to correct the condition; if the abdominal cavity is too small to contain all of the intestines, the protrusion is covered with a synthetic material and the skin slowly stretched to cover the organs. The outcome depends on which portion and how much of the intestines and other organs protrude outside the abdominal wall. *See also* BIRTH DEFECT.

Exophthalmos

Bulging of the eyeball, due to swelling in the tissue of the socket.

The eyeball rests on fatty tissue in the eye socket (orbit). When these tissues become swollen, the eyeball is pushed forward, causing it to protrude and force the eyelids open. This swelling cuts off some of the eyeball's ability to move, which limits vision or may cause double vision. If the eyelids cannot close, the cornea is constantly exposed and dries out, causing blurred vision. If the swelling is extreme, the optic nerve may not get enough blood, which can lead to blindness.

CAUSES

Swelling of the tissue behind the eye may occur because of a swollen artery (aneurysm); inflammation of the tissues due to infection; eye tumors; or an overactive thyroid gland (hyperthyroidism). Hyperthyroidism may occur due to a number of reasons, such as a tumor in the thyroid gland, a lack of a necessary mineral such as iodine, or a malfunction in the pituitary gland, which directs the production of the thyroid hormone.

TREATMENT

Treatment of the underlying cause will help to relieve the symptoms, especially if diagnosed early. In some cases, surgery may be necessary to decrease the pressure on the optic nerve and restore vision. *See also* EYE; HYPERTHYROIDISM; *and* THYROID GLAND.

Exotoxin

A protein released into the surrounding medium by certain bacteria; often the primary cause of disease.

Bacteria cause disease by releasing poisonous substances into the body of the person they have invaded. Two types of toxins are produced by bacteria.

Endotoxins are part of the cell wall of the bacteria and are not released into the host unless the bacteria are destroyed. They are resistant to heat and generally cause only mild symptoms, such as fever.

Exotoxins are proteins that are secreted into the bacteria's surroundings. They are extremely powerful—only a tiny concentration is enough to cause disease. Tetanus , anthrax, and botulism are examples of diseases in which symptoms are caused by exotoxins. Symptoms caused by exotoxins can include fever, irregular heartbeat (arrhythmia), destruction of blood ves- sels, diarrhea, and shock. Despite their potency, exotoxins are easily inactivated by heat. *See also* BACTERIA; FEVER; *and* TOXIN.

Expectorants

Drugs that stimulate coughing and loosen phlegm.

Expectorants are over-the-counter drugs that loosen phlegm or mucus that is blocking the airways, allowing it to be expelled more effectively through coughing. They work mainly by stimulating lungs to produce watery secretions that dilute the phlegm; some expectorants also act directly to make the phlegm less sticky. Expectorants should not be taken for a dry cough, in which coughing is not accompanied by phlegm. *See also* COUGH.

Exploratory Surgery

Surgery used to aid in the diagnosis of a disorder.

Exploratory surgery is used to diagnose a disease or disorder when less invasive testing is ineffective or when time constraints prevent such testing. Surgery may be used to explore the extent of damage following trauma, to diagnose intestinal dysfunction, or to determine the cause of an infection or fever. Exploratory surgery may be performed alone or in conjunction with surgery to repair the problem.

In laparoscopic exploration, a common form of exploratory surgery, two or three small incisions are made, and a surgeon uses a rigid viewing tube (laparoscope) to view the abdomen. This surgery causes minimal tissue damage and generally heals quickly. *See also* LAPAROTOMY, EXPLORATORY.

Expressing Milk

Manually releasing milk from the breast.

Most commonly, milk is expressed for the purpose of putting it into a bottle for later feeding, allowing the nursing mother to combine the benefits of providing her child with breast milk with some of the conveniences associated with bottle-feeding. Breast milk will keep fresh in a refrigerator for a few days, and for up to two weeks in a freezer.

How to Express Milk

First wash hands thoroughly. Position the hand so the thumb is above and the forefinger below the edge of the areola, and then press the fingers together, squeezing gently and rhythmically for about five minutes. The milk is caught in a cup or other clean receptacle. Repeat the procedure twice on each breast, alternating between breasts. Milk can also be expressed with a manual or battery-operated pump.

There are a number of other reasons to express milk, all of which pertain to the mother's or baby's health or comfort:
- The breast is too firm for the baby to easily grasp in his or her mouth.
- The mother's breast is infected—milk from an infected breast can be discarded and nursing can be continued from the other breast until the infection clears up.
- The mother or baby is hospitalized.
- A premature baby cannot yet nurse.
- Nipples are sore or inverted.

Extraction, Dental

Removal of a tooth or teeth.

Extraction is done to treat severely decayed, abscessed, or broken teeth. Crowded, improperly aligned, or impacted teeth are also occasionally treated by removal.

The area around the tooth is anesthetized with a local anesthetic, and the tooth is grasped with dental forceps and slowly rocked loose. Occasionally the tooth is removed in smaller pieces with the aid of a dental drill. Other times the tooth is exposed by moving the gums out of the way and removing some of the surrounding bone. After removal, the extraction site is cleaned and stitched closed. *See also* TOOTH.

Extradural Hemorrhage

Also known as epidural hemorrhage

Uncontrolled bleeding into the space between the inner surface of the skull and the dura mater, the outer layer of the tissue that covers the brain.

Extradural hemorrhage can be caused by a blow to the head that fractures the skull and ruptures blood vessels on the upper side of the dura mater. These vessels bleed profusely, and a pool of blood (hematoma) can rapidly develop, pressing against the brain and causing severe damage.

ALERT

When to See a Doctor

A headache that occurs after a head injury, accompanied by symptoms such as drowsiness, vomiting, and seizures, may indicate an extradural hemorrhage. Any head injury that causes loss of consciousness calls for an examination by a doctor.

The injured person may lose consciousness briefly and then appear normal. Symptoms may not appear for hours or even days. An extradural hemorrhage can be diagnosed by a physical examination and CT scanning of the head. It is treated by craniotomy, surgery in which an opening is made in the skull so that the blood can be drained and also injured blood vessels repaired. *See also* HEAD INJURY *and* HEMATOMA.

Extrapyramidal System

The system of nerve pathways important in controlling voluntary movement.

The extrapyramidal system is a sequence of nerve highways that connect nerves in the cerebrum, the basal ganglia (structures deep within the brain), and the brain stem. These pathways are used to carry and modify electrical impulses sent from the brain to the skeletal muscles.

Injury to any part of the extrapyramidal system can impede voluntary movements and affect muscle tone. It can cause the emergence of involuntary movements such as tremors and spasms, as can be found in Parkinson's disease, Huntington's chorea, and cerebral palsy. Phenothiazine drugs, used to treat psychiatric disorders, can also produce abnormal movement. *See also* ANTIPSYCHOTIC DRUGS; BRAIN; *and* CHOREA.

Exudation

When fluids such as blood, plasma, or lymph fluids ooze or leak out of tissue.

Exudation may occur as a response to any number of injuries or infections. On the skin, trauma by a blow, burn, or infection causes the blood vessels to dilate and increase flow of blood to the area. The area becomes inflamed—reddened and warm to the touch. Dead and dying red and white blood cells accumulate and form a pus-filled pocket of fluid (blister or abscess) or engorge the surrounding tissues. The surface of the skin may become porous, permitting the accumulated fluids to ooze out of the tissue.

Exudation may also occur internally. For example, if the large intestine becomes inflamed or ulcerated, as may occur with tuberculosis or cancer, it can exude mucus, blood, and lymph fluids, producing diarrhea and severe discomfort.

Exudation is also used to refer to the fluid that is emitted from the body through this process. *See also* ABSCESS; BLISTER; BURN; CANCER; *and* TUBERCULOSIS.

Eye

The organ of vision, which captures images and converts them into neural signals, which are sent to the brain to be interpreted.

The eye begins to form in the third week of embryonic growth. Nerve tissue forms a crude lens and cuplike structure, the optic cup, linked to a slender cord, the optic nerve. The inside of the optic cup forms the retina; the outside forms three layers, called tunics, that form the wall of the eyeball. By the fifth month, the lens thickens and clarifies, and the eye's structure becomes more clearly established. Links to the brain grow more complex.

The retina is not completely developed at birth, so newborns cannot focus. Usually the eyes wander until after the first month; then growth accelerates rapidly during the first year. Growth then slows considerably and, after puberty, is negligible.

STRUCTURE

Five muscles attached by ligaments to the outer layer of the eyeball and one muscle attached to its back control movement. Another muscle controls the eyelid.

The Tunics. The outermost layer of the eye consists of the cornea and the sclera, the white of the eyeball. The next layer, the vascular tunic, consists of the pigmented iris; the ciliary body, which forms the fluid that nourishes the eye (aqueous humor); and the choroid, a structure rich in blood vessels that regulates blood flow to the retina. The innermost layer, the nervous tunic, includes the retina and the optic nerve.

The pupil is the dark opening in the middle of the iris. Clear, jellylike vitreous humor fills most of the eyeball behind the eye's exposed features.

The lens is made of clear crystalline proteins and is located immediately behind the pupil. Working with the transparent cornea, it focuses the light rays of an image onto the retina. The lens can change in thickness and curvature in order to adjust where it is focused, in a process called ac-

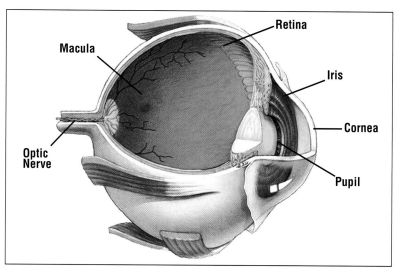

commodation. If the eyeball is of abnormal length or the cornea is abnormally curved, the image on the retina can be blurred; this can be treated with corrective lenses.

The retina consists of cells that are sensitive to light; they are called rod and cone cells based on their shapes. These cells are made of three parts: a light-detecting outer segment (shaped like a rod or cone), an energy-transducing inner segment, and a terminal that relays the visual signal to the next cell in the pathway to the brain.

FUNCTION

Rod and cone cells absorb light and react to it, thus producing signals that can be sent to the brain. Light induces chemical changes in molecules (photopigments) in the outer segments of rods and cones. Rods recognize intensity, rather than the color, of light. Cones contain either red, green, or blue pigment, each of which responds most strongly to a particular color of light. The combination of rod and cone pigments provides the necessary aspects of visual information that can be interpreted by the brain into color vision.

Topics related to the Eye *that are discussed elsewhere include* Blindness; Blurred Vision; Optic Atrophy; Retinal Artery Occlusion; *and* Vision Tests. *Entries related to the anatomy of the eye include* Lens; Optic Nerve; Pupil; Retina; Retinal Detachment; *and* Retinopathy. *Also see the discussions of* Ophthalmology *and* Optometry.

Retina.
Shown above, a diagram of the eye, at the rear of which is the retina which consists of rod and cone cells that are sensitive to light. The eye focuses light rays to form an image on the retina, *(below),* which then converts this image into a pattern of nerve impulses that are transmitted to the brain.

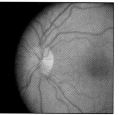

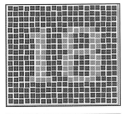

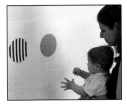

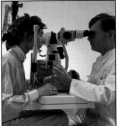

Eye Examinations.
Various tests, above, are used to assess the external and internal condition of the eyes, either as part of a standard vision test or to make a diagnosis. During an eye exam, the physician checks eye movement (middle), visual acuity, visual field (bottom), and color vision (top). Eye exams can determine the cause of vision problems, and determine if a patient may need glasses or contact lenses, or a more radical corrective.

Eye, Artificial

A silicone, plastic, or integrated implant used to maintain normal appearance if an eye is lost.

Some artificial eye implants available today can be attached to the eye muscles, thereby allowing them to move like a normal eye. After the implant is placed, a thin layer of pink tissue, called conjunctiva, is sutured over it so that the implant will not be seen. A prosthesis is then placed over the implant. *See also* PROSTHESIS.

Eye Drops

A medication or diagnostic fluid that is dripped into the eyes.

Liquid drugs that can be squeezed from a dropper into the eye are useful in the treatment or diagnosis of eye disorders. The lower lid is gently pulled away from the surface of the eye; the dropper does not touch the eye or eyelid, to avoid contamination. Antibiotics, antihistamines, and glaucoma drugs can be administered as eye drops, as can examination aids that dilate or constrict the pupil. *See also* EYE.

Eye, Examination of

Inspection and testing of the eyes to check vision, diagnose eye disorders, and evaluate treatment.

Examination of the eyes is performed by an ophthalmologist or optometrist. An ophthalmologist specializes in disorders of the eye, while an optometrist specializes in correcting vision through eyeglasses, contact lenses, and other nonsurgical means.

VISION TESTS
The doctor usually begins by evaluating visual acuity. With each eye, the patient examines an eye chart (a Snellen chart) from a distance of 20 feet, reading the smallest line of letters he or she is able to. With normal vision, the subject should be able to read letters that are 3/8 inch high from 20 feet away (20/20 vision). After eyesight is

Presbyopia

As the lens of the eye loses some of its elasticity and ability to bring close objects into sharp focus, eye strain or fatigue may result while viewing close objects, particularly while reading. This condition is known as presbyopia, and some degree of it is common with age. Glasses or contact lenses generally correct the condition, and reading and doing other close work under proper lighting can limit fatigue.

tested at a distance, the physician tests near visual acuity by using a test card held close to the eyes. These tests can readily diagnose nearsightedness, farsightedness, astigmatism, and age-related inability to focus on objects, known as presbyopia.

Central and peripheral vision are checked through a visual field test. The patient tracks a moving object with the eyes. Distortions in central or peripheral vision can sometimes indicate a disorder, such as glaucoma, retinitis pigmentosa, or a tumor.

PHYSICAL EXAMINATION
The external features of the eyes, including the rims of the orbits, eyelids, lashes, and tear ducts, are examined for irregularities. The movement of the eyes (ocular motility) is checked, and pupils are examined to check for proper shape, size, and response time to changes in light.

The eye may be examined microscopically with a device known as a slit lamp, which may be used to diagnose infection or inflammation within the eye, corneal disorders, and cataracts. Other instruments that may be used include a tonometer, which is designed to measure fluid pressure within the globe of the eye, and an ophthalmoscope, which enables a physician to see the back of the eye through the pupil to the retina, blood vessels, and optic nerve. These tests assess the health and strength of the eyes and may assist in diagnosing disorders, particularly some neurological disorders with symptoms that manifest through irregular appearance or movement of the eyes.

There is an important discussion of EYE EXAMINATIONS *under* EYE. *Other related discussions include* BLINDNESS; EYE, FOREIGN BODY IN; EYE INJURIES; *and* OPTIC NERVE.

Eye, Foreign Body in

An object that is touching or has entered the eye.

Any foreign object that has entered the eye can cause tearing, blurred vision, light sensitivity, or swelling of the eyelid. The white of the eye can become red and irritated. The object may scratch the eyeball's transparent tissue (cornea). Scratched eyes may become infected by bacteria.

WASHING THE EYE

Sometimes the eye's own tears are enough to wash away the object. If they do not, the eye should be flushed with clear water or saline solution for fifteen minutes. Contact lenses should be left in place. The head should be held to one side, and the eyelids held open, although the eye itself must not be touched. If both eyes are involved, the person may wish to use a shower, holding the face up to the shower head and allowing a gentle flow of water into the eyes. Alternatively, the person may immerse his or her head in a large bowl of water until the eyes are covered. The eyes should remain open—blinking repeatedly may scratch the cornea.

REMOVING OBJECTS

Sometimes a foreign body can be removed. If the object is visible, it may be possible to remove it with a cotton swab or the corner of a clean cloth. However, too much pressure may cause the object to become more deeply embedded. **Removal of a foreign body should not be attempted if it is on the cornea. Never attempt to remove an object that is embedded in the eye.**

If the object cannot be removed easily, the entire eye should be covered with a light bandage, and medical attention should be sought. The doctor will examine the eye with a microscope and remove the object with a tweezer, needle, or other instrument. An antibiotic ointment will be applied to fight infection, and drops will be put into the eye to relax the muscle. An eye patch may be put in place to protect the eye from further injury and to keep the eyelid

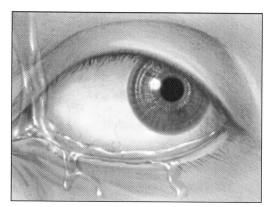

Foreign Body in the Eye.
When a foreign body irritates the eye, it generally causes pain, redness, tearing, and blepharospasm (uncontrollable eyelid contractions). Left, washing out a speck from the lower eyelid.

closed while it heals. If an object has penetrated the eye, it must be removed by an ophthalmologist.

Occasionally a small irritation, known as a stye, may swell into a bump on the inner surface of the eyelid; this may feel like a foreign object. The doctor will roll the eyelid over a thin stick to examine the inner surface of the eyelid to see if a stye is responsible. An antibiotic ointment and rest, with an eye patch in place, usually eliminates this irritation. *See also* EYE INJURIES *and* STYE. *See* EAR, FOREIGN BODY IN *for an example of removing a foreign object from another orifice.*

Eye Injuries

Trauma to the eye, including foreign objects in the eye, chemical damage, and burns.

Injuries to the eye are almost always accompanied by pain or intense itching; some may impair vision. Bleeding, redness, or fluid discharge may occur. The person may become extremely sensitive to light and develop a headache. The pupils of the eye may appear to be different sizes.

Trauma. All trauma to the eye should receive treatment from trained medical personnel. Both eyes should be lightly covered until medical treatment occurs. Pressure should never be applied to the eye, and the victim should not rub the injured area. An object that has penetrated the eye should not be removed. Contact lenses should not be removed unless medical assistance is delayed.

Chemical Burns. If the eye has come into contact with chemicals, it should be flushed as quickly as possible with large amounts (at least three to five quarts) of saline solution or clean water. If a household chemical is involved, the label should contain emergency instructions. If no instructions are available, water should be used. Contact lenses should be removed after rinsing.

Burns. Eye burns may result from fireworks, gas explosions, or even sunlight or sunlamps. If the skin around the face has peeled or blistered, and sunglasses designed to filter out ultraviolet radiation have not been used, the eyes have probably been damaged. A cool compress gently placed over both eyes may reduce pain. Emergency medical help should be contacted.

Abrasions. A scratch on the cornea may come from a foreign object in the eye or from rubbing the eye with a finger or fingernail. Contact lenses that trap an object under them or lenses that fit poorly and have been worn for too long may also damage the eye. The eye should be kept closed and should not be rubbed. Because all corneal abrasions carry the risk of deeper injury and infection, they should be examined by a medical professional.

Black Eye. With a black eye, purple bruising appears around the eye and on the eyelid from burst blood vessels. There may be swelling of the eyelid. Over time, the color changes to yellow and green. This is essentially an external injury, though frequently the eye itself is also injured. Cool compresses applied gently but immediately will reduce pain and swelling. Normally, a black eye will not require a doctor's attention unless there is continued pain, double vision, or light sensitivity, or if the discoloration does not subside in a few days.

> EYE INJURIES *and related issues are also discussed in* BLACK EYE; BLINDNESS; BLURRED VISION; BURNS; OPTIC ATROPHY; RETINAL ARTERY OCCLUSION; *and* TRAUMA. *Anatomical topics that relate to* EYE INJURIES *are included in* EYE; LENS; OPTIC NERVE; PUPIL; *and* RETINA. *Also refer to* COMPRESS; CORNEA; *and* EYE, FOREIGN BODY IN.

Eye Tumors

> Benign and malignant growths arising in the eye.

Eye tumors are rare. The great majority are painless but malignant.

TYPES

Malignant Melanoma. The most common eye tumor is malignant melanoma, a form of skin cancer that arises in the choroid, the layer of tissue between the sclera and the retina. Malignant melanoma of the eye generally occurs later in life; excessive exposure to sunlight may be a risk factor. As it grows, the cancer can cause the retina to become detached, inhibiting vision.

Basal Cell Carcinoma. Another malignant eye tumor is basal cell carcinoma, which originates in the eyelid. The risk of this cancer is increased by prolonged exposure to sunlight. It does not usually spread outside the eye.

Retinoblastoma arises in the retina and is seen early in life; a tendency toward developing retinoblastoma may be inherited. The tumor can affect one or both eyes and can interfere with vision, causing a child to squint or have crossed eyes.

SYMPTOMS

Often, eye tumors do not show any symptoms in early stages. Over time, vision may be gradually lost, and the eyes may bulge. In some cases a tumor may be visible on the eyelid or through the pupil of the eye.

TREATMENT

Small tumors of the eye can be removed by freezing (cryosurgery), laser treatment, or radiation. If the cancer is large or has spread, removal of the entire eye is often necessary to prevent the cancer from spreading to the brain and elsewhere.

> *Background information about* TUMORS *can be found in* BENIGN; CANCER; GERM CELL TUMOR; MALIGNANT; MELANOMA; RETINOBLASTOMA; TROPHOBLASTIC TUMOR; TUMOR; *and* TUMOR-SPECIFIC ANTIGEN. *Articles about the* EYE *include* LENS; OPTIC NERVE; PUPIL; *and* RETINA. *See also* BLINDNESS; BLURRED VISION; *and* OPTIC ATROPHY *for related details.*

Eyelash Disorders

Abnormal growth or development of the eyelashes.

Two rows of eyelashes, curving outward, line each lid. Eyelashes contain sensitive nerve endings that trigger blinking, which protects the eye from foreign bodies.

Trichiasis. Injury or infection can cause eyelashes to grow inward, a condition known as trichiasis. This irritates the eyeball and can damage the cornea. The eyelashes grow back if removed unless the follicle is destroyed by electrolysis, freezing, or—through a recent, unperfected procedure—a laser. *See also* TRICHIASIS.

Blepharitis, a mild chronic eyelid inflammation, can destroy lash roots. Loss of many eyelashes can increase vulnerability to foreign bodies and infection. Mild soap and topical antibiotics can prevent or treat the infection. *See also* BLEPHARITIS.

Pediculosis and phthiriasis are licelike infestations that may deposit visible reddish-brown feces around the eyelashes, causing blepharitis and conjunctivitis. Symptoms include lashes bound by a moist crust, itching, and irritation. They may be treated with a medicated shampoo. *See also* PEDICULOSIS *and* PHTHIRIASIS.

Entropion, in which an eyelid becomes lax and forces the lashes against the cornea, can cause scratching and infection. Treatment involves manipulating the eyelid and lashes away from the cornea, lubricating the eye, and using antibiotics. *See also* ENTROPION.

Stye. Infection near the eyelashes can cause a stye, a pus-filled abscess that causes irritation and may impair vision. Warm compresses encourage pus drainage, and antibiotics prevent recurrence. *See* STYE.

Alopecia Areata. There is a very slight chance that several eyelashes disappearing and not growing back may be a sign of alopecia areata, a progressive autoimmune skin disease in which white blood cells mistakenly destroy hair follicles. It can result in total body hair loss. Treatments achieve modest success only in mild cases by restimulating hair growth. *See also* ALOPECIA.

Eyelid

The protective layer of skin that can cover the eye.

The eyelid is made of the tarsal plate, a thin fibrous tissue covered with thin skin, which secretes and spreads the oily element of tears that keeps the eyes from drying and the eyelids from sticking together. Ligaments attached to the eye sockets control eyelid muscles. The larger, upper eyelid is more mobile because its muscle is larger. The eyelids blink reflexively every three to seven seconds, pushing back the eyeball each time to protect it. Eyelashes line each eyelid and contain highly sensitive nerve endings; by sensing incoming objects, including air gusts, these nerves trigger the eyelids to close, protecting the eye. *See also* EYE *and* LACRIMAL APPARATUS.

Eyestrain

Aching or discomfort in the eyes.

While not a medical term, eyestrain is often used by the general population to refer to strain, aching, throbbing, fatigue, dryness, or other eye discomfort associated with intense or extended use of the eyes in a particular task. There are a number of measures that can be taken to reduce eyestrain, including using proper lighting, taking frequent breaks, wearing corrective lenses, using tinted computer screens and various color backgrounds, and placing monitors by windows (to rest the eyes periodically by exercising far sight). While such measures may bring positive results and are generally healthy working habits, doctors do not believe the eyes can become damaged from use. *See* ACCOMODATION *and* EYE.

Resources on Vision and the Eyes
Brown, Evan L,. and Kenneth Deffenbacher, *Perception and the Senses* (1979); Peninsula Center for the Blind, *The First Steps: How to Help People Who are Losing Their Sight* (1982); Schmidt, Robert F., *Fundamentals of Sensory Physiology* (1986); Wolf, K.P., *Eyewise: Eye Disorders and Their Treatment* (1982); American Foundation for the Blind, Tel. (800) 232-5463 (AFB-LINE), Online: www.afb.-org; National Fed. of the Blind, Tel., (410) 659-9314, Online: www.nfb.org; Prevent Blindness America, Tel. (800) 331-2020, Online: www.pba.org.

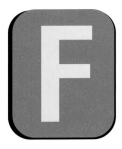

Face-Lift

Also known as rhytidectomy

A type of cosmetic surgery performed to tighten and smooth out the skin of the face.

As a natural part of the aging process, the skin develops wrinkles, hangs more loosely, and develops fat deposits. A face-lift is a way to surgically remove these characteristics and make the face appear younger.

PROCEDURE

A face-lift is usually performed as an outpatient procedure, with sedation and a local anesthetic. The surgery lasts two to four hours. The plastic surgeon makes incisions around the face's perimeter, behind hairlines, along natural creases where possible, and around the ears. Excess facial fat is removed, muscles tightened, and excess skin is removed. The incisions are closed using fine sutures, and the face is bandaged.

A facelift may be performed at the same time as eyelid surgery (blepharoplasty) or nose reshaping (rhinoplasty).

RECOVERY

After surgery, the face is bruised and swollen. The stitches are removed after a week, and it takes another one to two weeks for the bruising and swelling to heal. The scars tend to be hidden in the hairline and the face's natural creases, and they fade over time. The effects of the face-lift may last five to ten years.

Complications are rare. The most common complication is the pooling of blood under the skin (hematoma), which requires draining and may result in scarring.

ALTERNATIVES

Cosmetic surgery alternatives to face-lifts include carbon dioxide laser resurfacing, chemical peels, collagen injections, forehead lifts, and wrinkle injections.

> **For further information related to this topic see** COSMETIC DENTISTRY; COSMETIC SURGERY; ELECTIVE SURGERY; HAIR TRANSPLANT; PLASTIC SURGERY; *and* SURGERY. *Articles about related subjects include* LIPOSUCTION *and* RHINOPLASTY.

Resources on Facial and Cosmetic Surgery

Converse, J.M., *Reconstructive Plastic Surgery* (1977); Engler, Alan, *Body Sculpture: Plastic Surgery of the Body for Men and Women* (2000); Grazer, F.M. and J.R. Klingbeil, *Body Image: A Surgical Perspective* (1980); Henry, Kimberly A., et al., *The Plastic Surgery Sourcebook: Everything You Need to Know* (1999); Rudolph, Ross, et al., *Skin Grafting* (1979); American Society of Plastic Surgeons, Tel. (888) 475-2784, Online: www.plasticsurgery.org; American Society for Aesthetic Plastic Surgery, Tel. (800) 364-2147, Online: surgery.org; www.nycornell.org/ent/.

Facial Pain

A feeling of discomfort in part or all of the face.

Facial pain may be a result of actual injury to the face, teething in a baby, wisdom tooth eruption in an adult, or partial dislocation of the jaw. Less commonly, facial pain may originate from another point in the body (referred pain) or may arise for no apparent reason.

Infection. Commonly, inflammation of the nasal passages (sinusitis) can cause acute pain near the eye sockets and in the cheekbones. An infected toothache or abscess can cause pain that spreads to the face, as can a boil or other inflammation in the nose or ear.

Nerve Damage. Damage to the nerves of the face can cause pain, which sometimes occurs on one side of the face (trigeminal neuralgia) and may also involve facial tics (tic doloreaux). Facial palsy, or Bell's palsy, is a disorder in which the main facial nerve becomes damaged, causing weakness of the face. Shingles (herpes zoster) may also damage the main facial nerve, causing pain and blistering.

Cardiac Causes. If face pain occurs with chest, shoulder, neck, or arm pain, it may indicate a heart attack. Emergency medical help should be sought immediately.

Treatment. Analgesics can be prescribed for temporary pain relief. In general, the underlying cause should be diagnosed and treated. *See also* ABSCESS; FACIAL PALSY; HEART ATTACK; SHINGLES; SINUS INFECTION; TIC DOLOREAUX; *and* TRIGEMINAL NEURALGIA.

Facial Palsy

Also known as Bell's palsy

A nerve disorder that produces weakness and possibly paralysis on one side of the face.

There are two facial nerves that are positioned at each side of the skull. If a facial nerve becomes inflamed, it can cause pain, weakness, or paralysis on the affected side of the face. It is unknown why the nerve becomes inflamed or why only one of the two nerves is usually affected.

Symptoms. The main symptom of facial palsy is weakness on one side of the face. The eyelid and the mouth may sag, and it becomes difficult to frown, smile, or close the eye. There may be pain around the ear. The taste buds may be damaged, and noise can appear louder than it is.

Treatment. Facial palsy is not dangerous and can occur at any age; the condition is usually temporary. No specific treatment has been proven effective. Treatment with corticosteroids or a pituitary gland hormone, corticotropin, all of which reduce inflammation, may speed recovery. If the patient is unable to close the eye, it must be protected from excessive dryness with lubricating eye drops and an eye patch. If paralysis continues for at least a year, a healthy nerve can be grafted to the facial muscle. *See also* ANTI-INFLAMMATORY DRUGS; FACIAL PAIN; NERVE INJURY; *and* PALSY.

Facial Spasm

Also known as facial tic

Involuntary twitching of the facial muscles.

In adults, facial spasm is a rare condition in which the muscles that are supplied by the facial nerve jerk or twitch. It occurs close to the eye and affects only one side of the face. Research suggests that the facial nerve is irritated by an artery migrating into a position that causes pulsating blood to repeatedly strike the nerve. The nerve then sends signals to cause the muscles on one side of the face to contract. Facial spasm appears mainly in middle-aged women.

In children, transient facial tics are fairly common and may be caused by head injuries, stimulant drugs, or stress. They range from simple grimacing to complex vocalizations. In most cases, the child grows out of the tic and requires no treatment.

Treatment. In adults, injections of botulinum toxin can control facial spasms 90 percent of the time. The injection may need to be repeated after three months. In acute cases, a neurosurgeon may correct the condition by surgically moving the offending artery away from the facial nerve. *See also* SPASM; STIMULANT DRUGS; *and* TIC.

Fahrenheit Scale

A temperature scale in which the freezing point of water is set at 32 degrees and its boiling point at 212 degrees.

Body temperature, generally measured with a thermometer, is usually given in the Fahrenheit scale. Normal body temperature hovers around 98.6°F. While most thermometers used to measure body temperature are calibrated in the Fahrenheit scale, the Celsius, or centigrade, scale is also sometimes encountered. Normal body temperature in the Celsius scale is 37°C. Body temperature above or below normal is a diagnostic indicator of illness.

To convert from Celsius to Fahrenheit, multiply by 9/5 and add 32. To convert from Fahrenheit to Celsius, subtract 32 and multiply by 5/9. *See also* CELSIUS SCALE; FEVER; TEMPERATURE; *and* THERMOMETER.

Failure to Thrive

Term used when an infant or child does not gain weight or grow in height at a normal rate.

Failure to thrive occurs when a child does not get enough nutrients or is too sick to digest food. In infants, this is usually due to problems with breast feeding or difficulties digesting formula. Lack of adequate nutrition may result from insufficient caloric intake, gastrointestinal disease, malabsorption, birth defects, or endocrine problems.

Malabsorption disorders can prevent growth, because digested food cannot be absorbed by the small intestine. Enzymes may be missing, either through heredity or disease. The cells may be impaired by disease that affect the tissue, permitting extra bacterial growth or blocking the normal passageways. If much of the small intestine has been surgically removed, malabsorption may occur, usually because there is not enough intestinal surface left.

Another cause of failure to thrive is lack of emotional nourishment. If an infant is neglected, abused, or does not have a close relationship with a concerned and loving parent, the infant may become depressed,

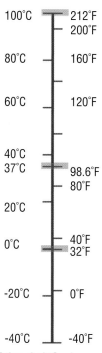

Fahrenheit Scale. Above, the Fahrenheit scale is a temperature scale named for the German Physicist Gabriel Fahrenheit. On this scale normal body temperature is 98.6°F and the boiling point of water is 212°F. To convert Fahrenheit to Celsius, subtract 32 and then multiply by 0.56 (or 5/9).

causing a loss of appetite and listlessness. Sometimes the mother may simply be inexperienced in feeding a baby and needs to attend classes in newborn care. Families that neg-lect children because of a drug or alcohol problem should seek counseling and treatment for those addictions.

DIAGNOSIS

If failure to thrive is suspected, there are several tests that may be performed to find the cause. A complete blood count (CBC) will be performed to detect anemia. A urinalysis may also detect problems. The doctor may perform thyroid function tests and other hormonal studies. Hemoglobin electrophoresis can determine conditions such as sickle cell disease.

Background information about this topic can be found in BIRTH DEFECT; BOTTLE FEEDING; BREAST FEEDING; NUTRITION; *and* HORMONES. *Related topics include* ALCOHOL DEPENDENCE; DEVELOPMENTAL DELAY; *and* PREGNANCY, DRUGS IN.

Fainting

Temporary loss of consciousness due to a lack of oxygen in the brain.

Weakness, nausea, or dizziness may precede fainting. The vagus nerve regulates breathing and circulation; in a vasovagal attack, fear, stress, or pain may overstimulate the vasovagal nerve and cause fainting. Sitting for long periods and suddenly standing causes blood to collect in leg veins, depriving the heart of blood to send to the brain and possibly resulting in fainting. When bloodflow through the neck and brain is obstructed, this may cause fainting, preceded by difficulty speaking or weakness in the limbs. Stokes-Adams syndrome, in which the heartbeat is irregular, may also be a cause.

After fainting, a person should lie down for up to fifteen minutes. If a person feels lightheaded, sitting can prevent fainting. Recurrent fainting or a delay in regaining consciousness demands immediate medical attention. *See* LOSS OF CONSCIOUSNESS.

Falls, Preventing

Accidents are the sixth leading cause of death in the United States; among those over 65, falls are the leading cause of injury-related deaths. One-quarter to one-third of all people over 65 fall each year. Up to a third of those falls result in broken hips or other fractures; bruises and head injuries are also common. Of the more than 200,000 older adults who fracture a hip, nearly a third die withing a short period, and fewer than half regain full mobility, with many requiring long-term care.

CAUSES

Many conditions can lead to an increased incidence of falls, particularly in the elderly. Vision often degenerates with age, resulting in a lessened ability to judge distances or see small objects that may cause an individual to trip. A number of prescription drugs, including tranquilizers and antidepressants, may cause dizziness or drowsiness. Some medical conditions, such as heart disorders, lung disorders, and arthritis, may also lead to a greater likelihood of falling.

Many causes of falls are less directly age-

Preventing Falls at Home

Several adjustments in the home can lower the risk of falling:
- Provide adequate lighting.
- Avoid clutter on the floor or electric wires running across high traffic areas. Use a cordless phone or several phones to avoid long phone cords.
- Do not use loose area rugs. Place non-slip mats under rugs. Repair frayed carpet edges.
- Clean up spills.
- Install grab bars in the bathroom and kitchen.
- Install seats in shower stalls or bathtubs.
- Store objects in easy reach, so that a person does not need to stand on a ladder or chair.
- Buy long-life bulbs to limit the number of times they need to be changed. If possible, another person should install new light bulbs.
- Avoid staircases if possible; a younger person can offer support when climbing stairs. Install handrails for additional support.
- Consider an alarm system that will call for aid from family or a service in times of emergency.

---

related. Alcohol consumption can impair balance and coordination. Diseases such as Parkinson's, dementia, stroke, and general muscle weakness may also increase the chances of falling.

Prevention. Quick reflexes and strong muscles are the best defense against falling. Regular exercise can help maintain muscle tone, and frequent social interactions and mental activities can sustain alertness. Reducing activity due to fear of falling is not an effective preventive measure; less activity leads to decreased fitness and thus can actually increase the chances of falling. A balanced diet, especially one that includes adequate calcium and vitamin D to enhance bone strength, may also help prevent accidents. *See also* AGING; GERONTOLOGY; *and* INJURIES.

Familial Mediterranean Fever

Also known as periodic fever

An inherited disease characterized by periodic attacks of fever accompanied by inflammation of the membranes of the abdomen and lungs.

Familial Mediterranean fever occurs mainly in people of Sephardic Jewish, Armenian, and Arabic descent. It is usually an inherited illness, although no family history can be found in up to half of all cases.

People with familial Mediterranean fever may also have arthritis, skin lesions, or amyloidosis, a disorder characterized by the accumulation of a starch-like substance in different parts of the body.

Symptoms usually begin between age five and 15, although they may start later in life. The duration and frequency of attacks have no set pattern. A fever usually lasts 24 to 48 hours, but some may last for as long as 10 days. Attacks tend to occur every few weeks but may be as infrequent as once or twice a year. Severity may decrease with age.

There is no specific treatment; the drug colchicine, which is used to treat gout and amyloidosis, has been found to reduce the incidence of attacks. *See also* AMYLOIDOSIS; ARTHRITIS; FEVER; PERITONITIS; *and* PLEURISY.

Family Planning

The attempt to control the number and spacing of children within a family.

Family planning usually involves the use of contraception to temporarily avoid pregnancy or the use of surgical sterilization as a permanent solution. Contraception options include barrier methods, such as the use of condoms; hormonal methods, such as the use of a birth control pill or implant; and natural methods.

In natural family planning, a couple tracks the woman's body temperature or cervical mucus to determine when in the month she is ovulating and likely to conceive; the couple then abstains from intercourse during that time. If done carefully, natural family planning methods may have a very high success rate; however, they and hormonal methods of contraception provide no protection against sexually transmitted disease and should be used only by long-term monogamous couples.

Surgical sterilization procedures involve severing the fallopian tubes in a woman or the vas deferens in a man.

Although not intended for such a purpose, abortion can be used to end an unwanted pregnancy. *See also* CONTRACEPTION.

Family Practitioner

Also known as general practitioner or family physician

A physician who provides basic, ongoing care for individuals and families.

Family practitioners provide continuing and comprehensive medical care for individuals and families. They frequently serve as the first point of contact for an individual in need of medical care.

Family medicine is a specialty that integrates biological, clinical, and behavioral science. Within the medical realm, family practitioners must possess knowledge of all organ systems. They must be able to diagnose a range of conditions and refer patients to appropriate specialists. Family practitioners also serve as the primary health advocate for patients. *See also* DOCTOR.

Family Therapy

A form of therapy in which two or more members of a family attend psychotherapy together.

Family therapy is usually employed to address problems of children and adolescents; it may be combined with individual therapy. The underlying idea of family therapy is that the family unit has a powerful impact on the individual child and that a child's problems will improve not just through individual insight but through an improved family situation.

Problems within the family, including sibling rivalry, marital discord, and parenting problems, can present themselves in the context of the family's interaction in the course of therapy. The therapist addresses the issues that come up in the group, attempting to define the behavior patterns and help establish more appropriate, supportive interactions between family members. The therapist offers alternatives to detrimental behavior, including teaching communication skills, such as active listening, and discouraging verbally abusive communication.

Family therapy can help with individual problems such as depression, anxiety, behavioral disorders, and eating disorders. It may also be a vital part of treatment for child abuse and substance abuse.

PARTICIPATION

As many members of the family as possible should participate in the therapy. The success of family therapy is limited when one or more members of the family choose not to be involved or do not cooperate with therapy. An unwilling family member may miss appointments, fail to attend a session, or not participate. When this occurs, it may be possible to continue therapy with the remaining members of the family.

FAMILY THERAPY *receives further discussion in relation to such topics as* BEHAVIOR THERAPY; COGNITIVE-BEHAVIORAL THERAPY; INSIGHT PSYCHOTHERAPY; PLAY THERAPY; PSYCHIATRY; *and* PSYCHOANALYSIS. *See also the relevant articles on* CHILD ABUSE *and* SUBSTANCE ABUSE.

Fanconi's Syndrome

A kidney disorder in which important body chemicals such as amino acids are excreted in the urine.

Fanconi's syndrome is a rare disorder of the kidneys that can occur as the result of a birth defect or as a consequence of a number of inherited conditions. In some cases there is no identifiable cause.

In Fanconi's syndrome, certain nutrients that are imperative to the body's overall functioning are not absorbed or circulated through the body but are instead passed in the urine. These nutrients may include amino acids, phosphates, potassium, and calcium. The result is stunted growth, an overall feeling of illness, failure to thrive, and the development of some bone disorders.

In some cases, a specific abnormality of body chemistry can be identified and treated. Some patients can benefit from a kidney transplant. But often the underlying condition cannot be treated, and kidney function deteriorates progressively, resulting in death early in life. *See* AMINO ACIDS; CALCIUM; FAILURE TO THRIVE; KIDNEY TRANSPLANT; PHOSPHATES; *and* POTASSIUM.

Farmer's Lung

A lung condition caused by allergic hypersensitivity to a plant fungus or mold.

Farmer's lung is an occupational form of allergic alveolitis, an inflammation of the minute air sacs in the lungs. It occurs when an individual working or living on a farm inhales mold or fungi growing on grain stored under damp conditions. The resulting symptoms include shortness of breath, fever, headache, and muscle pains resembling those of influenza. A single exposure for a person allergic to the mold or fungus can cause an attack lasting as long as two days. Chronic exposure for a sensitive individual can result in permanent lung damage.

Diagnosis. Farmer's lung is diagnosed by first determining whether the patient has been exposed to mold or fungi found on farms, followed by a physical examination that can include a chest x-ray and a blood test to detect particular infection-fighting cells (antibodies) that act against the agent causing the symptoms.

Treatment. Corticosteroid drugs can be prescribed to relieve the symptoms, but the best measures are preventive, notably keeping grain and hay dry during storage and keeping storage areas well ventilated. Persons prone to farmer's lung can wear protective masks to limit exposure to molds and fungi. Prognosis is good if exposure can be limited. *See also* ALVEOLITIS.

Fascia

Band of connective tissue that supports and binds together many structures in the body.

The superficial fascia surrounds the entire body (except the face) as part of the tissue directly underneath the skin. Thicker tissues in the palm of the hand and sole of the foot serve to cushion the bones beneath.

The deep fascia covers muscles within the body that are separated and divided into different groups. The deep fascia also supports the soft organs of the body, such as the liver, kidneys, and stomach.

Fasciotomy

Surgery used to detach or cut a segment of connective tissues (fascia) surrounding a muscle or group of muscles in order to relieve pressure.

A fasciotomy is generally performed when trauma has caused a muscle to greatly swell, as in crush syndrome, or when a muscle is constricted by surrounding tissues. In a fasciotomy, some fascia around the affected muscle are surgically severed, allowing it to bulge through and thus relieve pressure. Fasciotomies are often performed to correct alignment problems of the foot, such as heel spur syndrome and planar fasciitis. A related treatment for carpal tunnel syndrome involves cutting the fascia in the wrist to relieve pressure on the median nerve. *See also* CARPAL TUNNEL SYNDROME; CRUSH SYNDROME; FASCIA; *and* PODIATRY.

Fasting

Eating no food or severely limiting the diet for a period of time.

In the course of modern living, people are exposed to a number of sources of toxins, such as pollutants in the air and water and pesticides in food. According to supporters of fasting, these substances accumulate in the body and lead to ailments such as fatigue, depression, skin problems, arthritis, and problems with digestion; fasting allows the body to eliminate accumulated toxins, or detoxify, more efficiently.

Types. In a water fast, a person consumes only water for two or three days. In a juice fast, only freshly made vegetable and fruit juices are consumed for a similar time period. Some detoxification therapists may supervise a longer fast.

Procedure. The day before a fast, a person eats lightly and has a final meal of fresh, raw vegetables or fruits. During the fast, a person should allow time for plenty of rest and should not engage in overly strenuous activities. Mild exercise, such as walking, may be recommended. Afterwards, food is reintroduced slowly. Processed foods, refined sugars, alcohol, and caffeine should be avoided.

Benefits of fasting are supported by anecdotal evidence but are not clinically proven. They are claimed to include anything from greater energy and overall well-being to the alleviation of ailments such as arthritis and irritable bowel syndrome.

Precautions. Infrequent, brief fasts are generally safe for people in good health, but prolonged or repeated fasting may lead to a deficiency in necessary nutrients and thus cause illness. People who should not fast include diabetics, pregnant women, children, and people who are malnourished or otherwise ill.

As with many complementary therapies, fasting should not be pursued to the exclusion of conventional treatment, because this may cause a treatable illness to remain undiagnosed and untreated. *See also* ALTERNATIVE MEDICINE; DETOXIFICATION; *and* JUICING.

Fats and Oils

Organic compounds found in many foods; the most concentrated source of food energy.

Fats and oils used in the diet vary greatly in their effects on health. Fat and oils can be saturated, polyunsaturated, or monounsaturated, which is is marked by the structure of the molecules and often by their form (liquid or solid) at room temperature. Although fats have been much maligned, they are in moderation essential to the diet in several ways. They are necessary for the absorption of the fat-soluble vitamins A, D, E, and K. Individuals on extremely low-fat diets may suffer from a deficiency of these vitamins. Fats also provide essential fatty acids, required for many of the body's chemical and hormonal processes.

The caloric values of oils and fats do not differ significantly according to the degree of saturation—all fats contain nine calories per gram. Twenty to thirty percent of daily caloric intake should consist of fats, but saturated fats should not exceed 10 percent.

TYPES OF FAT

Saturated fats are generally solid at room temperature; they can be found in animal fats and butter, as well as plant sources, such as coconut oil, cocoa butter, and palm oil. Saturated fats raise the blood cholesterol level; too much cholesterol can clog the arteries, leading to heart disease.

Hydrogenation

A polyunsaturated fat that is normally liquid or soft may be converted into a harder, more saturated fat by the process of hydrogenation. Hydrogenation also tends to change the shape of the fatty acid molecule from a folded shape (cis) to an extended (trans) shape. These fatty acids may make up between five and 35 percent of a product like margarine. Trans fatty acids often behave like saturated fats, raising low-density lipoprotein (LDL) levels and lowering high-density lipoprotein (HDL) levels. While LDL contributes to an accumulation of cholesterol, HDL aids in eliminating cholesterol. As a result, hydrogenated fats should be consumed cautiously by anyone on a cholesterol-lowering diet.

Unsaturated fats are usually liquid at room temperature. They can be found in olive, canola (rapeseed), sunflower, safflower, and soybean oils. In general, plant oils are higher in polyunsaturated fats than animal fats, with the exception of coconut oil, palm oil, and cocoa butter, which are among the most saturated of all fats. Conversely, cod liver oil and other fats found in fish have high levels of unsaturated fats. Olive and canola oils especially contain high levels of monounsaturated fats and low levels of polyunsaturated fats and thus help lower blood cholesterol. However, these oils are still high in calories and should be consumed in limited quantities, particularly by those on low-fat diets.

Fats, oils, and other related substances are also brought up in GLYCEROL; LIPID DISORDERS; LIPID-LOWERING DRUGS; LIPIDS; *and* FATTY ACIDS. *Other important subjects to keep in mind include* DIET AND DISEASE *and* NUTRITION.

Fatty Acids

Primary component of fat; pivotal in chemical processes and tissue formation in the body.

Fatty acids are one of the primary components of fats; they are either acquired in the diet or created in the body. In addition to being useful in various chemical functions throughout the body, fatty acids are critical in brain development and functioning. Several fatty acids, such as linoleic acid, linolenic acid, and arachidonic acid, are essential to the diet, although isolated deficiencies are rarely seen in healthy adults.

Fats are composed of an alcohol molecule (glycerol) and one to three fatty acids. The structure of the fatty acid determines whether a fat is saturated, monounsaturated, or polyunsaturated. During digestion, glycerol can be detached from the fatty acids and burned for quick energy, similar to the way sugar (glucose) is used.

FATTY ACIDS SHOULD be discussed in GLYCEROL; LIPID-LOWERING DRUGS; LIPIDS; *as well as* FATS AND OILS *because they affect the* BRAIN; INTESTINES; KIDNEY; *and* LIVER. *Also see* DIET AND DISEASE *and* NUTRITION.

Fecal Impaction

A hardened mass of feces that cannot be eliminated by a normal bowel movement.

Fecal impaction can occur after a long period of constipation. It is most common in young children who postpone bowel movements and in older people, especially those who are bedridden and have fiber-poor diets. The main symptoms are an intense desire to have a bowel movement and pain in the anus, rectum, and the center of the abdomen. An enema can correct the problem, although manual removal is sometimes necessary. Preventive measures include a high-fiber diet, drinking a lot of water, and having regular bowel movements. *See also* ENEMA *and* FECES, ABNORMAL.

Feces

Also known as stool

Waste material that is the end product of the digestive process and is discharged through the anus.

Feces consist of water; the undigested residue of food, notably dietary fiber; dead cells from the lining of the intestinal tract (epithelium); waste material from the blood; mucus and other secretions from the intestine; bile from the liver; and bacteria, which can represent up to half the total weight. Bile causes feces to appear brown. Physicians often examine the color, consistency, and odor of feces, as well as the possible presence of bacteria, blood, pus, or other abnormal contents, which are important factors in the diagnosis of intestinal disorders. *See also* FECES, ABNORMAL.

Feces, Abnormal

Feces whose content, color, consistency, or odor are out of the ordinary.

CAUSES
Bleeding in the gastrointestinal tract can result in blackened or bloody feces; darkened feces may also result from a large intake of iron. Bloody or darkened feces could be a sign of cancer or diseases such as

ulcerative colitis and should be brought to the attention of a doctor. Unusually light-colored feces can be the result of a disease such as celiac sprue, which reduces the absorption of fats in the intestinal tract. Ulcerative colitis and other intestinal disorders, as well as an infection such as gastroenteritis, may change the consistency of feces, causing them to be very loose and liquefied. Diarrhea is an obvious cause of loose, liquid feces and can also cause them to be abnormally light in color. Constipation can result in unusually hard feces and fewer than normal bowel movements.

DIAGNOSIS
A number of tests can be done to identify the cause of abnormal feces. Samples can be tested for the presence of specific bacteria and other infectious agents. If there is blood in the stool, a physical examination can help determine if the blood originates from hemorrhoids, intestinal growths, or another disease. *See also* CELIAC SPRUE; CONSTIPATION; DIARRHEA; GASTROENTERITIS; HEMORRHOIDS; *and* ULCERATIVE COLITIS.

Fee for Service

A medical billing system in which the patient pays a specific price per service rendered.

At one time, fee for service was the prevailing billing system in Western healthcare. With the rise of managed care, however, fee-for-service billing has declined. Managed care often offers billing systems under which the doctor may receive a given amount per patient (capitation) or a mix of capitation and fees for specific services.

There is much debate over whether fee for service is superior to other payment systems. Some studies have found that the fee-for-service model results in more patient visits and greater continuity of care. Other studies have found that patients are less satisfied with access to their physicians under fee-for-service billing than they are with fixed payment and other payment systems. *See also* ACCESS TO CARE; HEALTH INSURANCE; *and* HEALTH MAINTENANCE ORGANIZATION.

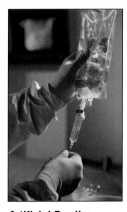

Artificial Feeding.
Intravenous or artificial feeding, above, can provide all the nutrients necessary to meet a patient's daily requirements. Nutrients are administered through a tube inserted into the stomach, or small intestine. Artificial feeding is usually done when a patient is unable to swallow, has tubes in their lungs, or is brain injured.

Feeding, Artificial

Providing nutrients intravenously or through a tube to the stomach or small intestine.

Artificial feeding is performed when a patient is unable to eat enough or at all, which may occur if patients are unable to swallow, have tubes in their lungs, are paralyzed or brain injured, or have an inability to adequately digest or absorb dietary nutrients. Two major types of techniques exist. One is parenteral nutrition, in which nutrients are delivered by a needle through a vein (intravenously). The other is enteral nutrition (tube feeding), in which a nutrient mixture is delivered directly into the stomach or small intestine via a tube. Artificial feeding can be done on a temporary or permanent basis.

Temporary feeding tubes involve a tube threaded into the nose and extended into the stomach (nasogastric tubes), into the top of the small intestine (nasoduodenal tubes), or into the second section of the small intestine (nasojejunal tubes). Permanent types of tubes include those placed directly into a surgical opening (stoma) in the stomach or intestines.

Artificial feeding can be done in a hospital setting or at home. It is important to include the patient in meals by feeding him or her with the rest of the household—eating together is an important social ritual. *See also* HYPERALIMENTATION.

Feeding, Infant

Providing nutrition to a baby through breast milk or milk or soy formulas.

Doctors agree that the healthiest way to feed a newborn is to give the child breast milk exclusively for the first six months. Some solid foods should then be added, along with water, while breast-feeding continues. Ideally, cow's milk should be avoided until the baby is no longer nursing.

BREAST-FEEDING
Colostrum. Breast milk contains every nu-

Infants and a Vegetarian Diet

The American Dietetic Association has approved vegetarian diets as healthy and nutritionally complete, as long as they are properly planned. However, it is important not to be too restrictive with children of age two and younger, as infants need great amounts of essential fatty acids, which exist primarily in meat. It is, however, suitable to avoid meat during pregnancy and breast-feeding.

trient that a baby will need in the first few months of life. Colostrum, the milk produced for the first few days after birth, is higher in protein and lower in fat and sugar than the breast milk produced later. It contains antibodies, providing protection against infection. It is important that a mother breast-feed an infant during the first few days of life, regardless of whether she chooses to later on.

Benefits. Recent reports have shown that bacterial meningitis in infants may be prevented by breast-feeding. There is also evidence that adults who were breast-fed as babies have lower rates of several chronic disorders, such as diabetes, celiac disease, lymphatic cancers, inflammatory bowel disease, asthma, and allergies. They also have a lower incidence of liver disease, chronic lung disorders, heart disease, and obesity than adults who were bottle-fed as infants.

Breast-feeding the newborn also has benefits for the mother. Women who nurse describe a unique feeling of closeness and bonding with their babies. It is easier for a woman to lose weight after delivery if she breast-feeds. Also, breast-feeding is convenient, requiring no mixing, heating, or sterilization, and is much less expensive than using formulas.

BOTTLE-FEEDING
There are many reasons why a mother may decide against breast-feeding. Between one and five percent of women do not produce sufficient milk. Some women may have had breast surgery that removed some of the glandular tissue of the breast. For some women, particularly if they work outside the home, breast-feeding may be difficult

to fit into a schedule. In these cases, commercial formula may be the better choice.

Commercial formulas have similar nutritional values to breast milk. Some formulas, however, are designed for a specific purpose. Most formulas are made out of modified cow's milk, with vitamins added. For infants who are lactose intolerant, soy-based formulas may be used. There are also formulas designed for the nutritional needs of premature infants. Formulas should be used with a doctor's supervision.

PROBLEMS

Many problems with infant feeding are relatively benign or disappear over time. Colic decreases as a baby gets older. Vomiting may be caused by overfeeding, which can be stopped by reducing the amount of formula or milk. An inadequate nipple, in which the nipple is too small for the baby to get enough breast milk, can be enlarged. Formula intolerance may be due to a food allergy or malabsorption; it may be ameliorated by identifying and removing the substance that is causing the reaction.

Gastroesophageal reflux, in which the stomach contents come back into the esophagus, may cause an infant to refuse to eat or vomit frequently. Reflux is sometimes accompanied by hiatal hernia, in which a part of the stomach protrudes above the diaphragm. Symptoms of reflux include crying, refusing to eat, gulping milk or formula for a few seconds and then stopping, and not gaining weight. Most infants outgrow reflux by the age of 12 months.

If the doctor rules out the above problems with feeding, he or she may look for signs of a physical difficulty. A cleft lip and palate or large adenoids may affect feeding. Normal swallowing may be affected by cerebral palsy. Infants with metabolic disorders may feel pain and cramps when fed certain foods and thus refuse to eat at all.

INFANT FEEDING *is a topic that is well complimented by the discussions of* BOTTLE FEEDING; BREAST FEEDING; BREAST PUMP; CHILD BIRTH; COLIC, INFANTILE; CRYING IN INFANTS; FAILURE TO THRIVE; NUTRITION; POSTMATURITY; *and* PREGNANCY COUNSELING. *Other important related articles include* DIET, ATKINS; DIETARY, FIBER; *and* VEGETARIANISM.

Feldenkrais Method

A method of bodywork that views an individual's awareness of his or her own movement as essential for changing bad habits and optimizing movement range and style.

Developed by the engineer and physicist Moshe Feldenkrais, this method combines elements of martial arts, physiology, psychology, and neurology to alter or improve movement patterns. In order to learn how to change an individual's manner of movement, a person must first develop an awareness of his or her own self-image, or distinct way of moving. The Feldenkrais method aims to reverse or "interrupt" any negative or uncomfortable patterns of movement to generate a more fluid range of motion. To achieve this, the therapy involves two approaches: Awareness Through Movement, or group movement courses, and Functional Integration, which involves a skilled practitioner and hands-on touch as a method for retraining the body. The program is ideal for those suffering from specific physical conditions (i.e., a stroke, spinal disorders, or arthritis), or for healthy individuals seeking improved physical performance. *See also* BODYWORK.

Femoral Nerve

The nerve of the thigh.

The femoral nerve is made up of nerve fibers that originate in the lower spinal cord, emerge from the lower vertebrae, and continue down to the thighs. These nerves supply sensation for and activate the muscles that assist in the bending and straightening of the knee. In addition, femoral nerves supply sensation to the front of the thigh.

Femoral nerve dysfunction can impair movement or sensation in the thigh, often making it difficult to straighten the knee. Nerve damage may be caused by direct trauma, by prolonged pressure on the nerve, or by a tumor. It is often seen as a result of a slipped disk in the spine or a dislocated hip. *See also* NERVE INJURY.

Femur

The thigh bone, stretching from the hip to the knee.

The femur is the longest bone in the body. The ball-shaped head of the femur fits into a socket in the pelvis, forming the hip joint. This ball-and-socket-type joint allows the bone to move in all directions and rotate. A section of bone near the top, where several large muscles attach, is known as the greater trochanter. The head of the femur is connected to a small section of bone that attaches to the long part of the bone, known as the shaft. The shaft meets the tibia, or the shin, and forms the hinge-like knee joint. The bone at this end splits into two bumps, called the condyles, that help to carry the weight on the knee joint.

Femur, Fracture of

A break in the long bone that extends from hip to the knee.

Femoral fractures occur at the neck of the femur or in the shaft, which runs down the leg. Fractures at the neck occur near the hip, where the head joins to the shaft or between the main part of the neck and the protruding bone known as the greater trochanter. These injuries are most common in older people, who tend to have more brittle bones, but they can happen to anyone as a result of an accident or severe trauma. Femoral fractures may require plates or rods to hold the bone in place while healing. Serious fractures may require replacement of the neck and head of the femur with an artificial part, which allow for a full recovery of movement.

Fractures across the shaft are usually caused by sudden extreme force on the bone. The danger in these cases is that a large amount of blood may be lost, due to the many veins that supply the shaft. A fractured shaft needs to be realigned, splinted, and kept in traction while healing. During this process, exercise of the joints is necessary in order to prevent them from stiffening. *See also* FEMUR; FRACTURE; *and* INJURY.

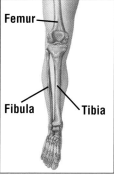

Fractured Femur.
The diagram above shows a fractured femur, a break in the thigh bone, which extends from the hip to the knee. Complications of a fractured femur can occur if the bone has broken across the neck (the short section between the top of the shaft and the hip joint) or across the shaft.

Fertility

The ability to have children.

Women begin their reproductive years with the first menstrual period (menarche), and end at menopause. Men become fertile at puberty and can sire children even into old age, barring health problems.

Fertility depends on several factors:
- production of healthy sperm;
- production of healthy eggs;
- unblocked fallopian tubes;
- ability of the sperm to penetrate and fertilize the egg;
- ability of the fertilized egg to implant in the uterine wall;
- sufficient embryo quality to ensure a successful pregnancy.

A woman's most fertile period is in her 20s, with fertility beginning to decline after age 30. Women over age 35 are three times more likely to have difficulty conceiving than women in their 20s. After age 35, age becomes a risk factor in pregnancy, due to an increased chance of chromosomal anomalies. Most "defective" eggs are not fertilized; if they are, the pregnancy usually results in a miscarriage or stillbirth. If such a pregnancy goes to full term, there is a greater chance of birth defects.

The number of eggs also declines with age. A female fetus has between six and seven million developing egg cells; she is born with about two million. At puberty, 300,000 to 400,000 remain to mature on a monthly basis. The thousands that do not mature gradually degenerate. By menopause, no eggs remain.

Women in their 40s who use donor eggs have the same chance of carrying a pregnancy to term as much younger women, thus indicating that egg age is the main factor in infertility in older women.

Infertility evaluations are recommended for younger women who have not been able to conceive after a full year. Due to the increased difficulty that older women experience, it is recommended that they undergo testing after only six months. *See also* INFERTILITY *and* PREGNANCY.

Fertility Drugs

Medications that stimulate ovulation in the treatment of an inability to become pregnant.

One of the more common causes of infertility is a problem with ovulation. Medications can be used to stimulate ovulation; with the use of these drugs, more than one egg often matures at a time, increasing the chances of a multiple pregnancy.

Clomiphene, also known as Clomid, is one of the more popular drugs used to induce ovulation. It has also been used to increase a man's sperm count, but it does not improve the sperm's ability to move or reduce the number of abnormal sperm.

Usually a woman undergoes six treatment cycles with clomiphene. If ovulation does not occur after treatment, increasing doses are used. Between 75 and 80 percent of women ovulate after receiving clomiphene; of those, 40 to 50 percent become pregnant. Five percent of pregnancies that result from clomiphene-induced ovulation are multiple pregnancies.

Side effects include hot flashes, abdominal swelling, breast tenderness, nausea, vision problems, and headaches. A small percentage of women develop ovarian hyperstimulation syndrome, in which the ovaries enlarge and the abdomen retains fluid.

Human menopausal gonadotropin, known more commonly as Pergonal, may be also be used. Pergonal, however, is expensive and often has severe side effects. It is injected into the muscle to stimulate ovarian follicles to mature, after which a second chemical, human chorionic gonadotropin, is used to trigger ovulation. More than 95 percent of women who receive this treatment ovulate; 50 to 75 percent become pregnant, with 10 to 30 percent of those pregnancies multiple. Side effects include ovarian hyperstimulation and a risk of developing ovarian cancer.

> *Topics related to this issue include* FERTILITY; FERTILIZATION; IN VITRO FERTILIZATION; OVULATION; *and* PREGNANCY, MULTIPLE. *Anatomical issues that should come under consideration include* UTERUS *and* VAGINA.

Fertilization

Also known as conception

The union of sperm and egg.

Fertilization takes place in the upper third portion of the fallopian tube. When ejaculation occurs, hundreds of millions of sperm are released and swim up through the uterus to the fallopian tubes in search of the egg. Not all of them survive the journey. The sperm that survive swarm over the egg's surface, but only one succeeds in entering. The sperm penetrates the egg by releasing an enzyme that dissolves the egg's firm outer layer, called the zona pellucida. Immediately after, a chemical change occurs in the egg's outer membrane, barring entry to all other sperm.

Once inside, the chromosomes of the sperm unite with those of the egg to form the zygote. This cell promptly begins undergoing multiple rounds of cell division.

Fertility Drugs and Multiple Births

Because fertility drugs stimulate multiple ovulations, they also increase the likelihood of multiple pregnancy. A multiple pregnancy increases the mother's weight during pregnancy; strains her body, causing muscle and skeletal problems; worsens pre-existing conditions; and increases the chance of premature birth and defects.

Twins are the most common multiple birth. One of the fetuses usually lies crosswise, increasing the mortality rate of the second delivery. Risks also include uterine bleeding and dangerously exhausting labor, although a Cesarean section eliminates most delivery dangers. The more fetuses in the uterus, the lower the likelihood that all will survive.

In vitro fertilization refers to a laboratory process in which fertilization occurs outside the body. The ovaries are stimulated to produce eggs, which are then retrieved and placed in a special nutrient solution with sperm. Once the embryos reach a particular level of development (usually 8 to 16 cells), they can be implanted in the woman's uterus. *See also* CHILDBIRTH; FERTILITY; INTERCOURSE; OVULATION; PREGNANCY; *and* REPRODUCTIVE SYSTEM.

Resources on Fertility
Eli Y. Adashi, Eli Y., John A., Rock, and Zev Rosenwaks, eds., *Reproductive Endocrinology, Surgery, and Technology (*1998); Breitkpf, Lyle J. and Marion Gordon Bakoulis, *Coping with Endometriosis* (1988); Laucella, Linda, *Hormone Replacement Therapy: Conventional Medicine and Natural Alternatives, Your Guide to Menopausal Health-Care Choices* (1999); Older, Julia, *Endometriosis* (1984); Endometriosis Assoc., Tel. (800) 992-3636, Online: www.endometriosisassn. org; Endocrine Web, Online: www.endocrineweb.com;www.nycornell.org/medicine/edm/index.html.

Fetal Alcohol Syndrome

Birth defects often seen in offspring of women with a history of heavy alcohol use during pregnancy.

Because alcohol easily passes through the placenta, alcohol use during pregnancy can have severe effects on the development of a fetus. Alcohol use increases the risk of miscarriage and of infant mortality. Infants who survive are at risk for a number of physical and mental defects, with the severity of the defects rising with increasing alcohol use. Fetal alcohol syndrome is seen in 2.2 out of 1,000 live births.

SYMPTOMS

Defects associated with fetal alcohol syndrome include:

- **Low Birth Weight.** Infants born to mothers who consumed alcohol during pregnancy have an average birth weight of four pounds, compared to a normal birth weight of seven pounds.
- **Short stature** and general delayed physical growth.
- **Small head size** with abnormal facial features, such as a short upper jaw and pronounced epicanthal folds around the eyes.
- **Heart Defects.**
- **Mental retardation,** ranging from mild to moderate.
- **Behavioral problems,** such as attention deficit hyperactivity disorder.

TREATMENT AND PREVENTION

Children born with fetal alcohol syndrome can require varying levels of treatment. Defects in the heart or other vital organs may require surgery; mental and behavioral problems may require educational and behavioral intervention.

Fetal alcohol syndrome can be prevented by avoiding alcohol when trying to conceive and during pregnancy. There is no established safe level of consumption. *See also* AL-COHOL DEPENDENCE; BEHAVIORAL PROBLEMS IN CHILDREN; HEART DISEASE, CONGENITAL; *and* MENTAL RETARDATION.

Fetal Circulation

The flow of blood in a fetus.

During pregnancy, the fetus' bloodstream is connected to the mother's through the placenta, which provides oxygen and nutrients and carries off wastes. The two blood systems are completely separate, although occasionally some mingling does occur.

The baby's blood type can be completely different from the mother's. This usually does not present a problem, except in the case of Rh incompatibility, in which case maternal antibodies might cross into the baby's bloodstream and attack the baby as if it were a virus. The globulin RhoGam, however, can be given to the mother to prevent her from forming antibodies against the baby's tissue in the first place.

An important feature of fetal circulation is the blood vessel known as the ductus arteriosus. This blood vessel bypasses the lungs, which are not used until birth. After birth, the ductus arteriosus is closed off to permit normal heart-lung circulation. *See also* FETUS; PREGNANCY; *and* RH INCOMPATIBILITY.

Fetal Distress

When a baby experiences trouble during labor, usually from a lack of oxygen.

There are several signposts for fetal distress, the most important of which is based on fetal heart monitoring. The normal fetal heart rate is between 120 and 160 beats per minute. During a contraction, the blood supply to the fetus is temporarily reduced and the heart rate increases. A low or high fetal heart rate can indicate distress. In another method, a sample of fetal blood is obtained from the scalp and tested to determine the pH. If the fetal blood is too acidic, there is too much carbon dioxide in it, indicating that the fetus is not receiving sufficient oxygen.

Treatment. Fetal distress may require immediate medical intervention, such as a Cesarean section. *See* CHILDBIRTH, COMPLICATIONS *and* CESAREAN SECTION.

Fetal Heart Monitoring

Recording a baby's heartbeat during labor.

In recent years, electronic fetal monitoring has become routine in most hospitals as a way to track the baby's health during childbirth. Belts are placed around the mother's abdomen to detect contractions and the fetus' heartbeat, and the information is displayed on a nearby monitor.

During childbirth, the normal fetal heart rate is between 120 and 160 beats per minute. When a contraction occurs, the baby's blood supply is temporarily reduced and its heart rate increases. If the rate is too low or too high, the fetus may be in distress and may require emergency intervention. *See also* FETAL DISTRESS.

Fetoscopy

A prenatal diagnostic procedure in which a doctor can view a fetus and obtain tissue samples.

Fetoscopy is a rarely used prenatal test in which a lighted telescope-like instrument called a fetoscope is inserted through the abdomen into the uterus. The doctor is able to view the fetus through the fetoscope and may even withdraw blood and tissue samples to test the fetus for suspected disorders.

Use. Fetoscopy enables experimental intervention for unusual conditions. *See also* AMNIOCENTESIS.

Fetus

An unborn baby from approximately the eighth week of pregnancy until birth.

Before the eighth week after conception, a developing baby is known as an embryo. At eight weeks, a fetus is about one inch long and is recognizably human, with the beginning development of facial features, fingers, toes, eyes, and ears. The earliest a fetus is able to survive outside the uterus is approximately 23 weeks. *See also* CONCEPTION; EMBRYO; GESTATION; *and* PREGNANCY.

Fever

An elevated body temperature, usually in response to an illness or infection.

Body temperature is controlled by the hypothalamus, which acts as a natural thermostat, keeping temperature within a normal range. Normal body temperature ranges from 97° to 99°F, with an average of 98.6°F. Body temperature follows a 24 hour cycle, reaching its peak at around 4 P.M. and its lowest level in the early morning. During a fever, the hypothalamus works to maintain body temperature a few degrees above normal; after a fever breaks, the range returns to normal.

CAUSES

Fever is one of the body's generalized responses to infection. Substances that trigger a fever are known as pyrogens; they include bacteria and other microorganisms, as well as the toxins they produce. Body temperature becomes elevated during an illness, because microorganisms do not survive well in an environment that is too hot. It may not be necessary or even wise to bring a fever down quickly, unless body temperature rises to a dangerous level.

In addition to infection, fevers may be caused by dehydration, heat stroke, reac-

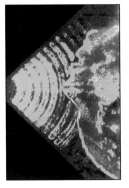

Fetoscopy. The image from a fetoscopy, above, allows a physician to view a fetus by inserting a lighted telescope-like instrument through the abdomen to the uterus.

ALERT

Emergency Situations

A fever is considered an emergency if it is accompanied by a severe headache, a stiff neck, severe swelling in the throat, or mental confusion.

A very high fever can also be an emergency. The temperature at which a fever becomes dangerous varies according to age:
- In infants from newborn to six months of age, a fever over 100.5°F is cause for concern, and above 101°F is serious.
- In children and adults, a fever of 103°F is serious, and a fever of 105°F or more is considered dangerous and potentially fatal.

If a fever is 101º F and persists for three days or more, or if a low-grade fever persists for several weeks, a doctor should be consulted.

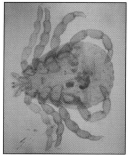
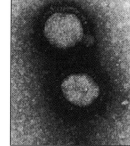
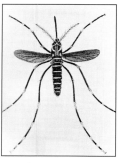

Fever.
Above, are magnifications of bacteria and insects that cause fever. A fever can be caused by bacterial or viral infections such as influenza, or tonsillitis. In such cases, proteins called pyrogens are released when the body's white blood cells fight the microorganisms responsible for the illness. The proteins raise body temperature to try to destroy the invading microorganisms.

tions to medication, autoimmune reactions, hormonal disorders, and cancer. They may also have no known cause.

SYMPTOMS

A fever can often be felt as a warmth and flushing of the skin, as blood vessels near the surface of skin dilate to eliminate excess heat. A person with a fever may also experience chills.

A fever may regularly fluctuate, with the body temperature rising and falling in a regular pattern. This is accompanied by the alternating chills and flushing experienced in many illnesses. A spike in temperature occurs when temperature elevates sharply within a very short period of time. In small children, it is not uncommon for a fever to spike suddenly at the beginning of an illness.

When a fever breaks, the patient often sweats profusely, which helps to lower the temperature.

TREATMENT

Over-the-counter medications such as aspirin, ibuprofen, and acetaminophen, are effective at lowering a fever. Aspirin should not be given to children, because Reye's syndrome, a potentially life-threatening condition, may develop in children with viral infections who have taken aspirin.

Cold compresses and sponging with lukewarm or cool (never cold) water can lower a fever and make the patient feel more comfortable. A person with a fever should rest and drink plenty of fluids.

FEBRILE SEIZURES

A febrile seizure is a seizure caused by a fever. There is a brief period of unconsciousness and the seizure may be accompanied by convulsions.

Febrile seizures occur in approximately two to five percent of all children under the age of five. The tendency for febrile seizures runs in families. In most cases, a child prone to febrile seizures usually outgrows them.

Febrile seizures usually occur when the temperature is either falling or rising rapidly. If a serious disease such as meningitis or encephalitis has been ruled out and the period of unconsciousness lasts only a few minutes, the seizure should not be a major cause for concern.

Anticonvulsant medication may be prescribed to reduce the likelihood of future occurrences.

Taking a Temperature

Body temperature can be measured with a thermometer. Thermometers come in many varieties, and measure temperature in degrees Fahrenheit and Centigrade. Some have a digital readout.

The most common type of thermometer is the oral thermometer. It is placed under the tongue for three minutes, and then removed and read.

For an infant or young child, who may not be able to hold a thermometer in the mouth for three minutes, rectal thermometers are the preferred choice. The bulb end of the thermometer is lubricated and inserted gently into the anus. It should not be forced, and the parent should not let go of the other end while it is inside. If the child protests or is otherwise uncomfortable, the thermometer can be removed after only one minute, as the majority of the temperature registers by that time. Temperatures obtained rectally are usually 1° warmer than those obtained orally. For this reason, it is important to tell the child's physician how the temperature was obtained.

A thermometer can also be placed in the child's armpit. This temperature reading usually produces results that are 1° cooler than those obtained orally.

Newer models of thermometers can be placed in the ear; the temperature registers in less than a minute. There is some evidence, however, that suggests that the ear thermometers are not very accurate.

Issues related to the incidence of a FEVER include BACTERIA; DIAGNOSIS; FUNGUS; INFECTION; INFLUENZA; SEIZURE; SEIZURE, FEBRILE; and VIRUS. The entries LASSA FEVER and RELAPSING FEVER are also available for review.

Fever Blister

Also known as a cold sore

An infection of the Herpes simplex virus that appears as small blisters, which are usually located around the lips.

Fever blisters are extremely contagious. The *Herpes simplex* virus can be transmitted during an outbreak through kissing or other direct contact with the blisters. It remains contagious until the blisters crust over and begin to heal.

There is no cure for the *Herpes simplex* virus, but the antiviral drug acyclovir, in tablet or ointment form, may reduce the blistering and promote healing. Common side effects of acyclovir include rash, hives, mild burning or stinging at the application site, headache, and lightheadedness. *See also* ANTIVIRAL DRUGS *and* COLD SORES.

Fiber, Dietary

Essential component of many carbohydrates, comprised of the structural materials of plants largely not directly digestible by humans.

Dietary fiber is often found in the cell walls of plants. It comes in two forms: soluble and fermentable on the one hand; insoluble and poorly fermentable on the other.

SOLUBLE FIBERS

Soluble fibers form a gel when mixed with water. Examples include guar, pectin, mucilages, and the fiber in barley, oat bran, beans, and other legumes. Soluble fibers are also fermentable. This means that in the lower small and upper large intestine, they are broken down (fermented) by bacteria into short-chain fatty acids, which aid in chemical processes and provide energy after they are absorbed.

Overconsumption of Fiber

Too much fiber can be dangerous, especially if it is obtained through bran and fiber supplements. It can cause bowel obstructions, which, in extreme cases, can require surgical removal. An excess of fiber can also impede the absorption of nutrients and may result in deficiencies of calcium, zinc, and iron.

INSOLUBLE FIBER

Insoluble fiber passes generally unchanged through the digestive tract and absorbs as much as fifteen times its weight in water. This softens and increases the size of the stool. The added bulk promotes peristalsis, the wave-like contractions of the muscles of the intestinal wall, and decreases the amount of intestinal muscle pressure necessary to move the stool through the bowel.

BENEFITS

Soluble fibers lower blood cholesterol and sugar. Insoluble fibers prevent constipation by reducing the amount of time stool stays in the lower intestine; they also aid in the treatment of diverticular disease by lowering the likelihood that fecal matter will fill the pouches in the intestinal wall and lowering the intestinal pressure that leads to diverticulae.

In addition, a high-fiber diet is helpful in treating irritable bowel syndrome. High-fiber foods also play an important role in a healthy weight-loss program, since they are usually low in calories and their bulk can enhance the sense of fullness after eating.

High-fiber foods or supplements in excessive amounts, however, appear to reduce the absorption of some nutrients, perhaps because they cause food to be moved through the digestive tract more quickly.

RECOMMENDED CONSUMPTION

The daily fiber consumption for an adult should be no less than 20 grams, and no more than 35 grams. Among the best sources of dietary fiber are bran, dried apricots, prunes, peas and beans, and whole-grain breads and cereals.

The sudden addition of large amounts of fiber to the diet can cause gastrointestinal problems, ranging from sensations of gas and bloating to cramps and diarrhea.

DIETARY FIBER *is an issue that is closely related to issues such as* DIET AND DISEASE; FATS AND OILS; FATTY ACIDS; *and* NUTRITION. *Important issues are also related in* CARBOHYDRATES; CHOLESTEROL; *and* DIVERTICULITIS. *Also refer to* CRAMPS; DIARRHEA; DIGESTIVE SYSTEM; *and* INTESTINE.

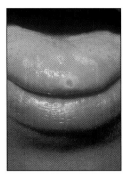

Fever Blister.
Above, is a small fever blister caused by the *Herpes simplex* virus. These blisters are usually located in and around the mouth.

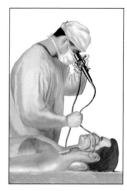

Fiberoptics.
Fiberoptic instruments such as the endoscope above, allow surgeons to view organs within the body. Fiberoptics is the transmission of images through bundles of thin, flexible, glass or plastic threads, which uses light by internal inflection. Microelectronics is replacing fiberoptics in such instruments.

Fiberoptics

A technology using flexible glass or plastic fibers to channel light.

In fiberoptics, light passes through thin strands of plastic or glass. The material used in fiberoptics has optical properties such that once light passes through the center of the fiber, it is reflected off the sides. Thus, even if the fiber is bent, the light remains inside the fiber. Looking through a fiberoptic tube can allow a person to see an image that is around a corner or is otherwise difficult to see.

MEDICAL APPLICATIONS

Fiberoptics has many medical applications. Since fiberoptics allow one to see around corners and in constricted spaces, they prove ideal for studying internal anatomy. A variety of fiberoptic endoscopes have been developed that allow a physician to observe, photograph, and even operate on many internal structures in the body. Fiberoptic endoscopes may be inserted through an incision or into a natural body orifice in order to view the gastrointestinal or respiratory tract, or other areas of the body.

> FIBEROPTICS *is a kind of medical technology that incorporates topics such as* BIOMECHANICAL ENGINEERING; ENDOSCOPY; *and* IMAGING TECHNIQUES. FIBEROPTICS *are used for viewing the* DIGESTIVE SYSTEM; INTESTINES; *and* STOMACH.

Fibrillation

A vibration or tremor in a muscle characterized by independent and irregular pulsating actions of the muscle fibers.

Fibrillation often occurs when a nerve that supplies a particular muscle is destroyed. As a result of the nerve damage, the muscle atrophies and "quivers" uncontrollably. Fibrillation occurs spontaneously and is localized to specific muscle filaments. Unlike fasciculation (a similar pulsating of the muscle), it is not visible under the skin, but can be detected through an electromyogram (EMG) or electrocardiogram (EEG).

FIBRILLATION OF THE HEART
Atrial or ventricular fibrillation is an instance where the heart muscle degenerates because the normal functioning of the electrical conduction system of the heart is disrupted. This results in a disorder of the heart rate in which the atria or ventricles in the heart are stimulated to contract in a rapid and asymmetric manner, producing a weak and irregular pulse. *See* ATRIAL FIBRILLATION *and* VENTRICULAR FIBRILLATION.

Fibrinolysis

The process of dissolving a blood clot after healing has begun.

When clots form to stop blood loss, they block the unwanted flow of blood. When healing begins, the body must safely dissolve the clots so they do not travel to other parts of the body and clog necessary flow. This process of dissolving the clot is called fibrinolysis.

PROCESS
Two opposing elements are involved in the formation and dissolution of blood clots. The coagulation process starts with the platelets sticking to the edges of the break and building a web across the opening. The web or fibrin protein attracts other platelets until a plug is formed and the bleeding stops. When the break in the blood vessel begins to heal, another protein called plasmin breaks down the fibrin and makes it soluble so that the blood clot dissolves harmlessly.

FIBRINOLYTIC DRUGS
Fibrinolytic drugs are often administered after heart attack, along with aspirin and heparin, to thin the blood and reduce the likelihood of blood clots forming and floating dangerously through the system. Stroke victims may be also treated with this combination of drugs. Note that, as with all agents that inhibit clot formation, the danger of excessive and uncontrollable bleeding is present and the patient must be closely monitored. *See also* BLOOD CLOTTING.

Fibrocystic Disease

A term for cystic fibrosis or for a benign condition characterized by lumps in the breast.

Most women with fibrocystic breast disease have some general lumpiness in their breasts, usually in the upper or outer regions. Cysts may develop and some breast pain may occur. The presence of cysts does not mean an increased risk of developing breast cancer for the majority of women.

Breast lumps may increase in size or tenderness right before menstruation. This is due to the dilation of the milk ducts and the surrounding areas, which in turn form cysts. The surge in hormones increases the amount of fluid present in the cysts. Any new or suspicious lump should be brought to the attention of a medical practitioner.

Fibrocystic breast disease occurs most often in women over age 30, but generally stops by menopause. Hormone replacement therapy can prolong the condition.

Generally there is no need to do anything about fibrocystic breast disease. If the condition causes severe discomfort, medication can be given to reduce cyst formation. Cysts can be aspirated. *See also* BREAST, LUMP IN THE *and* CYSTIC FIBROSIS.

Fibroid

Also known as myoma or fibromyoma

A nonmalignant tumor of the uterus.

Fibroids are growths that arise from the muscles and connective tissue of the wall of the uterus. Fibroids usually are round, ranging in size from a quarter of an inch to four inches. They sometimes become attached to neighboring organs. As fibroids grow, they can distort the uterine cavity, giving it an irregular, lumpy appearance.

Up to 20 percent of women over the age of 30 develop fibroids.

CAUSES

Fibroids are believed to be caused by an abnormal response to estrogens, the female sex hormones. The hormonal stimulus during pregnancy can cause fibroids to become large enough to interfere with delivery of the baby.

SYMPTOMS

Many fibroids cause no symptoms, but a fibroid that grows enough to erode the lining of the uterine cavity can cause prolonged or heavy menstruation. A very large fibroid can exert pressure on the bladder, causing a frequent need to urinate, or on the bowel, causing constipation. Large fibroids can also distort the uterus enough to cause difficulty in conceiving or early miscarriage. Some women experience pain if a fibroid becomes twisted.

DIAGNOSIS

Fibroids generally are detected during a routine pelvic examination. The diagnosis can be confirmed by a computerized tomography scan, an ultrasound examination, or a dilatation and curettage, a minor surgical procedure in which tissue is scraped from the lining of the uterus.

TREATMENT

If the bleeding caused by fibroids is intense, medication such as injections of the hormone medroxyprogesterone can be given to stop menstrual bleeding.

While small, symptomless fibroids generally can be left alone, a myomectomy, surgical removal of the fibroids, may be recommended for women of childbearing age to prevent them from interfering with pregnancy. Caesarean delivery may be recommended for such a pregnancy. For other women, a hysterectomy, total removal of the uterus, may be recommended if there are a large number of fibroids, since myomectomy is a major operation and has a higher rate of complications than a hysterectomy.

Emergency surgery may sometimes be necessary if a fibroid attached to the uterine wall becomes so twisted that it is starved for blood and oxygen. The result is a sharp pain low in the abdomen, intense enough to require surgery. *See* HYSTERECTOMY; MYOMECTOMY; PREGNANCY; TUMOR; *and* UTERUS.

Fibroma

A nonmalignant tumor of connective tissue, which supports the structures in the body.

Fibromas arise in the cells that make up the connective tissue—tissue that supports various structures in the body. For example, a fibroma can form in the cells around the follicles in the ovary where eggs (ova) develop and are released for possible fertilization; these are called ovarian fibromas. Fibromas may also form in the tissue surrounding nerve fibers. Multiple fibromas of the nervous system can form in an inherited disorder called neurofibromatosis. Fibromas can sometimes be unsightly, but they are not life-threatening. *See also* NEUROFIBROMATOSIS *and* TUMOR.

Fibrosarcoma

Cancer arising from cells of connective tissue, which supports various structures in the body.

Fibrosarcomas are a rare cancer. They usually occur in the connective tissue surrounding a bone in an arm or leg, but can also originate in a bone or in the tissue around nerve cells. Some fibrosarcomas develop when a fibroma, a benign tumor, turns cancerous. They can be life-threatening if they spread to other tissues.

A fibrosarcoma is detected by the swelling that it causes or by the abnormal appearance of veins lying above it. Fibrosarcomas are treated by surgery or radiation, which can be effective if the cancer is detected early. *See also* CANCER *and* TUMOR.

Fibrosis

Thickening and excessive growth of body tissues.

Fibrous, or scar, tissue can form as a result of injury or infection. It may also form as part of a hereditary disease, or it may develop for unknown reasons. Fibrous tissue impedes the normal functioning of nearby organs or muscles; the extent of damage it causes depends on where it is located.

TYPES

Pulmonary fibrosis is the buildup of fibrous tissue in the lungs, causing the lungs to become stiff and making breathing difficult. Pulmonary fibrosis often results from infection or the inhalation of mineral or organic dust, such as silica, metal dust, molds or bird droppings; or toxic fumes, such as chlorine or sulfur dioxide. The patient has less stamina and is short of breath after exercise. Other symptoms include loss of appetite, coughing, weakness, and chest pain. Pulmonary fibrosis is treated with corticosteroids. Some patients die after only a few months; others may live for years.

Myelofibrosis is a progressive disease of unknown cause in which fibrous tissue slowly replaces the bone marrow, resulting in the production of abnormal red blood cells, causing anemia and an enlarged spleen. There is no cure for this disease.

Cystic fibrosis is a hereditary disease in which the body produces an excess of mucus that clogs the lungs and results in repeated infections. Mucus also blocks the ducts from the pancreas to the small intestines, which compromises the digestion of fats, leading to chronic diarrhea and malnutrition. The immune system is weakened, leaving the individual vulnerable to disease. There is no cure for this condition and treatment is restricted to addressing the symptoms and diseases to which the sufferer is vulnerable. The median age of survival for sufferers of cystic fibrosis is 31. *See also* CYSTIC FIBROSIS *and* IMMUNE SYSTEM.

Fibrositis

Muscle pain and stiffness; often used to describe nonspecific back pain.

Unexplained complaints of pain and stiffness are sometimes given the name fibrositis. The term, however, is not recognized by all physicians, as many physicians believe that it does not describe any true inflammation of the muscles.

Most cases of fibrositis seem to be related to bad posture, tension, or extensive periods of time spent sitting in a cramped position. The pain related to fibrositis is commonly felt in the back, neck, shoulders, chest, buttocks, and knees. Typically experienced by older and middle-aged people, fibrositis may worsen in cold, damp weather or after exercise to which the body is not accustomed. Painkillers, massages, and hot baths may help the pain. Exercises to strengthen muscles and improve posture may help to prevent further attacks of the condition. *See also* ANALGESIC DRUGS; EXERCISE; *and* MASSAGE.

Fibula

A long, thin, outer bone in the lower leg.

Fastened on each end by ligaments, the fibula runs from just below the knee to the ankle and holds muscle. Its support of body weight is negligible, making it an ideal candidate for a bone graft and one of the more likely bones to fracture, a fracture that, de-

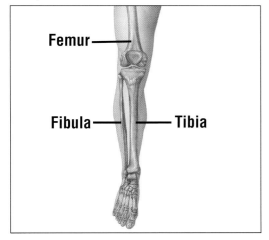

Femur

Fibula — Tibia

pending on the age of the person and magnitude of the break, may take up to six weeks to heal. The fibula often breaks above the ankle when the ankle is violently twisted; the ankle itself may sprain or dislocate, and the tibia, or shin bone, may also break. Once a fracture of the lower fibula is confirmed by x-ray, the lower leg is cast in plaster. A mid-bone fracture does not need a cast to heal. Severe breaks and breaks coupled with ankle dislocation often require surgery to reattach shards of bones or implant metal pins. *See also* FRACTURE.

Fifth Disease

Also known as erythema infectiosum

A viral infection that causes a red, patchy rash on the face or cheeks.

Fifth disease is transmitted mainly by body fluids, including drops from a sneeze or cough, as well as blood.

Symptoms of the disease appear between four days and two weeks after exposure. Fifth disease is usually mild. The most common symptoms are mild respiratory symptoms, malaise (a generalized feeling of illness), and a rash. Fifth disease is an infection of the parovirus, and manifests itself as red, raised patches that appear on a patient's face, trunk and extremities. The face appears as if it has been slapped. Also present is circumoral pallor, or a pale ring around the lips. The parovirus has been known to cause anemia, aplastic crisis in patients with sickle-cell anemia, and hydrops—fluid overload and heart failure in a developing fetus. These conditions are extremely rare, however.

Treatment. There is no vaccine for fifth disease. It will usually clear up within ten days, but a pediatrician should examine the child to make sure the rash is fifth disease and not another illness. The condition has a tendency to recur. *See also* ANEMIA.

Fight-or-Flight Response

Reaction to stress produced by the adrenal glands and autonomic nervous system.

During times of stress, fear, or anxiety, the body reacts by preparing its systems to either fight back or flee from the danger. Epinephrine and norepinephrine, hormones produced by the adrenal glands, speed up the sympathetic nervous system; the heart rate increases in order to get more oxygen into the body, more blood flows to the muscles allowing them to operate better, and the pupils dilate to improve the vision. This physical preparation for danger is common to animals as well as humans. *See also* ADRENAL GLANDS *and* AUTONOMIC NERVOUS SYSTEM.

Fibula.
The diagram at left shows the fibula, a long thin bone in the outer leg that is used to hold muscle. Bone is often taken from the fibula for grafting in other parts of the body.

Filariasis

General term for infestation by any of several types of parasitic worm of the family *Filarioida*.

Infestation by filarial worms begins with a bite from a blood-sucking insect. While adult worms range in size from three-quarters of an inch to 20 inches, the eggs and larvae (microfilariae) are microscopic. When a mosquito or midge feeds on an infested person, these microscopic offspring can be picked up and transported by the insect. Filiarial worms and their larvae are the source of various diseases and affect over 120 million people worldwide, primarily throughout tropical and subtropical regions of South America, Asia, the Pacific Islands, and Africa.

TYPES

Lymphatic filariasis affects the lymphatic system and its vessels. Infestation of this type results in localized accumulation of fluid in the tissues (edema), and an eventual thickening, darkening, and hardening of the affected skin (elephantiasis) after prolonged and repeated infestation.

Onchocerciasis affects the eye. The larvae of this type congregate near the skin in order to be transmitted by a blood-sucking insect. If they congregate near the eye, they can cause blindness.

Calabar swelling affects the skin of the human host. The infestation initially produces a crawling sensation in the skin. This sensation is followed by irritation and pain, as well as edema.

SYMPTOMS

While generally not fatal, infestation of filarial worms produces serious symptoms, including acute fever, enlargement of the scrotum (hydrocele), elephantiasis, and other pulmonary bronchial asthmatic conditions. When left untreated, filariasis can lead to severe deformities of the skin, vision, and lymphatic system. Early detection and treatment with anthelmintic drugs offer the best prognosis for those afflicted with this illness.

DIAGNOSIS

Two tests are commonly used to diagnose filariasis. The first, known as circulating filariae antigen detection, uses a blood specimen from a finger prick collected with filter paper and processed by simple lab techniques. The second method examines a blood smear to identify microfilariae. Early detection and treatment are essential to avoid permanent injury.

TREATMENT

Filariasis is treated with anthelmintic drugs, which kill adult worms, or microfilaricidal drugs (such as ivermectin), which kill microfilariae. Diethylcarbamazine is mostly used as a microfilaricide but also has macrofilaricidal effects (for adult worms).

PREVENTION

Although there is no vaccine against filariasis, diethylcarbamazine can be taken in preventive doses. Use of mosquito netting and insect repellent also reduces the chances of infestation.

In order to understand the nature of this disorder articles on FLATWORM; FLUKE; INFECTION; PARASITE; RINGWORM; *and* TROPICAL DISEASES *should be consulted.* BITES; MOSQUITO BITES; SAND-FLY BITES; TSETSE FLY BITES; *and* VENOMOUS BITES AND STINGS *should also be referred to.*

Filling, Dental

Procedure of repairing decayed areas of the teeth.

After a decayed area of a tooth is located, it is cleaned to stop deterioration and filled to restore the tooth's proper function and prevent future bacterial invasion. Removing the decayed area with a small drill completes the cleaning stage. Then the cavity is filled with a pliable substance. The most common filling material for back teeth is an alloy of silver and other metals known as silver amalgam. Front teeth, and occasionally back teeth, are filled with a tooth-colored material.

Some people have questioned the safety of metal fillings. Others dislike them for cosmetic reasons. Modern dentistry has made available composite resins, plastic-like materials composed of glass and resin that can be colored to match a tooth. They are not quite as durable as metal fillings but are steadily improving.

Fillings can last for long periods of time, although as they age they can become brittle; many individuals with fillings in their teeth know all too well the unpleasant experience of chewing an apple or a piece of candy and losing a filling. Occasionally, even a filling that appears intact has worn down enough that the seal between it and the tooth has been broken. The result is that bacteria can get under the filling and attack the rest of the tooth. When dentists find this problem, they replace the filling. See also CARIES, DENTAL.

Finger Joint Replacement

Surgery in which a finger joint is replaced by an artificial joint.

A finger has three bones joined at joints by ligaments and crossed by tendons that bend and straighten the finger. The muscles work without friction because the tendons, sheathed in synovium membrane and filled with fluid, glide instead of pulling.

Finger joint replacement usually becomes necessary when the joint has deteriorated due to disease, such as rheumatoid arthritis or osteoarthritis. When the cartilage, bone, and lining of the joints are destroyed by arthritis, joint replacement can strengthen and stabilize the finger. Osteoarthritis may also require finger joint replacement in order to reduce pain and restore mobility.

The artificial joint, usually made of metal and plastic or silicone rubber, is attached to the bones of the finger. Joint replacement usually succeeds in reducing pain, and, with exercise, restoring mobility. Completely normal movement may not be possible, as the disease may have destroyed tissue surrounding the joint. See also HAND; JOINT; OSTEOARTHRITIS; PROSTHESIS; and RHEUMATOID ARTHRITIS.

First Aid

Immediate assistance offered during an emergency situation.

When a sudden illness or accident occurs, the first people on the scene will most likely not be medically trained. First aid is the assistance that is offered until trained medical personnel arrive on the scene. The goal of first aid is to preserve a victim's life and to prevent further harm.

Everyone should learn the basics of first aid, because responding to an emergency demands preparation, and almost everyone encounters an emergency sometime during his or her life.

An important first step in an emergency is to remain calm—effective first aid cannot be administered in a state of panic. Another basic step in first aid is assessing the situation—who is hurt, how badly, what sort of help is needed, and what sort of help can be offered. Key concerns in assessing the severity of an emergency include presence or absence of heartbeat, adequate breathing, any source of bleeding, and appearance or loss of consciousness. If the victim is not breathing or has no pulse, CPR (cardiopulmonary resuscitation), should be administered while someone else calls for emergency medical help. It is important to know that dialing 911 in the United States accesses the nearest emergency dispatch station. If a person is bleeding profusely, blood loss should be controlled by applying direct pressure to the wound.

Preparation is the first step in providing adequate first aid. Everyone should take a first aid class and keep a first aid kit and fire extinguisher at home, in the car, and at work. It is very important to remain calm in emergency situations. Panic can endanger both the victim and the rescuer. Act only if it is safe to do so.

> *Whenever considering issues of* FIRST AID *it is important to keep in mind topics such as* CARDIOPULMONARY RESUSCITATION; DIAGNOSIS; EMERGENCY, FIRST STEPS OF; EMERGENCY MEDICINE; *and* HEIMLICH MANEUVER; *especially when treating* CHOKING; CONCUSSION; HEAT STROKE; *and* HYPOTHERMIA.

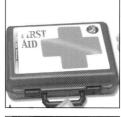
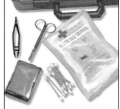
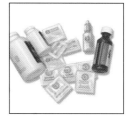
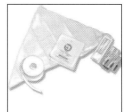

First Aid.
A first aid kit, above, generally consists of bandages, aspirin, tweezers, antiseptics and more. First aid is treatment for minor injuries such as small wounds, cuts, sprains, or minor burns. For a minor injury, first aid is administered to prevent the condition from worsening.

Fitness.

Many daily practices can help contribute to a high level of physical fitness, including walking (*top*) and cycling (*bottom and right*).

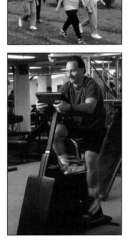

Resources on Fitness

Costill, David L., Inside Running: Basics of Sports Physiology (1986); McArdle, William D., et al., Exercise Physiology: Energy, Nutrition, and Human Performance (1996); Vliet, Elizabeth Lee, Women, Weight and Hormones (2001); National Osteoporosis Foundation, Tel. (800) 223-9994, Online: www.nof. org; President's Council on Physical Fitness and Sports, Tel. (202) 690-9000, Online: www.fitness.gov; Women's Sports Foundation, Tel. (800) 227-3988, Online: www.lifetimetv.com/WoSport; https://public1.med.cornell.edu/cgi-

Fitness

The ability to perform work and daily activities without becoming exhausted.

Fitness is a measure of how healthy a person is. A fit person is able to increase the lifespan, avoid chronic diseases, improve work capacity, and enjoy an overall better quality of life.

The term fitness includes several aspects of physical health. The best known and most basic is cardiovascular fitness, which is the ability of the heart to use oxygen in an efficient way. Good cardiovascular fitness,

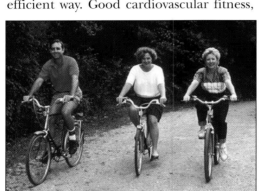

increases a person's endurance and allows for the completion of tasks with minimum wear. Flexibility, or bending, stretching, and twisting, can increase the ability to perform tasks without excess exertion. Strength, which is required for pushing, pulling, and lifting, helps a person to do more.

All of these elements of fitness feed off of each other. Increasing muscle strength will help with endurance. Flexibility and stretching can help to prevent injuries while participating in sports or other activities. The best ways to increase fitness are to keep active on a daily basis, as well as to find exercises that will help with improving cardiovascular fitness, flexibility, and endurance.

Background material on FITNESS *can be found under titles such as* AEROBICS; AGING; EXERCISE; *and* FITNESS TESTING. *Important related subjects include* DIET AND DISEASE; MULTIVITAMIN; NUTRITION; *and* VITAMIN SUPPLEMENT. *See specific topics such as* KEGEL EXERCISES; MUSCLE; SALT; SPRAIN; STRAIN; WALKING; *and* WALKING AIDS.

Fitness Testing

Tests that measure a person's fitness level.

Doctors may conduct fitness testing for several reasons. The tests can help to determine an appropriate exercise program for an individual, and then to monitor that person's progress. Fitness tests are also a good way of testing the heart, to see how it performs. In this case, the testing may reveal problems or weaknesses that are not apparent in the resting heart, such as insufficient oxygen or blood flow during stress.

Fitness testing is usually done in a doctor's office, often as part of a general physical examination that includes blood tests, body fat analysis, and measure of height and weight. The resting heart rate is taken, and then an activity, such as walking on a treadmill or riding a stationary bicycle, is performed. The heart rate is tracked as the work intensifies. When the exercise is finished, the length of time necessary for the heart to return to its resting rate is also measured. Based on this information, a doctor can prescribe an exercise program that the person can perform, and then increase, in order to improve overall fitness.

Fixation

A Freudian term indicating arrested emotional development in one of the three stages of childhood sexual development.

Freud theorized that the key markers of childhood development are sexual stages, where the child's concerns focus on physical gratification. In the oral stage, the child is concerned with putting things in his mouth. An individual fixated in this stage may, for example, become a compulsive overeater. The anal stage occurs during the time of toilet training, and fixations in this stage tend toward aggressive behavior and obsessive compulsive disorders. The phallic stage refers to a period of sexual awakening and masturbation. Sexual fantasies and obsessions are thought to be fixations at the phallic stage of development. *See also* CHILD DEVELOPMENT.

Flail Chest

Incorrect breathing motion as a result of a chest injury.

A flail chest results when a violent injury causes the ribs to fracture such that a portion of the chest wall becomes isolated. The isolated part of the chest functions abnormally as a result, moving in when inhaling and out when exhaling (the opposite of normal breathing). Breathing becomes disrupted, and the condition may lead to respiratory failure. It may also cause pain when breathing or coughing, greater susceptibility to infection, and lung collapse.

Turning a person onto the injured side may help in an emergency. Once seen by a physician, local anesthetic and pain-relievers will be given to help the patient ventilate. A firm chest wrap will also help the ribs to heal and, in some instances, oxygen supplementation may be required. In most cases, surgery is not necessary. The condition usually clears up once the ribs are healed. *See also* EMERGENCY FIRST STEPS *and* RESPIRATORY FAILURE.

Flatfoot

A foot without an arch.

All people are born without arches. Feet are flat until the ligaments and muscles that help to support the feet develop, usually by age six. For some people, however, this support structure is weak and the feet remain flat. In most cases, there is no known reason for this, though sometimes it does appear to have a hereditary link. As an adult, the arches may fall, sometimes because of a sudden increase in weight, or a weakening of the muscles due to disease. Flat feet may cause pain when standing or walking for long periods of time. Many people with flat feet have no complaints.

The most common way to reduce pain from flat feet is either to put insoles or orthotics into shoes. Insoles are cushioned inserts that can usually be purchased in drug stores or athletic shoe stores. They reduce shock, and provide support for heels and arches. However, these usually only fit in one shoe and tend to wear out quickly. Orthotics are a better long-term solution. For a pair of orthotics, a podiatrist makes a plaster cast of the foot, and then the orthotics are made from leather and cork. They can be put into most pairs of shoes, and can last up to ten years. *See also* FOOT *and* ORTHOPEDICS.

Flatulence

Production of excessive amounts of intestinal gas.

Intestinal gas consists of oxygen, nitrogen, hydrogen, carbon dioxide, and methane. Small traces of other gases, such as hydrogen sulfide and ammonia, are the sources of the odor that is characteristic of this gas. Some of the gas comes from inhaled air; other components are produced by chemical reactions within the intestines, including fermentation performed by bacteria within the large intestine.

Foods such as peas, beans, wheat, oats, bran, brussels sprouts, cabbage, and corn may contribute to excess gas. Lactose intolerance can also be a factor.

Flatulence is not a serious condition from a medical point of view. A change in diet, which includes the avoidance of certain foods, may help alleviate the problem. *See also* COLON; FLATUS; INTESTINE; LACTOSE; *and* LACTOSE INTOLERANCE.

Flatus

Gas or air that is located in the intestines.

Flatus is produced in the colon. It is composed of oxygen, nitrogen, hydrogen, carbon dioxide, methane, and small traces of hydrogen sulfide and ammonia. The hydrogen sulfide and ammonia are the source of the characteristic odor of the gas. Some of the components of flatus come from inhaled air. Others are produced by fermentation resulting from the activity of bacteria within the large intestine. *See also* COLON; FLATULENCE; *and* INTESTINE.

Flatworm

Parasitic worms medically referred to as platy-helminthes.

Flatworms capable of causing human illness are the tapeworms (cestodes) and the flukes (tremetodes).

Types. Common tapeworms include *Taenia saginata* (beef tapeworm) and *Taenia solium* (pork tapeworm). Victims of tapeworm infestation may not experience symptoms, but in some cases there is abdominal cramping, diarrhea, nausea, muscle spasms, and pain.

Flukes infest animals and humans. Once infested, these worms can cause damage to the liver, and to the intestines and bladder (schistosomiasis). Symptoms in the early stages of infestation may cause itching and a rash. Later symptoms involve fever, chills, abdominal pain or pain during urination, and lymph node enlargement.

Prevention. Tapeworm infestation is prevented by thoroughly cooking meat and carefully washing hands when preparing food. Fluke infestation is prevented by diligent sanitation measures, testing of natural bodies of water, and prohibition of swimming in unsafe areas.

Treatment for tapeworm is through antihelmintic drugs. Intestinal flukes infestation is equally treated with an antihelmintic drug (praziquantel). *See also* ANTIHELMINTIC DRUGS; FLUKE; ITCHING; LIVER FLUKE; PARASITE; SCHISTOSOMIASIS; *and* TAPEWORM INFESTATION.

Floaters

Faint images that float across the field of vision.

Clumps of gelatinous protein in the vitreous humor, the jellylike substance of the eyeball behind the lens, cast extremely faint shadows on the retina that dart away elusively when the eye tries to follow them and drift in peripheral vision when the eye remains still. They usually go unnoticed and do not impair vision or harm the eye.

The vitreous liquefies, pulls away, and shrinks from the retina with age. This process—posterior vitreous detachment—causes floaters, and their appearance may be disturbing, but they do not impair vision or harm the eye. However, if they are extremely annoying, during reading, for instance, and do not go away after you move your eyes, it is prudent to see the doctor. Sudden dark clouds of floaters and flashes of light may be signs of retinal detachment, while vitreous hemorrhage is likely at the sight of a large red floater. Both demand medical attention. *See also* EYE, DISORDERS OF: LENS; RETINA; RETINAL DETACHMENT; *and* VITREOUS HEMORRHAGE.

Flossing, Dental

Preventative dental procedure involving soft nylon or silk thread.

Flossing is as important to good dental health as brushing the teeth. A toothbrush can clean the surface of each tooth, but even the most sophisticated of toothbrushes cannot get between the teeth to remove particles of food. When these food particles remain in place for long periods of time, they can start the process that leads to tooth decay. Moreover, food particles attract bacteria that cause gum disease (periodontitis) and bad breath (halitosis).

Flossing should be done at least once a day for the best chance of having healthy teeth and gums. The proper method is to cut off a strip of floss and run it between each tooth, taking care to remove any food that may be caught. Some people prefer finer floss, especially if their teeth are particularly close together. Others prefer a wider floss; floss even comes in ribbon form. Some companies market floss packets in which each piece of floss comes attached to its own plastic handle.

Many people neglect to floss because they fail to understand its importance, or because they think flossing is difficult. Getting into the habit of regular flossing is a critical step in making sure the teeth and gums remain healthy. *See also* HALITOSIS *and* PERIODONTITIS.

Flow Cytometry

The measuring and counting of cells as they flow past a focused beam of light.

Flow cytometry is a means for counting and measuring cells, using a device known as a cytometer. Thousands of cells may be studied as they flow one at a time through a focused light beam, generally a laser. The automated technique is especially useful for analyzing the arrangement and amount of DNA content of tumor cells. This test is helpful in identifying benign from malignant cells, as the pattern of DNA in cancer cells differs from normal cells. Flow cytometry can be used to diagnose lymphomas and leukemia, evaluate the immune system, assess the growth rates of cells—a critical factor in the diagnosis of cancers, and monitor the effects of anticancer drug treatment. *See also* CANCER; CELL; CYTOLOGY; IMMUNE SYSTEM; LEUKEMIA; *and* LYMPHOMA.

Fluctuation

A term that means varying and unstable; used as a diagnostic indicator.

Fluctuation refers to a variation in fluid pressure or fluid flow, which a doctor may locate simply through feeling and pressing on the body (palpation). When fluctuation is detected in the lower abdomen, ascites—an accumulation of fluid within the abdominal cavity—is usually present. A fluctuation in a more limited region may indicate abscess or cyst formation. *See also* ABDOMEN; ABSCESS; ASCITES; *and* CYST.

Fluke

Parasitic worm belonging to the class *Trematoda*.

Flukes constitute a wide range of worms that infest humans, and are responsible for causing serious damage to internal organs. Most people who contract a fluke infection will not experience any symptoms. When there are symptoms of fluke infestation, these symptoms are non-specific to the disease (i.e., headache, abdominal pains, nausea) and may be difficult to diagnose.

TYPES
• **Blood Flukes.** Flukes of the genus *Schistosoma*, known as blood flukes, live in the veins of the pelvic region and cause the disease schistosomiasis. The disease produces scarring of the liver and walls of the intestine or bladder. Blood may also appear in the urine. It is contracted through contact with freshwater.

• **Intestinal flukes** that infest humans cause abdominal pain, diarrhea and intestinal obstruction. They are acquired by eating contaminated freshwater fish or contaminated vegetation.

• **Lung flukes** inhabit certain crabs and crayfish and may be passed to humans, producing respiratory ailments and hemorrhaging.

• **Liver flukes** are contracted though the ingestion of freshwater vegetation (typically watercress). These worms infest the liver and bile-ducts, often producing inflammation of the gallbladder and acute abdominal pain.

Treatment. All are treated with antiparasitic (antihelmintic) medications. *See* ANTIHELMINTIC DRUGS; LIVER FLUKE; PARASITE; SCHISOTSOMIASIS; *and* WORM INFESTATION.

Fluorescein

Also known as Fluor-I-strip, Fluorescite, and Funduscien.

A red crystalline substance used for diagnostic purposes.

Fluorescein sodium is a red crystalline powder, generally used to detect lesions or foreign bodies in the cornea of the eye, as well as certain retinal abnormalities. The chemical enhances details of the veins and other features in the retina when it is injected intravenously (fluorescein angiography).

USES
Fluorescein is used to detect retinal defects that include formation of new blood vessels (choroidal neovascularization), diabetes-related retinal disorder (proliferative diabetic retinopathy), and light toxicity.

PROCEDURE

Following dilation of the pupil with a special agent, a fluorescein dye may be injected, which is passed into the eye's blood circulation. The natural fluorescence of the dye may then be seen and photographed by means of a special camera. *See also* ANGIOGRAPHY; CORNEA; EYE, DISORDERS OF; *and* RETINA.

Fluoridation

Supplementing fluoride content of water as preventive dentistry.

Programs designed to supplement the level of fluoride in drinking water were begun in the mid-1900s, when it was discovered that the mineral fluoride was responsible for preventing dental cavities, or caries, in the populations of industrialized areas. It has since been proven that the right amount of fluoride in water, 0.7 to 1.2 parts per million, reduces the incidence of dental caries and extractions, especially during a person's formative years.

Many studies have confirmed the effectiveness and safety of water fluoridation. However, excessive ingestion of fluoride can cause problems such as tooth discoloration. A dentist should be able to advise whether fluoride supplements are needed if drinking water is not flouridated. *See also* CARIES, DENTAL *and* FLUORIDE.

Fluoride

Mineral that occurs naturally in soil and water and is useful in formation of teeth.

Fluoride is a form of the chemical element fluorine and is best known for its ability to help prevent tooth decay. Fluoride is found naturally in water, although sometimes it is in such low concentration that more must be added (fluoridation) to make it effectively protective for the teeth. It can also be added to toothpaste, mouthwash, and other dental solutions, as well as some other food substances. Fluoridation is mostly done in industrialized countries.

Fluorine in its gaseous phase probably does not occur in the Earth's crust. It occurs as compounds in rocks and soil. As water runs over the rocks and soil, it washes over these compounds and releases the fluoride ion. Because fluorine is a common element, it is found in virtually all bodies of water.

When people ingest fluoride through water, it goes through the bloodstream and into the saliva. It bathes the teeth constantly and keeps them protected against decay. This is particularly important for young children, whose teeth are just beginning to form. Fluoride that is ingested in this manner is known as systemic fluoride.

In areas in which too little fluoride is found in the water, fluoride can be added to the water, or in some cases to other substances—not just toothpaste or mouthwash, but also milk and salt, for instance. This is known as topical fluoride. *See also* FLUORIDATION *and* TOOTH DECAY.

Folic Acid

One of the vitamins that make up the B complex.

Folic acid (folate) and vitamin B_{12} function together in the synthesis of DNA and in cell production, particularly in the production of blood cells. Therefore, a deficiency of folic acid can result in anemia.

Folates are found in leafy green vegetables, liver, legumes, yeast, strawberries, and oranges. Large amounts of folic acid can be obtained by eating fresh fruits or vegetables daily. It should be noted, however, that cooking damages folic acid content, and antacids reduce folic acid absorption. Supplemental folic acid is absolutely essential before and during pregnancy, since sufficient amounts of folic acid can prevent neural tube birth defects, such as spina bifida. All women of child-bearing age should receive adequate amounts of folic acid, either by diet or by supplements.

Megadoses of folic acid may mask symptoms of vitamin B_{12} deficiency in certain susceptible individuals. *See also* NUTRITION; SPINA BIFIDA; *and* VITAMIN B.

Follicle

A small body cavity out of which hair grows.

An example of a follicle is a hair follicle, which is the site where body and scalp hairs are attached to the skin. The total number of hair follicles for an adult human is five million, with one million of these on the head and 100,000 on the scalp. The only places on the body that are devoid of hair follicles are the soles of the feet, the palms of the hands, and the mucous membranes of the lips and genitals. *See also* ELECTROLYSIS; HAIR; HAIR GROWTH; *and* HAIR REMOVAL.

Follicle-Stimulating Hormone

A hormone that regulates the sex glands.

Follicle-stimulating hormone, or FSH, is one of the hormones produced by the anterior pituitary gland. One of the gonadotropin hormones, FSH regulates fertility and sexual development. In women, FSH stimulates the ovaries to cause maturation of the egg during the menstrual cycle. The levels of FSH vary throughout a woman's monthly cycle. In men, FSH stimulates the production of sperm. A test to measure the levels of FSH in a woman can determine reasons for infertility or whether or not a woman is experiencing menopause. *See also* GONADOTROPIN HORMONES *and* PITUITARY GLAND.

Folliculitis

Inflammation of the hair follicles.

Folliculitis is a term used to refer to a group of skin conditions that occur when hair follicles become inflamed. Symptoms usually include a rash or raised bump on the skin above the hair follicle, although they vary depending on the condition.

Causes of folliculitis include infection by bacteria, yeasts, and fungi, and irritation from hair removal. Bacterial infections causing folliculitis are usually due to the *Staphyloccus aureus* bacteria. Boils are an example of a symptom of this infection. Yeast infections due to folliculitis are most commonly caused by the *Pityrosporum ovale* yeast. Pityrosporum folliculitis is an itchy type of folliculitis usually affecting young adults. Ringworm of the scalp is caused by a fungus and may cause folliculitis, resulting in scaling and hair loss. Shaving, waxing, and certain moisturizers may cause folliculitis, as may chemicals such as coal, tar, and cutting oils. Another cause of the disorder is the overuse of topical steroids.

Treatment. Bacterial infections are treated with soap and water, antiseptics, and antibiotics. Treatment for yeast infections includes propylene glycol, or antifungal lotions, creams, or tablets. Fungal infections are treated with prescription oral antifungal agents. *See also* ANTIFUNGAL DRUGS; BACTERIA; FUNGI; *and* YEASTS;

Fomites

Inanimate objects that become the vehicle by which a disease is transmitted.

The fomite has itself been contaminated by contact with a person or other carrier of disease. It may be microscopic in size, such as a dust particle, or larger, such as a piece of clothing, a tool, or a doorknob. While many diseases are transmitted via airborne particles or droplets of water, a number of diseases (i.e., AIDS) can be transmitted by contaminated needles, or instruments in a doctor's office. *See also* INFECTIOUS DISEASE.

Fontanelle

Also known as a soft spot

Space on a baby's head where the bones of the skull have not yet fused together.

The fontanelles allow a baby to fit through the birth canal more easily, and also leave room for the brain to grow. There are two fontanelles, one located towards the front of the head (anterior) and one located towards the back of the head (posterior). The fontanelles generally close between the ages of seven and 19 months.

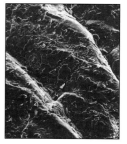

Hair Follicle.
Above is a scanning electron micrograph of the surface of human skin from which a hair grows. There are millions of follicles such as this one located all over the body.

Food Additives

Substances that do not naturally occur in foods, such as chemical preservatives.

Food additives are used to prevent or delay spoilage; to enhance color, flavor, or texture; to increase nutritional value; or to replace nutrients lost in processing.

There are approximately 3,000 intentional additives, most of which have been approved for use by the Food and Drug Administration and classified as Generally Recognized as Safe (GRAS). In addition to these are the more than 10,000 indirect additives that enter the food supply unintentionally, and include substances present during growing, processing, or packaging, as well as environmental pollutants. Most additives are used in such small quantities that they present little or no risk to health, are considered safe by doctors and nutritionists, and may even help to reduce illness caused by foodborne material that may cause disease (pathogens).

Sometimes basic minerals and vitamins are added to foods to prevent deficiencies. For example, iodine has long been added to bread in order to prevent goiter and other deficiency-caused diseases, and vitamin D is added to milk and other beverages to enable proper calcium absorption. Some food additives, such as BHT and BHA (often added to cereals), have significant health benefits.

Other additives, however, may pose problems for some consumers. Sugar additives may pose a risk for diabetics. Sulfur-based compounds (sulfites) are used as preservatives in food and certain over-the-counter medications, but also cause life-threatening allergic reactions in asthmatics. Use of sulfites in the United States has been reduced by the government, although they are still added to foods like dried fruit and shrimp, and may be formed naturally in most wines.

> *It is also important to understand* ARTIFICIAL SWEETENERS; CHINESE RESTAURANT SYNDROME; *and* NUTRITION. *Also refer to* DIET AND DISEASE; FOOD CONTAMINATION; *and* NITRITES.

Resources on Food and Nutrition

Groff, James L. and Sareen S. Gropper, *Advanced Nutrition and Human Metabolism* (1999); Heim-burger, Douglas C. and Roland L. Weinsier, *Hand-book of Clinical Nutrition* (1997); National Academy Press Food and Nutrition Board, Recommended Dietary Allowances(1989); Shils, Maurice E., et al., Modern Nutrition in Health and Disease (1999); American Dietetic Association, Tel. (800) 366-1655, Online: www.eatright.org; Center for Nutrition Policy and Promotion, Tel. (202) 418-2312, Online: www. usda.gov/cnpp; Food and Drug Adminis-tration, Tel. (888) INFOFDA, Online: www.fda.gov; www.nycornell.org/medi-cine/nutrition/index.html.

Food Allergy

An allergic reaction caused by a component in food.

As in any other type of allergic reaction, the immune system of a person with a food allergy will treat relatively innocuous molecules as foreign invaders and will mount a response, complete with the release of histamines and antibodies designed to specifically combine with and neutralize the invader. A food allergy is not the same thing, chemically speaking, as a food intolerance, although they may share some of the same symptoms.

Fewer than one percent of the general public has a true food allergy. Children have a higher percentage of allergies than adults, but most of these allergies are outgrown by age six. It is very unusual to develop a food allergy past age 30.

Causes. The foods most likely to provoke an allergic response are cow's milk, egg whites, peanuts and other legumes, nuts, and wheat. The tendency to have food allergies, though not the specific allergy itself, runs in families.

Symptoms of food allergy include nausea and vomiting; diarrhea; hives; swelling of the lips, eyes, face, and tongue; nasal congestion; breathing difficulties; convulsions; and even anaphylactic shock, a severe and life-threatening allergic reaction involving a sudden drop in blood pressure.

The seriousness of a food allergy varies greatly according to the individual. Some people find them a source of mild distress; others have increasingly severe symptoms. In the most severe cases, an individual may go into anaphylactic shock and death may result without immediate medical intervention. As with any allergy, more than one exposure to the allergy-causing agent (allergen) is required for a reaction. In most instances, digestive symptoms from dairy products are caused by a lactose intolerance, not an allergy.

Diagnosis. Determining the cause of the allergic reaction often takes time, as it is necessary to isolate each suspected food and eliminate it from the diet.

Treatment. Antihistamines can be administered to alleviate the majority of symptoms, including hives. However, if a person is having a severe allergic reaction, medical attention should be sought.

Prevention. Once a food allergy has been established, that particular food should be avoided. *See also* ALLERGEN.

Food and Drug Administration

Federal agency that regulates the purity, efficacy, and safety of food and medicines.

The Food and Drug Administration (FDA) enforces the Food, Drug, and Cosmetic Act and related public health laws. It does this by regulating commercially produced food, prescriptions and over-the-counter medicines, cosmetics, animal foods, veterinary drugs, and medical devices.

For drug approval, the FDA usually examines tests and trials done or commissioned by pharmaceutical companies; a certain number of tests and research are done in their own laboratories. In deciding approval of both drugs and medical equipment, the benefits and risks are carefully assessed in order to determine whether the product in question will be safe and effective for the public. Devices that are implanted, such as pacemakers, and those that are life-supporting or sustaining must also be approved before they can be sold. After approval, the FDA monitors safety by maintaining records of cases.

The FDA is responsible for the purity of the country's blood supply, inspecting all aspects of blood banks, and is also in charge of vaccines and insulin, which are prepared from living organisms and their products.

In regulating food safety, FDA scientists test food samples for the presence of unacceptable levels of contaminants, such as bacteria and pesticide residues. All foods are subject to regulation except for meat, poultry, and eggs, which are principally regulated and inspected by the U.S. Department of Agriculture. However, it is the FDA that sets acceptable levels for drug residues in meat, poultry, milk, and eggs, and for certain chemical contaminants in fish. It also sets limits for pesticides in all foods, and tests, with the exception of poultry, for pesticide residues and other such contaminants. The FDA oversees all food labeling, except for that of eggs, poultry, meat, and alcohol.

If a product or company is found in violation of the FDA's regulations, the company can either voluntarily recall the product, or (in cases of non-cooperation) the FDA can seek legal action to implement the regulations and have the unsafe product seized and destroyed. *See also* FOOD CONTAMINATION *and* FOOD POISONING.

Food Contamination

A situation in which pollutants, bacteria, spores, or other microorganisms enter the food supply.

Sources of food contamination usually result from disease-causing (pathogenic) microorganisms or environmental pollutants.

The most pervasive of food-borne pathogens seems to be the bacteria *Escherichia coli*, which has been identified in a potentially lethal strain. This strain has contaminated meat in the United States and Japan, and has caused outbreaks traced to undercooked hamburgers and other meat products. In children under the age of ten, it can cause hemolytic-uremia syndrome, a potentially deadly form of kidney failure. Adults are less likely to develop such severe symptoms, but may develop blood clots and become comatose.

The globalization of the food industry and the importation of out-of-season produce has resulted in outbreaks of hepatitis A and cyclospora. Health officials have also found harmful bacteria in vegetables and fruits. Fresh fruits and vegetables should be thoroughly washed before consumption.

POLLUTANTS
Environmental contaminants can include pollutants, pesticides, and residues of antibiotics and hormones given to livestock.

Fish and seafood are sometimes contaminated by high levels of pollutants from their environment, especially heavy metals such as mercury, levels of which are amplified in predator fish, such as bluefish. Minamata disease (caused by mercury poisoning in fish and shellfish) is a primary example of the catastrophic effects environmental toxins can cause when they enter the food chain. (In 1997, over 12,000 people consumed contaminated fish from Japan's Minamata Bay; over 1,000 of those individuals died.)

PREVENTION

Since it is nearly impossible for regulatory forces to stop all contamination, one way to reduce risk of exposure to food contaminants is to eat a varied diet. If you do hunt or fish, follow guidelines set by local environmental agencies for eating fish or game from a polluted habitat.

While organic foods are no more nutritious than nonorganic foods, they are an option for people worried about pesticide residues, hormones, and antibiotics. Organic foods are labeled as such only after stringent certification procedures. Some authorities do not feel that organic foods are safer than nonorganic foods.

FOOD CONTAMINATION *is closely allied with such topics as* CHINESE RESTAURANT SYNDROME; FOOD ALLERGY; FOOD AND DRUG ADMINISTRATION; *and* FOOD INTOLERANCE. *Illnesses caused by this include* HEPATITIS *and* MENINGITIS. *See also* ENVIRONMENTAL MEDICINE *and* PUBLIC HEALTH.

Food Fad

Severe and often unhealthy restrictions of the diet.

The term food fad refers to any preference for or aversion to, a particular food or foods that is carried to extremes. Such fads are common in toddlers, adolescents, chronic dieters, and people suffering from stress. Extreme preferences or aversions of this type are usually short-lived. In some cases, however, the condition can affect a person's health and develop into an eating disorder (anorexia nervosa or bulimia).

The term food fad may also refer to the "fad diets" that comprise a significant portion of the multibillion dollar diet industry. Studies suggest that repeatedly going on extremely low calorie diets (in essence, periods of semistarvation) causes an increasing cycle of weight loss and weight gain. The body reacts by lowering its energy processing (metabolic) rate, which may result in weight gain. Most consequential is that these diets can be extremely dangerous to health. Fad dieting can also cause nutritional imbalances, loss of muscle tissue (including heart muscle), and even bio-chemical imbalances. Current high-fat, high-protein diets are believed to be unsafe and, in addition to inducing ketosis, can also raise cholesterol levels. *See also* ANOREXIA NERVOSA; BULIMIA; DIET AND DISEASE; EATING DISORDERS; KETOSIS; *and* METABOLISM.

Food Intolerance

A negative reaction to a food that is not caused by food poisoning or psychological factors.

Although often confused with food allergy, food intolerance is a different condition. In a true allergy, a person has a response to a specific food, involving the production of histamines, which irritate the gastrointestinal and respiratory systems as well as the skin. These produce symptoms ranging from digestive upset, to difficulty in breathing, to the appearance of hives and rashes. In a food intolerance, there may be similar symptoms but the symptoms are not caused by the body's histamines. Usually food intolerance is due to the absence of an enzyme that is needed to properly and completely digest a particular food.

Symptoms of food intolerance vary in type and intensity depending on the individual and his or her physical and emotional makeup. Some common, although nonspecific, symptoms include: adbominal pain; asthma; bloating; constipation; difficulty swallowing; fatigue; irritable bowel syndrome; muscle aches and pains; headaches; itchy and puffy eyes; anxiety; hyperactivity; and disorientation.

Sufferers commonly have difficulty digesting foods such as lactose (the sugar found in milk); gluten, which is found in wheat; monosodium glutamate (MSG), which is a common flavor enhancer; sulfites, which are used as preservatives; tartrazine, which is a yellow dye used in food, drugs, and cosmetics; and salicylates, which are found in a wide variety of fruits.

Treatment. It may be necessary for the person to work with a physician to isolate the suspect food and eliminate it from his or her diet. *See also* FOOD ALLERGY; GLUTEN; IRRITABLE BOWEL SYNDROME; LACTOSE; *and* LACTOSE INTOLERANCE.

Food Poisoning

Result of contamination by a variety of bacteria that have entered the food supply.

Food poisoning is generally caused by endotoxins, that is, toxic substances produced by bacteria such as *Salmonella, Campylobacter, Staphylococcus aureus, Listeria,* or *Escherichia coli.* These bacteria contaminate the food before or during preparation, and survive the cooking process. Sometimes food poisoning occurs because foods are left unrefrigerated for prolonged periods of time. If live bacteria inhabit food that is consumed, they may continue to multiply in the intestines and make the sufferer very sick. *Salmonella, Campylobacter, E. coli,* and *Listeria* are all present in uncooked food and thrive in the gastrointestinal tract. *Staphylococcus aureus* and *Clostridium botulinum* bacteria, for example, produce toxins that can cause anaphylactic shock and, in rare cases, death.

Food may be tainted after cooking by cooks who do not wash their hands after touching raw meat and then handle the finished dish.

Symptoms of food poisoning generally pass so quickly that the organism responsible is rarely identified. Symptoms are usually abrupt in onset and generally include stomach cramps and abdominal pain, diarrhea, vomiting, and general weakness. Fever usually does not occur in cases of food poisoning—if fever is present, another diagnosis is more probable.

Food poisoning usually lasts only between 24 and 36 hours and concludes without treatment. It can, however, be life-threatening in the very young, the very old, and those with compromised immune systems. Infection by *E. coli* is particularly dangerous for these individuals.

Preventing Food Poisoning

Although not every case of food poisoning can be prevented, measures can be taken to reduce risks:
- Cook food thoroughly.
- Wash hands and utensils with warm water and soap before and after each step of food preparation.
- Use a separate cutting board for poultry, meat, and fish, and disinfect cutting boards with a solution of two teaspoons of bleach to one quart of hot water. Wash the cutting board after disinfecting.
- Never return cooked meat to a cutting board where it was prepared before cooking.
- Macaroni, potato, and tuna salads should be refrigerated immediately after serving.
- Leftovers should generally not be kept longer than one or two days.
- Keep prepared foods at safe temperatures, particularly foods containing animal ingredients—bacteria can multiply and produce toxins in a few hours.
- Raw meat or fish and undercooked eggs present a high risk of food poisoning.

If you suspect severe food poisoning in a high-risk individual, immediately contact your doctor or go to the emergency room. If you or someone you know has food poisoning and is unable to stop the diarrhea or vomiting, is feeling dizzy or faint, or is having difficulty breathing, call a doctor.

Drinking water (hydration) is essential in situations of prolonged vomiting or diarrhea. In severe cases, it may be necessary to inject fluids into the veins (intravenously) or to have prescription medicine inserted (suppository) in the rectum—such as promethazine (Phenergan) or prochlorperazine (Compazine).

For background information about FOOD POISONING **see** FOOD CONTAMINATION; PTOMAINE POISONING; SALMONELLA; **and** STAPHYLOCOCCAL INFECTIONS. **Further details can also be found in** ENDOTOXIN; ENTEROTOXIN; **and** PARASITE.

Foot

The structure that supports and propels the body.

One-eighth of the skeleton's bones are in the feet—26 bones per foot. The calcaneus, or heel bone, joins the second largest bone in the ankle, the talus. Five smaller bones take up the instep: the navicular, the cuboid, and a row of three bones called the cuneiforms. The last four join the metatarsals, which extend to the phalanges, or bones of the toes. Two bones comprise the big toe; three comprise each of the rest.

Nerves and blood vessels are located in front of and behind the inside of the ankle joint. Muscles that control the foot and toes connect to tendons that wrap around the ankle. Muscles and ligaments support a natural arch. Fat, fascia—fibrous tissue—and tough skin comprise the sole.

Common injuries include fractures of the heel bone, usually from a fall, and of the toes and metatarsals. Clawfoot, flatfoot, and clubfoot are common deformities affecting the foot. *See also* MUSCLES.

Footdrop

Inability to raise the foot correctly.

Footdrop is diagnosed when the foot hangs from the ankle and drags on the ground, making it difficult to walk. Footdrop is a symptom of another condition, such as an inflammation or injury of a nerve that affects the foot, or diseases, such as diabetes or multiple sclerosis. Spinal cord injury, such as a disk prolapse, can also cause a lack of control in the foot. Rupture of the anterior tibialis tendon is a rare cause of footdrop.

Treatment. The condition that causes footdrop must be treated first, after which treatment of any remaining weakness in the foot must be addressed. An orthopedic brace known as a drop foot splint can help to keep the foot in the correct position while walking. *See also* BRACE; DISK PROLAPSE; *and* ORTHOPEDIC.

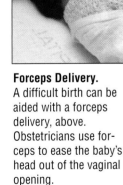

Forceps Delivery. A difficult birth can be aided with a forceps delivery, above. Obstetricians use forceps to ease the baby's head out of the vaginal opening.

Forceps

A surgical instrument that resembles a pair of tweezers or tongs and is used during various surgical procedures.

Forceps are used for grasping body tissues or other materials, such as gauze, during surgical procedures. Varying in size and design, forceps may have long or short jaws, locking handles, scissor-like handles, or fine teeth, depending on their purpose. For example, forceps used for holding body tissue have fine but rounded teeth at the tips of their blades to prevent damage. Obstetrical forceps have wide, cupped blades to delicately hold the sides of a baby's head. Other forceps include bone-holding forceps, sinus forceps, forceps with claw-like hooks (volsella), and dissecting forceps. *See also* CHILDBIRTH.

Forceps Delivery

The use of a curved, tong-like instrument to aid in vaginal births.

The use of forceps during delivery is considered if there are indications that the baby is being deprived of oxygen, if there are other signs of fetal distress, or if the mother does not have the energy or ability to push the baby out.

In the past, when doctors used forceps during a delivery, they often had to reach high into the vaginal tract, which could cause bruising or lacerations to the mother. Currently, forceps are only used once the cervix is completely dilated and the baby's head is within two inches of the vaginal opening. The use of forceps may still result in bruising and swelling of the baby's face and scalp, however, these injuries usually heal without complications within a few days.

Vacuum Extraction. Vacuum extraction can be used as a replacement for forceps delivery. This method involves a plastic cup that fits over the baby's head and the application of a vacuum pump to gently pull the baby out of the birth canal. Vacuum extraction may also cause slight bruising to the baby's head, which will heal in a short period of time. *See also* CHILDBIRTH COMPLICATIONS *and* VACUUM EXTRACTION.

Foreign Body

An object or particle in the human body that does not belong in the location in which it is found.

A foreign object in the body may obstruct function and could jeopardize a person's health or life. Generally, foreign objects are introduced into the body accidentally, but they are sometimes introduced deliberately by certain individuals. Children and people under the influence of alcohol and other drugs are most likely to deliberately inhale, swallow, or otherwise introduce a foreign object into their systems.

Airway Obstruction. A foreign object may become lodged in the airways and cause choking, which may require application of the Heimlich maneuver. If the object becomes lodged in the lungs, it may cause pneumonia or collapse of the lung. Foreign objects in the airway require emergency medical intervention.

Foreign Objects in the Gastrointestinal Tract. An estimated 80 to 90 percent of foreign bodies in the gastrointestinal tract pass through the digestive system spontaneously and without complications. Another 10 to 20 percent of foreign bodies require medical assistance and less than one percent require surgical intervention. Sharp objects require removal from the stomach to prevent perforation of the intestines.

Foreign Objects in the Ear. A foreign object in the ear should be removed by a physician, as attempting to remove it without proper instruments could have the opposite effect, pushing the object further into the ear canal.

Other Common Foreign Object Obstructions. Foreign bodies also commonly become lodged in the urethra, rectum, and vagina. Splinters in the skin are also considered foreign bodies. *See also* FIRST AID *and* HEIMLICH MANEUVER.

Forensic Medicine

The area of medicine that deals with the law.

Forensic medicine, also known as legal medicine or forensics, is the branch of medical science that examines questions of law. Forensic medicine uses applicable medical principles, as well as various dental, psychological, biological, chemical, and mechanical techniques, to investigate such legal questions as the cause of a person's death, or the context of a crime involving death or injury.

History. While forensic medicine was first recognized as a medical specialty early in the 19th century, medical testimony has been used in legal cases for more than 1500 years. Great Britain first established a coroner system in 1194. The government (Crown) appointed officials to examine each death and assess whether any were due to suicide, as this was against the religion of the Church. These "crowners" evolved into the modern coroner, who today investigates deaths thought to be from unnatural causes.

The first systematic presentation of forensic medicine was given by Fortunatus Fidelis, an Italian, in 1598. Earlier, the purpose of forensic medicine had been to determine whether or not a given death was the result of suicide. Over time, simple inspection of a corpse for that specific purpose broadened into a more scientific examination of the dead body, which became the modern practice of autopsy.

DNA Evidence

A common forensic technique is DNA analysis. Forensic experts use this technique to establish the identity of a deceased person, or to prove that a particular suspect was present at a crime scene. The forensic specialist might, for example, identify foreign skin fragments under the fingernails of the deceased person. Using a technique called polymerase chain reaction (PCR), the specialist can take even small, broken fragments of DNA, compare the DNA to a sample from the suspect, and determine whether the skin particles came from the suspect.

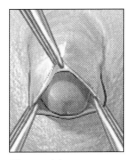

Circumcision.
Above, is the removal of the foreskin of the penis during a circumcision. The procedure is generally performed on newborn male babies.

The American colonies adopted the British coroner system in the 17th century. In 1915, New York City instituted a medical examiner system that became the model for other such departments throughout the country. The medical examiner's office developed laboratories for toxicology, blood grouping, and other procedures. Currently, the medical examiner decides if there is a need to perform an autopsy on a body. This individual also investigates deaths that are due to criminal violence, accidents, or suicides, as well as those that occur when a person is apparently in good health and is unattended by a physician.

Procedure. The primary tool of forensic medicine is the autopsy, a postmortem examination of a body. In modern forensic medicine, the autopsy has become an effective way for a forensic physician to determine the cause of death. If, for example, a weapon was responsible for the patient's death, the doctor can often determine, in detail, the type of weapon used and the context of its use. The doctor may even be able to determine the angle and distance from which a gun was fired.

The examiner's role in the medical investigation of unnatural death, especially in a suspected homicide, begins with an examination of the scene of death before the body is disturbed. The body and clothes, as well as the surrounding environment, are searched for evidence. The body is then transferred to the examiner's morgue, where an autopsy is performed and body fluids and organ samples are sent to specific laboratories for analysis.

Among the tools used by forensic medicine are DNA analysis, blood typing (matching blood types), fingerprint analysis, and facial reconstruction. Once all the data has been examined, the examiner attempts to ascertain the cause and context of death.

> *Other topics related to* FORENSIC MEDICINE *can be found in* AUTOPSY; BLOOD; BLOOD GROUPS; DEATH; DNA; GENE; POSTMORTEM EXAMINATION; *and* TESTS. *Subjects that inform this science include* DENTISTRY; GENETICS; ONCOGENES; SPOUSAL ABUSE; *and* SUBSTANCE ABUSE. *See also* FORMALDEHYDE.

Foreskin

Also known as the prepuce

The loose skin around the head of the penis.

The foreskin, or prepuce, loosely shrouds the head of the penis. During arousal, the foreskin retracts. Six months after birth, the foreskin slowly detaches from the head (glans) of the penis. It may remain taut in boys three or four years of age. Unless proper cleaning of the glans is hindered, there is no need to see a doctor. Circumcision, the removal of the foreskin, is a religious or hygienic practice in some cultures.

Formaldehyde

A chemical used as a preservative, disinfectant, or fumigant.

Formaldehyde is a colorless, pungent gas that may be prepared in a liquid solution for use as a preservative or astringent, or to clean and disinfect dishes, instruments, or fabrics used medically. Because of its hardening effect, formaldehyde is often used to preserve tissues for study.

Though widely applied, particularly for preservation and study of tissues, formaldehyde is a carcinogen (cancer-causing agent). It should always be used in a ventilated area. Contact with the skin should be minimized and direct inhalation avoided.

Symptoms of formaldehyde poisoning include irritation of the eyes, nose, throat and mouth; dizziness; abdominal pain; stupor; convulsions; and kidney damage. Immediate medical attention should be sought if formaldehyde poisoning occurs. *See also* CARCINOGEN *and* HISTOLOGY.

Formication

A feeling of insects crawling under the skin, usually seen in people experiencing withdrawal from certain drugs.

Formication should be distinguished from a delusion, where a person falsely believes they are experiencing the same feeling.

Fracture

An injury that causes a break in a bone.

A fracture occurs when more force or pressure is applied to a bone than it can bear. The force may come from a direct blow or torsion applied to the bone. The weight of a person's own body can cause a fracture if the person steps or falls at an angle at which bone must suddenly bear the weight of the whole body.

TYPES

The speed, angle, and weight of the responsible object determines just how the bone will break. Bones usually break at an angle, but they may also split lengthwise from torsion. Fractures are organized into two categories, closed and open. Within these two main categories are many different types of fracture.

Closed (or simple) fractures are fractures in which the broken bone remains below the skin. Because the surface has not been breached, there is little chance of infection.

Open (or compound) fractures occur when the ends of the bones break through the surface of the skin and are exposed. In these cases, there is a great risk of infection, as the bones and tissues are exposed to the typically nonsterile environment.

Spiral fractures are caused by twisting of the bones, such as those that may occur in skiing accidents.

Transverse fractures are horizontal breaks directly across the bone. Stress fractures, which are caused by a repetitive, damaging motion, such as running or jumping, are usually transverse.

Greenstick fractures, usually the result of sudden force, are characterized by a splintering of the top layer of the bone; they resemble a piece of bark peeled from a tree. They are most common in children.

Comminuted fractures are those in which the bone shatters into fragments. Comminuted fractures are caused by severe force, such as that experienced in a car accident.

SYMPTOMS

The following signs suggest a fracture:
- A limb that is visibly deformed or out of place—an open fracture is obvious as the ends of the bone can be seen;
- Limited movement, or movement that intensifies the pain;
- Swelling;
- Tenderness;
- Bruising;
- Inability to bear weight.

Even if a fracture is not immediately obvious, a doctor should be consulted. A break that is not easily detectable can still heal incorrectly and cause problems in the future if it is left to heal on its own.

TREATMENT

Bones begin to heal very rapidly, so it is important that a fracture be treated by a physician in order to ensure that the bones heal in the correct position. Until a physician can be reached, however, the following temporary measures may be taken:
- The injured person should be moved as little as possible;
- If the person must be moved, the affected area should be splinted in order to immobilize it;
- The injured person should not be given food or water; this can impede the function of anesthetia if surgery is deemed necessary.

The first thing a doctor will do to treat a fracture (usually after x-rays) is to move the bone ends back together; this process is called a closed reduction. A splint or cast may be applied after the closed reduction. If an operation is necessary, then it is called an open reduction. After an open reduction, the injured area must be immobilized so that the bones will stay in place as they heal. This may be done with a plaster cast. In more serious cases, pins or screws may have to be inserted to stabilize the bone.

When a bone heals, a blood clot is first formed to seal the ends of the blood vessels. Thus, for a period of time, painkillers that inhibit the clotting of blood should not be given to patients with bone frac-

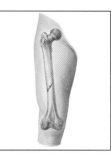

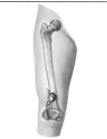

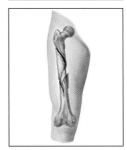

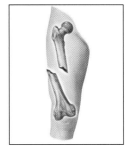

Fracture.
Breaks in bones that occur in fractures can be of varying types, as shown in the diagrams above. A bone is usually broken across its width, but it can also be broken lengthwise, obliquely, or spirally.

tures. After the ends of the blood vessels are sealed, the body begins to dispose of any debris from the break that is left in the injured area, and a mesh-like layer forms between the bone ends to provide a base for the new bone. A callus of new bone then fills into the fracture and bone ends, and over a period of weeks denser and stronger bone with calcium builds on top.

Bone grafts may be necessary if the bone ends cannot meet adequately. If a bone heals incorrectly, surgery may be needed to rebreak and reset the bone so it can heal properly.

REHABILITATION

A fracture takes a number of weeks to heal. During the healing period, the injured area must remain immobilized. Depending on the severity and location of the break, physical therapy may be necessary to restore strength and movement in the injured area.

FRACTURE *is further discussed in entries such as* BANDAGE; DENTISTRY; TRAUMA; *and* TRAUMATOLOGY. *Different kinds of* FRACTURES *include* COLLES' FRACTURE; FEMUR, FRACTURE OF; FRACTURE, DENTAL; HIP, FRACTURED; JAW, FRACTURED; MARCH FRACTURE; MONTEGGIA'S FRACTURE; POTT'S FRACTURE; RIB, FRACTURED; SKULL, FRACTURED; *and* STRESS FRACTURE.

Fracture, Dental

Breakage of a tooth.

Tooth enamel is extremely hard, but it is also susceptible to cracking if it is struck by a hard object.

Treatment. Bonding, using plastic resin, is the smoothing over of essentially superficial chips and breaks in the teeth, and usually suffices for the mending of fractures to the enamel or the hard material surrounding tooth pulp—the dentin. Damage to the pulp of the tooth generally requires a root-canal procedure. Severe fractures to the tooth must be treated with crowns. Fractures deep in the root and vertical fractures typically result in total removal of the affected tooth. *See also* BONDING; ROOT CANAL; *and* TEETH.

Fragile X Syndrome

The most common inherited cause of mental retardation, resulting from an abnormality in the X chromosome.

Fragile X syndrome results in varying mental impairment and characteristic physical features. It is identified by a break or weakness on the long arm of the X chromosome. Because females have two copies of the X chromosome and males have only one copy of this chromosome, fragile X syndrome predominantly affects males.

INCIDENCE

Approximately one in every 1,000 males has fragile X syndrome. The prevalence of carriers of the disorder in the general population is approximately one in 600.

SYMPTOMS

Symptoms of fragile X syndrome vary greatly in severity. Some children with the condition exhibit no impairment to intelligence, while others are severely retarded. This range in impairment is not completely determined by sex; some boys with fragile X syndrome may have normal intelligence, while some girls who have one normal and one abnormal X chromosome may be mentally retarded.

Other Symptoms. The physical features associated with fragile X syndrome include a long, narrow face, and prominent ears, jaw, and forehead. The testicles may be enlarged (macrochordism). Many young children may not exhibit these physical features until puberty, although prominent ears are seen in approximately two-thirds of children with fragile X syndrome. Loose finger joints are also quite common among children with the disorder. These physical features are often more subtle in females with the syndrome.

In order to obtain a greater understanding of FRAGILE X SYNDROME *please refer to the entries on* BIRTH DEFECTS *and* MENTAL RETARDATION; *For deeper knowledge of the genetic factors see* CHROMOSOME; CHROMOSOME ANALYSIS; CHROMOSOMAL ABNORMALITIES; DNA; GENE; *and* GENETICS.

Freckle

Also known as an ephelis

Flat, round, brown spot on the skin, which contains an excess of melanin, the human skin pigment.

People are genetically predisposed to developing freckles. The flat brown spots generally develop following exposure to sunlight or another ultraviolet light source. Freckles result from increased production of melanin, the human skin pigment. They fade after exposure to light has ended.

Freckles are not dangerous, and do not develop into skin cancer. *See also* MELANIN.

Friedreich's Ataxia

A degenerative genetic disease related to coordination disorders.

Friedreich's ataxia causes progressive damage to the nervous system, resulting in symptoms ranging from muscle weakness and speech problems to heart disease. Particularly affected are the spinal cord and the nerves that control muscle movement in the arms and legs.

Symptoms of Friedreich's ataxia usually begin when patients are between the ages of five and 15, but symptoms can appear in patients as young as 18 months or as old as 30 years of age. The first symptom of the condition is usually difficulty in walking and moving the arms. Deformities of the foot may be an early sign of the disease. Rapid, rhythmic, involuntary movements of the eyeball are common. Most people with Friedreich's ataxia develop scoliosis, the severe form of which may impair breathing. Other symptoms of the disorder include chest pain, shortness of breath, and heart palpitations.

Treatment. There is currently no cure for Friedreich's ataxia. Treatment is mostly concerned with alleviating the symptoms, and physical therapy attempts to help patients maintain optimal functioning as long as possible.

Prognosis. Approximately 20 years after the appearance of the first symptoms of Friedreich's ataxia, the patient is confined to a wheelchair. In later stages of the disease, the patient may become completely incapacitated. Heart disease is the most common cause of death among patients with the condition. *See also* NERVOUS SYSTEM.

Frostbite

Damage to the skin and underlying tissue caused by exposure to extreme cold.

Symptoms. Frostbite is distinguished by the cold, hard, pale appearance of skin that has been exposed to cold for an extended period of time. The area may feel numb, but there is also usually a sharp, aching pain. Any part of the body may get frostbite, but the hands, feet, nose, and ears are the most commonly affected areas.

The first symptom of frostbite is usually a "pins and needles" sensation, followed by numbness. The skin is hard and has no feeling. As the affected area thaws, the skin will become red and painful. While the area is warming, it is common to feel pain and tingling, a sensation called chilblains or pernio. In severe cases of frostbite, blisters may appear. Frostbite is often found in conjunction with hypothermia, a lowering of the body's core temperature. Symptoms of hypothermia include slurred speech, shivering, and memory loss.

Treatment. Rapid warming of the affected area is recommended, such as in water of 104 to 105°F. The affected area should not be rubbed with snow, as this may cause further damage to the area. Affected areas should be rested and protected from any trauma.

Risk Factors. People who take beta-blockers, which decrease blood flow to the skin, are particularly susceptible to frostbite. People with atherosclerosis—thickening and hardening of the arteries—are also at high risk. Other factors that increase the chances of frostbite include smoking, exposure to windy weather, diabetes mellitus, and peripheral neuropathy or Raynaud's phenomenon. *See also* AMPUTATION; GANGRENE; *and* RAYNAUD'S PHENOMENON.

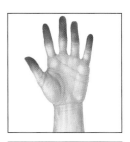

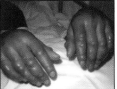

Frostbite.
Frostbite can be extremely damaging to the hands and extremities. The diagram and photo above shows frostbite's effects on the hands after exposure to severely cold temperatures—below 32°F (0°C).

Frozen Section

The slicing of a thin segment of tissue from a frozen specimen to aid in diagnosis.

A frozen section is generally used during surgical procedures to gain additional information for diagnosis. The tissue to be examined is frozen within a synthetic material and sliced finely with an instrument known as a cryostat. The resulting sample is then stained and examined under a microscope to determine pathology.

A physician examines a frozen section under a microscope while the patient is still anesthetized, and chooses a course of treatment based on the findings. Tissue may be evaluated by a frozen section for presence and nature of malignancy, or to examine tissue type. The procedure can be completed in 15 minutes. In contrast, a histological test for identifying malignancy and tissue type takes several days to complete because of the need to embed tissue in paraffin prior to sectioning. *See also* Histology *and* Malignant.

Frozen Shoulder

Extreme shoulder pain and stiffness, sometimes leading to immobility.

Frozen shoulder occurs when the shoulder joint becomes inflamed, and the lining in the capsule that covers the joint thickens. Frozen shoulder generally has no known cause, however, the condition may develop as a result of stroke, chronic bronchitis, or angina pectoris. Another cause of the condition may be reduced use of the shoulder due to a painful injury; when a motion becomes painful, a person may avoid it. Limited use of the shoulder may cause stiffening of the area.

Painkillers, anti-inflammatory drugs, and ice on the affected area can treat the condition. Physical therapy and stretching may help to restore use of the shoulder, although the rehabilitation process can be long. Arthroscopic surgery may be of value. *See also* Physical Therapy.

Fugue, Dissociative

A mental health disorder characterized by sudden wandering with a loss of identity or assumption of a new identity.

Dissociative fugue is a disorder characterized by running away from home, loss of memory, and possibly delirium. Attacks of dissociative fugue can last for hours, days, or months; the patient does not remember the incident.

Incidence. Dissociative fugue is more common in people who have experienced war or other extremely traumatic situations. About two out of every 1000 people are affected by dissociative fugue.

Causes. Dissociative fugues often occur in conjunction with mental illness, such as other dissociative disorders, post-traumatic stress disorder, or depression. They may relate to an individual's deep desires to escape a difficult situation at work or at home. They can also have a physiological cause, such as head injury, temporal lobe epilepsy, or dementia.

Symptoms. A person in a state of dissociative fugue may flee from home and begin life again in a new locality as a different person. The person may appear to be normal, but usually displays hallucinations, mood swings, and inability to remember details of life. These symptoms can continue for a few months, but most dissociative fugues are short-lived. When the dissociative fugue ends, the person retains no memory of the events that led to his or her disappearance. *See also* Amnesia; Delirium; *and* Dissociative Identity Disorder.

Fulminant

An illness that comes on suddenly and with great severity.

A number of illnesses can have very short onsets and serious consequences. One example of such an illness is fulminant hepatic failure, which not only destroys liver cells but also destroys brain cells within two weeks of the onset of the disease. Fulminant myocarditis starts with flu-like symptoms but is followed quickly with a severe inflammation of the muscle wall of the heart. The heart is then unable to contract and move blood through the arteries. Fulminant meningococcemia is an attack on the nerve cells by the meningococcus bacterium. All of these illnesses require immediate and critical care or the patient will die. *See also* HEART; HEPATITIS; *and* LIVER.

Fungal Infections

Diseases caused by the proliferation of fungal organisms.

Fungi are more like plants than they are like bacteria. People eat some fungi, such as mushrooms. Their spores can be found in the air we breathe and the food we eat. Most often they are harmless, but sometimes fungi cause infections that can be very difficult to combat.

A healthy immune system is normally able to control fungal infections easily. People with AIDS, those who are undergoing chemotherapy or radiation therapy for cancer, or people who have had an organ transplant can develop serious fungal infections, as the normal response of their immune systems is inhibited. Fungal infections develop very slowly; thus it may be months or even years before symptoms of a fungal infection become serious enough to require medical attention. Treatment is correspondingly slow to be effective.

TYPES

Candida. The most common fungal infection is called thrush or candida. Candida is a yeast that lives naturally in the mouth, gastrointestinal tract, and vagina. Usually it causes no symptoms. When the fungus becomes active, white or red patches appear in the mouth. Candida infection can cause a sore throat, pain when swallowing, and nausea. If mild, the infection can be treated by rinsing the mouth with a weak solution of hydrogen peroxide.

Infection may also occur in the vagina. Symptoms of vaginal candidiasis include

---

Preventing Fungal Infections

Fungi are all around us; however, few simple steps can help prevent fungal infections:

- Keep skin clean and dry, particularly under arms, in the groin, and between the toes;
- Do not walk barefoot on wet public areas like bathrooms or swimming pools;
- Do not borrow napkins, towels, combs, or hair brushes from others;
- Wear cotton, not nylon, socks;
- Wear open-toed shoes if your feet are especially prone to sweating.

---

itching, burning, and a thick, white discharge. A number of over-the-counter drugs are available to treat this infection, commonly referred to as a "yeast infection."

Cryptococcal meningitis is a fungal infection of the meninges, the tissues that cover the brain and spinal cord. Symptoms of cryptococcal meningitis include fever, vomiting, headache, nausea, fatigue, loss of appetite, and malaise (a generalized feeling of illness). This infection is treated by intravenous injection with the antifungal medication amphotericin B.

Histoplasmosis is an infection that starts in the lungs when the spores of the fungus *Histoplasma capsulatum* are inhaled. It may be a fairly mild infection that feels like a bad flu and from which sufferers recover quickly. If the infection spreads throughout the body, it can attack the liver, spleen, brain, heart, and adrenal glands. It is treated with oral antifungal medications.

Blastomycosis infects the lungs, resulting in a dry, hacking cough, chest pain, a fever, chills, and sweats. It is treated with the antifungal drug amphotericin B.

Skin and Nail Infections. White spot, ringworm, and athlete's foot are common fungal skin and nail infections. Fungal infections of the skin are treated with various topical antifungal agents.

FUNGAL INFECTIONS *are further discussed in the entries on* BLASTOMYCOSIS; CANDIDIASIS; CRYPTOCOCCOSIS; FUNGUS; MENINGITIS; *and* HISTOPLASMOSIS. *A broad overview of topics related to* FUNGAL INFECTIONS *can be found in* CHEST X-RAY; *and* INFECTION. *Interesting related articles include* MYCOSIS FUNGOIDES; *and* SEXUALLY TRANSMITTED DISEASE.

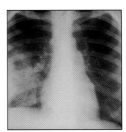

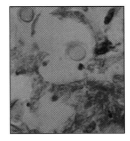

Fungal Infections. Above, a chest x-ray shows meningitis caused by a fungal infection. Fungal infections are diseases of the skin and other organs caused by the growth and spread of fungal organisms. Bottom, a micrograph of a pathogenic fungus.

Resources on Fungal Infections
Despommier, Dickson D., et al., Parasitic Disease (1995); Donaldson, Raymond Joseph, ed., *Parasites and Western Man* (1979); Klein, Aaron E., Nauss, Ralph Welty, *Medical Parasitology and Zoology* (1944); www.ny-cornell.org/medicine/infectious/index.html.

Fungus

Simple parasitic organism.

There are over 100,000 species of fungi (the plural of "fungus") in the world, including mushrooms, toadstools, yeasts, rusts, smuts, puffballs, molds, and mildews. Few of these organisms are harmful to the human body and many are quite useful; many mushrooms and truffles are culinary delicacies, some molds are the source of antibiotic drugs, and yeasts are used in brewing and baking. A fungus is like a plant but lacks chlorophyll and depends upon a host organism for nourishment, absorbing nutrients through osmosis from organic soil, food, or excrement. Mycology, the study of fungi, has yielded discoveries about the nature of fungi and about those fungi that are responsible for a number of illnesses, some of them fatal.

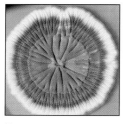

Fungus.
Fungi are simple parasitic life-forms, including molds, such as the penicillin mold above, mildews, yeasts, mushrooms at right, and toadstools. There are more than 100,000 different species of fungi worldwide.

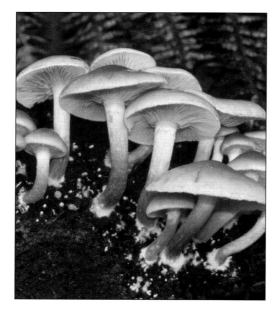

STRUCTURE

Yeasts, in particular, are made up of clusters of individual cells. Other fungi are comprised of hyphae—antler-shaped blooms of tubelike filaments produced by cell division and arranged into a complex network called a mycelium (pl., mycelia). Mushrooms and toadstools are examples of the large fruit-like structures formed by the mycelia of fungi that live in soil. Tiny seeds called spores are produced by many fungi and can become airborne; if they land in a nutrient-rich area of ideal temperature, such as healthy soil or the surface of food, a new mycelium may grow and, eventually, form a colony of mycelia and generate its own spores. Spores are a constant presence in air and soil.

DISEASES ASSOCIATED WITH FUNGI

Some fungi that live in soil, such as mushrooms, contain poisonous toxins that can cause illness or be lethal. Food-poisoning often occurs when crops become infected with fungi that produce harmful toxins. A fungus that infects rye (a cereal) creates ergot, a dangerous toxin that is rarely ingested today, as reliance on rye as a food source has decreased. Aflatoxin is a poison produced by a fungus that clings to groundnuts. In some parts of Asia and Africa, consuming moldy groundnuts may cause liver cancer. Other fungi are responsible for common skin diseases, such as athlete's foot.

Allergic Reactions. Alveolitis is an allergic reaction in the lungs to the inhaled spores of some fungi; when the fungi are inhaled, yeast forms and infects the blood. Breathing in the spores from moldy hay produces such a reaction, in the form of coughing and labored breathing. Asthma and rhinitis are also often the result of inhaling fungal spores.

A mycelium, or several mycelia, can form in the lungs, in or beneath the skin (through a cut), or in tissues throughout the body. The immune system usually prevents fungal infection, but when it is not at its strongest (such as in people with AIDS, chemotherapy and radiation therapy patients, or those who have recently had an organ transplant), illness—from skin irritation to severe or fatal infection—can result.

Ideas presented in this article are vital to an understanding of BLASTOMYCOSIS; CANDIDIASIS; FOOD POISONING; FUNGAL INFECTIONS; *and* HYGIENE. *Specific topics related to* FUNGUS *can be found in* ALLERGY; COUGHING; COUGHING UP BLOOD; *and* LUNG. *See also* SEXUALLY TRANSMITTED DISEASE.

G6PD Deficiency

A common inherited disorder caused by defective formation of the enzyme glucose-6-phosphate dehydrogenase (G6PD).

Two hundred to 400 million people worldwide have G6PD deficiency, with the highest incidences of the disorder in Africa and the Middle East.

CONDITIONS CAUSED BY G6PD DEFICIENCY

Two conditions caused by G6PD deficiency are neonatal jaundice and hemolytic anemia. Jaundice, which results in a yellowish discoloration in the whites of the eyes, skin, and mucus membranes, is caused by the deposition of bilirubin, a byproduct of the breakdown of hemoglobin. This is a direct result of a problem with the G6PD enzyme in the liver. Jaundice is common in newborns, but when it persists past a few days, G6PD deficiency is suspected. The condition may be severe enough to cause death or permanent neurologic damage.

Hemolytic anemia occurs when red blood cells are destroyed too quickly to be replaced. The symptoms of the condition include fatigue, paleness, shortness of breath, fast heartbeat (tachycardia), dark or red colored urine, fever, and an enlarged spleen. In G6PD deficient individuals, hemolytic anemia can be caused by exposure to certain drugs or foods, or by infection. Hemolytic anemia can be fatal if not treated.

TREATMENT

G6PD deficiency cannot be cured, but hemolytic crises can be avoided if patients avoid triggering substances. Infants with neonatal jaundice receive phototherapy—exposure to bright light. Hemolytic anemia is treated with the administration of oxygen and bed rest. Sometimes a blood transfusion is also performed.

Background material on G6PD deficiency can be found in GENETIC DISORDERS. *For further information, see* ANEMIA; ANEMIA, HEMOLYTIC; GENE; GENETICS; *and* INHERITANCE. *See also* GENETIC ENGINEERING *for more on research.*

GABA

Abbreviation for gamma-amino-butyric acid
A chemical released from nerve endings.

Nerve cells (neurons) communicate by releasing and receiving neurotransmitters. GABA is the most common inhibitory neurotransmitter; it prevents the passing of signals, decreasing the intensity of a message between neurons. As many as one-third of the synapses in the brain use GABA.

GABA is manufactured in the brain and spinal cord. It inhibits the release of neurotransmitters that stimulate nerve activity, such as norepinephrine and dopamine.

Anticonvulsants and benzodiazepine drugs increase the activity of GABA, limiting the passing of nerve signals and inhibiting involuntary spasms. Scientists speculate that patients with Huntington's chorea, a condition marked by spasms, lack a sufficient amount of GABA-producing nerve cells in the areas of the brain directly responsible for movement. *See also* HUNTINGTON'S CHOREA *and* NEUROTRANSMITTER.

Galactorrhea

Lactation in anyone not pregnant or nursing.

During pregnancy, the pituitary gland increases the production of a hormone called prolactin, inducing the body to produce milk. Disorders that increase the production of prolactin in people who are not nursing can cause secretions of breast milk.

Causes. Galactorrhea may be the result of a benign tumor in the pituitary gland or an underactive thyroid (hypothyroidism). Side effects from some drugs can also cause the disorder, as can brain conditions, such as meningitis. Frequently, the cause of galactorrhea is unknown.

Treatment. If the condition is related to a tumor, the drug bromocriptine, which stops the production of prolactin and shrinks the tumor, may be administered. Surgery may be necessary if the tumor continues to grow despite medication. *See also* BROMOCRIPTINE *and* PITUITARY GLAND.

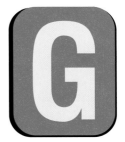

Galactosemia

A rare enzyme deficiency that affects the body's ability to metabolize galactose, a sugar formed from the breakdown of the milk sugar lactose.

Galactosemia is a hereditary disorder in which the affected individual lacks the enzyme that breaks galactose down into glucose. If the condition is left untreated, galactose begins to accumulate in the body, resulting in brain damage, cataracts, and liver problems.

One in 50,000 to 70,000 babies is born with galactosemia. As a result, it is one of the conditions for which newborns are routinely screened. Symptoms of the disorder may not be apparent at birth, but within a short time the baby develops jaundice, vomits often, and does not grow normally.

Infants with galactosemia must be fed a diet that is free of galactose. They are unable to digest milk or milk products. Seaweed and some fruits also contain galactose. If dietary restrictions are followed, the affected infant will go on to develop normally. *See also* DIET AND DISEASE.

Gallbladder

A pear-shaped sac underneath the liver.

The gallbladder stores bile secreted by the liver through the cystic duct. While in the gallbladder, the bile concentrates as water is absorbed from it through the gallbladder wall. When food enters the first section of small intestine (the duodenum), gastrointestinal hormones signal the gallbladder to contract, releasing bile into the common bile duct to the duodenum, where it breaks down fat. Fibrous tissue connects the gallbladder to the liver. Its inner walls are lined with mucosa, a mucous membrane; a thin membrane of cells called the serous coat allows water to drain.

The digestive system can actually function without the gallbladder, which may be necessary if repeated gallstones or other disease necessitates the removal of the gallbladder. *See also* BILE *and* DIGESTIVE SYSTEM.

Gallbladder.
Above, the gallbladder is a pear-shaped organ located under the liver. Its function is to secrete bile, a fluid that breaks down fat in the duodemum during the digestive process.

Gallbladder Cancer

Malignant tumor of the gallbladder.

Gallbladder cancers are rare and appear in individuals with gallstones. Most gallbladder cancers are adenocarcinomas and originate in the inner lining of the organ.

Gallbladder cancers often cause no symptoms until later stages. The symptoms that do appear include jaundice, a lump in the right side of the abdomen, weight loss, fever, nausea, and dark-colored urine. Gallbladder cancers often spread to the liver, the pancreas, and the small intestine. As much of the tumor as possible is removed surgically. If the cancer has spread, surgery alone will not be effective as a remedy. *See also* ADENOCARCINOMA *and* JAUNDICE.

Gallbladder Disorders

Conditions affecting the gallbladder.

The gallbladder is a small organ that is located adjacent to the liver. Its function is to store bile. Bile is a digestive enzyme that is produced in the liver. Once produced, the bile is then carried into the small intestine by means of the bile ducts.

Disorders of the gallbladder include the development of gallstones or other bile duct obstructions, biliary colic, cholecystitis, and gallbladder cancer.

Bile Duct Obstructions. Bile duct obstruction is caused most often by the presence of gallstones in the cystic or common bile duct or by inflammation. However, the liver still continues processing bilirubin, the main pigment in bile, which enters the bloodstream and is then deposited in the skin and urine, resulting in jaundice.

Biliary Colic. Biliary colic is pain resulting from an obstructed flow of bile. An attack of biliary colic may last for hours. The location of the pain may vary, but it is most often felt in the right upper portion of the abdomen, extending to the right shoulder blade. Other symptoms may include nausea, vomiting, chills, fever, and jaundice.

Cholecystitis. Cholecystitis is an inflammation of the gallbladder. It may be acute or chronic. Acute cholecystitis is usually caused by a gallstone in the cystic duct, but occasionally results from a bacterial infection. It can lead to gangrene or perforation of the gallbladder. Chronic cholecystitis is a result of scarring and other accumulated damage as the result of previous episodes of acute inflammation.

Gallbladder Cancer. Cancer of the gallbladder is associated with gallstones and is difficult to cure surgically once symptoms have started to appear. Fortunately, this condition develops in at most one percent of people with gallstones, and the risk of the disease is not generally considered an indication for surgical removal of the gallbladder in patients who are otherwise asymptomatic (without symptoms).

> *For background information on gallbladder disorders, see* Digestive System; Gastrointestinal Tract; *and* Metabolism. *Related information can be found in* Bile-Duct Obstruction; Fats and Oils; Fatty Acid; Gallbladder; Gallbladder Cancer; Gallstones; *and* Liver.

Gallstones

> Accumulations of crystallized minerals that form in the gallbladder or in its ducts.

Normally, gallstone formation is inhibited by bile acids. However, if cholesterol levels are high, the cholesterol crystallizes and forms stones. Stones in the gallbladder itself may not cause any problems, but stones that lodge in the cystic duct (which leads from the gallbladder to the bile-duct) or bile-duct can cause pain and inflammation.

Gallstones may be smooth or rough, and can range in size from small grains to stones the size of golf balls. Most gallstones are composed of cholesterol; up to 20 percent of gallstones, however, are made up of calcium salts from bile.

Incidence. Approximately one in ten people develop gallstones. Women have a higher incidence of gallstones than men.

Symptoms. A gallbladder attack is known as biliary colic. The symptoms of bil-

iary colic are a sudden sharp pain on the upper right side of the abdomen (occasionally migrating to the shoulder blade), nausea, vomiting, fever, and jaundice. Jaundice is usually an indication that the stone has become lodged in the common bile duct. Fever is attributed to inflammation of the gallbladder or infection of the bile duct, in addition to the obstruction.

Treatment. Surgical removal of the gallbladder, called a cholecystectomy, can be performed after an acute episode of biliary colic has been resolved. This is the preferred method for treating gallbladder disease, and is usually performed by laparoscopy rather than open surgery. Stone dissolution, in which stones consisting of cholesterol are broken down chemically, is a newer alternative. Biliary lithotripsy is the use of high-frequency sound waves to shatter the stones, but the procedure is seldom used any longer.

Noninvasive treatments for gallstones include the administration of a medication called urodeoxycholic acid, which can dissolve cholesterol gallstones. However, this drug works best for small stones that have not formed obstructions. It takes several months for the drug to dissolve the stone, and the chance of recurrence is high. *See also* Gallbladder Disorders.

Gamma Globulin

> A component of blood containing a number of different proteins, especially antibody molecules, designed to attack foreign invaders like viruses, fungi, or bacteria.

Gamma globulin is prepared from pooled human blood to protect people with defective immune systems. It is also used as a preventive drug against certain diseases, such as infectious hepatitis. Injections of gamma globulin can provide protection for several weeks for those with deficiencies of antibodies, such as those using immunosuppressant drugs, cancer patients, and people with HIV. It is also used to treat certain autoimmune diseases, including thrombocytopenia and hemolytic anemia. *See also* Autoimmune Disorders.

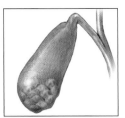

Gallstones.
Above, gallstones accumulate in the gallbladder or its ducts and are made up of crystallized cholesterol. Stones located in the gallbladder are not as serious as stones in the ducts, which may result in a blockage of bile.

Resources on Gallbladder

Blumgart, L.H., *Surgery of the Liver and Biliary Tract (*1994); Krames Communications, *The Gallbladder Surgery Book* (1991); Levine, Joel S., ed., *Decision Making in Gastroenterology* (1992); Berkson, D. Lindsey, et al., *Healthy Digestion the Natural Way* (2000); Sachar, David B., et al., *Pocket Guide to Gastroenterology* (1991).

Ganglion Cyst

A tumor or swelling found most commonly on the wrist or the foot.

A ganglion cyst is a fluid-filled bump that forms beneath the skin. Ganglion cysts are most common on the back of the wrist and on the fingers. They can also form on the shoulder, foot, elbow, and knee.

Causes. A ganglion cyst develops as a consequence of inflammation of the tissues that surround certain joints. The tissues swell up with mucus-like lubricating fluid and increase in size. The cysts can be tiny, or they can grow to the size of a golf ball. Larger ganglion cysts may cause tenderness and restrict movement. Ganglion cysts are associated with rheumatoid arthritis.

Treatment. Ganglion cysts may spontaneously disappear. If the pain is severe, the fluid may be aspirated, although ganglion cysts recur in 70 percent of cases. If the ganglion cyst reappears, surgical removal may be required. *See also* CYST *and* RHEUMATOID ARTHRITIS.

Gangrene

Damage or death of body tissue due to poor blood supply.

Any injury, surgical wound, or disease that restricts or stops the flow of blood to tissue can cause the tissue to die. This process is called gangrene. Injuries that occur on the body's surface, such as bedsores, chemical and deep burns, and frostbite, can result in gangrene. Decreased bloodflow within the body can also result in gangrene.

TYPES

"Dry" gangrene is usually associated with diabetes or arteriosclerosis. Gangrene complicated by bacterial infection is considered "moist" or "wet," and is not as common as dry gangrene.

SYMPTOMS

One of the earliest signs of either type of gangrene is a reddening of the dying tissue.

Gangrene.
Gangrene is the death of body tissue caused by poor blood supply to the area. Above, top, a normal wound can be contrasted with a gangrenous wound, above, bottom. The first sign of gangrene is generally a reddening of the dying tissue.

Initially, dry gangrene is painful, but the area becomes increasingly numb. The skin turns purple and then black. Moist gangrene may begin with blisters and swelling. The infection spreads quickly, causing bruise-like discolorations as the tissue dies. The infection may also release a foul smell, and immediate hospitalization is necessary to treat the condition.

TREATMENT

Antibiotics are administered as soon as gangrene is suspected. Damaged tissue must be removed surgically. Individuals suffering from moist gangrene may be put into a hyperbaric chamber, in which oxygen under pressure helps to kill the bacteria causing the infection.

> *Background material on gangrene can be found in* INFECTION. *For further information, see* ATROPHY; COMPLICATION; *and* DIABETES MELLITUS. *See also* AMPUTATION *and* DEATH *for more on possible consequences if a severe case of gangrene is left untreated.*

Ganser's Syndrome

A rare disorder in which an individual consciously or unconsciously presents symptoms of dementia.

Ganser's syndrome is sometimes called the disorder of approximate answers, because an individual will respond to mental status tests with an answer that is obviously wrong but is close to the correct answer. For example, an individual who is asked how many fingers there are on each hand may respond with the number six. The fact that the answer is so close to the correct answer indicates that there was a deliberate attempt to respond deceptively.

Ganser's syndrome is a psychological response to extreme stress. It may also result from untreated emotional or physical abuse in childhood. The condition appears suddenly; it was originally described in prison inmates and was first known as "prison psychosis." It is known as a fictitious disorder, because the symptoms are invented to imitate a real illness. *See also* MUNCHAUSEN'S SYNDROME.

Garderella Vaginalis

Bacterium found in the abnormal vaginal discharge of women with vaginitis (vaginal inflammation).

Garderella vaginalis infection produces a grayish frothy discharge with a characteristic fishy odor. Unlike other types of bacteria, *Garderella vaginalis* does not cause itching or irritation. The bacterium is not transmitted through sexual contact. Treatment is with antibiotics. *See also* SEXUALLY TRANSMITTED DISEASES.

Gastrectomy

The surgical removal of part or all of the stomach.

Gastrectomy is an operation that is performed on patients with a perforated or bleeding stomach ulcer, scar tissue that obstructs the passage of food, or a cancerous growth. In a gastrectomy, part or all of the stomach is removed.

TYPES

If all of the stomach is removed, the procedure is called a total gastrectomy. If only part of the stomach is removed, the operation is referred to as a partial gastrectomy. Partial gastrectomy is more common than total gastrectomy; however, both operations are very serious and require postoperative rehabilitation.

RECOVERY

After a gastrectomy, whether partial or total, the digestive process is affected. There is no longer a storage area for food, but the small intestine is capable of handling the preliminary breakdown of proteins that normally takes place in the stomach. Some dietary adjustments are necessary in patients that have had a gastrectomy. The major change is the necessity of eating small amounts of food at more frequent intervals during the day. Failure to do so results in dumping syndrome, in which food passes too rapidly into the upper intestine, causing discomfort, sweating, dizziness, and nausea.

Gastrectomy and Obesity

Gastrectomy is increasingly being viewed as a viable treatment for severe obesity. The removal or reduction of the size of the stomach severely restricts patients' caloric intake. Patients undergoing a gastrectomy are able to lose tremendous amounts of weight in a relatively short period of time. More importantly, they are able to keep the weight off, a clear advantage over conventional methods of weight loss. However, dietary restrictions must be adhered to on a permanent basis, and the long-term effects of the operation on obese individuals is not yet known.

COMPLICATIONS

Complications are more likely in patients who have had a total gastrectomy. These complications include:

Malabsorption. Malabsorption is a reduction in the ability of the body to absorb food, vitamins, and minerals. Supplements, especially of vitamin B_{12} and iron, must be given to patients who have had a gastrectomy, as the small intestine cannot absorb all the nutrients the body needs.

Gastroparesis. Gastroparesis involves the loss of the stomach's normal ability to contract, resulting from the severing of the vagus nerve during gastrectomy. This nerve is responsible for transmitting signals for muscle contractions to the stomach. When gastroparesis occurs, the stomach empties more slowly. Patients often report acid reflux, bloating, and a feeling of fullness after eating only a small amount of food.

OUTLOOK

The outlook for patients who have had a gastrectomy is generally good. Only 10 percent of patients who have had the operation suffer serious complications. Some patients experience abdominal pain and heartburn after they have had a gastrectomy for an ulcer. These symptoms may be caused by recurrent ulcers in the remainder of the stomach and may not necessarily be due to the gastrectomy itself.

For background information on gastrectomy, see DIGESTIVE SYSTEM; GASTROINTESTINAL TRACT; *and* STOMACH. *Further information can be found in* GASTRITIS; OBESITY; PEPTIC ULCER; STOMACH CANCER; *and* STOMACH ULCER.

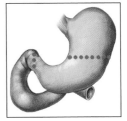
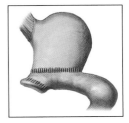

Gastrectomy.
In a gastrectomy, part or all of the stomach is removed and the intestine is reattached to the remaining area. Above, the stomach before a gastrectomy; below, the stomach after the procedure.

Gastric Erosion

A break that develops in the stomach lining.

Gastric erosions affect the innermost layer of the lining of the stomach (the mucosa). If the lesions extend deeper into the stomach lining, they are then called gastric ulcers or peptic ulcers. The causes of gastric erosions are not clear, but they are similar to the causes of peptic ulcers. These causes include the ingestion of alcohol, iron, or drugs known as NSAIDS—nonsteroidal anti-inflammatory drugs. Serious illnesses may cause stress that can also result in the development of gastric erosions. *See also* NONSTEROIDAL ANTI-INFLAMMATORY DRUGS *and* PEPTIC ULCER.

Gastric Lavage

Washing out of the stomach.

A gastric lavage is a procedure that is performed in a hospital in order to empty the contents of the stomach. This is done in cases of drug overdose or accidental ingestion of a poison. In a gastric lavage, a flexible rubber tube is introduced through the mouth and moved along the esophagus into the stomach. Saline solution is fed through the tube to flush out the matter in the stomach, and the fluid (along with the ingested toxins) is removed via the tube. *See also* DRUG OVERDOSE *and* POISONING.

Gastritis

Inflammation of the stomach lining.

Gastritis may be acute, in which the patient suffers from sudden attacks, or it may be chronic, in which the condition develops over a long period of time.

Types. There are several types of gastritis, each of which has distinct symptoms:

Atrophic gastritis, in which the stomach lining becomes atrophied, is seen in the elderly and patients whose stomachs do not produce enough acid. It may be an end-product of *Helicobacter pylori* infection.

Acute stress gastritis is caused by severe illness or injury. The illness or injury do not have to affect the stomach directly for gastritis to develop.

Chronic erosive gastritis can be caused by medicines, especially aspirin and other nonsteroidal anti-inflammatory drugs (NSAIDs). It can also be caused by other conditions, such as Crohn's disease or bacterial and viral infections. This form of gastritis develops slowly. Gastric (peptic) ulcers may result from this condition.

Causes. Causes of gastritis include infection by *Helicobacter pylori* or other bacteria; viral infections; NSAIDs; stress. burns, or other severe injuries; Crohn's disease; and vitamin B_{12} deficiency.

Symptoms. Common symptoms of gastritis include nausea, vomiting, upper abdominal discomfort, and loss of appetite.

Diagnosis. Gastritis is diagnosed by a barium x-ray of the stomach or a gastroscopy, in which a tube is passed into the stomach so that the doctor can view the stomach lining.

Treatment. Antacids and other medications that limit acid production in the stomach are used to treat mild cases of gastritis. If the problem is caused by other underlying conditions, those conditions should be treated first.

Background information on gastritis can be found in GASTROINTESTINAL TRACT *and* STOMACH. *For related information, see* ACID REFLUX; GASTRECTOMY; GASTROSCOPY; PEPTIC ULCER; *and* STOMACH ULCER. *See also* DIET AND DISEASE *for more on connections between diet and gastritis.*

Gastroenteritis

Inflammation in the gastrointestinal tract.

Gastroenteritis is commonly referred to as stomach flu or intestinal flu. It is characterized by sudden, acute attacks. Gastroenteritis can range from a mild condition to one that is more severe.

Incidence. Children and the elderly are particularly at risk for contracting gastroenteritis, as are individuals with suppressed immune systems.

Causes. Gastroenteritis is most often caused by viruses or bacteria, including rotavirus, norwalk virus, cytomegalovirus, campylobacter, salmonella, shigella, *Escherichia coli, Giardia lamblia, Entamoeba histolytica*, and *Cryptosporidium.*

Symptoms. Attacks of gastroenteritis usually last only for a few days. The symptoms include loss of appetite, diarrhea that may be watery or bloody, cramps, abdominal pain, low-grade fever, nausea, and vomiting. The major problem from gastroenteritis is the loss of excessive amounts of fluid due to diarrhea or vomiting, which may lead to dehydration. Dehydration can upset the body's electrolyte balance and can result in shock or coma if not treated.

Treatment. Although mild cases of gastroenteritis usually pass without treatment, antibiotics may be prescribed if the cause is determined to be bacterial in origin. Replacement of lost fluids is important to treat the dehydration that is often a result of gastroenteritis. If dehydration is severe, hospitalization may be necessary to replace fluids intravenously.

> *For background information on gastroenteritis, see* GASTROINTESTINAL TRACT *and* INFECTIOUS DISEASE. *Further information can be found in* ANTIBIOTIC DRUGS; BACTERIA; DIARRHEA; DIGESTIVE SYSTEM; ENTERITIS; *and* WATER SAFETY.

Gastroenterology

The field of medicine dealing with the gastrointestinal tract, or digestive system, and the various ailments and conditions that affect it.

Major organs studied by gastroenterologists are the mouth, esophagus, stomach, duodenum, small intestine, large intestine, colon, and rectum. Disorders affecting the liver, gallbladder, and pancreas are also part of this medical specialty.

Gastrointestinal Bleeding

Bleeding in the gastrointestinal tract, which includes the mouth, the esophagus, the stomach, and the intestines.

The appearance of blood or hemoglobin in the feces is the sign of a disease or abnormality within the gastrointestinal tract. Upper gastrointestinal bleeding involves a source near the lower outlet from the stomach (pyloric valve). Lower gastrointestinal bleeding involves a source farther down in the intestines.

Causes. Gastrointestinal bleeding can occur at any age, and for a number of different possible reasons. In children, the appearance of blood in the feces is most commonly due to swallowed blood from a nosebleed, milk allergies, or disorders such as intussusception or Meckel's diverticulum. Adolescents and young adults may suffer from gastrointestinal bleeding as the result of bleeding ulcers, Crohn's disease, and colitis. Middle-aged and older adults are susceptible to disorders like colon cancer and diverticulitis, which may cause gastrointestinal bleeding.

Symptoms. The symptoms of gastrointestinal bleeding include blood in the stools and vomiting blood or material that looks like coffee grounds. Gastrointestinal bleeding can range from occult or microscopic bleeding (where the amount of blood is so small that it can only be detected by laboratory testing) to massive hemorrhaging. Prolonged occult bleeding can lead to severe iron loss and subsequent anemia. Acute massive bleeding can lead to shock and death.

Treatment. Gastrointestinal bleeding may be indicative of an underlying cause requiring immediate medical intervention. If blood is noticed in the feces or in vomit, medical help should be sought as soon as possible. Intravenous fluids and medications, blood transfusions, drainage of the stomach through a nasogastric tube, and other medical measures may be required. Once the condition is stable, the doctor will attempt to ascertain the cause by means of various diagnostic tests, and treat the underlying condition.

> *Background material on gastrointestinal bleeding can be found in* DIGESTIVE SYSTEM *and* GASTROINTESTINAL TRACT. *For related information, see* ANEMIA; COLON CANCER; CROHN'S DISEASE; FECES; GASTROENTERITIS; INTUSSUSCEPTION; MECKEL'S DIVERTICULUM; PEPTIC ULCER; *and* VOMITING BLOOD.

Resources on the Gastrointestinal Tract

Levine, Joel S., ed., *Decision Making in Gastroenterology* (1992); Berkson, D. Lindsey, et al., *Healthy Digestion the Natural Way* (2000); Sachar, David B., et al., *Pocket Guide to Gastroenterology* (1991); Thompson, W. Grant, *The Ulcer Story: The Authoritative Guide to Ulcers, Dyspepsia, and Heartburn* (1996); Windhager, Erich E., *Handbook of Physiology* (1992); Crohn's and Colitis Foundation of America, Inc., Tel: (800) 932-2423, Online: www.ccfa.org; Digestive Disease Nat. Coalition, Tel. (202) 544-7497, Online: www.ddnc.org; National Institute of Diabetes and Digestive and Kidney Diseases, Tel. (301) 496-3583, Online: www.niddk.nih.gov; www.nycornell.org/medicine/digestive/index.html.

Gastrointestinal Hormones

Group of hormones designed to regulate the functions of the digestive organs.

Special endocrine cells in the stomach, pancreas, and intestine release gastrointestinal hormones to regulate the secretion of certain digestive enzymes.

Gastrin is produced in the stomach and helps to govern acid secretion. As food enters the stomach, gastrin is released and enters the bloodstream. When gastrin comes in contact with the glands in the stomach that produce hydrochloric acid, it acts as a signal to start secretion of that acid. Gastrin also controls the secretion of pepsinogen, which is converted into pepsin, an enzyme that breaks down protein.

While fairly rare, the condition known as Zollinger-Ellison syndrome occurs when a tumor, located on either the pancreas or the wall of the intestine, secretes the hormone gastrin. In response, the stomach and duodenum produce large amounts of acid, resulting in ulceration.

Secretin is produced by the small intestine. It enters the bloodstream and circulates to the pancreas, where it stimulates the production and secretion of pancreatic enzymes. These enzymes enter the intestine through the pancreatic duct and shift the pH of the contents from acidic to basic. They also break down fat, carbohydrates, and proteins. *See also* PANCREAS.

Other hormones produced by the gastrointestinal tract include cholecystokinin, motilin, neurotensin, and enteroglucagon.

Gastrointestinal Tract

Group of organs in the body that control digestion.

The gastrointestinal tract is another name for the digestive system. It consists of the mouth, pharynx (throat), esophagus, stomach, and small and large intestine. It does not include the liver, gallbladder, or pancreas. *See also* DIGESTIVE SYSTEM.

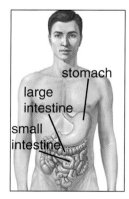

Gastrointestinal Tract. The gastrointestinal tract, above, consists of all the organs that participate in digestion. These organs are the mouth, the pharynx, the esophagus, the stomach, and the small and large intestine.

Gastrojejunostomy

Also called the Billroth II procedure or a gastric bypass

Surgical procedure in which the stomach is connected to the jejunum—the second portion of the small intestine.

A gastrojejunostomy is performed to treat a duodenal ulcer (an ulcer on the lower end of the stomach) or obstruction of stomach outflow from a tumor. Ulcers are caused by increased acid secretion, reduced mucus production, or substances that irritate the lining of the stomach (i.e., caffeine). By connecting the stomach to the small intestine, a gastrojejunostomy enables food to pass directly into the intestine, avoiding the duodenum, where a large percentage of chemical digestion occurs.

A gastrojejunostomy requires the creation of a small gastric pouch that empties directly into the jejunum. Often this procedure is performed in conjunction with a procedure to remove the lower part of the stomach (gastrectomy). After stitching the jejunum to the lower part of the stomach, an opening is made to allow food to pass through. *See also* GASTRECTOMY.

Gastroscopy

Examination of the stomach and abdominal cavity using an endoscope.

Procedure. In a gastroscopy, a flexible endoscope (thin fiberoptic tube) is inserted through the mouth and fed through the esophagus into the stomach. The endoscope is attached to a video monitor, allowing the physician to detect abnormalities that might not be visible on x-ray.

What to Expect. A gastroscopy takes about 30 minutes, and is generally safe. Though it involves some discomfort, a gastroscopy is usually painless. Generally the patient should not eat after midnight before the day of the test. A sedative is administered to relax the patient before the endoscope is inserted into the throat, as this can be uncomfortable and anxiety-producing. A sore throat and occasionally mild bleeding may follow for a few days after the exam. These effects usually are not dangerous and heal without difficulty.

Risks. There is some danger of perforation, stomach bleeding, and aspiration of gastric fluids into the lungs. Although these risks are minimal, they should be discussed thoroughly with the physician prior to the procedure.

> *For background information on gastroscopy, see* DIAGNOSIS; DIGESTIVE SYSTEM; *and* STOMACH. *Related information can be found in* COLONOSCOPY; GASTRITIS; GASTROINTESTINAL TRACT; *and* PEPTIC ULCER.

Gastrostomy

> A surgically-produced opening in the stomach, connected to the outside of the abdomen so that food can be introduced through a tube.

Often permanent, gastrostomy may be performed on patients who are unable to eat. This inability to eat may be due to cancer of the esophagus, stroke, or neurological impairments that make it difficult to chew.

Procedure. A surgeon pushes a flexible viewing tube (endoscope), guide wire, and feeding tube down through the patient's esophagus into the stomach. An opening in the abdomen is then created. The tube is anchored in place with a mushroom-like ending that hugs the stomach lining and cannot be accidentally pulled out. *See also* DIGESTIVE SYSTEM.

Gauze

> A thin, open-weave fabric, usually made of absorbent 100 percent cotton, used as a dressing for wounds and held in place by bandages.

Gauze may be applied dry or soaked in an antiseptic cream or fluid. It is used to cover wounds and during surgery to absorb blood and other fluids. *See also* WOUND.

Gauze is rarely used on open wounds on the skin because it sticks to moist tissue and disturbs healing tissue when removed. Some gauzes used internally are made of material that can be absorbed by the body.

Gavage

Also known as tube feeding

> The act of providing nutrients through a tube inserted into the gastrointestinal tract.

Gavage is used to maintain a person's nutritional status over a period of time or as a treatment for malnutrition. Patients may require gavage due to the side effects of chemotherapy or radiation therapy, or as a means of obtaining nourishment after severe burns, sepsis (a bacterial infection of the blood), or malabsorption syndromes (conditions resulting from an impaired ability to absorb nutrients from food). Other conditions that may require tube feeding include surgery, trauma to the esophagus, impaired swallowing ability following a stroke, and paralysis.

The term "gavage" can also refer to hyperalimentation, or "excessive feeding." This method is used to treat people suffering from wasting diseases, such as AIDS, cancer, or lupus. *See also* AIDS; CANCER; *and* LUPUS ERYTHEMATOSUS.

Gender Identity

> An identification with maleness or femaleness.

Fixed within the first two to three years of life and reinforced during puberty, gender identity rarely changes. The fact that it can, however, demonstrates that it is not inextricably tied to biological sex. A person can experience extreme ambivalence about his or her gender identity. A man, for example, may identify with femaleness to the extent that physically being a man causes daily inner conflict and presents extreme difficulty in satisfying the need for intimacy and sexual gratification. Such feelings of discomfort may be a sign of transsexualism.

Some individuals with gender identity ambivalence seek hormonal or surgical sex-change treatment, which requires psychological testing to rule out delusion and prevent postoperative trauma. Afterwards, the patient's sex drive is low and reproduction is not possible. *See also* SEX CHANGE.

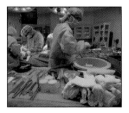

Gauze. Above, gauze is commonly used during surgery to absorb blood and other fluids. It is not generally used to cover open wounds, as it can disturb healing tissue.

Gene

A portion of a chromosome that carries genetic information.

Genes are the pieces of hereditary information we carry in our cells. They control or influence various characteristics, from our physical appearance to our intellectual capabilities. However, genes do not only operate in a vacuum; environment plays an important role in how the genes are actually expressed.

STRUCTURE

On the molecular level, a gene is a segment of DNA. The double helix structure of DNA can be envisioned as a twisted ladder, with rungs that are made up of a repeating sequence of small units known as nucleotides. There are four types of nucleotides, represented by the letters A, G, C, and T. The order in which the four nucleotides are arranged is essentially a code containing detailed information that tells the body how and when to create proteins. These proteins are used for various purposes, ranging from creating actual physical structures of the body (muscles, skin, and body organs) to controlling processes that occur within the body. Each human cell contains between 80,000 and 100,000 genes, and each gene is comprised of approximately 1500 nucleotides.

Each gene contains the information needed to make a specific protein. The proteins produced determine the chemical activities of a cell, and by extension the entire organism. All of the members of a species have the same genetic sequence, or types of genes. What makes each person unique, however, are the tiny varia-

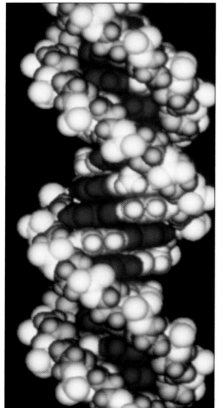

DNA.
Below, a model of the DNA molecule. DNA has the structure of a ladder, with each rung made up of a repeating sequence of nucleotides. The four types of nucleotides are adenosine (A), cytidine (C), guanosine (G), and thymidine (T).

tions within the code. If a gene is defective, the resulting protein will not function properly, leading to a variety of symptoms.

The approximately 100,000 genes in the human genome (the full DNA sequence) are distributed among 23 pairs of chromosomes. Of those pairs, 22 are regular chromosomes (autosomes), and the remaining are sex chromosomes.

DOMINANT AND RECESSIVE GENES

Because genes come in pairs, two genes control the expression of each trait. Generally one gene will be dominant over the other, recessive, gene. For example, suppose that height is affected by a single pair of genes. A dominant gene T would cause a person to be tall, whereas a recessive gene t would cause a person to be short. If the two genes that determine height are both T, then the person will be tall. If the two genes consist of one T and one t, then the person will also be tall (since T is dominant over t). However, a person with T/t genes may be able to have children who are short. Only if both genes are t will the person be short.

Many disease-causing genes are recessive. Thus, a person with one normal and one abnormal gene is a carrier; he or she may be physically normal, but can pass on the disease-causing gene to offspring.

Dominant and recessive genes also play a role in human eye color. Two pairs of genes are responsible: one to produce the pigment, the chemical that gives the iris its color, and the other to deposit it in the proper site. Brown eyes are dominant and blue eyes are recessive. Yet two brown-eyed parents could have a blue-eyed child, providing that both parents had one dominant brown gene and one recessive blue gene.

GENETIC DISORDERS

Genetic disorders are abnormalities caused by the presence of a defective gene. Symptoms of the disorder may be present from birth (congenital) or may develop later in life. A genetic disorder may result from an abnormality of an entire chromosome, as is the case with Down's syndrome, or it may be caused by an abnormality in one or

The Human Genome Project

In February 2001, the Human Genome Project published a draft sequence and initial analysis of the human genome—the genetic blueprint for a human. Begun formally in 1990, the project is a 13-year effort coordinated by the United States Department of Energy and the National Institutes of Health. The project originally was planned to last 15 years, but rapid technological advances have accelerated the expected completion date to 2003.

Project goals are to identify all the approximately 30,000 genes in human DNA, to determine the sequences of the three billion chemical bases that make up human DNA, to store this information in databases, to develop faster, more efficient sequencing technologies and tools for data analysis, and to address the ethical, legal, and social issues that may arise from the project.

more genes. While most genetic disorders are inherited, a genetic abnormality may also occur as a result of prenatal exposure to a harmful agent such as a drug, chemical, or radiation, as these may trigger a gene's DNA sequence to change (mutate). The seriousness of genetic disorders varies widely. Some conditions can be fatal or seriously debilitating, others can be managed with appropriate care, and still others may cause few or no symptoms whatsoever. Even within a single abnormality, there can be a wide range of response.

Family history is the single most important piece of information in determining a couple's risk for having a child with a genetic disorder. If parents think they are carriers for a genetic disease, they may be able to have their blood tested to determine if this is the case. Genetic tests are available for an ever-increasing number of disorders.

GENETIC ENGINEERING

Genetic engineering involves "tinkering" with the genes of an organism—inserting genes from one cell into another. Since the mid 1970s, scientists have been able to transfer human genes, such as those responsible for producing insulin, into bacteria. The bacteria's rapid rate of multiplication results in an abundant supply of the desired protein.

In recent years, genetically engineered foods, such as tomatoes that resist rotting, have appeared in supermarkets. Various other crops have been made more resistant to disease or have had their nutritional content "boosted" by utilizing genes from other species. This has been a source of concern for some people, who worry that adding genes from one species to another may have unforeseen effects.

Genetic engineering is also being considered as a method of treating various genetic diseases, particularly autosomal recessive diseases (such as cystic fibrosis), which are caused by the presence of two recessive genes. Insertion of a "good" copy of the gene could theoretically result in a permanent cure. This same technology would also make possible the insertion of "designer" genes into sperm or eggs, resulting in genetically engineered children.

Background material on gene can be found in GENETICS. For further information, see CHROMOSOME ANALYSIS; GENETICS; and INHERITANCE. See also CHROMOSOMAL ABNORMALITIES and METABOLISM, INBORN ERRORS OF for more on diseases resulting from genetic mutations.

Resources on Genes
Davies, Kevin, *Cracking the Genome: Inside the Race to Unlock Human DNA* (2001); Moore, Keith L., *Before We Are Born: Essentials of Embryology and Birth Defects* (1998); Nussbaum, Robert L., et al., *Thompson & Thompson Genetics in Medicine* (2001); Pollack, Robert, *Signs of Life: The Languages and Meanings of DNA* (1994); Ridley, Matt, *Genome* (2000); Alliance of Genetic Support Groups, Tel. (800) 336-GENE, Online: www.medhelp.org/geneticalliance; Easter Seals, Tel. (800) 221-6827, Online: www.seals.org; National Center for Biotechnology Information, Tel. (301) 496-2475, Online: www.ncbi.nih.gov; Office of Rare Diseases, Tel. (301) 402-4336, Online: rarediseases.info.nih.gov/org; http://www.med.cornell.edu/research/cores/genetherapy/index.html.

"General Paralysis of the Insane"

The name for the cognitive and physical degeneration in the last stages of the sexually transmitted disease syphilis.

When syphilis is left untreated, the disease progresses to the nervous system. Sufferers slowly develop symptoms that include convulsions, paralysis, and difficulty in speaking. Behavioral changes follow as the brain is further affected. The sufferer has difficulty concentrating, has memory loss and impaired judgment, and ignores personal hygiene. Headaches, insomnia, low energy levels, irritability, and depression are also experienced. The prognosis is poor for sufferers who reach this stage in the disease, as the bacteria that cause syphilis can be killed but the damage that has already been done to the brain cannot be reversed. *See also* SYPHILIS.

Genetic Code

Information that is carried in the DNA and passed from parent to offspring, containing blueprints for the structure and function of an organism.

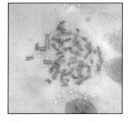

Chromosomes. Above, the chromosomes of a human cell undergoing mitosis. When something goes wrong during this complex process, the result is a genetic disorder.

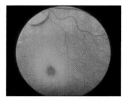

Tay-Sachs Disease. Above, Tay-Sachs disease is a genetic disorder that is recessive and primarily affects the nervous system. Above, a cherry-red spot appears in the macula of the eye, with a lipid deposit in the retinal cells. The result is usually blindness.

The smallest pieces of genetic information are called nucleotides. If the double helix of DNA is envisioned as a twisted ladder, the nucleotides are the rungs of the ladder. There are four types of nucleotides, represented by the letters A, C, T, and G. The order, or sequence, of the nucleotides provides the information necessary for the body to create proteins, which are the structural and functional bases for the body and its processes. The sequence of all the nucleotides in the DNA of an organism is its genetic code.

Genes are made up of a sequence of nucleotides. Each gene contains the information needed to make a specific protein. The proteins that are produced determine the chemical activities of a cell, and, thus, the entire organism. Chromosomes are made up of a number of genes. All members of a species have the same number of chromosomes, containing the same types of genes. It is different details within the genes that make each individual unique. For example, in every person, the same genes control eye color. The exact sequence of the nucleotides in those genes, however, determines the actual color of the eyes. *See also* GENE.

Genetic Counseling

Guidance based on a family's genealogy.

Genetic counseling, typically performed by a clinical geneticist, pediatrician, or family physician with genetics experience, involves the creation of a family tree inclusive of blood relationships, history of diseases and miscarriages, and information from death certificates. Analyzing this pedigree, including interviewing or examining either ill or healthy family members, can help a genetic counselor predict occurrence or recurrence of illnesses and disorders.

Such analysis can provide a couple with an abnormal child with a prognosis for that child. It can also determine the risk and severity of recurrent abnormalities in the couple's subsequent children. *See also* GENE *and* GENETIC DISORDERS.

Genetic Disorders

Abnormalities caused by the presence of defective chromosomes or genes.

Genes contain information for producing various proteins. If a gene is defective, the protein produced as a result of the information in the gene will also be defective. A genetic disorder may result from an abnormality in the chromosomes, such as one too many or one too few chromosomes, or it may be caused by a single defective gene. Genetic abnormalities may be inherited, arise spontaneously, or occur as a result of prenatal exposure to a harmful agent, such as a drug, chemical, or radiation.

The severity of genetic disorders varies widely. Some conditions can be fatal or seriously debilitating, others can be managed with appropriate care, and still others may cause few or no symptoms whatsoever. Even within a single abnormality, there can be a wide range of response. Symptoms of a genetic disorder may be present from birth (congenital) or may develop later in life.

Autosomal Recessive Disorders. The majority of genetic disorders are caused by autosomal recessive genes. This means that the disorder will occur only if the defective gene is inherited from both parents. Examples of autosomal recessive disorders include cystic fibrosis, Tay-Sachs disease, sickle cell anemia, and thalassemia (a blood disorder). If a person has only one defective gene, he or she will have no symptoms but will be a carrier of that disease and may pass the disease on to offspring. If two carriers have children, each of their children has a 25 percent chance of inheriting the condition.

Autosomal Dominant Disorders. Disorders caused by autosomal dominant genes are less common. In this case, a person only needs to inherit a defective gene from one parent in order to have the condition. For this reason, most patients also have an affected parent. Rarely, an autosomal dominant disorder occurs through a spontaneous mutation. An example of this is achondroplasia, a form of dwarfism. Eighty percent of affected individuals have normal parents.

Locating Defective Genes. In recent years, due to work done on the human genome, the genes responsible for several disorders have been "discovered"; their location on a particular chromosome has been identified. Among these disorders are Huntington's chorea, cystic fibrosis, Marfan's syndrome, sickle cell anemia, thalassemia, Gaucher's disease, G6PD deficiency, and Tay-Sachs disease. Knowing the location of a gene for a given disorder can help in properly diagnosing that disease. In the future, this knowledge may lead to the ability to cure these diseases by replacing the defective gene with a healthy one.

Treatment. Treatment of genetic disorders is a largely experimental field. Current treatments are aimed at preventing the transmission of genetic disease and treating individuals in order to avoid, alleviate, or compensate for symptoms.

Gene therapy, inserting correct copies of the gene into the appropriate cell, is a potential way to cure genetic diseases. However, it is a very new technique and so far has enjoyed only limited success in the treatment of diseases such as hemophilia (a blood clotting disorder) and squamous cell carcinoma (a form of skin cancer).

Prevention. Family history is the single most important piece of information in determining a couple's risk for having a child with a genetic disorder. If parents suspect they may be carriers for a genetic disorder, it is advised that they seek genetic counseling. They may be able take a blood test to determine the presence or absence of the responsible gene.

Prenatal screening techniques can reveal if a fetus already conceived is suffering from a genetic disorder. For example, the alphafetoprotein test and amniocentesis can determine the presence of Down's syndrome. Having the information, however, does not determine a course of action.

For background information on genetic disorders, see GENE *and* GENETICS. *For further information, see* CHROMOSOMAL ABNORMALITIES; CYSTIC FIBROSIS; DOWN'S SYNDROME; *and* METABOLISM, INBORN ERRORS OF. *See also* GENETIC ENGINEERING *for more on research.*

Genetic Engineering

The process of altering the genetic makeup of an organism.

Since the mid 1970s, scientists have been able to transfer human genes into bacteria. Often, a gene that produces a specific protein (such as insulin or growth hormone) is inserted, or spliced, into the DNA of bacteria or other quickly reproducing microorganisms, such as viruses. The microorganisms then reproduce rapidly, producing many copies of the gene and thus a large supply of the desired protein.

In recent years, genetically engineered foods, such as tomatoes that resist rotting, have appeared in supermarkets. Various other crops have been made more resistant to disease, or have had their nutritional content boosted, by the insertion of genes from other species. This has been a source of concern for some scientists and consumers, who worry about the effects of cross-species genetic "swapping."

Genetic engineering is also being considered as a method of treating various genetic diseases, particularly autosomal recessive diseases (such as Tay Sachs disease), which are caused by the presence of two recessive genes. Insertion of a healthy copy of the gene would result in a permanent cure. Theoretically, the same technology makes possible the insertion of "designer" genes into sperm or eggs, resulting in genetically engineered children.

Background material on genetic engineering can be found in CHROMOSOMES; GENE; *and* GENETICS. *For related information, see* CHROMOSOME ANALYSIS; CONGENITAL; GENETIC DISORDERS; *and* INHERITANCE.

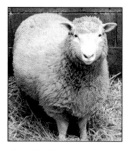

Genetic Engineering. In genetic engineering, scientists alter the genetic makeup of an organism. Results of genetic engineering are most striking in the case of Dolly the sheep, above, who was created in the laboratory by the process of cloning.

Resources on Genetic Disorders
New, Maria, *Genetics of Endocrine Disorders* (2001); Pollack, Robert, *Signs of Life: The Languages and Meanings of DNA* (1994); Alliance of Genetic Support Groups, Tel. (800) 336-GENE, Online: www.medhelp.org/geneticalliance; Easter Seals, Tel. (800) 221-6827, Online: www.seals.org; National Center for Biotechnology Information, Tel. (301) 496-2475, Online: www.ncbi.nih.gov; Office of Rare Diseases, Tel. (301) 402-4336, Online: rarediseases.info.nih.gov/ord; http://www.med.cornell.edu/research/cores/genetherapy/index.html.

Genetic Probe

Also known as a DNA probe

A method for detecting microorganisms by using genetic material.

A genetic probe is used to detect and identify microorganisms by causing them to bind to a specially prepared combination of genetic material and chemicals. Included in the mixture is a marker—either a radioactive material or a vitamin component known as biotin—that can be easily detected and tracked. The material is prepared so that it only binds to one type of microorganism; thus, when body tissue or fluids are exposed to this genetic probe, only the selected organism will bind to it, revealing the presence, amount, and location of the material.

Genetic probes can be used to determine if a person has a specific disease, often chlamydia or gonorrhea, by testing for the presence of the microorganism that causes the disease. *See also* MICROORGANISM.

Genetics

The study of how traits are passed on from parents to offspring.

Many human characteristics are determined or influenced by genetic makeup. Some physical characteristics, such as eye color, are solely determined by genetics, while others, such as intellectual ability, are influenced by genetics and environment.

The study of genetics is the study of how traits are passed through generations. This includes the study of underlying biochemical processes, the study of inheritance patterns in groups of people, identifying and locating genes responsible for particular traits, and the study of the treatment and prevention of genetic disorders.

Treating Genetic Disorders. Many disorders are caused by or are affected by a person's genetic makeup. Genetic disorders may be caused by irregularities in a person's chromosomes, as is the case with Down's syndrome, or in one or more genes, as with cystic fibrosis. The likelihood of developing conditions such as heart disease, cancer, and diabetes can also have a genetic component.

Much of current genetics research focuses on identifying the location and purpose of every gene in the human body. This information will be instrumental in allowing geneticists to figure out how to prevent, and ultimately cure, genetic diseases. Currently, treatment is aimed at preventing the transmission of diseases and controlling symptoms. Individuals affected by a genetic disorder, with a family history of genetic disorders, or who have already had a child with a genetic disorder are advised to seek genetic counseling before having more offspring. With genetic counseling, prospective parents can figure out the likelihood of having children with a given disease, learn how that disease may impact an affected child and the entire family, and decide on what course of action they feel is best.

For background information on genetics, see CHROMOSOMES *and* GENE. *Further information can be found in* CHROMOSOMAL ABNORMALITIES; CHROMOSOME ANALYSIS; CLONE; CONGENITAL; *and* INHERITANCE.

Genital Ulceration

Sores or ulcers on the genitals, indicating a sexually transmitted disease.

Genital ulceration is generally a sign of syphilis, chancroid, lymphogranuloma venereum, or genital herpes.

Syphilis. One of the earliest signs of syphilis is a painless ulcer or chancre at the infection site—usually the penis, vulva, or vagina. The ulcer begins as a small, red, raised area and then turns into an open sore. The ulcer is not painful and doesn't bleed, but leaks a clear fluid. It usually heals in 3 to 12 weeks.

Chancroid. Chancroid begins with small painful blisters on the genitals and anus that rupture and form ulcers. These may enlarge and merge into one large sore. The ulcers may heal spontaneously, but often become infected by bacteria.

Lymphogranuloma venereum also begins with genital blisters that turn into ulcers. These sores often go unnoticed and may heal on their own.

Genital herpes begins with itching and soreness in the genital area, and then a redness that develops painful blisters. These blisters break and merge to form painful ulcers. The sores crust over and eventually heal, until the next outbreak.

Treatment. Many genital ulcers heal without medical intervention. Various medications can be given to both help the healing process, as well as to cure the underlying sexually transmitted disease. *See also* CHANCROID; HERPES, GENITAL; LYMPHOGRANULOMA VENEREUM; *and* SYPHILIS.

Germ

> A microorganism capable of causing illness in people or animals.

At the request of a French winemaker, Louis Pasteur researched the fermentation process and discovered that microbes were the agents of fermentation and lived without air. This led to the discovery of the germs that cause septicemia and gangrene, both of which were major diseases in the late nineteenth century. The discovery also led to the germ theory of disease. Pasteur invented pasteurization as a technique for keeping milk from fermenting by heating it to the point where the microorganisms living in it were killed. Joseph Lister was later to apply the same thinking to the disinfecting of wounds and medical instruments used in surgery. *See also* MICROORGANISM.

Germ Cell Tumor

> A tumor of the cells that form sperm and ova.

When germ cells turn malignant, it is often in the very early stages of their development. In men, 95 percent of testicular cancers arise from the sperm-forming germ cells. About 40 percent of these tumors are classified as seminomas. Seminomas are made up of a single type of cell, while other tumors of the testes (nonseminomas) can consist of several different types of cells. Seminomas are treated by surgical removal of the affected testicle and are curable if treated early. Radiation therapy is used if the tumors have spread beyond the testicle. Nonseminoma germ cell tumors are treated with surgery and chemotherapy. Prognosis is excellent. *See also* TESTIS, CANCER OF.

Gerontology

> The study of the physical, psychological, and social consequences of aging.

Modern medicine and the benefits of an affluent society have extended life spans dramatically over the last century. Between 1960 and 1990, the total population of the United States rose 39 percent, with the number of people over 65 growing 89 percent and those 85 and over growing 232 percent. Individuals today live longer, healthier, and more productive lives. With preventive health care, exercise, and a balanced diet the effects of aging can be minimized, and people may lead rich and active lives well into their 80s and beyond.

THEORIES OF AGING

A person's genetic make-up, lifestyle, and environment all contribute to the rate at which the body ages. Most research on aging has shown the upper limit of the human lifespan to range from age 95 to 110. No one knows exactly why aging occurs. Some scientists think the body has an internal clock that makes cells stop reproducing after a given number of cell divisions. Others point to a gradual decline in the functioning of major organs and the immune system, making people more vulnerable to disease as they age. Some alternative medicine advocates claim that aging results from an accumulation of toxins, radiation damage, or free radicals, although these theories are not clinically supported.

PHYSICAL ASPECTS OF AGING

In approximately the latter third of life, the body's cells cease to be able to replicate

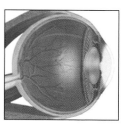

The Aging Eye. Above, as the eye ages, changes occur. The iris fades, and the cornea becomes less sensitive. The pupil shrinks, and the lens becomes yellowed and cloudy. These factors contribute to a decrease in visual acuity.

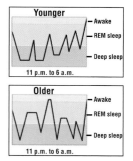

Sleep Patterns. Sleep patterns also change as a person ages. Above, top, a younger person gets more deep sleep and less REM sleep. Above, bottom, an older person gets more REM sleep and less deep sleep.

Estimated Life Expectancy at Birth
In years by race and sex for the United States, 1997.

ALL RACES		WHITE		BLACK	
Both Sexes	76.5	Both Sexes	77.2	Both Sexes	71.1
Male	73.6	Male	74.3	Male	67.2
Female	79.9	Female	79.9	Female	74.7

from the National Center for Health Statistics,
National Vital Statistics Report, Vol. 47, No. 28, Dec. 13, 1999.

Nursing Home Residents
Number and distribution of nursing home residents aged 65 and over in the United States.

Age of Admission	# Residents	Percentage
total	1,385,400	100.0
65-74 years	242,000	17.5
75-84 years	586,300	42.3
85 years and over	557,100	40.2

from the Center for Disease Control
1995 National Nursing Home Survey

Resources on Gerontology and Elder Care
Cassel, Christine, *Geriatric Medicine* (1990), Fries, James F., *Aging Well* (1989); Rossman, Isadore, *Looking Forward: The Complete Medical Guide to Successful Aging* (1989); Schneider, Edward L. and John W. Rowe, *Handbook of the Biology of Aging* (1996); Weiss, Robert, et al., *Complete Guide to Health and Well-Being After Fifty* (1988); American Assoc. of Retired Persons, Tel. (800) 424-3410, Online: www.aarp.org; American Geriatrics Soc., Tel. (212) 308-1414, Online: www.americangeriatrics.org; National Council on Aging, Tel. (800) 424-9046, Online: www.ncoa.org; www.nyc-ornell.org/medicine/geriatrics/index.html; www.cornellaging.org/.

themselves as promptly and healthily as they once did, resulting in a loss of functioning in the body's systems. The skin loses some of its fat layer, becomes drier, and loses elasticity. Fat in the body as a whole lessens, reducing the ability of the body to adjust to changes in environmental temperature. The blood vessels lose elasticity, and plaque builds up in the arteries, restricting the flow of blood. The body tries to compensate for this by raising the blood pressure. The ligaments and cartilage that smooth the action of the joints grow less flexible. The bones lose strength and density and are more easily fractured. Lungs lose some of their ability to absorb oxygen and expel carbon dioxide. Short term memory may become less effective. Vision may also deteriorate.

PSYCHOLOGICAL ASPECTS OF AGING
Some researchers argue that phases of aging are determined more by ability than by age. For instance, many people well into their early 70s do not experience any significant signs of aging. They may be capable of keeping up with the mental and physical tasks they performed 10 years earlier. Most people, however, do begin to slow down noticeably by their middle to late 70s. Many often suffer from feelings of depression and loss as a result. Leaving a job, declining health, and loneliness can have adverse effects on people in their senior years. In addition, studies have shown that among the elderly, those who are emotionally isolated and have less contact with people often have shorter life-spans than those who are socially involved. Part-time or volunteer jobs can help the elderly stay active and involved. Physical activity of any sort can also aid in relaxation, quality of life, and overall sense of well-being. In instances of serious depression, antidepressant medications may be prescribed, although they are not a cure in themselves.

SOCIAL ASPECTS OF AGING
As the population ages, and particularly as the number of men and women over 65 increases in proportion to people in their prime earning years, there will be less financial and social support for the elderly. In the United States, during the year 2000 there were approximately 4.6 persons aged 20 to 64 for every person 65 and older. By 2030 there are expected to be only 2.6 persons for every senior. For the Social Security system, there are going to be far fewer workers supporting more retirees. Since Social Security is dependent on current income, the cost will be almost insupportable unless major changes are made.

The elderly account for almost half of all days spent in the hospital and a third of the country's cost of health care, but many believe that older Americans do not receive adequate medical care. Many physicians refuse to accept Medicare recipients outright, pointing to low pay schedules and red tape. Of the country's 126 medical schools, only eight require courses in geriatric medicine. Because of wrong prescriptions or incorrect dosages, more than half of all deaths resulting from drug reactions occur among the elderly. Conversely, about a third of acute hospital procedures performed on older patients are believed to be unnecessary. There is, however, no conclusive evidence that adequately offers reasons for this phenomenon.

Background material on gerontology can be found in AGING. *For further information, see* ANTIDEPRESSANT DRUGS; ELDERLY, CARE OF THE; *and* GENETICS. *See also* ALZHEIMER'S DISEASE; DEGENERATIVE DISORDERS; DEPRESSION; *and* FALLS IN THE ELDERLY *for more on conditions affecting elderly individuals.*

Gestation

The length of time during pregnancy that a fertilized egg cell develops into a baby.

The gestation period for a human is about nine months (280 days). The gestational period is divided into three stages (trimesters), with developmental milestones marked at specific weeks. Knowing how far into gestation a fetus is provides important information for monitoring its growth. If a baby is born too soon before its due date, it may not be developed enough to survive well outside the uterus; it often has respiratory and neurological problems. If a fetus remains in the uterus well after its due date, the placenta may cease to function, preventing the fetus from receiving oxygen and nutrients. *See also* PREGNANCY.

Giardiasis

Parasitic Infestation by the microscopic organism *Giardia lamblia*.

Giardiasis is caused by the single-celled parasite (protozoan) *Giardia lamblia*. It may be contracted by consuming water or food contaminated with cysts passed in the stool or through direct contact.

Symptoms. Generally, giardiasis produces no symptoms, but symptoms may include nausea, increased gas and flatulence, abdominal pain and discomfort, diarrhea, and foul-smelling stools. Weight loss may occur in severe cases.

Diagnosis. Diagnosis is confirmed by laboratory identification of the parasite in the patient's stool or secretions of the upper part of the small intestine (duodenum). Periodic stool examination may be required for diagnosis, as the parasites are passed in the fecal matter intermittently.

Treatment. Minor cases of giardiasis clear up without treatment. For severe cases, the antibiotic drug metronidazole can effectively treat infestation. Those living in close contact with persons infected with giardiasis should be tested for the disease. *See also* PARASITE *and* PROTOZOA.

Gigantism

Unusual growth, due to excess production of the growth hormone.

Growth hormone, produced by the pituitary gland, is responsible for growth and development through the production of a protein called IGF-1. Increased production of this hormone leads to increased growth. If too much growth hormone is produced during childhood, a child may experience rapid and unexpected growth, achieving height beyond the norm.

Causes. In most cases, a tumor in the pituitary gland is responsible for the release of too much growth hormone.

Diagnosis and Treatment. Once it is determined that unusual growth is not due to other harmless causes, such as simple heredity, imaging of the pituitary and blood tests can detect if there is a tumor present. The tumor may be irradiated and surgically removed; the drug octreotide is sometimes, but rarely, used to counteract the effects of the tumor. The height, however, will not be lost.

For background information on gigantism, see GROWTH HORMONE. *Further information can be found in* CHROMOSOMAL ABNORMALITIES; BROMOCRIPTINE; CANCER; CHROMOSOMES; CONGENITAL; GENE; GENETIC DISORDERS; INHERITANCE; METABOLISM, INBORN ERRORS OF; MRI; *and* PITUITARY GLAND. *See also* GROWTH, CHILDHOOD *for more on accepted standards in child development.*

Gilbert's Syndrome

An inherited liver disease characterized by elevated levels of bilirubin.

In Gilbert's syndrome, due to an enzyme deficiency, the liver is unable to process bilirubin into a form that can be excreted through the bile, resulting in jaundice. Gilbert's syndrome is believed to be the most common cause of hyperbilirubinemia. Jaundice is relatively mild but may be exacerbated by fasting. The syndrome does not lead to liver damage and does not require treatment. *See* HYPERBILIRUBINEMIA.

Gilles de la Tourette's Syndrome

Generally referred to as Tourette's syndrome

A rare, inherited neurological disorder distinguished by repetitive involuntary movements and sometimes vocalizations.

Tourette's syndrome begins during childhood and is characterized by tics of the head, neck, arms, legs, and trunk. Tics can be sudden movements that involve one muscle group or complex coordinated patterns of successive movements involving several muscle groups. Symptoms worsen during times of stress. Tourette's syndrome affects males three to four times more often than females. It is estimated that 100,000 Americans are permanently afflicted with Tourette's syndrome.

Causes. Tourette's syndrome is a disorder of the central nervous system. Research suggests that it is caused by an abnormality in the brain's uptake of essential neurotransmitters—chemicals in the brain that transfer signals between nerve cells.

Symptoms. Symptoms of Tourette's syndrome range from simple facial or vocal tics, such as blinking the eyes, grimacing, or grunting, to complex vocal tics, such as involuntarily uttering obscenities or mimicking other people. Tics may also involve the neck and shoulders. In some cases, especially in females, the syndrome is accompanied by obsessive-compulsive behavior.

Diagnosis. Tourette's syndrome is underdiagnosed, because its symptoms mimic those of psychiatric disorders and other neurological disorders. Diagnosis often involves ruling out other disorders before Tourette's syndrome is recognized.

Treatment. Antipsychotic drugs can reduce the frequency and severity of tics. Patients with Tourette's syndrome can help keep symptoms under control by avoiding stress and fatigue, which exacerbate the tics. Support from family and friends and psychotherapy can help patients with Tourette's syndrome cope with the social isolation that often accompanies the disorder. *See also* CENTRAL NERVOUS SYSTEM *and* TIC.

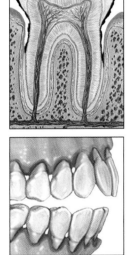

Gingivitis. Above, top, gingivitis is an inflammatory condition of the gums that results when plaque and bacteria irritate and damage the gums and the connections from the gums to the roots of the teeth. Above, bottom, the disease causes the gums to recede from the roots of the teeth.

Gingivectomy

Procedure for removing part of the gums.

A gingivectomy is performed when the gums have become so diseased that healing or restoration is impossible. Gum infection can affect the health of the teeth. In milder cases of gum infection, the gums can be cleaned or cut back slightly, but when the damage is severe, much more of the gums must be removed.

In a gingivectomy, the gums are numbed, trimmed, reshaped, and treated with antibacterial medication. The healing process lasts several weeks and those who fail to take proper care of their teeth during this period can suffer a recurrence of infection. *See also* DENTISTRY *and* GINGIVITIS.

Gingivitis

Inflammation of the gums.

Like the teeth, the gums (gingiva) are affected by plaque buildup. Failure to brush and floss properly can result in an infection with bacteria that destroy the gums and the bones and teeth around them.

Most people pay insufficient attention to their gums and may be unaware of any trouble in this area until symptoms occur. In the early stages of gum disease (gingivitis), the gums bleed easily during toothbrushing. There may be pain and tenderness, the gums may be swollen, and there may be a discharge of pus, especially as the disease progresses.

Gingivitis can often be reversed simply through proper dental hygiene, including brushing regularly and flossing carefully. The use of either dental floss or interdental stimulators is essential in keeping the gums healthy and strong. Failure to take care of the teeth and gums can result in a worsening of the inflammation, to the point that the damage is no longer reversible and more extreme measures must be taken. The gums can recede to the point that even healthy teeth can loosen and fall out. *See also* FLOSSING, DENTAL *and* PERIODONTITIS.

Gland

One of several organs that produces and secretes chemicals to be used within the body.

The glands create and release chemicals, including hormones, that help the body carry out everyday functions. Hormones also activate tissues and organs and coordinate activities within the body.

Types. There are two types of glands. Endocrine glands release chemicals directly into the bloodstream. The chemicals then travel through the body to the organ or tissue in which they operate, which may be located far from the gland. The glands of the endocrine system include the pituitary gland, thyroid gland, parathyroid glands, adrenal glands, pancreas, ovaries, and testes. The pituitary gland coordinates many of the activities of the other endocrine glands.

Exocrine glands secrete chemicals into ducts, tubelike passageways that lead directly into organs or tissues, such as the mouth, eyes, or skin. Salivary glands, sebaceous glands, sweat glands, and lacrimal glands, which release tears, are examples of exocrine glands.

> Background material on gland can be found in EN-DOCRINOLOGY. *For related information, see* ADRENAL GLANDS; ENDOCRINE DISORDERS; ENDOCRINE GLAND; EXOCRINE GLAND; HORMONES; HYPOTHALAMUS; LYMPHATIC SYSTEM; PARATHYROID GLANDS; PITUITARY GLAND; *and* THYROID GLAND.

Glands, Swollen

An enlargement of the lymph nodes or glands, generally a clear sign of infection.

Background. The lymph system parallels the blood circulatory system. Just as blood flows through the blood vessels, lymphatic fluid moves through the tissues of the body and the spaces between cells. Lymphatic fluid is a clear, watery fluid that acts as an intermediary between the blood and the cells. The fluid moves through a network of vessels the thickness of a single hair. Dead or damaged white and red blood cells are

> ## Physical Examination
>
> In a physical examination, one of the first things a physician will examine is the area under the patient's jaw and neck. If there is an infection in the body, the lymph glands in this area will be swollen. The physician will also check other areas of the body in which glands are present to determine if those glands are swollen as well. If an infection is present, the glands will be enlarged and firm to the touch. The location of the swollen glands points to the part of the body that is infected, though it does not indicate the specific underlying cause of the infection.

allowed through the porous walls of the vessels. These substances then accumulate in the glands.

The glands are grouped in various areas throughout the body. Areas where the glands can be felt include the armpits, the groin, under the jaw, the neck, and behind the ears.

Causes. The most common cause of swollen glands is infection. Glands play a crucial role in the body's response to infection by bacterial, fungal, and viral pathogens (disease-causing agents). The glands can become swollen even if the infection is so small as to go undetected by the infected individual. If a person is infected by a pathogen, the gland will swell and become painful to the touch.

A less common cause of swollen glands is cancer. Leukemia and Hodgkin's disease are two types of cancer that can cause swelling of the glands. If the glands enlarge slowly and painlessly, it is possible that a cancerous tumor may be the cause.

Treatment. Swelling of the glands caused by infection generally disappears spontaneously if the underlying infection is treated. It may take up to a couple of weeks for the glands to return to normal size after an infection. If the cause of the swelling is cancer, the cancer must be treated with radiation therapy or chemotherapy.

> For background information on swollen glands, see LYMPHATIC SYSTEM. *Further information can be found in* CANCER; EXAMINATION, PHYSICAL; GLAND; *and* INFECTIOUS DISEASE. *See also* CHEMOTHERAPY *for more on treatment.*

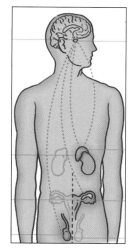

Endocrine System. Above, the endocrine system consists of many glands, all of which send and receive hormonal triggers.

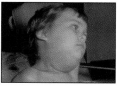

Swollen Glands. The glands usually swell when there are infectious agents present in the body, such as fungi, viruses, or bacteria. Certain diseases, such as the mumps, above, are characterized by swollen glands.

Glaucoma

Damage that is caused by the high pressure of fluid in the eye.

A certain level of pressure holds the eyeball together, but an excess of that pressure may damage blood vessels or the optic nerve, resulting in impaired vision or blindness. Glaucoma rarely afflicts those under the age of 40. The damage often occurs before symptoms become apparent.

Description. The aqueous humor is a fluid that nourishes the cornea and lens. It flows from behind the iris, through the pupil, and into the space in front of the iris. Then it passes into the bloodstream. All of the aqueous humor secreted is normally reabsorbed. In the case of a disorder such as glaucoma, however, drainage is partially or completely blocked, and pressure builds. The cause is unknown.

Types. Chronic simple glaucoma accounts for 95 percent of cases. Chronic secondary glaucoma arises from complications of another eye problem, such as infection, swelling, allergy, injury, a tumor, or a cataract. Chronic simple and secondary glaucoma cause similar damage.

Acute glaucoma, rare and sudden, can occur within hours. In this case, the drainage of aqueous fluid is entirely blocked, resulting in such great pressure that the increased hardness of the eyeball can be felt. Symptoms include severe headaches, nausea, and vomiting. Only immediate medical attention can avert blindness. Acute glaucoma is either "simple" or "secondary": the former when the drainage is chronically low; the latter when it is brought on by another cause.

Congenital glaucoma is rare. Present at birth, it results in defective aqueous fluid drainage canals, which makes the small eyes of an infant bulge.

Diagnosis and Treatment. An annual eye exam after the age of 40 detects any sign of glaucoma. If caught in time, treatment is highly successful. Pilocarpine, the first glaucoma drug in the form of eye drops, constricts the pupil, drawing it away from the drainage angle, increasing drainage and decreasing pressure. Timolol maleate decreases the secretion of aqueous fluid and thus limits pressure. Dipivefrin influences both secretion and drainage to relieve pressure.

> *Background material on glaucoma can be found in* EYE *and* EYE, DISORDERS OF. *For related information, see* AGING; BLOOD PRESSURE; CORNEA; HEADACHE; NAUSEA; OPTIC NERVE; VISION, LOSS OF; *and* VOMITING.

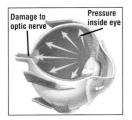

Glaucoma.
Above, in patients with glaucoma, pressure inside the eye radiates towards the back of the eye and causes damage to the optic nerve.

Resources on Glaucoma
Eden, John, T*he Physician's Guide to Cataracts, Glaucoma, and Other Eye Problems* (1992); Kronfeld, P.C., *The Hu-man Eye in Anatomical Transparencies* (1943); Schmidt, Robert F., *Fundamentals of Sensory Physiology* (1986); Wolf, K.P., *Eyewise: Eye Dis-orders and Their Treat-ment* (1982); Glaucoma Research Foundation, Tel. (800) 826-6693, Online: www.glaucoma.org; National Association for the Visually Handicapped, Tel. (212) 889-3141, Online: wwww.navh.org.

Glioblastoma Multiforme

A type of malignant brain tumor.

Glioblastoma multiforme belongs to the family of cancers called gliomas, which arise from glial cells—cells that compose the supporting tissue of the brain. Glioblastomas are common and highly malignant, growing quickly within the brain. Most of these cancers are found in the cerebrum, the main mass of the brain. The symptoms can include loss of vision, speech disturbances, impaired mental functioning, and muscle weakness, depending on the site of the tumor. Treatment includes surgery, radiation therapy, and chemotherapy, but the prognosis is limited. *See also* CANCER; CHEMOTHERAPY; *and* RADIATION THERAPY.

Glioma

A tumor of certain cells of the brain.

Fifty to 60 percent of brain tumors are gliomas, tumors of the glial cells. Glial cells provide support and nourishment to the nerve cells of the brain. The most common form of glioma is the astrocytoma, which usually develops in the cerebrum, the part of the brain that handles thought, memory, and speech. A subgroup, glioblastoma multiforme, is fast-growing and accounts for about a third of all brain tumors. Other gliomas include medulloblastoma, oligodendroglioma, and ependymoma. *See also* ASTROCYTOMA; EPENDYMOMA; GLIOBLASTOMA MULTIFORME; MEDULLOBLASTOMA; *and* OLIGODENDROGLIOMA.

Globulin

Any of a large group of proteins found in the blood and tissues of plants and animals.

There are many different types of globulins, including alpha globulins, beta globulins, and gamma globulins. The most important globulins for immunity are the gamma globulins, which serve as the primary stimulant of the immune system. Gamma globulins can be filtered out of the blood of healthy donors who have developed antibodies to diseases. They can then be given to a recipient with a deficient immune system to create temporary immunity. *See also* ANTIBODY *and* IMMUNITY.

Glomerulonephritis

Destructive inflammation of the filtering units of the kidneys (glomeruli).

A number of conditions can cause glomerulonephritis, including infections. The immune system responds to infections by making antibodies to attack the infectious agent. In some cases, the antibodies can combine with molecules that trigger the immune response (antigens). The resulting antibody-antigen complexes can stimulate an inflammatory process in which enzymes and inflammatory cells attack and destroy the glomeruli.

Symptoms. Bloody, foamy, or cola-colored urine; swelling of the feet, legs, and sometimes the hands, often accompanied by joint pain; and abdominal discomfort can result from an acute attack of glomerulonephritis. Those symptoms often follow a streptococcal infection, such as strep throat. Chronic glomerulonephritis may cause no symptoms and may be detected in a routine blood test. At the other extreme, a sudden attack of acute glomerulonephritis that causes kidney failure may result in an abnormally low production of urine.

Diagnosis. A urinalysis using a microscope can detect red blood cells and other debris derived from the glomerulus. The

---

> ## Dietary Changes to Limit Glomerulonephritis
>
> Dietary changes in older persons with glomerulonephritis are designed to delay or prevent the onset of kidney failure. In many cases, a diet low in protein and phosphate may be advised to reduce the workload on the kidneys. Careful control of blood sugar levels in diabetic patients is also very important to keep the kidneys functioning adequately for as long as possible.

presence of glomerulonephritis and its probable cause can often be determined by a careful urinalysis and additional blood tests. Often a biopsy, a sample of kidney tissue, is taken for examination under a microscope. Several blood and urine samples can be taken to see how well the kidneys are functioning and how they are responding to treatment.

Treatment. Treatment depends on the underlying cause of the condition. Children experiencing glomerulonephritis after a streptococcal infection may get well with little or no treatment. Adults often will be given immunosuppressive drugs, such as corticosteroids, to reduce the activity of the immune system.

Drugs that reduce the high blood pressure caused by glomerulonephritis may also be prescribed, along with salt restrictions and other dietary measures. If these measures fail to stop the progression of the condition, dialysis (the removal of waste products and excess fluid from the body) may be necessary to supplement the work of the kidneys.

In some cases, a blood-purifying technique called plasma exchange may be performed to remove the damaging immune complexes from the body. If these measures do not work and kidney failure occurs, permanent dialysis or a kidney transplant are the life-saving options.

For background information on glomerulonephritis, see KIDNEY. *Related information can be found in* ABDOMINAL PAIN; ANTIGEN; BIOPSY; CORTICOSTEROID DRUGS; DIALYSIS; IMMUNE SYSTEM; IMMUNITY; IMMUNOSUPPRESSANT DRUGS; KIDNEY TRANSPLANT; *and* STREPTOCOCCAL INFECTIONS.

Glomerulosclerosis

Scarring of the glomeruli, the filtering units of the kidney.

The glomerulus, a channel through which blood flows in the kidney, can be damaged by the normal process of aging. Since normal life is possible even with a third or less of normal kidney function, and since the deterioration causes no symptoms, the condition may go unnoticed. However, extensive glomerulosclerosis is more serious and can result from a number of medical conditions, including inflammation of the glomeruli (glomerulonephritis), diabetes, high blood pressure (hypertension), and intravenous drug abuse. Extensive scarring of the glomeruli may reduce kidney function enough to require external removal of waste products and excess fluid from the body (by dialysis) or a kidney transplant. *See also* DIALYSIS; GLOMERULONEPHRITIS; *and* KIDNEY TRANSPLANT.

Glossectomy

Surgery to remove the tongue.

A glossectomy may be required in cases of tongue cancer; sometimes the removal of a portion of the tongue will suffice, but in other cases the whole tongue may need to be removed. Partial removal will impair speech, and a complete removal will result in a loss of speech and eating ability, in which case the patient will have to be fed through a feeding tube. Radiation treatment is the preferred method of treatment for this type of cancer. *See also* SPEECH; TONGUE; *and* TONGUE, CANCER OF.

Glossitis

An inflamed tongue.

The tongue is the organ responsible for speech and for breaking down food. A mass of muscles and nerve cells, the tongue can be adversely affected by conditions that affect the mouth or other parts of the body.

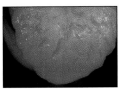

Glossitis.
Above, the red and swollen tongue of a patient with pellagra, a disorder caused by a niacin deficiency.

Glossitis, an inflamed tongue, is not a condition that exists on its own, but is rather a symptom of another disorder.

Causes. Common causes of glossitis are anemia resulting from iron deficiencies, pernicious and megaloblastic anemia (usually indicating a lack of vitamin B_{12}), and nutritional deficiencies, such as a lack of vitamin B, vitamin E, niacin, and riboflavin. Mouth disorders or irritations can also result in glossitis, as can herpes simplex, dehydration, irritation from dentures, and overuse of alcohol, tobacco, and hot spices.

Symptoms. The primary symptom of glossitis is a swollen tongue, which loses its papillae (the small protuberances on the tongue enabling taste), becoming red and smooth. It may be accompanied by pain and soreness.

Treatment. Treatment for glossitis consists of diagnosing and remedying the underlying disorder. *See also* ANEMIA; HERPES SIMPLEX; VITAMIN B; *and* VITAMIN E.

Glucagon

Hormone that converts glycogen to glucose.

Two of the hormones secreted by the pancreas are insulin and glucagon. During digestion, carbohydrates are broken down into glucose (a simple sugar), which the body either uses for energy or stores as glycogen. When glucose levels in the blood rise, the pancreas releases insulin, which causes the cells to take up glucose. When food does not enter the body, such as between meals, during sleep, and during periods of starvation, blood glucose levels drop. The alpha cells of the pancreas then secrete glucagon, which converts glycogen into glucose. This glucose then travels back into the bloodstream, where it is used for energy.

MEDICAL USE

Glucagon can be used to revive diabetics whose blood sugar has gotten too low (hypoglycemia). *See also* DIABETES MELLITUS; HUNGER; HYPOGLYCEMIA; INSULIN; METABOLISM; *and* PANCREAS.

Glucocorticoids

Hormones that aid in processing and using nutrients for energy (metabolism).

The adrenal cortex, the outer layer of the adrenal glands, secretes hormones that help the body break down fats, proteins, and carbohydrates into energy. These hormones, called glucocorticoids, have many functions, including the regulation of carbohydrate metabolism. The rate at which the glucocorticoids are released is determined by the pituitary gland, which receives instructions from the hypothalamus. The most important hormone in this group is hydrocortisone. *See also* ADRENAL GLANDS; DIGESTIVE SYSTEM; HORMONES; HYPOTHALAMUS; METABOLISM; *and* PITUITARY GLAND.

Glucose

A form of carbohydrate, known as a simple sugar, and the primary source of energy for cell function.

The body metabolizes dietary forms of carbohydrates into glucose. It is the primary type of carbohydrate that the body can use instantly for energy, and is also the main form of energy that can be used by the nervous system and brain. After the glucose is metabolized by a cell, its original source (i.e., bread or candy) is immaterial.

Uses. Glucose can be used instantaneously, releasing water, carbon dioxide, and energy. If energy is not needed immediately, the liver and muscle convert glucose into glycogen, which is stored in the liver and can be turned back into glucose when necessary. After liver glycogen stores have been expended, fat deposits are utilized as an alternate source of energy.

If a surplus of glucose exists and glycogen reserves are full, the liver and other organs convert excess glucose into fat. The resulting fatty acids are a far less efficient energy source than glucose, and are used when glucose stores become depleted. *See also* CARBOHYDRATES; DIABETES MELLITUS; *and* GLYCOGEN.

Gluten

Protein found in wheat and other grains, which produces an allergic reaction in some people.

Gluten is a protein found in wheat, rye, barley, and other cereal grains. In individuals with celiac disease (known as celiac sprue), gluten prompts an allergic reaction, causing the lining of the small intestine to become inflamed, so that minute hair-like projections (villi) shrink or disappear, preventing absorption of nutrients.

Diet and Celiac Disease

Individuals with celiac disease should read ingredient lists carefully and be aware that gluten is often used in processed foods as a thickener and in medications to bind pills together. Those with celiac disease who continue to consume gluten increase their chances of cancer, particularly intestinal lymphoma. Buckwheat, which is actually a fruit related to rhubarb, is a gluten-free alternative with a protein quality higher than that of wheat, oats, rice, or soy.

Symptoms. Symptoms of celiac sprue include weight loss, diarrhea, bloating, and foul-smelling stools, and, as the disease progresses, may lead to malabsorption. The only way for those with celiac disease to prevent further damage to their intestines is to avoid all foods or medications containing gluten. *See also* CELIAC SPRUE.

Glycerol

Organic compound belonging to the alcohol family, and a primary component of fat.

When linked to one of three fatty acids, glycerol makes up fats. The type of fats bonded to the glycerol determine what type of main dietary fat is formed. When one, two, or three fatty acid molecules bond to glycerol, they are called monoglycerides, diglycerides, and triglycerides. Dietary fats are broken down by the body into these components. The glycerol molecule can also be detached and used as a source of energy, similar to the way that the body utilizes glucose (sugar). *See also* GLUCOSE.

Goiter.
Above, a goiter is an enlarged thyroid gland that is generally caused either by an iodine deficiency or by an autoimmune disorder.

Resources on Goiter and Thyroid Disorders

Nuland, Sherwin B., *The Wisdom of the Body* (1997); Greenspan, Francis S., et al., *Basic & Clinical Endocrinology* (2000); Shin, Linda M., et al., *Endocrine and Metabolic Disorders Sourcebook* (1998); Arem, Ridha, *The Thyroid Solution* (2000); Rosenthal, M. Sara, *The Thyroid Sourcebook for Women* (1999); Hypoglycemia Support Foundation, Tel. (518) 272-7154, Online: www.hypoglycemia.org; Thyroid Foundation of America, Tel. (800) 832-8321, Online: www.tsh.org; American Thyroid Association, Tel. (718) 882-6047, Online: www.thyroid.org; www.nycornell.org/medicine/edm/index.html.

Glycogen

Form in which carbohydrate energy is stored in the muscles and liver.

When glucose (sugar) is not needed for immediate energy, it is converted into glycogen by the liver or muscles, and remade into glucose when necessary. Glucose released from glycogen produced by the liver can be used anywhere in the body; glycogen produced by the muscles is released later. The liver can store only half a day's supply of glycogen. After 24 hours without food, the carbohydrate reserves of the liver are usually exhausted, and the body must use fat or protein stores for energy. *See also* CARBOHYDRATE *and* GLUCOSE.

Glycosuria

The presence of the sugar glucose in the urine.

Glucose is removed from the blood by the kidneys, only to later be reabsorbed. Glycosuria may be caused by the abnormally high blood sugar levels associated with diabetes or by damage to the channels (tubules) in the kidneys where glucose and other substances are absorbed. Glycosuria can be caused by the hormonal changes that take place during pregnancy and may occur in those who have normal kidneys. The damage may also be the result of a congenital condition (originating from birth), side effects of a drug, or metal poisoning. Treatment depends on the type and degree of accompanying symptoms and the diagnosis of an underlying disorder. *See also* DIABETES.

Goiter

An enlarged thyroid channel.

The thyroid gland releases thyroid hormones that help to regulate metabolism. If the thyroid gland is unable to secrete enough of these hormones (hypothyroidism), it may enlarge in an effort to produce more of the hormones under the influence of thyroid stimulating hormone from the pituitary gland.

Types and Causes. A variety of conditions can lead to a goiter.

Endemic goiters are related to a lack of iodine in the diet. In the United States, the widespread use of iodized table salt has decreased the likelihood of this type of goiter. This is not the case in other parts of the world, where a lack of dietary iodine can cause the residents of a whole village to be marked by the telltale goiter noted by swelling of the neck below the Adam's apple.

Sporadic goiters result from ingestion of excess iodine or from growth-stimulating factors. Certain foods, known as goitrogens, may promote the growth of goiters. Large amounts of the drugs lithium, cobalt, and iodides can also cause goiters.

Grave's disease and Hashimoto's thyroiditis are both autoimmune disorders in which the body's own immune system attacks itself. These diseases cause overactivity of the thyroid, and can cause the thyroid to swell.

Symptoms. The best-known symptom of a goiter is swelling at the base of the throat below the Adam's apple. The size of the goiter may range from a barely perceptible lump to a huge enlargement due to multiple large lumps. The size dictates the other symptoms. Large goiters can press on the trachea and esophagus, causing breathing and swallowing problems.

Treatment. Goiters caused by iodine deficiency may be treated by eating iodine-rich foods. Thyroid hormone can be used to suppress TSH from further stimulating the growth of a goiter. If the thyroid produces normal to low amounts of thyroid hormone, TSH can be suppressed with thyroid hormone. If a goiter is causing severe breathing or swallowing problems, or if the gland is very damaged, it may need to be totally or partially removed.

> *Background information on goiter can be found in* THYROID GLAND. *For related information, see* HYPOTHYROIDISM *and* PITUITARY GLAND. *See also* GRAVE'S DISEASE; HASHIMOTO'S THYROIDITIS; *and* IODINE *for more on causes.*

Golfer's Elbow

Inflammation of the inner part of the elbow, leading to pain and tenderness in the area.

The forearm muscles, which help to bend the wrist and fingers, are attached to a bony prominence located on the inner side of the elbow. Playing golf with a faulty grip or swing is often the cause of inflammation of this inner portion of the elbow. Other activities that involve gripping and twisting, for example, using tools, are also causes of golfer's elbow.

Treatment usually consists of rest from the activity that caused the condition. Painkillers and anti-inflammatory drugs are also used, and the affected area is iced. Correcting the faulty technique that caused the inflammation can prevent recurrence, as can exercises to build strength in the region. *See also* EPICONDYLITIS.

Gonadotropin Hormones

Hormones that activate the ovaries or testes.

The ovaries and testes are responsible for female and male sexual development. The gonadotropins are a group of hormones that stimulate these glands to work. The gonadotropins themselves are secreted by another gland—the pituitary gland, located at the base of the skull called the sella turcica. The anterior lobe of the pituitary produces two gonadotropins, follicle-stimulating hormone (FSH) and luteinizing hormone (LH). These hormones stimulate the ovaries and testes to produce estrogen and androgen hormones.

Disorders in the pituitary gland can lead to overproduction or underproduction of gonadotropins. This can cause early onset of puberty or a lack of pubertal sexual development.

A synthetic form of LH can be used to treat early puberty. Another gonadotropin, human chorionic gonadotropin (HCG), which is produced by the placenta, can be produced synthetically to treat infertility. *See also* PITUITARY GLAND.

Gonadotropin, Human Chorionic

Also known as HCG

A hormone secreted during pregnancy.

Four days after becoming fertilized, an egg begins to secrete human chorionic gonadotropin, or HCG, which then spreads through the mother's body. The hormone is detected early and in high levels in the blood, but within a short time may be detected in the urine as well. Most home pregnancy tests detect the presence of HCG in urine. Outside of a normal pregnancy, HCG is also produced by a rare benign growth known as a hydatidiform mole. *See also* HORMONES; HYDATIDIFORM MOLE; MOLAR PREGNANCY; *and* PREGNANCY.

Gonads

Either the female ovaries or the male testicles.

The gonads (ovaries in women and testicles in men) are the sex organs where the smallest building blocks of creating a baby—the gametes or germ cells—are produced. The gonads are glands that are vital to reproduction. They also play an important role in establishing bodily and motivational differences between males and females. These differences are achieved by the gonads' production of various hormones: higher levels of testosterone in men and higher levels of estrogen and progesterone in women.

In women, the ovaries are located in the abdominal cavity. In men, the testicles or testes are located in the scrotum. Outside of the abdomen, the scrotum adjusts its distance to the body in order to achieve the necessary temperature required for sperm production. The sex organs of a fetus develop during the third month of pregnancy, but mature eggs and sperm are not produced by an individual until puberty. *See also* CONCEPTION; ERECTION; GENDER IDENTITY; OVULATION; REPRODUCTION, SEXUAL; *and* SEXUAL INTERCOURSE.

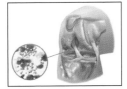

Gonorrhea. Above, gonococci bacteria, which cause gonorrhea, may also cause arthritis in one or both knees. A culture of the fluid in the affected knee will test positive for gonococci.

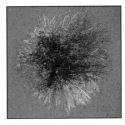

Gout. Above, intracellular urate crystals from a patient with gout, photographed in polarized light. The crystals form in the joints, soft tissues, and kidneys of gout patients.

Resources on Gonorrhea

Grist, Norman R., et al., *Diseases of Infection: An Illustrated Textbook* (1992); Shaw, Michael, ed., *Everything You Need to Know About Diseases* (1996); Rosenwaks, Zev, *Gynecology: Principles and Practice* (1987); Centers for Disease Control and Prevention, Tel. (800) 311-3435, Online: www.cdc.gov, STD hotline: (800) 227-8922; Infectious Disease Society of America, Tel. (703) 299-0200, Online: www.idsociety.org; National Institute of Allergy and Infectious Disease, Tel. (301) 496-5717, Online: www.niaid.nih.org; https://public1.med.cornell.edu/cgi-.

Gonorrhea

Also known as "the clap"

Sexually transmitted disease of widespread incidence that responds well to antibiotics.

The gonococcus bacterium likes warm, moist places in the body, such as the cervix, urethra, mouth, or rectum. Infection is transmitted by sexual contact, through either intercourse, oral sex, or anal sex. The risk of infection rises in people with many sexual partners or who do not use a condom or diaphragm.

Symptoms. Initial symptoms of gonorrhea are mild enough to go undetected. The first symptoms appear two to ten days after exposure. In men, there is a thick whitish or yellowish discharge from the penis and a burning sensation during urination. As the infection spreads up the urethra, there is an urge to urinate frequently. The first symptoms in women are a painful burning sensation during urination and an abnormally thick vaginal discharge. Both men and women may experience a rash in the palms or a mild sore throat. Men are more likely to suffer early symptoms than women. A pregnant woman can also transmit the disease to her child, as it can pass through the birth canal to cause blindness.

Diagnosis. Gonorrhea is diagnosed with either a microscopic examination of the urethral or cervical discharge, or by laboratory culture of the discharge for a couple of days, followed by microscopic examination of the culture. Both methods are often used to reduce the chance of error.

Treatment. Gonorrhea used to be treated with penicillin. As resistance of the bacteria to this antibiotic rises, however, other antibiotics are preferred. Very often, individuals who do not practice safe sex can contract other sexually transmitted diseases, such as chlamydia or syphilis, in addition to gonorrhea.

For background information on gonorrhea, see SEXUALLY TRANSMITTED DISEASES. *Related information can be found in* ANTIBIOTIC DRUGS; BACTERIA; CHLAMYDIA; INFECTIOUS DISEASE; PENICILLIN; SYPHILIS; *and* VISION, LOSS OF.

Complications of Gonorrhea

If gonorrhea is allowed to progress untreated, women may experience abdominal pain, bleeding between periods, vomiting, and fever, indicating a serious infection of the reproductive organs. The disease can scar the fallopian tubes, making the woman infertile and increasing the dangers of ectopic pregnancy (when an egg implants in the fallopian tube instead of the womb), which can be life-threatening.

In both men and women, if the infection enters the bloodstream, it can affect the joints, the heart valves, the liver, and the brain. Men may also experience swelling and inflammation of the reproductive system, narrowing of the urethra (possibly leading to urinary tract infection and kidney failure), and inflammation of the rectum (proctitis).

Gout

An inflammatory disease of the joints caused by deposits of uric acid (a compound found in urine), which takes the form of a salt when found in joints.

Gout has been known to doctors for many centuries. Patients with gout are at risk for uric acid renal calculi. It is much more common in women than men until menopause, when the gender difference narrows. Gout occurs as the result of the buildup of uric acid in the blood. This may happen when the kidneys do not remove uric acid effectively, because of an inherited condition or because of kidney damage. In a minority of cases, uric acid buildup results from the overproduction of urate, a salt of uric acid.

Symptoms. In more than half of all cases, the first sign of gout is pain in the first joint of the big toe, a condition known as podegra. Other joints, including the knee, ankle, wrists, and hands, can also be affected. The joint becomes red, swollen, and painful. Tender red nodules, called tophi, form under the skin near the joint. Some people have only a single attack of gout, while others can experience attacks over a period of years.

Diagnosis. When an attack of gout is reported, the doctor will do a blood test of uric acid levels and will also ask if there is a family history of gout, since kidney disease that causes gout can be inherited.

Treatment. In an acute attack of gout, anti-inflammatory drugs such as indomethacin are prescribed to relieve the pain. Colchicine, once the standard gout medication, is now less commonly used because of side effects such as nausea and diarrhea. Longer-term treatment after an attack is aimed at reducing levels of uric acid in the blood and addressing any underlying kidney disease that may cause this symptom. Medications to increase excretion of uric acid, such as probenecid, or to reduce the production of uric acid, notably allopurinol, can also be prescribed. With dietary measures, prompt use of drugs during an attack can usually keep the condition under control. *See also* Anti-Inflammatory Drugs *and* Uric Acid.

Graft-versus-Host Disease

A complication that sometimes occurs in bone marrow transplants, when donor white blood cells attack the recipient's tissues, particularly the skin, liver, and gastrointestinal tract.

Graft-versus-host disease is the opposite of a transplant rejection, in which the recipient's own immune system recognizes the transplanted tissue as "foreign" and attacks it. In graft-versus-host disease, the donor cells attack the recipient's tissue. Very rarely, graft-versus-host disease can also develop after a blood transfusion. White blood cells in the donated blood attack the host's tissues and destroy them. This form of graft-versus-host disease is seen primarily in patients with impaired immune systems.

As in transplant rejection, the chances of developing graft-versus-host disease are reduced when the donor and the recipient share close genetic markers, which prevents either from identifying the other as foreign. All bone marrow transplant patients also receive medications to suppress their immune systems in order to reduce the possibility of graft-versus-host disease.

Graft-versus-host disease is marked by fever, rash, low blood pressure, and shock. Prevention is preferable to treatment. *See also* Autoimmune Disorders *and* Rejection.

Grafting

Surgical transplantation of tissue to repair defects.

Tissue for grafting may be taken from another part of the body (autografting), another person (homografting), or an animal, such as a pig (xenografting, sometimes used in heart valve transplants). It is used to restore function in areas of damaged or missing tissue. Grafting may be used to promote healing, replace a diseased body organ, improve function, guard against infection, or for cosmetic purposes.

Skin Grafts. The most commonly grafted tissue is skin. Other tissues and organs that may be grafted include bone, connective tissues such as ligaments and tendons, cartilage, muscle, fat, blood vessels, nerves, and organs (such as the heart, lungs, liver, stomach, and kidneys). In addition to live tissue, synthetic material may be used to repair organs such as blood vessels.

One of the key challenges facing grafting surgery is the body's immune response to foreign tissue. The body often recognizes tissue from another person or animal as undesired and attempts to destroy it in a reaction known as rejection. To prevent this type of reaction from occurring, grafting is best done with tissue simply moved from one part of the body to another, or with a donation from an identical twin.

In the event that grafting from another person is necessary, physicians attempt to find tissue that is as similar to the recipient's tissue as possible, through a process known as tissue typing. This minimizes the risk of rejection of the transplanted tissue. In many cases, particularly following organ transplantation, medications that suppress the immune system, including corticosteroids such as prednisone, are used to protect the grafted tissue from immune system attack and destruction.

Background material on grafting can be found in Surgery. *For further information, see* Bone; Cartilage; Cosmetic Surgery; Graft-Versus-Host Disease; Immune System; Immunosuppressant Drugs; Ligament; Nerve; Rejection; Skin Graft; Tendon; *and* Xenografting.

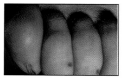

Gout. Above, a toe with gout, a disease characterized by the formation of monosodium urate crystals in the joints, soft tissues, and kidneys.

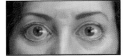

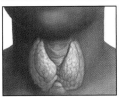

Grave's Disease.
Grave's disease is a common cause of hyperthyroidism (an overactive thyroid gland), which causes exophthalmos (bulging eyes), above, top, and enlargement of the thyroid gland. Above, bottom, the purple area represents the area of the thyroid gland that has become enlarged.

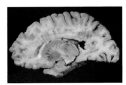

Gray Matter.
Above, the very outermost layer of brain tissue is the cerebral cortex, which is made up of wrinkled gray matter. This gray matter contains the nuclei of nerve cells (neurons), while the white matter further inside the brain contains the axons of these cells.

Granulation Tissue

Small, red granular foci that bleed easily in healing tissue.

Granulation tissue can be seen in the base of skin wounds when the overlying scab has been picked off. This tissue appears as clusters of fragile capillary blood vessels, which grow into damaged tissue.

After a wound has occurred, the damaged area begins to be replaced by granulation tissue, which has a bright red color. The tissue will eventually form a dense, fibrous scar. *See also* SCAR.

Granuloma

Chronic inflammation that causes concentric layers of cells to form a distinctive lesion.

Granuloma is caused by either a foreign body or a persistent microorganism that evades destruction by the chronic inflammatory response of the body.

The cause of non-infectious granuloma not associated with a foreign body is unknown and treatment may not be necessary. If treatment is desired, topical or injected corticosteroid drugs may be beneficial. *See also* CORTICOSTEROID DRUGS.

Granuloma Inguinale

Sexually transmitted disease, caused by the bacterium called *Calymatobacterium granulomatis*, which affects the genital region.

Granuloma inguinale is more common in tropical climates. It is a chronic bacterial infection of the genitals that produces red, pus-filled lumps on the penis, scrotum, and thighs of affected men, and around the vagina and nearby skin of affected women. The lumps may appear as soon as one day or as late as 80 days after exposure. If allowed to progress untreated, the disease may spread to the bones, joints, and liver, causing fever and anemia. Granuloma inguinale is treated successfully with antibiotics. *See* SEXUALLY TRANSMITTED DISEASES.

Grave's Disease

Overactivity of the thyroid gland, caused by an autoimmune disorder.

Grave's disease is caused by an autoimmune disorder, in which the body's own immune system attacks healthy tissue. In this case, the targeted area, the thyroid, responds to the immune system by producing excess thyroid hormone. It can swell, causing a large bulge at the neck. Other symptoms include unexplained weight loss, increased heart rate, sweating, and bulging of the eyes, which, in severe cases, can lead to paralysis of the eyeball. Treatment may include antithyroid medication, surgery to remove part of the thyroid, or doses of radioactive iodine. *See also* AUTOIMMUNE DISORDERS; HYPERTHYROIDISM; *and* THYROID HORMONES.

Gray Matter

The grayish tissue in the brain and spinal cord that contains closely packed nerve cells (neurons).

Gray matter is differentiated from white matter in that it contains clusters of the nuclei of nerve cells, while white matter contains the long, fiber-like projections of the cells (axons). The gray matter in the brain lies in the outer layers of the cerebrum (the upper portion of the brain, responsible for mental functions such as speech and memory), while the core of the cerebrum consists of white matter. The inner core of the spinal cord also contains gray matter. *See also* BRAIN *and* WHITE MATTER.

Grippe

A term that usually refers to influenza.

Influenza is an upper respiratory viral infection affecting the nose, the sinuses, the throat, the trachea, the bronchial tubes, and the lungs. Symptoms are chills and fever, muscle aches, a dry cough, a sore throat, hoarseness, a runny nose, a headache, fatigue, and malaise (a generalized feeling of illness). Specific antiviral agents can be used to treat this infection if they are initiated within the first 48 hours of symptoms. A flu vaccine is available, and annually updated vaccinations are advised for the elderly and for other high risk populations. *See also* INFLUENZA.

Groin, Lump in the

A swelling or lump in the region of the groin.

A swollen lymph gland is the most common cause of a lump in the groin area. A gland can swell due to infection, allergy, or some types of cancer, including Hodgkin's disease, lymphoma, and leukemia. Treatment depends on the underlying cause. Antibiotics may be given for a bacterial infection, antihistamines for an allergy, and radiation therapy or chemotherapy for cancer.

Another common cause for a lump in the groin is an inguinal hernia. This results from the stretching or rupturing of the inguinal canal, located where the scrotal sacs join the abdomen. Too much strain on the canal, particularly due to heavy lifting, can stretch or rupture this canal. In the early stages, the lump causes little pain and may elude detection. If detected early enough, the condition can be repaired with surgery. *See* HERNIA; HERNIA REPAIR; *and* INTESTINE.

Groin Strain

Pain in the groin, usually caused by overstretching the muscles.

The groin, located between the top of the thigh and lower abdomen, can become aggravated by extreme movement, such as in sports. The muscles most affected flex and pull the inner thigh. Other possible causes that can be mistaken for the condition include osteoarthritis, inflammation of the pubic bones, or a hernia in which the intestine bulges through the abdominal wall.

Treatment in most cases is simply physical therapy. If the muscle has splintered or broken off a segment of pelvic bone, surgery may be required. *See also* STRAIN.

Group Therapy

Psychotherapy in a group setting.

The interaction of a group of patients under the guidance of a psychotherapist is therapeutic for certain psychological problems. Group therapy may or may not be prescribed in conjunction with conventional single patient-therapist meetings.

Usually, eight to ten patients comprise a group. For an hour once or twice a week, group members and the therapist meet and discuss their problems. Alcohol and drug dependence, anxiety and eating disorders, depression, and personality problems are often treated with group therapy. *See also* PSYCHOTHERAPY.

Growing Pains

Mild aches and pains affecting children between the ages of six and twelve.

Growing pains are typically felt in the limbs and occur at night. There is no apparent cause, and, despite the name, no definite link to the growth process. The pains may interrupt sleep, but usually require no medical treatment. They generally dissipate with age. *See also* CHILD DEVELOPMENT.

Growth, Childhood

The physical and mental development of a child as he or she turns into an adult.

New parents eagerly monitor the growth of their infant, as their baby seems to change before their eyes. But the fastest period of growth during the life cycle has already taken place, during the development of the embryo in the womb. After birth, the growth process begins to slow, until full height and proportion is reached sometime around age 18.

After the infancy period, children need between 11 and 12 hours of sleep during a 24-hour period. It is common for children to resist bedtime, but sleep is important for their healthy development.

Heredity and environment both play crucial roles in determining a person's size. The height and build of the parents undoubtedly affect the growth of the child, but environment can interfere with the hereditary factors. Children who are malnourished, in poor health, or do not have adequate exercise will not reach the size to which they are genetically predisposed. Still, there are averages that can be applied to most cases. Boys grow faster than girls until about age seven months, then girls grow faster until age four. At this point the speed of growth between the sexes remains the same until puberty.

A baby grows about ten inches in the first year, tripling in weight. After age two, growth slows to about two inches per year, and usually continues at that rate until adolescence. Growth may not be as steady as this, however, and may occur in spurts, most notably during puberty.

For background information on childhood growth, see GROWTH HORMONE. *Further information can be found in* CHILD DEVELOPMENT; EXERCISE; GENE; GENETICS; GROWING PAINS; HEREDITY; HYPOTHALAMUS; INFANT; NUTRITION; PITUITARY GLAND; *and* PUBERTY.

Growth Hormone

Hormone that stimulates the body to grow.

One of the most important hormones secreted by the pituitary gland is growth hormone. The hypothalamus in the brain secretes hormones that can both stimulate and inhibit the pituitary gland's release of growth hormone. The amount of growth hormone that is released can be influenced by other factors, including blood glucose levels, stress, exercise, and sleep.

When released, growth hormone signals the liver to produce the protein IGF-1, which aids in the increase of the size and growth of cells. Growth hormone also helps regulate the body's metabolism. It stimulates the body's production of protein and decreases fat stores, while inhibiting sugar uptake into the cells.

The most intense period of growth takes place before birth, during the first few years of life, and during puberty. During the adult years, growth hormone is mainly used to maintain lean body mass. Disorders of the pituitary gland, such as a tumor, can lead to abnormal growth hormone secretion. The release of too much of the growth hormone can result in overgrowth (gigantism or acromegaly). A lack of the hormone can lead to short stature. Synthetic forms of the growth hormone may be used as a treatment for short stature. *See also* HYPOTHALAMUS *and* PITUITARY GLAND.

Guided Imagery

Practice of conscious visualization to evoke a positive physical response.

Guided imagery is a method that uses the imagination as therapy and as a means of promoting relaxation. While the body is at rest, a person will take several deep breaths and begin imagining a place, an image, or an event that evokes a positive feeling.

The three primary types of guided imagery are receptive visualization, programmed visualization, and guided visualization. During receptive visualization, the individual chooses a problem and allows the solution to come to him or her in the form of an image. During programmed visualization, a person consciously imagines achieving a goal. Guided visualization combines receptive and programmed forms of visualization and is the most commonly used. *See also* ALTERNATIVE MEDICINE.

Guillain-Barré Syndrome

Disorder that damages the peripheral nerves, resulting in spreading numbness and tingling in the fingers and toes, as well as muscle weakness.

In Guillain-Barré syndrome, antibodies attack the nerve tissue, causing damage. The syndrome causes inflammation and the destruction of the myelin sheaths covering the nerve fibers.

Cause. The cause of Guillain-Barré syndrome is unknown; however, the majority of cases develop after a viral infection. Five to ten percent of all cases occur after a medical procedure, such as an operation.

Symptoms. The first symptoms of Guillain-Barré syndrome may occur within a few days of an infection. Tingling sensations are eventually followed by muscle weakness in the arms, legs, and face. Symptoms that can signal an emergency situation include widespread numbness and difficulty in breathing. In severe cases, paralysis may result.

Treatment. Plasmapheresis, the removal of damaging antibodies, is often performed on patients with Guillain-Barré syndrome. However, treatment mostly focuses on relieving pain and regaining muscle strength. Recovery often takes several months, with some impairment remaining in approximately ten percent of patients. The mortality rate for Guillain-Barré syndrome is between three and four percent. *See also* AUTOIMMUNE DISORDERS.

Guinea Worm Disease

Also known as dracunculiasis

Disease caused by the parasitic round worm *Dracunculus medinensis* or "guinea worm."

Guinea worm disease threatens nine out of ten people living in Africa, South America, the Caribbean, the Middle East, and India. The worm is ingested with impure drinking water. Stagnant water may contain small crustaceans known as cyclops, which act as intermediary hosts for the guinea worm larvae. Once killed by the parasite, cyclops are ingested by humans drinking contami-

nated water. Stomach acids break down the cyclops, liberating the worm larvae, which puncture the victim's intestine and enter the body tissue. The disease tends to recur annually during the agricultural season.

Symptoms. *Dracunculus medinensis* is the largest of the tissue parasites affecting humans. Females may grow up to one meter in length and two millimeters across, and lay between one and three million embryos. Guinea worms migrate through the victim's body, causing severe pain, particularly in the areas around the joints. Eventually the worm emerges, usually through the feet, causing fluid to collect in the tissues (edema), blistering, and a painful ulcer. When the worm perforates the skin, extreme pain is accompanied by fever, nausea, and vomiting. At this point, the condition can be definitively diagnosed.

Treatment. Treatment includes removal of the worm with the drugs niridazole and thiabendazole, along with antibiotics to reduce secondary infection and immunization against tetanus.

Prevention. As no vaccination exists against the disease, eradication of the cyclops or their removal through careful filtering of the drinking water using fine mesh is essential to prevent infestation. *See* ANTIHELMINTIC DRUGS; PARASITE; ROUNDWORMS; *and* WORM INFESTATION.

Gumma

A tumor in late stage syphilis.

Gummas are soft growths of tissue appearing during late, or tertiary stage syphilis. Each usually contains a mass of dead and inflamed fibrous tissue. Gummas occur most frequently in the liver but may also appear in the brain, testis, heart, skin, and bone. Tertiary syphilis can last for years or decades and typically occurs long after the person has forgotten previous bouts with primary or secondary syphilis. Penicillin is the treatment for all stages of syphilis. Early detection and treatment have made tertiary syphilis less frequent, affecting three out of every 10,000 people. *See* SYPHILIS.

Guthrie Test

Diagnostic test used to screen for increased levels of phenylalanine, an amino acid.

The Guthrie test is performed on babies 8 to 14 days after birth. It screens the blood for elevated levels of the amino acid phenylalanine and low levels of tyrosine, another amino acid. These are associated with a disease known as phenylketonuria (PKU), a hereditary disorder. Infants suffering from phenylketonuria lack the enzymes that process and eliminate phenylalanine in the blood. Without this enzyme, dangerous levels of phenylalanine accumulate in the bloodstream. The disease may produce mental retardation, due to the toxic effect of phenylalanine on the brain.

Phenylketonuria must be treated early to prevent mental retardation, which can be severe. If the disorder exists in the family, prenatal screening through amniocentesis or chorionic villus sampling are advised. Treatment involves limiting the dietary intake of phenylalanine, which is found in artificial sweeteners. *See* Amniocentesis; Chorionic Villus Sampling; Mental Retardation; *and* Phenylketonuria.

Gynecology

Study of reproductive health concerns of women.

A woman relies on her gynecologist for care relating to the sex organs, birth control, pregnancy, and other related issues. Most gynecologists are also trained in obstetrics—reproductive medicine.

It is recommended that a woman see her gynecologist once a year, especially after becoming sexually active. A routine gynecologic evaluation starts with taking a gynecologic history, which includes questions about the frequency and duration of the menstrual periods, as well as questions about sexual activity to assess the possibility of injuries, infection, and pregnancy. Birth control is also discussed, as is the woman's reproductive history. This is followed by both a pelvic exam and a breast exam.

One of the most common diagnostic procedures in gynecology is the pap smear, in which cells are scraped from the cervix to check for possible cancer. If the results are abnormal, a biopsy is performed. Past the age of 40, it is recommended that women have a base-line mammogram, followed by additional screenings every other year and annually after age 50.

For the woman entering menopause, the gynecologist is still very important. He or she can help the patient deal with symptoms. The gynecologist may recommend estrogen replacement therapy to alleviate the symptoms of menopause and also to prevent heart disease and osteoporosis. *See also* Breast Self-Examination; Mammography; Pap Smear; *and* Pelvic Examination.

Gynecomastia

Development of breasts in males.

Men produce some estrogen, the hormone that leads to secondary sex characteristics in women. If a man produces an excess of estrogen, it can lead to breast enlargement. It can initially start as a swelling on one side and then progress to bilateral gynecomastia (swelling of both breasts).

Causes. Gynecomastia could be the result of several conditions. Cirrhosis of the liver can inhibit the liver's ability to break down estrogen. A tumor in the testis can cause estrogen levels in the blood to rise. It can also be the side effect of drugs that expose men to improper amounts of androgen and estrogen hormones.

Symptoms and Diagnosis. The symptoms of gynecomastia are swelling and pain in one or both of the breasts. While trying to determine the cause, tests may be done to investigate the condition of the liver and hormone levels in the blood.

Treatment. Treatment for gynecomastia depends on the underlying cause. Swelling takes some time to subside, even as long as a few years. If the condition is noticeable and causing embarrassment, cosmetic surgery may be performed. *See also* Breast *and* Estrogen.

Resources on

Dechnery, William, *Current Obstetric and Gynecological Diagnosis and Treatment* (1991); Jones, Howard W., III, et al., *Novak's Textbook of Gynecology* (1988); Tyler, Sandra L., et al., *Female Health and Gynecology: Across the Lifespan* (1982); Rosenwaks, Zev, et al., *Gynecology: Principles and Practice* (1987); American Board of Obstetrics and Gynecology, Tel. (212) 871-1619, Online: www.abog.org; American Society for Reproductive Medicine, Tel. (205) 978-5000, Online: www.asrm.org; Planned Parenthood Federation of America, Inc., Tel. (800) 829-7732, Online: www.plannedparenthood.org; www.ivf.org/home.html; www.nycornell.org/obgyn/ www.nycornell.org/medicine/womenshealth/index.html.

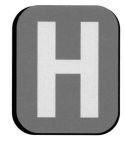

Hair

A protein strand that grows from a hair follicle in the skin.

A normal hair will grow, depending on location, for up to three or more years, after which time it will fall out and be replaced by a new hair. The amount of hair on a person's body and head is determined by genetic factors.

Color. Hair color changes over the life cycle. Aging causes the follicles to produce less melanin, the pigment that is responsible for hair color. Hair starts to become gray at different times for different people. Some people experience some degree of hair graying in their 30s. By the age of 40, about 40 percent of people have some gray scalp hair. Body, facial, and pubic hair may start to turn gray later, or not at all.

Texture. As people age, the rate of hair growth slows. Hair strands become thinner and less coarse. About 25 percent of men begin to show signs of baldness by the time they are 30 years old. About 66 percent of men are either bald or have a balding pattern by the time they are 60 years old. Men usually lose hair in a typical pattern, first from the front and top of the scalp. Women also lose hair in a typical pattern; hair becomes less dense all over, and the scalp may become visible through the thinning hair. Most types of baldness cannot be cured, though the drug minoxidil promotes hair growth in some people. *See* HAIR GROWTH.

Hair Growth

The development and extension of hair from the hair follicles.

Hair growth, texture, and color differs across people of different races, ages, and genders. However, there are some very basic explanations for the rate and variation of human hair.

The outer layer of the skin contains many hair follicles, which produce a protein called keratin. New hair, specifically that which is found on the head, is made of this protein and pushes the old cells (which have a longevity of about three years) through the hair shaft at the rate of approximately six inches each year.

The number of hair follicles a person has and the shape of the follicles are determined before birth. Round follicles traditionally produce straight hair, while curved follicles produce curly hair. These follicles experience alternating phases of growth and rest, resulting in 100,000 or more hairs on the scalp at one time. However, the average person may lose many of these hairs, shedding anywhere from 100 to 150 hairs a day.

Hair Loss. Natural thinning of the hair occurs as people age. This condition is also known as alopecia. Male and female pattern baldness, called androgenic alopecia, is a genetically predisposed condition affecting men as early as their teens. Most women experience signs of hair thinning (especially at the base of the crown) much later.

There are a few methods of stopping hair loss and regrowing hair. In a hair transplant operation, small plugs of hair and the surrounding glands and hair shaft are moved from one part of the head to another. The drug minoxidil, also known by the brand name Rogaine, stops hair loss in some people and increases hair growth in a small proportion of individuals. This treatment must be used continuously or the new hair will fall out. The oral agent finasteride can also induce new hair growth in some men with androgenic alopecia. It can cause birth defects and should never be used by women.

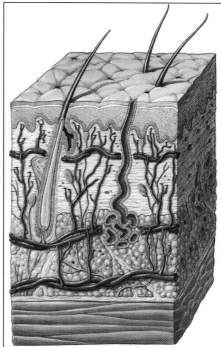

Hair Follicle.
Above, hair is made up of a protein called keratin and grows from below the skin through follicles. The shape and size of the follicles influences the texture of the hair.

Background material on hair growth can be found in HAIR. **For further information, see** AGING; ALOPECIA; HAIR TRANSPLANT; KERATIN; **and** PROTEINS. **See also** PREGNANCY **for more on other drugs to avoid while pregnant.**

Resources on Hair and Hair Loss

Feinberg, Herbert S., *All About Hair* (1978) Norwood, O'Tar T., and Richard C. Shiell, *Hair Transplant Surgery* (1984); Stough, Dow, B., and Robert S. Haber, *Hair Replacement: Surgical and Medical* (1996); National Alopecia Areata Foundation, Tel. (415) 456-4274, Online: www.alopeciaareata.com; www.nycornell.org/dermatology.

Hair Removal

Removing body hair from the skin.

Hair removal is usually performed for purely cosmetic reasons. There are many methods of removing unwanted hair. The area may be shaved with a razor, which is a simple way of eliminating body hair. Waxing is a more long-lasting method of removing hair, but hair must grow to about half an inch in order to be removed effectively by waxing. Electrolysis is an even more permanent way of removing hair. An electrolysis technician uses electricity to kill the hair follicle, preventing hair from returning. Several types of lasers are also effective for removal of hair. Recently, a topical cream that decreases hair growth in some women became available. *See also* Electrolysis *and* Follicle, Hair.

Hair Transplant

Surgical relocation of hair-bearing scalp, usually from the back or side of the head, to hairless areas in the front or on top of the head.

There are several methods for transplanting hair. The major types of hair transplant procedures are punch grafts (plugs), strip grafts, flap grafts, scalp reduction, and tissue expansion.

Punch grafting, the most common procedure, involves a punch graft or plug about one-fourth of an inch in diameter that is punched out of the donor site. The plug, containing about 15 hairs and surrounding tissue, is transplanted into a hole in the bald area. Mini-plugs (half the size of regular plugs) and microplugs (one-fourth the size of regular plugs) are used for smaller spaces. Repeat transplantation sessions are scheduled at four-month intervals until the desired effect is reached.

Strip grafting involves long strips of bald skin being replaced by strips of hairy scalp. A flap graft, used to form a new hairline, is similar to a strip graft, except that flaps of hairy skin on the back or side are lifted, repositioned, and sewn to adjacent skin.

Scalp reduction involves an area of bald skin being removed and the two remaining sides of skin stitched together, reducing the area of baldness.

Tissue expansion is performed by inserting a balloon under hair-bearing scalp and gradually inflating it with a saline solution on a weekly basis, until the skin has stretched enough for the expanded tissue to be repositioned over the bald area. *See also* Hair Growth.

Halitosis

A disagreeable breath odor.

Halitosis refers to bad breath. It may be caused by a variety of factors, including the condition of the mouth, eating food with strong odors, and certain diseases.

Causes. Any dental infection can result in bad breath, as can throat or lung infections. Smoking may cause a chronic form of bad breath. Foods such as onions or garlic and alcoholic beverages may be the source of bad breath, as substances found in those foods and drinks are carried through the bloodstream to the lungs, where they are expelled from the body.

Impaired motility of the stomach may result in bad breath due to fermentation of the stomach contents. Esophageal reflux can also contribute to the problem.

Lung disease may also result in halitosis. Kidney failure can cause a urine-like odor, whereas liver failure may produce a fishy smell. Diabetics may have acetone in their breath, resulting in a fruity odor.

Treatment. Ammonia, fecal, or fruity odors will be accompanied by other symptoms and may indicate treatable disorders, such as infections. Good oral hygiene is the most effective way to combat halitosis that is not the result of an underlying disorder. This includes frequent brushing and flossing, as well as keeping the mouth moist by drinking water. Avoiding foods such as garlic and onions can help prevent halitosis. Brushing teeth and using mouthwash can only mask odors from food; it cannot eliminate them entirely. *See also* Oral Hygiene.

Hallucination

A mental state in which an individual perceives something that is not actually present.

In a healthy individual, the mind may misinterpret sensory data and form an illusion; for example, that the bending of light in the desert atmosphere is an oasis. A hallucination, however, involves perceptions of sounds, images, and sometimes tactile perceptions when there is nothing for the mind to interpret. This may be a symptom of deeper psychophysiological problems.

Hearing voices and seeing images, often of a highly frightening nature, is a symptom of schizophrenia; it may also be caused by manic-depressive illness and certain physiological brain disorders. People with high fevers, in states of delirium from shock, or in alcohol withdrawal sometimes experience hallucinations.

Hallucinations of smell may be indicative of tumor-induced frontal-lobe epilepsy. Hallucinations of touch and smell are only common in schizophrenia, where the sufferer may experience sensations like insects crawling on the body or may smell excrement or burning substances. Hallucinations may also be induced by substances such as mescaline and LSD, by anticholinergic drugs used to treat Parkinson's disease, and by extreme stress and prolonged sensory deprivation. *See also* DELIRIUM.

Hallux Valgus

Bowing of the big toe.

In hallux valgus, the big toe overlaps the one next to it and the base of the big toe extends past the normal profile of the foot. The bump where it protrudes is called a bunion and may cause pain. Hallux valgus is present in some individuals at birth, but also often results from wearing high-heeled shoes with narrow toes.

Treatment. Proper footwear is essential. In extreme cases, surgery may be performed to realign the bones and remove excess bony tissue. *See also* BUNION *and* TOE.

Hamartoma

A nonmalignant growth that resembles a tumor.

A hamartoma results from the faulty development of an organ. It is composed of an abnormal mixture or portion of tissue elements. Most hamartomas occur in the skin, but they also can grow in the heart, kidneys, or lungs. They generally do not result in the damaging compression of neighboring tissues caused by cancers. Hamartomas generally do not require treatment, as they are not dangerous. *See also* BENIGN.

Hammer Toe

A clawlike or clenched appearance to the toe as a result of misalignment of the toe joints.

In hammer toe, the toes remain in a permanently bent position, resulting in pain and difficulty in movement. The second toe is most commonly affected, though the condition may affect any toe.

Hammer toe can result from wearing shoes that cramp the foot. In some cases it can be a result of long-term diabetes or other diseases that cause muscle and nerve damage. Hammer toe is treated with an orthopedic device to position the toes properly and relieve pain. In extreme cases, surgery may be performed to straighten the toes. Properly fitting footwear can prevent the condition. *See also* HALLUX VALGUS.

Hand

The body's tool for holding and manipulating objects.

The hand is the most flexible part of the skeleton. Muscles in the palm control movement, achieved by tendons sheathed in lubricating fluid that reduces friction. The ulnar artery, near the little finger, and the radial artery, near the thumb, carry blood into the hand; veins on the back of the hand take it away. Ulnar, radial, and median nerves register sensation and determine movement. *See* NERVOUS SYSTEM.

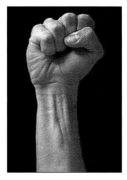

Hand.
Above, the hand is the most flexible part of the skeleton. The fingers can close tightly to grasp objects.

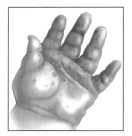

Hand-Foot-and-Mouth Disease. Above, hand-foot-and-mouth disease infects babies and young children and causes a distinctive rash on the palms of the hands.

Hand-Foot-and-Mouth Disease

A common, relatively mild infection caused by a Coxsackie virus and affecting babies and young children.

Hand-foot-and-mouth disease is caused by one of a number of Coxsackie viruses. The disease usually lasts from five to seven days. Early symptoms are fever, poor appetite, sore throat, and malaise (a generalized feeling of illness). Sores later appear in the mouth, on the palms, between the fingers, and on the soles of the feet. There is no treatment for hand-foot-and-mouth disease other than rest. Isolation of infected people is recommended, since the disease is contagious through direct contact with their stool or with discharges from their noses and throats. *See also* VIRUSES.

Handedness

The preferential use of one hand over the other.

Most people show a preference for performing coordinated activities, such as writing or tying their shoes, with a specific hand. Ninety percent of the adult population is right-handed. The remainder exhibit a preference for left-handedness or ambidexterity (equal use of both hands).

Handedness is linked to the brain. Each side of the brain controls the functions on the opposite side of the body. If a person is right-handed, then the left side of the brain is dominant—a greater number of nerves connect to that side of the brain. If a person is left-handed, then the right side of the brain is dominant.

Sources. Heredity is probably the most influential factor in determining handedness. Research suggests that, even in infants, there is dominance of one side of the body over the other, causing a greater quantity of nerves to travel to the corresponding side of the brain.

The left hemisphere of the brain is responsible for speech in the majority of right-handed individuals. The brain's right hemisphere is the center for speech in most left-handed individuals. If a right-handed individual suffers a stroke on the left side of the brain that is responsible for his centers of speech, it will result in a speech impairment (aphasia), while a left-handed person usually develops aphasia from damage to the right side of the brain.

The left hemisphere of the brain is connected to verbal ability and analytical reasoning, while the right hemisphere is connected to emotional intuitiveness and spatial ability. However, no data exists that strongly links handedness to ability in any of these areas. *See also* APHASIA; BRAIN; SPEECH; SPEECH DISORDERS; *and* STROKE.

Hashimoto's Thyroiditis

An autoimmune disease in which antibodies are produced that injure or destroy the thyroid gland.

Hashimoto's thyroiditis is the most common cause of hypothyroidism, a condition in which the thyroid gland produces insufficient amounts of thyroid hormone. In patients with the condition, the thyroid gland is often enlarged. The disease is progressive, as the functioning areas of the gland are gradually destroyed.

Incidence. Hashimoto's thyroiditis is most common in women. Women are eight times more likely to have Hashimoto's thyroiditis than men.

Symptoms. The first symptom of Hashimoto's thyroiditis is usually a painless enlargement of the thyroid gland, located in the neck. Approximately 80 percent of patients still have normal thyroid function when they are diagnosed. Some patients have other autoimmune endocrine disorders, resulting in diabetes or underactive adrenal or parathyroid glands. They may also suffer from other diseases, such as rheumatoid arthritis or lupus.

Treatment. No specific treatment is available to halt the progression of Hashimoto's thyroiditis. As hypothyroidism develops, thyroid hormone replacement therapy is required. *See* HYPOTHYROIDISM.

Headache

Pain or discomfort in the head.

A headache is a very common medical problem, and it is most often not a sign of a serious disorder. Headaches may occur infrequently or chronically, and the pain can range from mild discomfort to harsh, debilitating pain. As many as 45 million Americans suffer from headaches.

The brain itself does not have any pain receptors. A headache is the result of pain signals caused by interactions between the brain, blood vessels, and surrounding nerves. The pain comes from nerves surrounding the skull, strain in muscle tissues, and changes in blood vessels in the head, skin, and neck. Headaches can be triggered by factors such as stress, poor posture, too little or too much sleep, overeating, or loud-noise conditions.

TYPES

Headaches may be primary or secondary. A primary headache is an actual disorder and not a side effect of another disorder. Primary headaches include migraines, tension headaches, and cluster headaches. Secondary headaches are the side effects of other medical disorders, such as dental disorders, sinus infections, allergies, head injuries, or brain tumors.

Tension Headaches. Tension headaches are caused by muscle tension in the neck, shoulders, and head. These headaches may be the result of uncomfortable posture, stress, or fatigue. They may persist for a few brief moments or last for days. The pain is often described as crushing and concentrated and may range from mild to moderate intensity. Tension headaches are felt on both sides of the head and do not get worse with physical activity. The pain is centralized above the eyes or in the rear of the head, but can travel from the head down to the back of the neck and shoulders. Tension headaches begin in the morning and grow worse during the day.

Migraine. A migraine headache usually persists for one day and recurs at least once

ALERT

When to See a Doctor

If headaches are chronic and severe, especially if they are accompanied by nausea or vomiting, they may indicate a severe underlying cause and should be brought to the attention of a physician.

a month. The classic migraine headache is a pulsating, moderate to severe pain that worsens with activity and is associated with nausea and sensitivity to light or noise. It is usually concentrated on one side of the head and can be accompanied by visual, neurological, or gastrointestinal changes. Some patients experience a neurological disturbance (aura), such as flashing lights, tunnel vision, or an unpleasant smell, before the onset of the headache.

Sinus Headaches. These are caused by sinus congestion and infections and are quite common. Pain is located in the front of the head and is worse in damp weather.

Rebound Headaches. Extended use of painkillers can lead to dependency, producing headaches when drug levels in the body decrease. Suddenly ceasing intake of caffeine may also cause a headache.

CAUSES

It is unknown exactly why some people are more prone to headaches than other people; the exact cause of chronic primary headaches, such as migraines, also remains unknown. However, headaches do tend to run in families, and researchers have found that children of migraine sufferers are more likely to experience the pain of migraine headaches.

Whatever the underlying cause, headaches are often triggered by environmental or dietary factors. If a person knows what will trigger a headache, the best way to avoid the headache is to avoid the trigger. Common environmental triggers for headaches include stress, pollution, noise, very bright light, weather changes, and odors. Common dietary triggers for headaches include nitrates and monosodium glutamate (MSG), alcohol (particularly red wine and champagne), artificial sweeteners (such as

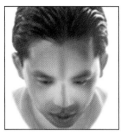
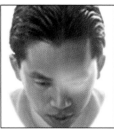
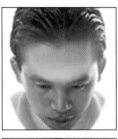
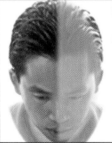

Headache.
Above, top, in a sinus headache, the pain is behind the cheekbones. Second from the top, in a cluster headache, the pain is in and around an eye. Third from the top, in a tension headache, the pain is like a band squeezing the head. Bottom, in a migraine, there is nausea or photophobia (light sensitivity).

saccharin and aspartame), caffeine, chocolate, and some types of medications.

The monthly fluctuation of hormone levels in women can trigger headaches. Some women regularly experience migraine headaches before, during, or a few days following menstruation.

Alternative Treatments for Headache Pain

Nondrug alternatives can also be used to treat headache pain. Biofeedback therapy electronically monitors the body's senses, such as temperature and muscle tension. By observing their bodies' involuntary responses, people can learn to gain some control over these responses and reduce tension and pain. Cognitive therapy teaches a person to reduce negative thought processes, and stress management skills can help prevent responses to stress and tension that might trigger a headache.

TREATMENT

Preventive therapies, such as avoiding triggering factors, can reduce the frequency of headaches. Pain relievers (analgesics), especially if taken as soon as pain begins, can reduce the severity of the headache. Medication may also be effective in reducing other symptoms of an attack, such as nausea, vomiting, and sensitivity to light or noise. If all other methods fail, a physician may take a more aggressive approach, such as intravenous injections or intramuscular injections to ease the pain.

PREVENTION

Lifestyle changes can reduce the frequency of headaches. Long periods of fasting can cause swings in blood sugar levels that may trigger headaches, and should be avoided. A well-balanced diet and limiting or eliminating caffeine, alcohol, and smoking can prevent headaches. Regular exercise and a healthy amount of sleep can also help.

For background information on headache, see CENTRAL NERVOUS SYSTEM. Further information may be found in ANALGESIC DRUGS; AURA; BRAIN TUMOR; GENETICS; MIGRAINE; and NERVE. See also ALLERGY; ARTIFICIAL SWEETENERS; CAFFEINE; DIET AND DISEASE; DRUG DEPENDENCE; HEAD INJURY; SINUSITIS; and STRESS for causes of headaches.

Resources on
Bakal, Donald A., *The Psychobiology of Chronic Headache* (1982); Rapoport, Alan M., and Fred Sheftell, *Headache Relief* (1991); Raskin, Neil, *Headache* (1988); Saper, Joel R., et al., eds., *Handbook of Headache Management* (1993); American Council for Headache education, Tel. (800) 255-ACHE, Online: www.achenet.org; Nat. Headache Foundation, Tel. (800) 843-2256; www.med.cornell.edu/neuro.

Head Injury

Damage to the scalp, skull, or brain as a result of a blow to the head.

Head injuries may occur as a result of any blow to the head. In minor head injuries, the skull protects the brain from damage. A significant blow to the head may fracture the skull or cause brain damage. In addition, injured blood vessels in the brain can bleed (hemorrhage), and significant brain damage can result.

CONCUSSION

A concussion is a form of injury to the brain that is sometimes associated with a brief loss of consciousness. Symptoms of a concussion may include loss of memory, dizziness, nausea, and headache.

Progressively worsening symptoms may indicate a more serious head injury, and medical attention should be sought.

SKULL FRACTURES

Skull fractures may damage arteries and veins, causing bleeding around the tissue of the brain. The fractures may allow foreign material into the brain, leading to bacterial infection.

SERIOUS INJURIES

More serious injuries result in damage to the brain itself. Bruising or tearing of brain tissue can result in permanent loss of brain function. Pools or clots of blood between the brain and the skull can put pressure on the brain, causing swelling and destruction of brain tissue. Symptoms such as severe headache, dizziness, repeated vomiting, visual changes, pupils of different sizes, and diminished consciousness may indicate serious head injury; anyone who exhibits such symptoms requires immediate medical treatment.

Brain damage may be indicated by an extended loss of consciousness, followed by memory loss (amnesia) of the period before or after the injury . The longer the period of unconsciousness or memory loss, the more severe the damage may be. Damage to the brain may result in symptoms such as muscular weakness (paralysis), speech impairment (aphasia), or changes in mental capabilities or personality.

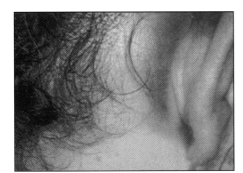

TREATMENT

Patients who become dizzy or unconscious should be placed under medical supervision. Blood clots and severe skull fractures, which can be life-threatening, require surgical repair. Serious, progressive brain damage along with loss of consciousness always requires emergency intervention, often involving life support and surgery.

PROGNOSIS

The survival rate of patients who have had major head injury has improved. However, some head injuries cause permanent physical or mental incapacity or personality changes. There is also an increase in the chance of seizures after a head injury. Recovery can be slow; improvement can take years after injury.

Background material on head injury can be found in ACCIDENTS *and* HEADACHE. *For related information, see* APHASIA; BLEEDING; BRAIN DISORDERS; CONCUSSION; CONFUSION; EPILEPSY; PARALYSIS; *and* SKULL, FRACTURED.

Head Lag

The backward flop of an infant's head when placed in a sitting position.

Prior to four months of age, an infant's neck muscles are weak and the head must be supported at all times. Past four months, the infant can hold the head up. The new strength is a sign of proper muscle development, as a child must be able to control the head to be able to learn how to sit properly. *See also* CHILD DEVELOPMENT.

Head, Neck, and Back Injuries

Injuries in areas vital to human function.

The head, neck, and back contain the central nervous system—the brain and spinal cord. Falls, sports injuries, and other traumas can cause damage to these areas.

A severe blow to the head can fracture the skull, causing brain damage and amnesia. Prolonged unconsciousness can cause paralysis and brain damage. The survival rate after major head injury has improved, but recovery is slow.

An injury at birth or skin contracture—shrinkage of scar tissue owing to burns or injuries—can cause wryneck, or torticollis, where the head is permanently twisted to one side. Paralysis or death may result from dislocations, fractures, or whiplash of neck vertebrae. Strangulation can cut off breathing and blood flow, while lacerations to the jugular vein or carotid artery can cause serious blood loss or death.

Severe injury to the spine may cause paralysis. Heavy lifting and carrying, prolonged sitting in the workplace, and obesity can cause muscle pulls and tears, ligament strains, and spinal or nerve damage, making life a daily struggle.

For background information on head, neck, and back injuries, see BRAIN; CENTRAL NERVOUS SYSTEM; *and* SPINAL CORD. *Further information can be found in* FRACTURES AND DISLOCATIONS; OBESITY; PARALYSIS; *and* TORTICOLLIS.

Head Injury. Skull fractures are commonly found in children and are caused by abuse or accidents. At left, Battle's sign appears several days following a fracture at the base of the skull. Blood may have come from the ear soon after the fracture.

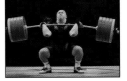

Head, Neck, and Back Injuries. Head, neck, and back injuries can be caused by improper form during heavy lifting. Above, a weight lifter at the 2000 Olympics shows proper form, which can help prevent head, neck, and back injuries.

Health

Physical and mental well-being.

Broadly defined, health is the absence of disease, disorder, and injury. The World Health Organization further defines it as the opportunity to grow physically and mentally without the pitfalls of malnutrition, environmental hazard, and rampant infectious disease. Fulfilling genetic potential could be seen as the fullest expression of health. Health can also refer to the ability to perform social, occupational, and family roles, deal with stress, or even handle illness or injury.

The capacity of a group to achieve a collective balance in the health of its members can be measured. For example, scientific advances have helped Americans live longer, healthier lives. Life expectancy in 1920 was just over 54 years. Americans born today will not only live twenty years longer, but will live free of many of the diseases that once endangered health and life. *See also* PUBLIC HEALTH.

Health Food

Variety of products marketed for their nutritional value, minimally processed and often grown without the use of pesticides.

The term health food can refer to a range of foods or supplements, often sold at so-called health food stores. The benefits of specific supplements have not often been proven, and most physicians agree that a varied and balanced diet should be the primary way to provide nutrients sufficient for the healthy maintenance of the body.

Consultation with a physician is recommended before taking supplements of any sort; some herbs and other health food supplements act like drugs and can interact with prescription medications. While organically grown foods have not been proven to be more nutritious, pesticide residues are minimized, and more sustainable agricultural practices may thus indirectly influence human health. *See also* DIET AND DISEASE *and* HERBAL MEDICINE.

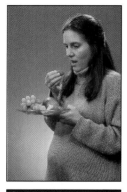

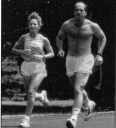

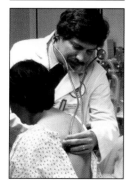

Healthy Practices. Many healthful habits can help to prevent disease or injury in an individual. Above, top, healthy eating is very important, especially in preventing obesity and its related diseases (such as heart disease and type II diabetes). Second from the top, daily exercise can also help to prevent weight gain and improve mental and emotional outlook. Bottom, regular physical examinations by a medical professional can provide early detection for diseases, and thus improve the chances for survival.

Health Hazard, Public

Communal site, physical structure, or substance that poses a health risk to the community.

Any substance, geographic site, or physical structure poses a health risk to a population or a group within that population if it exposes people to carcinogenic or otherwise toxic conditions. The hazard may be food prepared at a certain factory that is sold in a region of the country, a toxic waste dump sending fumes into a residential neighborhood, or a manufacturing plant spilling hazardous waste into a state's water supply. Though the size of the population and the source of the problem vary, there are several criteria commonly used to define a public health hazard.

Public Health Hazards and Children

The biological sensitivity of children places them at special risk for harm from exposure to toxic substances. Children are more sensitive because of differences in how they absorb and respond to environmental chemicals and radiation. Children also risk greater exposure to harmful pesticides, because they consume more of certain fruits, such as apples, that retain pesticide residue. As a result, the Children's Environment Health Network recommends that legislators take steps to strengthen regulations regarding air quality and pesticide control, and that clinicians remember to consider environmental exposure when diagnosing illness in children.

Definition. The U.S. Department of Health and Human Services deems that a public health hazard exists when a site or substance exposes people to toxic material. First, there must be evidence that people have been exposed to the hazard's harmful effects, are currently being exposed, or are likely to be exposed in the future. Second, there must be reason to believe that people are exposed to the toxic material at a high enough concentration to cause symptoms over a period of time greater than a year. Alternatively, there must be community-specific data indicating that the site or substance has an adverse effect on human health sufficient to require intervention.

Testing. It is not always possible to establish a causal relationship between a public health hazard and the health of the exposed population. However, statistical analysis can uncover an unusual concentration of a disease or disorder within a segment of the population. The finding might be a higher prevalence of birth defects or leukemia near a toxic waste dump or in a population that has been exposed to contaminated water. The incidence of the disease may greatly exceed the prevalence within a comparable group that is not exposed to the hazard. Exposure to airborne hazardous waste often causes sensory irritation, irregular heartbeats, and damage to the respiratory system. Other types of hazards cause different symptoms, including blurred vision, persistent cough, diarrhea, and even cancer.

Background material on public health hazard can be found in PUBLIC HEALTH. *For further information, see* ASBESTOSIS; CARCINOGEN; *and* MESOTHELIOMA. *See also* ARRHYTHMIA, CARDIAC; BIRTH DEFECTS; CANCER; COUGH; LEUKEMIA; RESPIRATORY TRACT INFECTION; *and* VISION, LOSS OF *for more on symptoms caused by toxins in the environment.*

Health Insurance

An organized plan to cover health care costs.

Health insurance is a contract that requires the insurance provider to cover all or part of an individual's health care costs in exchange for a monthly premium paid to the insurance provider by the individual, the individual's employer, or both.

Types. Indemnity (fee-for-service) insurance is the traditional form of medical care. Managed care is the alternative. Under indemnity insurance, the insured consults a doctor and the insurance company covers all or part of the cost. Indemnity insurance generally offers an unlimited selection of hospitals and doctors, but the cost may be higher than managed care insurance. Also, some indemnity plans do not cover visits to a doctor's office, or they cover fewer prescriptions or diagnostic tests than managed care plans.

Terms. According to the typical terms of an indemnity contract, the insured individual must pay a certain amount of the costs each year. This is called the deductible, the amount of which varies widely. The insurance company begins coverage once the insured individual has spent his or her own money in the amount of the deductible. Some deductibles are enforced on a per charge basis for each family member.

Usually, once the deductible is satisfied, the indemnity insurer pays 80 percent and the insured 20 percent. Less commonly, the insured and the insurer each pay 50 percent of costs. A stop-loss clause is a limit on the amount the insured must copay. After this limit is attained, the insurer covers the cost at a 100 percent rate up to an amount called the lifetime cap—the total amount an insurer will pay on the insured's behalf in the latter's lifetime.

"Reasonable and customary" charges are those common to a specific geographic region. Indemnity insurance providers establish these limits; some medical providers will accept them, while others demand the patient pick up the difference. Thus the insured must always verify in advance what procedures or medications will be covered by the insurer and to what degree.

The individual or individual's employer pays the monthly premium, which is determined by the insurer. A plan that pays 80/20 may demand a higher premium than that of a 50/50 plan, but the cost of each visit, after satisfying the deductible, will be less under the former. Plan specifics must be weighed against likely costs, which is never an easy prediction.

The Self-Employed. Since insurance companies do most of their business with groups, individual rates tend to be high. In addition to formal research, individuals should inquire among friends about plan recommendations. Perhaps a society or other group offers its members health insurance coverage. The self-employed may be able to buy insurance through affiliation with organizations such as the National Association for the Self-Employed or the National Association of Retired Persons.

Resources on Public Health Hazards

Basch, Paul F., *Textbook of International Health* (1999); Fletcher, Robert H., et al., *Clinical Epidemiology: The Essentials* (1996); Moeller, D.W., *Environmental Health* (1997); National Research Council, Committee on Environmental Epidemiology, *Public Health and Hazardous Wastes* (1991); Timmreck, Thomas C., *Introduction to Epidemiology* (1994); Turnock, Bernard, *Public Health: What It Is and How It Works* (2000); U.S. Public Health Service, Tel. (202) 619-0257, Online: phs.os. dhhs.gov/phs/phs.html; www.med.cornell.edu/public.health/.

Resources on Health Insurance

Bove, Alexander A., Jr., *The Medicaid Planning Handbook: A Guide to Protecting Your Family's Assets from Catastrophic Nursing Home Costs,* 2nd Rev Ed (1996); Chan, Paul D., *Family Medicine* (2001); Rowell, Joann C., et al., *Understanding Health Insurance: A Guide to Professional Billing* (2001); American Academy of Family Physicians, Tel. (800) 274-2237, Online: www.aafp.org; American Hospital Association, Tel. (800) 242-2626, Online: www.aha.org; National Health Information Center, Tel. (301) 565-4167, Online: nhic-nt.health.org; www.nycornell.org/ent/.

Capitation. Capitation is a means of reimbursement sometimes used by insurance companies. This method is based on a flat fee per patient in a given group rather than on varied fees from each patient based on services rendered by the physician.

For background material on health insurance, see FOOD AND DRUG ADMINISTRATION; HOSPITALS, TYPES OF; MEDICAID; MEDICARE; *and* PUBLIC HEALTH. *Further information can be found in* HEALTH; HEALTH MAINTENANCE ORGANIZATION; INPATIENT TREATMENT; *and* OUTPATIENT TREATMENT. *See also* DIAGNOSIS *for more on procedures covered under insurance.*

Health Maintenance Organization

Also known as an HMO

Health plan that offers comprehensive prepaid medical coverage.

A health maintenance organization, or HMO, offers a health plan that provides comprehensive prepaid health coverage for hospital and physician services. The HMO requires members to use authorized health care providers. Generally, members choose a primary care physician from a list of preapproved choices. The primary care physician acts as a gateway for access to medical specialists; the HMO only pays for specialty services that are recommended by the primary care doctor.

Types. There are four main types of HMO. In an independent practice association (IPA), physicians participate in a prepaid healthcare plan. The physicians practice in their own offices, charge agreed-upon rates to enrolled patients, and bill their patients on a fee-for-service or fixed-per-patient basis. A staff-model HMO consists of a group of physicians who are salaried employees of the HMO or of a group within the HMO. Medical care is delivered at HMO-owned facilities. In a network-model HMO, the HMO contracts for services within a network of multi-specialty medical clinics. In the group-model HMO, the health maintenance organization contracts with a specific group of physicians to deliver medical care.

Terms. HMO plans usually require a co-payment for services. The patient pays a fixed, predefined amount per visit to a doctor or hospital. The amount varies depending on the service provided. Some critics have charged that since HMOs are often for-profit organizations, medical decisions are made for financial reasons. They also charge that the HMO structure takes too much power out of the hands of physicians and patients.

Background information on health maintenance organization can be found in HEALTH INSURANCE; MEDICAID; *and* MEDICARE. *For related information, see* HOSPITALS, TYPES OF; INPATIENT TREATMENT; *and* OUTPATIENT TREATMENT.

Hearing

The process of sensing and interpreting sound.

The ear is the organ of hearing. Sound is amplified slightly by the external portion of the ear (pinna) and then travels through the outer-ear to the eardrum (tympanic membrane)—a thin, taut membrane that vibrates in response to sound waves. The vibration is transferred through three small bones in the middle-ear known as the hammer (malleus), the anvil (incus), and the stirrup (stapes). The stirrup touches the membrane leading to the inner-ear, where tiny, sensitive hairs convert the vibrations into electrical impulses, which are carried by nerve fibers to the brain. The brain then interprets the signals into sound.

DISORDERS OF THE EAR

Disorders of the ear may result in hearing loss or an impaired sense of balance. Disorders can be the result of birth defects, injuries, or diseases.

Birth Defects. Approximately 35 percent of all congenital (present-at-birth) hearing defects are genetic. Defects in the development of the outer-ear, eardrum, or middle-ear can often be corrected surgically. A pregnant woman who contracts German measles during the first trimester of pregnancy may give birth to a baby with a defective inner-ear.

Injury. Blows to the head and burns near the head can cause damage to the outer-, middle-, or inner-ear, resulting in temporary or permanent hearing loss. Sudden pressure changes also can damage the ear; scuba divers must take precautions to prevent damage to their ears when diving. Extremely loud noises can rupture the eardrum, and continual use of certain drugs can cause damage to the ear.

Diseases. Middle-ear infection (otitis media) is a common illness in young children. It is caused by an infection in the ear or the nose that spreads to the middle-ear. This may occur as a side effect of an allergy, respiratory infection, or infection of the adenoids. The infected ear fills with pus and is painful. Although middle-ear infections can be treated with antibiotics, in some cases infection is severe and recurrent, leading to a ruptured eardrum. The eustachian tube, which connects the middle-ear to the back of the throat, may become blocked.

Otosclerosis is a disease in which a growth around the stirrup hampers its movement. The disease begins in childhood and gradually worsens, resulting in progressive hearing loss. It can be treated by surgical replacement of the stirrup with an artificial stirrup.

Acoustic neuroma is a tumor of the auditory nerve. It causes a gradual deterioration of hearing ability and ringing in the ears (tinnitus). The tumor can be removed.

Ménières' disease is a disorder in which fluid accumulates in the inner-ear, resulting in vertigo, hearing loss, and tinnitus. Medication can be prescribed to treat this condition. If the disorder persists, surgery may be necessary to drain the excess fluid and reduce the pressure in the ear.

Presbycusis is a gradual loss of hearing that develops as a person ages. The first sign is a difficulty in hearing high-pitched sounds. There is no cure for presbycusis, but the patient usually can benefit from a hearing aid. *See also* BALANCE *and* EAR.

Hearing Aid

Small battery-operated electronic device worn to amplify sound and mitigate a hearing impairment.

Hearing aids can assist individuals with hearing loss by amplifying sound. There are hundreds of different models of hearing aids currently on the market. Every hearing aid includes a microphone to pick up the frequency of the sound, an amplifier to increase the intensity of the sound, a receiver or speaker to transfer the sound to the ear, and a battery to power the device. A hearing aid can be worn in one ear (monaural) or in both ears (binaural).

How it Works. A microphone in the hearing aid gathers sound and converts it into an electric current. The amplifier intensifies the strength of the current and sends it to the earpiece, which converts it back into an amplified sound.

Types. There are two kinds of hearing aids. Air conduction hearing aids amplify sounds and direct them to the ear. People whose ears cannot transmit sound from the outer- to the inner-ear use bone-conduction devices. These carry the sounds to the bones behind the ear, which transmit the vibrations directly to the inner-ear.

Hearing aids vary according to how they are worn and what types of hearing loss they are targeted for.

A completely-in-the-canal hearing aid (CIC) is the smallest hearing device. It is

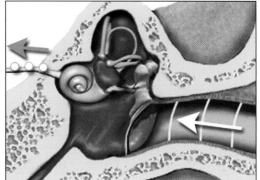

Hearing. Above, when sound waves vibrate the eardrum, nerve impulses in the ear change and are carried to the brain, which interprets the sound.

Resources on Hearing

Davis, Hallowell, and S.R. Silverman, *Hearing and Deafness* (19078); Jerger, James, *Hearing Disorders in Adults* (1984); Pender, Daniel J., *Practical Otology* (1992); Stevens, S., and H. Davis, *Hearing: Its Psychology and Physiology* (1983); Strong, W.J., *Music, Speech, Audio* (1992); National Association of the Deaf, Tel. (301) 587-1788 (voice), -1789 (TTY), Online: www.nad.org; American Academy of Neurology, Tel. (651) 695-1940, Online: www.aan.com; American Board of Neurological Surgery, Tel. (713) 790-6015, Online: www.abns.org; www.med.cornell.edu /neuro/.

practically invisible and is appropriate for mild to moderately severe hearing loss.

An in-the-canal hearing aid (ITC) is a small and cosmetically attractive custom device and is appropriate for a wide range of hearing loss.

An in-the-ear hearing aid (ITE) is a custom-made ear shell that is fixed to the outer-ear and offers options, such as tone controls with which the user can adjust the sound of the hearing aid.

A behind-the-ear hearing aid (BTE) is connected to a custom-made ear shell that offers increased hearing power and the versatility for telephone use.

A body hearing aid is stored in a portable case that is carried in a shirt pocket. A cable connects the hearing aid to a receiver in the ear. It is the most powerful hearing aid and used for patients with severe hearing loss.

> *For background information on hearing aid, see* DEAFNESS; EAR, DISORDERS OF; *and* HEARING. *Further information can be found in* AGING; COCHLEAR IMPLANT; EAR EMERGENCIES; EAR, EXAMINATION OF; EAR FOREIGN BODY IN; *and* EAR TUBE. *See also* HEALTH INSURANCE *and* MEDICARE *for more on paying for a hearing aid.*

Hearing Tests

Various physical tests to assess the ability to hear.

Hearing deficit is measured through audiometry—an examination of hearing designed to assess the degree and nature of hearing loss.

TYPES

Audiogram. By means of an audiogram, the audiologist can determine if hearing loss occurs in one or both ears. Hearing loss due to mechanical abnormalities in the ear canal or middle-ear is said to be conductive. When the inner-ear, the auditory nerve, or the pathways of this nerve in the brain are involved, the deficit is said to be sensorineural.

During an audiogram, sounds of varying intensity are presented through earphones. Normal hearing can detect intensities of as low as 10 to 20 decibels (dB). This general range is used by the audiologist to assess hearing loss. For example, a person who is unable to hear sounds below an intensity of 50 dB is said to have a 30 to 40 dB hearing loss. A vibratory device can be placed behind the mastoid process—a bony region of the skull behind the ear—to test sensorineural hearing, bypassing the outer- and middle-ear.

Speech Threshold Audiometry. This is designed to test for speech comprehension. During this test, the patient listens to a series of two-syllable words spoken at specific volumes. The spondee threshold is the intensity at which the subject can repeat half of the words presented.

Discrimination. This measures a subject's ability to tell closely related words apart. During this type of test, pairs of similar one-syllable words are presented. When hearing loss is purely conductive, scores on a discrimination test are often normal. Should hearing loss be due to sensory disorder, however, discrimination will be somewhat impaired. Severe impairment of discrimination usually indicates neural involvement in hearing loss.

Tympanometry. This seeks the underlying cause of conductive hearing loss by measuring the resistance to pressure—the impedance—of the middle-ear. During this test, a small microphone is placed in the ear canal. The test then measures the amount of sound that passes through the middle-ear versus how much sound is reflected back. Results can identify blockage of the Eustachian tube, fluid in the middle-ear, or irregularities in the ossicles—bones that mechanically transmit sound to the middle-ear.

Other Tests. Additionally, a battery of sophisticated tests exist to evaluate irregularities of the auditory processing regions of the brain.

> *Background material on hearing tests can be found in* EAR, EXAMINATION OF *and* HEARING. *For related information, see* CENTRAL NERVOUS SYSTEM; BRAIN; EUSTACHIAN TUBE; *and* MIDDLE-EAR EFFUSION, PERSISTENT. *See also* DIAGNOSIS *for more on diagnosis hearing problems.*

Heart

The organ that pumps blood.

The body is dependent upon nutrient-rich blood, and the heart is the organ that delivers it. As the center of the cardiovascular and circulatory systems, the heart beats automatically from the time of its creation in the embryo until death.

Composition. The heart is enclosed in a protective membrane of lubricating fluid —the pericardial sac. Located in the middle of the chest cavity between the lungs, an individual's heart is the size of an adult human fist and is made of cardiac muscle cells that pump blood out of the heart and maintain the heartbeat. This heavily muscled layer of cells is called the myocardium, and is covered by an outer layer called the epicardium.The heart's inner layer—the endocardium—continues inside all the body's blood vessels.

Structure. The heart has four chambers. The small upper chambers are called atria (singular, atrium); the larger, lower chambers are called ventricles. The right and left sides are divided by a wall of muscle—the septum—that keeps the blood of either side from mixing with the other. Valves among the chambers keep blood from flowing backwards.

Function. Blood delivers oxygen and other nutrients to cells throughout the body and takes carbon dioxide, along with other waste products, back to the heart via the veins. This oxygen-poor blood is dark red. It flows into the right atrium of the heart via the superior and inferior vena cava and through the tricuspid valve into the right ventricle, which pumps the blood through a one-way valve into the pulmonary arteries that lead to the lungs. There, the blood deposits carbon dioxide (which is exhaled) and picks up oxygen. The oxygen-rich blood turns bright red and flows back to the heart via the pulmonary veins to the left atrium, through the bicuspid valve, and into the left ventricle, the heart's strongest chamber, which

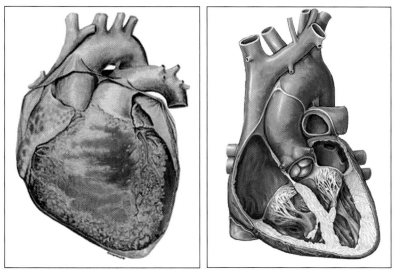

pumps the blood through valves into the aorta. From the aorta, the blood travels into the arteries, the smaller arterioles, and the capillaries, where blood pressure has faded and the exchange of oxygen and carbon dioxide between blood and cells takes place. The blood loses its oxygen and turns dark red, and is then pulled back to the heart by the action of muscles surrounding the veins.

The heart coordinates its beats; the atria pump together to send blood into the ventricles, and the ventricles pump together to send blood to the lungs and body. This synchronicity is achieved via electrical impulses conducted by the cells of the heart.

The heart's pacemaker, the sinoatrial node, located in the right atrium, controls the electrical impulses that contract the atria. The atrioventricular node relays the same impulses through Purkinje's fibers—conductive heart muscle—resulting in contraction of the ventricles. An individual's heart rate is higher when he or she exerts physical or emotional energy. Using neurotransmitters, the autonomic nervous system controls the heart rate according to the need of the body.

The Heart. Above, left, an illustration depicts the outer structure of the heart. Above, right, a cross-section of the heart clearly shows each of the four chambers (the two atria and the two ventricles), as well as the valves that are located between the chambers, and the large pulmonary artery and vena cava.

For background information on heart, see CARDIOLOGY *and* CIRCULATORY SYSTEM. *Related information can be found in* ATRIAL FIBRILLATION; ATRIAL FLUTTER; CARDIAC ARREST; CARDIAC OUTPUT; CARDIAC STRESS TEST; HEART ATTACK; HEART DISORDERS; HEART SOUNDS; *and* VENTRICLE.

Resources on the Heart
Debakey, Michael E. and Antonio M. Gotto, *The New Living Heart* (1997); Gotto, Antonio, *A Patient's Handbook of Cholesterol Disorders* (2000); Gould, Lance K., *Heal Your Heart: How You Can Prevent or Reverse Heart Disease* (2000); Neill, Catherine A., *The Heart of a Child: What Families Need to Know About Heart Disorders in Children* (1992); Ameri-can Heart Association, Tel. (800) 242-8721, Online: www.amhrt.org; Heart Information Network, Tel. (973) 701-6035, Online: www.heartinfo.org; www.nycornell.org/ cardiothoracic.surgery/ www.nycornell.org/medicine/cardiology/html.

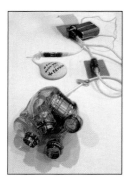

Artificial Heart.
Above, the self-contained artificial heart pump and power supply that was implanted into the chest of Robert Tools, a man with end-stage heart failure, in July 2001.

Heart, Artificial

An implantable mechanical device designed to take over the function of the heart when it fails completely, usually as a temporary measure to keep the recipient alive until an organic heart transplant can be performed.

History. Work with artificial hearts in animals began in 1958. The first implantation of an artificial heart device in a human occurred in 1969. The device supported the patient's circulation for 64 hours, during which time a heart transplant was performed. The patient died 32 hours after the heart transplant.

Starting in 1982, several artificial hearts of a type called Jarvik 7 were implanted, with the intention that these artificial hearts would serve as permanent replacements. All the patients died within months because of complications related to the device, such as infections and fatal strokes. The Jarvik 7, once designed to be a permanent heart replacement, has largely gone out of use today.

Current Use. Artificial heart devices currently in use are designed to perform the function of the left ventricle, which pumps blood to most of the body. A left ventricular assist device is powered by an external source. It is connected by electrical lines running through the chest wall of the patient. These devices have kept patients alive for days or weeks while they await heart transplants. However, they are not currently intended for permanent use. *See also* HEART DISORDERS; HEART SURGERY; *and* HEART TRANSPLANT.

Heart Attack

Also known as a myocardial infarction

The death of heart tissue caused by interruption of the supply of oxygen-rich blood to the heart.

The immediate cause of a heart attack is the blockage of a narrowed coronary artery. The section of heart muscle that loses its blood supply can die in minutes. The risk to a person's life depends largely on which part of the heart is affected.

ALERT

Heart Attack Warning Signs

Every year thousands of deaths can be prevented by heeding the warning signs of heart attack. Often, people believe discomfort will pass and the waiting costs them their lives. Others either fail to recognize the signs or consider them not severe enough to warrant a visit to the doctor. Know the many forms a heart attack can take. Anyone suffering from any of the following symptoms must receive emergency medical treatment as soon as possible: crushing or squeezing pain in the chest beneath the sternum (breastbone); chest pain and vomiting or nausea; chest pain and a cold sweat or damp, sticky skin; chest pain and pale, blue skin, especially around the lips; chest pain and extreme anxiety—a feeling of imminent death; pain that spreads from the chest into the arm, neck, back, shoulders, or jaw; lightheadedness, dizziness, breathlessness, giddiness, or fainting; and a heartbeat that feels strange or out of sync.

Death of tissue that controls the electric impulse system (heartbeat) can precipitate lethal heart rhythm irregularities. If a less vital part of the heart muscle is affected, survival is possible, even if 30 percent or more of the heart muscle dies.

SYMPTOMS

Chest pain is perhaps the most noticeable symptom of a heart attack, but chest pain can occur in different ways: as a severe, crushing feeling in the center of the chest; as a persistent but dull ache; or as pain that spreads from the chest to the shoulders and sometimes to the arms, neck, and jaw. Chest pain is occasionally ignored because it is similar to the symptoms of indigestion. In some cases, a heart attack can occur without pain.

Other symptoms of a heart attack include cold sweats, dizziness, or weakness (sometimes enough to cause fainting); nausea and vomiting; shortness of breath; and a shallow, irregular pulse. When these symptoms occur, medical help should be sought at once by calling 911. Prompt treatment can be life-saving and can limit the damage to the heart. While quick treatment of any kind is vital for survival and recovery, the best source of medical help is a

Emergency Balloon Angioplasty

A newer treatment for a heart attack is an emergency balloon angioplasty. In this procedure, a thin tube, called a catheter, with a balloon at its end is threaded through a blood vessel (in a process called cardiac catheterization) to the site of the blockage. Then the balloon is inflated to reopen the blocked artery. Balloon angioplasty is widely used in non-emergency treatment for narrowed coronary arteries, although many medical centers are now using it during the actual heart attack.

hospital emergency department that is associated with an intensive care unit specializing in cardiovascular crises.

DIAGNOSIS AND TREATMENT

The diagnosis of a heart attack may require an electrocardiogram that shows abnormal electrical activity of the heart, as well as blood tests that can detect the molecules secreted by dying heart cells.

In the most severe cases, if the heart is fibrillating, normal rhythm can be restored by transmitting an electrical impulse from a defibrillator to the heart muscle through electrodes held to the chest. If the heart has stopped, emergency department personnel will try to maintain the pumping action by performing cardiopulmonary resuscitation (CPR) and administering various medications. Because most heart attacks are caused by blood clots, patients will often be treated with reperfusion therapy, which may involve the injection of thrombolytic (clot-dissolving) drugs into a vein, or a direct intervention, such as balloon angioplasty performed via cardiac catheterization. Experience has shown that thrombolytic therapy can dissolve clots and salvage heart tissue if it is given in the first few minutes or even hours after a heart attack occurs. In addition to thrombolytic agents, the patient will also be given aspirin and heparin, both of which are drugs that reduce clotting in the body.

PROGNOSIS

After emergency department treatment, patients usually go to a coronary care unit (CCU), an area of the hospital staffed by specially trained doctors, nurses, and technicians. A CCU will have sophisticated electrocardiogram equipment and a variety of devices that allow minute-by-minute monitoring of the patient's condition. This equipment will recognize any heart irregularities and sound an alarm. The CCU will also be equipped with defibrillators and other life-saving equipment on hand for immediate use.

Patients typically stay in a CCU for several days, until the heart and other vital organs are functioning regularly. At that point, the patient may be moved to a regular hospital room. The duration of the hospital stay for a heart attack victim depends on the degree of damage detected by electrocardiograms, blood tests, cardiac stress tests, and other diagnostic procedures.

ALERT

Heart Attack Risk Factors

Each year, 1.5 million Americans suffer heart attacks, and more than 500,000 of these people die. Smoking, an unhealthy diet, obesity, and lack of exercise place people at serious risk for a heart attack. The most important fact about heart attack symptoms is that 60 percent of deaths occur before a patient reaches a hospital. Sometimes this happens because death is sudden, but often treatment is not sought in time because the symptoms of a heart attack are not recognized or are ignored.

A second heart attack can occur in up to 25 percent of first heart attack patients. If the risk is high, bypass surgery or balloon angioplasty may be performed to maintain blood flow to the heart.

Full recovery from a heart attack usually takes several months. A rehabilitation program to enable restoration of normal or near-normal activity, accompanied by drug treatment that can include aspirin, heparin, and beta-blockers, is successful in a large percentage of cases.

Background material on heart attack can be found in CARDIOLOGY; CIRCULATORY SYSTEM; and HEART. For further information, see CARDIAC ARREST; CARDIAC STRESS TEST; ECG; HEART DISORDERS; HEART FAILURE; HEART IMAGING; THROMBOSIS; and VENTRICLE.

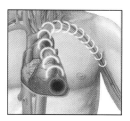

Heart Attack. Above, pain in the chest or radiating from the chest down the left arm may be a warning sign of a heart attack.

Resources on Heart Attack

Berne, Robert M., et al., *Cardiovascular Physiology* (2001); Debakey, Michael E. and Antonio M. Gotto, *The New Living Heart* (1997); Gould, Lance K., *Heal Your Heart: How You Can Prevent or Reverse Heart Disease* (2000); Wallwork, John, and Rob Stepney, Heart Disease (1976) American Heart Association, Tel. (800) 242-8721, Online: www.amhrt.org; Heart Information Network, Tel. (973) 701-6035, Online: www.heartinfo.org; National Heart, Lung, and Blood Institute, Tel. (301) 496-4236, Online: www.nhlbi.nih. gov; www.nycornell.org/ cardiothoracic.surgery/ www.nycornell.org/medicine/cardiology/html.

Heartbeat

Contraction of the heart muscle that pumps blood to the lungs and the rest of the body.

On average, the heart beats about 72 times every minute and about 100,000 times a day in a healthy adult, although this rate can be affected by a number of factors. During physical exertion, the heart beats faster to meet the body's increased demand for the oxygen-rich blood. The heart also beats faster during times of emotional or psychological stress.

Phases. There are two phases of each heartbeat, contraction and relaxation. The period of contraction is called systole, and occurs when blood flows from the heart to the body. The two upper chambers of the heart are called atria, and the two lower chambers are the ventricles. Oxygen-depleted blood returns from the body and flows into the right atrium. From there it is pumped to the right ventricle, which pumps blood to the lungs to pick up oxygen and drop off carbon dioxide. This blood then travels to the left atrium and is pumped to the left ventricle, which sends it out to the body through the aorta, the main artery from the heart. Each heartbeat sends two to three ounces of oxygen-rich blood out through the aorta. Each contraction is followed by diastole, or relaxation, during which the heart muscle expands so that its chambers fill with blood again. The heartbeat is controlled by electrical impulses sent out from a bundle of specialized cells, known as the sinoatrial node, which are located near the right atrium.

Assessment. The heartbeat is most noticeable on the left side of the chest. It is easy to measure the heartbeat by checking the pulse, feeling the expansion and contraction of a blood vessel near the surface of the skin, often in the wrist and neck. A more accurate assessment of the heartbeat can be made through a stethoscope placed on the left side of the chest. Either method can detect abnormalities of the heartbeat.

Abnormalities. During a routine physical, a physician will listen for heartbeat abnormalities. Tachycardia is an abnormally fast heartbeat, usually defined as more than 100 beats per minute. Bradycardia is an abnormally slow heartbeat, usually of less than 60 beats per minute. An ectopic

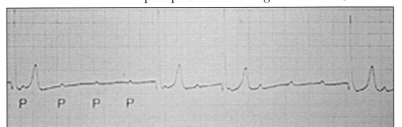

Heartbeat. At right, in a heartbeat, oxygen-poor blood enters the right side of the heart. The right ventricle then pumps the blood to the lungs, where it becomes oxygenated. The left ventricle then pumps the oxygen-rich blood to all parts of the body; once the oxygen has been used, the blood returns to the heart. Above, an ECG (electrocardiogram) chart, which records the activity of the heart.

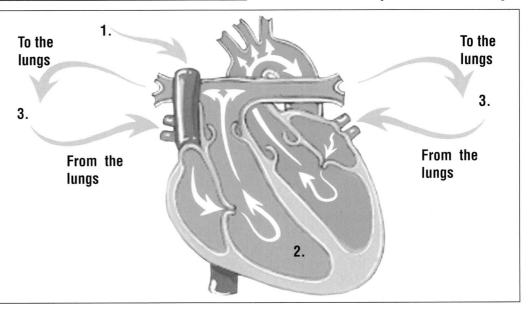

heartbeat is a heartbeat that does not have a regular pattern of contraction and expansion. The presence of bradycardia, tachycardia, or ectopic heartbeat can indicate functional problems of the heart that call for detailed diagnosis and may require further treatment. *See also* HEART.

Heart Block

Interruption of the electrical impulses that travel from the sinoatrial node in the upper chambers of the heart (atria) to the lower chambers (ventricles), causing them to contract abnormally.

Heart block is an interruption of the electrical impulses that cause the heart to beat. The disorder causes the ventricles to beat less often or out of rhythm with the atria.

Types. There are three degrees of heart block. In first-degree heart block, the least serious, electrical impulses in the heart are slowed but not interrupted. The contractions of the chambers are only slightly out of rhythm. First-degree heart block can be detected by an electrocardiogram, but the condition usually causes no symptoms.

In second-degree heart block, some of the electrical impulses do not reach the ventricles. The rhythm of the heart becomes slower and less regular. Second-degree heart block can cause dizziness or fainting spells.

Third-degree heart block, also known as complete heart block, is when electrical impulses do not reach the ventricles at all. The atria and ventricles beat without their normal coordination. The atrial beat will vary according to the person's level of physical activity, while the ventricles may beat at a steady rate of about 40 beats per minute. Third-degree heart block prevents the brain from getting enough oxygen-carrying blood, consequently resulting in symptoms such as severe fatigue, lightheadedness, fainting, or seizures.

Causes. No specific cause of heart block can be found in a large percentage of cases. One common cause that can be identified is a previous heart attack. Heart block can also occur in persons with atherosclerosis (thickening and hardening of the walls of

the arteries) and those with enlargement of the heart caused by untreated rheumatic arthritis or hypertension. Other causes of heart block include endocarditis (inflammation of the lining of the heart and the heart valves) and abnormalities of the mitral or aortic valve. Heart block can be a congenital condition (present at birth) or it can be a side effect of some medications prescribed for heart conditions.

Diagnosis and Treatment. Heart block can be diagnosed by the patterns shown on an electrocardiogram. If the condition is intermittent, determining the proper diagnosis may require the patient to wear a Holter monitor—an all-day electrocardiogram device. Treatment of heart block depends on the severity of the condition. First- or second-degree heart block may call for nothing more than periodic monitoring by a physician. Third-degree heart block that causes severe symptoms may be treated by an implanted pacemaker to ensure a regular heartbeat.

Background material on heart block can be found in CARDIOLOGY; CIRCULATORY SYSTEM; *and* HEART. *For related information, see* CARDIAC STRESS TEST; FAINTING; HEART DISORDERS; HEART FAILURE; HEART IMAGING; *and* SEIZURE.

Heartburn

A burning sensation behind the breastbone.

The burning chest pain that characterizes heartburn may travel from the tip of the breastbone to the throat. It may also be accompanied by regurgitation or excessive salivation. Heartburn occurs when the lower esophageal sphincter relaxes, allowing the acidic contents of the stomach to back up the esophagus. Unlike the stomach, the esophagus does not have a protective lining. Refluxed stomach acid causes pain and inflammation in the esophagus.

Treatment and Prevention. Antacids can alleviate the burning chest pain of heartburn. To prevent heartburn, acid production of the stomach can be blocked by various medications, such as ranitidine or omeprazole. *See also* ACID REFLUX.

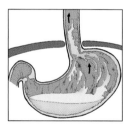

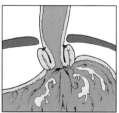

Heartburn.
Above, top, heartburn occurs when acid from the stomach backs up into the esophagus. Above, bottom, fundoplication is a surgical procedure that is used to treat heartburn. The stomach lining is folded to reinforce the barrier between the esophagus and the stomach.

Heart Disease, Congenital

Malformation of the structures or surrounding blood vessels of the heart of a newborn baby.

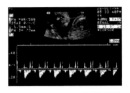

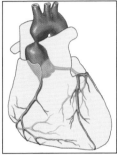

Congenital Heart Disease. Since congenital heart disease is present at birth, it can often be detected in the fetus by a coronary ultrasound, above, top. Above, bottom, one serious congenital heart defect is coarctation of the aorta, in which part of the aorta is constricted.

Congenital means "present at birth." Congenital heart disease occurs when the heart develops abnormally before birth. The cause of most congenital heart disease is unknown. One cause of congenital heart defects is rubella (German measles) contracted by women in the first three months of pregnancy. Vaccination has virtually eliminated this problem in the United States. Another cause is fetal alcohol syndrome—birth defects resulting from a pregnant woman drinking heavily. Congenital heart defects are found in one-third of babies born with Down's syndrome. These heart abnormalities are often accompanied by other physical defects.

Types. There are many forms of congenital heart defects. They can affect the heart wall, the main blood vessels of the heart, the heart valves, or several structures at once.

The tetralogy of Fallot is a congenital defect that causes four abnormalities: ventral septal defect, a hole in the wall between the ventricles; pulmonary stenosis, obstruction of the artery going to the lungs; hypertrophy, or thickening, of the right ventricle; and abnormal location of the aorta, the main artery from the heart. Each of these defects can occur individually in some babies.

Some defects affect the vessels around the heart. Transposition of the great vessels is a defect in which the positions of the two main arteries of the heart, the pulmonary artery and the aorta, are reversed, so that oxygen-carrying blood that should travel to the body goes back into the lungs. Coarctation of the aorta is narrowing of the aorta, reducing the flow of blood to the body.

Congenital defects can also affect the valves of the heart. In aortic stenosis, the valve between the left ventricle and the aorta is deformed. This prevents the valve from opening and closing properly to control the flow of blood. Congenital defects of the mitral valve, controlling blood flow between the left atrium and left ventricle, are rare but cause serious problems. There can be congenital mitral stenosis, narrowing of the valve. There is also congenital atresia, in which there is no opening at all in the pulmonic valve. A congenital defect of the pulmonic valve, which controls flow between the right ventricle and the pulmonary artery, consists of severe narrowing of the valve that restricts blood flow out of the heart to the lungs.

Symptoms. Symptoms of congenital heart disease depend on the nature of the abnormality. If the defect causes oxygen-poor blood to be pumped from the heart, cyanosis—a bluish appearance—can result. Eating problems and poor growth can occur. In some cases, symptoms do not appear for years. Children and adults with congenital heart disease may experience breathlessness during physical activity.

Diagnosis. A congenital heart defect that is not detected before birth is often diagnosed later by the distinctive sounds a doctor hears through a stethoscope. The exact nature of the disorder can be determined by tests such as ultrasound, electrocardiogram, magnetic resonance imaging (MRI), and angiography, depending on the nature of the disorder.

Treatment. Many congenital heart defects can be repaired by surgery. Several operations may be needed in some cases. Some defects require immediate treatment. The only alternatives for hypoplastic left heart syndrome are a complex series of operations or a heart transplant. Other defects can be treated surgically later in life. The success rate of surgery has increased steadily over the years, and many children with congenital heart disease can lead normal or near-normal lives, although they must be monitored constantly.

For background material on congenital heart disease, see CARDIOLOGY; CIRCULATORY SYSTEM; and HEART. Related information can be found in CONGENITAL; CYANOSIS; ECG; HEART DISORDERS; HEART FAILURE; HEART IMAGING; and MRI.

Heart Disease, Ischemic

Deficiency in oxygen supply to the body resulting from reduced blood flow due to narrowing or obstruction of the coronary arteries.

In ischemic heart disease, the flow of oxygen-carrying blood through the arteries is reduced by atherosclerosis, in which deposits called plaque, made of cholesterol, fat, and fibrous tissue, build up in the inner wall of the blood vessels. This buildup reduces blood flow and can result in blockage of an artery, causing a heart attack.

Symptoms. For many people, the first symptom of ischemic heart disease is angina pectoris—chest pain that is usually felt first during periods of physical exertion, when the narrowed arteries can no longer deliver an adequate supply of oxygen-carrying blood. Angina becomes worse as the disease progresses, so that it can occur during moderate exercise or even at rest. Other symptoms can include shortness of breath and fatigue. Some people with ischemic heart disease do not have any symptoms at all.

Diagnosis. The existence and extent of ischemic heart disease is determined by electrocardiography, which gives a record of the electrical activity of the heart; echocardiography, which uses ultrasound to get an image of the heart; a stress test; or angiography, x-ray images of the arteries made after injection of a special dye.

Treatment. A variety of drugs can be prescribed to ease the symptoms of ischemic heart disease. These increase blood flow and help manage the irregular heartbeats (arrhythmias) that often accompany the disease. Angiotensin-converting enzyme (ACE) inhibitors, beta blockers, and calcium channel blockers are commonly used medications. Balloon angioplasty, in which a balloon is opened inside the artery at a narrowed place, is often performed, as is coronary artery bypass surgery, in which a blood vessel taken from another part of the body is used to create a new pathway for blood flow around one or more narrowed or blocked areas. *See also* HEART DISORDERS.

Heart Disorders

Conditions that affect the ability of the heart to supply the body with an adequate amount of blood.

Like any part of the body, the heart is subject to a number of diseases and abnormalities, some of them congenital, some acquired. Disorders of the heart are the most common cause of death in the United States and other industrialized nations.

Disorders That Impair Blood Flow. This class of heart disorder includes the major causes of death, such as heart attack. The cause of most of these conditions is deterioration of blood flow through the coronary arteries, which supply blood to the heart.

Over time, the coronary arteries can become narrowed and less flexible because of atherosclerosis—the buildup of fatty deposits in the walls of the blood vessels. As all or part of the heart muscle is deprived of its normal blood supply, it must work harder to maintain blood flow to the body. One result can be congestive heart failure—a weakening and enlargement of the heart muscle. Another can be angina pectoris— the pain that occurs first during exertion and then, as deterioration of the heart continues, even at rest. The heart can experience an arrhythmia (disturbance of its normal beating pattern), which in extreme cases can lead to fibrillation (a complete loss of heart rhythm). Also, an artery can become blocked, causing a heart attack, the death of part of the heart tissue, which can result in sudden death.

Congenital Disorders. This group of disorders consists of abnormalities in the structure of the heart or its major blood vessels that are present from birth. It includes septal defects, "holes in the heart," and malformations of the heart valves, such as stenosis or prolapse.

Infection. A bacterial, fungal, or viral infection of the heart can cause endocarditis—inflammation of the tissue lining the inside of the heart muscle. Very often, such an infection damages the mitral and aortic valves that control blood flow between the chambers of the heart and out of the heart.

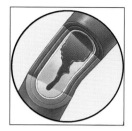

Heart Disorders.
One serious heart disorder is blockage of the coronary artery from atherosclerosis, above. In patients with this disease, fatty deposits, or plaques, build up in the walls of the arteries, impeding blood flow. The arteries may become so narrow that a heart attack results.

The result can be conditions including mitral insufficiency, in which the mitral valve does not close properly, and mitral stenosis (narrowing of the opening of the valve). These valve defects are often caused by rheumatic fever, an immune system disorder caused by a bacterial infection.

Muscle Disorders. These disorders are known under the general name of cardiomyopathy, a reduced ability of the heart to pump blood because the heart muscle is weakened. Cardiomyopathy can be caused by a congenital condition, a viral infection, overconsumption of alcohol, or a bacterial infection. Another muscle disorder is myocarditis—an inflammation of the heart muscle that can result from a bacterial or viral infection. Less frequently, myocarditis can be a side effect of a medication or of radiation therapy.

Injuries. Many highway fatalities are caused by blunt injuries to the heart, as the driver impacts the steering wheel hard enough to compress the heart between the breastbone and the spine. A mild compression can just bruise the heart, but a severe impact may result in complete and fatal rupture of the heart muscle. The introduction of seat belts and air bags has reduced the incidence of these injuries, but many drivers fail to follow instructions to buckle their seat belts on the road.

Nutritional Disorders. The most common nutritional disorder affecting the heart is obesity, which leads to high blood pressure, atherosclerosis, and an excessive demand on the heart's pumping ability. A disorder that was more common in the past was beriberi, a deficiency of vitamin B_1 that leads to heart failure. While most Americans get enough vitamin B_1 from their diet to prevent beriberi, it is still a major problem for chronic alcoholics. Chronic alcoholism can damage the heart by causing cardiomyopathy.

Background material on heart disorders can be found in CIRCULATORY SYSTEM *and* HEART. *For further information, see* ANGINA PECTORIS; ATHEROSCLEROSIS; ATRIAL FIBRILLATION; AUTOMOBILE SAFETY; CARDIOMYOPATHY; CONGENITAL; HEART ATTACK; HEART FAILURE; MYOCARDITIS; *and* OBESITY.

Resources on Cardiovascular Disorders

Debakey, Michael E. and Antonio M. Gotto, *The New Living Heart* (1997); Gotto, Antonio, *A Patient's Handbook of Cholesterol Disorders* (2000); Gould, Lance K., *Heal Your Heart: How You Can Prevent or Reverse Heart Disease* (2000); Neill, Catherine A., *The Heart of a Child: What Families Need to Know About Heart Disorders in Children* (1992); American Heart Association, Tel. (800) 242-8721, Online: www.amhrt.org; Heart Information Network, Tel. (973) 701-6035, Online: www.heartinfo.org; www.nycornell.org/cardiothoracic.surgery/ www.nycornell.org/medicine/cardiology/html.

Heart Failure

Chronic condition in which the heart muscle becomes weakened, progressively reducing its ability to pump blood to the body.

The most common cause of heart failure is coronary artery disease—narrowing of the arteries that supply blood to the heart muscle. Other causes can be uncontrolled hypertension, abnormalities of the heart valves, cardiomyopathy, endocarditis, alcohol or drug abuse, and hormonal abnormalities such as hyperthyroidism. In heart failure, the strength of the heart's contractions decreases and less blood can reach the body. The heart must work harder to meet the body's need for oxygen, so it may become enlarged and its valves may begin to leak blood.

Symptoms. In the early stages of heart failure, there can be few or no symptoms. As the condition progresses, it causes shortness of breath, weakness, fatigue, a chronic cough, and decreased exercise tolerance. Heart failure can also result in fluid retention. If this fluid buildup is caused by weakness of the right chambers of the heart, the legs, the ankles, and the abdomen become swollen. If the left side of the heart is weakened, fluid builds up in the lungs, contributing to breathing problems.

Treatment. A first measure in treatment of heart failure can be dietary change to reduce the intake of salt; the sodium in salt contributes to the buildup of fluid in the body. A diuretic can be prescribed to help the body get rid of excess fluid. Digitalis may be prescribed to strengthen the ability

Risk Factors for Heart Failure

Age is a risk factor for heart failure. As the heart ages, its tissue becomes less flexible. Heart failure is most common in people over the age of 70. Incidence in the elderly is increasing and fewer people are dying young from other heart diseases. Someone who survives a heart attack is vulnerable to heart failure because the heart has been damaged. Smoking, poor diet, and lack of exercise can all contribute to the development of heart failure over time.

of the heart to pump blood. Other medications for heart failure include vasodilators such as angiotensin-converting enzyme (ACE) inhibitors, which take some burden off the heart by widening the arteries, and beta blockers, which improve the heart's ability to pump blood to the body. If heart failure is caused or worsened by a faulty heart valve, surgery may be done to repair or replace the valve. Surgery can also be done to repair a congenital (present-at-birth) defect causing heart failure. A last resort for severe heart failure is a heart transplant, but a shortage of donor organs rules out this option for most patients.

> *Background material on heart failure can be found in* CARDIOLOGY; CIRCULATORY SYSTEM; *and* HEART. *For further information, see* HEART DISORDERS. *See also* ALCOHOL DEPENDENCE; ATHEROSCLEROSIS; CARDIOMYOPATHY; DRUG DEPENDENCE; *and* ENDOCARDITIS *for more on possible causes.*

Heart Imaging

Various techniques for directly visualizing the human heart for diagnostic purposes.

Heart imaging consists of techniques that allow the physician to directly view the heart and other cardiovascular structures. Imaging techniques, including chest x-rays, computed tomography (CT) scanning, fluoroscopy, echocardiography, and magnetic resonance imaging (MRI) have become widely favored for their combination of high resolution and noninvasive process.

TYPES

Chest x-ray is usually the first imaging exam in cases where heart abnormality or disease are suspected. Here, the size and shape of the heart are clearly seen, as well as the outline of blood vessels in the lungs. Heart valve problems or heart failure tend to increase the size of the heart. Abnormalities of the lung arteries may suggest cardiac disease or lung disease.

Echocardiography is one of the most common techniques for imaging the heart. It is painless, noninvasive, and widely available. In echocardiography, high frequency sound waves are emitted by a transducer and reflected from structures in the heart and accompanying blood vessels, creating a moving image that appears on a video screen. For a more detailed picture or in order to visualize structures behind the heart, a probe may be passed down the patient's throat in a procedure known as transesophageal echocardiography. Ultrasound studies of the heart are capable of detecting irregularities in the motion of the heart wall, the volume of blood pumped by the heart, pericardial diseases, and fluid accumulations.

CT or Computed Tomography Scanning (also known as CAT) is a special type of x-ray technique allowing greater precision and better resolution of cardiac structures. The CT scan combines x-ray technique with computer enhancement to provide images of tissue sections or tomograms, through the living heart. Recent advances in CT technology are able to provide three-dimensional visualization of the heart.

MRI (Magnetic Resonance Imaging) uses a magnetic field to provide images with extraordinary detail. Like echocardiography, MRI is safe, painless, and noninvasive. The subject is placed in a tube containing a powerful magnet that causes the atomic nuclei within the cells of living tissue to vibrate. These signals are converted by computer into two- and three-dimensional images.

Preventing the Need for Heart Imaging. In addition to a healthy lifestyle, which never includes smoking and in which alcohol is only consumed in moderation, and a diet that is varied, high in fiber, and low in fat and cholesterol, other lifestyle changes can promote a healthy heart, such as:

- regular exercise;
- an active lifestyle; and
- stress reduction.

> *For background information on heart imaging, see* CAT SCAN; ECHOCARDIOGRAPHY; MRI; *and* X-RAY. *Related information can be found in* ANGIOGRAPHY; PET SCAN; *and* RADIONUCLIDE SCANNING. *See also* HEART DISORDERS *for more on disorders for which heart imaging is needed.*

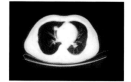
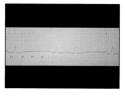

Heart Imaging.
There are many different techniques that can be used to visualize the heart. Above, top, a computed tomography (CT) scan of the chest, in which the heart is visible. Above, bottom, an ECG (echocardiography) track, which records heart activity.

Heart-Lung Machine

Device that performs the function of the heart and lungs temporarily during open-heart surgery, which often involves a heart transplant or the repair or replacement of a damaged heart valve.

A heart-lung machine consists of an oxygenator, which adds oxygen to and removes carbon dioxide from the blood, and a pump that sends the oxygenated blood to the rest of the body.

Before surgery, tubes called cannulas are inserted into the main veins leading to the heart and either the aorta (the major artery carrying blood from the heart) or another major artery. Blood flows through the cannulas into the oxygenator, which removes carbon dioxide and adds oxygen to the blood through a thin membrane. The blood loses heat in its passage through the oxygenator, but is warmed in a heat exchanger before it is pumped back into the body; it is sometimes kept cool to lower the body temperature and to give the surgeon more time to operate. Since a heart-lung machine does not work as efficiently as the body's own organs, it can be used for only a few hours. *See also* HEART SURGERY.

Heart-Lung Transplant

Radical surgery in which the heart and lungs of a patient are replaced by those of a donor.

A heart-lung transplant is a final measure to save the life of someone with an end-stage medical condition, such as chronic emphysema, cystic fibrosis, or sarcoidosis. The tissue type of donor and patient must be matched carefully to prevent rejection by the patient's immune system.

Procedure. After the donor organs are removed, the patient's chest is opened with an incision down the breastbone. The patient is connected to a heart-lung machine, and both lungs and the heart are removed and replaced by donor organs. The blood vessels linking heart and lungs are left in place. Connections are then made to the trachea (which carries air between the head and lungs) and to appropriate veins and arteries. If the patient receiving the transplant suffered from a condition that primarily affected the lungs, the heart that is removed may be transplanted to a patient with end-stage heart disease. *See* CYSTIC FIBROSIS; EMPHYSEMA; *and* SARCOIDOSIS.

Heart Rate

Pace at which the heart contracts to pump blood to the lungs and the rest of the body.

Heart rate is faster in childhood than in adult life and tends to become slower with age. An infant's heart rate may be 120 beats per minute. Most adults in good physical condition have a heart rate between 60 and 100 beats per minute. The rate generally is lower in athletes or persons who regularly engage in strenuous physical activity. A trained athlete may have a heart rate as low as 40 or 50 beats per minute.

The heart rate is generally at its slowest during sleep and increases with physical activity, as the heart responds to the body's demand for more oxygen-carrying blood. A fast walking pace can increase the heart rate by 20 to 30 beats per minute, while the normal rate may double during sexual intercourse. The heart rate may also be increased substantially at times of stress. During a panic attack, the heart rate may reach 170 beats per minute, as the body responds to the rush of adrenaline (epinephrine) that is secreted by the adrenal gland. Some persons trained in meditation techniques, such as yoga, can slow their heart rate voluntarily. *See also* HEARTBEAT.

Heart Sounds

Sounds produced by the structures of the heart and movement of blood, used for diagnostic purposes.

Heart sounds are routinely listened to by physicians in the course of a general checkup to help evaluate the health of the cardiovascular system. The process of listening, known as auscultation, is generally carried out with the aid of a stethoscope.

The doctor will listen to the strength, quality, and rhythm of the heartbeat, noting peculiarities such as abnormal sounds (murmurs) detected over the heart or blood vessels, caused by various abnormalities of the heart valves.

Irregularities in various heart sounds suggest specific underlying causes. For example, certain murmurs result from the seepage of blood from heart valves that do not thoroughly seal. Similarly, constricted or narrowed heart valves may be identified by murmurs. It is important to note that many non-life-threatening causes exist for irregular heart sounds. These include pregnancy, natural aging of the heart, and heart irregularities occurring in infancy and early childhood.

Those over the age of 50 should have regular heart checkups. Early detection of heart irregularities or disease offer the best hope for proper treatment.

> Background material on heart sounds can be found in AUSCULTATION; DIAGNOSIS; and HEART. For related information, see AGING; HEARTBEAT; HEART DISORDERS; HEART IMAGING; HEART VALVE; and PREGNANCY.

Heart Surgery

> Operation performed to repair a defect of the heart or to replace a severely damaged heart with a transplanted organ.

The first successful human heart surgery, repair of a valve defect, was performed in the early 1950s, using a machine that kept blood circulating during the procedure. The widespread use of heart surgery became possible in the 1970s, with development of a heart-lung machine—more formally, a cardiopulmonary bypass machine—that performs the functions of both the heart and the lungs, supplying oxygenated blood to the body. Another innovation making it possible to perform extended surgery on the heart is hypothermia—reducing the stress on the heart by lowering its temperature. Today, hundreds of thousands of Americans undergo heart surgery each year for various conditions.

> **Minimally Invasive Surgery**
>
> After several decades, the field of heart surgery is undergoing continuing expansion and development. Minimally invasive techniques eliminate the need to saw open the breastbone and reduce the size of the incision needed for an operation. Some procedures, such as bypass surgery, can now be done without stopping the heart.

TYPES

Coronary artery bypass surgery is done to provide new channels for the flow of blood around sections of coronary arteries that are partially or totally blocked by atherosclerosis. A section of another blood vessel, most often a vein from the leg, is stitched into place to loop around the blocked area.

Valve repair or replacement can be performed either on the mitral valve, which controls flow between the chambers of the heart, or the aortic valve, which controls blood flow out of the heart. A valve that has been damaged by disease, deterioration, or a congenital condition can be repaired surgically or replaced by a mechanical valve or one made of animal tissue.

Arrhythmia surgery is done to correct abnormal heartbeats. If arrhythmia originates in one specific segment of the heart, or if it results from an abnormality in the heart's own system of electrical pathways, surgery can be performed. A defibrillator device can be implanted for severe, life-threatening arrhythmias.

Aneurysm surgery is done to remove, replace, or repair a weakened, bulging region of an artery that could otherwise rupture or hemorrhage.

Heart Transplant. A heart transplant replaces an otherwise untreatable, failing heart with an organ from a donor whose death was not caused by a heart condition. Some severely ill patients undergo heart-lung transplants, in which both organs are replaced in a single procedure.

> For background information on heart surgery, see CIRCULATORY SYSTEM; HEART; and SURGERY. Further information can be found in ANEURYSM; HEART-LUNG MACHINE; HEART TRANSPLANT; HEART VALVE SURGERY; and HYPOTHERMIA.

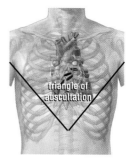

Heart Sounds.
When a medical professional listens to the sounds of the heart through a stethoscope, the process is known as auscultation. The area in which the stethoscope is placed is often called the "triangle of auscultation."

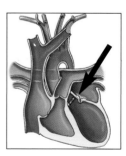

Heart Surgery.
Valve replacement can be performed on either the mitral valve, which controls the flow of blood between the chambers of the heart, or the aortic valve (above), which controls the flow of blood out of the heart.

Heart Transplant

Replacement of all or part of a diseased or damaged heart with all or part of a healthy heart taken from a donor.

Donor and Recipient. The recipient of a heart transplant is generally an individual under 60 years of age whose heart is failing, who has no other serious medical conditions (such as cancer or lung disease), and whose heart failure cannot be treated in any other way. The donor heart comes from a healthy young person who has suffered brain death from an injury, stroke, or other incident, and whose heart has not been damaged. Donor and recipient must be matched for the size of the organ, blood type, and tissue type, to reduce the risk of rejection by the recipient's immune system. At any given time, several thousand Americans are awaiting a heart transplant.

Procedure. When a suitable donor is found, the recipient is placed on a heart-lung machine (cardiopulmonary bypass) that will supply oxygen-carrying blood to the body. The surgeon then removes almost all of the heart, usually leaving only the back walls of the two atria (the upper chambers of the heart) in place. In some cases, more of the heart will be left in place, depending on the amount of damage that is present. The sections that are replaced are the two ventricles, which pump blood to the lung and the rest of the body, and the valves controlling blood flow in and out of the heart.

During the operation, the donor heart is kept cool to prevent damage. The donor heart is sewn into place and is connected to the pulmonary artery, through which blood flows to the lungs, and the aorta, which supplies the rest of the body. When the connections are complete, the transplanted heart is gradually brought up to body temperature, the patient is taken off the heart-lung machine, and the heart begins its new function.

Risks and Prognosis. The major danger after heart transplant surgery is rejection of the transplanted organ. Drugs that suppress the immune response, such as cyclosporine and azathioprine, must be taken indefinitely by the recipient to prevent rejection. Tissue samples of the transplanted organ are taken for the first 3 to 6 weeks after surgery and then less frequently for years afterward to detect signs of rejection. Since immunosuppressive treatment reduces the body's defense against infection, antibiotics are part of postoperative therapy. The recipient is also monitored for other complications, such as coronary artery disease (which can develop in half of all patients) and damage to the kidneys and other organs. The one-year survival rate for heart transplant surgery is now over 85 percent, with the five-year survival rate at over 60 percent.

Background information on heart transplant can be found in CIRCULATORY SYSTEM *and* HEART FAILURE. *For further information, see* ANTIBIOTIC DRUGS; HEART-LUNG MACHINE; IMMUNE SYSTEM; *and* REJECTION. *See also* ACCIDENTS *and* STROKE *for more on conditions affecting the donor.*

Heart Valve

A structure that controls the passage of blood between the chambers of the heart.

Heart valves are key to the proper pumping of blood. They allow blood to pass from chamber to chamber and keep it from flowing backwards.

There are four heart valves. Blood enters the right atrium, which pumps it into the right ventricle via the atrioventricular, or tricuspid, valve, which has three triangular flaps that open and join. The right ventricle pumps blood into the pulmonary artery via the semilunar, or pulmonary, valve. Oxygen-rich blood returns from the lungs, enters the left atrium, passes the mitral, or bicuspid valve, which has two flaps, into the left ventricle, which pumps blood via the aortic valve throughout the body.

When the ventricles contract, the tricuspid and mitral valves prevent the backflow of blood into the atria. Pulmonary and aortic valves keep the blood from reentering the ventricles. *See* HEART VALVE SURGERY.

Heart Valve Surgery

A procedure done to repair or replace a faulty heart valve when the symptoms it causes cannot be controlled by drug treatment.

Many heart valve disorders can be treated by drugs that increase the ability of the heart to pump blood, or reduce the load on the heart by widening blood vessels or reducing blood pressure. Surgery on the heart valves becomes necessary when the symptoms of a heart valve abnormality are worsening despite drug therapy. Heart valve surgery is a major operation that is done under general anesthesia.

Repair. Surgical repair of a heart valve is possible if the damage to the valve is not very severe. If the problem is stenosis (narrowing of the opening of the heart valve), the leaflets of the valve can be stretched and widened using a procedure called a balloon valvuloplasty. In this procedure, a thin tube (catheter) with a balloon on one end is inserted into a vein and through that vein into the heart. Once the catheter is inside the heart valve, the balloon is inflated, widening the opening of the narrowed valve. If a heart valve is torn, it can be sewn together surgically. If the leaflets of a valve do not close completely, the base of the valve can be changed to facilitate more complete closure.

Replacement. When a heart valve is damaged beyond the possibility of repair, it can be replaced. Replacement surgery is

Minimally Invasive Heart Valve Surgery

Until recently, all heart valve procedures were done by sawing a vertical opening eight to ten inches long in the breast bone and puling the segments apart to give the surgeon access to the heart. In recent years, however, a technique called minimally invasive surgery has become available. It allows the surgery to be done through a vertical opening four or five inches wide, reducing the length of the hospital stay and recuperation. Since minimally invasive surgery requires a high degree of skill on the part of the surgeon and the operating room staff, it is available at only a limited number of medical centers.

most often done on the two major valves of the heart: the mitral valve and the aortic valve. The mitral valve prevents a backflow of blood into the chambers of the heart. The aortic valve prevents backflow to most of the body. A replacement valve may be a mechanical device made of metal or plastic. A mechanical valve can last for as long as 20 years, but any patient who receives such a valve must take an anticoagulant drug (to prevent the formation of blood clots) and must be monitored regularly.

The alternative to a mechanical valve is a biological valve, made of animal or human tissue. Since few human valves are available, specially processed pig valves serve as substitutes. Biological valves are less likely to require anticoagulant therapy and monitoring, but they are less durable than mechanical valves. A majority must be replaced after a decade. A patient's age can thus help determine the choice between a mechanical or biological valve replacement, since valve replacement may not be an issue in a very old patient.

For background material on heart valve surgery, see CIRCULATORY SYSTEM; HEART VALVE; *and* SURGERY. *Further information can be found in* AGING; ANESTHESIA, GENERAL; ANTICOAGULANT DRUGS; AORTIC STENOSIS; MITRAL STENOSIS; STENOSIS; THROMBOSIS; *and* XENOTRANSPLANTATION.

Heat Cramps

Severe muscle spasms caused by the loss of salt from the body.

Strenuous activity and extreme heat can cause the body to sweat too much salt and water, bringing on painful muscle spasms in the calves, feet, or hands. Heat cramps especially affect those who are not used to exercising in hot weather, particularly the elderly and young children.

Heat cramps can be treated by drinking water with a small amount of salt (1/4 teaspoon per 1 quart of water), or sports drinks. They can be prevented by staying hydrated when exercising and trying to exercise in the cooler parts of the day (early morning or evening). *See also* HEAT STROKE.

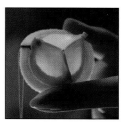

Artificial Heart Valve
Above, replacement heart valves for humans are made by attaching heart tissue from a calf to a plastic core. Either the mitral valve or the aortic valve may be replaced.

Heat Disorders

Abnormalities in the way the body deals with heat.

There are many different types of heat disorders, including miliaria and heat intolerance; Grover's disease is also related.

Miliaria. Miliaria, also called prickly heat, is a common problem caused by blocked sweat glands. It is caused by exposure to heat and humidity. As a result of exposure to heat, sweating increases until the pores are blocked. This results in decreased sweating, causing prickly heat. This condition causes itchy, sore, red papules (small elevations in the skin). Treatments for miliaria include using an air conditioner, using topical steroids to reduce itching, increasing fluid intake, and using oral antibiotics if the area has become infected. The most important therapeutic technique is to cool the skin.

Heat Intolerance. Heat intolerance is the inability of the body to remain comfortable when external temperatures rise. Heat intolerance causes heavy sweating and an overheated sensation. The disorder usually comes on slowly and persists for a long period of time, sometimes for life. There are many causes of heat intolerance. Two possible causes are amphetamines, such as diet pills, and thyrotoxicosis, a condition in which excess thyroid hormone increases the basal metabolic rate, causing a rise in body temperature.

Grover's Disease. Heat exposure has also been implicated as a factor that may worsen Grover's disease, also called transient acantholytic dermatosis, though it is not technically a heat disorder. Grover's disease is a skin disease that causes soreness and the formation of itchy papules. The papules form on the shoulders, neck, thighs, and scalp. They may be rough and crusty. Sunburn, sweating, fever, radiation treatment, and cancer are also thought to cause Grover's disease. Treatment for Grover's disease involves topical steroids, vitamin A, and isotretinoin (a drug that inhibits the function of the sebaceous glands in the skin). *See also* MILIARIA.

Heat Exhaustion

Excessive sweating and a drop in blood pressure as a result of exposure to high heat conditions over a period of time.

Heat exhaustion usually follows a period of strenuous exercise in hot weather when fluids in the body are not replaced. Salt lost through sweating is also a factor, upsetting the balance of sodium and potassium in the bloodstream. The elderly are particularly vulnerable to heat exhaustion, as are chronic alcoholics, the obese, and those taking medications such as antihistamines and antipsychotic drugs.

Symptoms of heat exhaustion include: fatigue; weakness; hot, moist, and flushed skin; nausea; dizziness; and headache. The pulse is rapid and weak. Breathing may be fast and shallow. The victim may be confused and may faint.

Treatment is aimed at cooling the affected person off and replacing lost fluids. Shade, air conditioning, a cool wet towel, and immersion in cool water are all means of treatment. The victim should be given sport drinks, electrolyte beverages, or water. Emergency medical personnel may provide fluids with salt directly into the bloodstream (intravenously). Recovery is usually rapid. *See also* AGING; FAINTING; FIRST AID; HEADACHE; HEAT STROKE; NAUSEA; *and* TACHYCARDIA.

Heat Stroke

A body temperature high enough to incapacitate the body's cooling mechanisms.

Heat stroke is the most severe of the heat-related syndromes. It results from excessive exposure to very high temperatures and is accelerated by heavy exertion and direct sunlight. Especially on very humid days, the victim cannot sweat enough to reduce body temperature. Diabetes, alcoholism, vomiting, and diarrhea add to the risk of heat stroke in hot weather.

Symptoms of heat stroke include a body temperature of above 105°F, headache, ver-

Preventing Heat Stroke

Heat stroke is a potentially dangerous medical situation. The following simple measures can help to prevent heat stroke:

- Do not leave a child or elderly person in a closed, parked car during hot weather.
- Do not leave an elderly person in a closed room or apartment without air conditioning during summer heat waves.
- At the first signs of heat exhaustion, move to a shady area and drink cool liquids.
- Do not exercise during the hottest times of the day (between 12 and 3 PM).
- Wear light, loose-fitting clothing and a hat.
- Drink lots of liquids and monitor urine color. Urine should be clear or light yellow. Sip often; do not drink large quantities at once.
- Limit time in a hot tub or sauna to fifteen minutes during summer months.
- Limit consumption of alcoholic beverages or caffeinated beverages in hot weather.
- Do not wrap an infant in blankets or heavy clothing in hot weather, as the cooling system of infants is not fully developed.

tigo, and fatigue. The affected individual does not sweat. The skin is red, hot, and dry. The pulse is weak and rapid, breathing becomes fast and shallow, and the pupils are often dilated. The victim is likely to be confused and may experience convulsions and lose consciousness. Heat stroke can be fatal if left untreated.

Treatment and Recovery. If the temperature of a victim of heat stroke is not reduced quickly, permanent brain damage may result. The victim should be wrapped in cool wet sheets or immersed in cool water. Emergency medical assistance (911) should be called immediately. The body temperature should be monitored constantly to make sure it is not lowered too far. Drugs may be administered to control convulsions. The body temperature of the victim may vary erratically for days or even weeks afterward.

For background material on heat stroke, see FEVER; HEAT DISORDERS; *and* HEAT EXHAUSTION. *Further information can be found in* EMERGENCY FIRST STEPS; FIRST AID; HEADACHE; SEIZURE; *and* TEMPERATURE. *See also* ELDERLY, CARE OF THE *and* INFANT *for more on high risk groups.*

Heat Treatment

Heat as a means of treating an injury or disease.

Heat encourages blood flow to an injured area, which is believed to help tissues heal more quickly. It can relieve pain and stiffness caused by arthritis or overexertion of a muscle or joint. Heat can also help to drain pus from an infected area.

Heat may be applied to the body in either moist or dry form. Moist heat involves soaking in a hot bath or putting a compress (a piece of fabric that has been soaked in hot water) on the affected area. Heating pads, hot water bottles, or heat lamps are ways to apply dry heat. Ultrasound treatment, which is the use of sound waves to stimulate blood flow, is also considered a type of heat treatment.

Heat should not be used immediately after an injury, as it may cause damaged blood vessels to bleed. Ice should be used first to reduce inflammation. *See also* ARTHRITIS *and* ICE PACKS.

Heavy Metals

A group of metallic elements that includes gold, mercury, platinum, lead, and silver.

There is abundant evidence that heavy metals are toxic to the body. Exposure to high levels of heavy metals has been linked with developmental retardation, cancer, and, in high concentrations, even death. Exposure to high levels of mercury and lead has also been associated with the development of autoimmune disorders, in which the immune system starts to attack its own cells. However, gold is sometimes used in the treatment of rheumatoid arthritis, an autoimmune disorder.

Since the Industrial Revolution, production of heavy metals has increased for purposes such as plumbing and insecticide. Lead is specifically a problem in developing countries. In some of these areas, the majority of children under the age of two have dangerously high blood lead levels. *See also* LEAD POISONING.

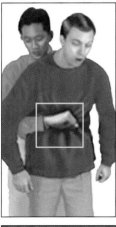

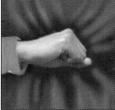

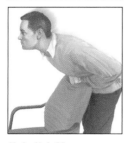

Heimlich Maneuver.
Above, top, a choking adult should be firmly grasped around the abdomen from behind. A fist should be placed just under the breast bone, and pulled up and in quickly to dislodge the blockage. If the object is not dislodged, chest compressions should be given. Bottom, if choking when alone, a person should thrust his or her body weight on the back of a chair.

Heimlich Maneuver

Method for clearing an obstruction from the air passages.

The Heimlich maneuver is only applied to a conscious adult or child older than one year of age with complete airway obstruction. Patients with complete airway obstructions will be unable to speak and may use the universal sign of choking, placing their hands around their throats. If these signs are present, the victim should be approached from behind and "hugged" below the ribs, just above the navel. With one fist grasped by the other hand, five thrusts are delivered in quick succession, pulling inward and slightly upward. The thrusts should be firm and sharp. If the obstruction is not removed, the process is repeated. If the airway is cleared and the victim is not breathing, emergency help must be called and artificial respiration started immediately.

A child victim requires gentler thrusts to prevent injury. If the victim is an infant, he or she should be held face down with one hand supporting the chest, and the head held slightly lower than the body. With the heel of the other hand, the child should be struck between the shoulder blades five times in quick succession. If this does not clear the obstruction, the baby should be turned on his or her back. Using the forefinger and second finger, five thrusts should be made to the breastbone. If the object can be seen, it should be removed. If not, careful attention should be paid not to push the object further down the throat. Emergency help should always be summoned. *See also* CHOKING.

Helicobacter Pylori

Also known as *H. pylori*

Bacteria that thrive in the mucus-secreting cells of the stomach lining.

Helicobacter pylori are the only bacteria that can survive in the acidic environment of the stomach. However, many types of bacteria are able to grow in the stomach if the stomach does not produce enough acid.

Associated Conditions. *Helicobacter pylori* are considered a major cause of peptic ulcers, particularly in people with a history of chronic gastritis—inflammation of the lining of the stomach. It is not known how the bacteria promote ulcers. They may inflame the gastrointestinal lining, or it is possible that they stimulate excessive acid production by the stomach. Weight loss and malnutrition in elderly patients, known as geriatric failure to thrive, is also associated with *Helicobacter pylori* infection.

Treatment. *Helicobacter pylori* infections are treated with a number of medications, including bismuth, antibiotics, and antiulcer drugs. Completely eliminating the bacteria can be difficult at times, but treatment can reduce the recurrence rate of ulcers to less than 20 percent. Patients who carry the *Helicobacter pylori* bacterium but have not developed ulcers or gastritis should not be given antibiotic therapy, since this treatment has not proven beneficial as preventive therapy. *See also* GASTRITIS.

Hellerwork

A method of bodywork, using verbal dialogue and deep touch, designed to improve body alignment and flexibility.

Developed by Joseph Heller and based on the ideas of Ida Rolf, Hellerwork is a technique that involves working with a practitioner on deep-tissue bodywork (deep localized massage) and movement education. Verbal exchanges and video feedback help the patient or client to understand the natural design of his or her body, and how the body may be realigned for a more efficient use of energy. In a series of eleven 90 minute sessions, a Hellerwork practitioner will work with the individual to discuss emotional and physical concerns related to breathing, will assist the client in releasing tension from different parts of the body, and will attempt to retrain over time how the client sits, stands, and walks. *See also* ALTERNATIVE MEDICINE; BIOFEEDBACK; BODYWORK; *and* ROLFING.

Hemangioblastoma

A type of brain tumor.

Hemangioblastoma is a rare, slow-growing benign tumor found in children, young adults, and, most often, middle-aged individuals. In some people, hemangioblastoma is related to Von Hippel-Lindau disease, a genetic disorder. Comprised of capillary vessel-forming endothelial cells, it typically arises as cysts in the cerebellum and it does not usually spread to other parts of the brain. The cyst or cysts slowly develop into a tumor that causes headache, vomiting, incoordination, and involuntary rapid eye movement. Because the tumor is normally clearly defined from the surrounding tissue, it can usually be removed surgically, which, in most cases, completely cures the disease. *See also* BENIGN *and* CYST.

Hemangioma

A birthmark caused by an abnormality of the blood vessels.

When a child is born, hemangiomas and other birthmarks may be present, or, may appear shortly after birth. They are classified as tumors but are very rarely dangerous; although they may be considered unsightly—and rather large—they can be removed easily. There are several types of hemangiomas, which can be flat or raised.

Strawberry or Cherry Hemangioma is a raised birthmark. As its name implies, it is a reddish discoloration. A strawberry or cherry hemangioma can be less than the size of a dime or as large as several inches across. Strawberry hemangiomas are the result of an abnormal distribution of blood vessels in the skin. They are more common in baby girls than in baby boys and usually first appear in the two months after birth. They often grow rapidly for one to three months and then stop growing and begin to lose their distinctive appearance, sometimes vanishing completely after the first year of life. Some may remain for years, but 90 percent of them will fade by age nine.

Port-Wine Stains. A port-wine stain, or nevus flammeus, is a hemangioma that tends to be permanent, which is composed of expanded capillaries. Port-wine stains are flat and appear as a purple or reddish mark. They can appear anywhere on the body, but since about half of them appear on the face. Since port-wine stains do not disappear with age, early treatment is recommended and low-power lasers provide a safe and effective method of removal.

Some hemangiomas develop deeper in the skin. These appear as spongy lumps that may have a purple top layer. They can occur anywhere on the body, but most often are on the back, chest, face, or scalp.

Eliminating Spider Veins

Spider-vein removal is rarely a necessary treatment, but it can relieve some aching and embarrassment; for most people, it is a cosmetic procedure. Sclerotherapy eliminates unsightly spider veins by injecting a saline solution or detergent directly into the blood vessels, after which a compressive bandage is worn over the treated site. This causes the veins to clot or group together and to fade away after a short period of time. Several injections over a period of weeks may be required in some cases. The success rate ranges from 50 to 90 percent.

Spider Veins. The hemangiomas that appear later in life include spider veins. These are collections of small blood vessels that form a visible spot on the skin, often on the leg or thigh. They usually pose no medical problem but are generally considered unsightly. They can be removed by laser therapy or a technique called sclerotherapy.

Waiting watchfully is recommended for most hemangiomas because removing them may leave a permanent scar. Removal may be advised in some special cases, such as when a hemangioma is on the lip or tongue, when its location causes it to interfere with sight or other basic functions (such as defecation), or when it bleeds persistently. Removal can be accomplished by cryosurgery, which uses extreme cold to eliminate tissue; laser treatment; or conventional surgery. *See also* BIRTHMARK; COSMETIC SURGERY; *and* LASER SURGERY.

Resources on Cardio vascular Disorders

Debakey, Michael E. and Antonio M. Gotto, *The New Living Heart* (1997); Gotto, Antonio, *A Patient's Handbook of Cholesterol Disorders* (2000); Gould, Lance K., *Heal Your Heart: How You Can Prevent or Reverse Heart Disease* (2000); Neill, Catherine A., *The Heart of a Child: What Families Need to Know About Heart Disorders in Children* (1992); American Heart Association, Tel. (800) 242-8721, Online: www.amhrt.org; Heart Information Network, Tel. (973) 701-6035, Online: www.heartinfo.org; www.nycornell.org/ cardiothoracic.surgery/ www.nycornell.org/medicine/cardiology.html.

Hemarthrosis

Blood flow into the joint that causes swelling.

Joints are enclosed by a protective capsule. If the ligaments or the joint sustains an injury or if the capsule is torn, blood may enter the capsule, swelling the area around the joint. Blood disorders such as hemophilia, in which blood does not clot, may also lead to hemarthrosis, since even a slight injury or bump can cause bleeding.

Hemarthrosis causes injuries to swell immediately. It may also cause a spasm that stiffens the joint into a locked position. Ice applied to the affected area can reduce the pain and swelling. A medical practitioner will manipulate the joint to examine the nature of the swelling (ballottement). Fluid withdrawn from the swollen area can confirm the diagnosis of hemarthrosis, as well as reduce the swelling.

Raising the joint to an elevated position and reducing or eliminating any heavy activities that affect the joint will ease the pain and alleviate the condition. Eventually cells in the joint will absorb any excess blood into the capsule. *See also* BLOOD; BRUISE; HEMOPHILIA; *and* JOINT.

Hematology

The study of the blood, its primary functions, and its functional disorders.

The circulatory system is the body's main transportation system. The fluids and cells carried in the blood take oxygen to the tissues. They also collect and carry carbon dioxide and other waste products to the lungs or the kidneys for removal.

Blood is a complex mixture of elements. Plasma is the fluid that carries the blood cells while holding hormones and proteins in solutions that may be absorbed by various sorts of tissue. Red blood cells take oxygen from the lungs and deliver it to the rest of the body. The white blood cells act to protect the body from disease and attack foreign viruses, bacteria, and fungi. The platelets are the coagulating mechanism when there is damage to the vast network of veins and arteries.

Blood disorders divide themselves into distinct categories, among which are bleeding and clotting disorders, bone-marrow disorders (including leukemia, cancers of the bone marrow, and aplastic anemia), anemias, platelet disorders, and malignant cancer of the lymphoid tissue (lymphoma and Hodgkin's disease). Hematologists are specially trained physicians that take care of patients with blood disorders.

> *Further information related to Hematology can be found in* BLOOD; CIRCULATORY SYSTEM; *and* DIAGNOSIS. *Related anatomic issues are discussed in* ARTERIES, DISORDERS OF; KIDNEY; LUNG; *and* VEIN. *See also* HODGKIN'S DISEASE.

Hematoma

An accumulation of blood that leaks out of the circulatory system through damaged blood vessels.

When blood escapes from a damaged vein or artery, it may flow out through a break in the skin, or it may push aside adjacent tissues, forming a pocket until it can be reabsorbed and removed in the healing process. If the hematoma forms under a fingernail, the nail may blacken and fall off entirely. If it does not, the physician may need to puncture the nail in order to relieve the pressure.

If the blood is trapped in the head, as it might be if the leak is in the skull (subdural hematoma), pressure against the underlying brain tissue can produce very serious consequences, such as the loss of neural function. This condition occurs in about one of 10,000 people, affecting mainly the elderly and infants. When there is bleeding in the skull, it is usually under the dura mater—one of the tissue layers that surround the brain. Symptoms and signs of this disorder include:

- headaches in varying degrees of intensity and duration;
- confusion or dementia;
- anxiety, apathy, irritability, and tension;
- weakness or malaise;
- impaired or awkward movement;

- a loss of motility that may be complete or may affect only one side of the body; and
- a numbness that may affect only one side of the body; and
- paralysis and coma.

If any of these symptoms appear after a fall or blow to the head, medical treatment must be sought at once.

Background information about Hematoma can be found in BLEEDING; BLOOD; CIRCULATORY SYSTEM; *and* HEMATOLOGY. *Also see* ANXIETY; COMA; *and* PARALYSIS; *and* TRAUMA.

Hematuria

Blood in the urine.

Hematuria refers to urine that is colored differently from the usual pale yellow, or urine that is cloudy or blood-tinged. Some common causes of hematuria include:

- various sorts of medications;
- urinary tract infections; and
- bladder or kidney cancer.

Cancer related hematuria is a serious condition that needs immediate diagnosis and treatment. Other diseases affecting the bladder may also result in hematuria. Exercise may also cause it, but that type of hematuria will go away in a day or so.

Any significant changes in urine color, that cannot be linked to the consumption of a food or medication should be reported to the doctor immediately. This is particularly important if it happens for longer than a day or two, or if there are repeated episodes. Blood tests and urinalysis may be performed if the color cannot be attributed to any ingested food or medication. Liver tests or cystoscopic examination may be performed as well.

Treatment. Hematuria due to food or drugs is temporary and requires no treatment. Any underlying conditions resulting in hematuria, such as those affecting the bladder or kidneys, are treated accordingly.

Related articles for consideration include BLOOD; INTERNAL BLEEDING; HEPATITIS; *and* URINE. *More information about this topic can be found in* URINARY TRACT INFECTION.

Hemianopia

A loss of half the field of vision in each eye.

Caused by damage to the brain, optic nerve, or nerve tracts, the loss of vision occurs in either the outer or inner halves of the visual fields. It may occur in older people suffering from transient ischemic attacks —stroke symptoms lasting less than 24 hours—or in younger people suffering from migraine. A stroke, tumor, injury, or infection that damages the back of the brain may inflict hemianopia. *See* BRAIN.

Hemiballismus

Uneven flinging motions of the arm or leg that occur only on one side of the body.

Hemiballismus is characterized by throwing or splaying of the limbs on one side of the body. It is caused by disease in the basal ganglia, the area of the brain responsible for controlling movement. Hemiballismus movements are involuntary, sudden, and violent. Hemiballismus is perhaps the most violent form of involuntary movement (dyskinesia) known. It involves both limbs and muscles and often advances to uncontrolled twitching (chorea) or writhing (athetosis) movements. The timing and force of the limbs' movements are random and unpredictable and may cause injury to the affected person or people nearby. The most effective drug used to treat the symptoms is the antipsychotic drug haloperidol (Haldol). *See also* BRAIN *and* MUSCLES.

Hemicolectomy

The surgical removal of about half of the colon.

Hemicolectomy refers to a surgical procedure in which approximately half of the colon is removed. The remaining segments of the colon are then joined together, usually with sutures. This surgery is usually performed as a treatment for Crohn's disease or ulcerative colitis. *See also* COLON; COLON CANCER; COLECTOMY; *and* SURGERY.

Hemiplegia

Total paralysis or fragility of the arm, leg, and trunk on the same side of the body.

Hemiplegia is often characterized by an abnormal muscle tone, rigidity or spasticity (spastic hemiplegia), and limp and wasted muscles (flaccid hemiplegia). If the legs are rendered unstable then it may be unsafe to walk, since balance can be easily lost. The impairment of motor ability impedes an individual's ability to control the timing and intensity of muscle actions.

The most common causes of hemiplegia include:
- head injury;
- brain tumor;
- inflammation of the brain;
- psychological causes;
- multiple sclerosis and meningitis.

Childhood hemiplegia has a number of causes including:
- infant or pediatric stroke or bleeding in the brain;
- premature birth;
- brain tumors; and
- infections.

Children with hemiplegia may develop speech and language disorders in addition to seizures and impaired muscle coordination on one side of the body. The disorder does not affect mental ability.

The most effective method of treating hemiplegia is to identify and treat the underlying causes. Physical therapy can strengthen weak muscles. *See also* Encephalitis; Paralysis; *and* Spasticity.

Hemochromatosis

A relatively common inherited disorder characterized by the accumulation of iron in the body.

Excess iron can have adverse affects on several organs. Damage to the pancreas can ensue, resulting in bronze-colored skin and it can later develop into cirrhosis, liver cancer, diabetes, and heart failure. Iron deposits in the joints cause arthritis, and in the testes they can result in impotence and sterility. Hemochromatosis is transmitted by one or two genes. The condition is more common among men; women are thought to be less susceptible to the condition due to regular blood loss through menstruation. Between the ages of 40 and 60, symptoms usually begin to appear; they include weakness, weight loss, and impaired sexual performance. Treatment involves phlebotomy, the removal of a unit of blood once or twice a week until iron levels become normal. Maintenance treatment three or four times a year may be necessary. The prognosis for this condition is good with early detection, as treatment prevents the development of complications. *See* Iron.

Hemocysteine

Usually spelled homocysteine

An amino acid in the blood that is an important risk factor contributing to heart attacks and strokes.

Hemocysteine is a by product of the metabolic processes when a person digests meat. Low intake of vitamins B_6, B_{12}, and folic acid also increase the production of this acid. In the past, levels as high as 20 micromoles of hemocysteine per liter were considered normal and safe. Recent research indicates that the danger of heart attack or stroke rises even at levels as low as nine micromoles per liter. *See also* Amino Acids.

Hemodialysis

A filtering process used to treat kidney failure.

In hemodialysis, a person whose kidneys have stopped functioning is connected to a machine that filters wastes from the blood and excess fluid from the body. Blood from the patient flows to the artificial kidney through a shunt (vascular channel) connecting an artery to a vein. Patients can be kept alive for years by hemodialysis while they await a kidney transplant. Hemodialysis is also performed in emergency situations involving poisoning or a drug overdose. The alternative method is peritoneal dialysis, which uses the abdominal cavity as the site of filtering. *See also* Kidney.

Hemoglobin

The compound in the blood that takes oxygen from the lungs and delivers it to the body's tissues while removing waste products.

Each red blood cell contains millions of molecules of hemoglobin. Hemoglobin is made up of red, iron-rich heme and the globin protein. Each molecule of heme combines with a molecule of oxygen in the lungs and then exchanges the oxygen for carbon dioxide in the functioning tissues of the body. When a red blood cell nears the end of its useful life, the spleen and liver absorb it and recycle the iron and globin. The amount of hemoglobin in the blood is carefully controlled by the body; too little leaves the tissues oxygen-poor. An individual may become anemic and experience chronic fatigue, pallor, dizziness, and weakness. Malformed and malfunctioning red blood cells can be inherited, as in hemophilia or sickle cell anemia, or acquired through the impact on the blood of certain drugs or toxins in the environment. *See also* BLOOD; BLOOD CELLS; *and* LUNGS.

Hemoglobinopathy

Disorders in red blood cells caused by genetic abnormalities of hemoglobin. They are often family- and race-related.

People with sickle cell anemia have red blood cells that are misshapen and often clog small blood vessels so that oxygen cannot be delivered to the tissues. It results in pain, breathing difficulties, vulnerability to infection, kidney problems, and stroke. People with one normal hemoglobin gene and one abnormal gene will not suffer from the symptoms; however, they can pass the abnormality to their children.

Thalassemia is a condition in which the red blood cells carry a smaller amount of hemoglobin than normal due to a genetic disorder. There are two main types of thalassemia (alpha and beta) the seriousness of the disease depends on whether the person has two affected genes or one. The symptoms are similar for both: anemia,

jaundice, enlarged spleen, and gallstones.

Other hemoglobinopathies are identified by the letters C, S-C, and E. The symptoms are similar to those of sickle cell anemia or thalassemia but milder. Treatment for all hemoglobinopathies is usually limited to antibiotics, lifestyle choices that minimize the anemia, and good hygiene to control infection. Hydroxyurea is now used to treat some forms of sickle cell disease, and frequent red blood cell transfusions are used to treat severe thalassemia. *See also* ANEMIA; BLOOD; GENE; *and* THALASSEMIA.

Hemoglobinuria

Hemoglobin in the urine.

Only a small amount of hemoglobin (the molecule that carries oxygen in the red blood cells) is normally present in blood plasma (the fluid in the blood containing important nutrients). When the hemoglobin in red blood cells breaks down abnormally (hemolysis), this releases the hemoglobin into the plasma; this excess hemoglobin is then excreted into the urine.

Hemoglobinuria may result from the tissue damage or a severe burn. Strenuous exercise can have the same result, as can a bout of malaria, or (in rare cases) exposure to very cold weather. Some individuals are born with a disorder known as nocturnal hemoglobulinuria, which results in the release of excess amounts of hemoglobin into plasma during sleep. *See also* BLOOD; BLOOD CELLS; MALARIA; *and* URINE.

Hemolysis

A condition in which red blood cells are destroyed or damaged prematurely.

Every red blood cell exists for about three months. If the cells are deformed or damaged, the bone marrow attempts to compensate by producing additional red blood cells. If production lags behind, a person will suffer from hemolytic anemia. This form of anemia is rarer than bone marrow disorders that impede the normal production of red blood cells. Red blood cells can be damaged in an enlarged or diseased spleen, in their passage through malfunctioning heart valves, or by obstacles in blood vessels; they also can be destroyed in an autoimmune reaction if the white blood cells do not recognize red blood cells and attack them. *See also* IMMUNITY.

Cancers, such as lymphoma, will destroy red blood cells, and a number of drugs have the same effect. Inherited abnormalities in hemoglobin, in the red blood cell membrane, or in enzymes can also cause hemolysis. The symptoms are the same as with anemia: weakness, pallor, and chronic fatigue. If the onset is quick and severe, a person may experience chills, fever, jaundice, nausea, and lowered blood pressure. *See* ANEMIA; BLOOD CELLS; *and* CANCER.

Hemolytic Disease of the Newborn

Also known as erythroblastosis neonatorum

A serious disease of the infant caused by production of maternal antibodies to fetal red blood cells.

This disease develops in newborns when the mother's blood is Rh-negative, the father's blood is Rh-positive, and the baby's is Rh-positive. Such an incompatibility may lead to newborn hemolytic disease. The mother produces antibodies against the fetus's blood. As a result of the incompatibility, the mother's antibodies treat the unborn child's red blood cells as invaders and attack them. Some cells rupture, producing the disease. Bleeding in the mother during pregnancy increases her risk of developing the potentially dangerous antibodies. If bleeding occurs in a woman at risk for hemolytic disease of the newborn, she is given $Rh_o(D)$ immune serum globulin, which combines with and destroys any antibodies. To prevent hemolytic disease, a pregnant woman who is Rh-negative is checked for antibodies every two months—sometimes more often—during pregnancy. After delivery, if the baby is Rh-positive, $Rh_o(D)$ antibodies are given to the mother within 72 hours. *See also* ANTIBODY.

Resources on Hemophilia & Genetic Disorders
Bloom, Arhtur L, *The Hemophilias* (1982); Jones, Peter, *Living with Hemophilia* (1995); Pollack, Robert, *Signs of Life: The Languages and Meanings of DNA* (1994); Alliance of Genetic Support Groups, Tel. (800) 336-GENE, Online: www.medhelp. org/geneticalliance; Easter Seals, Tel. (800) 221-6827, Online: www.seals.org; National Hemophilia Foundation, Tel. (800) 42-HANDI, Online: www.hemophilia.org. Office of Rare Diseases, Tel. (301) 402-4336, Online: rarediseases.info. nih.gov/ord; http://www. med.cornell.edu/research/ cores/genetherapy/.html.

Hemolytic-Uremic Syndrome

A disorder in which the number of platelets in the blood drops sharply, red blood cells are damaged, and the kidneys stop functioning.

Hemolytic-uremic syndrome is characterized by a change in platelet function in the small blood vessels. This rare disorder occurs most often in children following a diarrhea-causing infection. In an adult woman, it may occur shortly after delivery.

Causes. The precipitating factor may be a bacterial infection, but it can also be seen as a reaction to chemotherapy drugs.

Symptoms of a mild attack are similar to those for most forms anemias. More serious cases will experience kidney failure and elevated blood pressure. Adults are often likely to be at risk of heart failure or stroke. Treatment for children includes preventative measures, simply as a precaution against kidney failure; otherwise, the disease is self-limiting. In adults, the doctor may prescribe plasmapheresis, in which the plasma is filtered out of the blood and replaced. *See also* ANEMIA; ANEMIA, MEGALOBLASTIC; BACTERIA; KIDNEY; *and* INFECTION.

Hemophilia

An inherited disease in which a person bleeds easily and excessively, even from minor cuts or bruises.

Sometimes called the royal disease (because Queen Victoria of England passed it on to much of the European nobility), hemophilia is caused by defective coagulation factors VIII or IX in the blood. Proper blood coagulation involves more than a dozen different substances; 12 of these are identified by number, and two are specifically involved in hemophilia. Factor VIII is called the antihemophilic factor because it promotes proper blood clotting. Factor IX is called the Christmas factor. The factors produce slightly different forms of hemophilia, although the symptoms and treatment are the same. Type A is called classic hemophilia, it is caused by a lack of factor

VIII. Type B, called Christmas disease, is caused by a shortage of factor IX.

While an episode of excessive external bleeding in a hemophiliac patient will get quick attention, the more ominous problem of internal bleeding may not be noticed or dealt with promptly. The joints are particularly vulnerable because the continual flexing leads to wear and tear on their ligaments. Bleeding in the joints can result in osteoarthritis or crippling deformities as the ligaments are destroyed.

Gastrointestinal bleeding is also possible and may not be observed until it becomes chronic and dangerous. Bleeding in the muscles or other tissues puts pressure on the nerves, causing pain and reducing sensation. This can cause permanent nerve damage. Bleeding in the tongue can make it swell and impair breathing. What may seem to be a minor bump on the head can cause bleeding within the skull (known as a subdural hematoma), with consequent pressure on the brain.

In mild cases, the tendency to bleed may not be noticed until an individual has a tooth extracted, is in a traumatic accident, or undergoes surgery. In the most severe cases, the disease will be observed very early in life if an infant bruises easily or bleeds copiously after minor injury, or an immunization shot produces a large bruise that disappears slowly.

SYMPTOMS

Symptoms of hemophilia include poor or slow clotting from cuts or other injuries to the blood vessels, blood in the urine or in the stool that will turn it black, and swelling of the joints. Blood tests will reveal if there is ineffective or abnormal factor VIII or factor IX in the blood.

The initial diagnosis will be made based on observation of the excessive bleeding and testing for blood factors VIII and IX. There are drugs that assist in the clotting function, at least temporarily (such as desmopressin). Transfusions of plasma or plasma concentrates that carry the clotting factors may also be prescribed.

In the early 1980s, much of the blood

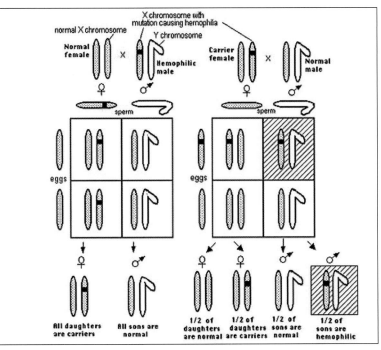

available for transfusions was contaminated with the HIV virus, so 90 percent of American hemophiliacs contracted the AIDS virus. In the past decade, screening has become more effective, and transfusions are again a safe treatment that can be very effective during serious bleeding epi-sodes. After transfusions, the clotting factor responds immediately to form clots at blood vessel breaks. Within six to eight hours, the clotting factors will have been used up, but hopefully the necessary clotting has taken place. Within 24 hours, the efficacy of the transfusion will have been exhausted.

TREATMENT

In general, treatment of hemophilia includes attention to lifestyle. People with hemophilia should avoid medications like aspirin, heparin, warfarin, and anti-inflammatory drugs because they thin the blood. Hemophiliacs must also avoid contact sports and other situations in which even minor injury is likely.

Further information can be found in AIDS; BLEEDING; BLEEDING DISORDERS; BLOOD; BRUISE; *and* INTERNAL BLEEDING. *Also see* HERITABILITY; HIV; *and* INHERITANCE. *See also* GENE; GENETICS; HERITABILITY; *and* INHERITANCE.

Hemophiliac Inheritance. Mothers pass the hemophiliac gene on to their sons on the inherited X chromosome. The Y chromosome that determines the sex of boys does not have the gene that carries the instructions to create factor VIII or factor IX, and so the boy-child with these XY chromosomes will probably be diagnosed with hemophilia. It is often quite unlikely that a newborn girl will have two X chromosomes that carry the gene for the disease.

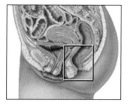

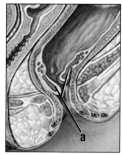

Where Hemorrhoids Occur. Above, top, hemorrhoids are little more than enlarged veins within the tissue of the rectum or anus. They occur due to excessive straining while passing wastes or in women who experience prolonged pregnancy. Above, bottom, they may occur either externally or internally (a). Internal hemorrhoids are found above the anal sphincter—external hemorrhoids occur outside of the anal canal.

Hemorrhoidectomy

The surgical removal of varicose veins in the rectal and anal region (hemorrhoids) that have reached the bleeding stage or cause extreme discomfort.

It is estimated that almost 50 percent of the adult population over the age of 30 has hemorrhoids. Most people learn to live with them by eating the right foods (such as a high-fiber diet), avoiding strenuous physical activity (especially lifting and straining), and using topical ointments to ease the discomfort. In some cases, however, hemorrhoids are excessively painful or bleed significantly and may be treated surgically.

Types. The various medical procedures employed to treat hemorrhoids include injection sclerotherapy, rubber-band ligation, surgical excision, cryosurgery, infrared coagulation, electrocoagulation, and laser surgery.

With injection sclerotherapy, the hemorrhoid is injected with a saline solution, which produces scar tissue and obliterates the varicose vein. In rubber band ligation, a tight rubber-band is wrapped around the base of the hemorrhoid with a specialized instrument called a ligator. The hemorrhoid fades away from a depleted blood supply, and the rubber-band falls off.

Other methods include cryosurgery, in which the hemorrhoid is frozen with liquid nitrogen and removed; infrared coagulation, in which radiation from a halogen projection bulb causes the vein to shrink; electrocoagulation, in which electric current is used; and laser surgery.

Rubber-band ligation is currently the most popular method for internal hemorrhoids; some proctologists estimate that 90 percent of cases can be treated this way. External hemorrhoids usually do not require surgical treatment unless they are inflamed with a protruding blood clot.

Recovery. Given the location and sensitivity of the problem, the recovery period is especially important for the patient. Pain and discomfort are usually treated with non-narcotic painkillers; narcotic medications cause constipation and can exacer-

bate the postoperative condition. The patient takes laxatives, such as mineraloil, to soften stools and facilitate bowel movements. Warm baths are also recommended to ease discomfort. Complete recovery takes about three to six weeks. *See also* HEMORRHOIDS *and* MINERAL OIL.

Hemorrhoids

Clusters of swollen veins in the lining of the anus.

Hemorrhoids are a variation of varicose veins. Because they are thin and prone to rupture, bleeding can occur during a normal bowel movement. Some people have an inherited predisposition towards weak veins that makes them particularly vulnerable to hemorrhoids. They are common during pregnancy and after childbirth. Hemorrhoids can occur inside the anal canal, at the anal opening, or can protrude outside the anus.

Symptoms. Most hemorrhoids force themselves on the patient's attention by the bleeding and pain they cause during defecation. Blood may be seen on the stool, on toilet paper, or in the toilet bowel. The most severe pain occurs when a blood clot forms in a hemorrhoid outside the anus. This can also create a painful lump at the opening of the anus. Any rectal bleeding should be reported to a physician, because it may also indicate the presence of intestinal cancer. *See also* CANCER.

Diagnosis. Hemorrhoids can be diagnosed by an examination of the affected area. The doctor will usually perform a proctoscopy, which gives a view of the rectum. This procedure enables the physician to rule out a cancer as the cause of bleeding. The examination may also include a barium enema or a colonoscopy, which produces images of the intestinal tract.

Treatment. A hemorrhoid that causes moderate discomfort can be treated with a non-prescription ointment or cream, or with pads containing witch hazel or a local anesthetic. Daily warm baths or showers can also help reduce discomfort by keeping the area free of fecal material. Increasing the intake of fluids and fiber-rich foods can also ease symptoms by making stools softer. An inflated cushion when sitting down for long periods may also be helpful.

For more painful external hemorrhoids, tiny, tight rubber-bands can be used to tie them off; the treated hemorrhoid usually will disappear in a few days. Other forms of treatment for bothersome hemorrhoids include cryosurgery, which uses extremely cold liquid nitrogen or carbon dioxide to eliminate them; injection of a shrinking agent into the vein; and photocoagulation, which destroys the hemorrhoids with powerful beams of light. *See also* Barium X-Ray; Cryosurgery; Intestine, Cancer of; *and* Varicose Veins.

Hemosiderosis

Also known as pulmonary alveolitis

A disease in which hemosiderin, an iron-containing pigment, accumulates in the lungs.

The primary form of this disease is found among children under ten years of age, either on its own or in conjunction with heart disease. There is evidence that an allergy to milk may be involved. Symptoms include coughing, spitting up blood, and wheezing. Sometimes an affected person will have spells of vomiting and diarrhea. Long-term symptoms include episodes of pulmonary bleeding, fever, and a rapid heartbeat. Treatment in acute cases includes oxygen, blood transfusion, and medication. Avoiding milk or milk products may offer some help. *See also* Iron *and* Lungs.

Hemostasis

The cessation of bleeding internally or externally.

The body has an elaborate system to control bleeding. First, the injured blood vessels constrict in an attempt to reduce the flow of blood. Next, platelets near the injury build a web across the break. At the same time, the platelets enlarge and become sticky so that they cling to the edges of the break and form a mesh pattern. Then the coagulation system activates, re-

sulting in a fibrin (a threadlike insoluble protein) clot that, with the platelet plug, stops the bleeding. After healing repairs the injured blood vessel, the clot dissolves, and the used-up platelets are scavenged by white blood cells. *See* Bleeding *and* Blood.

Hemostatic Drugs

A family of drugs used to control bleeding during surgery or after a traumatic accident.

A number of drugs have been developed to reduce blood loss by improving the blood's clotting ability. The mechanism of drug action differs depending on the drug. Aprotinin is a protease inhibitor derived from cows' lungs that blocks the clot-dissolving system. Desmopressin treats mild hemophilia and some platelet disorders; Amicar mouthwash decreases bleeding after dental procedures in hemophiliacs. Forms of blood factors VII, IX, and XIII treat bleeding hemophilia patients with these specific deficiencies. *See* Anemia *and* Hemophilia.

Hemothorax

A condition in which blood enters the pleura from a broken vessel and inhibits normal lung expansion.

The pleura are two thin membranes, one of which lines the outside of the lungs, the other covers the inside of the surrounding chest wall. The pleura slide smoothly against each other so that the lungs can expand and contract without friction. If blood leaks into the space between the two membranes, usually due to a chest injury or cancer, it is called hemothorax.

Symptoms are rare but if there are any, they usually include shortness of breath and chest pains. A diagnosis of hemothorax can be confirmed either by a chest x-ray or an ultrasound exam. Health care professionals may also make a visual examination of the lung passages with a specialized device called a thoracoscope. A sample will be taken with a needle introduced into the accumulated fluid to check for bacteria, fungi, and cancer. *See* Abdomen *and* X-Ray.

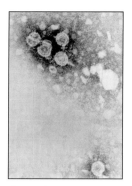

Hepatitis B. Above, a transmission electron micrograph of hepatitis B virions, also known as Dane particles, which have a diameter of about 42 nanometers. Hepatitis B is a sexually transmitted disease that causes a set of liver disorders and kill over 5,000 people per year. Hepatitis B can be prevented with the proper use of barrier contraceptives and a vaccination.

Primary Causes of Chronic Liver Disease. Below, a representative sample of the primary causes of chronic liver disease from Jefferson County, Alabama. Although more than half of the cases of liver disease are caused by hepatitis viruses, there are still many cases where the reason for its incidence is as yet unknown.

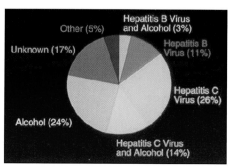

Treatment. If the condition is mild and the bleeding has stopped, the problem will usually be self-limiting, as the normal body processes reabsorb fluid. If the bleeding is considerable or if it continues, a catheter may be used to drain the blood. If the accumulated fluid is too thick to flow freely through a tube, surgery may be necessary. *See also* ENDOSCOPY *and* LUNGS.

Hepatectomy

Surgical removal of a part or the whole liver as a treatment for disease, trauma (partial), or the first stage of a liver transplant operation (total).

Partial Hepatectomy. Because the liver has extraordinary regenerative powers, as much as three-quarters of the organ may be removed, and it can still function and grow back. Benign liver tumors usually require a partial hepatectomy. Liver cancer is usually treated with surgery as well. Damage from tapeworm larvae (hydatid disease) may also call for a partial hepatectomy. Auto and motorcycle accidents and other trauma may cause enough liver damage to require partial removal.

Total Hepatectomy. Adults with advanced cirrhosis and children with missing or malformed bile-ducts (biliary atresia) or alpha-antitripsyn deficiency, a genetic defect that can lead to cirrhosis, are often candidates for liver transplants. About 4,000 hepatectomies are performed a year. *See also* CIRRHOSIS; LIVER; *and* LIVER TRANSPLANT.

Hepatitis

A swelling of the liver from various causes.

The liver is critical to the digestive process because it takes nutrients out of food and converts them into amino acids, glucose, and proteins to be used by the organs and tissues. The liver also plays an important role in the neutralization of toxins that are released by bacteria or ingested with food or drink. Alcohol in any form is toxic to the liver. The effects of alcohol on the liver accumulate over time so that alcohol abuse eventually enlarges, inflames, and scars the liver to the point where it can no longer function properly.

Causes. Hepatitis is a general term for a condition that may be caused by a number of different agents, including viruses, bacteria, parasites, toxic drugs, toxins, or diseases of the immune system. Five viruses have been identified that specifically attack the liver and produce hepatitis A, B, C, D, and E. Infectious mononucleosis may cause hepatitis. Certain toxic chemicals and insecticides have also been shown to cause hepatitis.

Symptoms. Hepatitis can be acute (short-term) or chronic (long-term). People usually recover from acute hepatitis in a period of months. All forms of hepatitis share similar symptoms, including dark urine, appetite loss, fatigue, bloating, jaundiced skin coloring, yellowing of the whites of the eyes, nausea and vomiting, and low-grade fever.

Diagnosis. Liver function tests include the measurement of specific enzymes that seep into the blood if the liver is inflamed. The bilirubin test measures the amount of this pigment in the blood. A level above three mg/dl indicates a liver disorder, though this test does not indicate the cause of that disorder. *See also* DIGESTIVE SYSTEM; HEPATITIS, CHRONIC ACTIVE; HEPATITIS, VIRAL; *and* MONONUCLEOSIS.

Hepatitis, Chronic Active

A severe form of hepatitis that may develop from a virus or an autoimmune reaction.

If an individual with hepatitis remains symptomatic for more than a few months, the condition is considered chronic. The person may experience few symptoms (chronic persistent hepatitis) or many symptoms; about half of patients with hepatitis B or C experience no symptoms at all. Symptoms of chronic active hepatitis include jaundice, fatigue, nausea and vomiting, dark urine, and pain in the vicinity of the liver. About a third of all individuals with viral hepatitis progress to the chronic active form. Additionally, a compromised autoimmune system may result in a condition where the immune system attacks and destroys liver cells as if they were foreign invaders. A biopsy will reveal the type and course of the disease. *See also* BIOPSY.

TREATMENT

When the source of the viral infection is hepatitis B or C, chronic active hepatitis may respond to interferon, a drug used to stimulate the immune system. Interferon is not a cure for hepatitis B or C, but it is an effective treatment. Side effects of interferon are common and include headache, depression, and flu-like symptoms. Other antiviral drugs (such as ribavirin) are sometimes used in combination with interferon to treat hepatitis C. *See also* IMMUNE SYSTEM.

Corticosteroids, such as prednisone, are used to treat autoimmune chronic hepatitis. Results of this course of treatment have been positive, with patients experiencing reduced symptoms and improved liver function. Prednisone has its own undesirable side effects, including weight gain, hypertension, and diabetes, and the drug is not always effective. As a last resort, a liver transplant may be the only option.

Untreated, chronic active hepatitis will often end in deterioration of liver function and, eventually, death. *See* CORTICOSTEROID DRUGS; HEPATITIS; *and* HEPATITIS, VIRAL.

Hepatitis, Viral

Hepatitis caused by a virus.

The majority of cases of hepatitis are caused by viruses, some of which are specific for hepatitis; others produce hepatitis as a related consequence. Five types of hepatitis virus are recognized and diagnosed as specifically causing the liver inflammation known as hepatitis. They are called hepatitis A, B, C, D, and E. Symptoms are similar for all of these viruses and include dark urine, appetite loss, fatigue, jaundice of the skin and whites of the eyes, bloating and abdominal cramps, low-grade fever, pale or clay-colored stools, and fatigue. Diagnosis in most cases is guided by blood tests, which reveal antibodies, specific to one of the forms of hepatitis, or elevated liver enzymes. *See also* HEPATITIS.

TYPES OF VIRAL HEPATITIS

Hepatitis A is acquired by consuming materials (usually by drinking or eating foods) contaminated with fecal matter from an individual who already has the disease. It is usually communicated as the result of poor hygiene or through personal contact. Shellfish can acquire the virus when sewage is dumped into coastal waters; they can then transmit the virus to anyone who eats them. The virus can survive at normal room temperature for hours on a hard surface like a toilet seat. The incubation period for hepatitis A lasts about two to six weeks, so the disease can spread widely before countermeasures are taken. The body is slow to destroy the virus that causes the disease but most patients will recover within a few months. Complications are possible among the elderly, those with compromised immune systems, and those who already have liver problems, such as alcoholics.

Hepatitis B is spread through infected body fluids like blood, semen, saliva, suppurating sores, or breast milk. It does not spread by simple physical contact, from droplets coughed or sneezed into the air, or by eating food prepared by someone who has the disease. The incubation period for hepatitis B lasts from one to six months, so it is usually impossible to tell how it was acquired. Some people will go on to develop chronic hepatitis. Infants and small children are particularly vulnerable, but most recover from the disease, albeit slowly. Once recovered, the infected person will be immune to any later reinfection with this particular virus, although he or she may contract one of the other hepatitis viruses. Someone infected with hepatitis B may fully recover and have no symptoms and yet remain a carrier capable of infect-

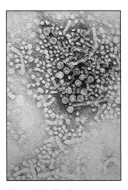

Hepatitis B. Above, an electron microscope image of hepatitis B virus, which is also known as serum hepatitis. This form of hepatitis is rather rare in the United States. It is, however, endemic in parts of Asia, where millions of individuals are affected. This type of hepatitis is spread through infected blood and fluids, as well as from mother to child. Small children and newborns develop chronic hepatitis B more often than adults.

ing others through sexual contact, shared hypodermic needles, and shared food or drinks. A pregnant woman can pass the virus to her unborn child so all babies should be vaccinat- ed for hepatitis B at birth.

Hepatitis C. Many individuals who are infected with hepatitis C have no symptoms whatsoever and never realize that they have the disease. Most people with hepatitis C become chronically infected. People with strong immune systems may recover spontaneously from hepatitis C without treatment. In about 50 percent of patients with evidence of chronic hepatitis C, interferon alpha plus ribavirin cures the disease. Those with chronic hepatitis C who are not treated or not cured by treatment may live normal lives, but they remain carriers of the disease and can infect others. Some people with chronic hepatitis C develop complications like cirrhosis, liver failure, or liver cancer.

Hepatitis D attacks individuals who have already had hepatitis B. The virus does not cause the disease by itself but worsens infections of hepatitis B; a person may get the two forms of hepatitis at the same time. It is transmitted through the same routes as hepatitis B, through bodily fluids from shared IV needles or unprotected sex. Hepatitis D is usually suspected when the condition of someone with hepatitis B suddenly becomes severely worse. It is diagnosed with tests that reveal hepatitis D antibodies in the blood.

Hepatitis E is almost nonexistent in developed countries; it is found mainly in sub-Saharan Africa and in Asia. It is similar to hepatitis A and spreads primarily through contaminated water supplies, with an incubation period that lasts from about two to six weeks. It is not transmitted by sexual contact, contaminated blood, IV needles, or other bodily fluids. Most people with hepatitis E recover from it on their own within a few months.

Resources on Hepatitis
Johnson, P.J., and I.G. McFarlane, *The Laboratory Investigation of Liver Disease* (1989); Zakim, David, and Thomas Boyer, Hepatology: A Textbook of Liver Disease (1996); American Liver Foundation, Tel. (800) GO-LIVER, Online: www.liverfoundation.org; Hepatitis Foundation International, Tel. (800) 891-0707, Online: wwwhepfi.org; http://www.med.cornell.edu/research/cores/genetherapy/index.html.

Information that develops this topic can be found in IMMUNE SYSTEM; IMMUNITY; SEXUALLY TRANSMITTED DISEASES; *and* VIRUS. *Further aspects of this illness are discussed in* FEVER; JAUNDICE; PUBLIC HEALTH; *and* TROPICAL DISEASES.

Hepatomegaly

An enlarged liver.

The liver is involved in many bodily functions and is affected by a variety of conditions, many of which result in hepatomegaly. Hepatomegaly is primarily caused by anemias, bacterial and viral infections, Baylor cirrhosis, cancer, leukemia, hepatitis A and B, toxic states, and heart disease. Each of these needs to be treated in its own way in order to affect the hepatomegaly. *See also* HEART DISEASE; INFECTION; *and* LIVER.

Herbal Medicine

Medical treatment utilizing herbs, plants, roots, and flowers for curative purposes.

Herbal medicine utilizes plants and plant derivatives as remedies for various illnesses and conditions. While they may be sold as fresh leaves and roots, herbs are also frequently marketed as tablets and powders. They can be swallowed, mixed into drinks, rubbed on the skin, or inhaled.

Common Herbal Medicines

Many different kinds of herbal preparations are available to consumers. A few of the most commonly used herbal remedies are alfalfa, echinacea, chamomile, feverfew, ginger, ginkgo biloba, ginseng, hawthorn, senna, valerian, saw palmetto, and oil of evening primrose. Since herbs are not strictly regulated by the Food and Drug Administration (FDA), a physician should be consulted before any herbal remedy is taken.

Herbal Ingredients in Common Medications. While herbal medications are readily available in health-food stores, many common pharmaceutical drugs contain herbal ingredients as well. Penicillin, an antibiotic, is made from mold; digoxin, a common heart medication, comes from foxglove; morphine and codeine, popular painkillers, are derived from the opium poppy. These are only a few of the more than one hundred commonly prescribed pharmaceutical drugs that are at least partially derived from plant sources. In addition, drug companies have sent representatives around the world to work with local peoples to analyze herbal remedies.

International Use of Herbal Preparations. Due to the high price of pharmaceutical drugs, over three-quarters of the world's population relies on herbal healing. Also, the status of herbs is growing in American society, as Americans spend an ever growing amount of money on herbal remedies. This leads to questions about the effectiveness and reliability of the various herbal preparations that are available.

The Dangers of Herbal Medicine

Large amounts of some herbal remedies are highly toxic. Illness following the consumption of any herbal medicine demands medical attention; the sufferer should bring the packaging to the doctor as well. Ephedra plant extracts, for example, contain large amounts of ephedrine, a powerful stimulant that can cause irregular heartbeat and death. *Glycyrrhiza glabra* (licorice), is also a controversial herbal remedy because of its effects on the body's hormonal homeostasis, especially in relation to levels of the hormone aldosterone, which controls levels of potassium. *Glycyrrhiza* will affect aldosterone in such a way as to deplete potassium levels.

Regulation of Herbal Remedies. Unlike pharmaceutical medications, herbal remedies are not strictly regulated by the Federal Food and Drug Administration (FDA). The producers of these preparations do not have to disclose all the possible side effects of the herbs, and there is no standard for purity in herbal remedies. Claims may be made about the supposed effects of the herbs without scientific substantiation. For this reason, it is very important for individuals, especially pregnant women, to consult a physician before taking an herbal preparation. It is also important to learn as much as possible about the herbal remedy before it is ingested or applied.

Background information about Herbal Medicine can be found in ALTERNATIVE MEDICINE; CHINESE MEDICINE; *and* NATUROPATHY. *Also see* STRESS; *and* STRESS ULCER.

Hereditary Spastic Paraplegia

A set of disorders, the primary feature of which is progressive and severe lower extremity spasticity.

Hereditary spastic paraplegia (HSP) is also known as familial spastic paraparesis and Strümpell-Lorrain syndrome. It is not a single disease but rather a group of clinically and genetically diverse disorders. The majority of patients begin to experience symptoms when they are around eight years old, although it can appear earlier or later. HSP is labeled as "uncomplicated" if the symptoms are limited to lower, extremity weakness, bladder disturbance, and, to a lesser extent, impaired position sense in the legs. HSP is categorized as "complicated" when added neurological disorders are involved. An individual may develop a stiffness in the leg and stumble when walking as a result of weakened foot and hip muscles. Additional symptoms may include urinary urgency that may progress to a stage of urinary incontinence. *See also* SPASTICITY.

Heredity

The transmission of genetic traits from parents to their offspring.

Genes, comosed of deoxyribonucleic acid (DNA), are located on chromosomes in the nuclei of each and every cell. Human beings inherit a full set of genes—with half coming from the mother and half from the father—from the egg and sperm cells that conceived them. Thus half of every human's genes are passed on to his or her offspring. The combination of these two parts determines the individual's inherited traits. These may include the risk or likelihood that they will contract certain diseases or disorders, or the diseases and disorders themselves may be passed on through a family's generations. *See also* CONGENITAL; DNA; FAMILIAL; GENE; GENETIC CODE; GENETIC DISORDERS; GENETIC ENGINEERING; HERITABILITY; *and* INHERITANCE.

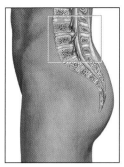

Where a Hernia Appears in the Back. Above, the position of a herniated lumbar disk. This is a relatively common condition caused by excessive weight, bad posture, improper weightlifting and other sorts of back trauma. Herniated disks are treated with rest and anti-inflammatory drugs, unless the condition is sever, in which case a diskectomy may be necessary.

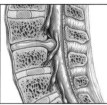

Herniated Disk Repair. Below, a herniated disk will be removed from the back near the spine, however, surgery is not often done. About half of all cases of herniated disks repair themselves with the proper rest and stretching. Surgery is only done when the pain persists and the symptoms are debilitating.

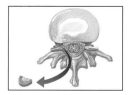

Heritability

The measure of the degree to which a trait is genetically determined and the degree to which it can be changed by environmental factors.

Heritability is, at best, an approximation of how genetically determined a trait is. There is a complex interplay between nature and nurture to determine the characteristics of an individual. Further complicating the explanation are the genes themselves, in that they interact in complicated ways. Additive genes combine their effects, dominant genes mask traits that would otherwise be caused by recessive genes. Often, traits are the result of interaction between a number of genes, each of which has only a small effect. Some traits—such as blood groups and disorders such as cystic fibrosis—are entirely inherited. Others, such as occupational diseases, are entirely environmental. Most, however, lie somewhere in between. *See also* CYSTIC FIBROSIS; DNA; GENES; GENETICS; *and* INHERITANCE.

Hermaphroditism

Having both male and female reproductive organs.

True hermaphrodites have both male and female internal reproductive organs. This condition is extremely rare. Most children with ambiguous genitals are pseudohermaphrodites—they have either ovaries or testicles, but not both. Internally, pseudohermaphrodites are either male or female, and surgery is used to correct the appearance of the external genitals; psychological development also needs to be considered.

Hernia

The protrusion of an organ through a weak spot in the tissues containing or enveloping it.

Caused by congenital weakness in the containing tissue, a hernia typically applies to a frailty or opening in the abdominal wall that draws in part of the intestine. It can also refer to herniated organs elsewhere in the body, such as the brain. Lifting heavy objects, surgery, weight gain, severe coughing, and straining to defecate may cause or enlarge a hernia that shrinks when the sufferer is lying down.

A hernia in the abdomen can form a visible bulge that may or may not resist being pushed back inside the abdominal wall. It can cause discomfort or severe pain, particularly when it resists efforts to be repositioned. Hernia diagnosis may involve blood tests, a lymph-node examination, and tests on liver and kidney function. The intestine may be trapped (a strangulated hernia), which demands immediate medical attention. Hernias that resist all external repositioning efforts often require surgery.

Anatomical information related to this article can be found in ABDOMEN; INTESTINE; KIDNEY; *and* LIVER. *Treatment and other options are discussed in* HERNIA REPAIR; HIATAL HERNIA; *and* SURGERY. *See also* BLOOD TESTS.

Hernia Repair

Surgically repairing a hernia and, if necessary, strengthening the abdominal muscles.

A hernia occurs when a portion of the intestine, bladder, or fat bulges out of the abdominal cavity. Various types of hernias may require repair, but the most common is repair of an inguinal hernia, in which the intestines protrude into the inguinal canal, the area from which the testicles descend. Inguinal hernia repair is one of the most common surgical operations; over 500,000 are performed in an average year.

Sometimes, hernias disappear naturally. This is especially common with umbilical hernias in children, and a doctor may simply be able to push the intestines back into their proper place. However, if the hernia is large or cannot be pushed back, surgical intervention may be necessary. If the intestine becomes twisted and blocked (strangulated hernia), emergency surgical repair is needed.

Hernia repair may be done under local, regional, or general anesthesia. After making an opening in the abdomen, a surgeon pushes the intestines back into the abdomen or the surgeon may remove the strangulated portion of intestine and rejoin the healthy sections. The muscles, ligaments and tissues are closed and fortified with stitches. In some cases, mesh or wire may be used to reinforce the area.

Laparoscopic hernia repair, a procedure in which a viewing tube (endoscope) and surgical instruments are inserted through tiny incisions to the site of the hernia and used for repair, is less invasive and abbreviates recovery time. However, it is a more costly procedure and usually requires general anesthesia. *See also* HERNIA.

Herpangina

A disease of childhood caused by the Coxsackie virus.

Like hand-foot-and-mouth disease, herpangina produces blisters in the mouth. These blisters are located toward the back of the palate, on the tonsils, and in the throat. The virus is transmitted by saliva and by droplets in the air from coughing or sneezing. Symptoms of herpangina include a fever and sore throat that last several days. Treatment includes: fever reducing medications and fluids to avoid dehydration. *See also* BLISTER; DEHYDRATION; FEVER; HAND-FOOT-AND-MOUTH DISEASE; *and* VIRUSES.

Herpes

A set of viruses that cause diseases often resulting in eruptions on the skin such as cold sores, fever blisters, chickenpox, shingles, and genital sores.

The main categories of the herpes virus are herpes simplex and herpes zoster. Cytomegalovirus is a herpes virus that attacks individuals who have contracted AIDS. Herpes simplex is either Type 1 or Type 2. Type 1 produces fever blisters around the mouth, fever, fatigue, and swollen glands. Type 2 produces painful sores on the genitals or anus. Herpes zoster causes chickenpox and shingles, which produce a painful rash that changes into fluid-filled blisters.

Treatment. The herpes virus cannot be eliminated from the body. There are antiviral drugs (acyclovir and its derivatives) that reduce its impact and bolster the body's immune system if they are applied early in the course of the disease. These drugs reduce the severity and duration of acute outbreaks. The herpes virus affects one-sixth of the population of the United States. Individuals with this disease should eat a regular and healthy diet, exercise regularly, and avoid stress, all of which strengthen the immune system. Affected areas should be kept clean and dry but should not be touched until the sores have healed. Hands should be washed with soap and warm water frequently, especially if the sores are touched.

For more information on Herpes see Viruses; Antiviral Drugs; Cold Sores; *and* Chickenpox. *Articles about related conditions include* Cytomegalovirus; Herpes Simplex; Herpes Zoster; *and* Herpes Genital.

Herpes, Genital

The herpes simplex type 2 virus is the cause of genital herpes, which is transmitted most often by sexual contact.

It is estimated that one in ten adults in the U.S. has genital herpes; up to one million new cases are diagnosed each year. The incubation period for the virus is about five days, and the course of the disease takes about three weeks from the first appearance of symptoms to the healing of sores. Once infected, a person carries the virus in dormant form for the rest of his or her life. There may be recurrences of the disease from time to time when the immune system is compromised or when the person experiences emotional or physical stress.

Symptoms. People with genital herpes usually experience flu-like symptoms during the initial stages; later, small bumps will develop. These will itch and cause some measure of pain. The bumps open into suppurating sores on the penis, in the vulva and vagina, on the cervix, around the anus, and on the buttocks.

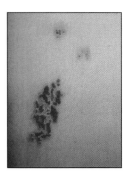

Herpes. Above, type 1 herpes (HSV-1) causes small sores on the skin. These sores are mostly cosmetic problems, although they may cause some measure of minor irritation and aggravation.

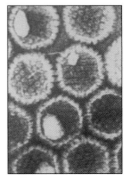

Genital Herpes. Below, a micrograph image of herpes simplex virus type 2 (HSV-2), better known as genital herpes. This virus, which is spread thorough sexual contact, affects more than 45 million Americans over the age of 12. About one in every five people are affected, with a slightly higher incidence among women than among men. The prevalence of this disorder has increased steadily since the 1970s.

Resources on Herpes

Grist, Norman R., et al., *Diseases of Infection: An Illustrated Textbook* (1992); Shaw, Michael, ed., *Everything You Need to Know About Diseases* (1996); Rosenwaks, Zev, *Gynecology: Principles and Practice* (1987); Centers for Disease Control and Prevention, Tel. (800) 311-3435, Online: www.cdc.gov, STD hotline: (800) 227-8922; Infectious Disease Society of America, Tel. (703) 299-0200, Online: www.idsociety.org; National Institute of Allergy and Infectious Disease, Tel. (301) 496-5717, Online: www.niaid.nih.org; https://public1.med.cornell.edu/cgi-.

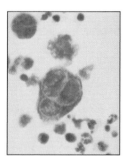

Herpes Simplex. Above, a microscopic image of the herpes simplex virus. Type 1 and type 2 look similar under microscopic and micrographic analysis; however, too few people undergo this type of analysis at any time. Millions of Americans are infected carriers, and they will never know it.

Treatment. Genital herpes is a highly contagious disease for which there is no cure. The best treatment is prevention. Sexual contact with persons with unknown histories should be avoided and a condom should always be used, though uncovered areas of the body are also vulnerable. The physician may prescribe the antiviral drug acyclovir if the disease is diagnosed within the first 72 hours to resolve the acute attacks. Otherwise, sores should be kept clean with warm, soapy water, and should be allowed to dry and form a scab. If episodes occur frequently (over six times per year), daily suppression with agents such as acyclovir can prevent recurrences while taking the medication.

Topics related to Genital Herpes include HERPES; SAFE SEX; SEXUALLY TRANSMITTED DISEASE; PENIS; *and* VAGINA. *Other important information is included in articles on* SKIN; VAGINITIS; *and* VIRUS. *See also* GENITAL ULCERATION.

Herpes Gestatonis

A skin rash that occurs during pregnancy.

Despite its name, herpes gestatonis is not caused by the herpes virus or any of the other related viruses. It is thought to be an autoimmune reaction, and can appear any time after the 12th week of pregnancy.

Symptoms. The rash is extremely itchy and includes small blisters known as vesicles, as well as larger swellings known as bullae. It often begins on the abdomen and then spreads to other areas, often covering a ring-shaped area. The rash intensifies after delivery and disappears within a few weeks or months. It often recurs with subsequent pregnancies or if the mother is taking oral contraceptives. The newborn may also exhibit a similar rash.

Treatment. Treatment is designed to alleviate the itching and prevents the formation of new blisters. Corticosteroids are used, either as a topical application for a mild rash or taken orally in more severe cases. *See also* ABDOMEN; ALTERNATIVE MEDICINE; BLISTER; DELIVERY; HERBAL MEDICINE; IMMUNE SYSTEM; PREGNANCY; *and* RASH.

Herpes Simplex

A viral infection causing small, painful blisters on the skin and mucous membranes.

The herpes simplex virus has two types, type 1 and type 2. Herpes simplex types 1 and 2 look the same under the microscope, but type 1 usually attacks above the waist and type 2 attacks below. Once infected, an individual will carry the virus for the rest of his or her life; however, outbreaks may be fairly frequent at first and slowly subside over a period of years. *See also* VIRUS.

During the latent or inactive periods, the virus retreats to the nerve cells that serve the affected areas. Even when the disease is inactive, the virus may be present on the skin's surface and may spread to others during intimate contact. Activation of the virus may be caused by other infections, sunburn, or almost any situation that causes emotional or physical stress.

A herpes simplex outbreak usually starts with flu-like symptoms and fever. Soon after, there will be a tingling or itching sensation, and then the appearance of small blisters with a red circumferential ring, either on the lips and in the mouth (type 1), or on the penis, in the vulva, in the anus, or on the buttocks (type 2). The blisters usually appear in clusters that combine to make large, painful sores.

The best treatment for herpes simplex is to keep the affected areas clean and dry. Antiviral creams and pills like Acyclovir are sometimes helpful if started early in the outbreak. *See also* ANTIVIRAL DRUGS; HERPES; INFLUENZA; *and* HERPES, GENITAL.

Herpes Zoster

Also known as shingles

A disease caused by the same virus that causes chickenpox.

After a childhood attack of chickenpox, the virus, varicella-zoster, may remain dormant in the nerves, only to reactivate much later in life. The infection travels back up the nerve to the area of the skin that the nerve serves. The reactivation is probably caused by a compromise of the immune system that allows the virus to multiply in people such as the elderly, those with AIDS, those being treated for cancer, or those who have had an organ transplant. However, the majority of patients with shingles have no apparent underlying disease or abnormality of the immune system. A sufferer of shingles may transmit the virus to another by direct contact. If the receiver has not had chickenpox, she or he may well develop that disease.

Herpes Zoster and the Elderly

Researchers are not certain why the varicella-zoster virus, the virus that causes chickenpox and shingles, reactivates in some individuals and not others. About 20 percent of those who have chickenpox will develop shingles later in life. About 30 percent of all cases occur in people over 55. However, the elderly are most vulnerable to the initial pain as well as the continued discomfort it causes after the virus runs its course. Post-herpetic neuralgia, a more long-lasting nerve pain following the disease, affects one quarter to one half of all patients over 50 and may continue for months or sometimes even years after infection.

SYMPTOMS

Herpes zoster may start with symptoms such as chills and fever, nausea, diarrhea, and painful urination. In later stages, when the virus reaches the nerve endings, there will be a rash, blistering, and sometimes burning pain. The rash will later turn to fluid-filled blisters with red rings around them. The rash may follow the path of the nerve on one side of the face and spread to the neck, or on one buttock and travel down the leg. The blisters are very sensitive to the touch and painful. The blisters will take a week or more to scab over and begin to heal, but the area may remain sensitive and painful for weeks or even months after the blisters have healed.

Once an individual has been infected with and recovered from herpes zoster, he or she will have developed an immunity to the virus and rarely will suffer another attack. There are no long-term effects of the disease, although if the sores are large there may be some scarring. If the disease attacks the face and eye, there may be permanent vision damage.

TREATMENT

Treatment should be started as quickly as possible after the onset of the disease. The doctor will prescribe antiviral medications, such as acyclovir, if the patient is diagnosed with herpes zoster within 72 hours of the appearance of the rash. The blisters should be cleaned with soap and warm water; antibiotic ointment should be used to reduce the likelihood of bacterial infection.

Articles that develop topics mentioned in relation to Herpes Zooster include AIDS; CHICKENPOX; HERPES; IMMUNITY; *and* VACCINATIONS. *Further information about symptoms includes* AGING; BLISTER; DIARRHEA; *and* FEVER.

Heterosexuality

The physical attraction to individals of the opposite sex.

Depending on the culture, like other sexualities, heterosexuality is associated with set patterns of behavior specific to either males or females. However, normal human sexuality is thought to span a wide spectrum, ranging from exclusively heterosexual to exclusively homosexual. Some believe that many individuals experiment with same-sex activities during adolescence or early adulthood, but then form exclusively heterosexual relationships in later adulthood. *See also* BISEXUALITY; HOMOSEXUALITY; SEX; *and* SEXUALITY.

Hiatal Hernia

A condition in which part of the stomach presses into the abdomen through a hole in the diaphragm.

Researchers do not understand the cause of a hiatal hernia, but think it is a congenital condition with links to smoking and obesity. A reflux of gastric acid may accompany this condition, so symptoms may include burping, heartburn, and chest pains. Treating weight issues and smoking habits usually alleviates this disorder. *See* HERNIA.

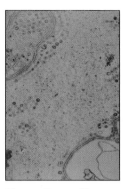

Herpes Zoster. Above, an electron micrograph of the herpes zoster virus inside the nucleus of a cell. This is a virus that causes lesions. Herpes zoster can occur only in people who have contracted chickenpox; and only about 20 percent of those who have had chicken pox will contract herpes zoster. In almost all cases, herpes zoster appears only once in a lifetime, if at all.

Herpes Zoster Lesions on the Back. Below top, the lesions that herpes zoster (also known as shingles) makes on the back. This is the classic color and pattern for herpes zoster blister clusters. Below bottom, a dermatone pattern is also common among those who suffer from shingles.

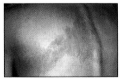

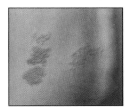

Hiccup

Spasm of the lungs and vocal cords, producing a sound resembling a chirp.

A hiccup is the sudden, involuntary movement of the breathing muscles (diaphragm), followed by the sudden, involuntary closure of the vocal cords. Hiccups usually occur in clusters and can be caused by sudden excitement, a surge of emotion, cigarette smoking, excess alcohol intake, or sudden stress. *See also* STRESS.

Chronic hiccuping is much more serious; it can be due to a number of conditions, including pregnancy, gout, asthma, injury, pneumonia, and gastric ulcer. Some drugs, including steroids, barbiturates and benzodiazepines can also cause chronic hiccups. Severe chronic hiccuping can result in exhaustion, insomnia, inability to eat, and cardiac abnormalities. Medications such as baclofen, chlorpromazine or phenytoin can help in some cases. Acupuncture or hypnosis have been reported to be effective for some patients. If all else fails, the nerve controlling the diaphragm can be blocked by surgery. *See* DIAPHRAGM.

High Colonic

Also known as colonic or colonic irrigation

The flushing of toxic waste and impacted feces out of the colon.

High colonics involves the insertion of a tube into the rectum through which water, or a saline solution at body temperature, is flushed into the colon. An additional tube carries the water and residual colonic matter out of the body. The aim of the therapy is to eliminate certain toxins and impacted fecal matter from the body. High colonics are often prescribed by naturopaths (practioners of natural healing techniques) for those suffering from constipation or the symptoms of "toxicity" (such as acne, fatigue, insomnia, and weight problems).

Risk Factors. This form of treatment still poses many risks.

- An improperly inserted rectal tube can tear the rectum's lining;
- Repeated irrigation of the bowel with 5 to 25 gallons of water can stretch the bowel and impair the body's ability to eliminate waste;
- Large amounts of water can potentially be absorbed by the body, causing water intoxication and fatality;
- Perforations in the colon can result from high water pressure.

Due to possible complications resulting from high colonic therapy, many health care professionals advise their patients against undergoing this form of naturopathic treatment.

HIGH COLONIC *is a form of* ALTERNATIVE MEDICINE, *other forms include* BIORHYTHMS; BIOFEEDBACK; HERBAL MEDICINE; MASSAGE; *and* NATUROPATHY. HIGH COLONIC *may adversely affect the* COLON; *and thus the* INTESTINE.

Hip

The joint between the thigh bone and the pelvis.

The rounded upper end of the thigh bone, or femur, lodges snugly in a cup-shaped cavity in the lower pelvis. Strong ligaments form the attachment and allow a wide range of movement, making the hip a classic example of a ball-and-socket joint. It is strong and stable enough to carry the weight of the upper body and withstand the force of running and jumping. *See also* BOWED LEG *and* HIP REPLACEMENT.

Hip, Congenital Dislocation of

The abnormal development of one or all parts of the hip joint, resulting in the top of the femur being located outside the hip socket.

Congenital dislocation of the hip may be detected at birth or shortly afterward. Usually, the hip socket is too shallow for the head of the femur (thigh bone) to fit properly, making the joint more susceptible to dislocation. This abnormality may lead to altered shapes of the bones making up the joint. If this is detected in infancy, a brace or splint is used to properly position the head of the femur in the hip socket. The procedure is generally successful within six to eight weeks, and further development and walking are normal. If this condition is not treated in infancy, it may require extensive surgical repair later in life and may lead to long-term problems with walking. *See also* HIP *and* HIP, FRACTURED.

Hip, Fractured

A fracture involving the hip joint.

What is commonly referred to as a hip fracture is actually a fracture of the thigh bone, or femur, which meets the pelvis to form the hip joint. Elderly people are the most common sufferers, usually owing to a fall. Surgery is required if the upper end, or neck, of the femur is displaced. If it is impacted, the person must be kept bedridden for a few weeks and undertake daily exercises in bed to facilitate natural healing.

Hip Replacement

Also known as hip arthroplasty, a surgical procedure to replace all or part of a diseased hip joint with artificial parts.

The most common reasons for hip replacement surgery are osteoarthritis, which wears down the hip joint; rheumatoid arthritis, which causes joint pain, stiffness, and swelling; avascular necrosis, the loss of bone caused by insufficient blood supply; bone tumors; and traumatic injury. According the American Academy of Orthopedic Surgeons, about 200,000 hip replacement operations are performed each year.

When Considering Hip Replacement. Before recommending hip replacement, the orthopedic surgeon must consider all other options, such as medication (usually a nonsteroidal anti-inflammatory medication or corticosteroids), a physical therapy regimen, and walking aids. Sometimes a surgical repositioning of the joint (osteotomy) is recommended as a simpler procedure that may relieve pain. The key factors in deciding on hip replacement are

the degree of pain, the amount of bone and cartilage damage, the amount of reduction of activity, and the age and overall health of the patient.

Those not usually recommended for hip replacement include people who have Parkinson's disease or severe muscle weakness, because there is a higher likelihood of dislocating an artificial hip. People with weakened immune systems or who are in poor health are less likely to recover well. People under 60 years of age are also not good candidates for hip replacement, because the life span of an artificial hip joint is 10 to 15 years.

PROCEDURE

During a hip replacement operation, the surgeon removes the diseased bone tissue and cartilage from the hip joint, and saws off the top two parts (the ball and the trochanter, to which muscle and tendon are attached) of the thigh bone (femur). The surgeon then widens the socket of the hip and inserts an artificial socket that is usually made of a plastic cup in a metal casing. A hole is cut into the femur, and a metal or ceramic prosthesis (ball and shaft) is inserted. Both are then cemented into place, and the new ball is inserted into the new socket. The trochanter is reattached with wires, and the incision is sutured. The operation normally takes about two to three hours.

RECOVERY

The patient is encouraged to begin walking with aids within a day of the operation, but he or she has to be careful not to disturb the joint, which takes about one to two weeks to become stable. Possible infection is a concern because the new joint does not receive a sufficient blood supply. The patient is given antibiotics and afterwards must receive antibiotics whenever any infection is present in the body. Blood clots may also cause a complication. Many patients also require surgery in the other hip. If the patient is in good health, it may be replaced in the same operation or delayed for eight to twelve weeks.

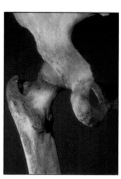

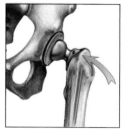

The Hip Bone and a Prosthetic Hip Replacement. Top, after a lifetime of use, the hip bone may become weak, crack, or break. One of the most highly successful kinds of surgery has been the hip-bone replacement. The prosthesis can either be cemented (as is the case in the lower picture) or, in a newer procedure a porous cementless prosthesis is inserted. Bone grows into the porous material, making the replacement stronger. The cementless replacement is often used for younger patients.

Resources on Hip replacement & Elder Care

Cassel, Christine, *Geriatric Medicine* (1990), Fries, James F., *Aging Well* (1989); Rossman, Isadore, *Looking Forward: The Complete Medical Guide to Successful Aging* (1989); Schneider, Edward L. and John W. Rowe, *Handbook of the Biology of Aging* (1996); Weiss, Robert, et al., *Complete Guide to Health and Well-Being After Fifty* (1988); American Assoc. of Retired Persons, Tel. (800) 424-3410, Online: www.aarp.org; American Geriatrics Soc., Tel. (212) 308-1414, Online: www.americangeriatrics.org; National Council on Aging, Tel. (800) 424-9046, Online: www.ncoa.org; www.nyc-ornell.org/medicine/geriatrics/index.html; www.cornellaging.org/.

PROGNOSIS.

The operation has a high success rate; 90 to 95 percent of patients report improvement in pain and mobility. After 10–15 years, the cement that holds the prostheses to bone starts to loosen, causing pain and possibly requiring further surgery. A recent response to this complication has been to develop shafts that are porous allowing bone to grow through them, thus further cementing them in place. *See also* BONE; BONE, DISORDERS; DISLOCATION, JOINT; FRACTURE; HIP; HIP, CONGENITAL DISLOCATION OF; HIP, FRACTURED; *and* OSTEOPOROSIS.

Hirschsprung's Disease

Also known as megacolon

A disease that occurs when a section of the large intestine lacks the nerves to control the normal rhythmic contractions.

As a result of Hirschsprung's disease, an infant is unable to excrete feces and gradually develops a large and twisted colon. Hirschsprung's disease accounts for 33 percent of all neonatal intestinal obstructions.

Symptoms of this disorder include the failure to pass the meconium stool, vomiting, abdominal distention, and the failure to have normal bowel movements. Dehydration and weight loss are also common. In some instances, infants with this condition may alternate between constipation and diarrhea. A definitive diagnosis is made with a rectal biopsy. *See* INTESTINE.

Hirschsprung's disease is treated with a temporary colostomy (an incision in the abdomen to drain waste), so fecal material passes into a disposable pouch; it is closed when the child is about 12–18 months old. At that time, the abnormal section of the intestine is removed and the remainder is reconnected. *See* COLON *and* COLOSTOMY.

Hirsutism

Excessive body or facial hair in women.

Hirsutism resembles the male hair growth pattern on a female. This condition may be the result of an underlying illness. It is usually caused by increased production of androgens (male hormones); androgen disorders affect between 5 and 10 percent of females. Excess body hair in women can also be a normal familial trait. Treatment of hirsutism involves removing unwanted hair, which can be done temporarily by shaving, waxing, depilatories, or through electrolysis. *See also* FOLLICLE *and* HAIR.

Histiocytosis X

A group of rare childhood disorders involving the proliferation of abnormal immune cells.

In histiocytosis X, immune cells—in particular, histiocytes and eosinophils—multiply in the bones and lungs and cause scarring. Histiocytosis X diseases include Letterer-Siwe disease, Hand-Schüller-Christian disease, and eosinophilic granuloma. Recovery from Hand-Schüller-Christian disease and eosinophilic granuloma may occur spontaneously. All these disorders can be treated with corticosteroids and cytotoxic drugs. In severe cases, possibly fatal respiratory or heart failure may result. *See also* BONE; HEART FAILURE; IMMUNE SYSTEM; IMMUNITY; LUNG; *and* SCAR.

Histocompatibility Antigens

Proteins that are normally found in body tissue, and that function in the immune system.

Histocompatibility, the presence of compatible tissue, is used to determine the success in transplanting tissues or organs from one person to another. Histocompatibility is determined by the major histocompatibility antigens, called human leukocyte antigens (HLA).

Function in Transplants. HLA types are specific markers that the immune system uses to identify foreign cells as opposed to self cells. If the histocompatibility antigens of the transplanted tissue do not match the histocompatibility antigens of the rest of the body tissue, the transplanted tissue will be attacked by the recipient's body. It is important, therefore, to ensure that transplant donor tissue has HLA types that are similar to those of the body tissue of the transplant recipient. There are six HLA proteins used to test for histocompatibility. They are found on the surface of the white blood cells, as well as on other cells in the body. The greater the number of HLA matches, the greater the chance for a successful transplant.

Function in the Immune System. Histocompatibility antigens are located on most cells in the body. They function as a guide for T cell lymphocytes (a specific type of white blood cell) in the immune system. These antigens help T cells identify and destroy foreign disease-causing agents in the body. They also help T cells to recognize and fight tumor cells. *See also* ANTIGEN; DONOR; IMMUNITY; IMMUNE RESPONSE; IMMUNE SYSTEM; *and* TRANSPLANT SURGERY.

Histoplasmosis

A respiratory disease caused by the parasitic fungus *Histoplasma capsulatum.*

Histoplasmosis is a fungal infection associated with exposure to the feces of birds and bats, or soil contaminated with these feces. In the Mississippi and Ohio river valleys of the United States, 80 percent of the population may have been exposed to this common fungus through the inhalation of spores. Many such cases will be without symptoms, although the disease can be severe and even fatal in others, particularly those with immune system disorders such as HIV and AIDS.

Any of the following could indicate the presence of a histoplasmosis infection: chills, fever, headache, cough, chest pain, lumps in the leg, enlargement of the liver and spleen, ulceration of the tongue or palate, and shortness of breath. Exposure to, or the presence of, the disease may be identified through an analysis of blood, urine, or sputum; or by means of a skin test, examination of ulcerated tissue, lymph nodes, liver tissue, or bone marrow.

Three forms of the illness exist and vary widely in severity. The first, known as primary acute histoplasmosis, is usually self-limiting and goes away in a matter of weeks. Symptoms are similar to those of a severe cold or flu. Progressive disseminated histoplasmosis is spread widely throughout the body via the lungs into the bloodstream, requires treatment with oral antifungal medications, and can involve the liver and spleen, as well as producing ulcers of the throat and mouth. Additionally, the brain, adrenal glands, and heart may be affected, and this form is 90 percent fatal. Chronic pulmonary histoplasmosis produces symptoms resembling tuberculosis: coughing up bloody phlegm and severe shortness of breath. *See also* AIDS; FEVER; FUNGI; HIV; INFECTION; *and* TUBERCULOSIS.

Histrionic Personality Disorder

A personality disorder characterized by feelings of emptiness, coupled with an intense need to be liked, and to be the center of attention.

Individuals with histrionic personality disorder usually express themselves with seductive and flirtatious behaviors aimed at gaining approval and attention. Dramatic and expansive behavior often appears as outgoing. Attention to personal appearance is excessive and may take an inordinate amount of time. Relationships are often rocky and marked by ups and downs. Individuals with this disorder tend to become intimate very early in relationships and misjudge them as being closer and more important than they are.

Cause. As with other personality disorders, histrionic personality disorder is probably a result of both inborn tendencies and environmental influences. This personality disorder usually manifests itself in early adulthood; this has been attributed to an unstable family environment in which one or both parents were continually experienced as manipulative or seductive. *See also* PERSONALITY DISORDER.

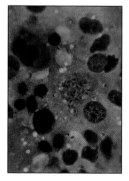

Histoplasmosis. Above, a microscopic image of the fungus that causes histoplasmosis. According to the Centers for Disease Control, in regions where the fungus that causes histoplasmosis is found, up to 80 percent of the population is often infected. The National Institute for Occupational Safety and Health Publications Dissemination (NIOSH/ NCID) provides information for workers who may need protective equipment to reduce the risk of infection.

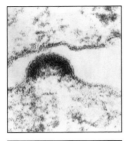

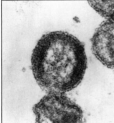

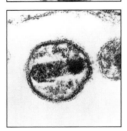

HIV-1. Top, the budding HIV cell—budding is how HIV replicates— is the first stage in which it is visible. HIV buds when viral proteins accumulate under the cell membrane. Middle, the bud begins to constrict, constituting a connected sphere with a viral nucleoid center. Bottom, as constriction continues, the virus pinches itself off and becomes a free infectious virus outside of the cell; the bar shape in the center of the bottom image is used to discriminate HIV-1 from HTLV-2 and HTLV-3. HTLV is a family of human T-lymphotrophic viruses—thus the name—that were discovered at the same time as HIV.

HIV

Also known as human immunodeficiency virus

The virus that causes AIDS.

One of the most virulent new diseases to attack humankind is the Acquired Immunodeficiency Syndrome, or AIDS. Two forms of the virus that causes AIDS, HIV-1 and HIV-2, have been identified. HIV-1 is most prevalent in Europe, Asia, and the Americas. HIV-2 is largely limited to sub-Saharan Africa. The virus penetrates a healthy cell (often one of the white blood cells that provide a substantial part of human immunity) and incorporates itself into the DNA of the infected cell. The cell is destroyed and discharges new copies of the virus to infect other cells. The process continues slowly over a period of months or years until enough damage has been done so that the sufferer is vulnerable to any one of a number of other infections.

HIV is transmitted through body fluids: blood, semen, vaginal secretions, and breast milk. The virus is also present in saliva and tears but at greatly reduced levels. Transmission of the virus can take place during sexual relations, including intercourse, oral or anal sex. It can be transmitted by shared IV needles or by other contact with contaminated blood, such as during transfusions. A person is particularly vulnerable to HIV if there is a cut or abrasion on the skin into which the virus can penetrate. *See also* AIDS; AUTOIMMUNITY; HERPES; INFECTIOUS DISEASES; IMMUNITY; PUBLIC HEALTH; *and* SEXUALLY TRANSMITTED DISEASES.

Hives

Also known as urticaria

Raised red welts on the surface of the skin that are usually associated with allergies.

Hives usually occur in batches. Histamine and other factors in the skin cause itching and swelling of hives. They are more common among individuals who suffer from fever or asthma. There are many substances that can trigger hives outbreaks through allergic reactions. These include: medications, certain foods (such as some kinds of fruit, berries, shellfish, nuts, eggs, and milk), pollen, animal dander, and insect bites. Exposure to water or sunlight, as well as stress may also cause hives in some individuals. There are also many infections or illnesses that may trigger outbreaks of hives. These include: dermographism, cold urticaria, lupus erythematosus, dog tapeworm, hereditary angioedema, Henoch-Schonlein purpura, mononucleosis, hepatitis, and mastocytosis. Symptoms of hives may include itching and swelling of the skin into welts, which may enlarge and join together to form large, raised areas.

Hives may be treated with antihistamines, epinephrine, terbutaline, cimetidine, corticosteroids, sedatives, and tranquilizers to reduce itching and swelling. When hives occur in the throat, they may obstruct the airway and must be treated. Although hives are uncomfortable, they are usually not serious and may disappear on their own.

> *For background information about this topic see* ALLERGIES; ANTIHISTAMINE DRUGS; BITES; DERMATITIS; HEPATITIS; MONONUCLEOSIS; *and* SKIN. *Information about doctors who treat* HIVES *can be found in* DERMATOLOGY.

Hoarseness

A condition resulting in a husky, rasping voice.

The vocal cords are strands of elastic tissue covered by mucous membranes that stretch across the larynx and attach at each end of the thyroid gland. These cords produce sound when air from the lungs passes over them, causing them to vibrate. When they become irritated or strained, the sound is distorted, producing a raspy, croaking tone. *See also* LARYNGITIS.

Causes. The most common causes of hoarseness include acute laryngitis, or inflamed vocal cords due to infection. Overuse can also cause hoarseness by straining the muscles of the larynx. Chronic hoarseness can be the result of activities that irritate the vocal cords, such as smoking, drinking alcohol, or regular exposure to harsh chemicals, as may occur in the workplace. Acid reflux, or the flow of stomach acid back into the throat, can also irritate the vocal cords.

Treatment. The immediate treatment for hoarseness should be to rest the voice. If the hoarseness is caused by an infection, medication may help. Home care, such as drinking plenty of fluids or steaming the face, may also help. Avoiding alcoholic drinks and smoking will also reduce the irritation of the vocal cords. Persistent hoarseness, lasting beyond two weeks, should be investigated by a physician; it may indicate a serious condition such as cancer of the larynx. *See also* LARYNX; THROAT; VOICE, LOSS OF; *and* VOCAL CORDS.

Hodgkin's Disease

A malignant condition of the lymph system.

Hodgkin's disease is rare, with an incidence of 3 per 100,000 Americans per year. It generally occurs in young people between the ages of 15 and 34, with another peak after age 55. It is named for Thomas Hodgkin, the British physician who described it in 1832.

SYMPTOMS

Hodgkin's disease causes an overgrowth of lymphocytes, the blood cells involved in the body's immune defense system. Lymphocytes are present in the lymph system, a network of vessels that extends throughout the body. Lymphocytes collect in the lymph nodes, small structures that occur throughout the lymph system. The overgrowth of lymphocytes in Hodgkin's disease causes the lymph nodes to swell, usually in the neck, under the arms, or in the groin. Other symptoms include fever, weakness, weight loss, night sweats, shortness of breath, and chest discomfort.

DIAGNOSIS

An essential step in the diagnosis of Hodgkin's disease is a biopsy, a tissue sample taken from lymph nodes to detect the proliferation of lymphocytes. Other tests can include x-rays of the chest, liver, and spleen; a bone marrow biopsy; a computerized tomography (CAT); or magnetic resonance imaging (MRI) and a liver biopsy.

Hodgkin's Disease and Fertility
The reproductive system can be affected by treatment for Hodgkin's disease, especially among men. Various treatments and when they are taken have different affects on the ability to conceive a child; if radiation is used alone, about half of all families were able to conceive, but that number declines when radiation and drug treatments are taken together.

TREATMENT AND PROGNOSIS
When Hodgkin's disease is diagnosed at an early stage or when only a single lymph node or single organ is involved, radiation therapy is usually the treatment, and it may be combined with chemotherapy. Radiation therapy may be directed at the single site of occurrence or at larger segments of the body. When the condition has spread somewhat, the emphasis is on chemotherapy, using a combination of three, four or more drugs. The regimen is different for children, with lower-dose radiation therapy supplemented by chemotherapy. The prognosis for most patients with Hodgkin's disease is good, with five-year survival rates of up to 90 percent when the condition is detected and treated early. Even when the disease has spread, five-year survival rates are as high as 60 to 80 percent.

COMPLICATIONS
Radiation therapy and chemotherapy can increase the risk of other cancers, most notably non-Hodgkin's lymphoma, another cancer of the lymph system. Patients thus are advised to have periodic examinations for several years after treatment, with x-rays, blood tests, and other examinations that diagnose other cancers or a recurrence of Hodgkin's disease.

Issues related to HODGKIN'S DISEASE *and its symptoms are discussed in* BLOOD; FEVER; LYMPHATIC SYSTEM; *and* LYMPHOCYTE. *Related diagnostic techniques include* BIOPSY; CAT SCAN; MRI; *and* X RAY. *Similar disorders include* BURKITT'S LYMPHOMA; LYMPHANGITIS; *and* LYMPHOMA.

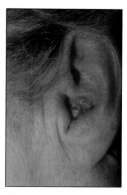

Hodgkin's Disease. Above, skin lesions on the ear of an individual with Hodgkin's disease. Such skin disorders do not usually occur in people with Hodgkin's disease until late in the development of the disease. Many patients with Hodgkin's disease choose to take part in clinical trials of new treatments and medications in hopes of being part of the research that leads to a cure.

Resources on Hodgkin's Disease
Kampe, W. A., G. B. Humphrey, and S. Poppema, *Hodgkin's Disease in Children: Controversies and Current Practice* (1999); Lacher, Mortimer J., and John R. Redman, *Hodgkin's Disease: The Consequences of Survival* (1990); Williams, Stephanie F., Ramaz Farah, and Harvey J. Golomb, *Hodgkin's Disease* (ongoing); National Cancer Institute, Tel. (301) 435-3848, Online: www.nci.hih.gov; Cancer Information Service, Tel. (800) 4-CANCER, Online: http://cis.nci.nih.gov/; www. ny-cornell.org/medicine/hematology/index.html.

Holter Monitor

A portable ECG machine worn by a person in order to record heart activity.

The Holter monitor is a portable device for recording up to 24 hours of the heart's electrical activity. It is particularly useful in detecting cardiac arrhythmias, which may not be identified during a standard electrocardiogram (ECG) of only a few minutes duration. *See also* DIAGNOSIS.

The Holter monitor, powered by batteries, is worn over one shoulder. By means of four chest electrodes, it monitors heart activity continuously while the person engages in any normal day's activity. Since abnormalities of heart rhythm and blood flow may occur briefly and sporadically, the monitor offers better chances of catching such irregularities. The person wearing the Holter device will be asked to keep a diary of any symptoms he or she may experience, and record the time of day they occur.

The Holter 24-hour record will be entered into a computer that subsequently analyzes the electrical impulses of the heart (ECG), identifying any changes in rhythm or heart rate. The ECG may then be compared with the patient's diary entries. It is also possible to connect the Holter monitor directly to the hospital through telephone lines, for an immediate record of symptoms as they occur. Other Holter monitors are capable of simultaneously recording brain electrical activity by electroencephalogram (EEG) while monitoring heart ECG. *See also* ARRHYTHMIA; BLOOD; CARDIAC; HEART; *and* ELECTROCARDIOGRAM.

Homeopathy

A method of treating illness by prescribing weak doses of substances that enhance the body's natural immunological response to the illness.

Homeopathy seeks to cure rather than merely treat the symptoms of an illness. Its basic philosophy is: that which causes the symptoms of a disease may also cure it. Homeopathic medicine consists only of naturally occurring, nontoxic substances derived from the mineral, plant, and animal kingdoms; these further stimulate the body's natural defenses against the disease by causing the symptoms. Finding such remedies has required an informed process of trial and error, however, since homeopathy was first considered as a science in the late 18th century, standard compendiums of remedies and cross-referenced symptoms are at the homeopath's disposal. In general, a homeopathic remedy, when given to a healthy person, causes the same symptoms suffered by an ill person. To prevent exacerbating the symptoms, only small amoungs are perscribed, enough to boost the body's fight aginst the disease.

The Homeopathic Controversy

Although homeopathy has counted among its supporters several well-known personages—the British royal family, John D. Rockefeller, Mark Twain, and Thomas Edison, just to name a few—and had a practitioner and champion in the U.S. Congress in the person of Senator Royal Copeland. It still remains a subject of controversy among physicians. in the view of some, the American Medical Association (AMA) was founded mainly in response to the creation of the American Institute of Homeopathy in 1844. Homeopaths accuse the medical community of persecuting their discipline at the behest of the pharmaceutical companies, whose profits are threatened by the popularity of homeopathic remedies. Physicians are just as adamant in challenging the scientific basis for the claims made by homeopathy. In recent years, homeopaths have endeavored to work with physicians in treating patients; in addition, physicians have increasingly examined homeopathy for cures and approaches involving difficult cases. These initiatives have been taken in an effort to encourage collaboration and reduce animosity between the disciplines.

Homeopathy is not meant to replace conventional medicine, but it seeks to provide additional perspective whose application might achieve a cure unattainable by using conventional medicine. Rejected by most doctors, homeopathy aspires to restoring not just one aspect of a person's health but also a holistic state of physical, emotional, and mental well-being. Toward this end, homeopaths take into consideration the person both as a whole and as a unique individual, so that treatment may be tailored accordingly.

HOMEOPATHIC MEDICINE

More than half of homeopathic medicines are derived from plants. Salts and metals comprise most mineral remedies. Animal venoms, secretions, insects, musk, and squid ink are in many remedies. All substances are harvested in their natural or purest state and diluted by straining with alcohol or by grinding with lactose, then combined with sugar from cow's milk and cast into tablets of a texture that dictates their delivery into the body. For example, some pills dissolve quickly under the tongue, while others must be chewed. Why such small amounts of homeopathic medicines achieve success may have something to do with resonance in a person's system. Frequency, not size of dosage, is crucial. Prescriptions rarely vary with age.

The History of Homeopathy

"Homeopathy" comes from the Greek: "homoios" means "similar" and "pathos" means "suffering." The concept of seeking remedies that produce the same symptoms suffered by a disease is the "Law of Similars," an observation that goes back 25 centuries to Hippocrates. But only in the nineteenth century was practical knowledge finally written down, when the German physician Christian Friedrich Samuel Hahnemann published Organon of Homeopathic Medicine, and the Materia Medica Pura. Homeopathy came to the United States in the early nineteenth century and increased in popularity until the mid-twentieth century, when all homeopathic colleges were closed owing to the perception that they provided poor education. In the 1990s, approximately 500 to 1,000 medical doctors employed homeopathic practices, although homeopathy has been experiencing rebirth.

The danger of homeopathic medicine is in worsening a person's symptoms or muddling them, further obscuring the underlying cause. The benefits include the fact that there are few or no side effects, and no chance that an infection will develop resistance to the medicine, as it can to antibiotics. The United States does not subject homeopathic medicine to the safety and effectiveness trials that conventional drugs must undergo to be approved. In 1938, the FDA approved every medicine in the Homeopathic Pharmacopoeia of the United States; both prescribed and non-prescribed homeopathic medicine continue to be exempt, though those sold as over-the-counter must treat only self-limiting maladies, such as headaches, and must have labels detailing indications and ingredients.

Issues related to HOMEOPATHY *include* ALTERNATIVE MEDICINE; AMERICAN MEDICAL ASSOCIATION; FOOD AND DRUG ADMINISTRATION; *and* HERBAL MEDICINE. *Related information can also be found in* IMMUNITY *and* IMMUNE RESPONSE;

Homocystinuria

Also known as cystinuria

An inherited disorder in which the kidneys do not reabsorb certain amino acids adequately, so excessive amounts of these substances are present in the urine.

The symptoms of homocystinuria include blood in the urine, kidney stones, and extreme pain. These kidney stones will often contain the amino acid cystine. Damage to the kidneys may result from stones that cause urethral obstruction or infection. However, homocystinuria seldom results in kidney failure or severe damage. This disorder occurs in about 1 of 10,000 people.

Homocystinuria cannot be cured, but it can be managed. A large fluid intake is recommended, particularly of water. Different solutions or medications can be given to keep the urine alkaline and decrease cystine excretion. *See also* KIDNEY *and* URINE.

Homosexuality

Being physically attracted to members of one's own sex.

Homosexuality was once considered abnormal. Today it is recognized as a sexual orientation present from birth and early childhood. However, depending on the culture, certain patterns of lifestyle are still associated with homosexuality.

Normal human sexuality is thought to span a wide spectrum, ranging from exclusively heterosexual to exclusively homosexual. It is estimated that between six to ten percent of adults are involved in exclusively homosexual relationships. A much higher percentage experiment with same-sex activities during adolescence or early adulthood, but are later exclusively heterosexual. No particular hormonal, genetic or psychological causes have been proven to determine an individual's particular sexual orientation. What is clear is that homosexuality often appears not to be the result of a deliberate choice.

Some homosexuals, male and female, form long-lasting monogamous relationships. Others have multiple sexual contacts with different partners. This last type of behavior puts one greater at risk for contracting a sexually transmitted disease, regardless of orientation. *See also* BISEXUALITY; HETEROSEXUALITY; SEX; *and* SEXUALITY.

Hookworm Infestation

Infection by either of two species of intestinal parasitic roundworm.

Hookworm infestation is caused by contact with soil contaminated with larvae of either *Ancylostoma duodenale* or *Necator americanus*. These parasites' eggs are discharged with feces into the soil, hatching after about two days. Parasite larvae live in the soil before they penetrate the skin of those walking barefoot through fields. Traveling through the lymphatic vessels and the bloodstream, the hookworm larvae reaches the lungs. Larvae climb the respiratory tract and are swallowed, after which they penetrate the small intestine, attach themselves to the lining, and commence sucking blood.

Symptoms. Symptoms of hookworm infestation include an itchy rash near where the larvae penetrated the skin. Migration of the larvae through the lungs may produce fever, coughing, and pneumonia. When worms reach adult age they may produce abdominal discomfort, as well as iron deficiency anemia and intestinal bleeding.

Diagnosis is done by examining a stool sample, where the eggs of the hookworm are visible under a microscope. Treatment includes antihelminthic drugs, such as pyrantel pamoate or mebendazole. Treatment of anemia may require iron supplements, or in severe cases, blood transfusion. The best preventive measures are diligent sanitation and wearing footwear. *See also* ANEMIA; BLOOD CELLS; *and* PARASITE.

Hormone Replacement Therapy

Treatment of disorders with either synthetic or natural hormones.

Artificial and naturally obtained hormones can be used to treat a number of disorders. Androgen drugs may be given to males who lack the hormone needed for sexual development. Synthetic growth hormone may be used to stimulate normal growth in those who do not produce enough naturally. The gonadotrophins, follicle stimulating hormone (FSH) and lutenizing hormone (LH), may be used to treat infertility. The most common type of hormone replacement therapy, however, is the use of estrogens in post-menopausal women. *See also* HORMONES.

Estrogen replacement therapy is used to treat symptoms of menopause, such as hot flashes, night sweating, and vaginal dryness. However, its more important long-term effects are the prevention of atherosclerosis, or narrowing of the arteries, and osteoporosis, softening of the bones. By itself, estrogen can increase the potential for uterine cancer, so the estrogen is combined with doses of progesterone. The drugs are given either orally or via a patch applied to the skin. Common side effects of hormone replacement therapy may include breast tenderness, water retention, and weight gain. *See also* ANDROGEN HORMONES; ATHEROSCLEROSIS; DIAGNOSTICS IN WOMEN'S HEALTH; ESTROGEN DRUGS; ESTROGEN HORMONES; HOT FLASHES; MENOPAUSE; *and* PERIMENOPAUSE.

Hookworms. Below, these are the mouth parts of the hookworm, known medically and biologically as *Ancylostoma braziliense*. Dogs and cats are often infected by this particular species of hookworm. These are not uncommon in the Southeastern region of the United States, especially around Louisiana and Florida. The arrows in the top picture point to the 2 pairs of ventral teeth. Although hookworms are rarely life-threatening, dermatitis, pneumonia, and enteritis are all signs of a hookworm infestation.

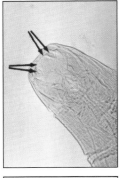

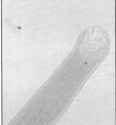

Hormones

Chemical substances that help the body carry out and maintain normal functions.

The endocrine system is composed of glands and organs that secrete chemical substances called hormones. While the nervous system uses nerve impulses to relay information, the hormones signal one another to commence or end their activities. Hormones travel through the bloodstream to the tissues or organs they control. Hormones often act in series, with complex interrelationships.

THE HYPOTHALAMUS AND THE PITUITARY GLAND

The hormonal chain of command begins in the brain, with the hypothalamus. The hypothalamus and the pituitary gland are connected through a small stalk containing blood vessels and nerves. When the hypothalamus detects stimuli that the body needs to react to in some way, it releases a hormone to the pituitary gland. That signals the pituitary to begin to release its own hormones, which will in turn set off others throughout the body and those will set off others, et cetera. These hormones, produced in the amount directed by the pituitary gland and hypothalamus, then travel to the organs and tissues they control. Some may activate other hormones while on the way.

EFFECTS OF HORMONAL DISORDERS ON THE BODY

Since hormones are closely related to one another, a single disorder can have an effect on numerous other bodily systems. A tumor in the pituitary gland, for example, may cause it to overproduce or underproduce any of its hormones, leading to a breakdown in such functions as metabolism, fluid balance, and sexual activity.

EXAMPLES OF HORMONES

Some hormones found in the body, as well as their functions are listed below:

- **ACTH** (adrenacorticotropic hormone). Released by pituitary gland; controls the production of corticosteroid hormones, mainly hydrocortisone, in the adrenal cortex, which help the body use its stores of fats, proteins, and carbohydrates; speeds up production of these hormones in response to stress, injury, heightened emotion, or other trauma.
- **ADH** (antidiuretic hormone). Produced by the pituitary gland; helps kidneys maintain balance of water in the body.
- **Aldosterone.** Released by the adrenal cortex, the exterior of the adrenal glands; maintains sodium levels in the blood.
- **Androgens.** Released by the testes, ovaries, and the adrenal cortex; androgens help produce secondary sexual characteristics in males and body hair in females.
- **Calcitonin.** Produced by the thyroid; maintains levels of calcium in the blood.
- **Chorionic Gonadotropin.** Produced by the placenta; helps the body maintain pregnancy.
- **Epinephrine & Norepinephrine.** Synthesized by the adrenal medulla, in the adrenal glands; helps the body handle stress by speeding up body's systems.
- **Erythropoietin.** Released by the kidneys; helps stimulate production of red blood cells.
- **Estrogen and Progesterone**. Produced in ovaries; helps develop female sexual characteristics; also maintains menstrual cycles and pregnancy.
- **FSH** (follicle stimulating hormone). Released by the pituitary gland; a gonadotropin hormone; stimulates activity in the gonads (ovaries or testes).
- **Gastrin, Secretin, & Cholecystokinin.** Produced by the gastrointestinal system; they help the stomach and gallbladder digest food, acting in response to fats and acids.
- **Glucagon**. Produced by the pancreas; helps to break down glycogen into glucose, a source of energy.
- **Growth Hormone.** Produced by the pituitary gland; helps cells grow and develop, and maintain lean body mass.

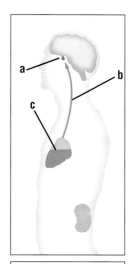

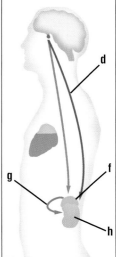

ACTH and Hormone Function. ACTH is a hormone that directs the adrenal gland in its hormone-releasing function. Top, (a) the pituitary gland is signaled via the vagus nerve (b) of low blood volume (c). The pituitary gland then produces vasopressin (d), the hormone that slows kidney filtration. Renin from the kidney (h) causes the adrenal glands (f) to produce aldosterone (g), which signals the kidney to retain salt.

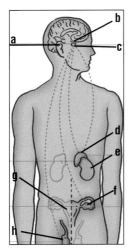

The Major Glands that Produce the Hormones. Above, hormones are produced in glands throughout the body. The hormone producing pineal gland (a), hypothalamus (b), and pituitary gland (c) are all found in and around the base of the brain. The adrenal gland (d) and the kidney (e)—are both located in the lower abdomen. These organs produce hormones that regulate absorption and release during digestion. The ovaries (f), uterus (g), and (in men) the testes (h) produce sex specific hormones.

- **Hydrocortisone.** Released by the adrenal cortex, the exterior of the adrenal glands; helps the body use fats, proteins, and carbohydrates for energy.
- **Insulin.** Synthesized by the pancreas; helps maintain glucose levels in blood.
- **LH** (luteinizing hormone). Released by the pituitary gland; a gonadotropin hormone, responsible for release of androgen and estrogen hormones.
- **MSH** (melanocyte-stimulating hormone). Released by the pineal gland; helps the skin produce melanin.
- **Oxytocin.** Produced by the pituitary gland; helps the uterus contract during labor, and helps lactation after delivery.
- **Parathyroid Hormone.** Released by the parathyroid glands; helps maintain normal levels of calcium in the blood.
- **Prolactin.** Released by the pituitary gland; stimulates the production of milk after childbirth.
- **Renin.** Produced by the kidneys; helps regulate aldosterone production and blood pressure.
- **Somatostatin**. Synthesized in the hypothalamus and the pancreas; balances the intestine's absorption of nutrients and regulates growth hormone secretion.
- **Testosterone**. Produced in the testes; aids growth and sexual development in males.
- **Thyroid Hormone.** Produced by thyroid; helps regulate metabolism, also necessary for growth and development.
- **TSH** (thyroid-stimulating hormone). Produced by the pituitary gland; stimulates release of thyroid hormones—regulating metabolism and growth.
- **Vitamin D.** Helps maintain levels of calcium and phosphates in the body.

Background material on Hormones may be found in ENDOCRINE SYSTEM; and GLANDS. Additional information regarding specific Hormones may be found in GROWTH HORMONE; LUTENIZING HORMONE; PROGESTERONE HORMONE; and FOLLICLE STIMULATING HORMONE. Hormones are also discussed in HORMONE REPLACEMENT THERAPY; INSULIN; GLUCAGON; PARATHYROID GLANDS; PITUITARY GLAND; PINEAL GLAND; THYROID GLAND; and VITAMIN D.

Horner's Syndrome

A group of physical manifestations that affect one side of the face.

Horner's syndrome is identified by a breach or break in a sympathetic (involuntary) nerve going to the face. This is often caused by accidental injury or damage as a result of surgery in the neck region. Symptoms include constriction of the pupil (miosis), drooping of the eyelid (ptosis), and a lack of facial sweating (anhidrosis).

Damage to the nerve fibers in the lower part of the neck is often an early sign of disease in the region. If the nerves in the neck are attacked by lung cancer, Horner's syndrome is often a side effect. *See also* NERVOUS SYSTEM *and* CENTRAL NERVOUS SYSTEM.

Horseshoe Kidney

A congenital malformation of the kidneys in which the bottom ends of the two organs are connected in a U-shape.

Horseshoe kidney usually causes no problems with kidney function, but it can result in complications, such as blood in the urine, kidney stones, urinary obstruction, and increased susceptibility to infection. The condition rarely causes kidney failure, and any resulting complications can usually be treated. Often, this condition remains undetected. *See also* KIDNEY; KIDNEY FUNCTION TEST; *and* KIDNEY, POLYCYSTIC.

Hospitals, Types of

Different categories of institutions designed to diagnose and treat sick individuals.

A hospital is an institution equipped to treat the sick and injured and house patients while they are treated. The most well-known type of hospital is a general hospital. These institutions offer a variety of services to the community by means of departments equipped with specially trained staff and a variety of sophisticated equipment. General hospitals are only one type of hospital, however. There are many other types, and two main ways to classify them; hospitals differ by ownership and type of by service offered.

OWNERSHIP

Some hospitals are owned by local or national governments, while others are owned by private institutions. Government-owned hospitals are supported by tax revenue. Nongovernmental hospitals further divide into two categories. Proprietary hospitals are operated on a for-profit basis for private gain. Other nongovernmental hospitals are operated on a nonprofit basis for the communal good. Hospitals in the latter category are often operated by churches, fraternal orders, universities, or independent associates. They are called voluntary hospitals.

Outside the United States, most hospitals are government-owned. In most countries, however, a few small proprietary institutions exist, often with a capacity of fewer than 50 beds. Nongovernmental hospitals account for less than five percent of the hospitals in the world.

SERVICES

Hospitals may be classified as general or special. A general hospital, as described above, treats most types of medical and surgical cases. General hospitals also provide maternity service and treatment for children. Special hospitals, however, provide services for only one or two classes of patients, or types of illness. Some hospitals treat only mental illnesses, contagious diseases, or cancer. Special hospitals account for nearly 1,000 of the 6,500 hospitals in the United States.

There are also a number of other ways to classify hospitals. Hospitals are civilian or military institutions. Military hospitals treat sick or wounded soldiers. Military physicians and their assistants provide treatment. Some military hospitals are known as mobile field hospitals. Staff and equipment for these hospitals follow the movement of troops to provide emergency treatment to the wounded.

Some hospitals affiliated with universities are teaching hospitals. Doctors train at these hospitals by providing treatment as part of their medical schooling or post-medical school training. Teaching hospitals are more likely to have cutting-edge technologies and experimental treatments than most other types of hospitals.

Information relevant to a discussion of Types of Hospitals is included in AMERICAN MEDICAL ASSOCIATION; DOCTOR, CHOOSING A; ETHICS, MEDICAL; MEDICAID; MEDICARE; *and* PUBLIC HEALTH. *Special related topics include* EMERGENCY HOSPITALIZATION; *and* MENTAL HOSPITAL.

Hot Flashes

Brief sensations of heat, a common symptom of menopause.

Changes in hormonal levels can often cause unpleasant side effects while the body tries to adjust. The loss of estrogen caused by menopause, ovary removal, or in men the removal the testes, can lead to the symptom known as hot flashes. This usually consist of a feeling of heightened body temperature, accompanied by reddening of the face, neck, and upper body, along withexcessive sweating. The flashes usually last about two or three minutes. They are most likely to occur at the end of the day, overnight, or during times of stress. Hot weather, food, or beverages may exacerbate them.

Hot flashes may continue to occur for as long as it takes the body to adjust to its new level of hormones. Until then, some measures may be taken to reduce their effects. Avoiding alcohol and caffeine can help, as can exercise and other methods of stress reduction. If the hot flashes are severe and disruptive, estrogen replacement therapy may be recommended for women and testosterone for men if there is no medical reason to withhold the therapy. Estrogen or testosterone may be taken orally or released through a transcutaneous patch. *See* DIET AND DISEASE; ESTROGEN HORMONES; HORMONE REPLACEMENT THERAPY; MENOPAUSE; PERIMENOPAUSE; *and* STRESS;.

Huntington's Chorea

Also known as St. Vitus' disease

A progressive degenerative neurological disorder.

Huntington's chorea is an inherited disease that causes cells in the cerebrum to waste away. The prevalence in the population is 1 to 2 per 25,000. Huntington's chorea is caused by an abnormal gene that is passed on to children. Symptoms do not appear until late in life, so affected individuals have children without realizing that they have the disease. In the past, it was impossible to determine if an individual had Huntington's chorea before the onset of symptoms; now, those who suspect they may have inherited Huntington's chorea can be tested for the presence of the gene.

Symptoms usually appear between the ages of 35 and 50. These include involuntary twitching, difficulty walking, personality changes, intellectual deterioration, and hesitant speech. The disease develops slowly, and the severity depends upon the degree of cell loss. Personality changes may be one of the earliest symptoms. Severe chorea and dementia appear as the disease progresses. Death occurs after many years—typically 15 and sometimes up to 30. There is no cure or treatment to halt progression of the disease, but medication may be prescribed to reduce the effects of the chorea. *See also* BRAIN *and* DEMENTIA.

Hurler's Syndrome

A collection of severe birth defects caused by a genetic anomaly.

Hurler's syndrome is seen in approximately 1 in every 10,000 births. It is characterized by dwarfism, mental retardation, curved spine, short and thick arm and leg bones, thick lips, large tongue and small malformed teeth. The cause is believed to be a chromosomal anomaly. Children with Hurler's syndrome generally live until their early teens. *See also* BIRTH DEFECTS; CHROMOSOME; CHROMOSOMAL ABNORMALITIES; DNA; *and* GENETIC ABNORMALITIES.

Hydatid Disease

Rare parasitic disease caused by the larvae of an intestinal tapeworm.

Hydatid disease occurs through the implantation of *Echinococcus granulosus* larvae in the liver, lungs, or the brain and the development of cysts. The disease primarily affects those living in a region where sheep are herded with the aid of dogs.

The close contact of dogs and sheep sustains a continual infestation within the dog and the sheep population. The eggs of the worm are passed in the dogs' feces. Any ingestion of soil contaminated with the eggs results in infestation. In human populations, children are the usual victims of this sort of infestation. *See also* JAUNDICE.

After migrating to the liver, lungs, or brain, the larvae cause cysts. These grow slowly, and symptoms of their presence may not be exhibited for years. In many cases, symptoms never become present. The severity of the resulting hydatid disease is dependent on the size and location of cysts.

A cyst in the liver may become a sensitive lump that obstructs the bile duct and results in jaundice. A cyst in the lungs may obstruct the airway and result in bronchitis. Cysts in the brain function like brain tumors, causing headaches, vision disturbances, seizures, paralysis, or death. Wherever they are implanted, cysts of this sort sometimes rupture and result in coughing up blood (hemoptysis) or a life-threatening allergic reaction (anaphylactic shock). *See also* ANAPHYLACTIC SHOCK.

People with hydatid disease may remain asymptomatic for decades, before abdominal pain and a palpable mass develops. Diagnosis is usually made after symptoms are reported, followed by x-ray or CT scanning. Treatment usually requires surgical excision of the cysts and worms, and administering anti-parasite mediations. Repeated worming of dogs in sheep-raising areas, as well as destruction of sheep offal and carcasses, offer the best prevention against the disease. *See* CYST; INTESTINE; LIVER; TAPEWORM INFESTATION; *and* WORM INFESTATION.

Hydatidiform Mole

An abnormal cluster of cells that develop in the uterus instead of the placenta.

The tissue around a fertilized egg normally develops into the placenta, which provides a link between the fetal and maternal bloodstreams for the exchange of nutrients, minerals, and waste materials. Sometimes, however, this tissue develops into an abnormal grape-like cluster of cells instead. This structure, called a hydatidiform mole, continues to grow even after the fetus, if there was one, degenerates. *See also* FETUS.

The mole produces the pregnancy hormone human chorionic gonadotropin (hCG), resulting in a positive pregnancy test. The uterus continues to grow, but larger than expected according to the dates. Hydatidiform moles are more common among older women. They occur in approximately 1 in 2,000 pregnancies in the United States, with a higher incidence in other parts of the world. *See also* UTERUS.

An early warning sign is usually some vaginal bleeding, often followed by the passage of grape-like material. The absence of a fetal heartbeat is also an indication that the pregnancy is abnormal. Ultrasound can determine if there is a normal sac present in the uterus. Any placental tissue left in the uterus after childbirth or after a miscarriage has the potential of becoming a mole. Other than that, the cause of hydatidiform moles is largely unknown.

Treatment involves surgical removal, usually by D&E (dilation and evacuation), followed by monitoring of hCG levels for 12 months afterwards. For this reason, it is recommended that a woman avoid pregnancy until the year is up. *See* D AND C.

Eighty percent of all hydatidform moles are benign. However, 15 percent become invasive, growing into the uterine wall, and five percent develop into a choriocarcinoma, a form of cancer. The hCG levels should fall to normal within eight weeks, unless a cancerous growth develops. Even if that is the case, the cure rate is high. *See also* CANCER; HYSTERECTOMY; *and* UTERUS.

Hydramnios

Swelling caused by the accumulation of excessive amounts of amniotic fluid during pregnancy.

Amniotic fluid acts as a cushion and "shock absorber" around the developing baby during pregnancy. The amount of fluid in the uterus is regulated by the fetus, which begins to urinate and swallow amniotic fluid during the second trimester. Hydramnios is sometimes associated with birth defects involving the central nervous system or gastrointestinal tract. The fetus may be unable to swallow amniotic fluid or else is producing an abnormally large amount of urine. Hydramnios may also occur in diabetic women and in pregnancies involving multiple fetuses. Symptoms include breathlessness, nausea, abdominal distention and pain, and premature labor.

Only in about 1 in every 1,000 pregnancies is the condition severe enough to cause pain. If the hydramnios is slight, treatment may consist of nothing more than additional rest. If the pain is severe, however, hospitalization may be necessary. Various medications may be administered to relax the uterus and prevent premature labor. Sometimes amniotic fluid is withdrawn in a procedure similar to amniocentesis in order to relieve the pressure. However, this amniotomy must be repeated several times and may trigger premature labor. *See also* AMNIOCENTESIS; CONCEPTION; DELIVERY; PREGNANCY; *and* UTERUS.

Hydrocele

An accumulation of fluid under the membrane that surrounds the testes.

The membrane that surrounds the testes can become filled with fluid. Sometimes this is apparent at birth but, more often it occurs later in life. The condition is neither painful nor dangerous, though the accumulation can become large enough to be rather uncomfortable, in which case it is drained surgically. *See also* PENIS; REPRODUCTIVE SYSTEM, MALE; SURTERY *and* TESTES.

Hydrocephalus

Also known as water on the brain

An accumulation of cerebrospinal fluid in the cranial cavity.

An uncommon disorder, hydrocephalus is caused by fluid absorption in the head. This causes great amounts of fluid to accumulate, the head to swell, and the bones of the skull to slowly spread apart. If this serious disorder is not treated, it can cause brain damage and increase the risk of a dangerous infection. Hydrocephalus is caused by an infection in the mother during pregnancy, or a developmental problem, such as aqueductal stenosis. After birth, the cause may be tumors, cysts, infection, or bleeding. *See also* CYST *and* SKULL.

The disorder can be treated depending on the cause, thereby preventing permanent brain damage. The most common treatment is surgically inserting a shunt to drain the excess fluid from the brain to the abdominal cavity. The head size will gradually return to normal as the baby grows up. The shunt should be monitored to ensure it is working correctly. *See also* BRAIN; INFECTION; SHUNT; SWELLING; *and* TUMOR.

Hydronephrosis

Enlargement of the kidney resulting from the accumulation of urine.

Urine flows out of a kidney and into the bladder through two channels, the ureters. That flow can be reduced if a ureter is blocked or narrowed by a stone, a tumor, a blood clot, or an enlarged prostate gland. A severe, sudden blockage can cause acute pain, but slowly progressing hydronephrosis may cause no symptoms. Untreated, the condition can result in a kidney infection or kidney failure. The problem is usually treated through surgery to remove the blockage, but occasionally a kidney is damaged so badly that it must be removed. *See also* BLADDER; KIDNEY; KIDNEY STONE; PROSTATE GLAND; URINARY DIVERSION; *and* URINARY TRACT INFECTION.

Hydrops

Fetal swelling or edema.

Hydrops is a rare fetal abnormality that has many causes. It may occur as a result of fetal anemia due to Rh disease (when mother and child have different Rh blood factors). This condition requires evaluation by a maternal-fetal medicine specialist.

Hydrotherapy

Use of water as a form of therapy or treatment for disease.

Hydrotherapy consists of any form of treatment that involves water, either taken internally or used externally to promote healing. This includes many forms of bathing, wraps, douches, saunas, and water exercise.

Water has been used for many centuries and by many cultures for therapeutic purposes; however, it was reintroduced and became quite popular in European curative spas in the nineteenth century. Most of these spas featured water cures that used natural spring water at very hot or cold temperatures. Hot water is thought to slow the activity of the internal organs, relaxing

Hydrotherapy Precautions

Otis G. Carroll developed hydrotherapeutic treatment method, called constitutional hydrotherapy, in 1908. His method added electrostimulation to the more traditional use of hot and cold packs and compresses. He believed that the electricity was supposed to stimulate the nervous system, while the application of hot and cold compresses enhanced the constitution of tissues and cells. Today, practitioners believe that this sort of therapy increases the body's white blood cell count, thus benefiting the immune system. However, critical researchers point out that nearly anything, from a good night's rest to a cold shower, can increase the number of white blood cells. There are some people that should not undergo hydrotherapy at all; individuals with asthma, kidney disease, a weak heart (especially if a pacemaker has been implanted), blood disorders, metal implants, and those who have lost feeling in part of their body should avoid intensive hydrotherapy treatments.

the body, while cold water increases the activity of the internal organs and invigorates the body.

TYPES OF HYDROTHERAPY

Baths. Herbal, mineral, as well as foot and arm baths are often used to alleviate stress and to treat specific bone and muscular ailments. Sitz baths (hip baths) involve using hot and cold water together.

Whirlpools and Exercise. Water in motion, using therapeutic water activities or whirlpools, can massage the body and alleviate muscle tension.

Douches. Douches involve the alternation of hot and cold water sprayed on different parts of the body.

Compresses and Packs. A compress is made from an absorbent material soaked in either hot or cold water, then applied to a part of the body. Packs are usually larger and are used to wrap an entire portion of the body.

Enemas. Water enemas require an individual to consume mineral water in order to cleanse the lower intestine and eliminate toxins. This method is often used to treat constipation or fecal impaction.

HYDROTHERAPY *should be discussed in relation to* ALTERNATIVE MEDICINE; NATUROPATHY; WATER; *and* WATER SAFETY. *Also relevant are articles detailing* DOUCHE; ENEMA; EXERCISE; *and* MASSAGE. *Also refer to* SITZ BATH *and* WAX BATH.

Hygiene

Cleanliness as a means of preserving health.

Hygiene is technically the practice of preserving health, but is most commonly associated with cleanliness. Hygiene in relation to issues of public health refers to the study of those factors that affect health, such as sanitary water, housing, and workplaces. Poor hygiene can enable the spread of infectious diseases, ranging from common colds, flu, and athlete's foot to serious diseases such as Lyme disease or Hanta virus.

Good hygiene that prevents disease begins with as simple a measure sucha as regularly washing the hands with warm soapy water. Keeping household areas, especially the kitchen and dining room, and wherever else food is prepared and served, clean and disinfected—is another easy way to prevent the spread of bacteria and germs.

Soap and hot water will remove most germs and dirt, but in areas that are prone to high amounts of dangerous germs, disinfectants (such as bleach and other widely available commercial products) will kill germs on surfaces that otherwise appear to be completely clean. Germ "hot zones" include the kitchen and bathroom. Careful, regular cleaning of these areas will cut down immensely on the spread of germs that cause disease.

For background information related to Hygiene *see* GERM; *and* ORAL HYGIENE. *An in depth perspective of issues concerning* Hygiene *can be found in* ENVIRONMENTAL MEDICINE; PUBLIC HEALTH; *and* PUBLIC HEALTH DENTISTRY. *See also* BACTERIA; INFECTIOUS DISEASES; *and* WATER.

Hygroma, Cystic

Also known as lymphangioma

An inborn tumor of the lymphatic system.

Cystic hygroma is characterized by a large sac filled with lymph fluid. This sack protrudes either from the skull or at the nape of the neck. A cystic hygroma often feels as though it is filled with water but there is no need for any serious worry because it is always benign. *See also* SKULL.

This condition occurs almost exclusively in small children and infants; cystic hygroma is present in about 1 of every 6,000 births. Researchers have discovered a relationship between the incidence of cystic hygroma and cases of Turner and Down's syndrome. *See also* CRYING IN INFANTS.

The large lymph sac rarely causes any major physical problems, unless it puts pressure on the airway, but it is usually cosmetically unpleasant because the hygroma may cover a significant area. For that reason, surgical removal is always recommended. *See also* DOWN'S SYNDROME; LYMPH; LYMPH NODE; LYMPHATIC SYSTEM; SURGERY; *and* TURNER SYNDROME.

Hymen

A membrane located across the vaginal opening.

The hymen partially or fully blocks or encircles, the vaginal opening. An intact hymen does not impede menstrual flow. In many cases, the hymen is torn during the first incidence of penetrative sexual intercourse, although it can also rupture due to other causes. A small amount of bleeding may occur when the hymen is torn. The degree of tightness varies among women, so the hymen may be pliable enough that it does not tear during intercourse. *See also* VAGINA.

Hyperacidity

The stomach's oversecretion of hydrochloric acid.

Hyperacidity occurs when the stomach secretes an excessive amount of hydrochloric acid. This condition was once believed to be the sole cause of heartburn. Recent evidence, however, indicates that hyperacidity alone is not sufficient; heartburn also results from excessive gastric secretions whenever esophageal reflux occurs.

Hyperacidity is a contributing factor in the development of duodenal ulcers and some gastric ulcers. Other types of ulcers, however, are not associated with excessive acid levels. *See also* ULCER *and* STOMACH.

Hyperactivity

A general tendency toward restlessness or excessive movement usually found in children with minimal brain dysfunction or hyperkinesis.

There have been some recent reports that have linked certain foods to Attention Deficit Disorder (ADD). Food dyes, additives, and sugar have all also been accused of causing certain degrees of hyperactivity in young children.

Children who are hyperactive may also develop hyperkinetic syndrome, a disorder of childhood that is characterized by excessive energy, emotional instability, significantly short attention span, and an absence of fear and shyness. Occasionally, the syndrome develops in children with brain injury, mental defects, or epilepsy.

Hyperactivity may also exist in children with ADD, in which case it is known as Attention Deficit Hyperactive Disorder (ADHD). These children display short attention spans, as well as highly impulsive and hyperactive behavior.

There are no laboratory tests to diagnose the condition; each child must be evaluated separately. Young boys are ten times more likely to be diagnosed with ADD than young girls.

The Myth About Sweets

Teachers and parents often claim that giving children sugary snacks causes them to be hyperactive. However, scientists have not found any increase in movement or discipline problems in children after they have eaten candy or sweets. Sugar does not make unaffected children hyperactive, and it does not make hyperactive children more energetic. There is no need to limit sugar due to worries about hyperactivity. However, sugar is the major cause of tooth decay in children.

Treatment includes counseling, special schools or classes, and sometimes drug therapy. Methylphenidate, a central nervous system stimulant, is the most common drug prescribed. Recently, there has been controversy over alleged over prescription practices. *See* ATTENTION DEFICIT DISORDER.

Hyperaldosteronism

Also known as aldosteronism

The excess production of aldosterone.

Aldosterone, a hormone secreted by the adrenal cortex, regulates levels of sodium in the blood, which helps to maintain normal blood pressure and blood volume. A tumor in the adrenal gland (Conn's syndrome) or any other disorder that slows down blood flow to the kidney, such as heart failure or cirrhosis of the liver, may cause the overproduction of aldosterone. Symptoms include high blood pressure, tiredness, and weakness. Treatment may consist of drugs to prevent the effect of aldosterone on the kidneys, along with a salt restricted diet. If a tumor is the cause, it may be surgically removed; most individuals usually recover completely and quickly. *See also* ADRENAL GLANDS; ALDOSTERONISM; BLOOD PRESSURE; CONN'S SYNDROME; HORMONES; KIDNEY; LIVER; SODIUM; TUMOR; SURGERY; *and* WATER.

Hyperalimentation

Now called parenteral nutrition

Delivering nutrients directly into the bloodstream.

Hyperalimentation is given when a person is unable to eat or eat adequately and is instead fed through a catheter directed into the bloodstream. Short term parenteral nutrition is generally given through a vein in the hand or arm. In some cases, the intravenous solutions cause the vein to become irritated and clots develop; when this happens, a new vein must be found. Long-term parenteral nutrition is administered via an intravenous catheter placed in a large vein close to the heart. There, the increased amount of blood flow allows for the feeding solution to be diluted, so that the site can be used for a longer duration. This method for feeding, however, poses substantial risks and generally it is used when feeding through a tube is ineffective. *See also* ARTIFICIAL FEEDING; NUTRITION; INTRAVENOUS INFUSION; VEIN; *and* CATHETER.

Hyperbaric Oxygen Treatment

The use of pressurized oxygen in a chamber to treat certain diseases.

Hyperbaric oxygen treatment can be administered in two ways. In one method, the patient lies on a stretcher, which is slid into a chamber and sealed. Pure oxygen is then used to pressurize the chamber. The second method is to treat several patients at once in a large chamber. Each patient breathes the oxygen through a face mask or a hood. Both types of treatment are equally effective. There are several approved conditions for which hyperbaric oxygen treatment may be prescribed to treat. These conditions include gas embolism, carbon dioxide poisoning, crush injury, decompression sickness, gas gangrene, certain wound problems, severe anemias, necrotizing infections, osteomyelitis, radiation tissue damage, compromising skin grafts, thermal burns, intracranial abscess, and diabetic sores. *See also* ABSCESS; ANEMIA; BURNS; RADIATION; OSTEOMYELITIS; SKIN; *and* WOUND.

Hypercalcemia

An increased plasma concentration of calcium

Hypercalcemia has many causes, not the least of which is cancer. Between 10 and 20 percent of all cancer patients develop this condition. It is especially a concern for cancer patients older than 65.

The calcium levels in the blood are regulated by three major hormones: calcitonin, calcitrol, and parathyroid hormone. If any of these hormones falls out of balance, due either to over- or underproduction (as can caused by cancer for example), then the calcium levels can increase to levels that may cause a crisis.

Calcium is usually absorbed by the intestine and stored in the bones. Sometimes the overabsorbtion of calcium can be mediated by the kidney, which absorbs calcium, and the condition will remain mild and go unnoticed.

Symptoms. Symptoms tend to depend on how high the calcium levels are raised. Slight increases are hard to detect and symptoms generally do not develop. Greater calcium level increases are marked by nausea, vomiting, abdominal pain, constipation, depression, and headache. The highest levels can result in coma.

Many people die within a month of treatment. The survival rate after one year is also quite low. *See also* AGING; BONE; CALCIUM; CANCER; CONSTIPATION; DIGESTIVE SYSTEM; HORMONES; HYPERPARATHYROIDISM; INTESTINE; KIDNEY; *and* MILK.

Hypercapnia

An excess of carbon dioxide in the blood.

If the carbon dioxide concentration in the blood is high, a person with hypercapnia will become confused and sleepy; the body will try to rid itself of the carbon dioxide by deep, rapid breathing. Hypercapnia may be caused by slowed breathing, as in an alcohol-induced stupor; by inhaling polluted or inadequately oxygenated air; or by a lung disorder caused by disease. Oxygen is used to treat the immediate symptoms; underlying conditions need to be assessed and treated appropriately. *See also* SLEEP.

Hypercoagulable State

A state in which there is a propensity for blood clots to form in the body.

In a hypercoagulable state, the body is more likely to form blood clots. The cause of the blood clots depends on the specific illness. Several inherited, acquired, and genetic conditions including pregnancy and inflammatory disorders, may cause hypercoagulability. There are several anticoagulation drugs available that will thin an individual's blood. *See also* THROMBOSIS.

Hyperemesis

Excessive vomiting during pregnancy.

Hyperemesis usually occurs in the first trimester of pregnancy, and it is different from the more common "morning sickness." This condition is related to hormone production and may be aggravated by stress. Other symptoms include an inability to eat, nausea, and persistent retching.

This will cause dehydration, fevers, and (in some cases) jaundice; the blood may contain bile, and acute cases of starvation may result. Since the dehydration and nutrient deficiencies can be severe, intravenous nutrient administration is not uncommon. Sedatives may also be administered. *See also* PREGNANCY.

Hyperglycemia

When the blood sugar is abnormally high, often a consequence of diabetes.

In a normal digestive system, carbohydrates and sugars are converted into glucose. The pancreas releases a hormone called insulin to regulate blood glucose. When the blood glucose level goes up, the pancreas secretes insulin, which moves the glucose into the body's cells and tissues to be used for energy.

ALERT
Diabetic Emergencies

High blood sugar (hyperglycemia) can lead to coma, and low blood sugar (hypoglycemia) can lead to shock. Either can render a person unconscious. These are potentially fatal emergencies and must be dealt with immediately. A person who is known to be diabetic and has fruity breath is suffering from diabetic ketoacidosis caused by hyperglycemia. The person may seem to be inebriated, or may be unconscious; he or she may be feeling extremely thirsty; urinating frequently; or breathing heavily. If a person is sweaty, he or she may be suffering from hypoglycemia. People suffering from hypoglycemia may sweat heavily and act paranoid or belligerent. Consuming sugary food should lead to recovery—if a person is unconscious, emergency assist- ance must be contacted immediately.

People with diabetes produce too little insulin (if they produce any at all) or they produce insulin at inappropriate times. Without the control that insulin provides, the glucose level in the blood gets too high. Without the necessary insulin in the blood, the body begins to break down fat in order to supply energy to the cells. Too much fat breakdown can raise blood acid levels, leading to an emergency situation.

Medications and home therapy devices are available to regulate blood glucose. Insulin can be taken by injection; drugs that enhance insulin production or action may also be taken orally. An individual with diabetes must learn to regulate his or her treatment in order to avoid hyper- or hypoglycemia. *See also* DIABETES INSIPIDUS *and* DIABETES MELLITUS.

Hyperhidrosis

Abnormally excessive sweating.

In most cases, hyperhidrosis manifests itself by unusual sweating from the palms, soles, and armpits. It may occur on its own, or as part of a group of symptoms indicating a disorder in the nerves of the peripheral system. Perpetually damp palms may hinder the ability to carry out normal activities, both professional and social. In addition, the cellular material produced by the glands in the armpits and feet can lead to body odor, if left on the skin's surface. While the condition may clear up on its own, anticholinergic drugs, including benztropine and trihexyphenidyl, which affect the autonomic nervous system, may also be prescribed. *See also* SWEAT.

Hyperkeratosis

Thickening of the outer layer of skin due to increased amounts of keratin.

Corns and calluses are the most common forms of hyperkeratosis. These are caused by prolonged rubbing or friction of the skin with another object. Plantar warts also involve hyperkeratosis. The term is also used to describe the thickening of the nails due to fungal infections and psoriasis.

Hyperlipidemias

A condition in which the fat content of the blood is abnormally high.

Two major categories of fats are present in the bloodstream. Cholesterol and triglycerides attach themselves to proteins (called lipoproteins), and are one of the main sources of energy for the muscles of the body; these are also used in the structure of other tissues. Both are necessary for good health, yet an overabundance of these fats creates the danger of heart disease and stroke because of clogging of the arteries.

The body attempts to control the amount of fat in the blood by curtailing the production of lipoproteins or regulating their removal; however, a high-fat diet can override these vital mechanisms. In addition, it is evident that hereditary factors are involved in setting the baseline levels in people. *See also* CHOLESTEROL.

Good and Bad Cholesterol

Most of the body's cholesterol is manufactured in the liver. Vegetable and fish oils are rich in polyunsaturated fats; olive and canola oils are rich in monounsaturated fats, and meats and dairy products carry saturated fats. The polyunsaturated and monounsaturated fats are converted to high density lipoproteins (HDL), whereas the saturated fats are become low density lipoproteins (LDL) or very low density lipoproteins (VLDL). VLDL and LDL are "bad" cholesterols because they clog up the arteries and reduce blood flow to brain and heart. The "good" cholesterol, HDL, helps clear the arteries. The recommended maximum total cholesterol intake is 200 mg/dl, and minimum HDL is 45 mg/dl.

The main treatment for high triglyceride levels is simply making lifestyle changes: avoiding foods with saturated fats, not smoking, getting regular exercise, and weight loss, if necessary. If cholesterol levels remain high, and the person is at risk of heart disease or has already had a heart attack, a doctor may prescribe one of a number of cholesterol lowering drugs. *See also* ARTERY; BLOOD; DIET AND DISEASE; EXERCISE; FATS AND OILS; FATTY ACIDS; HEART; HEREDITY; PROTEINS; *and* STROKE.

Hyperparathyroidism

A condition caused by excess production of parathyroid hormone.

The parathyroid glands produce parathyroid hormone, which regulates the calcium in the blood. Calcium helps cells to function, muscles to contract, blood to clot and nerves to transmit and accept impulses. When calcium levels are abnormal, the production of the parathyroid hormone increases or decreases in order to signal the bones, intestines, and kidneys to adjust their calcium use to normalize circulating levels. If too much is secreted, then the balance of

Hyperparathyroidism. Below, the parathyroid glands are located behind the thyroid gland; they are very small, and produce the parathyroid hormone that controls blood calcium levels. About 1 in 1,000 people over 60 years old have hyperparathyroidism, but incidence has been declining in recent years, according to the American Academy of Family Physicians.

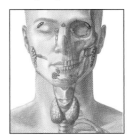

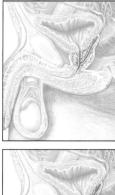

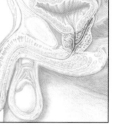

Prostate Hyperplasia.
Top, a normal prostate gland is shown in color. The prostate's cells have multiplied—possibly due to the overproduction of TSHs (thyroid stimulating hormones)—and produced the prostate with benign prostatic plasia, below.

calcium is disturbed and the organs malfunction. Bones thin as the intestines absorb too much calcium, and the kidneys release excess calcium; this causes stones to form.

The most common cause is a tumor in a parathyroid gland, or a glandular enlargement. Abnormally low levels of calcium in the blood can also cause excess hormone production. Symptoms include fatigue, back and joint pain, and fractures caused by fragile bones. Interference in the gastrointestinal balance of calcium absorption can cause abdominal pain, loss of appetite, and nausea. *See also* CALCIUM *and* KIDNEY.

The condition is diagnosed with blood calcium levels. Treatment may include surgery to remove the tumor and, if necessary, part or all of the gland. If the remaining parathyroid tissue does not produce enough parathyroid hormone (hypoparathyroidism), then that condition may be treated with vitamin D to help manage calcium absorption. *See also* BLOOD; BLOOD TESTS; GLANDS; HORMONES; HYPOPARATHYROIDISM; KIDNEYS; SURGERY; *and* VITAMIN D.

Hyperplasia

Increase in the size of a tissue or organ.

Hyperplasia is caused by the multiplication of an organ's cells, as opposed to hypertrophy, which is a growth due to the increase in size of the existing cells. Hyperplasia can be triggered by a hormone, either normally, as in changes in tissues during pregnancy, or abnormally, as may be caused by overactive hormone production by a gland.

Hyperpyrexia

Also known as malignant hyperthermia

A condition that causes a severe fever during anesthesia or while using muscle relaxants.

A predisposition toward this condition may be inherited by a child when only one parent has the genetic trait. It is also associated with muscular disorders, such as muscular dystrophy and central core diseases. Hyperpyrexia is usually diagnosed during the first

administration of anesthesia; a person develops a high fever and rigid muscles. Muscle tissue is destroyed, and re- leased myoglobin can damage the kidneys and cause acute renal failure. Volatile gas anesthetics—such as halothane, enflurane, isoflurane, sevoflurane, and desflurane, which induce general anesthesia—will cause hyperpyrexia in those with a disposition toward this disorder. If it is not treated promptly, the condition can be fatal. Hyperpyrexia can be prevented by administering a dose of dantrolene sodium before anesthesia. Before surgery, a family history should always be taken. *See also* FEVER.

Hypersplenism

A condition in which the spleen is enlarged and may destroy necessary blood cells.

The function of the spleen is to clean up the small particles of worn-out blood cells, bacteria, fungi, and viruses. The spleen enlarges in response to a number of different illnesses. An enlarged spleen traps more and more damaged cells. Eventually it gets clogged, and this begins a vicious circle: the larger the spleen, the more it traps; the more it traps, the more it enlarges, to the point where it begins to destroy normal cells. Hypersplenism refers to the situation in which the spleen takes too many blood cells out of the circulation.

Symptoms of hypersplenism are anemia, a lowered immune capacity due to a reduction in white blood cells, and poor blood clotting due to a loss of platelets. An enlarged spleen may press against the stomach, causing the individual to feel full even after a light meal. There may be back pain or abdominal pain. A physical examination will usually reveal the enlargement of the spleen. *See also* ANEMIA.

Treatment starts with the discovery of the underlying cause of spleen enlargement. If the spleen is destroying too many cells, then it will have to be surgically removed. Radiation may also be prescribed to reduce the size of the spleen. *See also* BLOOD; BLOOD CELLS; *and* SPLEEN.

Hypertension

Blood pressure that is dangerously high.

As blood flows through the body, it exerts pressure against the walls of the arteries, the vessels carrying oxygenated blood from the heart. Blood pressure increases when the heart contracts and decreases when the heart relaxes. Blood pressure is expressed in two numbers. Systolic pressure, the higher number that is written first or on top, is the pressure exerted on the arteries during the contraction of the heart. Diastolic pressure, the lower number that is written second or the number on the bottom, is the pressure when the heart relaxes (sometimes called resting pressure). Those two pressures are expressed as millimeters of mercury, mm Hg, referring to the height to which a column of mercury is raised in a sphygmomanometer (blood pressure measuring device).

An optimal blood pressure for a healthy young adult is about 120/80, although it can range from 110/70 to 140/90. Blood pressure tends to increase with age. A child will have readings lower than those of a young adult, and older persons will have higher readings. At any age, persistent elevation of blood pressure above 140/90 is regarded as hypertension.

Race and Hypertension

The incidence of hypertension is quite high in people of African descent. Research has shown that a high level of blood sodium, which raises blood pressure, is protective against malaria, a major threat in Africa. Early detection and treatment of hypertension in people of African ethnicity is essential to preventing stroke. Currently, African Americans are 50 percent more likely to die of stroke and twice as likely to have a nonfatal stroke than white Americans.

Treatment is essential because hypertension is a major risk factor for cardiovascular disease. About one-third of all heart attacks and strokes occur in people with hypertension. But while one in every four adult Americans has hypertension, only half of them are aware of the condition and being treated for it. In addition to the 50 million adults with hypertension, an estimated 34 million others have borderline blood pressure elevations, so fewer than half of all adults have blood pressure readings in the healthy range. Hypertension is more common in men than in women until early middle age, when the incidence is greater in women than in men.

CAUSES

Nine of every ten cases of hypertension are described as idiopathic, meaning that the cause is not known. There appears to be a genetic factor, since hypertension can run in families. Cigarette smoking and obesity are associated with idiopathic high blood pressure, as is a diet high in salt. The sodium in salt (which, chemically, is sodium chloride) causes the body to retain excess fluid, increasing blood pressure.

A lack of physical activity also increases the risk of hypertension. Persons who lead sedentary lives, without any regular exercise, have been found to be 50 percent more likely to develop hypertension than people who are active. Stress is also known to cause at least a temporary increase in blood pressure, although the overall role of stress and personality in hypertension remains a matter of some controversy.

Oral contraceptives may increase blood pressure above the normal level, and hypertension occurs in up to 10 percent of pregnancies. Generally, pressure returns to normal after birth. In 10 percent of cases, hypertension is caused by an underlying disorder, such as diseases affecting the kidneys or the adrenal glands.

SYMPTOMS

In most cases, hypertension causes no symptoms. Very severe hypertension may cause dizziness, but this is rare. Despite its dangers, hypertension generally is detected only during examination by a physician or through self-testing.

DIAGNOSIS

The most widely used way of diagnosing hypertension is by use of a sphygmomanome-

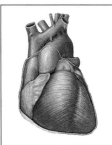

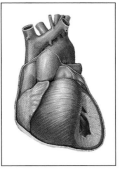

The Hypertensive Heart. Top, the normal heart that is not affected by hypertension has normal ventricular walls. The bottom image shows the hypertensive heart. The walls of the hypertensive heart have thickened. This causes the cardiac muscle to work harder, increasing the risk of a heart attack.

Resources on Hypertension

Berne, Robert M., et al., *Cardiovascular Physiology* (2001); Debakey, Michael E. and Antonio M. Gotto, *The New Living Heart* (1997); Gould, Lance K., *Heal Your Heart* (2000); American Heart Association, Tel. (800) 242-8721, Online: www.amhrt.org; Heart Information Network, Tel. (973) 701-6035, Online: www.heartinfo. org; National Heart, Lung, and Blood Institute, Tel. (301) 496-4236, Online: www. nhlbi.nih.gov; www.ny-cornell.org/cardiothracic. surgery/; www.nycor-nell.org/medicine/cardiol-ogy/index.html; www.nycornell.org/medi-cine/cp/index.html.

The Effects of Hypertension on the Kidneys. Below, the kidney is especially sensitive to the effects of hypertension. The kidneys filter wastes from the blood and excrete fluids when the pressure of the blood in the bloodstream forces blood through. High blood pressure causes the surface of the kidney to become bumpy as they continue their filtering operations under the stress of the intensified blood flow caused by hypertension.

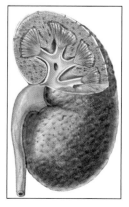

ter. An inflatable cuff is placed around the arm, and blood pressure is measured by the height to which a column of mercury rises. Blood pressure can vary from hour to hour and day to day. It can also be affected by events; even the anxiety of being in a doctor's office can raise blood pressure above normal levels. As a result, the diagnosis of hypertension often requires several readings, unless an initial measurement shows a very high pressure. When high blood pressure is suspected, a patient may be asked to monitor his or her blood pressure at home, using portable manual or semiautomatic devices.

> ## Processed Foods
>
> One reason why Americans have a high intake of sodium is that much of it comes from processed foods that are not believed to contain a lot of salt or do not have a salty taste. More than 80 percent of dietary sodium comes in such processed foods. For example, many sweetened breakfast cereal products have high sodium levels, and a single serving of some canned soups contain as much as 1,000 milligrams of sodium. All processed foods have nutritional labels listing the amount of salt they contain. Reading these labels is an important first step in controlling sodium intake and blood pressure.

TREATMENT

If an underlying disorder such as a kidney condition is identified as the cause of hypertension, high blood pressure is treated by treating that condition. For individuals with idiopathic hypertension, treatment almost always starts with recommendations for lifestyle changes. A hypertensive individual who is obese will be put on a weight-reduction diet. An individual who smokes will have to give up tobacco. A physically inactive person will have to exercise regularly—even a brisk walk for 30 minutes a day can achieve a highly beneficial blood pressure reduction.

Until recently, the standard recommendation was a diet that limited sodium intake to no more than 2,400 milligrams a day, about 1 1/8 teaspoons of salt. But new studies have shown that lower intakes are even more beneficial. In 2000, the federally sponsored DASH (Dietary Approaches to Stop Hypertension) study found that an intake of 1,500 milligrams a day produced the most beneficial lowering of blood pressure. The average American intake at that time was an estimated 3,500 milligrams a day. The DASH study found that 1,500 milligrams of sodium a day reduced systolic blood pressure by an average of 11.5 mm Hg for persons with hypertension—a reduction estimated to decrease the risk of stroke by at least 35 percent and the risk of heart attack by 15 to 25 percent.

Another lifestyle measure is to limit alcohol intake to no more than two drinks a day. An alcohol intake of three or more drinks a day has been linked to about seven percent of all cases of hypertension. In addition to raising blood pressure, alcohol interferes with the action of drugs prescribed to control high blood pressure.

MEDICATION

If lifestyle changes fail to reduce blood pressure or if blood pressure is dangerously high when hypertension is first diagnosed, there are a number of medications that can be prescribed to bring blood pressure down to safe levels. The choice of a specific drug for a specific patient can depend on a number of factors, including the patient's age, race, and general health. A doctor may prescribe a single drug, or may choose combination drug therapy to increase effectiveness while keeping side effects to a minimum. Medications for hypertension include:

Diuretics, or Water Pills. These are the oldest class of hypertension drugs, and reduce blood pressure by increasing the excretion of sodium, thus reducing the volume of blood that the heart has to pump. One advantage of diuretics is that they generally cost less than other hypertension medications.

Beta-Blockers. They act on the nervous system, slowing the heart rate and blocking the effect of some hormones that act to raise the blood pressure.

Calcium Channel Blockers. These block the entry of calcium into the muscle cells that control the width of blood vessels. Reduced activity of these muscle cells results in wider blood vessels, easier blood flow, and lower blood pressure.

Angiotensin-Converting Enzyme (ACE) Inhibitors. They interfere with the normal process by which angiotensin I, a normal body chemical, is converted to angiotensin II, which raises blood pressure by narrowing the blood vessels. It also decreases the body's secretion of sodium.

Alpha-Blocking Medications. These interfere with the activity of norepinephrine, a hormone produced by the adrenal gland that raises blood pressure by narrowing blood vessels in response to stress.

Vasodilators. They lower blood pressure by causing arteries to relax (dilate), becoming wider. Because a vasodilator can produce a very rapid drop in blood pressure, they sometimes are given by injection to treat a hypertensive crisis.

Peripheral Adrenergic Antagonists. Like alpha-blocking medications, they lower blood pressure by acting against norepinephrine, inhibiting its release by the adrenal gland or blocking its activity.

> *Issues related to* HYPERTENSION *are discussed in* BLOOD PRESSURE; DIET AND DISEASE; DIURETIC DRUGS; EXERCISE; *and* SALT. *The anatomy of* HYPERTENSION *is discussed through the articles* ARTERY; HEART; KIDNEY; *and* VEIN.

Hyperthermia

Also known as heat stroke or heat exhaustion

Extremely high body temperature.

Heat exhaustion often occurs to those working or exercising in high temperatures. Symptoms may include cool, moist, red or pale skin; nausea, headache or dizziness, and extreme fatigue. Heat stroke, which causes the body to stop sweating, is considered a medical emergency and must be treated immediately. Symptoms include hot dry skin, rapid pulse and breathing, or unconsciousness, and extremely high body temperature. The sufferer must be wrapped in a cold wet sheet or blanket constantly fanned. If conscious, the person must drink lightly salted water. *See also* HYPOTHERMIA.

Hyperthyroidism

A condition in which the thyroid gland overproduces the thyroid hormone, resulting in an elevated metabolic rate.

The two main forms of hyperthyroidism are Graves' disease and hyperfunctioning nodular goiter (HNG). In Graves' disease, the thyroid gland is stimulated by an abnormal antibody instead of by the normal thyroid stimulating hormone, produced by the pituitary gland. In addition to the symptoms listed above, patients may experience tremors in their hands. They may also develop an erratic heartbeat. The most characteristic physical symptom of Graves' disease is protruding eyes. In HNG, hyperfunctioning thyroid nodules result from the development of adenomas of the thyroid gland. Adenomas are portions of the gland that are walled off from the rest of the thyroid. The adenomas often produce large amounts of thyroid hormone, resulting in the development of all of the symptoms of Graves' disease, but without the effect on the eyes.

Symptoms of hyperthyroidism include increased heart rate, elevated blood pressure, muscle weakness, weight loss despite an increase in appetite, fever, rapid pulse, agitation, and delirium. If left untreated, it is potentially fatal, particularly if the heart rate is affected. *See also* HYPOTHYROIDISM.

Treatment. Hyperthyroidism is treated with an oral solution of radioactive iodine. The thyroid gland needs iodine to manufacture its hormone, so the solution is delivered to the gland and causes hormone production to slow down. A second dose of the solution may be needed a few months later. If the thyroid has been damaged or permanently shut down, thyroid replacement therapy may be needed. Another form of treatment is antithyroid tablets. This therapy needs to be carried out over the course of a year, and is not as effective as the iodine treatment. Surgery can also be performed to remove hyperfunctioning nodules. *See also* BLOOD PRESSURE; GOITER; GRAVES' DISEASE; *and* HORMONES.

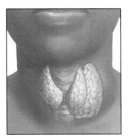

Hyperfunctioning Thyroid Gland. Above, in blue is the hyperfunctioning thyroid gland. A hyperfunctioning thyroid will usually produce a goiter. Such overproduction may be caused by tumors in the thyroid gland or the glands that stimulate the thyroid—the ovaries and the pituitary in particular, but this is quite rare.

Goiters and Hyperthyroidism. Below, a woman with a goiter caused by hyperthyroidism. About five percent of the population exhibits this condition. The most common cause of goiters is a lack of iodine, but other conditions that cause the thyroid to overproduce will also cause the condition.

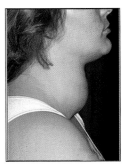

Hypertrichosis

An excessive amount of hair on the body, compared with other individuals of the same sex, age, and ethnicity.

Hypertrichosis tends to occur on areas of a person's body that are not usually covered with hair. It can be caused by the drug minoxidil, which is a common treatment for baldness, but it also has links with a genetic condition. It is usually treated with electrolysis or laser hair removal. Hypertrichosis should be distinguished from hirsutism, which is a disorder characterized by excessive hair in women. *See also* HIRSUTISM.

Hyperuricemia

Abnormally high blood levels of uric acid.

Uric acid is a waste product usually removed from the blood by the kidneys. Removal may be hindered by an inherited condition, excess uric acid from the destruction of cells by a disease such as leukemia, or by the side effects of certain drugs, such as diuretics. The resulting buildup of uric acid levels in the blood can cause the formation of urinary-tract stones or the development of gout. Hyperuricemia can be treated by drugs, such as allopurinol, that reduce the body's production of uric acid. Reducing intake of peas, beans, and other foods rich in purine (the compound that produces uric acid) will also reduce uric acid. *See also* KIDNEY.

Hyperventilation

Abnormally rapid or deep breathing caused by a medical condition or stress.

The immediate symptoms of hyperventilation include a sense of not being able to catch one's breath and feelings of panic or anxiety. Rapid, deep breaths may result in a high level of oxygen and low level of carbon dioxide in the blood. This causes increased blood alkalinity, which can causes numbness in the fingers and toes, as well as faintness and painful spasms of muscles in the hands and feet. These physical effects can add to the psychological effects, resulting in the mental distress called hyperventilation syndrome. Hyperventilation can be stopped by increasing the level of carbon dioxide in the blood. A person experiencing hyperventilation should breathe into a paper bag; a plastic bag should not be used because of the danger of suffocation. If someone faints from hyperventilation, breathing returns to normal almost immediately. *See also* LUNGS.

Hyphema

A condition in which blood collects in the eye.

Hyphema requires immediate medical attention. Blood pools between the iris and the cornea as the result of an injury—sometimes spontaneous and unnoticed—that ruptures a small blood vessel. Vision is impaired as aqueous fluid and blood mix, but improves as red blood cells settle. Pain and bloodshot eyes may also occur. The person must remain inactive, or else repeated bleeding may occur and cause permanent clouding, requiring a corneal transplant. Typically, the blood disappears and vision is fully restored within a few days; surgical drainage may necessary if the blood lingers. Some doctors prescribe eye drops, but analgesics should be avoided because they thin the blood. *See also* EYE *and* EYE DROPS.

Hypnosis

An induced state of heightened susceptibility to suggestion, resembling a trance.

Hypnosis may be induced by a hypnotherapist to treat a variety of problems. A hypnotherapist uses a soothing voice and relaxing phrases to guide a subject into a state of deep relaxation and an openness to suggestion. A person may also be taught to perform self-hypnosis. Some people are more hypnotizable than others, a quality that seems to be related to the ability to visualize images. Contrary to popular belief, the ability to be hypnotized does not necessarily relate to an individual's suggestibility. Hypnosis has been used successfully to treat panic disorders and acute anxiety, as an individual can learn to relax rather than become agitated in stressful times. Hypnosis has been used less effectively in weight-loss programs. It is considered controversial in retrieving repressed memories. *See also* ALTERNATIVE MEDICINE; BIOFEEDBACK; HIGH COLONICS; *and* HYPNOTHERAPY.

Hypnotherapy

Using hypnosis as a form of psychotherapy or to treat disease.

A trancelike state in which an individual is highly responsive to suggestion, hypnosis may be induced artificially in order to relax the subject and achieve a therapeutic effect. It effectively treats phobias, panic attacks, and anxiety; this is also used to encourage the cessation of unhealthy habits; to control pain related to cancer, menstruation, or childbirth; and to lessen symptoms, as in gastrointestinal disorders and asthma. Typically, a person must be comfortable with the process and trust the hypnotist to benefit from hypnotherapy. *See also* BIOFEEDBACK *and* HYPNOSIS.

Hypoaldosteronism

Low production of aldosterone.

One of the hormones secreted by the adrenal cortex, aldosterone helps the body maintain normal levels of blood pressure and blood volume by regulating the intake and output of sodium. Inadequate amounts of aldosterone, as well as the other hormones of the adrenal cortex, particularly cortisol, can result in Addison's disease, characterized by a high loss of water and sodium through urination, increased potassium, weakness, and low blood pressure. Treatment may include drugs to replace the deficient hormones. *See also* ADDISON'S DISEASE; ALDOSTERONISM; ADRENAL GLANDS; *and* HORMONES.

Hypochondriasis

The overwhelming personal terror that one suffers from a serious illness, in the face of evidence to the contrary.

An individual suffering from hypochondriasis is highly sensitive to even the most insignificant of bodily signs, amplifying their significance to life-threatening levels. A mole may be assumed to be the beginning of skin cancer, a cough can be taken as the first sign of tuberculosis, and feeling breathless after climbing the stairs is interpreted as an indication of heart disease.

Although there is no serious disease underlying the symptom, and family members and friends reassure the sufferer, and although doctors may run tests, no amount of hard evidence or support is comforting to a hypochondriac. Although most people worry from time to time that they may suffer from a serious illness or disorder, when the fear of disease hinders the ability to function at work or to have a social life, hypochondriasis is diagnosed.

People with hypochondriasis tend to be intensely self-involved; their constant worries elicit attention, concern and help from family, friends, and doctors. However, over time, these supportive people tire of the complaints. The worries of a person with hypochondriasis are so self-focused that, often, little attention is paid to others.

Treatment. Hypochondriasis may be a way for an individual to avoid attending to the emotional difficulties that he or she may be experiencing. For this reason, recognizing and treating anxiety and depression with medication and psychotherapy may be a proper method of treating this illness. Cognitive and behavioral therapy are also used to modify a person's view of the physical symptoms and to begin dealing with them. In addition, a routine of forced activity and thinking of others besides oneself (including taking part in a program of physical, social, and intellectual activities) may help redirect one's focus outward. *See also* ANXIETY; COGNITIVE-BEHAVIORAL THERAPY; DEPRESSION; *and* PSYCHIATRY.

Hypoglossal Nerve

The twelfth cranial nerve; it controls the tongue.

The hypoglossal nerve fibers begin in the brain stem and travel through the neck to the throat and tongue muscles. This nerve is purely a motor nerve; it does not serve any sensory function. Damage to its neurons leads to atrophy of the muscles on that side of the tongue, causing the tongue to deviate to the side of the injury. If the hypoglossal nerve is damaged as a result of a stroke, one side of the tongue is paralyzed.

Hypoglycemia

The lack of sufficient glucose in the blood.

Hypoglycemia will compromise many body functions. The brain, whose main energy source is glucose, is most vulnerable. Several drugs can lower blood sugar, but the most common is insulin. This can be a problem for people with diabetes who regulate their blood sugar with insulin injections. Hypoglycemia can also occur when there are problems in the pituitary gland, where glucose is regulated, or the liver, where glucose enters the bloodstream. *See* DIABETES.

Hypoglycemics, Oral

A family of drugs used to control the blood sugar levels in people with diabetes.

In type 1 diabetes, no insulin is produced at all, so regular insulin replacement injections are necessary. However, in type 2 diabetes (maturity-onset diabetes), drugs can be used that stimulate the pancreas to produce more insulin or that increase the effectiveness of insulin already present. These drugs are prescribed when diet and exercise do not adequately control the level of glucose in the blood. They are taken in the form of pills, usually once in the morning, and they include acarbose, acetohexamide, miglitol, rosiglitazone, tolbutarnide, and many others. Hypoglycemics interact negatively with a number of drugs, including over-the-counter drugs such as aspirin. Anyone using hypoglycemics should consult a physician before taking any other drugs. *See also* INSULIN.

Hypohidrosis

Abnormally low sweat production.

Hypohidrosis is related to a disorder in the autonomic nervous system, which controls sweat production. There are several possible causes of hypohidrosis, including ectodermal dysplasia, which is an inherited disorder, with symptoms including, dry skin, and hair, and brittle nails. Anticholinergic drugs, which may be prescribed for other conditions affecting the autonomic nervous system, can lead to hypohidrosis, as may some forms of dermatitis. *See* SWEAT.

Hypomania

Abnormally elevated mood.

Hypomania is less severe than mania; it is part of a pattern of moods characteristic of bipolar II disorder, a variant of manic-depressive illness in which full-blown manic episodes (as seen in bipolar I disorder) do not occur. In this disorder, long-term periods of severe depression alternate with periods of mild elation. Hypomania may be distinguished from a "good mood" in that people will show other features associated with mania, such as a decreased need for sleep, hyperactivity, and racing thoughts. These features must persist for at least four days to be considered clinically important. In contrast to full-blown mania, hypomania does not interfere significantly with an individual's ability to function effectively in work, school, or social situations. *See also* BIPOLAR DISORDER; DEPRESSION; *and* MANIA.

Hypoparathyroidism

Deficiency of the parathyroid hormone.

The parathyroid glands, located behind the thyroid gland, produce the parathyroid hormone; it regulates the levels of calcium in the bloodstream. If the gland secretes an inadequate amount of parathyroid hormone, the bones, intestines, and kidneys will not engage in the normal processes of releasing and absorbing calcium.

Hypoparathyroidism is usually caused by the removal of the parathyroid glands. This may occur during surgery on the nearby thyroid gland or if the parathyroid gland has to be removed as a remedy for hyperparathyroidism (excessive production of the parathyroid hormone). In some very rare cases, a person may be born without parathyroid glands or they may cease working on their own. *See* PARATHYROID GLANDS.

The symptoms of hypoparathyroidism (resulting in hypocalcemia) are muscle seizures and spasms, usually in the face, hands, and feet. There may also be numbness and a burning sensation around the lips and fingers, restlessness, fatigue, and depression. Diagnosis is confirmed by blood tests to measure the levels of calcium and parathyroid hormone. *See* HYPOCALCEMIA.

Hypoparathyroidism cannot be treated by administration of the parathyroid hormone itself, so vitamin D, which also aids the body with calcium absorption, is used instead. Simple vitamin D supplements and calcium usually remedy the condition, though calcium levels should continue to be monitored on a regular basis. *See* CALCIUM.

Hypophysectomy

The elimination of the pituitary gland through surgery, with radioactive implants, or by chemical injection.

Usually a hypophysectomy is performed because of a tumor in the pituitary gland that causes it to malfunction. The procedure is also performed to treat specific types of cancer, including breast, ovarian, and prostate cancer, which are exacerbated by the hormonal secretions from the pituitary gland. *See also* HORMONES.

Growths that may require hypophysectomy include: ACTH-producing tumors, which can cause Cushing's disease; prolactin-producing tumors, the cause of milk production in non-childbearing females; impotence in men; growth hormone-producing tumors, the cause of acromegaly or gigantism; and recurrent pituitary tumors.

Any tumor that puts pressure on nearby areas of the brain (the pituitary gland is near the nasal passages). *See also* TUMOR.

Procedure. After the patient is given a general anesthetic, the surgeon usually removes the gland through the nose unless the tumor is especially large, in which case the skull must be cut open to provide access to the gland. Following removal of the pituitary gland, the patient subsequently takes hormone replacement drugs, including sex hormones such as estrogen and testosterone. *See also* BRAIN; BREAST CANCER; CUSHING'S DISEASE; HORMONES; PITUITARY GLAND; SURGERY; *and* TUMOR.

Hypoplastic Left Heart Syndrome

A developmental defect in the heart's left ventricle.

The left ventricle of the heart is responsible for pumping blood into the aorta and through the body's major arteries. When the left heart chambers and valves are underdeveloped or completely absent, normal blood flow cannot occur. At birth, a duct connecting the aorta and the pulmonary artery allows blood to flow from the right ventricle to the rest of the body. However, in hypoplastic babies, this duct closes a few days after birth, and the infant develops heart failure. Most infants with this syndrome die, although a heart transplant may be attempted. *See* VENTRICLE.

Hypospadias

A condition found in boys in which the opening of the urethra is in the wrong place.

Hypospadias occurs in 1 in 500 males. In its most severe form, the opening may be located near the scrotum. Severe hypospadias results in curvature of the penis. Ten percent of boys born with this condition also have undescended testes. Severe hypospadias can lead to difficulties in urination and sexual activity.

Treatment. Hypospadias can be corrected surgically. The opening is moved closer to the tip of the penis and the penis is straightened. Circumcision is usually not performed, as the foreskin is used for skin grafts. The operation is usually performed during the first year. *See also* PENIS; TESTIS; TESTIS, UNDESCENDED; *and* URETHRA.

Hypotension

Dangerously low blood pressure.

While hypertension (high blood pressure) is a major cardiovascular risk factor if it is uncontrolled, hypotension generally is not a cause for concern, although its symptoms can be rather bothersome. Those symptoms occur only when blood pressure is so low that the brain does not get an adequate supply of blood. Hypotension can occur naturally in some younger persons whose heart and blood vessels are normal but who have below normal blood pressure. In older people, it may be a side effect of medications taken for high blood pressure.

DIAGNOSIS

A resting blood pressure reading of less than 90 over 50, or a drop in blood pressure of more than 20 mm/hg when getting up from sitting or lying down is sufficient to diagnose hypotension.

CAUSES

If blood pressure falls enough to reduce blood flow to the brain, dizziness or fainting will occur. Hypotension is classified by the occasions when it occurs. Orthostatic hypotension, the most common type, occurs when someone stands up after being in a stooped or reclined position. Normally, blood vessels in the legs contract to keep the supply of blood to the heart and brain constant. In orthostatic hypotension, this reaction does not occur, and the result is a temporary period of dizziness or near-fainting. This can also occur when someone gets up very quickly after sitting or lying down for a long period. Orthostatic hypotension is also a side effect of some antidepressant drugs.

ALERT

Sudden Hypotension
Sometimes hypotension can be a sign of a serious, even life-threatening, condition. A sudden onset of unusually low blood pressure can be due to an injury that has caused severe loss of blood, or by burns that cause a major reduction in blood volume. A heart attack or failure of the adrenal glands are among the major crises that can bring on a sudden reduction in blood pressure. Any unexpected, severe and sudden attack of hypotension is a clear signal that immediate medical help should be sought, either by going to a hospital emergency room or by calling the emergency medical service.

Postural hypotension occurs while standing. It is common among older people who are taking medications, such as beta-blockers, to treat hypertension. Sometimes the medication works too effectively, widening the arteries and slowing the heartbeat so much that the brain does not get enough blood even during moderate activity. Postural hypotension can also be caused by a neurological disorder that limits the ability of the autonomic nervous system to control the activity of the organs or the blood pressure. One such disorder is Shy-Drager syndrome, a widespread degeneration of the autonomic nervous system function that causes serious problems throughout the body. A condition called idiopathic orthostatic hypotension (the word idiopathic means unknown cause) is quite a bit more common.

Hypotension can result from the body's inability to produce enough norepinephrine, the hormone made by the adrenal gland that maintains adequate blood pressure by constricting the arteries. Hypotension sometimes affects teenagers and young women because of an imbalance in the blood's saline content. Sweating during exercise can lead to a temporary condition of low pressure.

Sometimes hypotension is caused by a disease. Diabetes, for example, can bring on hypotension by damaging the nerves that control blood pressure.

Frequent Hypotension

Some people experience the symptoms of hypotension almost every time they stand up. This vasodilator syncope (fainting) can be caused by a failure of the heart's normal control system. The heart can contract so much that it triggers autonomic nervous system signals that decrease the heart rate and blood pressure too much. Frequent vasodilator syncope can be a sign of chronic fatigue syndrome.

TREATMENT

Medical help should be sought if the symptoms of low blood pressure become troublesome. If hypotension is a side effect of a medication, it should be reported to the doctor so that the prescription can be altered. Often, low blood pressure can be treated with common sense. If it occurs during exercise or physical activity, care should be taken to be sure the body gets enough water and salt to replace what is lost through perspiration. There are a number of sport drinks designed to meet those particular needs.

Someone who consistently experiences the symptoms of orthostatic hypotension can follow a routine of getting up slowly after lying down, sitting for a short period with the legs dangling before standing up. A chair, table, or other support should be close at hand to provide support if dizziness does occur.

Related issues are expanded upon in AGING; BLOOD PRESSURE; HYPERTENSION; *and* SHY-DRAGER SYNDROME. *Information about specific aspects of this disorder can be found in* DEGENERATIVE DISORDERS; HORMONES; *and* NERVOUS SYSTEM.

Hypothalamus

Area of the brain that controls the nervous system.

Located behind the eyes and below the thalamus, the hypothalamus is a small portion of the brain that reacts to incoming stimuli from other parts of the brain, and gives directions to the endocrine system and sympathetic nervous system in order to react to those stimuli. The sympathetic nervous system, part of the more inclusive autonomic nervous system, handles stimuli by causing the actions of the organs to speed up. The other part of this system, the parasympathetic system, slows down the various bodily functions. When the body is under stress or alarmed, it is the hypothalamus that helps the body handle these feelings by speeding up the heart, breathing, and blood flow to the muscles, so that a person can fight or flee the cause of stress. The hypothalamus participates in the maintenance of the body through sleep, helps to stimulate sexual activity, and regulates moods and appetite.

The same signals that the hypothalamus uses to direct the nervous system are also used to control the endocrine system. The hypothalamus is connected to the pituitary gland, which secretes its own hormones; they in turn cause the release of other hormones. When the hypothalamus detects stress, heightened emotion, or injury, it tells the pituitary to release adrenocorticotropic hormone (ACTH), which causes the adrenal glands to secrete the corticosteroid hormones that use or store food as a source of energy, suppress inflammation, and handle some of the actions of the immune system. Epinephrine and norepinephrine, hormones that work like the sympathetic nervous system by speeding up the organs during stress, are also part of the chain of actions directed by the hypothalamus. The thyroid, which releases energy, and the gonads, or sex glands, are also under the control of the hypothalamus.

The hypothalamus helps to control body temperature by directing nerve cells that are sensitive to either heat or cold. If the blood flow to the brain becomes hotter or cooler, the hypothalamus reacts by having the body sweat or shiver, so that a person becomes aware that it is time to adjust the body temperature. If the blood is low on glucose (a source of energy, especially for the brain) or water, the hypothalamus tells the body to get food and drink.

A brain hemorrhage can disrupt the activities of the hypothalamus. Disorders in the pituitary gland, such as a tumor, means that the body will not receive signals sent by the hypothalamus, causing a malfunction of many of the systems controlled by the sympathetic nervous system.

The function of the Hypothalamus in relation to other organs is discussed in Brain; Hormones; Nervous System; *and* Thalamus. *Related disorders are discussed in* Brain Hemorrhage; *and* Brain Tumor.

Hypothermia

Dangerously low body temperature.

Hypothermia is the condition in which the body is incapable of maintaining a temperature greater than 95°F. Individuals with poor circulation, such as those with diabetes, congenital heart failure, and alcoholics, are especially susceptible. Prolonged exposure to icy water, or exposure to environments with cool temperatures and high humidity (especially when coupled with drinking alcoholic beverages in such environments), can cause hypothermia.

SYMPTOMS

The onset of hypothermia is slow and subtle. A person's reaction time slows; the or she may become confused, loose coordination, and may even begin to have hallucinations. The affected person often bescomes sleepy and unmotivated. For example, if hypothermia sets in while a person is in icy water, he or she may cease trying to swim or struggle and simply drown. In the most extreme cases, the muscles can become rigid, heartbeat can become irregular, and the person with hypothermia becomes drowsy and has difficulty speaking. If help is not provided, the person soon becomes unconscious, lapses into a coma, and may die.

TREATMENT

Whenever possible, move the victim to a warm environment; all wet clothing should be removed and replaced with warm, dry

ALERT

Hypothermia Mortality in the Elderly

The risk of mortality by hypothermia is five times greater for a person over 75 than it is for middle-aged and young people. The metabolism of the elderly is slower and less capable of keeping the body temperature stable. There is less fat and muscle tissue, and the blood vessels near the surface of the skin are less able to constrict and thereby preserve heat. Moreover, the shivering response and an awareness of the cold are reduced in the elderly. In addition, many conditions of the elderly can themselves lower the body temperature or leave people vulnerable to hypothermia. These include malnutrition, thyroid disease, stroke, Parkinson's disease, diabetes, and congestive heart failure.

clotting. The victim should be wrapped in a blanket. If he or she is awake and alert, warm beverages, without caffeine or alcohol, may be given. If the or she is not breathing and has no pulse, cardiopulmonary resuscitation (CPR) should be administered, and emergency help should be summoned immediately *See also* Cold Injury; Frostbite Treatment; First Aid *and* Cardiopulmonary Resuscitation.

Hypothermia, Surgical

The intentional cooling of a heart patient's body temperature to slow down the heart action, blood flow, and metabolic rate in order to permit a surgeon to have more time to operate safely.

Hypothermia decreases the metabolism of body cells and tissues, and therefore it reduces the amount of oxygen needed during surgical procedures. Surgical hypothermia also reduces the metabolic activity within the brain an estimated five percent per degree of cooling. Surgical hypothermia is usually induced for surgical procedures performed on the heart, but it is also used when an organ is being removed and preserved for transplantation.

Modern open-heart surgery is usually performed with a heart-lung machine that maintains blood circulation. Mild hypothermia (to about 82° to 88°F or 28° to 31°C) is generally induced as a safety precaution to allow for complications in longer operations. It is estimated that some form of surgical hypothermia is used in a majority of the over 400,000 heart-bypass procedures performed every year.

A heat exchanger, connected to the heart-lung machine, is regularly used to cool the blood before it returns to the body. To keep the heart cold and prevent damage from lack of oxygen, a continuously circulating cold (about 40°F or 4°C) saline solution is passed through the open chest cavity. After the operation, the individual is carefully rewarmed and switched from use of the heart-lung machine to the use of the restarted heart.

> For information regarding the HEART as it relates to Surgical Hypoithermia see HEART; HEART BEAT; HEART FAILURE; HEART RATE; HEART SURGERY; HEART TRANSPLANT; HEART DISORDERS; and HEART-LUNG MACHINE. The articles on HYPOITHERMIA and METABOLISM are also informative.

Hypothyroidism

An underactive thyroid gland condition.

The thyroid gland secretes hormones that help with the metabolism of nutrients and maintain calcium levels. The thyroid hormones help the body release energy and create substances such as proteins. If the level of hormone production is too low, it causes all of these activities to slow down, and the body begins to function inefficiently. This is known as hypothyroidism.

Cause. The most typical causes of hypothyroidism are autoimmune disorders, in which antibodies are created that attack the body's own healthy systems. Other possible causes include surgery that removes part of the thyroid, usually performed to reduce the effects of hyperthyroidism. The complete absence of the thyroid at birth is possible, though quite rare.

Symptoms of hypothyroidism are fatigue, weakness, and cramps. There may be a depressed heart rate, dry skin, and hair loss. Weight gain, or myxedema, may occur. While trying to compensate for the lack of hormone production, the thyroid may be-

come overworked and swell, producing a goiter. In children, undiagnosed hypothyroidism may inhibit growth and brain development. Treatment usually consists of lifelong doses of thyroxine, a thyroid hormone replacement. *See also* GLAND; GOITER; HORMONES; HYPERTHYROIDISM; METABOLISM; MYXEDEMA; *and* THYROID GLAND.

Hypotonia

A severe loss of muscle tone in which the muscles feel soft and doughy.

Tone is the level of tension in muscles that allows them to maintain position, oppose gravity, and still be able to move smoothly. Hypotonia, a severely reduced degree of tension in the muscle, is a symptom of many cerebral, spinal, genetic, and muscular diseases. They include: Guillain-Barré syn- drome, muscular dystrophy, meningitis, encephalitis, and Huntington's chorea. Hypotonia can also be caused by injury or trauma. *See also* MENINGITIS *and* MUSCLE.

Hypotonia in Infants

Also known as floppy infant syndrome

A severe loss of muscle tone in an infant, with or without weakness.

Infants with hypotonia, or little muscle tone, are like rag dolls; they are limp and have little resting tone in their muscles. In severe cases of hypotonia, some infants even have trouble breathing. Infant hyptonia is believed to be caused by a neurological or muscle problem, and it is usually related to other conditions such as botulism, Down's syndrome, myasthenia gravis, and many others. *See also* BIRTH DEFECTS.

Hypovolemia

The loss of 20 percent or more of the body's total blood volume.

The cause of hypovolemia can often be a traumatic accident in which a person sustains an injury that bleeds copiously. It can be caused by internal bleeding from the

How to Tell. Hypotonic baby's sleep with elbows and knees loosely extended. Head motion control is often absent. Attempts to stimulate the muscles will show the baby's lack of movement control; he or she will offer no resistance to stay up straight.

stomach, or intestines (known as gastrointestinal hemorrhage), or even by diarrhea and vomiting, if fluid loss is extreme enough and liquids not replenished fast enough. Burns can produce hypovolemia when they result in an excessive loss of body fluids from the brined skin surface.

Symptoms. A person suffering from hypovolemia exhibits classic symptoms of shock. He or she is initially tired, light headed or confused. Blood pressure is low, the pulse is weak and fast, and the respiration rate is high. The skin becomes cool, pale, and clammy.

Treatment is first aimed at finding and treating the cause of the fluid loss. The person should be kept warm and placed in a horizontal position with her or his legs elevated. As soon as possible, emergency medical technicians should be summoned. *See also* BLOOD CELLS; BLOOD PRESSURE; BURN; DEHYDRATION; SHOCK; *and* TRAUMA.

Hypoxia

A condition in which the blood has little oxygen, resulting in oxygen-starved tissues.

When there is too little oxygen in the tissues of the body to maintain normal metabolic processes, the condition is called hypoxia. Hypoxia can be caused by over-exercising, carbon-monoxide poisoning, impaired breathing, anemia, and the excessive (or simultaneous) intake of alcohol or narcotics. It also occurs in mountain climb-ers and individuals in high-flying aircraft when cabin pressure is compromised (altitude sickness).

Symptoms. In the earliest stages of hypoxia, respiration rate and depth increase, pulse rate increases, and blood flow from the heart increases. In the later stages, the individual will be exhausted and have a headache but will also be euphoric ("euphoria of the depths" is a well-known experience of divers). Vision may be impaired, and the person may be confused, slow, and unaware that there is any problem. Judgment is poor, and reaction time is slowed. If the person loses consciousness, it may last

for days or even weeks. There may be seizures and muscle spasms, and the patient may complain of neck stiffness.

Treatment. In the case of altitude sickness, a quick descent to below 10,000 feet should return a hypoxia sufferer to normal. In other cases, more serious and immediate treatment may be required. If oxygen must be administered, the air passages to the lungs must first be clear. A heart-lung machine can assist in the breathing. Unless the cause of the hypoxia is disease or infection, there are no particular medications that can help.

Oxygen Starvation

Hypoxia specifically applies to situations in which the oxygen in the blood is inadequate. Ischemia is the term used when blood circulation is reduced either from accident, disease, or exposure to extreme cold, heat, or shock. As with hypoxia, the blood then supplies an inadequate amount of oxygenated blood to the tissues, especially the heart and the brain. Both hypoxia and ischemia are particularly dangerous and must be treated promptly, because the brain is soon damaged when deprived of oxygen. The destruction of brain cells is irreversible.

Prognosis depends a great deal on how long the hypoxia lasts and how severe the lack of oxygen was. Since the brain is most vulnerable, neurological problems are likely, with dementia or psychosis at worst, and confusion, hallucinations, or memory loss at best. *See also* ALTITUDE SICKNESS; BLOOD; DEMENTIA; HEART-LUNG MACHINE; HEMOGLOBIN; ISCHEMIA; *and* LUNG.

Hysterectomy

Surgical removal of the uterus, with or without removal of the fallopian tubes and ovaries.

Hysterectomies are one of the most frequently performed operations in the United States; approximately 670,000 are performed each year.

The uterus may be partially removed, completely removed, or removed along with the cervix, fallopian tubes, ovaries, and other parts of the pelvic area.

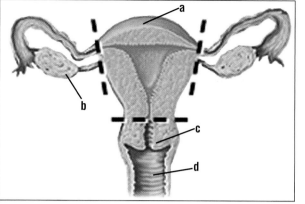

TYPES

Partial or subtotal hysterectomy is the removal of the upper part of the uterus, leaving intact the base of the uterus and the entire cervix.

Total hysterectomy is the removal of the entire uterus and the cervix. A total hysterectomy with bilateral salpingo-oophorectomy is the removal of the uterus, cervix, fallopian tubes and ovaries.

Radical hysterectomy is the removal of the uterus, fallopian tubes, and ovaries, in addition to the pelvic lymph nodes and upper part of the vagina. This is usually performed to treat advanced cancer of the uterus or cervix.

WHY IT IS DONE

There are many acceptable reasons why gynecologists recommend hysterectomies, but the presence of a cancer of the uterus, ovaries, or cervix makes it imperative, because the patient's life is at risk. A hysterectomy may be performed to treat fibroid or benign tumors of the uterus if they are large, rapidly growing, or cause excessive bleeding or pelvic pain or bladder pressure. About one-third of all hysterectomies are due to fibroid tumors.

Endometriosis, a condition in which tissue from the uterine lining grows outside the uterus and causes pain or bleeding, may be an indication that hysterectomy is desirable if less invasive treatments, such as hormone therapy or D&C, are not successful. Hysterectomies may be recommended to relieve heavy or persistent menstrual bleeding (menorrhagia) that cannot be controlled by any other methods, and for severe, long-term infections (salpingitis or pelvic inflammatory disease).

A hysterectomy may also be performed to remove a severely prolapsed uterus, in which the uterus has descended into the vaginal canal due to weakening of pelvic muscles. This condition causes urinary stress incontinence, pelvic pain, or bowel movement problems.

This operation may also be performed after the delivery of a child by Cesarean section if there are major complications, such as uncontrolled bleeding or widespread infection, or if cancer of the cervix has been ascertained in the course of the delivery.

RECOVERY

The operation may take one to two hours under general anesthesia. The average hospital stay lasts from three to five days, and the recovery period is usually three to six weeks. Sexual intercourse can be resumed about a month after the surgery.

After a hysterectomy a woman is unable to conceive children, does not menstruate, and needs no contraception. If the ovaries have been removed, hormone replacement therapy is usually prescribed.

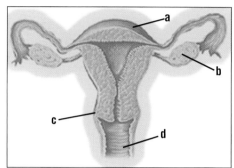

The Types of Hysterectomy. Top left, a partial hysterectomy; in this only the top of the uterus (a) is removed. Top right, a total hysterectomy whereby the entire uterus(a) and the cervix (c) is removed. Above right, a radical hysterectomy, where the uterus (a), all of the connected tubes, the ovaries (b), the pelvic lymph nodes, and the cervix (c), and the upper part of the vagina (d) is removed. The type of hysterectomy performed is based on the condition being treated. Hysterectomy is not an emergency operation, so an individual has time to think over the surgical options.

> *Related information is found in* CERVIX; CERVIX, CANCER OF THE; DIAGNOSTICS IN WOMEN'S HEALTH; *and* UTERUS. *Important issues are discussed in* D AND C; ENDOMETRIOSIS; FIBROID; GYNECOLOGY; MENOPAUSE; *and* VAGINAL BLEEDING.

Hysterosalpingography

Also known as hysterogram or uterotubography

A radiographic examination of the uterus and oviducts following an injection of a radiopaque substance.

Hysterosalpingography involves the inspection of the uterine cavity and fallopian tubes with radiography. A special dye injected through the cervix makes these structures visible in x-ray photographs. Many women say that this test feels similar to a pap smear. The technique is primarily used to diagnose possible causes of infertility.

Hysterosalpingographies have been used successfully to diagnose:

- lesions in the uterine cavity;
- endometrial polyps;
- birth defects of the uterus;
- tubal adhesions;
- foreign bodies;
- fallopian tube obstruction;
- pregnancy outside the uterus;
- traumatic injury;
- scarring; and
- endometrial cancer.

Abnormalities in either the structure or the function of the fallopian tubes may be due to endometriosis, infection (for example; certain common sexually transmitted diseases, including chlamydia, gonorrhea, syphilis, trichomoniasis, and others); or surgical intervention, such as a tubal ligation. All of these treatments may result in infertility. The doctor will request that a hysterosalpingography be performed shortly after the regular menstrual period ends. The radiocontrast dye helps outline the size, shape, and the closed or opened condition (patency) of the fallopian tubes, masses in the uterus, and fibrous tissue (adhesions). This test should not be taken by individuals who have pelvic inflammatory disease (PID) or if there is any unexplained vaginal bleeding or discharge of an unknown origin.

Should such adhesions be identified, the physician may request a further examination of the uterus using a viewing device known as a hysteroscope, which may also be used to help break up the adhesions, enhancing the likelihood of pregnancy. Further diagnostic information may be gathered with a laparoscope—another viewing device, inserted into the pelvic cavity through an incision in the abdominal wall.

Important information about this topic can be found in CERVIX; CERVIX, CANCER OF THE; ENDOMETRIOSIS; FALLOPIAN TUBE; INFERTILITY; OVARIAN CYST; PELVIS; RADIOPAQUE; SEXUALLY TRANSMITTED DISEASES; UTERUS; *and* VAGINA. *Diagnostic and treatment options are discussed in* LAPAROSCOPY; LIGATION; PAP SMEAR; *and* PELVIC EXAMINATION.

Maintaining Reproductive Health

Reproductive health is maintained through preventative measures, particularly periodic pelvic examination, and pap smears, as well as regular gynecological visits during the reproductive years and through the perimenopausal years (the years approaching menopause). Regular examination is essential for the early detection of infections of the uterus, cervix, vagina, or fallopian tubes, as well as ovarian tumors, cysts, and cervical cancer, all of which can lead to infertility. These conditions are treatable if they are detected early.

Iatrogenic

Any mental or physical disorder brought on by the effects of diagnosis or treatment.

Iatrogenic disorders are those brought about by the diagnosis or intended treatment of an illness. Into this general category fall widely differing ailments.

A patient may take on symptoms of a mental or physical disorder that the physician has misdiagnosed and described to the patient, a so-called psychosomatic illness. A misdiagnosis of a serious physical ailment can sometimes produce actual symptoms of disease, although the process remains very poorly understood.

A more straightforward class of iatrogenic illnesses are hospital infections during surgery or subsequent convalescence. For example, a patient who has gone into the hospital to have a bone fracture repaired and contracts tuberculosis through unsterile conditions has acquired an iatrogenic illness. The term however, more often applies to the ill effects of treatment by the physician, such as illnesses produced by drugs prescribed by a doctor. *See also* PSYCHOSOMATIC ILLNESS.

Ice Packs

A means of applying ice in order to reduce pain or swelling, and aid in healing.

Cold can help treat injuries in a number of ways. It lessens pain or inflammation, and stops bleeding by causing the blood vessels to contract, which decreases the flow of blood. Applied immediately after an injury, ice packs can reduce pain and swelling. Ice packs are best used for bruises, sprains, injuries that swell, arthritic joints, and reducing pain after surgery or during physical therapy. Ice packs should not be used on areas of skin that lack sensation due to diseases, such as diabetes or paraplegia, or areas where injury or surgery have caused an inadequate blood supply. After intense exercise, ice baths may be used to minimize muscle soreness. *See* HEAT TREATMENT.

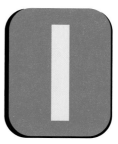

Making an Ice Pack

Ice should not be applied directly to the skin, but should be placed in some kind of container, such as a bag or cup, or wrapped in a cloth. Do not leave on for more than 15 or 20 minutes, and apply every two hours, more or less, depending on the severity of the injury. Do not apply directly on the nerve at the elbow or heel as this may lead to temporary nerve palsy.

To make an ice pack, mix 1/3 cup of rubbing alcohol with 2/3 cup water. Put into a recloseable plastic bag and leave in the freezer until frozen to a slush. This pack may be refrozen and reused.

Ichthyosis Vulgaris

A hereditary disorder causing dry, scaly skin.

Ichthyosis vulgaris, which is normally most severe on the legs, causes the skin to become dry and scaly. The arms, hands, and body trunk are also susceptible.

Symptoms of ichthyosis vulgaris usually develop before a child is four years old. Symptoms worsen in the winter months, and may clear up in warmer weather. The disorder may clear up in adulthood, but may recur in the elderly. The presence of many fine lines on the palm of the hand is associated with ichthyosis. The disorder may also be associated with skin conditions, such as *atopic dermatitis* and *keratosis pilaris.*

Treatment may include intensive moisturizing and, possibly, bathing with non-drying soap. There is no cure for the disorder, although it usually can be successfully controlled. *See also* DERMATITIS *and* KERATOSIS PILARIS.

Ileostomy

An operation to create an artificial opening (stoma) from the bottom of the small intestine (ileus) to the outside of the abdomen.

Removal of all or a portion of the intestines may be required if they are chronically inflamed or have precancerous growths, and when other treatments are not effective. Diseases that may warrant removal of the intestines include Crohn's disease, colitis, and familial adenomatous polyposis.

If only part of the intestines are removed, or if the intestines are damaged due to illness or trauma and need time to heal, a temporary ileostomy may be performed in which a section of the intestine is removed. Normal functioning is usually restored once the intestines have healed. If the entire colon and rectum are removed, a permanent ileostomy is performed.

Procedure. An ileostomy is performed under general anesthesia and requires hospitalization. The affected portion of the intestines is removed, and the end of the small intestine is brought to the surface of the abdomen and stitched to the skin.

Recovery. Following surgery, the patient is not allowed to eat until the intestine begins to function. For several weeks afterward, diet is restricted until the intestines return to their normal function. Specifically, high-residue foods, which are hard to digest, such as nuts and corn, are avoided. Some further dietary restrictions may also be recommended after a full recovery.

After an ileostomy, digested food wastes pass through the stoma and collect in a plastic bag. The material will be primarily liquid, as it has not passed through the colon, which removes excess water from normal stool before it is expelled. Supplemental salt may be added to the diet, as well as additional fluids, to prevent dehydration. A patient with a new ileostomy will receive training on how to care for the stoma. It is essential that the area around the stoma be kept as clean as possible in order to avoid irritation or infection.

Alternatives to Ileostomy

When the intestines are removed, an external ileostomy is not the only option. In a Kock pouch procedure, an internal pouch is made out of part of the small intestine, and a nipple-like valve, which will be covered with a gauze patch, is created on the skin. Stool collects in the internal reservoir until it is emptied by hand through a catheter. It must be emptied several times a day.

A more recent technique is the ileanal pouch procedure. After removing the colon, the end of the small intestine is fashioned into a pouch and connected to the anus to allow for normal defecation.

Resources on Imaging Techniques

Cullinan, John Edward, *Illustrated Guide to X-Ray Techniques* (1980); Kee, Joyce LeFever, *Handbook of Laboratory and Diagnostic Tests with Nursing Implications* (1994); Nuland, Sherwin, *Doctors: The Biography of Medicine* (1995); Ravin, Carl E., ed., *Imaging and Invasive Radiology in the Intensive Care Unit* (1993); Segen, Joseph, C., and Joseph Stauffer, *The Patient's Guide to Medical Tests* (1998); American Hospital Association, Tel. (800) 242-2626, Online: www.aha.org; The American Board of Radiology, Tel. (520) 790-2900, Online: www.theabr.org; American Healthcare Radiology Administrators, Online: www.ahra.org; www.ny-cornell.org/radiology/.

For background material on ileostomy, see DIGESTIVE SYSTEM *and* INTESTINE. *Further information can be found in* ANESTHESIA, GENERAL; COLITIS; COLOSTOMY; CROHN'S DISEASE; INTESTINE, CANCER OF; INTESTINE, OBSTRUCTION OF; *and* INTESTINE, TUMORS OF.

Ileus, Paralytic

Also known as adynamic ileus.

A temporary condition in which the routine contractile movements of the intestinal wall cease.

When the intestinal walls cease to contract, the passage of the contents of the intestines is prevented. Unable to pass gas and stools, the bowel becomes blocked, resulting in persistent pain and possibly fever. An excess of gas is produced, resulting in distended intestines and abdomen. An inflated abdomen squeezes the chest cavity and can impair breathing.

Paralytic ileus may be caused by an infection of the abdominal wall (peritonitis), inflammation of the pancreas (pancreatitis), an abdominal blood clot, or a reduction of blood supply and thickening in the intestinal wall (atherosclerosis). It is often the result of a damaged artery or vein, kidney failure, perforated ulcer, abdominal surgery, cancerous growth of the colon, or abnormal electrolytic levels.

The condition is treated by sucking out the intestinal contents by extending a tube from the nasal passages or the mouth into the intestine. Normal contractions usually resume on their own. *See also* ATHEROSCLEROSIS; PANCREATITIS; *and* PERITONITIS.

Imaging Techniques

Techniques for creating medical pictures of internal organs for diagnostic use.

A battery of imaging techniques has evolved, offering enormous versatility in the diagnosis of illness and abnormality. Newer techniques using sound waves (ultrasonography) or magnetic fields (magnetic resonance) rather than x-rays have found widespread application. Medical imaging continues its rapid advance, with many new imaging technologies in the experimental stages.

TYPES OF IMAGING

X-ray is the most common form of imaging. It is used to diagnose conditions as varied as bone fractures, abnormal tissue in the heart and lungs, or dental caries and abscesses. The technique relies on differing absorption of the high-energy x-radiation due to differing bone or tissue density due to the specific content of fat, water, muscle, and air. The black and white x-ray image can clearly indicate bone fractures, whether hairline or more substantial. It is also sometimes capable of imaging diseased tissue—for example, in standard x-rays of the lung, diseased tissue appears lighter than its normal counterpart. Pneumonia, emphysema, and lung cancer may be diagnosed in this way. Occasionally contrast material (dye) is injected into the blood vessels or introduced into hollow organs to improve detail.

CT scan (computerized axial tomography, also known as CAT scan) is a more sophisticated x-ray technique employing computers to compose an image from repeated x-ray samplings gathered from differing angles. Information from narrow beams of x-rays, projected through the body at different angles, are used to make up a single, detailed image. CAT scanning provides a great increase in resolution over conventional x-ray, and is capable of identifying lesions of less than 2 mm in diameter.

The CT scanning machine's doughnut-shaped apparatus surrounds a moveable table on which the patient lies. Radiation is recorded by detectors on either side of the body from the x-ray source; both rotate about the body as it scans. Iodinated "dye" may be injected intravenously as part of the test. The procedure generally takes about 15 minutes.

Ultrasound or ultrasonography, uses high-frequency sound to image organs or tissues in the body. The echo of sound waves from structures of differing densities is translated into an image. Two of the most common uses of ultrasound are for studies of the heart and during pregnancy. Echocardiography is used to visualize the size, shape, and general condition of the heart, as well as the pressures associated with the accompanying blood flow. Several forms of ultrasonography enable the cardiologist to see all cardiac valves, the dimensions of each ventricle, and the atria. Ultrasound scanning is also the preferred technique for observing the development of the fetus, as it is noninvasive and will not expose the mother or fetus to harmful radiation.

MRI, which stands for magnetic resonance imaging, makes use of strong radio frequency magnetic fields that act on the hydrogen atoms contained in human cells. The atoms are lined up under the influence of a magnetic field and then relax when the field is turned off. As they do so, they emit a signal, which is relayed to a computer and reassembled into an extremely high-resolution image. An MRI scan requires 30 to 45 minutes, and is carried out with the patient lying within the MRI machine—a tube-shaped unit. MRI is free of harmful x-ray effects. Though MRI is expensive, its use is becoming widespread particularly where high-resolution imaging of the brain is desired.

PET, or positron emission tomography, uses a short-lived radioactive particle known as the positron. A substance, such as glucose, is labeled radioactively and injected. The radioactive molecules follow the course of the blood flow, and are pinpointed by a detector. Thus metabolism, may be visualized. Portraits of abnormal cerebral metabolism recorded by PET may help in the diagnosis of AIDS, dementia, epilepsy, and other disorders. PET also offers insight into brain functioning, indicating areas engaged in particular tasks, and therefore requiring increased blood flow. The main use of PET currently, however, is in the diagnosis of cancer.

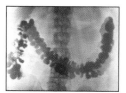

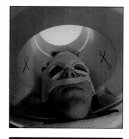

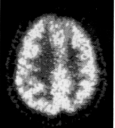

Imaging Techniques. Improved imaging techniques have enabled physicians to diagnose and treat problems with a greater rate of success. Top, a barium x-ray of the large intestine. Middle, a man places his head in an MRI scanner. Bottom, a PET scan of a human brain.

> *Background information on imaging techniques can be found in* DIAGNOSIS. *For related material, see* AIDS; ANGIOGRAPHY; BRAIN DISORDERS; CT SCAN; DEMENTIA; EMPHYSEMA; EPILEPSY; LUNG CANCER; MRI; PET SCAN; PNEUMONIA; *and* ULTRASOUND SCANNING.

Immersion Foot

A condition in which the feet lose color and pulse due to a prolonged period in warm or cold water.

Most commonly suffered by soldiers or people involved in shipwrecks, immersion foot is first characterized by feet that are pale and lack a pulse. The feet then regain a pulse and become inflamed, swollen, and painful.

Initial treatment for immersion foot is usually a gradual, careful rewarming of the foot (for cases involving cold water). If the feet are already at the reddened stage, with a pulse, then they need to be slowly cooled down. Cases of immersion foot that are not treated may lead to gangrene, skin ulcers, or weakness. *See also* GANGRENE *and* ULCER.

Immobility

Loss of movement.

Immobility is the result of another disorder. It is usually partial, affecting one limb or area; total immobility occurs only when a severe trauma, such as a stroke, brain tumor, or head injury, leads to a coma. Partial immobility may happen during a period of recovery from illness, or as the result of nervous system disorders, such as multiple sclerosis, Parkinson's disease, or hemiplegia.

Reduced mobility may be caused by an underlying medical condition, such as asthma or angina; it may be exacerbated by physical activity. Arthritis or recovery from an injury may lead to stiffness in the joints that limits mobility. Immobility can also be part of the treatment of an injury, such as splinting or putting a fractured limb in a cast while the bones knit.

Complications. Immobility can lead to bedsores, contracture (healing skin shrinks and lessens mobility), or even pneumonia. Edema, or buildup of fluid in the body, may also occur. The most likely complication of immobility are stiffness and deterioration of muscle tissue due to lack of use. The best way to prevent this is to begin physical therapy as soon as possible. Exercise and stretching can help to maintain muscle strength and flexibility. *See also* ASTHMA; ANGINA; BEDSORES; EDEMA; HEMIPLEGIA; MULTIPLE SCLEROSIS; PARKINSON'S DISEASE; PHYSICAL STROKE; *and* THERAPY.

Immune Response

The body's specific means of defending against invading pathogens (disease-causing agents).

Specialized lymphocytes (white blood cells), known as helper T cells, trigger a "two-pronged attack" on disease-causing pathogens, consisting of a cell-mediated response and an antibody-mediated response. In the cell-mediated response, killer T cells attack and destroy infected cells, as well as other body cells that have become abnormal. In the antibody-mediated response, other lymphocytes, known as B cells, produce antibodies that bind to the pathogens and either inactivate or destroy them. *See also* IMMUNE SYSTEM.

Immune System

A group of cells and proteins within the body that are designed to protect the body from invasion by foreign substances or organisms.

The components of the immune system are designed to distinguish between "self" and "non-self"—that is, what belongs in the body and what does not. It is believed that this recognition system occurs by detection of antigens—protein, lipid, or carbohydrate markers—on the surface of cells.

INNATE IMMUNITY

Innate immunity refers to the immune response that is present in all people at birth and does not have to be learned. Innate immunity involves barriers that keep foreign invaders from entering the body. The skin is the body's first line of defense against infection. As long as the skin remains unbroken, it is a solid barrier that microorganisms cannot penetrate. The regular body openings—the eyes, ears, nostrils, mouth, urethra, anus, and vagina—are lined with mucus and other fluids (for example, wax or tears) to wash away or trap any particles that enter. However, if a break occurs in the skin, resulting in a cut or sore, foreign invaders can easily enter into the bloodstream and can travel from there to anywhere in the body.

Similarly, the acid produced by the stomach creates an environment that is unfriendly to microorganisms. If the stomach does not produce enough acid, for whatever reason, foreign invaders can reproduce there and travel to infect other parts of the body.

The inflammatory response is also part of innate immunity. When part of the body is damaged by foreign antigens or by injury, chemicals, including histamine, bradykinin, and serotonin, are released by the damaged tissue. These chemicals cause blood vessels to leak fluid into the damaged area, resulting in swelling, which isolates the foreign invaders from the rest of the body. In addition, the chemicals also attract white blood cells, which identify the antigens, then engulf and destroy them.

ACQUIRED IMMUNITY

Acquired immunity develops after a person's body has been exposed to various antigens. A specific type of while blood cell called a lymphocyte is involved in acquired immunity. T cells and B cells are the two types of lymphocytes.

T Cells. The T cell is a type of white blood cell produced in the bone marrow. T cells mature in the thymus gland.

There are many different types of T cells, with each variety capable of responding to a particular type of antigen. When the antigen is detected, those specific lymphocytes become activated, or sensitized, and increase in size. The lymphocytes then divide rapidly to form hundreds of cells. Some of the newly formed cells will be killer T cells, which directly destroy the invaders. Some will become helper T cells, which enhance responses. Some will be suppressor T cells, which inhibit defenses several weeks after the infection is over. A few sensitized T cells will remain in the

lymph nodes as memory cells in the event that the same antigen invades the body another time at a later date.

B Cells. Another type of white blood cell called the B-lymphocyte, is responsible for antibody immunity. When a specific type of B cell responds to its particular antigen, the sensitized B cells also divide rapidly. Most of the new cells will differentiate into plasma cells, which produce antibodies. Others will become memory cells and behave similarly to T memory cells.

Antibodies. Immunoglobulins, also known as antibodies, are produced by B cells in response to specific antigens. Antibodies "recognize" antigens according to shape, but a perfect fit is not required to form an antigen-antibody complex.

There are five different classes of antibodies: IgM, IgG, IgA, IgE, and IgD. IgM is produced upon initial exposure, within two weeks of the introduction to the antigen, in what is known as the primary antibody response. IgM is found in the blood, but not in the organs.

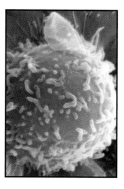

Immune System Response.
Bits of infectious material, shown here, covering a B-lymphocyte, stimulates an immune response.

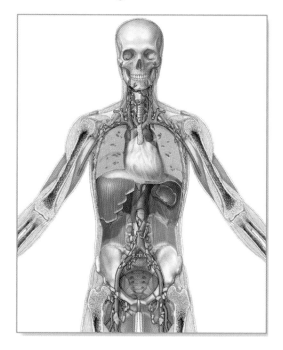

Immune System.
The immune system, left, acts as the body's defense against foreign particles.

The majority of antibodies belong to the IgG class. These antibodies are produced after subsequent exposure to an antigen. The secondary antibody response occurs much more rapidly than the primary response. IgG is found in the blood, as well as in body tissues, and can cross the placenta to the fetus. (These maternal antibodies provide passive immunity for the baby until its own immune system matures.)

IgA is found in the blood, as well as in body secretions. It helps to protect against microorganisms that enter through the mucous membranes. IgE is the antibody involved in allergic reactions. It is also thought to play a role against various parasitic diseases. IgD is present only in small amounts in the blood, and its function is largely unknown.

The immune system also produces various antiviral substances, the best known of which is interferon. Interferon stimulates cells to produce other antiviral proteins to prevent the production of more viruses within host cells.

Effects of Acquired Immunity. The antigen-antibody complex involved in acquired immunity results in one of three outcomes:

- The antigen is destroyed outright;
- The antigen is inactivated, but not destroyed;
- The antigen becomes more susceptible to phagocytosis by white blood cells called neutrophils or macrophages.

After the infection is over, some antibodies remain in circulation to prevent further infection. This is referred to as immunity.

ACTIVE AND PASSIVE IMMUNITY

Active immunity occurs when an individual has been exposed to an antigen and develops antibodies in response. Exposure to the antigen may come about as a result of having a disease, or receiving a vaccine against a particular disease. Many viral diseases, such as measles, mumps, diphtheria, hepatitis A, meningitis, and chicken pox, can now be prevented by receiving an inoculation. The shot contains weakened or "killed" versions of the virus, or antigens from its protein coat, which stimulate the body's immune system against it without actual infection with the disease. Vaccinations are given in a set schedule during

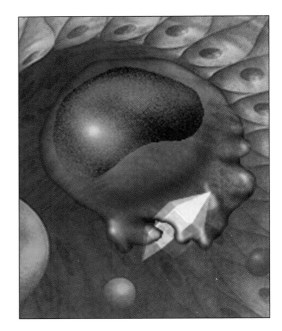

Immune System.
Right, an illustration depicting a white blood cell (shown in purple) attacking a virus (shown in white).

childhood, and periodic boosters are required several years later to ensure continued immunity against the viral agent.

Passive immunity occurs when an individual receives someone else's antibodies against a disease, which temporarily protects against the illness but which will not result in permanent immunity. The most common example of passive immunity is in a newborn baby. The infant receives antibodies from its mother's blood during pregnancy and for the first few months or so is protected against various diseases. Additional antibodies are transmitted through the breast milk. However, the antibody levels eventually drop, and the child must be exposed to the antigens and develop his or her own antibodies for permanent immunity.

IMMUNE SYSTEM DISORDERS

An allergy is an example of the immune system overreacting to a relatively innocuous molecule. An allergen is a substance that is treated as a harmful antigen in particular individuals. In these individuals, the body unleashes a full immune system response to the allergen, including inflammation, redness, and swelling. It is actually the immune response that is the problem, not the allergen itself. For example, in individuals with hay fever, pollen is the allergen "mistaken" for an antigen. The immune response is a release of IgE from sensitized plasma cells. IgE combines with mast cell receptors in the nasal passages. The mast cells cause the release of histamine, which causes dilation of blood vessels and increased permeability. This in turn causes the congestion, increased fluid output, and itchy/scratchy feelings in the respiratory pathways and often eyes and ears. Certain drugs known as antihistamines can tone down this response by counteracting the effects of the histamine. The allergen can be a food or other chemical as well, but the result is the same. Sometimes the immune response can be so severe it can become life-threatening—the air passageways can become blocked, or the swelling can reach dangerous proportions. Other symptoms of allergic responses are nausea, vomiting, and the appearance of hives (raised, itchy bumps on the skin).

Autoimmune diseases are those in which the immune system begins attacking the body's own tissues. It is unknown what stimulates the immune system to begin producing these abnormal antibodies. Immune reactions normally result in inflammation. In the case of autoimmune disease, the inflammation is chronic and results in long-term damage. The most common targets of autoimmune disease are connective tissues located in and around the joints, as well as elsewhere in the body. The muscles can also become inflamed, as can the membrane coverings around the heart and lungs. The brain can be affected as well.

Each autoimmune disease has a particular set of symptoms. Sometimes these symptoms overlap, making it difficult to diagnose precisely from which autoimmune disease a patient is suffering. Analyzing the abnormal antibodies can be helpful in the diagnosis of autoimmune diseases.

Immunodeficiency disorders are diseases caused by the improper functioning of the immune system. Immunodeficiency may be a congenital condition. It may also be acquired, due to a disease such as AIDS or by medications used to treat cancer or to prevent transplant rejections. Immunodeficiency disorders are characterized by severe, recurring infections that last longer than they would in healthy individuals. These infections usually do not respond to antibiotics.

For background material on immune system, see CELL *and* INFECTIOUS DISEASE. *Further information can be found in* ALLERGY; ANTIBODY; ANTIGEN; B-CELL; FEVER; GAMMA GLOBULIN; IMMUNOGLOBULINS; INFLAMMATION; INTERFERON; MICROORGANISM; LYMPHOCYTE; PLACENTA; T-CELL; *and* VACCINATION.

Immunity

Resistance to a particular disease or antigen.

Immunity against certain diseases is achieved by the continued presence of antibodies and memory cells in the body even after the infection has subsided. This ensures that if the specific antigen is encountered again in the future, it will be dealt with swiftly. Everyone is born with a certain degree of natural immunity against infectious agents. As children develop and mature, their systems are exposed to a number of foreign microorganisms for which they must establish defensive antibodies. Immunization is another preventative measure in which immunity to a particular disease is achieved through an inoculation. *See also* IMMUNE SYSTEM *and* IMMUNIZATION.

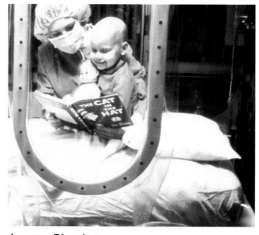

Immune Disorders.
Children with suppressed immune systems may need to utilize a laminar airflow system (above). The system allows air to escape the bubble, but does not permit germs to enter.

Resources on the Immune System
Clark, William R., *At War Within: The Double-Edged Sword of Immunity* (1997); Mims, Cedric A., *The War Within Us: Everyman's Guide to Infection and Immunity* (2000); Kendall, Marion D., *Dying to Live: How Our Bodies Fight Disease* (1998); Ravicz, Simone, *Thriving With Your Autoimmune Disorder: A Woman's Mind-Body Guide* (2000); American Academy of Allergy, Asthma & Immunology, Tel. (800) 822-2762, Online: www.aaaai.org; American Autoimmune Related Diseases Association, Tel. (800) 598-4668, Online: www.aarda.org; www.nycornell.org/

Immunization

A process in which immunity against a particular disease is achieved through an inoculation.

Immunization ensures the presence of certain antibodies in the body in an effort to prevent the individual from contracting a contagious disease. Once immunized against that disease, the body is able to deal swiftly with the antigen when it is encountered again in the future.

Active immunity refers to the state in which an individual has been exposed to an antigen and develops his or her own antibodies in response. This exposure may occur as a result of either having a disease or receiving a vaccination to prevent one. Many viral diseases can be prevented altogether by receiving an inoculation. The shot contains weakened or killed versions of the virus, or antigens from its protein coat, which sensitize the body's immune system. Vaccinations are given on a set schedule during childhood, and periodic boosters

Immunization Schedule for Infants and Children

Age	Vaccine
2 months	DPT/Tetramune and OPV (oral polio virus)
4 months	DPT/Tetramune and OPV
6 months	DPT/Tetramune
15 months	MMR (measles, mumps, rubella)
18 months	DPT/Tetramune and OPV
4–6 years	DPT/Tetramune and OPV
14–6 years	Td (adult tetanus toxoid and diphtheria) booster

are required as a follow-up to insure continued immunity against the viral agent.

Passive immunity refers to the state in which an individual receives someone else's antibodies. This temporarily protects against the illness, but it will not result in permanent immunity. The most common example of passive immunity is found in the case of a newborn baby. The infant receives antibodies from its mother's blood during pregnancy and for the first few months is protected against various dis-

eases. If the mother breast-feeds, more antibodies are transmitted through the milk. However, the antibody levels eventually drop, and the child must be exposed to the antigens and develop its own antibodies to ensure permanent immunity.

Another instance of passive immunity occurs when an individual is exposed to a disease which would be dangerous for that person to contract and for which he or she has not been immunized. Examples of this include hepatitis, or German measles for a pregnant woman. These individuals can receive an injection of gamma globulin, which may provide temporary immunity for up to several weeks. However, this method is not foolproof, and the person may still contract a mild case of the disease.

The vaccine used for active immunization may consist of either killed or live attenuated viruses or bacteria. It may also be a toxoid—an inactivated bacterial product or a specific single component of bacteria. It may even be a recombinant DNA segment, as in the case of hepatitis B. The vaccine is usually grown on other substances, either to add other components, such as proteins, or to reduce the chances of the vaccine itself causing disease.

Active immunization with living organisms induces a more long-lived immune response than using killed organisms. A single dose is often sufficient for complete immunization. Multiple immunizations are recommended when there is a factor present that interferes with a person's successful primary immunization. All immunizing agents must be stored properly to retain their effectiveness.

Primary active immunization develops more slowly than the incubation periods of most diseases. Therefore, immunization must occur prior to exposure in order to provide protection. Boosters "reimmunize" a previously immune individual. This secondary immunization provides a much more rapid increase in immunity.

Depending on the type, vaccines are administered either orally or by injection. Sometimes injections may need to be done subcutaneously, or under the skin, or else deep within the muscle tissue. Timing between primary immunization and booster injections is also very important.

It is possible to administer different antigens simultaneously, such as measles, mumps, and rubella (MMR) or diphtheria, pertussis, and tetanus (DPT). Live virus vaccines are usually given one month apart.

RISKS

Even though all vaccines approved and licensed in the United States have been proven to be safe and effective, each has been associated with adverse reactions ranging from minimal to severe. Live vaccines in particular have a potential for harm if given to a pregnant woman or to those with impaired immune systems or taking immunosuppressive drugs. Early versions of the measles vaccine used to cause high fever and rash in a significant proportion of patients. Allergic reactions may occur upon exposure to egg protein, such as are used in the preparation of measles, mumps, influenza, and yellow fever vaccines. Patients may also show sensitivity to antibiotics or certain preservatives used in the vaccines. *See* IMMUNIZATION SCHEDULE.

Background information on immunization can be found in IMMUNE SYSTEM *and* VACCINATION. *For related material, see* ALLERGY; ANTIBODY; ANTIGEN; DIPHTHERIA; GAMMA GLOBULIN; HEPATITIS; MEASLES; MUMPS; RUBELLA; *and* TETANUS.

Immunoassay

Any variety of diagnostic tests designed to evaluate the antigen–antibody response of an individual's immune system.

Several techniques exist to assess the health of the immune system. This can be done by testing the effectiveness of the antigen–antibody response—the cornerstone of immunity. Immunoassays vary in their sensitivity and specificity to a given antigen.

TYPES OF IMMUNOASSAY

ELISA, an acronym for enzyme-linked immunoassay, is a diagnostic test used to identify the presence and quantity of a variety of antigens and antibodies. ELISA binds an antibody to a specific region of a complementary antigen, by means of an enzyme. The method can help identify a range of viral and bacterial antibodies and antigens.

ELISA is a commonly applied test for allergies, as the allergic reaction typically involves an immune response. Additionally, ELISA is widely used as a test for antibodies associated with exposure to HIV, the causative agent of Acquired Immune Deficiency Syndrome (AIDS). A colorless compound is added to the solution containing the antibody–antigen enzyme. If an immune reaction takes place, the enzyme acts on the compound in the solution, producing a color change diagnostic of the immune response. The intensity of this change can be precisely measured using a device known as a spectrophotometer.

Should the results of an ELISA test prove positive, a more sensitive immunoassay, known as the Western blot (also known as immunoblot) may be requested. This test is designed to measure, with great specificity, minute quantities of antibodies that indicate the presence of labeled proteins within the antigen. Proteins associated with Lyme disease may also be identified by means of Western blot.

Antigen Capture Assay is designed to measure small amounts of antigen in the serum. A small bead is coated with a purified antibody to the antigen in question. The fluid suspected of containing the antigen is then washed over the bead's surface and, if present, is then captured. A second antibody that has been attached to an enzyme marker is then added. If the antigen is present, the enzyme-antibody will cause a reaction, identifying the captured antigen.

Complement Fixation is a general immunoassay, relying on the lysis (destruction) of red blood cells by complement proteins present in serum, during the uniting of antibody and antigen. Complement fixation has been used to diagnose divergent immune reactions; it also is the basis for several tests used to diagnose syphilis.

Immunoassay is a safe, painless procedure for diagnosing immune response and identifying a range of immune disorders. A small sample of blood or other fluid is used for such tests. No preparation on the patient's part is required. While false positives or negatives are possible, refinement of immunoassay techniques has made the percentage of such errors extremely low.

> *For background information on immunoassay, see* DIAGNOSIS *and* IMMUNE SYSTEM. *Related material can be found in* AIDS; ANTIBODY; ANTIGEN; ELISA TEST; GAMMA GLOBULIN; HIV; IMMUNE RESPONSE; IMMUNOGLOBULIN; LYME DISEASE; *and* SYPHILIS.

Immunodeficiency Disorders

A group of diseases caused by the improper functioning of the immune system.

Immunodeficiency disorders are characterized by severe, recurring infections that last longer than usual. These infections usually do not respond readily to treatment with antibiotics. Immunodeficiency may be a congenital condition or may occur as the result of a disease, such as AIDS. Medications used to treat cancer or prevent transplant rejections may also predispose the body to these recurrent infections.

TYPES

More than 70 congenital immunodeficiency disorders have been identified. In some disorders, either the numbers or functionality of the white blood cells is affected. In others, components of the immune system, such as the antibodies are involved. Some of the more prominent immunodeficiency disorders include:

- X-linked agammaglobulinemia affects only boys and involves decreased numbers of B lymphocytes;
- Common variable immunodeficiency results in low antibody levels despite normal B lymphocytes, and may also include abnormal T cell function;
- Selective antibody deficiency affects a single class of antibodies, usually IgA;
- Severe combined immunodeficiency disorder results in deficient B cells, T cells, and antibodies;
- Wiskott-Aldrich syndrome affects only boys, and involves a combined deficiency of B and T cells;
- Ataxia-Telangiectasia affects the nervous and immune systems;
- Hyper-IgE syndrome, also called Job-Buckley syndrome, involves very high levels of IgE antibodies;
- Chronic granulomatous disease affects mostly boys; in this disorder the white blood cells are incapable of destroying certain bacteria and fungi;
- Transient hypogammaglobulinemia of infancy involves low antibody levels; the disorder usually begins around three months of age and may last six to eighteen months;
- DiGeorge anomaly children are born without a thymus gland, which is where the T cells mature; it also may include missing parathyroid glands and heart problems;
- Chronic mucocutaneous candidiasis involves poorly functioning white blood cells.

Acquired immunodeficiency disorders are more common. Some diseases may cause only a minor problem, whereas others may disable the immune system completely.

TREATMENT

Individuals with an immunodeficiency disorder must exercise care and avoid exposure to infectious disease (or to individuals carrying an infectious disease). At the first sign of an infection, a physician should be consulted and antibiotics administered, if bacteria are the cause. An immunostimulant drug is sometimes given to boost the immune system. In severe cases, a bone marrow transplant may be the best option to improve immune system functioning.

> *Background information on immunodeficiency disorders can be found in* AUTOIMMUNE DISORDERS; IMMUNE RESPONSE; *and* IMMUNE SYSTEM. *For further reading, see* AIDS; ANTIBIOTIC DRUGS; ANTICANCER DRUGS; B-CELL; INFECTIOUS DISEASE; *and* T-CELL.

Resources on Immunodeficiency Diseases

Clark, William R., *At War Within: The Double-Edged Sword of Immunity* (1997); Mims, Cedric A., *The War Within Us: Everyman's Guide to Infection and Immunity* (2000); Kendall, Marion D., *Dying to Live: How Our Bodies Fight Disease* (1998); Ravicz, Simone, *Thriving With Your Autoimmune Disorder: A Woman's Mind-Body Guide* (2000); American Academy of Allergy, Asthma & Immunology, Tel. (800) 822-2762, Online: www.aaaai.org; American Autoimmune Related Diseases Association, Tel. (800) 598-4668, Online: www.aarda.org; www.nycornell.org/

Immunologic Memory

A phenomenon in which white blood cells retain a memory of invading organisms. This memory enables the body to deal with antigens more efficiently when they are next encountered.

Immunologic memory occurs after the immune system responds to an antigen (a foreign invader). A specific type of white blood cell called a lymphocyte is responsible for this phenomenon. The two types of lymphocytes are T cells and B cells.

T cells destroy antigens and thus are responsible for cellular immunity. There are many different types of T cells, and each variety is capable of responding to a specific type of antigen. When an antigen is detected, the specific T cells that respond to that antigen become activated (or sensitized) and increase in size. They then divide rapidly to form hundreds of cells. After the infection has been cleared from the body, a few sensitized T cells will remain in the lymph nodes as memory cells in the event that the antigen is encountered again at a later date.

B lymphocytes are responsible for antibody immunity. When a specific type of B cell responds to its particular antigen, the sensitized B cells also divide rapidly. Most of the new cells will differentiate into plasma cells, which produce antibodies. Some B cells will become memory cells and will behave similarly to T memory cells. After the infection is over, a small percentage of antibodies will remain in circulation in the event that the antigen is encountered again. *See also* ANTIBODY; ANTIGEN; IMMUNE RESPONSE; IMMUNE SYSTEM; *and* IMMUNIZATION.

Immunoglobulin

Antibodies made up of proteins found in the blood and tissue fluids.

Immunoglobulins are commonly produced in response to specific antigens (foreign substances invading the body). Antibodies "recognize" antigens according to shape, but a perfect fit is not required to form an antigen–antibody complex.

The antigen–antibody complex results in one of three outcomes: the antigen is destroyed outright; the antigen is inactivated, but not destroyed; the antigen becomes more susceptible to phagocytosis by white blood cells called neutrophils or macrophages. After the infection is over, some antibodies remain in circulation.

There are five different classes of antibodies: IgM, IgG, IgA, IgE, and IgD. IgM is produced upon initial exposure, within two weeks of introduction of the antigen, in what is known as the primary antibody response. IgM is found in the blood, but not in the organs.

The majority of antibodies belong to the IgG class. These antibodies are produced after subsequent exposure to an antigen. IgG is found in the blood as well as in body tissues, and can cross the placenta to the fetus. These maternal antibodies provide passive immunity for the baby until its own immune system matures.

IgA antibodies are found in the blood, as well as in body secretions. These antibodies help to protect against microorganisms that enter through the mucous membranes. IgE is the antibody that is involved in allergic reactions. It is also thought to play a role against various parasitic diseases. IgD is present only in small amounts in the blood; its function is unknown. *See also* ANTIBODY; ANTIGEN; BLOOD CELLS; IMMUNE RESPONSE; IMMUNE SYSTEM; *and* IMMUNODEFICIENCY DISORDERS.

Immunology

The study of the immune system.

The immune system protects the body against environmental hazards and foreign invaders, such as viruses and bacteria. Proteins, carbohydrates, fats, and nucleic acids stimulate immune responses. White blood cells actively seek out and destroy infectious agents. *See also* IMMUNE RESPONSE; IMMUNE SYSTEM; IMMUNITY; IMMUNIZATION; *and* IMMUNODEFICIENCY DISORDERS.

Immunostimulant Drugs

Drugs designed to improve the functioning of the body's immune system.

Immunostimulant drugs are medications that are given to individuals with immunodeficiency disorders in order to boost the immune system. Some of the more prominent drugs are cytokines—chemicals normally produced by T cells that can be taken to stimulate the immune system. They include IL2, IFN2, IFN alpha and beta, G-CSF, and GM-CSF. Immune globulin, administered as either an injection or an infusion, can raise antibody levels. Interferon-gamma is used to treat chronic granulomatous disease.

The best hope for someone with a severe immunodeficiency disorder is to receive a bone marrow transplant. Gene therapy is still in the experimental stages, but is showing increasing promise. *See* IMMUNE SYSTEM .

Immunosuppressant Drugs

A family of drugs used to reduce the body's natural antipathy to organ transplantation and to control autoimmune disorders.

The body's immune system is essential in preventing infection and destroying foreign or diseased cells. Sometimes, however, healthy functioning of the immune system may have an undesired effect, as in the case of the rejection of a transplanted organ. Sometimes the immune system attacks and damages healthy cells, resulting in an autoimmune disorder. Immunosuppressant drugs are used to reduce the functioning of the immune system, thus preventing organ rejection or alleviating the symptoms of autoimmune disorders.

Corticosteroids are among the most widely used immunosuppressants. They are used to treat autoimmune disorders (such as rheumatoid arthritis). They suppress the immune system by decreasing the effectiveness of white blood cells. Long-term use of corticosteroids can result in se-

rious side effects, however, so it may be necessary for other immunosuppressants to be prescribed over the long term.

Cytotoxic Immunosuppressants prevent the growth of harmful white blood cells. They are used when corticosteroids are ineffective or as a long-term treatment. They are also used to treat some kinds of cancers and to prevent transplant rejection. Side effects may include nausea and hair loss.

Cyclosporine and Tacrolimus are used to prevent transplant rejection or when other immunosuppressants are ineffective. They prevent white blood cells from operating effectively. Side effects include high blood pressure and damage to the kidneys.

Dosage

Immunosuppressant drugs are instrumental in making organ transplants possible. However, in compromising the immune system, these drugs leave the patient vulnerable to a host of infections. For this reason the drugs are generally administered in large doses intravenously just before and after a transplantation, and smaller doses are continued after the transplant.

Small doses are likely to be continued indefinitely, leaving the patient more vulnerable to infection for the rest of his or her life. Similarly, immunosuppressants used to treat an autoimmune disorder may also be necessary indefinitely.

Side Effects. Because immunosuppressants make the immune system less effective, people who take them are more vulnerable to infection. Individuals taking immunosuppressants who experience signs of infection, such as a fever, a cough, or any abnormal bleeding or bruising, should consult a doctor.

Drug Interactions. Immunosuppressant drugs do not mix well with most other drugs. They may enhance or reduce the effects of other drugs or interfere with the immunosuppressant. It is important to discuss with a physician possible interactions before taking any other drug.

For background information on immunosuppressant drugs, see IMMUNE RESPONSE *and* IMMUNE SYSTEM. *Related material can be found in* ANTIBODY; ANTIGEN; AUTOIMMUNE DISORDERS; *and* CORTICOSTEROID DRUGS.

Immunotherapy

A treatment designed to suppress or stimulate the immune system to treat allergies or disease.

Immunotherapy is a medical regimen whose purpose is to suppress or stimulate the effects of the immune system. It is often used in the treatment of allergies. When immunotherapy is used for this purpose, a small amount of the allergen is injected to stimulate the body to begin producing an antibody to neutralize the allergic response. Immunotherapy is also used in the treatment of certain cancers (such as Kaposi's sarcoma and leukemia) and autoimmune diseases (such as rheumatoid arthritis and Crohn's disease).

The drugs most commonly used in immunotherapy are interferon and interleukin and agents that neutralize TNF. These drugs either suppress or stimulate the function of the immune system, depending on the dosage. *See also* ALLERGY; CROHN'S DISEASE; IMMUNE SYSTEM; *and* RHEUMATOID ARTHRITIS.

Impaction, Dental

A tooth embedded in tissue or bone at the time it should erupt.

A structural development or defect may impede a tooth from emerging fully, or at all, from the gum. Overcrowding of teeth, improper direction of growth, and dense bone may all cause impaction.

Impacted wisdom teeth are common but should pose no problems, unless they delve into the gum, leaving a flap of soft tissue over the crown, allowing debris and bacteria to become stuck between tooth and gum. Pain, swelling, inability to open the mouth, and inflamed lymph nodes in the upper neck may result.

Depending on the teeth involved, orthodontics, extraction, and antibiotics may be necessary, while some symptoms may be allayed by taking pain-relievers and rinsing with warm salt water. *See also* BRACE *and* EXTRACTION, DENTAL.

Impetigo

A highly contagious inflammatory pustular skin disease, caused by bacteria.

This skin infection is characterized by rapidly spreading red, oozing, crusty sores. Impetigo may be particularly severe in infants and children. In babies, the streptococci and staphylococci bacteria that cause the condition need to exist in skin that is already compromised in order to survive. An infant's skin is weaker than an adult's skin, and so babies and young children are at a higher risk for developing the disease. Thus, a preexisting skin problem, such as diaper dermatitis, may lead to impetigo.

Treatment consists of prescription antibiotics, such as erythromycin or penicillin, and washing with soap and water. A topical antibiotic, Bactroban, is usually effective in mild cases of impetigo. All bedding, clothes, and personal articles that have touched infected skin are contagious and must be cleaned. Impetigo may look serious, but scarring is very uncommon. If treated, it will usually go away. *See also* DERMATITIS; STAPHYLOCOCCAL INFECTIONS; *and* STREPTOCOCCAL INFECTIONS.

Implant

The insertion of tissue or other material into the body in order to restore or improve function, or for other medical or cosmetic purposes.

Tissue or artificial material may be implanted in the body either permanently or temporarily for many reasons. A few of the many types of implants include:

Brain implants involve the transplantation of nervous tissue in an attempt to restore functioning after damage due to degenerative illnesses.

Cochlear implants can be utilized when hearing loss is caused by damage to the inner ear. The implant is a device capable of converting sounds into electrical impulses that are sent to the brain.

Tooth implants are now often used in place of dentures and braces. They consist of

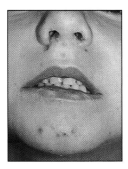

Impetigo.
Red, crusty sores (above) are characteristic of impetigo, a contagious skin infection that is most common in children.

porcelain, metal, or plastic attached to a post that is surgically embedded in the jawbone.

Hormonal implants are made of biodegradable materials that dissolve slowly in the body. They release a steady supply of hormones, providing long-term contraceptive protection.

Penile implants. In the case of permanent impotence, sexual function may be restored using a penile implant, a semirigid or inflatable prosthetic device that is surgically implanted under anesthetic.

Cosmetic implants. Implantation may also be used for cosmetic purposes. For example, in breast enhancement, silicone or other material is surgically added to the breast tissue. *See also* BREAST SURGERY; COCHLEAR IMPLANT; CONTRACEPTION; *and* PENILE IMPLANT.

Implantation, Egg

> **The attachment, penetration, and embedding of the embryo in the wall of the uterus (the first stage of pregnancy).**

This event occurs approximately seven days after the sperm has entered the egg cell (conception). The fertilized egg immediately begins to undergo multiple rounds of cell division until it forms a hollow ball of cells known as the blastocyst. The trophoblast cells, or outer layer of the blastocyst, secrete enzymes to erode an area of the uterine wall just large enough to accommodate the tiny embryo. Slowly, the embryo works its way down into the underlying connective tissues. *See also* CONCEPTION *and* OVUM.

Impression, Dental

> **A mold of the teeth, the gums, and (occasionally), the palate.**

An aid in the study of the placement of teeth and the structure of the mouth, and in the design of orthodontic appliances, a dental impression is a cast model that may serve as the foundation or cast for a bridge, denture, inlay, or onlay.

The mold is made by putting a custom-designed form over the area of the mouth

in question and pouring in a quick-setting rubber compound or alginate. The material hardens and, once removed, is filled with plaster of Paris, which forms the base upon which an appliance can be built to correct irregularities.

> *Background material on dental impression can be found in* DENTAL EXAMINATION *and* TEETH. *For further information, see* BRIDGE, DENTAL; DENTURE; ONLAY, DENTAL; *and* ORTHODONTIC APPLIANCES.

Impulse Control Disorders

> **A group of disorders characterized by the inability to control one's need for immediate gratification, tendencies toward reckless behavior, and an inability to tolerate frustration.**

A person suffering from an impulse control disorder exhibits self-destructive, illegal, or aggressive behavior. Types of impulse control disorders include stealing (kleptomania), setting fires (pyromania), pathological gambling, and uncontrolled outbursts of anger or rage (intermittent explosive disorder).

Impulsive behaviors are not motivated by anger, financial gain, or revenge, which typically motivate such behaviors, but by a desire to achieve an emotional payoff. A kleptomaniac, for example, achieves a feeling of euphoria or a reduction in stress as a result of stealing and usually is not interested in the intrinsic value of the stolen items.

Cause. Although it is difficult to determine the exact cause of such conditions, during times of stress and in uncomfortable circumstances, those suffering from impulse control disorders experience strong- er urges that increase their activities. Impulse control disorders seem to be a maladaptive way of relieving anxiety. They frequently occur among children and young adults.

Treatment may involve a combination of group therapy, psychotherapy, and, in some cases, medication to relieve intense feelings of anxiety. With guidance and counseling, many children outgrow the disorder. *See also* STRESS.

In Situ Carcinoma

A Latin term describing a less dangerous cancer.

In situ is a Latin phrase meaning "in place." Carcinoma in situ is a phrase that describes cells in the earliest stage of cancer, cells that are beginning to become abnormal but have not yet formed a definitive invasive cancer. It is assumed to be the precursor of an invasive cancer. It is completely surrounded by normal cells, without sign of spreading to neighboring tissue. Carcinoma in situ is found in the skin, the cervix; and the breast. Mammograms often detect ductal carcinoma in situ. *See also* CANCER; CARCINOMA; *and* MAMMOGRAM.

In Vitro Fertilization

Surgical placement of a healthy fertilized egg in a woman's uterus.

The term *in vitro* means literally "in glass" and may refer to any procedure carried out on biological material in a test tube. In vitro fertilization, specifically, is a technique used by infertile couples who are attempting to conceive. The ovaries are stimulated into producing several eggs, which are then retrieved and fertilized with the partner's sperm in a laboratory. The resulting embryos are implanted in the woman's uterus.

A combination of clomiphene, human menopausal gonadotropins, and a gonadotropin-releasing hormone is used to stimulate egg production. After identifying the mature eggs by means of ultrasound, they are retrieved with a needle inserted through the vagina or abdomen. The eggs are placed in a petri dish together with washed sperm (a sample containing only the most active sperm).

Embryo transfer occurs approximately 40 hours later. Usually three or four embryos are transferred, in order to maximize the chances of a successful implantation in the uterus. The remaining embryos can be frozen for later attempts. The success rate of in vitro fertilization is only around 25 percent for each attempted episode of embryo transfer. *See also* CLOMIPHENE; GONADOTROPIN HORMONES; INFERTILITY.

Incest

A form of sexual abuse defined by sexual contact between relatives.

It is estimated that in the United States, between 15 and 40 percent of children under age 14 have been sexually abused, with ten percent of these cases involving incest. Incest occurs in families at every level of society, regardless of race, educational background or income. The abuse is most commonly perpetrated by fathers, brothers, stepfathers, and stepbrothers, but mothers have also sexually abused their children. Parents who commit incest often have histories of childhood sexual abuse as well.

Incest can begin at any age, but most typically begins with inappropriate fondling when a child is between eight and 12 years of age. When the victim reaches puberty, the abuse usually escalates to include sexual intercourse.

The physical effects of incest include scarring and permanent damage to the genitals, rectum, mouth, and throat. Death may even result. Abused girls are at risk for contracting sexually transmitted diseases. After puberty, pregnancy is also a risk.

Long-term effects include depression, substance abuse, self-destructive behavior, and eating disorders. Many abused children grow up with distorted self-images and feel as though they were responsible for the abuse. Psychosomatic disorders are also common. Therapy is usually the recommended treatment. *See also* SEXUAL ABUSE.

Incision

A surgical cut made with a scalpel or other surgical instrument.

The incision is one of the most basic and common surgical procedures, serving a great variety of needs. Incisions in the chest, abdomen, and other areas of the

Resources on Fertility
Eli Y. Adashi, Eli Y., John A., Rock, and Zev Rosenwaks, eds., *Reproductive Endocrinology, Surgery, and Technology (*1998); Breitkopf, Lyle J. and Marion Gordon Bakoulis, *Coping with Endometriosis* (1988); Laucella, Linda, *Hormone Replacement Therapy: Conventional Medicine and Natural Alternatives, Your Guide to Menopausal HealthCare Choices* (1999); Older, Julia, *Endometriosis* (1984); Endometriosis Assoc., Tel. (800) 992-3636, Online: www.endometriosisassn. org; Endocrine Web, Online: www.endocrine-web.com;www.nycornell.org/medicine/edm/index.html.

body allow a surgeon access to the heart, lungs, and other internal organs for diagnosis or repair. Incisions may also be used to drain fluid from abscesses or other types of infection or wound. These incisions are generally made with a scalpel.

Some extremely delicate surgeries require other instruments to create the incision, such as laser surgery to correct disorders of the eyes.

A physician will attempt to make as small an incision as possible, in order to speed healing, lessen the threat of infection, and minimize scarring. Laparoscopic surgery, in which a surgeon uses small incisions to insert a viewing tube and other instruments into a cavity, minimizes incision size but is not possible for all procedures. *See also* LAPAROSCOPY *and* LASER SURGERY.

Incompetent Cervix

Weakness of the cervix.

The cervix is the neck of the uterus and usually remains closed until the onset of labor. The weight of the growing fetus can force a weak, incompetent cervix to open beginning in the 12th week of pregnancy, possibly resulting in a miscarriage.

Ultrasound scanning or an internal pelvic examination can reveal the widening of the cervical opening. One-fifth of women who have experienced two or more post-14th-week miscarriages have an incompetent cervix. The problem can be solved with a procedure called cerclage, in which the cervix is literally stitched closed. At the beginning of the ninth month, the stitches are cut so childbirth can occur. *See also* CERVIX *and* CERVIX, DISORDERS OF.

Incontinence

An involuntary bowel movement or release of urine.

FECAL INCONTINENCE
The inability to retain feces (human waste product) in the rectum can be caused by a number of conditions. These include de-

fective function of the muscles of the anus or rectum, a fecal impaction that lodges in the rectum, and medical conditions such as diabetes, myasthenia gravis, multiple sclerosis, or spina bifida in children. Mental impairment may also contribute to the condition. The incidence of fecal incontinence does not increase with age, although older people are more likely to experience the condition because of fecal impaction or loss of muscle function.

Treatment. Many persons do not seek treatment for fecal impaction because the condition is embarrassing and because they believe it is not treatable. But treatment aimed at the underlying cause can be effective in many cases. A high-fiber diet can prevent fecal impaction. Muscle function can be improved by an exercise regimen. Biofeedback, using a monitor that measures the contraction of the sphincter at the end of the anus, can be effective over time. In the case of nerve injury, enemas can be used to excrete feces on a regular schedule. In those cases where the anal sphincter is damaged, surgery may be able to correct the defect.

URINARY INCONTINENCE
There are several forms of urinary incontinence:

• Urge incontinence is the inability to control the function of the bladder accompanied by an urgent need to urinate. It is often triggered by a sudden change of position, but can occur while walking.

• Stress incontinence is the release of a small amount of urine due to a cough, a laugh, or physical exertion.

• Overflow incontinence is a consequence of urine retention, a condition in which the bladder cannot be emptied normally and becomes overfull.

• Total incontinence is a complete lack of bladder control caused by failure of the sphincter, the muscles controlling the flow of urine from the bladder.

Causes. Incontinence may be due to a variety of factors. Urge and stress incontinence are often largely associated with nervous system disorders, diet, and weakness

Resources on Urology and Incontinence

Campbell, Meredith F., & E. Darracott Vaughan, *Campbell's Urology* (2002); Hinman, Frank, *Atlas of Urologic Surgery* (1989); Tanagho, Emil A. and Jack W. McAninch, eds., *Smith's General Urology* (1995); National Kidney Foundation, Tel. (800) 622-9010, Online: www.kidney.org; American Association of Kidney Patients, Tel. (800) 749-2257, Online: www.aakp.org; American Foundation for Urologic Disease, Tel. (800) 242-AFUD, Online: www.af-ud.org; National Institute of Diabetes and Digestive and Kidney Diseases, Tel. (301) 496-3583, Online: www.niddk.nih.gov;www.nycornell.org/medicine/nephrology/index.html; www.cornellurology.com/

in the sphincter and urethral muscles. In some cases, the bladder may prove to be abnormally small or may need to be trained to retain larger amounts of fluid. Men suffering from an enlarged prostate, and women, after multiple pregnancies, are often more likely to experience incontinence, as are the elderly.

Diagnosis. A urinalysis will be done to determine or rule out any evidence of blood or infection. A physical examination can be done to look for disorders or malformations of the urinary tract. Other tests include taking x-rays of the kidney and ureters (the tubes that carry urine from the kidney to the bladder), measuring the pressure within the bladder (cystometrics), performing a cystoscopy, an examination of the urethra (which carries urine out of the bladder), and viewing the bladder through a viewing tube.

Treatment. Treatment depends on the nature of the urinary incontinence in a given individual. Stress incontinence in older women can be treated with estrogen creams to counter the thinning of tissue that can occur with low estrogen levels. Medications to strengthen urethral muscle tone can help, and surgery can be done to increase pelvic support of the bladder. Some patients can learn how to insert a catheter to drain urine from the bladder. Treatment of urge incontinence is aimed at making the muscles of the bladder less spastic and the urethra stronger. Total incontinence often requires surgery.

If incontinence is due to a fistula—an abnormal opening between the bladder and the surface of the skin or vagina—surgery can be done to correct the malformation. If the bladder has been damaged by an injury, a previous operation, or cancer, surgery can help repair the damage and create an access port through which urine can be removed by catheterization.

For background information on incontinence, see DIGESTIVE SYSTEM. *Related material can be found in* AGING; BIOFEEDBACK; DIABETES MELLITUS; FECAL IMPACTIONS; FECES; FECES, ABNORMAL; MULTIPLE SCLEROSIS; MYASTHENIA GRAVIS; PREGNANCY; PROSTATE, ENLARGED; *and* SPINA BIFIDA.

Incubation Period

The latency period between exposure to infection and the appearance of the first symptoms of a particular illness.

Infectious diseases have a characteristic time lag between exposure to the pathogen and the onset of illness. This incubation period can vary in length from a matter of hours—as is the case with the common cold, food poisoning (salmonellosis), and toxic shock syndrome—to months or years. The precise incubation period for AIDS following exposure to the HIV virus is still not known but in some cases may be a decade or more. Long incubation periods for contagious diseases are of particular concern to epidemiologists as they allow for the widespread dissemination of the disease during this asymptomatic latency phase. *See also* AIDS; ASYMPTOMATIC; COLD, COMMON; FOOD POISONING; HIV; INFECTION; INFECTIOUS DISEASE; SALMONELLA; *and* TOXIC SHOCK SYNDROME.

Indigestion

Upper abdominal discomfort often due to difficulty digesting food.

Indigestion is a general term used to describe a number of symptoms referring to upper abdominal discomfort. Also called dyspepsia, this condition occurs most often after eating.

Causes. Specific causes can rarely be found, but certain foods—particularly those that are unfamiliar or highly spiced—can provoke an attack of indigestion. Habits, such as eating too fast or too much, may also cause indigestion. Excessive amounts of alcohol can also be a factor. Some individuals experience indigestion on a regular basis; others, only occasionally.

It is important to note that indigestion, while not a serious condition, can be a symptom of another disorder, such as cholecystitis, gallbladder disorders, gastritis, pancreatitis, peptic ulcer, stomach cancer, or a ruptured appendix.

Resources on the Digestive System

DLevine, Joel S., ed., *Decision Making in Gastroenterology* (1992); Berkson, D. Lindsey, et al., *Healthy Digestion the Na-tural Way* (2000); Sapolsky, Robert M., *Why Zeb-ras Don't Get Ulcers: An Updated Guide to Stress, Stress-Related Diseases, and Coping* (1998); Sachar, David B., et al., *Pocket Guide to Gastroenterology* (1991); Thompson, W. Grant, *The Ulcer Story: The Authoritative Guide to Ulcers, Dyspepsia, and Heartburn* (1996); Crohn's and Colitis Found. of America, Inc., Tel: (800) 932-2423, Online: www. ccfa.org; Digestive Disease National Coalition, Tel. (202) 544-7497, Online: www.ddnc. org; Gastro-Intestinal Research Found., Tel. (312) 332-1350, Online: www. girf.org; National Institute of Diabetes and Digestive and Kidney Diseases, Tel. (301) 496-3583, Online: www.niddk.nih.gov; www. nycornell.org/medi-cine/digestive/index.html.

Symptoms. Common symptoms of indigestion include:

- Bloated feeling and/or gas;
- Generalized discomfort;
- Heartburn;
- Nausea;
- Unpleasant sensation of fullness.

Diagnosis. Diagnosing the condition is difficult, even through barium x-rays of the gastrointestinal tract, endoscopy, or an abdominal ultrasound. However, these tests can rule out a more serious problem.

Treatment. Antacids or other medications that limit the production of stomach acid may be useful in treating indigestion. Metoclopramide is an anti-nausea drug that enhances stomach motility and the emptying of the organ's contents.

Prevention. If specific foods are suspected of causing the condition, they should be avoided or consumed in moderation. Persons suffering from indigestion should also be mindful of the amount of food they eat and should try to eat slowly.

Background material on indigestion can be found in ACID REFLUX; DIGESTIVE SYSTEM; HEARTBURN; *and* STOMACH. *For further information, see* APPENDICITIS; CHOLECYSTITIS; GALLBLADDER, DISORDERS OF; GASTRITIS; PEPTIC ULCER; AND STOMACH CANCER; ULTRASOUND SCANNING; *and* X-RAY.

Induction of Labor

Bringing about the onset of labor through chemical or other means.

Induction of labor is generally indicated if the health of the mother or baby is in danger from continuation of the pregnancy. It is most often done under the following circumstances:

- **Postmaturity**—after 42 weeks, there is a danger that the placenta has become senile and is no longer performing its tasks adequately;
- **Maternal diabetes**—diabetic mothers tend to have very large babies, who may have difficulty passing through the birth canal;
- **Preeclampsia or eclampsia**—these are two life-threatening conditions that

can be helped by delivery;

- **Premature rupture of membranes around the fetus at term**—if labor has not begun within 24 hours after the membranes rupture, it is often induced;
- **High blood pressure**—this is usually related to eclampsia.

Methods of Induction. Labor can be induced by several methods. A chemical known as pitocin, a synthetic form of the naturally occurring hormone oxytocin, may be administered. Pitocin can cause contractions to begin, or it can cause them to intensify and strengthen once they have already begun, thereby speeding up the progress of labor. Also, prostaglandin hormones—found in seminal and menstrual fluids—may be administered, as they will usually induce uterine contractions. Doctors may also attempt to induce labor by rupturing the membranes around the fetus; this procedure alone is often enough to stimulate labor.

For background information on induction of labor, see CHILDBIRTH, COMPLICATIONS. *Related material can be found in* DIABETES MELLITUS; ECLAMPSIA; HYPERTENSION; PREECLAMPSIA; *and* RH INCOMPATIBILITY. *See also* PREGNANCY *for more on the timeline of fetal development.*

Infant Mortality

Infant mortality refers to the number of infant deaths per 1,000 live births.

Neonatal mortality is defined as the death of an infant that occurs before the infant is 28 days old. The Neonatal Intensive Care Unit (NICU) facilities have greatly reduced this number since 1950. Postneonatal mortality refers to infant deaths that occur between the 28th and 364th day of life. Most deaths, sixty-six percent, occur during the neonatal period. Thirty-four percent occur in the postneonatal period.

The infant mortality rate in the U.S. was 7.1 in 1997. Some reduction in infant mortality is due to more available prenatal care and the increasing availability of NICUs. The WIC, a program for women, infants, and children, provides low-cost prenatal care for economically disadvantaged families.

Infant deaths have devastating effects on the families of the lost infant. Infant mortality is a public health issue; it is often used as the indicator of the health status of a country. The rate of infant mortality is directly related to the mother's health, the quality and access to public medical care, and socioeconomic status.

There is some disparity between the infant mortality rate for white babies and babies of other races. In 1997, the white infant mortality rate was 6.3, while the rate in the U.S. for all races was 7.2. Economic and social factors are blamed for this disparity. *See* SUDDEN INFANT DEATH SYNDROME.

Infant Pyloric Stenosis

A narrowing of the pylorus (the part of the stomach leading to the small intestine) that prevents food from properly passing through the stomach.

The first symptom of this disorder is sudden, forceful vomiting, which is caused by a narrow pylorus opening in the bottom of the stomach. Because food cannot enter the small intestine properly, the stomach contents are ejected. It is more common in baby boys than girls; one in 150 newborn boys show symptoms, compared with one in 750 baby girls. Babies may lose weight and become dehydrated because of the continual vomiting after feeding.

After the dehydration is corrected, the doctor can correct this condition with surgery. A few children have been treated successfully using antispasmodic drugs, but surgery is the usual treatment. It corrects the problem easily and permanently.

Infantile Spasms

Also known as West Syndrome.

A rare seizure disorder of infancy and early childhood.

Infants with this disorder experience sudden, brief contractions of one or more muscle groups. The contractions involve the neck, the trunk of the body, and the extremities. Other characteristics of the disorder are hypsarrhythmia (abnormal, chaotic electroencephalogram) and mental retardation. Congenital abnormalities, cerebral atrophy, and hydrocephalus are also common in babies with infantile spasms.

Infants may be treated with adrenocorticotropic hormone or prednisone. Overall, the prognosis of children with infantile spasms is poor, because although spasms stop during childhood for most patients, the neurological problems persist. *See also* PREDNISONE *and* EEG.

Infection

Any invasion of the body by a pathogen that causes disease.

Most pathogens may be classified as bacteria, viruses, fungi, or parasites. Other pathogens that are more difficult to classify also cause disease, such as prions, which are protein particles that cause mad cow disease. There are billions of these microscopic organisms (microorganisms) everywhere, so it is impossible and impractical to protect the body from invasion by all of them. Fortunately, most microorganisms are not pathogenic—they do not cause illness in humans, plants, or animals. Many are also beneficial to the human body since they aid in the digestion of food and clean up the dead cells on our skin.

Microscopic organisms that do make us ill do so in various ways. Some produce toxins (poisons) that cause diseases like tetanus or cholera. Toxins may also be produced outside the body and, when ingested, cause diseases such as botulism. Some diseases are caused when the multiplication of microorganisms overwhelms the body's immune system, or when the immune system itself is weakened. It must then be assisted with drugs or surgery.

Background information on infection can be found in INFECTIOUS DISEASE *and* MICROORGANISM. *For further reading, see* BACTERIA; CHOLERA; FUNGI; IMMUNE RESPONSE; IMMUNE SYSTEM; PARASITES; PATHOGEN; TETANUS; *and* VIRUSES.

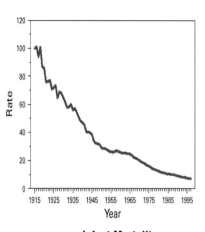

Infant Mortality.
In 1997, the infant mortality rate in the U.S. was 7.1 deaths for every 1,000 births. Above, infant mortality rate in the U.S by year, 1915 to 1995.

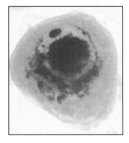

Infection.
Infections are caused by pathogens, which include viruses, bacteria, fungi, and parasites. Below, image of a virus in a cell in urine.

Infection, Congenital

An infection that exists at or before birth, as a result of heredity or environmental influences.

There are numerous types of disorders that can develop in a growing fetus, many of which can cause severe defects and abnormalities in the baby. Some disorders are due to substances ingested by the mother during pregnancy, some are caused by environmental contaminants, and still others are the result of hereditary illness. Drugs, (both illicit and prescription), alcohol, and smoking can all cause permanent damage to a developing fetus. Disorders may be chromosomal, gastrointestinal, spinal, or a result of maternal diabetes or rubella.

Sepsis is a severe bacterial infection that spreads through the body of the newborn during the first month of life. It causes listlessness, slow heart rate, fluctuating body temperature, poor feeding, and difficulty breathing. Treatment with intravenous antibiotics helps, but even so, 30 percent of babies die in the first few weeks of life.

Congenital rubella is an infection with the virus that causes German measles. It is believed to be transmitted by the inhalation of viral particles in the air or close contact with an infected person. The virus enters the bloodstream of the mother and spreads throughout the body, including the placenta. Miscarriage, heart and eye defects, and deafness often occur as a result. Sometimes women with rubella are given immune serum globulin, but its effectiveness is still uncertain. A rubella vac-cination before pregnancy may be effective in preventing the infection.

Herpes is another viral infection that can cause serious damage to a developing baby. It can infect the major organs of the body, resulting in permanent damage or death. Without treatment, 85 percent of infected babies die. With treatment consisting of antiviral drugs, the death rate decreases by 50 percent.

Congenital toxoplasmosis is caused by the parasite *toxoplasma gondii,* which is passed from a pregnant woman to her developing fetus. The toxoplasma infects cats, and the parasite's eggs are passed from the cat in its feces. It also occurs in people who eat undercooked meat, such as beef, pork, or lamb. Pregnant women with cats should not clean the litter box. They should also avoid any undercooked meats. Babies born to mothers with toxoplasmosis may have birth defects, such as blindness or neurological damage, or they may die.

Syphilis is a chronic sexually transmitted disease. It usually begins with a sore on the genitals, skin lesions, and then progresses to neurological and cardiac symptoms if it is not treated. Babies born to mothers with syphilis can have congenital syphilis and experience symptoms, such as bone lesions, rashes, and runny nose.

Tuberculosis is a highly infectious disease, most common in areas of poverty. It is transmitted by breathing air laden with infectious particles, usually in confined living spaces. Children or infants with tuberculosis experience fever, cough, fatigue, weight loss, low appetite, and general pneumonia-like symptoms that do not respond to antibiotics. However, many children do not have any symptoms. When the child's central nervous system becomes infected, tuberculosis becomes tuberculomeningitis, characterized by high fever, headache, and personality changes. When left untreated, it can result in coma or death.

Congenital Rubella

Congenital rubella is rare now due to increased immunizations and testing for the disease. But nonimmunized pregnant women are at risk for the disorder, which can cause serious physical abnormalities in the developing fetus. Symptoms of the disorder include rash, low birth weight, microcephaly, bulging fontanelle, cloudy or white appearance of eyes, simian crease, and motor or mental retardation. Adequate prenatal care is essential in preventing the severe effects of rubella.

For background material on congenital infection, see CONGENITAL. *Further information can be found in* ALCOHOL DEPENDENCE; DRUG DEPENDENCE; GENETICS; SEPSIS; RUBELLA; SYPHILIS; TOXOPLASMOSIS; *and* TUBERCULOSIS.

Infectious Disease

The term used when a pathogen (disease-causing agent) invades a healthy body or when the immune system is weakened, permitting a previously dormant pathogen to cause illness.

An infectious disease may be so mild as to be asymptomatic or so serious as to be life-threatening. The severity depends on the body's immune system, the numbers of germs that invade the body, and the toxicity (amount of poison) of the pathogen.

TYPES OF PATHOGENS

Bacteria are living cells that multiply very rapidly by cell division. The more there are in the body, the more dangerous the disease. Bacteria do damage in two ways: They produce toxins that destroy human cells, and they compete with the body for the nutrients necessary for life.

Viruses cannot reproduce on their own, but they can invade healthy cells and use the cells' reproductive power to make new copies of themselves.

Fungi are particularly dangerous because if they find themselves in a hostile environment, they produce spores that are practically indestructible. The spores travel unchanged until they land in a welcoming environment, at which time they turn into the fungus and attack the host.

Parasites are self-contained living organisms that may be as small as a single cell or as large as a 30-foot-long worm. They can cause swelling of the extremities (edema) or allergic reactions to toxins that they produce. They steal nutrients from the host and may invade the intestinal wall or other organs of the body.

TRANSMISSION

The ability of a pathogen to survive as it travels from one host to the other is the factor that determines its capabilities for infection. Most disease is transmitted by contact. An infected person touches an uninfected person, and the microorganism moves to the new host. Alternatively an infected person sneezes or coughs, and the germ travels with the droplets onto the skin or into the lungs of the new host. A germ can be left on a door handle, a tool, an eating utensil, or on the food itself. If a person touches the object, or eats or drinks the food, the germ has a new host.

Dust particles can carry bacteria, viruses, or fungal spores, or these pathogens can float in the air without a vehicle. If they can survive without the benefit of a host for a short time, they may find a new host by landing on the skin or by being inhaled.

Finally, vector transmission occurs when an intermediary ("middle man") carries the microorganism to the new host. The intermediary may be an infected mosquito or tick that bites or stings and leaves a few microorganisms at the site.

THE IMMUNE SYSTEM

The immune system consists of different cells and proteins that fight germs and the toxins they produce. The first line of defense is the skin. However, if there is a break in the skin, such as a scratch or a cut, the pathogen may be able to find its way into the body. Another protective mechanism is the mucous membrane that lines the airways and the gastrointestinal tract. The membrane is constantly exposed to external invasions from the air or food, but it has the ability to produce enzymes that attack pathogens. Internal secretions in the stomach and intestines also help to destroy and eliminate microorganisms that have found their way into the body. Finally, men have a long urethra, which discourages invasion of microorganisms, and women secrete an acid in the vagina that destroys most microorganisms.

Injury triggers other defense mechanisms. Inflammation increases the flow of blood to a damaged area, allowing for an accumulation of white blood cells to attack invading germs. White blood cells called B-lymphocytes reside in the blood stream and produce chemicals called antibodies that seek out microorganisms and destroy them. Other white blood cells, known as T-lymphocytes, find human cells that have been invaded by viruses and eliminate them.

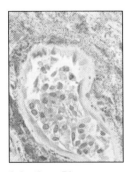

Infectious Disease. Some infectious diseases, such as the Ebola virus, above, can be life-threatening and are extremely contagious. Others may be mild and cause few, or even no symptoms.

Vaccinations for Children

The Food and Drug Administration suggests the following vaccinations for children:

- HIB protects against Haemophilus influenzae type B, which causes meningitis and can infect the blood, joints, bones, throat, and heart.

- DPT is a combination against diphtheria, tetanus, and pertussis (whooping cough). Diphtheria produces a sore throat, a fever, hoarseness, and extreme fatigue. Tetanus can attack the facial and jaw muscles, causing lockjaw. Untreated tetanus is fatal. Pertussis produces a characteristic cough with possible damage to the lungs and complications of pneumonia.

- Hepatitis B protects against the disease of the same name, a viral disease that can cause liver failure and death.

- Polio protects against the disease of the same name, which was epidemic in the 1950s. It starts with a fever, a sore throat, and a headache, but eventually progresses to paralysis of the legs. There is no cure for this disease.

- MMR protects against measles, mumps, and rubella (German measles). Measles causes a high fever, a cough, and a rash. Mumps causes painful swelling of the salivary glands, a fever, and a headache. It can progress to meningitis and deafness. Adult males suffering mumps may experience painful swelling of the testes. Rubella is especially dangerous for pregnant women because their babies may develop heart disease, blindness, hearing loss, or brain damage.

- Chickenpox can be prevented by a vaccine. The disease is caused by the varicella virus, which produces an itchy, uncomfortable rash and a mild fever. The real danger is in secondary infections of the open sores by streptococci or complications of pneumonia or meningitis.

[1] When a child receives a vaccine is as important as the vaccine itself. See Immunization for a recommended schedule of childhood vaccinations.

An increase in body temperature (fever) improves the ability of the body to fight infection, although in extreme situations it may be very uncomfortable or even dangerous to the brain. A doctor will need to decide whether reducing the fever, either with medication or by actually cooling the body physically—is better for the patient than allowing the fever to do its job.

Immunization prepares the body for an infection by teaching the immune system to produce antibodies specific to particular diseases. Tetanus shots, for example, are now routinely given every ten years. Most children get a series of vaccinations against tetanus, pertussis, influenza, polio, measles, mumps, rubella, and chickenpox. Adults at risk can be protected against anthrax, cholera, encephalitis, meningitis, hepatitis A and B, pneumonia, rabies, typhoid, and yellow fever.

MEDICATIONS

There are antibiotics (drugs that combat bacteria), antifungal drugs, antivirus drugs, and antiparasite drugs. Antibiotics in particular have been remarkably successful in combating many bacteria-based diseases. However, certain bacteria have developed strains resistant to the drugs, forcing the pharmaceutical industry to continually seek out ever new formulations.

Antibiotics are not specific to any particular bacteria. Most bacteria are identified by their shape, but they can also be identified as gram-positive or gram-negative, depending on how they respond to a laboratory technique called Gram's stain. If the bacteria stain pink, they are called gram-negative; if they stain blue, they are gram-positive. The color is an indicator of the type of cell wall the bacterium has. This is important, as many antibiotics interfere with the ability of the bacterium to repair its cell wall.

Gram-positive bacteria are controlled by penicillins, tetracycline, or erythromycin. Anthrax is an example of a gram-positive bacterial infection, as are staphylococcus and streptococcus infections.

Gram-negative bacteria have a double membrane, which can resist attack by many antibiotics. Gram-negative bacteria also have the ability to exchange DNA with other bacteria and thus "learn" how to be resistant to drugs. Treatment for gram-negative disorders (such as urinary tract infections or meningitis) requires certain types of antimicrobial drugs to target the underlying bacteria causing the condition.

There are fewer drugs that fight viral diseases. (Indeed, there are no drugs to combat such viral diseases as the common cold or infectious mononucleosis.) Influenza can be treated with four antiviral agents to shorten the course and severity of the disease. These agents are available if they are started within the first 48 hours of symptoms. For most viral diseases, however, a person's recovery depends on the body's immune system. Similarly, infections caused by the herpes virus have no cure. Acyclovir or other medications may

Pneumococci Infections

A form of streptococcus bacterium, pneumococci can cause a number of different sicknesses, depending on where the bacteria first lodge.

- Pneumonia is probably the most common infection caused by pneumococci. It attacks the lungs of people with weakened immune systems, such as those with Hodgkin's disease, lymphoma, multiple myeloma, and sickle cell disease. It also may develop after bronchitis or another viral infection of the lungs, such as influenza.
- Otitis is a middle-ear infection most often seen in children. If untreated, the infection can spread to the brain and spinal cord.
- Bacterial meningitis is an infection of the covering of the brain and the spinal cord.
- Bacteremia is an infection of the blood that can spread to the heart.
- Endocarditis is an infection of the heart valves which, if the valves rupture, can lead to heart failure.
- Peritonitis is an infection of the abdominal cavity.
- Arthritis is an infection of the joints.

assist in controlling the acute episodes.

Human immunodeficiency virus (HIV) has become widespread only in the last 20 years, but it is so severe an illness that many millions of dollars are being spent in search of a cure. Many drugs are available to slow the progress of the disease, but the virus usually develops a resistant strain if only one drug is used.

Antifungal medications are also fairly limited. Fungal infections may take a long time to show symptoms and their cure is often an equally lengthy process.

Antiparasite medications kill parasites, such as protozoa or worms, that live inside the body. There is a selection of amebicides that will kill parasites in the intestinal tract. Malaria, for example, is a parasitic infection of the blood caused by plasmodium, a single-cell microorganism. It is treated with chloroquine, quinine, or other similar drugs, but none is completely effective against the disease.

Background material on infectious disease can be found in IMMUNE RESPONSE and IMMUNE SYSTEM. For related information, see ALLERGY; BACTERIA; B-CELL; EDEMA; FEVER; FUNGI; HIV; IMMUNIZATION; PARASITE; PATHOGEN; T-CELL; VACCINATION; VECTOR; and VIRUSES.

Inferiority Complex

A neurotic state of mind in which an individual is haunted by persistent feelings of inadequacy and worthlessness.

Feelings of inferiority often have their source in childhood, when an individual was chastised, ridiculed, or demeaned by parents, other adult figures, or peers. Physical or psychological abuse in childhood often results in feelings of self-loathing and unworthiness that express themselves as an inferiority complex.

Questions about one's worth and abilities are normal, particularly in adolescence. The complex becomes serious and should be treated when it expresses itself in violence and aggression, or when it causes an individual to become overzealous in activities to the detriment of his or her personal welfare. *See also* SUPERIORITY COMPLEX.

Infertility

The inability to have a baby by natural processes.

Infertility is diagnosed after a full year of sexual intercourse without contraception. The condition affects approximately 5.3 million people in the United States, which is about nine percent of the population of reproductive age. Infertility affects both men and women in equal numbers. Approximately one-third of infertility cases can be attributed to the male partner, and about one-third to the female partner. For the remaining couples, infertility is believed to be caused by problems with both partners. However, not all cases of infertility can be explained medically.

Fertility depends on several factors:
- production of healthy sperm;
- production of healthy eggs;
- unblocked Fallopian tubes;
- ability of the sperm to penetrate and fertilize the egg;
- ability of the fertilized egg to implant itself in the uterine wall;
- sufficient embryo quality to ensure a successful pregnancy.

Resources on Infectious Diseases

Despommier, Dickson D., et al., *Parasitic Disease* (1995); Fields, Bernard, et al., *Fields' Virology* (1996); Grist, Norman R., et al., *Diseases of Infection: An Illustrated Textbook* (1992); Radetsky, Peter, *The Invisible Invaders: The Story of the Emerging Age of Viruses* (1994); Shaw, Michael, ed., *Everything You Need to Know About Diseases* (1996); Centers for Disease Contol and Prevention, Tel. (800) 311-3435, Online: www.cdc.gov; Infectious Disease Society of America, Tel. (703) 299-0200, Online: www.idsociety.org; Nat. Institute of Allergy and Infectious Disease, Tel. (301) 496-5717, Online: www.niaid.nih.org; Office of Rare Diseases, Tel. (301) 402-4336, Online: rarediseases.info.nih.gov/ www.nycornell.org/medicine/infectious/index.html

An egg is able to be fertilized for approximately 24 hours after ovulation. It is released into the abdominal cavity, then enters the fallopian tube and begins its journey toward the uterus. Sperm can survive for two to four days after being released into the female reproductive tract. The encounter with the egg will take place in the upper third of the fallopian tube. The fertilized egg immediately begins undergoing a series of cell divisions; when it implants in the uterine wall about a week later, it consists of a multicell embryo.

Causes. Infertility rates have increased in recent years due to the increase in sexually transmitted disease and the accompanying rise in pelvic inflammatory disease. The trend toward delayed childbearing is also responsible, as fertility decreases significantly with age. Women aged 35 to 44 are twice as likely to be infertile as women between the ages of 30 and 34.

Other factors, such as cigarette smoking, use of recreational drugs, and exposure to occupational and environmental hazards can affect fertility in both men and women. Some women experience temporary infertility if their body-fat level falls below a certain percentage, causing them to stop ovulating. Conditions such as endometriosis, uterine polyps, and fibroids can all interfere with conception and implantation. Ten to 30 percent of infertility cases have more than one cause. Thus, even if a specific problem is detected relatively early, further testing is usually done.

Male Infertility. The most common male infertility factors involve sperm production. A normal sample of semen contains between 400 million and 600 million sperm. Azoospermia refers to the absence of any sperm cells. Sometimes sperm are produced, but their number is too low to ensure fertilization. Although only one sperm can possibly fertilize an egg, a large number of sperm is generally needed to guarantee the egg will be fertilized. Most of the sperm released will not reach the final destination, as the journey is long and rigorous. The mobility of the sperm is also a factor in achieving fertilization.

Diagnosis and Treatment. Sperm analysis is one of the first tests done when a couple is unable to conceive. A semen sample is obtained and assessed regarding the volume, number, mobility, and shape of the sperm. A problem with the quantity or quality of sperm is usually caused by low hormone levels, injuries, infection, or a (reversible) reaction to a prescription drug. Sometimes, the remedy involves avoiding tight underwear or hot tubs, as sperm require a lower temperature to develop properly (which is why the testicles are located in the scrotum outside the abdomen). An enlarged vein in the scrotum (variocele) that impairs fertility can be easily corrected with surgery.

If the problem is a low sperm count, artificial insemination is an option, especially with "washed sperm" in which only the most active sperm have been selected for use. If there are no sperm or they are not viable, donor sperm is an option.

Female Infertility. The most common female infertility factor is an ovulation disorder. Other causes include blocked fallopian tubes, congenital abnormalities involving the uterus, and hormonal imbalances.

Diagnosis and Treatment. Failure to ovulate accounts for 20 percent of all female infertility problems. A woman can determine the date of ovulation by checking her resting (basal) body temperature throughout the month. Ovulation can then be confirmed with tests that measure the progesterone levels in the bloodstream, which peak about a week after ovulation.

If ovulation is not occurring, a number of drugs can be administered to induce ovulation, such as Clomid (clomiphene) or Pergonal (human menopausal gonadotropin). Usually a woman is started off with a relatively low dose and with each cycle is given a progressively larger dose until ovulation occurs. Side effects of these drugs include ovarian hyperstimulation syndrome, in which the ovaries become enlarged.

Damaged or blocked fallopian tubes account for 30 percent of infertility cases. The blockage may be due to adhesions or scar tissue. The test that determines if there is a blockage (and also shows the shape of the interior of the uterus) is known as a hysterosalpinogram. Surgery can attempt to clear the tubes of any obstruction, although the success rate is low. A woman with damaged tubes may be a candidate for in vitro fertilization.

Cervical factors such as the thickness and quality of the cervical mucus can also contribute to infertility. The amount and quality of the mucus normally varies during the cycle, becoming thinner, clearer, and more copious around ovulation. If the mucus is scant, too thick, or too dry, the sperm will not be able to travel through it on their way to the egg.

Unexplained infertility occurs in about 20 percent of all cases.

Treatment of infertility depends on the underlying cause. In 90 percent of all cases, the treatment involves medication or surgery. In vitro fertilization (IVF), gamete intrafallopian transfer (GIFT), and zygote intrafallopian transfer (ZIFT) all involve stimulating the ovaries to produce multiple mature eggs and then retrieving them.

In IVF, fertilization takes place in a laboratory. After 40 hours the embryos are transferred to the uterus. In GIFT, the sperm and eggs are placed together inside the fallopian tubes, where fertilization will take place. In ZIFT, fertilized eggs, which have already undergone a few cell divisions, are placed directly in the fallopian tubes.

In all of these procedures, which account for only five percent of all fertility treatments, multiple births are very likely to result, as more than one egg or embryo is transferred to increase the chances of pregnancy. Each attempt takes at least ten days and is quite costly. The risks include ovarian rupture, bleeding, and ectopic pregnancy. The success rates depend on where the procedure is performed; more experienced clinics and practitioners tend to have higher success rates.

> *Background material for infertility may be found in* RE-PRODUCTIVE SYSTEM, MALE *and* Reproductive Syem, Female. *See also* Artificial Insemination; Fertility; *and* Fertilization *for more on artificial techniques.*

Inflammation

Swelling; the response of living tissues to damage.

The acute inflammatory response involves three main functions. A material called exudate is released in the area of the wound, carrying proteins, fluids, and cells from blood vessels into the damaged area to mediate defenses. If an infecting agent, such as bacteria, is found in the damaged area, the exudate can get rid of it. The damaged tissue can then be broken down.

Acute inflammation occurs as the result of physical damage (bruises, broken limbs, internal injury), exposure to chemicals and microorganisms, and any number of other causes. Inflammation results in changes in blood flow, increased permeability of blood vessels, and the escape of cells from the blood to the tissues. Acute inflammation lasts only for a few days. If it lasts longer, it is referred to as chronic inflammation.

Treatment varies depending on the underlying cause. For minor injuries suffered to external tissue, ice packs may be beneficial. *See also* ICE PACKS *and* SWELLING.

Inflammatory Bowel Syndrome

Disorders that cause an inflammation of either the small or large intestine.

Inflammatory bowel disease is the general term for two disorders of the gastrointestinal tract: Crohn's disease and ulcerative colitis. Generally, there is no known cause although it has some ties to genetic inheritance. Chronic inflammation is present in both disorders; they vary as to which parts of the gastrointestinal tract are affected, as well as to specific symptoms. Crohn's disease and ulcerative colitis share a set of symptoms that include abdominal pains, such as bloating and cramps; constipation; diarrhea; fever; and fatigue. *See* CROHN'S DISEASE; INTESTINE; IRRITABLE BOWEL SYNDROME; *and* ULCERATIVE COLITIS.

Resources on Infertility
Eli Y. Adashi, Eli Y., John A., Rock, and Zev Rosenwaks, eds., *Reproductive Endocrinology, Surgery, and Technology (*1998); Breitkopf, Lyle J. and Marion Gordon Bakoulis, *Coping with Endometriosis* (1988); Laucella, Linda, *Hormone Replacement Therapy: Conventional Medicine and Natural Alternatives, Your Guide to Menopausal Health-Care Choices* (1999); Older, Julia, *Endometriosis* (1984); Endometriosis Assoc., Tel. (800) 992-3636, Online: www.endometriosisassn.org; Endocrine Web, Online: www.endocrineweb.com;www.nycornell.org/medicine/edm/index.html.

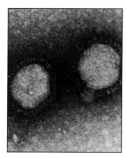

Influenza.
Influenza is a common viral infection of the upper respiratory tract. Above, the influenza virus.

Influenza

A viral infection of the upper respiratory tract.

TYPES

There are two main families of influenza virus, referred to as types A and B. Type A mutates every year, so antibodies that attack last year's strain are usually ineffective against this year's version. Type B is a little more stable, meaning that it does not mutate as often as type A; therefore, antibodies against last year's strain may be helpful against this year's version. Every 20 years or so, a completely new strain appears and can cause widespread disease and even death. The Spanish flu pandemic of 1918 was the worst influenza epidemic ever reported. Almost half a million people died from this strain of the influenza virus in the United States alone.

SYMPTOMS

Influenza is spread when an infected person coughs or sneezes, releasing water droplets that carry the virus into the air which is then breathed by others. The virus infects the mucous membranes of the nose, throat, and lungs, causing inflammation and swelling. Within 24 to 48 hours of exposure the sufferer will experience chills and a fever of 102°F to 104° F. Other symptoms include weakness, loss of appetite, muscle aches (particularly in the back and legs), headache, sore throat, and burning eyes. During the first couple of days the symptoms are mild, but as the disease progresses the patient will develop a severe cough that brings up sputum. Some individuals (mainly children) may also experience nausea and vomiting.

For previously healthy people the fever may last two or three days, but the coughing and bronchitis may persist for ten days. Swelling of the airways and weakness and fatigue may last for weeks. For the ill or elderly, the disease can be severe and even fatal. Furthermore, elderly individuals are often vulnerable to complications, especially bacterial infections that attack the body in its weakened condition.

PREVENTION

Vaccination is the best preventive option and is usually successful. The influenza vaccine is updated each year to combat the current strain of virus. Most people have no reaction to the vaccine, though some will develop a red and tender area around the site of injection. A few children may develop a low fever, a headache, and feel a little sick. The condition of people who already have a respiratory disease may worsen. Allergic reactions to the vaccine are possible in people who are sensitive to egg protein, as the vaccine is cultivated in an egg base. These people should not be vaccinated.

TREATMENT

Two antiviral drugs, amantadine and rimantadine, are available to combat influenza A. They do not work against type B. These drugs should be taken for two or three weeks following vaccination or throughout the winter season if the vaccination cannot be given. The drugs have side effects, including nervousness, confusion, hallucination, dizziness, and headaches, especially among the elderly or those with brain or kidney disease.

A new family of drugs was approved in 1999 by the Food and Drug Administration for use in treating influenza. These are neuraminidase inhibitors, and the first of

---

Risk Factors

The following people are at special risk of contracting influenza and should be vaccinated every year:

If you have:
- Lung diseases such as asthma, emphysema, chronic bronchitis, tuberculosis, or cystic fibrosis;
- Heart disease;
- Kidney disease;
- Diabetes or other metabolic problems;
- Severe anemia;
- Lowered immunity or AIDS;
- Recently had an organ transplant.

If you are:
- Living in a nursing home or other care facility;
- Over 50 years old;
- A doctor or a nurse;
- Employed in a high-exposure-risk profession.

these drugs to become available are called zanamavir and oseltamivir. The drugs are prescribed only for adults who have had the symptoms of influenza for less than 48 hours. They work against both type A and type B influenza. Early trials indicate that they reduce the duration of the illness and the severity of the symptoms. The inhaled drug zanamavir may cause increased asthmatic symptoms in people with asthma.

Most people with influenza are directed to stay in bed until the fever has subsided, which usually is a couple of days. Aspirin and acetaminophen may help control the fever. It is important to remember not to give aspirin to children, who are in danger of contracting a serious disease called Reye's syndrome, which is caused by the combination of aspirin and a virus. There are also many over-the-counter drugs that will treat the symptoms of influenza, such as nasal decongestants, cough suppressants, and steam inhalers.

COMPLICATIONS

Complications are likely for people with compromised immune systems, such as those undergoing chemotherapy, those who have had a recent organ transplant, or those who are suffering from AIDS. Young children and the elderly are at particular risk for influenza, both for the consequences of the disease itself, and for the possible complications. In these people, the development of bacterial infections is possible. Any secondary bacterial infection should be treated with antibiotics.

> **For background information on influenza, see INFECTIOUS DISEASE and VIRUSES. Related material can be found in AGING; AIDS; ANTIBIOTIC DRUGS; ANTIVIRAL DRUGS; ASPIRIN; AUTOIMMUNE DISORDERS; BACTERIA; CHEMOTHERAPY; IMMUNIZATION; and VACCINATION.**

Infrared

> **A low-frequency portion of the electromagnetic spectrum, beyond visible red.**

Infrared rays are a portion of the electromagnetic spectrum. Such radiation includes radiant heat; radio, TV, and microwaves; visible and ultraviolet light, and x-rays and gamma rays.

Sources of infrared radiation include the sun, electric heating elements, and incandescent lights. As infrared energy is readily converted to heat, infrared sources are often used therapeutically for the stimulation of circulation and for pain relief. Long wave length infrared radiation is emitted by all heated bodies, particularly those at relatively low temperature, such as heating pads or hot water bottles. Shorter wave length infrared is emitted by all incandescent sources. *See also* RADIATION; RADIATION HAZARDS; RADIATION SICKNESS: RADIATION THERAPY; RADIOACTIVITY; THERMOGRAPHY; *and* X-RAYS.

Ingrown Toenail

> **A condition in which the edge of the toenail grows into the skin of the toe.**

Ingrown toenails are most common on the big toe, but can occur on any toe. The skin around the toenail becomes red, and possibly infected. Having curved toenails, wearing shoes that fit poorly, and trimming the toenails improperly can result in ingrown toenails, which can be painful.

Home treatment of ingrown toenails includes trimming the nail and soaking the foot in warm, saltwater. If the nail cannot be trimmed or an individual experiences severe pain, swelling, or redness, a doctor should be contacted.

If an infection is present, ingrown toenails can be treated with antibiotics. A doctor or other health-care professional can trim the toenail around the ingrown edge. Soaking the area in warm saltwater several times a day can help to relieve pain. If ingrown toenails occur chronically or recurrently, they can be treated with certain surgical procedures.

Ingrown toenails can be prevented by wearing shoes that fit, trimming toenails straight across and to an appropriate length, and keeping feet dry and clean. *See also* ANTIBIOTICS; SWELLING; *and* TOE.

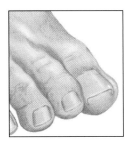

Ingrown Toenail. Above, an ingrown toenail, a painful but minor condition in which the edge of the toenail penetrates the skin of the toe.

Resources on the Influenza

Kolata, Gina, *Flu: The Story of an Epidemic* (1999); Grist, Norman R., et al., *Diseases of Infection: An Illustrated Textbook* (1992); Shaw, Michael, ed., *Everything You Need to Know About Diseases* (1996); Fettner, Ann Guidici, *The Science of Viruses: What They Are, Why They Make Us Sick, How They Will Change the Future* (1990); Centers for Disease Con-tol and Prevention, Tel. (800) 311-3435, Online: www.cdc.gov; Infectious Disease Society of America, Tel. (703) 299-0200, Online: www.idso-ciety.org; National Institute of Allergy and Infectious Disease, Tel. (301) 496-5717, Online: www.niaid.nih.org.

Inhaler

Device for administering medicine to treat respiratory tract disorders.

There are three kinds of inhalers: aerosols, nebulizers, and turbo-inhalers. An aerosol inhaler delivers the drug as a spray. A nebulizer delivers a drug as a mist, through a face mask. A turbo-inhaler delivers a powdered drug. Some devices are metered-dose inhalers, which deliver a specific amount of medication. Conditions treated by inhalers include asthma, bronchitis, and alveolitis, and the drugs that are given through an inhaler include vasodilators, which help to open airways, and steroids, which reduce inflammation.

The user of any inhaler should first wash the hands and then sit or stand with the head tilted back. For a nasal inhaler, one nostril should be held closed by a finger. The inhaler should be inserted about one-half inch into the other nostril, inhaling as the medicine is dispensed. For a mouth inhaler, the nozzle should be put into the mouth, with the user breathing as the top of the inhaler is pressed to release the medication. If the inhaler is used for asthma, all the directions should be followed exactly for the medication to reach the lungs. *See also* ALVEOLITIS; ASTHMA; BRONCHITIS; INFLAMMATION; NEBULIZER; STEROID DRUGS; *and* VASODILATOR DRUGS.

Inheritance

The transmission of traits from parents to off-spring.

Inheritance is the transmission of genes and the traits they create from one generation to the next. Genes, located on chromosomes in cell nuclei, are the units that carry hereditary information. Because chromosomes are paired, so, too—almost unanimously—are genes. These gene pairings are called alleles. Alleles contain information for the encoding and production of proteins responsible for the hereditary traits that define an individual.

There are approximately 100,000 genes in each human cell, distributed among 23 pairs of chromosomes. Twenty-two pairs are regular chromosomes, called autosomes, and the remaining pair are the sex chromosomes–they determine a person's gender: Females have two X chromosomes, while males have one X chromosome and one Y chromosome. On the autosomes, genes occur in pairs, thus two genes govern the production of any given protein and affect the same physical characteristic. Genes on the X and Y chromosomes, however, are not necessarily paired.

TYPES OF INHERITANCE

Dominant-Recessive Inheritance. Two genes for a particular trait are inherited, one from each parent. These gene pairs are the alleles; in most cases, one allele is dominant—it codes for a particular trait while masking the trait coded by the other (recessive) allele. The dominant allele is symbolized by a capital letter; the recessive is designated by a lowercase letter.

Consider for example, the paired genes that control the pigments that determine eye color. The dominant allele, B, codes for brown eyes, and the recessive allele, b, for blue eyes. If the pair of genes controlling eye color consists of dominant alleles—or BB—the person will have brown eyes. If one dominant and one recessive allele—Bb—constitute the pair of genes, the allele for brown eyes will dominate and mask the allele for blue eyes, and the person's eyes will be brown. However, this brown-eyed person still possesses an allele for blue eyes—the "b" in "Bb"—and may pass it on to offspring. Only two recessive alleles—bb—will result in blue eyes. It is impossible to determine by simple physical observation whether an individual with a dominant trait (say, brown eyes) has two dominant alleles (BB) or one dominant and one recessive allele (Bb).

Intermediate Inheritance. Some traits show incomplete dominance, in which one allele, though dominant, does not completely mask the code of the other. This results in a unique trait different from either the entirely dominant or the entirely recessive gene pair. For example, inheritance of the sickling gene causes the substitution of a single amino acid in a polypeptide chain of hemoglobin. While receiving two sickling alleles (ss) causes sickle-cell anemia, those who receive only one sickling allele (Ss) have a condition called sickle-cell trait. While generally healthy, they make both normal and sickling hemoglobin and are susceptible to dangerous drops in blood oxygen. Those with two dominant alleles (SS) are normal.

Multiple-Allele Inheritance. In this case, one pair of genes is responsible for the trait, but there are more than just two alleles. Human blood groups fall into this category. Blood type is dependent upon the presence of a specific protein called an antigen. Type A blood has antigen A, comprised of either two A alleles or one each of A and O. Type B blood has antigen B, comprised of either two B alleles or one each of B and O. Type O has neither A nor B antigens and is always comprised of two O alleles. Type AB has both A and B antigens, made up of an A allele and a B allele. The A and B alleles are co-dominant; either one of them may dominate the O allele.

Sex-Linked Inheritance. Sex-linked traits are determined by genes on X chromosomes. The Y chromosome carries only a few genes, most related to the perpetuation of the Y chromosome. Many genes on the X chromosome do not have a matched gene on the Y chromosome and thus cannot be masked by another dominant gene.

All eggs carry an X chromosome. Half of all sperm carry an X chromosome, and the other half carry a Y chromosome. When an X chromosome–carrying sperm combines with an egg, the resulting zygote —the cell produced when a sperm fertilizes an egg—will carry two X chromosomes and thus be female (XX). When a Y chromosome-carrying sperm combines with an egg, the zygote will carry an X chromosome and a Y chromosome and thus be male (XY). Fathers always pass on a Y chromosome to a son and an X chromosome to a daughter. Therefore, they cannot pass on

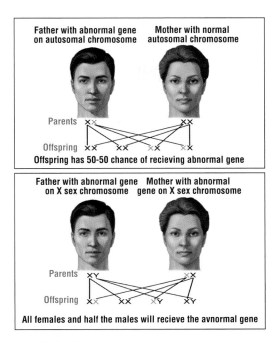

Father with abnormal gene on autosomal chromosome   **Mother with normal autosomal chromosome**

Parents   xx   xx

Offspring   xx   xx   xx   xx

Offspring has 50-50 chance of recieving abnormal gene

Father with abnormal gene on X sex chromosome   **Mother with abnormal gene on X sex chromosome**

Parents   xY   xx

Offspring   xx   xx   xY   xY

All females and half the males will recieve the avnormal gene

Autosomal Genes.
Top: Genes on the autosome occur in pairs, which means that two genes can affect the same physical characteristics.

Sex-linked inheritance.
Bottom: Genes on X chromosomes determine sex-linked traits such as hemophilia and color blindness.

sex-linked characteristics to their sons, only to their daughters. Mothers pass on an X chromosome to all of their offspring and can therefore pass on sex-linked characteristics to any child.

Common human sex-linked characteristics include hemophilia and color blindness. They are recessive traits, meaning they will occur only when there are no dominant genes involved. A woman can have two dominant normal genes, two recessive genes, or one dominant and one recessive. If she has two dominant genes, she will not have the trait or pass it on to any offspring. If she has two recessive genes, she will have the trait and pass it on to offspring. If she has one dominant allele and one recessive, she herself will not exhibit the condition, but she may pass the recessive allele on to her offspring. She is therefore a "carrier."

In contrast, a male has only two options. He can carry one dominant or one recessive allele on his X chromosome. If it is dominant, he is normal. If it is recessive, he has the condition. There are no male carriers of a sex-linked characteristic.

Polygene Inheritance. Polygenes are a set of several genes responsible for a particular trait. For example, four gene pairs determine height. Because of the increased

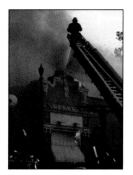

Injury.
Firefighters, above, risk burns and fractures daily in order to do their jobs. External harm or injury to the body can also come in forms such as bites, sprains, joint dislocation, and stings.

range of possibility allowed by the greater number of genes and alleles, polygene inheritance makes it possible for average parents to have tall children.

PREDICTING INHERITANCE

The probability of an offspring inheriting a specific trait can be derived from parental genetic makeup. For example, if it is known that both brown-eyed parents have the alleles Bb, then there is a 75 percent chance the child will have brown eyes—via BB, Bb, or bB alleles—and a 25 percent chance the child will have blue eyes, via bb alleles. However, in the case of a trait like height, environment, nutrition, and disease may all make predictions more difficult.

Other Factors. Inheritance is also affected by mosaicism, a condition in which some cells in a person's body have one genetic blueprint and the remaining cells have another. The usual cause is a defect in early embryonic cell division. A common form of mosaicism is the random inactivation of one of the two X chromosomes in women, which allows some cells to express the genes on the X chromosome inherited from the mother, and other cells to express the genes on the X chromosome inherited from the father.

INHERITANCE AND DISEASE

Genetic diseases can, to an extent, be predicted based on patterns of inheritance. Most genetic disorders are recessive. For example, cystic fibrosis is an autosomal recessive condition that is passed on in the same pattern that blue eyes are transmitted. Hemophilia is a recessive sex-linked disease that predominantly affects males.

In general, if a person has family members with a genetic disorder and wishes to have children, he should receive genetic counseling to determine whether he has the gene for that disorder and what the chances are of passing it on to offspring.

> *Background information on inheritance can be found in* CHROMOSOMAL ABNORMALITIES; CHROMOSOME; GENE; GENETICS; *and* HEREDITY. *For related material, see* ANEMIA, HEMOLYTIC; COLOR VISION; CONCEPTION; CYSTIC FIBROSIS; DOWN'S SYNDROME; HEMOPHILIA; *and* SPERM.

Injury

A trauma to any part of the body.

The term injury covers a wide variety of circumstances that can result in harm to the body. They generally are considered problems that are due to some kind of external attack, rather than diseases (which tend to come from within the body). Injuries may include: fractures, sprains, strains, joint dislocations, cuts, burns, cold-related trauma, bites, stings, and sickness from poison.

All injuries need to be treated according to the specifics of their condition. Some general rules include:

Fractures and Sprains. Immediate care for suspected fractures or sprains is commonly called RICE: Rest the injured part; Ice the area; Compress with a bandage; Elevate the injured part to help the blood flow away from the area.

Animal Bites and Scratches. Apply pressure with a clean bandage or towel to stop bleeding. Clean the area, and call a physician to find out if antibiotics or shots, such as tetanus, may be needed; try to note as

Prevention

Many common injuries can be prevented. The majority of accidents take place in the home, so safety measures taken in the house can help to decrease injury, especially when small children are present.

Following simple rules like these, as well as just using common sense, can help to decrease the potential for injury:

- Keep cleaning materials and anything else potentially poisonous locked up and out of the reach of children.
- Do not leave objects that could be tripped over on the floors.
- Keep all knives, utensils, and tools locked up.
- Make sure that all medicines are clearly labeled, not out of date, and out of reach of children.
- Do not leave stoves unattended during cooking; check that gas burners are completely off when stoves are not in use.
- Check smoke detectors regularly to ensure that they function properly.
- Keep all firearms locked up; make sure that the owner knows how to operate them safely, and that children understand that they are not toys.

many details as possible about the animal that caused the wound.

Poison. Find out what the victim has swallowed or find out how he or she has been poisoned. Call for an ambulance, or the local poison control center.

Burns. For minor burns, run the injured part under cold water or apply an ice pack until pain subsides. Clean and bandage the burned area to avoid the possibility of infection. *See also* BITES, ANIMAL; BURNS; DRUG POISONING; EMERGENCY FIRST STEPS; FIRST AID; FRACTURES; POISON; *and* SPRAINS .

Inoculation

The administration of a vaccine, which is a solution of weakened viruses that stimulates the production of antibodies (protective proteins).

Active immunity against a disease can be artificially induced by immunization, the injection of a vaccine. The body launches an immune response against the antigens (foreign substances) contained in the vaccine and develops memory cells so that future encounters with the same pathogen will be dealt with swiftly. Some vaccines, like polio, can be administered orally, as well as injected. *See also* ANTIGEN; IMMUNE SYSTEM; *and* IMMUNIZATION.

Inoperable

Any irregular physical condition not amenable to treatment by surgery.

There are many possible reasons that a particular ailment may be deemed inoperable. A patient may simply be too weak or frail to safely withstand a treatment that would be otherwise safe. In some cases, the location of an irregularity (for example a tumor), may make it inaccessible to the surgeon's instruments, or it may appear in a region that presents inordinate risk, as is the case with inoperable tumors of the brain.

Inoperable may also be used to describe conditions that will not be significantly improved by surgery, as in cases where disease has spread throughout the body. *See also* BRAIN TUMOR *and* SURGERY.

Insect Bites

Any bites, caused by insects, that may produce swelling, irritation, itching, or disease.

Most insect bites do not require medical attention, though a few can lead to serious, even fatal, results. Many common insects can produce anaphylactic shock in persons with heightened allergic sensitivity to insect saliva or venom. A number of insects are carriers for viral, parasitic, and bacterial infections, some are grave. Identifying symptoms and, whenever possible, the insect responsible for the bite or sting will help in recommending treatment.

Types of Insect Bites:

• Mosquito bites are among the most common insect bites. Generally, the small, itching bumps subside quickly, posing no threat to health. Some species of mosquito do, however, transmit serious diseases, including malaria, dengue fever, encephalitis, and yellow fever;

• Common flea bites acquired through contact with dogs or cats produce irritation and itching. Some species of fleas, however, may carry diseases such as plague and murine typhus;

• Bedbugs are likewise often benign, irritating pests, but may carry Chagas' disease;

• Spiders, though not truly insects, sometimes inflict painful bites on humans. While generally nonthreatening, some species, including the black widow and brown recluse, inject a highly toxic venom;

• Various species of louse may infest the head, body, or pubic area, producing an itching, excoriated skin rash; in some cases they transmit diseases such as trench fever, epidemic typhus, or relapsing fever.

Treatment. Insects should be removed from the skin and the area cleaned. Where itching, pain, or irritation are severe, an ointment containing antihistamine and corticosteroid will reduce swelling and offer pain relief. In cases of bedbug or flea infestation, an entire residence may need to be treated with insecticides. For lice, insecticidal lotions effectively treat infestation. *See also* INSECTS AND DISEASE.

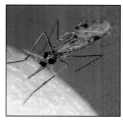
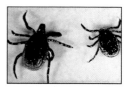

Insect Bites.
Insects such as the Lyme tick, top, and mosquito, bottom, can pose some serious health risks to humans. Lyme disease is a bacterial infection transmitted to humans by lyme ticks that live on deer. Symptons of the disease include headache, fever, lethargy, and muscle aches. Mosquito bites can be life-threatening to humans because they transmit diseases such as dengue fever, malaria, and encephalitis.

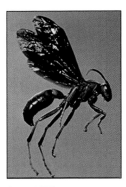

Insect Stings.
Wasps, above, are not known to carry human diseases, but allergic reactions to their venom and to the venom of insects such as yellow jackets and bees, can cause reactions in humans ranging from mild to fatal.

Insect Stings

Perforation of the skin by stinging insects such as wasps, bees, yellow jackets, ants, and hornets.

A small number of stinging insects are known to attack humans. While stings of wasps, ants, bees, yellow jackets, and other insects are often painful, they are by and large not a serious risk to health. It's not the piercing of the skin, but the insect's injection of a swelling and irritation–inducing liquid (venom) that causes pain. This discomfort is usually minor and lasts one to two days. However, some people exhibit severe allergic reactions in addition to the characteristic swelling, redness, and discomfort normally associated with such stings. In cases of allergy, these individuals may experience anaphylactic shock, a potentially life-threatening condition.

Bees and Wasps. In the United States, bee and wasp stings are common. In general, a person may withstand ten such stings per pound of body weight without risk of serious complication. Attacks involving multiple stings can cause circulatory collapse or cardiac arrest. Those with severe allergy to such stings may lapse into anaphylactic shock from a single sting. Certain aggressive species of bee, such as the Africanized honeybee, or killer bee, pose another threat due to their tendency to attack in swarms with little provocation.

Fire ants produce painful, occasionally fatal stings and are common to the American South. Such stings produce immediate pain, followed by swelling and blistering. When the blister ruptures after 30 to 70 hours, a secondary infection may develop and in some cases the entire limb may swell. Fire-ant stings are likewise capable of inducing anaphylactic shock, which acts to constrict the air passages and lower blood pressure, although this reaction occurs in fewer than one percent of those stung.

Treatment. Bees, fire ants, and wasps may leave a stinger embedded in the skin following attack. Care must be taken to gently remove the stinger without squeezing it, which will inject more venom into the skin. Scraping with a dull table knife or credit card against the skin next to the embedded stinger will help to remove it. Tweezers should be avoided. Ice may be applied to reduce the pain. Antihistamine or corticosteroid cream is helpful in reducing swelling and for pain relief. It is critical that the area be repeatedly washed during the healing process to avoid infection. Consult a physician if an infection develops.

Alert. Individuals known to have allergies to stinging insects should carry allergy kits including antihistamines and syringes for injecting epinephrine to improve breathing and circulation. Symptoms of (whole-body) reaction to insect stings include nausea; hives; facial swelling; shortness of breath and wheezing; difficulty swallowing; light-headedness and fainting; chest and throat tightness; and swell- ing or redness over most of the body. The onset of symptoms can occur anywhere from within minutes to several hours later. A doctor should be contacted immediately.

> *For background information on insect stings, see* INSECTS AND DISEASE. *Related material can be found in* ALLERGY; ANAPHYLACTIC SHOCK; ANTIHISTAMINE DRUGS; CARDIAC ARREST; CORTICOSTEROID DRUGS; EPINEPHRINE; *and* VENOMOUS BITES AND STINGS.

Insects and Disease

Disease spread through bites, stings, or other activities of insects.

Insects, though generally innocuous, transmit serious illnesses, especially in developing countries. The following list describes some of the ways in which insect-related disease is transmitted.

Venom. A small number of insects cause illness by venomous stings. Stings are usually a form of defense on the part of the insect. While most stings cause temporary pain or discomfort, allergy or extreme potency of venom can result in severe tissue damage, breathlessness, irregular heartbeat, and death. Extreme allergy can lead to a life-threatening allergic reaction (anaphylactic shock). Black widow spiders and scorpions have especially toxic venom.

Hygiene. Insects and bugs, such as flies and roaches, that interact with feces, decomposed matter, and food proposed for human consumption transmit disease. When restaurants or living environments are not kept clean or sanitized, the areas may attract insects. The legs of these insects carry disease-causing organisms. Typhoid fever, shigellosis, and other intestinal infections are spread by these insects, which land on food, cooking and eating utensils, and skin.

Blood-Sucking. The largest group of disease-causing insects consists of those that suck blood. Parasitic disease-causing organisms are contracted by the insect when it feeds on an infected host. The infected insect then transmits the organism to the new host through the blood.

Some species of mosquito are carriers of malaria, dengue fever, encephalitis, yellow fever, and other illnesses. Tick bites can transmit a number of illnesses, particularly Lyme disease. Flea bites acquired through contact with dogs or cats produce irritation and itching. Some species of fleas, however, may carry diseases, such as plague and murine typhus. Sand flies in the Middle East can transmit the spleen-and-liver disease called kala-azar.

Skin and Hair Infestation. Yet another class of insect are those that simply live on the host. They attach themselves to the skin or hair and suck blood. These insects often cause varying levels of irritation and discomfort. Chiggers, itch mites (the source of scabies), and lice are common sources of this infestation.

Treatment. Most insect bites are quickly identified due to the immediate pain or irritation caused by the bite. Identifying the insect responsible will allow for speedy diagnosis and treatment. Resulting diseases, however, require specific care above and beyond treatment of the bite or sting itself.

Background material on insects and disease can be found in INFECTIOUS DISEASE. *For further reading, see* ANAPHYLACTIC SHOCK; CHAGAS' DISEASE; DENGUE; ENCEPHALITIS; KALA-AZAR; LEISHMANIASIS; LICE; LYME DISEASE; MALARIA; MOSQUITO BITES; TSETSE FLY BITES; TUMBU FLY BITES; TRENCH FEVER; TRYPANOSOMIASIS; *and* YELLOW FEVER.

Insight Psychotherapy

Also known as psychodynamically oriented psychother-

A form of psychotherapy that aims to relieve emotional conflict by helping the patient understand the cause of a conflict.

The idea behind insight psychotherapy is that a person experiences emotional and mood disorders because of unconscious psychological conflicts. Behavior that is a reaction to an unconscious conflict tends to be maladaptive, because a person tries to work out unresolved issues from the past in ways that may not be appropriate or relevant to what is happening in the present. Becoming aware of the cause of these conflicts can break the cycle of inappropriate behaviors and relieve the symptoms.

Insight psychotherapy allows for a stable and supportive relationship with a physician, in which a person can express fears and thoughts that may not otherwise be acceptable to share with another person. This relationship can itself be healing.

Insight psychotherapy has been used for a large range of disorders, including long-standing behavioral problems, phobias, and obsessive-compulsive behaviors. It is often used in combination with other therapies. *See also* PERSONALITY DISORDERS *and* PHOBIA.

Insomnia

Episodic or chronic inability to attain sufficient sleep.

Almost everyone has suffered a bout of transient insomnia when worried about a problem or when feeling fearful. Even happy events can lead to a few nights of poor sleep. When problems persist for upwards of a month, however, a person may be experiencing insomnia.

It is not just the quantity of sleep but the quality that is important in feeling refreshed the next day. If a person spends eight hours in bed tossing and turning, sleeping and waking up, he or she will not benefit as much as from fewer hours of sound sleep.

Causes. Insomnia has a variety of physi-

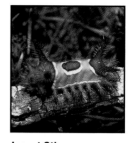

Insect Stings.
The sting of a saddle-back catepillar, above, can be both painful and harmful.

Sleep and Aging

As we age, we require less sleep. A newborn sleeps 16 hours a day, the average middle-aged person sleeps seven hours a day, and the average amount of sleep continues to decrease as we age. It is not uncommon for older people to sleep fewer hours each night than they did in their youth and to awaken for a variety of reasons during the night. As a person ages, it may take longer to get to sleep. Older people may also wake up more often and wake at an earlier hour.

If less sleep at night does not cause fatigue or decreased alertness during the day, then it may not be indicative of insomnia. Realizing that as people age they will need less sleep can reduce frustration and worry. But because insomnia may indicate a medical problem, it is important to rule out other causes before deciding that one simply needs less sleep.

cal, psychological, substance-related, and environmental causes. A sleep problem can be caused by external stimuli, such as noise or too much light in the room. A recent move from an urban to a rural area, or vice versa, may result in changed sleep patterns.

A number of substances may contribute to difficulty falling asleep. By far the most commonly used substance that affects sleep is caffeine. It is wise to eliminate intake of caffeine in the afternoon and evening. The use of alcohol, sedatives, and sleeping pills, which initially may aid in sleeping, can cause the opposite effect when used over time. For this reason, sleeping pills should be taken only as prescribed and never for longer than a two-week period. Other medications that can interfere with sleep are antidepressants, decongestants, amphetamines, and most illegal drugs.

Certain medical conditions contribute to sleeping problems, including those that cause pain (such as arthritis), coughing, and kidney problems or any illness that causes frequent urination. Parkinson's disease and Alzheimer's disease, which impact the brain, can also cause sleep disruption. Sleep apnea, common in overweight people, and narcolepsy, the uncontrollable need to sleep during the day, can also result in insomnia.

Psychological disorders can also cause insomnia. People with depressive disorder tend to have trouble falling asleep, wake often during the night, or awaken early in the morning, often before sunrise. The manic episodes of manic-depressive disorder result in high energy levels that do not subside at night, causing significantly fewer hours of sleep. Insomnia, including the onset of nightmares, may precede a psychotic episode and help predict its onset.

Treatment. It is important to first determine if there is an underlying medical cause for insomnia and to treat the problem. A review of all medications and substances, consumed including caffeine and over-the-counter medications, as well as prescription drugs—is important to determine if any of these is contributing to problems with sleep. If an emotional problem, such as depression or anxiety, is causing the lack of sleep, the disorder should be recognized and treated with psychotherapy, medication, behavior therapy, or relaxation therapy to see if the insomnia can be alleviated.

How to Fall Asleep

- Do not go to bed if you are not tired, since staying in bed when you are wide awake can cause additional anxiety and fears of not falling asleep, which snowball and make sleeping more difficult.
- Avoid substances that may contribute to sleep problems and try to make the sleep environment as comfortable as possible.
- Keep the room dark, and make sure the bed is comfortable. Sometimes indulging yourself with particularly comfortable bedding can be a stimulus to better sleep.
- Sleeping pills should be taken only under the direction of a physician; also they should be used judiciously, and never for extended periods of time.
- Thirty minutes of daily exercise can also help a person fall asleep and sleep more soundly.

Taking naps can help when pain or breathing problems due to asthma or a cold are causing unavoidable sleep disturbances, but naps should be avoided as a means of achieving a regular pattern of sleeping and waking.

For background material on insomnia, see SLEEP *and* SLEEP DEPRIVATION. *Further information can be found in* ALCOHOL DEPENDENCE; ARTHRITIS; CAFFEINE; DRUG DEPENDENCE; OBESITY; PSYCHIATRY; *and* SUBSTANCE ABUSE.

Insulin

A hormone produced by the pancreas that helps to maintain blood glucose levels.

When the body takes in food, the digestive system breaks down proteins into amino acids and starches, sugars into simple sugars, and fats into fatty acids. Glucose, the main source of energy in the body, comes from the digestion of sugars and carbohydrates. As the blood glucose levels in the body rise, the pancreas releases insulin. This hormone helps send the fats and proteins into the parts of the body that need them, and stops the liver's production of glucose. This helps the body maintain the necessary amount of blood glucose for the tissues and organs to function effectively. Insulin also makes sure that the fat stored in the adipose tissues is not broken down and used when it is not necessary.

LACK OF INSULIN

When little or no insulin is produced, glucose accumulates in the blood, causing the condition known as hyperglycemia. The excess glucose is excreted by the kidneys, causing excessive urination and dehydration. The fat stores in the body break down, causing rapid weight loss. The longer a person goes without insulin, the more complications ensue. A lack of insulin caused by the inability of the pancreas to produce enough (or any) insulin results in a disease known as diabetes mellitus.

INSULIN THERAPY.

Although a proper diet and exercise will help stabilize blood glucose levels, Type I diabetics, who do not have any insulin in their bodies, must receive some from an external source.

Insulin cannot be taken orally, because the digestive juices in the gastrointestinal tract will destroy it. Therefore, insulin must be administered through injection—either under the skin, into a muscle, or into a vein. Monitoring of blood glucose levels will help determine when and how often shots are necessary.

Types of Insulin

There are four types of insulin, each with a different duration of effectiveness. Most people use a combination of the different kinds to maintain a normal blood glucose level.

- **Rapid-Acting Insulin:** Should be taken within 15 minutes of a meal; lasts 2–5 hours;
- **Short-Acting Insulin:** Peaks within 2 hours; has a duration of about 8 hours;
- **Intermediate-Action Insulin:** Peaks within 6 hours; can last up to 24 hours;
- **Long-Acting Insulin:** Peaks within 4–14 hours; duration of about 36 hours.

Complications. Hypoglycemia is the most common complication resulting when too much insulin is injected. If a friend or family member takes insulin for the treatment of diabetes, it is important to be aware of the symptoms of hypoglycemia. These include: a racing pulse, head- ache, clamminess, hand tremors, hunger, tingling, and confused thought. Treatment involves helping to raise blood glucose by giving the individual fruit juice or small amounts of food. Glucose or dextrose tablets also should be kept handy.

Background information on insulin can be found in DIABETES INSIPIDUS; DIABETES MELLITUS; *and* PANCREAS. *For related material, see* DEHYDRATION; GLUCOSE; HYPOGLYCEMIA; *and* METABOLISM.

Insulinoma

A nonmalignant tumor of the pancreas.

An insulinoma arises in the cells of the pancreas that secrete insulin. These tumors are rare. While they are not cancerous, they produce abnormally large amounts of insulin, which can produce hypoglycemia—dangerously low levels of sugar in the blood. Extreme hypoglycemia can be life-threatening. When low blood-sugar levels caused by an insulinoma are detected, those levels can be kept near normal by drug treatment. The insulinoma then can be removed surgically. *See also* HYPOGLYCEMIA; INSULIN; PANCREAS; *and* TUMOR.

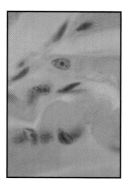
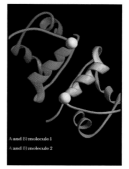

A and B molecule 1
A and B molecule 2

Insulin.
At top, a magnification of the insulin-producing Islest of Langerhans in the pancreas. Bottom, the molecular structure of insulin.

Resources on Diabetes
Groff, James L. et al., *Advanced Nutrition and Human Metabolism* (1999); New, Maria, *Genetics of Endocrine Disorders* (2001); Walker, Elizabeth A., et al., *American Diabetes Association Complete Guide to Diabetes* (2000); American Diabetes Association, Tel. (800) 342-2383, Online: www.diabetes. org; The Juvenile Diabetes Foundation International, Tel. (800) JDF-CURE, Online: www.jdfcure.org; National Institute of Diabetes and Digestive and Kidney Diseases, Tel. (301) 496-3583, Online: www.niddk.nih.gov; www.nycornell.org/.

Intelligence

The ability to reason and to understand concepts.

The observation that some people seem smarter than others has led to attempts to measure intelligence differences, with controversial results. One consequence of such testing is that intelligence has come to be regarded as a single ability (like muscle strength), whereas all indications are that a number of complex factors are involved in an individual's mental navigation through the problems and challenges of life. Some psychologists regard three factors as critical to overall intelligence: problem-solving; learning; and speed of thought. Others divide the components of intelligence into seven factors, and others into as many as a hundred. The fact that an individual's acuity in performing some task or solving a particular type of problem is high or low compared with the scores of other individuals should not, in and of itself, be any indication of higher or lower relative intelligence.

Currently, the trend is toward recognizing that there are three very distinct and different areas of mental acuity and ability that play a critical role in determining an individual's success: abstract intelligence, which involves the ability to understand and manipulate concepts and symbolic representations (as in mathematics); practical intelligence, which involves the ability to solve physical problems and manipulate the physical world (as in assembling or repairing machinery); and social or emotional intelligence, which involves dealing wisely and effectively with other people in a social context. Another area that is sometimes added is creative or imaginative intelligence, which involves the ability to manipulate forms and images in an evocative manner. These four "intelligences" have been recognized since antiquity, but it is only in very recent times that the bias toward purely abstract reasoning as the sole measure of intelligence has given way to an appreciation of other mental abilities and talents as deserving of the label of intelligence. *See also* INTELLIGENCE TESTS.

Intelligence Tests

Tests that purport to indicate an individual's mental ability, specifically the intelligence quotient (IQ).

The numerical measure that is the result of intelligence tests is called an intelligence quotient, or IQ. Children are often tested around the age of six or seven (sometimes earlier) to determine their IQ, on the supposition that an individual's intelligence is virtually fully formed by that age. Studies have repeatedly cast doubt on this assumption and have indicated that, like physical development, intellectual development occurs in fits and starts throughout youth until the late 20s.

TYPES OF TESTS

There are several types of tests generally administered. The most widely used are the Wechsler tests—the Wechsler Adult Intelligence Scale (WAIS) for adults and the Wechsler Intelligence Scale for Children (WISC)—which measure verbal ability, general knowledge, and spatial manipulation. A test that focuses on learning ability and is thus used more for educational assessment is the Stanford-Binet test, a revised version of the oldest intelligence test, which was devised by the French researcher Alfred Binet (1857–1911).

HOW INTELLIGENCE TESTS WORK

In most cases, the IQ is arrived at by dividing the mental age (as indicated by the test) of the person tested, by the person's chronological age (hence the term "quotient"), and multiplying by 100. The tests have been administered many times and are devised to ensure that three-quarters of the population test within the IQ range of 80 to 120. Individuals who test below 65 are deemed in the lower one percent of the population, and those who test above 135 are deemed in the upper one percent. Scores lower than 70 have been used to render legal definitions of mental retardation and diminished mental capacity, and educational advantages have frequently been given to individuals testing above 140.

Yet, the only judgment that can be rendered definitively from such tests is that it is an activity in which a vast majority of the population performed more or less equally. It is questionable whether the test is really a good measure of a person's intelligence or the intelligence of the population against which he or she is being compared.

RELIABILITY

Further problems with the reliability of intelligence tests has arisen from the recognition that many social biases, of which the devisers of the test are unaware or unmindful, find their way into tests.

For example, Canadian students taking the test were penalized for not recognizing that a map of North America did not include the Florida Peninsula, but American students taking the same test were not penalized for failing to recognize that the same map omitted Hudson Bay. Similar disparities have been found among different ethnic groups and nationalities—even the ability to solve simple problems involving telling time will be influenced by a culture's attitude toward the value of punctuality. Such differences make any attempt to judge the intelligence of one race or group against any other an exercise in utter nonsense and pseudo-science.

> *Background information on intelligence tests can be found in* CHILD DEVELOPMENT *and* MENTAL RETARDATION*. For further reading, see* PSYCHIATRY*. See also* DOWN'S SYNDROME *for more on chromosomal abnormalities causing mental retardation.*

Intensive Care

Closely monitored health care given to patients with life-threatening conditions.

Intensive care is specialized care given to critically ill patients. These patients are closely monitored in case their condition deteriorates rapidly. Intensive care is given in a specially equipped unit of a hospital or other health care facility called the intensive care unit (ICU).

In an intensive care unit, patients are monitored with electronic equipment that continually assesses their vital signs, such as blood pressure, heart rate, and breath rate. Intensive care units have a high ratio of medical staff (doctors and nurses) to patients, and the staff members are specially trained in resuscitation. The majority of intensive care units in hospitals are overseen by specialists.

Patients who most often need intensive care are those who are on artificial ventilation, in which a machine helps them to breathe. These patients may not be able to breathe on their own due to a respiratory illness or because they are unconscious from an injury. Other patients needing intensive care include those who have suffered a myocardial infarction (heart attack), heart transplant or bypass surgery, those who are in shock and are unresponsive to emergency medical treatment, and those who are suffering from renal (kidney) failure. *See also* ARTIFICIAL RESPIRATION; *and* HOSPITALS, TYPES OF.

Intercourse, Painful

Also known as dyspareunia.

Pain during the act of sexual intercourse.

This condition can occur in women who do not get enough stimulation or are suffering from a sexual disorder. It is estimated that one in five women suffers from dyspareunia at some point in her life.

Causes. Dyspareunia is most often caused by insufficient lubrication, or where the penetrating penis puts pressure on tissue within the abdomen. Other causes can include:
- infections of the vagina, vulva, cervix, or urinary tract;
- pelvic inflammatory disease;
- sexually transmitted diseases;
- endometriosis;
- scar tissue from an episiotomy.

Another contributing factor is insufficient estrogen production, seen most often in women who are breast-feeding or postmenopausal. Their vaginal tissue becomes thinner and drier. Rarely, a retroverted uterus, which is tilted backward and down instead of forward, can result in pain with deep penetration.

Treatment depends on the underlying cause. Any infections are treated with medication. If thinning vaginal tissue is the problem, water-soluble lubricants, such as K-Y Jelly, may help alleviate the discomfort. Estrogen replacement therapy is recommended for women past menopause. If deep penetration and thrusting are causing pain, couples may benefit from a change in position. Counseling is helpful in cases of lack of sufficient stimulation or of sexual dysfunction disorder. *See also* ENDOMETRIOSIS; EPISIOTOMY; SEXUAL DISORDERS; *and* SEXUALLY TRANSMITTED DISEASES.

Interferon

> A chemical naturally produced by the body to protect against disease.

Interferon helps prevent a virus from infecting new cells and sends chemical messages to activate the immune system. Interferon is called a biological response modifier. It is secreted by cells in response to viral infection. It can be duplicated in the laboratory and has proved effective in treating cancers like Kaposi's sarcoma, several forms of leukemia, multiple myeloma, and some types of lymphoma. Manufactured interferon has also been used to treat chronic hepatitis B and C and HIV. Interferon works by stimulating cells of the body to resist the viral attack. It stops cells from dividing and therefore inhibits the spread of the virus in the body.

Manufactured interferon has various side effects, including fever, vomiting, diarrhea, sleepiness, back pain, depression, and insomnia. These side effects are mostly related to the amount of the dosage and are reversible when the dosage is reduced or when administration of the drug is stopped entirely. Since side effects diminish with time, patients should continue taking the drug until the unpleasant effects subside. *See also* AIDS; CANCER; HEPATITIS; HIV; *and* IMMUNE SYSTEM.

Internal Bleeding

> Bleeding that occurs inside the body or from any of the internal organs.

Internal bleeding is a potentially hidden danger. Injury, illness, or a disorder can cause bleeding within the body—from blood vessels, tissues, and organs into cavities, other tissues, or organs—that is not immediately or visibly apparent. It must be suspected after a vehicular accident, fall, or major blow to the head or body.

Symptoms. Pain in the chest, abdomen, or pelvic region; abdominal muscle spasms; a weak, rapid pulse; clammy skin; spitting, vomiting, or coughing up blood or extremely dark sputum; bleeding from orifices; or blood in the stool or urine can all be signs of internal bleeding. However, there may also be no symptoms whatsoever. Days or even weeks may pass before any signs appear, thus the need for immediate medical examination following cases of impact—even those that seem mild—to the body. A failure to seek prompt attention may be life-threatening. Until help arrives, if there is no risk of spinal injury, lay the person down and elevate the feet. Monitor breathing and pulse. *See also* EMERGENCY FIRST STEPS *and* EMERGENCY ROOM.

Internist

> A physician who specialized in the medical management of diseases in adults.

An internist specializes in the diagnosis and treatment of diseases in adults. This medical specialty is called internal medicine. A minimum of seven years of medical school and postgraduate training is required for internists.

Intersex

> A child, born with ambiguous genitals, whose sex is not obvious.

In this condition, the gonads, or internal sex organs, may be completely normal.

True hermaphrodites, which are rare, are children that have both male and female internal reproductive organs. Most children with ambiguous genitals are pseudo-hermaphrodites and have one or the other but not both kinds of reproductive organs.

A female pseudohermaphrodite is a genetically normal female with the sex chromosomes XX. Her clitoris is larger than normal and resembles a small penis. Her internal organs are female. This condition is caused by prenatal exposure to high levels of male hormones. The fetus usually has enlarged adrenal glands that overproduce male hormones or else a chemical problem, such as a missing enzyme, that prevents the conversion of male hormones to female ones. In some cases where the mother took progesterone during pregnancy or has a tumor that increases hormone production, the male hormones may come from her bloodstream.

A male pseudohermaphrodite is a genetically normal male with the sex chromosomes XY. He may be born with a very small penis, or missing one entirely. This condition is caused by the inability of the fetus to produce sufficient quantities of male hormone, or an inability to respond properly to the hormones produced. The latter is known as androgen resistance syndrome.

Treatment. Once the child's sex has been correctly identified, the child should be raised as a child of that gender. Surgery to correct the appearance of the genitals is usually done around the time of puberty.

> *For background material on intersex, see* GENDER IDENTITY; REPRODUCTIVE SYSTEM, FEMALE; *and* REPRODUCTIVE SYSTEM, MALE. *Further information can be found in* ANDROGEN HORMONES; CLITORIS; ESTROGEN HORMONES; HERMAPHRODITISM; PENIS; *and* PROGESTERONE.

Interstitial Pulmonary Fibrosis

> The stiffening and scarring of interstitium, the tissue between air sacs of the lung.

Interstitial pulmonary fibrosis can be caused by exposure to environmental pollutants such as asbestos, rock dusts, and chemical fumes; by radiation exposure; or by infections such as tuberculosis, allergic alveolitis, and sarcoidosis. But in most cases, it is considered idiopathic—that is, there is no known cause. These cases are believed to be due to an autoimmune reaction, in which the body's defense system against infection attacks its own tissues. This form of the condition can occur at any age, but it is most common in older persons, those in their 60s and 70s.

Symptoms and Complications. The stiffening of lung tissue causes breathing to become more difficult and results in progressively worsening shortness of breath, a persistent cough, chest pain, and clubbing of the fingers. Progression of the condition leads to worsening of the symptoms and can result in heart failure or other life-threatening complications.

> ### Prevention
> While idiopathic pulmonary fibrosis cannot be prevented, protective measures can be taken by persons exposed to industrial pollutants that can cause the condition. One basic measure is to avoid cigarette smoking, a major cause of lung damage in its own right and an irritant that worsens the effects of other pollutants. The use of personal protective equipment, such as face masks that cover the mouth and nose, and knowledge about the dangers of industrial materials can reduce lung damage.

Diagnosis is based on symptoms, and is confirmed by a chest x-ray or an examination of a sample of tissue (biopsy) taken from the lung. Treatment of interstitial pulmonary fibrosis of unknown cause relies on corticosteroids and other drugs to suppress the activity of the immune system. If the condition can be traced to an underlying disease, treatment is aimed at that disease. In the most severe cases, a lung transplant can be a treatment of last resort.

> *Background information on interstitial pulmonary fibrosis can be found in* AUTOIMMUNE DISORDERS *and* RESPIRATORY SYSTEM. *For related material, see* ALVEOLITIS; BIOPSY; IMMUNE SYSTEM; LUNG CANCER; SARCOIDOSIS; TUBERCULOSIS; *and* X-RAY.

Interstitial Radiation Therapy

Radiation therapy used to eradicate cancer of the interstitial tissues.

Radiation therapy (along with chemotherapy) remains a primary weapon in the fight against cancer. The intercellular connective tissue known as interstitial tissue can experience various forms of malignancy. Radiation therapy for interstitial cancers calls for decisions to be made as to the choice of therapy, specifics of dose, and timing of treatment, which depends on the location, severity, and progress of the malignancy. In treatment, high-speed radioactive particles are directed at irregular cells or tissues, destroying them by destroying their DNA.

Interstitial therapy is usually carried out using a linear accelerator, capable of producing a narrow, focused beam of radiation that may be accurately directed at the site of malignancy. Such external beam radiation therapy is sometimes called teletherapy. Radiation may also be directed at malignancy from within the body by means of a surgically implanted source. This technique is known as brachytherapy. Both forms have met with some success in the treatment of many cancers, including Hodgkin's disease, squamous cell cancer, and tumors of the brain and spinal cord.

The value of interstitial (and other) radiation therapies is offset by the potential damage to healthy tissues and cells in the neighborhood of the diseased tissue. Side effects of radiation therapy can sometimes be acute, and include lethargy and nausea, inflammation, soreness, and ulceration. Occasionally, secondary cancers are produced by the radiation therapy, which can cause healthy cells to mutate if they receive sub-lethal doses in the process of tumor irradiation. Improved methods of radiation therapy are constantly evolving, helping to reduce the threat to healthy tissue. *See also* BRAIN TUMOR; CANCER; CHEMOTHERAPY; MALIGNANT; *and* RADIATION.

Intestine.
The diagram at right shows the 27-foot intestine that extends from the stomach to the anus. It is divided into two sections—the small intestine and the large intestine—which together break down food, absorb water and nutrients, and carry waste from the body.

Intertrigo

An inflammation of the top layers of skin, caused by the presence of moisture and bacteria in between the skin folds.

Intertrigo is most commonly found in people who are obese. The condition usually develops on the inner thighs and armpits, and on the underside of the breasts. *See also* INFLAMMATION *and* OBESITY.

Intestine

The primary section of the digestive tract.

The intestine, which is divided into small and large sections and is 27 feet in length, extends from the stomach to the anus. It breaks down food, absorbs water and nutrients, and passes waste from the body.

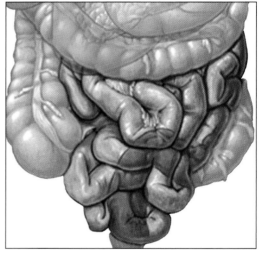

With a diameter of an inch and a half and a length of 21 feet, the small intestine has three parts. The first, the duodenum, is a curved segment exiting the stomach, followed by two longer, coiled segments, the jejunum and ileum. The latter two move freely, while the duodenum is attached to the back abdominal wall.

Peristalsis, the contraction of the intestinal muscle in rings, squeezes along food against a slick inner lining that easily allows its passage. This lining, the mucosa, contains legions of finger-shaped villi composed of millions of fronds—palm-leaf-shaped wisps—that expand the surface area exponentially and take in nutrients and water for absorption into the blood.

The small intestine is surrounded by the large intestine. At six feet by two inches, the large intestine's outer shape is a blend of consecutive bulges, like a caterpillar. Muscles are structured in bands and contain no villi. Its major segment is the colon, divided into the ascending, transverse, descending, and sigmoid colons. Material not absorbed by the small intestine enters the large intestine, which takes in any remaining vitamins, mineral salts and water, with the residual feces—comprised of fat, fiber, digestive secretions, and bacteria—entering the rectum. *See also* FECES.

Intestine, Cancer of

Malignant tumors of the intestinal tract.

Cancer of the small intestine, the upper segment of the intestinal tract, is rare, but cancer of the large intestine, consisting of the colon and rectum, is the third most common cancer of Americans. It is frequently called colorectal cancer. As many as 95 percent of these cancers are adenocarcinomas, which arise in the mucosa, the innermost lining of the colon. Many of them originate as polyps, nonmalignant tumors called adenomas. Large adenomas whose cells have a greater degree of abnormal development are more likely to become cancerous. Early detection and removal of polyps is a basic preventive measure for cancer of the intestine.

Types. A commonly used method of classifying colorectal cancers is the Dukes system, named for a British cancer specialist. The Dukes A cancer may have grown from the mucosa to partially invade the muscle wall of the intestine. The Dukes B cancer extends all the way through the muscle wall, and a Dukes C cancer has spread to nearby lymph nodes.

Symptoms and Diagnosis. The early symptoms of colorectal cancer are similar to those of indigestion or a gastrointestinal illness. They include persistent constipa-

> ## Lifestyle and the Intestines
> The role of lifestyle and diet in cancer of the intestine is an unsettled issue. People who eat a diet high in saturated fat are believed to be at greater risk. For many years, a diet rich in fiber was recommended as a preventive measure, but several studies have found no reduction in risk associated with dietary fiber intake. A low-fat, high-fiber diet including fresh fruits and vegetables is still recommended, primarily for general health and for prevention against cardiovascular disease.

tion or diarrhea, unusually narrow stools, bloating of the abdomen, and occasional pain. The symptoms of rectal cancer include diarrhea, unusual straining at bowel movements, and a feeling that the bowel has not been emptied properly. But the most significant symptom of colorectal cancer is the passage of blood with stools. The presence of blood calls for diagnostic tests, such as sigmoidoscopy, an inspection of the colon through an instrument called an endoscope; colonoscopy, inspection of the entire colon with a similar instrument; and a barium enema x-ray examination.

Risk of Metastasis. Colorectal cancers usually grow slowly, but they will eventually penetrate the intestinal wall and invade neighboring tissues, usually by spreading to nearby lymph nodes. These cancers can send metastases, or colonies, to the lungs, liver, and brain. Cancer of the rectum can spread throughout the pelvic area, to the ovaries, prostate, and other organs.

Treatment. Surgery to remove the growth is common treatment for cancer of the intestine. The extent of the surgery depends on the stage at which the cancer is detected. Simple removal of an early cancer may be sufficient, while more extensive surgery is necessary if the cancer has spread. In addition to surgery, chemotherapy and radiation therapy may also be administered to attack the cancerous cells.

> *For background material on cancer of the intestine, see* COLON CANCER; DIGESTIVE SYSTEM; *and* INTESTINES. *Further information can be found in* ADENOMA; COLONOSCOPY; CONSTIPATION; DIARRHEA; DIET AND DISEASE; METASTASIS; OBESITY; POLYP; *and* SIGMOIDOSCOPY.

Intestine, Obstruction of

A partial or complete blockage of the small or large intestine.

The passage of the contents of the intestine can be hindered by a number of conditions. In some cases, blockage can be purely physical, resulting from a tumor, impacted feces, food, or gallstones. Other conditions that affect the passage of substances through the intestine include: inherited disorders that cause narrowing of the intestinal tract; bands of scar tissue (called adhesions) that sometimes form after surgery; and the twisting or knotting of the bowel (a condition known as volvulus). Medical conditions, such as Crohn's disease or diverticular disease, can also result in blockage of the intestine. But in many cases, there is an unexplained failure of peristalsis, the regular muscle contractions that move contents through the intestine. Depending on the location of the blockage, symptoms can include abdominal pain, swelling, constipation (or diarrhea), and vomiting.

Diagnosis is based on symptoms, usually confirmed by x-rays that show the nature of the blockage and where it occurs. The blocked contents can be removed through a tube inserted into the intestine via the throat. Surgery is necessary if the blockage is caused by a physical obstruction; the type of surgery depends on the extent and location of the blockage. *See also* CROHN'S DISEASE; DIVERTICULAR DISEASE; GALLSTONES; IMPACTED FECES; *and* VOLVULUS.

Intestine, Tumors of

Growths in the lower part of the digestive tract.

Tumors of the intestine can be malignant or benign. They can occur in any part of the intestine, including the duodenum, the jejunum, the ileum, the colon, and the rectum. Most cancers occur in the large intestine, the segment running from the ileum (the lowermost part of the small intestine) to the rectum. *See* INTESTINE *and* TUMOR.

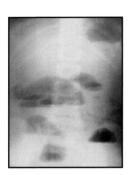

Intestinal Obstruction. X-rays of the abdomen, above, are important in diagnosing the presence of small bowel obstruction, a blockage that hinders passage through the small or large intestines.

Noncancerous growths, or polyps, often occur in the colon. Polyps emerge from the lining of the colon. Polyps can be hyperplastic (benign), which become adenomatous (malignant). Some polyps can be detected by a hemoccult stool test, which looks for blood in the feces. Many polyps, however, are too small to cause bleeding. They may be seen on visual examination of the colon, such as through a colonoscopy or sigmoidoscopy. Once these polyps are detected, they can be removed by minor surgery.

The follow-up to detection of these growths in the intestine depends on their nature and number. Hyperplastic polyps may require little or no follow-up. The presence of adenomatous polyps will require regular examinations, with a colonoscopy done at least every three years. *See also* COLONOSCOPY; INTESTINE, CANCER OF; SIGMOIDOSCOPY; *and* TUMOR.

Intracavitary Therapy

The placement of radioactive material or a drug in a body cavity to treat cancer.

Intracavitary therapy allows treatment of a cancer by exposing it directly to a therapeutic substance. The technique is applied primarily for treatment of cancers of the cervix, vagina, rectum, or uterus. If a radioactive material is to be used, it generally is inserted in the form of wires and small tubes, under general or local anesthesia. It is left in place for a period sufficient to produce its effects. This radioactive material is sometimes implanted to treat cancer of the prostate.

Intracavitary therapy can also be used to introduce drugs into the abdominal cavity or the space around the lungs in cases where there is a flow of fluid containing cancerous cells from a primary tumor. This is done by passing a needle into the abdomen or chest under local anesthesia. After fluid is drawn off through the needle, the anti-cancer drug can then be injected, through the needle or a catheter. *See also* CANCER *and* RADIATION THERAPY.

Intracerebral Hemorrhage

Bleeding into the brain from a burst vessel, causing a stroke.

More than 10 percent of all strokes are caused by intracerebral hemorrhages. The blood that flows from the ruptured vessel presses against the brain, destroying tissue and disrupting cerebral function.

Symptoms of an intracerebral hemorrhage include sudden headache, weakness and confusion. Often there is loss of consciousness, and the person collapses to the ground. Symptoms require immediate medical attention. Either a call for emergency medical help or a trip to the nearest hospital emergency room should be made.

Diagnosis is made by a physical examination and tests of body and brain functions, such as walking, hearing, vision, reading, and understanding spoken language. The diagnosis can be confirmed by a computerized tomography scan or magnetic resonance imaging, both of which produce an image of the brain.

Treatment generally consists of measures to maintain bodily function, reduce blood pressure, and relieve pressure within the skull. Surgery may be performed to remove a clot that has formed near the surface of the brain.

Persons at higher risk of this type of hemorrhage include those with uncontrolled hypertension or atherosclerosis and those with diabetes. The prognosis depends on the location and extent of the bleeding. *See also* ATHEROSCLEROSIS; CT SCAN; DIABETES; *and* EXAMINATION, PHYSICAL.

Intrauterine Device (IUD)

A small, flexible plastic device inserted into the uterus to prevent pregnancy.

The intrauterine contraceptive device (abbreviated as IUD or IUCD) is used by about 100 million women. Of the 20 percent of those who use any contraceptive, the IUD is the most popular form of reversible birth control in the world. It has one of the high-

ALERT

Safety Issues

Women who might be pregnant and women who are at risk for or may have sexually transmitted infections should not use IUDs. It is also not advised for women at higher risk for ectopic pregnancy, or those with certain cervical and uterine abnormalities.

est effectiveness rates of any type of contraception. Two types of IUDs are currently available in the United States. They are both T-shaped, plastic devices about an inch long that are inserted into the uterus.

The Copper T type releases copper, which attracts white blood cells to the uterus. White blood cells fight infections and destroy parasites, dead tissue, and any foreign substance. Sperm is a foreign substance to the female body. The extra white blood cells destroy the sperm before they reach the egg. Once the copper IUD is inserted, it can be left in place for up to 10 years.

The Progestasert releases the hormone progesterone, which may thicken the cervical mucus, thereby preventing sperm from entering the uterus. It may also prevent implantation of the fertilized egg into the lining of the uterus. The IUD begins working immediately upon insertion and stops affecting fertility upon removal. The progesterone IUD must be replaced each year.

Side effects of the IUD include cramps, heavier-than-usual periods, and midcycle bleeding. These problems usually disappear within a few months. If they persist, or if the woman is experiencing any other difficulty, she should contact her physician.

Precautions. A woman with an IUD should check periodically to make sure the device is still in place. She should contact her physician if she is unable to locate it or suspects it may have become dislodged. If she becomes pregnant while using an IUD, the device should be removed.

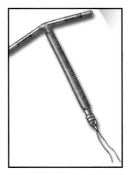

IUD.
More than 100 million women use the IUD, above, as a contraceptive. This small plastic devise is inserted into the uterus.

Background information on intrauterine device can be found in CONTRACEPTION. *For related material, see* IMMUNE RESPONSE; PARASITE; REPRODUCTIVE SYSTEM, FEMALE; *and* SEXUAL INTERCOURSE.

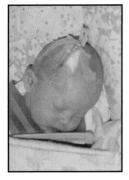

When intravenous fluids, antibiotics, and other medications must be given to an infant, the scalp provides accessible veins. In the photo, above, a small intravenous catheter has been inserted into a scalp vein and antibiotics are being given.

Intrauterine Growth Retardation (Restriction)

A condition diagnosed when a fetus is exceedingly small for its age, usually occurring because the fetus does not receive adequate nutrition through the placenta.

The possible causes for intrauterine growth retardation include inadequate maternal diet; maternal cigarette or drug use; heavy exposure to alcohol; maternal chronic conditions, such as heart disease; abnormalities of the placenta; abnormalities of the umbilical cord; fetal infections; and the presence of multiple fetuses.

If a doctor suspects intrauterine growth retardation, an ultrasound exam will be performed to confirm the diagnosis.

Prevention of intrauterine growth retardation consists of the mother eating properly, avoiding harmful substances, and receiving adequate prenatal care.

Treatment is aimed at the underlying cause. If the growth retardation is due to inadequate prenatal care or maternal diet, that can be rectified. Any diseases or infections are treated and brought under control as much as possible. Abnormalities affecting the placenta or umbilical cord, or the presence of multiple fetuses, are not easily remedied.

If the uterine environment is deemed harmful, an early delivery may be necessary; the doctor will weigh the danger of allowing the pregnancy to continue, with the problems a premature baby will face.

Due to its small size and possible prematurity, a baby who suffers from intrauterine growth retardation will, at birth, lack a normal layer of body fat and will be unable to maintain its body temperature and blood sugar levels properly. Such babies usually must receive special care after birth, possibly including placement in an incubator and close monitoring by a physician.

Babies with intrauterine growth retardation may grow slowly throughout their childhood and may experience delayed intellectual development as a result of the condition. Because intellectual outcome is usually normal, the term intrauterine growth restriction is now preferred to intrauterine growth retardation because intellectual outcome is usually normal. *See also* BIRTH; PREGNANCY; PREMATURITY; *and* PRENATAL CARE.

Intravenous Infusion

The addition of blood or medication to the circulatory system through a needle that penetrates one of the veins.

In order to introduce blood or drugs into the circulatory system, a vein in the crook of the elbow or the back of the hand is chosen. A needle is inserted, and the fluid is pushed into the vein with a small pump or dripped into the vein from an elevated sac.

Intravenous infusion of blood is called transfusion. Depending on what the patient needs, a transfusion may consist of red blood cells, platelets, plasma, or, more rarely, white blood cells. The major concern in blood transfusion today is avoiding the introduction of bacteria or viruses along with the blood component. In the 1980s, numerous instances of the transmission of AIDS via transfusion were reported. Modern testing methods have pretty much eliminated this problem, but there is still a danger of allergic reactions or infection. Blood of matching type must be used, and recipients with rare blood types may have a difficult time in finding a donor.

When drugs are to be administered, intravenous infusion offers precise control of the quantity and timing of the administration. Some drugs can be administered only intravenously, since they do not survive the digestive process. *See also* AIDS; BLOOD; *and* BLOOD TRANSFUSION.

Introitus

The opening to the vagina.

This part of the vagina is bordered by protruding flaps of skin called the labia major and the labia minor. Bartholin's glands, which provide lubrication, are located beside the introitus. *See* BARTHOLIN'S GLANDS.

Intubation

The insertion of a tube into the windpipe or into the intestinal system.

Intubation most often is done to deliver oxygen to the lungs when normal breathing is not possible, because of a condition such as a severe respiratory disease, or when general anesthesia is necessary.

The procedure is done by an anesthesiologist. The first step is inspection of the throat through an instrument called a laryngoscope. This is done to determine the location of the vocal cords, which could be damaged in the procedure. The next step is insertion of the tube, called an endotracheal tube, into the mouth or the nose. Then the tube is maneuvered down the throat, past the vocal cords, into the main airway (trachea) leading to the lungs. The tube sometimes is fixed in place by an inflatable cuff inside the trachea. The part of the tube outside the body is usually held in place by tape.

A different use of intubation is for suctioning or artificial feeding. In artificial feeding, the tube can be inserted surgically into the stomach or the intestinal tract. Controlled amounts of nutrients then can be administered through the inserted tube. *See also* ARTIFICIAL RESPIRATION; FEEDING, ARTIFICIAL; *and* HYPERALIMENTATION.

Intussusception

A condition in which the intestine telescopes into another section of itself.

Intussusception is a relatively rare condition in which part of the intestine telescopes into another segment. Usually, the small intestine is involved. This is the most common cause of intestinal obstruction in young children. It affects more boys than girls, and it occurs most often before a child's first birthday.

Cause. The cause is unknown, but certain viral infections are known to increase susceptibility to the condition.

Symptoms. Intussusception often occurs suddenly, with no advance warning. The first indication of a problem is severe pain that occurs at frequent intervals. Gradually, a child becomes weaker and lethargic. A fever will also develop. Vomiting, with bile present in the vomit, may occur as well.

Diagnosis. A physical examination may reveal a mass in the abdomen. X-rays or barium x-rays of the affected area are used to diagnose the condition and distinguish it from other types of abdominal pain.

Treatment. If left untreated, intussusception can be very serious. The barium enema used for diagnosing the condition may be enough to force the telescoped segment of intestine back into its normal position, although the condition may recur in many cases. Surgery is often necessary. *See also* ABDOMINAL PAIN; BARIUM X-RAY EXAMINATION; *and* INTESTINE.

Involuntary Movements

Unconscious and unintentional body movements.

Involuntary movements are uncontrollable motions of the body such as twitching, trembling, or grimacing. These spontaneous movements may involve the head, limbs, or trunk. They can be sluggish and circuitous (athetosis); jerky and unsteady (chorea); or fidgety and affecting only one side of the body (tic). Involuntary movements may be symptomatic of an underlying disorder (i.e., Huntington's chorea or Parkinson's disease), or arise as side effects of some psychotherapeutic medications.

The following conditions may produce involuntary trembling and body shakes but do not indicate an underlying disease:
- fatigue, anxiety, and tension;
- sudden alcohol withdrawal;
- excess of caffeine (consumption of at least ten cups of coffee or tea in a 12-hour period).

If an individual develops any uncontrollable movements that are not the result of a fatigue, alcohol withdrawal, or caffeine, a physician should be consulted. *See also* ATHETOSIS; CHOREA; DYSKINESIA; *and* TIC.

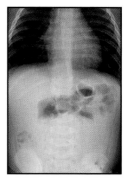

Intussusception. The abdominal x-ray above shows an intestinal condition in which one section of the bowel has slipped into another section. This rare condition causes swelling, reduced blood flow, obstruction, and tissue damage.

Iodine

An element essential to proper thyroid function.

Iodine is necessary for the production of thyroid hormones. If a person has a deficiency of iodine, generally as a result of a dietary lack, the thyroid cannot produce enough hormones. It may then enlarge to compensate, resulting in a goiter, which appears as a swelling in the front of the neck. Iodine can be found in iodized salt, seafood, and dairy products. Because these foods are common in developed countries, iodine deficiency is rare among people in the developed world.

Radioactive iodine may be administered as a treatment for an enlarged, overactive thyroid. The iodine is taken in by the thyroid, where the radioactivity damages the tissue and reduces it to a more normal size. *See also* GOITER; HYPERTHYROIDISM; HYPOTHYROIDISM; *and* THYROID GLAND.

Ion

An electrically charged atomic particle.

Ions are formed when a neutral atom either gains or loses electrons. Atoms that lose one or more electrons are positively charged, and are called cations; those that gain electrons form negatively charged particles called anions. Simple ions consist of a single charged atom, while complex ions comprise a number of ions with a net charge.

Function. Ions play a key role in the neurological functions of the body, since they are instrumental in the transmission of nerve impulses. A key example of the importance of ions in the body is the sodium-potassium pump, which is essential in the transmission of nerve impulses. Sodium and potassium ions are instrumental in bridging the synapses between nerve cells.

Electrolytes—solutions that are able to conduct electrical charges—contain ions. Ions also play a key role in the body's acid–base balance. Sodium and chloride ions, which are the components of table salt, are essential to health; they contribute to maintaining both the fluid and acid–base equilibria in the body.

Because ions aid in many bodily functions, it is important that their levels be maintained. If these levels drop, certain disorders may result (i.e., hypokalemia, which causes muscle weakness). In addition, dehydration can cause the ions in the body to become more concentrated, resulting in symptoms such as muscle cramps, dizziness, and thirst.

Ionizing radiation, which includes x-rays, alpha and beta particles, gamma rays, and neutrons, is a type of energy that converts atoms into ions. This type of radiation occurs naturally in radioactive minerals, is generated by the products of nuclear reactions, and is also produced by x-ray machines. Ionizing radiation has sufficient energy to affect the molecular structure of living cells; in large doses it causes cancer and severe tissue damage in humans. Certain medical procedures involve exposure to ionizing radiation as well, such as radiation therapy to kill cancer cells.

For background information on ion, see CENTRAL NERVOUS SYSTEM *and* NERVOUS SYSTEM. *Related material can be found in* ANGIOGRAPHY; ELECTROLYTE; POTASSIUM; RADIATION THERAPY; SODIUM; *and* X-RAYS.

Ipecac

A substance used to induce vomiting in cases of poisoning.

Syrup of ipecac is an emetic—that is, a substance that induces vomiting. It is used to bring about vomiting in the case of accidental poisoning. It should be an essential component of the medicine cabinet, especially if there is a child under the age of 12 in the house. Syrup of ipecac should be used only on the advice of a doctor, pharmacist, or poison control center, since certain poisons can cause further damage if they are vomited. Never use ipe-cac if the person has swallowed lye, as it may cause severe esophageal erosions. *See also* DRUG POISONING *and* POISONING.

Iron

A mineral that aids in the formation of hemoglobin (carrier of oxygen in red blood cells) and myoglobin (fuel for muscles).

When the body's reserves are low, absorption increases; in general, about ten percent of the iron in one's diet is absorbed. Iron is crucial to the formation of red blood cells. Sources of iron include meats, dried beans and peas, fortified cereals, grain and pasta products, dark green leafy vegetables, and dried fruits and nuts. Eating foods rich in vitamin C with foods that contain iron aids in their absorption.

Most balanced diets supply a person with sufficient amounts of iron. Iron supplements should not be taken unless prescribed by a medical professional, after blood tests have determined that a deficiency exists. Symptoms of deficiency include fatigue, pallor, and headache. Many pregnant women also take iron supplements to ensure the healthy development of the fetus. *See also* ANEMIA; CHLOROSIS; *and* IRON DEFICIENCY.

Irrigation, Wound

Flushing a wound or body cavity with saline water, antiseptic fluid, or other medical solutions.

The goal of irrigation is to reduce the risk of infection by removing bacteria and other foreign matter from a wound. Various solutions—including saline water and antiseptic fluid—have proven highly effective Irrigation floods the wound with copious amounts of cleansing fluid.

The most common method of wound irrigation is the forced syringe irrigation technique, which utilizes a syringe or tube to flush fluid into and out of the desired area. Wound irrigation can be performed under duress in situations where there is an extreme emergency, but it is always best to call emergency medical technicians and receive treatment from an emergency medicine specialist. *See also* EMERGENCY, FIRST STEPS; BLEEDING, TREATMENT OF; WOUND.

Irritable Bladder

Uncontrollable contractions of the bladder (the sac used as a receptacle for urine before it is released from the body).

Sometimes caused by a urinary tract infection, an irritable bladder can produce a need for urination so acute that there is not enough time to get to a bathroom. Though the person may not feel any irritation while urinating, the urge itself is indicative of abnormal functioning of the bladder. Other causes can include an enlarged prostate gland or a stone in the bladder.

Diagnosis starts with a urine sample that is tested for signs of infection. A special type of x-ray may be taken during urination to reveal any abnormalities, such as stones or tumors. If an infection is found, it will be treated by an appropriate antibiotic. If no specific cause is identified, drugs can be given to relax the muscles that make the bladder contract, or to reduce the activity of the nerves controlling contraction. A urologist may also try to "retrain" the bladder by gradually increasing the amount of fluid the person is able to retain. *See also* PROSTATE, ENLARGED; STONES; *and* URINARY TRACT INFECTION.

Irritable Bowel Syndrome

Spasms caused by an overreaction of the bowel (intestinal) muscles.

There is no identifiable cause of irritable bowel syndrome, which is also called spastic colon or irritable colon syndrome. Even a mild stimulus such as eating, gas, or even the presence of stool causes the muscles of the large intestine to contract. It is a common condition, which is believed to account for half of all visits to gastroenterologists. It occurs twice as often in women as in men, with the onset generally in the early or middle years of adult life. Irritable bowel syndrome is not known to lead to a more serious condition, but it can have an adverse effect on an individual's career, social life, and travel. *See also* COLON.

Symptoms. Some persons experience diarrhea; others have constipation. Still others may have constipation alternating with bouts of diarrhea. Other possible symptoms include abdominal pain and swelling, gas, chronic flatulence, and mucus in the feces, as well as small stools or flat, ribbon-shaped stools.

Diagnosis. A number of tests can be done to exclude other causes of the symptoms. The doctor will ask about dietary habits to detect possible food intolerance. Feces will be studied for parasites. A sigmoidoscopy may be performed to examine the colon. A tissue sample will be taken to look for conditions such as ulcerative colitis. Irritable bowel syndrome will be diagnosed when all other possible causes of the symptoms have been ruled out.

Treatment. The extent of treatment can depend on the severity of the symptoms and how much they interfere with the patient's life. An antispasmodic drug, such as dicyclomine or hyoscamine, may be prescribed. Some patients may be prescribed an antidepressant drug, while others will be given medication for anxiety. Laxatives or medications for diarrhea are prescribed with care taken to avoid dependence. Dietary measures may also be recommended. Some patients will be told to increase their intake of foods rich in fiber, to take fiber supplements, and to reduce intake of fatty foods, such as cheese, butter, whole milk, and meats. Patients may be asked to keep note of the foods they have eaten before symptoms occur, to identify possible dietary causes of those symptoms. Ultimately, treatment of irritable bowel syndrome is re-

strained because the condition is known not to be life-threatening or to be the prelude to a more serious condition.

> *Background material on irritable bowel syndrome can be found in* Digestive System *and* Intestine. *For further information, see* Colon Cancer; Constipation; Crohn's Disease; Diarrhea; Parasite; *and* Ulcerative Colitis.

Ischemia

A condition in which the blood supply to an organ or muscle is restricted because of a constriction or a blockage in a blood vessel.

The blocking factor may be a blood clot alone, but it is likely that an artery is partially obstructed by buildup of plaque on the walls of the blood vessel. A piece of plaque (an embolus) or a blood clot may break loose from a healing wound or surgical procedure and find its way to the blood vessels of a critical organ, which then may become starved for oxygen. If the organ affected is a lung, for example, this may result in pulmonary thrombosis; if the brain, it may cause a stroke; if the heart, it may cause a heart attack.

Aspirin and other blood-thinning drugs are prescribed for people in danger of excessive blood clotting. If the patient is restricted to bed and has little opportunity to exercise, he or she must make a special effort to move the limbs and breathe deeply since the blood will tend to pool in the lower parts of the body and promote the production of blood clots. *See also* Blood Clotting *and* Blood-Clotting Tests.

Isolation

A technique in which a hospital patient is prevented from infecting others or is protected from infection by others.

An isolated individual is kept in a hospital room apart from other people, aside from doctors and nurses. This procedure prevents the patient from infecting others. It also prevents the patient from becoming infected by others. *See also* Hospital.

Treatment Option

One treatment for irritable bowel syndrome is to relieve stress. While the exact relationship between stress and the syndrome is not clear, it is known that the contractions of the colon are partially controlled by the nervous system. Individual patients may be told to try stress reduction and relaxation techniques, and perhaps to try biofeedback (a method that measures specific body responses to ascertain the causes of behavioral disorders).

Jaundice

A yellowing of the skin and eyes that derives from elevated levels of bilirubin.

Jaundice, a condition in which the skin and the whites of the eyes take on a yellowish cast, is a symptom of a variety of disorders affecting the liver and gallbladder. The coloration is caused by the presence of excessive amounts of bilirubin.

Bilirubin is an orangish-yellow pigment found in bile, which is produced by the liver and stored in the gallbladder. Bilirubin is a by-product of heme, a component of the hemoglobin in red blood cells; it is formed when these cells are broken down.

CAUSES

• Acute or chronic liver disease, such as is produced by viral hepatitis, autoimmune liver disease, alcohol- or drug-induced liver disease, or genetic liver disease. In hepatitis, jaundice is more common with acute liver disease; in chronic hepatitis, jaundice occurs only with severe damage.

• Infant jaundice occurs when the relatively immature liver of a newborn causes a temporary increase in bilirubin levels and a mild form of jaundice. Most infant jaundice is resolved on its own, as the baby's feeding and bowel function improve. Very high levels of bilirubin can lead to kernicterus, a type of brain damage.

• Gilbert's disease is a hereditary condition in which mild jaundice occurs. This condition does not require treatment once it is recognized, as the jaundice is not serious and there are no other symptoms.

• Obstruction of the bile ducts produced by gallstones or by tumors of the pancreas, bile duct, or elsewhere.

DIAGNOSIS

Bilirubin levels may be measured in the blood as part of diagnostic tests for liver function. Elevated levels of bilirubin may be an indication of a number of conditions, including an obstruction in the bile duct, liver damage, or the breakdown of an excessive number of red blood cells.

TREATMENT

Jaundice is usually an indication of a problem in the liver, bile ducts, pancreas, or gallbladder, and the underlying disorder must be diagnosed and treated by a physician.

For background information on jaundice, see BILIRUBIN. *Related material can be found in* ANEMIA; BILE DUCT OBSTRUCTION; CHOLESTASIS; CORTICOSTEROID DRUGS; GALLBLADDER DISORDERS; GALLSTONES; GILBERT'S SYNDROME; *and* LIVER DISEASE, ALCOHOLIC.

Jaw, Dislocated

Condition in which the lower jaw is out of its joint.

The mandible, or lower jaw bone, is connected to the base of the skull by the temporomandibular joints. The bone can be disconnected from these joints by sudden force, or even by yawning. Signs of a dislocated jaw are pain in front of the ear on the side that has suffered the injury. The jaw will project, and the mouth will not close.

To replace the jaw, a person should place a thumb on each side of the lower back teeth and press down. The lower jaw should then click into place. Frequent recurrences of a dislocated jaw may require surgery to stabilize the joint. *See also* DISLOCATION, JOINT; *and* JAW, FRACTURED.

Jaw, Fractured

Breaking of the jaw bone (mandibula).

A fractured jaw may be caused by a direct blow, a fall or other accident. Symptoms of a fracture range from swelling, tenderness, and bruising to tooth damage, impaired movement, and loss of feeling in the lower lip.

Minor fractures may heal on their own, but for more severe injuries, surgery may be needed to place the bone fragments together. To immobilize the jaw during the healing process, upper and lower sets of teeth may be wired together. In some cases, holes may need to be drilled into the jaw bone, and wire inserted. Wires usually remain in place for about six weeks. *See also* FRACTURE *and* JAW, DISLOCATED.

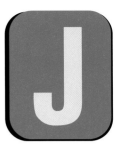

Jealousy (Delusional)

Preoccupation with the belief that a partner is unfaithful, with no evidence that this is the case, accompanied by behavior that ranges from controlling to violent.

A person suffering from delusions of jealousy becomes obsessed with the idea that a partner is unfaithful and will seek out any evidence of this idea. The individual may follow the partner, go through his or her belongings, make phone calls to check up on the partner, threaten those with whom the partner associates, interrogate the partner incessantly about his or her behavior, and even threaten or act violently toward the partner.

If the preoccupation with suspicion and jealousy is a factor no matter what relationship the individual has, the person should seek the help of a psychiatrist, since it may be indicative of an underlying personality disorder. *See also* PERSONALITY DISORDERS.

Jejunal Biopsy

The removal of a small tissue sample from the jejunum (middle portion) of the small intestine, for the purpose of diagnosis.

The small intestine is composed of the duodenum, jejunum, and ileum. A gastroenterologist may observe the condition of the upper gastrointestinal (GI) tract by means of a fiber-optic instrument known as an endoscope, in a process known as upper endoscopy. Such flexible endoscopes allow tissue samples to be removed from the jejunum for biopsy and examination in the laboratory.

The role of the jejunum (and ileum) is to absorb fats and nutrients from food in the digestive tract. The surface of the small intestine is patterned with projections of villi and microvilli as well as multiple folds that aid in the breakdown and digestion of food from the stomach.

A number of disorders of the small intestine may be diagnosed through upper endoscopy and removal of jejunal tissue by biopsy. So-called malabsorption disorders result when nutrients are improperly or incompletely absorbed into the bloodstream from the small intestine. Weight loss and diarrhea are the primary symptoms of malabsorption. The diagnostician will test the biopsied tissue for enzyme activity to establish the nature and cause of the disorder.

Many other irregularities of the jejunal tissue may also be evaluated through biopsy. Some of these include sugar intolerance, gluten intolerance (Celiac Sprue), and Whipple's disease, a severe bacterial infection of the intestine, capable of spreading from the small intestine to the lung, brain, heart, eyes, and joints. Antibiotics are usually prescribed to treat the disease. *See also* CELIAC SPRUE *and* WHIPPLE'S DISEASE.

Jellyfish Stings

Painful, itching stings caused by marine jellyfish.

Jellyfish are a type of coelenterate equipped with specialized stinging cells capable of penetrating human skin. Such cells are concentrated in the jellyfish's tentacles. Contact with the jellyfish or its tentacles typically produces a painful, raised rash appearing in a linear pattern. Jellyfish stings may be quite painful and are usually accompanied by itching. The rash may yield to raised, pus-filled blisters, which eventually rupture. Additional symptoms include nausea, muscle spasms, headache, breathing difficulty, and heart irregularities. The sting of one type of jellyfish, the Portuguese man-of-war, is potentially lethal.

Jellyfish stings may be treated with vinegar for 30 minutes to neutralize the toxin. Embedded spines or tentacles should be removed with sterile tweezers. Baking soda may be used after the wound is cleaned, to relieve pain. Ointments containing antihistamine and corticosteroid may be applied to reduce swelling and alleviate discomfort. Antivenom treatments exist for some but not all coelenterates. Seek medical help if there are signs of an allergic reaction (i.e., difficulty breathing or loss of consciousness); CPR may be necessary.

Jet Lag

Also known as jet fatigue and circadian dyschronism

A condition that occurs following long flights spanning across different time zones, due to the conflict between environmental cues and the body's internal biological clock.

Jet lag afflicts travelers who take long flights over different time zones. The internal biological clocks of these individuals are disrupted, resulting in a wide variety of psychological and physiological effects that often include fatigue and irritability.

Incidence. The experience of jet lag differs widely from individual to individual. Generally, people over 30 years old who are used to a daily routine are most susceptible to jet lag. Moreover, symptoms grow worse as more time zones are crossed. Jet lag is usually more severe when moving eastward (shortening the traveler's day) rather than westward (lengthening the traveler's day). Women have reported a relationship between jet lag and their menstrual cycle.

Causes. Jet lag is caused by a temporary dissociation between environment time and internal biological time. In a jet-lagged individual, environmental cues temporarily conflict with the internal rhythms of the body. The internal pacemaker of the body is controlled by a group of cells in the hypothalamus of the brain. However, the body's internal clock takes its cues from the environment. These cues include the light/dark cycle, the availability of food, and the body's level of activity.

Symptoms. The chief symptom of jet lag is a feeling of fatigue or tiredness that may occur in the middle of the day, along with an inability to sleep during the night. Other common symptoms include headache, irritability, loss of concentration, general weakness, dizziness, and gastrointestinal disorders such as indigestion, loss of appetite, and bowel irregularities.

The symptoms of jet lag are different for different individuals. Vacationers complain that they are not enjoying themselves, pilots may become prone to errors in judgment, and athletes can be plagued by a reduced motivation to train.

Melatonin and Jet Lag

Evidence suggests that the hormone melatonin can alter the phase of the body clock. Ingestion of melatonin in the afternoon advances the body clock (the internal time is later), whereas melatonin consumed in the morning has the opposite effect. For that reason, some travelers take melatonin to help control their internal clocks and prevent jet lag. While some studies have suggested that melatonin can be effective for this purpose, other studies have found that melatonin has no effect on jet lag.

Treatment. Over time, the body's internal clock and the environment become re-synchronized. In the meantime, individuals affected by jet lag are advised to get sufficient sleep. Short naps may help the sufferer avoid drowsiness. Long naps, however, will only prolong the time it takes the body to adjust.

Prevention. To prevent jet lag, travelers should choose flights that arrive as close to night time as possible. In addition, they should avoid sleep deficits prior to departure, which may compound sleep loss due to jet lag. Travelers should always drink sufficient water and eat nutritious foods during and after flights.

Background material on jet lag can be found in AVIATION MEDICINE. *For further information, see* AGING; GASTROINTESTINAL TRACT; INDIGESTION; NUTRITION; PUBLIC HEALTH; SLEEP; *and* SLEEP DEPRIVATION. *See also* MENSTRUATION, DISORDERS OF *for more on other problems that may affect women's menstruation.*

Jogger's Nipple

Soreness of the nipples in people who jog, caused by constant friction of clothing rubbing against the skin; that may result in bleeding during long distances.

Men who experience jogger's nipple can put bandages over the nipples to prevent soreness. Women who wear comfortable, cotton jogging bras and other clothing will usually not experience irritation. A soothing cream or petroleum jelly may help alleviate soreness after long runs. *See also* AEROBIC *and* EXERCISE.

Joint

The meeting point of two bones.

Lined with cartilage and fluid-filled synovial membrane, which prevents friction, a joint is the junction of bone ends or edges.

TYPES

There are two types of joints—fixed and mobile. Secured by fibrous tissue, fixed joints allow very limited movement (as in the case of spinal vertebrae) or none at all (as in the borders of the bones of the skull). Bone surfaces are covered by smooth, slick cartilage. Synovial fluid—clear, sticky, and contained within a membrane—seals and lubricates the joint. Over-extension of the joint is prevented by ligaments; muscles, attached to the bone by tendons on either side of the joint, control movement.

Hinge Joint. The most basic joint is the hinge joint, allowing bending and straightening. These include fingers, knees, and elbows, though the latter two also allow some limited rotation.

Pivot Joint. The joint between the first and second vertabrae, in the neck, is an example of a pivot joint. Allowing only rotation, a pivot joint is constructed either of a ring pivoting around an axis or of a pointed bone pivoting within a ring.

Ellipsoidal Joint. An elliptic cavity houses the oval-shaped end of a bone in an ellipsoidal joint. As is the case with the wrist, it allows a full range of movement except for pivoting.

Ball-and-Socket Joint. The ball-and-socket joint is the most sophisticated and dextrous, allowing rotation and backward, forward, and sideways movement. The hip and shoulder are examples.

DISORDERS

Injury or birth defect may cause full or partial dislocation, a dislodging of the bone end from a joint. Bone-end fractures, which are uncommon, may cause bleeding into the joint hemarthrosis or the buildup of synovial fluid (synovitis). Arthritis—i.e., swelling—often afflicts joints, as do sprains, cartilage damage, and tears of ligaments or the joint capsule

Background information on joint can be found in BONE; CARTILAGE; LIGAMENT; MUSCLE; *and* TENDON. *For related material, see* ELBOW; HIP; KNEE; NECK; SHOULDER; SKULL; *and* SPINE. *See also* ARTHRITIS; DISLOCATION, JOINT; HEMARTHROSIS; *and* SPRAIN *for more on various disorders affecting the joints.*

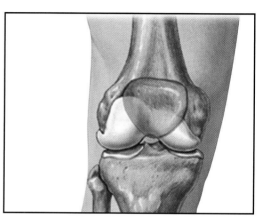

Jumper's Knee

The inflammation of the tendon below the kneecap (patella).

Pain, swelling, and tenderness running from the kneecap to the leg that intensifies with activity are indications of jumper's knee. This condition, considered an overuse injury, is caused by stress on the attachments of the tendons to the kneecap (patella), which leads to tiny tears in the tendons. Participants in sports in which there is constant running and jumping; such as basketball, volleyball, long-distance running, and track—are more likely to be affected by jumper's knee.

Ice packs and anti-inflammatory drugs can reduce the pain associated with jumper's knee. Exercises that strengthen the thigh muscles can help to protect the knee from this type of overuse injury. *See also* ICE PACKS.

Types of Joints.
The human body contains two types of joints — fixed and mobile. Fixed joints allow very limited movement, while mobile joints such as fingers, knees, at right, elbows, and wrists allow bending and straightening.

Resources on Joints
Lee, Thomas F. *Conquering Rheumatoid Arthritis: The Latest Breakthroughs and Treatments* (2001); McArdle, William D., et al., *Exercise Physiology: Energy, Nutrition, and Human Performance* (1996);Warren, Russell F., The Unstable Shoulder (1998); American Physical Therapy Association, Tel. (800) 999-APTA, Online: www.apta.org; National Osteoporosis Foundation, Tel. (800) 223-9994, Online: www.nof.org; American College of Rheumatology, Tel. (404) 633-3777, Online: www. rheumatology.org/aca/; American Academy ofOrthopaedic Surgeons, Tel. (800) 346-AAOS, Online: http://othoinfo. aaos.org/fact/; https://public1.med.cornell.edu/cgi-.

Kala-azar

Also known as assam fever and leishmaniasis

Parasitic disease affecting the spleen and liver.

Kala-azar is caused by a single-celled microorganism (protozoan). It occurs mostly in Africa, the Mediterranean, and India.

The disease is transmitted by the bite of a sand fly. The fly sucks the blood of one infected host, contracts the protozoa, and infects another person.

Symptoms usually appear two months or more after infection and include fever, weight loss, reduction in the number of white blood cells, and enlargement of the spleen and liver.

The disease can be fatal if left untreated. Kala-azar, and other forms of leishmaniasis, are treated with compounds of antimony, such as sodium stibogluconate. Controlling the sand fly population is the best way of preventing the spread of the disease. *See also* LEISHMANIASIS.

Kaposi's Sarcoma

A skin cancer often seen in AIDS patients.

Classically, Kaposi's sarcoma was a , non life threatening cancer occurring in older men and was characterized by purple, red, or brown lesions, usually on the skin of the lower legs. A different form of Kaposi's sarcoma is seen in AIDS patients; it occurs earlier in life, usually in the 30s.

Kaposi's sarcoma tumors can break out on the trunk, arms, head, and neck , as well as the mouth or genitals. Tumors can also arise in the intestinal tract and the lungs, where they can cause serious internal bleeding. Other symptoms depend on the site of the tumors and can include diarrhea, cramps, weight loss, fever, cough, and shortness of breath.

Classic, mild Kaposi's sarcoma can be treated successfully with low-dose radiation. Some symptoms of AIDS-associated Kaposi's sarcoma can also be relieved by low-dose radiation. A combination of chemo- therapy with interferon and a variety of other anti-cancer agents, such as bleomycin, doxorubicin, vincristine, and zidovudine, can help about 80 percent of patients, but the long-term prognosis can be poor due to complications. *See* AIDS.

Kawasaki Disease

Also known as mucocutaneous lymph node syndrome

A childhood disease most common in Asia, characterized by fever, conjunctivitis, redness in the tongue and mouth, and swelling of the lymph nodes in the neck.

The first symptom of Kawasaki disease is a sudden high fever. Three to five days later, redness of the lips, tongue, and throat appear, as well as a deep red rash and swollen lymph nodes in the neck. Arthritis or swelling of the joints may occur. Some children will develop aneurysms of the coronary arteries. There is no known cause for this disease—scientists suspect, however, that Kawasaki disease is caused by an unidentified virus or bacteria.

Treatment requires hospitalization, aspirin, and gamma globulin therapy to reduce the risk of heart complications, such as aneurysms. *See also* LYMPHATIC SYSTEM.

Kegel Exercises

Exercises that strengthen the pelvic floor.

Connecting the base of the spine (coccyx bone) to the pubic bone, the pubococcygeious muscle is also known as the pelvic floor. In women, its strength is important during pregnancy and the second stage of labor. Incontinence and flatulence can also be controlled by a stronger pelvic floor.

The contraction of the muscle can be felt by halting urination mid-stream. A pulling can be felt around the anal (and, in women, vaginal) sphincters. Kegel exercises consist of slowly tightening the muscles, holding for a four-count, then slowly relaxing. One must use only the pelvic floor muscle and not the muscles of the legs, buttocks, or abdomen. Four sets of ten repetitions each day are performed. *See also* PELVIC FLOOR EXERCISES.

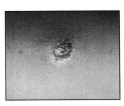

Leishmaniasis. A sand fly can deposit leishmania parasites in the skin where they cause a small sore or ulcer before creating further tissue damage throughout the body.

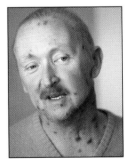

Kaposi's Sarcoma. A type of malignant tumor that is a common complication of AIDS but is otherwise rare. The lesions of Kaposi's sarcoma appear on the skin as slightly raised, purplish nodules,

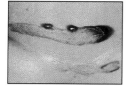

Keloid. Most common in young women and people of color, keloid is an overgrowth of scar tissue. Though not dangerous, severe cases may limit mobility and cause changes in appearance.

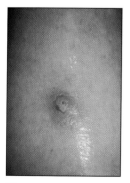

Keratoacanthoma. A skin growth similar to squamous cell carcinoma. It is more common among smokers.

Keloid

Similar to hypertrophic scar

An overgrowth of scar tissue at the site of a skin injury.

Most keloids will become less noticeable over time. If rubbed against clothing, they may become irritated. Severe cases sometimes limit mobility and cause changes in physical appearance.

Keloids can result from surgical incisions performed as a result of wounds, vaccinations, burns, chicken pox, acne, and scratches. They are most common in young women and people of color.

Keloids usually do not require treatment. Cryotherapy (freezing at the site) can reduce large keloids, as can corticosteroid injections, radiation, and surgical removal. The condition is not dangerous, but may cause psychological stress if the keloid significantly affects the patient's appearance. *See also* ACNE; CHICKEN POX; SCAR.

Keratin

A fibrous, resistant protein that makes up most of the material of the skin, hair, and nails.

Hair is made of keratin, the same material that comprises nails and the durable barrier at the surface of skin. It resists damage from a variety of physical and chemical agents. Cells present at the root of hair produce keratin. When these cells die, hair takes up the keratin that is left behind, adding color and texture. *See also* SKIN.

Keratitis

An inflammation of the cornea.

Caused by infection, prolonged wear of contact lenses, or the virus that causes cold sores—herpes simplex virus type 1. Keratitis spawns red eye, irritation, blurred vision, sensitivity to light, pain, and watering of the eyes. Antifungal or antibacterial drops or oral antibiotics are usually effective as treatment for the condition.

Prevention and Prognosis. To prevent keratitis, it is important not to wear contact lenses while sleeping. Cases that do not respond to treatment immediately may demand long-term care. *See also* CONTACT LENS *and* CORNEA.

Keratoacanthoma

A small, round growth on the skin that is firm except for the center, which may be scaly.

Keratoacanthoma is a type of skin growth similar to squamous cell carcinoma. It grows quickly and is more common among men and people who smoke. It is thought to be caused by ultraviolet radiation or perhaps a trauma to the skin.

Traditional treatment requires surgical removal of the growth. In cases where the growth is quite deep, surgery may prove to be disfiguring, particularly to the face. More recently, these skin growths have been successfully treated with injections of corticosteroids or flurouracil chemotherapy. *See also* CORTICOSTEROID DRUGS *and* SQUAMOUS CELL CARCINOMA.

Keratoconjunctivits

A disorder of the cornea, usually caused by a virus.

Epidemic keratoconjunctivitis is the most common form of keratoconjunctivitis, which is associated with conjunctivitis. Symptoms may include redness, inflammation, a whitish membrane over the conjunctiva, and painful swelling of a lymph gland in front of the ear. Snowflake-like spots develop in the cornea. Specific treatment does not exist, though corticosteroid drugs may diminish the spots.

Keratoconjunctivitis sicca is caused by deficient tear production (dry eye) and persistent corneal and conjunctival dryness, which may have a variety of causes. Symptoms of the condition include a gritty, irritated sensation and oversensitivity to light. The best treatment is frequent use of artificial tears. If it fails, a doctor should be consulted. *See also* CORNEA; EYE; EYE, DISORDERS OF; *and* VIRUS.

Keratoconus

Abnormal bowing of the corneas, which causes them to become thinned and conical in shape.

Keratoconus results in thinned corneas bulging into cones. It has no known cause, but may be hereditary. Affecting more females than males, it usually occurs in both eyes and begins in the teens or twenties. Symptoms include distorted and blurred vision, pain, tearing, clouding, and sensitivity to light. Rubbing may exacerbate its progression. Various corrective contact lenses can solve the problem in its early stages, but a minority of sufferers develop corneas that have become too scarred or conical. Treatments include transplants or grafts of donor corneas. *See also* EYE; *and* EYE, DISORDERS OF.

Keratomalacia

The final phase of corneal damage owing to a lack of vitamin A.

Keratomalacia occurs rarely in developed countries, and afflicts extremely malnourished children. Long-term vitamin A deficiency dries out the eyes and forms foamy patches on the corners of the conjunctiva. Symptoms include over sensitivity to light and a gritty irritation under the eyelids. Large doses of vitamin A can cure early symptoms, but if left untreated, the condition may progress into keratomalacia. Ulcers and opacity cloud the cornea, cause infection, and may lead to loss of the eye. *See also* CORNEA *and* EYE, DISORDERS OF.

Keratopathy

A general term for disorders of the cornea.

In actinic keratopathy, sunlight, a sunlamp, a welding torch, or some other source of ultraviolet light strips off the cornea's outer layer, revealing nerves and inflicting extreme pain.

An impairment of the blink reflex and reduction in tear film can cause exposure keratopathy. It may occur in cases of facial palsy, outward turning of the eyelid (ectropion), or soft tissue inflammation in the eye socket (exophthalmos). *See* EYE.

Keratosis, Actinic

A precancerous skin growth usually associated with sun exposure.

Visible signs of the condition include flat, scaly, wart-like areas on the skin. These growths usually occur on areas that have been exposed to sunlight. The lesions are localized, and occur on the face, scalp, back of the hands, chest, and other areas. Some of those who suffer from keratosis will develop skin cancer.

Actinic keratosis occurs most commonly in those with fair skin, especially in the elderly and young people. The skin growths should be examined by a trained physician to guard against any possible malignancies.

Growths are usually surgically destroyed or removed to eliminate the potential for any cancer to develop. Keratosis can be prevented by minimizing exposure to the sun, wearing protective clothing, and regularly using sunscreen with an SPF of 15 or above. *See also* KERATOSIS PILARIS; SKIN CANCER; *and* SQUAMUS CELL CARCINOMA.

Keratosis Pilaris

A skin condition, common in children and the obese, where keratin collects by the hair follicles.

Keratosis pilaris usually manifests as rough, goosebump-like skin. It commonly occurs on the outer upper arm and upper thighs, but can also appear anywhere on the body. The affected areas feel like sandpaper. Individual lesions develop around hair follicles. Keratosis pilaris most commonly occurs in the winter and clears up in the summer months.

Treatment for keratosis pilaris consists of using moisturizing lotion to soothe the affected areas. In serious cases, creams containing urea or lactic acid are prescribed. *See also* KERATIN; LESIONS; *and* SKIN.

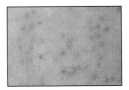

Keratosis Pilaris. A condition where goosebumps appear on the skin, keratosis pilaris is caused by an excess of keratin, a protein that makes up most of the skin, hair, and nails.

Keratotomy, Radial

A surgical procedure to correct or reduce myopia (nearsightedness).

In a radial keratotomy, a series of deep surgical incisions are made in the cornea to flatten the area over the pupil. This procedure reduces the nearsightedness of the patient and may even correct it completely. The procedure is called a radial keratotomy because the incisions resemble the radii of circles.

After the patient is given a relaxant and eye drops containing an anaesthetic, the ophthalmologist measures the thickness of the cornea to determine how deep to make the incisions. The doctor then makes four to sixteen incisions with a calibrated diamond blade, making sure to avoid the optical (center) zone, through which the patient sees. The procedure usually takes fifteen to thirty minutes.

Introduced in 1978, radial keratotomy was one of the most commonly performed eye operations. Research indicates that after operations about 85 percent of patients can pass a standard driver's license eye exam that requires 20/40 vision (without glasses or contact lenses). New types of surgery such as LASIK (laser in situ keratomileusis) and PRK (photorefractive keratectomy) have now replaced radial keratotomy. *See also* MYOPIA.

Kernicterus

Also called nuclear jaundice

A severe form of jaundice of the newborn, characterized by high levels of unconjugated bilirubin in the blood, the appearance of yellow skin, and lesions in the cerebral gray matter.

An excess of the pigment bilirubin in the blood finds its way into brain cells, causing those cells to die. Premature infants are at high risk for kernicterus.

An infant in danger of developing kernicterus will show signs of jaundice during the first few days of life. The baby may become inactive or drowsy, have poor feeding, vomit, arch the back and neck repeatedly, rolled-up eyes, and seizures.

Kernicterus is preventable if the jaundice is treated appropriately and promptly. Without treatment, a newborn will probably die at the end of its first week. Kernicterus is a serious condition that can lead to mental retardation, damage to the brain, abnormal muscle control, deafness, paralysis of upward eye movements, and death. *See also* JAUNDICE.

Ketosis

Accumulation of fatty acids (ketones) in the body as the result of a lack of glucose (sugar).

Ketosis is a dangerous metabolic imbalance that occurs when the diet lacks sufficient carbohydrates or when a person has type I diabetes. When glucose and glycogen stores are depleted by high-protein, low carbohydrate diets or fasting, protein is metabolized to supply the body with the necessary glucose. The degradation of the body's protein in the organs and muscles would cause death in several weeks, so the body attempts to preserve protein by utilizing an alternative fuel source. Fats are partially burned as a substitute for glucose. Sustained breakdown of fat leads to a buildup of ketones in the bloodstream.

Symptoms of ketosis include loss of appetite, nausea, vomiting, sweet-smelling breath, and abdominal pain. If the condition is suspected, medical assistance should be called immediately; untreated, the disorder can prove fatal. *See also* CARBOHYDRATES; FAD FOODS; FASTING; *and* FATTY ACIDS.

Ketogenic Diets

Recently, ketogenic diets have gained attention due to weight loss that occurs soon after starting the diet. This is water loss, as the kidneys rid the system of ketones and protein byproducts. Weight is quickly regained when carbohydrates are reintroduced. Ketosis increases the acidity of the blood, affecting chemical equilibrium and leading to side effects like nausea, dizziness, fatigue, headache, and bad breath. Ketogenic diets are dangerous for diabetics and pregnant women in particular.

Kidney

The organ that excretes waste and excess water and filter the blood.

Fist-sized and bean-shaped, the two kidneys are located underneath the liver and the spleen. Each kidney's function and structure is almost identical. In addition to its role in the urinary tract, the kidney is a primary organ of the circulatory system. It regulates the environment of cells in the body.

The body is about 56 percent water; two-thirds is found inside cells, and the remaining third is present outside the cells. The kidneys regulate the amount and composition of this water by acting on the blood.

The aorta is linked directly to the kidneys, by arteries which ramify into arterioles, and end in twisted masses of capillaries called glomeruli. These filter waste and fluid from blood and pass the resulting fluid into tubules that lead into the medulla. The glomeruli and tubules together are called nephrons, and are the kidney's main filtering mechanisms, which number one million per kidney.

Every minute nearly two pints of blood arrive in the kidneys through the renal arteries. The glomeruli's porous walls allow waste, electrolytes, nutrients, and some water to pass into the tubules. Water, minerals, nutrients, and salts essential to the body are reabsorbed by the bloodstream. Proteins and most red blood cells remain in the bloodstream. Each day, approximately 180 liters of fluid pass from the glomeruli into the tubules.

Between the tubular fluid of the tubules and the blood in the surrounding vessels, processes take place that determine which substances are excreted and which are reabsorbed. Blood acidity, water, salt, and mineral content is regulated. Blood exits the kidneys through the renal veins while urine passes from the tubules to larger tubes called calyces, through the renal pelvis and the ureter to the bladder.

Working continuously, the kidneys produce about one to two liters of urine each day, depending on liquid consumption.

Kidneys pass water when it is in excess and conserve it when water is depleted.

The kidneys also generate hormones. One, erythropoietin, controls red blood cell production and release from the bone marrow. When blood pressure drops, the kidney releases the enzyme renin, which reacts with a blood protein to produce angiotensin, which both contracts arteries and regulates the excretion of potassium and the reabsorption of sodium.

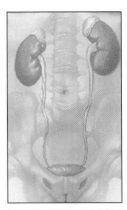

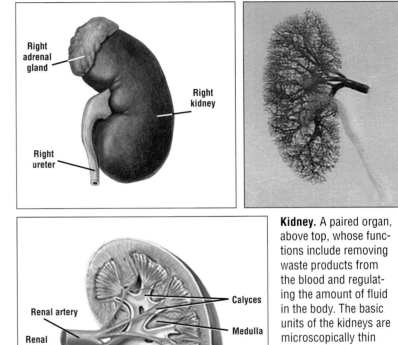

Kidney. A paired organ, above top, whose functions include removing waste products from the blood and regulating the amount of fluid in the body. The basic units of the kidneys are microscopically thin structures called nephrons, above bottom, which filter the blood and cause wastes to be removed in the form of urine. On the left is a diagram of the parts of the kidney, which serves as an intrical part of the body's urinary system.

Background material on Kidney can be found in BLOOD AND CIRCULATORY SYSTEM. *Related information is contained in* AORTA, ENZYME, NUTRIENTS, PROTEIN, RENAL DISEASE, SODIUM, TOXOCOLOGY, AND URINARY SYSTEM. *See also* BLADDER AND WATER *for more on Kidney.*

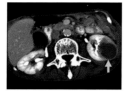

Kidney Cancer. Above is an x-ray of a cancerous kidney. The yellow arrow indicates a dark spot where the tumor may be growing. Blood in the urine is a warning sign of this condition.

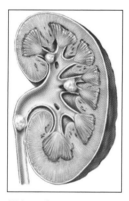

Kidney Stones. Kidney stones are small, crystallized substances, such as calcium, that form in the kidney or other parts of the urinary tract. Smaller kidney stones can pass out of the body on their own, although this can be painful. Larger stones may require surgery.

Kidney Cancer

Malignant tumor of the kidney.

About 85 percent of kidney cancers are adenocarcinomas, which arise in the lining of the tubules, the tiny passageways in which waste products are filtered out of the blood. Blood in the urine is the most common symptom of this ailment, which often spreads to other organs by the time it is detected. Most other kidney cancers are fibrosarcomas, which develop in the shells that surround the two kidneys. A third kind of kidney cancer, Wilms' tumor (nephroblastoma), occurs mostly in children under the age of four and accounts for about 20 percent of all childhood cancers. If detected early, 50 to 80 percent of all children survive this ailment.

Aside from Wilms' tumor, most kidney cancers occur in people 50 and older. Women are twice as likely as men to develop kidney cancer. Environmental exposure to carcinogens is known to increase the risk. These carcinogens include asbestos, lead acetate, and potassium bromide. Workers in the rubber, textile, leather, dye, petroleum, and plastic industries are exposed to carcinogens that can increase their risk of kidney cancer.

Symptoms. The most common symptom of kidney cancer is blood in the urine, which sometimes is present only in microscopic amounts. Other symptoms include fever, fatigue, loss of appetite, and pain in the side of the lower back.

Diagnostic tests include urinalysis to detect blood and abnormal cells, ultrasound examinations, tomography or magnetic resonance imaging scans, and x-rays. These x-ray examinations include intravenous pyelography, in which a special contrast injected into the bloodstream allows a series of images to be obtained, and nephrotomogram, which provides images of cross-sections of the kidney.

Treatment and Prognosis. Surgery to remove an affected kidney usually can be curative if the cancer has not spread beyond the organ. The surgeon can perform a partial nephrectomy (removing only part of a kidney in which an early cancer has been detected), a simple nephrectomy (removing the entire affected kidney), or a radical nephrectomy (removing the kidney and some surrounding tissue). The odds that cancer will be found in the other kidney are about 20 percent.

The Phenacetin Risk

Phenacetin is an ingredient used in many over-the-counter pain relief products. After suspecting a link between the ingredient and kidney cancer, the Food and Drug Administration has taken action against phenacetin. Anyone who consistently used a product containing phenacetin should be aware of the possible increased risk and consult a physician about possible damage.

If cancer is detected at a more advanced stage, radiation therapy may be given before or after surgery. Kidney cancer is not usually treated with chemotherapy because the organs' ability to process drugs is reduced by the disease. The survival rate for kidney cancers that are detected early is high. The survival rate is far lower for cancers detected at a later stage, especially if they have spread to other tissues. *See also* CANCER; KIDNEY; KIDNEY FUNCTION TESTS; *and* NEPHRECTOMY.

Kidney Cyst

A fluid-filled cavity within a kidney.

Kidney cysts are common, occurring in half of all people over the age of 50, and usually cause no symptoms, although they sometimes give rise to pain in the back. They often are detected by x-ray examinations administered for other conditions. Detection is followed by further tests, such as a computerized tomography (CT) scan or ultrasound, as kidney cysts are rarely associated with cancer. If no cancer is found and the cyst causes no symptoms, treatment consists of monitoring the cyst. *See also* COMPUTERIZED TOMOGRAPHY SCAN; KIDNEY; KIDNEY CANCER; *and* ULTRASOUND.

Kidney Function Test

Any diagnostic test designed to test the efficiency or health of the kidney.

Kidney function is generally assessed through urine and blood. The most basic kidney function test is urinalysis, where urine is collected, examined under a microscope, and, in some cases, cultured. There are also a number of kidney imaging techniques. Depressed or elevated levels of serum creatinine, a waste product produced during the kidney's activity of filtering blood; blood nitrogen urea or BUN, found in urine; and other indicators indicate the condition of the kidneys.

TYPES OF TEST

A creatine clearance test estimates creatine levels in samples of blood, based on the patients age, sex, and weight. Precise values may be obtained by monitoring urine output over a 24 hour period. Sudden elevation of creatine and BUN, as well as high levels of potassium and acid, low calcium, high phosphorus, and elevated blood pressure may suggest varying degrees of acute kidney failure. Tests of the kidney by auscultation—listening through a stethoscope—will detect a scratchy sound.

Infection of the kidneys can be diagnosed with kidney function tests. The bacteria or other pathogen is extracted from a urine sample. then cultured and identified. Such infections produce an elevated number of white blood cells.

A variety of diseases affect the nephrons' ability to purify the blood. One such ailment, chronic interstitial nephritis, causes edema in the feet and ankles and hypertension. Kidney function tests of urine will show elevated protein, glucose, blood potassium, phosphate, and bicarbonate. For certain kidney disorders, additional tests such as biopsy may be performed.

Background material on Kidney Function Test can be found in KIDNEY CANCER AND KIDNEY IMAGING. Related information is contained in AUSCULTATION, BLOOD, HYPERTENSION, KIDNEY, AND URINALYSIS.

Kidney Imaging

Techniques for visualizing the kidney as an aid to diagnosis.

X-ray studies of the abdomen identify the size and shape of the kidney. Using an injected substance, usually a dye, to help outline structures on x-ray, intravenous urography allows visualization of the kidneys and urinary tract. More accurate measurements can be obtained using ultrasound (high frequency sound waves, which are reflected by tissue in the kidney to yield an image). Ultrasound imaging is also considered desirable because no x-rays are used. Unlike intravenous urography, it can be used effectively even in cases of poor kidney function.

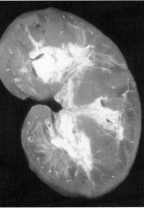

Kidney. A diagnostic image of a healthy human kidney.

CT (computed tomography) is a more sophisticated form of x-ray. CT can distinguish solid from liquid masses, is useful for tumor identification, and may also help a medical professional to evaluate the extent of malignant growth beyond the kidney.

Angiography, like intravenous urography, involves the injection of a radiocontrast or radiopaque solution, in this case into an artery, and then following the dye's course by x-ray. More recently, angiography has been used with CT scanning, which offers clearer imaging with small amounts of the dye injected intravenously.

MRI, or magnetic resonance imaging, is a more recent and sophisticated technique that employs a magnetic field. It is often preferred because, like ultrasound, the technique is completely safe, using no harmful radiation. The atomic nuclei within tissues are induced to resonate, sending a signal to the MRI detectors, which can then create a highly detailed image. Kidney tumor shape can be assessed through three-dimensional imaging. Additionally, MRI is an ideal means of imaging blood vessels and other structures surrounding the kidneys. *See also* ANGIOGRAPHY; CAT SCAN; KIDNEY; KIDNEY CYST; MRI; RADIOPAQUE; *and* X-RAY.

Kidney Transplant

Surgical procedure in which failed kidneys are removed and replaced with a kidney from a donor.

If the kidneys fail as a result of disease, a successful kidney transplant can restore normal kidney function. Each year in the U.S. approximately 11,000 kidney transplant operations are completed, making it the second most common transplant surgery after cataract surgery. A transplant is a major medical intervention, however, and can only be performed on people who are otherwise in good health.

If a patient is determined to be a good candidate for transplantation, a donor must then be located. A person with two healthy kidneys can donate one kidney without impairing his or her own kidney function. The donor's tissue must be as similar to the recipients as possible to minimize the chance of rejection, a reaction in which the recipient's immune system recognizes the donated kidney as foreign material and attempts to destroy it. Close family members usually provide the best tissue match for transplantation.

Removal of donor kidneys is now performed through laparoscopic nephrectomy, in which the kidney is extracted through a very small incision. The technique requires far less hospital time than conventional surgery, and healing is rapid.

If a living donor cannot be found, then it is possible to use a kidney from a person with healthy kidneys who has recently died. The kidney must be immediately removed from the body and can be stored in a cold saline solution for up to two days before it must be transplanted. This has a slightly lower success rate than a transplant from a living donor, and the demand for donated kidneys greatly exceeds supply, resulting in waiting times of two to three years.

Procedure. A transplant operation is performed with the patient under general anesthesia and generally lasts two to three hours. An incision is made in the abdomen, and the kidney is placed into the lower left or right side of the abdomen.

The kidney's new blood vessels are connected to the blood supply of the leg, and a ureter connecting the kidney to the bladder. A drain may be inserted to siphon excess fluid from the abdomen, and the wound is then stitched.

Rejection. After the new kidney is implanted, the patient is given immunosuppressant drugs, such as prednisone, cyclosporin or imuran, to prevent the immune system from attacking the kidney. Despite tissue typing for compatibility and the use of drugs to suppress immune response, rejection episodes following surgery are common. Symptoms of tissue rejection include fluid retention leading to weight gain, tenderness and inflammation at the transplant site, and fever.

If rejection occurs, the type or dosage of immunosuppressant drugs may be modified. If these efforts fail to reverse the rejection, the organ is often left in place, and dialysis is resumed. The risk of rejection increases with each additional attempt.

Long-Term Side Effects. After transplantation, the patient must remain on immunosuppressant drugs indefinitely. This makes the patient more susceptible to illness and infection. Kidney transplant patients are at considerably higher risk for some forms of cancer. Lymphoma, for example, is about 30 times more common in kidney recipients—likely a byproduct of immune suppression. These risks, however, are usually considered acceptable for a procedure that has a high and growing success rate and can restore an active life to people who suffer kidney failure.

Prognosis. For transplant patients, the rate of success after one year is close to 90 percent. Between three and eight percent of these patients experience kidney failure each subsequent year following surgery, but kidney transplants can function well for over 30 years.

Background material on Kidney Transplant can be found in KIDNEY CANCER AND TRANSPLANT SURGERY. *Related information is contained in* ABDOMEN, CANCER, FEVER, IMMUNOSUPPRESSANT DRUGS, KIDNEY CYST, KIDNEY TUMORS, LAPAROSCOPY, LYMPHOMA AND TISSUE TYPING.

Resources on Nephrology and Urology

Cameron, Stewart, *Kidney Disease: The Facts* (1986); Legrain, Marcel, et al., *Nephrology* (1987); Campbell, Meredith F., & E. Darracott Vaughan, *Campbell's Urology* (2002); Hinman, Frank, *Atlas of Urologic Surgery* (1989); Tanagho, Emil A. and Jack W. McAninch, eds., *Smith's General Urology* (1995); National Kidney Foundation, Tel. (800) 622-9010, Online: www.kidney.org; American Association of Kidney Patients, Tel. (800) 749-2257, Online: www.aakp.org; American Foundation for Urologic Disease, Tel. (800) 242-AFUD, Online: www.afud.org; National Institute of Diabetes and Digestive and Kidney Diseases, Tel. (301) 496-3583, Online: www.niddk.nih.gov;www.nycornell.org/medicine/nephrology/index.html; www.cornellurology.com/.

Kidney, Polycystic

An inherited disorder in which the kidneys develop multiple cysts.

The cysts that develop in polycystic kidney disease result in enlarged kidneys with impaired function. Polycystic kidney appears to be a genetic disorder. In some cases, the cysts may appear in the liver and other organs. The condition is more common in adults, but also afflicts children. In adults, complications include pain, blood in the urine (hematuria), kidney stones, and high blood pressure (hypertension). In children, high blood pressure, anemia, kidney failure, and liver disease are common difficulties. The majority of people with the condition reach end-stage renal disease in their 40s or 50s, necessitating dialysis or a kidney transplant. Children with the disorder may die in infancy or early childhood.

There is no way to prevent cyst formation, but the symptoms and complications of the disorder can be treated. Controlling high blood pressure as well as treating any urinary infections is important in preventing damage to the kidney. *See also* DIALYSIS; HYPERTENSION; KIDNEY; KIDNEY CYST; *and* KIDNEY TRANSPLANT.

Kidney Tumors

Benign or malignant growths arising in the kidney

Nonmalignant kidney tumors, unlike kidney cancers, are not life-threatening and often cause no symptoms. They include fibromas, which arise from connective tissue; leiomas, arising from smooth muscle; and lipomas, arising from fatty tissue. Another nonmalignant kidney tumor, hemangioma, affects blood vessels and may cause bleeding. A hemangioma may grow large enough to be mistaken for a kidney cancer. Benign tumors of the kidney do not require treatment unless they become unusually large or cause pain, loss of function, or other symptoms. *See also* BENIGN; HEMANGIOMA; KIDNEY; KIDNEY IMAGING; *and* KIDNEY FUNCTION TESTS.

Kilocalorie

Measure of energy the equivalent of 1,000 calories; however, in dietetics and medicine, the unit is equal to one calorie.

A kilocalorie, or nutrionist's calorie, is the unit of energy necessary to raise the temperature of one kilogram of water one degree centigrade. The scientific calorie measures the amount of heat (energy) to raise one gram of water one degree. A nutritional calorie, therefore, actually refers to a kilocalorie measurement. The kilocalorie is used to describe the energy content of food by representing the amount of human metabolic energy that is generated by burning that particular food. Kilocalories are used to calculate the 'appropriate food intake necessary to meet the metabolic needs of an individual. *See also* CALORIE; ENERGY; *and* METABOLISM.

Klinefelter's Syndrome

A chromosomal abnormality in which a male has an extra X chromosome.

Normally, females have the sex chromosome XX, and males posess the chromosome XY. Individuals with Klinefelter's syndrome have an XXY chromosome. This anomaly occurs in approximately 1 in 700 male births. The chance of having a baby with Klinefelter's syndrome is much higher in older mothers.

The physical characteristics vary, but males with Klinefelter's syndrome tend to be tall and thin, with somewhat feminized bodies, including moderate breast development. Their testes are small and they usually cannot produce sperm, causing them to be sterile. Boys with this syndrome usually have normal intelligence, although there is a chance of mental retardation. However, they often exhibit speech and reading disabilities. There is no treatment for this condition, but hormone treatment can sometimes help develop secondary sex characteristics, such as facial hair. *See also* CHROMOSOMAL ABNORMALITIES.

Klumpke's Paralysis

Paralysis of the lower arm accompanied by the decay of muscles in the hand and numbness of the fingers (but not the thumb) and the inner forearm.

Klumpke's paralysis is the result of damage to the first thoracic nerve, a spinal nerve located behind the shoulder blade. A dislocated shoulder generally causes paralysis in the arm and hand.

At times, this injury is accompanied by Horner's syndrome, a type of nerve damage affecting the face with symptoms including a constricted pupil, drooping upper eyelid, and a lack of perspiration on one side of the neck and face.

The condition frequently remains permanent. Exercise is recommended to preserve the mobility of the joints, although it is not a cure. *See also* BRACHIAL PLEXUS *and* HORNER'S SYNDROME.

Knee

The joint between the thigh bone (femur) and the shin (tibia).

Capable of bending, straightening, and slight rotation, the knee is a modified hinge joint covered by the kneecap (patella). Between bones, cartilage minimizes friction. Ligaments on either side of the joint provide support and prevent excessive lateral movement. Within the joint, cruciate ligaments support by resisting deep bending, overextension, and the sliding of bone ends against one another. The thigh muscles (quadriceps) straighten the knee, while the muscles of the back of the thigh (hamstrings) bend it. *See* ARTHOSCOPY; BIOMECHANICAL ENGINEERING; FITNESS; KNEE JOINT REPLACEMENT; PROSTHESIS; *and* JOINT.

Knee Ligament Surgery. Right, when one of the many ligaments in the knee is damaged, surgery is needed to repair it. Usually, a surgeon will drill several holes into the knee to insert the instruments needed for the surgery; sometimes, a camera, or viewing scope, is used for viewing the damage and the repair.

Knee Joint. Below, a healthy human knee joint.

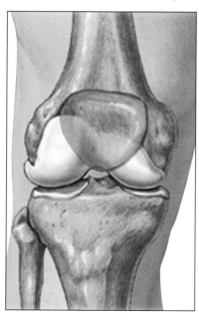

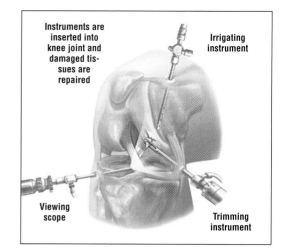

Knee Joint Replacement

Replacement of the knee joint to treat severe, disabling degeneration of the joint.

Knee replacement is usually performed in response to severe arthritis or osteoarthritis. These degenerative disorders wear away at the bones of the knee and cause the surface of the knee joint to become rough and irregular, interfering with smooth and painless flexing of the knee joint. If these conditions do not respond to conventional therapy, and if pain is acute and interferes with the ability to walk, joint replacement surgery becomes an option. The procedure is a major surgery and thus carries certain risks. The possibility should be discussed in detail with a qualified orthopedic surgeon trained in knee joint replacement.

PROCEDURE

The surgery is conducted under general anesthesia. An incision is made over the knee and the kneecap (patella) is removed. Next, the heads of the femur and tibia are shaved smooth to remove rough edges and allow the replacement materials to cement strongly to the bone. A metal prosthesis is cemented to the thigh bone (femur) and a plastic or metal prosthesis to the front shin bone (tibia). The parts are designed to slide over each other frictionlessly, allowing the knee to bend easily. A small drainage tube is inserted to allow fluid to be drained from the knee during surgery. The skin is stitched up, and the wound is dressed.

After surgery, the leg is placed in a continuous passive motion (CPM) device—a mechanical brace that flexes and extends the knee at a programmed rate. The amount of flexing will gradually be increased as the treated area heals and strengthens. In addition to strengthening the knee, the CPM device speeds recovery, decreases postoperative pain, and guards against blood loss and infection.

COMPLICATIONS

Blot clots in the veins of the legs are the most common postoperative complication of knee joint replacement. Occasionally these clots become dislodged and travel to the heart or lungs, causing an embolism, which can be life-threatening. The risk can be reduced with blood thinning drugs after surgery and by moving the legs.

Risk of infection in knee joint replacement is higher than for many other surgeries (about one–half percent). Special precautions are taken, including the use of a laminar flow operating room, with specially filtered, bacteria-free air. Surgeons wear sterile suits, which enclose the entire head and body. Antibiotics given before, during, and after the surgery also reduce infection risk.

After surgery and recovery, precautions should be taken against any wound infection, and infection should be treated aggressively if it occurs.

PROGNOSIS

The vast majority of patients are able to walk without assistance after recovery from a knee replacement. The extent of success depends in large part on the physical therapy following surgery, in which mobility is gradually returned to the knee and the muscles are gradually strengthened. A prosthetic knee can last 15 to 20 years, although highly strenuous activity may cause it to loosen earlier. *See also* ARTHRITIS; EMBOLISM; KNEE; ORTHOPEDICS; *and* OSTEOARTHRITIS.

Knock-Knee

Inward curvature of the legs that causes the knees to touch and the feet to separate at a wider distance than normal.

Many children show some inward or outward curving of the legs between the ages of three and five, but in most cases this clears up without treatment as the child grows. In some cases, the condition may be caused by a disease that softens the bones, such as rickets or osteomalacia. Between ages five and six, the legs begin to straighten, and by puberty, most children have overcome the problem and can stand with both knees and ankles touching.

Causes in adults may include injuries to the knee or upper or lower leg that do not heal properly. Diseases that soften the bones, such as rickets, rheumatoid arthritis, and osteoarthritis also may cause the knees to turn in.

If knock-knees in children persist beyond age 10, joint strain in the lower leg may result. Heel supports in the shoes may correct the line of the leg. An osteotomy, surgery in which the tibia is cut and realigned, may be needed to straighten the leg. In extreme cases, knee joint replacement is necessary if arthritis has developed. *See also* RICKETS.

Koplik's Spots

Small white spots with red rings on the inner surfaces of the cheeks; an early sign of measles.

The first sign of measles is a red rash that begins behind the ears and spreads down the neck to eventually cover most of the body. The sufferer will have flu-like symptoms of a runny nose, a sore throat, a fever, reddened eyes, and coughing. A few days after the onset of these symptoms, tiny white spots with red rings will appear on the tongue and in the lining of the mouth, particularly on the insides of the cheeks opposite the molars. Koplik's spots, when seen, are considered diagnostic of measles. *See also* MEASLES.

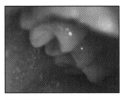

Koplik's Spots. The first signs of measles, a red rash that may begin behind the ears.

Kuru

A New Guinean disease of the 1950s and 1960s, now believed to have been caused by a newly discovered infectious agent called prions.

Kuru is characterized by a loss of coordination followed by dementia. The disease was consistently fatal. It is now believed that kuru was transmitted through ritual cannibalism and caused by infectious agents called prions. Symptoms may not appear for months, or even years after the virus has entered the body. Prions multiply by inducing normal protein molecules to change their shape and are also believed to be responsible for mad cow disease (technically called bovine spongiform encephalopathy because it causes the brain to be riddled with tiny holes). *See also* CREUTZFELDT-JAKOB SYNDROME *and* DEMENTIA.

Kwashiorkor

A severe form of malnutrition in infants and young children, resulting from inadequate protein intake.

This condition appears primarily in tropical and subtropical areas and in countries experiencing severe economic problems, famine, or war. In the United States, cases of kwashiorkor are rare.

Early symptoms of malnutrition include fatigue, irritability, and lethargy. As the lack of protein in the diet continues, an infant or child with Kwashiorkor may experience anemia, edema, growth failure, decreased immunity, a large potbelly, dermatitis, depigmentation of the skin, loss of hair, and hypoalbuminemia, and may produce bulky stools containing undigested food.

Improving protein intake and calorie consumption will correct the condition if treatment is initiated early enough. If the malnutrition is not treated, coma and death will result.

A child who has had Kwashiorkor will never reach adult height and weight. Severe forms of the condition can leave the child with permanent physical and mental problems. *See* ABDOMEN *and* PROTEINS.

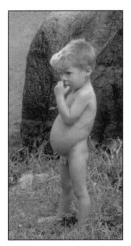

Kwashiorkor. A boy with a swollen abdomen from the parasitic infection schistosomiasis. In underdeveloped countries, such sights are often the result of severe malnourishment.

Kyphoscoliosis

Backward curvature of the spine combined with a curve to one side.

This form of scoliosis may be congenital, showing up at birth, or as a result of a musculoskeletal disorder such as paralysis, muscular dystrophy, or polio. The condition is the combination of scoliosis and kyphoscoliosis, resulting in both an outward curvature of the spine and a curve to one side. Kyphoscoliosis may develop on its own over time, becoming apparent during puberty, most commonly in girls. Indications of kyphoscoliosis are the same as other forms of scoliosis: one shoulder higher than the other or uneven hips. There may be pain or fatigue in the lower back. Tests by a physician will determine the type and extent of scoliosis. Treatment may involve a brace or the insertion of rods in order to straighten the back while growing. *See also* KYPHOSIS *and* SCOLIOSIS.

Kyphosis

Excessive outward curve of the spine.

Kyphosis is a deformity of the thoracic spine in which the normal curve is greatly exaggerated. This causes the spine to curve outward, leading to either a hump or rounded back. The condition seems to be caused by osteoarthritis, disease, injury, fracture of a vertebra, rapid growth during adolescence, a tumor on the vertebra, or poor posture. Kyphosis can also develop following some spinal surgeries.

Signs of kyphosis are a gradual rounding of the back, back fatigue, stiffness, and pain. Treatment consists of exercises to strengthen the back, a firmer mattress, or, in more severe cases, a brace to keep the spine straight.

Kyphosis in young people can disappear if treated correctly, but may not heal if it is caused by a degenerative bone disease. In rare instances, surgery is necessary to restore proper form to the spine. *See also* ORTHOPEDIC BRACE *and* SCOLIOSIS.

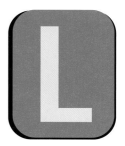

Labial Adhesions

Scar tissue between the labia.

Often mistaken for a congenital absence of a vagina, labial adhesions afflict prepubertal girls and postmenopausal women. Though related to low levels of estrogen, the cause is unknown.

Often, children will not display symptoms from labial adhesions. When they do, the scar tissue has blocked the urethra, causing burning during urination and, in the case of severe adhesions, urine retention. Severe symptoms necessitate the application of a thin film of conjugated estrogen twice daily for a week to ten days. The labia usually separate on their own or with slight traction. Otherwise, surgical separation followed by the conjugated estrogen cream application regimen is necessary. Recurrence is common and can be prevented by proper hygiene. *See* VAGINA.

Labile

Term meaning changeable, either chemically or emotionally.

The term labile has varied uses in medicine. It can apply to structures that are not fixed, unsteady, or rapidly changing. When associated with emotions, it implies a rapidly shifting state, one prone to disorder. Chemically, labile describes that which is readily altered or decomposed by heat—also known as thermolabile.

Labyrinthitis

Disorder of the labyrinth causing vertigo, nausea, and hearing loss.

The inner-ear is composed of two different types of organs; the cochlea (the spiral cavity in the inner-ear) helps with hearing, and the vestibular labyrinth is responsible for maintaining balance. Named for its twisting, turning shape, the labyrinth is made up of different sections that are filled with fluids. As the head and body move, the fluids in the chamber shift, sending signals to the brain, which then reorients the body. This allows the body to maintain equilibrium, balance, and eye position. If a disorder strikes the labyrinth, the body loses these abilities.

Causes. Labyrinthitis is usually caused by an infection. Viruses such as the flu, measles, or mumps can result in labyrinthitis. Bacterial infections that lead to labyrinthitis are commonly the result of an untreated middle-ear infection (otitis media). Bacteria may also reach the inner-ear from another part of the body by travelling through the bloodstream. An infection of the inner ear causes inflammation in the tissues, which disrupts the flow and movement of the fluids that maintain balance.

Symptoms. The primary symptom of labyrinthitis is vertigo, or a sense of spinning, either as if you are spinning while everything around you is stationary, or that you are still while the world around you spins. This essentially causes motion sickness, nausea, dizziness, or vomiting. Attacks of vertigo associated with labyrinthitis are triggered by head motion, and may last anywhere from one day to a few weeks. It may make walking or standing difficult, and even lifting the head up from the pillow can become a chore. Labyrinthitis also may cause some temporary hearing loss and tinnitus, or ringing in the ears, but this is not very common.

Treatment. Labyrinthitis, if caused by a viral infection, will usually disappear on its own. If the condition is the result of bacteria, antibiotics will be necessary to clean out the infection. In both cases, medication can help with some of the difficult symptoms, such as nausea. Bed rest may be recommended, in order to eliminate head motion that can exacerbate the condition. Over-the-counter motion sickness medication may also help. The symptoms will disappear gradually, but if they persist for more than a few weeks, or if hearing loss and tinnitus persist, a physician should be consulted. *See also* EAR; EAR, DISORDERS OF; MOTION SICKNESS; *and* VERTIGO.

Laceration

An irregular tear in the skin, which heals more slowly than a straight cut.

Often, a laceration in the perineum (the area of skin between the vagina and anus) is incurred during the birth process. The skin around the vagina stretches tremendously to accommodate the passage of the baby's head; however, sometimes the strain is too great and a small rip appears. If there is a likelihood of this occurring, the doctor will usually perform a procedure known as an episiotomy, in which a small cut is made in the area between the vagina and the anus. This cut is closed afterwards with sutures and heals better and more rapidly than a laceration. *See also* EPISIOTOMY.

Lacrimal Aparatus

System of glands and ducts that creates and disposes of tears.

The lacrimal apparatus is the system responsible for tears, a fluid composed of salt and water. The most important purpose of tears is to moisten the cornea, the thin lens-like cover over the eyeball, and conjunctiva, the membrane that covers the white of the eye. The moisture provided by tears, as well as fluids secreted by the membrane of the conjunctiva, help keep the cornea transparent and prevent corneal ulcers. Tears also constantly clean the eye as well; they contain lysozyme, a naturally-occurring antibiotic, and also rinse small pieces of debris and foreign matter away.

The lacrimal apparatus are epocrine glands, or glands that use ducts to send their secretions directly into organs or to the surface of the skin. Like many systems in the body, the lacrimal apparatus works to maintain a balance of fluids; the glands secrete the fluid, and the ducts dispose of it. The main lacrimal glands are located on the outer edge of the eye socket, or orbit. These glands secrete tears when the eye becomes irritated, or during crying. The accessory glands are located in the con-

junctiva; their role is to provide the eye with its necessary layer of moisture.

The lacrimal glands are run by the parasympathetic nervous system, a part of the autonomic nervous system. The parasympathetic nervous system regulates seemingly automatic tasks such as heart beat, pupil contraction, and tear manufacture. A constant supply of tears is necessary to keep the eye moist; the parasympathetic nerve maintains a regular flow. The accessory lacrimal glands handle this task under normal circumstances; while the main lacrimal glands secrete tears when there is need for more than usual. When tears are released by the accessory lacrimal gland, they drain into the puncta, which are openings located at the inside end of the eye, towards the nose. The tears then flow into lacrimal sacs, which lie along the eye socket, next to the nose. Muscles around the sacs contract when the eye blinks, and this causes the lacrimal sacs to empty into the nasolacrimal ducts, which then open into the nose. Excess tears, such as those produced during crying, run directly out of the eye.

Disorders include watery eye, or overproduction of tears, and keratoconjunctivitis sicca, dry eyes caused by a lack of tear production. *See also* KERATOCONJUNCTIVITIS; PARASYMPATHETIC NERVOUS SYSTEM; TEARS; *and* WATERY EYE.

Lactase Deficiency

A lack of lactase, causing lactose intolerance.

Lactase is an enzyme that is essential in the body's ability to break down lactose, a sugar that is found in milk. Lactase is found in the small intestine. If the enzyme is not present, then the body is not able to digest lactose or food products that contain it. As a result, the lactose ferments in the intestines, causing abdominal cramps, bloating, flatulence, and diarrhea.

A person may be born without lactase, or a deficiency sometimes develops later in life. Lactase can be absent at birth, but appear soon after, which eliminates the possi-

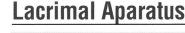

Lacrimal Gland. Each eye also has a tear gland, or lacrimal organ, situated at the outside corner of the eye. The salty secretion of these glands lubricates the forward part of the eyeball when the eyelids are closed and flushes away any small dust particles or other foreign matter on the surface of the eye.

bility of lactose intolerance. A lactase deficiency may also develop as a result of an intestinal disease, such as gastroenteritis or celiac sprue, (gluten gluten).

African Americans and Asians make up 80-90 percent of lactase deficiency cases. Five to 15 percent of sufferers are white. A lactose-free diet is suggested, although medication that breaks down lactose may be taken. If the lactose-free diet is followed, calcium intake must be ensured by eating other calcium-rich foods, such as shellfish, tofu, spinach, and broccoli, or by taking calcium supplements. *See also* ALLERGIES *and* GLUCOSE.

Lactic Acid

Acid produced by cells due to insufficient amounts of oxygen during glucose metabolism.

During intense exercise, muscles rely on stored glucose (glycogen) in liver and muscle for energy. Since the first steps of glycogen breakdown do not require oxygen, Glucose is broken down into lactic acid, which may accumulate in muscles causing fatigue and pain. The goal of the athlete is to supply the muscles with enough oxygen to completely utilize the glucose, thus preventing lactic acid from collecting. However, during strenuous exertion, some lactic acid buildup is inevitable, as the heart is unable to pump enough blood to supply the muscles with sufficient oxygen. After exercise, when oxygen is more available, lactic acid is broken down by the liver. *See also* GLYCOGEN *and* GLUCOSE.

Lactose Intolerance

A reaction to the sugar contained in milk.

Lactose is a disaccharide, composed of two linked monosaccharides, glucose and galactose, which are simple sugars.

Lactose intolerance is caused by a lack of the enzyme lactase (necessary for the digestion of lactose), which is a hereditary condition. Populations likely to carry the gene include Central and South Americans, Asians, those of African ancestry, Mid-

dle Easterners, American Indians, Ashkenazic Jews, central and southern Europeans, and Mediterranean. Lactose intollerance can also be acquired during the course of certain gastrointestinal diseases.

ALERT

Individuals with extreme intolerance to lactose should be aware that lactose is used as a binder for pills in thousands of medications.

Many lactose-intolerant individuals are able to digest several ounces of dairy products without reaction. The lactose content of yogurt and cheeses is low, and may therefore often be tolerated. Products such as lactase enzymes can be taken with dairy products to aid digestion, and reduced-lactose dairy products also exist. *See also* LACTASE DEFICIENCY.

Lactulose

Also known as D-galactose

Form of laxative used to treat constipation.

Lactulose is a synthetic disaccharide used as a laxative. When ingested, lactulose causes water to be absorbed by the feces via the intestinal blood vessels, resulting in softer stools that are easier to eliminate. Lactulose is not absorbed or metabolized by the gastrointestinal tract. In some instances, it may be used to treat liver failure in order to eliminate toxins, such as ammonia, from the body. *See also* LAXATIVE DRUGS.

Lamaze Method

A technique used to suppress pain during pregnancy without the use of drugs.

In the 1950s, the French obstetrician Ferdinand Lamaze modified for use in Western culture a Russian childbirth method called psychoprophylaxis. Using distraction to alter the perception of pain, Lamaze claimed that his method rendered childbirth painless, and while this may be an exaggeration, studies have shown that a more relaxed pregnant woman may experience a swifter and less painful labor. Techniques include massage; controlled deep breathing; concentration on an object, such as a photograph; and guidance provided by a supportive, proactive coach—the unborn baby's father, or the mother's significant other.

The Lamaze method is based upon the notion that childbirth is a healthy, natural, awesome human event and that the woman has innate wisdom that can be further coaxed forth by caregivers and loved ones to help her feel prepared to handle the rigors of childbirth. Cultivating her inner strength, calm, and relaxation, the woman may fear the process less and, in fact, relish the experience.

Much of the method's appeal and popularity is due to its emphasis on the couple's teamwork. It does not preach for or against painkillers during labor. Intimidation by the modern technology of obstetrics is tempered by an emphasis on the human element. By educating parents on all aspects of childbirth—from labor stages to parenting techniques—the Lamaze method seeks to turn mother and father into authoritative participants in the process so that they can make informed decisions. *See also* CHILDBRITH *and* PREGNANCY.

Laminaria

A type of seaweed.

Used to induce labor for over 100 years, laminaria "tents" are made out of the dried stems of laminaria digitata, also called oarweed, a fan-shaped brown seaweed that grows up to 50 meters in length along the British and Pacific coasts.

Laminaria tents may also be used to induce abortion. Whether inducing abortion or child labor, one or more tents are inserted into the cervix 12 hours before the procedure. The stem swells to three to four times its original diameter and dilates the opening during the six to 12 hours it is in place. This is one of the least invasive methods of cervix dilation. Some possible side

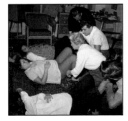

Lamaze. A natural childbirth class. Soon-to-be mothers lying on the ground are practicing breathing while being assisted by an instructor.

effects are pain, cramping, and fever. *See also* ALTERNATIVE BIRTH METHODS.

Laminectomy

A surgical procedure to remove part or all of a lamina (the bony arch of a vertebra) or laminae, thereby exposing the spinal cord and relieving pressure.

Laminectomy is the most common surgical response to spinal stenosis (narrowing of the spinal passage) caused by osteoarthritis. It relieves pressure on a herniated vertebral disk in the lumbar spine.

In a laminectomy, the neurosurgeon or orthopedist makes an incision in the patient's back to expose the problem lamina(e) and removes the necessary bone and cartilage. If whole laminae have been removed, the spine is fused with metal rods or bone grafts to provide stability. *See also* NEUROSURGEON; OSTEOARTHRITIS; ORTHOPEDIST; *and* SPINAL STENOSIS.

Lance

To surgically pierce, incise, or prick a body part (such as a vein or fingertip) or growth (such as a boil or abscess).

Having a lesion, such as a boil or abcess, lanced is a minor and common surgical procedure. It is often performed using a small, pointed, double-edged scalpel called a lancet. *See* ABCESS; BOIL; *and* LESION.

Lanugo Hair

Fine dark body hair that may cover a newborn's back, shoulders, or parts of the face. It usually falls out within a few weeks.

Lanugo hair is most commonly seen in babies that are born prematurely. The soft, downy hair appears on the fetus by the fourth or fifth month, but usually disappears by the ninth. Lanugo hair can also appear in adults suffering from cancer, particulary cancer of the breast, lung, kidney, and intestines. It is also common in patients dealing with anorexia nervosa.

Lanugo hair may also reappear as a side effect of some drugs. *See also* HAIR.

Laparoscopy

Exploration of the abdominal region using a specialized endoscope known as a laparoscope.

Laparoscopy allows the physician to directly visualize internal organs contained within in the abdominal wall (or peritoneal cavity). The liver, ovaries, and other organs are seen using a viewing instrument known as a laparoscope, a flexible tube with a small camera to allow structures to be seen on a video monitor during the procedure. The laparoscope is inserted into the body cavity through a small incision, usually under one—half inch. As an aid to diagnosis, laparoscopy has largely replaced laparotomy, the surgical opening of the abdominal cavity. Causes of pelvic pain may be diagnosed by laparoscopy, particularly when the liver is involved.

The laparoscope is also equipped to preform surgical techniques, including liver or ovarian biopsy, lysis of adhesions (the destruction of abnormal tissue), removal of foreign bodies, and treatment of endometriosis. Other surgical procedures include cholycystectomy (removal of the gallbladder), resectioning of the small bowel or colon and tubal ligation (sterilization using the laparoscope to sever the fal-

lopian tubes and tie them off).

Laparoscopy has revolutionized adrenalectomy, the removal of the adrenal glands when tumors or disease (such as Cushing's syndrome) are present. Once a major, invasive surgery, it is now carried out with laparoscopy through four small incisions. The diseased adrenals are identified, separated from surrounding tissue, and removed through one of the incisions.

Laparoscopy is performed in a hospital setting and may be carried out with either general or local anesthesia. During the procedure, the peritoneal cavity is distended using carbon dioxide or nitrous oxide, displacing the organs and allowing a clear area for the laparoscope to be inserted. It is usually completed in about an hour, depending on the particular procedure.

Background material on Laparoscopy can be found in ABDOMEN *and* ENDOSCOPE. *Related information is contained in* ANESTHETIC, BIOPSY, CHOLYCYSTECTOMY, CUSHING'S SYNDROME, ETIOLOGY, LAPAROTOMY, NONINVASIVE, LAPAROTOMY, *and* TUMORS

Laparotomy, Exploratory

The opening of the abdomen by surgery, in order to perform diagnostic study.

Many types of exploratory surgery exist to attempt to diagnose disorders of unknown or uncertain etiology. Laparotomy involves the opening of the abdominal wall or peritoneal cavity by surgical incision in order to identify and evaluate abnormalities of the kidney, pancreas, stomach, liver, bowels, or other organs. Often, tissue will be removed from the site of concern for laboratory analyses.

Advances in medical imaging have replaced this type of surgery to a great extent. Such noninvasive means of diagnosis are often more precise and avoid the trauma, threat of infection, and recovery time associated with surgery. Where surgery is required following diagnosis by imaging, it may be carried out using a technique known as laparoscopy, which requires only a small incision.

Laparoscopic Testing

Laparoscopy requires local or general anesthetic and is carried out in a hospital. Following inflation of the abdominal cavity using nitrous oxide or carbon dioxide, the fiberoptic laparoscope is inserted and guided to the region of interest. In addition to helping to visualize internal organs, laparoscopy allows for extensive surgical repair with minimum invasiveness, reducing trauma, increasing the precision of surgery, and reducing recovery time. Laparoscopy is usually completed in under an hour, and is considered a low-risk procedure, though some potential for internal bleeding, infection, injury to bile ducts, or perforation exists.

Laparoscopy may also be used for exploratory diagnosis, eliminating the need to surgically open the abdominal cavity. Laparotomy is now often reserved for special or emergency situations. *See also* ETIOLOGY; LAPAROSCOPY; *and* NONINVASIVE.

Larva Migrans

Infection caused by the larvae of certain parasitic worms.

Larvae are worms at the stage between egg and adult. Larva migrans (also known as toxocariasis) is an infection caused by hookworms that normally infest the gastrointestinal system of dogs and cats.

The disease takes two forms: visceral larva migrans and cutaneous larva migrans. Both are characterized by symptoms caused by movement of the larvae. Infection is caused by contact with soil, sand, or material contaminated with animal feces containing worm eggs. After hatching, the larvae move to the skin, roam, and create itchy red lines that are sometimes accompanied by blistering.

Treatment of larva migrans includes a course of medications specially targeting parasitic worm infestation. *See also* ANTIHELMINTIC DRUGS *and* TOXOCARIASIS.

Laryngectomy

Removal of the larynx.

The larynx, or voice box, aids in sound production by carrying air over the vocal cords, which causes them to vibrate and create sound. Cancer of the larynx may require the removal of the voice box, although radiation therapy is preferred.

When the larynx is removed, the end of the windpipe, which once was connected to the voice box, is attached to an opening in the neck, allowing the patient to breathe. Therapy may help a person regain what is known as esophagal speech. This requires breathing in a controlled manner to produce a noise that the tongue can turn into gruff sounds that resemble speech. Elec-

tronic voice boxes are another alternative. The device is placed near the throat and produces a buzzing noise that converts breaths into speech. *See also* CANCER OF; LARYNX; LARYNX *and* SPEECH.

Laryngitis

Inflammation that occurs in the mucous membranes of the larynx.

Most cases of acute laryngitis will fade away on their own in a few days. Drugs may be prescribed to bring down a fever, or, in cases of bacterial infections, antibiotics may be applied. To relieve the symptoms, a person should avoid speaking; avoid alcohol and cigarette smoke; drink fluids such as water, juice, and warm tea with honey; use a humidifier; or apply steam by putting the face over a bowl of hot water for a few minutes at a time. Do not gargle or whisper; both produce sounds that will irritate the vocal cords.

Chronic laryngitis can be cured by remedying the underlying cause: avoiding smoke or alcohol; wearing a mask in the workplace to diminish inhalation of chemicals; resolving acid reflux through dietary changes or medication.

If acute laryngitis does not disappear on its own after a few days, a physician should be consulted to test for other causes of the condition. *See also* HOARSENESS *and* LARYNX.

Laryngoscopy

Techniques for observing the interior of the larynx.

Laryngoscopy, or study of the larynx, may be indirect or direct. In indirect laryngoscopy, the interior of the larynx is examined with the aid of a mirror. Direct laryngoscopy is more sophisticated, employing a laryngoscope, a flexible viewing instrument similar to an endoscope. The device is threaded down the throat and allows the diagnostician to directly examine structures of the larynx. Using the laryngoscope to see into the larynx by means of fiberoptic light, the physician may observe

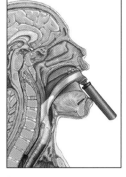

Laryngoscopy.
Laryngoscopy is the study of the larynx. A device may be threaded down the throat and allows the diagnostician to examine the structure of the larynx.

strictures, lesions, or foreign bodies that may be lodged in the larynx.

The procedure is usually performed using a local anesthetic that is sprayed into the mouth. The patient may be seated or supine during the course of the examination. In addition to viewing the larynx, certain surgical procedures such as removal of nodules or polyps, as well as sampling tissue for study through biopsy, are possible during larygoscopy. *See also* Biopsy; Endoscopy; Fiberoptic; Larynx; *and* Polyp.

Larynx

Also called the voice box

The tube between the windpipe and upper airway.

The larynx delivers air to and from the lungs, generates voice, and prevents the entry of food into the airway during swallowing. It is constructed of cartilage, membrane, and ligaments.

The entire larynx is lined with a mucous membrane of squamous cells. Covered by a taste bud, the epiglottis remains upright, leaving the larynx open to breathe, until food or liquid is swallowed, when it flops down over the larynx and food passes on either side and into the esophagus. Anything other than air that enters the larynx spurs the cough reflex to expel the object.

Vocal ligaments, joining the arytenoid cartilages to the thyroid cartilage, form mucosal, or vocal, folds, called true vocal cords. In speech, air from the lungs vibrates the vocal cords and the tongue while palate and lips manipulate the sound produced to create spoken words. The glottis is the opening between the vocal cords through which the air passes. *See* Speech.

Larynx, Cancer of

Malignant tumor of the voice box.

Cancer of the larynx is associated with smoking and heavy drinking. It occurs most often after the age of 60 and is more common in men than in women.

The most obvious symptom is persistent hoarseness, which occurs when the tumor develops on the vocal cords. A tumor that develops elsewhere in the larynx may not cause hoarseness but can cause throat discomfort, swallowing difficulties, and difficulty breathing, as well as coughing up of blood.

Diagnosis. The diagnosis is made by laryngoscopy, an examination of the larynx that enables a physician to see the tumor, and can be confirmed by removal of a tissue sample (biopsy) to determine if the growth is cancerous.

Radiation therapy is an effective treatment if a cancer is detected in its early stages. Cancers that do not respond to radiation therapy usually require laryngectomy, surgery in which part or all of the larynx is removed. After this operation, a patient must learn new ways of producing speech. The prognosis is poor if the cancer has spread beyond the larynx to other parts of the throat, but survival can be prolonged by radiation therapy and chemotherapy. *See also* Cancer; Chemotherapy; Larynx; Radiation Therapy; *and* Throat.

Laser

Acronym for light amplification by stimulated emission of radiation

A device used in diagnosis and surgery.

Lasers are instruments for converting light of various frequencies into a single coherent and intense beam of uniform frequency radiation. Laser light has wide application in medicine, both for therapy and diagnosis.

A variety of laser surgeries exist to treat a myriad of disorders. Eye abnormalities such as farsightedness, nearsightedness, and astigmatism, for example, may be corrected by techniques of refractive surgery such as radial keratotomy, photorefractive keratectomy, and LASIK (laser in situ keratomileusis). Laser surgical techniques are also used for coronary artery disease, cervical disorders, and skin resurfacing. *See also* Astigmatism; Cervix, Disorders of; Coronary Heart Disease; Glaucoma; *and* Laser Treatment.

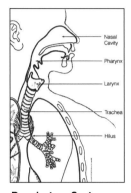

Respiratory System. The diagram shows the parts of the respiratory system, including the larynx, the tube that separates the windpipes and the upper airway.

Laser Treatment

Use of laser light for surgery or treatment of illness

Lasers are applied in medicine as a precise way of cutting (incising or excising) and sealing off (cauterizing) tissue. The highly focused beam of light heats up a small number of cells, causing them to vaporize, while minimally affecting surrounding cells. Advantages to laser surgery include extreme precision, reduced blood loss, and minimized pain and trauma.

Several types of laser exist, each with a precise function. Common lasers include carbon dioxide lasers, argon lasers, and YAG (yttrium aluminum garnet) lasers.

USES

Lasers can be used for a variety of purposes. They are frequently used in ophthalmic, neuro, thoracic, and plastic surgeries. They can:
- target and destroy diseased tissue, such as tumors in the brain or liver;
- stop bleeding in tiny blood vessels;
- reduce scarring from surgeries;
- seal off lymph nodes to reduce swelling and impede the spread of diseased cells;
- seal off nerve endings to reduce postoperative pain;
- remove tattoos or birthmarks and otherwise alter the appearance of skin.

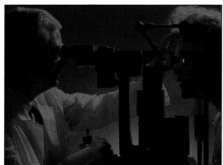

Surgeon Performing Laser Eye Surgery. A surgeon performs laser cataract eye surgery on a teenage patient, above.

Laser Eye Surgery. Refractive eye surgery is used to treat common eye disorders including nearsightedness (myopia), farsightedness (hyperopia), and distorted vision (astigmatism). The laser is rapidly replacing many conventional types of surgery for refractive errors due to the extreme precision and control it allows the ophthalmologist.

A special device known as the excimer laser is now used for the correction of moderate nearsightedness in a procedure called photorefractive keratectomy (PRK), as well as in a recently developed technique called laser in situ keratomileusis or LASIK.

With PRK, the cornea is reshaped by using ultraviolet light to remove tissue from the outer surface.

The precision of the beam allows surgical cuts as fine as 39 millionths of an inch. The technique is performed with local anesthetic and completed in a matter of minutes.

LASIK is a more sophisticated procedure than PRK and can correct a wider range of nearsightedness, although it requires greater skill on the part of the surgeon. A tiny cut is made in the cornea, and tissue is then removed from under the resulting flap with a laser. *See also* ASTIGMATISM; HYPEROPIA; LASER; OPHTHALMOLOGY; *and* VISION, DISORDERS OF.

Lassa Fever

A highly contagious disease produced by a virus carried by a type of rat.

Lassa is carried by a small rat that is widespread in Africa. The virus is most often passed to humans through inhalation of the rat's urine or contact with urine-contaminated food, but is also communicable between humans through such agents as infected urine, feces, saliva, vomit, or blood.

Symptoms appear gradually, with hospitalization usually required within four to five days of onset. Early symptoms include sore throat, fever, headache, chill, and malaise. This is followed by diarrhea, vomiting, and pains in the abdomen. Symptoms typically intensify during the second week, leading to shock, impaired mental condition, agitation, and, occasionally, grand mal seizures. Mortality rates for the disease vary between 25 and 35 percent.

Diagnosis and Treatment. Lassa is diagnosed by blood test. An antiviral drug is used to treat the disease but must be administered within six days of onset. If treatment is not available, death may result. *See also* BLOOD TEST; INFECTIOUS DISEASE; SALIVA; URINE; *and* VOMIT.

Laurence-Moon-Biedl Syndrome

Also known as Laurence-Moon-Bardet-Biedl or Bardet-Biedle

A rare inherited condition that affects several of the body's systems.

This disorder is caused by a recessive gene, which means that it occurs only when a child inherits the abnormal gene from both parents. Four different gene defects have been implicated.

CHARACTERISTICS

Characteristics of Laurence-Moon-Biedl syndrome include:

- rod/cone dystrophy—a progressive eye condition that can lead to blindness;
- polydactyly—extra fingers or toes;
- hypogenitalism—underdeveloped genitals;
- obesity.

Other, less commonly seen symptoms include kidney malformations and renal dysfunction, developmental delay, speech difficulties, diabetes, hepatic fibrosis, and other hormonal deficiencies. *See also* DEVELOPMENTAL DELAY; DIABETES; GENETIC DISORDERS; *and* OBESITY.

Laxative Drugs

Drugs and dietary supplements used to counteract the effects of constipation.

Constipation can be caused by a number of different things, including lack of exercise, inadequate fiber in the diet, and disease. Many drugs cause constipation, particularly narcotics, which relax the muscles of the bowels. Laxatives include high-fiber foods like bran, stool softeners that retain water in the bowels, mineral oil that softens the stool and eases its passage, osmotic agents that keep water in the intestinal tract, and stimulants that irritate the bowels into producing a semisolid bowel movement. Excessive use of laxative drugs can cause diarrhea. *See also* DIET; FIBER, DIETARY; *and* STOOL.

Lead Poisoning

Damage to the brain nerves, red blood cells, and digestive system, usually acquired by the swallowing or iinhalation of lead or lead salts.

Lead poisoning can either occur over a short period of time and in large amounts (acute poisoning) or over a long period of time and in small amounts (chronic). In both cases, symptoms of poisoning are not always detectable. Signs of acute poisoning can be severe stomach pain, diarrhea, vomiting, weakness in limbs, and seizure. Lead poisoning is sometimes fatal. Chronic poisoning carries the same symptoms as the acute form, but may also result in loss of memory, erratic moods, physical instability, headaches, and blindness.

Incidence. Lead poisoning is one of the most serious health problems facing American children. Paint chips with high lead content, common in older homes, are often the cause. Children either eat the lead-based paint chips or inhale the dust.

Adults are usually affected by lead poisoning at their jobs. Instances of poisoning occur in smelting, battery manufacturing, and other industries where workers might inhale lead fumes. Nearby inhabitants of such industrial plants can also be affected. The exhaust of cars that use lead-based gasoline is another source of poisoning.

High levels of lead are found in drinking water that flows through deteriorating pipe. Today, only lead-free pipes and solder may be used, but older pipes may be made of lead or copper with lead soldering.

TREATMENT

Treatment for severe cases of lead poisoning involves removal of lead from the body using substances that combine with and neutralize the lead (chelating agents).

Several steps can be taken to diminish lead present in drinking water. After extended periods of non-use, run the cold water until it has become as cold as possible. This will flush out any water that has absorbed lead while standing in the pipes.

Avoid using hot tap water for human

consumption, since more lead is likely to dissolve in hot water. Do not use water softeners, or use them only on the hot water line, since softened water leaches much more lead than hard water does.

> *Background material on Lead Posoning can be found in* CHELATING AFENTS AND CHILD DEVELOPMENT *Related information is contained in Attention Deficit Disorder,* Brain, Blindness, Digestive System, Learning Disabilities, Poisoning, Water and Vomitting.

Learning Disabilities

Developmental disorders that limit the ability of individuals with at least average intelligence to store, produce, or process information.

Learning disabilities are believed to be caused by neurological problems or damage in the areas of the brain that are responsible for processing language. The disability may be caused by genetic factors or by any condition affecting the brain, such as an injury (prenatal or postnatal), encephalitis, or meningitis.

Estimates of how many people suffer from learning disabilities vary widely, from two percent to 20 percent of school children in the United States. It is difficult to accurately diagnose a learning disability because it must first be differentiated from other causes of learning problems. These include mental limitations, poor motivation and study skills, poor teaching, visual or auditory problems, physical disability, or emotional problems.

TYPES OF LEARNING DISORDERS
Dyslexia, a reading disorder, is the most common of learning disorders. A child with dyslexia will have problems seeing words as they appear on the page, often transposing letters or adding syllables.

Dyscalculia is a disorder that results in problems recognizing numbers, counting, and grasping basic mathematical concepts.

Dysgraphia is a writing disorder that involves difficulty forming letters, writing legibly, composing sentences, spelling, punctuating, and using proper grammar.

Dyspraxia involves problems with the body's motor coordination.

Symptoms. A child who has learning disabilities will exhibit some or all of the following signs. However, these should only be considered indications, and further investigation by a professional can determine if the child has a learning disorder:

• Poor reading comprehension and the tendency to reverse letters, for example, to mistake a "d" for a "b" or a "p" for a "q";

• Inability to put simple, whole structured sentences together by age two;

• Math problems, especially reversing numbers;

• Poor memory;

• Trouble telling time or writing;

• Trouble with coordination. By kindergarten, a child should reach certain milestones that include the ability to tie shoes, button clothing, and use scissors;

• Difficulty following a schedule;

• Extreme disorganization;

• Problems following simple directions.

Diagnosis. Because so many factors can contribute to a child's difficulty in school, it is important to see the appropriate professional (and possibly several different professionals) to determine why a child is significantly behind others of the same age in achieving reading, writing, or mathematical skills. To complicate matters, a child who has a learning disability, which is a neurologically-based problem, may develop secondary problems that are behavioral, psychological, or social in nature. Because of this, the sooner the diagnosis is made, the better. A child who grows to adulthood with an undiagnosed disorder may suffer from continual feelings of failure, which can frequently result in delinquency and departure from school.

A physician should test a child's vision and hearing and general health to make sure that the problem is not physical in origin. A learning disability tends to present itself in the first grades of school when a child is learning to read and write. If it is discovered later, however, other problems may have developed because of the child's discomfort about the learning disability. If a child exhibits problems socializing with others, emotional difficulties, or conduct problems, a physician may refer the child to a psychiatrist or psychologist. A psychologist can also perform intelligence testing.

Attention Deficit Disorder (ADD) is an inability to control distractions and results in a constellation of symptoms that include impulsivity, fidgeting, and excessive activity in general. It may coexist with a learning disorder and is often considered a learning disorder. The treatment for this disorder is different from the treatment for other learning disabilities, although learning difficulties are consistent with the diagnosis. A pediatrician may recommend further testing if a child may have ADD.

Treatment of learning disabilities is highly individualized, depending on the nature and severity of the child's disability. Usually, treatment consists of educational and home intervention aimed at helping the child learn to the best of his or her abilities and maintain high self-esteem. Educational interventions may range from giving a child extra time to complete assignments or using varied teaching methods in the classroom to having the child work one-on-one or in a small group with a special education teacher. The state is required to provide appropriate public education for children with developmental disorders and learning disabilities between the ages of three and 21. Parents can help a child with learning disabilities by working closely with the school to develop the best educational program for the child, as well as providing emotional and practical support at home. *See* ATTENTION DEFICIT DISORDER; CHILD DEVELOPMENT; *and* DYSLEXIA.

Leeches

> **Bloodsucking parasitic worms.**

Leeches are annelid worms with specialized suckers at either end of their bodies, one for attaching to their host, the other for consuming blood. They are found on land in tropical areas and in bodies of warm water. Over 650 species of leech exist.

The salivary juices of the leech contain an anticoagulant substance known as hirudin (sometimes extracted for use in medicine to prevent blood clotting). The anticoagulant allows the blood to flow freely, and the leech to feed. The mouth parts of the leech are able to pierce the host's skin (usually without being noticed), allowing the injection of hirudin. The leech will then feed until satiated and drop off, leaving a wound that may bleed for a number of hours.

Leeches are removed by stunning them with alcohol, salt, a lit match, or vinegar. The resulting wound will have to be bandaged to staunch excess blood (due to the anticoagulant). Some leeches manage to attach themselves internally and have to be removed surgically.

Leeches are occasionally used for medicinal purposes. They can be utilized to drain a collection of partially clotted blood (hematoma) from wounds. *See also* ALTERNATIVE MEDICINE; BLOOD; *and* PARASITE.

Leg Ulcers

> **Open sores on the legs or feet that are usually caused by poor circulation.**

When either the arteries or veins in the legs are blocked, tissues are starved for oxygen and leg ulcers develop. Ulcers also strike diabetics who suffer from poor circulation in the legs and arms. Usually, the sores are located on the inner sides of the ankles and shins. The ulcers become infected and exude pus. Arterial ulcers develop between and under the toes and around the outside of the ankles. They are likely to be painful, particularly if the patient is lying down with the legs elevated.

Treatment should address the underlying cause of the ulcers. Bandages should be changed two or three times a week with great care so as not to tear new skin. The sores may be cleansed with warm soapy water. The best treatment is to apply pressure bandages and elastic stockings to promote circulation. Exercise, heat, and massage may help. *See also* ULCER.

Resources on Learning Disabilities
Cordoni, Barbara, *Living with a Learning Disability* (1990); Hallahan, Daniel P., *Introduction to Learning Diabilities* (1996); MacCracken, Mary, T*urnabout Children: Overcoming Dyslexia and Other Learning Disabilities* (1986); Snowling, M. J., and M. E. Thomson, eds., *Dyslexia: Integrating Theory and Practice* (1991); Learning Disabilities Association of America. Tel. (412) 341-1515, Online: www.ldanatl.org.

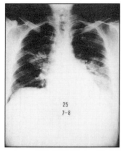

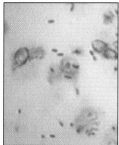

Legionnaires' Disease. A severe form of pneumonia, characterized by headache, chest pain, lung congestion, and high fever. Above, top, a chest x-ray of the bacteria. Above, bottom, the bacterium that is most commonly transmitted through contaminated water sources.

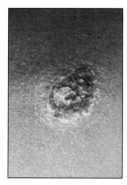

Leishmaniasis. A sand fly can deposit leishmania parasites in the skin where they cause a small sore or ulcer before going through the body for further tissue damage.

Leg, Shortening of

A shortened leg, usually due to injury or disease.

A shortened limb may be apparent at birth, due to a congenital condition such as dwarfism (achondroplasia), or as the result of a disease like polio. An injury to the thigh or shin bone that has not been properly set may also cause shortening of the leg. A deformity of the hip or spine may displace the leg and make it appear shorter.

If the difference in length is dramatic, a limp may develop. In these cases, lifts in the shoe or a raised heel will make walking easier. Surgical lengthening can be performed in extreme cases. *See* AMPUTATION.

Legionnaires' Disease

A form of pneumonia caused by *Legionella pneumophila* bacteria.

Since the first identified outbreak of Legionnaires' disease in 1976. previous outbreaks have been recognized, dating as early as the late 1940s. Over 700 cases are reported each year, but there may be more, as the disease is often misdiagnosed as pneumonia.

Legionnaires' disease is caused by the *Legionella pneumophila* bacterium, which multiplies in the air conditioning systems of hotels and hospitals and infects humans when they inhale the air. It is not transmitted from person to person.

Symptoms. Early symptoms of Legionnaires' disease resemble influenza, with a high fever, fatigue, a headache, a dry cough, and chills. Later stages are characterized by shortness of breath, diarrhea, a wet cough, and confusion.

People with compromised immune systems are most vulnerable to Legionnaires' disease, including people with AIDS, those who have had a recent organ transplant, or those who are being treated with chemotherapy. The elderly, smokers, and people taking corticosteroids are also at increased risk for this disease.

Treatment. Early treatment of Legionnaires' disease with antibiotics such as erythromycin can control the disease, though recovery is slow. About 15 percent of people who contract the disease die from respiratory failure. There is no vaccination available for the disease. *See also* ANTIBIOTIC DRUGS; IMMUNE SYSTEMS; *and* INFLUENZA.

Leiomyoma

A nonmalignant tumor of smooth muscle.

Leiomyomas arise in smooth tissue such as the walls of blood vessels and the uterus. In the uterus are also called fibroids, a name derived from the fact that they eventually are replaced by fibrous tissue. Up to 40 percent of women develop such leiomyomas by the age of 40, but they usually do not cause symptoms. If a woman does have symptoms such as a bleeding abnormality, surgery can be preformed to remove the tumor. More serious cases may require hysterectomy if fertility is not an issue. *See also* HYSTERECTOMY *and* TUMOR.

Leishmaniasis

Disease caused by parasitic protozoa, transmitted through the bite of sand flies.

Leishmaniasis is a disease caused by leishmania, single-cell microorganisms (protozoa) living in sand flies and transmitted to humans through the sand fly bite. The sand fly deposits the leishmania parasites in the skin, where they cause a local sore or skin ulcer before migrating though the body, causing considerable tissue damage.

Symptoms. Leishmaniasis damages the immune system, impairing the body's ability to ward off infection. As the disease progresses, weakness increases and the skin may appear dark or grayish and flaky. The disease often proves fatal within two years, with the cause of death usually from complications associated with infection coupled with impaired immune response.

Leishmania infection can cause skin disease (cutaneous leishmaniasis) and affect the mucous membranes. The skin ulcers of the cutaneous form sometimes resemble leprosy, skin cancer, or fungal infection. Visceral leishmaniasis, in which the parasite migrates to the bone marrow, spleen, and lymph nodes, is a potentially fatal condition. Children stricken with the disease exhibit symptoms including vomiting, diarrhea, chills, cough, and fever. Symptoms in adults are less specific, usually beginning with a long fever accompanied by fatigue and loss of appetite.

Leishmaniasis initially causes a slow-healing, ulcerated wound. Additional lesions may form around this area. The systemic form of the disease may cause fever, anorexia, abdominal pain, vomiting, scaly grayish skin, and thinning hair. Where mucous membranes are involved, nasal congestion, runny nose, and difficulty breathing are common.

Diagnosis may be made through biopsy of involved tissues (skin, spleen, lymph, or bone) or through immunofluorescent antibody test. The disease is treated with antimony-containing compounds including meglumine antimonate and sodium stibogluconate. Prognosis for a cure is good providing that treatment is undertaken before immune system damage occurs. In the case of mucocutaneous leishmaniasis, where the illness has produced severe facial lesions, reconstructive plastic surgery may be required. Visceral leishmaniasis often impairs the functioning of the spleen and, in drug-resistant cases of the disease, removal of the organ (splenectomy) may be required.

Protection from sand fly bites though the use of insect repellents, screens and netting, and protective clothing is the best defense against leishmaniasis. Health measures aimed at sand fly eradication are also of critical importance. There are no preventative drugs or vaccines for leishmaniasis. Prevention also involves reporting to a doctor symptoms of leishmaniasis in those who have traveled outside the U.S. and been exposed to sand fly bites. *See also* IMMUNE SYSTEM; INSECT BITES; PARASITE; PROTOZOA; *and* SPLEEN.

Lens

Part of the eye responsible for focus.

The lens and cornea of the eye operate in tandem to form an image on the retina, allowing the eye to see. Supported by the delicate fibers from the ciliary body and located behind the iris, the lens is transparent, elastic, and a trifle less convex on its front than its back. The lens enables correct focusing of the eye on objects of varying distance by adjusting the degrees of curvature on its surface. *See also* CORNEA; EYE; LENS DISLOCATION; *and* RETINA.

Lens Dislocation

A shifting of the lens from its normal position.

Lens dislocation typically occurs when the delicate fibers that join the lens to the ciliary body rupture due to injury. The lens may slide backward or down into the vitreous humor, resulting in extreme distortion or double vision. Forward dislocation often closes the drainage angle and causes glaucoma, which, if severe, may require lens removal. *See also* EYE, DISORDERS OF.

Leprechaunism

Also called Williams Syndrome

A rare genetic disorder resulting in characteristic facial features, mild to moderate mental impairment, and heart problems.

Leprechaunism occurs in one in 20,000 births and is caused by missing portions of chromosome seven. Individuals with this condition have characteristic facial features, including a small upturned nose, long upper lip, wide mouth, small chin, and puffiness around the eyes. Blue and green-eyed children with Williams syndrome often have a prominent starburst pattern on their iris.

Other symptoms include:
- heart or blood vessel problems;
- elevated blood calcium levels;
- extreme irritability or colic in infancy;

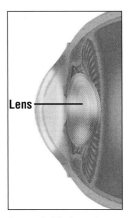

Lens. A thin layer in the eye that works with the cornea to form viewable images. The lens also regulates focusing, by adjusting its own curvature.

- low birth-weight;
- small stature as adults;
- problems with kidney structure or function (or both);
- poor muscle tone and joint problems.

Williams syndrome involves some degree of intellectual impairment. Young children often experience developmental delays with milestones such as walking, talking, and toilet training. However, sufferers exhibit a very outgoing social personality and good language skills. *See* CHROMOSOME.

Leprosy

Also known as Hansen's disease

An infection caused by *mycobacterium leprae*.

Mycobacterium leprae, the bacterium that causes leprosy, does not attack the brain or spinal cord, but only the nerves of the skin, mucous membranes, eyes, and testes. The affected areas become insensitive and therefore vulnerable to cuts and bruises that go unnoticed by the sufferer.

Transmission. Leprosy is most often transmitted through close contact with an infected person, though it may be acquired from the soil, armadillos, bedbugs, or mosquitoes. The disease is most common among young men in Asia, Africa, Latin America, and the islands of the Pacific. In the U.S. there are about 5000 cases in Hawaii, California, and Texas, but most of these patients have immigrated from other countries. More than 95 percent of people can develop a natural immunity to the bacteria that cause leprosy and doctors and nurses who treat people with leprosy are not at risk of contracting the disease.

Types. People with healthy immune systems develop paucibacillary (tuberculoid) leprosy when they are exposed to *Mycobacterium leprae*. Paucibacillary leprosy is relatively benign and is not infectious. Seventy to 80 percent of leprosy sufferers have this form of the disease. Those without the natural immunity to *Mycobacterium leprae* may develop multibacillary leprosy.

Symptoms. The first symptom of leprosy is the appearance of flat or slightly raised patches on the skin. These patches are reddened and numb. In the multibacillary form of the disease, the patient may lose hair, including the eyebrows and eyelashes. If untreated, the bacteria will infect the peripheral nerves, the inner lining of the nose, and all the other organs of the body. Further symptoms of leprosy include numbness, muscle weakness, and paralysis.

Treatment. The deformities produced by secondary infections have led to ostracism of infected people. Leprosy patients were isolated into distant colonies in the past and still are in the countries where the disease is more common. Today multiple drug therapy (MDT), a combination of three drugs, can stop the progress of the disease and can even affect a cure. Early treatment can prevent mutilations and deformities but treatment will have to be continued for many months and even years in some patients. *See also* INFECTIOUS DISEASE.

Lesion

Tissue altered by an abnormality within a circumscribed area, injury, or wound, or region of infected skin in a skin disorder.

Lesions may take many forms including tumors, infections, wounds, and chemical or hormonal reactions.

Types of Lesions. Diffuse lesions are those that spread over a large area, while focal lesions are more localized. When many systems in the body are affected, the lesion is said to be indiscriminate. Toxic lesions result from poisonous microorganisms. Vascular lesions are those affecting blood vessels.

While many lesions are benign and self limiting, others are serious and potentially life-threatening, particularly those that occur in the brain. Among nervous system lesions are local lesions and peripheral lesions (which affect nerve endings).

Treatment. Surgery, radiation, and drug therapy are all used to treat lesions, depending on the individual need of the patient. *See also* BRAIN, DISORDERS OF.

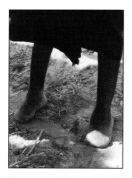

Leprosy. An example of the effects of lepromatous leprosy is shown. This Tanzanian woman's feet have been deformed by her body's reaction to the lepromatous bacterium.

Leukemia

Cancer of the white blood cells.

There are two broad categories of leukemia: acute and chronic. Both affect the bone marrow, in which blood cells are formed: the red cells, or erythrocytes, which carry oxygen through the blood; platelets, which form clots in case of injury; and white cells, or leukocytes, which protect against infectious agents. In acute leukemia, immature white cells multiply abnormally, crowding out mature white cells and interfering with the production of red cells and platelets. The immature white cells can accumulate in organs and tissues, disrupting their function.

There are subcategories of both classes of leukemia. Acute myeloid leukemia affects a kind of white cell that carries distinctive granules (granulocytes). Its incidence rises with age. Acute lymphoid leukemia affects white cells that do not have granules (called lymphocytes). It is the most common cancer of children. Chronic myeloid leukemia affects mature granule-containing white cells, and chronic lymphoid leukemia affects mature cells that do not contain granules. A subtype of chronic lymphoid leukemia is hairy-cell leukemia, named for the distinctive appearance of the affected white cells.

Risk factors for both kinds of leukemia include long-term exposure to radiation, such as x-rays; exposure to some organic chemicals, such as benzene; and a genetic predisposition.

The risk of chronic leukemia is also related to exposure to some viruses, such as the human T-lymphocyte virus. Most patients with chronic myeloid leukemia are found to have genetic abnormalities. It is unknown whether this is a cause of the condition or a result of it.

Symptoms of both classes of leukemia are fatigue and weakness, weight loss, fever, enlarged lymph nodes, skin rash, pain in joints, and frequent infections. Tests used to diagnose leukemia include a physical examination to detect symptoms such as swollen lymph nodes and an enlarged liver or spleen, blood tests to detect cell abnormalities, bone marrow tests and tissue samples, studies of genetic material to detect abnormalities, and tests of immune function.

Prognosis of leukemia depends on the type and the stage at which it is detected. The prognosis is better for acute leukemia than for chronic leukemia. Long-term remissions of acute leukemia can be achieved in many patients; the five-year survival rate for children is 70 to 80 percent, and averages about 45 percent for adults.

The average time of survival for chronic lymphoid leukemia detected early is 10 years or more; if diagnosed at a late stage, the average survival is about two years.

Up to 20 percent of patients with hairy-cell leukemia have long-term survival without treatment, and treatment can prolong life for such long periods that physicians cautiously refer to the disease as "curable."

Treatment for acute leukemia usually involves chemotherapy with a combination of drugs, given first to achieve remission and then to prolong it. A bone-marrow transplant, using marrow from a close relative, may be performed if prolonged remission is achieved. Treatment for leukemia also centers on chemotherapy combined with blood transfusions, and infusions of immunoglobulins and antibiotics to strengthen defenses and attack infections.

The discipline of treatment for the different leukemias is evolving continuously as physicians try different combinations of medications. One new agent used in treatment of leukemia is interferon, a protein secreted by immune system cells. One type of interferon has been approved by the FDA for treatment of chronic myeloid leukemia, but the side effects can be severe, including fever, weakness, and aches.

> *Background material on Leukemia can be found in* BLOOD and CANCER. *Related information is contained in* BONE MARROW, CHRONIC MYELOID LEUKEMIA, FEVER, GENETICS, GRANULOCYTES, IMMUNE SYSTEM, JOINTS, LIVER, LYMPH NODES, LYMPHOCYTES, OXYGEN, PROTEIN, RASH, SPLEEN and TRANSPALNT SUREGRY..

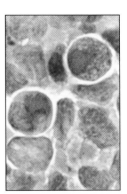

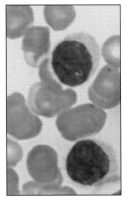

Leukemia Cells. Above, top, human cells with acute myelocytic leukemia (AML) in the pericardial fluid, shown with an esterase stain at 400 magnification. Above, bottom, a histological slide of hairy-cell leukemia.

Leukemia, Chronic Lymphoid

A blood cancer of immune system cells.

Chromic lymphoid leukemia results from uncontrolled reproduction of white blood cells called lymphocytes, which are important in the immune defense system.

There are several subtypes of chronic lymphoid leukemia. The most common type involves B-cells, which produce antibodies to fight invading bacteria or viruses. A second type involves T-cells, which regulate the activity of B-cells. A subtype is hairy-cell leukemia, in which both T-cells and B-cells have a characteristic hairy appearance when seen under a microscope.

Symptoms. The lymphocytes that are overproduced in this leukemia accumulate in lymph nodes and cause swelling. The liver may also become enlarged, causing jaundice and abnormal lymph tissue. Other symptoms include fever and night sweats. The lymphocytes cannot fight infectious agents, leaving the patient vulnerable to infections.

Diagnosis and Treatment. Almost all chronic lymphoid leukemia patients are over the age of 50 The condition is diagnosed by blood tests that detect the abnormal proliferation of lymphocytes, and by taking a sample of bone marrow (bone marrow biopsy). If the disease is mild and slow-moving, no immediate treatment may be given.

Treatment consists of chemotherapy, at times accompanied by radiation therapy. Blood transfusions and injections of infection-fighting immunoglobulins may also be given. The treatment is aimed at controlling the symptoms, since there is no cure.

Prognosis. Fatal bacterial or viral infection is the greatest determining factor for prognosis. Over 50 percent of patients survive for five years after the condition is diagnosed. Eventually, infection overcomes the victim and results in death. *See also* BIOPSY.; BLOOD; CHEMOTHERAPY; IMMUNO-GLOBULINS; *and* LEUKEMIA.

Resources on Leukemia
Margolies, Cynthia P., and Kenneth B. McCredie, *Understanding Leukemia* (1993); Mazza, Joseph J., *Manual of Clinical Hematology* (1988); Miller, Benjamin Franck and Claire B. Keane, *Bloodstream Infections: Laboratory Detection and Clinical Considerations* (1988); Seeman, Bernard, American Red Cross, Tel. (800) HELP-NOW, Online: www.red-cross.org; Leukemia Society of America, Tel. (800) 573-8484, Online: www.leukemia. org; The National Hemophilia Foundation, Tel. (800) 42-HANDI, Online: www.hemophilia.org; www.nycornell /medicine/hematology/index.html.

Leukemia, Chronic Myeloid

Cancer of white blood cells called granulocytes.

Granulocytes are a class of white blood cells that fight infection. In chronic myeloid leukemia, there is uncontrolled overproduction of these cells. In their uncontrolled state, they inhibit the oxygen- and nutrient-carrying capabilities of red blood cells, as well as attack organs.

This cancer is uncommon in young people. In most cases, there is a slow onset of symptoms, which can last for several years. These symptoms include fatigue, weight loss, night sweats, and fever. Symptoms usually become more severe when the disease enters a more active, or acute phase, and can include problems with vision and abdominal pain.

> ### Philadelphia Chromosome
> One genetic abnormality related to chronic myeloid leukemia is called the Philadelphia chromosome. It affects two chromosomes of the 22 pairs found in human cells. A piece of chromosome nine is attached to chromosome 22. This section of chromosome nine is known to contain a gene which plays a role in cancer. This translocation alters the expression of the gene.

Diagnosis is made by blood tests that detect an abnormal number of granulocytes in the blood and bone marrow. A genetic test may be done to detect the Philadelphia chromosome. Chemotherapy is effective if the disease is detected early. Rarely, excess granulocytes are removed in a process called apheresis. Bone marrow transplant is effective for eligible patients. *See also* LEUKEMIA.

Leukocytes

White blood cells.

Granulocytes, lymphocytes, and monocytes are the three main kinds of leukocytes. These are the cells affected in a patient with leukemia. *See also* LEUKEMIA.

Leukodystrophies

A group of hereditary nervous system disorders known as demyelinating diseases.

Myelin is a lipid-like substance that surrounds the nerves of the brain and peripheral nervous system and is instrumental in the transmission of signals through the nervous system. In a demyelinating disease, there is abnormal formation or maintenance of myelin, which can affect motor, sensory, and mental processes.

Specific leukodystrophies include adrenoleukodystrophy, metachromatic leukodystrophy, spongy degeneration (Canavan), globoid cell (Kra-bbe) leukodystrophy, Alexander disease, Pelizaeus Me-rz-bacher disease, and Cockayne syndrome.

These disease vary in age of onset, severity, and prognosis. Symptoms include impaired speech, blindness, paralysis, seizures, and death. Most treatment is aimed at controlling the symptoms. *See also* MYELIN; *and* NERVOUS SYSTEM.

Leukoplakia

White clusters on the mucous membranes of the mouth or vulva.

These white patches usually form on the mouth in response to the thickening of tissue that commonly occurs in the elderly or from a chronic irritation such as that arising from dentures, smokeless tobacco, or alcohol abuse. They are cancerous or precancerous in a small percentage of cases. Other than the patches themselves, leukoplakia generally causes no discomfort. The cause of vulvar leukoplakia is unknown.

Leukoplakia is diagnosed by a process of elimination. Patches on the mouth are most common in men over the age of 45. Treatment of leukoplakia requires the removal of the patch by traditional or laser surgery, but there is a high incidence of recurrence. Microscopic examination of the tissue will reveal any malignancy in the tissue. *See also* AGING *and* DENTURES.

Liability Insurance, Professional

Insurance that protects physicians against lawsuits filed by patients.

Professional liability insurance protects against claims that allege physician negligence, resulting in the patient's injury. This type of insurance is typically purchased by physicians. Due to a broadening definition of negligence, many insurance companies have raised premiums and some have stopped offering coverage altogether *See* HEALTH INSURANCE; HYPOCRATIC OATH; *and* MALPRACTICE, INSURANCE.

Lice

Wingless insect parasites of the head, body, or pubic area.

Lice are tiny insect parasites that suck blood from their hosts and also infest garments, bedding, and other personal items. Lice infestation, also known as pediculosis, produces intense itching and irritation to the skin. Scratching may break the skin surface, leading to bacterial infection.

Types. Three common species of louse are known to prey on humans.

Head lice inhabit the hair and scalp, but also occasionally the eyebrows, beard, or mustache. Such lice are readily spread from person to person through sharing of combs, brushes, hats, or other personal items, or through human contact.

Body lice have a similar shape as head lice but are somewhat larger. They may attach themselves to nearly any part of the body, often favoring the shoulders, abdomen, and buttocks. In addition to causing severe itching, some body lice are vectors for diseases, including trench fever, relapsing fever, and typhus. Body lice are generally the result of poor hygiene or overcrowded conditions.

Pubic lice are tinier insects. Their rounded, broader appearance makes them resemble crabs, from which they derive the popular name crab lice.

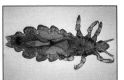

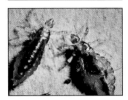

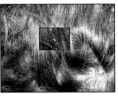

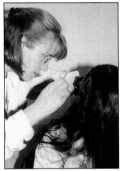

Lice. Lice are tiny parasites that suck blood from their hosts. Most commonly, they are known to infest the hair, above top. The lice also infests the body, second from top. Generally the lice will set up nests in hair, second from bottom, where they will multiply and spread throughout the infested area. Often, lice are found during routine checks of the hair, bottom. Most lice can eventually be washed away with special soaps and shampoos.

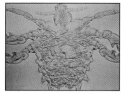

Pubic Lice. This breed of lice is tinier than other lice.Their rounded, broader appearance makes them resemble crabs, from which they derive the popular name crab lice. They tend to cause more intense itching, around the penis, vagina, or anus.top, a skin disorder where skin cells are mistaken for foreign objects and are attacked causing an itchy rash.

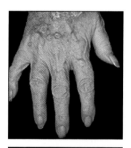

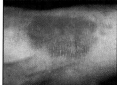

Lichen Planus. Above top, a skin disorder in which skin cells are mistaken for foreign objects and are attacked causing an itchy rash.
Lichen Simplex. Above, bottom, a skin problem in which a person scratches an itchy or irritated area, resulting in thick itchy patches forming on the skin.

Symptoms. In addition to intense itching, lymph glands in the neck may become swollen due to scalp infection. Sometimes, head lice go unnoticed. Body and pubic lice tend to cause more intense itching, the latter around the penis, vagina, or anus. Further, female lice of all three species lay tiny whitish-gray eggs, known as nits, which may be observed clinging to body hair. In the case of body lice, eggs may also be found in the seams of clothing that is in close contact with the body. Pubic lice leave behind excrement that appears as tiny dark brown specks on clothing. As pubic lice are the smallest, their detection may be difficult. Often, they appear as tiny bluish specks on the skin. Their nits are laid on hairs close to the body and are likewise difficult to locate.

Treatment. Medications are effective in killing all three forms of lice and their eggs, but it is essential that clothing, bedding and personal items that may harbor lice or nits be thoroughly cleaned in hot, soapy water or discarded. Permethrin is the medication of choice, with few side effects. Another medication, lindane, may be applied as a lotion, cream, or shampoo, but is not suitable for treating children. These and other medications may cause irritation to the skin. A repeat application is necessary after 10 days to ensure all lice and eggs have been destroyed. *See also* HAIR; HYGENE; PARASITE; PUBIC LICE; SCALP; SKIN; *and* TYPHUS.

Licensure

The granting of a license to practice medicine.

Doctors must be licensed by the state in which they practice medicine. Each state has different qualifications that must be met for a license to be granted. Generally, an internship lasting one year is required of doctors once they finish medical school. Once the internship is over, the doctor must pass a state licensing test. The license is then granted by the state licensing board. This board also has the power to suspend or revoke the license. *See also* INTERN.

Lichen Planus

A common condition in which inflammatory cells enter the skin and cause a particular type of rash.

The onset of lichen planus is slow. The condition usually clears up within 18 months, but may last longer.

The definitive cause of lichen planus is unknown, but some believe it is caused by a viral infection that creates an abnormal immune system reaction. Others hypothesize that it is an autoimmune disorder.

This rash is characterized by shiny, flat-topped, itchy bumps smaller than a centimeter in diameter. They are usually purplish with white lines running through them. They may be close together or form lines or rings. The condition usually affects the front of the wrists, the lower back, the forearms, and the ankles. Lichen planus can usually be treated with a corticosteroid cream. *See also* SKIN.

Lichen Simplex

Also called neurodermatitis

A common skin problem, caused by scratching or rubbing an itchy or irritated area, which results in the development of one or more itchy patches on the skin.

The stimulus to scratch may be a mosquito bite, stress, or just a nervous habit. The condition most often affects adults and seems to occur more in women. Itchy patches usually develop on the nape of the neck, the scalp, the shoulder, the wrist, or the ankle. Occasionally the genitals are affected as well.

Skin affected by lichen simplex looks thick and may develop groups of small bumps. The condition is persistent and has a tendency to recur as the itchy patches invite more scratching and rubbing.

Treatments for lichen simplex include steroid creams and moisturizers. Scratching should be avoided. Antihistamine pills will lessen the itch. Phototherapy (ultraviolet light treatment) may help to heal serious cases. *See also* CORTICOSTEROID; PHOTOTHERAPY; *and* SKIN.

Lichenification

A disorder in which the skin becomes leathery, thick, and the lines in the skin are accentuated.

Lichenification most commonly results from repeated scratching of an irritated area of skin. This scratching is often an attempt to relieve the itching sensation that accompanies skin disorders such as eczema and lichen simplex. *See* ECZEMA *and* SKIN.

Lid Lag

A delay in the normal downward movement of the eyelid.

Lid lag can usually be seen when the eye looks downward. The delay often accompanies eophthalmos, or a protrusion of the eyeball. Lid lag is a common characteristic symptom of thyrotoxicosis. *See also* EYE *and* THYROTOXICOSIS.

Life Expectancy

The average length of a person's life, based on statistics.

Life expectancy is the average amount of time, in years, a person can expect to live. The number is determined by statistics.

Nationality and Life Expectancy. The average life expectancy in western countries is generally over 70 years. For example, in the United States, the estimated life expectancy in the year 2000 was 77.12 years for the total population; 74.24 years for men, and 79.9 years for women. Life expectancies in some developing countries can be as low as 40 years; however, this statistic is misleading since the infant mortality rate in these countries is so high.

Gender Differences. In general, women have longer average life expectancies than men. This has been the case since 1900, when life expectancy data first began to be compiled. Before that time, women actually lived for a shorter period of time on average than men, because of the large number of deaths during childbirth. How-

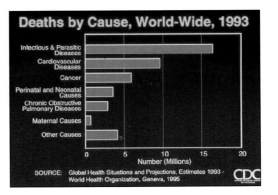

ever, improvements in obstetrics have resulted in safer deliveries and longer life expectancies for women.

The gender gap in life expectancy since 1900 is largely the result of an increase in male mortalities as a result of the widespread adoption of smoking by men and resultant increase in male deaths from smoking related illnesses, such as lung cancer and heart disease, during this time period.

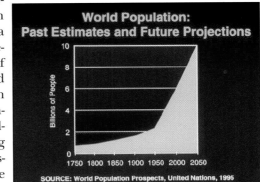

The gender gap has narrowed since 1970, however, as women began to take up smoking. In recent years, both sexes have begun to make healthier lifestyle choices, resulting in increased life expectancy overall. *See also* NICOTINE *and* PUBLIC HEALTH.

Life Support

Process in which a person is kept alive artificially with a ventilator, to maintain breathing, and/or a pacemaker, to sustain the heart beat.

Life support devices are used for a short period to keep a victim alive in times of emergency, or for a lengthier time in the event of serious illness. Life support is designed to supply oxygen, food, and water to the patient. It is also used to maintain body temperature, blood pressure control, carbon dioxide disposition, and the proper removal of waste. *See* TERMINAL HEALTH CARE.

Ligament

Elastic tissue that binds the joints and bone ends.

In addition to binding joints together, ligaments are also important to joint composition because they prevent excessive movement that can result in injury.

Overextending a joint can often result in damage to the ligaments. These injuries are most common to the ankles and knees. A minor sprain can be treated with a cold compress, ice, a bandage, or physical therapy. If the injury has resulted in a partial or complete tear of the ligament, the joint must be immobilized by a cast or splinted. In severe cases, surgery may be necessary to repair the damage. *See also* JOINT.

Knee Ligament. Many ligaments run between the femur and the tibia in the knee joint. The ligaments of the knee joint include the anterior cruciate ligament, the posterior cruciate ligament, and the meniscal ligaments.

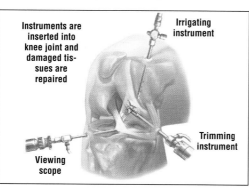

Instruments are inserted into knee joint and damaged tissues are repaired

Irrigating instrument

Trimming instrument

Viewing scope

Ligation

The surgical procedure of tying off (ligating) a blood vessel, tube, or duct with thread to prevent bleeding or to close a duct or tube.

Sperm ducts are ligated in vasectomies and in testicular cancer operations. Varicose veins can be effectively treated by ligation. Gallbladder operations involve ligation of the cystic duct. Emergency surgery, especially on accident victims, often requires ligation of blood vessels to stop bleeding.

The term is also used in the names of various surgical procedures. Tubal ligation is a popular form of sterilization in which the fallopian tubes are tied off. Elastic-band ligation is used to treat hemorrhoids. *See also* FALLOPIAN TUBES; GALLBLADDER; *and* HEMORRHOIDS.

Ligature

Surgical thread, suture, nylon, or wire used to ligate (tie off) a blood vessel, tube, or duct.

A ligature is a length of thread, suture, nylon, wire, or other material used to tie off a blood vessel, duct, or tube. It may be used in several of procedures, such as hemhorroid removal, in which a hemhorroid is "strangled" by a ligature to cut off its blood supply and eventually falls off. *See* LIGATION.

Light Therapy

The use of light to treat a variety of disorders.

Exposure to various forms of light is used to treat a variety of medical conditions. Sunlight seems to trigger the release of certain chemicals in the body. Most notably, the lack of light at the end of the day triggers the production of melatonin, one of many chemicals that regulate how signals are passed through the nervous system. Melatonin seems to be connected to sleep and regulation of the body's rhythms. Sunlight is also a source of vitamin D, necessary for healthy bones and teeth.

USES OF LIGHT THERAPY

The primary use of light therapy is in treating seasonal affective disorder (SAD), a type of depression that occurs only in the winter months, characterized by depressed mood, sleepiness, and cravings for sugar. The main treatment for SAD is exposure to a broad spectrum light in the early morning and evening. This light contains nearly the entire spectrum of sunlight, except for ultraviolet rays. While being exposed to the light, a person can read, watch television, or participate in another quiet activity, but the eyes must remain open.

Broad spectrum lights are available commercially and can be used at home. However, a physician should first be consulted in order to diagnose SAD, as light is not an effective treatment for other types of depression or mood disorders.

Side Effects. Side effects include headache, slight nausea, glare, eye irritation, and hyperactivity. These temporary effects can be avoided by reducing the amount of time spent in front of the light. If side effects persist, a physician should be consulted.

Infants born with severely high levels of bilirubin may be treated by being placed under a bright light, which helps the body process the bilirubin.

Psoriasis can be treated by exposure to ultraviolet light after administration of the drug psoralen. This causes a reduction of the scaly, itchy areas of skin. Prolonged exposure to ultraviolet light can increase the likelihood of skin cancer.

Scientists have experimented with using light exposure in combination with drugs or topical acids to treat certain kinds of skin cancer or precancerous growths. Also, there have been some indications that exposure to a type of ultraviolet light can alleviate the symptoms of lupus, a serious autoimmune disease.

Light therapy has also been said to be helpful in treating insomnia, jet lag, prolonged menstrual cycles, and nonseasonal depression. However, these uses are not clinically proven. In the case of depression, a physician should be consulted. These diseases are very serious, but they can often be effectively treated with professional counseling and antidepressant drugs. Further, light therapy should not be used in the case of bipolar disorder. *See also* DEPRESSION; JAUNDICE; MELATONIN; LUPUS; *and* PSORIASIS.

Lightening

When a fetus enters the pelvic cavity during the final weeks of pregnancy.

The fetus drops from its initial position into a lower part of the uterus in preparation for birth. Its head then pushes against the cervix, which may subsequently cause some discomfort or minor pain for the mother. First-time mothers may mistake this sensation for labor contractions. Mothers often bond more with the fetus with the lightening experience. *See also* CHILDBIRTH.

Limb Defects

Abnormalities involving the arms or legs that are present at birth (congenital).

The cause of limb defects may be genetic or may be due to an environmental factor, such as maternal exposure to toxins. Limb defects include congenital amputation (absence of an entire limb or just part of it), congenital dislocation of the hip, femoral torsion, knee dislocation, and clubfoot (talipes).

Limb defects, other than a missing limb, can be corrected with surgery or orthopedic procedures in the first few months after birth. *See also* BIRTH DEFECTS; HIP, CONGENITAL DISLOCATION OF; *and* TALIPES.

Limb, Artificial

A prosthetic device used to replace missing or diseased limbs.

An artificial limb consists of an extension, which consists of foam rubber encased in metal, wood, or leather, and is made to match the limb it is replacing. The artificial joint is composed of plastic and metal, and is mechanized to simulate the natural movement of the part it replaces. While prostheses can be found ready made, they generally fit, function, and appear better when custom-made to suit the individual.

An artificial limb operates by mimicking the process that moved the natural body part. The brain is still sending the instructions that moved the limb to the stump. Electronic circuitry in the prosthesis picks up the impulses at the nerve endings in the stump and moves the artificial limb.

Artificial limbs have improved greatly in recent years. They can be equipped with sophisticated electronics and can allow an individual to run and participate in some sports. Sometimes, artificial limbs are placed for cosmetic purposes. *See also* PROSTHESIS.

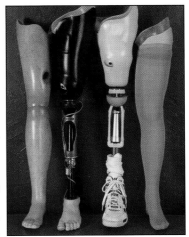

Prosthetic Legs. Prosthetic legs at the Sabolich Center in Oklahoma City. They show different materials and coverings.

Limbic System

Area of the brain that plays a role in body functions, emotions, and sense of smell.

The limbic system plays a major role in the autonomic nervous system (ANS), which is responsible for regulating body functions. The area is located in the center of the brain and appears to be a ring of nerve cells connected in clusters. The limbic system is quite large and contains several different structures, including the hippocampus, which is essential to long-term memory. *See* Brain *and* Nervous System.

Like much of the brain, the limbic system is usually studied by examining patients or animals known to have damage to that particular section of the brain. People who have experienced damage to the limbic system often exhibit inappropriate and excessive crying or laughing, bad tempers, anxiety, fear, and depression.

Linear Accelerator

Device for producing high speed radiation, often used for radiation therapy.

Accelerators are machines designed to speed up charged particles (electrons), producing x-radiation and neutrons in the process. As the name implies, linear accelerators speed particles along a straight path, as opposed to ring-shaped accelerators, which speed particles in a circular path. Linear accelerators are widely used for medical purposes, particularly for radiation therapy to treat cancerous malignancies.

Using an accelerator, a narrow beam of high-speed radiation may be directed at the tumor or other abnormal tissue in an effort to destroy it while doing a minimal amount of damage to the surrounding tissue. A patient's radiation schedule will depend on the depth and extent of tumor growth, the overall health of the patient, the nature of the malignancy, and other factors. *See* Cancer; Malignant; Radiation Hazards; Radiation Therapy; *and* Tumor.

Resources on Lipids
Berne, Robert M., et al., *Cardiovascular Physiology* (2001); Debakey, Michael E. and Antonio M. Gotto, *The New Living Heart* (1997); Gotto, Antonio, *A Patient's Handbook of Cholestorol Disorders* (2000); American Heart Associ-ation, Tel. (800) 242-8721, Online: www.amhrt.org; Heart Information Network, Tel. (973) 701-6035, Online: www.heartinfo.org; Nat. Heart, Lung, and Blood Inst., Tel. (301) 496-4236, Online: www. nhlbi.nih. gov; www.nycornell.org/ cardiothora-cic.surgery/; www.nycornell.org/medi-cine/cardiology/html.

Lip Cancer

Malignant tumor of the lip.

Lip cancers, like other oral and nasal cancers, are almost all squamous cell cancers, affecting cells in the surface layer of tissue. They usually arise on the lower lip and almost always occur later in life. Risk factors include prolonged exposure to sunlight and a history of smoking.

A lip cancer usually is first detected as a whitish area that forms a yellow, scaly crust. The affected area may become ulcerous. A lip sore that persists for many weeks calls for a visit to a physician.

Without treatment, the cancer can spread to the jaw and then to the neck. The diagnosis is made by taking a tissue sample, and the standard treatment is removal by surgery followed by radiation therapy.

In recent years, the use of chemotherapy before surgery for large lip cancers has increased, and a number of studies evaluating different combinations of surgery and chemotherapy are underway. *See also* Squamous Cell Carcinoma.

Lipid Disorders

An excess or deficiency of fat in the blood stream.

Fat is critical to the metabolic process. It is the body's main source of energy, and the body calls on stored fat in times of hunger, as well as to help fight infection and heal wounds. Too little fat leaves a person vulnerable to disease and extremes of heat or cold, and leaves vital organs and bones less protected in the event of accident or injury.

LOW LIPID LEVELS

Low blood lipids (fats) are a symptom of a number of inherited enzyme diseases that can be very serious and difficult to treat. Lowered lipid levels in the blood stream may indicate an overactive thyroid, malnutrition, or cancer. A number of inherited diseases affect the way fat is broken down by enzymes in the digestive process.

Tangier disease, for example, is an inherited condition in which the person has very low levels of high density lipoproteins (HDL).

HIGH LIPID LEVELS

Too much fat, a common result of inherited disease, poor diet, or both, is much more common and even more dangerous. It builds up plaque on the inner surfaces of the arteries, making the heart work harder to pump the blood to the cells and tissues. Further, the plaque that builds up in the arteries can break off and travel to other parts of the body, where it can block smaller passages or clog already constricted blood vessels. The result may be pulmonary thrombosis, heart attack, or stroke.

Lipids are of two kinds, cholesterol and triglycerides. Either kind attaches to proteins in the bloodstream to produce lipoproteins that flow through the circulatory

---

Lipids and the Elderly

The elderly are at increased risk of developing diabetes and high blood pressure. At the same time they have been collecting plaque in their arteries for 50 years or more, so the arteries are clogged and less flexible. Strict diet control will not only reduce the build-up of plaque; recent studies indicate that low cholesterol levels can actually remove plaque from arteries.

---

system. The tendency toward hyperlipidemias can be inherited, and a baseline level of cholesterol and triglycerides is established by each individual's metabolism. However, fat content is also strongly influenced by diet. Saturated fats are converted into low-density lipoproteins ("bad" cholesterol), while polyunsaturated and monounsaturated fats found in fruits, vegetables, and oils like olive oil are converted into high density lipoproteins ("good" cholesterol).

Background material on Lipid Disorders can be found in BLOOD PRESSURE AND CHOLESTEROL. *Related information is contained in* AGING, ANEMIA, ARTORY, BLOOD, HYPERLIPIDEMIAS, LIPIDS, LIPID LOWERING DRUGS, OBESITY, PLAQUE, PULMONARY THROMBOSIS AND TANGEIR DISEASE.

Lipid-Lowering Drugs

A number of relatively new drugs that reduce the levels of lipids in the blood.

Lipids including cholesterol are fats that can clog arteries and lead to heart disease, stroke, and pulmonary thrombosis. In many cases, levels of blood lipids can be controlled through diet and exercise, but sometimes, especially if a person has a family history of high cholesterol and heart disease, drug treatment is necessary. Lipid-lowering drugs may function in several ways to lower harmful forms of cholesterol (LDLs) and raise the levels of beneficial cholesterol (HDLs).

The main types of lipid-lowering drugs include statins, anion-exchange resins, fibrates, and nicotinic acid. Each drug treats a specific type of excess lipid. *See* CHOLESTEROL; LIPID DISORDES; *and* LIPIDS.

Lipids

Group of organic compounds comprising the chief component in cell membranes.

Lipids are substances that are not soluble in water, but can be dissolved by an organic solvent. These substances include fats, oils, sterols, esters, and waxes. Lipids, in moderate quantities, are essential to health. Two types of lipids can be distinguished: dietary lipids and blood lipids. Lipids serve as a source of energy for sustaining metabolism. Stored body fat is essential in providing the body with stores of energy. Lipids also provide important fatty acids and are carriers of fat-soluble vitamins. *See also* MEMBRANE, CELL.

Lipoatrophy

Fat loss under the skin.

An insulin allergy is believed to cause lipoatrophy in diabetics, even though the skin dents that characterize the disorder occur in areas where insulin is not injected. Other possible causes of the disorder are fat absorption and metabolism problems.

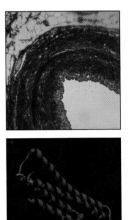

Lipids. Above, top, a cross section micrograph of a blood vessel shows a large artheroma—a lipid deposit—that can decrease blood flow. Above, bottom, a three-dimensional computer model of an apolipoprotien. A lipid combined with an apolipoprotein forms a lipoprotein. The green spiral ribbons are alpha-helix amino acid strings.

Lipoma

Common nonmalignant tumor of fatty tissue composed of mature fat cells.

Lipomas are most often are found on the trunk, thigh, or shoulder, where they are seen as slow growing masses. They are more common in women than men. A lipoma usually does not cause any symptoms, but some may be painful. While they rarely become cancerous, a biopsy is recommended for unusually fast growing lipomas to rule out malignancy. Bothersome lipomas can be removed by liposuction or surgery. *See also* TUMOR.

Liposarcoma

A cancer arising in fatty tissue.

Liposarcomas are uncommon forms of cancer that generally develop in late-middle age. They can occur in any fatty part of the body, but tend to appear on the abdomen or thigh, where they cause visible swelling. Under a microscope, a liposarcoma visibly consists of immature cells of varying sizes with bizarre nuclei. When detected, they usually can be removed surgically, but often recur. *See also* CANCER.

Liposuction

Also known as suction-assisted lipectomy and lipoplasty

A surgical procedure in which excess body fat is suctioned out of a specific problem area through a small cut in the skin.

Liposuction is especially appropriate for body areas where fat deposits are not often reduced by diet or exercise, particularly the chin, upper arms, abdomen, chest, buttocks, hips, and thighs.

The three main types of liposuction are dry, tumescent, and ultrasound-assisted liposuction (UAL). Dry liposuction involves significant blood loss, thus tumescent liposuction, in which saline solution, lidocaine (an anesthetic), and epinephrine (a hormone) are injected, has increased in popularity. Ultrasound-assisted liposuction utilizes a small, heated probe that produces ultrasonic vibrations to liquefy fat cells, which are then suctioned out. *See also* COSMETIC SURGERY; *and* LIPIDS.

Lipreading

A way to comprehend speech by watching the movement of the speaker's lips.

Lipreaders use an aggregate of visual cues to decipher the meaning of speech. While lipreaders watch the lips of the speaker to decipher the words being spoken, they also consider the speaker's mood, the movement of the tongue and lower jaw, the state of the eyes and eyebrows, and any meaningful gestures. Lipreaders also observe the natural flow and rhythm of the words.

Hearing loss can make speech sound quieter or distorted. Lipreading is a valuable tool for people with moderate hearing loss, and is often essential for the deaf.

Some people find lipreading difficult, and even the most skilled lipreader cannot accurately identify every word. Fast speech, poor pronunciation, bad lighting, and moustaches can make lipreading difficult or even impossible. *See also* HEARING.

Lisp

A common speech defect in which "s" and "z" are pronounced as "th."

Lisping is often seen in young children learning to speak, as the "s" and "z" sounds are difficult to produce. Most children outgrow immature speech before they begin grade school.

Causes. A lisp is caused by the protrusion of the tongue between the teeth when enunciating syllables. Often, it is not associated with any anatomical irregularity, although a cleft lip and palate, in which the lip and roof of the mouth are not fully joined together, generally causes lisping. If the child's parents lisp, there is an increased tendency to develop irregular speech patterns. A child who has lost his or her front teeth may lisp temporarily. Hearing loss or damage to the palate, mouth, or teeth can cause a delay in a child's speech development.

Treatment. If the lisping is caused by an anatomical irregularity, that must be fixed before the lisp can be corrected. If the lisp has no anatomical cause, it usually disappears without treatment by grade school. If lisping continues, a speech-language pathologist can teach a child techniques to enable proper speech. *See* SPEECH DISORDERS.

Listeriosis

An infection caused by listeria bacteria and acquired by consuming contaminated dairy products or raw vegetables.

Listeria can attack any organ of the body. The elderly, small infants, and those with compromised immune systems are most vulnerable. Infection with the listeria bacteria usually takes place in the summer months and often attacks the meninges (the covering of the spinal cord and the brain). In patients with listeriosis, brain abscesses form and meningitis produces a stiff neck and fever. Left untreated, the disease can cause confusion, coma, and death. The bacteria also attack the eyes, the lymph nodes, the blood, and even the valves of the heart. Listeriosis is treated with penicillin and other antibiotics. *See* MENINGITIS.

Lithium

A drug used to treat bipolar mood disorder (manic-depression).

Lithium is an effective mood stabilizer used to even out the mood swings of bipolar disorder, reducing manic periods and elevating depressed periods. Side effects include thirst, hand tremor, nausea, irregular heartbeat, muscle twitches, dizziness, slurred speech, confusion, hair loss, fatigue, and impotence. The side effects are reduced over long-term use and can be minimized by careful monitoring. Arthritis drugs and thiazide diuretics may interfere with lithium elimination and raise levels in the blood to toxic levels. Thiazide diuretics may also raise lithium levels.

Lithotomy

Surgical removal of a stone from the urinary tract.

Once the standard method of removing a stone from the kidney or another part of the urinary tract, lithotomy now has been replaced in more than 95 percent of cases by other methods, such as cystoscopy (a procedure in which stones are crushed and removed with basket forceps) and lithotripsy. Lithotomy is now only performed in instances when large stones lodged within the kidney must be removed. During the procedure, an incision is made in the right or left side of the back to remove a kidney stone. *See also* CYSTOSCOPY; LITHOTRIPSY; *and* STONE.

Lithotomy Position

A particular position assumed by a patient during a medical examination.

The patient lies on his or her back with knees bent and legs wide apart. Stirrups usually support the feet and legs.

The term lithotomy is used to describe the surgical removal of stones from the bladder; the position was originally used for patients undergoing this type of operation. Today, it is commonly used for pelvic examinations and childbirth, as well as various types of pelvic surgery.

Lithotripsy

The use of shock waves to break up calculi (stones) into pieces so that they are passed out of the body.

The main types of lithotripsy are extracorporeal shock wave lithotripsy (ESWL) and intracorporeal lithotripsy. In ESWL, a physician locates the stone with a fluoroscope and uses a lithotriptor against the patient's back to generate shock waves. In percutaneous lithotripsy, a type of intracorporeal lithotripsy, the doctor inserts a specialized endoscope (nephroscope) into the kidney and uses an ultrasonic probe to break up the stones. *See* LITHOTRIPTOR.

Lithotriptor

The machine used to disintegrate small calculi (stones) in the surgical procedure called extracorporeal shock wave lithotripsy (ESWL).

Approved by the FDA in 1984, the lithotriptor has enabled millions of patients to avoid the four day hospital stays surgery once required. It is used to break up stones in the various organs, such as the kidneys and the gallbladder. One type of lithotriptor requires the patient to be in a water bath while shock waves are transmitted. Another type has a soft cushion or membrane on which the patient lies. A drawback of the lithotriptor, however, is its inability to reach stones in the lower half of the ureter due to their location behind the pelvic bones. New laser alternatives may be used to break up these hard-to-reach stones.

Livedo Reticularis

A bluish mottling of the skin that usually develops on the legs.

Livedo reticularis may be a benign condition. However, it is sometimes associated with serious underlying conditions, such as vasculitis and connective tissue disorders. It should always be properly evaluated.

Liver

Organ responsible for regulation of chemicals in the blood and some chemical production.

The liver is the internal organ that regulates the main chemicals in the blood. Located in the upper-right quadrant of the abdominal cavity, the liver is cone-shaped and is the largest internal organ.

Structure. The liver is divided into two main lobes. The larger right lobe is subdivided into two smaller lobes. The organ is almost completely shielded by the ribs, which aid in protection. The liver cells, known as hepatocytes, secrete bile, a fluid that exits the liver through a series of ducts. After leaving the bile ducts, the fluid is

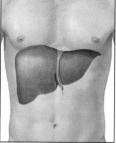

Liver. The largest internal organ, the liver is located in the upper abdomen, above. The dual lobed organ, above right, regulates chemicals in the blood and produces several essential chemicals.

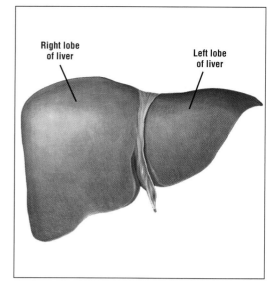

Right lobe of liver   Left lobe of liver

then stored in the gallbladder until required for digestion.

One unique feature of the liver is that it receives blood from two different sources. Blood enters through the hepatic artery, which delivers the blood through normal systemic circulation. Blood also reaches the organ from the portal vein, which collects the blood that has already passed through the small intestines and received nutrients from the digestive system.

Functions. The liver has several important functions. The organ is essential to the production of proteins for blood plasma. These proteins include: albumin, which regulates water levels in blood and tissue; complement, which is important in the immune system's defense against infection; coagulation factors, which are necessary for clotting in the event of damage to blood vessels; and globulin, which aids in carrying oxygen to the bloodstream. The liver also produces cholesterol and other fat-carrying lipids.

A second function of the liver is to absorb glucose that the body's cells do not immediately need and store it in the form of glycogen. When more energy is required by the body, the liver converts the glycogen back into glucose, which is then released back into the bloodstream.

The liver is also essential in regulating the blood level of amino acids, the main component of proteins. When there is an excess of amino acids in the blood, the liver converts the acids into glucose, proteins, or other amino acids. They may also be converted into urea, which is then passed to the kidneys for disposal in the urine.

The liver and the kidneys also work together to remove poisons and drugs from the bloodstream. The process begins when the liver absorbs the undesirable substances and converts them into a water soluble form. They are then excreted in the bile and carried out of the liver.

The liver is unique among internal organs in its ability to regenerate in the event of injury or illness. It is estimated that, in a healthy individual, an injured liver can regenerate as much as 80 percent of the total size of the organ. There are a number of serious liver diseases, classified as congenital liver disorders, viral and non-viral infections, drug-induced and toxin induced disease, vascular disorders, metabolic disorders, iron accumulation, alcoholic liver disease, and tumors.

> *Background material on Liver can be found in* BILIARY SYSTEM AND BLOOD *Related information is contained in* ABDOMEN, ALCOHOLIC LIVER DISEASE, AMINO ACID, CIRRHOSIS, LIVER ABSCESS, LIVER BIOPSY, LIVER IMAGING, LIVER FUNCTION TEST, PROTEIN, TUMORS AND WATER.

Liver Abscess

A pus-filled pocket on or near the liver, caused by bacteria or amoebas.

When pathogens (disease-causing agents) invade the body, the immune system sends white blood cells to attack and swallow them. The white blood cells then die and may accumulate to form a pocket of pus. Such an abscess in or on the liver may cause long-lasting fever, chills, weight loss, nausea, diarrhea, weakness, and abdominal pain. The patient may become jaundiced (yellow). The abscess will usually be diagnosed by blood tests. If the cause is found to be amoebic, the abscess will be treated with medications. If the cause is found to be bacterial, the abscess will be drained, followed by a long course of antibiotics. *See also* ABSCESS; ANTIBIOTIC DRUGS; *and* JAUNDICE.

Liver Biopsy

Removal of tissue from the liver for purposes of diagnosis.

Samples of liver tissue for diagnosis are obtained by inserting a fine needle through the skin and drawing out a small piece of the tissue for further analysis. The region from which the biopsy sample is taken is often first identified by computerized tomography or ultrasound scanning.

A liver biopsy is generally carried out on an outpatient basis under local anesthesia, though the patient will be asked to wait at the hospital or doctor's office for several hours following biopsy to ensure that there are no complications. These complications are unusual, but may include lacerations (tearing) and bleeding. Additionally, there is a danger of leakage of bile from the liver into the abdomen, causing an inflammation known as peritonitis. The patient undergoing liver biopsy should remain near a hospital for an additional two weeks after the biopsy in case of subsequent bleeding.

Liver biopsy may also be performed through the veins. In this procedure, a fine catheter (tube) is inserted into a vein in the neck and threaded through the heart. Finally, it is guided into one of the hepatic veins, which leaves the liver. The biopsy needle is then inserted through a catheter, through the hepatic vein, and into the liver, where it extracts a tissue sample.

This technique results in less bleeding and is considered safer to the liver than the alternate procedure. Biopsies are also occasionally performed during exploratory surgery (surgery undertaken to find the source of a problem).

> *Background material on Liver Biopsy can be found in* BILIARY SYSTEM AND EXPLORATORY SUREGRY. *Related information is contained in* BILE, BILE DUCT, BLOOD, CIRRHOSIS, HOSPITAL, LIVER, LIVER FUNCTION TESTS, LIVER IMAGING, PERITONITIS, PREVENTATIVE MEASSURES, AND WATER.

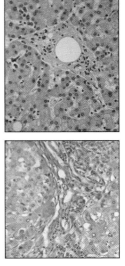

Liver Cells. Above, top, epatocytes–liver cells–clustered around a central vein. Above, bottom, liver cirrhosis is characterized by the presence of fibrous septa and regenerative nodules.

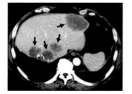

Liver Cancer.
Hepatocellular carcinoma accounts for 80 to 90 percent of all liver cancers. It occurs more often in men than women, and occurs mostly in people 50 to 60 years old. The cause of liver cancer is unknown.

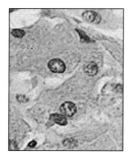

Alcohol Induced Liver Disease. Alcoholic hepatitis usually occurs after years of excessive drinking. The longer the duration of alcohol use and the larger the consumption of alcohol, the greater the probability of developing liver disease.

Liver Cancer

A malignant tumor of the liver.

Like most cancers, liver cancer can be classified as primary, meaning that it originates in that organ, or secondary, meaning that it is a metastasis, or colony, of cancers arriving from elsewhere in the body. Liver cancers are generally secondary. While primary liver cancers account for less than two percent of liver cancers in the United States, the incidence is higher in some parts of Asia, the Middle East and Africa, as they are associated with viral hepatitis, which is common in those regions. About 75 percent of primary liver cancers are hepatomas, which arise in the parenchymal cells that perform the basic blood-filtering processes of the liver. A much smaller percentage are cholangiocarcinomas, which arise in the bile-duct cells within the liver. Secondary liver cancers can originate in the stomach, large intestine, or pancreas.

Symptoms. The symptoms of both primary and secondary liver cancer include weight loss, weakness, loss of appetite, abdominal swelling and pain, fever, and nausea. As the cancer progresses, it can cause yellowing of the skin (jaundice) and an accumulation of fluid in the abdomen.

Diagnosis. Diagnostic tests for liver cancer include x-rays of the chest and abdomen, liver function assays, computerized tomography or magnetic resonance imaging, and ultrasound scans. The diagnosis can be confirmed by examination of a tissue sample (biopsy). Because many liver cancers cause an increase in the production of alpha-fetoprotein, a protein produced in the liver, a test may be done to detect elevated levels of that protein.

Treatment depends on whether a primary cancer is confined to one area of the liver or has spread through the liver and perhaps to other parts of the body. In many cases, surgery to remove a localized tumor and some surrounding tissue can be curative. But surgery may not be possible for a localized tumor where so much tissue must be removed that liver function is severely

impaired. In such cases, chemotherapy and radiation therapy may be performed. Sometimes, the entire liver may be removed and replaced in a liver transplant procedure. Chemotherapy and radiation therapy are treatments designed to prolong life in cases of secondary liver cancer, with therapy aimed at the liver cancer and the original cancer. *See* CANCER *and* LIVER.

Liver Disease, Alcohol- or Drug-Induced

Damage to the liver caused by prolonged substance abuse, resulting in cirrhosis and death.

Among its many functions, the liver serves to cleanse the body of toxins. A continual barrage of toxins such as alcohol can eventually ravage the organ. Alcohol abuse can result in several types of damage to the liver, which, if left unchecked, can progress to cirrhosis and, finally, liver failure.

Alcohol- or drug-induced hepatitis is an inflammation of the liver caused by exposure to alcohol, illegal drugs, over-the-counter or prescription medicines, some health food store products, and chemicals such as carbon tetrachloride or chloroform. While heavy, long-term use of alcohol (more than two drinks per day) is the most frequent cause, it can sometimes result from moderate drinking.

> **ALERT**
>
> Acetaminophen, the active ingredient in over-the-counter painkillers such as Tylenol™, can cause severe liver damage when taken in combination with alcohol. It may also affect the liver without the presence of alcohol.

Symptoms of alcohol or drug induced-hepatitis include jaundice, light-colored stools, lingering fatigue that may last for weeks or months, loss of appetite, and flu like symptoms (fever, nausea, and vomiting). Some individuals with alcoholic hepatitis are asymptomatic (no symptoms).

Decreased consumption of alcohol is the best way to avoid to alcoholic liver disease. In most patients, the inflammation of the liver lasts approximately two weeks. Alcoholic hepatitis can be fatal in rare cases, particularly if there is prior liver damage.

Treatment involves ceasing consumption of alcohol or other substances that caused the hepatitis, in order to allow the liver to heal itself.

Fatty liver, or steatohepatitis, is another liver disorder that may be alcohol-induced, occurring when fat permeates the liver. Its exact causes are not known, although scientists theorize that a damaged liver may be less capable of processing (metabolizing) fat, causing it to accumulate. Fatty liver has no particular symptoms of its own, but rather is seen in combination with conditions like alcohol abuse, diabetes, tuberculosis, obesity, poor diet, and the use of corticosteroids. It is reversible; as soon as drinking ceases alcohol the fat will subside. It is not associated with scarring or inflammation of the liver.

Cirrhosis, or fibrous scarring, results from chronic liver disease or severe damage to the liver, in which the blood flow is obstructed and the liver is unable to perform its functions.

Liver failure is the final stage of cirrhosis. Toxins build up in the body, and the effects of alcohol and drugs become cumulative. There is no cure for liver failure, except for a transplant.

> *Background material on Alcohol or Drug Induced Liver Disease can be found in* ALCOHOL DEPENDENCE AND CIRRHOSIS. *Related information is contained in* **Acetomin-phen, Jaundice, Liver Failure and Liver Transplant.**

Liver Failure

Extreme impairment of liver functioning, resulting from acute inflammation of the liver (hepatitis) or the advanced stages of cirrhosis.

Liver failure occurs as the result of an excessive build-up of scar tissue in the liver. In addition, a lack of healthy liver cells makes it impossible for the liver to perform its key functions. Toxins accumulate in the blood, and the body becomes even more sensitive to the effects of drugs and alcohol.

Liver failure has catastrophic effects on other body organs as well. The kidneys begin to fail. Huge, swollen blood vessels (varices) develop in the esophagus and stomach as blood flow is rerouted around the liver. These varices are very susceptible to bleeding and can be the source of a major hemorrhage and subsequent blood loss. Fluids can also build up in the brain, causing swelling, coma, and eventually death.

Symptoms. The symptoms of liver failure are virtually identical to those of advanced cirrhosis and hepatitis. They include fatigue, jaundice, vomiting, abdominal pain, disorientation, and fever. When the liver is unable to break down and remove substances, such as ammonia, from the blood, signal transmission through the nervous system breaks down and brain dysfunction results. In such circumstances, agitation, restlessness, and drowsiness may occur. In addition, coma (hepatic encephalopathy) may result. Other complications may also arise when liver failure accompanies cirrhosis. These include fluid retention in the abdomen and internal bleeding. In this instance, the onset of brain dysfunction occurs more slowly.

Diagnosis and Treatment. Liver failure is usually diagnosed through a series of liver function tests and tests for specific viruses in conjunction with a patient's medical history and a physical examination. While there is no exact cure for the condition, certain medications can reduce levels of toxicity of the blood.

A liver transplant can also be an alternative if the patient meets the right criteria. Until recently, liver transplants did not meet with much success. Today, however,

> ## Liver Transplants
>
> 85 percent of all people who receive liver transplants are alive five years later. The primary drawback to liver transplantation is the scarcity of donor organs. In 1997, less than 4,000 people in the United States received liver transplants, while there were over 25,000 cases of cirrhosis. It is possible, however, for two people to benefit from one donated liver, as the body does not require the entire organ to function.

because of better surgical techniques, improved methods for preserving the donor organ, and medications designed to help the body accept the transplant, the outlook for those who undergo the procedure is much more positive.

> *Background material on Liver Failure can be found in* CIRRHOSIS AND HEPATITIS. *Related information is contained in* ALCOHOL AND DRUG INDUCED DISORDERS OF THE LIVER, BILE, BILIARY SYSTEM, COMA, HEMORRHAGE, FATIGUE, FEVER, JAUNDICE, LIVER CANCER, AND LIVER TRANSPLANT.

Liver Fluke

Disease-causing parasitic flatworm of the class trematoda.

The human liver fluke causes 20 to 30 million cases of infection per year, primarily in Southeast Asia, Japan, Korea, Taiwan, and China. Liver flukes infest the human pancreatic and biliary ducts.

The parasite's eggs are passed with feces, continuing their development in a species of snail, which acts as an intermediate host. Larvae known as cercaria emerge from the snails to infest numerous species of freshwater fish, where they further develop into a durable metacercarian form. Eating uncooked fish infested with larvae also causes the disease.

Symptoms. Consumption of under 100 parasites may produce no symptoms. Heavy infestation, however, causes diarrhea, abdominal pain and enlargement of the spleen (splenomegaly).

In severe cases, fever, acute pain in the liver, and enlargement of the liver may accompany jaundice, tachycardia, and weight loss. While the disease itself is rarely fatal, complications include metaplasia, often leading to cancer of the biliary tract.

Diagnosis and Treatment. Liver fluke is diagnosed through detection of eggs in the feces, as well as obsercation of liver enlargement in endemic areas. The drug praziquantel is effective in treating infestation by liver fluke. *See also* FEVER; FLUKE; JAUNDICE; LIVER; SPLEEN; TACHYCARDIA; WEIGHT LOSS; *and* WORM INFESTATION.

Resources on Liver
Heimburger, Douglas C. and Roland L. Weinsier, *Handbook of Clinical Nutrition* (1997); Johnson, Alan G., and David R. Trigie, *Liver Disease and Gallstones* (1987); National Academy Press Food and Nutrition Board, *Recommended Dietary Allowances* (1989); Shils, Maurice E., et al., *Modern Nutrition in Health and Disease* (1999); American Dietetic Association, Tel. (800) 366-1655, Online: www. eatright.org; Center for Nutrition Policy and Promotion, Tel. (202) 418-2312, Online: www. usda.gov/cnpp; Food and Drug Administration, Tel. (888) INFOFDA, Online: www.fda.gov; www.nycornell.org/medicine/nutrition/index.html.

Liver Function Tests

Various blood tests used for diagnosis, to evaluate the performance of the liver, and identify disorder or disease.

Liver problems may be diagnosed by measuring various factors in the blood indicative of liver malfunction. This is accomplished through a variety of tests.

An enzyme, alkaline phophatase, is produced in the liver (as well as bone and placenta). Following illness or injury, this enzyme floods into the bloodstream, where it may be detected. Its presence may suggest liver injury, obstruction of the bileducts, and certain forms of cancer.

Analine transaminase is also an enzyme that sometimes occurs in the blood when liver cells have been injured. Its presence may be used to diagnose ailments involving these cells, such as hepatitis.

A bilirubin test, which measures this component of bile juices produced by the liver, can help diagnose obstructions of bile flow and destruction of the red blood cells from which bilirubin is made, an indicator of liver damage.

Alpha fetoprotein is a protein produced by the fetal liver and testes. Positive results of this test may indicate severe hepatitis, liver cancer, or testicular cancer.

Mitochondrial antibodies may be examined in the blood. These antibodies attack mitochondria, a central cell component involved in energy production. Positive results may indicate autoimmune disorders, including chronic active hepatitis and biliary cirrhosis.

A number of other tests on blood may be performed to assess and analyze liver function, depending on the type of ailment suspected. Liver function tests may be followed by or supplemented with liver imaging and biopsy.

> *Background material on Liver Fuction Tests can be found in* LIVER BIOPSY AND LIVER FAILURE. *Related information is contained in* ANTIBIOTICS, BILE, BILE DUCTS, BILIARY SYSTEM, BLOOD, ENZYME, HEPATITIS, LIVER CANCER, PROTEINS, AND TESTES, CANCER OF.

Liver Imaging

Techniques used to visualize the liver, assess its condition, and diagnose any liver problems.

Proper and accurate diagnosis of the liver may require blood analysis, as in liver function tests, or the direct observation of liver tissue by means of one or more imaging techniques.

TYPES OF LIVER IMAGING

Ultrasound scanning directs very high frequency sound waves at the area of interest. These ultrasound waves are then reflected back at differing rates, depending on the density of the structures they encounter. In the case of the liver, ultrasound is ideal for detecting abnormal masses such as tumors. Cirrhosis and other more widespread irregularities of tissue may require the use of other imaging techniques. Ultrasound is favored because it does not involve surgery, and for its clarity of image and safety.

Radionuclide imaging relies on a radioactive chemical, which is injected into the body and taken up by the organ in question. The location of radioactivity within the cells of the liver is recorded by a radiation detector, which relays the information to a computer that is able to compose an image from this data.

Among other imaging techniques, one of the most powerful (and safest) is known as MRI or magnetic resonance imaging. The patient is placed in a tube-like machine under a strong magnetic field, causing cells in the liver tissue to resonate. This information is then translated by a computer into a vivid image.

Additional imaging techniques include computer tomography (CT or CAT), endoscopic study (involving a flexible optical instrument), and cholangiography (in which an opaque substance is injected into the bile ducts), as well as the standard x-ray.

Background material on Liver Imaging can be found in CAT SCAN *and* LIVER FAILURE. *Related information is contained in* CHOLANGIOGRAPHY, ENDOSCOPY, LIVER, LIVER FUNCTION TESTS, MRI, RADIONUCLIDE SCANNING, *and* ULTRASOUND.

Liver Transplant

Replacement of a diseased or damaged liver with a healthy donor organ.

The liver is responsible for cleansing and filtering toxins from the blood. Failure of this organ may be caused, in adults, by cirrhosis or liver cancer and, in children, by malformed bile ducts (biliary atresia) or an enzyme deficiency (alpha1-antitrypsin deficiency, which can lead to cirrhosis). End-stage liver disease is not reversible and is in time fatal; the only way to prolong life is through liver transplant surgery.

As in many other organ transplants, the possibility of liver transplant depends on whether the person is otherwise healthy enough to withstand the rigors of major surgery and whether a donor liver is available. Factors affecting the success of surgery include the presence of other illnesses or disorders, age, and, in adults with alcoholic liver disease, whether alcohol use has been stopped.

The supply of available livers is far lower than the number of people who need a transplant. Thus, not everyone who can benefit from a liver transplant receives one. People who need a liver transplant are placed on a national computerized waiting list, UNOS. Interim transplant candidate medical care is aimed at keeping the patient as healthy as possible.

The most commonly performed liver transplant is known as adult cadaveric liver transplantation. In this procedure, the entire liver of the recipient is removed and replaced with a healthy liver from a recently deceased person. The donor organ is usually obtained from a person who has suffered brain death, with the consent of the next-of-kin. Unlike many other types of transplant surgery, which require complex matching of tissue types, liver transplants only require that the donor and recipient are approximately the same size and of compatible blood types. Because the liver is able to regenerate to a great extent, a cadaveric liver is often split in two and transplanted into two people, thus increasing the supply of available livers. The half-liver soon grows to full size and becomes fully functional.

More recently, tissue from living donors has been used successfully for transplantation. Living-donor liver transplantation helps avoid the lengthy wait for a donor organ. In this procedure, a section of healthy liver tissue is taken from a living donor and transplanted into the recipient. The unique nature of liver tissue allows this transplanted tissue to grow, eventually regenerating a complete, healthy liver to replace the diseased one. Living donors are selected on the basis of compatible blood type and likelihood of full recovery from the procedure. Risks to donors include infection, bleeding, bile leakage, and even death.

Procedure. Before surgery, the patient is given a battery of tests to make sure he or she is healthy enough for surgery, and is administered immunosuppressant drugs in order to suppress the immune system and minimize the chance of rejection.

The procedure is performed under general anesthesia. If a full liver is transplanted, the diseased liver is removed and the new one implanted. If a part of a liver is transplanted, the diseased liver remains in place until the new liver has grown and begun functioning, at which point another operation is performed to remove the diseased liver.

Recovery. The surgery requires a hospital stay of five to seven days. Patients generally resume normal activity in four to seven weeks.

Complications. Risks common to all major surgeries include bleeding and infection. The immunosuppressant drugs increase the risk of infection.

Further complications may arise as a result of the difficulty of the transplant. A blood clot may form in the artery leading to the liver, or bile may leak from sutured bile-ducts, causing infection. Both of these possibilities are monitored and, if necessary, treated after surgery.

The most common complication is rejection, in which the immune system recognizes the new liver as foreign material and attempts to destroy it. This usually occurs within a few months after surgery and can be treated with immunosuppressant drugs.

Immunosuppressant drug treatment must be continued indefinitely, although physicians attempt to use as low a dose as possible, as the drugs cause increased susceptibility to infection and disease.

Prognosis. Liver transplantation has a fairly high success rate, especially for children. Approximately two-thirds of adults and 80 to 90 percent of children survive transplantation and can be discharged from the hospital.

Any serious complications generally occur within the first year after transplantation. After the first year, good health can continue indefinitely.

Background material on Liver Transplant can be found in LIVER FAILURE AND TRANSPLANT SUREGRY *Related information is contained in* ASCITES, BILIARY SYSTEM, HEPATITIS, HEMOCHROMATOSIS, IMMUNE SYSTEM, LIVER CNCER, LIVER FAILURE, AND LIVER FUNCTION TESTS.

Lobectomy

The surgical removal of a diseased, abscessed, or cancerous lobe in the brain, lungs, liver, or thyroid

Their are several reasons for performing a lobectomy. Prefrontal lobotomies in the brain were common in the 1940s and 50s to correct mental illness but are now rarely performed. A lung lobectomy may be performed to remove a malignant tumor. A hepatectomy may be performed on the liver in the event of severe injury or illness. Another common lobectomy is the thyroidectomy. Thyroidectomies are performed in cases of thyroid cancer, incidences of thyrotoxicosis (abnormally high level of thyroid hormone), on goiters that are causing breathing difficulties, or on benign tumors. *See also* BRAIN; CANCER; GOITER; HEPATECTOMY, PARTIAL; LOBECTOMY, LUNG; THYROID CANCER; THYROIDECTOMY; *and* TUMOR.

Lobectomy, Lung

The surgical removal of one of the lobes of the lung, usually performed by a thoracic surgeon.

A lobectomy is usually performed to extract a malignant lung tumor. The procedure is also used to treat bronchiectasis (a widening of the bronchi or air passages), a lung abscess that has not responded to drug treatment, emphysema, uncontrolled inflammation, and severe lung injuries.

After making an incision in the chest from the armpit to the back of the ribcage, the surgeon separates the ribs (sometimes removing one), ties off the blood vessels and bronchi leading to the diseased lobe, and removes the lobe along with adjacent lymph nodes. The remaining lung tissue will expand to fill the space. *See* LOBECTOMY.

Lochia

Vaginal bleeding seen for the first three to six weeks after giving birth.

Lochia is composed of the uterine lining, which helped sustain the baby over the nine months of pregnancy and is later discarded. The flow starts out as a red, heavy discharge, resembling a heavier than usual menstrual period, and gradually decreases in volume and changes in color to brown and then yellow. A sudden increase in the flow is a sign that the woman is over-exerting herself and should cut back on her activities. An unusually heavy discharge, or one accompanied by a strong odor, is a sign of infection. *See also* VAGINA.

Lockjaw

Stiffness of the jaw muscles, one of the symptoms of tetanus infection.

Tetanus is caused by the bacterium *Clostridium tetani,* which has spores that can remain dormant for many years in the soil or the feces of animals and can activate when lodged in an open wound. As the bacteria multiply, they excrete a toxin that pro-

duces tight muscles in the jaw, face, neck, and back, and difficulty in breathing and swallowing. Muscle spasms are common in patients with tetanus. After infection, an antitoxin can be used to neutralize the toxin or the tetanus vaccine can be administered. It is preferable, however, to receive the tetanus vaccine and its boosters before any infection occurs. *See also* TETANUS.

Loose Bodies

Fragments of bone, cartilage, or capsule lining that shift within a joint.

Deterioration of bone, cartilage, or component of a joint can result in pieces breaking away and entering the joint. If caught between joint surfaces, they may interrupt movement and lock up the joint. Pain and swelling will follow. The pain may subside, but the fragments may find their way into the joint again. Loose bodies may be felt, or they can be pinpointed with x-rays. Doctors can usually remove loose bodies during arthroscopic surgery.

Loss of Consciousness

A state of being unable to respond to external stimuli resulting from reduced brain activity.

Someone who has lost consciousness may be suffering from something as minor as fainting, or as serious as a stroke. Unconsciousness can result from injuries to the head, shock, stroke, a loss of blood to the brain, hypotemia which is too little oxygen in the blood, hypoglycemia which is too little sugar in the blood or other chemical changes, or drug overdoses or exposure to toxins. *See* DRUG OVERDOSE *and* FIRST AID.

The first step in dealing with an unconscious victim is to check the victim's airways to make sure he or she is breathing. If the victim is not breathing, remove any obstruction from the airways and begin artificial respiration or CPR if necessary. Call for medical help, but try not to leave the unconscious person unattended. Do not give food or drinks to anyone who is unconscious.

Ludwig's Angina

A bacterial infection of the mouth and throat that causes swelling that may block the air passages.

Ludwig's angina often follows an infection of the roots of the teeth, such as a tooth abscess. It affects the neck and the surrounding areas. Symptoms include neck pain, swelling and redness, fever, weakness, fatigue, and difficulty in breathing. Close examination may reveal a swollen tongue that is pushed up and back because of the swelling of the neck. The doctor first makes sure the air passages are clear and the breathing is normal. Penicillin is administered intravenously until the swelling subsides and orally afterwards. While this disease is life-threatening when untreated, it is easily medically controlled without complications. *See also* INFECTION.

Lumbar Puncture

Also known as a spinal puncture or spinal tap

Puncture of the spinal cord using a fine needle; used to extract spinal fluid for diagnosis or to inject drugs.

A lumbar puncture is used to remove fluid from the spinal cord for diagnosis. During the procedure, a long needle is inserted into the space between the third and fourth vertebra of the spine. *See* SPINE.

A lumbar puncture is performed in a hospital setting with the patient seated or lying down and with his or her back arched as much as possible. The spinal fluid that is removed during the procedure may then be tested for proteins, glucose, and other chemicals. It may also be cultured and analyzed in a microbiology lab or examined by a doctor for cell abnormalities.

Irregularities of spinal fluid may indicate an infection or cancer (detected in an elevated white blood cell count). Meningitis or leukemia may also be discovered.

After the procedure the patient should rest for the next 12 hours. This prevents additional fluid from seeping from the puncture, resulting in the characteristic headache that follows this procedure.

Lumbosacral Spasm

A prolonged, disproportionate flexing of the muscles that encircle the lower section of the spine.

Lumbosacral spasm causes lower back pain and may sometimes result in an abnormal curvature of the spine (scoliosis). Treatment includes bed rest, painkillers (analgesic drugs), muscle relaxant drugs, joint manipulation by pain management and sports medicine specialists, injections of local anesthetic to treat small areas of muscle spasm, physical therapy and, laser infrared treatment, which has anti-inflammatory and analgesic properties. *See* SPINE.

Lung

The organ that supplies the body with oxygen and removes carbon dioxide from the blood.

The two lungs lie within the ribcage of the chest. Each lung is enclosed in a friction-reducing double membrane, the pleura, within which the lungs expand on inhalation and contract on exhalation. Air enters the lungs through the windpipe (trachea), which divides into two passages (bronchi): right and left. Within the lungs, the bronchi branch into smaller air passages called bronchioles. These end in tiny sacs called alveoli, whose thin walls allow oxygen from the air to diffuse into the blood, while carbon dioxide, the waste product of respiration, passes from blood into the lungs and is expelled. *See also* OXYGEN.

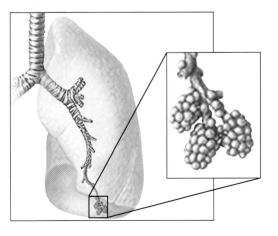

Lungs. The primary organ of the respiratory system, the lungs (at right) supply the body with oxygen. The trachea divides repeatedly into bronchi until each branch reaches the air sacks, the alveoli.

Lung Cancer

Malignant tumor of the lung.

About half of all lung cancers are squamous-cell carcinomas that arise in the lining of the bronchi, the larger airways of the lung. Other types include adenocarcinomas, which arise at the outer edges of the lungs, and large-cell carcinomas, which appear in the smaller bronchi. About a quarter of lung malignancies are classified as small-cell lung cancer. These tend to grow most rapidly and thus are more deadly.

Cause and Incidence. Lung cancer is the second most common cancer in the United States, behind breast cancer, and provides perhaps the clearest cause-and-effect relationship in the study of tumors (oncology). Smoking has been linked to the great majority of lung cancers. Men who smoke are 10 to 17 times more likely to develop lung cancer than non-smokers; women who smoke are five to 10 times more likely to develop lung cancer than non-smokers. The difference in risk between male and female smokers is due to the fact that women tend to smoke fewer cigarettes than men; the risk of developing lung cancer is directly related to the number of cigarettes smoked.

Non-smokers are also at risk if they are exposed to second-hand smoke. Studies have shown that cigarette smoke that is not inhaled and thus passes into the environment is more carcinogenic than smoke that is inhaled. Most cases of lung cancer that are not directly related to cigarette smoking are due to environmental exposure to other substances that damage the lungs. Workers who have been exposed to asbestos have a seven-fold greater risk than the general population. Other environmental pollutants, such as those contained in smog, are also related to the risk of lung cancer.

Early Detection. Lung cancer generally occurs in the later years, most often after 50, because it takes years of exposure to lung-damaging substances to develop the condition. No routine screening test has been found effective in detecting lung cancer at an early stage, but doctors will order periodic sputum analyses or x-ray examinations for smokers in an attempt at early detection.

Symptoms of lung cancer start with breathing difficulty, such as wheezing, coughing, shortness of breath, and the distinctive harsh sound (stridor) that is present in every breath. There may be a persistent cough, hoarseness, coughing up of blood, fatigue, and loss of appetite and weight. The cancer also causes periodic bouts of respiratory diseases, such as pneumonia or bronchitis; bone pain; and persistent headaches.

Diagnosis of lung cancer can start with a physical examination to detect swollen lymph nodes in the neck and neighboring regions, and respiratory sounds that reveal breathing abnormalities. Chest x-rays, computerized tomography (CT) scans, and magnetic resonance imaging (MRI) scans can establish the existence, size, and location of a tumor. With the guidance of these devices, a sample of lung tissue to determine malignancy may be obtained with a needle.

Treatment. For lung cancer detected at an early stage, surgical removal of the tumor and of neighboring tissue to which it may have spread often is effective. Lobectomy, in which the affected part of the lung is removed, or total removal of a lung may be necessary. If surgery is not possible because of a patient's medical condition, radiation therapy may be effective.

Most lung cancers are detected at later

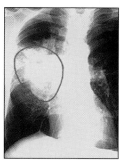

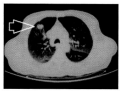

Lung Cancer. Above top, a chest x-ray shows a growth in the lungs. Above, bottom, the CAT scan clearly shows a tumor.

Lung Cancer Clinical Trials

A number of clinical trials using different combinations of surgery, chemotherapy, and radiation therapy are underway at any given time in an effort to find regimens that will improve the survival rate of individuals with lung cancer. Persons diagnosed with lung cancer can ask their physicians about participation in such trials, which can include experimental treatments using new agents developed through biotechnology. The National Cancer Institute and the American Cancer Society are just two sources of information about such clinical trials.

Resources on Lung and Lung Cancer

Crystal, Ronald G., *The Lung: Scientific Foundations* (1997); Crystal, Ronald G., and John B. West *Lung Injury* (1998); Murphy, G., et al., *Informed Decisions: The Complete Book of Cancer Diagnosis, Treatment, and Recovery* (1997); Renneker, Mark, ed., *Understanding Cancer* (1988); Steen, R. Grant, *A Conspiracy of Cells: The Basic Science of Cancer* (1993); Steward, Clifford T., ed., *Cancer: Prevention, Detection, Causes, Treatment* (1988); American Cancer Society, Tel. (800) ACS-2345, Online: www.cancer.org; National Cancer Institue, Tel. (800) 4-CANCER, Online: www.nci.nih.gov; www.nycornell.org/medicine/hematology/index.html.

stages, when surgery will not be effective. In these cases, patients may have surgery followed by radiation therapy, but the majority will have radiation therapy alone or with chemotherapy.

Small-cell lung cancers are treated with combination chemotherapy. A number of different drugs are in clinical use, but studies have not shown a clear difference in results among the various regimens. Patients with small-cell cancers that respond to chemotherapy often experience recurrence of the cancer in a drug-resistant form within several years. The prognosis for most lung cancers that are not detected at a very early stage is not good.

Background material on Lung Cancer can be found in CANCER AND SMOKING. *Related information is contained in* ASBESTOS, BRONCHITIS, CARCINOMA, CHEMOTHERAPY, EMPHYSEMA, LYMPH NODES, MALIGNANT, MRI, ONCOLOGY, SQUAMUS CARCINOMA, STRIDOR AND X-RAY *See also* ADDICTION, BREAST CANCER, PNEUMONIA, PREVENTATIVE MESSURES, PREVENTATIVE MEDICINES, AND RESPIRATORY SYSTEM.

Lung Disease, Chronic Obstructive

Persistent airway obstruction that worsens progressively.

Chronic obstructive lung disease can result from a number of diseases, most notably emphysema and bronchitis. Almost all cases of emphysema are caused by cigarette smoking, which results in the destruction of the smallest working units (alveoli) of the lungs. The results include chronic cough, increasing breathlessness, weight loss, and loss of appetite. Bronchitis, chronic inflammation of the lungs, is also more common in smokers. The symptoms include continued coughing, wheezing, and breathlessness. Emphysema can be relieved by medications (bronchodilators) that widen the airways of the lung. Bronchitis can be treated by inhalant anti-inflammatory drug. Prevention, notably not smoking, is the best treatment. *See also* ANTI-INFLAMMATORY DRUGS; BRONCHITIS; BRONCHODILATOR DRUGS; EMPHYSEMA; *and* NICOTINE.

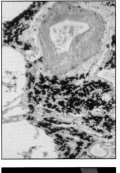

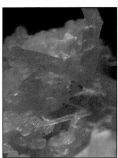

Lung Disease. Above, bottom, bronchioles are the smallest tubes of the lungs. They bring air to the alveoli, where gas exchange occurs. Lung tissue that has been polluted with coal dust particles, top, has been characterized as "black lung" tissue, and is associated with lung cancer.

Lung Imaging

Techniques for directly visualizing the lungs for evidence of disease or disorder.

The most basic lung imaging procedure is the chest x-ray, which can reveal serious ailments of the lung including pneumonia, lung tumors, collapsed lung, fluid in the pleural space (located between the lung and the chest wall), and emphysema.

CT or CAT scanning is an advanced x-ray in which an image of the lung is assembled by computer after a fine radio beam repeatedly scans the tissue from varying angles. Sometimes a dye will be injected to outline features in the subsequent x-rays.

MRI, or magnetic resonance imaging, makes use of a magnetic field rather than x-rays. The subject is placed horizontally in the MRI machine, a tube-like structure in which a magnetic field is generated around the patient. This field causes the nuclei of cells to vibrate. A computer translates this resonance into a high-resolution image.

Ultrasound scanning also uses no x-rays. Sound waves are directed at the lung and reflected back to detectors. Differing tissue density causes variations in the returning ultrasound waves. This technique is used to identify fluid in the pleural space between the lung and chest wall.

Nuclear lung scanning relies on short-lived radioactive particles to image the flow of air and blood through the lungs. Such visualization is ideal for the detection of blood clots in the lungs as well as for screening of the lungs in cancer patients.

Angiography evaluates the blood supply to the lungs. A special dye, which is visible on x-ray, is injected into a blood vessel and its course through the arteries and veins of the lungs is recorded. The technique is used to diagnose pulmonary embolism, a blood clot in the pulmonary artery, which pumps blood from the heart to the lungs.

Background material on Lung Imaging can be found in LUNG AND X-RAY *Related information is contained in* BLOOD CLOTS, CAT SCAN, EMPHYSEMA, MRI, TISSUE SAMPLES, AND ULTRASOUND.

Lung Tumors

Benign or malignant growths in the lung.

Most lung tumors are cancerous and are caused by smoking. Nonmalignant lung tumors are not associated with smoking and generally occur in young adults. The most common form of benign lung tumor is a bronchial adenoma, a growth in the lining of a small airway (bronchiole) of the lung. The symptoms include difficulty breathing and coughing up blood. Less common are lung fibromas, which arise in fibrous tissue, and lipomas, originating in fatty tissue. Severe symptoms are treated by surgical removal of the tumor. *See* LUNG *and* TUMOR.

Lupus Erythematosus

A chronic disease that primarily affects the connective tissue of the joints, although it may manifest in other body systems as well.

The exact origin of lupus erythematosus is unknown, but it is a type of autoimmune disease in which the immune system attacks the synovial membranes found in the joints, causing pain and inflammation. Antinuclear antibodies are found in the blood of all lupus patients. There are two types of the disease: discoid lupus erythematosus (DLE), the milder, begins as a rash and eventually results in scar tissue; systemic lupus erythematosus (SLE) is the more severe form, which affects the joints as well as other systems of the body.

Symptoms. Symptoms of lupus erythematosus include joint pain, swelling, redness, rashes, chest pain, fatigue, fever, and sensitivity to sunlight. Patients generally contract the disease between the ages of 15 and 35. In addition, women are ten times more likely to have the condition.

The severity of lupus ranges from mild to severe, and in some instances it can be fatal. Complications of the disease include internal bleeding, reduced resistance to infection, kidney disease, and severe damage to the joints. It is possible that every system in the body may be affected. There may be periods in which the disease flares up and other times when it appears to be dormant.

Treatment. Corticosteroids and other anti-inflammatory drugs are administered to lessen the swelling and pain in the joints. However, there is no known cure for the condition and the disease can be fatal if the kidneys are affected. Early treatment, especially for those with SLE, is believed to increase life expectancy. *See also* AUTOIMMUNE DISEASE *and* CORTICOSTEROID DRUGS.

Lupus Vulgaris

One of a number of forms of lupus; a chronic, progressive disease that attacks and destroys skin tissues.

Lupus is a term that is used to refer to any chronic skin disease. Lupus vulgaris is a bacterial disease that is rarely seen today. The disease did appear in Europe in the early years of the 20th century. Most of the lesions associated with lupus vulgaris appear on the face and neck. The skin is gradually eroded, leading to serious disfigurement. Ultraviolet light was used to cure the disease around the turn of the 20th century and, more recently, antibacterial drugs have proven effective in its treatment. *See also* ANTIBIOTIC DRUGS; *and* ULTRAVIOLET LIGHT.

Luteal Phase Defect

A defect in the functioning of the corpus luteum that may prevent a fertilized egg from implanting in the uterus.

Once the ovary releases a follicle, the empty shell becomes the corpus luteum. The corpus luteum is responsible for producing progesterone after the embryo implants. Once the placenta matures, it takes over progesterone production. However, if the corpus luteum fails to produce enough of the hormone before this point, a miscarriage occurs. If a woman experiences a miscarriage for this reason, progesterone suppositories should be administered in future pregnancies to prevent reccurrence. *See also* PREGNANCY.

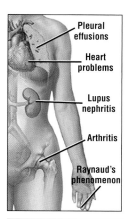

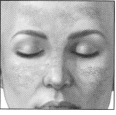

Lupus Erythematosus. A chronic disease that primarily affects the connective tissue of the joints, but can also affect the heart and respiratory systems, above top.
Lupus Vulagaris. A form of lupus that destroys skin tissue, above bottom.

Luteinized Unruptured Follicle Syndrome

The inability of a follicle to release the fertilized egg even after the corpus luteum has formed.

This syndrome occurs when enough luteinizing hormone (LH) is released to cause the follicle to produce progesterone, but not enough LH is present to release the egg through ovulation. In this event, the follicle acts as the corpus luteum. This syndrome often results in luteal phase defects. *See* LUTEINIZING HORMONE *and* OVULATION.

Luteinizing Hormone

One of the gonadotropin hormones.

The gonadotropin hormones are the group of hormones that stimulate activity in the ovaries and testes. Luteinizing hormone (LH), along with follicle-stimulating hormone (FSH), are found in the anterior lobe of the pituitary gland, and are secreted into the blood stream. The hypothalamus begins the chain of events by releasing gonadotrophin releasing hormone (GRH), which is also known as luteinizing hormone-releasing hormone (LH-RH). This activates the pituitary gland, which releases the gonadotrophins. In women, FSH stimulates the development of the follicle and estrogen production; in men it stimulates sperm production. In women, LH helps cause the production of progesterone, and in men it stimulates testosterone. The hypothalamus releases GRH rhythmically after puberty; in women, it bases the timing on the menstrual cycle. Estrogen levels increase throughout this period, and when a certain amount is in the system, LH is released. In men, testosterone levels determine the secretion of GRH and LH. Measurement of LH levels can be used to diagnose the cause of hypogonadism (underactive gonads). High amounts of LH indicate a problem in the ovaries or testes; low levels indicate a problem in the pituitary gland or hypothalamus. *See also* GONADOTROPIN HORMONE.

Luteinizing Hormone-Releasing Hormone

Hormone that causes the secretion of luteinizing hormone.

Luteinizing hormone-releasing hormone (LH-RH) or gonadotrophins (GNRH) is the hormone that causes the release of luteinizing hormone (LH), follicle-stimulating hormone (FSH), the gonadotrophin hormones made in the pituitary. The hypothalamus secretes LH-RH, which stimulates the pituitary gland to release luteinizing hormone and FSH. This hormone then directs the ovaries and testes, the glands responsible for sexual development, to produce estrogen hormones and androgen hormones. The LH-RH is released in rhythmic pulses, based on the levels of estrogen and progesterone in women and the amount of testosterone in men.

A synthetic form of LH-RH is used to treat conditions such as hypergonadism (premature sexual development). The synthetic LH-RH causes an overload of the hormone, which lowers the secretion of GNRH and estrogen and androgen hormones in an attempt to correct the body's balance. LH-RH may also be used as a treatment after surgery to remove uterine fibroids because of its ability to suppress GNRH and estrogen. LH-RH may have some use as a male contraceptive, or as a treatment for prostate and breast cancer.

Luxated Tooth

Dislocated tooth.

A tooth can be knocked loose or even out of its socket from a sharp blow. The sooner the tooth is put back in its correct position, the better the chance that proper healing will take place.

Treatment of a luxated tooth involves manipulation into proper position, application of a dental splint, and in the case of severe damage to the nerve of the tooth, root-canal treatment. *See also* ROOT-CANAL TREATMENT *and* TEETH.

Lyme Disease

Bacterial disease, transmitted through the bite of an infected tick.

Lyme disease is an infection of a spiral-shaped bacterium or spirochete, carried by infected ticks of the ixodes variety, also known as deer ticks. Lyme disease is particularly prevalent along the East Coast of the U.S., although areas of the Midwest and West Coast also have a high incidence.

The ixodes tick, as well as the smaller nymphal tick and even smaller larval tick, may all carry and transmit the spirochetes that produce lyme disease. The smaller ticks are more difficult to detect on the skin and, because of this, are likely to be responsible for the greatest number of transmissions. The longer the bloodsucking parasite is attached to the skin, the greater the chance of disease.

Symptoms. Victims may be unaware of a tick bite. A characteristic rash around the site of the tick bite (erythema migrans) appears in some cases a few days to a few weeks after the bite, and is a key diagnostic indicator of the disease. The rash may expand for several days and show a central clearing. The rash will fade but in some cases recur. As the bacteria spread in the blood and lymphatic system, satellite rashes may appear on different parts of the body. Symptoms are similar to those of many other diseases, making proper diagnosis difficult. Flu-like symptoms sometimes accompany the early phase of lyme disease, including fever and chills, fatigue, headache, stiff neck, sore and aching muscles and joints, backache, nausea and vomiting, sore throat, and swollen glands. Later symptoms may include abnormalities in the brain, nervous system, heart, digestion, reproductive system, and skin. In some cases, the symptoms abate, in others they persist or recur following a period of latency. Diagnosis is based on symptoms and the prevalence of ticks in a given geographic area.

Treatment. Oral antibiotics are often used, though in some cases, intravenous antibiotics are needed. Early treatment may prevent later, more serious, complications. Unfortunately, not all patients respond well to treatment.

Prevention. Long sleeves and pants should be worn in tall grass or brush. Use an anti-tick spray, such as permetherin or DEET, and check the body and clothing frequently. Ticks are often found on the thigh, groin, underarms, backs of knees, behind the ears, and on the neck at the hairline. Immediately remove any attached tick with tweezers. Grasp the tick as close to the skin as possible and carefully pull it straight out. Avoid squeezing the tick, as this will inject bacteria into the skin. Apply antiseptic to the bite and save the tick for identification. *See also* BITE *and* GLANDS.

Lymphangiography

X-ray examination of the lung following the injection of a contrast dye.

Lymphangiography allows the diagnostician to examine the lymphatic system by means of an oil-based dye, which is visible on x-ray. The dye is injected into the hand or foot of the patient, depending on whether the intended object of visualization is located in the upper or the lower section of the body.

The primary use of lymphangiography is to chart the progress of cancers of the lymph, or lymphomas. After the contrast dye has been injected, its course is followed as the lymphatic vessels are filled. The patient may experience tenderness at the point of injection following the procedure, although this discomfort should quickly lessen. Abnormal results of the study, such as incomplete filling of the lymph nodes by the solution, may indicate obstruction of the lymphatic system in the form of lymphatic or metastatic (secondary) tumors. Lymphangiography has been used for assessing the stage of lymphomas due to Hodgkin's disease, though CT or CAT scanning is now the preferred method for performing this assessment. *See also* CANCER; CAT SCAN; *and* LYMPHOMA.

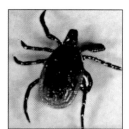

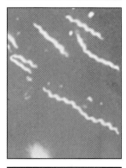

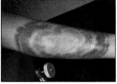

Lyme Disease. Lyme disease is a bacterial disease usually transmitted through the bite of a tick, above top. The bacteria, above middle, first shows up as a rash, near the initial bite, above bottom, but can later effect the heart and nervous system.

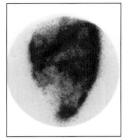

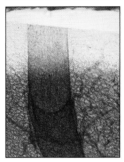

Monoclonal Antibody. Above top, this gamma camera scan was injected with a monoclonal antibody that recognizes colorectal, ovarian, and breast carcinoma (cancer).
Lymph Vessel. Above bottom, the valve preventing backflow is barely visible.

Lymph node tissue. Below, site of frequent skirmishes between the body's defenses and toxic invaders.

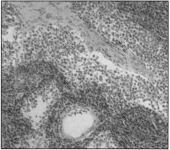

Lymphangioma

Benign lymph-based tumor or lesion that appears on the skin.

Lymphangiomas, like other angiomas, usually are congenital and appear shortly after birth. They are composed of abnormally widened vessels of the lymph system, sometimes intermingled with small blood vessels. Puncturing these vessels produces a colorless fluid.

There are two forms of lymphangioma. In one common form, the growth appears just below the skin, creating a whitish swelling. They usually appear on the neck and can grow large enough to be disfiguring. They are removed surgically in the early years of life. The other class of lymphangioma consists of a cluster of blisters that sometimes is not visible at birth, but becomes apparent as a child grows.

An injury can release blood into the lymphangioma, giving it a reddish tint. Treatment starts with watchful waiting, since many of these lesions disappear spontaneously. If the lesions persist, they can be removed surgically. *See also* ANGIOMA; BENIGN; CONGENITAL; *and* LESION.

Lymphangitis

A bacterial infection of the lymph vessels that carry lymph fluid between the tissues and the lymph nodes.

Bacteria, such as streptococci or staphylococci, can enter the lymph system through a break or cut in the skin or from a skin infection, usually on the arm or leg. They multiply rapidly and produce red streaks that run from the site of infection to the nearest lymph nodes. The lymph nodes become enlarged and sensitive to the touch. If the disease is left untreated, the victim becomes feverish, with chills, a fast heart rate, and headache. The infection progresses rapidly throughout the body. Lymphangitis can usually be treated easily with antibiotics. *See*

also ANTIBIOTIC DRUGS; BACTERIA; INFECTION; *and* LYMPHATIC SYSTEM.

Lymphatic System

The system of vessels and nodules that move extravascular fluids from tissue to the bloodstream.

The lymphatic system plays a major role in the immune system, helping to defend the body against infection and cancer. The system contains many vessels carrying lymph, a fluid made of substances that accumulate outside the blood vessels, including water, excess proteins and other factors, and some foreign substances.

Lymph nodes, which act as filters, lie along the vessels and ducts of the lymphatic system. These nodes remove microorganisms and foreign substances from the lymph. The lymph nodes contain white blood cells known as lymphocytes, which are designed to control or destroy harmful bacteria and viruses. When a part of the body becomes inflamed or affected by illness, the lymph nodes become tender and swollen, sometimes irritated, while they control the spread of the disease.

Disorders. Cancer can be spread through the lymphatic system. A tumor may invade the lymph and send fragments

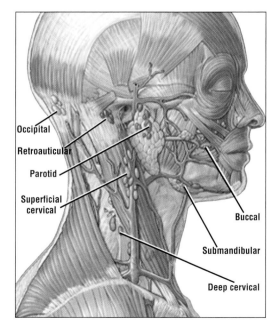

to the lymph nodes, causing the growth of additional tumors. This occurs often in cases of breast cancer, in which the cancer tends to quickly spread to the lymph nodes of the armpit and surrounding areas.

In the condition called lymphedema, the lymphatics become blocked or obstructed, causing one of the limbs to become tense and swollen. *See also* CANCER; LYMPHEDEMA; LYMPHOCYTES; LYMPHOMA; *and* LYMPHOMA, NON-HODGKIN'S.

Lymphedema

Swelling due to obstruction of the lymphatic system.

The lymphatic system contains many vessels that carry lymph, a fluid made of substances that accumulate outside the blood vessels, such as water, excess proteins and other factors, and some foreign substances. The amount of lymph produced increases as a result of injury or burns. When the lymphatic system cannot remove all of it, the area swells, which is known as edema. Usually, such swelling is temporary, because the tissues heal and the blood vessels no longer leak excessively. If the lymphatic system becomes damaged or blocked, however, protein continues to accumulate in the tissues from the blood capillaries, building to dangerous levels when the lymphatics fail to drain, causing chronic swelling. This decreases the amount of oxygen in tissues, disrupts their normal functioning, and impairs the healing process. Tissue often becomes fibrous as a result, and the impaired region feels hot. Stagnant protein combines with the overheated condition to foster bacterial and fungal infections.

Lymphedema typically occurs in the leg or arm, though any region may be affected, including the genitals, the gut, the lungs, and the liver. The disorder may be minimal and persist for many years without complications, but in severe cases it may decrease mobility and may even be life-threatening.

Diagnosis. The condition may allow easy diagnosis from obvious and consistent symptoms. Confirmation can be made through an imaging technique known as lymphoscintigraphy, in which a contrast dye is injected and observed on x-ray as it passes through the lymphatic system.

Symptoms of lymphedema include feeling of constriction and heaviness in the limb; aching buttocks (in leg lymphedema) or pain behind the shoulder (in arm lymphedema); prickling sensation or flashes of pain in the limb; tenderness in the elbow, leg, groin, or knee; pain resembling arthritis in joints; swollen or inflated abdomen (if the leg is affected); and the sensation of warmth in affected areas.

Treatment. Lymphedema is a chronic condition, which can never be completely cured. Treatment is aimed at causing improvement in the limbs. One treatment strategy is known as combined lymphatic therapy, in which several physical therapy techniques are supplemented with drugs known as benzopyrones. Skin care, include massage to release fluid and open passages, bandages, and compression garments to reduce the limb size, are all part of combined lymphatic therapy, as is exercise. If the limbs are disabled, surgery may be needed to remove the swollen tissue and some of the skin around the affected area.

Background material on Lymphedema can be found in LYMPHATIC SYSTEM AND SWELLING.. *Related information is contained in* ALTERNATIVE MEDICINE, Arthritis, Burns, Edema, Liver, Prickly Heat, and Veins, disorders of.

Lymphocytes

White blood cells that move between the lymph system and the blood circulatory system and protect the body against bacteria, viruses, and fungi.

Lymphocytes are among the longest-lived cells of the body. They survive and function for years, if not decades. Lymphocytes move from the lymph system to the blood circulatory system and back in their function as the main part of the body's immune system.

The lymphocytes are the most important of the white blood cells in fighting disease. There are three main types of lymphocytes. B-lymphocytes are made in the bone marrow and produce antibodies, which mark the infectious agents as a danger and then signal other white blood cells to attack and kill the enemy. T-lymphocytes are made in the lymph nodes, thymus, and spleen. They produce antitoxins that counteract the toxins given off by bacteria. Natural killer lymphocytes are cells that attack and destroy target cells identified by the other lymphocytes. *See* LYMPHATIC SYSTEM.

Lymphoma

A malignant tumor of the lymphatic system.

The lymphatic system consists of vessels that carry lymph, a body fluid that plays an important role in the body's immune defense system. Lymphoma is the term that describes an uncontrolled growth of cells of lymphoid tissue. Lymphomas appear most often in the lymph nodes or spleen.

Lymphomas are classified by cell type, the degree of differentiation of the cells, and the pattern of occurrence. Two special forms of lymphoma are Hodgkin's disease and Burkitt's lymphoma. All other forms are referred to as non-Hodgkin's.

The cause of most lymphomas is unknown, but evidence suggests that a virus may be involved. Hodgkin's disease usually occurs in late childhood or after age 60; the incidence of non-Hodgkin's lymphoma increases with age. *See also* CANCER; HODGKIN'S DISEASE; *and* LYMPHATIC SPLEEN.

Lymphoma, Non-Hodgkin's

A cancer of lymphoid tissue.

Lymphomas, cancers of the lymph system, are divided into two broad groups. If certain abnormal cells, called Reed-Sternberg cells, are present, the cancer is classified as Hodgkin's disease; if those cells are not present, it is classified as non-Hodgkin's lymphoma. In turn, non-Hodgkin's lymphoma is classified as low-, medium- or high-grade, depending on the rate of growth. Rate of growth is not necessarily associated with prognosis; some high-grade cases respond better to treatment than some low-grade lymphomas. The incidence of non-Hodgkin's lymphoma has increased substantially in recent decades, primarily because it often occurs in persons whose immune defenses are weakened by HIV, the virus that causes AIDS.

Symptoms. The first symptom of non-Hodgkin's lymphoma is often painless swelling of lymph nodes in the neck, the groin and under the arms. Subsequent symptoms vary according to the parts of the lymph system that are affected. General symptoms can include persistent fever and fatigue, night sweats, and weight loss. In advanced stages of the disease, the liver and spleen become enlarged. If the gastrointestinal tract is involved, symptoms include nausea, vomiting, and abdominal pain. If the bone marrow is involved, symptoms resemble those of anemia, such as fatigue, rapid heartbeat, pallor, and recurrent infections. Urinary tract involvement can result in kidney failure, anemia, fatigue, and loss of appetite.

Diagnosis of non-Hodgkin's lymphoma is achieved through examination of tissue samples from lymph nodes; blood tests; x-rays of the chest, liver, bones and spleen, CT scans; and lymphangiography, x-rays of the lymph nodes.

Treatment depends on the classification of the disease and the stage at which it is detected. Localized low-grade lymphoma can be treated with radiation therapy of the affected area, which sometimes is enough to bring about long-term remissions or cure. Chemotherapy, using single agents or a combination of drugs, may be done in combination with radiation therapy. For medium-grade lymphoma, radiation therapy usually is combined with chemotherapy, using a combination of drugs. High-grade lymphoma is treated with an aggressive combination chemo-therapy. The five-year survival rate for non-Hodgkin's lymphoma is about 50 percent. *See also* CANCER; CAT SCAN; LYMPHOMA; *and* LYMPHATIC SYSTEM.

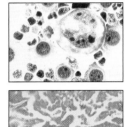

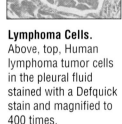

Lymphoma Cells.
Above, top, Human lymphoma tumor cells in the pleural fluid stained with a Defquick stain and magnified to 400 times.
Follicular Lymphoma.
Above, bottom, micrograph of a follicular non-Hodgkin's lymphoma, cancer of lymph tissue.

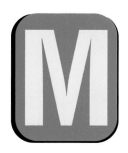

Macrobiotics

Group of vegetarian based diets with varying restrictions.

Macrobiotics refers to a variety of diets in which permitted foods vary, although there is often an emphasis on grains, and local, unprocessed produce. The focus of most macrobiotic diets is vegetarian; specific dietary restrictions vary greatly. Extreme forms that permit only rice or other grains and limit liquids are dangerous and nutritionally unbalanced, and can cause malnutrition if followed for an extended period. People following an extremely rigid macrobitoic diet benefit from vitamin supplements. Less restrictive forms generally allow for more balanced nutrition, although vitamin B_{12} and B_2, calcium, and iron may be lacking. *See also* DIET *and* DISEASE.

Macroglossia

An enlarged tongue.

An abnormally large or swollen tongue is usually a feature of conditions such as Down's syndrome or of hormone disorders such as acromegaly or hypothyroidism. Tumors on the tongue may also lead to macroglossia, as can amyloidosis, a rare condition that causes the buildup of a substance called amyloid (a mixture of protein and starch) in the organs and tissues.

The only treatment for macroglossia is to resolve the underlying condition. *See also* ACROMEGALY; DOWN'S SYNDROME; TONGUE; TONGUE, CANCER OF; *and* SWELLING.

Macular Degeneration

A progressive retinal disorder that causes vision loss.

Age-related macular degeneration (AMD) is a painless condition that affects 10 million Americans. One out of five adults between the ages of 60 and 75 develop macular degeneration. After age 75, one in three people develop the disorder.

Macular degeneration results from the destruction of light-sensitive cells (photocells) in the centrally-located macula region of the retina of the eye. The photoreceptors in the macula are responsible for fine, sharp vision, essential for reading and driving. Both eyes are usually affected, either simultaneously or separately.

TYPES

There are two types of macular degeneration. In the wet type, circular scar tissue forms, often surrounded by a hemorrhage. Degradation begins with an incomplete breakdown of the insulating band between the retina and the choroid strip of blood vessels behind the retina. Fluid begins to leak, and newly replaced blood vessels destroy the retinal nerve tissue, leaving scar tissue. A blind spot develops and enlarges, causing partial obliteration of the central field of vision.

In the dry (atropic) type, a pigment is deposited in the macula unaccompanied by scars, leakage, or blood

Amsler Grid

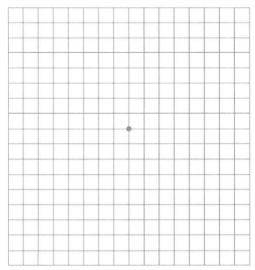

CAUSES

The cause for macular degeneration is unknown. Its prevalence in some families, indicates that the disease has a possible genetic component. Smoking is considered a risk factor.

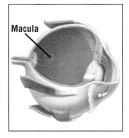

Macular Degeneration. An Amsler grid is used to check for macular degeneration, a condition that destroys light-sensitive cells in the macula (see diagram left). To test yourself, place this page on a flat surface in good light. Wearing reading glasses or contact lenses, cover one eye and look at the dot at the center of the grid from 12 to 15 inches away; repeat with your other eye. If any of the lines on the grid appear wavy, the condition should be discussed with an opthamologist.

TREATMENT

In early stages of the disease, laser treatment may prevent new blood vessels from growing around the macula, limiting the progression of the disease. There is no specific treatment, although regular monitoring of the disease by an ophthalmologist is recommended.

There is no effective prevention for macular degeneration either, but regular eye exams can help maintain a healthy retina. People with a family history of macular degeneration should avoid smoking. *See also* BLIND SPOT; BLURRED VISION; EYE; LASER; LASER TREATMENT; *and* VISION.

Magnesium

Mineral that makes up part of every cell and aids in carbohydrate metabolism

Magnesium is essential to the function of every living cell. It plays a key role in the manufacture of DNA and protein, bone building, muscle function, and the transmission of nerve impulses. It is also instrumental in releasing energy from glycogen stored in the muscles.

The recommended daily allowance of magnesium is 400 milligrams. Sources include leafy green vegetables, dried peas and beans, soybeans, seeds, nuts, whole grains, meat, poultry, fish, and eggs, as well as drinking water (except for soft water). Magnesium is often taken with calcium.

Deficiency. Because of its abundance in numerous food sources, magnesium deficiency is quite unusual. It occasionally occurs in individuals who have an underlying disorder that impairs magnesium absorption or metabolism, such as alcoholism, severe diabetes mellitus, liver disease, kidney disease, or prolonged diarrhea or vomiting. Heavy use of diuretics may also lead to magnesium deficiency.

Symptoms of deficiency include depression, insomnia, muscle weakness, tremor, nausea, irregular heartbeat, a prickly or burning sensation, and convulsions.

Overdose. A toxic dose of magnesium is 6000 milligrams. An overdose can cause calcium and phosphorus depletion. Symptoms include fatigue, diarrhea, slurred speech, profuse sweating, unsteadiness, decreased tendon reflexes, abnormal heart rhythms and, occasionally, paralysis. Toxic intake rarely occurs unless as a result of the ingestion of excessive amounts of magnesium-based antacids, laxatives, or megadoses of supplements. *See also* MINERAL.

Magnetic Therapy

Applying magnets to areas of the body in order to relieve pain and promote healing.

Magnetic fields can be found, among other places, in magnets, such as those found on refrigerators, and in electromagnetic devices that send a charge through a coil. These fields affect and are affected by anything with an electric or magnetic charge.

All living things contain cells with weak electric charges. Nerve signals are actually small electrical impulses passed along nerve pathways, and the maintenance of a proper balance of water and other substances in the cells is controlled in part by the exchange of charged particles of sodium and potassium.

It is certain that the application of a magnetic field has some effect on the body. Magnetic resonance imaging (MRI) scanning is based on measuring minute reaction of cells in the body to an applied magnetic field. In magnetic therapy, practitioners use the body's response to an applied magnetic field as a medical therapy. In general, the magnetic field is supposed to increase blood flow and relax muscles.

Magnetic therapy is touted to relieve pain, particularly pain associated with muscle cramps and spasms.

Magnets are, for the most part, free of side effects, although it is not known whether they have any adverse long-term effects. People with pacemakers or defibrillators should not wear magnets or go very near a person wearing magnets, as they may interfere with the functioning of these electronic devices. *See also* ALTERNATIVE MEDICINE; MRI; *and* MUSCLE.

Malabsorption

Inability of the body to absorb essential nutrients as the result of a variety of medical conditions.

In malabsorption, ingested foods enter the small intestine, are inadequately absorbed, continue through to the colon, and are excreted. As a result, the body does not receive enough nutrition from the vitamins, minerals, carbohydrates, fat, and protein in the diet.

SYMPTOMS

The most frequent indicator of malabsorption syndrome is steatorrhea, stools containing excess fat, which are oily, frothy, and foul-smelling. Deficiencies of nutrients such as calcium, folic acid, and vitamins A, D, E, and K will develop if the malabsorption is not treated. Symptoms can include scaling of the skin (hyperkeratosis) from vitamin A deficiency; bruising and blood in the urine from vitamin K deficiency; and bone pain, muscle spasms, numbness, tingling, and even bone fractures from vitamin D and calcium deficiencies.

CAUSES

While symptoms of malabsorption syndrome are fairly similar, causes for the disorder may vary. Some of the more common causes include:
- celiac sprue, in which the small intestine becomes damaged as a result of an inability to digest gluten;
- food intolerances;
- bacterial overgrowth in the intestine;
- amyloidosis, in which the body accumulates abnormal amounts of the protein amyloid;
- whipple's disease, a bacterial infection of the intestine;
- crohn's disease, chronic inflammation of the intestine;
- short-bowel syndrome, in which more than half of the small intestine is diseased or has been surgically removed;
- cystic fibrosis; and
- chronic pancreatitis.

TREATMENT

Treatment involves identifying and addressing the underlying disorder. Fat-soluble vitamins and other nutritional supplements may ameliorate some symptoms.

Information about related disorders can be found in AMYLOIDOSIS; CELIAC SPRUE; CROHN'S DISEASE; CYSTIC FIBROSIS; FOOD INTOLERANCE; *and* WHIPPLE'S DISEASE. *Treating underlying causes involves* FOLIC ACID, VITAMIN CALCIUM A; VITAMIN D; VITAMIN E; *and* VITAMIN K.

Malalignment

Abnormalities in teeth organization.

Malalignment can consist of rotation, overlapping, or abnormal spacing of the teeth. The teeth may not meet when the jaw closes, or the top or bottom teeth may jut out. Sometimes, the teeth meet but are individually crooked. Teeth can be malaligned for any of a number of reasons. Most often, they simply grow in crooked— a condition known as malocclusion. Injuries to the teeth or jaw and jaw growth problems can also cause malalignment.

Orthodontics can improve the alignment of teeth and the bite (occlusion). Occasionally, an orthodontist works with an oral and maxilofacial surgeon to realign the jaws and teeth. *See also* MALOCCLUSION *and* ORTHODONTICS.

Malar Flush

Heightened color over the cheekbones that is accompanied by a bluish tinge.

Malar flush is a diagnostic indicator of mitral stenosis, the narrowing of the heart valve that controls blood flow between the left ventricle and the left atrium of the heart. This condition reduces the oxygen content of the blood, causing the unusual tinge of the facial tissue. Malar flush alone is not a conclusive sign of mitral stenosis; malar flush can occur in people without mitral stenosis, and, likewise, mitral stenosis may not always manifest malar flush. *See also* MITRAL STENOSIS.

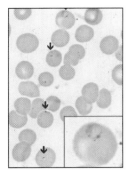

Malarial cells.
Pictured above is a magnification of a malarial cell. Malaria is commonly transmitted by a mosquito bite, affects the red blood cells, causing aches, chills, and fever.

Malaria

Tropical disease caused by a protozoan parasite, transmitted by mosquito.

Malaria is a tropical disease that affects the red blood cells. It is caused by any of four species of *plasmodium*, a single-celled parasite known as a protozoan. The four species of plasmodium—*falciparum, vivax, ovale,* and *malariae,* produce four variants of malaria with somewhat distinct symptoms.

If promptly diagnosed and treated, malaria is curable, though the emergence of multi-drug resistant strains of the parasite hampers eradication in some areas. The disease is of particular danger to pregnant women, as it can cause severe anemia and sometimes maternal death.

TRANSMISSION

Malaria can be spread through infected blood transfusions or contaminated needles, but the primary means of transmission is through the bite of an infected anopheles mosquito. The presence of infected mosquitoes in a geographic region often coincides with the rainy season. Over 90 percent of all malaria cases are now confined to sub-Saharan Africa.

The cycle of malaria begins when a female mosquito bites someone who carries the disease. The parasites are taken up with ingested blood into the mosquito's salivary gland. The disease may then be passed to the next person bitten by the mosquito. Once in the human bloodstream, the parasites migrate to the liver, where they multiply. After maturing in the liver over a period of two to four weeks, the parasites then emerge and enter the victim's red blood cells. Here they continue to multiply, eventually causing the blood cells to rupture.

SYMPTOMS

Malarial symptoms begin from 10 to 35 days after the plasmodium parasite enters the system. Early symptoms may be mistaken for the flu; they include a low fever, headaches and muscle aches, chills, and

general malaise. Subsequent symptoms vary with the type of malaria.

Vivax and ovale malaria symptoms often begin suddenly, with aching and chills followed by sweating and intermittent fever. Periods of fever last one to eight hours, and attacks tend to recur every 48 hours. These forms of malaria remain in the liver if untreated; mature parasites are released periodically into the bloodstream, causing a relapse of symptoms. In vivax malaria, delirium sometimes occurs due to high fever.

Falciparum malaria also begins with chills. Body temperature gradually rises and then suddenly plummets. The initial attack may persist for 20 to 36 hours before subsiding; it then recurs every 36 to 70 hours. Symptoms are similar to vivax and ovale malaria but tend to be more severe. Falciparum parasites leave the liver but may remain for months in the bloodstream if not properly treated. Patients infected by plasmodium falciparum may develop cerebral malaria, a potentially fatal illness characterized by high fever, drowsiness, delirium, and confusion.

Malariae malaria begins suddenly, with symptoms resembling vivax malaria but recurring every 72 hours. If left untreated, this form of malaria can remain in the bloodstream for years, causing periodic renewed attacks.

All four forms of malaria produce an increase in white blood cells (lymphocytes and monocytes), as well as anemia and low platelet counts. If untreated, jaundice and enlargement of the spleen and liver may develop. Vivax, ovale, and malariae cases subside on their own in 10 to 30 days but may recur periodically. Untreated falciparum is fatal in 20 percent of cases.

DIAGNOSIS

Where malaria is endemic, flu-like symptoms without definite cause suggest infection. Enlargement of the spleen is also indicative.

Diagnosis is confirmed through a blood test that identifies the presence of the specific plasmodium parasite. The test may be repeated if they are inconclusive, as the blood level of plasmodium varies over time.

TREATMENT

The regimen of treatment for malaria is dependent on the specific strain, taking into account any drug resistances. Generally, quinine, taken either orally or intravenously (quinidine), remains the treatment of choice for falciparum malaria. Other forms usually require chloroquine followed by primaquine.

PREVENTION

When traveling to regions known for malaria, the following preventative steps should be taken: wear protective clothing, leaving as little exposed skin as possible; use long-lasting insect repellents; and use nettings and screens to keep mosquitoes out of sleeping areas. Drugs such as chloroquine may be taken to prevent malaria, though certain strains of falciparum are resistant. Vaccines against malaria are currently in development.

Signs of malaria in areas of infestation should be reported to a doctor at once. Initially, those suspecting infection may treat themselves with pyrimethamine-sulfadoxine until medical help is found.

> *Background information about Malaria can be found in* INFECTIOUS DISEASE; TRAVEL MEDICINE; *and* TROPICAL DISEASE. *Vital information about treatment options is included in the entries on* PUBLIC HEALTH; TRAVEL IMMUNIZATION; *and* VACCINATION. *Related topics are discussed in* TRAVELER'S DIARRHEA; TSETSE FLY BITES; *and* YAWS.

Malignant

Resistant to treatment, progressively worsening, and life-threatening.

Malignant is a term used to categorize a condition that tends to worsen steadily, often resulting in death. The term is most commonly used in describing cancer. In the study and treatment of abnormal growths (oncology), the term is applied to tumors that grow uncontrollably, invade neighboring tissue, and send colonies to other parts of the body. It is contrasted with benign disorders or tumors, which remain mild and controllable. *See also* CANCER.

Mallet Toe

A toe that curls under itself.

The cause of mallet toe is unknown. It may affect more than one toe, but usually is not found in the big toe. Pressure from shoes may cause corns to develop on the curled toe's tip. Though orthopedic pads can help this condition, surgery is usually the best way to correct this condition. *See also* FOOT.

Mallory-Weiss Syndrome

Laceration or tear of the lower esophagus and the upper part of the stomach, causing the retching of blood.

Mallory-Weiss Syndrome occurs as a result of forceful vomiting. Excessive bouts of drinking followed by vomiting can increase the risk of this occurrence, along with violent coughing attacks, or epileptic convulsions. Such attacks can cause severe contractions in the diaph-ragm, resulting in damage to the lower esophagus. Mallory-Weiss syndrome is the cause of five percent of all cases of upper gastrointestinal bleeding.

Symptoms. The primary symptoms of Mallory-Weiss Syndrome are the vomiting of blood or the passage of tarry black stools, which indicate bleeding in the upper intestine.

Treatment. Most episodes of bleeding stop on their own, but sometimes it is necessary to tie off an artery or inject vasopressin (also known as anti-diuretic hormone) to constrict the blood vessel. The tear usually heals in about ten days without special treatment, but will occasionally need to be repaired using an endoscope. Acid-suppressing medications may be administered, as will blood transfusions in the event of severe blood loss.

Prevention. Efforts to minimize coughing and vomiting, as well as avoiding large amounts of alcohol, may prevent Mallory-Weiss syndrome. *See also* ESOPHAGUS; GASTROENTEROLOGY; GASTROINTESTINAL BLEEDING; GASTROINTESTINAL TRACT; *and* VOMITING.

Resources on Malaria & Infectious Diseases

Butcher, G.A., *Malaria: The Intelligent Traveller's Guide* (1990) Despommier, Dickson D., et al., *Parasitic Disease* (1995); Litsios, Socrates, *The Tomorrow of Malaria* (1996); Shaw, Michael, ed., *Everything You Need to Know About Diseases* (1996); Centers for Disease Contol and Prevention, Tel. (800) 311-3435, Online: www.cdc.gov; Infectious Disease Society of America, Tel. (703) 299-0200, Online: www.idsociety.org; Nat. Institute of Allergy and Infectious Disease, Tel. (301) 496-5717, Online: www.niaid.nih.org; Office of Rare Diseases, Tel. (301) 402-4336, Online: rarediseases.info.nih.gov/ www.nycornell.org/medicine/infectious/index.html

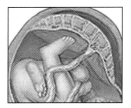
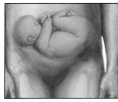
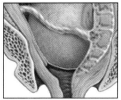
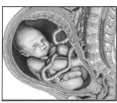

Malpresentation.
A Cesarean section is often performed because of a malpresentation. Above, several of the ways a fetus can be malpresented: Top, an instance of placenta previa, in which the placenta has torn away from the uterine wall; second from top, transverse position; third from top, placenta abruptio, in which the placenta is blocking the area of the birth canal; bottom, breech position, in which the fetus is head up, reversed from the normal fetal position in the womb.

Malocclusion

Misalignment of the teeth.

In a well functioning bite, or occlusion, the upper and lower teeth are properly aligned and fit well together when the jaw is closed. When the teeth don't fit together comfortably, often because of crowding or excessive spacing, dentists call it malocclusion.

Underbite and overbite are the two most recognizable types of malocclusion. In underbite, the bottom teeth jut out, while in overbite, the top teeth are prominent. Malocclusion can also refer to top and bottom teeth that do not close properly when the jaw closes.

Not all malocclusion is cause for concern or results in problems such as inflammation, soreness, or excessive wearing of the teeth, but many may interfere with proper functioning. From a medical standpoint, malocclusion is serious when the misalignment does not allow proper function of the teeth. Where malocclusion does not interfere with proper functioning, treatment may be chosen for cosmetic reasons.

Most malocclusion problems are treated by orthodontists. Teeth may be straightened through braces or other devices that gradually work the teeth into a different position (orthodontics). If a tooth is crowding other teeth into misalignment, it may be removed. Occasionally, surgical alignment of the jaws may also be needed. *See also* ORTHODONTIC APPLIANCE.

Malpresentation

An abnormal position of a fetus in the uterus.

From about the seventh month of pregnancy until birth, most babies are positioned head down and are born head first with the face toward the mother's back, a position known as occiput anterior.

A baby in the breech position is situated so that its feet or buttocks are located near the cervix. As a result, these are the first body parts to emerge from the birth canal in a breech birth.

In the occiput posterior, the baby is positioned head down but its face is turned toward the mother's front, making delivery difficult as the baby passes through the birth canal.

Transverse presentation is when the baby is positioned sideways in the uterus, with its head on one side of the mother's abdomen and its feet on the other. The shoulder is usually blocking the birth canal, making vaginal delivery impossible.

Treatment. In cases of malpresentation, a doctor may try to shift the baby's orientation. A forceps delivery or a Cesarean section may be necessary. *See also* DELIVERY.

Mammalgia

Also known as mastodynia or mastalgia

Pain or discomfort in one or both of the breasts.

Most causes of mammalgia are benign, such as breast tenderness during puberty, pregnancy, and menopause. Breast pain may also occur as a side effect of some drugs or be a symptom of disorders such as herpes zoster or alcoholic liver damage. If breast pain is severe or accompanied by discharge from the nipples, a physician should be consulted. *See also* BREAST.

Mammary Duct

Tubes in the breast that carry milk to the nipples.

After giving birth, a woman produces breast milk (lactates) and may choose to breast-feed her infant. Milk is secreted from glandular tissue in the breasts known as lobules and travels through the mammary ducts to the nipples. About 20 ducts open onto each nipple. The mammary ducts also have wider areas (reservoirs) where milk can be stored. The lobules and ducts form the glandular tissue of the breast; they are covered by a layer of fatty tissue, which contributes to the breast's smooth appearance. Spontaneous discharge from the mammary ducts can be a sign of a serious underlying condition. *See also* BREAST; MILK; *and* NIPPLE.

Mammography

An x-ray examination of the breast performed to screen for breast cancer.

Mammography is a screening technique for the early detection of breast cancer; it is also used to search for breast cancer in the event of observed breast abnormalities. This non-invasive procedure uses low-level x-rays to examine breast tissue for possible signs of malignancy. The low radiation dose is not believed to pose significant long-term health risks. Since mammography is highly sensitive to abnormalities, subsequent tests, including ultrasound, MRI, and removal of tissue for analysis (biopsy), are often required if a possible cancer is detected.

Many physicians recommend regular mammogram tests for women after age 40. Between the ages of 35 and 40, women are encouraged to have a mammogram to establish a baseline, which allows for more accurate evaluation of later examinations. Healthy women below age 30 rarely receive a mammogram, since the risk of cancer at this time is generally low.

Women with one or more risk factors for breast cancer should regularly perform self-examination and receive mammography. Along with the risk of contracting breast cancer with age, women who have previously had breast cancer, or have first degree relatives with cancer, have been diagnosed with certain benign breast abnormalities, are of African American descent, or become

pregnant after age 35, are considered to be at a higher risk for breast cancer.

Procedure. The breasts are examined individually with equipment specifically designed for mammography. A breast is compressed between a film plate and a special paddle; the compression enables a more accurate reading.

Effectiveness. When performed regularly at one and two year intervals, mammography can reduce breast cancer deaths by 25 to 35 percent. In addition to (but not replacing) mammography, monthly breast self-examination can help with early detection of lumps or irregularities of the breast.

Treatment. Detection of malignancy generally requires removal of the cancerous tissue in a process known as lumpectomy. During this surgery, tissue is also removed from the lymph nodes, to see if the cancer has spread.

See also BIOPSY; BREAST; BREAST CANCER; BREAST LUMP; BREAST TENDERNESS; BREAST, DISORDERS OF; *and* MALIGNANT; *for more information about breasts and related disorders. Breast diagnostic procedures are also discussed in* BREAST SELF-EXAMINATION; THERMOGRAPHY; ULTRASOUND; *and* ULTRASOUND SCANNING. *See* GYNECOLOGY.

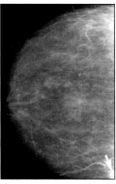

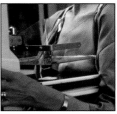

Mammography.
The x-ray above shows a mammogram of a fatty breast with an obvious cancer indicated by an arrow. The photo below, shows a woman's breast being compressed to get the optimum mammographic image.

Screening Recommendations for Individuals with Breast Cancer

The National Cancer Institute provides the following recommendations for mammography screenings:

- Women age 40 or older should receive screening mammograms every one to two years.
- Women at increased risk for breast cancer may benefit from earlier or more frequent screening. They should consult a physician about when to begin mammograms and how often to be screened.
- Starting at around age 20, women should receive clinical breast exams as part of regular, routine health care.

Mammoplasty

Cosmetic surgery performed on breasts.

Mammoplasty may be performed to reduce breast size (reduction mammoplasty), to increase breast size (augmentation mammoplasty), to raise the breasts' center of gravity (mastopexy), or to reconstruct one or both breasts after damage from an accident or after removal by a mastectomy.

Mammoplasty is performed under general anesthesia and requires a two-night hospital stay. The incisions produce scars that are highly visible for about a year and then fade somewhat; care is taken to make incisions in minimally visible areas, such as along the bottom contour of the breasts. In addition to the standard risks of surgery and general anesthesia, there are risks of scarring, loss of sensation, and an inability to breast-feed. *See also* BREAST SURGERY.

Mania

An episode of heightened mood characterized by improved self-esteem, increased energy, decreased need for sleep, impulsiveness, poor judgment, and grandiosity.

During a manic episode, an individual's mood is high, energy is increased, and need for sleep is reduced. The mood elevation can range from mild to extreme, but the primary characteristic is that mania is out of control, with destructive elements that can lead to problems with relationships and work. A person in a manic period may feel infallible, exhibit out-of-control spending, engage in unprotected sex, or take on projects well above his or her limits. At its most extreme, a mania may result in drug abuse, financial disaster, severe (or life-threatening) aggression, and social or professional recklessness.

Manic episodes tend to begin in young adulthood and recur more often if left untreated. The duration of these episodes varies from a few days to a few months. Most patients who experience manic episodes also experience alternating periods of depression, in a condition known as bipolar disorder. Mania is most dangerous when it alternates or becomes intermixed with periods of depression without intervening normal moods. Manic or depressive episodes that occur four or more times per year are known as rapid cycling and can be especially difficult to treat.

Mania occurs in about one to two percent of the population. There is no laboratory test for diagnosing mania, making its diagnosis dependent on its visible clinical and behavioral features. Because the feelings of elation are usually pleasurable, mania may be considered by the sufferer to be simply a desirable and normal change of mood. The destructive aspects of mania and the fact that the mood represents a chemical imbalance make it important to seek treatment, which usually consists of a combination of psychotherapy and drug treatment.

When mania occurs for the first time later in life, it may be a sign of problems with medication or brain disease. Some of the symptoms of mania may also indicate an impulse control disorder.

See also BIPOLAR DISORDER; DEPRESSION; IMPULSE CONTROL DISORDERS; *and* MOOD DISORDERS DEPRESSION *for background information. Articles on treatment options include* ANTIDEPRESSANT DRUGS; PROZAC; *and* PSYCHOTHERAPY.

Manometry

Technique for determining liquid or gaseous pressure in the body.

Manometry is done with a an instrument known as a manometer, which may consist of a glass tube filled with water, oil, or mercury. It may also come in the form of a coiled spring, a diaphragm, or an electrical device. Manometers measure blood pressure and fluid pressure in the skull and spine. Most often, the instrument is used to determine esophageal pressure as a means of diagnosing abnormalities in the contractions of the esophagus, the organ used to propel food to the stomach. It is also possible during manometry to test the esophagus for pH levels. *See also* ACID REFLUX; BLOOD PRESSURE; ESOPHAGUS; *and* PH.

Marasmus

An advanced type of protein and calorie malnutrition (PCM) characterized by progressive wasting.

Marasmus is the single greatest health danger to children worldwide. Approximately half of all children in underdeveloped countries suffer from primary protein and calorie malnutrition.

Marasmus usually occurs in infants under one year old who are not breast-fed, and whose bottle-feeding is insufficient. This may be due to the use of contaminated water or of diluted, improperly sterilized, or unrefrigerated formula. Marasmus may also occur as as a secondary result of an acute disease (especially one involving chronic diarrhea), a malabsorption syndrome, or failure to thrive.

An infant with marasmus usually develops chronic, profuse diarrhea and mineral imbalances. Children with the condition appear emaciated and are often apathetic and hypersensitive. If marasmus is prolonged and severe, surviving children often suffer lasting developmental impairment. *See also* DIARRHEA; FAILURE TO THRIVE; KWASHIORKOR; *and* MALABSORPTION.

March Fracture

Break in the foot (metatarsal) bone due to repeated jarring.

The metatarsals are the long bones in the foot that connect the heel to the toes. The march stress fracture is so named because it is a common injury for soldiers on long marches. It is usually caused by extended periods of running or walking on hard surfaces. The second and third metatarsal bones are the ones most often affected. Symptoms include pain and swelling. Rest and immobilization of the foot in a cast are the usual treatments. *See also* FRACTURE.

Marfan's Syndrome

A hereditary disorder of varying severity that results in weakened connective tissues in the body.

Marfan's syndrome is inherited as an autosomal dominant trait; a child who inherits the gene for the disorder from only one parent will exhibit the disorder. It may also appear spontaneously. The incidence for Marfan's syndrome is about one in 10,000.

The most recognizable characteristics of Marfan's syndrome affect the skeletal system. Most individuals have tall, lanky frames with long arms, as well as long, spidery fingers (arachnodacytly), and a sunken or protruding breastbone.

Like some other diseases associated with skeletal abnormalities, Marfan's syndrome causes the white of the eye to appear blue. Other eye abnormalities include nearsightedness and lens dislocation. Cardiovascular abnormalities pose the most serious problems and may include:

- enlargement of the base of the aorta;
- aortic regurgitation, in which some blood washes back into the left ventricle when the heart pumps;
- prolapsed mitral valve, in which the mitral valve is loose or malformed;
- dissecting aortic aneurysm, in which the aorta becomes so thin that it rips, requiring immediate surgical repair.

There is no cure for Marfan's syndrome. Treatment is primarily focused on correcting vision and treating and preventing complications from heart abnormalities. Depending on the severity of heart problems, surgery may be necessary and can extend life expectancy. *See also* HEART; SKELETON; *and* VISION.

Marijuana

An illegal drug that causes a feeling of calm and relaxation.

Marijuana is made from the dried leaves and flowers of a species of hemp plant. It is a mind-altering drug whose psychoactive ingredient is THC (tetrahydrocannabinol). Lower doses cause a feeling of calm, while higher doses may result in anxiety or paranoia and, sometimes, trigger a psychotic episode. Marijuana is not physically addictive, but long-term use is linked to a lack of motivation.

Marijuana has been found to be a useful anti-nausea drug for people undergoing chemotherapy or receiving treatment for AIDS. As a result, some states are legalizing it for this medicinal purpose. *See also* AIDS; CHEMOTHERAPY; *and* DRUG ABUSE.

Marital Counseling

Therapy for married couples or long-term partners that aims to improve communication between individuals and resolve relationship difficulties.

As opposed to individual therapy, marital counseling often sets aside personal problems of the individuals in a relationship in order to focus on their relationship and its dynamics. This is sometimes seen as a hin-

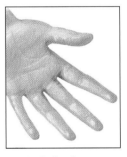

Marfan's Syndrome. The diagram, above shows long, spidery fingers (arachnodacytly), one of the characteristics of Marfan's syndrome. Marfan's is an inherited disorder that affects the skeletal system.

drance to progress and has led to accusations that marital counseling is a superficial form of therapy. Yet studies indicate that a therapeutic environment is conducive to transforming patterns of communication, clarifying core issues, and revealing each partner's participation in relationship dynamics. Usually, couples attend sessions together, though at times a counselor may find it beneficial to meet with either partner separately. *See also* PSYCHOANALYSIS.

Marsupialization

A surgical procedure used to drain an abscess or cyst.

In marsupialization, an incision is made to open an abscess or cyst and the edges of the incision are stitched together to form a pouch. The pouching keeps the wound open until it heals. This procedure is used on the Bartholin's gland (located on either side of the vaginal entrance) and on certain pancreatic cysts. *See also* CYST.

Masochism

A form of sexual behavior in which a person is aroused by being physically injured or humiliated.

While most sexual deviations, including exhibitionism, pedophilia, and voyeurism, occur more often in men, masochism occurs more often in women. The point at which normal behavior becomes dysfunctional is difficult to discern in sexual matters. Generally, if both partners are adults and consent to play a role that is not physically or emotionally harmful to either one, the behavior is not considered dysfunctional.

Most masochists tend not to seek treatment, as they consider the deviation to be an integral part of their behavior, and a passion that is undesirable to eliminate. Behavior in a child that may be viewed as masochistic or self-harming, such as self-cutting, is not a sign of masochism but rather indicates another, serious problem, such as depression or abuse. *See also* SADISM.

Massage Therapy

Rubbing and kneading the muscles and joints to reduce stiffness and pain.

Massage is a therapeutic technique employed to increase the circulation of blood to the muscles and joints. It uses modified amounts of pressure and friction, depending on the circumstances. It is usually performed manually. Massage can relieve stress and anxiety and can increase blood supply to the tissues. It is effective in promoting general health and energy levels, rehabilitating muscle and sports injuries, and relieving painful muscle spasms.

Massage can be a useful in treating a nerve-damaged patient. It reduces pain by the application of counter-pressure and can alleviate the irritation of nerve endings in the skin. Researchers have suggested that infant massage increases the development of the nerves, brain, and muscles. In a similar manner, massage therapy is gaining increasing popularity for neurologically impaired adults. *See also* ALTERNATIVE MEDICINE *and* MUSCLE.

Mast Cell

A type of cell, present in most areas of the body, that is involved in allergic reactions.

In an allergic reaction, antibodies bind with an antigen in the body. Mast cells are then stimulated to release several biologically active substances, including the chemical histamine. Histamine causes the sneezing and the itchiness and watering of the eyes that is associated with respiratory allergies. *See* ALLERGY; ALLERGEN, *and* ANTIGEN.

Mastectomy

A surgical operation to remove part or all of one or both breasts.

Mastectomy is generally performed to treat breast cancer. The amount of breast tissue that is removed depends on the stage of cancer, the severity of the disease, the patient's age, and her or his overall health. The surgery aims to minimize tissue loss while maximizing the chances of removing all of the cancerous tissue. The operation is usually followed by other cancer treatments such as chemotherapy. If the patient desires, reconstructive surgery may be performed for cosmetic reasons. Counseling and support groups can also address emotional issues.

TYPES AND PROCEDURE

The categories of surgery are, in order of severity, lumpectomy, partial mastectomy, total mastectomy, modified radical mastectomy, and radical mastectomy. All types of mastectomy are performed with the patient under general anesthesia.

Lumpectomy is removal of the cancerous tumor, sometimes along with some surrounding tissue. It is usually performed if the tumor is small and localized. The entire lump is then analyzed by a pathologist to determine if further surgery is needed.

Partial mastectomy, also known as a "wedge resection," is when a wedge-shaped piece of tumor and tissue is removed.

Total or simple mastectomy is one in which the whole breast and no other tissue or nodes is removed.

Modified radical mastectomy is when the entire breast and some auxiliary nodes are removed.

Radical mastectomy is removal of the whole breast, including lymph nodes and muscle tissue. Postoperative radiation therapy is usually not necessary .

RECOVERY

After a lumpectomy or partial mastectomy, an individual can usually leave the hospital after one or two days and can resume normal activities about two weeks later. After a more extensive operation, the hospital stay will last about a week. The individual undergoing treatment is given analgesics (pain-killers) for at least a week after the operation. Long-term complications of radical mastectomy may include lymphedema (accumulation of lymph fluid under the skin and resultant swelling) and stiffness of the arm, shoulder, and pectoral region.

PROSTHESES AND RECONSTRUCTIVE OPTIONS

The patient may choose to wear a temporary prosthesis (artificial breast) after surgery and, upon full recovery, may get fitted for a permanent device. Other options include reconstructive mammoplasty (plastic surgery on the breast area). *See also* BREAST.

> *Background information about mastectomy can be found in* BREAST SURGERY; BREAST LUMP; GYNECOLOGY; *and* SURGERY. *Articles containing information about related conditions include* BREAST DISORDERS *and* BREAST TENDERNESS.

Mastication

Process of chewing food.

The primary function of the teeth is to chew food so that it can be swallowed and digested properly. Diseased, improperly aligned, or missing teeth can make chewing difficult. Improperly aligned teeth can cause strain to the joint of the jaw, the teeth and their supportive structures. *See also* DENTURE *and* TEETH.

Mastitis

An inflammation of the breast tissue usually caused by a bacterial infection.

Mastitis often affects women who are breast feeding. Bacteria that are in the baby's saliva or present on the skin can enter through a break in the skin of the nipple and move up the milk ducts to the milk glands, where they multiply. Symptoms of mastitis include redness and tenderness of the breast, fever, and enlarged lymph nodes on one side.

Women with mastitis can continue to breast feed, since this will decrease the risk of developing an abscess, but they should be careful not to let the nipples become cracked. Warm compresses can be applied to the breast to help relieve the pain. Mastitis usually responds well to antibiotics, though the treatment may have to be continued for a time to prevent recurrence of the infection. *See also* ABSCESS; ANTIBIOTIC DRUGS; BACTERIA; *and* BREAST.

Mastocytosis

Also known as urticaria pigmentosa

A disease in which an increased number of mast cells in the skin causes skin lesions that become itchy and form hives when they are rubbed.

The cause of mastocytosis is unknown. The main types of mastocytosis include: mastocytoma (which consists of a single lesion); urticaria pigmentosa (in which the lesions affect much of the skin); and systemic mastocytosis, (in which lesions also appear on internal organs).

The lesions appear as tan to light brown spots on the skin. The lesions contain cells that produce histamine. When rubbed, they release histamine into the body, causing the lesions to itch and swell and produce headaches, diarrhea, rapid heartbeat, and lightheadedness. Antihistamines may reduce the itching. In most cases mastocytosis disappears by adulthood. *See also* ANTIHISTAMINE DRUGS; MAST CELLS; *and* SKIN.

Mastoiditis

A bacterial infection of the mastoid, the bone behind the ear.

Mastoiditis usually follows a bacterial infection of the middle ear (otitis) that spreads into the mastoid bone, which has a structure like a honeycomb. Until the discovery of antibiotics, mastoiditis was one of the leading causes of death in children.

Symptoms include pain in and behind the ear, redness of the area, fever (which may spike quite high), headache, and pus drainage from the ear. The diagnosis will be made from the symptoms, but a culture of the drainage may show bacteria. A skull x-ray or CAT scan may indicate an abnormality in the bone.

Treatment. Preventive treatment starts with prompt and proper handling of otitis, since most cases of mastoiditis start in the middle ear. If the infection does travel to the mastoid, intravenous antibiotics will normally control the infection, but if the antibiotics do not work, surgery may be

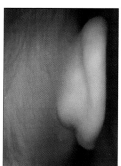

Mastoiditis.
The child (above), has noticeable swelling and redness behind his right ear because of mastoiditis. Mastoiditis is an infection of the bony air cells in the mastoid bone, located just behind the ear. It is rarely seen today because of the use of antibiotics to treat ear infections.

necessary to drain the abscess. A full course of antibiotic treatment may take two weeks or more. Complications from mastoiditis include recurrence of the infection, hearing loss, destruction of the mastoid bone, and spread of the infection to the brain or elsewhere in the body. *See also* ABSCESS.

Masturbation

Also known as autoeroticism

The action of stimulating one's own genitals in order to produce a feeling of sexual pleasure.

Masturbation is estimated to have been practiced at least once by over 97 percent of all men and 80 percent of women. Masturbation is considered a normal sexual activity, and, in fact, is recommended as a way of practicing safe sex. *See also* SEXUALITY.

Maternal Mortality

Death of a woman related to or resulting from pregnancy or childbirth.

Maternal mortality is not as widespread as it once was, due to improved nutrition and prenatal care. Women are in better health before becoming pregnant, and family planning is increasingly used to allow the mother time to recover between pregnancies. Nevertheless, conditions still exist which may cause maternal mortality.

In the past, mothers most often died from postpartum infections or severe hemorrhage. With proper hygiene and antibiotics, most infections are now dealt with

Age and Risk

Age can be an important consideration in determining the safety of a pregnancy. Teenage girls often do not receive proper prenatal care or nutrition, thereby putting them at greater risk for complications and reducing their chances of having healthy babies and bodies afterwards. Women older than 35 tend to develop diabetes and hypertension more frequently than younger women. They also have higher rates of miscarriage, stillbirth, and placenta previa. At all ages, proper prenatal care and close medical supervision can maximize the chances for a safe pregnancy.

easily. Ensuring that all of the placenta has been removed can minimize bleeding, as can medications that strengthen uterine contractions. Occasionally, severe or protracted bleeding may necessitate tying off one or more of the major uterine vessels, or more rarely, an emergency hysterectomy must be performed.

The major causes of maternal mortality today are physical trauma from an accident, eclampsia, and untreated ectopic pregnancy. Even if the mother has a preexisting condition such as diabetes or heart problems, careful monitoring by a physician can maximize the mother's health. *See also* ECLAMPSIA; ETOPIC PREGNANCY; *and* UTERUS.

McArdle's Disease

One of a group of muscle-related enzymatic deficiencies known as glycogen storage diseases, characterized by weakness, fatigue, and severe muscle cramping and pain after exercise.

McArdle's disease is caused by a defective gene. Because of the missing enzyme, glucose cannot be released from glycogen stored in skeletal muscles to create energy, and the body breaks down muscle instead.

Symptoms include exercise intolerance, decreased stamina, and fatigue, cramping, pain, tenderness, weakness, wasting, swelling, and stiffness of the muscles. The severity of symptoms vary widely. The effects are less severe in children.

Treatment involves exercise management, diet management, and Vitamin B_6 supplements, often injected directly into the bloodstream. *See also* DNA *and* MUSCLE.

Measles

Also known as Rubella

A highly contagious viral infection.

Measles is spread in droplets of water that come from the sneeze or cough of an infected person. The incubation period for the virus is from ten days to two weeks, after which time flu-like symptoms may develop, including nasal stuffiness and discharge, sneezing and coughing, irritated eyes, and

a sore throat. The symptoms persist, and a profound malaise accompanies a fever that may spike to as high as 104° F and remain at that level for a week. A few days after the onset of symptoms, tiny white spots with red rings appear on the tongue and the lining of the mouth, particularly on the insides of the cheeks opposite the molars. These spots are called Koplik's spots.

COMPLICATIONS

People with measles may be susceptible to additional infections. Complications from bacterial infections can lead to pneumonia and middle ear or brain infections, particularly among the very young, the elderly, and others with compromised immune systems.

TREATMENT AND PREVENTION

Treatment focuses on making the person as comfortable as possible while the immune system deals with the virus. Bed-rest and plenty of fluids are standard recommendations. Acetaminophen may ameliorate pain and fever. Over-the-counter medications can suppress cough, though it is important to spit up mucous and phlegm that may collect in the lungs. Using a vaporizer that generates moist air or standing in a hot shower may ease breathing.

A person who has had measles gains lifelong immunity to the disease. An immune mother transfers antibodies to her child for the first year of the child's life. Children are routinely vaccinated against measles; this has largely eliminated the epidemics that used to sweep the country every two or three years. The first dose of the measles, mumps, and rubella (MMR) vaccine is given to a child between the twelfth and fifteenth month of life. College and university students, doctors, nurses, and people who travel internationally are considered at increased risk for measles and should receive two doses of the MMR vaccine for total protection.

For information related to this subject see BACTERIA; INFECTIOUS DISEASES; *and* VIRUSES. *Prevention is discussed in* IMMUNITY; PUBLIC HEALTH; *and* VACCINATION. *Related disorders include* MUMPS *and* RUBELLA.

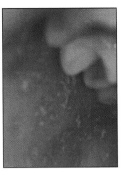

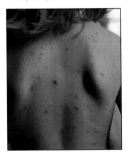

Measles.
Koplik spots, above, are seen with measles. They are small, white, often on a reddened background that occur on the inside of the cheeks early in the course of the measles. Measles outbreaks still occur in the U.S. It is a fairly serious childhood infection that is recognized by the rash, below, Koplik spots, red eyes and photophobia, and coughing.

Mebendazole

A broad spectrum antihelminthic drug, used to treat various parasitic worm infections.

Mebendazole, also known as Vermox, is an antihelminthic drug used to treat parasitic infections from tapeworms, roundworms, hookworms, pinworms, and whipworms. The drug is taken in pill form and should be taken with food. Destruction of all parasitic worms generally takes several days.

Warnings. The drug should be avoided by pregnant women, those who are breast feeding, or patients suffering from any of the following: Crohn's disease, inflammatory bowel disease, liver disease, ulcerative colitis, or an allergy to mebendazole or other substances, including preservatives or dyes. Additionally, some other medications can adversely interact with mebendazole. Side effects may include fever or chills, sore throat, rash, itching, and weakness. *See also* ANTIHELMINTHIC DRUGS; ASCARIASIS; HOOKWORM INFESTATION; PARASITE; ROUNDWORMS; TAPEWORM INFESTATION; *and* WORM INFESTATION.

Meckel's Diverticulum

Congenital condition in which a small sac (diverticulum) forms from the wall of the intestine; it may become the source of gastrointestinal bleeding.

Meckel's diverticulum generally forms in the ileum, the lower part of the small intestine, and is about two inches long. Usually there are no symptoms unless the diverticulum becomes inflamed. In severe cases, the intestine can become obstructed or even perforated, resulting in bleeding. Bleeding can also result from the formation of an ulcer at the site of the diverticulum's attachment to the lining.

Meckel's diverticulum is rare. Symptons usually occur in children and young adults. In cases of extreme and sudden bleeding, an immediate blood transfusion and surgery are necessary. Complications of the disorder that result in infection or a twisting or telescoping of the small intestine are treated by a surgical removal of the sac. *See also* INTESTINE.

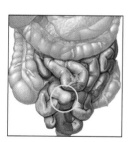

Meckel's Diverticulm. The diagram above details Meckel's Diverticulum, a rare condition that occurs when a small sac, shown in circle, forms from the wall of the intestine.

Meconium

The sticky, greenish or blackish discharge from the bowels of a newborn baby.

Meconium, which accumulates in the fetal intestine, is the breakdown of swallowed amniotic fluid, fetal hair, gastrointestinal secretions, and mucus. Meconium comprises the first stools passed by a newborn.

Meconium Aspiration Syndrome. If meconium is expelled into the amniotic fluid during birth and inhaled by the baby, it can irritate the lungs, leading to respiratory problems. This condition is called meconium aspiration syndrome (MAS).

This can cause severe respiratory distress. If meconium is seen in the amniotic fluid during birth, a doctor will use a suction device to remove the discharge from the baby's nose, mouth, throat, and trachea. If meconium inhalation is serious, mechanical means of respiration and suction may be used. *See also* RESPIRATORY SYSTEM.

Mediastinoscopy

Technique for examining the organs and tissues separating the lungs, known as the mediastinum.

Mediastinoscopy involves the use of a flexible fiberoptic endoscope known as a mediastinoscope. This instrument is inserted through an incision in the chest wall and is used to directly examine structures around the lungs; the lungs themselves, lymph, heart, trachea, esophagus, and thymus.

The procedure is used to assess potentially cancerous tissues (neoplasia), masses, or other irregularities. It is most often employed to diagnose enlarged lymph nodes or to evaluate the extent of lung cancer. Mediastinoscopy is also used as a staging technique to track the progress of malignancy and treatment.

If an abnormality is detected, it is possible to use the endoscope to extract a small sample of tissue (biopsy) for further testing to evaluate possible malignancy. This is done by passing biopsy devices through a hollow channel in the endoscope.

WHAT TO EXPECT

Prior to mediastinoscopy, food should be avoided for about eight hours. The procedure is done under general or local anesthesia in a hospital setting. An incision is made above the breastbone, and the mediastinoscope is inserted into the chest. The technique may precede more invasive surgery of the chest, known as thoracotomy. *See also* BIOPSY; ENDOSCOPE; ESOPHAGUS; FIBEROPTIC; HEART; LUNG CANCER; MALIGNANT; NEOPLASIA; THYMUS; *and* TRACHEA.

Medicaid

Public assistance programs, run jointly by states and the federal government, for people of any age who cannot afford to pay for their own health care.

Unlike Medicare, Medicaid is need-based. Each state administers Medicaid, so the regulations vary widely from state to state. Also unlike Medicare, people can qualify for Medicaid at any age, and Medicaid can cover long-term nursing care. Medicaid also covers many drug expenses and typically does not require payment of deductables and co-payments. Older people in need of nursing care are often housed in nursing homes at their own expense until their assets fall below the level at which they qualify for Medicaid, which then continues to pay for the care. People age 65 and older who meet eligibility requirements can possibly qualify for both Medicare and Medicaid. *See also* HEALTH INSURANCE; MEDICARE; *and* PUBLIC HEALTH.

Medicare

A federally managed health insurance program for people with some disabilities and for those over the age of 65.

Medicare is a federal program that funds some 65 percent of health care costs of citizens 65 years of age and older. It also covers younger individuals, provided they are disabled and have been receiving Social Security Disability payments for at least 24 months. Enrollment in Medicare is not automatic; those eligible must enroll, but nearly every U.S. citizen age 65 or older is eligible. Information on eligibility and enrollment can be obtained free of charge by calling (800) 638-6833.

There are two types of Medicare coverage: Medicare Part A covers hospitalization, home, and hospice health care, provided that deductables and co-payments have been paid and the patient's need for medical services has been properly certified. Medicare Part B requires that enrollees pay a monthly premium, but provides a wider variety of health services than Part A, including outpatient hospital visits, diagnostic testing, ambulance services, and equipment such as wheelchairs and home oxygen equipment. So-called Medigap insurance that covers a portion of medical expenses not covered by Medicare is available from a number of private insurance companies. *See also* HEALTH INSURANCE; INPATIENT TREATMENT; *and* OUTPATIENT TREATMENT.

Medicine Chest

A cabinet used primarily for the storage of medications and first-aid items.

A medicine chest or cabinet is a convenient storage space for common household medical supplies. It is a good idea to stock a medicine chest with important prescription drugs, over-the-counter medications, vitamin supplements, and contraceptives. Simple first-aid supplies, including bandages, tweezers, non-mercury thermometers, and antiseptics, should also be among the items available in a medicine cabinet. Review and clean the medicine chest regularly to eliminate any expired medications.

The conventional medicine chest is located in the bathroom, which may not be the best place to store medications, as it is often hot, humid, and accessible to small children who should never be at the medicine chest without supervision. It may be best to choose a secure, cool, and dry location, such as a bedroom closet, for your medicine chest. *See also* BANDAGE; FIRST AID; *and* VITAMIN SUPPLEMENTS.

Resources on Learning Disabilities

Bove, Alexander A., Jr., The Medicaid Planning Handbook: A Guide to Protecting Your Family's Assets from Catastrophic Nursing Home Costs, 2nd Rev Ed (1996); Chan, Paul D., *Family Medicine* (2001); Rowell, Joann C., et al., *Understanding Health Insurance: A Guide to Professional Billing* (2001); American Academy of Family Physicians, Tel. (800) 274-2237, Online: www.aafp.org; American Hospital Association, Tel. (800) 242-2626, Online: www.aha.org; National Health Information Ctr., Tel. (301) 565-4167, Online: nhicnt.health.org.

Meditation

A form of relaxation that can relieve stress, reduce anxiety, and lower blood pressure and stress.

In meditation, a person sits quietly and comfortably and allows the mind to relax. While there are many forms of meditation, most of them begin with sitting with the spine vertical, breathing slowly and deeply, and allowing the mind to empty. In concentrative meditation, a person focuses on the breath or on a word or phrase (mantra) to the exclusion of all external stimuli. In mindful meditation, a person remains receptive to all stimuli and simply lets them pass through the mind without reaction.

Transcendental Meditation

Based on Eastern teachings, meditation has been observed to be an effective means of relieving stress, treating stress-related illnesses, and promoting a sense of calm and well-being. In the late 1950's, a South Asian monk, Maharishi Majesh Yogi, popularized a form he called Transcendental Meditation: it promoted a state of placid restfulness which researchers found has some therapeutic value for cardiac, and stress-related illness.

Successful, meditation can lead to a state of rest that is deeper than sleep. A single session of meditation typically lasts 15 to 20 minutes, although some practitioners may meditate for several hours at a stretch.

Meditation can be used as a general lifestyle aid to reduce stress and anxiety. Over the long term, it has been shown to reduce blood pressure, lower heart rate, and lower the rate of oxygen use. In addition, it can be used as a supplementary treatment to control chronic pain and anxiety disorders. Meditation does not cure these disorders, but by allowing the body and mind to relax, it enables a person to better cope with the illness, and may stave off symptoms triggered by stress and anxiety.

Meditation is closely related to topics such as ALTERNATIVE MEDICINE; NATUROPATHY; MASSAGE THERAPY; *and* STRESS. *It can be used in conjunction with* ACUPRESSURE; HERBAL MEDICINE *and an understanding of* DIET AND DISEASE.

Megacolon

Extreme enlargement of the colon, resulting in the inability to move feces.

A congenital or acquired condition, megacolon can develop in all age groups. The most common cause is damage to the colon or rectum.

Hirschsprung's disease is a congenital condition in which a child is born without ganglion nerve cells in a segment of the rectum, which can result in megacolon. The child is unable to have any bowel movements and develops abdominal distention and malnutrition.

Psychogenic megacolon is sometimes seen in children who resist toilet training, and, as a result, exhibit severe and chronic constipation.

Chagas' disease, a parasitic infection prevalent in Latin America, destroys the ganglion cells of the rectum and can result in megacolon. Hirschsprung's disease is treated surgically.

Other causes of megacolon include spinal cord injury, Parkinson's disease, and certain medications, including narcotics.

Any underlying condition that has caused the development of megacolon should be treated as well. For the treatment of constipation caused by megacolon, enemas or laxatives may be prescribed to help retrain the bowel to function normally. *See also* CHAGAS' DISEASE; COLON; HIRSCHPRUNG'S DISEASE; *and* TOILET TRAINING.

Megalomania

An exaggerated feeling of importance.

Megalomania is not formally a psychiatric disorder, but it becomes serious and worthy of therapeutic attention when the individual is deluded, thinking he or she is, in some sense, a famous individual (such as Napoleon or Joan of Arc), or has utterly unrealistic and impractical plans. Often, megalomaniacal impulses mask feelings of inadequacy and inferiority. Megalomania may also be a characteristic of a manic phase in someone with bipolar disorder. *See also* BIPOLAR DISORDER; INFERIORITY COMPLEX; *and* SUPERIORITY COMPLEX.

Meibomianitis

Inflamed glands in the eyelid.

Inside each eyelid are approximately 30 meibomian glands. These glands manufacture and release an oily substance that keeps the lids from sticking together during long periods of closure, such as sleep. In meibomianitis, an eyelid becomes inflamed, causing a thickening of the oily secretion. It typically affects those with blepharitis, an inflammation of the eyelid, and may then lead to cysts on the eyelid known as chalazions. *See also* BLEPHARITIS; CHALAZION; *and* EYE.

Meigs' Syndrome

Fluid accumulation resulting from an ovarian tumor.

In unusual cases, a fibroma or other tumor of the ovary can cause excess fluid either in the abdominal cavity (ascites) or in the lungs (pleural effusion). The most common symptoms are breathlessness and pain. The condition is diagnosed by a physical and examination and is treated by surgical removal of the tumor. *See also* OVARY.

Melanin

The primary agent of normal coloration of the skin, hair, and the iris of the eyes.

Melanin is produced by cells called melanocytes, which react to a hormone, melanocyte stimulating hormone, that is secreted by the pituitary gland. The amount of melanin normally present in the body is under genetic control. Localized areas of increased melanin production result in darker patches on the skin, such as moles and freckles. When the skin is exposed to sunlight, melanin production increases, producing a suntan. This helps protect the skin from damage from the sun's rays.

In albinism, a genetic defect results in the partial or complete absence of the pigment melanin from the body, resulting in very light coloration. *See also* ALBINISM.

Melanoma

A skin tumor that arises in melanocytes, the cells that produce the pigment melanin.

There are two main types of melanomas: juvenile and malignant. Juvenile melanomas usually are benign, while malignant melanomas are often cancerous.

Spitz nevus (a benign skin lesion) appears in early childhood and is usually seen on the face or on the leg. The tumor forms as a result of overactivity of melanocytes or from an abnormal collection of blood vessels in the skin. A Spitz nevus can grow to one inch in diameter and has a reddish-brown color. It can be surgically removed if there is a possibility that it may become cancerous or for cosmetic reasons.

Malignant melanoma is less common than the other forms of skin cancer, squamous cell carcinoma and basal cell carcinoma, but it is potentially the most deadly. The incidence of malignant melanoma increases with age and with extended exposure to sunlight; persons with a history of severe, blistering sunburns are at especially high risk.

Symptoms. A large percentage of melanomas develop from a mole or other dark spot on the skin. The signs that a mole has become cancerous are an asymmetrical appearance, unusual color, and increasing size.

Diagnosis. Melanomas can spread quickly throughout the body; early diagnosis and treatment is essential. Diagnosis is made by biopsy, in which a tissue sample is examined microscopically for cancerous traits. Adjacent lymph nodes may also be analyzed if the melanoma is believed to have spread.

Treatment is surgical removal of the melanoma and surrounding tissue, possibly followed by radiation or chemotherapy. Lymph nodes may also be removed. *See also* CANCER; CANCER SCREENING; MELANOMA; SKIN; SKIN CANCER; *and* TUMOR.

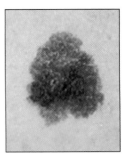

Melanoma.
Above is an image of a melanoma, or skin tumor, formed due to an abnormal collection of blood vessels in the skin. Juvenile melanomas tend to have a reddish brown appearance and can be surgically-removed.

Melanosis Coli

Deposits of brown pigment in the lining of the colon.

Long-term, persistent use of laxatives for real or imagined constipation, can often result in a condition known as melanosis coli. One characteristic of melanosis coli are the black and brown discolorations on the lining of the colon . The condition can usually be detected by a colonoscopic examination or by a biopsy (when a sample of tissue is taken from the colon). Melanosis coli is most often seen in older persons and usually produces no symptoms. The laxatives most commonly associated with melanosis coli are cascara, rhu-barb, and senna. *See also* BIOPSY; CANCER; COLONOSCOPY; CONSTIPATION; *and* LAXATIVE DRUGS.

Melena

Black, tarry stool caused by bleeding in the gastrointestinal tract.

Blood found in stool may be caused by bleeding in the upper intestinal tract—the esophagus, stomach, or duodenum. The most common cause is a bleeding peptic ulcer. The blood is blackened by the action of secretion during digestion. Melena may also indicate another intestinal tract or stomach disorder and should be investigated promptly. Abdominal pain that is relieved by antacids or food intake is usually indicative of a peptic ulcer. Stools can also appear black as a result of iron, licorice, or bismuth intake. *See also* COLON CANCER; DIVERTICULITIS; DUODENUM; ESOPHAGUS; INTESTINE, CANCER OF; PEPTIC ULCER; STOMACH; STOMACH, DISORDERS OF; *and* WEIGHT LOSS.

Melioidosis

A bacterial infection found predominantly in Southeast Asia and Northern Australia.

Melioidosis is an infection caused by the bacterium *Pseudomonas pseudomallei*, which is transmitted through contaminated soil and surface waters. It enters the body if contaminated dust is inhaled or when there is contact with contaminated soil, particularly through skin abrasions. The infection most often settles in the lungs, forming abcesses, though it can spread to affect the heart, liver, kidneys, and eyes.

Symptoms of melioidosis include headache, fever, chills, cough, chest pain, and loss of appetite.

Melioidosis is treated with antibiotics; orally if the symptoms are mild, intravenously if they are more severe. Treatment can take as long as three to twelve months. *See also* ANTIBIOTIC DRUGS.

Membrane, Cell

The fatty layer at the outside edge of a cell responsible for its structural integrity.

The cell membrane consists of two layers of fatty material and proteins. In addition to forming the cell's structural wall, the membrane also functions as a filter, regulating the passage of material into and out of the cell. The semipermeable membrane allows necessary matter, such as oxygen and nutrients, to enter the cell and waste material, such as carbon dioxide, to exit it. Very small molecules are able to pass freely through the membrane. However, larger molecules can only pass through under certain conditions. *See also* B-CELL; CELL; DNA; MEMBRANE; PROTEINS; PROTEIN SYNTHESIS; *and* PROTOZOA.

Membrane, Cell. At right, a diagram of cell membrane which consists of two layers of fatty materials and proteins. The membrane allows oxygen and nutrients to pass into the cell and filters out waste materials.

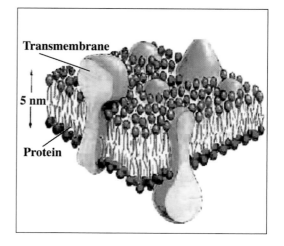

Transmembrane

5 nm

Protein

Memory

Fundamental cognitive process that allows individuals to acquire, retain, and recall information and experiences.

It is not known where in the brain the actual memory process takes place. However, damage to the lower side portion of the brain (temporal or limbic lobes) produces memory loss. In addition, studies in which electrical stimulation is applied to the temporal lobe have been successful in evoking different memories.

TYPES

Memory retention can be described in three stages: understanding (sensation lasting less than a second), short-term, and long-term.

Short-term memory lasts from a few seconds to a few minutes. Remembering a telephone number long enough to dial it exemplifies use of short-term memory. Unless transferred to long-term memory, the information will vanish almost immediately after the last digit is dialed.

Long-term memory consists of memories from a few hours to many years in the past. For example, long-term memory is used for recalling childhood experiences.

MECHANISM

Memory is a neurophysiological process involving complex molecular, cellular, and electrical (synaptic) changes. The process of memory can be divided into three stages: encoding, storage, and retrieval.

Encoding consists of processing incoming information for storage. During the encoding process, information is acquired and consolidated.

Storage follows encoding; information is stored for short-term or long-term use.

Retrieval is the process of bringing stored information to the conscious level.

LEARNING

Memory is linked to the process of learning. Learning can be described as obtaining knowledge, whereas memory is used for the storage of that knowledge.

Memory Loss and The Elderly

A decline in neural function often leads to some form of short-term memory loss among the elderly. The use of notes, calendars and diaries can help combat this common forgetfulness.

Long-term memory is generally preserved, however, any significant loss of the ability to recall familiar facts should be cause for concern. Long-term memory loss in the elderly is usually not a result of aging, but rather a symptom of what is often a dementing illness, such as Alzheimer's disease. If you or someone in your family appears to be suffering from severe memory loss, contact your physician immediately. The doctor will ask some basic questions about the nature of the memory loss and perform some diagnostic tests, possibly including angiography, CAT scan, EEG, or blood tests.

A good memory is essential for learning. Some individuals display an exceptional photographic (eldetic) memory, in which they can remember information and events with uncanny clarity. This sort of memory, however, is not necessarily linked with the ability to process or understand the stored information; there have been numerous cases of individuals with autism or mental retardation who have remarkable memories.

DISORDERS

A malfunction at any of the stages of memory formation can result in memory loss. Most memory disorders are a result of a malfunction in either retention or recall.

Memory loss appears in different forms and is seen in many clinical conditions, including amnesia, Alzheimer's disease, and Wernicke-Korsakoff syndrome. Thiamine deficiency damages the brain and results in mild to severe memory loss. Patients suffering from depression or bipolar disorder are believed unable to properly encode information because the constant influx of manic and depressed thoughts disrupts the process of long-term storage.

Information vital to an understanding of memory can be found in AGING; BRAIN; CENTRAL NERVOUS SYSTEM; *and* CEREBRUM. *Memory disorders include* ALZHEIMER'S DISEASE; AMNESIA; *and* WERNICKE-KORSAKOFF SYNDROME. *Also see* BRAIN DAMAGE; BRAIN HEMORRHAGE; *and* BRAIN ABSCESS.

Resources on Memory
Damasio, Antonio R., *Descartes' Error: Emotion Reason and the Human Brain* (1994); Herman, Judith, *Trauma and Recovery* (1992); Restak, Richard, *The Secret Life of the Brain* (2001); Schachter, Daniel L., *Searching for Memory: The Brain, The Mind, and the Past* (1996); West, Robin L. and Jan D. Sinnott, eds., *Everyday Memory and Aging* (1992); National Mental Health Association, Tel. (800) 969-NMHA, On-line: www.nmha.org; Alzheimer's Disease Education and Referral Center, Tel. (800) 438-4380, On-line: www.alzheimers.org; www.ny-cornell.org/medicine/neurology/index.html;www.nyp.org/css/.

Menarche

The first menstrual period.

Menarche indicates the beginning of a young woman's reproductive maturity. It normally occurs between the ages of nine and 16. On average, American girls begin menstruating at age 13. Over the past century, the average age of menarche has decreased by three or four months per decade, most likely due to improved nutrition.

Puberty, which signals the beginning of the physical changes from childhood to adulthood, begins approximately two years before menarche. *See also* ADOLESCENCE; MENSTRUATION; *and* PUBERTY.

Menière's Disease

Inner ear disorder characterized by vertigo, tinnitus and hearing loss.

Deep within the inner ear is the labyrinth. It is composed of two parts, the bony labyrinth and the membranous labyrinth; the latter is a set of passageways responsible for maintaining balance. Fluid in the membranous labyrinth, called endolymph, moves as the body moves, touching nerve receptors that signal the brain that the body has changed position. The brain then directs the rest of the body to adjust its position. In Menière's disease, the functioning of the membranous labyrinth is impaired, adversely affecting balance and the body's sense of position.

Menière's Disease.
A build-up of fluid in the inner ear that affects the body's sense of position, causing dizziness, imbalance, and vertigo.

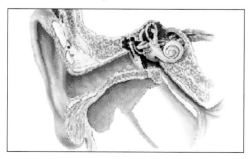

CAUSES
Menière's disease seems to result from an increase in the amount of fluid in the membranous labyrinth, which causes the labyrinth to become distorted or enlarged. This may be due to a break in the membranous labyrinth, causing endolymph, to flow into the area between the membranous labyrinth

and the bony labyrinth. The endolymph then mixes with the perilymph, the inner ear fluid that usually occupies that space. The nerve receptors in the labyrinth become overloaded with signals. Not knowing which signal is correct, the brain tries to react to all of them, causing a sense of dizziness or vertigo. The exact cause of this disruption in the membranous labyrinth is not known; some cases have been connected to head injuries and syphilis.

SYMPTOMS
The characteristic symptom of Menière's disease is vertigo, or dizziness. Vertigo associated with Menière's disease may occur as infrequently as once a year, or there may be periodic phases of unsteadiness that last for days. Accompanying vertigo are symptons associated with motion sickness, such as nausea, vomiting, and sweating. Tinnitus may also accompany the vertigo, as may slight hearing loss. The intensity of the symptoms varies with individuals.

TREATMENT
There is no completely effective cure for Menière's disease at this time. A tube may be inserted in the inner ear to drain fluid. The vestibular nerve can be severed, which cuts down on confusing signals to the brain. In both of these operations, though, nerves in the area, such as the auditory and facial nerves, may be damaged. A total removal of the labyrinth can cure Menière's disease, but it causes complete hearing loss in one ear.

Nonsurgical options can be used to treat the symptoms. Any drug that can reduce fluid retention, such as allergy medication, may help. Dietary changes that reduce the amount of fluid in the body, such as cutting back on salt, alcohol, and caffeine, may also lessen attacks.

For background information about Menière's Disease see BRAIN; EAR; LABYRINTHITIS; ORGANS OF BALANCE; TINNITUS; HEARING; *and* VERTIGO. *Treatment opteions deal with issues such as* BIOMECHANICAL ENGINEERING; DIZZINESS; *and* HEARING AIDS. *See* NAUSEA *and* VOMITING.

Meningioma

A benign tumor of the tissue covering the brain.

Meningiomas arise in the middle layer of the meninges, the protective tissue surrounding the brain. These tumors are not cancerous, but they can cause problems as they expand and put pressure on the brain.

Symptoms usually caused by the pressure the tumor places on the brain, can include impaired mental function, headaches, vomiting, and altered function of speech or vision. The growth may also invade the bone and cause an external bulge on the skull.

Diagnosis is made by X-rays, CAT scanning and magnetic resonance imaging of the skull. Most meningiomas can be removed by surgery, but some may also require radiation therapy. *See also* BRAIN.

Meningitis

Inflammation of the meninges, the membranes that surround the brain and the spinal cord.

There are three layers of meninges that enclose the brain. The tough outer layer is called the dura; the lacy web-like middle layer is called the arachnoid; and the fibrous inner layer is called the pia. The pia contains many of the blood vessels that serve the brain and the spinal cord.

CAUSES

Meningitis is a quickly progressing, and sometimes fatal, infection that is produced when bacteria, viruses, or fungi proliferate in the space between the meninges. Pathogens may reach the meninges from elsewhere in the body, through a head injury, or through surgery. The bacteria that most often cause meningitis are *Neisseria meningitidis, Streptococcus pneumoniae,* and *Haemophilus influenzae.*

Meningitis most often infects children under the age of two, or adults with high risk factors for the disease. Risk factors include alcohol abuse, chronic nose and ear infections, pneumonia, and sickle cell disease.

Vaccination

A vaccine is available to prevent some types of *neisseria meningitidis* meningitis; however, it is most often used during an epidemic or for people who have been in close contact with someone infected with the disease. Children should be routinely vaccinated against *haemophilus influenzae*, the bacteria that causes the type of meningitis most common among children.

TYPES

Acute bacterial meningitis is life-threatening and must be treated immediately to prevent brain damage or death. Symptoms of acute bacterial meningitis include fever, severe headache, nausea and vomiting, stiff neck, sensitivity to light, and irritability. There may also be speech impairment, hallucinations, facial paralysis, chills, drowsiness, rapid breathing, and a red or purplish skin rash. While a spinal tap will often show whether the spinal fluid contains bacteria, treatment of acute bacterial meningitis cannot be postponed for test results since the results may not be available for three to five days, during which time the illness will worsen considerably.

Chronic meningitis is diagnosed when the swelling of the meninges lasts for a month or more. It is most common among people with compromised immune systems and is caused by slower-growing bacteria or fungi. The symptoms are the same as for acute bacterial meningitis, except that they appear over a longer period of time.

Viral meningitis is milder than bacterial meningitis and usually clears up by itself.

TREATMENT

Antibiotics or antifungal drugs are administered to combat the specific infectious bacterial or fungal agent. Anti-inflammatory drugs may be prescribed to control swelling and treat convulsions or shock.

Information related the treatment and effects of Meningitis can be found in ANTIBIOTIC DRUGS; ANTIFUNGAL DRUGS; BACTERIA; INFECTION; INFECTIOUS DISEASE; *and* VIRUS. *Articles with anatomical relevance include* BRAIN; BRAIN DAMAGE; DIAGNOSIS; PARALYSIS; RASH; *and* SWELLING.

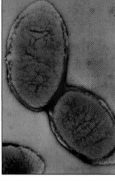

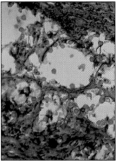

Meningitis. The different strains of meningitis are magnified, above. Meningitis occurs when bacteria viruses or fungi invade the meninges, the membranes that surround the brain and spinal cord.

Meniscectomy

Surgical removal of part or all of a damaged meniscus (crescent-shaped cartilage) from a joint.

Most problems with the meniscus of a joint result from sports injuries or prolonged stress due to athletic activity. Symptoms include pain, swelling, clicking, popping, snapping, and locking. Meniscectomy is performed to remove part or all of a damaged meniscus (usually in the knee), to relieve pain, and to "unlock" the joint.

PROCEDURE

In open meniscectomy, an orthopedist makes an incision at the side of the patella (kneecap) and opens it to repair the meniscus. After a hospital stay of a few days, the patient returns home; the splint is removed several days later. The joint takes about four to six weeks to fully heal.

Arthoscopic surgery has replaced open surgery as the preferred method of meniscectomy. In an arthoscopic meniscectomy, an orthopedic surgeon confirms the location of the torn meniscus with magnetic resonance imaging (MRI) and then with an arthoscope (a fiberoptic viewing tube), which is inserted in a small incision near the joint. The surgeon removes the torn part of the cartilage through the arthoscope with forceps or by suction, and any injured ligaments are sewn together. The patient can go home the same day and can usually walk without the aid of crutches in three to seven days.

Both open and arthoscopic surgery are effective in relieving symptoms of meniscus damage. The scar for open surgery is larger, because the incision in this type of surgery is larger. Joggers may have to switch to walking after a meniscectomy. Meniscectomy may also increase the odds of premature osteoarthritis in the joint.

Further information on meniscectomy can be found in MRI; ORTHOPEDICS; OSTEOARTHRITIS; OSTEOCHONDRITIS DISSECANS; *and* JOINT. *Specific concerns are dealt with in* EXERCISE; KNEE; SPORTS MEDICINE; STRESS FRACTURE; *and* WALKING.

Menopause

The end of a woman's menstrual periods and, consequently, of reproductive ability.

Menopause, sometimes referred to as climacteric, is not a single event, such as occurs at the start of reproductive maturity, but rather spans a number of years in which the body gradually changes.

Menopause may occur any time between the ages of 42 and 58, with the average age being 51. Menopause is considered premature if it occurs before age 40; this may occur naturally or due to surgical removal of the ovaries. Smokers undergo menopause an average of two years earlier than nonsmokers. As many women continue to ovulate for some time after menstruation ceases, contraception is necessary until one year after the last menstrual cycle.

Perimenopausal transition is the term used to describe the five to ten years before the menstrual periods stop completely. Changes in the menstrual cycle at this time may include shorter periods, irregular cycles or heavy menstrual flow. Medical attention may be needed if a woman experiences vaginal bleeding more often than every 21 days, or if the flow is unusually heavy or lasts longer than seven days. These symptoms may indicate abnormal growths in the uterus, such as fibroids, polyps, or endometrial cancer.

SYMPTOMS

Symptoms related to menopause can be directly linked to changing hormone levels. During the perimenopausal phase, there is a gradual decline in estrogen production, which accelerates as menopause nears. Since estrogen affects the vagina, uterus, bladder, breasts, bones, heart, and brain, changes occur in all of these body tissues. Symptoms associated with estrogen loss affect 75 percent of women who experience natural menopause and 90 percent of women whose menopause is brought on by surgical means.

Hot flashes are feelings of warmth unaccompanied by a measurable change in body temperature. Flushing and sweating may follow. They occur more commonly at night than during the day. Night sweats may cause insomnia, which can lead to other symptoms such as mood swings, irritability, depression, and fatigue, all of which have in the past been identified as symptoms of menopause itself.

Vaginal dryness, which includes the drying and thinning of the tissues of the vagina and urethra, is another common occurrence. This may lead to inflammation, inadequate lubrication, and painful intercourse. Vaginal atrophy may also result in symptoms that resemble a urinary tract infection. Loss of muscle tone in the pelvis may result in episodes of incontinence and increase the risk of developing a prolapsed uterus or bladder.

Other Symptoms. Lower estrogen levels may cause increased growth of facial hair and thinning of scalp hair. Women prone to adult acne may find it worsening.

There is no evidence that menopause itself causes depression, though the changes associated with menopause may contribute to depression.

Severity of Symptoms. There is a large variation in the way women experience menopause. It is estimated that only five to 15 percent experience significant problems. A woman should notify her doctor if hot flashes, insomnia, or any other symptoms are severe enough that they interfere with normal daily activities.

HORMONE REPLACEMENT THERAPY

Hormone replacement therapy (HRT) has been proven effective in alleviating many of the symptoms of menopause and in preventing osteoporosis; it may also provide protection against heart disease. HRT should not be prescribed if a woman has a history of breast or uterine cancer, active liver disease, or active thrombophlebitis. Treatment may not be needed if symptoms are mild.

> *Background material on menopause can be found in* AGING; HORMONE REPLACEMENT THEORY; HORMONES; *and* PERIMENOPAUSE. *Further related issues are dealt with in* DEPRESSION; DIAGNOSTICS IN WOMEN'S HEALTH; *and* GYNECOLOGY.

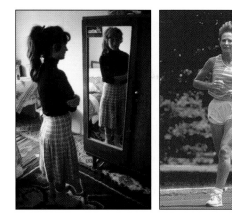
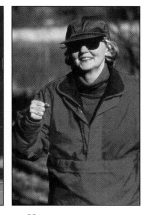

Menorrhagia

Prolonged and excessive bleeding during the menstrual cycle.

Menorrhagia usually occurs late in the child-bearing years or after menopause; it occasionally occurs in girls near puberty.

Causes. Menorrhagia may be caused by cancerous or fibroid tumors in the uterus or ovaries, polyps in the uterus, or thickening of the uterine lining. It may also be caused by hormone disorders, birth control methods or drugs, or by complications of pregnancy.

Symptoms include excessive and prolonged menstrual bleeding, usually accompanied by cramps and the passing of blood clots. The individual may also experience fatigue, diarrhea, and nausea.

After menopause, any cramps or vaginal bleeding should be brought to the attention of a physician.

Treatment. In order to diagnose the cause, a physician will perform a biopsy. Treatment then depends on the underlying cause. If cancer or precancerous cells are discovered, the tumors can be surgically removed and a dilatation and curettage (D&C) performed. If the cancer is advanced, a hysterectomy may be suggested.

> *Menorrhagia and related issues are also discussed in* DIAGNOSIS; D AND C; HYSTERECTOMY; MENOPAUSE; *and* MENSTRUATION. *Similar symptoms and illnesses are discussed in* BIOPSY; GYNECOLOGY; *and* VAGINAL BLEEDING.

Menopause.
Menopause is only one transition in a woman's life, marking the point at which the ovaries stop releasing eggs, and the body decreases the production of female hormones. It is important for women to maintain an active lifestyle throughout life so that this transition does not (as it ought not) mean a cessation of productive and enjoyable activity.

Resources on Menopause

Adashi, Eli Y., John A. Rock and Zev Rosenwaks, *Reproductive Endocrinology, Surgery and Technology* (1987); Krimsky, Sheldon and Lynn Gold-man, *Hormonal Chaos: The Scientific and Social Origins of the Environmental Endocrine Hypothesis* (1999); Laucella, Linda, *Hormone Replacement Therapy: Conventional Medicine and Natural Alternatives, Your Guide to Menopausal Health-Care Choices* (1999); Endocrine Web, Online: www.endocrineweb.com; www.nycornell.org/medicine/edm/index.html.

Menstrual Extraction

A form of early surgical abortion.

In a menstrual extraction, the contents of the uterus are suctioned out without prior dilation of the cervix. This method is best performed between five and seven weeks of gestation. Menstrual extraction is sometimes referred to as a preemptive abortion if it is performed prior to a positive confirmation of the pregnancy. The procedure can be done without anesthesia and is safer than a later surgical abortion. However, the failure rate is higher. *See also* ABORTION.

Menstruation

From the Latin word mensis which means month; the cycle of events leading up to and after the monthly release of an egg into a woman's reproductive tract.

Fertility in women follows a monthly cycle. During the cycle, the inner lining of the uterus (the endometrium) builds up in preparation for receiving a fertilized egg. If the egg is not fertilized, the egg and the lining (consisting of tissue and blood) disintegrate and are discharged through the vaginal opening. The first day of the menstrual flow marks the first day of the menstrual cycle. An average cycle is 28 days, but this varies from one woman to the next and sometimes from cycle to cycle. Most women experience a cycle of 21 to 35 days.

The menstrual cycle is regulated by the interaction of the nervous and endocrine systems. A variety of hormones, produced by several different organs, are involved. Each step in the cycle depends on changing levels of the different hormones. As may be expected, the control is not very precise, which contributes to the wide variability of the cycle.

THE PROCESS OF MENSTRUATION

At the start of the menstrual flow, hormones produced by the ovaries (estrogen and progesterone) are at a very low level. This causes a gland in the brain (hypothalamus) to release gonadotropin-releasing hormone (GnRH), which stimulates the pituitary gland to release follicle-stimulating hormone (FSH) and leutinizing hormone (LH), which act on the ovary. FSH causes an egg to start maturing inside its follicle, and FSH and LH stimulate the maturing follicle to release estrogen into the bloodstream. Estrogen affects the uterus, causing an increase in the blood supply and a thickening of the lining.

The effects of FSH, LH, and estrogen build up slowly for about 14 days, although the amount of time is highly variable. Just before day 14 of the menstrual cycle, a sudden increase of LH from the pituitary gland causes the follicle to burst and release the egg. This is ovulation.

The ruptured follicle has not finished playing an active role; it develops into a structure called the corpus luteum, which releases estrogen and progesterone. These hormones stimulate additional buildup of the uterine lining.

Meanwhile, the hypothalamus detects the increased levels of estrogen and progesterone and lowers the amount of GnRH accordingly. This causes the pituitary to decrease the amount of FSH and LH it is releasing. Progesterone is now the hormone found in the greatest concentration.

If the egg is not fertilized while traveling through the fallopian tube on its way to the uterus, the corpus luteum starts to degenerate, and the levels of estrogen and progesterone begin to fall. The drop in these hormone levels causes a decrease in the blood supply to the uterine lining. Menstruation begins as the blood-filled uterine tissues disintegrate and begin to be discharged. This marks the beginning of the next cycle.

Although the events leading up to ovulation may occur over a variable amount of time, ranging from one to three or four weeks, once ovulation has occurred, menstruation will follow in 13 or 14 days, provided the egg is not fertilized.

LIFE PHASES

Menarche refers to the first menstrual period; it normally occurs between the ages of nine and 16. On average, American girls begin menstruating at age 13. Over the past century, the average age of menarche has decreased by three or four months per decade, most likely due to improved nutrition.

It is not uncommon for the menstrual cycle to be erratic during the first few years. Most women settle into a regular pattern, although some may continue to have erratic cycles throughout their reproductive years. The menstrual cycle can be affected by illness, stress, and travel.

Menstruation does not occur at all when a woman is pregnant. The absence of menstruation is therefore considered one of the major indicators of pregnancy. Amenorrhea is the absence of any menstrual periods; it occurs in premenopausal women who are not pregnant, and may be caused by a variety of factors.

Menopause marks the end of a woman's reproductive years. It is not an abrupt "event," but rather a process that takes place over the course of a few years. Gradually, the amount of time between menstrual periods lengthens until no periods occur at all. It is not uncommon to skip periods during this time, and then briefly resume menstruating once more.

> **Further reading on menstruation can be found** FERTILIZATION; MENOPAUSE; PERIMENOPAUSE; SEX; SEXUALITY; VAGINA; and VAGINAL BLEEDING. **Menstruation is also discussed in relation to** DELIVERY; HORMONES; and PREGNANCY. **See also** MENSTRUATION, DISORDERS OF **for more information.**

Menstruation, Disorders of

AMENORRHEA

Amenorrhea is the absence of any menstrual periods in premenopausal women who are not pregnant.

Primary amenorrhea is diagnosed in young girls who have not begun menstruating by age 16. Menarche can be delayed in athletic or very thin girls whose body fat level is below a certain percentage.

Secondary amenorrhea is defined as the absence of menstruation for six months or

longer in adult women who are not pregnant. Secondary amenorrhea has a variety of causes, including sudden weight loss and prolonged bouts of exercise. Stress and either too few or too many fat cells in the body can prevent the ovaries from producing estrogen in a normal cycle. Taking oral contraceptives can often affect a woman's monthly cycle, even for a few months after discontinuing use. Nursing mothers often fail to menstruate for several months. As a woman approaches the age of menopause, it is normal to begin skipping periods.

It is important to note that even if a woman isn't menstruating, she may still be ovulating and may still get pregnant.

Treatment. If amennorhea is caused by an underlying disorder, that should be treated. Estrogen therapy may be recommended. A sufficient level of estrogen is needed for the prevention of bone weakness (osteoporosis) later in life.

DYSMENNORHEA

Dysmenorrhea refers to painful menstrual periods. More than half of all women experience mild cramps during the first few days of a period. Dysmenorrhea, which occurs in about ten percent of women, involves severe pain that cannot be tolerated without medication.

Primary Dysmennorhea. If the pain is not a sign of another gynecological problem, the condition is called primary dysmenorrhea. It is caused by excessive levels of prostaglandins, chemicals that are found in menstrual fluids and semen which trigger uterine contractions. Severe cramps may also be due to internal "gridlock;"a lot of fluid and tissue attempting to exit all at once through a relatively small opening. Pain therefore persists until enough material has been expelled. After a woman has given birth, the opening has been somewhat stretched, and this problem may cease.

Secondary dysmennorhea is caused by an underlying condition such as abnormal growths in the uterus (fibroids, adenomyosis, endometriosis) or a sexually transmitted disease.

OLIGOMENORRHEA

Oligomenorrhea is diagnosed when a woman experiences fewer menstrual periods than the usual 11 to 13 per year. Some women never have regular periods; others may suddenly begin to experience irregular cycles for no apparent reason. This irregularity is not related to approaching menopause but may be caused by an insufficient amount of estrogen. If erratic menstrual cycles are accompanied by acne and an increase of body and facial hair, the cause may be an excess of male hormones known as androgens.

Treatment. In most cases, oligomenorrhea presents no health threat unless a woman is trying to become pregnant. If the condition is due to insufficient estrogen production by the ovaries, hormone supplements should restore normal menstruation. Oligomenorrhea caused by an excess of androgens is treated depending on the underlying cause.

MENORRHAGIA

Menorrhagia refers to abnormal menstrual periods that last longer than seven days or involve unusually heavy bleeding. Heavy periods may be caused by hormonal disturbances in a woman's cycle, fibroids, pelvic infection, endometriosis, or the presence of an IUD. A one time heavy period which arrives late may be due to a miscarriage.

Menorrhagia may result in anemia, due to heavy blood loss, but is otherwise not considered a serious condition.

Treatment. A combination of estrogen and progesterone, usually in the form of oral contraceptives, are prescribed to reduce bleeding. A physician may also wish to perform a D&C (dilatin and cutterage) to determine if there are any other causes. Bleeding due to fibroids or endometriosis is treated by those conditions. An IUD that causes bleeding must be removed.

Disorders of menstruation are also discussed in the articles detailing D AND C; INTRAUTERINE DEVICE; MENORRHAGIA; MENSTRUATION; OGLIOMENORRHEA; *and* VAGINAL BLEEDING. *Other vital issues include* FIBROID *and* PREGNANCY. *See also* PRECOCIOUS *and* PUBERTY PUBERTY.

Resources on Menstruation
Adashi, Eli Y., John A. Rock and Zev Rosenwaks, *Reproductive Endocrinology, Surgery and Technology* (1987); Golub, Sharon, *Periods: From Menarche to Menopause* (1992); Krimsky, Sheldon and Lynn Goldman, *Hormonal Chaos: The Scientific and Social Origins of the Environmental Endocrine Hypothesis* (1999); Laucella, Linda, *Hormone Replacement Therapy: Conventional Medicine and Natural Alternatives, Your Guide to Menopausal Health-Care Choices* (1999); Endocrine Web, Online: www.endocrineweb.com; www.nycornell.org/medicine/edm/index.html.

Mental Hospital

An institution specializing in the treatment of mental illness.

Patients suffering from severe mental illness maybe admitted to a mental hospital when they become a danger to themselves or others. Hospital staff provide medical treatment, individual and group therapy, and a controlled, safe environment for long-term care.

The first mental hospitals, more commonly known as insane asylums, were massive buildings constructed in the 19th and early 20th centuries. They served as little more than warehouses and resembled prisons in that patients' stays were marked by brutality, neglect, and life-long terms. A notable exception was the hospital taken over by the Frenchman Phillippe Penel, who in the 18th century was one of the first medical authorities to promote the humane treatment of patients.

While there are some court-ordered hospitalizations today, most patients voluntarily admit themselves when they experience crisis and need the round-the-clock care that only a mental hospital can provide. Length of stay varies depending on the patient.

Psychosis, schizophrenia, and dementia, which are dangerous outside of a clinic, are the most common psychiatric illnesses that require hospitalization. *See also* HOSPITAL; MENTAL ILLNESS; *and* NURSING HOMES.

Mental Illness in America

At any given time, more than 20 percent of hospital beds are filled with individuals who are admitted for psychological reasons; psychiatric conditions are the top reason for hospital admissions in America. About one-fifth of all families will have to deal with a person suffering from major mental illness in the family. However, many people (especially those who need it most) are not being treated. Nearly a quarter of a million people with mental illnesses are homeless or living in shelters where they do not have access to the necessary treatments. The success rates for treating mental illnesses are much higher than those for treating physical illnesses, when an individual gets the proper care.

Mental Illness

A disorder that disrupts a person's mood, emotions, cognitive, or social abilties.

Mental health is the capacity to love and to work and the ability to continue to do so while experiencing the normal range of life's sadnesses and anxieties. A mentally healthy person is able to function, perform everyday activities, and handle responsibilities necessary to sustain life, such as holding a job, caring for family, and communicating with others. Such a person develops and maintains relationships with family, friends, and coworkers, and has realistic perceptions about other people.

Mental illness compromises these abilities. Types of mental illness vary greatly and range in severity. Some forms of mental illness may be subtle, so that others may not even perceive a problem, while others, such as schizophrenia, can impair the most basic ability to function in society.

THE STIGMA OF MENTAL ILLNESS

While we have progressed beyond the point where we believe (as people did as recently as the early 1900's) that mentally ill people are possessed by the devil, mental illness still tends to be hidden by sufferers and their families. As recently as 25 years ago a person suffering from mental illness tended to keep such a diagnosis quiet. Mental illness remains little understood by the public and is still an issue that is rarely discussed.

American society tends to view mental illness with discomfort, shame, and a lack of tolerance. To compound the problem, there are people who tend to blame the sufferer for his or her behavior. Because mental illness makes it difficult for people to function in their everyday lives, they may be stigmatized as being unsuccessful, weak, or undisciplined.

Beyond the stigma that society places on mental illness, there is a practical limitation placed on treatment by health insurance companies. Even before managed care placed severe limitations on the cost

Types of Mental Illness

- *ANXIETY DISORDERS.* Anxiety is a common response to an uncomfortable experience, self-doubt or apprehension of an upcoming event. Persistent feelings of fear and uncertainty that impair capacity for enjoyment and ability to function for extended periods of time, may indicate an anxiety disorder. These include panic disorder, obsessive-compulsive disorder, phobias, and generalized anxiety disorder.
- *COGNITIVE DISORDERS* are characterized by problems with the thought processes including memory, orientation as to time and place, ability to follow a train of thought, and focusing attention. Motor skills may also be affected. These disorders include delirium, dementia, Alzheimer's Disease, and amnesia.
- *EATING DISORDERS* are characterized by a preoccupation with food, distorted body image, eating or alternating between near starvation and large binges, and either extremely low body weight or severe obesity. Eating disorders include anorexia or bulimia.
- *GENDER IDENTITY DISORDER* involves a person's discomfort with his or her biological gender, and a desire to appear or behave as a person of the opposite sex. The disorder is diagnosed only when an individual's discomfort with his or her birth gender is extreme and interferes with emotional or social well-being.
- *IMPULSE CONTROL DISORDERS* involve ongoing, persistent, and extreme lapses inn judgement due to the inability to control behavior. Impulse control disorders may lead an individual to break laws or harm others, or themselves. They include intermittent explosive disorder, kleptomania, and compulsive gambling.
- *MOOD DISORDERS.* People experience a range of moods that vary depending on situation and temperamental makeup. When the mechanism in the brain that regulates mood is out of balance, a person may experience persistent feelings of unhappiness, euphoria or irritability, or out-of-control mood fluctuation. Mood disorders include depression, mania, and bipolar disorder.
- *PERSONALITY DISORDERS.* While there is a wide range of "normal" behavior that is part of the diversity of human life, a personality disorder is a set of behaviors that makes it difficult to interact with others, have realistic perceptions of oneself and others, and control impulses. People with personality disorders find it extremely difficult to adapt to new situations or make necessary adjustments to behavior patterns. These disorders include obsessive-compulsive disorder, borderline personality disorder, and paranoid personality disorder, among others.
- *PSYCHOSES AND SCHIZOPHRENIA* involve a loss of connection with reality, manifesting in delusions, hallucinations, or bizarre behavior. Those suffering from these disorders may experience disorganized thought processes and exhibit disorganized speech patterns, either putting together words that do not make sense or changing the subject without completing a thought.
- *SEXUAL DISORDERS* involve extremely low levels of sexual interest, problems achieving sexual satisfaction, or uncontrollable sexual behaviors. A category of disorders known as paraphilias encompasses a number of behaviors considered to be deviant, including the use of objects to become sexually aroused (fetishism), the use of pain or humiliation for sexual excitement (sadism or masochism), exhibitionism, voyeurism, and desire for sexual activity with a child (pedophilia). Paraphilias that involve consenting adults and do not impair daily functioning are usually not considered dysfunctional. However, any nonconsensual activity, especially involving children, is both highly dysfunctional and illegal.
- *SLEEP DISORDERS* are often a symptom of a mental disorder and may be the impetus for a person to seek treatment. These disorders include insomnia, the inability to fall asleep or stay asleep; sleepwalking, a severe sleep disturbance in which a sleeping person gets out of bed and walks around or even attempts to eat or drive; and nightmare disorder, which involves persistent, frequent nightmares.
- *SUBSTANCE ABUSE* involves alcohol, prescription, or illegal drug use in a fashion that is excessive, out-of-control, and interferes with the ability of a person to function daily, because of their dependence on the substance.

Signs of Mental Illness

Answering yes to one or more of these questions may indicate a possible mental illness. If you are concerned about your emotional or mental well-being or that of your child, seek the advice of a physician or qualified therapist.

1. Do you feel sad much of the time? Do you have difficulty finding enjoyment in life? Do you have persistent feelings of hopelessness or thoughts of suicide?
2. Has there been a substantial decline in your performance at work or in school?
3. Are you using drugs or alcohol to feel better or to cope with problems, and is your substance use affecting your ability to perform daily activities? Is it out of control, causing problems in your relationships or with your work?
4. Do you have significant mood swings, feeling hyperactive and overly optimistic some of the time and down and blue at other times? Has your behavior during optimistic times caused financial problems or problems with your relationships or daily activities?
5. Are you persistently troubled by events from your past or worries about the future? Do these worries or fears cause you to avoid activities and people to the extent that you are unable to function?
6. Have you had significant changes in sleeping or eating habits?
7. Do you have problems with sexual functioning?
8. Do you frequently feel angry or behave aggressively to others in ways that feel out of control? Do you often feel embarrassed or sorry about such behavior later?
9. Does your child have behavior problems or delays in development (toilet training, learning, coordination, communication, or social problems)?
10. Do you have thoughts or images that keep intruding on your mind and become preoccupations, such as coming in contact with germs, leaving the door unlocked, or causing harm to people? Do you have compulsive behaviors such as counting or washing, which seem to help relieve comfortable feelings or fears?
11. Do you have trouble making sense of what other people are saying, have difficulty remembering or feel persistently confused or upset by the behavior of others?
12. Are your relationships with others usually plagued by difficulties?
13. Have you seen your family doctor and a number of specialists in attempts to diagnose and treat physical symptoms without receiving relief or treatment? (Although a mental illness may be indicated, there may simply not have been a clear diagnosis of a physical problem.)

and amount of treatment that one could expect for mental health treatments, mental illness was typically reimbursed at a rate of 50 percent compared to 80 percent for most physical illnesses.

SYMPTOMS

Symptoms and complaints about physical illness can be specific and localized. A pain, swelling or discoloration appears in a particular place. A doctor can perform tests that indicate specific problems, such as a high white blood cell count, or impaired kidney function. The complaints that one presents when describing difficulties with mental health, on the other hand, are less localized and cannot be so easily tested. Emotional distress is not located in a specific area and cannot be measured by physical tests. A person may feel out of control, worried, afraid, or hopeless. The patient may consult a physician when these feeling cause physical symptoms, such as heart palpitations, stomach pain, or breathing difficulties, but a mental illness affects an individual's whole life and experience. A mental illness must be assessed in the context of a person's life.

DIAGNOSIS

A diagnosis of mental illness must take into account a number of factors related to a person's personality and life situation. People vary greatly in their behaviors. Distinctive, even eccentric behaviors are part of what make us unique, human, and interesting to one another. Thus mental illness cannot be diagnosed simply by cataloging a set of thoughts and behaviors; rather they must be viewed in context. For example, exaggerated, enthusiastic, and agitated behavior may be normal range for a person who is outgoing, but they signal a problem for someone who is consistently sedate and low-key.

In general, mental suffering that persists for a long period of time, interferes with the ability to function in everyday life, or causes problems with physical health, or makes it necessary to take medication that may be prescribed for mental illness.

Sometimes, an emotional difficulty will dissipate over time with counseling by an empathic person or a mental health professional or therapist. When problems persist, however, it may be necessary to seek medical treatment. Generally, the place to begin is with one's primary care physician, particularly when that physician has known and treated an individual over a period of years, and may be more likely to notice a trend in current behavior or attitudes, that is inconsistent with past behavior. In addition, the onset of physical symptoms that were not present in the past, such as sleeplessness, anxiety, depression, mood swings, severe headaches or chest pains, can be examined and evaluated for a physical or mental cause.

TREATMENT

Beyond the stigma that society places on mental illness, there is often an unfortunate limitation placed on treatment by health insurance companies. In recent years, there have been significant advances in drug treatments and the development of more specific therapies for mental illnesses. Medications address chemical imbalances in the brain and may provide relief for anxiety, depression, panic disorder, and a number of other psychiatric problems. Providing a pill alone, however, is often not the best solution to treating a mental health problem; a combination of therapy and medication may be the most effective treatment for dealing with a problem. Psychotherapy and behavioral therapy, may be employed either with or without medication, to treat problems from obsessive-compulsive disorder to depression. Self-help and support groups may also be useful in treating some forms of mental illness.

For background information about mental illness see ANXIETY DISORDER; EATING DISORDER; PERSONALITY DISORDER; *and* PSYCHOTHERAPY. *Specific disorders are discussed in* DEPRESSION; OBSESSIVE-COMPULSIVE BEHAVIOR; PSYCHOSIS; SCHIZOPHRENIA; SEXUAL DYSFUNCTION; SLEEP DISORDER.

Mental Retardation

Intelligence below an IQ of 70, with limitations in adaptive functioning, that begins in childhood.

Mental retardation is not a disease but rather an extreme in the wide range of human intelligence. Approximately three percent of the population suffers from mental retardation, and one out of 10 American families has a family member who is mentally retarded. It is equally likely to affect people of all racial, ethnic, and economic backgrounds.

About 80 to 85 percent of those with mental retardation have a mild form. Their skills are near average, and although they may learn more slowly than peers, with proper educational and family support they can function independently as adults. Those with moderate retardation, 10 percent, need added support and may need to live in a group home, which provides a mixture of support and limited independence. The five percent with more severe mental retardation, will have more difficulty functioning in society and may require additional support to be able to manage day-to-day activities.

CAUSES

The causes of mental retardation are not always known. However, some common causes can be determined:

Genetic conditions result from abnormalities in an individual's genetic makeup. Some forms of mental retardation, especially mild forms, run in families.

Down's syndrome is the most common genetic cause of mental retardation. It is caused by an extra chromosome. The incidence of Down's syndrome increases significantly from one in 1000 births in mothers under the age of 30 to one in 50 to 100 births in women over the age of 40. The characteristic physical features of a child with Down's syndrome are slanted eyes, thickened tongue, short neck and extremities, and a broad, flat face. Mental retardation can range from mild to severe; some children with Down's syndrome can grow up to function nearly independently.

Fragile X syndrome is the second most common genetic cause of mental retardation. Its effects vary greatly, ranging from no noticeable symptoms to severe mental retardation. It is more common in males than in females.

PKU (phenylketonuria) is a genetic disorder that results in problems with the metabolism of the amino acid phenylalanine. If phenylalanine builds up in the body, it can cause damage to the brain and other parts of the body. Many states mandate testing for this disorder at birth, since the ill effects can be prevented by avoiding foods with phenylalanine.

Prenatal Conditions. The chances of

Resources on Mental Illness
American Psychiatric Association, *Diagnostic and Statistical Manual of Mental Disorders, 4th Edition* (1994); Barchas, Jack D., *Psychopharmacology: From Theory to Practive* (1977); Beckham, E. Edward and William R. Leber, eds., *Handbook of Depression: Treatment, Assessment, and Research* (1985); Wender, P.H. and D.F. Klein, *Mind, Mood, and Medicine: A Guide to the New Biopsychiatry* (1981); Nat. Depressive & Manic-Depressive Association, Tel. (800) 82-NDMDA, Online: www.ndmda.org; National Mental Health Association, Tel. (800) 969-NMHA, Online: www.nmha.org; www.ny-cornell.org/psychiatry/.

giving birth to a mentally retarded child increase when the mother is exposed to rubella, syphilis, and certain other infections during pregnancy. Maternal malnutrition, ingestion of alcohol, exposure to lead, and possibly smoking can also increase a child's risk of mental retardation.

Problems at Birth. Premature or low birth weight infants, as well as any babies that have suffered significant trauma during or shortly after birth, have increased incidence of mental retardation.

Diseases in Early Childhood. Mental retardation may be a complication of certain childhood diseases, such as measles, chicken pox, and whooping cough. These diseases can be prevented with vaccinations.

Toxins. Although adults may not suffer from the effects of exposure to lead, childrenexposed to these and other toxins may suffer mental deficits.

DIAGNOSIS

Two factors are evaluated to determine whether or not a young child is mentally retarded: IQ (intelligence quotient) and adaptive skills.

IQ. A child with an IQ below 70 may be considered mentally retarded. Although the results of IQ tests can be affected by factors unrelated to intelligence, such as cultural biases, language problems, motivation, and test conditions, an individually administered IQ test is necessary to determine mental retardation, and can be used as a measure in young children.

Adaptive skills, the second measure of mental retardation, include a thorough evaluation of skills needed to function in day-to-day activities: communication, taking care of oneself, self-direction, ability to navigate from place to place, and interaction with others. The Vineland Adaptive Behavior Scale (VABS) provides a formal measure of adaptive function.

Adaptive skills can be taught, modified, and improved throughout a person's lifetime, so that a child once considered mentally retarded can manage successfully enough in his or her environment that the diagnosis no longer applies.

Resources on Mental Retadation

Clarke, Ann. M., Alan D.B. Clarke, and Joseph M. Berg, *Mental Deficiency: The Changing Outlook* (1985); Dudley, James R., *Confronting the Stigma in their Lives: Helping People with a Mental Retadation Label* (1997); National Alliance for the Mentally Ill, Tel. (800) 950-6264, Online: www. nami.org; National Mental Health Association, Tel. (800) 969-NMHA, Online: www. nmha.org; www.nycornell.org/psychiatry/.

TREATMENT

Mental retardation should be diagnosed and treated as early as possible. Children with undiagnosed mental retardation may experience ostracism, discomfort, and frustration as they try to adapt to an environment that is ill-suited to them. In the United States, federal legislation guarantees diagnostic and treatment services to children with handicapping conditions, including mental retardation, from birth to 21 years of age. Programs in the various states are administered by Departments of Health (DOH) for children up to three years of age, and by Departments of Education thereafter. Programs in public schools depend on the severity of the retardation, and may range from extra help within the classroom, to supplemental activities, to placement in a special school. The goal of treatment is to afford a person with mental retardation an opportunity to develop the most of his or her potential. Ideally, a child will be able to improve adaptive skills and live within society as successfully as possible. Training includes activities to improve vocational, communication, math, and social skills.

Mental and emotional disorders are present to a greater degree in mentally retarded than in non-retarded persons. Mental retardation produces challenges to daily living that can result in frustration and exacerbate emotional problems. Aggressive and self-destructive behavior and sensitivity to overstimulation and crowding are more common in those with mental retardation than in the general population. Behavior modification has been used effectively to reinforce desirable behavior and discourage aggressive or destructive behavior. Medications may augment the efficacy of behavioral programs. This should be done under the care of a psychiatrist.

Aspects of mental retardation are discussed in BIRTH DEFECT; DOWN'S SYNDROME; FRAGILE X SYNDROME; INTELLIGENCE; INTELLIGENCE TESTS; *and* PHENYLKETONURIA. *Relevant specifics can be found in the entries on* FETAL ALCOHOL SYNDROME; TOXINS; *and* WITHDRAWAL, EMOTIONAL. *See also* CHICKENPOX; MEASLES; *and* WHOOPING COUGH.

Meperidine

Also known as Demerol

A narcotic painkiller (analgesic).

Meperidine is a prescription drug for moderate to severe pain. Because of the potential of addiction and interactions with other medications, it is important that a physician know a patient's other medications and health conditions before prescribing this medication.

Like all powerful analgesics, excessive use can lead to increased tolerance and addiction. In combination with MAO-inhibitor (MAOIs) antidepressant drugs, such as Nardil, Parnate, and Marplan, meperidine is extremely dangerous, potentially leading to agitation, fever, seizure, coma, and even death.

If taken with alcohol, it can increase the affects of alcohol and cause problems in concentration and coordination.

Side Effects. Taken alone, side effects may include dizziness, lightheadedness, nausea, vomiting, and sweating. *See also* ANALGESIC DRUGS *and* NARCOTIC DRUGS.

Mercury

Metallic element used in the manufacture of a number of products.

Mercury is a heavy metal. In elemental form, it exists at room temperature as a silver liquid; it also exists in the form of salts (inorganic compounds) and as a component of organic compounds. It causes skin irritation and is a toxin that can have lethal effects on the central nervous system.

Mercury has been used historically in hatmaking and in glassmaking, and is currently used in many other industries. Both elemental and inorganic forms of mercury are used in manufacturing electrical equipment, scientific instruments, dental amalgams, disk batteries, felt, disinfectants, and caustic soda. The compound methylmercury is used as a fungicide on grain. *See also* CHELATING AGENTS; MERCURY POISONING; *and* MINAMATA DISEASE.

Mercury Poisoning

Complex of symptoms caused by exposure to mercury or compounds containing mercury.

Mercury has long played a significant role in industrial production and craft, and mercury poisoning has accompanied such work. The phrase "mad as a hatter" refers to the psychosis that hatmakers in the nineteenth century exhibited due to exposure to toxic levels of mercury.

Exposure to mercury generally occurs from environmental pollution, including atmospheric fumes from refining, smelting, mining, or from the burning of fossil fuels. Marine environments are often contaminated by industrial runoff and dumping of mercury-containing materials. Organic mercury compounds are found in fish, shellfish, and in grains treated with the fungicide methylmercury.

Mercury and its compounds may be ingested, absorbed through the skin, or inhaled. Ingestion or inhalation of mercury can be fatal. If mercury exposure is suspected, call a poison control center and seek immediate medical attention.

Symptoms of acute mercury poisoning include a metallic taste, stomach pain, coughing, chest tightness, and breathing trouble. Pneumonia may develop, which can be fatal. Exposure to inorganic mercury compounds can cause nausea and vomiting, diarrhea (possibly bloody), and kidney damage.

Symptoms of chronic mercury poisoning include loose teeth, excessive salivation, painful or numb limbs, and emotional and mental changes, possibly including mood swings, irritability, loss of motivation, inability to concentrate, hallucinations, and memory loss.

The prognosis for mercury poisoning depends on the amount of mercury involved, length of exposure, and speed of treatment. Acute exposure may result in complete recovery, but it may be fatal. Fetuses and young children are particularly at risk for permanent developmental impairments. *See also* MERCURY *and* MINAMATA DISEASE.

Mesenteric Lymphadenitis

An inflammation of the lymph nodes in the abdominal membrane.

The cause of mesenteric lymphadenitis is not known, but has been linked to viral infections such as tuberculosis. The first symptom of this condition is lower abdominal pain. The disorder may also cause fever, night sweats, weakness, vomiting, tenderness, or rigidity. A mesenteric cyst may also be present; this is usually treated by draining the cyst. The disorder usually disappears after a short time. If symptoms persist for longer than half of a day, surgery may be necessary to observe the lymph nodes. If they are yellow in color, a carcinoid tumor is suspected. *See also* ABDOMEN.

Mesothelioma

Tumor of the tissue lining the lungs and chest cavity.

Mesotheliomas can be benign or malignant. There is a strong association between malignant mesotheliomas and long-term exposure to asbestos; up to 80 percent of malignant mesotheliomas occur in persons with a history of asbestos exposure.

A mesothelioma grows as a thick sheet over the lining of the lungs and chest cavity (mesothelium). It is composed of spindle cells or fibrous tissue which may enclose gland-like spaces.

Symptoms of a mesothelioma include shortness of breath, coughing, wheezing, chest pain, and bloody sputum. Diagnosis is made by chest x-rays, CAT scanning, and examination of fluid from within the chest cavity to detect abnormal cells.

Treatment. Most nonmalignant mesotheliomas can be surgically removed. Treatment of malignant mesothelioma can include surgery, radiation therapy, and chemotherapy, alone or in combination, but these measures generally can only alleviate symptoms. Prevention by protection against exposure to asbestos is strongly recommended. *See also* ASBESTOS *and* CANCER.

Metabolism

Combination of physical and chemical processes necessary for the maintenance of life.

Primarily, there are two types of chemical reactions are part of the metabolic process. An anabolic reaction uses energy to create complex molecules from simpler ones. Conversely, a catabolic reaction produces energy through the breakdown of complex molecules into simpler ones. The combination of these two processes supplies the body with the energy and some of the materials it needs for day-to-day activities.

The Resting Metabolic Rate (RMR) is the balance of caloric (energy) needs and energy expenditure by the body in a state of rest. Metabolic rates increase with more physical activity, or when certain hormones are released due to fear, illness, or stress.

While muscular activity accounts for most of an individual's energy consumption, regular exercise can increase the RMR, so that more calories are burned while at rest. In contrast, crash dieting (periods of severely restricted-calorie diets) without medical supervision can reset the Resting Metabolic Rate so that the body functions on extremely few calories. People who go through cycles of such dieting can actually reset their metabolisms so that they ultimately gain weight on as few as 800 or 900 calories per day.

Metabolic rates gradually decline with aging, in part due to decreased in muscle mass. This corresponds to an approximately two percent decrease in caloric requirements per decade after the age of 30. The decrease of the resting metabolic rate over time means that, while portion sizes must decrease, nutrient requirements remain fairly constant. Foods that comprise the diet must, therefore, be dense in nutrients and well-balanced.

For more in depth materials on metabolism see BASAL METABOLIC RATE; METABOLISM, INBORN ERRORS OF; CALORIE, KILOCALORIE, ENERGY; *and* ENERGY REQUIREMENTS. *Further related informatijon is contained in* DIET AND DISEASE; EXERCISE; *and* NUTRITION. *Also refer to* AMINO ACIDS.

Metabolism, Inborn Errors of

Genetic diseases that affect the body's ability to perform its normal chemical reactions.

In metabolic disorders, defective enzymes cause either a buildup of harmful substances or else prevent the body from producing the materials it needs. This can cause organs to function improperly and lead to a variety of symptoms. Phenylketonuria (PKU) and galactosemia are common examples of metabolic disorders.

The enzyme for phenylalanine breakdown is defective in individuals with PKU, Causing an excessive amount to accumulate. Phenylketonuria results from the build-up of an amino acid phenylalanine, found in many proteins. If left untreated, PKU can lead to mental retardation. Newborns are routinely screened for this disorder while still in the hospital; people with PKU can avoid symptoms by avoiding foods that contain phenylalanine.

Galactosemia is a form of lactose intolerance. Lactose is the primary sugar found in milk and dairy products. The body breaks down lactose into glucose and galactose, which are used for energy. In galactosemia, the enzyme responsible for converting galactose is defective, resulting in a buildup of the substance. This can lead to brain damage, digestive problems, and infections. Treatment consists of strictly avoiding all foods that contain milk or milk products. Infants can be fed with soy-based or other lactose-free formulas.

Other metabolic disorders include tyrosinemia (inability to metabolize the amino acid tyrosine), glutaric acidemia (buildup of glutaric acid), homocystinuria (inability to properly metabolize the amino acid methionine), and biotinidase deficiency (inability to process biotin). These are treated through diet management.

> *Disorders related to inborn errors of metabolism include* PHENYLKETONURIA; GALACTOSEMIA; *and* HOMOCYSTINURIA. *Issues that are related include* AMINO ACIDS; ENZYMES; *and* METABOLISM. *Also see* DNA; GENETICS; GENETIC COUNSELING; GENETIC DISORDERS; *and* GENETIC PROBE.

Metabolite

Any substance resulting from a metabolic (energy and nutrient processing) reaction.

A metabolite is a substance that has been transformed or changed after being metabolized by the body. Examples of metabolites include chemicals or toxins that have been transformed by the body into substances that are more easily excreted by the kidneys. *See also* METABOLISM *and* TOXIN.

Metaplasia

Abnormal transformation of one adult tissue into another type.

Metaplasia can occur in a number of organs. For example, fibrocystic disease of the breast can cause some skin cells to change so that they resemble sweat gland cells. Metaplasia often occurs in the tissue that lines various organs, such as the bladder, the intestine, and the bronchi. The transformation usually is not harmful, but may be pre-cancerous. Myeloid leukemia is sometimes preceded by metaplasia affecting the spleen, liver, and blood. *See* CANCER.

Metastasis

A malignant tumor that develops from cancer elsewhere in the body.

A metastasis is a malignant colony of cells originating from a primary cancer. The cancerous cells can travel through the lymphatic system, the bloodstream, or neighboring tissue. The sites in which a metastasis occurs depend on the location of the original cancer. For example, kidney cancer usually spreads to the lungs, liver, and bones, while prostate cancer spreads to the spine and pelvis. Chemotherapy and radiation therapy are prescribed after surgery (for a primary cancer) to attack metastases that may be too small to detect. A cancer that causes metastases is consider aggressive and dangerous, requiring quick and drastic measures in treatment. *See also* CANCER.

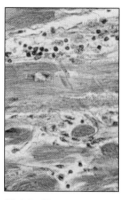

Metabolite.
The magnified image above, shows a substance metabolized or changed by the body into a substance more easily excreted by the kidneys.

Resources on Metabolism

Feek, C.M., and C.R. Edwards, *Endocrine and Metabolic Diseases* (1988); Groff, James L. and Sareen S. Gropper, *Advanced Nutrition and Human Metabolism* (1999); Heimburger, Douglas C. and R. L. Weinsier, *Handbook of Clinical Nutrition* (1997); Shils, Maurice E., et al., *Modern Nutrition in Health and Disease* (1999); American Dietetic Association, Tel. (800) 366-1655, Online: www.eatright.org; Center for Nutrition Policy and Promotion, Tel. (202) 418-2312, Online: www.usda. gov/cnpp; Food and Drug Admin., Tel. (888) INFOFDA, Online: www.fda.gov; www.nycornell.org/medicine/nutrition/index.html.

Metatarsalgia

Pain on the bottom of the foot felt while standing.

The long bones of the foot (metatarsals) meet the toe bones at the ball of the foot. Pain in this area may be caused by injury, arthritis, bone inflammation, foot strain, uncomfortable shoes, or abnormal bone structure in the foot. Calluses may form, and the muscles may weaken if underlying factors factors persist for long periods of time.

A physician should be consulted if the pain persists or if calluses form. Correcting the way in which the foot bears weight helps remove the pressure on the metatarsal heads. *See also* ARTHRITIS *and* CALLUS.

Methanol

Toxic form of alcohol.

Methanol (methyl or wood alcohol) is a volatile, colorless liquid used in products such as antifreeze, windshield fluid, canned heat, paint strippers, varnishes, and dyes. Exposure occurs via ingestion, inhalation, or skin absorption.

A low dose can cause nausea, fatigue, headache, and temporarily or permanently blurred vision. A larger dose may produce dizziness, stomach pain, vomiting, confusion, and slowed heart rate and breathing. Temporary or permanent blindness may occur several days later. A high dose can cause rapid breathing, coma, and death. Chronic inhalation may result in blurred vision progressing to complete blindness.

If exposure occurs, get emergency help quickly. The outlook depends on the amount of exposure and speed of treatment. *See also* ACCIDENT *and* ANTIFREEZE POISONING.

ALERT

Methanol Poisoning

Methanol is exceedingly toxic. A fatal dose can be as little as two to eight ounces for an adult, and only two tablespoons for a child. If methanol exposure is suspected, contact 911 or a poison control center immediately. Do not induce vomiting.

Methotrexate

A drug used for cancer and, recently, for serious cases of psoriasis and rheumatoid arthritis.

Prescribed for many forms of cancer, methotrexate is administered for rheumatoid arthritis when other drugs have proven ineffective. It is a very powerful drug and is to be taken only once a week for rheumatoid arthritis or psoriasis. Taking this drug more frequently can lead to fatal overdose.

SIDE EFFECTS

Side effects include abdominal pain, chills, fever, dizziness, fatigue, mouth ulcers, and nausea. Methotrexate affects the immune system, leaving the recipient vulnerable to other infections. It is not to be taken during pregnancy or by individuals suffering from alcoholism or liver disease. *See also* IMMUNE SYSTEM; *and* PSORIASIS.

Microcephaly

An abnormally small head in a newborn baby.

Microcephaly, an unusually small head is generally associated with poor brain growth. The majority of children afflicted with microcephaly are mentally handicapped.

CAUSES

This disorder is caused by chromosomal errors, improper implantation of the embryo during early pregnancy, infection, malnutrition, or the maternal use of certain drugs.

Women who have a history of miscarriages or infertility have a higher risk of giving birth to a baby with microcephaly. Exposure to rubella or x-rays during pregnancy also place the baby at risk.

SYMPTOMS

The primary indication of microcephaly is a head circumference below average range. Microcephaly can result in problems, such as cerebral palsy and seizures. *See also* BIRTH DEFECTS *and* DNA.

Microorganism

Any living entity that is microscopic or sub-microscopic in size.

Microorganisms include bacteria, fungi, protozoa, viruses, and other living things that are invisible to the naked eye. The medical community refers to microorganisms that cause disease as pathogens. Less technical terms used to refer to disease-causing microorganisms are germ and microbe.

A microorganism, however, need not be pathogenic. Indeed, many of the bacteria that reside on and in the body are actually helpful; some, for example, perform activities essential for digestion and clean up debris from the skin. *See also* BACTERIA; FUNGI; INFECTIOUS DISEASE; PATHOGEN; *and* VIRUS.

Microscope

Optical instrument used to magnify objects; used medically for the study of tissues and cells.

Microscopes of varying types are used to study tissues and cells, often for diagnostic purposes. The size, shape, number, and characteristics of cells may be analyzed and subcellular structures may be examined. The clarity of a microscopic image depends on its magnification, resolution, and contrast. Magnification increases the apparent size of the object under examination; most microscopes view objects at varying degrees of magnification. Resolution refers to the microscope's ability to distinguish between closely neighboring objects or structures. Contrast allows different cell structures to be clearly seen, often through the use of selective stains or dyes.

TYPES

Light microscopes, the most common types of microscopes use standard incandescent light to illuminate the object of study. Magnification may vary greatly (roughly between 25 and 1,000 times unaided vision) and the illumination source may be modified. Most light microscopes in medical use today have several lenses of varying magnification. Immune reactions, for example, may be evaluated using a fluorescent light source. Contrast is often enhanced through the use of staining techniques. Different materials within cells absorb colored stains at different rates.

While light microscopes can have very high magnifications, their resolving power is limited to about 500 times the unaided eye. While this is sufficient for most types of diagnostic examination of tissues and cells, examination of smaller subcellular structures requires even greater resolution.

Transmission electron microscopes replace the incandescent light source with a beam of electrons (the negatively charged subatomic particle that orbit the nucleus of an atom). Electrons pass through the specimen and strike a photographic plate, producing an image of the material. The instrument is capable of resolving objects 10,000 times better than the naked eye and has dramatically advanced the understanding of the microscopic world.

Scanning electron microscopes are a more recent and sophisticated variant. While the standard transmission electron microscope requires extensive preparation and sectioning of the specimen into ultra-thin slices before observation, a scanning electron microscope (SEM) can image the entire specimen by causing secondary electrons to be emitted by the specimen's surface. Through point-by-point mapping of the emission, a highly detailed three-dimensional image is created.

USES

Specialized microscopes, which display an enlarged image on a television screen, are used for surgery on tiny vessels and tissues, for example in the inner ear or fallopian tubes. The primary use of microscopes in medicine, is as a diagnostic tool.

Microscope analysis is vital for a physician to make a well informed DIAGNOSIS *or perform proper* DIAGNOSTICS IN WOMEN'S HEALTH; *which is related to* GYNECOLOGY. *Other imaging sources for information include* IMAGING TECHNIQUES.

Microsurgery

Highly precise surgery on delicate tissues using a microscope and, often, micromanipulators.

Microsurgery employs a high-powered binocular microscope and specialized instruments to perform surgical operations requiring extreme precision.

During microsurgery, surgeons can view the operating field magnified from six to 40 times, providing a functional look at nerves and blood vessels too small to see clearly with the naked eye. Operating microscopes are equipped with several binocular eyepieces, so more than one person can view the tissue and participate in surgery. Often, the field of view is also sent to a television monitor, allowing other members of the surgical team to observe the procedure.

USES

Microsurgery is used for a wide variety of delicate surgeries, including:
- connecting tiny nerves, blood vessels, and other tissue during the grafting of a severed limb;
- repairing the retina and other parts of the eye;
- performing a coronary bypass;
- removing brain and spinal cord tumors;
- transplanting muscles, tendons, or organs.

With microsurgery, tiny blood vessels with external diameters of 0.08 inches, known as microvessels, may be surgically rejoined, as may micronerves. The surgeon is often able to reestablish sensation by repairing or replacing severed and damaged peripheral nerves. Microsurgery requires supreme hand-eye coordination.

Among the more startling possibilities provided by microsurgery is the ability to restore severed tissue. Under favorable conditions, whole limbs may be replaced.

BENEFITS

Advantages of microsurgery include diminished blood vessel and nerve damage (due to the precision of the instruments), and greater visibility of the surgical area. Decreased tissue damage often leads to faster healing and fewer complications. Microsurgery has lowered mortality rates for serious diseases, including cancer and heart disease, and its supplemental use has improved the results of conventional surgical procedures. The technique has been extended to the cell and embryo.

For background information about microsurgery please see CORONARY ARTERY BYPASS; EMBRYO; *and* MICROSCOPE; *and* SURGERY; *Related anatomical information can be found in the entries* ARTERY; EYE; HEART; *and* NERVE. *Also refer to* ORGAN DONATION *and* TUMOR.

Middle-Ear Effusion, Persistent

A buildup of fluid in the middle ear.

The middle ear is the location of most ear infections. An accumulation of fluid in the middle ear that presses against the eardrum causes the pain and pressure known as otitis media. When the middle ear fills with a sticky fluid, causing stuffiness and hearing loss, the condition is known as a persistent middle-ear effusion, or otitis media with effusion (OME). This condition is rarely painful and is most common in children. It may affect one or both ears.

CAUSES

Middle-ear effusion usually follows within three to 16 weeks of an episode of acute otitis media. Some tests link the condition to bacteria—perhaps leftover from the otitis media. The most identifiable cause, however, is a malfunctioning eustachian tube.

On-Screen Microsurgery

A new technique known as three-dimensional on-screen microsurgery system (TOMS) allows surgeons to perform microsurgery without looking through a microscope. Two cameras in a video microscope are used to project a magnified three-dimensional image on one or more television monitors. The technique allows increased visibility of tissue under operation and reduces eye strain.

The tube may exert pressure on the middle ear, which then lets in fluid from the surrounding capillaries. The fluid buildup then interferes with the bones in the middle ear that pass sound vibrations to the inner ear. Eustachian tube problems may be the result of previous exposure to a virus, second-hand smoke, injury, or congenital disorders that cause the tube to function abnormally. Middle-ear effusion is also common in children who are prone to asthma, sinus infections, or allergies.

SYMPTOMS

One of the difficulties with middle-ear effusion is its lack of symptoms. The primary sign is some loss of hearing, but as the condition most commonly affects young children, they may be unaware of this or unable to describe it. Parents or teachers may notice before the child realizes there is a problem. Children may complain of stuffiness or a stopped-up feeling in the ears.

DIAGNOSIS AND TREATMENT

Middle-ear effusion may first be suspected as a result of a hearing test. After that, the eardrum is examined for changes that indicate the condition.

Middle-ear effusion often clears up on its own, perhaps with the aid of decongestants to help unblock the eustachian tubes. If the infection persists and there is a concern about long-term hearing loss, antibiotics may be prescribed, usually for 14 to 21 days. Some physicians may extend the course of antibiotics in order to prevent recurrence, but there actually is little evidence that this works. Increasingly, the medical community is questioning whether antibiotics are of any use at all for this condition. There is also additional concern about overmedication creating mutated strains of viruses that are becoming increasingly resistant to antibiotics. In extreme and persistent cases of middle-ear effusion surgery known as a myringotomy may be performed to drain the fluid from the ear. *See also* EAR; EARACHES: EAR, DISORDERS OF; EUSTACHIAN TUBE; MYRINGOTOMY; *and* OTITIS MEDIA.

Mid-Life Crisis

A crisis of confidence about a person's life choices, usually occurring in middle age.

A mid-life crisis is often triggered when a person reaches a certain age or starts to feel a decline in health or sexual function. At the bottom of such a crisis, whether conscious or not, is a realization of mortality and a questioning of the worth of one's life. Often in the 30s or 40s, a person starts to question whether he or she is leading the life that was envisioned in earlier years or that lives up to its potential. A person may have doubts along with an impulsive desire to make changes.

Questioning one's life can be disruptive or useful. It may provoke either needed and healthy changes or may lead to unnecessary and counterproductive changes. A person suffering from a mid-life crisis may suddenly feel extremely bored, tired, or irritable, have sexual affairs, or behave in ways that make him or her feel younger. A person may also handle a mid-life crisis in a way that is healthy for both the individual experiencing it and to others connected with that life.

It is healthy to evaluate one's life, to spend some time alone, and to be aware of the direction that life is taking. Assessing core values is important at this time. Perhaps previous goals were unrealistic. Perhaps small changes can be made, rather than disruptive, life-shattering changes. While they may be an increased desire to make major changes, they should be considered carefully, as they may be irreversible.

Committing oneself to a healthier lifestyle, without the illusion of becoming younger, can be quite beneficial. Recommitting to a spouse or to children can also be beneficial. Sometimes, a dissatisfying relationship can be revitalized or transformed through honest communication or counseling. Trying new activities, taking classes, and making an effort to meet new people may also be effective ways of improving one's life and reaching a fuller potential. *See also* AGING *and* DIET.

Midwifery

A form of health care focused on pregnancy and childbirth.

Midwives, most of whom are women, are health care practitioners specially trained to assist with childbirth. There are two basic kinds of midwives: certified nurse-midwives and lay, or independent, midwives. Midwives' training and experience varies widely, as does the setting in which they practice. They also differ in their procedures and approaches to childbirth.

Midwives generally are involved in a woman's care throughout pregnancy and remain with her during the course of childbirth. They also provide maternal postpartum care and teach basic infant care.

Many midwives view childbirth as a natural process and have a conservative approach to medical interventions. Some use modern techniques, such as administering pitocin to strengthen contractions. Generally, midwives are not licensed to perform forceps deliveries.

Midwives usually are involved in uncomplicated births. It is recommended, however, that a midwife have medical supervision and a professional connection to a medical facility in case any problems arise.

HISTORY OF MIDWIFERY

Until the 20th century, midwives were the primary health care providers for childbirth. In the past century, childbirth increasingly fell under the purview of medical doctors. At the same time it became removed from the home setting, and relocated to the hospital. A revival in the use of midwives began in the late 1960's, and by 1971 the American College of Obstetricians and Gynecologists began officially recognizing certified nurse-midwives.

Midwives were early advocates of natural (drug-free) childbirth, as well as innovations such as independent birth centers, and the use of birthing rooms and birthing chairs in a hospital setting. They also encouraged the movement of "rooming in" to promote mother and child bonding.

When to Use a Midwife

The use of a midwife should only be considered if the mother has no preexisting conditions, such as heart disease or diabetes, and if there are no complications in the pregnancy. Additionally, women over the age 35 are not good candidates, as they may experience more problems than younger women. Women interested in using a midwife should also make sure that there is conventional medical backup available.

TYPES OF MIDWIVES

Nurse-midwives are individuals who belong to a specialized category of advanced nursing that focuses on pregnancy, childbirth, and postpartum care including issues such as the care of the newborn, family planning, and other gynecological and family medical needs. Nurse-midwives are required to have a registered nursing degree and a certificate of midwifery from the American College of Nurse-Midwives, which stipulates a year of training in obstetrics and gynecology. Some go on to get a master's degree as well after a year of internship.

Nurse-midwives mostly practice in hospitals and clinics or in birth centers. They may assist medical doctors or have their own group or private practices. There are currently 4,000 certified nurse-midwives in the United States, and they are increasing in popularity.

Lay midwifery is very different from nurse-midwifery; many of the practices of lay-midwives may conflict with standard obstetric care and ideas. Most lay midwives assist in home births only and are not affiliated with any medical facilities. The use of a lay midwife is illegal or discouraged in many localities and is generally not covered by insurance. The Midwives Alliance of North America (MANA) is currently trying to develop national certification guidelines for lay midwives.

Further information about midwifery can be found in the entries on DELIVERY; NURSE; PLACENTA; and PREGNANCY. Important related details are included under the entries for FORCEPS; FORCEPS DELIVERY; and POSTPARTUM HEMORRHAGE. ECTOPIC PREGNANCY and FETUS are also quite vital.

Migraine

Severe form of headache, usually recurrent and affecting only one side of the body.

Migraines can affect anyone at any age. Most migraine sufferers begin to get migraines between the ages of ten and 30 and continue until the age of 50. Twenty-five percent of women and eight percent of men complain of migraine headaches. The majority of migraine sufferers have close relatives who also suffer from migraines, indicating that there may be a genetic predisposition for these headaches.

Cause. The reason for migraines is not understood. Two theories exist for the physical process of migraines. One is that the arteries to the brain narrow (constrict) and then widen (dilate), triggering pain receptors that produce the migraine. The second, and latest, theory surmises that proteins are released in the brain, inflaming blood vessels and nerves, resulting in pain.

Symptoms. There are two forms of migraines: migraines without an aura (a set of symptoms preceding the migraine) and migraines with an aura. An aura may consist of an alteration in vision, numbness in the face, arms, and hands, muscle weakness, or difficulty speaking. Aura symptoms last no longer than one hour and affect only one side of the body.

Whether a migraine is preceded by an aura (classic migraine) or is not (common migraine), symptoms may include:

- pulsing pain centralized on one side of the head that can curtail the ability to function;
- at least five attacks per year that last four to72 hours;
- pain upon physical exertion;
- nausea or vomiting; and
- light sensitivity or sound sensitivity.

Before a physician can diagnose a migraine, he or she must ascertain that the patient has no other diseases that could produce the same symptoms.

Treatment. If migraine attacks occur more than once a month, the patient should determine what triggers his or her attacks and avoid the triggers, thus limiting the number of attacks.

Aspirin or acetaminophen, along with an anti-nausea drug, can treat a mild migraine. An acute migraine may need to be treated with ergotamine—a vasoconstrictor that narrows blood vessels, preventing the dilation that causes pain. Medications for high blood pressure and heart disease, such as beta blockers and calcium-channel blockers, have also been found to provide relief in some sufferers of migraine.

> *Interesting treatment options are listed under* AURA; ALTERNATIVE MEDICINE; BIORYTHMS; *and* BIOFEEDBACK/BIOFEEDBACK TRAINING. *Further information can be found in articles on* HEADACHES; PAIN; *and* PAIN RELIEF. *See also* NAUSEA.

Milia

A cluster of cysts in the skin or a mucus membrane.

Milia is often seen in newborns. It appears as small, white bumps, most commonly across the cheeks, nose, chin, and forehead. These bumps may also develop on the gums or roof of the mouth. This condition occurs when dead skin, normally brushed off of the skin naturally, is trapped underneath the surface. When irritated, the area around these bumps becomes red, although the center is still white. Sometimes milia is incorrectly called "baby acne."

No treatment is necessary. As the surface of the cysts wear off, the dead skin is lost and the milia disappear. *See also* CYST.

Triggers

Although the underlying cause of migraines is unknown, the attacks are often triggered by specific conditions. A variety of situations can produce a migraine attack in a vulnerable individual:

- Anxiety;
- Climatic changes;
- Ingestion of chocolate, aged cheese, red wine, nuts, and fried food;
- Loud noises, intense smells, and strong lights;
- Menstrual cycle and birth control pills; and
- Smoking and fatigue.

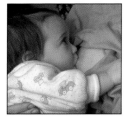

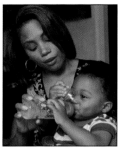

Milk.
Breast feeding, above, top, provides babies with the right balance of nutrients and antibodies to help fight illness and infection. As children get older, bottle feeding, above, bottom, replaces breast feeding.

Milk

Nourishing, white liquid secreted by female mammary glands.

Breast milk is the ideal food for infants. It contains just the right balance of nutrients such as protein, carbohydrates and fat, as well as maternal antibodies that help babies fight off illness and infection until they develop their own antibodies. However, breast milk can occasionally be a source of toxins. Infants can be exposed to prescription or illicit drugs in breast milk. Most chemicals are metabolized rapidly, so that they only appear in breast milk after recent exposure. Yet, with supplemental iron, the benefits of breast feeding far outweigh the risks.

Animal's milk is a food source in many areas of the world, and each type varies in nutritional makeup. Cow's milk is the most popular, particularly in the United States. It may also be a source of contaminants, since cows are often treated with chemicals or antibiotics. It is essential that milk be pasteurized, as raw milk often contains illness-causing bacteria. Cow's or goat's milk should not replace breast milk in the diets of infants under the age of one.

Many adults lose the ability to produce the enzyme lactase and become lactose intolerant. For those who can tolerate it, milk is an excellent source of calcium; it provides approximately 72 percent of the calcium in the American diet. *See also* BREAST-FEEDING; LACTOSE INTOLERANCE; *and* PASTEURIZATION.

Milk-Alkali Syndrome

A condition of excess alkali in the blood which can lead to nausea, headache, and fatigue.

People with peptic ulcers often consume excessive amounts of milk or antacids, such as sodium or calcium bicarbonate, to relieve pain and promote healing. These antacids quickly neutralize the acid in the stomach, but they are absorbed into the bloodstream where they change the pH balance and can lead to alkalosis. Milk-alkali syndrome has, however, become rare.

Symptoms of alkalosis include nausea, headache, and kidney damage from calcium deposits in the tissue. Antacids should not be taken by peptic ulcer sufferers for more than a few days at a time. The disease can be treated with a number of other drugs. A change in diet, reducing alcohol consumption, and eliminating smoking are recommended. *See also* ALKALOSIS.

Milk of Magnesia

A type of laxative.

Milk of magnesia may alleviate constipation and can serve as a possible treatment for symptoms of heart-burn. *See* ACID REFLUX.

Minamata Disease

Form of mercury poisoning.

This severe type of mercury poisoning is named after the original outbreak site in Japan, where more than 100 people were affected, 46 of whom died from damage to the central nervous system, brain lesions, and brain atrophy.

The syndrome was traced to a nearby chemical plant that dumped inorganic mercury wastes into the waters of Minamata Bay. These wastes were converted into methylmercury by aquatic microorganisms, which then contaminated the local seafood, affecting the local population who ate the tainted fish.

Children born to women who had eaten the contaminated fish developed severe neurological and anatomical deformities, even when the mothers themselves did not exhibit any signs of toxicity. These babies usually appeared normal for the first six months, then developed symptoms including limb deformities, stunted skeletal growth, muscle weakness, disturbed cognitive development, and convulsions. Minamata disease thus offers a sobering lesson on the consequences of introducing toxins into the food chain.

The largest outbreak of Minamata disease occurred in 1971 in Iraq, where a shipment of methylmercury-treated grain from Mexico was mistakenly made into bread instead of being used only for planting, as intended. Tragically, 6,530 people around the entire country were stricken, and 459 died. *See also* BIRTH DEFECTS; BRAIN; FOOD CONTAMINATION; MERCURY POISONING; *and* MUSCLE.

Mind-Body Medicine

Term used to refer to the many alternative therapies that emphasize the interrelationship between the mind and body.

The mind-body, or the psychophysiological approach to medicine, promotes the idea of the body as a whole entity. Practitioners of this approach view certain conditions, such as migraines, asthma, digestive disorders, and eczema, as directly related to an individual's mental and emotional health. These therapies aim to stimulate the health of the mind in conjunction with the body (for example, techniques such as yoga) in order to alleviate various symptoms and generate an overall sense of well-being in the individual .

Mind-body practitioners work to reduce stress, anxiety, and other mental health conditions by treating the body in a "holistic" manner using techniques less familiar to Western physicians. By targeting the psychological factors underlying a specific disorder, practitioners will suggest any one of a number of therapies designed to improve the function of the nervous and endocrine systems and promote relaxation.

Mind-body medicine includes techniques such as biofeedback, guided imagery, hypnotherapy, meditation, relaxation response, and support groups. Some other alternative healing therapies grounded in this approach include acu-puncture, acupressure, herbal medicine, massage, and yoga.

Mind-Body Medicine is a type of ALTERNATIVE MEDICINE *closely allied with* ACUPUNCTURE; ASTON PATTERNING; HERBAL MEDICINE; HOMEOPATHY; QIGONG; ROLFING; *and* SHIATSU.

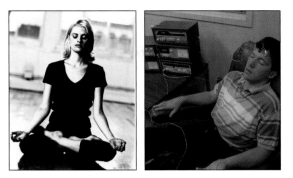

Mind-Body Medicine.
Techniques such as yoga, above, and biofeedback, at right, have become some of today's most popular ways to reduce stress, alleviate certain illnesses, and enhance a person's well-being.

Mineral

Elementary, inorganic substance that originates in water and soil and is incorporated into animal and plant life.

Certain minerals are essential, in small amounts, to many body process. They play important roles in every cell; in oxygen transport, in the maintenance of chemical and fluid balances, in regulating heartbeat, and in controlling enzyme and hormone activity. The major minerals, required in quantities of hundreds of milligrams per day, are calcium, magnesium, and phosphorus. A variety of trace minerals, those required in minute amounts, such as zinc, are also essential to health. A balanced and diverse diet should provide all the necessary minerals; supplementation is necessary only in some special circumstances. *See also* CALCIUM; IRON; MAGNESIUM; *and* PHOSPHORUS.

Mineral Oil

Type of stool softener obtained from petroleum.

Often used as a laxative, mineral oil softens stool and eases its passage from the body. It can be taken orally or administered as an enema and is usually recommended after severe bouts of constipation or painful bowel movements. Mineral oil should not be used over prolonged periods of time as it can prevent the absorption of vitamins, or be aspirated into the lungs. *See also* LAXATIVE DRUGS.

Miscarriage

Also known as spontaneous abortion

A sudden loss of pregnancy before the 20th week.

Approximately half of all fertilized eggs do not survive to become implanted in the uterus. After successful implantation, the miscarriage rate is approximately 20 percent. Loss of pregnan-cy after the 20th week is known as a stillbirth.

CAUSES

Quite frequently, it is impossible to state what causes a miscarriage to occur. The most common reason is a genetic or chromosomal anomaly in the embryo or an abnormality in the placenta or uterus. Other contributors to miscarriage include environmental factors such as exposure to drugs, chemicals, radiation, and heavy metals. Additionally, any physical trauma sustained by the mother may lead to a loss of the pregnancy. The rate of miscarriage increases with maternal age.

More than half of all miscarriages occur in the first eight weeks of the pregnancy; this is during the early phases of development for all the major organs.

SYMPTOMS

The most common symptom of a miscarriage is vaginal bleeding. The bleeding may be accompanied by cramps, which can vary in severity. Eventually the cervix dilates and the woman starts passing large clots and tissue.

It is important to note that not all vaginal bleeding is indicative of a miscarriage. There are a variety of other reasons for vaginal bleeding that need not result in a miscarriage. However, a doctor should be consulted immediately for any signs of bleeding.

Another possible indication of a miscarriage is the lack of fetal growth from one prenatal visit to the next, or the inability to hear the fetal heartbeat after it was detected, or past the time when it should be heard for the first time (between the 12th and 16th weeks).

TREATMENT

A woman who suspects a miscarriage should go to a doctor for evaluation. In addition to a physical exam, this includes listening for a fetal heartbeat as well as the use of ultrasound to help rule out an ectopic pregnancy. If the physician determines that a miscarriage has occurred, it is important to make sure that all fetal material is expelled. A dilation and curettage (D&C) may need to be performed.

Incompetent Cervix

The cervix is the opening from the uterus to the vagina; it usually remains closed until the onset of labor. In a condition known as incompetent cervix, the weight of the fetus forces the cervix open, resulting in a miscarriage. This form of miscarriage can be prevented with cerclage, a procedure in which the cervix is stitched closed. At the beginning of the ninth month, the stitches are cut so childbirth can occur.

PREVENTION

Other than ensuring that the mother receives good nutrition and prenatal care, there is little that can prevent a miscarriage. If there is any bleeding during pregnancy (threatened miscarriage), a doctor will usually advise a patient to forgo exercise and sexual intercourse. Bed rest may be recommended as well. Certain circumstances may require hospitalization.

RECOVERY

A woman should wait a few weeks after a miscarriage before resuming sexual relations and two menstrual cycles before attempting to conceive. In addition to the physical recovery, many women find a miscarriage emotionally difficult and may require treatment.

Sometimes after a late miscarriage, a woman's breasts begin producing milk as they normally would after giving birth. The breasts will dry up within a few weeks. Medication can be given to facilitate this as well.

Background material on this topic can be found in CERVICAL INCOMPETENCE; EMBRYO; PREGNANCY, FALSE; *and* VAGINAL BLEEDING. *Vital anatomical information can be found under* CERVIX; UTERUS; *and* VAGINA; *See also* ABORTION.

Mites and Disease

Diseases caused by parasitic arachnids.

Many mites are associated with human disease. The scabies mite *(Sarcoptes scabiei)*, produces an infestation of the skin, often between the fingers, on the front of the wrists, and in the folds of the elbows, armpits, buttocks, and genitals. Chiggers (larvae of the thombiculidae family) and similar mites cause intense itching. They may be diagnosed by examining skin scrapings under a microscope. Most mites are transmitted by human contact and cannot survive more than a few days in the absence of a human or animal host.

Treatment for mite diseases should follow positive identification, as the symptoms can mimic other diseases. Treatment entails application of insecticidal cream, lotion, or solution, accompanied by thorough washing of garments and bedding. Many mite diseases are readily transmissible through skin contact. It is therefore advised that all those in close contact with someone positively diagnosed seek treatment as well. *See also* CHIGGER BITE; INSECTS AND DISEASE; SCABIES; *and* STING.

Mitral Insufficiency

Also known as mitral regurgitation or incompetence

Failure of the mitral valve to close sufficiently as it controls the flow of blood between the left atrium and left ventricle of the heart.

When the mitral valve does not close properly, some of the blood that is supposed to flow into the left ventricle leaks into the left atrium, an upper chamber of the heart. This leakage causes the heart to work harder than normal. Both the left atrium and the left ventricle may become enlarged.

CAUSES

The most common cause of mitral insufficiency is mitral valve prolapse. It can also be due to rheumatic heart disease or other inflammatory conditions, such as systemic lupus erythematosus (a congenital defect) or infective myocarditis.

ALERT

Acute Mitral Insufficiency

Sudden (acute) mitral insufficiency can occur when one of the tendons holding the valve in place ruptures. The result can be pulmonary edema, a quick and dangerous buildup of fluid in the lungs; and cardiogenic shock, a swift drop in blood pressure as the heart loses its ability to pump blood to the body. Acute mitral insufficiency requires emergency treatment.

SYMPTOMS

Symptoms may not appear for years. First, there is shortness of breath during periods of heavy exertion. As the condition worsens, breathlessness is experienced with less and less exertion. Fatigue and weakness may occur without shortness of breath. Growing pressure on the airways may lead to a chronic cough. An accumulation of fluid may cause swelling of the arms, legs, and sometimes the abdomen. Over the years, untreated mitral insufficiency can lead to atrial fibrillation and can increase the risk of embolism and endocarditis.

DIAGNOSIS AND TREATMENT

Chronic mitral insufficiency can be diagnosed by the abnormal sound (heart murmur) that it causes and that can be heard through a stethoscope. The diagnosis will be confirmed and the extent of the problem determined by a chest x-ray, an electrocardiogram, and an echocardiogram. These will show the nature of the valve defect and its effect on the heart.

Mild mitral insufficiency may require only careful monitoring. For severe cases, treatment can include antibiotics to reduce the risk of endocarditis and medications to prevent atrial fibrillation and the formation of embolisms. Medications such as vasodilators or diuretics may be prescribed to decrease the workload of the heart. If the condition continues to worsen, surgery can be done to repair a damaged mitral valve or to replace it with an artificial valve.

Vital information about this vital organ can be found in CARDIOLOGY; CONGENITAL HEART DISEASE; EMBOLISM; ENDOCARDITIS; *and* MITRAL STENOSIS. *Related anatomical articles include* BLOOD; HEART; HEART VALVE; *and* VENTRICLE.

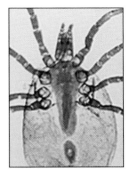

Mites.
Shown above is a magnified image of a mite. Mites are carriers (vectors) of many important diseases including typhus (scrub and murine) and rickettsiapox.

Mitral Stenosis

Narrowing of the valve that controls blood flow from the left atrium to the left ventricle of the heart.

The narrowing associated with mitral stenosis reduces the blood pressure through the valve. As a result, the left atrium works harder to move blood sufficiently. Over the years, the left atrium may suffer heart failure. This failure, an inability to pump enough blood to satisfy the needs of the body, eventually causes a buildup of fluid in veins and tissues.

Causes and Symptoms. The most common cause of mitral valve stenosis is scarring of the valve due to an untreated bout of rheumatic fever during childhood. Symptoms generally remain dormant for many years. The primary symptoms of mitral stenosis are shortness of breath and fatigue, experienced first during exertion and then at times of rest as the condition worsens. Untreated, mitral stenosis can lead to atrial fibrillation, an arrhythmia that is potentially life-threatening.

Mitral stenosis is diagnosed by a physical examination followed by tests such as electrocardiography, echocardiography, a chest X-ray, and stress testing. Drug treatments, such as diuretics and antiarrhythmic medications, can often keep the condition under control. Some patients may need surgery to repair the damaged valve. If the valve requires a replacement, either a mechanical device or a valve made of animal tissue is used. *See also* HEART; HEART DISEASE; *and* HEART VALVE SURGERY.

Mitral Valve Prolapse

A slight deformity of the valve between the left atrium and the left ventricle of the heart whereby a bulge causes blood to leak into the atrium.

Mitral valve prolapse is the most common heart valve abnormality, affecting up to five percent of American adults. It causes a distinctive murmur, sometimes accompanied by a clicking sound, that can be heard through a stethoscope. Mitral valve prolapse almost always relates to a congenital condition that is present from birth and is more common in women than men. It usually causes no symptoms, although some persons with the condition may experience shortness of breath, palpitations, and some chest pain while at rest.

Mitral valve prolapse often requires no treatment, but medications, such as beta blocking drugs, may be prescribed if symptoms are present. Physicians recommend taking antibiotics before seeing a dentist or undergoing minor surgery to reduce the risk of infection. Serious complications are unusual. In rare cases, abnormal heart rhythms may develop as well as endocarditis (inflammation of the lining of the heart). Severe leakage may lead to heart failure; sometimes surgery is needed to correct the valve abnormality. *See also* HEART; HEART DISEASE; *and* HEART VALVE SURGERY.

Mittelschmerz

Abdominal pain that occurs in the middle of the menstrual cycle, around the time of ovulation.

Mittelschmerz is sometimes accompanied by slight vaginal bleeding. It is believed to be related to ovulation. When the follicle ruptures, releasing the egg, some fluid leaks into the abdominal cavity and acts as an irritant. The bleeding may be due to the drop in estrogen levels that accompany ovulation. Mittelschmerz usually only lasts a day or two. Rarely is the pain severe. *See also* MENSTRUATION *and* REPRODUCTIVE SYSTEM.

Mobilization

Restoration of movement in body parts.

Mobilization usually refers to the process of helping to restore movement to a body part that may have been injured or affected by disease. Exercises and physical therapy can increase mobilization by alleviating stiffness or retraining a body part for a movement that it may have lost. In surgery, the term mobilization refers to freeing an organ or body part from its connective tissue. *See also* EXERCISE *and* PHYSICAL THERAPHY.

Molar Pregnancy

A form of miscarriage in which the tissue around the fertilized egg, instead of developing into a normal placenta, forms an abnormal structure known as a hydatidform mole. The mole keeps growing even after the fetus has deteriorated.

Because a hydatidiform mole produces the hormone human chorionic gonadotropin (hCG), which is produced during pregnancy, a pregnancy test will be positive. However, it soon becomes apparent that the uterus is growing more quickly than expected. There may be vaginal bleeding or passage of a grape-like cluster of tissue, but often the first symptom is the lack of a fetal heartbeat. Ultrasound can be used to distinguish between a molar pregnancy and a normal one. *See also* HYDATIDFORM MOLE.

Mold

A microscopic organism that produces spores that are light enough to float in the air.

Mold growths appear as discolorations on warm, damp areas of wood, paper, or leaves. They produce and release spores that flourish when they land on other warm, damp areas. While mold spores are not themselves considered disease-causing (pathogenic), inhalation of a large concentration of spores can produce allergic reactions, asthma attacks, infections, and other respiratory problems. Molds can be controlled by cleaning, disinfecting, and drying the moldy area. *See also* ALLERGY MICROORGANISM; *and* PATHOGEN.

Moles

Also known as nevus (singular) or nevi (plural)

Common, harmless, dark spots on the skin.

Moles vary in color; they may be pink, brown, bluish-gray, or black. They can be present at birth or develop after sunlight exposure. Moles begin to grow in infancy, but new moles develop at any age. During pregnancy, spots may become darker. In old age, moles may disappear completely.

A congenital pigmented nevus is a mole that is present at birth, in about one baby in 100, and may range in size from a few millimeters in diameter to a spot that covers half a baby's skin. A congenital mole should be evaluated by a doctor to see if the mole presents a risk of becoming cancerous. A halo nevus is a white ring surrounding a mole. It is not dangerous, and will disappear in time. An atypical nevus is a mole with unusual features, such as an irregular border. Although it may resemble a cancerous mole, it is benign. However, any atypical-appearing mole should be evaluated by a physician to be certain it is not malignant.

Although typical moles are harmless and usually require no treatment, they may need to be removed. A mole that has bled, has an unusual shape, has changed color, or is growing rapidly should be checked by a doctor to be certain it is benign. Moles that are either unsightly or irritated by the rubbing of clothing can be removed. *See also* BIRTHMARK; DERMATOLOGY; MOLAR PREGNANCY; SKIN; *and* SKIN CANCER.

Molluscum Contagiosum

A contagious viral infection of the skin that produces wart-like growths.

The wart-like growths associated with molluscum contagiosum usually appear on the chest, arms, abdomen, or groin and may be from one-half inch to 1.5 inches in diameter. These growths have a smooth, shiny surface with a depression in the center.

The virus that causes molluscum contagiosum is transmitted by direct contact with an infected person or by contact with clothes, towels, or washcloths that have been used by an infected person.

The growths associated with the condition often disappear on their own if the sufferer has a normal immune system, but may also be treated with over-the-counter wart preparations. Cryosurgery (freezing of the affected area) can remove the growths, though this surgery may leave a scar. *See also* Virus *and* WART.

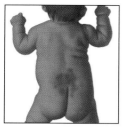

Mongolian Spot.
Mongolian blue spots, above, are flat bluish gray skin markings commonly appearing at birth or shortly after. They appear at the base of the spine, on the buttocks, and shoulder.

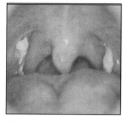

Mononucleosis.
Infectious mononucleosis, cause a sore throat, large lymph nodes and fatigue. The throat above may appear red and the tonsils covered with a whitish material (exudate).

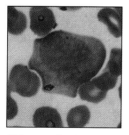

This so-called **"Downy cell"** is typical of lymphocytes infected by the Esptein-Barr virus in infectious mononucleosis. Downy cells may be classified as types I, II, or III. The cell above is a type II.

Mongolian Spot

Also known as mongolian blue spot

Flat, blue or bluish gray marks, commonly appearing at birth or shortly thereafter.

Mongolian spots have an irregular border and shape. They appear on the base of the spine, buttocks, and back. These pigmented lesions are benign and are not associated with any other condition or illness.

The condition is commonly associated with darker-skinned individuals, especially Asians, East Indians, and Africans. The spots may appear similar to a bruise. The blue area has a normal skin texture and may cover a large portion of the back. Usually, Mongolian spots disappear by the time a child is ten years old. *See* Bruise *and* Skin.

Monitor

Device designed to measure bodily functions and alert a physician in the case of irregularity or failure.

Many types of medical monitors exist to measure and keep track of critical health indicators (vital signs). Some monitors are used for a patient only during a hospital stay, particularly those used for medical evaluation during and after surgery. Others may be used on an outpatient basis to provide early warning of irregular conditions or track the progress of ongoing treatment.

Among the more common types of monitor are those for blood pressure, cardiac function, fetal heartbeat, and other prenatal functions, and the Holter monitor, a mobile device used to record a patient's electrocardiogram over an extended period. *See also* Blood pressure; Cardiology; ECG; Fetal Heart Monitoring; Heart *and* Holter Monitor.

Monoarthritis

Arthritis that affects only one joint.

This specific, highly localized sharp pain and stiffness can be the result of osteoarthritis, gout, or an infection. *See also* Arthritis; Gout; *and* Osteoarthritis.

Mononucleosis

An infection of the Epstein-Barr virus, one of the family of herpes viruses.

The Epstein-Barr virus enters the body through the nose and throat and moves quickly to the B-lymphocytes (white blood cells). Since the virus is usually transmitted through saliva from the mouth, mononucleosis is popularly referred to as the "kissing disease." It may take as long as four to eight weeks for symptoms of mononucleosis to appear. The disease is not especially contagious and the incidence of infection peaks in the early teen years.

The Epstein-Barr virus has been detected in people with compromised immune systems, such as those with AIDS or who are being treated for cancer with chemotherapy, but the exact role of the virus in these situations is not known at this time.

Symptoms of mononucleosis are usually mild and include a fever that rises from 102° to 104° F, a sore throat, swollen glands, loss of appetite, and (most characteristic of the disease) fatigue and weakness that may last for weeks. The throat and tonsils become very red and the tonsils may have a whitish coating. A small percentage of patients develop a red rash on their bodies. A third of the people who contract mononucleosis develop strep throat or an enlarged spleen. Other complications of the disease include hepatitis, encephalitis, and myocarditis (an inflammation of the heart).

Acyclovir

The antiviral drug Acyclovir reduces the spread of the Epstein-Barr virus. However, once infectious mononucleosis takes hold, the drug does not seem to affect the symptoms or prognosis.

Treatment. Since mononucleosis is caused by a virus (against which medications are not generally effective), it is treated with rest, plenty of fluids, and an attempt to maintain normal eating habits even though the sufferer may not be hungry. A nonsteroidal anti-inflammatory drug can reduce fever and relieve muscle aches.

Aspirin is not advised for children because of the danger of Reye's syndrome, a dangerous condition caused by the combination of aspirin and a virus in children. If the air passages are swollen and breathing is difficult, the patient may be given corticosteroids. Most symptoms of mononucleosis abate in ten days to two weeks. At that point, recovered patients can resume most of their normal activities. However, fatigue may persist for weeks or even months after other symptoms have disappeared. *See also* AIDS; B-CELL; EPSTEIN-BARR; IMMUNE SYSTEM; REYE'S SYNDROME; *and* VIRUS.

Monteggia's Fracture

Break and dislocation of the forearm bones.

A break in the inner forearm (ulna) occasionally leads to the dislocation of the outer forearm bone (the radius). This condition is known as Monteggia's fracture and is usually the result of injury such as a fall or direct blow.

Surgery to repair Monteggia's fracture requires incisions on both sides of the forearm in order to replace the radius into the joint. The broken ends of the ulna may then be rejoined and immobilized with plates, screws, or a plaster cast in order to heal correctly. *See also* FRACTURE.

Mood Disorders

Persistent mood disturbance that is marked either by a cyclic pattern of depression and euphoria.

The two major groups of mood disorders are: major depression and bipolar disorder, also know as manic-depression. Major depression affects about 10 percent and bipolar disorder affects 1.2 percent of adults at some point during their lifetime.

While all individuals experience occasional everyday unhappiness, people with major depression sustain a depressed mood for two weeks or more. Other symptoms include low self-esteem, poor concentration, feelings of hopelessness and helplessness, lack of pleasure, low energy, and changes in sleep patterns and appetite. Depressions often begin during or after stressful events like the death of a loved one, divorce, moving, or job loss. Later, depressive episodes may recur without any clear stressor. While some people have only one episode of depression, the majority of sufferers will have multiple depressive episodes or persistent depression.

Several problems can imitate depression, like undiagnosed medical illness, adverse drug reactions, and alcohol and drug abuse. Anyone who has depressive symptoms for two or more weeks should seek medical evaluation and treatment.

Bipolar disorder is marked by alternating periods of depressed moods and euphoric or irritable moods. The manic phase is characterized by sharply increased energy, grandiose or idealized thinking, decreased sleep, increased sexual drive, and excessive spending.

Both major depression and bipolar disorder are serious illnesses, not only due to the painful symptoms and impaired functioning that result, but because they are associated with a high risk of suicide.

There are effective and safe treatments for mood disorders including antidepressant medication, mood stabilizers such as lithium and valproic acid, electroconvulsive therapy (ECT), as well as various forms of psychotherapy. The combination of a biological therapy, such as a prescription medication with psychotherapeutic treatment is very effective.

Mood Disorders are further discussed in relation to ANTIDEPRESSANT DRUGS; DEPRESSION; BIPOLAR DISORDER, SUICIDE; *and* POSTPARTUM DEPRESSION. *Also refer to entries detailing* ACTING OUT; ALCOHOL DEPENDENCE; DELIRIUM; INSECURITY; MENTAL ILLNESS; *and* PSYCHIATRY.

Morbidity

Term used to describe a state of illness or disease.

The term morbidity is used to indicate the presence of disease in tissues or organs. Additionally, the term morbidity rate is sometimes used in place of "incidence" to denote the number of diseased people within a given population over time. This variable is sometimes compared with the number of deaths in a given population or region, known as the mortality rate. *See also* DEATH *and* MORTALITY.

Morning After Pill

Also known as ECP, emergency contraceptive pill or post-coital pontraception

Coloquialism for high doses of oral contraceptives taken to prevent pregnancy after a single act of unprotected sex.

An emergency contraceptive pill (ECP) must be taken within 72 hours of intercourse to be effective. Physicians prefer not to use the term "morning after pill," as it implies that the pill can be used often and should only be taken in the morning, neither of which are advisable. While the failure rate of ECP's is low, it is still higher than that of oral contraceptives, making them ineffective and unreliable as conventional contraceptive alternatives.

ECP's are not to be confused with so called abortion pills such as mifepristone (RU 486); which induce miscarriage. ECP's prevent conception by thickening the cervical mucus, making it difficult for sperm to pass through, and by thinning the endometrial lining, thereby decreasing the chances that an egg will implant. Side effects include nausea, breast tenderness, and an irregular menstrual cycle. *See also* ABORTION; BIRTH CONTROL; *and* CONTRACEPTION.

Morning Sickness

Nausea and vomiting early in pregnancy.

Usually, morning sickness occurs early in the day. Although its exact cause is un-

known, it may be caused by either hormonal changes or low blood sugar. Morning sickness occurs in about half of all pregnancies and is not usually a cause for alarm. A doctor should be consulted if vomiting is severe and persistent or if an affected woman vomits blood or loses more than two pounds of body weight. *See also* EMBRYO; MULTIPLE BIRTHS; *and* PREGANCY.

Morphea

Disease of unknown cause in which hard, oval patches form on the skin.

Morphea is a form of localized scleroderma, an autoimmune disease that affects the skin in which body tissue hardens. Hard, whitish patches with a purple ring around them form on the skin. They are most often found on the trunk, but can also occur on the face, legs, and arms. In generalized morphea, the patches spread throughout the entire body. In this form of the disease, the underlying muscles may tighten and atrophy. However, generalized morphea does not usually affect the internal organs. The disease often improves on its own after two or three years. *See also* IMMUNE RESPONSE; IMMUNE SYSTEM; *and* SCLERODERMA.

Morphine

A powerful opioid pain relief (analgesic) drug that is effective in controlling pain.

Almost all of the strongest painkillers are based on morphine, a natural substance extracted from poppies. Synthetic morphines are also available. Morphine is available in injectable form, as pills, and as sustained-release pills.

Side Effects. Morphine is a highly addictive drug. Long-term users develop a tolerance to it; over time, they need increasingly higher dosages to get the same effect. Withdrawal may be difficult unless the dosages are reduced slowly over time. It is likely to produce constipation in the elderly, and high doses make most people sleepy. *See also* ANALGESIC DRUGS.

Mortality

Rate of death.

Mortality is calculated by the number of deaths per year in a particular population relative to the population as a whole. It is often measured per 100,000, 10,000, or 1,000 people. Analyzing mortality rates in different countries or among specific groups in the same country provides information for the study of death and dying. For instance, infant mortality is comprised of the rate of death of live-born infants within the first year, and perinatal mortality is the percentage of infant deaths within the first week. Comparative mortality can also measure the safety of a certain occupation or reveal risks or dangers specific to particular socioeconomic groups. *See also* DEATH.

Mosaicism

A condition in which some cells have one genetic makeup while others have a different makeup.

Mosaicism is usually caused by mistakes during cell division when the chromosomes are being replicated. Mosaicism can also be caused by mutations in embryonic cells during early development.

One of the more common forms of mosaicism is the random inactivation of one of the two X chromosomes in women. During embryonic development, each cell inactivates one of its X chromosomes, so that roughly half of the cells express the maternal X chromosome, and half express the paternal X chromosome.

Mosaicism can lead to the appearance of chromosomal and genetic abnormalities if some cells carry an abnormal gene or chromosome. For example, if some cells in a person's body contain 46 chromosomes, and other cells also contain the extra chromosome responsible for Down's syndrome, the person may exhibit symptoms of Down's syndrome. The severity of symptoms, however, can very greatly and is often less than if all the cells contain the abnormality. *See also* DNA *and* GENETICS.

Mosquito Bites

Mosquitoes are a species of winged, parasitic insect found throughout the world. Female mosquitoes lay eggs in bodies of water, usually in warmer regions. Eradication programs often focus on these areas.

Females of the subfamily *Culicinaein* are specialized for sucking blood and are equipped with a long, slender proboscis that acts like a tiny hypodermic needle. These mosquitoes inject an irritating saliva under the skin and then siphon blood from the penetration.

Saliva from biting mosquitoes causes a characteristic reaction of swelling, irritation, and itching. Even common household mosquitoes may produce severe reactions in people who are allergic to certain antigens contained in mosquito saliva.

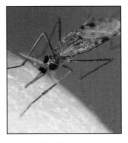

Mosquito Bites.
Above, a mosquito uses its long, slender proboscis to inject the skin and then extract blood from the penetration. A mosquito's saliva can cause reactions such as swelling and itching.

> ## Prevention
> Insecticides, particularly those containing DEET, offer good defense against mosquito bites, especially when their use is combined with protective clothing and the use of Permethrin-treated mosquito netting in living and sleeping areas. Some drugs offer defense against malaria in endemic areas, though none are a guarantee, as drug-resistant strains of plasmodium exist.

MOSQUITO-BORNE DISEASES
Many types of mosquito carry disease-causing microorganisms that can be transmitted through their bite. The Asian tiger mosquito, found in the U.S., may carry encephalitis or dengue fever. Species found elsewhere are responsible for dengue fever, yellow fever, filariasis, and malaria.

Among these, malaria, a potentially fatal disease that affects red blood cells, is the most prevalent. It is transmitted by a female mosquito of the genus *Anopheles*. Worldwide, one in 17 people die every year from mosquito-borne illnesses.

> *This subject is closely related to issues detailed under* DENGUE FEVER; ENCEPHALITIS; FILARIASIS; MALARIA; *and* YELLOW FEVER. *An intimate understanding of* INSECTS AND DISEASE; INSECT BITES; TROPICAL DISEASES; *and the* TSETSE FLY *may also be beneficial. Also see* MICROORGANISM.

Motion Sickness

Nausea and uneasiness that accompanies car, air or sea travel in particular individuals.

Motion sickness occurs when the inner ear is overly sensitive to motion of traveling. It can be described as a feeling of dizziness, headache, or nausea and may lead to excessive sweating, salivation, or vomiting. Children suffer more from motion sickness than any other segment of the population. Most children will naturally outgrow it.

CAUSE

Motion sickness may occur because the brain is receiving conflicting messages from sensory organs. The inner ear, which is responsible for balance, sends one message to the brain, while the eyes transmit a conflicting message. During a trip, there is a constant change of body position that causes conflicting messages to be sent to the brain. For example, reading in a moving vehicle causes nausea because the eyes relate a fixed picture to the brain, while the body relates a message of motion.

TREATMENT

The best way to remedy motion sickness is to halt the activity that causes nausea. If this is impractical, medications can offer relief. Physicians suggest over-the-counter anti-nausea pills whose main ingredient is dimenhydrinate, which decreases the sensitivity of the motion-detecting nerves in the ear. The pills are most effective if used an hour before a trip. Most drugs should not be taken with alcohol or sleeping pills. A skin patch of time-released scopolamine is sometimes prescribed for severe motion sickness. In addition, ginger has been used to treat motion sickness for centuries and has fewer side effects. *See also* EAR; INNER EAR; *and* VERTIGO.

Resources on Motor neuron Disease

Calne, Donald B., *Neurodegenerative Diseases* (1994); Leigh, P. Nigel, and Michael Swash, eds, *Motor Neuron Disease: Biology and Management* (1995); Ringel, Steven P., *Neuromuscular Disorders: A Guide for Patient and Family* (1987); National Institute of Neurological Disorders and Stroke (NIH), Tel. (301) 496-4000, www.ninds.nih.gov/health_and_medical/disorders/motor_neuron_diseases.html; Muscular Dystrophy Association, Tel. (800)572-1717, Online: mda@mdausa.org; National Organization for Rare Disorders (NORD), Tel. (800) 999-NORD (6673), orphan@rarediseases.org.

Preventing Motion Sickness

Motion sickness can be reduced if certain travel strategies are used. Before embarking on a journey, always make sure that you are well rested and in good health. Limit the intake of alcoholic beverages, carbonated soft drinks, and the consumption of greasy or spicy meals. While traveling, keep the windows open and avoid focusing on close objects, as in reading. It may help to close your eyes or stare out into the horizon. It may also help to sit in an area where the motion is least felt, such as the front seat of a car. Crackers, olives, fresh lemon, or a sip of ginger ale may ease symptoms.

Motor Neuron Disease

Rare disorders in which the nerves that are responsible for muscular activity degenerate within the brain or spinal cord.

Motion is regulated by the nervous system. Though nerves are connected throughout the body, they originate in the brain and are concentrated in the spine. A nerve dysfunction anywhere along the path that a nerve travels from the brain to the muscle can result in motor disorders. If the muscles are not continuously stimulated by messages from the brain, the muscles can shrink (muscle atrophy) and possibly become paralyzed. The cause of motor neuron disease is unknown.

TYPES

Examples of motor neuron disease include Lou Gehrig's disease (amyotrophic lateral sclerosis or ALS), progressive muscular atrophy, progressive bulbar palsy, primary lateral sclerosis, and progressive pseudobulbar palsy. Infantile progressive spinal muscular atrophy (Werdnig-Hoffman paralysis) is an example of an inherited, childhood motor disease. Acute muscle weakness advances rapidly and results in death. Chronic spinal muscular dystrophy can exist in a benign form that starts during childhood and produces muscle weakness, but never becomes degenerative.

SYMPTOMS

Motor neuron degeneration generally begins in the hands and arms. Eventually, the diseased side of the body becomes weak and gradually wastes away. Other symptoms of the disease include difficulty swallowing, breathing, and walking, and muscle cramping and stiffness.

Lou Gehrig's Disease

A motor neuron disease that affects about 1 in 100,000 people, amyotrophic lateral sclerosis (ALS), also known as Lou Gehrig's Disease (after the famed Yankee baseball player),involves the shrinking of nerves that control the muscles, resulting in loss of muscle control. ALS affects men more than woman, seems to run in families, and symptoms do not usually appear until after the age of 50. It is invariably fatal. The cause is unknown and no cure is known.

DIAGNOSIS

EMG is a diagnostic tool that measures the electrical action of the muscle and thus determines whether or not the nerves are functioning properly. Other useful diagnostic tools include muscle biopsy, blood tests, CT scanning, and MRI.

TREATMENT

There is no specific cure for motor neuron disease. Treatment is directed at alleviating the symptoms and enabling the patient to remain independent for as long as possible. During the later stages of the disease, the patient may need assistance dressing and eating. He or she may develop difficulties swallowing food and need supervision or medical intervention to prevent choking. The disease is complicated by the fact that the patient's intelligence and reasoning are intact. He or she is aware of what is happening, but may be unable to speak.

Background information about motor neuron disease; can be found in the entries for AMYOTROPHY; NERVE INJURY; *and* NERVE, TRAPPED. *Related anatomical information can be found in* BRAIN; *and* SPINAL NERVE.

Mouth

The oral cavity.

The inside of the mouth, excluding teeth, is covered by a mucous membrane which extends outside the mouth to form the lips. Food is taken in through the mouth, where it is moistened by saliva and chewed before being swallowed. Breathing occurs through the mouth and the nose, and the mouth is also necessary for speech. *See also* TEETH.

Mouth Cancer

Malignant tumor of the oral cavity.

Mouth cancer most often arises on the lips or the tongue, although it can affect the floor of the mouth, the cheeks, the salivary glands, and the gums. Almost all mouth cancers are squamous cell carcinomas, originating in the surface layer of tissue lining the mouth; the major exception is cancer of the salivary glands, which is an adenocarcinoma.

Most mouth cancers are related to tobacco and alcohol use; pipe and cigar smokers are at greater risk than cigarette smokers, and the combination of smoking and heavy drinking greatly increases the risk. Mouth cancers generally occur in people 40 years of age and older, and are twice as common in men as in women. Risk factors include inadequate diet, poor oral hygiene, and, for lip cancer, long-term exposure to sunlight. Exposure to radiation and environmental pollutants are also factors.

SYMPTOMS

Symptoms of cancer inside the mouth include canker sores that persist for more than two weeks, raised white patches called leukoplakia, or red patches called erythroplasia. There may be pain and soreness, especially if the tongue is affected. Lip cancer commonly starts as a white patch. As the patches, or plaques, become cancerous, they may form bumps or become ulcerous, often causing bleeding.

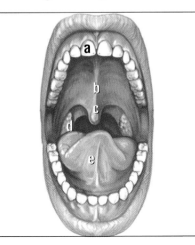

Mouth.
The mouth is the origination of the digestive tract. The teeth and salivary glands aid in breaking down food for digestion. The tonsils aid against infections. Inside the mouth are the incisors (a); the soft palate (b); the uvula (c); the tonsils (d); and the tongue (e).

DIAGNOSIS

Because mouth cancers cause no symptoms in their early stage, they often are first detected by dentists. Confirmation that a plaque or ulcer is malignant is done by microscopic examination of a tissue sample (biopsy). A CAT scan may be done to determine whether the cancer has spread to the bone. A specialized x-ray examination using a revolving camera may be performed to get a detailed view of the cancer.

TREATMENT

Mouth cancer can be treated by surgery and radiation therapy. Surgery is performed when the cancer can be removed without major damage to function or appearance. Techniques include ordinary surgery, or removal by laser, electric current (electrocoagulation), or freezing (cryotherapy). Chemotherapy is preferred for cancer of the lip because surgery can cause major scarring. A large mouth cancer, or one that has spread to nearby lymph nodes, may be treated by surgery followed by radiation therapy. Chemotherapy is done only when surgery and radiation therapy have not resulted in complete removal of the cancer.

PROGNOSIS

The outlook depends on the stage at which the cancer is detected and its location. The overall five-year survival rate for all mouth cancers is 90 percent, but the rate drops steadily for cancers that are diagnosed at an advanced stage.

Mouth Ulcer.
Mouth ulcers are caused by many disorders. These include canker sores, leukoplakia, gingivastomatitis, oral cancer, oral lichenplanus, oral thrush, and similar disorders.

Background material on this topic can be found in BENIGN; CANCER; CARCINOGEN; METAPLASIA; MOUTH; MOUTH ULCER; *and* TUMOR. *Further information about* CANCER *related issues is included in* METASTASIS; MUTAGEN; ONCOLOGY; POLYP; *and* PREMOLAR. *See also* TOBACCO SMOKING.

Mouth, Dry

Lack of saliva production in the mouth.

The mucous membranes that line the mouth contain three sets of salivary glands. Saliva helps lubricate the mouth, break down food, and aid in swallowing. Saliva also helps prevent food buildup that can cause tooth decay. A disorder in the salivary glands affects all of these activities.

Most cases of dry mouth are temporary. They may be part of a brief reaction, such as to fear or a drug, or may be related to an infection of the salivary glands. Radiation therapy for mouth cancer can also impair the salivary glands.

The best known example of long-term dry mouth is Sjögrens syndrome, an autoimmune disorder in which the immune system reacts against the glands that are responsible for producing lubricating secretions. Dry mouth, as well as dry eyes, are notable symptoms.

Treatment. In severe cases, artificial saliva sprays may help. Careful attention to dental care can help to wash out food debris that can lead to tooth decay. *See also* MOUTH CANCER; MOUTH; SALIVA; SALIVARY GLANDS; *and* SJOGRENS SYNDROME.

Mouth Ulcer

Open wound in the mucous membrane of the mouth.

The mouth is lined with mucous membranes that, with the help of the salivary glands, keep the mouth lubricated. Breaks in the mucous membrane are known as mouth ulcers. Mouth ulcers are usually round spots that may be white, gray, or yellow, surrounded by a red ring. They are painful, and the pain can be exacerbated by food or drink, especially if salty or acidic.

Mouth ulcers may be caused by a variety of conditions. The most common ulcers are canker sores, which are usually found on the inside of the cheeks and lips, or sometimes on the tongue. Other possible causes include the herpes simplex virus (which also causes cold sores around the outside of the mouth), oral thrush, leukemia, syphilis, tuberculosis, and anemia.

Treatment should be aimed at the underlying cause. Symptoms can be relieved by keeping the area clean and avoiding foods that can irritate the ulcer. Topical corticosteroids, histamines and antacids may help relieve pain. If the mouth ulcer does not clear up in three to four weeks, a physician should be consulted to ensure that it is not an early sign of mouth cancer. *See also* ANEMIA; CANKER SORE; COLD SORES; CORTICOSTEROIDS; HERPES SIMPLEX; LEUKEMIA; MOUTH; MOUTH CANCER; THRUSH; SYPHILIS; *and* TUBERCULOSIS; .

Mouthwash

Fluid that is used as a rinse for the mouth.

Some mouthwashes simply freshen the taste inside the mouth, while others contain antiseptics. Antiseptic mouthwashes may be used to treat bad breath (halitosis), but they are a short-term solution, as they do not treat the underlying cause. A mouthwash that contains hydrogen peroxide can act as a cleanser for inflamed teeth and gums (gingivitis) that are too painful for brushing. Mouthwashes made of warm water and salt can reduce inflammation caused by problems, such as impacted wisdom teeth. Fluoride mouthwashes can help to prevent cavities. *See also* HALITOSIS.

Movement

Action that changes the position of bones, soft tissues, or body organs.

All movement is activated by muscles. To change the position of two bones, the muscle attached to those bones contracts across the joint, pulling the bones into another location. More complex motions may involve coordinated action of large groups of muscles, joints, and bones, while skin, ligaments, and tendons stretch to accommodate the new position. Sometimes, groups of muscles work in opposi-

---

Movement Disorders

Movement disorders occur when the nervous system's ability to control movement is disrupted.

PARKINSON'S DISEASE is a loss of control of movement that may begin with mild shaking, then evolve into trouble walking, or executing simple tasks with the hands, arms, and sometimes face. Caused by the deterioration of the basal ganglia region of the brain, which controls many common, automatic movements, Parkinson's disease is currently not curable, although medication may help control symptoms.

TOURETTE'S (GILLE DE LA TOURETTE'S) SYNDROME is a disease in which there is an increase in involuntary movement, known as motor tics. These may include facial twitching or jerking of body parts, or uncontrolled bursts of sound or words. The disorder is probably genetic, and the symptoms may be controlled with medication and therapy.

INJURY OR DETERIORATION of the muscles, joints and bones also impair movement. Diseases like osteoarthritis interrupt the ability of joints to operate smoothly. Injuries to bones or muscles can interrupt movement temporarily or permanently.

---

tion, some working to initiate the movement, others working to keep the motion smooth and steady. Movements that do not involve the bones include eye and tongue.

Voluntary movement is the result of instructions sent from the brain. A portion of the brain (the motor cortex) sends a signal to the nerve fibers that run down the spinal cord. These signals are routed to the nerve fibers that direct the appropriate muscle group. Sensory nerve receptors help control the movements by sensing and recording the degree of muscle contraction necessary for each motion. That data is stored in portions of the brain (cerebellum and basal ganglia) so that the movement can be executed with more efficiency.

Involuntary movements are not willed and occur in reaction to certain kinds stimuli. Reactions like blinking when bright light shines in the eyes, are usually less controlled and complex. Organ movements, such as the heartbeat, are also involuntary.

Information related to this topic can be found in INVOLUNTARY MOVEMENTS; PARKINSON'S DISEASE; TOURETTE'S SYNDROME; *and* TRAUMA. MOVEMENT *issues are also central to understanding* AGING; ELDERLY, CARE OF THE; GERONTOLOGY; *and* SENILITY. *See also* HEART ECTOPIC *and* HEART BEAT.

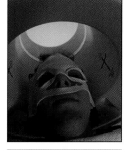

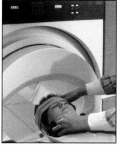

MRI. Above one woman is undergoing an MRI scan(top), while (bottom) a patient's head is being secured by a technician preparing for a magnetic resonance image.

MRI

Acronym for Magnetic Resonance Imaging

Non-invasive diagnostic technique used to visualize internal organs, tissues, and structures.

MRI is a powerful technique for high-resolution examinations of anatomical features of the body. It is used to diagnose illness throughout the body as well as to chart the course of treatment. MRI, unlike x-ray or CT scan, uses no harmful radiation. Instead, it relies on a principle known as magnetic resonance. When the atomic nuclei within cells are subjected to a strong magnetic field, they vibrate or resonate, emitting a radio signal. This is then translated by computer to form an image of spectacular clarity. The computer is able to translate the magnetic resonance into either a two- or three-dimensional picture. MRI provides greater contrast between normal and diseased tissue, making it an ideal diagnostic tool. It is used most often to image the abdomen, blood vessels, bone, brain, spinal cord and canal, and joints.

An MRI machine consists of a large cylindrical apparatus housing a powerful magnet. The patient lies flat on a movable table that positions him or her correctly inside the tube; the patient must remain still during the course of the MRI. Before a patient is placed inside the unit, all metallic objects must be removed, as they are unsafe within the powerful magnetic field. As the horizontal table moves forward, successive slices of tissue are scanned by the MRI. These thin sections may then be projected as either two-dimensional or three-dimensional images.

Open MRI units avoid the confining tube-like construction that some patients find claustrophobic, though such open units are not as precise as closed MRI's and are not sufficient for all situations.

Uses

While an MRI may be used to help visualize any part of the body, it has proven particularly useful in the examination of the brain and musculoskeletal regions.

Nervous System. Brain tumors, abscesses, nerve damage, bleeding or edema, and other irregularities affecting the fluid content of tissue are clearly visualized, as are diseases and abnormalities of the spine, including herniated disks and spinal cancers. Irregularities of the brain stem and cerebellum and certain degenerative diseases of the nervous system, like multiple sclerosis, may be diagnosed with MRI.

Musculoskeletal System. A variety of musculoskeletal disorders are also evaluated through such imaging, including bone death due to insufficient blood supply (avascular necrosis) and sports injuries of joints such as the knee and shoulder.

Cardiovascular System. Injection of a contrast dye accompanying MRI is very useful in cardiovascular diagnoses, particularly for aortic aneurysms and other blood vessel abnormalities. Blood vessels of the head and neck may be studied in a procedure known as MRA, or magnetic resonance angiography. MRA has become a favored test to detect the presence of arterial blockage.

Other Uses. Magnetic resonance imaging may also be useful for the diagnosis of kidney and liver masses. Tumor shape can be assessed in three-dimensional MRI images, and solid masses distinguished from hollow or cystic ones.

PRECAUTIONS

An MRI scan requires more time to complete (usually between 30 and 45 minutes) than a traditional x-ray. An MRI may not be used for patients with pacemakers and some types of metal clips or prostheses. Conditions that may preclude the use of MRI include pregnancy and special life-support requirements. Patients suffering from claustrophobia may find the MRI chamber uncomfortably confining.

Although there are many related issues some of the most important include ABSCESS; ANGIOGRAPHY; BONE IMAGING; BRAIN MAGING; CAT SCAN; CHEST X-RAY; COMPUTER AIDED DIAGNOSIS; COLONOSCOPY; HEART IMAGING; IMAGING TECHNIQUES; KIDNEY IMAGING; PET SCANNING; RADIOPAQUE; SPECT; SPINAL ULTRA-SOUND; *and* X-RAY. *All of these can be used in the diagnosis of* BRAIN DISORDERS; KIDNEY TUMORS; MULTIPLE SCLEROSIS; NECROSIS; *and* NERVE INJURY.

Mucopolysaccharidosis

A type of hereditary disease in which mucopolysaccharides, a type of organic compound, cannot be broken down and thus accumulate in the body.

Mucopolysaccharidosis is caused by a deficiency of the enzymes needed to break down mucopolysaccharides. There are ten such known enzyme deficiencies, each linked to a different gene. These genes are all recessive; a child must receive the abnormal gene from both parents in order to have the disorder. Some of the defective genes are located on regular (autosomal) chromosomes, and others are located on sex chromosomes (in which case a male only needs to receive the gene from his mother).

SYMPTOMS

The severity and age of onset of symptoms varies depending on the type of mucopolysaccharidosis. The mucopolysaccharides accumulate in the arteries, skeleton, eyes, joints, ears, skin, and teeth, producing potentially severe effects in these areas. Possible symptoms include:

- developmental delay;
- intellectual impairment;
- behavioral problems;
- coarse facial features;
- stiffness in joints;
- chronic respiratory tract infections;
- recurrent otitis media;
- corneal clouding, leading to visual impairment; and
- hearing impairment.

TREATMENT AND PROGNOSIS

No treatments have been identified for any of the mucopolysaccharidoses. For some diseases, the prognosis is very poor, with death occurring in childhood or adolescence, while other diseases are mild enough that an affected person can live a relatively normal life.

Background material on mucopolysaccharidosis can be found within the articles on AMINO ACIDS; DEVELOPMENTAL DELAY; ENZYMES; GENETIC PROBE; HEREDITY; HERITABILITY; and JOINTS. It is also important to understand topics such as CHROMOSOME ANALYSIS and CHROMOSOMAL ABNORMALITIES.

Multiple Personality Disorder

Also known as Dissociative Identity Disorder

A disorder in which two or more distinct identities alternately control a person's behavior.

Usually caused by extremely traumatic childhood experiences—often severe sexual or physical abuse—dissociative identity disorder is a defense first used by the sufferer to survive the trauma. Dissociation, in which a person loses awareness of all or part of his or her self or surroundings, is a common defense mechanism that is easily used by children. When a child dissociates repeatedly over a long period of time, he or she may develop one or more alternate personalities, they usually are not aware of each other. The personalities are distinctly different and have their own patterns of relating to the world and may manifest different facial expressions, tone, or dress.

SYMPTOMS AND DIAGNOSIS

The realization that an individual suffers from dissociative identity disorder often happens when another person notices a shift in personality taking place, or when it becomes apparent that there are frequent gaps in memory that cannot be explained by normal forgetfulness. As an individual with dissociative identity disorder is rarely aware of the different personalities, the disorder is often first recognized by others.

TREATMENT

Treatment for multiple personaility disorder involves intensive psychotherapy, in which the individual confronts and deals with past abuse, learns to integrate the personalities, and learns new coping skills. Antidepression or antianxiety drugs may be prescribed as an adjunct to therapy; however, they are in no way a substitute for therapy.

Issues related to multiple personality disorder can be found in articles regarding AVOIDANT PERSONALITY DISORDER; FUGUE, DISSOCIATIVE; GENDER IDENTITY; PERSONALITY TESTS; and TRAUMA. Other important topics include PSYCHOANALYSIS; RAPE; and SCHIZOID PERSONALITY DISORDER.

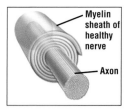

Multiple Sclerosis.
In multiple sclerosis, a central nervous system disorder, the myelin sheath which is a single cell whose membrane wraps around the axon, see above, is destroyed with inflammation and scarring.

Multiple Sclerosis

Chronic, progressive nervous system disorder in which the nerves in the eye, brain, or spinal cord lose their myelin covering.

Multiple sclerosis (MS) is a disease that attacks the brain and spinal cord. It is characterized by degeneration and replacement by scar tissue of the myelin sheath that covers the nerve tissue. Frequently, MS involves partial or complete paralysis, muscle spasms, speech disorders, and hand tremors. The varied symptoms may make it difficult to diagnose the disease in its early stages. The disease worsens over time. Multiple sclerosis sufferers have periods of active disease and periods of remission.

CAUSES

Nerve fibers in the brain and spinal cord are covered in a myelin sheath, which insulates the nerves and enables electrical impulses to be passed quickly along. Inflammation or loss of the myelin sheath impairs nerve transmission. Although the cause of MS is unknown, researchers suggest that the body's immune system may be responsible for the destruction of the myelin sheaths. A virus or other substance may trigger the body to build up infection-fighting cells against its own myelin, exacerbating inflammation and causing a gradual destruction of the myelin in the brain and spinal cord.

Risk Factors for MS

Heredity may have a small influence in determining who develops multiple sclerosis. Approximately five percent of sufferers have siblings who also have MS; 15 percent have another affected relative. Women are more likely than men to suffer from the disease.

Climate is also a factor in the development of MS. People who live in a temperate climate during their first years of life have a greater likelihood of developing multiple sclerosis than people who live in a tropical climate.

SYMPTOMS

The onset of multiple sclerosis usually occurs in early adulthood. The symptoms vary depending on where the scar tissue develops. Damage to the spinal cord causes loss of balance and tingling, weakness, or numbness in an arm or leg. Damage to the white matter in the brain may produce vertigo, fatigue, muscle weakness, double or blurred vision, and numbness and weakness in the face. The patient may develop recurrent muscle contractions (spasticity) and stiffness, spontaneously drop things, or drag a foot. Other symptoms include an unsteady gait (ataxia) and slurred speech. Sometimes, there is difficulty with bowel or urinary control.

The development of the disease is unpredictable. The disease may be in remission for long periods of time. Hot weather or a fever can intensify symptoms, and an infection can trigger a relapse. As the symptoms become more frequent, there is an increased chance that they will persist.

DIAGNOSIS

Diagnosis is based on the symptoms. Each case must be examined on an individual basis. Blurred vision and motor or sensory abnormalities that flare up and then disappear may be a common pattern. The physician will look for other signs that the nervous system is not functioning properly, such as uncoordinated eye movement. Magnetic resonance imaging (MRI) may be used to search for scar tissue in the brain. A spinal tap may be performed to examine the cerebrospinal fluid. An evoked potentials test is used to measure the electrical response of the brain to stimulation of given nerves.

TREATMENT

There is no cure for multiple sclerosis. The goal is to allow the patient to enjoy an active lifestyle. Regular exercise, emphasizing both cardiovascular and weight training is recommended. Physical therapy can lessen muscle spasticity. Multiple sclerosis patients may tire easily and are therefore encouraged to listen to their bodies and rest when necessary. An injection of beta-interferon can decrease the frequency of relapses. Corticosteroids can also be administered to alleviate symptoms.

DEMYELINATION; BRAIN DISORDERS; NERVE ; VERTIGO; *and* VIRUS *explain the basics of this topic.* BRAIN; BRAIN STEM; IMMUNE SYSTEM; SPINAL CORD; *and* NERVOUS SYSTEM *expand on the basics with additional anatomical information. Articles including* BLURRED VISION; FATIGUE; *and* SCAR *are also important to understanding this topic.*

Multivitamin

Nutritional supplement that contains one or more vitamins.

Some people may benefit from taking a multivitamin, including older adults, those on strict weight-loss diets of under 1,000 calories a day, those whose diet is limited by food allergies, those with diseases of the digestive tract affecting nutrient absorption, heavy drinkers, as well as pregnant or lactating women. In these situations, a physician can recommend the proper supplement.

When taking a multivitamin, choose one whose components are no more than 100 percent of the daily recommended allowance; high doses can have toxic effects. Check expiration dates, since vitamins and minerals may lose potency over time. The label should carry words like "proven release," "release assured," or the initials "USP" (the testing organization United States Pharmacopeia) to ensure that the supplement will be properly absorbed. *See also* DIET; MINERAL; NUTRITION AND VITAMIN.

ALERT

Supplements and Medications

Vitamins and supplements should not be used for self-medication for a health problem. Also, supplements may interfere with some prescription medications. Therefore, it is best to notify a physician about any supplements you are taking and ask about possible interactions with prescribed medications.

Mumps

A contagious, acute virus that causes painful enlargement of the salivary (parotid) glands.

Mumps is caused by the *paramyxo* virus and is spread from person to person through saliva, articles in contact with saliva, and airborne droplets. The incubation period ranges from 12 to 24 days.

Children between the ages of two and 12 are the most commonly infected group, although the infection can occur in teenagers and adults. About 4,000 cases of mumps were diagnosed in the U.S. in 1991.

Symptoms. The most common symptons of mumps are facial pain, swollen glands, fever, headache, sore throat, and swelling of temples or jaw. The salivary glands behind the jaw and ear (parotid glands) almost always become enlarged and painful. In males, testicle pain, lumps, and swelling may also occur.

Treatment. There is no treatment for mumps. Alternating ice and heat, acetaminophen, salt water gargles, and extra fluids may help relieve symptoms. After having mumps, the body develops a lifelong immunity to the disease.

Vaccination. The MMR vaccine protects against measles, mumps, and rubella. It is usually given to toddlers when they are 12 to 15 months old. *See* VACCINATION *and* VIRUS.

Munchausen's Syndrome

A psychiatric condition in which a person who is not ill fabricates symptoms for the purpose of emotional rather than financial gain.

In order to convince medical practitioners and others of an illness, a person with Munchuasen's syndrome often fabricates a medical history or actually induces symptoms to feign illness. The emotional reward is attention and support, particularly from medical professionals. The patient is often self-educated or even trained in one or more areas of medicine.

A chronic patient who has been difficult to diagnose and appears to have extraordinary symptoms representing relatively rare or fatal illnesses may have Munchausen's syndrome.

Munchausen's syndrome by proxy has received a lot of media attention. In this case, a parent, usually the mother, deliberately causes injury or symptoms in a child. The parent is often a health professional and enjoys relationships with those in the medical profession. Often, the problem presented is apnea, which can lead to crib death or SIDS. For this reason, whenever there is more than one death from SIDS in a family, the parents may be investigated. *See also* PSYCHOANALYSIS *and* PSYCHIATRY.

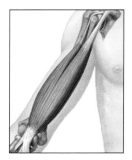

Muscle.
The diagram above, show the tendons that connect muscle to their bony origins and insertions.

Resources on Muscle
Germain, Blandine C., *Anatomy of Movement* (1993); Nuland, Sherwin B., *The Wisdom of the Body* (1997); Olson, Todd R., *A.D.A.M. Student Atlas of Anatomy* (1996); Parker, Steve, *Eyewitness: The Human Body* (1999); American Medical Association, Tel. (312) 464-5000, Online: www.amaassn.org; Human Anatomy and Physiology Society, Inc., Tel. (800) 448-HAPS, Online: www.hapsweb.org; National Institutes of Health, Tel. (301) 496-4000, Online: www.nih.gov; www.med.cornell.edu/cell.biology/; www.ny-cornell.org/medicine/gim/index.html; http://physiology.med.cornell.edu/.

Murmur

An abnormal sound caused by turbulent blood flow, detected by a physician using a stethoscope.

Although some murmurs do not indicate a problem, most are caused by a disturbance of blood flow due either to a defective heart valve or a narrowing of a chamber of the heart. For example, a "whooshing" noise can indicate an abnormal back flow from the left ventricle to the left atrium because the mitral valve, which controls flow between the two chambers, does not close properly when the ventricle contracts.

Murmurs can be caused by inflammation of the valves related to infection. Other causes include septal defects (holes in the wall between chambers), pericarditis (inflammation of the membrane around the heart), and patent ductus arteriosus (a congenital birth defect).

The nature and the location of the murmur, combined with its timing in relation to the normal sounds of the heart and other symptoms, enable a cardiologist to make an initial diagnosis of a specific problem. The diagnosis can be confirmed by echocardiography or one of many other tests of heart anatomy and function. *See also* BLOOD; HEART; HEART ATTACK; INFECTION; PATENT DUCTUS ARTERIOSUS; *and* PERICARDITIS.

Muscle

An organ responsible for movement.

There are three types of muscles: involuntary, voluntary, and cardiac. Involuntary muscles are composed of smooth muscle and are controlled by the autonomic nervous system (they are not consciously controlled). For example, the muscles in the digestive system are involuntary; they work whenever they are needed and cannot be forced to contract otherwise.

Voluntary muscles are made up of striated muscle and can be consciously controlled. For example, the muscles that move the arms and the legs are voluntary muscles; they can be controlled at any time and can perform an amazing number of functions for the body. These muscles are connected to the bones by tendons. There are also flat tendons called aponeuroses that attach muscles to other muscles.

The cardiac muscle, the heart, is made of a different type of striated tissue than that of voluntary muscles; it contracts and relaxes rhythmically for a persons entire life. *See also* HEART *and* SKELETON.

Muscle Spasm

Sudden contraction of a muscle that is involuntary and painful.

Common muscle spasms are caused by minor strain or injury. People often experience spasms after they exercise too hard, too long, or without sufficient warm-up. Sometimes, a person may experience a muscle spasm from sitting in the same position for a lengthy period of time. Spasms can also be brought on by stress.

More serious causes of muscle spasm may include brain damage due to a blow to the head, stroke, cerebral palsy, or other brain disorders. In addition, muscle spasms can be caused by pressure on a nerve from a prolapsed disk.

Muscle spasms cause abnormal hardness and inflexibility of the muscle. Moving an affected muscle can cause it to contract violently and is often accompanied by pain. The muscle may feel hard or rigid to the touch.

Pain in a leg can be temporarily relieved by standing and walking on it. An exertion-related spasm may be relieved by drinking a sports drink. Stretching, massaging, and applying heat to a spastic muscle might bring relief. Relaxation techniques and vitamin B complex and vitamin C supplements can provide adequate treatment for stress-related muscle spasms. If spasms are due to brain disorders, a neurologist and rehabilitation specialist (physical or occupational therapist) should be consulted. *See also* CRAMP; MUSCLE-RELAXANT DRUGS; OCCUPATIONAL THERAPY; PHYSICAL THERAPY; STRESS; *and* VITAMIN.

Muscle-Relaxant Drugs

A family of drugs used to counteract muscle spasms.

Muscle relaxants are usually used in combination with pain relievers (analgesics) and physical therapy. They are used to treat acute pain resulting from muscle spasms or chronic tightness of the muscles, or to control the symptoms of diseases such as muscular dystrophy. Dosage is critical, as too little will have no effect, and too much can lead to side effects.

Side effects can include hives, rash, faintness, weakness, and temporary loss of vision. Drowsiness and dizziness are common; constipation or diarrhea and nausea are less common. They must not be taken when breast-feeding. Adverse reactions among the elderly are likely to be more frequent and more severe. *See also* ANALGESIC DRUGS; MUSCLE SPASM; *and* MUSCULAR DYSTROPHY.

Muscular Dystrophy

A disease in which the muscles progressively grow weaker and decrease in size.

Muscular dystrophy is an inherited disease that can take several forms of varying severity. The cause of the loss of muscle strength and tissue mass is not understood.

In most cases of muscular dystrophy, the arms, legs, and spine of the affected person become increasingly deformed. By the teenage years, most patients are confined to a wheelchair. Death may result from pneumonia or other respiratory infection.

TYPES

Duchenne's muscular dystrophy is the most common form of muscular dystrophy, affecting 20 to 30 in 100,000 males. It affects only males. The onset of the disease is usually before age five. In Duchenne's muscular dystrophy, the protein dystrophin is not produced at all, leading to muscle weakness. One of the first symptons is when a toddler exhibits a decrease in mobility; the disease progresses throughout childhood.

Few affected children survive into their twenties.

Over half of all cases are inherited. The gene responsible for the disorder is recessive and located on the X chromosome. A female carrier has a 50 percent chance of passing the disorder on to her son.

Becker's muscular dystrophy, which affects three in 100,000, involves a different defect in the same gene. An abnormal form of the protein dystrophin is produced that does not function properly. It results in similar, but less severe, than Duchenne's muscular dystrophy.

Other, rarer forms of inherited muscular dystrophy include Landouzy-Dejerine, which is transmitted by an autosomal dominant gene and affects the shoulder and facial muscles; Leyden-Mobius, which affects the pelvis; and Erb's, which affects the shoulder. The latter two usually don't appear until adulthood. All three are rarely severe.

TREATMENT

There is no treatment available to halt or reverse progression of the disease. Treatment focuses on physical therapy to minimize the deformities. *See also* MUSCLE *and* SPINE.

Mushroom Poisoning

Adverse effects from eating toxic species of fungi.

Mushroom poisoning occurs frequently when novice mushroom hunters mistake a toxic species for an edible one. Children are also at risk for eating wild mushrooms. A wild mushroom should never be eaten unless there is complete certainty that it is edible—some species that are toxic enough to kill immediately if injested closely resemble non-poisonous varieties.

The effects of mushroom toxicity vary greatly according to species, and may even have diverse effects on different people who have eaten them.

There are four types of mushroom toxins (mycotoxins): gastrointestinal irritants that cause abdominal cramping, diarrhea, nausea, and vomiting; neurotoxins, whose

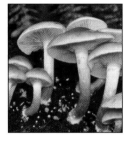

Mushroom.
Wild mushrooms (shown above), which are toxic, can easily be mistaken for those that are edible. The toxicity in some wild mushrooms can even cause death.

symptoms include hallucinations, spastic colon, depression, and agitation; protoplasmic poisons, which result in the destruction of cells, followed by organ failure; and disulfiram-like toxins, which are usually nontoxic unless alcohol is drunk within 72 hours of eating the fungi, causing a temporary toxic syndrome. *See also* POISONING.

Mutagen

Agent that causes a mutation in genetic material.

All processes in living cells are controlled by the genes in the cell nucleus. These genes are gathered in bodies called chromosomes and consist of sequences of deoxyribonucleic acid (DNA). A change in the DNA sequence of a gene, known as a mutation, affects the performance of that gene. The effects of mutations range from causing a gene to stop working entirely, to causing it to produce a different, possibly defective, protein, to causing a cell to begin reproducing without control (resulting in a cancer).

TYPES OF MUTGENS

Some mutations occur spontaneously, but many are caused by agents known as mutagens. Mutagens include x-rays, gamma rays, and alpha-and-beta radiation. Ultraviolet radiation in sunlight is a mutagen that can cause skin cancer. A number of chemicals are also mutagens, including chemicals in tobacco smoke and chemicals used in industrial processes, such as asbestos. Occupational exposure to mutagens including asbestos, benzene, styrene, some dyes, cadmium, and organic pesticides can increase the risk of cancer-causing genetic changes. *See also* CARCINOGEN.

Mutation

An alteration in the genetic sequence of a cell.

The characteristics of human beings and most other living things are governed by a molecule called deoxyribonucleic acid (DNA) which is found in the nucleus of a living cell. A DNA molecule consists of two intertwined chains made of sugar and phosphate groups, to which chemicals called bases are attached. A unit consisting of a base, sugar, and phosphate group is called a nucleotide.

Sections of a DNA molecule serve as templates that regulate the production of the proteins that carry out the functions of a cell; each such section is called a gene. In human cells, genes are carried in units called chromosomes; there are 23 pairs of chromosomes in the nucleus of each cell.

A mutation, a change in a gene or in a chromosome, can alter the function of the cell and that of the cells produced when the mutated cell divides. Further divisions produce a population of cells containing the mutation. In some cases, the change can be harmless or even beneficial; mutations are the underlying cause of evolution. But most of the time, the change is harmful—as in mutations that cause the uncontrolled growth of cells known as cancer.

Types. There are several types of mutations. A point mutation is a change in a gene, often resulting from a change in a single nucleotide, that can alter the protein whose production is governed by that gene. This mutation may result in the production of faulty proteins that disrupt the activity of cells. Sometimes, mutations affect entire chromosomes, causing parts of them to be erased, enlarged, or reordered.

Causes. Some mutations occur spontaneously, with no known cause. Some result from the action of mutagens, chemical or physical agents that act on genes and chromosomes. High-energy radiation of the sort emitted in nuclear reactors or used in x-rays is one such mutagen. A number of chemicals also can act as mutagens. These include the family of chemicals called poly-

Beneficial Mutations

Some mutations persist from generation to generation because they have a beneficial effect that counterbalances the damage they cause. An important example is the mutation that causes sickle-cell anemia. A child develops sickle-cell anemia when he or she inherits two copies of a gene containing that mutation. Children who inherit a single copy of the gene, however, are born with protection against malaria.

cyclic aromatic hydrocarbons, which are created when tobacco is burned and which are responsible for the lung cancer suffered by chronic smokers.

Effects. Mutations, spontaneous or inherited, are responsible for birth defects. Genetic mutations cause congenital conditions such as hemophilia and phenylketonuria. Chromosomal mutations cause conditions such as Down's syndrome and Turner's syndrome. While some mutations are unavoidable, the risk of harmful mutations is lessened by avoidance of known mutation-causing substances (mutagens) such as tobacco smoke and radiation.

Although mutations are discussed throughout the book, some of the most important entries include CARCINO-GENS; CHROMOSOME; DNA; GENE; GENETICS; GENETIC COUNSELING; *and* MUTAGEN. *Important related information is in* DOWN'S SYNDROME *and* TOBACCO SMOKING.

Mutism

Refusal or disinclination to respond or communicate verbally.

Selective mutism is a childhood disorder in which a child will not speak in one setting (such as at school or with adults outside of the home), but can speak normally otherwise. The onset is usually between the ages of three and eight years old and is often first manifested when the child goes to school. Selective mutism tends to occur in shy, anxious, and inhibited youngsters and is believed to be a type of anxiety disorder. Psychological factors are believed to play a role in the development of selective mutism, and include overprotective or controlling caretakers, frequent moves, and early

exposure to trauma (such as early hospitalization, abuse, or death of a loved one). Often, children with selective mutism have other developmental disorders including delayed onset of speech, articulation disorders, bed wetting, and soiling. Any child who develops selective mutism warrants a thorough evaluation by a physician, both to rule out other diagnoses which may masquerade as selective mutism, and to diagnose any other developmental disorders that may be present. Both psychological and behavioral modification are useful in the treatment of selective mutism.

The presence of mutism in an adult with a normal level of consciousness can be caused by many conditions. Many psychiatric conditions can result in mutism, including schizophrenia, catatonia, and depression. Additionally, adult mutism that is neurologically-based, such as from a brain tumor is referred to as "akinetic mutism." As with children, the development of mutism in an adult is not normal and should be assed by a physician. *See* SPEECH.

Myalgia

Medical term for muscular pain.

Myalgia is a basic symptom of conditions characterized by inflammation of muscles, joints, or fibrous tissue (rheumatism). Myalgia is manifested in many common viral infections and autoimmune diseases, such as rheumatoid arthritis, systemic lupus erythematosus, and polymyalgia rheumatica. It is the primary symptom of muscle tissue inflammation diseases, such as dermatomyositis and polymyositis.

Treatment. Anti-inflammatory drugs can be prescribed to reduce inflammation, and anti-spasmodic drugs can be effective in easing muscle tension. Circulatory stimulants, diuretics and analgesics can also offer relief. Dietary factors should be examined, as well as the patient's posture, stress, and work conditions. Alternative medicine techniques, such as a chiropractor's adjustment, massage, and herbal medication, may also provide relief. *See* MUSCLE.

Myasthenia Gravis

Abnormal neuromuscular transmission that results in muscular weakness.

Myasthenia gravis is a rare, progressive disease in which the muscles in the eye, face, throat, and limbs become weak. The typical patient has drooping eyelids, a blank expression, and labored speech. Most patients experience weak muscles and generalized fatigue.

The disease occurs more frequently in women than men. The onset of myasthenia gravis occurs between the ages of 20 and 40 in women and between 50 and 70 in men. The disease can develop gradually or rapidly, and its manifestation varies from patient to patient.

CAUSE

Although the cause of myasthenia gravis is not known, but there is some genetic element. Myasthenia gravis is an autoimmune disease in which the immune system attacks the body's own neuromuscular acetylcholine receptors. Under normal conditions, acetylcholine is released from the motor nerve terminal in a controlled quantity. In myasthenia gravis, the body destroys the acetylcholine receptors in the muscle. The membrane becomes less sensitive to acetylcholine, which decreases the muscle's ability to receive messages to produce movement.

Approximately 70 percent of people affected with myasthenia gravis involving the respiratory system exhibit thymus gland abnormalities. Ten percent of the patients have a thymic tumor.

SYMPTOMS

In most patients, the first symptom to appear is eye-related such as double vision and drooping eyelids. Another common symptom is muscle weakness in the face and neck, causing slurred speech, difficulty speaking, swallowing food, and the possibility of choking or regurgitating. In addition, muscle weakness in the limbs can cause simple acts like getting dressed or walking up a flight of stairs to become rigorous activities.

The most dangerous situation occurs when the respiration muscles in the chest cavity are affected, causing breathing difficulties (myasthenic crisis).

Patients often fluctuate between symptom-free days and days of active disorder. Infection, menstruation, some medications, and stress can intensify symptoms.

TREATMENT

Medications that may be administered include edrophonium, which increases the amount of acetylcholine released and temporarily increases muscle strength, and other drugs that can increase the level of acetylcholine, such as pyridostigmine or neostigmine. A patient may receive corticosteroids to inhibit the autoimmune response.

If drugs do not offer relief, a procedure called plasmapheresis is performed to eliminate hazardous antibodies from the blood.

If thymus abnormalities are involved, the thymus may be removed. If a thymus tumor is present, it can usually be removed; most such tumors are benign. *See also* ACETYLCHOLINE; NEUROTRANSMITTER; *and* NERVE DISORDER.

Mycoplasma

Microorganisms that can only live in a body cell (a characteristic of viruses), but which are roughly the same size as bacteria.

Mycoplasmas cause a variety of sicknesses, most of which affect the upper respiratory system. Mycoplasma pneumonia is called walking pneumonia because the sufferer experiences symptoms similar to those of a bad cold rather than to those of pneumonia. Symptoms of mycoplasma pneumonia may develop after as long as three weeks, while symptoms of other viral pneumonias can develop in as little as a few days. Mycoplasmas can also cause conjunctivitis; pink-eye and; otitis media, a middle ear infection. Mycoplasma infections can be controlled by antibiotics. Drugs that improve the immune system are also helpful in the treatment of mycoplasma infections. *See also* BACTERIA; VIRUSES; *and* PNEUMONIA.

Mycosis Fungoides

An uncommon lymphoma that develops out of mature T-lymphocytes of the skin.

Mycosis fungoides is a rare form of Non-Hodgkin's lymphoma that differs from other lymphomas (cancers of lymph tissue) because symptoms generally manifest very slowly. It may first appear as a chronic, reddish rash that can remain unchanged for months or years, or can spread slowly over most of the skin. Areas of skin may become thickened and ulcers can develop. The lymph glands become abnormally large.

Mycosis fungoides usually is diagnosed in persons over the age of 50. The diagnosis is confirmed by a biopsy, in which a sample of skin tissue is taken and examined. Mild cases are treated by long-wave ultraviolet radiation with psoralen drugs. Electron-beam radiotherapy is also effective. Thickened areas may be treated with sunlight and cortisone-like steroid drugs applied to the skin. More severe cases may require chemotherapy. *See also* LYMPHOMA.

Myectomy

Surgical procedure to remove part or all of a muscle.

Myectomies may be performed as treatment for urethral instability or urge-incontinence, congenitally enlarged colon (Hirschsprung's disease), crossed eyes (strabismus), enlargement and impairment of the heart (hypertrophic cardiomyopathy), benign tumors of the uterus (fibroids), and severely injured or infected muscles. *See also* MUSCLE *and* MYOMECTOMY.

Myelitis

Inflammation of the spinal cord.

The most common form of myelitis is called transverse myelitis because it affects one level (the transverse) of the spinal cord. The cause of myelitis is not certain, although a third of sufferers experience the first symptoms after a minor viral infec-tion. It is suspected that the symptoms result from an allergic or auto-immune reaction.

Symptoms start with acute back pain, followed by limb weakness and numbness, and loss of bladder and sphincter control. Normal recovery time for patients suffering from myelitis is one to three months. If the patient has not recovered by that time, the condition may become chronic. *See also* MYELOPATHY; *and* SPINAL CORD.

Myelocele

Birth defect in which the spinal cord is exposed through an opening in the lower vertebrae.

Myelocele is the most severe form of spina bifida, in which the spinal nerves, as well as the sac covering the spinal cord (meninges), bulge out from the spine. This results in a failure of the nerves to develop properly. Frequently children born with myelocele suffer from paralysis of the lower body. *See also* SPINE *and* SPINA BIFIDA.

Myelodysplastic Syndrome

A diseases in which the body cannot produce new blood cells.

Myelodysplastic syndrome (MDS) is sometimes referred to as pre-leukemia, because it progresses to acute leukemia. An indifudual who is living with myelodysplastic syndrome will have bone marrow that does not function properly, and thus does not produce enough new blood cells. There is no known cause for the disorder, although it may occur after radiation or chemotherapy to treat cancer. The primary treatment for myelodysplastic syndrome is bone marrow stem-cell transplantation. Topotecan, an antineoplastics medication, usually used to treat cancer, may also be perscribed. Depending on the type of myelodysplasia and how quickly it progresses to leukemia, the average survival time after diagnosis can range from five months to five years. *See also* BONE; BONE CANCER; CANCER; CHEMOTHERAPHY; *and* LEUKEMIA.

Myelography

X-ray examination of the spinal canal.

Myelography is used to examine the spinal canal, particularly the lower back region. A contrast medium is injected into the spinal canal, and the distribution of the dye allows a record of the spinal cord (myelogram) to be created. Myelography is used to diagnose irregularities of the spinal cord and canal, including dislocation of vertebrae, ruptured or herniated disks, abscesses, or tumor.

The patient must avoid food two to four hours before the test. A long, thin needle is inserted into the spine and a radiocontrast dye is injected. X-ray or computed tomography (CAT) is used to visualize the location of the contrast medium. Widening or narrowing of the spinal canal, seen in the distribution of dye, indicates disease or injury (pathology).

As myelography is an invasive procedure, some risk exists for infection, meningitis, hemorrhage, herniation of the brain, or seizures. The most common side effect is nausea or vomiting. Magnetic resonance imaging (MRI), a painless and noninvasive imaging technique, is largely replacing myelography. *See also* CAT Scan; Diagnostics; Lumbar Puncture; MRI; Noninvasive; *and* Tomography.

Myelomeningocele

A neural-tube defect related to spina bifida.

In myelomeningocele, a segment of a baby's spinal column is exposed and protrudes from the back in a sac-like structure. Neurological impairment below the sac, including paralysis, is common.

Other congenital defects associated with this disorder include syringomyelia, in which there is a fluid-filled cavity in the spinal cord, clubfoot, and hip dislocation. Meningitis may result if there is drainage from the spinal cord. Urinary tract infections are also likely to occur. Immediate surgery is recommended to repair the defect. *See also* Spinal Cord *and* Spinal Injury.

Myelopathy

Disorders of the spinal cord.

Damage to the spinal cord can result from a number of different causes, including inflammation, injury, arthritis, malformation of the vertebrae, bleeding into the spinal cord, fractured vertebra, osteoporosis (a disease causing brittle and weak bones), or an enlarged cyst in the spinal cord. Degenerative myelopathy is thought to be an autoimmune disease in which the immune system attacks the sheath that protects the spinal cord. Symptoms of degenerative myelopathy include pain, numbness and tingling of the extremities, and paralysis. Treatment for degenerative myelopathy is based on its underlying cause. *See* Myelitis; Spinal Injury; *and* Spinal cord.

Myelosclerosis

Also known as myelofibrosis

A disease of the bone marrow.

In myelosclerosis, the bone marrow becomes fibrous like scar tissue; eventually dominating the healthy bone marrow, and blood cell production is severely inhibited. Myelosclerosis is seen most often in people over fifty years old, peaking in occurrence between ages sixty and seventy.

Symptoms of myelofibrosis include lost appetite, anemia (fatigue and weakness), bone pain, fever, and night sweats. The anemia will be confirmed by blood tests showing low red blood cell counts, although platelet counts may remain high. The spleen and the liver may become enlarged.

Treatment is usually chemotherapy, to control the blood counts, and transfusions of red blood cells or platelets to counteract the inefficient production by the bone marrow.

On average, persons with this disease live five years after diagnosis, rarely more than ten. Death occurs from secondary infection or leukemia. *See also* Anemia; Blood; Blood Disorders; Bone Marrow; Erythrocytes; *and* Leukemia.

Myiasis

Infestation of tissue by the larvae of flies.

When maggots infest living tissue, the condition is known as myiasis. Over 50 species of fly can be responsible, and the disease may manifest in the skin, intestinal tract, or body cavities, including the nose, mouth, eye, vagina, sinuses, or urethra. Eggs or larvae (maggots) may be deposited in existing wounds, though many fly species are able to pierce flesh. Intestinal myiasis occurs when eggs or larvae previously deposited in food are swallowed and survive in the gastrointestinal tract. Some infested patients show no symptoms, while others experience abdominal pain, vomiting, and diarrhea.

Among the species that cause myiasis, especially troublesome are the tumbu fly (*Cordylobia anthropophaga*) in tropical regions, common to West Africa, and the human botfly (*Dermatobia hominis* or *torsalo*) found in Mexico and Latin America. Neither the tumbu fly nor the botfly require broken skin to deposit their eggs.

Treatment for myiasis usually involves the removal of the larvae. In many cases, this may be facilitated by covering the wound with an air-tight bandage or thick ointment until the larvae die or exit the wound. In the case of intestinal myiasis, a mild cathartic agent may be used to induce vomiting. Drugs are not effective against myiasis. Prevention involves controlling fly species responsible for the diseases *See also* ECTOPARASITES *and* INSECTS AND DISEASE.

Myocarditis

Inflammation of the heart muscle (myocardium).

Myocarditis is most often caused by a viral infection. The most common virus is Coxsackie type B, which infects the gastrointestinal tract, but cases have also been linked to the viruses that cause polio, rubella, and influenza. Other causes include bacterial or fungal infections and a number of diseases, including systemic lupus erythematosus, but these are rare.

Myocarditis may also be a side-effect of radiation treatment for cancer or of an adverse drug reaction.

SYMPTOMS

Mild cases of myocarditis may cause no symptoms because there is only minimal damage to the heart. In more severe cases, when the inflammation of the heart muscle is accompanied by inflammation of the outer membrane of the heart (pericardium), the patient may experience shortness of breath and fatigue. These are all symptoms of heart muscle dysfunction resulting from a reduced ability of the heart to pump blood efficiently. Because these symptoms can come on slowly, months or even years after the beginning of myocarditis, a patient may not seek medical help until heart failure is well advanced.

DIAGNOSIS

The diagnosis of myocarditis is made on the basis of a physical examination and tests including electrocardiogram and echocardiogram. A chest x-ray may show whether there is accumulation of fluid in the lungs (pulmonary edema). A tissue sample (biopsy) may also be examined.

TREATMENT

Treatment of myocarditis is aimed at the underlying condition. If, however, the cause cannot be determined, treatment is centered on relief of the symptoms. Steroids can be prescribed to reduce inflammation, and analgesics to reduce pain. Patients will be told to reduce physical activity until there is evidence that the inflammation and heart injury have healed. Diuretics, beta blockers or angiotensin-converting inhibitors may be given to improve blood flow.

In rare cases, untreated myocarditis can produce a severe form of pulmonary edema or a myocardial infarction that require immediate emergency care.

Background material on this topic can be found in HEART; INFECTION; INFLAMMATION; PERICARDITIS; *and* VIRUS. *Related disorders include* INFLUENZA; LUPUS; POLIO; *and* RUBELLA. *See also* HEART ATTACK.

Myoclonus

Brief, involuntary jerks or spasms of a muscle or group of muscles at rest or during movement.

Myoclonus characterizes a symptom of a disease rather than a diagnosis. Myoclonic twitches or spasms are caused by abrupt muscle contractions or a momentary decrease of muscle contractions. They can occur alone or in sequence, in a pattern or without pattern, infrequently or numerous times each minute.

Myoclonus is one of several symptoms in an array of nervous system disorders such as multiple sclerosis, Parkinson's disease and Alzheimer's disease. Myoclonus can occur in healthy people as well. Everyday examples include hiccups and the jerks that people experience while falling asleep. Acute cases of pathologic myoclonus can produce deformed movement and limit the ability to eat, talk, and walk. Myoclonus is common among epileptics.

Treatment for myoclonus includes the use of medications that reduce the symptoms, such as barbiturates, clonazepam, and sodium valproate. These drugs are also used to treat people with epilepsy.

Issues related to this topic include ALZHEIMER'S DISEASE; MUSCLE SPASM; EPILEPSY; *and* PARKINSON'S DISEASE. *Kinds of spasms include* ESOPHAGEAL SPASM; INFANTILE SPASMS; *and* LUMBOSACRAL SPASM. *See also* BARBITURATE DRUGS.

Myomectomy

Surgical removal of a non-cancerous tumor of a muscle (myoma), most often fibroids from the muscular wall of the uterus.

Fibroids can cause pelvic pain, excessive bleeding, infertility, and urinary problems. Myomectomy removes fibroid tumors without impairing reproductive ability. Laparoscopic myomectomy, which causes minimal scarring, is an option in some cases. Of the approximately 250,000 operations for fibroid tumors performed each year in the U.S., 25 percent percent are myomectomies and 75 percent are hysterectomies. *See also* FIBROIDS *and* HYSTERECTOMY.

Myopathy

A disease-group affecting the muscles.

Myopathies of the muscles are often progressive, inherited conditions, but may also be caused by immune-system disorders, poisoning, or drug side effects.

Steinert's disease (mytonic dystrophy) is an inherited disorder characterized by muscle weakness as well as tight, contracted muscles that are unable to relax normally. The hands are particularly affected; drooping eyelids are common. Symptoms can appear at any age and range from relatively mild to severe. The most severe cases are also associated with small testes, premature baldness, diabetes and mental retardation. Individuals with a severe form of myotonic dystrophy generally do not live past age 50.

Myotonia congenita, also known as Thomsen's disease, is a rare autosomal disorder characterized by stiff hands, legs and eyelids. Treatment is geared toward medications and physical therapy, to relax the muscles and relieve stiffness. *See also* MUSCLE-RELAXANT DRUGS *and* MUSCLE SPASM.

Myopia

Also known as near-sightedness

A condition in which the eye is too long, so that the person cannot clearly see objects far away.

Myopia is caused when the eyeball is too long from front to back, causing vision to focus in front of the retina rather than on the retina. Generally, myopia begins in childhood and progresses until about age 30, when it stabilizes. It can be easily treated with corrective lenses, such as glasses or contact lenses. In addition, a surgical procedure known as Lasik can reshape the cornea and improve vision. Lasik is performed under local anesthesia, usually a special form of eyedrops; during the procedure, the surgeon will use a laser to flatten the front of the eyeball, correcting the vision. Lasik is still a fairly new procedure, and the long term effects of the surgery have not yet been evaluated. *See also* OPHTHALMOLOGY.

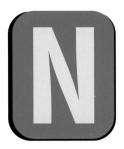

Nalidixic Acid

Antibiotic prescribed to prevent or treat urinary tract infections.

Nalidixic acid is one of the oldest antibiotics, introduced in 1963. It is effective against almost all of the bacteria that can infect the urinary tract, including some that have developed resistance to other antibiotics. Its action is concentrated in the urine, and it usually can cure a bacterial infection in several days. It is not generally prescribed during pregnancy, because of the risk of birth defects, or when a woman is breast-feeding, because it can pass into breast milk. Sometimes it increases sensitivity to sunlight, and it can give a false reading of high blood sugar levels. Other side effects include nausea, vomiting, blurred vision, drowsiness, and dizziness. *See also* IN-FECTION; URINARY SYSTEM; *and* URINARY TRACT INFECTION.

Narcissism

Personality disorder characterized by an inflated sense of self-importance and the devaluation of others.

A narcissist seeks excessive attention and admiration from others and uses relationships as an opportunity to exploit others to satisfy his or her needs. Such a person appears haughty and arrogant and believes that he or she is entitled to purchase, experience, associate with, and achieve only the best in life. Relationships tend to be shallow and are experienced only to the extent that the other person is viewed as enviable, inferior, or useful to the narcissist's goals.

Since a narcissistic person's self image is built on a faulty and fragile structure, such people will be extremely intolerant of criticism or indifference. It is not unusual for a narcissist to spend a great deal of time and emotional energy questioning the meaning behind another person's words or actions in an attempt to determine if these words or actions undermine his or her sense of self.

Such individuals are not capable of making sacrifices for others, of empathy, or of accepting others as they are, and thus experience particular failure at being parents, causing resulting emotional problems in their children. *See also* CHILD DEVELOPMENT; EMPATHY; PERSONALITY DISORDERS; PSYCHIATRY; *and* PSYCHOTHERAPY.

Narcolepsy

Chronic, uncontrollable bouts of severe daytime sleepiness.

Narcolepsy is an unusual sleep disorder whose cause is unknown. The disorder is found repeatedly in particular families, indicating a genetic predisposition. Although narcolepsy does not pose any medical risks, sudden spells of sleepiness can increase the possibility of dangerous accidents while performing tasks that require full attention. In addition, these episodes reduce the sufferer's productivity during normal waking hours.

Symptoms begin in adolescence or young adulthood. Narcoleptic attacks can occur many times a day, with each attack lasting from a few seconds to an hour; these attacks range from mildly irritating to hallucinatory. The attacks often occur during long meetings or lectures. Upon awakening the person feels temporarily reinvigorated, but can abruptly fall asleep again. Most narcoleptic patients experience paralysis without a loss of consciousness (cataplexy). A narcoleptic may drop something that is in his or her hand or become limp and fall to the floor.

Other symptoms include sleep paralysis or hallucinations that are more intense than regular dreaming.

Treatment. Diagnosis is based upon the symptoms and the results of an electroencephalogram (EEG). The patient may be sent to a sleep lab, if necessary. Treatment includes additional naps, stimulant drugs (such as ephedrine or amphetamine) to curb drowsiness and antidepressant drugs (such as imipramine) to control cataplexic attacks. *See also* CATAPLEXY *and* SLEEP.

Narcosis

Artificially induced deep sleep or drowsiness.

Narcosis is a condition of stupor and lethargy caused by the effects of narcotics or chemicals. It is similar to a period of sleep in that the subject is in a state of reduced awareness and experiences a decreased ability to respond to external stimuli. It can be differentiated from sleep in that the subject cannot be totally roused from this state. Narcosis is alleviated by counteracting the action or effects of the narcotics or chemicals responsible. *See also* DRUG *and* SUBSTANCE ABUSE.

Nasal Congestion

Partial blockage of the nasal passage.

The soft skin-like lining (mucous membrane) of the inside of the nose and respiratory tract is coated by a protective substance (mucous) that keeps it moist and traps inhaled particles. About one cup of mucus is produced every day under normal conditions. When the membrane becomes irritated and inflamed, the production of mucus increases. The result is a stuffy nose and often a flow of mucus down the back of the throat (postnasal drip).

The inflammation that causes nasal congestion can result from a number of conditions, the most common being allergies and infections. Excess mucous production can also lead to expansion of the blood vessels inside the nose, adding to the blockage and causing episodes of sneezing, stuffiness, and a runny nose.

Nasal congestion can be eased by heating a pot of water and inhaling the steam, loosening the mucus. Decongestant drugs are available in nasal sprays and over-the-counter drops, but overuse of these drugs can worsen congestion. Nasal steroid sprays such as beclomethasone can be prescribed for severe allergic cases of nasal congestion. *See also* DECONGESTANT DRUGS *and* POSTNASAL DRIP.

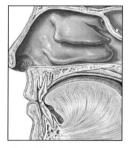

Nasal Anatomy.
The nasal passages, shown above, may become partially or completely blocked due to congestion, a foreign object, blood accumulating from an injury, or a deviated septum.

Nasal Discharge

Release of fluid through the nose.

The mucous membranes line the nasal passageways that run from the nostrils to the throat help to filter air and keep the area lubricated. When an infection is present, the mucous membranes become inflamed, which prevents airflow and causes stuffiness. They also produce more fluid, which can lead to nasal discharge, commonly known as a runny nose.

Types. There are primarily two types of nasal discharge. When the discharge is caused by a viral infection, such as a cold, or by allergies, the flow of mucous is usually clear. If the fluid becomes trapped in the passageways, such as may occur with sinus infections, the warm, moist environment permits the growth of bacteria. The result is a thicker, colored flow of nasal discharge. Another notable type of nasal discharge is a bloody nose; this is usually the result of an injury to the nose or, possibly, to another part of the skull.

Treatment. The best treatment for nasal discharge resulting from a cold, allergies, or sinusitis is to let it run its course. There are also over-the-counter mucous thinning medications available. Drinking plenty of liquids also may keep the mucous thin, which fascilitates easier flow. Humidifiers or nasal sprays can help relieve nostrils irritated by nose blowing or dryness associated with a stuffed nose. *See also* COLD; NASAL CONGESTION; NOSE; *and* SINUSITIS.

Nasal Obstruction

Blockage of the nasal passages.

The nasal passages, which run from the nostril to the upper part of the throat, allow the flow of air into the body. If they become blocked, breathing is impaired. The most common cause of nasal obstruction is nasal congestion, which is the result of inflammation of the mucous membranes in the nasal passages. Other types of obstruction of the nasal passages include a deviated, or twisted, septum (the combination of cartilage and bone between nostrils), nasal polyps, or a hematoma, which is an accumulation of blood clots resulting from a blow or other injury. Children may cause nasal obstruction by intentionally pushing objects into their noses. *See also* CARTILAGE; HEMATOMA; NASAL CONGESTION; NOSE; *and* POLYPS.

Nasogastric Tube

Narrow, flexible plastic or rubber tube that is passed into the stomach through the nose and esophagus.

A nasogastric tube is used to feed an ill patient who is unable to eat normally, to introduce medicine, and to remove fluid, poisons, waste, and other contents from the stomach.

Introduction of the tube may cause discomfort or trigger a gag reflex. To prevent this from occurring, it is coated with a lubricant gel that often contains a topical anesthetic such as lidocaine.

A possible risk of nasogastric feeding is aspiration pneumonia. In order to minimize this risk, proper placement of the tube is confirmed with x-ray and food is introduced into the tube slowly. *See also* PNEUMONIA *and* POISONING.

Nasopharynx, Cancer of

Malignant tumor at the top of the throat.

The nasopharynx is the passage that runs between the nasal cavity, which lies behind the nose, and the topmost part of the throat. Most cancers of the nasopharynx are squamous cell cancers, but some are cancers of the lymph system or other parts of the nasopharynx.

Incidence and Cause. Cancer of the nasopharynx is much more common in the Far East than in Europe and the United States. While some theories stress a connection between lifestyle and diet and the cancer, some indicate the Epstein-Barr virus as the cause.

Symptoms. The first symptoms of cancer of the nasopharynx include changes in speech, frequent nosebleeds, and a runny nose. The cancer can grow, spreading to the nasal cavity and sinuses and to lymph nodes in the neck, causing nosebleeds, double vision, loss of the sense of smell, partial facial paralysis, and pain.

Diagnosis and Treatment. Diagnosis requires a biopsy, in which a tissue sample is analyzed for the presence of cancerous cells, often followed by x-rays to determine the extent to which the cancer has spread. Since the nasopharynx is a difficult site for surgery, radiation therapy is recommended for localized tumors. Surgery to remove affected lymph nodes in the neck may be performed for more advanced cases, sometimes accompanied or followed by chemotherapy. *See also* CANCER *and* CHEMOTHERAPY.

Natural Contraception

The attempted prevention of pregnancy by the avoidance of sexual intercourse or the use of barrier contraceptives (such as a condom or diaphragm) during a woman's fertile period.

Natural contraception involves avoiding sexual intercourse at the times at which a woman would be most likely to conceive. Conception can only occur for five days before ovulation, during the day of ovulation itself, and for three days after ovulation. These days are known as "fertile" days. At other times of the menstrual cycle (known as "infertile" days), conception is not possible. Natural contraception involves the prediction of fertile days and the avoidance of intercourse or the use of barrier contraceptives during these days. On infertile days, no method of contraception is used.

The main problem with natural conception is that most women have irregular menstrual cycles, thus it is difficult to predict fertile days with any certainty. In addition, unless barrier contraceptives are also used, natural contraception provides no protection against sexually transmitted diseases (STDs). The use of natural contraception as the sole form of contraception is not recommended. *See* CONTRACEPTION.

Naturopathy

Alternative medical discipline that promotes pure air, water and foods and seeks to treat disease by encouraging the healing powers of the body.

Naturopathy, a term coined by Benedict Lust, a German emigré to the United States in the early 20th century, is a general term for various alternative medical therapies, among which are natural diet practices, acupuncture, homeopathic therapy, body-work therapy, herbal medicine, and light and sound therapies.

Basic Principles. The basic principles underlying naturopathic medicine are:

• The body has the power to heal itself. Self-healing is considered more effective than introducing chemical substances into the body. For some, the belief in this "natural healing force" or "vital force" may take on religious or mystical overtones.

• It is more important to treat the cause of a disease than its symptoms, which are viewed as the body's attempt to heal itself.

• The physician's or healing practitioner's first responsibility is to do no harm or violence to the patient during the course of treatment.

• Each individual is viewed as a unique whole comprised of integrated systems that interpenetrate one another, none of which can be treated in isolation.

• The chief aim of medicine is to prevent the occurrence of illness; this requires a healthy lifestyle supported by a healthy attitude and environment.

Cautions. These principles may present problems if taken to extremes or applied indiscriminately; for example:

• Some diseases or injuries require assistance from sources beyond the body to catalyze the healing process.

• A physician must recognize that there are cases where therapy may be painful, but is necessary in order to prevent deterioration, death, or the use of conventional methods (e.g., chemotherapy).

• Scientific method and clinical investigation demands that conclusions be drawn in which the application of a given therapy will produce an expected result. This premise contradicts the naturopathic notion that every person is wholly different from every other person.

• Even under the best of circumstances, where a person exercises the utmost caution and lives a healthy lifestyle, diseases and injury may occur requiring medical treatments that would not be characterized as natural or naturopathic.

• The control an individual has over his or her environment is often limited by social, political, economic, and other factors, at times beyond an individual's power. Relying on the creation of a healthy environment for a person's health and well-being may prove less than effective in many instances. *See also* ACUPUNCTURE; ALTERNATIVE MEDICINE; *and* BODYWORK.

Nausea

Abdominal sensation that leads to vomiting.

Nausea may be accompanied by retching, dizziness, abdominal pain, considerable salivation, clamminess, and lowered blood pressure. Nausea is a common symptom in many different diseases or conditions affecting the gastrointestinal system or the kidneys.

Causes. Any of the following may bring on nausea, which in turn is usually followed by vomiting: strong or unpleasant odors; medications; viral infections; sea-sickness or motion sickness; migraine headaches; morning sickness during pregnancy; food poisoning; food allergies; chemotherapy in cancer patients; emptiness of the stomach; heat exhaustion; or intestinal obstruction.

A person who is not pregnant and has experienced nausea for a prolonged period of time should consult a healthcare professional.

Treatment. When the cause of nausea and vomiting is known, the underlying disorder can be treated. If vomiting occurs, the patient should take in as much fluid as possible without upsetting the stomach further. Antiemetic drugs may be prescribed to suppress nausea. *See also* VOMITING.

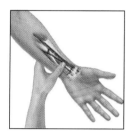

Acupressure for Nausea. There is some evidence that acupressure (above) is capable of relieving nausea. This technique can be practiced by grasping the patient's arm and applying pressure to the inside of the arm with the thumb.

Nebulizer

Device to deliver asthma and other respiratory medications in the form of a mist.

For people with asthma or other respiratory problems, a nebulizer allows medicine to be administered directly into the lungs, either through a face mask or a breathing tube. The nebulizer forces air or oxygen through a water-based mixture of the prescribed drug to form an inhalable mist. The mist is produced continuously, so the patient does not have to time the breathing with a machine's cycle. This is an excellent medication delivery mechanism for children under five years of age, patients who have difficulty using metered-dose inhalers, and patients with severe asthma or who are prone to suffering acute asthma attacks. *See also* ASTHMA *and* INHALER.

Neck

The connection between the head (along with the brain) and the body.

The neck supports the head and contains many structures vital to the functioning of the body. The spinal cord, which carries nerve impulses from the body to and from the brain, passes through the neck, as does the esophagus, which carries food from the mouth to the stomach, and the trachea, the windpipe through which air flows from the nose to the lungs. Many major blood vessels, such as the carotid arteries and the jugular veins, are also located in the neck. *See also* CENTRAL NERVOUS SYSTEM.

Neck Dissection, Radical

Surgical procedure to remove lymph nodes in the neck, designed to prevent the spread of a cancer of the head, face, or neck.

A radical neck dissection is performed to treat cancers of the neck, throat, and mouth that have either spread (metastasized), but are still contained in the neck region, or that have not responded to radiation treatment.

With the patient under general anesthesia, an incision shaped like a large "H" is made on the affected side of the neck. The skin is pulled back to expose the muscle just above the collarbone. The surgeon cuts through the muscle and removes the entire lymphatic system in the neck, the internal jugular vein, the lower salivary gland, and surrounding tissue. Removal of the voicebox (laryngectomy) may be necessary in some cases. A postoperative tracheotomy is occasionally performed to ensure passage of air.

Prognosis is variable. Depending on the amount of tissue removed, head movement may be impaired. *See also* CANCER.

Neck Rigidity

Immobility of the neck.

When muscles in the neck and spine clench in a spasm, they cause the neck to become rigid. Occasionally, the spasm may cause the neck to arch back.

Muscle spasms and rigidity of the neck can occur as a result of stress, injury, arthritis, or even from sleeping in an odd position. In many cases, pain can be relieved with anti-inflammatory drugs. Neck spasms and rigidity can be reduced by strengthening the muscles in the neck and upper back and adopting correct positions for sleeping and carrying heavy objects.

A patient with neck rigidity accompanied by numbness, tingling, or weakness should be attended to by a physician, as this may indicate a more serious injury. *See also* ARTHRITIS; IMMOBILITY; *and* NECK.

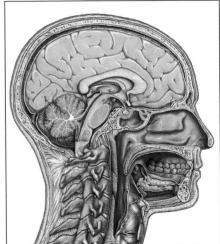

Cross-Sections of the Head and Neck.
The neck contains many vital structures, including (*above*) the spinal cord, the esophagus, and the trachea, as well as major blood vessels that carry blood to and from the brain. Below, the muscles in the neck allow for rotation and movement of the head, neck, and spine. When the muscles in this area tighten, the neck becomes rigid and unable to move. It may also arch backwards in some cases.

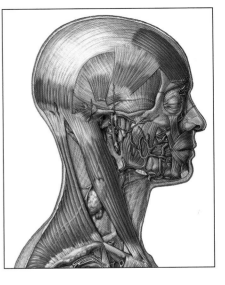

Necrolysis, Toxic Epidermal

Also known as TEN

Dangerous skin condition in which the top layer of the skin peels off.

Toxic epidermal necrolysis is often caused by a reaction to a drug. Drugs that can induce the condition include penicillin, sulfonamides, anticonvulsants, nonsteroidal anti-inflammatory drugs, and allopurinol.

Symptoms. The disorder generally begins with a painful red area of skin that sometimes begins to blister, followed by sloughing off of the skin and mucous membranes all over the body. Between 20 and 100 percent of the skin can be affected.

Treatment for toxic epidermal necrosis includes a two to three week course of prednisone. This will stop the damage, but will not restore skin that has already been lost to the disease. Treatment in a hospital burn unit may be necessary. The condition has a 30 percent mortality rate, generally as a result of infections that develop at the site of the damaged skin. *See also* ALLERGY.

Necrosis

The death of tissue or bone matter.

Necrosis is caused when the tissues and bones do not receive enough blood flow (ischemia). Trauma through extreme heat or cold, radiation, and chemicals can all cause necrosis. When larger areas of dead tissue form as the result of frostbite, for example, necrosis may then lead to gangrene. *See also* GANGRENE.

Neonatology

Branch of medicine dealing with the care, development, and diseases of newborn infants.

The neonatologist cares for infants up to the age of four weeks. After this time, the medical care of the child is transferred to a pediatrician. *See also* PEDIATRICS.

Neoplasia

The process of tumor formation.

Neoplasia occurs when the normal controls over cell multiplication are lost, because of a mutation of a cell's genetic material or an outside influence, such as a mutagen. The result is abnormal duplication of the cell in which the change occurred. The resulting neoplasm is not necessarily dangerous. Some neoplasms are malignant, spreading readily to other tissues, but others are benign, with limited, local growth. *See also* MUTAGEN *and* TUMOR.

Nephrectomy

Surgical removal of a kidney, usually one with a malignant tumor.

Other conditions that may require nephrectomy include severe infections, stones (calculi), injury, and hereditary polycystic kidney disease, in which cysts grow in the kidneys, causing failure. Cancer of the kidney often requires removal of the entire organ, its surrounding fat, lymph nodes, and the adjacent adrenal gland. Smaller tumors may only require removal of part of the kidney.

Laparoscopic nephrectomy for transplantation has been performed since the mid-1990s. It eliminates the large (12- to 18-inch) flank incisions from the navel to the middle of the back common in traditional kidney removal. Laparoscopic nephrectomy requires only several tiny incisions in and near the navel. After carbon dioxide is pumped through one of the incisions to expand the surgical area, airtight tubes are placed into the abdomen to create a passage for camera and instruments.

Recovery. After a kidney is removed, the patient's other kidney gradually takes over the workload of both kidneys and fully adjusts within six months. If both kidneys are removed, the patient requires a kidney transplant. *See also* DIALYSIS; KIDNEY TRANSPLANT; *and* LAPAROSCOPY.

Nephritis

Inflammation of the kidneys caused by infection, an immune disorder or a metabolic disorder.

Nephrons are the functional units of the kidneys. They consist of two subunits: glomeruli, which do the initial filtering of waste material from the blood; and tubules, which collect and regulate chemicals in the urine. These functions can be impaired by pyelonephritis, a bacterial infection, either acute or chronic. Acute pyelonephritis is more common in women, usually resulting from a bladder infection that spreads to the kidney. It is treated with antibiotics. Chronic pyelonephritis can be present from birth, often because of an inherited abnormality that leads to persistent infections. Surgery may be needed to correct the underlying cause.

Another form of nephritis is glomerulonephritis, an inflammation of the glomeruli that can result from an abnormal immune system response. Symptoms can range from high blood pressure to gradual kidney failure requiring artificial kidney treatment (dialysis) or a kidney transplant. The immune system disorder that causes nephritis can be treated by drugs that depress the immune response or by plasmapheresis (filtering of the blood to remove immune complexes). Glomerulonephritis can also be caused by tropical infections, such as malaria or schistosomiasis. *See also* DIALYSIS; GLOMERULONEPHRITIS; INFECTION; MALARIA; PLASMAPHERESIS; PYELONEPHRITIS; RENAL FAILURE; *and* SCHISTOSOMIASIS.

Nephrocalcinosis

Abnormal deposits of calcium in the kidneys.

Excess deposits of calcium in the kidneys can result from any condition that causes excess blood levels of calcium, such as overactivity of the parathyroid glands (the pea-sized glands located next to the thyroid gland in the neck), sarcoidosis (inflammation of the lymph nodes and other bodily tissues), Cushing's syndrome (overproduction of corticosteroid hormones by the adrenal glands), or renal tubular acidosis, in which the urine has lower than normal acidity. It also can occur in individuals who take excessive amounts of vitamin D or some antacid drugs.

The abnormal deposits of calcium gradually cause the kidney to calcify, or harden, interfering with kidney function. Treatment of the condition is aimed at the underlying cause. *See also* CUSHING'S SYNDROME; PARATHYROID GLAND; RENAL TUBULAR ACIDOSIS; *and* SARCOIDOSIS.

Nephrolithotomy

Surgical procedure to remove one or more stones from the kidney.

Kidney stones (calculi) are solid crystals that form and fall out of the urine solution. These painful stones may cause bleeding, infection, or damage to the kidney, and they should be treated aggressively. When kidney stones are too large to be dealt with through other means, such as shockwave treatment (lithotripsy) or medications, they may be surgically extracted by nephrolithotomy.

During a nephrolithotomy, an incision is made either in the abdomen or the side, depending on the nature of the kidney abnormality. The kidney stones are surgically extracted thorugh the opening, and the incisions are stitched up. *See also* CALCULUS; KIDNEY; LITHOTRIPSY; *and* URINARY TRACT.

Nephrology

The branch of medical science that deals with the kidneys.

Nephrology is a subspecialty of urology, which deals with the entire urinary tract. Nephrology is concerned with the normal functioning of the kidney and with the causes of kidney disease, their diagnosis, and their treatment. A nephrologist uses a variety of tests and imaging techniques to investigate kidney disorders. Treatments are aimed at several conditions, including

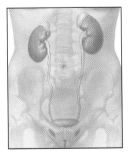

Kidney Location. Nephrology is the study of the kidneys. Above, the location of the kidneys in the abdomen.

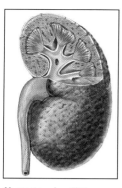

Hypertensive Kidney. One disease that may affect the kidneys is hypertension (high blood pressure). Above, hypertension causes a bumpy surface on the outside of the kidneys.

kidney stones, tumors, high blood pressure (hypertension), kidney infection, and kidney inflammation. Treatment can range from drug therapy to surgery and, in the case of kidney failure, dialysis (artificial kidney treatment) or kidney transplant. *See also* CALCULUS; DIALYSIS; HYPERTENSION; KIDNEY TRANSPLANTS; *and* TUMORS.

Nephropathy

Any condition that damages the kidneys, impairing their function.

Nephropathies include infections, congenital malformations, tumors, autoimmune disorders, and kidney damage resulting from diseases such as diabetes. Many of these conditions interfere with the flow of urine within or from the kidney. A tumor or kidney stone can result in obstructive nephropathy, blocking flow out of the kidney. Failure of one or both of the valves at the end of the ureters (the tubes through which urine flows to the bladder) can cause reflux nephropathy (a back flow of urine). Kidney function can also be damaged by toxins—poisons such as carbon tetrachloride—resulting in toxic nephropathy. *See also* CALCULUS *and* DIABETES .

Nephrosclerosis

Deterioration of kidney function resulting from the replacement of normal tissue with scar tissue.

Nephrosclerosis results from an inflammation of the kidney, which can be caused by a number of diseases. When such inflammation occurs, a tough fibrous protein (collagen) forms in place of normal kidney structures. This disorder generally occurs in the final stages of illnesses that cause kidney inflammation, such as hypertension diabetes, glomerulonephritis, and chronic pyelo-nephritis. Treatment of nephrosclerosis is aimed at relieving the underlying condition, which will halt the progress of nephrosclerosis. *See also* DIABETES; GLOMERULONEPHRITIS; INFLAMMATION; KIDNEY; *and* PYELONEPHRITIS.

Nephrostomy

Surgical procedure in which a small tube (catheter) is inserted into the kidney to allow for the drainage of urine, usually when the ureter is not functional or needs to heal.

A nephrostomy is commonly performed after a kidney operation, such as the removal of a kidney or ureter stone (calculus), to facilitate the healing process. A nephrostomy tube can also accommodate a nephroscope for viewing the kidney, and instruments can be inserted through it to help remove calculi.

Longer-term urine drainage by nephrostomy tube presents risks of infection and obstructions in the tube. *See* KIDNEY.

Nephrotic Syndrome

Symptoms caused by damage to the glomeruli, the filtering units of the kidney.

In the kidneys, blood passes through millions of tiny units (nephrons) where waste products are filtered out into the urine and normal levels of salts and water are maintained. Each nephron includes a filtering component called a glomerulus. In nephrotic syndrome, the pores that allow toxic substances to pass into the urine become enlarged because of damage to the glomerulus, so that abnormal amounts of protein leak into the urine. The decrease in blood protein leads to a build-up of fluid in the body (edema), which causes swelling. Difficulty breathing may also occur if fluid is in the lungs.

Causes. Nephrotic syndrome can be caused by diabetes, amyloidosis, glomerulonephritis, and other conditions.

Treatment of the disease is aimed at the underlying disease. In many cases, steroids such as prednisone can help to reduce the edema. If treatment fails to stop progression of the condition, artificial kidney treatment (dialysis) or a kidney transplant may be needed. *See also* AMYLOIDOSIS; DIABETES; DIALYSIS; EDEMA; GLOMERULONEPHRITIS; *and* PREDNISONE.

Nerve

A cordlike bundle of fibers made up of nerve cells through which impulses pass between the central nervous system and the rest of the body.

Each nerve is made up of a bundle of fibers called axons, which are the projections of individual nerve cells, called neurons. Nerves have a sensory function and a motor function. The sensory function is to carry information from receptors to the central nervous system (the brain and spinal cord). The motor function is to carry impulses from the central nervous system to a given muscle, organ, or gland. Most nerves conduct both sensory and motor impulses, although some only carry one type of impulse.

Nerve functions are affected by a number of factors, including temperature and pressure, and the nerves may be damaged by various injuries or disorders. The functioning of nerves throughout the body may be impaired by inflammation, infection, vitamin or mineral deficiencies, and metabolic conditions. *See also* NERVE INJURY.

Nerve Block

Injection of a local anesthetic into a nerve, resulting in loss of sensation to the part of the body served by that nerve.

In a nerve block, a local anesthetic is injected into an area around the target nerve, but at a point in that nerve that is far from the affected area of the body. For example, in epidural anesthesia, which is used during childbirth, an anesthetic is injected into the lower back and the entire lower half of the body is anesthetized as a result.

Nerve blocks are generally utilized when it is not feasible to inject the anesthetic directly. This may occur if the affected area is inflamed, if there is a risk of spreading infection, if the area is too large to anesthetize by other means, or if the area is inaccessible. *See also* ANESTHESIA, LOCAL *and* NERVE.

Nerve Injury

Damage or laceration to a nerve that severs all or a portion of its conducting fibers.

Nerve damage is often caused by accidents. Nerve injury can result from lacerations (open wounds), fractures, or crush injuries. In each case, nerve injury can result in a loss of feeling and muscular control in the affected area.

In a nerve injury, the individual nerve fibers within the peripheral nerve may be disconnected while the nerve trunk generally remains intact. The severed fibers at the point of injury may degenerate. If the ends of the nerve fibers remain intact, they can regenerate themselves.

Complete severance of a nerve is often caused by a power tool accident or a knife wound. If the nerves are completely disconnected, the nerve fibers cannot regenerate. A surgical procedure is the sole treatment for a severed nerve. Only the peripheral nerves, those existing outside the brain and spinal cord, can be surgically repaired. *See also* CRUSH SYNDROME; FRACTURES; MYELIN SHEATH; NERVE; *and* PERIPHERAL NERVE.

Nerve, Trapped

Compression or distention of a nerve, causing numbness, burning, or tingling.

If a nerve is immensely compressed or stretched, the majority of nerve signals are obstructed. A more mild compression may only partially block the transmission of nerve signals. A tingling sensation indicates nerve damage. Numbness, in which no pressure is felt, can indicate that the actual nerve is dead.

Causes. Many different types of injuries can result in a trapped nerve, including spinal cord compression, carpal tunnel syndrome, and crutch palsy.

Treatment. An injured nerve repairs itself over time. Only in the most painful cases is surgical decompression required. *See also* NERVE *and* NERVE INJURY.

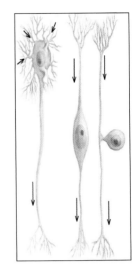

Nerves. Above, every nerve is composed of a bundle of nerve cells. Nerve impulses from the central nervous system enter the nerve through structures called dendrites. They then move down the length of the nerve to exit at projectile fibers called axons.

Nervous Breakdown

Nonscientific term used popularly to describe individuals who have suffered a mental collapse.

A nervous breakdown is generally accompanied by incapacitating anxiety, episodes of debilitating tearfulness and withdrawal, or bouts of shouting, hysteria, and paranoia. The term generally describes an individual who is suffering a mental crisis that is in immediate need of aggressive treatment, possibly including hospitalization. The term nervous breakdown carries a stigma insofar as it implies mental instability and pathological tendencies, but, in fact, many people experience an emotional crisis resulting in an inability to function normally for a period of time. *See also* ANXIETY; HYSTERIA; *and* PARANOIA.

Nervous System

The system in the body that perceives and analyzes changes in the conditions in and outside of the body and responds to these changes.

The body's most important need is to survive. The nervous system is responsible for many of the body's responses to threats to its survival, such as running from danger, shivering in response to cold temperatures, and quickly withdrawing a hand from a hot stove. Several of these responses are automatic; that is, they are not consciously controlled by the brain. However, the nervous system is also responsible for voluntary functions—those functions that are controlled by the brain.

STRUCTURE

The central nervous system (CNS) is made up of the brain and the spinal cord, each of which contains billions of connected neurons (nerve cells). The function of the CNS is to receive sensory information from receptors and organs and to send information to muscles, organs, and glands.

Sensory information travels to and from the CNS via nerves, which extend to every part of the body. These nerves are all made up of bundles of axons (projections) of many neurons, and together they comprise the peripheral nervous system. The peripheral nervous system consists of all of the nerves that connect the CNS to the rest of the body. The 31 pairs of spinal nerves connect to the spinal cord and the 12 pairs of cranial nerves connect directly to the brain.

In addition, the nervous system can be further divided based on the various functions of the nerves. Two of the most prominent of these divisions are the autonomic nervous system and the somatic nervous system. The autonomic system is responsible for regulating unconscious or automatic functions, while the somatic nervous system controls the muscles that produce voluntary movement.

FUNCTION

The nervous system mainly controls automatic responses to various stimuli (also called reflexes), although the more developed areas of the brain can initiate voluntary actions. The specific processes that are responsible for these voluntary actions are not well understood. In general, however, the actions of the nervous system have their

Nervous System.
At right, the pathway of a nerve impulse from the receptor nerves (often located just under the skin), which receive stimuli from outside the body, to the effector neurons (often located in the central nervous system), which formulate responses to stimuli.

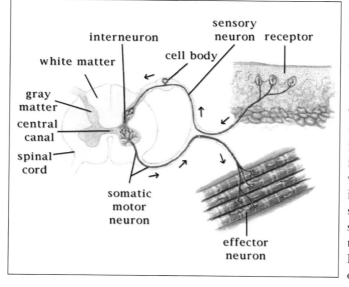

interneuron
white matter
gray matter
central canal
spinal cord
somatic motor neuron
cell body
sensory neuron receptor
effector neuron

foundation in the transmission of nerve signals through large and complex networks of neurons.

An Example of a Nervous System Response. When a hand touches a hot stove, receptors in the hand perceive the heat of the stove and send an impulse through what is called a sensory fiber (a fiber in a nerve responsible for sending information about perceived changes in the environment) to the spinal cord. The spinal cord then sends a signal via what is called a motor fiber (a fiber in a nerve responsible for sending information about movement) back to the muscles in the hand, causing these muscles to contract and move the hand off the source of the heat.

Since the nerve impulses did not pass through the brain, the person will not consciously control the response of the body. It is likely that pain will only be felt after the hand is already removed from the stove, because pain can only be perceived by the brain and the nerve impulses do not reach the brain until after the hand has been removed. This type of nervous system response is called a reflex. In contrast, when nerve impulses reach the brain, the response of the nervous system is conscious and voluntary.

DISORDERS

Various disorders may result from damage to or impairment of the various parts of the nervous system. Any disorder of the brain or spinal cord is a disorder of the central nervous system, while conditions that affect the nerves are disorders of the peripheral nervous system. These conditions may include disorders that affect any of the senses (hearing, sight, smell, taste, and touch), those that affect memory (such as amnesia), and those that affect movement (such as ataxia—the inability to coordinate voluntary movement of the muscles).

> *For background material on nervous system, see* NERVE. *Further information can be found in* AUTONOMIC NERVOUS SYSTEM; BRAIN; CENTRAL NERVOUS SYSTEM; MEMORY; SPINAL CORD; *and* SYNAPSE. *See also* ATAXIA; BRAIN DISORDERS; *and* NERVE INJURY *for more on nervous system disorders.*

Neuralgia

A sharp, intermittent pain along the route of a nerve, most commonly in the head or face.

Neuralgia is pain caused by a damaged or irritated nerve. The pain can be short-lived and mild, or persistent and oppressive. The pain lasts only for a few seconds but may occur repeatedly throughout the day.

Types. Neuralgia exists in many different forms, including:

• concentrated pain experienced in the ear, throat, and the back of the tongue (glossopharyngeal neuralgia)—triggered by chewing or yawning;

• lower back pain and pain on one side of the face only (trigeminal neuralgia);

• intense pain around the eye socket (migraine);

• damage to the peripheral nerves (peripheral neuropathy);

• pressure on the sciatic nerve; and

• burning and lingering pain accompanying the *Herpes zoster* virus (shingles).

Causes. It is not clear what causes glossopharyngeal neuralgia and trigeminal neuralgia. In the case of trigeminal neuralgia, researchers propose that the trigeminal nerve is compressed by a vein or an artery. In some cases, a physical injury causes the condition. In rare cases, tumors or multiple sclerosis can cause nerve damage resulting in facial neuralgia pain. Common over-the-counter pain medications usually do not offer enough relief for severe nerve damage discomfort.

Treatment. Milder episodes of neuralgia can be treated with aspirin or other over-the-counter pain-killing medications. Severe neuralgia may be treated with a stronger prescription pain reliever. In acute facial neuralgia, surgery may be required. Medications that can alter nerve conduction may be prescribed.

> *Background reading on neuralgia can be found in* NERVE *and* NERVOUS SYSTEM. *For related material, see* HERPES ZOSTER; INJURY; MIGRAINE, SCIATIC NERVE; SCIATICA; *and* TRIGEMINAL NEURALGIA. *See also* ASPIRIN; PAIN RELIEF; *and* SURGERY *for more on possible treatments.*

Resources on Nervous System

Kandel, Eric R., et al., *Principles of Neural Science* (1991); Kumin, Maxine, *Inside the Halo and Beyond: The Anatomy of a Recovery* (2000); Sanes, Dan Harvey, et al., *Development of the Nervous System* (2000); Sife, Wallace, *After Stroke, Enhancing Quality of Life* (1998); Epilepsy Foundation, Tel. (800) EFA-1000, Online: www.efa.org; Muscular Dystrophy Association of America, Tel. (800) 572-1717, Online: www.mda-usa.org; American Academy of Neurology, Tel. (651) 695-1940, Online: www.aan.com; American Board of Neurological Surgery, Tel. (713) 790-6015, www.abns.org;

Neural Tube Defects

Group of disorders resulting from the improper development of a fetus' neural tube.

The neural tube is the foundation of the entire nervous system, developing into the brain and spinal cord. The neural tube forms within the first few weeks after conception from the neural folds arising out of the cell layer known as the ectoderm. The neural tube then seals off, with the brain forming at the front of the tube, and the spinal cord in the back. Sometimes the tube fails to close properly, giving rise to a group of disorders known as neural tube defects (NTDs).

Types. The most common neural tube defect is spina bifida ("split spine"), which is characterized by the incomplete closure of one or more vertebrae. The condition ranges from mild to severe, with the spinal cord actually protruding in the most severe cases. Paralysis may result.

Other NTDs include anacephaly (the absence of most or all of the cerebrum) and hydrocephalus (excess fluid in the brain).

Causes. NTDs are congenital (present at birth) and are believed to be genetic in origin, although the fetus' environment does play a factor in whether or not the genes for the conditions are expressed. These defects affect about two out of every 1,000 babies born.

Diagnosis. Prenatal detection of NTDs is possible with the use of a blood test known as the alpha-fetoprotein (AFP) test. A fetus with nervous system problems will secrete large amounts of this protein into the mother's bloodstream. If high levels of AFP are found in the mother's blood, additional tests, such as ultrasound or amniocentesis, will be performed.

Prevention. In recent years, it has been found that NTDs can be largely prevented if the mother's diet contains sufficient amounts of the vitamin folic acid. In general, balanced diet and good prenatal care are also important in preventing NTDs. *See also* BLOOD TESTS; CONGENITAL; NERVOUS SYSTEM; *and* SPINA BIFIDA.

Neurapraxia

Nerve injury in which the nerve appears to be healthy, yet the functioning of conducting fibers is impaired.

Neurapraxia is the inability of an apparently healthy nerve to transmit signals to the muscles. It is a transient neurological condition common to ice hockey and football players who receive constant abuse to the network of nerves around the neck and shoulders (brachial plexus). Although cervical cord neurapraxia is benign, there is a high probability of recurrence.

Common symptoms of neurapraxia include a burning pain, numbness, and loss of sensation. Motor changes range from muscle weakness to a total paralysis. The episodes are short-lived, with total recovery within a few weeks. *See* PARALYSIS.

Neuritis

Inflammation of a nerve or nerves, causing pain, paralysis, disturbance of sensation, and/or loss of reflexes.

Nerve inflammation may be caused by a viral (*Herpes zoster*) or bacterial (Hansen's disease) infection. Optic neuritis is a condition in which the optic nerve becomes inflamed. Such conditions usually improve without treatment.

The term neuritis has taken on a generic meaning and is often applied to nerve injury or disease that results from causes other than inflammation. Neuritis is almost interchangeable with the term "neuropathy," which includes all peripheral nerve disorders. *See also* INFECTION; NEUROPATHY; *and* SHINGLES.

Neuroblastoma

Malignant tumor of the adrenal glands or sympathetic nervous system.

Neuroblastoma is the third most common cancer in children. Four of every five cases of neuroblastoma are diagnosed during the first ten years of life. Most neuroblastomas arise in the adrenal glands or in the part of the sympathetic nervous system (which controls automatic body functions) that is located at the back of the abdomen. However, this type of cancer can also occur in the chest, neck, or brain.

Symptoms. The symptoms of neuroblastoma include a growing mass in the neck, weight loss, generalized pain, irritability, loss of appetite, and a pattern of bruises around the eyes. The diagnosis is made by x-ray examinations, blood tests, and urine tests, sometimes accompanied by an examination of tissue samples (biopsy).

Treatment and Prognosis. Neuroblastoma can be treated by surgical removal of the tumor unless the tumor is located in an area in which the operation would harm the patient. Surgery is often followed by chemotherapy and radiation therapy, which are used alone when surgery is not possible. The prognosis depends on the stage at which the cancer is discovered. Prognosis is generally good for infants and younger children but not for older children in whom the cancer has spread (metastasized). *See also* ADRENAL GLANDS; CHEMOTHERAPY; *and* RADIATION THERAPY.

Neurocutaneous Disorders

Group of disorders in which cutaneous (skin-related) symptoms occur along with symptoms of brain disease.

Some examples of neurocutaneous disorders are neurofibromatosis, tuberous sclerosis, and Sturge-Weber syndrome. All of these disorders may be associated with seizures, developmental delay, and learning and behavioral problems, as well as with skin-related symptoms. Such skin-related symptoms may include discolored patches, raised nodules, and small swellings on the skin, depending on the condition affecting the patient. Treatment of neurocutaneous disorders is specific to the particular disorder. *See also* NEUROFIBROMATOSIS; STURGE-WEBER SYNDROME; *and* TUBEROUS SCLEROSIS.

Neurofibromatosis

Also known as von Recklinghausen's disease

Genetic disorder characterized by multiple growths of abnormal nerve tissue (neurofibromas), which appear in the skin and other parts of the body.

Neurofibromas are growths of the support cells surrounding the nerves of the body. The growths appear after puberty as lumps under the skin.

Symptoms. Approximately one-third of those with neurofibromatosis experience no symptoms. Many people with the condition have light brown patches of skin (called café au lait spots) over the chest, back, pelvis, elbows, and knees. These spots may be present at birth or may appear during infancy. The neurofibromas begin appearing between the ages of ten and fifteen and may range in number from less than ten to several thousand.

Neurofibromas may cause skeletal problems, such as abnormal curvature of the spine, rib deformities, enlarged bones of the arms and legs, and bone defects in the skull. The growths may also cause neurological problems, such as developmental delay and behavioral problems.

Neurofibromas may also exert pressure on the peripheral nerves, impairing their normal function. Various neurological complications can result, including blindness, deafness, and difficulties in coordination. Serious complications can result if there is pressure on the spinal cord.

Patients with Type 2 neurofibromatosis develop neurofibromas in the inner ear, leading to problems with balance.

Treatment. There is no way of preventing the formation of the growths or halting the progression of the disease. However, individual growths that are causing problems can be removed surgically or treated with radiation therapy.

Background information on neurofibromatosis can be found in NERVE; NERVOUS SYSTEM; *and* TUMOR. *For further reading, see* AUTONOMIC NERVOUS SYSTEM; BLINDNESS; CAFÉ AU LAIT SPOTS; CHILD DEVELOPMENT; DEAFNESS; HEARING LOSS; MENTAL RETARDATION; *and* PUBERTY.

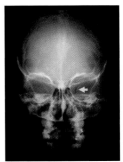

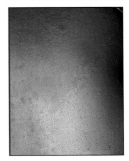

Neurofibroma. Neurofibromas are growths of abnormal nerve tissue that can be damaging to the nervous or skeletal system. Above, top, an x-ray of the skull of a child with neurofibromatosis. The child developed visual problems and a nerve tumor in the optic nerve was discovered. Above, bottom, a picture of a giant café au lait spot on a person with neurofibromatosis.

Neuroma

Nonmalignant tumor arising in nerve tissue.

A neuroma may arise in any of the nerves of the body. It may be the result of an injury, but in most cases the cause is unknown. A neuroma is usually not life-threatening, since it is not cancerous, but it can cause troublesome symptoms, depending on the specific nerve affected. One common symptom of a neuroma include pain in the region of the body served by the affected nerve. Numbness and weakness of the affected region may also occur. The remedy in such cases is surgical removal of the tumor. *See also* CANCER; NERVE; NERVE INJURY; *and* TUMOR.

Neuropathic Joint

Repeated damage to a joint due to numbness.

Neuropathy means a loss of sensation. The reflexes that indicate pain are not felt in a neuropathic joint. As a result, an excess of stress or strain can occur without any attempt to stop the damaging action. The wear on the joint can lead to osteoarthritis, swelling, and deformity in the area. Neuropathic joints may be a side effect of diabetes or untreated syphilis.

Due to loss of feeling, these injuries may not be detected until the deformity is visible. Once the injury is discovered, it may then be treated. The nerve damage in the joint, however, is not treatable. *See also* ARTHRITIS *and* DIABETES.

Neuropathy

Nervous system disorder that affects the peripheral nerves, which connect the central nervous system (CNS) to the nerves throughout the body.

Neuropathy is also referred to as peripheral neuropathy or peripheral nerve damage. Disease or injury to the peripheral nerves prevents them from transmitting messages from the brain and spinal cord to the organs, muscles, and glands. It is

Preventing Neuropathy

More than two million Americans suffer from the painful nerve disorder neuropathy. However, it is possible to prevent the condition. The suggested methods to prevent the onset of neuropathy are to avoid toxins, injuries, and alcohol, and to get plenty of exercise and sleep. Maintaining good nutritional habits will also help to prevent the disorder.

thought that neuropathy is a result of damage to nerve components such as axons or myelin sheaths. If an axon loses its myelin sheath, the electric signals will not be transmitted properly.

CAUSES

Peripheral nerves are extremely long and delicate and therefore easily susceptible to damage. Some of the more common causes of neuropathy include: diabetes mellitus; rheumatoid arthritis; exposure to toxins, such as arsenic, mercury, and lead; autoimmune diseases; viral and bacterial infections; cancer; cancer medications; vitamin B deficiencies; kidney disease; pressure on a nerve (carpal tunnel syndrome); liver disease; underactive thyroid; alcoholism; drug dependence; and certain hereditary conditions.

SYMPTOMS

The first symptom of neuropathy is usually numbness or tingling in the toes. Pain may develop in the toes, and may move upward and spread to the front of the thighs. Sometimes, the pain will travel to the fingers and hands. The symptoms vary in intensity, ranging from barely noticeable to almost unbearable. Some patients find that the symptoms are more severe at night.

Other common symptoms of neuropathy include tingling and numbness; burning or freezing pain; sharp, jabbing pain; the sensation that the patient is wearing an invisible sock; extreme sensitivity to touch; muscle weakness; loss of balance and coordination; a drop in blood pressure when standing; an upset stomach, ranging from diarrhea to constipation; incontinence; impotence; and night sweats.

TREATMENT

The goal of neuropathy treatment is to control the symptoms. The type and success of the treatment is dependent on the cause of the neuropathy. If the symptoms are triggered by medication, the physician may be able to alleviate the symptoms by prescribing another drug. Neuropathy from a compressed nerve can be treated with medications. Chronic diseases, such as diabetes, should first be controlled before attempting to manage the neuropathy. Over-the-counter pain relievers can treat mild symptoms of the condition. Burning pain is treated with tricyclic antidepressants. Jabbing pain can be treated with anti-seizure medication.

> *For background material on neuropathy, see* AUTONOMIC NERVOUS SYSTEM; CENTRAL NERVOUS SYSTEM; *and* NERVOUS SYSTEM. *Further information can be found in* ALCOHOL DEPENDENCE; BRAIN; CANCER; DIABETES MELLITUS; DRUG DEPENDENCE; GLAND; HYPOTHYROIDISM; INFECTIOUS DISEASE; NERVE; RHEUMATOID ARTHRITIS; *and* SPINAL CORD.

Neurosis

> **Mild psychiatric disorder in which the sufferer is distressed but not debilitated.**

The term neurosis is applied to a wide variety of symptoms and disorders that cause stress and anxiety and inhibit a person's ability to work or interact socially, but which do not totally debilitate or incapacitate that person. No physical abnormality has been shown to underlie any form of neurosis, and it does not typically develop into psychosis or a more extreme mental disorder.

Types. The categories of neuroses are:

• Dysthymsa—a mild form of depression that may be accompanied by lassitude (fatigue) and some momentary crying;

• Anxiety—mild phobias and obsessive-compulsive behaviors that do not result in withdrawal from the patient's routines of everyday life;

• Somatization—complaining about non-existent illnesses or symptoms, not resulting in prolonged hospitalization;

• Dissociation—inattentiveness and inability to focus on tasks, not resulting in the unawareness of self or of surroundings.

Treatment. In many instances, neurosis may be controlled by reducing social or work-related stress; through attending psychotherapy; and by adjusting diet, work, or sleep habits. Neurosis may also be treated with antidepressants. *See also* ANXIETY; ANXIETY DISORDERS; ANTIDEPRESSANT DRUGS; DEPRESSION; PSYCHOSIS; PSYCHOTHERAPY; *and* SOMATIZATION DISORDER.

Neurosyphilis

> **Infection of the spinal cord resulting from untreated syphilis.**

Syphilis is a sexually transmitted bacterial disease. First and second stage syphilis may stretch over a period of many years. In the small percentage of sufferers who reach the third stage of untreated syphilis, the bacteria infect the spinal cord and brain. This is called neurosyphilis. Symptoms include headache, stiff neck, irritability, confusion, visual disturbances, abnormal reflexes, incontinence, weakness, muscle atrophy, and uncoordinated movement. Neurosyphilis is treated with penicillin. If the sufferer has reached this third stage of syphilis without treatment, the prognosis is usually poor. *See also* SYPHILIS.

Neurotoxin

> **Chemical that damages the nervous system.**

Neurotoxins cause deterioration of nerve endings. Characteristic symptoms of such toxins are numbness, weakness, or paralysis of the section of the body being served by the affected nerve. Poisons from some spiders, snakes, scorpions, bees, and bacteria-act as neurotoxins. An example is the honey bee, whose sting releases apamin, which blocks potassium channels. Cayenne pepper releases capsaicin, which excites peripheral nerve endings. Arsenic and lead are chemicals that are neurotoxins. *See also* POISONING *and* TOXIN.

Resources on Neuroses

American Psychiatric Association, *Diagnostic and Statistical Manual of Mental Disorders, 4th Edition* (1994); Greist, John H. and James W. Jefferson, *Depression and Its Treatment* (1992); Solomon, Andrew, *The Noonday Demon: An Atlas of Depression* (2001); Wender, P.H. and D.F. Klein, *Mind, Mood, and Medicine: A Guide to the New Biopsychiatry* (1981); Nat. Depressive & Manic-Depressive Association, Tel. (800) 82-NDMDA, Online: www.ndmda.org; National Mental Health Association, Tel. (800) 969-NMHA, Online: www.nmha.org; www.ny-cornell.org/psychiatry/.

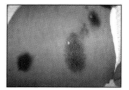

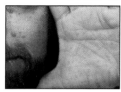

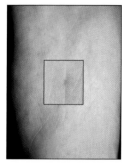

Nevus.
Many nevi (sing. nevus) are present at birth. Above, nevi come in many different varieties. The skin texture may be raised, and they are frequently darkly pigmented. Nevi have a greater chance of developing into skin cancer than other skin.

Nevus

A usually pigmented, sometimes hairy patch of skin that is present at birth (congenital) and may cover a significant area of the body.

The surface texture of a nevus may be smooth or bumpy, and the color varies from brown to bluish black. Visible signs of a nevus include a large, darkly pigmented lesion, which may or may not contain hair, with a smooth or warty looking texture. Because they are sometimes large and unsightly, they may eventually cause psychological stress. In addition, a giant nevus has a six percent chance of developing into skin cancer (malignant melanoma). Treatment involves surgical removal of the nevus and skin transplants, if necessary. *See also* MALIGNANT MELANOMA.

ALERT

The Risk of Skin Cancer

A doctor should be consulted immediately if an individual develops a new or changed mole, because of the risk of that mole developing into skin cancer.

Newborn

A baby who has just been born.

A normal, full-term baby is born between the 38th and 42nd weeks of pregnancy. Most full-term newborns weigh between five pounds, five ounces and ten pounds, and are between 18 and 22 inches long. During the first month of life, a baby gains about two pounds.

Tests. When a baby is born, he or she receives an APGAR score from the doctor. This reflects the baby's heart rate, respiratory effort, muscle tone, reflex irritability, and color. The baby is also tested for phenylketonuria, a metabolic disorder. Newborns with this disorder cannot ingest a substance called phenylalanine, which is present in most foods that contain protein. If buildup occurs, mental retardation and

brain damage can result. Babies are also tested for congenital hypothyroidism. If the newborn does not produce enough thyroid hormone, he or she may gradually show stunted growth. This condition is treated by giving the baby a tablet each day to replace the missing thyroid hormone. Another test newborns routinely receive is for galactosemia, a disorder in which the baby cannot process a certain sugar. If treated early enough, brain and liver damage can be prevented.

The First Days. Newborn babies, regardless of gender, may have swollen breasts and genitals because of the maternal hormones present at birth. There may be a milky discharge as well. Females may have a slight, bloody vaginal discharge, which is normal and will stop on its own.

A baby usually has its first bowel movement during the first 24 hours of life. It is normal for a newborn's stools to be tarry and black or green in color (meconium).

It is common for newborns to have birthmarks, such as strawberry hemangiomas, port-wine stains, salmon patches, mongolian spots, or milia. Many newborns have jaundice—a yellowing of the skin and whites of the eyes. This is usually not reason for concern.

Newborn babies tend to curl up in a fetal position during the days following birth. When a baby is on his or her stomach, her or she will be able to turn the head to one side. If held on the shoulder, a baby can lift his or her head. A newborn can see

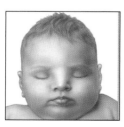

Newborn
Above, newborn babies tend to sleep a lot during the first few weeks of life. Later on, the baby will be awake for longer periods of time.

Reflexes in Newborns

Newborn babies are born with certain reflexes, which they outgrow by their third month of life. When stroked on one side of the mouth, a newborn baby will display the rooting reflex, turning the head in the direction of the stroke and opening the mouth. The gag reflex protects against choking. A baby will grasp an adult's finger with a great deal of strength. The "startle" or Moro reflex enables an infant to throw open the arms, stretch out the neck, cry, and then bring the arms and legs together, as if in a hug. Newborns also have a stepping reflex. A baby held up, as if standing, with feet touching the ground, will try to walk.

and follow objects that are eight to twelve inches directly in front of his or her face. The child's head will not be steady, causing it to roll back or to the side if not supported. Newborns can hear and distinguish between loud and soft sounds.

The First Weeks. During the first few weeks, a newborn will sleep between 14 and 18 hours a day. A baby should always be placed to sleep on his or her back, not on the stomach. This position reduces the chances of asphyxia, which some believe to be the cause of sudden infant death syndrome (SIDS). A baby will be alert for 30 minutes in every four-hour period. It is normal for a newborn to wake up during the night, sometimes several times, for a feeding. After one or two months, most babies will sleep for five or six hours straight.

Most newborns eat every two to five hours. After one month, a baby will consume about 25 ounces of breast milk or formula each day.

> *Background material on newborn can be found in* CHILD-BIRTH; CHILD DEVELOPMENT; INFANT; *and* PREGNANCY. *For related material, see* APGAR SCORE; ARTIFICIAL SWEETENER; GALACTOSEMIA; GYNECOMASTIA; HYPOTHYROIDISM; JAUNDICE; MECONIUM; MENTAL RETARDATION; PHENYLKETONURIA; *and* SUDDEN INFANT DEATH SYNDROME.

Nickel

Metal that can trigger allergic reactions and is a component in cancer-causing agents.

Nickel is a primary cause of allergic contact dermatitis. It is found in a variety of everyday objects, including coins, keys, jewelry, doorknobs, and tools. A spot test is now available so that people who are allergic may determine whether a substance contains nickel.

Occupational exposure to nickel and its compounds causes increased incidence of nasal, sinus, and lung cancers. Inhalation of nickel oxide fumes produces metal fume fever. Inhalation of nickel carbonyl may result in vertigo, nausea, headache, shortness of breath, and chest pain, and can cause fatality hours or days later. *See also* ALLERGY.

Niclosamide

Antihelmintic drug used to treat infections of parasitic cestodes.

Niclosamide belongs to the family of drugs called antihelmintics, used in the treatment of worm infections, including infectifish tapeworm, dwarf tapeworm, and beef tapeworm. Niclosamide is not effective against roundworms or pinworms. Taken orally, niclosamide kills tapeworms on contact. The worms are then passed with the stool. The medication is most effective when taken after a light meal. Some common side effects include abdominal or stomach pain, diarrhea, loss of appetite, nausea, or vomiting. Rare side effects include dizziness, drowsiness, rectal itching, skin rash, or an unpleasant taste in the mouth. It is important to take all of the medication prescribed to completely eliminate the infestation. *See also* ANTIHELMINTIC DRUGS; PINWORM INFESTATION; ROUNDWORMS; TAPEWORM INFESTATION; *and* WORM INFESTATION.

Nicotine

Clear, bitter liquid found in the leaves of the tobacco plant.

Nicotine is the primary active, addictive ingredient in cigarettes, cigars, and chewing tobacco. In large quantities, nicotine is extremely toxic and is thus used as an agricultural insecticide. Exposure to large quantities of nicotine can cause burning of the mouth, throat, and stomach, and may also cause convulsions, coma, and death.

Smoking. In small quantities, such as the amount inhaled in cigarette and cigar smoke, nicotine is a central nervous system stimulant, similar to amphetamines and cocaine. Nicotine causes elevated levels of dopamine in the body, a chemical that carries signals in the brain and is linked to arousal and excitement.

After inhaling from a cigarette, a smoker's heartbeat accelerates, blood vessels constrict, and a euphoric and relaxed state

Resources on Care of the Newborn
Apgar, Virginia and Joan Beck, *Is My Baby All Right?* (1972); Behrman, Richard E., *Nelson Textbook of Pediatrics* (1996); Gonik, Bernard and R. A. Bobrowski, *Medical Complications in Labor and Delivery* (1996); New, Maria, *Adrenal Disease in Childhood* (1984); American Academy of Pediatrics, Tel. (847) 228-5005, Online: www.aap.org; Fed. for Children with Special Needs, Tel. (800) 331-0688, Online: www.fcsn.org; Universe of Women's Health, Tel. (512) 418-2922, Online: www.obgyn.net; www.ny-cornell.org/obgyn/.

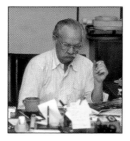

Some Cancer-Causing Chemicals in Tobacco Smoke

aminostilbene
arsenic
benz[a]anthracene
benz[a]pyrene
benzene
benzo[b]fluoranthene
benzo[c]phenanthrene
benzo[f]fluoranthene
cadmium
chrysene
dibenz[a c]anthracene
dibenzo[a e]fluoranthene
dibenz[a h]acridine
dibenz[a j]acridine
dibenzo[c g]carbazone
N-dibutylnitrosamine
2,3-dimethylchrysene
indeno[1,2,3-c d]pyrene
5-methylchrysene
5-methylfluoranthene
alpha-naphthylamine
nickel compounds
N-nitrosodimethylamine
N-nitrosomethylethylamine
polonium-210
N-nitrosodiethylamine
N-nitrosonornicotine
N-nitrosoanabasine
N-nitrosopiperidine

Tobacco Smoking.
Above, top, nicotine is the primary ingredient in cigarettes. It is a stimulant and is highly addictive, thus it is difficult to quit smoking. Above, bottom, a list of carcinogenic (cancer-causing) chemicals in tobacco smoke.

> ### ALERT
> #### Nicotine Poisoning
> Nicotine is extremely toxic for young children. Children may experience nicotine poisoning from ingesting cigarettes, loose tobacco, or nicotine gum, or from a nicotine patch that accidentally adheres to them. Symptoms of nicotine poisoning include dizziness, nausea, vomiting, and possible loss of consciousness. If a child exhibits symptoms of nicotine poisoning, remove the source of the nicotine and call a poison control center for instructions. Depending on the age of the child and the amount of nicotine ingested, symptoms of nicotine poisoning may pass fairly quickly; however, a doctor should still be consulted.

occurs. Nicotine also functions as an appetite suppressant, which helps explain why many people gain weight after they have quit smoking.

Nicotine is highly addictive, and withdrawal results in physical symptoms, which include rapid breathing, decreased blood pressure, sweating, and lowered heart rate. Other symptoms of withdrawal include anxiety, depression, insomnia, headaches, increased appetite, and weight gain.

Nicotine Replacement Therapy. Since quitting smoking is extremely difficult, both physically and psychologically, methods of nicotine replacement therapy have been developed. They include nicotine-containing chewing gums, skin patches, and nasal sprays, which help smokers gradually taper off levels of nicotine over a period of months. A smoker interested in quitting may wish to consult a physician about using nicotine replacement therapy. Some former smokers have had success with alternative methods of quitting, such as acupuncture and hypnosis.

Long-Term Health Effects. Tobacco smoking is associated with increased incidence of cancers of the mouth, respiratory tract, lung, and bladder, and with heart disease. Secondhand smoke is also a health concern. Secondhand smoke increases health risks for individuals, particularly children, who spend extended periods of time in smoky environments. *See also* CANCER *and* CARCINOGEN.

Niemann-Pick Disease

Rare, inherited metabolic disorder that affects newborn babies.

Niemann-Pick disease is the result of a deficiency of an enzyme called sphingomyelinase, which metabolizes a fatty substance known as sphingomyelin. The condition can be subdivided into Type A, Type B, Type C, and Type D.

Types. Both Types A and B result from an accumulation of sphingomyelin in the body, primarily in the liver, spleen, and lymph nodes. Approximately two-thirds of all infants with Niemann-Pick Type A disease are of Ashkenazi Jewish descent. Type B of the disease is a milder disorder with no brain involvement. Affected individuals usually come for medical attention during childhood due to distention of the liver and spleen. Type C results from an inability to metabolize cholesterol, which then accumulates in the body. Type D is an extremely rare variant of Type C and is only found in Nova Scotia, Canada.

Symptoms. As early as six months of age, babies affected with Niemann-Pick disease experience feeding complications, chronic vomiting, and enlargement of the spleen and liver, which causes the abdomen to appear distended. Some babies have a distinctive "cherry-red spot" in the retina of the eye. Also symptomatic of the disease are vertical eye movement difficulties, loss of muscle tone, slurred speech, and seizures, though these symptoms do not appear in patients with Type B of the disease.

Treatment. In recent years, bone marrow transplantation, enzyme replacement therapy, and gene therapy have proven successful in the treatment of Niemann-Pick Type B disease. There is currently no available treatment for Types A, C, and D.

Prognosis. Patients with Niemann-Pick Type A disease rarely live past three years of age. Niemann-Pick Type B sufferers may survive into late childhood or adulthood, and Type C and D sufferers generally live until their mid-teens. *See also* CONGENITAL *and* METABOLISM, INBORN ERRORS OF.

Night Blindness

Inability to see well in low-light situations

Individuals with night blindness cannot see well in dim light or at night. Most sufferers of the condition display no symptoms of eye disease, although some patients may have an inherited retinal defect. Vitamin A deficiency sometimes causes night blindness, as does the degenerative retinal condition retinitis pigmentosa and the acne drug Accutaine. *See* RETINITIS PIGMENTOSA.

Nightmare

Unpleasant dream that produces feelings of fear and is often clearly remembered upon awakening.

Nightmares occur in rapid eye movement (REM) sleep, during the middle and later parts of the sleep cycle. If the affected individual wakes up completely, the nightmare is generally remembered in its entirety.

Nightmares are very common, especially among children aged eight to ten. In children, nightmares can often be influenced by real-life events, such as watching a scary movie or television show, or when the child is anxious about being separated from parents. Painful or traumatic experiences, such as the death of a loved one or an injury due to accident, can also caused recurring nightmares.

In adults, the association between daytime events and nightmares is less specific. Most adults tend not to remember the content of nightmares upon awakening, or only remember small parts of these dreams. Nightmares in adults can result from excessive alcohol consumption. Eating before bed may also increase the incidence of nightmares in both children and adults, as it raises the body's metabolism.

Occasional nightmares are common and do not require treatment. Recurrent nightmares may be the result of anxiety or stress, and may be eased by a regular fitness program and stress-reducing techniques, such as relaxation therapy. *See also* SLEEP.

Night Terror

Sleep disorder, occurring mainly in children, in which an individual awakens suddenly in an agitated, almost terrified, state.

Night terrors generally occur in children between the ages of four and seven, disappearing gradually in adolescence. The arousal occurs between half an hour and three and a half hours after falling asleep (during the NREM, or non-rapid eye movement sleep). The sufferer may awaken screaming, not recognizing familiar faces or surroundings, and be incapable of being calmed. The sufferer usually has no memory of the incident the next morning. After some minutes of anxiety, the sufferer becomes calm and falls back to sleep.

Though distressing to parents, night terrors are not uncommon and generally disappear without any further intervention. For children who suffer from night terrors, care should be taken that late night snacking is eliminated and that the sleep environment is quiet and restful. Night terrors in adults may be an indication of a more serious anxiety disorder requiring professional attention. *See* ANXIETY DISORDERS.

NIH

National Institutes of Health.

Located in Bethesda, Maryland, the National Institutes of Health, part of the Department of Health and Human Services, include a research hospital, a computerized medical library, and 11 of the world's largest and most well-financed research centers. Created in 1887 as a one-room Laboratory of Hygiene, today the NIH dedicates an entire institute to the study of cancer; other institutes cover broader areas, such as the National Institute of Allergy and Infectious Diseases and the National Heart, Lung, and Blood Institute. As the predominant center of medical and dental research in the U.S., the NIH also funds research programs at universities, hospitals, and non-governmental organizations.

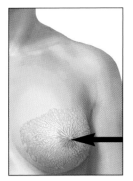

Breast Anatomy.
Above, the female breast is composed of fatty and connective tissue. The areola (the circular area around the nipple) is often a different color than the rest of the breast.

Nipple

Small prominence in the center of each breast.

Women's nipples contain small ducts through which milk can pass. The nipple and surrounding areola are both darker than the surrounding skin.

Disorders of the nipple include inversion, cracking, swelling, and discharge. Inversion may be caused by breast cancer. Cracking is generally the result of dry skin and is common during breast-feeding. Swelling may be the result of papilloma, a benign swelling. Discharge from the nipple can occur for many reasons. A discharge of milk from the breast of a woman who is not breast-feeding may be caused by a hormonal imbalance or a cyst. A bloody discharge may be a sign of breast cancer or breast abnormalities, and a discharge of pus is a sign of an abscess. *See also* ABSCESS; BREAST CANCER; *and* CYST.

Nitrites

Nitrogen compounds used as a preservative in meats and linked to cancer.

Nitrites are used in cured and processed meats as preservatives, in blood pressure and heart medications, and in fertilizers. When they are metabolized in the body, carcinogenic (cancer-causing) compounds known as nitrosamines are formed.

Nitrites are banned from many processed meats, while permissible levels have been lowered in others. Ascorbic acid (vitamin C) inhibits formation of nitrosamines, and thus it has been proposed that it be added to foods such as bacon that contain nitrites.

Acute exposure to nitrites causes vomiting, flushing, headache, dizziness, low blood pressure, blue skin, difficulty breathing, convulsions, and coma. Workers who handle nitroglycerin typically build a tolerance and stop experiencing its effects. However, abruptly ending exposure can cause heart attacks. *See also* HEART ATTACK.

Nitrogen

Element that makes up 80 percent of the air.

Nitrogen is a major component of air and is used in compressed air to dilute oxygen. It is colorless, odorless, and nontoxic, although it can act as an asphyxiant if it replaces oxygen in inhaled air.

Nitrogen bubbles in the bloodstream can cause the bends, a decompression sickness that affects people who work with compressed air, including scuba divers and miners. This can encompass a range of symptoms, including vertigo, itching, breathing difficulties, joint and muscle pain, paralysis, blindness, shock, and death. *See also* AIR *and* BENDS.

Nocardiosis

Bacterial infection that starts in the lungs but may spread to other organs.

Nocardia asteroides are bacteria that live in decaying matter in the soil. They are breathed or ingested by humans in soil dust and usually lodge in the lungs where they cause nocardiosis. People with compromised immunity are at maximum risk for contracting this disease. It spreads from the lungs to the brain and kidneys and may produce abscesses in these organs and underneath the skin. Initial symptoms of nocardiosis are similar to those of pneumonia and include a fever, chills, a cough, and shortness of breath. Only about half of all nocardiosis cases respond to treatment with antibiotics. *See also* ABSCESS; BACTERIA; *and* PNEUMONIA.

Nocturia

Also known as nycturia

Frequent need to urinate at night.

An average healthy person can sleep seven hours per night without needing to urinate. Older individuals suffer from frequent bathroom trips during the nighttime hours and urinate more than younger adults. It is common for urine to decrease in quantity and become increasingly concentrated at night. Nocturia is differentiated from involuntary urination at night (nocturnal enuresis).

Causes. Nocturia is common in the elderly because the kidneys are less able to consolidate the urine. The most common cause of nocturia is too much fluid intake before bedtime. Other causes include the consumption of coffee, caffeinated beverages, or alcohol before bedtime; diabetes mellitus; chronic or recurrent urinary tract infections; congestive heart failure; cystitis; drugs such as diuretics, lithium, and methoxyflurane; and excessive vitamin D.

Treatment. Medical attention is required if there is bed-wetting along with nocturia. The physician will ask the patient if he or she is in a period of added stress and perform diagnostic tests, such as a blood urea nitrogen test, urinalysis, and a urine concentration test. Most often, patients suffering from nocturia are advised to restrict their fluid intake after 7 P.M. and to reduce or eliminate their consumption of coffee and other caffinated beverages. If frequent urination is a result of medications, it might be advisable to take the medicine earlier in the day. *See also* AGING; URINALYSIS; URINARY TRACT INFECTION; URINATION, EXCESSIVE; URINATION, FREQUENT; *and* VITAMIN D.

Nocturnal Emission

Also known as a "wet dream"
Ejaculation that occurs during sleep, usually in conjunction with an erotic dream.

Though more common in boys undergoing the physical changes of puberty, a nocturnal emission may be experienced by males of any age. The individual may awaken just before or just after ejaculation, or may not discover the ejaculation until morning. In adult males with limited sexual activity, nocturnal emissions may result from an accumulation of semen. Nocturnal emissions are normal and are not cause for concern or medical attention. *See also* PUBERTY *and* REPRODUCTIVE SYSTEM, MALE.

Noise

Group of sound waves that is not periodic and is produced by irregular vibrations.

Noise is a sound that is not of a single frequency, but of many non-harmonic frequency components at randomly varying amplitudes. It is a disturbing signal that interferes with ordinary hearing.

Hearing can be damaged by loud noise, such as a jack hammer at a construction site or a jet engine. All workers are recommended to follow the Occupation of Safety and Health Administration (OSHA) guidelines and always wear protective earplugs in a noisy area. The hearing capability can be damaged by noise levels ranging above 90 decibels. A jet engine produces noise above 130 decibels. Loud music is usually at least in the range of 95 decibels. Ordinary conversation is about 60 decibels. The louder the noise, the less time is required to cause hearing loss. *See also* EAR; EAR, DISORDERS OF: ENVIRONMENTAL MEDICINE; HEARING LOSS; PUBLIC HEALTH; *and* TINNITUS.

Noninvasive

Medical technique or procedure that does not require incision or the introduction of a foreign object into the body.

Noninvasive techniques allow the physician to make critical diagnoses without inserting any instruments into the body. Techniques that require intravenous injection of contrast dye do involve a needle, but are still considered noninvasive.

Noninvasive diagnostic procedures eliminate the risk of infection because of surgery, require minimal preparation, are painless, and avoid the recovery period that follows invasive surgery. The most familiar noninvasive technique is x-ray. Other noninvasive techniques include computerized axial tomography (CAT or CT), MRI, and ultrasound. MRI and Ultrasound are safer than x-ray because potentially harmful radiation is not used. *See also* CAT SCAN; MRI; *and* ULTRASOUND.

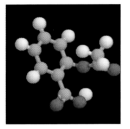

Aspirin Model.
Nonsteroidal anti-inflammatory drugs (NSAIDs) are medications taken for pain relief. Above, aspirin is one of the most popular NSAIDs.

Nonspecific Urethritis

Inflammation of the urethra (the tubular conduit that empties urine from the bladder) caused by an unknown pathogen (disease-causing agent) or trauma (injury).

Urethritis is usually caused by a chlamydial or gonococcal infection; however, it can also be caused by a virus such as *Herpes simplex*, injury to the urethra, surgery, and some chemicals.

Symptoms of urethritis are pain or burning during urination, an urgent need to urinate, blood in the urine, lower abdominal pain, and a yellowish discharge from the urethra. In men over 50, there may be incontinence. If urethritis is left untreated, there may be a narrowing of the urethra and the formation of an abscess around the duct.

Women are often asymptomatic (without symptoms) and therefore can unknowingly transmit bacteria, causing urethritis in sexual partners. In women the bacteria that can cause urethritis are more likely to infect the vagina, cervix, uterus, or ovaries than the urethra. If infected, the woman may experience pain during urination as the acidic urine passes over inflamed labia. She may also experience pain during sexual intercourse.

Treatment for urethritis is the same for both men and women. Antibiotics will be prescribed for a bacterial infection. If the cause is *Herpes simplex*, it may be treated with acyclovir. While undergoing treatment, the patient is advised to avoid alcohol and caffeine. *See also* CHLAMYDIA; GONORRHEA; SEXUALLY TRANSMITTED DISEASES; *and* URETHRA.

Nonsteroidal Anti-Inflammatory Drugs

Drugs used to control inflammation.

Inflammation is the body's response to injury of tissues or ligaments. In cases of mild to moderate pain resulting from inflammation, whether acute or chronic, nonsteroidal anti-inflammatory drugs (NSAIDs) may be used. Many different NSAIDs are available over the counter, and are much safer than steroid anti-inflammatories.

Function. NSAIDs work by reducing the production of the hormone prostaglandin, which is responsible for triggering blood vessels expansion and temperature elevation in response to infection or injury.

Types. Aspirin is perhaps the most well-known pain reliever and anti-inflammatory medication. Unlike other NSAIDs, its anti-inflammatory properties are relatively minimal. It is also used to reduce fever and prevent recurrence of heart attack or stroke. Aspirin can cause gastrointestinal ulcers and even bleeding, thus coated aspirins, which prevent the aspirin from dissolving until it is past the stomach, were developed. Aspirin reduces the ability of the blood to clot, making it somewhat dangerous for people with poor clotting ability. Aspirin is not recommended for people with asthma, since it can cause breathing difficulty. Children with influenza or chicken pox should not take aspirin because of the danger of Reye's syndrome.

Ibuprofen is a strong anti-inflammatory, but it may irritate the stomach and can cause indigestion, diarrhea, drowsiness, dizziness, and nausea.

Drug Interactions. Anti-inflammatories should not be taken with anticoagulant drugs, such as warfarin or heparin, except under medical advice. In addition, combining NSAIDs with alcohol increases the risk of stomach irritation. NSAIDs should also be avoided if a person is taking diuretics, diabetes medications, insulin, or steroids.

Any anti-inflammatory should not be used continuously for more than ten days to reduce pain or three days to reduce fever. People over 65 should only take ibuprofen every twelve hours.

For background reading on nonsteroidal antiinflammatory drugs, *see* PAIN RELIEF. *Further information can be found in* ASPIRIN; ASTHMA; DIARRHEA; FEVER; GASTROINTESTINAL BLEEDING; INDIGESTION; INFLAMMATION; NAUSEA; *and* REYE'S SYNDROME.

Norepinephrine

Hormone that aids in the body's response to stress.

Norepinephrine is primarily secreted by the adrenal medulla in the center of the adrenal glands. Along with epinephrine, it is released by the body during times of stress or anxiety. The release of these hormones is controlled by the sympathetic nervous system, which is one part of the autonomic nervous system. Norepinephrine and epinephrine help the body in preparing to either fight or flee; they speed up the heart and widen airways and blood vessels, causing a rise in blood pressure. The main function of norepinephrine is to prevent blood pressure from dropping, which is why it may be administered for shock or severe bleeding. *See also* ADRENAL GLANDS; FIGHT OR FLIGHT RESPONSE; *and* SYMPATHETIC NERVOUS SYSTEM.

Nosebleed

Also known as epistaxis

Bleeding from inside the nose.

Nosebleeds can occur frequently and without apparent injury. They are usually not an indication of a serious problem, but in rare cases may indicate that there is an urgent disorder.

Causes. Nosebleeds are more likely to occur in the dry winter months when the humidity is low and when mucous membranes are dry and brittle, cracked or split. Persistent nosebleeds may result from poor blood clotting or a blood disease such as hemophilia.

Nosebleeds frequently result from minor trauma, such as a blow or when a child puts a finger or an object in his or her nose and breaks the fragile blood vessels. Such nosebleeds generally occur in the forward part of the nasal passages and can be treated at home. Nosebleeds originating deeper in the nasal passages can bleed "backwards" down the throat. They are, as a consequence, more serious.

Treating Nosebleeds at Home

A person with a nosebleed should remain calm and sit with his or her head tilted forward slightly (to prevent the blood from draining back into the throat), breathing from the mouth. If there is nothing caught in the nostrils, they should be held shut, and a cold compress should be applied for five or ten minutes. If there is something caught in the nostril, the clear nostril should be pinched shut, and the person should breathe in through his or her mouth and blow out gently through the nose. Once the obstructing object has been removed, pressure and a cold compress should be applied to the area. If the bleeding continues for more than half an hour, medical attention should be sought.

When a person is taking a blood thinning medication, such as coumadin or heparin, or regular doses of aspirin, the blood may not clot properly. To stop a nosebleed, a doctor may apply a blood clotting agent to the bleeding area or apply cauterization. Packing the bleeding nostril with gauze or sponge will generally control the bleeding, but should only be done by trained medical personnel. *See also* ANTICOAGULANT DRUGS; ASPIRIN; *and* HEMOPHILIA.

Nose, Broken

A fracture of the nasal bone.

From the forehead, the nasal bones connect to the skull (cranium), and extend down to form the bridge of the nose, which is very difficult to fracture. The rest of the bridge is cartilage. When hit with a sharp blow from the side, the bones and cartilage may be displaced, while blows to the front of the nose will knock the bones outward, flattening the nasal structure.

Diagnosis and Treatment. Broken noses are common injuries, and are often not taken seriously. There usually is a great deal of swelling around the nose, and sometimes only x-rays can reveal the fracture. If a nose fracture is suspected, ice applied immediately will help to reduce the swelling and thus make diagnosis and treatment easier. If there appears to be a deformity or excessive bleeding, a doctor should be

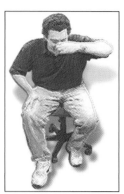

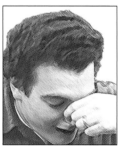

Nosebleed.
To treat a nosebleed, sit down and lean forward slightly (*above, top*). Pinch the nostrils closed and breathe through the mouth (*above, bottom*) until the bleeding has stopped.

called, as the nose may need to be reset. The manipulation and realignment may be conducted with only local anesthetic, except for in extreme cases, when general anesthetic may be necessary.

Prognosis. Most nose fractures heal without complication, but those that aren't treated properly may need to be surgically rebroken and reset in order to correct the problem. If the nose does not heal in proper alignment, it may eventually cause breathing problems or a susceptability to sinus infections. *See also* FRACTURE.

Nuclear Medicine

Area of medicine concerned with the use of radio-pharmaceuticals (known as radionuclides) for the diagnosis and treatment of disease.

Nuclear medicine generally involves the injection of a radiopharmaceutical, a sterile, pharmaceutically pure radioactively labeled compound that migrates through the blood to the site of disease either for treatment or, more commonly, in order to image abnormal regions for diagnosis. Radioactive tracers accumulate in regions of abnormal bone, blood, or tissue and are revealed through sensitive scanning using a device known as a gamma camera.

The radiopharmaceutical, following injection into a vein, is quickly distributed throughout the body. Various types of scanning are used depending on the area of study. Ailments of the heart may be diagnosed with radionuclide scanning, which can reveal narrowing of the coronary artery and help evaluate the heart's blood supply. Further, nuclear medicine may be used to assess recovery following heart attack (myocardial infarction) or to gauge improvement of blood supply after bypass surgery.

Radionuclide studies of bone are used to identify areas of inflammation, infection, hairline fractures, and bone cancer. Nuclear medicine has also proven useful in the diagnosis of respiratory disease, revealing the flow of blood and air through the lungs, as well as diseases and disorders of the liver and gallbladder.

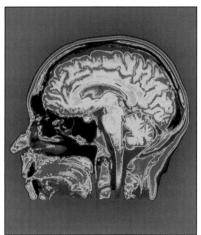

MRI of the Head.
MRIs are sometimes used in addition to radionuclide studies to image the brain and diagnose brain disorders. Above, an MRI of the head.

Background material on nuclear medicine can be found in DIAGNOSIS. *For further reading, see* BIOPSY; BONE CANCER; BYPASS OPERATIONS; CAT SCAN; CORONARY ARTERY BYPASS; HEART ATTACK; HEART IMAGING; HEART SURGERY; PET SCAN; RADIONUCLIDE SANNING; *and* X-RAY.

Numbness

Lack of sensation in part of the body due to interference with the transmission of nerve impulses along the sensory serves.

Numbness is manifested as either a loss of sensation or feeling, or a burning or tingling sensation in the body. Tingling is an indication of impairment or blockage of the nerves in the area. Unlike numbness, tingling suggests the nerve is not completely dead or severed, but rather just injured or temporarily blocked due to pressure. Numbness can also occur harmlessly, such as when a person's foot "falls asleep" because it was in a position that temporarily restricted blood flow.

Causes. The main causes for numbness are local injury to the nerves under the skin because of:
- lack of blood supply to the area;
- pressure on the nerves, caused by a herniated disk, tumor, or abscess;
- diabetes or other chemical abnormalities;
- vitamin B_{12} deficiency;
- hypothyroidism;
- carpal tunnel syndrome;
- stroke;
- multiple sclerosis because of damage to the nerve pathways in the central nervous system;
- long term radiation or chemotherapy drugs.

Treatment. A physician can determine the area of sensory impairment and the extent of nerve damage. The treatment corresponds to the extent and site of damage. *See also* NERVE INJURY.

Nurse

An individual trained in nursing.

Registered nurses (RNs) are trained and licensed by individual states in the care of sick individuals and the promotion of health. Not all nurses are licensed RNs, but all RNs are nurses. RNs may work in many places, including nursing homes, hospitals, clinics, doctors' offices, and the homes of patients. Certain RNs concentrate on a specific area of medical care, such as surgery or pediatrics.

Types. There are also many specific types of nurse, including nurse-midwives, nurse practitioners, licensed practical nurses (LPNs), and nurses' aides. Nurse-midwives and nurse practitioners are RNs, while LPNs and nurses' aides are not. Nurse-midwives are specially trained in prenatal care and in childbirth. Nurse practitioners provide health care, such as counseling or physical examinations, under the guidance of a doctor. LPNs provide initial patient care under the management of RNs and physicians, while nurses' aides provide support to nurses working in nursing homes, hospitals, and clinics.

Nurse, Home Care

Individual trained in nursing care who works with patients in their homes.

A home care nurse has a professional degree in nursing. Home care nurses work with patients in their homes in association with physicians and with others who are involved in the patients' care. Some home care nurses live with their patients, and some spend the majority of their time with their patients but live elsewhere.

Types. Home care nursing can be appropriate for patients of any age and any level of disability. Acute home care is temporary and is given to patients who need time to recover from an operation or a serious disease. Long-term home care is suitable for patients who suffer from a chronic condition, such as Alzheimer's or Parkinson's disease, and who will need nursing care for the rest of their lives. The majority of patients needing long-term home care are elderly. In both of these cases, a home care nurse is employed to provide nursing care for the patient.

Function. In addition to providing nursing care for their patients, home care nurses work as case managers to monitor and assess each patient's condition and progress. They work closely with patients and families to explain the disease or disability and its symptoms, and to create a treatment and care program.

Services. Home care nurses provide many services to patients and their families. Not all of these services are required by every patient. These services may include physical evaluations, neurological assessments, nutritional counseling, diabetic education and care, blood drawing, cancer care and chemotherapy, and pain management. Home care nurses may also administer injections and medications to patients when required.

Financial Considerations. Home care nursing involves considerable expenses, including the nursing care itself, as well as the various tests and medications required by the patient. For this reason, it is important to check with the patient's insurance company to see what is covered before employing a home care nurse. Acute home care may be covered by Medicare if it is only for a limited amount of time. Medicare will also cover certain types of skilled home nursing care. Financial assistance for home nursing care can also be procured from the Veteran's Administration, Champus (a program that provides insurance coverage for families of deceased veterans), and local Area Agencies on Aging.

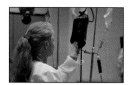
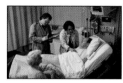

Nursing. Nursing care can either be given in the hospital or at home (by a home care nurse). Above, top, a nurse adjusts a hospital patient's IV drip. Above, bottom, a home care nurse at the bedside of her patient.

For background reading on home care nurse, see AGING; ELDERLY, CARE OF THE; *and* NURSE. *Further information can be found in* DEGENERATIVE DISORDERS; HOSPITALS, TYPES OF; PARALYSIS; *and* SENILITY. *See also* ACCIDENTS *and* INJURY *for causes of disorders for which a home care nurse would be appropriate.*

Nutrition

> The study of food, particularly what and how much people need to eat in order to stay healthy, and the science of how the body metabolizes food.

Proper nutrition involves a diet that includes a balance of macronutrients (carbohydrates, proteins, and fats), and micronutrients (essential vitamins and minerals). Emphasis should be placed on variety, drawing from all the basic food groups and from different categories within each group every day.

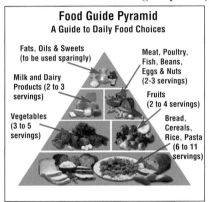

Food Guide Pyramid
A Guide to Daily Food Choices

Fats, Oils & Sweets (to be used sparingly)

Milk and Dairy Products (2 to 3 servings)

Vegetables (3 to 5 servings)

Meat, Poultry, Fish, Beans, Eggs & Nuts (2-3 servings)

Fruits (2 to 4 servings)

Bread, Cereals, Rice, Pasta (6 to 11 servings)

Food Pyramid.
Above, the Food Guide Pyramid illustrates the proportions of foods that should be consumed for a nutritious, balanced diet.

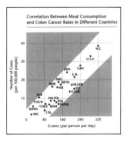

Correlation Between Meat Consumption and Colon Cancer Rates in Different Countries

Diets of Countries.
The graph above clearly demonstrates that there is a direct link between increased meat consumption and an increase in the incidence of colon cancer.

CARBOHYDRATES

Dieticians' guidelines suggest that adults should consume between six and eleven servings daily from the bread, cereal, rice, and pasta group. This food group provides carbohydrates, protein, dietary fiber, B vitamins, and minerals. Good sources include whole grains, legumes, lentils, and whole grain cereals. It is important to read ingredient labels for processed foods; added sugar, salt, and fats may be lurking, particularly in packaged cereals. *See also* CARBOHYDRATES.

FRUITS AND VEGETABLES

Foods from the fruit and vegetable group are generally low in fat and salt and contain ample amounts of vitamins, minerals, and dietary fiber. Adults should consume two to four servings of fruit daily, preferably fresh rather than canned or juiced. Vegetables should make up roughly three to five daily servings and are best when fresh or fresh-frozen. Overcooking vegetables can destroy nutrients—lightly steaming vegetables is an excellent way to preserve essential vitamins and minerals while retaining flavor. *See also* VEGETARIANISM.

PROTEINS

Adults should consume two to three servings daily of foods from the meat, poultry, dry beans, eggs, and nuts group. These foods are an excellent source of protein, iron, and B vitamins. Beans, skinless poultry, lean red meat, and baked, broiled or grilled fish are excellent low-fat selections from the protein group. *See also* PROTEINS.

DAIRY

The milk, yogurt, and cheese group (also known as the dairy group) should make up two to three servings per day. Foods in this category are sources of protein, calcium, and other minerals and vitamins. However, dairy products can be a source of saturated fats. To reduce saturated fat intake, try to consume skim milk and low-fat dairy products. *See also* CALCIUM.

WATER

Water makes up approximately 60 percent of our bodies and is essential to life. Adults should drink eight 8-ounce glasses of water each day, and very active people should drink even more. Coffee, tea, and caffeinated sodas do not count toward that total, as caffeine is a diuretic and causes the loss of water from the body. *See also* WATER.

DIETARY SUPPLEMENTS

Dietary supplements should not serve as a substitute for nutrients obtained from a variety of foods in the diet, although they may be beneficial as an addition to a balanced diet. In particular, women of all ages may wish to take calcium supplements to prevent osteoporosis. Whole foods may provide not just recognized vitamins and minerals, but also nutritional phytochemicals and elements that have not yet been identified. *See also* VITAMIN SUPPLEMENTS.

Fats and Oils

Some fats and oils are essential to the diet, but they should be eaten in limited quantities. Many high fat foods and junk foods like sweets, alcohol, soft drinks, and salty snacks (such as potato chips) provide "empty calories"—calories that are not accompanied by necessary vitamins and minerals. These foods should be eaten sparingly and not as a substitue for minimum serving requirements from the five basic food groups.

Nutrition and Diet, Alternative Therapies

Using food to promote health and to prevent or treat disease.

Both mainstream and alternative medicine hold that a balanced, healthy diet is essential for overall health and well-being. A balanced diet that is high in fruits, vegetables, and fiber and is low in fats, oils, and sugar is connected to a reduced risk of diseases such as heart disease and cancer. Also, this type of diet generally enhances a person's ability to fight infection and disease.

Diet plays an important role in many alternative therapies. As in mainstream medicine, diet is seen as a basis for good health and a complement to other treatments. Diet may also be used as a means of treatment itself. Specific types of diets, the use of supplements, and fasting may be used to prevent or treat specific diseases or undiagnosed ailments. Foods or specific components of food that allegedly provide medicinal or health benefits are referred to as nutraceuticals.

TYPES OF ALTERNATIVE DIETS

While there are many alternative diets, the two most common are vegetarian and macrobiotic. A vegetarian diet excludes most or all meat products. A macrobiotic diet also excludes most meat products. It is developed from Eastern philosophies and aims to balance a person's needs, environment, and choice of foods.

VEGETARIANISM. There are several types of vegetarian diets, including lacto-ovo-vegetarian, in which a person consumes milk products and eggs as well as plant-based foods, and veganism, in which a person avoids all animal products. A vegetarian diet may be pursued for any number of reasons, ranging from ethics to health.

Benefits. For the most part, a vegetarian diet is equally well-balanced and often better balanced than a diet that includes meat. Vegetables, grains, and legumes, which tend to form the basis of a healthy vegetarian diet, are naturally low in fat and high in fiber. Evidence suggests that vegetarians tend to be less obese and are less likely to develop heart disease, high blood pressure, type 2 diabetes, and alcoholism.

Precautions. For children and women who are pregnant or nursing, a vegetarian diet can be maintained, but special care should be taken to ensure that the diet provides enough protein and nutrients.

Vegans are at risk for developing a deficiency of vitamin B_{12}, which can be found only in animal sources. Thus, people who follow a vegan diet should take a vitamin B_{12} supplement.

MACROBIOTICS is a combination of diet and lifestyle that integrates awareness of the whole person, responsiveness to the environment, and ancient Chinese philosophies. A macrobiotic diet varies from person to person, but its basic emphasis is on eating locally grown, seasonal, organic foods in certain proportions.

In general, the balance of foods consumed in a macrobiotic diet consists of about 50 to 60 percent whole grains, 25 to 30 percent fresh vegetables, especially greens, five to ten percent legumes and seaweeds, and five to ten percent soy- and vegetable-based soups.

Benefits. Like a vegetarian diet, a macrobiotic diet is high in fiber and low in fat, a combination associated with decreased risk of heart disease and cancer. Proponents of the diet believe that it also can be used as a treatment for cancer and other diseases. While this is supported by anecdotal evidence, no clinical studies have proven that macrobiotics can cure cancer. Some studies have supported that the diet can help prevent cancer and heart disease.

Precautions. The main danger of a strict macrobiotic diet is that it may not provide enough essential vitamins and nutrients. Children and pregnant women are particularly at risk; some studies have found that children raised on a macrobiotic diet have slowed growth and development.

SUPPLEMENTS. Supplements of vitamins and minerals are given to treat vitamin deficiencies, and often children and adults take multivitamin supplements as an addition to a balanced diet. Some vitamins, minerals, and other supplements are also used therapeutically.

General Use. Proponents of nutritional supplements believe that many people suffer from mild to moderate nutritional deficiencies, which have less clear-cut symptoms than easily recognizable severe deficiencies, such as fatigue, anxiety, mood swings, lack of concentration, and insomnia. Identification of the insufficient nutrients and treatment with supplements is intended to alleviate symptoms and improve overall health.

Precautions. While many nutritional supplements are quite safe and may be beneficial, some vitamins and minerals are toxic at high doses. Also, the use of nutritional supplements as a replacement for conventional medical treatment can cause an illness to go undiagnosed and untreated. Thus, it is a good idea to consult a physician about taking nutritional supplements, especially if they are being taken in response to ill health.

ANTIOXIDANTS. Through the process of metabolism, the body produces electrically charged particles known as free radicals. These particles can cause damage to the cells, and such damage on a cellular or genetic level may be one of the factors that triggers cancer.

Antioxidants are substances that fight the effects of free radicals. They also improve detoxification enzyme levels and support the immune system. They are found in vegetables such as broccoli, carrots, and tomatoes. The vitamins A (in the form of beta carotene), C, and E, as well as the minerals magnesium and zinc, are a source of antioxidants, as are flavonoids. Studies have linked high doses of vitamin E to a decreased risk of coronary artery disease and stroke, and high doses of other antioxidants with decreased risk of cancer.

FASTING AND DETOXIFICATION. Some alternative therapies attempt to treat ailments by removing foods from the diet in an attempt to detoxify the body. The underlying theory is that people are exposed to a number of toxic substances in the course of modern living, and periodic fasting or alteration of the diet can help the body eliminate these toxins, promote overall health, and prevent various ailments.

Often, detoxification consists of a series of several two to three day fasts, during which only water or only fresh vegetable juices are consumed. In other cases, a diet of fresh, organic, unprocessed foods may be followed for a period of several weeks to several months. During and following detoxification, a person should avoid processed foods, refined sugars, alcohol, and caffeine.

Precautions. The benefits of detoxification are not clinically proven. Infrequent fasts of a couple of days are generally safe for people in good health, but prolonged or repeated fasting may lead to a nutrient deficiency and thus cause illness.

> *Background material on nutrition and diet, alternative therapies can be found in* ALTERNATIVE MEDICINE; DIET AND DISEASE; *and* NUTRITION. *For related information, see* CARBOHYDRATES; DIETARY FIBER; PROTEINS; *and* VEGETARIANISM. *See also* AIDS; CANCER; *and* HEART DISORDERS.

Nutritional Disorders

Health problems caused by a lack or surplus of one or more nutrients or by toxins in the diet.

There are three classes of nutritional disorders: those caused by a deficiency of nutrients; those caused by an excess of nutrients; and those caused by poisonous components of certain elements in food.

Nutritional Deficiency. Nutritional deficiency is characterized by a lack of nutrients in the body because of an inadequate intake of nutrients, disorders inhibiting the body's absorption of nutrients, loss of nutrients because of diarrhea or kidney failure, drug addition, or infection. Nutritional deficiency develops in stages, worsening over time. It is only after the body cells have undergone significant change that symptoms begin to appear.

People at increased risk for nutritional deficiency include infants and children,

Resources on Nutrition
Feek, C.M., and C.R. Edwards, *Endocrine and Metabolic Diseases* (1988); Groff, James L. and Sareen S. Gropper, *Advanced Nutrition and Human Metabolism* (1999); Heimburger, Douglas C. and R. L. Weinsier, *Handbook of Clinical Nutrition* (1997); Shils, Maurice E., et al., *Modern Nutrition in Health and Disease* (1999); American Dietetic Association, Tel. (800) 366-1655, Online: www.eatright.org; Center for Nutrition Policy and Promotion, Tel. (202) 418-2312, Online: www.usda.gov/cnpp; Food and Drug Admin., Tel. (888) INFOFDA, Online: www.fda.gov; www.nycornell.org/medicine/nutrition/index.html.

pregnant and breast-feeding women, the elderly, vegetarians and vegans, individuals addicted to drugs or alcohol, persons on fad diets, and those with chronic problems with nutrient absorption.

Diagnosis. The diagnosis of nutritional deficiency is based on patient history, a physical examination, and laboratory tests (such as measurements of plasma protein and electrolyte levels in the blood). Results of all of these tests are then compared with normal results for patients of that age and gender. Once a diagnosis is made, the nutritional deficiency is treated with appropriate methods, based on the cause of the condition.

Nutritional Excess. Nutritional excess can be the result of overeating, inadequate exercise, or excess vitamin intake. Obesity is the most common result of an excess intake of nutrients.

Causes of, or influences on an individual's tendency toward obesity include socioeconomic status, a large intake of food (especially fat), and an inactive lifestyle. Additional causes of obesity can include pregnancy, brain damage (particularly affecting the hypothalamus, the portion of the brain responsible for appetite), medications (such as antidepressants and antipsychotics), psychological factors, and hormonal imbalances (especially an excess of cortisol or thyroid hormone).

The diagnosis of nutritional excess and obesity is generally made using the body mass index (BMI) which represents the individual's weight (in kilograms) divided by the square of the height (in meters). Persons with a BMI of between 25 and 30 are considered overweight, and a BMI of greater than 30 indicates obesity.

Nutritional excess and obesity can be treated with a change in diet and exercise. Diet and behavioral modification in clinical settings are the most common treatments, while surgical procedures, such as gastric bypass (which reduces the volume of the stomach by creating a small pouch), are increasing in popularity.

Poisonous Elements. Nutritional disorders may also result from toxic or poisonous elements in food. These elements may be natural in origin, such as those found in fungi, or they may be artificially produced, such as pesticides, pollutants, or fertilizers. Toxicity may also result from the excess intake of vitamins and minerals, such as those found in supplements that are sold in drug and health food stores. Excess intake of many vitamins, including vitamins A, B_6, C, D, E, folic acid, and niacin, can result in toxicity. In addition, all trace minerals are toxic at high levels, and some (such as arsenic, nickel, and chromium) can eventually cause cancer.

> *For background information on nutritional disorders, see* DIET AND DISEASE *and* NUTRITION. *Further reading can be found in* METABOLISM, DISORDERS OF *and* VITAMIN SUPPLEMENTS. *See also* BERIBERI; OSTEOPOROSIS; *and* SCURVY *for more on specific disorders resulting from lacks of specific vitamins or minerals.*

Nystagmus

Disorder causing involuntary movements of the eyes, most often horizontally.

The movement of the eyes in nystagmus can be vertical or rotary, but is most often horizontal. The eyes usually move together.

Types. Congenital nystagmus is present at birth and is the most common form of the condition. Patients with congenital nystagmus may often not notice the eye movements until they are pointed out by others.

Acquired nystagmus is less common and is generally caused by a disease or injury of the brain. Any brain disorder can cause nystagmus if it affects the area of the brain controlling eye movements. Alcohol intoxication can also cause nystagmus.

Diagnosis. Diagnosis of nystagmus can often be made visually, but tests may also be performed, including electrooculography (a method of measuring eye movements with small electrodes).

Treatment. Most cases of nystagmus are not treatable, except for those caused by intoxication. Neither congenital nor acquired nystagmus can be reversed. *See also* ALCOHOL INTOXICATION.

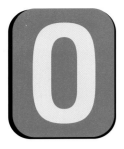

Obesity

An unhealthy excess of body fat.

Obesity is defined as a body weight more than 20 percent over what would be normal for a person's height. Approximately 25 percent of the population of the United States is considered obese, and that number is increasing, especially among children. Obesity increases the risk of heart disease, diabetes, certain types of cancer, arthritis, infertility, and sleep disorders.

Causes. Obesity occurs when the body takes in more food than it expends as energy. Oversized portions and the high fat and sugar content of snack, prepared, and fast foods have all contributed to unhealthy, high-calorie eating habits that cause weight gain and obesity. The sedentary lifestyle of industrialized cultures has also caused an increase in obesity cases. People sit all day at work, and travel by cars or trains rather than walking. Many are less active during their leisure time, watching television or playing video games rather than exercising or playing sports.

Inherited traits such as slow metabolism, fat distribution, or an inability to detect when a person has eaten enough may occasionally result in obesity. Diseases such as hyperthyroidism or Cushing's syndrome may also cause obesity. A doctor can diagnose these conditions and treat them with medication.

Treatment for obesity can simply be weight loss through reducing portion size and eating healthier, low-fat foods. Exercise is equally important; people who exercise are more likely to keep weight off. Losing weight slowly (at a rate that does not exceed two pounds per week) also increases the likelihood of sustaining weight loss. Fad diets that promise quick weight loss rarely maintain long-term success. Doctors, dieticians, or local health clubs can suggest appropriate weight loss programs.

The benefits of drug therapy for the treatment of obesity must be balanced against the risks of the various medications. Additionally, a number of surgical procedures can reduce the absorption of food from the gastrointestinal tract and can be of benefit to some patients with severe and disabling obesity.

> *Background reading material on obesity can be found in* DIET AND DISEASE; NUTRITION; *and* WEIGHT. *For further information, see* ARTERIOSCLEROSIS; ATHEROSCLEROSIS; CHOLESTEROL; HEART ATTACK; HEART DISEASE, ISCHEMIC; *and* HEART DISORDERS. *See also* WEIGHT REDUCTION *for more on various methods of weight loss.*

Obsessive-Compulsive Disorder

Also known as OCD

Uncontrollable, disturbing impulses and thoughts, and/or uncontrollable, repetitive, ritualized behaviors that overwhelm an individual's life.

A person suffering from obsessive-compulsive disorder usually experiences both obsessions and compulsions.

Obsessions are overwhelming and disturbing mental images that produce feelings of anxiety. The fears appear to be unconnected to what is actually occurring in a person's life and typically take the form of concerns about germs or cleanliness, disorganization, unacceptable and excessive sexual impulses, hostile thoughts, or a sense of foreboding and doubt. To be considered an obsession, these thoughts and feelings must interfere with the ability to perform the normal functions of life.

Compulsions are ritualized, repetitive behaviors that are undertaken in an attempt to relieve a feeling of anxiety. A person obsessed with a fear of germs may

---

Body Mass Index (BMI)

Obesity is determined by more than just weight. A person's body fat percentage is equally important. The body mass index (BMI) formula is one way to determine body fat. To find your BMI, multiply your weight in pounds by 703, then divide it twice by your height in inches.

Federal guidelines state that a person with a BMI of between 25 and 29.9 is overweight. A person with a BMI of over 30 is considered obese.

repeatedly wash the hands after touching anything that may be unclean. A person obsessed with doubt may check and recheck that the stove and the lights are off, the door is locked, and the faucets are turned off, to the extent that he or she is unable to leave the house.

Treatment. Several medications have been found to be effective in treating OCD, particularly the recently developed selective serotonin reuptake inhibitors (SSRIs), antidepressant drugs that include Paxil, Prozac, and Zoloft.

Behavior therapy may be effective as a treatment for OCD if it is used to expose the patient to the feared situation or object in a controlled situation, similarly to how phobias are treated. Insight psychotherapy can also be helpful. *See also* ANTIDEPRESSANT DRUGS; BEHAVIOR THERAPY; *and* PHOBIAS.

Occult Blood, Fecal

Blood in the stool that is not visible but can be detected by chemical analysis.

Bleeding in the intestines can be caused by a minor irritation, but can also be a symptom of serious disease, such as esophagitis, gastritis, stomach cancer, colon cancer, rectal cancer, and diverticular disease.

During a regular physical examination, the physician will collect a small amount of fecal material from the large intestine and test it for the presence of blood. Because the bleeding is not visible, it is called occult, and its significance can only be determined by additional tests to discover the source of the bleeding.

Follow-up tests for blood in the stool require the patient to collect a small sample from the stool at home over a period of three days. The samples are applied to a small circle of filter paper mounted on a card, which is then mailed back to the physician and tested for blood content. A test that reveals blood in the stool should be followed by a colonoscopy to determine the source of the bleeding. *See also* ANEMIA; ESOPHAGITIS; FECES, ABNORMAL; GASTRITIS; *and* RECTAL BLEEDING.

Occupational Medicine and Health

Area of medicine concerned with preventing and treating work related illnesses and diseases, and with encouraging good health in workers.

Occupational (work-related) illnesses and injuries are the concern of physicians who work in the area of occupational medicine and health. These physicians also try to promote the safety and general good health of workers.

History of Occupational Medicine. Although people have always encountered hazards at work, it is only within the last thousand years that occupational illness has been studied seriously. Occupational disease was first noticed in the middle ages in coal miners, who suffered from lung diseases as a result of breathing coal dust on the job. This realization led to attempts to ventilate the miners' work area to remove the dust. During the industrial revolution, occupational diseases and injuries became more prevalent due to an increase in pollution and poor working conditions. At that time, occupational medicine came into being and occupational physicians began to research the causes of work-related diseases and injuries.

In the past twenty years, occupational illnesses and injuries have dropped dramatically, in part due to the federal Occupational Safety and Health Administration (OSHA), which regulates workplace conditions. The strict controls placed on employers by the OSHA have led to increased employer concern for worker safety, resulting in cleaner workplaces, less lost time from employee illness or injury, and greater worker productivity. However, an average of 16 people still die each year in the United States from work-related causes.

Workplace Illnesses and Injuries. There are many types of work-related diseases and injuries. Due to the successful efforts of occupational physicians, some of these disorders are less common now than they were in the past. *See also* ENVIRONMENTAL MEDICINE *and* PUBLIC HEALTH.

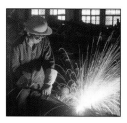

Protective Eyewear. Above, when working with hazardous or hot materials it is important to wear protective goggles to protect the eyes from injury.

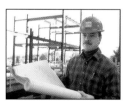

Occupational Medicine and Health. Depending on their job, people are subjected to different work hazards. People in jobs that require heavy labor, such as construction work (*above*) may be subjected to many hazards on the job. Such hazards may include excessive dust or noise, toxic chemicals, or repetitive strain injuries. On the other hand, employees in medical labs may be affected by infectious disease or radiation.

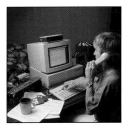

Repetitive Strain Injuries (RSIs). People who spend their workday at a computer screen may suffer repetitive strain injuries (RSIs), such as carpal tunnel syndrome. To alleviate the problem, it may be necessary to wear a wrist brace, however, this is not recommended except on the advice of a physician.

Dust diseases are lung conditions that result from the inhalation of various types of dust in the workplace. Some dust diseases include asbestosis, a lung disease associated with mining, milling, and shipbuilding, and alveolitis, a lung condition caused by the inhalation of organic material, often of fungal spores.

Toxic chemicals can cause injury or illness if they are inhaled or if they enter the body through other means. Lead and arsenic are poisonous and can damage the bone marrow, causing immune disorders. The fumes of cadmium, used in welding, and beryllium, used in high-tech industries, can cause lung damage. Some compounds used in plastics manufacturing, such as vinyl chloride and carbon tetrachloride, can harm the liver. Styrene, which is used in the manufacture of plastics and rubber, has been labeled as a possible carcinogen (cancer-causing agent) by the Environmental Protection Agency (EPA).

Skin diseases or disorders can be caused by allergic reactions to a number of chemicals used in many industries. Whenever a chemical is used in the workplace, contact with this chemical can cause dermatitis (skin inflammation). Burns to the skin are another potential workplace hazard.

Repetitive strain injuries (RSIs) are occupational injuries that result from repetitive, awkward, or forceful motions, or from direct pressure to body areas that are not strong enough to withstand such pressure. RSI is the fastest growing category of occupational injury. Carpal tunnel syndrome and tendonitis are examples of RSIs. This type of injury causes pain and inflammation, and can result in permanent disability if left untreated.

Radiation can cause illness in workers who work outdoors or in those who work with radioactive chemicals. People with occupations in which the majority of their time is spent outdoors are at risk of developing skin cancer. Individuals in the nuclear energy profession are at risk for radiation sickness and other disorders associated with radiation exposure, such as various cancers, organ failure, and cataracts.

Infectious diseases can be contracted at the workplace. People who work with livestock can acquire brucellosis or Q fever, while those who work with birds can acquire psittacosis. Sewer workers and miners, who often come in contact with rats, can contract leptospirosis from these animals. Individuals in certain health care fields who work with blood or blood products are at risk for infection from viral hepatitis or HIV.

Noise. Hearing loss can result from excessive noise in the workplace. Noise exposure creates a further safety hazard if employees are unable to hear instructions or warnings.

Stress can also result from the workplace environment. Job-related stress can cause increased absences from the job, and it also plays a part in job turnover rates. Factors that contribute to stress on the job include excessive monitoring by supervisors, sexual harassment, heavy workload, lack of recognition, lack of support from co-workers or supervisors, fear of job loss, or fear of death or injury on the job. Stressful situations at work can cause different psychological reactions in different people. Some individuals may suffer from anxiety and nervousness, while others may exhibit signs of depression. Physical symptoms, such as heart palpitations, gastrointestinal discomfort, headaches, backaches, hypertension (high blood pressure), insomnia, and muscle aches may also result from stress on the job. In addition, job-related stress can exacerbate preexisting conditions or disorders.

The Role of the Occupational Physician. Occupational physicians analyze patterns of absenteeism, injury, illness, and death in various parts of the work force. These doctors treat work-related illnesses and injuries. They also try to limit occupational health risks and promote healthy habits in employees.

Occupational physicians use epidemiological techniques to examine patterns of illness and injury in the work force. These techniques include compiling statistics about different parts of the work force. To compile these statistics, the incidence and prevalence of certain work-related disorders are recorded in terms of the age, occupation, sex, race, and marital status of the individuals studied. These observations can yield important findings about, for example, the link between a certain occupation and a given disease or injury.

Sometimes it is difficult for an occupational physician to ascertain the cause of a given illness or injury. At times the link between the occupation and the disease or injury is not obvious. The physician must take a full medical history of the patient and must try to determine if the cause of the disease or injury is work-related. At times, a full inspection of the patient's workplace may be necessary if the condition is suspected to have occupational causes. However, prevention, rather than treatment, is usually the key to eliminating illness and injury in the work force.

Occupational physicians use two techniques to try to limit job-related disease and injuries. Primary prevention involves attention to the workplace itself. Health hazards are removed, wastes are disposed of carefully and appropriately, and work areas are kept safe and dust-free. In secondary prevention, the workers themselves are tested for the first signs of work-related illness or injury. These testings are carried out regularly as a preventative measure. Such early signs of occupational disease or injury may include bacterial infections, allergies, or early stages of organ damage.

Occupational Health and Safety. There are many ways for employees to protect themselves against occupational illnesses and injuries. Protective equipment should be used at all times around dust. Such equipment may include protective clothing, masks, or respirators. This equipment will help to prevent dust diseases. When chemicals are used in the workplace, information about these chemicals and how to protect against them can be obtained from the employer. Health and safety training may also be available. Protective equipment, such as that worn to prevent dust diseases, should be worn when handling many of these chemicals. This equipment, along

with safety training, can also help protect against work-related skin disorders.

Risk for RSIs can often be reduced with a few simple adjustments. Some companies have consultants that are available to analyze the work area and work habits of employees. These consultants can make suggestions for modifications that can help to prevent against RSIs. Such suggested modifications may include taking more frequent breaks or changing work habits or posture. Individuals who are required to do a good deal of heavy lifting on a daily basis should start a strength conditioning program to build up their back, stomach, arm, and leg muscles. This will help these individuals to prevent back injuries. Orthopedic aids, such as braces or splints, should only be used under medical supervision, as they can be more harmful than helpful if they are not used correctly.

Radiation hazards can also be protected against. People who work outdoors should wear long sleeves and pants and should apply sunscreen with an SPF of 15 or greater to all exposed skin. Nuclear energy workers should wear the protective clothing that is supplied by their employers.

Infectious diseases can be prevented through the use of the proper safety equipment. Workers who come into contact with animals should be sure to wash thoroughly. Health care workers who work with blood or other bodily fluids need to protect their eyes and skin with the appropriate safety glasses and protective clothing.

Noise in the workplace can be abated through preventative measures. Employees can protect against hearing loss by wearing earplugs. Recreational activities with high noise levels should be avoided if noise exposure is high at work. Additionally, ear protection should be work at the workplace and during recreational activities with a high noise level.

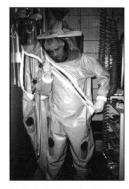

Safety Equipment . It is extremely important that anyone who must come into contact with hazardous materials wear protective clothing. Above, a worker wearing a suit used when Level Four hazardous materials must be handled. Below, three workers disposing of hazardous waste in specially marked containers.

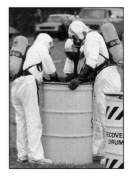

For background material on occupational medicine and health, see PUBLIC HEALTH. Further reading can be found in ACCIDENTS; CARPAL TUNNEL SYNDROME; NOISE; STRESS; and STRESS FRACTURE. See also HEARING LOSS for more on effects of excessive noise on hearing.

Occupational Therapy

The therapeutic use of productive or creative activity in the treatment or rehabilitation of physically or emotionally disabled people.

Occupational therapy is treatment, carried out by specially trained therapists, that is aimed at helping physically or emotionally disabled people relearn basic tasks. Such tasks may include dressing, walking, bathing, and grooming. The ultimate goal of occupational therapy, when possible, is to allow the patient to resume normal life and to take up some form of employment. Occupational therapy is usually started in the hospital and is later continued on an outpatient basis. *See also* THERAPY.

Oedipus Complex

Term in Freudian psychoanalytic theory describing the unconscious sexual attachment of a child to the parent of the opposite sex and the child's consequent jealousy of the parent of the same sex.

The term Oedipus complex was used by Sigmund Freud to describe a normal developmental phase by which a child comes to identify with the parent of the same sex and seeks sexual attachments with members of the opposite sex outside the immediate family. Sometimes, in the event of trauma or abuse, for example, an attachment to the same-sexed parent is blocked, the Oedipal phase may persist into adulthood and prevent the individual from establishing adult attachments with members of the opposite sex.

Freud named the Oedipus complex after the character Oedipus in Greek mythology, who unknowingly killed his father and then married his mother. In women, the complex is sometimes called the Electra complex, after another character in Greek mythology.

> *Background reading on Oedipus complex can be found in PSYCHOANALYSIS and PSYCHIATRY. For related material, see ACTING OUT; ADOLESCENCE; FAMILY THERAPY; PSYCHOTHERAPY; and PUBERTY. See also PSYCHOANALYST for more on a health professional that can treat Oedipus complex.*

Oligohydramnios

Condition in which there is an insufficient amount of amniotic fluid around a fetus.

Amniotic fluid is the liquid that surrounds a fetus in the uterus and acts as a "shock absorber." Normally, the amount of fluid is regulated by the fetus itself, which begins to urinate and swallow amniotic fluid during the second trimester. Too little fluid is associated with birth defects involving the urinary tract. It is also seen in cases of intrauterine growth retardation or fetal death. Early in the pregnancy, oligohydramnios usually results in a miscarriage. If it occurs later in the pregnancy and for a long duration, the pressure on the fetus rarely may, in rare cases, result in physical deformities. *See also* PREGNANCY.

Oligomenorrhea

Infrequent menstrual periods.

Oligomenorrhea may be caused by a variety of factors, ranging from anxiety or stress to the onset of menopause to a malfunction of the pituitary or thyroid glands. It is also sometimes caused by extreme exercise, combined with consumption of too few calories. Most of the conditions that cause oligomenorrhea will respond to treatment, which is aimed at the primary cause of the disorder. *See also* MENOPAUSE.

Oligospermia

An abnormally low sperm count.

A semen sample of from 1.5 to five milliliters normally contains between 400 million and 600 million sperm. Oligospermia, a sperm count of below 20 million sperm per milliliter, may be caused by a variety of factors, including inflammation of a testis (orchitis), failure of a testis to descend, stress, alcohol abuse, or cigarette smoking. In most cases, the condition can be treated. Oligospermia is one of the most common causes of infertility. *See also* INFERTILITY.

Oliguria

Decreased excretion of urine.

Urine production is sometimes lessened by natural body processes, for example, heavy sweating on a hot day without a substantial increase in fluid uptake. But oliguria can sometimes be a symptom of a serious, life-threatening condition. Certain medications can result in decreased urine production, such as diuretics, digitalis, anticholinergic drugs, sulfonomides, and methotrexate. Oliguria can also be a symptom of kidney failure, which may require dialysis (the removal of waste products from the body) or a kidney transplant. A major reduction in urine production, to less than one pint a day, is one of the most notable symptoms of kidney failure. *See also* Anticholinergic Drugs; Dialysis; *and* Kidney Transplant.

Onchocerciasis

Also known as river blindness

Condition produced by infestation with the worm *Onchocerca volvulus*.

Onchocerciasis is a tropical disease, affecting 30 to 50 million people. It is common over large areas in Africa and South America. It is caused by the parasitic worm *Onchocerca volvulus*, the larva of which are transmitted by the bite of *Simulium*, the black fly common to fast flowing rivers and streams. Such flies feed by bruising the skin of animals and drinking blood from the resulting wound. A larval stage of the *Onchocerca volvulus* worm develops within the insect, eventually penetrating the gut wall to infect the human host when the black fly feeds. The larval invaders require a year to develop into adults, producing unsightly, often disfiguring nodules in the skin.

Symptoms. The first symptoms of the infection are intense irritation and itching of the skin from an allergic reaction to the parasite. Secondary bacterial infection is common, with thickening and cracking of the skin occurring due to an inflammatory reaction by the body. Chronic onchocercia-sis infection often leads to blindness produced by the invasion of the eye by the larvae (microfilariae).

Diagnosis and Treatment. Diagnosis is usually made by immersing an infected skin sample in saline. In seconds, microfilariae larvae may be seen leaving the skin. Onchocerciasis is treated with the drug Ivermectin, which kills the microfilariae, though not the adult worms, which may require surgical removal. Efforts at preventing the disease center around aerial spraying and destruction of black fly populations in endemic areas. Travelers to areas in which onchocerciasis is prevalent should take precautions to ensure that they are not bitten by insects that may carry the larvae of the *Onchocerca volvulus* worm. *See also* Filariasis; Insect Bites; Insects and Disease; *and* Worm Infestation.

Oncogene

Gene that turns normal cells into cancerous cells, causing them to divide uncontrollably.

Oncogenes are either mutated versions of proto-oncogenes, genes that are found in every cell in the body and play a role in normal cell division, or they are carried into the cell by a virus.

An individual oncogene by itself cannot cause cancer, but it can increase the rate of cell division (mitosis) in the cell. Rapidly dividing cells, in turn, are at an increased risk for further mutations. When a cell accumulates several active oncogenes, it loses control over its mitosis and becomes a cancerous cell. These cells grow unrestrained and can invade normal body tissue.

The mutation of proto-oncogenes into oncogenes can be caused by various carcinogens (cancer-causing agents) in the environment, such as radiation, ultraviolet light, certain chemicals, certain viruses, cigarette and cigar smoke, and alcohol. It takes many different mutations to turn a normal cell into a cancerous cell; the number differs depending on the cell. *See also* Cancer; Carcinogen; Cell; Infection; Mutation; Nicotine; *and* Radiation Hazards.

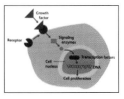

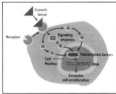

Oncogene.
Oncogenes are genes that induce normal cells to multiply uncontrollably. Above, top, in a normal cell, proteins called growth factors control cell growth and division. Above, bottom, an oncogene produces abnormal versions or quantities of growth factor, and the growth cycle of the cell speeds up.

Oncology

The medical specialty that deals with tumors.

Oncology also deals with benign tumors, but is particularly concerned with malignant types. Oncologists are specialists who deal with the causes of cancer, how cancers develop, the characteristics of different cancers, and the treatment of cancer.

The field of oncology includes a wide range of experimental techniques to determine the causes and characteristics of cancers, how they progress, how they can be prevented, and how they can be treated. In addition, it includes epidemiology work of the kind that helped establish the cause-effect relationship between cigarette smoking and lung cancer, and, increasingly, it also includes genetic studies to establish the underlying molecular mechanisms by which cells become cancerous.

Treatment of cancer usually requires a team approach, in which a physician specializing in oncology is assisted by personnel skilled in diagnostic techniques, surgery, radiation therapy, chemotherapy, and the supportive measures that are needed by cancer patients and their families. *See also* CANCER; CHEMOTHERAPY; DIAGNOSIS; *and* RADIATION THERAPY.

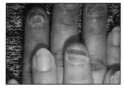

Onycholysis.
Above, in onycholysis the nails become loose and dirt and debris collect underneath them.

Onlay, Dental

Restorative application fixed to grinding surfaces of teeth.

A dental onlay is one of the three common methods of restoring a diseased or damaged tooth. It is more protective than an inlay, but less protective than a crown. Dental onlays can strengthen weakened teeth or may be used to compensate for small degrees of misalignment.

Dental inlays act essentially as silver alloy fillings, protecting or repairing small areas of a damaged tooth. Installing porcelain crowns involves reshaping the natural tooth before entirely covering it and the extensive damage or disease that had taken place prior to treatment. Dental onlay is made of gold or porcelain and covers part of the tooth, making it more durable than an inlay. An onlay does not require the complexity of reshaping and covering the entire tooth the way a crown would, however. A dentist can determine which restorative procedure is best for a particular condition. *See also* INLAY, DENTAL.

Onychogryphosis

Gross enlargement and curving of the nails, occurring mainly in the elderly.

Onychogryphosis can be an extremely painful condition—even the light pressure of a bed sheet can cause pain for those afflicted. Its cause is unknown, but it is believed to be the result of a fungal infection or poor circulation and can be treated by frequent trimming of the nails and the application of antifungal medications. Treatment usually takes a long time, and, if unsuccessful, the condition can be resolved by destroying the nail matrix on an outpatient basis using local anesthesia. *See also* ANTIFUNGAL DRUGS.

Onycholysis

A painless condition in which the nail loosens or separates from the underlying nail bed.

There are a number of reasons that cause this condition to develop. These causes can be either external or internal. External causes of onycholysis include household chemicals, such as nail polish, nail polish remover, and detergents. Jogging may also cause the condition, if the toenails repeatedly touch the tip of the shoes. Internal causes of onycholysis may include a primary skin disease such as psoriasis, or, less commonly, thyroid disease.

Prevention and Treatment. Onycholysis can be prevented by avoiding natural and chemical irritants. If microorganisms have invaded the separated nail area, and a secondary infection has developed, medication may be necessary to treat the infection. *See* PSORIASIS *and* THYROID DISORDERS.

Oophorectomy

Surgical removal of one or both ovaries.

An oophorectomy may be performed to treat ovarian cysts, tumors, abscess, cancer, endometriosis, or an estrogen-related disease, such as breast cancer.

The procedure can be performed under general anesthesia via an abdominal incision or by laparoscopy, in which the ovaries are removed by manipulating instruments through small incisions. The former is preferred when other variables, such as adhesions, may be present or when other procedures, such as a hysterectomy or removal of the fallopian tubes, will also be performed. These are sometimes performed on a preventive basis if the family medical history suggests risk.

Complications. Menstruation and childbearing ability may continue with the removal of one ovary, but removal of both ovaries ends both menstruation and reproductive ability.

Removal of both ovaries may cause symptoms similar to those experienced during menopause to occur, including changes in sex drive and hot flashes. Women who have both ovaries removed and do not take estrogen replacement therapy are at an increased risk for cardiovascular disease and osteoporosis. *See also* BREAST CANCER *and* OVARY, CANCER OF.

Open Heart Surgery

Operation in which the heart is stopped and a mechanical pump supplies blood to the body so that a cardiac condition can be corrected.

Open heart surgery became possible in the 1950s with the development of the heart-lung machine. Until then, only limited procedures could be carried out on a heart while it continued to beat. Consequently, few heart problems could be repaired by surgical means. Today, open heart surgery with cardiopulmonary bypass is performed for a variety of reasons: to create new channels for blood to flow around narrow or blocked arteries; to repair or replace defective heart valves; to repair a number of congenital heart defects; and for other heart conditions. During surgery, damage to the heart is kept to a minimum with a hypothermia technique that lowers the temperature of the muscles of the heart.

New Developments. Minimally invasive heart surgery is a significant development among the newer techniques that have expanded the range of procedures possible through open heart surgery. Minimally invasive heart surgery has made the surgery more effective and less traumatic. This revolutionary procedure can be done through an incision only four or five inches wide. With the aid of computer-guided instruments, the surgeon uses a control console to perform an operation that may last several hours, maximizing precision and minimizing injury.

For background information on open heart surgery, see HEART DISORDERS *and* HEART SURGERY. *Further material can be found in* CARDIAC ARREST; CARDIOVASCULAR DISORDERS; HEART; HEART ATTACK; HERAT DISEASE, CONGENITAL; HEART DISEASE, ISCHEMIC; HEART FAILURE; HEART TRANSPLANT; HEART VALVE SURGERY; *and* SURGERY.

Operable

A disease or condition for which a surgical procedure will result in a reasonable chance of improvement or survival.

Operable conditions can be treated by surgical means. Such methods may range from an outpatient procedure performed using only a local anesthetic to major surgery such as a heart transplant, which requires a general anesthetic and may last for many hours. Conditions that cannot be treated with surgery are deemed inoperable. This may be for various reasons, for example, the surgery may be determined to be too risky or physiologically impossible, the patient may not be healthy enough to withstand surgery, or the disease may have progressed to a point at which surgery will not be able to help the patient. *See also* NONINVASIVE *and* OPERATION.

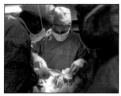

Breast Biopsy.
An operating room is specially designed and equipped for surgical procedures. Above, a surgeon performing a breast biopsy on a woman patient.

Resources on Ophthalmology

Davson, Hugh, ed., *The Eye* (1984); King, John Harry and Joseph A.C. Wadsworth, eds., *An Atlas of Ophthalmic Surgery* (1970); Vaughan, Daniel, et al., *General Ophthalmology* (1995); Wolf, K.P., *Eyewise: Eye Disorders and Their Treatment* (1982); American Council of the Blind, Tel. (800) 424-8666, Online: www.acb.org; American Foundation for the Blind, Tel. (800) 232-5463, Online: www.afb.org; Glaucoma Research Foundation, Tel. (800) 826-6693, Online: www.glaucoma.org; www.nycornell.org/op/.

Operating Room

A specially designed and equipped hospital room in which physicians perform surgical procedures on patients.

An operating room is designed to provide optimal conditions for surgeons to operate efficiently without bacterial contamination of themselves or the patients.

Basic elements of the operating room include power supply, lighting, ventilation, and water supply. The power supply is conventional electricity with emergency generator back-up, including some use of hydraulics and air compressors. The overall bright and diffuse lighting is supplemented by specific operating lamps to spotlight the operation site. A strong ventilation system provides a consistent supply of clean, filtered air to the operating room. There is a nearby stainless steel sink and water supply at which surgeons, assistants, and nurses can "scrub down" with bactericidal soaps and sterile brushes.

The focal point of the room is the operating table on which the patient is positioned. The instrument table (which holds sterile scalpels, dissectors, clamps, forceps, detractors, and other surgical tools) is located next to the scrub nurse, who dispenses the instruments to the chief surgeon. A circulating nurse provides additional assistance. A monitor screen shows the patient's vital signs (heartbeat, blood pressure, and brain waves), and a viewing screen or light box permits quick glances at x-rays and CAT or MRI scans. Two clocks show the actual time and the elapsed time of the operation, respectively.

The anesthesiologist, at the head of the table, carefully monitors the patient's vital signs and controls the amount of anesthetic and oxygen as needed. An intravenous drip to transfuse blood or other fluid by catheter is often necessary.

Transplants, heart bypasses, and brain surgery require additional, highly specialized equipment. Computers, robotics, and television screens are increasingly being used in operating rooms. *See also* SURGERY.

Operation

A surgical procedure usually performed in an operating room by a specialist, with surgical instruments and other equipment and with the help of other medical professionals.

An operation can be as simple as a general practitioner sterilizing and suturing a child's cut in a doctor's office or as complicated as open-heart surgery or a major organ transplant by a group of surgeons, operating room nurses, and anesthesiologist in the operating room of a top teaching hospital.

Some of the most common operations (in order of frequency) are: inguinal hernia repair; removal of the gallbladder (cholecystectomy); release of peritoneal adhesions; appendectomy; biopsy of breast tissue; excision and cleaning (debridement) of wounds, burns, or infections; mastectomy; removal of part of the large intestine (colectomy); hemorrhoidectomy; skin graft; hysterectomy; prostatectomy; and tonsillectomy. *See also* SURGERY.

Ophthalmology

The study of the eye and the diagnosis and treatment of conditions that affect the eye.

Ophthalmology does not only include the study of vision and the prescription of corrective lenses to remedy poor vision, but also the surgical treatment of such problems as glaucoma, macular degeneration, and cataracts.

Ophthalmologists often work in conjunction with other doctors because many problems that affect the eyes (especially the retina, located at the back of the eye) are the result of disorders elsewhere in the body. For example, hypertension (high blood pressure) can cause retinopathy (damage to the retina), as can atherosclerosis (narrowing of the arteries by increased cholesterol) and diabetes mellitus. Brain damage can also cause visual impairments. *See also* ATHEROSCLEROSIS; DIABETES MELLITUS; GLAUCOMA; *and* RETINOPATHY.

Ophthalmoscope

An instrument used to examine the interior of the eye, particularly the retina.

An ophthalmoscope consists of a light source (which may be strapped to the physician's head or held by hand) in a device consisting of mirrors and a magnifier. It is used to look at the back of the eye or fundus. With this device, the ophthalmologist can peer through the transparent pupil

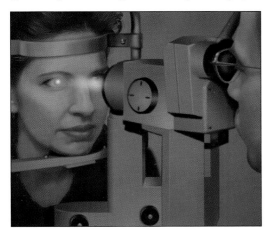

of the eye to the retina, observing the retinal blood vessels and the head of the optic nerve. Ophthalmoscopy is the only nonsurgical (noninvasive) means of examining the inside of the eye, the network of retinal blood vessels, optic disk, arteries and veins, foveal region, and the liquid vitreous humor. Ophthalmoscopy is a key diagnostic aid for the detection of diabetes, atherosclerosis (hardening of the arteries), and hypertension.

What to Expect. Prior to ophthalmoscopy, the physician often places drops in the eye to dilate the pupil for better viewing. Dilation takes 20 to 45 minutes. The patient should not attempt to drive following the procedure if eye drops have been used. It is also advisable to wear sunglasses after the procedure until the pupils have returned to their normal size, as the eyes will be more sensitive to light. Ophthalmoscopy is a safe, nonsurgical, and painless diagnostic test, generally performed in the doctor's office. *See also* OPHTHALMOLOGY.

Opiate

A drug either derived from, or chemically similar to, opium.

Opiates are chemically similar to, or derived from, opium, a chemical that is derived from the seeds of the poppy plant. Opiates include opium, codeine, and morphine, and are also called narcotic drugs. Opiates have an analgesic (pain-killing) effect, and work by combining with specific receptors on individual cells. These receptors are also referred to as opiates.

The following people should only take opiates if they are prescribed by a doctor: pregnant or breast-feeding women; people with epilepsy; asthmatics; those with liver, heart, kidney, gallbladder, or lung disease; people with inflammatory bowel syndrome; those with an enlarged prostate; or people with bleeding conditions. Opiates are habit-forming, and patients may become addicted to the drugs. Use of alcohol should be avoided by individuals taking opiate medications. *See also* ANALGESIC DRUGS *and* SUBSTANCE ABUSE.

Opportunistic Infection

An infection that does not normally infect people with healthy immune systems.

People with compromised immune systems are vulnerable to bacteria, fungi, viruses, or parasites that normally live harmlessly on or in the body. This category of people includes people with AIDS, people undergoing chemotherapy for cancer, or those who have recently had an organ transplant and are taking immunosuppressant drugs. It also includes people who have had severe burns. The elderly are at special risk because their immune systems are weakening with age, because they may already have a chronic disease such as diabetes or asthma, and because they may live in nursing homes or hospitals, where the risk of infection is much higher. *See also* BACTERIA; BURNS; IMMUNE SYSTEM; *and* IMMUNOSUPPRESSANT DRUGS.

Ophthalmoscope.
At left, an ophthalmoscope is a specialized magnifying microscope used to examine, treat (with a laser), and photograph (with a camera) the eye.

Optic Atrophy

Wasting away of the optic nerve, the nerve responsible for vision.

Optic atrophy can be the consequence of various conditions, and can result in varying degrees of vision loss. Optic atrophy is caused by disease or injury to the optic nerve. Such diseases or injuries may include optic neuritis (inflammation of the optic nerve) or optic disk ischemia (due to change in blood supply to the optic nerve, as in hypertension and stroke). Optic atrophy may also occur in patients with no previous symptoms of nerve disease. *See also* OPTIC DISK EDEMA *and* OPTIC NERVE.

Optic Disk Edema

Swelling of the head of the optic nerve, visible upon medical examination.

Optic disk edema can be seen by an ophthalmologist through an ophthalmoscope. The swelling may be caused by increased pressure of cerebrospinal fluid, a fluid located inside the skull, or it may be caused by problems with the optic nerve itself, such as damage to the nerve caused by a restriction in blood supply. It may be one of the first signs of a brain or orbital tumor. If left untreated, optic disk edema may progress to optic atrophy, the wasting away of the optic nerve. Optic disk edema caused by a rise in pressure in the skull is called papilledema. *See also* BRAIN TUMOR.

Optic Nerve

The nerve responsible for vision.

The optic nerve runs from the back of the retina (a layer of light receptors located at the back of the eye) to the brain, and transmits nerve impulses along that path. Optic nerves from each eye meet behind the eyes and cross over at the optic junction. As a consequence, nerve fibers from the right half of each retina pass to the right side of the occipital lobe, the area of the brain re-

Optic Nerve
At right, the optic nerve, located at the back of the retina, transmits visual information from the retina to the brain.

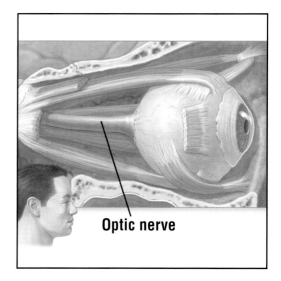

Optic nerve

sponsible for perceiving visual information. Similarly, nerve fibers from the left half of each retina pass to the left side of the occipital lobe.

Conditions affecting the optic nerve include optic disk edema, in which the head of the nerve swells because of pressure in the skull or damage to the nerve, and optic atrophy, in which the nerve wastes away, causing varying degrees of vision loss. *See also* OPTIC ATROPHY *and* OPTIC DISK EDEMA.

Optometry

The study of vision, including evaluation of quality and prescription of corrective lenses.

Specialists in optometry, called optometrists, examine the eyes and vision and supply corrective lenses, such as glasses or contact lenses, to individuals with poor vision. Optometrists are also responsible for supplying and adjusting corrective lenses. However, optometrists are not licensed physicians and do not perform laser surgery to correct vision problems. In addition, optometry does not include the performance of surgical procedures. Thus, more serious eye-related disorders are usually referred to ophthalmologists—licensed physicians who specialize in the care of the eyes. *See also* EYE; EYE, DISORDERS OF; OPHTHALMOLOGY; ORTHOPTICS; *and* VISION, DISORDERS OF.

Oral Contraceptives

Also known as birth control pills or "the pill"

Drugs containing the hormones estrogen and progesterone, used to inhibit ovulation.

In addition to preventing pregnancy, oral contraceptives offer other health benefits, such as reducing the severity of menstrual cramps and establishing a more regular menstrual cycle.

Types. The two types of oral contraceptive are the combined pill and the minipill. Combined pills contain both estrogen and progesterone, which prevent ovulation. Minipills only contain progesterone, and work by thickening the mucus in the cervix so that sperm cannot fertilize an egg.

Effectiveness. Both types of oral contraceptive are taken on a monthly cycle and must be taken consistently and regularly to be effective. If oral contraceptives are used correctly, they are more than 99 percent effective in preventing pregnancy. However, other medications, such as antibiotic drugs, anticonvulsant drugs, and barbiturates, may decrease their effectiveness.

Side Effects. Oral contraceptives containing estrogen (combined pills) can increase the risk of heart disorders, such as high blood pressure, and bleeding disorders, such as thrombosis (an abnormal blood clot). The incidence of these effects is increased in smokers or women over the age of 35. Medical studies have conflicted as to the relationship between the use of combined pills and breast cancer. However, it has been found that use of combined pills during reproductive years may decrease the risk of breast cancer after menopause. Less serious side effects of combined pills include weight gain, nausea, depression, changes in appetite, and headaches. If adverse effects of combined pills are severe, the dosage of estrogen in the pills may be reduced or the patient may instead be prescribed minipills. Side effects of minipills include bleeding between periods, irregular periods, and ovarian cysts. *See also* CONTRACEPTION, HORMONAL METHODS *and* PREGNANCY.

Oral Hygiene

Maintenance of healthy teeth and gums.

Oral hygiene is more than running a toothbrush across the teeth. Proper oral hygiene involves closely paying attention to the teeth, gums, and tongue. Neglecting any element of good oral hygiene can lead to tooth and gum disease.

Toothbrushing is the first step to proper oral hygiene. Brushing the teeth thoroughly at least twice a day removes food particles and harmful bacteria (plaque). Flossing is equally important; it serves to remove food that is trapped between teeth. There are several varieties of floss available on the market to accommodate all sorts of teeth; if nothing seems to work, a dentist can make a recommendation. The tongue must be kept clean as well, as it is a repository for bacteria. Brushing the tongue or using a tongue scraper keeps the tongue clean and healthy.

Oral hygiene also includes regular visits to a dentist. During a checkup, dental hygienists clean plaque and hardened buildup (calculus or tartar) from the teeth. Dental checkups may also include fluoride treatments, a preventive measure for strengthening the teeth. Similarly, polishing gives a pleasant appearance to teeth in addition to smoothing surfaces to which food and bacteria might adhere.

Background material on oral hygiene can be found in DENTAL EXAMINATION; HYGIENE; *and* TEETH. *For further information, see* CARIES, DENTAL; DISCOLORED TEETH; EROSION, DENTAL; GINGIVITIS; *and* PERIODONTAL DISEASE. *See also* FLOSSING, DENTAL; FLUORIDATION; *and* TOOTHBRUSHING *for more on oral hygiene practices.*

Oral and Maxillofacial Surgery

Surgical treatment of disorders of the mouth, jaws, and related parts of the face.

Oral surgeons provide many different services. They remove teeth, such as impacted or decayed third molars (wisdom teeth), and help save teeth by surgical root canals. They treat tooth and jaw infections, as well as cysts and tumors. They repair fractured top and bottom jaws and other injured facial bones. In addition, oral surgeons place dental implants and bone and other tissue grafts, and rebuild and correct facial and skeletal functional and aesthetic deformities (orthognathic surgery). *See also* CLEFT LIP AND PALATE; ORTHOGNATHIC SURGERY; *and* ROOT-CANAL TREATMENT.

Orbit

Deep cavity in the skull in which the eye is located.

In addition to the eyeball, the orbit contains muscles, blood vessels, fatty tissue, and nerves. The optic nerve passes from the back of the eyeball to the brain through a hole in the orbit. *See also* OPTIC NERVE.

Conditions Affecting the Orbit. The orbit may be fractured from a heavy blow, such as that which occurs in a car accident or sports injury. Such injuries usually do not affect the eyeball itself, as it is squeezed backwards during blinking. Such injuries usually heal on their own, although corrective surgery may be necessary if the face is deformed or if the eyeball is displaced.

In extremely rare cases, the fatty tissue of the orbit can become infected with bacteria, a condition known as orbital cellulitis. Pressure on the eye may cause damage, and the condition may spread backwards to the brain. Orbital cellulitis can be successfully treated with antibiotics.

Orchiectomy

The surgical removal of one or both testicles, usually to treat testicular or prostate cancer.

Though rare, testicular cancer is on the rise in the United States—approximately 7,000 American males were diagnosed with the disease in 2000, up about 50 percent since the early 1970s. Undetected, testicular cancer spreads to the liver, lungs, and lymph glands. However, early detection and treatment have greatly diminished the

mortality rate of the disease. Orchiectomy remains the best treatment, although radiation and chemotherapy are also given.

Orchiectomy can also be used to treat prostate cancer, which depends on male hormones to grow; thus, removing the supply of hormones limits the growth of the cancer. *See also* PROSTATE, CANCER OF.

Procedure. During an orchiectomy, a urologist makes a four-inch incision through the lower abdomen on the side of the affected testicle. (The scrotum, which tends to heal slowly and painfully, is no longer the site of incision.) The doctor pushes the testicle up through the pelvic region, removes it, and then ties off the spermatic cord. The lymph nodes in that area may also be removed. The removed testicle is replaced by a saline-filled testicular prosthesis (SFTP).

The average operating time is about 45 to 60 minutes, and an overnight stay in the hospital is suggested but not necessary.

Removal of one testicle does not adversely affect the patient's sex drive, potency, or ability to have children. A double orchiectomy requires hormonal therapy.

Orchiopexy

Surgical operation to relocate an undescended testicle from the abdominal cavity to the scrotum.

When one (unilateral) or both (bilateral) testicles fail to descend into the scrotum by birth, the condition is known as cryptorchidism. This is usually corrected surgically between the ages of one and five, as further delay may impede normal development, lead to infertility, and predispose the patient to testicular cancer.

In orchiopexy, a surgeon makes an incision along the lower abdomen on the side of the patient's undescended testicle and gently pushes the testicle down through the opening between the abdomen and scrotum (inguinal canal). The testicle is then stitched to the scrotum to prevent it from regressing back into the abdominal cavity. Recovery is usually uncomplicated and rapid. *See also* TESTIS, UNDESCENDED.

Orchitis

Inflammation of the testes caused by a bacterial or vial infection.

About 20 percent of men who contract the viral infection called mumps after puberty develop a painful inflammation of one or both testes. After recovery from the disease, the testes may return to normal, but in some cases there will be permanent damage such as infertility. Bacterial infections may also travel to the testes from the urethra or the bladder, causing inflammation. Orchitis is treated with antibiotics if the infection is bacterial. Treatment of orchitis caused by a virus is aimed at relieving the symptoms, as antibiotics are not effective against viral infections. *See also* BACTERIA; MUMPS; TESTES; *and* VACCINATION.

Organ Donation

The agreement of a person (or guardian or loved one) to give an organ or tissue for transplantation either while the donor is living (living donor) or after death (cadaveric).

If a person has a damaged or diseased organ but is otherwise in good health, an organ transplant may provide a longer life and a higher quality of life. Organ donations give thousands of people extensions on life, and there are now over 850 organ donation programs affiliated with 250 medical institutions in the United States. However, there are still many more people who need organ transplantations than there are organs available.

Most organs, such as hearts and lungs, can only be donated after death. Because organs deteriorate after they no longer receive a supply of oxygen, they are generally taken from people who have been diagnosed as brain dead but whose bodily functions are maintained with a heart-lung machine, which continues to supply oxygen to the organs. After an organ is taken from a body, it is cooled and can be stored for a short time before transplantation into the body of a recipient.

Other organs, such as kidneys, or tissues, such as bone marrow, can be taken from a living donor. Generally, these organs or tissues are taken from family member of the transplant recipient, as this increases the chance that the tissue types of the donor and the recipient will match. Also, this method of transplantation limits the possibility of organs being sold or otherwise obtained unscrupulously.

In order to donate organs, a person needs to give previous consent and, if applicable, obtain family consent. Often consent is given in the context of an advanced care directive, which is a verbal or written description of the care a person desires in the event he or she becomes terminally ill or injured. Organ donation consent can also often be included on an individual's driver's license.

Organ transplants from animal donors (such as pigs and baboons) to humans, a process known as xenotransplantation, is currently being researched in an attempt to compensate for the shortage of human organ donors.

The key coordinating organization for organ transplantation in the United States is the United Network for Organ Sharing (www.unos.org, 1-800-24-DONOR).

Organ Recipient Waiting List

Approximate number of people waiting for organ donations in the United States per year (1990-2000).

Organ	# of People
Kidney	46,000
Liver	16,000
Heart	5,000
Lung	4,000
Pancreas	1,500
Heart/Lung	250
Intestines	150

from the United Network for Organ Sharing (UNOS)

For background information on organ donation, see TRANSPLANT SURGERY. *Further material can be found in* HEART-LUNG TRANSPLANT; HEART TRANSPLANT; KIDNEY TRANSPLANT; LIVER TRANSPLANT; *and* SURGERY. *See also* GRAFT-VERSUS-HOST DISEASE *and* REJECTION *for more on transplant complications.*

Orgasm

The climax of sexual excitement, involving sudden rhythmic contractions of the pelvic muscles and genitals, along with intense feelings of sexual pleasure and a release of tension.

In women, the contractions of orgasm occur in the vagina, clitoris, and uterus. In men, orgasm results in ejaculation. The period after sexual climax is known as the resolution phase.

The intensity of an orgasm can vary. Women generally take longer and require more stimulation to climax than men. Many women require direct clitoral stimulation to reach orgasm. It is important to note that every sexual experience does not necessarily have to end in an orgasm in order to achieve sexual pleasure.

Multiple orgasms occur when an individual remains aroused after one orgasm and can climax again soon after without passing through the resolution phase. Men usually need a recovery period before they can have another orgasm. The amount of recovery time needed may vary from a few minutes to half a day, and the length of the recovery time period increases with age. *See also* SEXUAL INTERCOURSE.

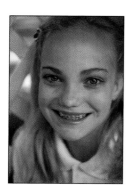

Braces.
Above, braces are an example of an orthodontic appliance, which is worn on the teeth to correct bite or alignment problems.

Ornithosis

Also known as psittacosis or parrot fever

Infectious disease passed from birds to humans.

Ornithosis is an infectious illness that results in flu-like symptoms. The cause of the disease is the bacterium called *Chlamydia psittaci*, which is associated with parrots and parakeets, as well as domestic birds. Ornithosis is acquired by handling the blood, tissues, feathers, or discharges (solid wastes and secretions) from infected birds. Breathing in dust particles from the dried droppings of infected birds can also cause the disease. It is rarely spread from person to person.

Symptoms of ornithosis usually begin ten days after exposure to the bacteria and include fever, headache, loss of appetite, vomiting, neck and back pain, muscle aches, chills, fatigue, and cough. Severe pneumonia is found in extreme cases and is potentially fatal.

Treatment. Ornithosis is treated with the antibiotic medication tetracycline. Oxygen and other forms of treatment for pneumonia are administered if that secondary disease develops. If birds are kept as pets, it is essential to clean the birdcages frequently to avoid dried droppings. *See also* CHLAMYDIA.

Orthodontic Appliances

Devices worn on the teeth to correct problems with bite or appearance.

Teeth that are aligned well and meet in a comfortable bite function best and are easiest to maintain and keep.

Orthodontics is a specialty of dentistry that deals with moving teeth and their supporting bone and gums, so that they may function better or are more aesthetically pleasing. Different types of appliances and braces can be used to move teeth. An orthodontist can improve the bite and smile of patients of all ages.

TYPES
Fixed Appliances. Fixed appliances are placed by a dental professional and can move the teeth in any direction. They are worn for extended periods of time, often for one to two years, and are used when many teeth have to be moved. Commonly, fixed appliances are fitted to either the front side or the back side of all of the upper teeth, all of the bottom teeth, or both the upper teeth and the bottom teeth. The portion of a fixed appliance that moves the teeth is the arch wire, which is threaded through, and held in place by, a bracket on each tooth.

The advantage to fixed appliances is that they give the orthodontist more strict control over the movement of the teeth. However, fixed appliances are more expensive than the alternative and take longer to shape and regulate. In addition, since brackets cover portions of most teeth, plaque (a sticky coating on the teeth composed of saliva, bacteria, and food debris) can accumulate.

Removable appliances effect more minimal changes on the teeth. They generally consist of a wire that fits in front of the teeth, connected to a plastic plate that covers the roof or the floor of the mouth. Teeth are moved by adjusting the tension on the wire, thus exerting force on the teeth.

The advantage to removable appliances is that they are easier to keep clean. However, they may interfere with speech, and some patients may remove them so frequently that they cease to be effective.

Background material on orthodontic appliances can be found in MASTICATION; OVERBITE AND OVERJET; *and* OVERCROWDING, DENTAL. *For further reading, see* DENTAL EXAMINATION *and* RESTORATION, DENTAL. *See also* DENTURE *and* WIRING OF THE JAWS *for more information on specific orthodontic appliances.*

Orthognathic Surgery

Surgical procedure to correct jaw deformities.

Orthognathic surgery is a hospital procedure performed under general anesthetic on jaws that are too long, too short, or otherwise out of alignment. This type of surgery requires an overnight stay in the hospital.

If a jaw is too long, it projects too far from the rest of the face. This can be corrected by surgically setting the jaw backward. A jaw that is too short can also be surgically corrected by sliding it forward. Splints are often required on the jaw until it heals. Pre- and post-surgical orthodontic appliances are also required to ensure proper healing.

Deformities of the jaw are often accompanied by severe malocclusion (an abnormal relationship between the top and the bottom sets of teeth). Both function and form are improved and corrected by orthognathic surgery. *See also* MALOCCLUSION *and* TEETH.

Orthopedics

The area of medicine that treats injuries and disorders of bones and joints, and the muscles, tendons, and ligaments affected.

Orthopedic surgeons, or orthopedists, are responsible for the treatment of a wide variety of musculoskeletal problems, often sustained by athletes. They reset broken bones, put on casts, and replace dislocated joints. They treat joint disorders, including all varieties of arthritis, and back problems, such as slipped disks. Orthopedic surgeons may repair or replace damaged hip, knee, shoulder or finger joints. Bone diseases, such as tumors or birth defects, are also handled by orthopedists. *See also* ARTHRITIS; ARTHROPLASTY; BACK PAIN; DISK PROLAPSE; DISLOCATION, JOINT; *and* FRACTURES.

Orthopnea

Discomfort in breathing when lying down on the back.

Orthopnea can occur because of the decreased ability of the heart to pump blood (heart failure). It is brought on by an increase in the flow of blood into the left ventricle, which cannot handle the increased workload. Other causes of orthopnea include accumulation of fluid in the lungs (edema), asthma, and chronic obstructive lung diseases, such as bronchitis or emphysema. The chest discomfort can be relieved by sitting or standing up. Nighttime orthopnea is called paroxysmal nocturnal dyspnea and can cause frequent waking from sleep.

Treatment of orthopnea depends on the cause of the disorder. In more advanced cases of heart failure, bed rest, a decrease in activity level, and/or weight loss may also be recommended to decrease the workload placed on the heart. Other conditions causing orthopnea, such as asthma or chronic obstructive lung disease, are treated by appropriate medications or surgery. *See also* BREATHING DIFFICULTY *and* HEART FAILURE.

Orthoptics

A subdiscipline of ophthalmology that focuses on the study of eye movements and on disorders relating to vision.

Orthoptists are eye muscle specialists who practice non-surgical treatment of eye-related conditions, including crossed eyes and decreased vision. Orthoptists work under the supervision of ophthalmologists on patients of all ages, although they primarily work in a pediatric setting. The majority of their patients are children, since many eye and vision disorders, such as crossed eyes (strabismus) and lazy eye (amblyopia), primarily affect young people. *See also* AMBLYOPIA; EYE, DISORDERS OF; OPHTHALMOLOGY; *and* STRABISMUS.

Osgood-Schlatter Disease

Enlargement of the tibial tuberosity, a prominence of bone located just below the knee.

The tibia, or shin bone, begins with a bony prominence called the tibial tuberosity, located right below the knee. This bump can become swollen and enlarged with repeated, excessive pulling of the quadricep muscle on the patellar tendon, which is attached to the tibial tuberosity.

Incidence and Symptoms. Osgood-Schlatter disease is most common in active, athletic boys age 10 to 14, as it results from overuse of the tendons in the leg before the connective tissue has matured. Symptoms include pain, tenderness, and, possibly, swelling around the kneecap, which increases with activity.

Treatment. Osgood-Schlatter disease usually clears up on its own. The most common treatments are rest, ice, and nonsteroidal anti-inflammatories (NSAIDs), along with a reduction in athletic activity. For severe cases, a cast to immobilize the area may be needed to allow the enlargement to subside. In extremely rare instances, surgery on the tibial tuberosity may be required. *See also* ANTI-INFLAMMATORY DRUGS *and* TIBIA.

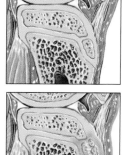

Osgood-Schlatter Disease. Above, top, the tibial tuberosity of a normal adolescent. Above, bottom, an Osgood-Schlatter lesion of the tibial tuberosity, with protruding bone fragments. The lump on the knee will be visible.

Osteitis

An inflammation of the bones.

There are three types of osteitis. Osteitis deformans is a progressive bone disease in which the bone breaks down and is regenerated in a weaker and more fragile form. The disease attacks the skull, spine, legs, collarbone, and pelvis. Osteitis fibrosa results from excess production of the thyroid hormone. This hormone softens the bones and replaces normal bone with cysts. Osteitis pubis often follows trauma, pelvic surgery, or childbirth. It is common among men in their thirties and forties. It causes pain in the groin, which is exacerbated by running, kicking, or even walking. Treatment for all of these forms of osteitis is rest, pain-relieving medication (analgesics), and, in some cases, hormone injections. *See also* ANALGESIC DRUGS; BONE DISORDERS; *and* THYROID HORMONES.

Osteoarthritis

Pain and stiffening of a joint or joints due to the loss of cartilage.

Joints are able to move smoothly and painlessly because of cartilage—a tough, elastic connective tissue found between the joints. If the cartilage is damaged or wears down, the joints become painful and swollen. This condition, known as osteoarthritis, commonly affects people over age 60. Unlike rheumatoid arthritis, which spreads systemically throughout the body, osteoarthritis attacks individual joints, often the fingers, knees, hips, feet, and spine.

Causes. The most common causes of osteoarthritis are age and wear, but other factors may lead to the condition as well. Genetic links have been found in people who experience osteoarthritis in the hands or knees; thus, these people may transmit the condition to their children. An injury to a joint may lead to early osteoarthritis. Many jobs that require repetitive motion of a joint also cause early cases of the condition. Some people may be prone to osteoarthritis because of structural mismatches in their joints, which lead to additional wear when moving.

Incidence. Up to 85 percent of people over the age of 65 may show some evidence of osteoarthritis when x-rayed, but less than 50 percent will experience symptoms. Men are more likely to have osteoarthritis in their hips, while women experience it more often in their fingers, hands, and, most commonly, knees.

Symptoms. Osteoarthritis sets in slowly. People under age 40 may experience the beginnings of the disease, feeling some passing pain and stiffness in joint areas. As cartilage becomes increasingly worn, symptoms increase in frequency and duration. Overuse of the joint causes pain, while inactivity leads to stiffness. The pain often occurs at night, even when the joint is at rest, and can interfere with sleep. Humid weather can exacerbate the condition. Cysts may appear around the joints, or the body may misguidedly attempt to heal itself by growing extra bone cells in the area, causing a deformity around the joint. Muscles that surround the joint may weaken if osteoarthritis pain causes a person to use that joint less.

Treatment. There is no cure for osteoarthritis, but the pain can be treated with anti-inflammatory drugs. Physical therapy, including exercise and stretching, can strengthen the muscles and help maintain mobility. If the joint is extremely damaged, surgical replacement with an artificial joint is an option.

Prevention. There is no sure way to prevent osteoarthritis, but maintaining a healthy weight can alleviate pressure on the joints. Exercise strengthens muscles. A calcium-rich diet will keep bones from weakening. Vitamins C, E, and beta carotene, all found in fresh fruit and vegetables, may also offer some protection.

For background information on osteoarthritis, see ARTHRITIS *and* ORTHOPEDICS. *Related material can be found in* AGING; BONE, DISORDERS OF; FINGER, JOINT REPLACEMENT; JOINT; LOOSE BODIES; *and* MOVEMENT. *See also* CERVICAL OSTEOARTHRITIS *for more on types of osteoarthritis.*

Osteochondritis Dissecans

Degeneration that causes bone and cartilage fragments to break free from the bone.

Osteochondritis dissecans usually sets in during adolescence, often affecting the knee. Its cause is unknown, though it may relate to injuries around small blood vessels beneath the joint, causing part of the surface of the joint to die and fragment. The bone and cartilage pieces (also known as loose bodies) occasionally reattach, but often float free in the joint.

Symptoms and Treatment. Symptoms of osteochondritis dissecans include pain and swelling; loose bodies may also get caught in the joint, causing it to lock. If such a bone fragment is still partially attached, then the area may be immobilized in a cast while healing. If there is complete separation, arthroscopy may be needed to clear out the area. *See also* LOOSE BODIES.

Osteochondritis Juvenilis

A disorder characterized by an inflammation of a growing section of bone in a child or adolescent.

The precise cause of osteochondritis juvenilis is not known, but it may be caused by disruption in the supply of blood to the affected bone. Various bones in the body, including the femur (thigh bone), the vertebrae, and bones in the wrist and foot, may be affected by the condition.

Symptoms of osteochondritis juvenilis include pain and tenderness, pressure, inflammation, restricted movement (if the affected bone is part of a joint), softening of the bone, and possible deformity.

Treatment and Prognosis. Osteochondritis juvenilis is treated with a brace or cast to immobilize the area and minimize the risk of deformity. In rare cases, an operation is needed to take pressure off the bone. Deformities may be permanent and patients with the condition are more likely to develop osteoarthritis later in life.

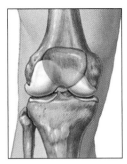

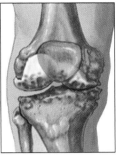

Osteoarthritis. Osteoarthritis is marked by loss of cartilage in the joints. Above, top, a normal knee joint. Above, bottom, a knee joint of a person with osteoarthritis. Note the wearing away of the cartilage and the spurring of the bone.

Osteochondroma

A nonmalignant bone tumor.

An osteochondroma is a bone tumor that consists of a stalk of bone covered with a cartilage cap. The tumor grows from the side of a bone, most often at the end of the long bones of the knee or shoulder. An osteochondroma usually begins to develop in the early adolescent years and grows until development of the skeleton is completed.

Incidence. Osteochondromas are the most common benign bone tumors. They occur most often in persons aged 10 to 20, who may develop one or many of the tumors. A tendency to have multiple osteochondromas can be genetic.

Treatment. In many cases, an osteochondroma causes no problems other than its effect on the patient's appearance. Surgery may be necessary for those osteochondromas that cause deformity of the skeleton or interfere with normal movement of tendons or a joint, however. *See also* BENIGN; BONE; BONE CANCER; BONE TUMORS; *and* TUMOR.

Osteodystrophy

Term that describes bone defects caused by body chemistry disorders.

The suffix "-dystrophy" refers to disorders caused by a lack of nutrients to a cell or structure. This leads to an interruption in growth and activity. Osteodystrophy, therefore, describes bones that are weak, soft, or stunted due to inadequate nutrition. An example of osteodystrophy is rickets, where a child's bones are deformed because of a lack of vitamin D, a condition called osteomalacia in adults. Osteoporosis is considered an osteodystrophy when caused by a chemical disorder such as Cushing's syndrome or an overdose of corticosteroids.

When the disorder that causes the lack of nutrition is treated, osteodystrophy is resolved. *See also* BONE, DISORDERS OF; CUSHING'S SYNDROME; DYSTROPHY; OSTEOMALACIA; *and* RICKETS.

Osteogenesis Imperfecta

Disorder in which the bones are unusually fragile.

Infants with osteogenesis imperfecta are usually born with several broken bones. In infants with this condition, the skull is so soft that the birth experience alone may result in trauma to the head and bleeding in the brain. It is not uncommon for children with this disorder to die suddenly within days or weeks after birth. While most children survive, they experience deformities and stunted growth due to multiple fractures. Mental development is normal, provided there is no trauma to the brain. *See also* BONE *and* BONE DISORDERS.

Osteoid Osteoma

Pain caused by an abnormal area of bone.

An osteoid osteoma is a benign tumor of the bone, about 0.2 inch, that causes deep pain. It usually affects long bones, such as the arm, leg, or spine, and is most often seen in children between the ages of five and 20. If the tumor is located on one side of the spine, scoliosis, a curvature of the spine, may result. The only way to diagnose the condition is with an x-ray. The pain, which often worsens at night, can be decreased with aspirin. Surgical removal of the affected bone area will alleviate the condition. *See also* BONE *and* BONE CANCER.

Osteoma

A nonmalignant bone tumor.

Osteomas may arise on any bone, and are generally slow-growing masses. An osteoma usually is small and harmless, but can cause troublesome symptoms if it presses against neighboring tissues. One common type is an osteoid osteoma, found in adolescents or young adults and diagnosed by x-ray. The pain usually can be relieved by aspirin alone, but surgical removal of the affected region is sometimes necessary. *See also* BONE DISORDERS *and* BONE TUMORS.

Osteomyelitis

A bacterial infection of the bone.

Bones can be infected by pathogens (disease-causing agents) in the bloodstream, by direct introduction of bacteria into the bone marrow during surgery or an accident, or by a transfer of pathogens from body tissues located adjacent to the bone. In patients with osteomyelitis, the body reacts to the infection by producing pockets of pus in the bone marrow. These pockets compress the blood capillaries in the marrow against the surrounding bone and press on the nerve endings, resulting in a considerable amount of pain.

Cause and Symptoms. The usual cause of osteomyelitis is the staphylococcus bacterium, which can then spread via the bloodstream to infect other organs of the body. Symptoms of osteomyelitis include pain and swelling of the affected bone, chills, and fever. In children, the disease usually attacks the ends of the leg and arm bones. In adults, the vertebrae are more likely to be affected. People undergoing kidney dialysis or those using intravenous drugs are most vulnerable to vertebrae staphylococcus infection.

Treatment. Osteomyelitis is generally treated with antibiotics. Treatment must sometimes continue for months to be successful. Abscesses in the bones may need to be drained surgically. If the disease is left untreated, or if it is treated with an ineffective antibiotic, bone can actually be destroyed. This may lead to chronic osteomyelitis, which is incurable and can produce painful symptoms for years. If osteomyelitis becomes chronic, the only effective treatment is to surgically remove the dead bone, amputating some or all of the affected limb.

> *Background material on osteomyelitis can be found in* BONE, DISORDERS OF *and* ORTHOPEDICS. *For further information, see* BACTERIA; BONE MARROW; IMMUNE RESPONSE; INFECTIOUS DISEASE; INFLAMMATION; PUS; *and* SURGERY. *See also* BLOOD POISONING *and* SEPSIS *for more on infections of the blood by bacteria.*

Osteopathic Medicine

A branch of medicine based on the idea that an individual's health can be restored through the manipulation of the skeleton and muscles.

Osteopathic medicine is a form of therapy that stresses the interrelatedness of the body's structures, organs, and systems. It aims to release tension, alleviate pain, and improve the overall functioning of the body by manipulating the bones, muscles, ligaments, and connective tissue. Osteopathic medicine has proven particularly useful for the treatment of a number of musculoskeletal disorders.

In the late 19th century, Andrew Taylor Still, an engineer and physician, developed the basic principles of osteopathy. Still's philosophy of medicine was based on the Greek notion that the condition of the musculoskeletal system is essential to an individual's overall health. Still deviated from the traditional practice of medicine in advocating the therapeutic and curative effects of osteopathic manipulative treatment. In 1892 he founded the American School of Osteopathy; in 1896, Vermont became the first state to license osteopathic physicians.

DIAGNOSIS

A practitioner of osteopathic medicine (referred to as a D.O., or Doctor of Osteopathy) will begin diagnosing the patient by asking the client a number of questions about his or her condition. The D.O. will evaluate the condition of the spine, hips, and legs and the mobility of the joints and connective tissue in what is known as active movement testing. During passive movement testing the practitioner will feel the body's response while sitting, standing, and walking to determine any tension or obstruction to the movement. X-rays are also used when necessary.

TREATMENT

The aim of osteopathic treatment is to correct the musculoskeletal dysfunction (if possible) in order to enable the body to

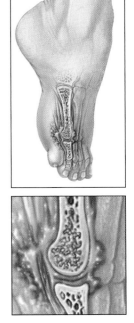

Osteomyelitis.
Osteomyelitis is an infection of the bone by bacteria. Above, top, an infected bone in the foot. Above, bottom, the bacteria attack the bone and pockets of pus are produced in the bone marrow, pressing on the surrounding nerve endings and causing pain.

heal itself. By manipulating the muscles, joints, and ligaments through a series of manual techniques, the D.O. attempts to return the body to a natural state of alignment. Diet and lifestyle changes may also be recommended. In some cases the D.O. may prescribe medication and even recommend surgical intervention.

The techniques used by an osteopath to treat the patient include:

• **Gentle Mobilization.** The joints are moved gently through their range of motion to free them from restrictions and increase circulation.

• **Articulation.** If joint motion or flexibility is restricted, a quick thrusting motion is applied. This technique is used especially for sports injuries; one such procedure, the McMurray maneuver, is used to replace the medial meniscus to the knee joint.

• **Release Assessment.** The patient is put in different positions to allow for muscle relaxation and assessment of healing following spasms or injury.

• **Muscle Energy.** Muscles are tensed and released to produce and evaluate muscle control and functioning.

• **Soft Tissue Manipulation.** Massage of deep tissues induces relaxation and releases impediments to muscle control.

CERTIFICATION

Osteopaths in the United States attend a medical college that grants its graduates degrees recognized by the medical community. These graduates are designated as D.O.s and may be granted admitting privileges in hospitals and practice medicine in any state in which they are licensed. Because a D.O. is trained and licensed as a physician, there is little risk that an osteopathic treatment would be used in place of another procedure necessary for recovery.

For background reading on osteopathic medicine, see ALTERNATIVE MEDICINE *and* BONE, DISORDERS OF. *Further information can be found in* BONE; JOINT; POSTURE; SPINAL CORD; *and* VERTEBRA. *See also* ACUPRESSURE; AYURVEDIC MEDICINE; *and* CHINESE MEDICINE *for more on other types of alternative medicine.*

Osteopetrosis

A hereditary disorder that increases the density of the bones and causes skeletal abnormalities.

Osteopetrosis literally means "marble bones." In this disorder, the body lacks a type of cell that prevents the bones from becoming too dense or large. There are a number of different osteopetroses of varying severity. Some forms of osteopetrosis may have no symptoms, while others may result in abnormal growth, anemia, and a greater likelihood of fractures. The most severe types are eventually fatal. Age of onset of the condition varies.

Treatment. There is no specific treatment for any osteopetrosis, although surgery can relieve related pressure on nerves or the brain. *See also* BONE DISORDERS.

Osteophyte

Also known as a bone spur

Bone outgrowth at the margins of a joint.

As osteoarthritis progresses, the body may make attempts to replace the worn out cartilage. The bones may try to fill in the area by producing dense, misshapen outcroppings at the edges of the joint. New cartilage may attempt to grow there, but the result is a swollen, gnarled growth that can restrict joint movement in the area. *See also* BONE *and* OSTEOARTHRITIS.

Osteoporosis

Loss of bone density, leading to bone weakness.

Osteoporosis is a condition marked by porous bones. Although we tend to think of the bones as pieces of solid, unchanging material, they are a constantly evolving organ. Every day, cells called osteoclasts break down bone, and osteoblasts then rebuild it. The processes keep pace with each other until about age 35, when the rebuilding slows, causing the bones to lose density. Resultant weakness can cause a loss of balance. Falls that might otherwise have been minor may now cause fractures. Posture is affected as the bones of the vertebrae begin to collapse.

TYPES

Osteoporosis falls into three categories.

Post-menopausal osteoporosis is caused by the loss of the reproductive hormone estrogen, which helps the body absorb calcium. This, of course, occurs more often in women, but men can develop this type of condition if they already have a hormonal deficiency.

Senile osteoporosis affects both men and women and is the result of the bone loss that can naturally occur with age.

Secondary osteoporosis is loss of bone density caused by an underlying condition, such as chronic renal (kidney) disease, hyperthyroidism (an overactive thyroid), some types of cancer, or partial gastrectomy (stomach removal).

CAUSES

Biological changes such as the loss of estrogen and the slow-down of the bone rebuilding process are common causes of osteoporosis. Other factors, however, such as lack of calcium in the diet, lack of exercise, smoking, and infrequent menstruation, can all contribute to lack of bone density. A diet too high in protein can cause an excessive loss of calcium in the urine, and an unusual excess of exercise may cause the release of too much B endorphin, which suppresses estrogen circulation and calcium absorption. Family history is also correlated to a tendency for osteoporosis.

SYMPTOMS

The most obvious signs of osteoporosis are loss of height, or in more advanced cases, the appearance of a hump where the weakened spine has begun to curve. A less apparent sign is when a simple fall causes a fracture where there might have been no damage when the bones were rebuilding at a faster pace.

DIAGNOSIS

X-rays can detect a decrease in bone density. Blood or urine tests can show if there is an increased level of byproducts from bone breakdown in the body. However, these methods usually can only detect osteoporosis once it is well advanced. A test called bone densiometry can detect the early onset of osteoporosis, and should be administered if a person is at risk for osteoporosis. Susceptibility for osteoporosis can be determined if a bone density test is done at menopause, and then repeated during the next few years to determine if bones are weakening at an excessive rate.

TREATMENT

Estrogen supplements are considered to be one of the most effective ways to treat osteoporosis; they help the body absorb calcium more efficiently and keep the calcium in the body. Calcitonin, a hormone that conserves calcium in the body, can be administered through daily injections. Calcitrol, a form of vitamin D, also helps with calcium absorption.

> ## Calcium-Rich Foods
>
> Most women require 1200 to 1500 milligrams of calcium a day. Many people are aware that dairy products contain calcium, however, certain non-dairy products, such as broccoli, are also excellent sources of calcium. Other calcium-rich, non-dairy foods include: seafood, including fish, shellfish, oysters, shrimp, salmon, and sardines; soy products, including soybeans and tofu; collard greens; navy beans; turnips; and calcium-enriched products, such as bread and orange juice.

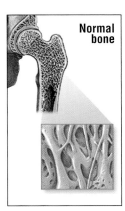

Normal bone

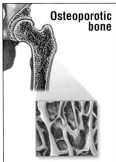

Osteoporotic bone

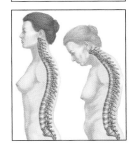

Osteoporosis. Osteoporosis is marked by the loss of bone density. Above, top, a normal bone can withstand some amount of force without breaking. Second from the top, an osteoporotic bone is porous and thus more vulnerable to fractures. At bottom, the posture of individuals with osteoporosis is poor, as the vertebrae deteriorate and are not able to support the body.

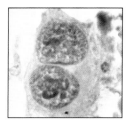

Osteosarcoma.
Osteosarcomas are the most common type of bone tumor found in children. Above, osteosarcoma cells taken from a tumor in the leg and magnified 400 times.

Resources on Osteoporosis
Bonnick, Sydney Lou, *The Osteoporosis Handbook: Every Woman's Guide to Prevention and Treatment* (2001); Costill, David L., *Inside Running: Basics of Sports Physiology* (1986); McArdle, William D., et al., *Exercise Physiology: Energy, Nutrition, and Human Performance* (1996); Vliet, Elizabeth Lee, *Women, Weight and Hormones* (2001); American Physical Therapy Association, Tel. (800) 999-APTA, Online: www.apta.org; National Osteoporosis Foundation, Tel. (800) 223-9994, Online: www.nof.org; President's Council on Physical Fitness and Sports, Tel. (202) 690-9000, Online: www.fitness.gov; Women's Sports Foundation, Tel. (800) 227-3988, Online: www.lifetimetv.com/WoSport; https://public1.med.cornell.edu/cgibin/orthopedics.

PREVENTION

There are ways to decrease the likelihood of developing osteoporosis. Eating a balanced diet with an adequate amount of calcium-rich foods is one of the simplest measures. There are over-the-counter calcium supplements available, but the body absorbs calcium from food more easily. Too much calcium can also be a problem, so the balance between dietary and supplement calcium intake should be carefully evaluated. Avoiding alcohol and cigarettes can also decrease the risk of osteoporosis. Alcohol is toxic to the cells that rebuild bones, and smokers tend to experience menopause earlier, which lessens their years of estrogen production.

THE PLACE OF EXERCISE. Exercise increases bone density. A good mix of aerobics and weight training makes the bones, and the muscles around them, stronger. It is important to keep in mind that it is never too late to begin an exercise program, and studies have shown that weight training can dramatically decrease the frequency of fractures in the elderly. A doctor or exercise professional should always be consulted before an exercise program is started. These professionals can help plan out an effective routine.

Background material on osteoporosis can be found in AGING; BONE, DISORDERS OF; *and* ORTHOPEDICS. *For further information, see* BONE IMAGING; CALCIUM; DIET AND DISEASE; MENOPAUSE; NUTRITION; NUTRITIONAL DISORDERS; *and* VITAMIN SUPPLEMENTS. *See also* FRACTURE *for more on the consequences of untreated osteoporosis.*

Osteosarcoma

A malignant tumor of the bone.

Osteosarcomas generally arise in the long bones of the arm or leg, or around the knee, hip, or shoulder joint. The cancer often invades neighboring tissues, either through the bone marrow or through colonies of cancerous cells that travel through the bloodstream to other parts of the body, most often the lungs.

Incidence and Symptoms. Osteosarcomas occur most often in young adults and the elderly. They are the most common bone tumor found in children. Although cases of the condition in the elderly are associated with Paget's disease, the cause of osteosarcomas in young adults is not fully understood. As an osteosarcoma grows, it distorts the bone, causing a lump that is often painful and accompanied by stiffness or tenderness. The bone becomes weakened, so it is easily fractured. This type of bone tumor can occur in any bone, but is most commonly found in the leg.

DIAGNOSIS AND TREATMENT

Diagnosis of an osteosarcoma is made by x-ray examination, computerized tomography, or magnetic resonance imaging scans and examination of a tissue sample.

Treatment for osteosarcomas starts with the surgical elimination of the cancer from the body, which often involves the removal of the entire bone. This might require the complete amputation of the affected limb or limbs. In many cases, a removed section of bone can be replaced by a metal prosthesis or bone graft. Surgery is usually followed by several months of chemotherapy aimed at eliminating the spread of cancerous colonies to other parts of the body. With treatment, an early stage cancer of this type is considered curable in 50 percent of cases. *See also* BONE CANCER; BONE TUMORS; CANCER; CHEMOTHERAPY; *and* PAGET'S DISEASE.

Osteosclerosis

Increase of bone thickness.

Osteosclerosis may occur for a number of reasons. An injury may cause the bone to grow overly dense in an area. Osteomyelitis can lead to increased density in the healthy bones surrounding the affected area. An benign bone tumor (osteoma) can result in a thick outgrowth of bone tissue. Most cases of osteosclerosis just affect one area of bone, but the disorder can also occur throughout the body, as in the case of a disease like osteopetrosis. *See also* OSTEOMA; OSTEOMYELITIS; *and* OSTEOPETROSIS.

Osteotomy

Surgical technique in which a bone is cut through.

Osteotomy is a surgical technique in which a bone is cut through (transected), allowing it to be repositioned. There are many applications and the procedure can be used on most bones in the body. Fractures may be reset, limbs either lengthened or shortened, and bent or bowed legs corrected. Osteotomies can be performed on even the tiniest bones, such as those of the middle-ear.

Osteotomy is commonly used in hip surgery, particularly for treating osteoarthritis of the hip. In this type of surgery, the surgeon alters the position of the thighbone. A recent technique known as Ganz osteotomy restores the hip socket using the patient's own bone and cartilage lining the hip joint.

In maxillofacial and craniofacial surgery, often used to alter the appearance of the face, replacement or repositioning of bones is often accomplished through osteotomy. Using a horizontal cut made through the jaw bone (mandible) with a bone saw or chisel, a surgeon moves the lower portion of the separated bone forward to the desired position. The surgeon is also careful to protect the facial nerves. The bone is then wired in place, the incision closed with sutures, and an external dressing applied. *See also* ARTHRITIS; COSMETIC SURGERY; HIP REPLACEMENT; JAW; MANDIBULAR ORTHOPEDIC REPOSITIONING; *and* MAXILLA.

Otitis Externa

Infection of the outer-ear.

The outer-ear (pinna) is a crescent-shaped piece of cartilage that collects sound waves and sends them through the outer ear canal to the eardrum. The eardrum then passes them on to the middle ear in the form of mechanical energy. Otitis externa is an infection, specifically located in the outer-ear canal.

Causes. The most common cause of otitis externa is water or moisture in the outer ear canal that allows bacteria or fungi to form and grow. Otitis externa is often referred to as swimmer's ear, because frequent swimmers are prone to the condition; water that flows into their ears while swimming may not always empty out, remaining in the outer ear-canal. The warm, dark, moist environment becomes a perfect place for bacteria to grow. Even those who are not swimmers may find themselves vulnerable to otitis externa, especially during the summer months, when heat and humidity in the atmosphere along with perspiration allow moisture to accumulate in the ear canal. Less commonly, otitis externa may be caused by eczema (skin inflammation).

Symptoms. The earliest symptoms of otitis externa are itching and pain in the ear. Scratching the ear may exacerbate the problem, however, as bacteria on the fingers can then enter the ear and worsen the infection. Itchiness, redness, muffled hearing, and a discharge from the ear may also result from the infection.

Treatment. The first part of treating otitis externa is to clean and dry the ear. Topical medications can then be applied. Antibiotics may be necessary to clear up bacerial infections. Corticosteroids can help to reduce inflammation and stop the urge to itch, which irritates the ear more. Fungal infections should respond to sulfanilamide powder and antifungal drops. With both types of infections, the most important part of treatment is to keep the ear clean and dry.

Prevention. To prevent otitis externa, the ear canal should be emptied after swimming. Each ear should be rested on a towel, and tugged gently to empty excess water. There are also over-the-counter drying ear drops that help remove moisture from the ear canal; a home version is to make a solution of equal parts vinegar and rubbing alcohol. A hair dryer on the lowest setting directed at the ear can also help to completely dry the ear. *See also* EAR; EARACHE; *and* EAR, DISORDERS OF.

Otitis Media

An infection in the middle-ear.

The middle-ear, which carries sound waves from the outer-ear to the inner-ear, is connected to the nose and throat passages by an airway called the Eustachian tube. This tube usually helps maintain equal air pressure between the air outside and inside the ear. When an infection or irritation is present, however, the Eustachian tube can become inflamed and constricted. Meanwhile, the mucous membranes that line the middle-ear produce more fluid, which accumulates and presses against the eardrum, causing the pain and pressure commonly referred to as an earache. The pressure may become so strong that it bursts the eardrum.

CAUSES

There are two main causes of otitis media; bacteria and viruses.

Bacteria. Bacterial infections are the most common cause of otitis media. Bacteria in the nose and throat can not only lead to inflammation in those areas, but infect the fluid in the ear as well, producing pus in the middle-ear.

Viruses. Flu, colds, and other upper respiratory tract infections inflame the Eustachian tube and encourage overproduction of mucous membrane. The fluid from viral infections is usually uninfected, but bacteria from the nose and throat can then infect it.

Other causes of otitis media include smoking and drinking alcohol, which can irritate and inflame throat and nasal passages. Severe allergies may cause some forms of earache, but this is fairly rare.

SYMPTOMS

The most common symptom of otitis media is an earache, and earaches are most commonly accompanied by pain and pressure in the ear. There may be some loss of hearing and a feeling of dizziness. Signs of an earache in very young children include irritability and pulling on the ear.

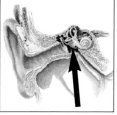

Otitis Media.
Otitis media is an infection of the middle ear, which is marked by an arrow in the image above. Causes of otitis media include bacteria and viruses.

TREATMENT

The most common forms of treatment for otitis media are antibiotics, to clear up infection, and painkillers. However, there is currently a great deal of concern about overmedication of young children. Stronger, earlier, and more frequent usage of antibiotics to treat infections in young children may be leading to the development of bacteria that are resistant to antibiotics. Countries that have cut back on early antibiotic use are showing success in lowering the number of resistant bacteria. There is also some question as to whether antibiotics are even effective or useful in treating otitis media. Recent studies have shown that up to 80 percent of ear infections may resolve on their own, which is close to the 95 percent cure rate from antibiotics. In less severe cases, over-the-counter painkillers may be recommended instead of prescription medications, while allowing the infection to run its course. If it persists, or if there is a risk of long-term damage to the ear, antibiotics are then prescribed.

For background information on otitis media, see EAR; EARACHE; *and* EAR, DISORDERS OF. *Related material can be found in* HEARING; OTORHINOLARYNGOLOGY; PEDIATRICS; *and* RESPIRATORY TRACT INFECTION. *See also* BALANCE *for more on symptoms of otitis media.*

Otoplasty

Plastic surgery performed on the external ears, usually to flatten protruding ears, but also to reform a missing or damaged external ear.

To flatten protruding ears, a surgeon makes incisions in the back of each ear, exposes the cartilage, creates a more pronounced fold inward in the central part (antihelix or anthelix) of the outer-ear (pinna), and may further sculpt the cartilage. The incision is then sutured, and the ear is bandaged. The operation, which may be as long as two hours in duration, may be performed under a local anesthetic, though a general anesthetic is recommended for children.

To form a missing or damaged ear, a

surgeon uses rib cartilage and possibly a skin graft to shape and set in place a normal-looking external ear, which may take several operations.

Ideally, otoplasty should be performed on a child after the age of four, when ear growth is near complete but the cartilage is still soft, making surgery and recovery easier. The child usually has to wear a ski-type headband for two to four weeks, especially while sleeping, to protect the ears. *See also* COSMETIC SURGERY.

Otorhinolaryngology

Medical specialty that deals with disorders of the ear, nose, and throat.

Otorhinolaryngology is the branch of medicine that is responsible for diseases of the closely connected ears, nose, and throat. Each of these areas are related to each other, and in many cases an infection, disorder, or injury in one of these areas can affect the other areas as well. The ears, nose, and throat act as one continuous plumbing system for the head; fluid from the ears drains into the throat, as do secretions from the nose and sinuses.

Probably the most common example of the interconnectivity of the ear, nose, and throat is a simple viral infection, such as the common cold. The cold will infect the upper respiratory tract, causing the mucous membranes in the tract to become inflamed. The swollen nasal passages then cause blockage in the sinuses. Fluid buildup in these cavities allows bacteria to thrive, so even after the cold has passed, sinusitis (bacterial infection of the sinuses) may linger. Meanwhile, the cold may also have caused inflammation in the cavities of the ear, blocking the route by which fluid from the mucous membranes in the ear drains. Bacteria can then accumulate in the ear, causing an ear infection. Otorhinolaryngologists, work to understand all three of these related areas of the body, and to prevent the spread of disease from one of these areas to another. *See also* EAR; NOSE; *and* THROAT.

Otosclerosis

Hearing loss caused by bone growth in the ear.

The stirrup is a tiny bone that is part of the chain that sends sound waves into the inner-ear. Sound vibrations from the eardrum travel across bones called the hammer, then to the anvil. The anvil then sends the vibrations to the stirrup, which connects to the inner-ear. Otosclerosis is a condition in which a spongy type of bone tissue grows around the stirrup, fixing it in place and preventing the sound vibrations from getting to the inner-ear. The result is a progressive loss of hearing.

Cause. There is no known cause for otosclerosis. It seems to affect women more often than men; it tends to strike in young adulthood, often during pregnancy.

Treatment usually consists of either a stapedotomy, an operation in which a small opening is made in the inner-ear to allow the sound to bypass the stirrup and the growth around it, or a stapedectomy, in which the defective stirrup and growth are removed and replaced with an artificial bone. *See also* BONE, DISORDERS OF; EAR; EAR, DISORDERS OF; *and* HEARING LOSS.

Otoscope

A diagnostic device used to examine the ear.

An otoscope is a simple device used for looking into the canal and eardrum of the ear. It may be used to locate foreign objects in the ear canal, identify accumulations of wax in the ear, and examine the eardrum for a variety of ailments or abnormalities.

An otoscope may be used to identify perforation of the eardrum, infection by cysts, or increased ear pressure associated with flying or diving (barotrauma). This common ailment is diagnosed by observing the retraction of the eardrum during otoscopy. In more severe cases, blood is seen behind the eardrum.

The otoscope is painless and safe. In addition to its use as a standard part of a physical exam, the otoscope is often used to

Resources on Otorhinolaryngology

Benjamin, Bruce, et al., *A Colour Atlas of Otorhinolaryngology* (1995); Cody, Thane, *Diseases of the Ears, Nose, and Throat* (1981); Morelock, Michael, *Your Guide to Problems of the Ear, Nose, and Throat* (1985); American Hearing Research Foundation, Tel. (312) 726-9670, Online: www.american-hearing.org; American Speech-Language-Hearing Association, Tel. (800) 638-8255, Online: www.asha.org; American Academy of Otolaryngology, Tel. (703) 519-1585, Online: www.entnet.org; www.nycornell.org/ent/.

rule out blockages and obstructions as a cause of observed hearing loss.

Abnormalities of the inner-ear require more sophisticated testing than that which can be accomplished with an otoscope. Hearing loss from a variety of causes may be assessed through an audiology exam, which uses tones of varying frequency and volume to test hearing. Usually, this is performed after the otorhinolaryngologist (ear, nose, and throat doctor) has used an otoscope to rule out inflammation or blockage as the source of hearing deficit. *See also* EAR; EAR, DISORDERS OF; HEARING TESTS; *and* OTORHINOLARYNGOLOGY.

Ototoxicity

Loss of hearing due to a reaction to medication.

Certain types of drugs are known to occasionally affect the hearing. The most common culprits are non-steroidal anti-inflammatory drugs, such as aspirin. Other ototoxic drugs include quinine, diuretics, and aminoglycoside antibiotics, such as streptomycin and chloramphenicol. Some anticancer drugs, such as antineoplastics, may also cause hearing loss.

Drug-induced hearing loss actually results from a toxic reaction of the nerves in the ear to the drug. Ototoxicity is not uncommon; about ten percent of all people taking aminoglycoside antibiotics may be affected. However, those who already have experienced some form of hearing loss, who have kidney disease or who are taking several ototoxic drugs are more likely to experience the condition. In these cases, regular hearing and blood tests should be administered in order to detect any hearing problems immediately.

Hearing loss due to ototoxicity is usually temporary, except when caused by aminoglycoside antibiotics, which may cause permanent loss of hearing in some individuals. For others, the hearing problems may be resolved if use of the drug is discontinued. *See also* ANTIBIOTIC DRUGS; ANTICANCER DRUGS; EAR; *and* NON-STEROIDAL ANTI-INFLAMMATORY DRUGS.

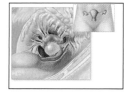

Ovarian Cyst.
Ovarian cysts are filled with fluid and are very common. Above, an artist's depiction of an ovarian cyst. This type of cyst is generally harmless, but may need to be removed surgically in rare cases.

Outpatient Treatment

Also known as ambulatory treatment

Medical care administered to patients who have not been admitted to a hospital.

Outpatient treatment is medical care that is given to people who are not confined to a hospital. Since these patients have not been admitted to a hospital, they are considered ambulatory, which literally means "able to walk about." *See also* HOSPITAL.

Ovarian Cyst

Abnormal fluid-filled sac in an ovary.

Ovarian cysts occur frequently, sometimes because of endometriosis or another medical condition, but often in the course of normal reproductive function.

Types. The most common type of ovarian cyst is a follicular cyst, in which the enlarged follicle that is supposed to release an egg at ovulation fails to rupture. The result is a fluid-filled sac on the surface of the ovary. Such a cyst usually subsides in a month or two, either on its own or with the help of treatment with oral contraceptives.

Another type of ovarian cyst is the dermoid cyst, which can occur after menopause and arises from deposits of cells that are left in the ovary in the earliest stage of fetal development and begin to multiply and spread.

Symptoms. Many ovarian cysts cause no symptoms and go away without treatment, but some can cause fever, vomiting, and sudden, severe pain that can be mistaken for appendicitis. A skipped, copious, or exceptionally painful menstruation can also be due to an ovarian cyst. Occasionally, cysts can become malignant.

Diagnosis. Ovarian cysts are diagnosed by a pelvic examination or by ultrasound scanning. Generally, they disappear without treatment. However, surgical removal of the cyst or the ovary may be necessary if symptoms are severe and chronic. *See also* AMENORRHEA; DYSMENORRHEA; ENDOMETRIOSIS; MENORRHAGIA; *and* OOPHORECTOMY.

Ovary

One of two glands located on either side of the uterus just below the opening of the fallopian tube.

Each ovary is shaped like an almond and is about 1.25 inch (30 mm) long and .75 inch (20 mm) wide. Ovaries contain many follicles (pockets) in which ovum (eggs) develop. The ovaries are also responsible for the production of the female sex hormones estrogen and progesterone. Disorders affecting the ovaries include abnormal development, inflammation (oophoritis), cysts, ovarian failure, and cancer. *See also* OVARY, CANCER OF.

Ovary, Cancer of

Malignant tumor of the ovary.

The ovary is the organ that serves two functions unique to females. The ovary produces the eggs that, when fertilized, develop into an embryo and eventually a baby. The organ also secretes the hormones necessary to the female reproductive cycle.

Cancer of the ovary is the fifth most common cancer in women. The mortality rate is high, probably because the lack of symptoms in its early stages results in diagnoses of the cancer only being made in advanced stages. Nearly 90 percent of ovarian cancer cases arise in the epithelium, the tissue lining the ovaries. The rest arise either in the egg-producing cells of the ovary or in its fibrous tissue.

Incidence. The incidence of ovarian cancer is high in women over the age of 50. A major risk factor is family history; a woman with a mother, daughter, or sister who has had ovarian cancer is at elevated risk. Having had one child reduces the chances of ovarian cancer by 30 to 60 percent, as does prior use of oral contraceptives, in each case because estrogen output is decreased. Each additional child reduces the risk for ovarian cancer by about 14 percent, and any pregnancy, whether or not it comes to term, also reduces the risk.

Recommendations For Women at High Risk

Three hereditary conditions that predispose a woman to ovarian cancer have been identified; genetic counseling is recommended for women with a first-degree relative (mother, daughter or sister) who has had this type of cancer. Tests recommended for women at high risk for ovarian cancer include periodic pelvic examinations, periodic transvaginal ultrasound tests, and blood tests to detect elevated levels of CA 125, a carbohydrate antigen that can indicate cancerous and benign tumors of the ovary.

Symptoms. As an ovarian cancer grows, it can cause abdominal pain and swelling due to accumulation of fluid, persistent indigestion and flatulence, loss of appetite, fatigue, a frequent urge to urinate, nausea, vomiting, and shortness of breath.

Diagnosis. Measures to diagnose cancer of the ovary include a pelvic examination in which the abdominal cavity is examined through a laryngoscope, blood tests for abnormal levels of ovary-related tumor markers, a pap smear, computerized tomography and magnetic resonance imaging scans, a urine test, and microscopic examination of tissue obtained by a laparotomy.

Treatment. If ovarian cancer is detected in its early stages, surgical removal of the affected ovary followed by chemotherapy and radiation therapy is often curative. If a woman is past child-bearing age, both ovaries may be removed. For women who want to bear a child and have one affected ovary, only that ovary may be removed. For ovarian cancers detected at a later stage, surgery will remove both ovaries, the fallopian tubes, and the uterus. Chemotherapy, administered either orally or directly into the abdominal cavity, follows surgery. For late-stage ovarian tumors, chemotherapy alone may be given to prolong survival, or chemotherapy may be used in conjunction with surgical removal of the tumor. The five-year survival rate for early stage ovarian cancer is as high as 90 percent, decreasing to 10 percent for cancers that have spread considerably before detection. *See also* CHEMOTHERAPY *and* RADIATION THERAPY.

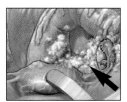

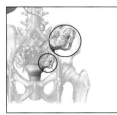

Ovarian Cancer.
Ovarian cancer is very hazardous because the ovaries are close to many other organs and the cancer can spread easily. Above, top, ovarian cancer cells are marked by an arrow. Above, bottom, cancerous cells can travel from the ovary to the lymph nodes and into other nearby organs.

Resources on Ovarian Cancer
Piver, M. Steven, *Myths & Facts About Ovarian Cance: What You Need to Know* (2000); Piver, M. Steven, and Gene Wilder, *Gilda's Disease: Sharing Personal Experiences and a Medical Perspective on Ovarian Cancer* (1998); Tilberis, Liz, *No Time to Die: Living With Ovarian Cancer* (1999); Ovarian Cancer National Alliance, Tel. (202) 331-1332, Online: www.ovariancancer.org/general/; American Cancer Society, Tel. (800) ACS-2345, Online: www.cancer.org; National Cancer Institue, Tel. (800) 4-CANCER, Online: www.nci.nih.gov; www.nycornell.org/medicine/hematology.html.

Overbite and Overjet

Overlapping of the upper and lower teeth.

Overbite refers to vertical overlap of the front teeth and overjet refers to horizontal overlap. When the overlap is too large then the front teeth are not able to function— bite and chew—as well as they should.

In a severe overbite, the top front teeth are too far in front of the bottom, and may even be called "buck teeth." An underbite is when the lower teeth are in front of the upper teeth.

Orthodontists, sometimes with the help of oral and maxillofacial surgeons, are able to treat these problems to create a healthy, functional, and pleasing bite and smile. *See also* ORAL AND MAXILLOFACIAL SURGERY.

Overcrowding, Dental

Lack of room for proper growth of teeth.

Overcrowding is the displacement of teeth by other teeth from normal positions of development. Typically, there are simply too many teeth to fit in a top or bottom jaw. Crowded teeth are harder to maintain and can be more prone to gum (periodontal) disease. Orthodontists correct dental crowding by moving the teeth into better alignment. Occasionally, it is necessary to remove a tooth or several teeth to create space into which other teeth are moved.

Overuse Injury

Muscle or bone injury caused by repetitive movement.

Overuse injuries are common in sports, but can also be the result of employment-related activity in jobs that call for repeated movements, such as those of musicians and assembly line workers. These injuries will often heal with rest and ice, and correcting faulty movement may prevent reoccurrence of the injury. *See also* EPICONDYLITIS, FRACTURES; GOLFER'S ELBOW; PERIOSTITIS; *and* TENDONITIS.

Ovulation

Release of an egg from a mature ovarian follicle.

The events leading up to ovulation begin in the hypothalamus, a structure in the brain that releases gonadotropin-releasing hormone (GnRH) into the blood vessels connecting to the pituitary gland. The pituitary, is then stimulated to release follicle-stimulating hormone (FSH) and leutenizing hormone (LH), which act on the ovary. Within the ovary, immature eggs are stored in fluid-filled sacs (follicles). FSH causes an egg to start maturing inside its follicle, which then grows.

FSH and LH also stimulate the follicle to release estrogen into the bloodstream. Estrogen affects the uterus, causing an increase in the blood supply and a thickening of the lining. The effects of FSH, LH, and estrogen build up slowly for about 14 days, although the amount of time is highly variable. Just before day 14 of the menstrual cycle, a sudden increase of LH from the pituitary gland causes the follicle to burst and release the egg into the abdominal cavity.

The egg is swept into the fallopian tube and travels to the uterus. The egg remains viable for about one day after ovulation. An encounter with viable sperm during this period will result in fertilization. *See also* CONCEPTION *and* OVARY.

Ovum

A mature egg cell.

During the third month of pregnancy, the ovaries of a female fetus contain millions of precursor cells, known as primary oocytes, which mature into secondary oocytes. Once the girl has reached puberty, a single secondary oocyte finishes its development and becomes an ovum approximately once a month. This mature egg cell is released at ovulation and travels through the fallopian tube to the uterus. The ovum is viable for only 24 hours. A meeting with viable sperm during this brief period will result in fertilization. *See also* CHROMOSOME.

Oxygen

Element present in air, necessary for respiration.

Oxygen is essential to every cell in the human body. Through the gas-exchange function of respiration—the inhalation and exhalation of gases—oxygen is drawn into the lungs and into the bloodstream. The oxygen enters the air sacs in the lungs (alveoli) and is dissolved into the bloodstream, where it binds to the hemoglobin in red blood cells and is then conveyed into cells throughout the body. The distribution of oxygen permits oxidation, a series of chemical reactions that enable the metabolism of food in order to release energy. Once oxygen has been used by a cell, the waste product carbon dioxide is released through exhalation.

> **ALERT**
>
> ## Oxygen Storage
>
> Oxygen is highly flammable. If supplemental oxygen is kept in the home, anything capable of producing flames, heat, or sparks, or any flammable material, including alcohol, should be kept away from the oxygen device.

Supplemental oxygen is often given to those who have markedly decreased levels of blood oxygen, primarily from chronic lung disease. Low blood oxygen levels put undue strain on the heart, since it must work harder to supply oxygen to the body's tissues. Supplemental oxygen must be prescribed by a doctor, as too much oxygen is also a risk. *See also* AIR *and* RESPIRATION.

Oxygen Therapy

The delivery of various forms of supplemental oxygen to cure disease and promote healing.

The body needs oxygen to survive. Oxygen is essential in the metabolism of food and the production of energy; body tissues that do not receive oxygen die within a matter of minutes.

For people whose breathing is seriously impaired or who are at very high altitudes, supplemental oxygen delivered through breathing tubes can maintain healthy functioning and prevent tissue damage.

Some other, less common, types of oxygen therapy include hyperbaric oxygen therapy, ozone therapy, and hydrogen peroxide therapy.

Hyperbaric oxygen therapy is a form of treatment in which a person is placed in a sealed chamber that is filled with pure oxygen at about twice the air pressure at sea level. Conventionally, hyperbaric oxygen therapy is used to treat:

- the bends—in deep sea diving, the formation of nitrogen bubbles in the blood as a result of rising too quickly;
- air embolisms—bubbles of air in an artery or vein that may block the flow of blood;
- carbon monoxide poisoning—carbon monoxide mimics oxygen in the body, entering red blood cells and preventing the delivery of oxygen to tissues;
- damage to tissues and blood vessels resulting from severe injury, burns, or radiation therapy for cancer; and
- bone infections.

Large amounts of oxygen at high pressure reduce the size of gas bubbles in the blood, quickly replace carbon monoxide in the body, provide oxygen to damaged tissues, and promote healing of damaged blood vessels and other tissues.

Complications of hyperbaric oxygen treatment may include seizures; pressure damage to the ear, lung, stomach, or other cavities; collapsed lung; air embolism; and, over the long term, cataracts. People with seizure disorders, emphysema, fluid build-up in the sinuses or other body cavities, or a history of collapsed lung should not be treated with hyperbaric oxygen therapy.

One of the greatest obstacles to hyperbaric oxygen treatment is its high cost and the limited availability of facilities.

Ozone and hydrogen peroxide therapy are both based around the theory that variant forms of oxygen (ozone is made up of three molecules of oxygen rather than two, and hydrogen peroxide is made of two molecules of hydrogen and two molecules of oxygen) break down quickly in the body and provide extra oxygen.

Both ozone and hydrogen peroxide are delivered in various ways. In ozone therapy, a common delivery system involves removing a pint of blood from the body, mixing it with ozone, and reinjecting it into the body. Hydrogen peroxide is often prescribed as a bath.

Neither ozone nor hydrogen peroxide therapy has been approved by the Food and Drug Administration (FDA) as a safe and effective treatment for any disease. Hydrogen peroxide, while safe in a very dilute three percent formula for cleaning minor cuts, has been determined to be unsafe for human use in concentrated form. *See also* ANTISEPTIC *and* OZONE.

Oxytocin

Hormone, secreted by the pituitary gland, which stimulates the uterus to contract during labor and the milk glands to provide milk after birth.

Release of oxytocin by the pituitary gland may be the precipitating factor in the beginning of labor. Oxytocin is used by physicians to induce labor when necessary. Usually, the drug is administered intravenously so that the effect can be monitored precisely. Oxytocin also induces the milk glands of the mother's breasts to release milk by contracting the small muscles in the breast. *See also* INDUCTION OF LABOR.

Ozena

Condition causing atrophy of the mucous membranes in the nose.

Rhinitis is an inflammation of the mucous membranes that line the nasal passages, and is most commonly associated with colds or allergies. Ozena is a very rare condition in which rhinitis causes these mucous membranes to waste away. This may result in a heavy nasal discharge that dries to a crust, and bad breath (halitosis). *See also* HALITOSIS *and* RHINITIS.

Ozone

Faintly blue gas made up of three bonded oxygen molecules; an essential part of the upper atmosphere and a respiratory irritant found in smog.

Ozone occurs naturally in the upper atmosphere and is a component of pollution in the lower atmosphere.

Upper Atmosphere. In the upper atmosphere, ozone blocks ultraviolet radiation from reaching the earth's surface. Recently, the ozone layer in the upper atmosphere has been thinning, either as a result of pollution, primarily from CFCs (chlorofluorocarbons), as a result of an unknown natural cycle or process, or both. Because of the reduced level of ozone in the upper atmosphere, greater amounts of harmful ultraviolet radiation reach the surface of the earth, resulting in a greater incidence of skin cancer and cataracts.

Lower Atmosphere. In the lower atmosphere, ozone is a respiratory irritant found in smog. Its effects vary, although it aggravates existing symptoms in those with lung diseases, such as asthma, emphysema, and bronchitis. People with such diseases, as well as young children, should avoid exposure to ozone if possible. Low levels of ozone in the air can cause symptoms, such as coughing during exercise. When higher amounts of ozone are present, chest pain, nausea, painful deep breaths, and shortness of breath can occur, persisting for several hours after exposure.

Background material on ozone can be found in AIR *and* POLLUTION. *For further reading, see* ASTHMA *and* BREATHING DIFFICULTY. *See also* CARBON MONOXIDE *for more on other kinds of pollutants.*

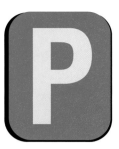

Pacemaker

A device, implanted under the skin, that can maintain normal heart rhythm by administering an electric impulse.

Some pacemakers regulate only the ventricles, and others regulate only the atria, while dual-chamber pacemakers serve both chambers. Conditions that require a pacemaker include atrioventricular block and sinus node dysfunction.

A pacemaker contains a power source about the size of a silver dollar that includes a battery, circuits to control activity, and wires called leads, which connect the power source to the chamber or chambers of the heart. Pacemaker implantation is a minor surgery done under local anesthesia requiring only a brief hospital stay.

The lithium batteries used in pacemakers can last up to ten years, and their replacement only requires a minor, local surgical procedure. Most pacemakers are programmable, meaning that after implantation, the pacemaker can be adjusted noninvasively with electrical signals transmitted through the skin. Pacemakers must be checked periodically, every six months, a procedure that sometimes can be done by telephone. *See also* HEART DISEASE.

Paget's Disease

An incurable form of bone cancer that often occurs in the elderly.

About one in twenty adults over the age of 75 suffers from this disease. It is characterized by abnormal bone development in which the affected bones are softer, more easily broken, and may tend to be deformed. Researchers believe the disorder may be genetically inherited and tends to affect more men than women. Also called osteitis deformans, Paget's disease most commonly affects the skull, leg, spine or pelvis but can also attack the bones in the middle ear causing deafness. The cause is unknown although it may be triggered by a viral infection.

Symptoms include joint pain in the hip or lower back, headaches, and tinnitus (ringing in the ear). Often, there are no early stage symptoms. In some cases, enlargement or changes to the skull may alter the bones of the face (producing a lion-like appearance). Diagnosis is commonly made through the use of x-rays and then confirmed by a bone biopsy.

Treatment. Pain associated with Paget's disease is usually treated with nonsteroidal, anti-inflammatory medications. Drugs for more advanced cases include the hormone calcitonin—to restore normal bone growth—and biophosphonates, to slow the progress of the attack. In the most severe cases, abnormal bones can be removed or restructured with bone transplants. If the disease attacks a hip or knee joint, the joint can be replaced. There is no known cure for this disease. *See also* BONE CANCER.

Pain

Unpleasant sensation alerting the sufferer that part of the body is injured or diseased.

Pain is produced by the stimulation of specialized nerve cells, pain receptors, in response to injury or disease. Pain is frequently localized and can range from mild to severe. Pain receptors are dispersed throughout the body; they transmit electrical nerve impulses along the nerves to the spinal cord and brain. The pain receptors may produce a reflex response in the spinal cord that sends an immediate signal back to the motor nerves to the point of pain, instructing them to contract. This is the type of reflex reaction that occurs when a person puts his or her hand on a hot stove. Such pain signals are also transmitted to the brain. At that moment, the person becomes conscious of the pain.

Throughout the body, there are different sorts of pain receptors; skin cells, for example, have pain receptors that are precise and can give accurate information in pinpointing the location and type of injury. The sense of pain as a result of a knife or gunshot wound is distinct from that which

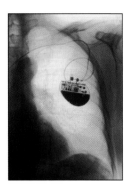

Pacemaker. This x-ray is of a person with an implanted pacemaker. The device is used to regulate a normal heart beat rate in individuals with dangerously slow and irregular heartbeat rates. Implantation does not require open heart surgery, and is performed under mild sedation and local anesthetic. A two-inch incision is made just below the collar bone, where the pace generator is surgically placed and the pace wires are inserted into a vein connecting to the heart.

is produced by intense cold, heat, or pressure. Intestinal pain, however, is more generalized. Thus it is difficult to determine the exact location of the injury or disease.

The ability to withstand pain, or the pain threshold, varies from person to person. There are also emotional factors involved. In general, the elderly protest less about pain than their younger counterparts. Having experienced physical suffering allows one to view it less traumatically.

Types. There are many different types of pain. Acute pain is experienced during childbirth or a scratched cornea. Chronic pain may linger for weeks after a serious infection or injury as a result of pain receptors that continue to transmit pain messages through the nervous system.

A referred pain is pain that is felt in a spot other than that of the disease or injury site. The sensory nerves converge and transmit confusing messages to the brain. Angina is one example, as it is pain caused by a reduction in blood flow to the heart which is often felt in the left shoulder.

The three most common forms of pain are:

- headache pain—40 million Americans suffer from headaches;
- lower back pain—15 percent of American adults suffer from lower back pain;
- arthritis pain—it affects about 20 million Americans.

Neuropathic Pain is the result of an abnormality occurring anywhere in the nerve pathway. The pain can be described as a deep ache or burning sensation. Shingles (or herpes zoster) is an example of an inflammatory infection, posttherapeutic neuralgia, that produces chronic neuropathic pain. Reflex sympathetic dystrophy is a type of neuropathic pain that is accompanied by swelling, sweating, and changes in blood flow and tissues, for example, atrophy or osteoporosis. A similar syndrome, named causalgia, may accompany a nerve injury.

Pain after surgery is commonplace. Pain that accompanies surgery can be constant or periodic, intensifying when the patient inhales deeply, moves, or laughs. Opiate analgesics are usually prescribed to relieve the pain. Cancer pain is either caused by an expanding tumor growing into the bones or nerves, or the result of radiation therapy. Physicians can prescribe medication, such as anti-inflammatory drugs or if needed, opiate drugs to alleviate the pain.

Treatment. In general, surgery should always be thought of as a last result. A surgical procedure that severs the nerve endings can be effective in reducing pain. However, surgery can also destroy other sensations as well. The most common procedure aimed at reducing pain is cordotomy, which is the severing of the nerve fibers on one or both sides of the spinal cord that travel to the brain. Cordotomy affects the sense of temperature as well as pain. Likewise, surgeons sometimes can relieve pain by severing nerve fibers outside the brain or spinal cord.

> *Background material on pain may be found in* Nerve; Nerve Injury; Nervous System; *and* Sensation. *Further information on treatment may be found in* Analgesic Drugs; Anesthesia; Cordotomy; *and* Pain Relief.

Pain Relief

Treatment of pain, especially with medication.

Pain relievers can be divided into various categories. Analgesics and anti-inflammatory drugs are sold over-the-counter; these include medications such as aspirin, ibuprofen, and acetaminophen. They are all safe for the short-term relief of minor aches and pains; most pain relievers should not be taken for more than ten days.

Narcotic Analgesics are opium-based. These are reserved for the treatment of intense pain. A narcotic drug is not used to treat chronic pain caused by cancer, head injury, or liver damage. Opiate-related compounds such as codeine, propoxy-phene (Darvon), morphine, and meperidine (Demerol) are much stronger than aspirin. These, like all drugs, have a potential for abuse, and may have unpleasant or harmful side effects. They should never be combined with other medicines or alcohol.

Resources on Pain

Cottrell, James E. and Stephanie Golden, *Under the Mask: A Guide to Feeling Secure and Comfortable During Anesthesia and Surgery* (2001); Kandel, Eric R., et al., *Principles of Neural Science* (1991); Rapoport, Alan M., and Fred Sheftell, *Headache Relief* (1991); American Academy of Neurology, Tel. (651) 695-1940, Online: www.aan.com; American Board of Neurological Surgery, Tel. (713) 790-6015, Online: www.abns.org;www.med.cornell.edu/neuro.

Certain antidepressants as well as antiepileptic drugs are used to treat several particularly severe pain conditions, notably the pain arising from shingles and facial neuralgias like tic douloureux. Researchers think that the antidepressant works because it increases the supply of the neurotransmitter, serotonin. A decrease in the amount of serotonin in the body is connected with depression.

Antiepileptic drugs have successfully been used to treat tic douloureux, a condition marked by attacks of facial pain that affects older adults by restoring the proper balance of incoming and outgoing nerve signals. Tic and other facial pains or neuralgias are often the result of injury to facial nerves when normal transmission of messages to and from the brain is hindered; this causes the nervous system to become hypersensitive. Antiepileptic drugs are effective in calming the excessive brain discharges associated with epileptic seizures.

Some non-drug treatments include: massage, ice packs, or heating pads as these may relieve localized pain that is associated with injury, muscle spasm, or inflammation. *See also* ANALGESIC DRUGS; ANTIDEPRESSANT DRUGS; AND OPIATES.

Painful Arc Syndrome

A disorder in which the sufferer's arm can not be raised between 45 and 160 degrees laterally.

While the person suffering from painful arc syndrome will experience pain within a certain range of motion, elevation of the arm to an angle outside of the 45-160° range usually can be performed without experiencing any painful side effects. Painful arc syndrome is caused by an inflammation of the bursae and tendons that are being pressed between the upper section of the shoulder blade, the scapula, and the upper bone of the arm (the humerus). The bursae are fluid-filled sacs that lie between the tendons or ligaments and the bone, whose sole capacity is to prevent the bone and tendon or ligament from rubbing against one another. *See also* BURSITIS.

Palpitation

A feeling that the heart beat is irregular, unusually strong or very rapid.

A palpitation can be felt after strenuous physical activity or in tense situations. Sometimes it is a product of the imagination, as the heart appears to skip a beat, jump, or race. A person who is overly concerned about the heart may feel palpitations when there is no underlying problem, while someone with a heart condition may be so accustomed to disturbances of the heart beat that no palpitation is realized.

Cause. A common physical cause of palpitation can be ectopic heart beats, which occur outside the normal rhythm of the heart. There can be a sensation of fluttering or thumping in the chest. Ectopic heart beats and the palpitations they produce need not be symptoms of a heart condition. They sometimes are linked to smoking, heavy drinking or a substantial intake of caffeine. An arrhythmia, such as atrial tachycardia, can produce palpitations that result in feelings of faintness, dizziness, and breathlessness. If these resulting symptoms persist for several days, a physician may seek to diagnose an underlying problem or disorder. One method of diagnosis is to have the person wear a Holter monitor, which gives a continuing record of heart function. *See also* ATRIAL FLUTTER; ECTOPIC HEART BEAT; *and* TACHYCARDIA.

Pancreas

A gland located behind the stomach near the spleen and duodenum that produces endocrine and exocrine secretions.

The principal role of the rather small triangle shaped pancreas is in the production of of the hormones glucagon and insulin. These two hormones, that are produced in the pancreatic islets—usually referred to as the islets of Langerhans—regulate the blood's glucose levels. During the digestion process, these hormones are released into the small intestine. *See also* INSULIN.

Pancreas. Top, this illustration shows the position of the pancreas in relation to the other abdominal organs. It is in the lower section just behind the liver. Middle, an illustration of the pancreas by itself; this is where insulin is produced. Bottom, the islets of Langerhans, these regulate the glucose levels in the blood.

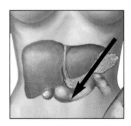

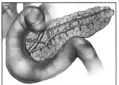

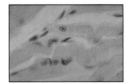

Pancreas, Cancer of

A malignant tumor of the pancreas.

The pancreas is a part of both the endocrine and the digestive systems. One segment of it produces insulin and glucagon, hormones that regulate blood levels of sugar. Another segment produces enzymes that help digest starches, fat, and protein. The great majority of cancers of the pancreas are ductal carcinomas, which arise in its exocrine (enzyme-producing) cells.

The incidence of pancreatic cancer has increased in recent years. Although evidence is inconclusive, it appears to be associated with a high intake of fats in the diet, as well as with heavy alcohol consumption and smoking.

Symptoms. Pancreatic cancer is not often detected in its early stages, because the first symptoms are not clear-cut. They include loss of appetite, a feeling of fullness after even light meals, nausea, vomiting, weight loss, yellowing of the skin and eyes caused by jaundice and changes in bowel function such as constipation or diarrhea. Sometimes a tumor that develops in the endocrine part of the gland causes clear symptoms because it affects the production of insulin or glucagon. The result can be abnormally low or high levels of insulin that affect major body functions.

Diagnosis. Tests for pancreatic cancer include a computerized tomography scan, ultrasound scans, blood tests to detect abnormal hormone levels, and tissue sample examinations. One specialized test is endoscopic retrograde cholangiopancreatography, in which a flexible tube is put through the intestinal tract to the pancreas, allowing an inspection of the gland.

Treatment. Surgery is the first line of treatment for cancer of the pancreas. A tumor in the exocrine section of the gland can be removed by what is called the Whipple restriction, which also removes part of the stomach, the gall bladder and other neighboring tissues. Surgery often is followed by combination chemotherapy.

Surgical removal of the entire pancreas has not been found to affect survival. If the cancer has spread so much that it cannot be removed surgically, creating bypasses around the tumor to improve digestive function may ease symptoms, and radiation therapy may be applied to reduce the tumor's size and relieve pain. The overall prognosis for cancer of the pancreas is not good, since most of these cancers are diagnosed at a late stage. *See also* CANCER; CAT SCAN; PANCREAS; *and* WHIPPLE RESTRICTION.

Dietary Adjustments

Diet can be part of the treatment for pancreatic cancer. Reducing the intake of fatty foods often reduces digestive symptoms that cause discomfort. Enzymes can be taken in tablet form to help improve digestive function, and special dietary supplements, available at most health food specialty stores, can provide the necessary calories and proteins. As with any dietary regulation, see a doctor or a nutritionist before making any drastic dietary changes.

Pancreatectomy

Surgical removal of all or part of the pancreas.

Variations of this procedure are performed to treat pancreatic cancer; cell carcinoma; pancreatitis, inflammation of the pancreas; carcinoma of the ampulla of Vater, where the common bile duct and pancreatic duct open into the duodenum; and insulinomas or benign insulin-producing tumors.

Types. In a total pancreatectomy, the surgeon removes the whole pancreas, part of the small intestine, part of the stomach, the bile duct, the gallbladder, spleen, and most of the lymph nodes in the area. For a subtotal pancreatectomy most of the gland is removed, leaving only a small part close to the duodenum.

With a Whipple Restriction, the surgeon removes the head of the pancreas, part of the stomach, and some tissue around it, leaving enough of the pancreas to continue producing digestive fluids, insulin and glucagon.

With a distal pancreatectomy only the tail of the pancreas is removed, and partial pancreatectomy requires only a relatively small portion of the gland to be removed along with the tumor.

A total pancreatectomy often causes diabetes, so insulin injections and a restricted diet are required as an integral part of ongoing treatment. A partial pancreatectomy may require oral supplements of pancreatic enzymes to aid digestion.

A relatively new surgical procedure called laparoscopic distal pancreatectomy with splenectomy is now being performed to excise a cystic tumor from the pancreas through a small abdominal opening, a procedure that saves days of hospitalization. *See also* WHIPPLE RESTRICTION.

Pancreatitis

An inflammation of the pancreas.

The pancreas is a small finger-sized organ located below the stomach, near the first loop of the small intestine (the duodenum). It has several critical functions including the secretion of digestive enzymes into the duodenum to assist in the digestive process and the production of insulin and glucagon to regulate the bloodstream and the body's ability to metabolize sugar. It also secretes bicarbonate to neutralize stomach acids that would otherwise flow into the intestinal tract.

The pancreas can become inflamed for a number of reasons. A gallstone may block the flow of pancreatic fluid in the main bile duct, resulting in severe inflammation of the pancreas. Backed up enzymes may leak out into the abdominal cavity causing peritonitis (inflammation of the peritoneum) and irritation of the other organs. Constant alcohol consumption blocks the ducts that drain the pancreatic fluid into the main bile duct, producing the same result.

Symptoms. The first symptoms of pancreatitis is the sensation of a severe pain in the upper abdominal region, possibly extending towards the back. The pain starts rather suddenly and reaches its peak quickly. It is steady and severe and may last for days. There is nausea, vomiting, fever, and weakness. If the cause is alcohol there may only be moderate pain. Other sufferers feel desperately sick, have a high fever, and have a rapid pulse rate.

There are no medications that are specifically designed to treat pancreatitis.

For Individuals Over Fifty

The elderly are at particular risk for pancreatitis because, while the small bile duct itself usually enlarges with age, the opening to the duodenum narrows significantly. Gallstones that accumulate over the years may grow large enough to block the duct. If pancreatitis does not resolve on its own, the first attempt to clear the problem is usually with endoscopy; a small tube that allows the surgeon to see and operate inside the bile duct and the duodenum. If endoscopy does not resolve the problem, surgery is recommended to remove the gall bladder and clear the pancreatic ducts.

An acute attack will put a person in the hospital, where he or she will be fed intravenously for two weeks or more and will be given medication to control the pain. Oxygen may also be administered if the amount in the blood stream is low. Infection of the pancreas after an acute attack of pancreatitis is a possibility. Infection would be characterized by symptoms that worsen after a week of treatment and by high white blood cell counts. Infection would be treated with antibiotics. *See also* GALLSTONE *and* PERITONEUM.

Pancreatography

Various procedures used to visualize the pancreas and bile ducts.

Pancreatography is a means of visualizing the pancreas for diagnostic purposes. There are several diferent methods of pancreatography, utilizing everything from advanced imaging techniques, such as magnetic resonance, to older techniques, such as endoscopy.

Endoscopic retrograde cholangiopancreatography (ERCP), is a form of pancreatography used to detect disorders of the pancreas, bile ducts, liver, and gallbladder. Blockages or stones can be diagnosed. A flexible endoscope is fed through the mouth and into the upper digestive tract. A smaller tube or cannula is then threaded through the endoscope. Through the cannula, an opaque dye is then injected into the bile and pancreatic ducts, where it is then taken up.

Recent advances in pancreatography include magnetic resonance (MR) pancreatography, a noninvasive alternative to standard pancreatography and ERCP. Similar to an MRI, an MR pancreatography subjects the patient to a strong magnetic field, causing the cells to vibrate at a frequency which can be rendered into a clear electronic image. MR pancreatography provides imaging of the pancreaticobiliary tract. Because this technique does away with ionizing radiation, sedation (invasive endoscopes), and the use of a contrast medium, it is considered much safer than traditional methods and is a promising tool for the detection of disorders such as: variant anatomy of the pancreatic duct; pancreatic duct trauma; and pancreatic neoplasia. *See also* BILE; BILIARY SYSTEM; CALCULUS; CANNULA; DUCT; ENDOSCOPY; ERCP; MRI; NEOPLASIA; PANCREAS; PANCREATITIS; *and* RADIATION.

Panic Disorder

A condition in which an individual, after having two or more panic attacks, avoids certain situations and activities in order to prevent the recurrence of these attacks.

A panic attack is a sudden, inexplicable experience of profound fear that may include dizziness, racing heart, hyperventilation, and severe anxiety with preoccupying ideas of disaster. It may resemble a heart attack because of the strong sensation of a quickly beating heart and possible chest pains. A panic attack starts with a single bodily sensation and develops as other physical symptoms of the "fight or flight" response mechanisms kick in. Panic disorder occurs when the fear of a panic attack escalates into a compounding fear of future panic attacks. This causes the person to avoid any situation that might trigger anxiety.

Causes. Those who believe that panic attacks are psychologically based do not feel that the panic attacks arose "out of the blue," as often reported by patients, but are the result of a period of prolonged stress, triggered by a significant life change in which significantly more responsibilities

must be assumed, such as marriage, birth or graduation.

Some researchers believe that there is also a biological trigger for panic attacks in which an individual may have a physical disposition to develop the fight or flight response under non-emergency situations. Those who experience panic attacks also tend to catastrophize even minor events.

Treatment. If a person starts to modify his or her lifestyle for fear of future attacks, it is a good idea to seek immediate treatment. A wide variety of treatments are available, and they are often used in combination. However, very little evidence exists about the effects of combined treatment. Cognitive and behavioral therapy help an individual to identify and reduce catastrophic thinking and deal with the physical sensations, by reproducing and alerting him or her to the symptoms of the disorder. Insight oriented psychotherapy may make a person feel more in control by providing an understanding of the underlying problems.

Medication, including antidepressants, are often used in combination with other therapies and may alleviate symptoms quickly. Although panic disorder is a chronic psychiatric problem, it is readily treatable with a variety of therapeutic techniques. *See also* ANTIDEPRESSANT DRUGS; ANXIETY; ANXIETY DISORDERS; PHOBIA; PSYCHIATRY; *and* PSYCHOTHERAPY.

Pap Smear

Also known as Pap test

A test that identifies abnormal cells on the cervix and other areas of the reproductive tract.

Regular Pap tests can identify precancerous changes in the cervix and uterus as well as cancer in its early stages. They can detect approximately half of all uterine cancers, as well as other noncancerous conditions.

The Pap test is done during a routine pelvic examination. A cotton swab is used to scrape a few cells from outside the cervix and inside the cervical canal. The cells are deposited on a slide—a smear—and then

Resources on Pap Smear and Cancer
Murphy, G.., *Informed Decisions: The Complete Book of Cancer Diagnosis, Treatment, and Recovery* (1997); Renneker, Mark, ed., *Understanding Cancer* (1988); Steen, R. Grant, *A Conspiracy of Cells: The Basic Science of Cancer* (1993); Steward, Clifford T., ed., *Cancer: Prevention, Detection, Causes, Treatment* (1988); American Cancer Society, Tel. (800) ACS-2345, Online: www.cancer.org; National Cancer Institue, Tel. (800) 4-CANCER, Online: www. nci.nih.gov; Nat. Alliance of Breast Cancer Organizations, Tel. (888) 80-NABCO, Online: www. nabco.org; www.nycornell.org/medicine/hematology/index.html; www.nycornell.org/medicine/cardiology/index.html.

analyzed in a laboratory.

The results of a Pap test are graded according to the nature of cell changes and according to how much of the cervix is affected. In order of increasing abnormality, they include:

- normal results that show no evidence of malignant cells;
- atypical cells of undetermined or undeterminable significance;
- a low-grade squamous intraepithelial lesioning;
- high-grade intraepithelial lesion and;
- invasive cancer.

These are classifications that follow the classic Bethesda system, thus they also include any changes associated with human papilloma virus (HPV), which has been linked to cervical cancer.

An abnormal Pap test does not necessarily lead to a cancer diagnosis. Abnormal cells may be due to infections of the cervix or vagina, or to cervical dysplasia. A repeat test is often recommended.

Colposcopy involves a close visual examination of the cervix and vagina and is performed after a second abnormal Pap test. Occasionally a small piece of tissue will be removed and examined under a microscope for evidence of cancerous changes.

Frequency. Pap tests are recommended from age 18 or when a woman becomes sexually active. After three or more consecutive negative tests, most practitioners feel a test every two years is sufficient. Women at high risk for cervical cancer and those with a family history of cancers should have the tests performed annually. Older women have an increased risk for developing cervical cancer; women over age 65 who have not had routine screening should have a Pap test.

Some procedures can interfere with the results of a Pap test, including cone biopsy, laser surgery, and cryosurgery.

> *Basic information on infections and diseases of the cervix and reproductive tract is contained in* Cervix, Cancer of; Cervicitis; Human Papilloma Virus; Inflammatory Disease; Pelvic Infection; *and* Uterus, Cancer of. *Further information may be found in* Colposcopy.

Papilledema

Also known as choked disk or swollen optic nerve

A swelling of the optic nerve that is caused by increased intracranial pressure.

Often, cancer in the nervous system causes papilledema, which is not a diagnosis but a sign of an underlying disorder. Hematomas and hemorrhaging have also been linked to optic nerve swelling. Symptoms of papilledema include an increase in the frequency of headaches (especially in the early morning or when rising), and nausea or vomiting caused by increased cranial pressure, which can lead to a loss of consciousness and death. A reduction in vision is rare, but some people will experience blurring or a transient graying out of the visual field. Diuretics are often prescribed while the underlying disorder is treated. *See also* Eye *and* Optic Nerve.

Papilloma, Intraductal

A small, benign tumor that grows within the milk duct of the breast.

This condition is uncommon and its causes are unknown. They occur most often in women over 50 years of age. Symptoms include, breast pain, nipple discharge from one breast only (watery or bloody discharge from a single milk duct may occur spontaneously), staining inside the bra, a breast lump, and breast enlargement.

After the condition is diagnosed, a breast biopsy is prescribed to rule out breast cancer. Breast self-examination may help detect the disorder. *See also* Benign; Breast; *and* Cancer Papilledema.

Papule

A skin lesion that is small, solid, and raised.

Papules are classified as skin lesions that are less than 0.4 of an inch in diameter. Acne and small pimples are examples of papules. Papules are usually caused by inflammation or growths of the skin. *See also* Lesion; Pimple *and* Skin.

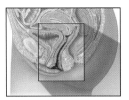

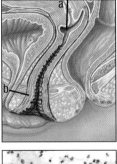

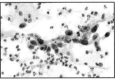

Pap Smear. Top, the site from which a pap smear is taken. Middle, close up of that sight: (a) the cervix and (b) the vagina. Bottom, a 200 times enlarged image of a pap stain showing cervical cancer; more specifically, squamous cell carcinoma. This is just one disorder that can be diagnosed with a pap test.

Paralysis

A lessening or loss of the ability to move or experience sensations in any part of the body caused by disease or injury to the nerves.

Paralysis is the loss of the capacity to move. It can be partial or total, and temporary or permanent. In addition, it may affect any number of muscles in the body, major and minor. The term paresis is used to describe muscle weakness and should be differentiated from muscle paralysis.

CAUSE

Muscle paralysis may be caused by an injury or disease affecting the central nervous system, the peripheral nervous system, or the muscles themselves. In a properly functioning system, muscles are stimulated to contract by nerve impulses from the motor cortex of the brain. The nerve impulses travel via the spinal cord or the peripheral nerves to the specific muscles. When these nerve impulses experience any disruption along their lengthy journey, paralysis may result. In addition, a muscle disorder can produce some forms of paralysis, even if there is no nervous system malfunction.

TYPES

Central Nervous System Disorders. Central nervous system disorders consist of those conditions which affect the brain and the spinal cord. A disease or injury that damages brain cells may paralyze the face, arm, or leg muscles on one side of the body (hemiplegia). The paralysis always appears on the side of the body that is opposite the site of the brain injury because motor fibers transverse at the brain stem. This type of brain damage often produces muscles that are inflexible (spastic paralysis).

Spinal Cord Disorders. Spinal cord disorders often occur as the result of automobile accidents that leave the victim's spine fractured. This form of injury to the spinal cord causes damage to the parts of the body below the spinal cord. For example, a spinal cord injury in the area of the neck can cause paralysis in the legs (paraplegia) or paralysis to both the arms and legs (quadriplegia). Damage to the brain stem, which links the brain to the spine can cause paralysis to the muscles that control breathing and swallowing. In addition, sustained pressure on the spinal cord (as the result of aging or injury for example) can result in disk prolapse or cervical osteoarthritis, which may lead to partial paralysis of the surrounding muscles. Paralysis may also result from the onset of certain diseases, which affect the nerves of the spinal cord; for example: multiple sclerosis, poliomyelitis, myelitis, Friedreich's ataxia, meningitis, and motor neuron disease.

Paralyzing Strokes

One of the most common causes of paralysis is a stroke. Strokes are the third leading cause of death in the United States, affecting more than 500,000 Americans each year; of these, 150,000 die within a few months of the occurrence. In the event of a stroke, bleeding or blood clotting occurs in the blood vessels that supply the brain. Depending on the type of stroke, the victim may experience either partial or total paralysis. There are few effective treatments after a stroke occurs, so the best measures are preventative: reducing or eliminating salt intake, avoiding alcohol use and smoking, normalizing weight with a healthy diet, and light exercise can all help. The elderly are most at risk for suffering strokes and they will usually need full time professional care in the wake of a paralyzing stroke.

Peripheral Nerve Disorders. Peripheral nerve disorders (or neuropathies) usually affect an individual muscle and in many cases cause temporary paralysis. These disorders are often caused by conditions such as: diabetes mellitus, liver disease, vitamin deficiency, cancer, excessive consumption of alcohol, and lead poisoning.

Muscle Disorders. These disorders cause weakness in the muscles which may lead to paralysis. Muscular dystrophy, an inherited condition, causes progressive muscular weakness that may result in paralysis. Another condition known as myasthenia gravis commonly affects the muscles of the eyes, face, throat, and limbs and can also result in temporary paralysis.

TREATMENT

If possible, the underlying cause of the paralysis should be treated first. Physical therapy is often suggested to minimize the possibility for joints to be locked into inconvenient positions and to strengthen muscles after a mild stroke. Electrical and mechanical stimulation may also be used to stimulate the affected muscle or muscles.

If an individual is completely paralyzed and confined to a wheel chair, nursing care is essential to prevent circulatory complication, to assist in excretory functions, and to turn the patient regularly to prevent bedsores. Therapy is often supplemented to help paralyzed individuals deal with the emotional side of experiencing paralysis. A high degree of motivation is critical for rehabilitation and recovery.

Background material on PARALYSIS *may be found in* BRAIN; NERVE INJURY; NERVOUS SYSTEM; *and* SPINAL CORD. *Information on specific types of paralysis is found in* BELL'S PALSY; PARALYSIS, PERIODIC; *and* SPASTIC PARALYSIS.

Paralysis, Periodic

A rare genetic disorder that causes unexpected bouts of muscle weakness and paralysis.

Periodic paralysis almost exclusively affects children and young adults. At the time of an attack, muscles do not respond to either standard nerve impulses or to those artificially produced. There is no known reasons as to why certain people experience periodic paralysis.

Potassium is essential for proper muscle functioning, thus, a drop in the blood's potassium levels may be somewhat responsible for this disorder. Hypokalemic-induced attacks may appear among twenty-year olds for the first time. They are harsher and last longer than what is termed a hyperkalemic attack. Furthermore, one who experiences a hypokalemic attack may have a higher incidence of paralysis on the day after eating a carbohydrate-rich meal or after a day of fasting.

A physician may prescribe acetazolamide to control the bloodstream's level of potassium. At the initial sign of muscle weakness, ingesting a potassium chloride tablet may prevent an attack. Restricting the intake of carbohydrate-rich meals and engaging in gentle exercise during the initial signs of muscle weakness may also reduce the frequency and intensity of these episodes. Ordinarily the disorder disappears before the age of 30 without any treatment. *See also* DIET; EXERCISE; GENES; MUSCLE; PARALYSIS; *and* POTASSIUM.

Paranoid Personality Disorder

A personality disorder characterized by unwarranted suspicions of others, including doubts about their honesty and loyalty, as well as a tendency toward maintaining long-held resentments and exhibiting a tendency toward retaliatory behavior.

Individuals affected by paranoid personality disorder tend to interpret the words and actions of others as intrusive, hostile and threatening, often believing that they are being followed or spied on. As a result of this pervasive distrust, such a person will rarely confide in anyone. He or she doubts even genuinely well-intentioned comments and is easily hurt or insulted. Talking to a person with this disorder, one may well feel uncomfortable, as though words need to be chosen with excessive care.

Unable to establish any strong sense of trust, a person with paranoid personality disorder may be particularly suspicious of the fidelity of a spouse or partner, determined, against all facts to the contrary, that the spouse is flirting, cheating or otherwise unfaithful. Because the sense of distrust and betrayal is unrelenting, there is a tendency to hold onto old resentments and to bring them up continuously. All of these behaviors create a distance from other people and a tendency to cause others to maintain their distance.

Antianxiety and antipsychotic drugs are sometimes prescribed in the most severe cases, but a broad program of psychotherapy is usually the only effective treatment. *See also* PERSONALITY DISORDER.

Resources on Paranoia
American Psychiatric Association, *Diagnostic and Statistical Manual of Mental Disorders, 4th Edition* (1994); Barchas, Jack D., *Psychopharmacology: From Theory to Practive* (1977); Beckham, E. Edward and William R. Leber, eds., *Handbook of Depression: Treatment, Assessment, and Research* (1985); Wender, P.H. and D.F. Klein, *Mind, Mood, and Medicine: A Guide to the New Biopsychiatry* (1981); Nat. Depressive & Manic-Depressive Association, Tel. (800) 82-NDMDA, Online: www.nd-mda.org; National Mental Health Association, Tel. (800) 969-NMHA, Online: www.nmha.org; www.ny-cornell.org/psychiatry/.

Paraphimosis

Painful constriction of the portion of the penis behind its tip.

Paraphimosis is the result of an extremely tight foreskin that has been pulled back. This causes the section of the penis behind the head (glans) to constrict, resulting in swelling and pain. The symptoms of paraphimosis can be relieved by local application of an ice pack followed by squeezing the glans. The condition can be treated by returning the foreskin to its normal position by hand. If this is not possible, surgery to cut the foreskin may be performed. Surgical removal of the foreskin (circumcision) prevents any possible recurrence of the condition. *See also* CIRCUMCISION.

Paraplegia

Weakness or paralysis of both legs, and frequently part of the trunk.

Paraplegia is caused by nerve injury in the brain or spinal cord. While the limbs and trunk are most commonly affected, paraplegia may also result in a loss of sensation and urinary control in the lower part of the body. Motor vehicle accidents, sports injuries, gunshot wounds, and a fall from a cliff, building site, or horse are the most common causes for this condition. Paraplegia occurs twice as often among males as females and is most likely to occur among young adults. *See also* PARALYSIS.

Parasite

An organism living upon or within a host without contributing to its survival.

Parasites may be single or multi-celled organisms, visible or invisible to the naked eye and living in or on the surface of the body, endo- and ectoparasites, respectively. While parasites such as lice may be little more than an irritating nuisance, other parasites produce severe, often fatal diseases, particularly in developing nations.

Endoparasites include the protozoans, whose cyst and trophozoite forms are found in feces and other tissues or excreta. They are acquired through drinking contaminated water or by insect bites. The plasmodium genus of protozoal parasites is spread through the bite of the anopheles mosquito and is responsible for malaria.

Common Parasitic Diseases

African Sleeping Sickness is caused by *Trypanosoma burcei*, transmitted by the tse-tse fly, and affects over 60 million people.
Amoebic Dysentery is caused by *Entamoeba hystolytica* and transmitted through infected food and water, especially fresh vegetables.
Babesiosis is caused by Babesia transmitted by tick bites and is often contracted with Lyme disease.
Chagas Disease is caused by *Trypanosoma cruzi* that are transmitted by the Chagas bug; it attacks the cardiovascular system through the blood stream.
Cryptosporidosis affects the small intestine and is caused by parasites of the Crypotosporidum genus.
Filariasis, also known as elepantiasis, is caused by *Wuchereria banerofti and* can be transmitted by ordinary mosquito bites.
Giardia: Also known as beaver fever, this disease is caused by parasites of the genus Giardia.
Leishmaniasis kala-azar is caused by protozoa of the leishmania genus (as is Leishmanisis Oriental Sore) transmitted by sand-fly bites.

Helminths or parasitic worms, including, tapeworms, roundworms, hookworms, pinworms and others, are responsible for a broad range of illnesses. For example, the beef tapeworm (*Taenia saginata*), and the pork tapeworm (*Taenia solium*) cause infections when contaminated meat is improperly cooked.

Ectoparasites generally live on the skin surface and include ticks, fleas, mites, bedbugs, leeches, and lice. Some ectoparasites are transmitters of more serious endoparasitic illnesses, such as Lyme disease, caused by a spirochete transmitted through the bite of an infected tick.

For more information about specific parasites see CHIGOE; CESTODES; ECTOPARASIDE; GIARDIASIS; LEECH; LICE; LIVER FLUKE; *and* TICKS AND DISEASE. *Articles about related disorders include* DYSENTERY; LYME DISEASE; *and* MALARIA.

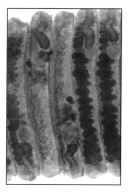

Parasite. Below, microscopic image of the body of a tapeworm. Tapeworm infestation usually results from the ingestion of raw fish or improperly-cooked food.

Parathion

An extremely hazardous insecticide.

Parathion and related products, including Malathion and Diazinon, are pesticides that work by acting as a stomach poison, killing insects that ingest them. Humans can be exposed to parathion from contaminated soil, water, air, and food. Parathion can be absorbed through inhalation, skin absorption or ingestion. It can be toxic, particularly to children, if not properly washed off foods.

Exposure to a toxic dose is generally indicated by breathing difficulties, gastrointestinal problems, visual disturbances, dizziness, nausea, vomiting, salivation, twitching muscles, and changes in pulse. Severe cases can result in loss of bowel control and diarrhea, deficiency of oxygen in the blood (cyanosis), convulsions, coma, and, if it is not treated quickly, death. Chronic exposure can cause severe cumulative effects.

Treatment consists of removing the chemical from the system by inducing vomiting, washing off contaminated skin, or other medical measures to support breathing. *See also* POISONING.

Parathyroid Glands

Glands that control blood calcium levels.

These structures are two pairs of these pea-sized, oval shaped glands, located on either side of and behind the thyroid gland. The main function of the parathyroid glands is to secrete the parathyroid hormone, which regulates levels of calcium in the body by acting on the bones, kidney and intestine.

Calcium is vital to the body because of its role in normal cell operations, as well as in carrying nerve impulses and the contraction of muscles. Abnormal levels of calcium, whether too low or too high, can affect all of these nerve and muscle operations.

Calcium is taken into the body through nutrients such as dairy products, eggs, and fish, as well as many green vegetables and fruit. When the parathyroid glands detect a drop in the levels of calcium in the blood, it releases parathyroid hormone (PTH). This hormone directs the kidneys to produce vitamin D, which helps the intestines absorb more calcium from incoming food. It also helps the kidneys reabsorb calcium from urine, further boosting calcium levels.

PTH then adds to calcium in the blood by decreasing the buildup of calcium in the bones, and accelerating the release of it. When the parathyroid gland finds an excess of calcium in the blood, it reverses these procedures so the kidneys do not produce as much Vitamin D, calcium is disposed through the urine, and allowed to accumulate in the bones.

PARATHYROID DISORDERS

The disorders that affect the parathyroid gland usually result in the over or under-production of PTH. Hyperpara- thyroidism, or the overproduction of the parathyroid hormone is characterized by symptoms such as muscle fatigues, weakness, abdominal pain, back pain, joint pain, and easily fractured bones. The most common cause is a benign tumor in the parathyroid gland, but this disorder may also be caused by hyper-functioning of all four hyperparathyroid glands. The usual treatment is removal of one or more of the affected parathyroid glands.

Hyperparathyroidism. Symptoms of hypoparathyroidism or the underproduction of the parathyroid hormone, include muscle cramps and aches, severe fatigue, numbness and a burning sensation in the area around the lips and fingers. This condition is often caused by the removal of much parathyroid glandular tissue during surgery. Hypoparathyrodism is usually treated with Vitamin D and calcium supplements.

Basic information on the role of the PARATHYROID GLAND *is contained in* CALCIUM; VITAMIN C; VITAMIN D; VITAMIN *and* VITAMIN SUPPLEMENTS. *Information regarding disorders of the parathyroid gland may be found in* ADENOMA; HYPERPARATHYROIDISM; HYPOPARATHYROIDISM; OSTEOPOROSIS; *and* PARATHYROID TUMOR. *For other related articles see also* HORMONES; PARATHYROIDECTOMY; *and* THYROIDECTOMY.

Parathyroid Tumor

A growth arising in a parathyroid gland.

There are four parathyroid glands, located in the neck, behind the thyroid gland. They secrete parathyroid hormone, which regulates the amount of calcium in the blood, thus helping keep bone and nerve function normal.

Parathyroid tumors are rarely malignant. Most are benign adenomas. They can cause the overproduction of parathyroid hormone, which leads to osteoporosis and weakening of the bones, as too much calcium is removed from them. Other symptoms of this condition, hyperparathyroidism, include fatigue, muscle weakness, bone pain, nausea, and vomiting.

Treatment of both benign and malignant parathyroid tumors is surgical; it includes the removal of the growth, which can result in a cure of a cancer if it is done early enough. Sometimes treatment for hypoparathyroidism, abnormally low levels of the parathyroid hormone, is necessary after surgery. *See also* ADENOMA; HYPERPARATHYROIDISM; *and* HYPOPARATHYROIDISM.

Parathyroidectomy

The surgical removal of one, some or all of the parathyroid glands, usually as a treatment for hyperparathyroidism and often due to the presence of a small, benign tumor or enlarged tissue.

If an adenoma (a tumor that is usually benign) is diagnosed, the affected gland is removed and the others are left intact. If the parathyroid tissue is enlarged or overactive, then the removal of most tissue is preferred. Usually at least one-half of one gland is left in to prevent hypoparathyroidism (when too little thyroid hormone is synthesized) because it creates low levels of calcium in the blood, muscle spasms, cramps, convulsions, and other symptoms. In some very rare cases, the surgeon will remove all of the glands and reimplant one in the forearm for easy access so that more tissue may be removed if necessary.

The patient is put under general anesthesia and an airway tube is inserted into the windpipe. The surgeon makes a horizontal incision in the neck just below the Adam's apple, where the parathyroid glands are located. Based on tissue analysis and presence of adenomas, the surgeon removes the appropriate tissue and then sutures up the wound. Statistically, 90 percent of hyperparathyroid patients have a non-cancerous tumor in one of the glands, and the remaining 10 percent have enlargement of all four glands. Cancer of the parathyroid glands is extremely rare.

The hospital stay usually lasts three to six days, and vigorous activity should be avoided for about a month. *See also* HYPERTHYROIDISM *and* THYROID.

Paratyphoid Fever

A mild form of typhoid fever caused by any one of three different species of salmonella bacteria.

There are over 2,000 species of salmonella bacteria. One of these species produces typhoid fever and three of them produce a milder form, called paratyphoid fever. Salmonella bacteria are found in water, contaminated shellfish, raw fruits and vegetables, raw milk, and eggs.

The distinguishing symptom of paratyphoid fever is the pink or rose-colored rash that appears on the the chest, stomach and abdomen. The onset of chills, diarrhea, fatigue, fever, and diarrhea are also symptomatic of this illness. Antibiotics may be effective in the treatment of paratyphoid fever, though the bacteria are increasingly resistant to these medications. An infected person may not exhibit symptoms of the disease and is then considered a carrier since he or she can infect others. Treatment should be sought as soon as possible as this can be a fatal condition. *See also* ANTIBIOTICS; RESISTANCE; *and* TYPHOID FEVER.

Paresthesia

Loss of feeling, sometimes accompanied by an experience of tingling in the skin.

Paresthesia is the medical term for the pins

and needles sensation. It is associated with an abnormal feeling of prickling, numbing, tingling, itching, or burning on the surface of the skin.

Temporary paresthesia is not uncommon. Either over-stretching or pressing on a nerve, or temporarily cutting off the blood supply can produce these symptoms. This causes a disruption in the conduction of nerve impulses that carry the information from the skin to the nerve center in the brain. A common example is the pins and needle sensation experienced after sitting in a cross-legged position for an extended period or immediately after awakening. The easiest way to remedy a foot that falls asleep is to change positions so as to remove the compression and massage the area and revive the diminished blood supply as discomfort is minimized.

Persistent paresthesia may be caused by a group of peripheral nerve disorders (neuropathy) and requires medical attention. An injured nerve may disrupt nerve sensation. In addition, the muscles supplied by the malfunctioning nerve may begin to weaken (muscle atrophy). In carpal tunnel syndrome, for example, compression of the median nerve produces paresthesia in the arm and shoulder. *See also* ATROPHY *and* NEUROPATHY.

Parkinson's Disease

A chronic brain disease that is characterized by muscle tremors, rigidity, and weakness.

Parkinson's disease is a gradually developing degenerative nervous system disorder that reduces muscle control. Its main symptoms include trembling when the muscles are at rest, difficulty initiating movement, an expressionless face, and an unbalanced walk. Parkinson's disease mainly affects members of the population between the ages of fifty and seventy years of old.

CAUSES

Parkinson's occurs as the result of a degeneration of the nerve cells within the basal ganglia inside the brain. When the brain begins to produce movement, such as lifting a leg, the nerve cells in the basal ganglia are responsible for creating smooth and coordinated movements. The basal ganglia interpret incoming signals and dispatch messages to the cerebral cortex via the thalamus.

Destruction or deterioration of the nerve cells result in a decline in the production of dopamine and a decrease in the electrical activity between the nerve cells

> ## Parkinson's and Nutrition
>
> Parkinson's disease slows down the speed at which food, liquids, and medications are digested in comparison to people of the same age without Parkinson's. Some of the medications for Parkinson's cause nausea, however, they should be taken before any substantial amount of food is eaten to aide absorption. Also, instead of three large daily meals, researchers recommend that multiple smaller meals be taken throughout the day. Some people with this disorder have trouble maintaining a healthy weight (which can hold off the development of Parkinson's symptoms), so nutritional supplements, especially multivitamins, are sometimes recommended in addition to exercise and a healthy diet.

and the muscles. Dopamine is the chemical (neurotransmitter) necessary for the nerve cells to communicate with the rest of the brain. The underlying cause of the damage to the nerve cells is unknown. The incidence of Parkinson's disease is higher among men and lower among smokers.

Drug Abuse. Among the known causes of Parkinson's disease is the use of recreational drugs (such as marijuana or ecstacy, MDMA), exposure to toxic quantities of carbon monoxide or manganese, and antipsychotic drugs used to treat paranoia and schizophrenia (such as thioridazine, flu-phenazine, haloperidol, and droperidol). Parkinson's results from the medication or toxins that block the action of dopamine on the neurons. The disease may be a side effect of brain inflammation of viral encephalitis.

SYMPTOMS

Parkinson's disease first appears as hand tremors, followed by symptoms occurring in the arm and leg of one side of the body, and later on the other side. The shakes may become more acute when the hand or leg is at rest; however, when the muscle is in use, the tremors cease. Advanced Parkinson's affects a person's gait, such that the sufferer will often shuffle, and adopt a soldier-like posture while walking. The affected individuals experience muscle fatigue, pain, and often balance complications. Parkinsonism may make certain basic tasks quite difficult, such as: buttoning one's clothes and signing one's name.

Facial muscles are affected, causing the patient's face to appear fixed and robot-like. The nerves, which are responsible for the facial muscles that produce the human grimace or frown often malfunction. There is an increased likelihood of depression. It is significant to note that Parkinson's disease can cause disability, but rarely does it result in death. Approximately one third of all patients may also suffer from varying degrees of dementia.

TREATMENT

Medication can alleviate some of the symptoms that accompany Parkinson's, such as stiffness and immobility; it is unable, however, to suspend the degeneration of the brain cells. Medications are usually not prescribed in the early stages of the disease. When needed, drug therapy strives to restore declining dopamine levels.

The drug levodopa (or L-dopa) is often prescribed to boost diminished dopamine levels. This drug requires constant medical supervision because its effectiveness tapers with persistent use. Another drug may be dispensed for a period, then levodopa reintroduced later can lead to greater success. Often levodopa will be prescribed in conjunction with carbidopa (Lodosyn, Sinemet, Sinemet CR), which assists the body in the up-take of levodopa. Long-term use of levodopa can cause complications, such as abnormal movements, sleeplessness, nightmares, and hallucinations. Medications, such as bromocriptine (Parlodel) and pergolide (Permax) are often used as effective alternatives to levodopa.

In many cases, anticholinergics, antihistamines, and antidepressants are prescribed to treat specific symptoms. Young patients in otherwise good health may undergo a surgical procedure that destroys part of the thalamus in order to reduce muscular tremors and rigidity. The transplantation of fetal brain tissue into the brain of those suffering from Parkinson's is an experimental procedure that some researchers claim as a viable and effective means of treatment. So far this procedure has only met with moderate success. Certain genetically engineered cells producing dopamines may help transplants gain wider acceptance.

Further information related to this can be found in AGING; BRAIN DISORDERS; *and* PARKINSONISM. *The anatomy of this disorder is discussed in* BRAIN *and* THALAMUS. *Articles relating to treatment options are included in* ANTIDEPRESSANT DRUGS *and* ANTIHISTAMINE DRUGS.

Parkinsonism

A neurological disorder typified by muscle rigidity, sluggishness, and a mask-like face.

The most common form of Parkinsonism is Parkinson's Disease. Symptoms include hand tremors, difficulty generating movements, muscle inflexibility and stiffness. In addition, there is muscle fatigue and muscular pain. Everyday tasks such as tying one's shoelaces or getting up out of a chair become increasingly more difficult as the disease progresses. Parkinsonism affects a person's gait to the degree that it no longer appears normal. The patient's face begins to lack natural human expressions and may appear robot-like.

These symptoms are predominately due to the fact that the facial muscles, which are responsible for human expression, are intensely affected by the neurological disorder. Causes of Parkinsonism have been attributed to cerebrovascular disease, encephalitis lethargica infection, antipsychotic drugs, recreational drug use, and carbon monoxide poisoning. *See also* BRAIN *and* PARKINSON'S DISEASE.

Resources on Parkinson's Disease

Carroll, David L., *Living with Parkinson's: A Guide for the Patient and Caregiver* (1992); American Academy of Neurology, Tel. (651) 695-1940, Online: www.aan.com; American Board of Neurological Surgery, Tel. (713) 790-6015, Online: www.abns.org; National Parkinson Foundation, Tel. (800) 327-4545, Online: www. parkinson.org; Parkinson's Disease Foundation, Tel. (800) 457-6676, Online: www.parkinsons-foundation.org; www.med.cornell.edu/neuro/; https://public1.med.cornell.edu.

Paronychia

An infection of the skin around the edge of a nail.

Paronychia is commonly caused by the staphylococcus bacteria or candida yeast. The condition is painful because the skin becomes swollen against the nail. Paronychia is very common in people who have diabetes or in people who have their hands in water for extended periods of time.

Treatment for nail infections includes hot water soaks (usually recommended three times daily) and antibiotics for bacterial infections or antifungal agents for candida infections. To prevent paronychia, toenails should be trimmed straight across instead of curved. *See also* CANDIDA *and* STAPHYLOCOCCAL INFECTIONS.

Passive-Aggressive Personality Trait

Behaviors that mask an unwillingness to comply to the will of others, and a generally hostile attitude.

No longer considered a personality disorder, the behaviors associated with this trait are displayed as chronic lateness, procrastination, and inefficiency. Individuals with this disorder may agree to perform tasks that they would rather not do and then undermine their own ability to complete the tasks, as a way of avoiding having to say no.

Passive behaviors are clouded ways of communicating a person's anger. They may include a tendency to obstruct the efforts of others, to put off a task until it must be handled by someone else, to be absent due to vague physical complaints, or to show up late for an event to avoid fully attending. A person with passive-aggressive personality traits will resist occupational and social obligations due to personal feelings of being hurt or victimized.

The angry reactions of others to this complex of thwarting behaviors may actually be satisfying to the passive-aggressive person, who is not able to openly express his or her own frustration and hostility. It is likely that such behaviors develop as a reaction to overbearing and controlling parents in a situation where their inflexibility and power of authority forced the covert responses characteristic of the passive-aggressive personality. *See also* PERSONALITY; PERSONALITY TESTS; *and* PSYCHIATRY.

Pasteurization

A process involving dairy products as well as beverages such as fruit juices that eliminates disease-causing organisms.

In pasteurization, food is heated to a moderate temperature and then quickly cooled. This process kills almost all disease-causing (pathogenic) organisms, and it extends the shelf-life of food.

Pasteurization does not sterilize food. In order to kill all organisms, sterilization must occur at a much higher temperature for a longer amount of time, which can destroy the food product. Because some organisms survive, pasteurized food products still spoil as bacteria and spores multiply.

It is unsafe to consume raw milk products and unpasteurized packaged fruit juices. Both have been linked to outbreaks of food-borne illnesses, such as tuberculosis, which have proved fatal. *See also* FOOD CONTAMINATION *and* FOOD POISONING.

ALERT
Food Irradiation

"Cold pasteurization" is a recently coined term that refers to the treatment of food with radiation that kills pathogenic organisms as well as insects and pests. Currently, this process is permitted in 37 countries but only about 25 of those regularly use it. Radiation also slows the foods ripening process, significantly extending the shelf life of many food products. This is an important development for the ever expanding needs that come with global demand for fresh foods. Unfortunately, irradiation does not kill viruses that may inhabit food. Also, irradiated foods have been found with reduced levels of Vitamin E and Vitamin C. Cold pasteurization is also a rather expensive process, so the benefits of food that can be stored for longer periods of time will only benefit consumers in developed countries. Scientists disagree about the ultimate consequences of food irradiation.

Patent Ductus Arteriosus

A congenital heart defect in which there is an abnormal channel between the pulmonary artery, which carries blood to the lungs, where it picks up oxygen, and the aorta, which carries oxygenated blood to the rest of the body.

A small defect of this sort may not cause symptoms, but if the opening is large, a newborn child's heart is overworked, leading to growth retardation, frequent chest infections, chronic shortness of breath, and heart failure. In most cases patent ductus arteriosus can be corrected surgically in the first few months of life. If surgery is delayed, permanent damage may result. *See also* CONGENITAL *and* HEART DISEASE.

Paternity Testing

Testing blood to determine if a particular man is the father of a particular child.

A paternity test is requested or court-ordered in the event of a dispute over who fathered a particular child. Blood taken from the potential father is compared to that of the child. Forensics specialists analyze proteins on the surface of red blood cells, other proteins in blood plasma, antigens, and short segments of DNA found in white blood cells. Referred to as DNA fingerprinting, the analysis reveals the wrongly named father in almost 100 percent of all cases. The chance of a merely coincidental match between the correlating father-suspect and the child is approximately one in 30 billion. *See also* BLOOD *and* BLOOD TESTS.

Pathogen

An organism or other substance that causes sickness or disease.

Pathogen is used to refer to an agent, often a living organism, such as bacteria, fungi, and other microorganisms, which have the potential to cause illness. Viruses are also referred to as pathogens even though they may not be viewed by some as living things. *See also* BACTERIA *and* VIRUSES.

Pathognomonic

Characteristic of a particular disease or condition.

Abnormalities and diseases are typically diagnosed by the symptoms exhibited by the patient. Such indicators may be revealed through tests including medical imaging, histology, blood or urine sampling, tissue biopsy or other diagnostic tests, are strongly recommended by the subjective report of the patient. When a symptom or array of symptoms is uniquely associated with a particular disease or affliction, they are said to be pathognomonic of that disease, and considered diagnostic indicators. *See also* BIOPSY; DIAGNOSIS; HISTOLOGY; IMAGING TECHNIQUES; *and* SYMPTOM.

Pathology

Either a condition produced by disease or the study of the nature and causes of disease.

Diseases are characterized by distinct changes in structure and function within the body. Such pathologies take many forms and are the domain of the pathologist—a physician trained in reading these signs of illness and abnormality. Microscopic changes caused by disease affect the number, size, shape, constituency or function of cells and belong to the study of cellular pathology. At the opposite extreme are diseases that produce gross physiological, anatomical, or behavioral changes.

Functional pathology refers to the study of changes in the function of organs, tissues, cells, etc., without accompanying structural changes. The study of pathology in the body's fluids is known as humoral pathology. The term pathology is sometimes also applied across fields of study; geographic pathology is concerned with the affect of climate and geography on the markers of disease.

Often tissues or cells extracted during biopsy or other surgery will be referred to a pathologist for analysis and diagnosis based on findings. *See also* ANATOMY; BIOPSY; CELL; HISTOLOGY; *and* MICROSCOPE.

Peak Flow Meter

A device used to measure the maximum airflow produced by forced exhalation.

Peak flow is an important diagnostic indicator of the health of the respiratory system, and it is one of a battery of common pulmonary function tests. It is measured with a special hand-held, calibrated meter.

Peak air flow is found to vary during the day in a characteristic pattern. It is lowest between four and six a.m. and highest around four p.m. The test will often be conducted at various points during the day in order to assess air flow and diagnose abnormalities. Asthma, bronchitis, and emphysema all decrease peak air flow by narrowing the airways, as does regular cigarette, cigar, and pipe smoking.

Measurement of peak flow can help diagnose various forms of asthma and also identify the cause of respiratory symptoms such as wheezing, coughing, and shortness of breath or labored breathing (known as dyspnea). The degree of individual or group disability (in the case of occupational respiratory hazards) as well as the progress of respiratory therapy may be evaluated with this technique.

A peak flow meter may also be used at home and is particularly useful for asthmatics. A person inhales deeply and then exhales as forcefully and rapidly as possible into a tube connected to a meter that registers peak air flow.

> *Background material on peak flow meters can be found in* BREATHLESSNESS *and* PULMONARY FUNCTION TESTS. *See also* ASTHMA; BREATHING; BREATHING, DIFFICULTIES; BRONCHITIS AND WHEEZE; COUGH; COUGH, SMOKER; *and* EMPHYSEMA.

Peau d' Orange

Also known as Erysipelas

A skin infection caused by streptococcus bacteria.

Peau d' orange is the result of bacteria entering the body through a break in the skin and causing an infection. The condition often begins with a bright red spot on the skin, which grows and spreads. It is accompanied by a fever, blisters, chills, and a headache. Peau d' orange causes a characteristic orange peel appearance.

Peau d' orange is generally treated with antibiotics, as it is a bacterial infection. Fever and pain are sometimes controlled by fever-reducing antipyretics. With treatment, the infection can be brought under control within a week. To prevent peau d' orange, any breaks in the skin should be kept as clean as possible. *See also* STREPTOCOCCAL INFECTIONS.

Pediatrics

The branch of medicine concerned with the development, care, and diseases of children.

Pediatrics is a wide ranging field, embracing many medical disciplines; generalists, neonatal care specialists, and behavior researchers monitor growth and mental development as well as various types of disease specialists who all do work specifically for children. Beginning at birth, and continuing through puberty, pediatric involvement centers itself around care in the earliest and most important stages.

Pediatric interventions begin at birth, as its practitioners take care of the health needs of the newborn and infants with congenital disorders and the very young who are susceptible to infectious diseases.

Childhood growth and development (physically, socially, and psychological) are monitored as necessary; the range of disorders tends to stay consistent throughout early childhood.

At puberty, a whole new set of possible ailments arises as new hormones enter a child's health profile and sex characteristics develop. Along with the prominent physical changes come the psychological developments of the young person, which are all taken care of by pediatricians.

> *See* CHILD DEVELOPMENT; NEONATALOGY; *and* PUBERTY *for a discussion of the foundations of pediatrics. Topics of concern to pediatricians are found in* DEVELOPMENTAL DELAY *and* CONGENITAL SEXUALLY TRANSMITTED DISEASES.

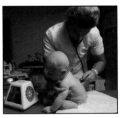

Pediatrics. Above, a pediatrician is treating an infant. The health of a newborn or a child is often the first thing on a new parent's mind.

Pedicle

A stem that attaches a tumor to normal tissue.

In oncology, a pedicle is a stalk-like extension through which blood flows to a tumor. The term is also applied to the bony bars that form the sides of the structure that surrounds the spinal column. In surgery, a pedicle is a stalk through which a skin flap receives nourishment until its transfer to another part of the body. *See also* BLOOD; CANCER; ONCOLOGY; *and* SKIN.

Pedophilia

A deviant sexual arousal pattern where an adult is aroused by sexual activity with a child.

This is a form of sexual dysfunction. It can be both abusive and criminal if ideas are acted upon. The sexual targets of a pedophile may be either girls or boys, although pedophiles are usually men. A pedophile may justify the behavior in his or her own mind as being protective or loving of a child, but a child is not able to consent to sexual acts of any sort and is always a victim of exploitation when sex is performed with an adult. Any sexual act with a minor is a statutory offense; it is illegal by virtue of statutes or law. Pedophilia is difficult to control, since it is often a driving force in an afflicted person's life. A very low rate of success is seen in treatment of pedophilia, although attempts have been made to treat it with behavior therapy and, ordered by a court, physical or medical castration. There may be a better chance of controlling pedophilia when the individual is in a relationship and is strongly motivated to change, although studies are inconclusive. *See also* SEXUAL OBSESSION.

Pellagra

A disease caused by a deficiency of niacin (vitamin B_3, niacinamide, nicotinamide, or nicotinic acid).

Pellagra can cause damage to nearly all of the body's cells, with the nerves, skin, and gastrointestinal tract most severely affected. Symptoms characteristic of pellagra are dermatitis, diarrhea, and dementia.

When pellagra sets in, the skin becomes scaly, rough, and brown in sun-exposed areas; the mucous membranes become painfully inflamed; and psychiatric prob-

ALERT

Niacin Overdose

While high doses of niacin in the form of nicotinic acid are prescribed as a cholesterol-lowering drug, care must be taken to minimize side effects and ensure that symptoms of overdose do not occur. Large supplemental doses of niacin can cause blurred vision; flushing, itching, and tingling; gastrointestinal problems including nausea and vomiting; abnormal blood levels of uric acid and sugar; an abnormal heart rhythm and rate; lightheadedness and liver damage. If these symptoms occur while on niacin treatment, the drug should be stopped at once. Large doses should not be taken without medical supervision. A niacin overdose can have lasting effects, damaging the liver.

lems may soon develop—these include anxiety, depression, apathy, memory loss (both short-term and long), psychosis, and delirium.

Pellagra is seldom seen in the United States today except in alcoholics, who frequently suffer from various nutritional deficiencies. Pellagra-like symptoms may also be caused by medications that affect niacin metabolism. These include certain types of antidepressants, anticonvulsants, antibiotics, and chemotherapy.

Diet. Generally a varied diet rich in high quality proteins is enough to treat pellagra. Good sources of niacin include meat (especially liver, either beef or calf), poultry, eggs, dairy products, fish, peanuts, and other legumes, and enriched grain products. Brewer's yeast, which is sold in many health food stores, is also an excellent source of niacin. Niacin, as well as the other B vitamins are affected, usually to deleterious ends, by exposure to sunlight and cooking, foods should always be eaten in the freshest form possible. *See* Alcohol RELATED DISORDERS; CELL; DEPRESSION; LIVER; SKIN; *and* VITAMIN B.

Pelvic Examination

Examination of the female pelvis, including reproductive organs, to assess gynecological health and diagnose possible disease or abnormality.

A pelvic examination consists of a series of observations and tests performed by a gynecologist. Women should have an exam annually beginning at age 18 or at the onset of sexual activity. A pelvic examination may be incorporated into a general checkup or may follow any particular gynecological complaint that is treated.

PRE-EXAM

After a clinical history is established, the examination process begins. The gynecologist palpates the abdominal region, presses gently around the belly and rib-cage, evaluates the size of the liver and spleen and feels for any abnormalities. Tapping with the fingers (a procedure referred to as percussion) is also used to sense the internal organs. Blood vessels in the abdomen as well as the activity of the intestine may be assessed using a stethoscope.

WHAT TO EXPECT

The pelvic exam is carried out with the patient lying on her back, with knees bent and feet held securely in stirrups at the base of the examining table. The doctor will inspect the pelvic area (vulva) for any signs of abnormality, including sores, inflammation, discoloration or discharge.

The next phase of the test involves a device known as a speculum, a plastic or metal instrument whose purpose is to hold the vagina open, allowing the gynecologist to clearly view the cervix and other internal structures. While insertion of the speculum often causes some anxiety, it should never be painful. The knees should be moved apart to allow insertion of the speculum, which is usually warmed and lubricated before use.

The clinician will note the position, size and general condition, of the cervix walls and the uterine opening before conducting a Pap smear. Cultures are collected with a cotton swab and sent to a laboratory to be tested. Chlamydia and gonorrhea may be diagnosed through a Pap smear as well as yeast and trichomonas infections. A test that returns positive results does not necessarily indicate cancer; it could also indicate precancerous cells; thus, proper pretreatment may prevent cancer from developing. The presence of herpes and other sexually transmitted diseases may also be detected. Any of these conditions may occur without

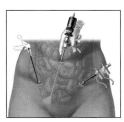

Pelvic Treatment.
Above, one of the more important forms of pelvic examination, and treatment, is a pelvic laparoscopy. It is less invasive than surgery, so the necessary recovery time is significantly shorter. Laparoscopy involves placing a telescope through the navel in order to examine the uterus, fallopian tubes; in many cases the causes of pelvic pain can be diagnosed. and treated, this way.

The Continuing Importance of Regular Testing

Doctors generally agree that annual gynecological visits should start around the age of 18 or whenever a woman becomes sexually active and they should continue just as regularly throughout the rest of a woman's life. Approximately 97 percent of all women get gynecological exams at some point in their lives, often just to check on general health matters, but also to learn about methods of birth control, how to avoid contracting a sexually transmitted disease, or in preparation for a pregnancy.

As women age, it becomes more important than ever to continue going to a gynecologist and receiving the necessary examinations. Even after a hysterectomy the pelvic tissue still needs to be checked, as it affects the overall health of an individual. In addition, cancers of the vulva and vagina are the most common in post-menaposual women. Annual check-ups are recommended not only for preventative healthcare but also so that updated information is constantly available to patients.

---

obvious symptoms in the patient.

Next, the speculum is removed and a bimanual exam is performed. A lubricated, gloved finger is inserted into the vagina to inspect the uterus and ovaries for size and shape as well as the presence of masses or other abnormalities. Pain during the bimanual exam may indicate an infection. The doctor may also insert a finger into the anus because, often, this is how colon can-

---

For related anatomical information see ABDOMEN; ANATOMY; CERVIX; OVARY; PELVIS; RECTUM; REPRODUCTIVE SYSTEM, FEMALE; UTERUS; *and* VAGINA. *Related conditions include* CHLAMYDIA; DISCHARGE; GONORRHEA; HERPES, GENITAL; PAP SMEAR; TRICHOMONIASIS; *and* VAGINAL DISCHARGE. *See also* PERCUSSION; SPECULUM; STETHOSCOPE; *and* GYNECOLOGY *for more diagnostic information.*

Pelvic Floor Exercises

Exercises to strengthen the pelvic floor.

The muscles and ligaments at the base of the abdomen help support the uterus, vagina, bladder, urethra, and rectum. These muscles and ligaments may stretch or lose strength as a result of childbirth or aging. This slackening may lead to prolapse of the uterus or incontinence.

One such exercise is to contract and relax the vagina during urination, starting and stopping the flow. Another is to place two fingers inside the vagina and practice contracting and relaxing the muscles. *See also* INCONTINENCE; KEGEL EXERCISES; PELVIS; *and* UTERUS, PROLAPSE OF THE.

Pelvic Infection

An infection of the pelvic region in women, usually caused by gonorrhea or chlamydia.

Pelvic infections are frequently the result of complications of a sexually transmitted disease, though they may also be the result of a vaginal delivery, a miscarriage, or an abortion. In women with pelvic infections, pus accumulates and may form an abscess in the fallopian tubes. There may be abdominal pain, nausea, vomiting, and fever. If the infection blocks the fallopian tubes, it can result in infertility. Antibiotics normally cure the infection, otherwise surgery is necessary to drain the abscess. If it ruptures without being drained, the infection can spread to other organs. *See also* INFERTILITY *and* SEXUALLY TRANSMITTED DISEASE.

Pelvic Inflammatory Disease

A severe or recurrent infection of the female reproductive organs, often following a sexually transmitted disease.

Pelvic inflammatory disease (PID) is caused by bacteria, usually the same ones that are responsible for the sexually transmitted diseases gonorrhea and chlamydia.

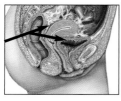

Pelvic Infections. Above, an illustration of where adhesions are found; infection, surgery, or trauma may cause the formation of pelvic adhesions. Because these adhesions cause connections between tissues that are not supposed to be connected, they can cause a variety of disorders—not the least of which is pelvic pain.

It can also be caused by bacteria that enter the reproductive tract via an intrauterine Device (IUD) or during an endometrial biopsy, miscarriage, abortion or giving birth. Nearly a million women in the United States develop PID each year. It is estimated that many more have the condition but are as yet undiagnosed.

Women most at risk are between the ages of 20 and 31; those who began having sexual intercourse at a young age; individuals who have multiple sexual partners; and people who engage in unprotected sex.

Complications. PID can affect the fallopian tubes, uterus, and ovaries. It can also lead to pelvic adhesions, which is scar tissue that forms between the internal organs and causes persistent pain. Untreated, PID can lead to infertility when the scar tissue affects the fallopian tubes, either sealing the entrance or distorting its shape. It also increases the likelihood of an ectopic pregnancy. More than 20 percent of women with PID caused by an STD will have difficulty conceiving.

Occasionally PID will result in an abscess, which, if it ruptures, will result in a life-threatening condition known as peritonitis. In this case, the infection spreads through the pelvic and abdominal areas. Blood poisoning may occur if the bacteria enter the bloodstream.

Symptoms of PID include:
- pain and tenderness in the lower abdominal region;
- foul-smelling vaginal discharge;
- fever;
- pain during sexual intercourse;
- heavy or irregular menstrual periods with cripplingly severe cramps.

Treatment. Most sexually transmitted diseases can be treated by antibiotics. Severe infections may require hospitalization. Surgery is sometimes performed to remove the adhesions and affected organs.

Basic information is contained in PELVIS; PELVIC EXAMINATION; PELVIC INFECTION; SEXUALLY TRANSMITTED DISEASES; *and* UTERUS. *More on the symptoms of pelvic inflammatory disease may be found in* ABSCESS; BLOOD POISONING; LESION; PELVIC PAIN, CHRONIC; *and* VAGINAL DISCHARGE.

Pelvic Pain, Chronic

Aches or pains that linger in a woman's pelvic area and last for six months or longer.

Doctors will diagnose Chronic Pelvic Pain (CPP) in women who experience a discomfort that lingers for six months or more. This condition occurs in many women for a variety of reasons. Whatever the cause, this type of pain can be both physically and emotionally debilitating.

Also, there are dozens of types of pelvic pain: it can be sharp or dull; it may increase in intensity during sexual intercourse or during bowel movements; or it may become better or worse at different points in a woman's menstrual cycle; it may be constant or it may fade in and out. The type of pain someone suffers from will usually correlate to the cause of the pain.

Symptoms of CPP do not always end with the pain; pelvic pain is often accompanied by irregular or heavy (or light) periods; vaginal discharges; stomach cramps or discomfort; and chronic diarrhea.

CAUSES

There are numerous causes for CPP. Sometimes the pain is related to a disorder in the reproductive system, sometimes other bodily systems are the cause. Some disorders in the reproductive system that may cause, or exacerbate, CPP include:

- uterine fibroid tumors or polyps;
- endometriosis;
- pelvic inflammatory disease;
- fibroids or endometriosis.

Disorders unrelated to the reproductive system that can affect the muscles in the pelvis or the excretory system and cause CPP include:

- overactive bladder;
- interstitial cystitis (an inflammation of the bladder wall);
- pelvic floor tension myalgia;
- stomach ulcers;
- hernias, slipped discs, and back sprains;
- urinary tract infections;
- appendicitis;

- kidney stones;
- irritable bowel syndrome.

Sometimes emotional states rather than physical states can cause CPP. Increased stress levels caused by work or relationships or family obligations; depression; hyperactivity; some kinds of neurosis; physical or psychological abuse all can lead to chronic pain. A condition can get worse with the onset of fatigue.

DIAGNOSIS

Because the pain's trigger may be emotional, doctors will often ask a number of personal questions about lifestyle choices and regular habits. This is to assess an emotional profile so that she or he can send you to the proper specialist.

A close external physical examination is also not uncommon. The stomach, back, groin and legs all need to be examined. Internal diagnostic tests may be much more thorough and intense than normal gynecological procedures. In cases that are especially hard to diagnose, a doctor and patient may decide on a laparoscopic examination. Laparoscopy involves inserting a thin tube with a light through a patient's abdomen so that the inside of the pelvis can be examined closely.

TREATMENT

Since there are so many possible causes for chronic pain, there is no single treatment. If there is an underlying physical disorder, that must be treated with the necessary medication, which may include antibiotics, hormones, painkillers or surgery.

If the underlying cause is emotional or psychological, then any of a number of possible psychiatric treatments may be recommended. Relaxation therapy, support groups, as well as individual counseling can all be effective, depending on an individual's particular case and personal treatment preferences.

Background material may be found in LAPAROSCOPY; PELVIS *and* PELVIS EXAMINATION. *More on possible causes of chronic pelvic pain is contained in* CYSTITIS; ENDOMETRIOSIS; PELVIC INFECTION; STRESS; *and* ULCER.

Pelvimetry

Measurement of pelvic proportions through manual observation or x-ray.

The pelvis is a structure composed of the innominate bones, the sacrum, the coccyx, and the ligaments connecting them. The purpose of the pelvis is to support the vertebral column of the spine and to facilitate the lower limbs in walking.

Pelvimetry is used to measure the pelvic proportions. This may be done in order to evaluate disease or injury (pathology) or to determine whether the birth canal is sufficiently wide enough for natural childbirth.

Standard pelvimetry makes use of a device known as the Colcher-Sussman pelvimeter, which can take measurements of the breadth and width of the pelvis or lateral orientation. More recently, both computed tomography (CT) and magnetic resonance imaging (MRI) have been used to diagnose cephalopelvic disproportion, the primary pelvic irregularity associated with complications in childbirth.

The diameters of the pelvis measured by pelvimetry are characteristically larger in the female than the male, owing to the requirements of reproduction. *See also* BIRTH CANAL; CAT SCANNING; CHILDBIRTH, COMPLICATIONS; COCCYX; FETUS; MRI; PELVIC EXAMINATION; PELVIS; REPRODUCTIVE SYSTEM, FEMALE; *and* VERTEBRA.

Pelvis

A skeletal bone structure composed of the coxae, pubis, sacrum, and coccyx; it rests on the lower limbs and supports the spine.

The pelvis attaches the lower limbs to the the upper body while transmitting the weight of the upper body to the lower limbs. This chiasmatic relation is true for both males and females even though there are striking differences in the size and structure of their pelvises; the female bone structure reflects a childbearing function—it is wider, lighter, rounder and shallower than that of a male's narrow, heavier,

larger, and less motile counterpart. At birth three parts of the pelvis (ilium, ischium, and pubis) are separate, but they fuse and become a single structure in time. *See also* CHILDBIRTH; COCCYX; PELVIC PAIN *and* PELVIMETRY.

Pemphigoid Bullous

A chronic autoimmune disease that most commonly affects people age 60 and older, causing blistering of the skin.

The blisters that are characteristic of bullous pemphigoid are large and can occur anywhere on the body. They are most common on the skin folds, such as the groin and underarms. The condition is not contagious. It results from the abnormal production of antibodies against normal constituents, at the basement membrane zone of the skin, which is responsible for adhesion of the top layer of the skin, the epidermis, to the bottom layer, the dermis.

Treatment for bullous pemphigoid includes prednisone, a corticosteroid drug. The condition sometimes gets better on its own and may disappear completely. *See also* AUTOIMMUNE DISORDERS; BLISTER; CORTICOSTEROID DRUGS; IMMUNE SYSTEM; PREDNISOLONE; *and* SKIN.

Pemphigus

An autoimmune skin disorder characterized by blistering of the skin and mucous membranes.

Pemphigus is the uncommon condition in which the immune system produces antibodies that erroneously attack proteins in the body's skin and mucous membranes. It results in intense blistering and exfoliation.

The cause of pemphigus is unknown, although certain drugs can induce a pemphigus-like reaction. Pemphigus occurs most commonly in middle-aged and older individuals. There is no cure, but this condition can be controlled with drugs. *See also* AUTOIMMUNE DISORDERS; BLISTER; GENETIC DISORDERS; IMMUNITY; PROTEINS; SKIN; *and* SKIN, DISORDERS OF.

Pelvis. Below, an illustration of the urinary bladder in the pelvis. The pelvis is a great work of design, strength, and balance. The male and female pelvic bones are slightly different, due to the child-bearing capability of the female.

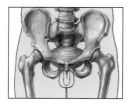

Penicillin Drugs

A family of antibiotic drugs used to combat bacterial infection.

In 1928 Alexander Fleming, a British bacteriologist, inadvertently discovered a fungus, penicillin, that killed certain bacteria. By 1941, penicillin was being widely used to control bacterial infections. Today, derivatives of penicillin remain among the most commonly prescribed antibiotics.

The original formulation had serious drawbacks. Its effectiveness as an antibiotic was compromised by stomach acid, so it could not be administered orally. Further, penicillin was only effective against a certain family of bacteria called gram-positive bacteria. Since then, dozens of variations of natural, semisynthetic, and synthetic penicillins have been developed to address these drawbacks, with varying degrees of success.

ANTIBIOTIC RESISTANCE

A problem with penicillin today is that many of the diseases penicillin had been able to cure are caused by bacteria that have mutated and become resistant to the antibiotic. The mechanisms of this resistance have only recently been understood, and there is hope that in the future penicillin variations can be developed that are as effective as they were originally.

SIDE EFFECTS

There are relatively few side effects of penicillin, however, some people become allergic to penicillin. They become sensitized after the first exposure, when the body identifies the penicillin as an invader and the immune system tries to eradicate what it interprets as a disease. Most allergic reactions are fairly mild. There may be hives or rashes on the skin or the lips, and the face or hands may swell. In some cases, though, a person can go into anaphylactic shock. The tubes leading to the lungs close down, blood pressure drops, the person may lose consciousness, and, if not immediately treated, death is possible. An allergic reaction will be observed within a few minutes after taking the drug. Alternative antibiotics are available that will not produce allergic reactions.

There is some evidence that penicillin counteracts the effect of birth control pills. Doctors strongly recommended that, if a woman is taking a penicillin drug, birth control methods other than birth control pills should be used.

> *For background information concerning penicillin drugs please refer to* ANTIBIOTIC DRUGS; ANTIBIOTIC RESISTANCE; BACTERIA; IMMUNITY; *and* RESISTANCE. *It may also be important to understand the nature of a related* ALLERGY. *See also* IMMUNE SYSTEM.

Penile Implant

A medical device that is implanted into the penis of a male with erectile dysfunction in order to achieve or simulate an erection.

There are two main types of implants: malleable and inflatable. The malleable version consists of a pair of semi-flexible plastic tubes or rods that can be flexed up or down by manipulation.

The inflatable type features a pair of inflatable plastic cylinders with a fluid reservoir and hydraulic pump inserted into the scrotum. The inflatable prosthesis is controlled by a bulb that, when squeezed, forces a saline solution into the cylinder and thereby causes an erection. Another variation of the device has the reservoir placed in the lower abdomen. Less invasive options such as drugs or injections should always be considered first because implants permanently damage erectile tissue and will destroy the natural erection reflexes.

The operation may take 40 minutes to an hour and a half, and is performed under general, spinal or local anesthesia. The surgery can be done on an outpatient basis or with a hospital stay of several days. The drug sildenafil citrate (Viagra) has significantly reduced the demand for penile implants. *See also* PENIS; SEX; SEX THERAPY; SEXUAL DESIRE, INHIBITED; SEXUAL DYSFUNCTION; SEXUAL INTERCOURSE; *and* SEXUALITY.

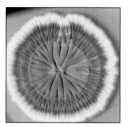

Penicillin Drugs. Above, a mold colony from which penicillin is produced. There are actually several varieties of mold that produce penicillin. Two of the most prominent include: Penicillium notatum and P. chrysogenum.

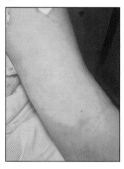

Penicillin Drugs. Above, a picture of a person affected by penicillin hypersensitivity. Some people have reactions similar to shock due to penicillin use, however, other drugs are available.

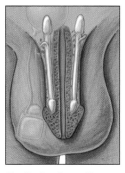

Penile Implant. Above, an illustration of a malleable penile implant. The flexible plastic rods can be seen clearly.

Penis

The male copulatory organ designed for sperm delivery and waste removal.

The male reproductive organ is an external structure that hangs suspended from the perineum. An attached root, a shaft, and an enlarged tip called the glans make up the three major components of the penis. A stretch of loose skin covering the glans called the prepuce or foreskin is often removed shortly after birth (circumcision).

The penis contains the urethra and three cylindrical bodies of erectile tissue. The erectile tissue consists of a network of connective and smooth muscle composed of vascular spaces that fill with blood during arousal. The corpus spongiosum surrounds the urethra and expands at the penile tip forming the glans. *See also* CIRCUMCISION *and* SEX.

Penis, Cancer of

A malignant tumor of the penis.

Cancer of the penis is rare. It generally occurs in elderly men who are not circumcised and have poor hygiene. Studies have found a possible association with infection by a human papillomavirus, specifically a virus that causes genital warts.

The cancer usually arises on the head of the penis (glans) or on the foreskin. It can cause a rash or be visible in the form of dry growths. Sometimes there is a small ulcer that bleeds easily. The cancer may grow quickly, spreading to the lymph glands of the groin and causing visible swelling.

However, cancer of the penis is usually slow-growing and can be cured by surgical removal of the affected area in its early stages. Diagnosis is made by a physical examination, a biopsy, and x-rays or computerized tomography (CT) scan to detect possible spreading to nearby tissues. Failure to detect and treat the cancer early could result in the surgical removal of part or all of the penis. *See also* BIOPSY; CANCER; CIRCUMCISION; GENITALIA; *and* PENIS.

Penis. Below, an illustration of the penis anatomy and the male urogenital organs. The parts include the: (a) glans; (b)urethra; (c) pubic symphysis; (d) the urinary bladder, which is made up of the apex, fundus, body, trigone, and neck; (e) prostate; and (f) testis.

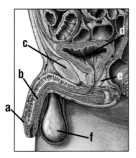

Peptic Ulcer

The loss of tissue in the lining of the lower esophagus, the stomach, or the duodenum.

The upper portion of the small intestine or the lower portion of the stomach are the most common locations for peptic ulcers. These ulcers develop as lesions or sores in the tissue walls that do not extend through to the muscle layers. When peptic ulcers heal, they often leave scar tissue at the site of the sore.

CAUSE

Most peptic ulcers are associated with increased acid production in the stomach. The two primary stomach acids are hydrochloric acid and pepsin. Pepsin is an enzyme that breaks down proteins; since the stomach wall is also made of protein, it will break that down too. *Heliobacter pylori*, bacteria that grow in the mucus-secreting cells of the stomach lining, are considered a major cause of peptic ulcer. Ninety to 95 percent of all patients with duodenal ulcerss, and 80 percent of those with gastric ulcers, are infected with *Heliobacter pylori*. They can inflame the gastrointestinal lining, stimulate excessive acid production, or do both.

Gastric ulcers are not associated with excessive acid levels. They are believed to form due to a deficiency in the stomach lining's protective mechanism. This makes it more susceptible to the perpetually present stomach acids.

Stress ulcers form in the lining of the stomach or duodenum following severe injury, infection, or shock. Small bruises may appear in the lining within hours of the injury and rapidly develop into ulcers. If recovery from the injury is prolonged, the ulcers may enlarge and begin bleeding. A stress ulcer differs pathologically and clinically from a chronic peptic ulcer. It is more acute and more likely to result in hemorrhage and perforation. Conditions often associated with stress ulcers include severe trauma, surgery, advanced malignancy, extensive burns, and brain injury.

Both gastric and duodenal ulcers tend to be passed along within families. Relatives of those with gastric ulcers are three times as likely to suffer from gastric ulcers. The same is true of duodenal ulcers. Drug-induced ulcers are most commonly caused by aspirin. Other drugs that are strongly suspected of being ulcerogenic include other nonsteroidal anti-inflammatory drugs (NSAIDs). Alcohol consumption also contributes to stomach lining erosion.

SYMPTOMS

The primary symptom of peptic ulceration is a burning, gnawing, or aching pain in the upper abdomen. It usually comes in waves and lasts for several minutes. The daily pattern of pain is related to the secretion of acid due to the presence of food in the stomach.

The pain tends to diminish in the morning when acid secretion is low and after meals when there is food present in the stomach. The pain is most severe before meals and at or around bedtime. It often appears for several days or weeks and then subsides only to reappear sometime later. Other symptoms of uncomplicated peptic ulcer include nausea, loss of appetite, and—in some cases—weight loss.

COMPLICATIONS

The three major complications of ulcers include hemorrhaging, perforation, and obstruction. Bleeding, which may result in vomiting blood or a substance resembling coffee grounds as well as tarry stools, varies from mild to severe.

Perforation results in the spilling of the gastric or intestinal contents into the peritoneal cavity. This is an emergency situation requiring immediate surgery, as it may develop into peritonitis.

The upper intestinal tract is sometimes obstructed because of scarring or damaged muscle tissue at the lower end of the stomach. Persistent vomiting will occur, often resulting in alkalosis (an excess of base in body fluids) because of gastric acid in the vomit. The obstruction is treated by surgically removing the scar tissue.

DIAGNOSIS

The most common technique used to diagnose peptic ulcers is endoscopy, which can confirm the presence of an ulcer, establish the site of bleeding in a gastric or duodenal ulcer, differentiate between benign and malignant ulcerations, and identify the presence of *H.pylori*, or another predisposing factor. Endoscopy involves inserting a small flexible tube with a camera down a patient's throat and into the stomach so that a doctor can evaluate its condition and take tissue samples.

TREATMENT

Antacids, such as magnesium hydroxide and aluminum hydroxide, relieve the pain by decreasing the levels of gastric acid. Cimetidine (Tagamet) is a histamine H2-receptor antagonist that inhibits gastric acid production, but it has some undesirable side effects, including male breast enlargement, confusion in elderly patients, and it delays the metabolism of other drugs. Sucralfate Carafate, which is not absorbed into the body, is an alternative drug with fewer side effects. Another drug, ranitidine, has an action similar to that of cimetidine, but is more powerful, can be taken less frequently, and has fewer side effects.

Most ulcers are treated without surgery, however, it is necessary in cases when there is scarring, recurrent bleeding, perforations, or extreme pain. Stomach ulcers are operated on more often that duodenal ulcers. The most common procedure is a partial gastrectomy, in which the ulcerous portion of the stomach is removed.

Dietary restrictions are usually limited to those foods identified with the onset or intensification of symptoms. Alcohol and caffeine intake should be limited, as they may induce gastritis and promote gastric erosion. Small amounts of food should be eaten frequently throughout the day, rather than two or three large meals.

Basic information is found in GASTRITIS *and* ULCER. *More on symptoms is contained in* ABDOMINAL PAIN *and* GASTROINTESTINAL BLEEDING. *Details on treatment may be found in* ANTACID DRUGS; ENDOSCOPY; *and* GASTRECTOMY.

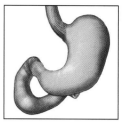

Peptic Ulcer. Above, the stomach and in red is the duodenum. Peptic ulcer disease is a serious health care problem in the United States. It costs American health care two to four million dollars every year, according to the *Physician's Assistant Journal.* Advances in treatment, however, are bringing those numbers down.

Resources on Ulcers and the Digestive System

DLevine, Joel S., ed., *Decision Making in Gastroenterology* (1992); Berkson, D. Lindsey, et al., *Healthy Digestion the Na-tural Way* (2000); Sapol-sky, Robert M., *Why Zeb-ras Don't Get Ulcers: An Updated Guide to Stress, Stress-Related Diseases, and Coping* (1998); Sachar, David B., et al., *Pocket Guide to Gastro-enterology* (1991); Thomp-son, W. Grant, *The Ulcer Story: The Authoritative Guide to Ulcers, Dyspep-sia, and Heartburn* (1996); Crohn's and Colitis Found. of America, Inc., Tel: (800) 932-2423, Online: www. ccfa.org; Digestive Disease National Coalition, Tel. (202) 544-7497, Online: www.ddnc. org; Gastro-Intestinal Research Found., Tel. (312) 332-1350, Online: www. girf.org; National Institute of Dia-betes and Digestive and Kidney Diseases, Tel. (301) 496-3583, Online: www.niddk.nih.gov; www. nycornell.org/medi-cine/di-gestive/index.html.

Perception

The intuitive manner in which sensations are understood, cognition.

A human being interprets the outside world using the senses of sight, sound, smell, taste, and touch (tactility). The ears react to mechanical vibrations. The eyes react to electromagnetic waves. The nose and tongue respond to chemicals. The sense organs in the skin respond to pressure, pain, and temperature. The sense organs in the muscles, joints, and tendons, respond to the motion and position of the body. This information is organized, interpreted and transmitted to the brain in the form of electrical nerve impulses.

Perception is the psychological process in which the energy of the outside world is converted into a specific representation of a person, an object, or an event. It is the body's interpretation of electrical impulses. The nerve impulses that stimulate the eyes do not see colors. Yet, the eyes do see in vivid color and can differentiate from light and darkness. Similarly, the ears are stimulated by vibrations that are neither music nor noise. The brain collates the nerve impulses from the eyes as light and color and from the ear as sound and pitch.

Various factors affect how something is perceived. Perceptions can be influenced by one's emotions, needs, and outlook. People of different cultures perceive pain, noise, music, and color differently. Individuals suffering from mental illness exhibit false perceptions or hallucinations; in such cases there is an absence of sensory stimuli. *See also* NERVOUS SYSTEM *and* SENSATION.

Percussion

Tapping the skin using the fingertips; used to evaluate size, shape and position of underlying structures or the presence of abnormalities.

Percussion is a simple, hands-on method for gaining information about internal structures using only the hands. By sharply tapping the skin surface, the physician is able to determine from the resulting vibration, sound, pitch, resonance and resistance, the location and density of internal (subcutaneous) organs, structures and possible abnormalities. Fluid and pus, for example, may be identified in this way.

Two main types of percussion are used. In the case of immediate percussion, the fingers tap the skin directly. Mediate percussion involves laying the palm of one hand against the skin of the patient and tapping the back of the wrist with the other.

Percussion has been found to have a high specificity for diagnosis, though the sensitivity is higher for palpation of the skin (a procedure in which the tissue is felt with the fingertips, without tapping). These two diagnostic procedures are therefore best applied in conjunction. Percussion is also frequently used with auscultation or listening with a stethoscope, to amplify the resulting sound and improve sensitivity. Diagnoses of abnormalities by percussion will typically call for further study, often by medical imaging. *See also* AUSCULTATION; IMAGING TECHNIQUES; PUS; STETHOSCOPE; *and* SUBCUTANEOUS.

Percutaneous

Having an effect through the skin.

Many treatments are said to be percutaneous—either carried out or having their effect through the skin layers. Ointments may be applied by friction so that they are absorbed into the skin. Injection or the removal of fluid by hypodermic needle is also considered a percutaneous operation, as are ultrasound studies designed to penetrate the skin for therapeutic treatment, as in the case of kidney stone destruction. Sampling (biopsy) of tissues or fluids by means of an aspiration needle, use of a tube (catheter) to drain an abscess or collect fluid, injections of drugs, vaccines or contrast materials to aid medical imaging are likewise regularly performed percutaneous procedures. *See also* BIOPSY; CATHETER; SKIN; ULTRASOUND SCANNING; *and* VACCINE.

Perforation

A hole or puncture in a body part or tissue due to disease, accident or injury.

Perforations from diseases include duodenal ulcer, colonic diverticulitis, and stomach cancer. A perforated eardrum is usually caused by a middle-ear infection or the accidental insertion of pointed objects.

Perforation of the uterus may be caused by an intrauterine device or by a curette during an abortion. Esophageal perforation can occur through endoscopy, and a gastroscope may perforate the stomach. Perforation of the nasal septum may be caused by trauma, drug abuse, or disease, and it is repaired by surgical closure or the insertion of a special septal "button." A kidney stone occasionally causes a perforation in the ureter. They are usually repaired surgically, but sometimes antibiotics or drugs may be used. *See also* ANTIBIOTIC DRUGS; DUODENAL ULCER; *and* EAR, DISORDERS OF.

Periarteritis Nodosa

Also known as polyarteritis nodesa

A disease that primarily affects the body's small and medium-sized arteries.

Arterial tissue affected by periarteritis nodosa becomes inflamed and is eventually destroyed. This pattern of destruction occurs in a particular spot along the course of each of the affected arteries, causing the development of nodules that can be felt during an examination.

Cause. The cause of periarteritis nodosa is unknown, but the disease may occur as a result of drug interactions or as a reaction to various vaccines. Viral and bacterial infections are also known to trigger the sometimes fatal inflammation. There is no way to prevent this disorder.

Incidence. Periarteritis nodosa usually develops in patients between 40 and 50 years of age. Men are three times more likely to have the condition than women. The five-year survival rate for people suffering from periarteritis nodesa is 50 percent.

Symptoms. The symptoms of periarteritis nodosa are mild at first, but as the disease progresses it can become a debilitating condition, and sometimes be fatal. The symptoms, depending on the area of the body affected, include fever, abdominal pain, numbness and tingling in the extremities, weakness, weight loss, kidney damage, high blood pressure, chest pain, muscle and joint pain, and even kidney failure and heart attack in some severe cases.

Treatment. As with other connective tissue diseases, there is no known cure for periarteritis nodosa. However, various treatments can alleviate the symptoms of the condition. Corticosteroids are chief among these and they may even prolong a period of remission. However, improvements in a person's condition is usually temporary.

> *Background material on periarteritis nodosa may be found in* ARTERY *and* ARTHRITIS. *Symptoms are discussed in* ABDOMINAL PAIN *and* CARDIAC ARREST. *More information on treatment is contained in* CORTICOSTEROID DRUGS. *See also* BACTEREMIA *for related information.*

Pericarditis

Inflammation of the pericardium, the membrane that surrounds the heart.

There are numerous causes of pericarditis. The acute form, which comes on very suddenly, can result from a bacterial, viral or fungal infection; or it can occur in association with a number of other diseases, including rheumatoid arthritis, rheumatic fever, kidney failure, scleroderma or systemic lupus erythematosus.

Pericarditis can also be caused by the spread of a cancer growing in the lung or in the breast, by a severe chest injury (trauma), or by a myocardial infarction (heart attack). One form of pericarditis occurs in the first few weeks following invasive heart surgery. In some cases, there is no apparent cause for the onset of acute pericarditis. Chronic pericarditis, which is less common, can be caused by a chronic infection, such as tuberculosis, and its symptoms will come on slowly.

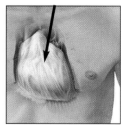

Pericarditis. Above, an illustration of the pericardial sac that surrounds the heart. When this is inflamed, the condition is known as pericarditis. Although this condition is caused by many so called "childhood" diseases, its incidence among the young is very low.

SYMPTOMS

The most common symptom of pericarditis is a sharp pain in the center of the chest, which can spread to the neck and shoulders. Sometimes it is severe enough to mimic a myocardial infarction (heart attack). The pain of pericarditis differs from that of angina pectoris or a myocardial infarction, because it is persistent and it worsens with deep breathing, changes in posture, or coughing.

Pericarditis caused by an infection can lead to the accumulation of pus and fluid in the space between the pericardium (the double-walled sac surrounding the heart) and the heart. A large accumulation of fluid can result in cardiac tamponade, compression of the heart, interfering with the activity of the heart, causing a steep drop in blood pressure.

Chronic pericarditis can produce symptoms resembling those of heart failure, such as shortness of breath and severe swelling of the abdomen. As the pericardium thickens it contracts so much that it interferes with the ability of the heart to pump blood. This condition is known as constrictive pericarditis.

DIAGNOSIS

Pericarditis usually can be diagnosed by a physical examination in which the physician detects the characteristic sounds accompanying the condition. The diagnosis can be confirmed by an electrocardiogram (ECG), a chest x-ray, and an echocardiogram. Blood and skin tests can be done to detect any related or underlying infections, and a sample of fluid may be taken for laboratory analysis.

TREATMENT

Painkillers such as aspirin and anti-inflammatory drugs—including ibuprofen (Advil™), naproxen (Anaprox™), fenoprofen (Nalfon™), or etodolac (Lodine™)—can be given to relieve the symptoms of pericarditis. Infections are treated by antibiotic drugs or other appropriate medications. An extreme accumulation of fluid can be removed by inserting a needle into the pericardial space. In severe cases of constrictive pericarditis, surgery can be done to remove the thickened pericardium.

While pericarditis can be a serious condition, most cases are not life-threatening. Symptoms of pericarditis should be reported to a physician as quickly as possible, since prompt treatment of an infection or other disorder causing the condition can be extremely effective.

See also CARDITIS; CARDIOVASCULAR DISORDERS; HEART; *and* MEMBRANE *to read about the foundations of pericarditis. Further information regarding treatment may be found in* ELECTROCARDIOGRAM; ECHOCARDIOGRAPHY; ANTIINFLAMMATORY DRUGS. *Related material is found in* TAMPONADE.

Perimenopause

The early onset of menopause symptoms; this condition occurs well before menopause sets in.

Women in their late 30s or 40s may experience menopause-like symptoms, including breast tenderness, diminished libido, an increase in the frequency of ovulation and occasional skipped periods; stress levels also acutely affect ovulation patterns in perimenopausal women. Other symptoms such as fatigue, low energy, and weight gain are normal for an aging body.

Hormone replacement therapy and low-dose birth control pills are both effective treatments, but these are also over-prescribed or prescribed too early in the perimenopausal process. Estrogen treatment, especially when there is too little progesterone, has links to uterine cancer; there is also a possible relation to breast cancer, however, research is ongoing.

The more general symptoms of perimenopause, those that come naturally with aging, are effectively overcome with healthy life-style choices, including regular exercise, decreased alcohol consumption and smoking, regular sleep, stress management and multivitamin supplements. Scheduling sex effectively renews the libidinal drive. *See also* AGING; DIAGNOSTICS, IN WOMEN'S HEALTH; FATIGUE; HORMONES; MENOPAUSE; *and* STRESS.

Perimetry

A diagnostic test used to evaluate the visual field.

Perimetry is a test used to measure the field of vision and to diagnose abnormalities and diseases of the optic nerve, retina and neuro-optic pathways. An individual will be asked to stare straight ahead into a device known as a perimeter. Then points of light are moved into the line of sight from the visual periphery until the patient indicates that they are visible.

Perimetry is most effective in the diagnosis of visual field deficit, which may be peripheral or central. In the case of central visual field deficit, isolated regions of defective sight are surrounded by areas of normal intact vision. Peripheral visual field deficit is the term for regions of defective sight surrounded by areas of healthy vision. *See also* OPTIC NERVE; RETINA; VISION; VISION, DISORDERS OF; VISION, LOSS OF; VISION TESTS; VISUAL ACUITY; *and* VISUAL FIELD.

Periodontal Disease

Disorders of the gum and bone that support teeth.

Periodontal disease is an acute or chronic infectious process of the gums and bone supporting the teeth. It typically occurs when the gums are not taken care of properly (in which case plaque develops on the teeth). Among the more common periodontal disease is the severe inflammation of the gums, known as gingivitis. Left untreated, this inflammation can develop into an infection of the tissue and bone that secure teeth (periodontitis).

Prevention of periodontal disease is like prevention of all dental disorders—a combination of proper dental hygiene and regular visits to the dental hygienist. There are various fluoride toothpastes and rinses on the market that claim to control or eliminate plaque, but these should not be treated as short cuts to proper dental care. *See also* DENTAL SURGERY; DENTISTRY; GINGIVITIS; GUMS; ORAL HYGIENE; PERIODONTITIS; PLAQUE; *and* TEETH.

Periodontics

Branch of dentistry that deals with the stabilizing structures of the teeth.

The supportive tissue (gum and bone) around the teeth are known as periodontium. A dentist who specializes in maintaining the periodontium is called a periodontist. Many people are unaware that proper dental care includes taking care not only of the teeth but the gums as well. If the gums become inflamed or begin to recede, the periodontist may need to initiate treatments including cleaning the gums, reshaping and removing excess and infected gums (gingivectomy), and reshaping of underlying bone or extraction of teeth. Periodontists use a variety of techniques to prevent, diagnose, and treat ailments of these structures. X-rays help sight bone erosions, and scaling and curettage remove harmful elements. *See also* GINGIVITIS; PERIODONTITIS; *and* SCALING, DENTAL.

Periodontitis

Infection of the gums and underlying bone.

Periodontitis is an inflammation of the gums and the surrounding tissue that most often results when gingivitis goes without adequate treatment and periodontal disease sets in. In its worst form, teeth may be lost despite surgery and other efforts.

CAUSE

The culprit that leads to periodontitis is plaque, the sticky substance that adheres to teeth when they are not brushed or cleaned properly. Plaque may not be visible, but the damage it does is severe. In periodontitis, plaque collects first on the teeth, and then in pockets between the teeth and gums. As the gums become inflamed, the pockets enlarge, and the teeth slowly separate from the gums. The pockets collect more plaque, and pus forms as a result of the growing infection. As the inflammation progresses, the ligaments and bone that hold the tooth in place are affected.

SYMPTOMS

The teeth and gums hurt, especially when hot, cold, or sweet food is eaten. The gums are either swollen or recessed, bad breath is present, and there may be bleeding while brushing or eating. There can be a discharge of pus around affected areas. The teeth will be loose, and in the worst case scenarios they could actually fall out. Because there is bone loss, it may be impossible to save diseased teeth.

TREATMENT

Treatment begins with nonsurgical steps. The teeth, gums, and root surfaces are carefully cleaned and the patient is put on a strict regimen of careful oral hygiene. Sometimes this is not enough to stop the disease, and surgery may be needed. Periodontic surgery involves removing or recontouring bone and gums. This includes careful and thorough cleaning of all affected areas. The recontouring is done to help prevent more pockets from forming where plaque can collect. Sometimes, bone must be grafted or augmented with a bone substitute to repair damage or deformities.

The patient is not immune to new attacks of periodontitis if he or she fails to adopt a strict practice of cleaning the teeth and gums regularly. Only good hygiene can keep periodontitis from recurring.

Background information about this subject can be found in DENTISTRY; INFECTION; ORAL AND MAXILLOFACIAL SURGERY; ORAL HYGIENE; *and* PERMANENT TEETH. *Articles related to this subject include* CARIES, DENTAL; DENTAL EXAMINATION; *and* GINGIVITIS *See also* PUBLIC HEALTH DENTISTRY.

Periostitis

Inflammation of the tissue covering a bone.

Bones are covered with a connective tissue called the periosteum. When a bone is struck by a direct blow, the area may become painful, swollen and tender. Rest, ice, and anti-inflammatory drugs should reduce the pain and swelling. Periostitis occasionally occurs from infections, such as syphilis. *See also* SYPHILIS.

Peripheral Vascular Disease

Impaired blood flow to the arms and legs due to arteriosclerosis, the thickening and narrowing of the blood vessels in the extremities.

As people get older, their blood vessels tend to become stiffer and harder. Peripheral vascular disease usually occurs in older individuals, a consequence of the hardening of the arteries that naturally occurs with aging. The progression of arteriosclerosis is accelerated by the risk factors associated with coronary artery disease: uncontrolled hypertension, high levels of blood cholesterol, weight, diabetes, poor or unbalanced diet, and cigarette smoking.

In the most extreme cases, peripheral vascular disease can result in a complete blockage of blood flow, causing ulcerous sores that do not heal or gangrene, a death of tissue that can regularly require amputation. Peripheral vascular disease that affects the blood vessels of the extremities can be caused by conditions such as Buerger's disease and Raynaud's disease.

SYMPTOMS

The classic symptom of peripheral vascular disease is intermittent claudication, severe pain, weakness, and tension that is most often present in the calves of the legs but sometimes can be felt all through the legs. These pains will often be accompanied by painful cramping in the affected extremity. The pain is usually most intense while walking, and it subsides at rest.

The onset and severity of the pain are indicators of the degree of reduced blood flow. In the most severe cases, the pain can occur even at rest, so that sleep becomes impossible unless the legs are dangled over the edge of the bed. The pain can be accompanied by dry, scaly skin and numbness of the legs. Symptoms of peripheral vascular disease also vary with age and gender, as well as with the location, duration, and aggravating and relieving factors that determine the nature of the pain.

DIAGNOSIS

Peripheral vascular disease can be diagnosed by a physical examination of the legs, abnormally low blood pressure readings, or an absence of pulse in the leg arteries. The doctor may take the femoral pulse (located at or slightly below the groin) to test blood flow. The diagnosis can be confirmed by ultrasound examination or an angiogram to determine the level of blood flow.

ALERT

After 50

Every older individual should be alert to symptoms of peripheral vascular disease in the earliest stages of their onset, because of the implications for life-threatening cardiovascular disease and closely related cardiovascular conditions. Statistics show that someone with intermittent claudication has at least double the normal risk of developing serious heart disease. Statistics also show that more that 20 percent of people with intermittent claudication will have a life-threatening myocardial infarction (heart attack) or a stroke.

TREATMENT

Lifestyle changes, such as a low-fat diet and giving up smoking, can slow the progression of peripheral vascular disease. Regular walking improves blood flow by stimulating the growth of new blood vessels. Depending on physical condition, up to one hour a day can be recommended. If intermittent claudication occurs, walking should be stopped until the pain subsides.

Thrombolytic therapy, or clot busting drugs, are used to dissolve blood clots that impede blood flow. In some cases, balloon angioplasty may be done to widen the affected arteries, endarterectomy may be done to remove the plaque that is blocking the blood vessels or bypass surgery can be performed to insert a section of vein or a synthetic blood vessel to loop around a blocked section of an artery.

Basic information is contained in ARTERIES, DISORDERS OF; ARTERIOSCLEROSIS; and MYOCARDIAL INFARCTION. Treatment options are discussed in ANGIOPLASTY, BALLOON; BYPASS; ELECTROCARDIOGRAM; and ENDARTERECTOMY.

Peritonitis

An inflammation of the peritoneum, the two-layered membrane that lines the abdominal cavity.

The peritoneum, the slick, friction reducing membrane that lines the abdomino-pelvic cavity, is usually extremely resistant to infection. Inflammation of the peritoneum, or peritonitis, will only develop if an infected organ continues to leak pathogens (disease-causing agents) into the abdominal cavity. Sources of infection may be perforations in the stomach, intestines, gallbladder, or appendix, or pelvic infection. If there is a failure of the liver or heart, accumulated fluid may become infected and spread to the peritoneum. In addition, surgery may release bacteria into the abdominal cavity.

Bacteria are not the only possible causes of peritonitis. Peritoneal dialysis is a procedure in which fluids are infused into the abdominal cavity to neutralize toxins that may be there. After a period of time, these fluids are drained, but they may carry bacteria to the abdominal cavity. Blood infections, cirrhosis, and peptic ulcer disease have also been found as causes

Symptoms. Symptoms of peritonitis include the accumulation of fluid in the abdomen, an inability to pass feces or gas, a low urine output, abdominal swelling and pain, a fever, nausea and vomiting, thirst, and the chills. If a person is undergoing dialysis, the dialysis fluid will often be cloudy. Someone suffering from peritonitis will often show excessive signs of guarding: refusing to let their abdomen be touched, and curling up in the fetal position as a protective measure.

Treatment. Peritonitis is normally treated with exploratory surgery, particularly if a burst appendix, peptic ulcer, or diverticulitis is suspected as the cause of the condition. A combination of antibiotics is administered, along with intravenous fluids to control dehydration. Treatment must be sought quickly, as this can be a fatal condition. *See also* APPENDICITIS; APPENDIX; PELVIC INFECTION; *and* PELVIC PAIN, CHRONIC.

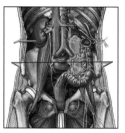

Peritonitis. Above, an illustration of the abdomen which is protected by the peritoneum. When the peritoneum becomes inflamed, the condition is known as peritonitis. Proper diagnosis of this condition may require an abdominal exploration.

Permanent Teeth

Second set of teeth for which there are no following sets.

The permanent (secondary) teeth are directly under the primary teeth. As the secondary teeth begin to push their way through (erupt), usually when a child is six years old, they push out the primary (baby) teeth. Most permanent teeth are in place before the child reaches adolescence, although back molars may come in later. The wisdom teeth (third molars), may emerge during the late teens or even young adulthood. In contrast to the 20 primary teeth, there are 32 permanent teeth. While the primary teeth are in place for less than 10 years, the permanent teeth are expected to function for much longer. Thus, proper care is vital to the long use expected of them. *See also* ERUPTION OF TEETH; ORAL HYGIENE; *and* PRIMARY TEETH.

Pernio

Also called chilblains

An inflammatory swelling or sore caused by extended exposure to the cold.

Pernios usually occur in areas previously affected by frostbite. The condition occurs most frequently on the hands, ears, and feet, although it can occur on any body area. There may be some local itching and swelling at the affected site. Only the most severe cases require medical attention. *See also* COLD INJURY.

Peroneal Muscular Atrophy

Also known as Charcot-Marie-Tooth disease

A hereditary disorder involving the nerves in the legs and arms.

In peroneal muscular atrophy, nerve fibers in the limbs or the myelin sheaths degenerate. This disease is inherited as a dominant genetic trait and is usually apparent before age 30. Symptoms include weakness in the legs, the absence of the stretch reflex, and possible foot deformities. Symptoms may also appear in the arms. Treatment usually involves leg braces or other orthopedic devices for walking. The disease progresses quite slowly and only affects the limbs. *See also* NERVOUS SYSTEM.

Personality

A general term for the sum of a person's traits, habits and behavior.

The concept of a personality derives from the ancient idea that how a person acts is determined by four specific fluids or "humors" that combined to make people choleric, melancholic, sanguine, and phlegmatic to various degrees. Today, the term is used to describe that aspect of a person's behavior that defies measurement, analysis or prediction. This would make the concept of personality of dubious use, except that there are instances in which people fail to cope with their environment in recognizable ways that seem related to their attitudes and behavior—in other words, to their personalities—and this gives rise to the notion of personality disorders.

Personality Tests. Useful as the categorization and treatment of personality disorders may be, there is significant controversy about whether tests for personality are appropriate to diagnose personality problems or personality traits. Personality tests have been routinely administered and decisions regarding the allocation of educational resources, hiring, and suitability for government service have been based on the results. The Goodenough-Harris test purports to measure both intelligence and personality on the basis of drawings of people made by a child. The test has been criticized for relying heavily on the conduct of the tester. The Minnesota Multiphasic Personality Inventory (MMPI) consists of more than 500 questions designed to reveal, among other things, psychopathological disorders (such as paranoia, schizophrenia, etc.), but the validity and reliability of such tests has yet to be demonstrated. *See also* RORSHACH TEST.

Personality Disorders

Persistent ingrained behavior patterns that cause ongoing conflicts with others and place severe limitations on one's potential for success.

The personality traits and behaviors that are present in personality disorders are noticeable to some extent in everyone. These traits may even be desirable or adaptive in moderation, especially if exhibited in appropriate ways. At times a perfectly healthy person may be controlling, dependent, reclusive, demanding, or impulsive.

For those suffering from a personality disorder, however, traits like these are intractable and persistent to the point of damage. While different situations demand an adjustment of behaviors, those with these disorders are not flexible or adaptable and relate in the same basic ways to most situations.

Nearly everyone knows people with personality disorders. They function at different levels than that for which they seem to have the potential, possess a distorted view of themselves and others, and they usually have trouble controlling their emotions. They often have stormy or unrealistic relationships with those around them.

These distorted views of self and others cause maladaptive behaviors. As a result, the exact response both feared and expected of others may be elicited. For example, in the case of histrionic personality disorder, the person behaves in a theatrical and overly demonstrative way in an attempt to gain attention and affection, which often turns people away from an individual who may be desperate. The person with paranoid personality disorder may be suspicious of a spouse and will hound the person mercilessly about his or her whereabouts and spy on the person, thereby driving the spouse away and ultimately causing the betrayal that is most feared by people with this disorder.

Personality disorders take a tremendous toll on an individual's personal life, work, and on society as a whole through medical costs and imprisonment. While at least one in twenty people suffers from a personality disorder, the number is far higher among the prison population.

Those diagnosed with a personality disorder are not likely to present this problem to a psychiatrist. Instead the problem is either turned away, redirected or presented as an overwhelming sense of dissatisfaction stemming from problems with family, friends or coworkers, or an inability to achieve a goal or a solution to problems.

CAUSES

Assessing the causes of these disorders raises the question of how much of someone's behavior is genetic and how much is determined by upbringing. Anyone who has raised a child knows that babies are born with a certain temperament, but environment is crucial in determining that child's personality. A powerless child faced with a manipulative, abusive, or unstable environment will develop coping mechanisms for survival during his or her formative years that will influence lifetime behavior patterns. Depending upon the temperament of the child and the severity of the family's problems, a personality disorder may result.

TREATMENT

Most personality disorders are difficult to treat. Medication may alleviate some of the symptoms of anxiety or depression, but the basic personality mechanisms often endure. For some of the disorders, psychotherapy may help the person gain a more realistic sense of self-awareness and understanding and a more realistic assessment of others. Even when the maladaptive behaviors are not totally alleviated, they may be significantly improved, and a difficult life situation may be improved in the process.

For Background information on personality disorders see ANXIETY and DEPRESSION. For more information on specific personality disorders see ANTISOCIAL PERSONALITY DISORDER; DEPENDENT PERSONALITY DISORDER; PARANOID PERSONALITY DISORDER; OBSESSIVE-COMPULSIVE PERSONALITY DISORDER; SCHIZOID PERSONALITY DISORDER; SCHIZOTYPAL PERSONALITY DISORDER; HISTRIONIC PERSONALITY DISORDER; and BORDERLINE PERSONALITY DISORDER.

Resources on Mental Illness

American Psychiatric Association, *Diagnostic and Statistical Manual of Mental Disorders, 4th Edition* (1994); Barchas, Jack D., *Psychopharmacology: From Theory to Practive* (1977); Beckham, E. Edward and William R. Leber, eds., *Handbook of Depression: Treatment, Assessment, and Research* (1985); Wender, P.H. and D.F. Klein, *Mind, Mood, and Medicine: A Guide to the New Biopsychiatry* (1981); Nat. Depressive & Manic-Depressive Association, Tel. (800) 82-NDMDA, Online: www.nd-mda.org; National Mental Health Association, Tel. (800) 969-NMHA, Online: www.nmha.org; www.nycornell.org/psychiatry/.

Personality Tests

Any of a number of diagnostic tests designed to evaluate personality and identify abnormality.

Many tests exist to assess aspects of personality. Personality disorders take extremely varied forms, with symptoms exhibited through behavioral irregularities. Tests used to diagnose such disorders may be visual, tactile, auditory or involve any combination of senses. Often such examinations involve a standardized set of written or spoken questions. Responses to such tests may be symptomatic of personality disorder or simply indicate general personality traits within the limits of a normal personality.

Personality disorders may involve sociopathic or violent behavior (as in the case of antisocial personality disorder), attention deficit, over dependency, a range of abnormal fears (phobias), passive-aggressiveness, and so forth. Other serious abnormalities include manic-depression and schizophrenia. Causes of personality disorders are also highly varied. With some ailments, there appears to be a strong genetic component, while others seem largely the product of upbringing and environment. Such disorders are still poorly understood. Personality tests are sometimes a beginning step in proper diagnosis and effective treatment, which may involve psychotherapy, drug treatment, a combination of these or, in rare cases, surgical intervention. *See also* AT-TENTION DEFICIT DISORDER; MANIC-DEPRESSIVE ILLNESS; MENTAL ILLNESS; PASSIVE AGGRESSIVE PERSONALITY DISORDER; PERSONALITY; PERSONALITY DISORDERS; PHOBIA; SCHIZOPHRENIA; *and* THOUGHT DISORDERS.

Perthes' Disease

Also called xoxa planta or Legg-Calve-Perthes disease

A deterioration of the top of the thighbone due to insufficient blood supply to the area.

Perthes' disease causes the top of the femur to become flat. Blood flow is interrupted, and the tip of the femur dies over a period of one to three weeks.

The disorder tends to occur mostly in boys between four and 10 years old. Perthes' disease is characterized by knee and thigh pain, atrophy of upper thigh muscles, asymmetry of legs, difficulty walking, and hip stiffness.

Bed rest and a splint or brace are recommended and, occasionally, surgery may be required. Patients may develop osteoarthritis later in life. *See also* ARTHRITIS; BRACE; BLOODFLO; *and* SPLINT .

Pessary

An object inserted into the vagina for therapeutic or contraceptive purposes.

A pessary may be placed in the vagina to help prop up the uterus in case of prolapse. It can also be used to alleviate discomfort caused by deep penetration during sexual intercourse. Another form of pessary is an inserted contraceptive device that provides a barrier to sperm. These include the diaphragm, contraceptive cap, and the contraceptive sponge. *See also* CONTRACEPTION PROLAPSE, UTERUS; SEXUAL INTERCOURSE; *and* VAGINA.

Pesticides

Pesticides are used on a variety of foods to minimize crop loss and damage.

While pesticides are by nature highly toxic substances, the danger to the consumer is minimal. Precautions should of course be taken to carefully wash all produce, a step

ALERT

Pesticide Fatalities

If you experience a reaction after handling any type of pesticide, immediately seek medical help. The following symptoms may indicate a reaction that could be lethal: breathing difficulties, salivation, nausea, diarrhea, vomiting, fatigue, headache, muscle tremors or twitching, numbness or allergic reactions affecting the skin, eyes, nose, mouth, and throat. To avoid lethal exposure, always be sure to wear proper protective clothing, gloves and goggles whenever handling pesticides.

that will not only remove most pesticide residues, but that also guards against infection by any pathogenic bacteria. A variety of pesticides are currently used on grains, fruits, and vegetables. The greatest risk is to those who work directly with pesticides, whether the work involves its production or its direct application to crops.

Pesticides applied around the house can pose an additional threat, especially when used improperly. Be aware that pesticide products labeled as "natural" or "biological" may be as toxic as synthetic substances and should also be used with care. If pesticides are used in or around the household, be certain to follow the directions carefully, and keep children and pets away from treated areas.

Background material on pesticides can be found in FOOD *and* POISON. *Some additional information is contained in* PHARMACOLOGY, PUBLIC HEALTH *and* ENVIRONMENTAL HEALTH, ONCOLOGY *and* TOXIN. *Information related to pesticides is available in* BREATHING DIFFICULTIES; DIARRHEA; FATIGUE; POISONING; *and* VOMITING

PET Scanning

Acronym for Positron Emission Tomography, a non-invasive imaging technique allowing transverse sectional images of tissue to be visualized.

HOW IT WORKS

Positron emission tomography, or PET, is an imaging technique used primarily to visualize the brain and heart. Positrons are positively charged, short lived, radioactive particles. The radioactive substance is either injected or inhaled by the patient. Easily traced by an imaging computer, the radioactive particles are carried to the regions of interest in the body by the process of the blood's exchange of fluids, nutrients, and waste products.

PET scanning does not provide detailed images of body anatomy as well as an MRI can; MRI scanning is best suited to anatomic profiling. PET scans represent the chemical activity of tissues and organs, or blood flow. A profile showing the distribution of blood (and therefore the most

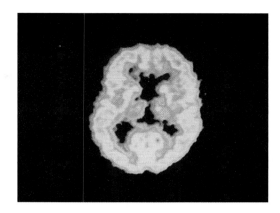

active areas of the heart muscle) is clearly observed in the resulting positron emission tomography scan. The computer is able to assemble the information into an three-dimensional image.

APPLICATIONS

PET is used for both clinical and research purposes.

Imaging the Heart. PET scanning of the heart, for example, follows the injection of a labeled, positron-emitting pharmaceutical that can show blood flow to the heart's muscle with unrivaled accuracy, as well as various aspects of heart metabolism.

Imaging Tumors. Abnormal growths (tumors) in the body typically consume a form of sugar known as glucose. Using a radioactive glucose solution makes PET scanning highly sensitive to tumors. Tumors of the lung, colorectal cancer, malignant melanoma, and malignant lymphoma may all be identified in this way. This is the most commun clinical use of PET.

Imaging the Brain. PET scans can monitor blood flow in the brain and aid in the diagnosis of a range of diseases including various forms of epilepsy, and degenerative diseases of the nervous system. PET's ability to chart brain activity has made it one of the most useful techniques for advanced brain research.

For information about other types of imaging see BRAIN; BRAIN, DISORDERS; BRAIN TUMOR; BRAIN IMAGING; CAT SCAN; GLUCOSE; HEART IMAGING; IMAGING TECHNIQUES; MRI; RADIONUCLIDE SCANNING; SCHIZOPHRENIA; *and* TOMOGRAPHY. *Imaging is a reliable* DIAGNOSTIC *technique.*

PET Scan. Above, an image of a PET (Positron Emission Tomography) scan. PET scans can pick up on the most subtle of brain injures because of the ultra-high resolution images that they produce. A nuclear medical expert is always consulted in order to determine the nature of the disorder that shows up in a PET scan.

Petachiae

A type of bleeding into the skin, subcutaneous tissues, and mucous membranes.

Bleeding that looks like pinpoint dots of blood is called petechiae. When pressed, petechiae does not become pale. There are numerous possible causes of petechiae, including local injury, allergic reaction, autoimmune disorders, viral infection, radiation or chemotherapy, bruising, aging skin, leukemia, certain drugs, and violent coughing and vomiting. If petechiae is experienced, or if there is persistent and unexplained bruising, consult a health care provider. *See also* BLEEDING.

Peutz-Jeghers Syndrome

A rare, inherited disease characterized by gastrointestinal polyps, brown spots around the lips, and a high risk for various tumors.

Dark brown spots on the lips and around the mouth that characterize Peutz-Jeghers syndrome are easily recognized during childhood but usually fade during adolescence. The polyps caused by Peutz-Jeghers syndrome do not usually cause any symptoms, but they may cause abdominal cramping, chronic bleeding (which may result in anemia), or an intestinal obstruction due to one portion of the intestine telescoping into another, a condition known as intussusception.

The polyps may also develop into malignant tumors, which is a serious complication. Thus, Peuts Jeghers syndrome can be fatal if it is left unchecked and untreated; monitoring is a permanent requirement.

Regular diagnostic tests, such as endoscopy, are recommended to monitor the polyps and ensure that it is not transforming into a malignancy. Polyps that are causing problems may be removed surgically. Peutz-Jeghers syndrome is related to familial polyposis, an inherited disorder, in which hundreds of polyps form in the colon and rectum. *See also* ANEMIA; INTUSSUCEPTION; POLYPOSIS, FAMILIAL; *and* POLYPS.

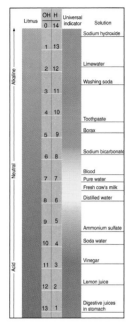

pH. Seven is considered neutral in the pH scale, as it is the value of pure water. When an antacid tablet is placed in water, its citric acid is neutralized by the sodium bicaronate base, thus releasing carbon dioxide and creating a "fizzing" effect. Magnesium hydroxide is another base used to relieve hyperacidity (heartburn) and neutralize stomach acid.

Peyronie's Disease

A condition in which fibrous tissue accumulates in the penis, resulting in a distorted erectile shape

In Peyronie's disease, the erect penis curves in a manner that may make sexual intercourse difficult or impossible. Erections may also be painful; in some cases, fibrous tissue extends into the erectile tissue, making erection impossible. This disease usually affects men between the ages of 40 and 60. The condition may resolve spontaneously. Injections of corticosteroids or ultrasound treatments may be helpful. Surgical removal of the fibrous material is a more common option, although the surgery may leave scar tissue that will make the condition worse and can also lead to impotence. *See also* PENIS.

pH

Scale used to measure balance of acids and alkalis in a fluid.

In chemistry, the actions of a solution are often determined by whether they contain more acids or alkalis(bases). The pH scale ranges from 0 to 14, with seven representing an equal balance of alkalis and acids. pH measures higher than seven indicate a solution contains more alkalis, and lower than seven mean that more acids are present. The human body functions best with a pH of 7.4. When the pH drops below that, the body is experiencing a condition called acidosis; when it rises above that, it is in a state of alkalosis. *See also* ACID.

Phagocyte

A type of white blood cell that engulfs and digests invading disease-causing agents (antigens).

The process by which phagocytes destroy antigens is called phagocytosis. Antigens coated with antibodies are produced by the immune system. They are easier for phagocytes to destroy than those not coated with antibodies. *See also* IMMUNE RESPONSE.

Phantom Limb

The persistent feeling that a limb is present after amputation.

When a limb has been amputated, it is not uncommon for a person to feel as if it were still present. This is due to the brain's misinterpretation of nerve impulses from the stump where the limb has been cut off. Though they are only from the remaining endings, the brain believes that they are from the whole limb, which leads to the feeling that the limb is still present.

Pharmacology

The field of drug research and application.

A medication is any substance used to combat disease or to counteract congenital or degenerative conditions. Pharmacology refers to the study, development, and use of available medications and the research into new drugs; the means of administering the drugs (by mouth, injection, inhalation, skin patch, etc.); the movement of the drug in the body (usually using the blood stream) so that it reaches the target site and is then disposed of properly; the efficacy of the drug; and side effects and interactions of a drug with other drugs. *See also* Drug.

Pharyngitis

Inflammation of the throat.

The pharynx, more commonly known as the throat, connects the oral cavity and nasal chamber to the esophagus. The throat, then, serves as an entry way for air on its way to the lungs and food traveling to the esophagus and stomach. The throat is lined with tissues that act as an immune system, sampling and analyzing bacteria and viruses as they enter the body. These tissues then prepare antibodies designed to fight them. The immune system tissues come together to form the two sets of tonsils, one pair at the back of the throat, and another at the base of the tongue. When there are many viruses or bacteria, the tonsils and linings of the throat become inflamed, causing a sore throat or pharyngitis.

Causes. Sore throats are most commonly caused by bacterial or viral infections. The most common infection that causes a sore throat comes from the bacteria streptococci, better know as strep throat. The characteristic symptom of this form of infection are tonsils that are not merely swollen and painful, but that also exhibit white patches or pus on their surface. A fever, headache, and swollen lymph nodes will usually accompany the infection. Diagnosis may be made either through a throat culture that takes a sampling of pus, or through a strep test.

Viral infections of the throat such as colds or flu, can also cause swollen tonsils, although in most cases they will not develop the pus or white patches common to strep throat. In cases of the mononucleosis virus, however, the tonsils may appear to be similar to those infected by bacteria; tested blood samples will be able to differentiate between the conditions.

Treatment. Pharyngitis must be treated according to its underlying cause, which is why it is important to determine the nature of the illness. If it is a viral infection, then antibiotics are not required, or particularly helpful; the body's own immune system is the best method for healing. If a bacterial infection, such as strep, is at the root of the problem, then a full course of antibiotics may be prescribed depending on the condition's severity. If the infection persists, or there is a frequent recurrence, then a doctor may recommend tonsil removal.

In both cases, the symptoms can be treated with home preparations such as a warm salt water gargle or over-the-counter throat sprays. Over-the-counter painkillers can also help relieve symptoms.

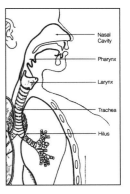

Pharyngitis. Above, an illustration of the respiratory system, with a detail of the pharynx (the throat). This can be caused by a bacterial or a viral infection, however, most cases are viral. This also occurs more frequently among children than among adults.

Basic anatomical information on pharyngitis is contained in Mononucleosis; Pharynx; *and* Tonsillitis. *More is contained in* Cold; Influenza; Sore Throat; Streptococcal Infections; *and* Strep Throat. *Details on surgical treatment is found in* Tonsillectomy.

Pharyngoesophageal Diverticulum

Pouch in the esophagus that can enlarge and become infected

A pharyngoesophageal diverticulum is a pouch at the top of the esophagus that protrudes outward. The pouch develops as the result of a failure of the sphincter (the muscle at the top of the esophagus) to contract when swallowing. The resistance of the throat muscles pushes the lining of the esophagus out, forming the pouch. It then will enlarge, allowing food particles to become trapped inside. This may lead to throat irritation, bad breath, swallowing difficulties and vomiting.

Treatment involves the surgical removal of the pouch, as well as the loosening of the sphincter to prevent recurrence. *See also* ESOPHAGEAL DIVERTICULUM; ESOPHAGUS; PHARYNX; SPHINCTER; SWALLOWING; *and* SWALLOWING DIFFICULTIES.

Pharynx, Cancer of

Malignant tumor of the throat.

The pharynx, or throat, is a muscular pathway between the mouth and nose and the esophagus; its structures include the vocal cords. Most cancers of the pharynx develop in the squamous cells that form inside its lining, and most of those cancers are related to tobacco and alcohol use. Any kind of tobacco—whether it is cigarettes, snuff, cigars, or chewing tobacco—can damage the genetic material of the cells of the pharynx, causing mutations that lead to uncontrolled growth. Alcohol also causes damage, and the risk of cancer of the pharynx is highest in persons who both smoke and drink.

Surviving Pharynx Cancer

A detailed follow-up usually is necessary after treatment for cancer of the pharynx because of its lasting effects on the body and on a person's lifestyle. The survivor will have to learn new techniques for eating, speaking and breathing after all or part of the larynx is removed. Therapists that specialize in teaching these techniques can also recommend specialized technology that enables nearly all cancer survivors to communicate effectively with their friends, family, co-workers, and doctors.

Symptoms. Symptoms of a cancer of the pharynx depend on its location. In general, squamous cell cancers start as plaques, symptomless white patches of abnormal cells. Unless they are detected early and removed, plaques can become cancerous, causing bumps and ulcers in the tissue lining the pharynx.

A tumor on a vocal cord can cause hoarseness; a tumor of the nasopharynx, the area behind the nose, can cause nosebleeds, hearing loss, ringing in the ears and pain; cancer of the laryngopharynx, the lowest part of the pharynx, can cause difficult or painful swallowing. General symptoms of cancer of the pharynx include a persistent sore throat, swollen lymph nodes in the neck, throat pain, bleeding, and weight loss.

Diagnosis. Diagnosis is made by physical examination of the pharynx through a laryngoscope, bronchoscope or esophagoscope and by removal of a tissue sample for microscopic examination (biopsy). A computerized tomography, CT, scan may also be done to precisely localize the tumor.

Treatment. Treatment depends on the location of the cancer and the stage at which it is detected. A cancer of the oropharynx, the region behind the throat, usually requires a combination of surgery and radiation therapy. Chemotherapy may be offered to a patient before surgery.

Cancer of the hypopharynx, the area behind and next to the voice box (larynx), usually necessitates surgery, because the difficulty in detecting such cancers means they usually are found at a more advanced stage. Both the larynx and pharynx may be removed. Radiation therapy and chemotherapy may be given after surgery. For cancer of the larynx that is detected at an early stage, radiation therapy is preferred because it can preserve the patient's ability to speak independently, without the use of a mechanical aide device.

Basic information is contained in BENIGN; CANCER; MALIGNANT; PHARYNX; *and* TUMOR. *Information about diagnosis and treatment lies in* ANTICANCER DRUGS; BIOPSY; CHEMOTHERAPY; RADIATION THERAPY; *and* TOMOGRAPHY.

Phenylketonuria

Commonly known as PKU

A hereditary metabolic disorder.

PKU is caused by a defective gene which in turn causes the production of a defective metabolic enzyme. In the absence of a functional enzyme to break it down, the amino acid phenylalanine accumulates in the blood. PKU occurs in most genetic groups, but is relatively rare among individuals of African descent and Jews of Eastern European origin. If left untreated, the buildup of phenylalanine can lead to mental retardation. Newborns are routinely screened for this disorder while still in the hospital with a simple blood test.

Symptoms. Symptoms of this disorder are usually absent in newborns. Children with phenylketonuria experience seizures, nausea, vomiting, hyperactivity, and sometimes psychiatric symptoms. There may be a particular body odor due to the presence of a phenylalanine by-product in body secretions. Untreated PKU in a pregnant woman can affect the developing fetus.

Treatment. Generally, treatment consists primarily of a carefully controlled diet to limit the intake of phenylalanine. Most proteins and natural foods contain phenylalanine, so a variety of synthetic foods must be substituted. Dietary restrictions must begin during the first few weeks of life. It used to be thought that once brain development was completed, the diet could be discontinued, but recent research indicates that a phenylalanine-restricted diet should be continued throughout a person's life. *See also* ARTIFICIAL SWEETENERS.

Pheochromocytoma

Also known as chromaffin tumor

A tumor of the adrenal gland which causes too much adrenalin, epinephrine, and norepinephrine to be secreted.

Adrenalin, epinephrine, and norepinephrine are the hormones partly responsible for regulating blood pressure and heart rate. People suffering from pheochromo-cytoma have trouble sleeping, tremors, sweats, regular and severe headaches, a very rapid heart rate and intense chest and abdomen pains. If the presence of abnormal blood tests identifies a malignancy, then a biopsy, an MRI, or a CT scan is used to locate the tumor(s); sometimes there are a few. As radiation and chemotherapy have proven ineffective against this type of cancer, the tumors must be removed. With surgery the survival rate is good, unless the tumor returns. There is no way known at present to prevent pheo-chromocytoma. *See also* CANCER.

Phlebitis

Inflammation of a vein, most commonly occurring in the legs and often associated with formation of a type of clot called thrombus.

Phlebitis can be the result of an injury caused by an accident (trauma), a medical procedure that damages a vein, or a drug that irritates the veins; infection association is also not uncommon. It occurs most often in the superficial veins, those lying nearest to the skin, and is somewhat more common in women than men.

Phlebitis is dangerous if it leads to the formation of a clot that blocks the smooth flow of blood through the vein back to the heart, a condition called thrombophlebitis. It causes symptoms including pain, swelling, redness and tenderness of the affected area. The condition usually can be diagnosed just by its appearance.

Because phlebitis of a vein close to the skin generally goes away in a week or two, it may not require treatment, but heating the affected extremity, elevating it, and taking aspirin or another anti-inflammatory drug can help relieve the symptoms. Thrombophlebitis occurring in a deep-lying vein is a much more serious condition, because the clot can break away and travel to the lung. Anticoagulant therapy under a doctor's care is absolutely necessary for deep-lying thrombophlebitis, also known as deep vein thrombosis or DVT. *See also* EMBOLISM; THROMBOSIS; *and* VEINS, DISORDERS OF.

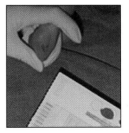

Phenylketonuria Test. Above, blood is routinely drawn from infants (often from their feet) in order to perform diagnostic tests. Taking blood from an infant's foot is commonly referred to as a "heel stick" as the blood is usually taken form the heel.

Phobia

A strong fear or aversion, that is often without rational explanation, of a thing or situation.

Despite being clearheadedly aware that a thing or situation presents no actual danger, it will inspire fear in an individual anyway. A phobic individual will not only recognize the fear, but he or she often also recognizes the irrationality of it. The object that incites fear is referred to as a phobic stimulus. Phobias are often referred to as the root fear with the suffix, phobia. Acrophobia (fear of heights), claustrophobia (fear of small confined places), xanthophobia (fear of the color yellow), and zoophobia (fear of animals) are a few of many phobias.

Phobias can often cause significant social problems. Social phobias are particularly prevalent; these are sometimes called phobic disorders and should be treated by a psychologist. *See also* PANIC ATTACK.

Phocomelia

Also known as Roberts Syndrome

A rare developmental disorder characterized by multiple abnormalities.

Phocomelia is transmitted as a recessive gene. It causes an error during cell reproduction, disrupting the normal chromosomal pairing. The manifestations of phocomelia include:

- symmetrical limb reduction, similar to that caused by thalidomide;
- craniofacial anomalies, such as cleft, lip and palate;
- nose and ear anomalies;
- severe mental and growth retardation;
- scant, silvery hair.

Other organs and body systems may also be affected. Survival beyond infancy is quite rare. Babies born with severe limb and facial defects are often stillborn or die shortly after birth. The recurrence risk for couples with a positive family history of this disorder is 25 percent. *See also* GENETICS *and* MENTAL RETARDATION.

Phosphates

Phosphates are compounds containing the element phosphorus. It is an essential ingredient in many life processes.

Elemental phosphorus (chemical symbol P), is usually referred to as white phosphorus when it is in a pure form; phosphates are compounds of phosphorous and other elements. Phosphorus compounds are widely used as in fertilizers and pesticides (organo-phosphates); either can be extremely toxic to humans and animals. In contrast, phosphate compounds are often used in medications. For example, sodium cellulose phosphate is used to prevent the formation of kidney stones by combining with dietary calcium before it reaches the kidneys; it also functions in bone metabolism, and a well-balanced diet will include approximately equal amounts of calcium and phosphate compounds. *See also* PHOSPHORUS POISONING.

Phosphorus Poisoning

Poisoning due to organic or inorganic phosphorus compounds.

Yellow phosphorus (which is a name for a type of phosphorus that can also be colorless) is often used in fertilizers, fireworks, and insect and rodent poisons. Phosphides and phosphorus gas are also toxic. Red phosphorus (phosphorus sesquifluoride), used on matches, is nontoxic.

Ingestion or inhalation of yellow phosphorus or toxic phosphide gases can cause fatigue, irregular heartbeat, nausea, vomiting and diarrhea, and a garlic-like breath odor. Severe kidney and liver damage can occur. Symptoms may temporarily subside, but coma and death can occur between a day and three weeks after the poisoning. Inhalation can also cause bronchitis and pneumonia. Treatment consists of washing out the stomach (gastric decontamination), eye irrigation injecting calcium, and treating kidney or liver failure. *See also* PHOSPHATES *and* POISONING.

Photocoagulation

A surgical process of coagulating (clotting) tissue by means of a precisely oriented, high-energy light source, such as a laser beam.

Photocoagulation has proven highly effective in treating small tumors, tiny blood clots, and certain types of optic damage. Small hemorrhages in or near the eyes and retinal damage can be treated with the argon laser often used in photocogulation. *See also* BLOOD *and* COAGULATION.

Photosensitivity

The sensitivity of the skin to light.

Photosensitivity is a reaction that occurs when skin is exposed to sunlight, fluorescent light, or suntan parlor lamps. Polymorphous light eruption is a type of photosensitivity that causes skin to become red, itchy, and bumpy as a result of the first few sun exposures of the summer. Other diseases, including lupus erythematosus, are photosensitive.

Certain medications, when combined with exposure to sunlight, cause a similar reaction. Medications that may contribute to photosensitivity include doxycycline, ciprofloxacin, and ofloxacin. Certain properties of limes, celery, and figs may cause localized photosensitivity in some people.

Medications and corticosteroids are used to treat photosensitivity. Avoiding sun exposure, especially during treatment, is essential, *See also* LUPUS ERYTHEMATOSUS.

Phototherapy

Use of natural sunlight or artificial light for therapeutic purposes.

Both natural and artificial light can be used in treatment for a variety of afflictions. Jaundice, a common disease in newborns, (also known as hyperbilirubinemia) may be treated with phototherapy. The disorder is due to abnormally high concentrations of bilirubin, a byproduct of hemoglobin, in the bloodstream. Jaundice typically gives the skin a yellowish appearance. The appearance of jaundice advances from the head to the feet. Phototherapy is used in protracted cases of the disease. An infant suffering from jaundice is placed under bright lights, which produce chemical changes in the bilirubin molecules of the body, causing them to be more effectively excreted by the liver.

Light can have a therapeutic effect on the skin, and phototherapy is sometimes used in cases of severe eczema or psoriasis. Ultraviolet radiation may supplement the use of sunlight or artificial light therapy.

Seasonal Affective Disorders. Some patients suffer depressive symptoms that are believed to be related to seasonal shortages of daylight. Such seasonal affective disorders are sometimes treated with phototherapy. Such therapy involves extending the day artificially in various ways. Occasionally, a computerized system of lighting in a patient's bedroom is used to simulate an early dawn and lengthened day. *See also* BILIRUBIN; BLOOD; DEPRESSION; ECZEMA; JAUNDICE; PSORIASIS; *and* ULTRAVIOLET LIGHT.

Physical Therapy

Post-injury treatment and rehabilitation through physical means.

Physical therapy is used to alleviate stiffness and strength loss caused by diseases, injuries, and disorders. Patients who have undergone an extended period of bed rest can benefit from physical therapy. Therapy can reduce pain and inflammation and help to reteach movements to joints and muscles that have suffered long-term immobilization, nerve injuries or strokes.

Physical therapy usually falls into two categories. In passive therapy, the therapist moves the parts of the body around in an effort to help increase flexibility and range of motion. Active therapy involves teaching the patient exercises, such as how to contract muscles groups or train muscles to perform certain movements. Physical therapy also includes therapeutic massage, heat or ice treatment, ultrasound, hydrotherapy, or the use of light and electrical currents. A qualified physical therapist should assess the patient's joint motion, muscle strength, endurance, and heart and lung functions in order to design an appropriate program for that individual. *See also* ARTHRITIS; EXERCISE; HEAT TREATMENT; ICE PACKS; INJURY; MOVEMENT; *and* PHYSICAL THERAPY.

Pica

A craving, brought on by a variety of conditions, for non-food items.

People with pica crave substances such as clay, soil, ice, coffee grounds, paint and plaster, laundry starch, paraffin, paper scraps, and ashes. Pica can be a symptom of a variety of diseases or conditions, particularly iron-deficiency anemia. Pregnancy can also cause pica. It is a cultural belief of some people in the southern United States, that consuming clay will ease pregnancy and ensure a healthy baby.

ALERT

Pica During Pregnancy

The practice of eating non-food substances can cause intestinal obstructions and possibly toxemia (which is also known as pre-eclampsia) in pregnancy. Increased newborn mortality and premature births have been linked to pica as well. Clay may also transmit gastrointestinal parasites. Since pica can be hazardous to health, depending on the nature of the craving, and can also indicate iron deficiency, it should be reported to a doctor for treatment.

Research has determined that iron deficiency has an influence on pica. Regardless of its origin, pica generally ceases when iron supplements are given to the victim. *See also* IRON DEFICIENCY *and* PREGNANCY.

Pigeon Toes

Also known as Intoeing

An inward rotation of the leg or foot.

A minor condition in which the toes point inward due to an abnormal set of the leg.

Common in toddlers, the condition usually corrects itself by age seven. Serious cases that last beyond that age and interfere with movement may require surgery. *See also* BONE DISORDERS.

Pigmentation

Skin color is determined by pigment, or melanin, found in the upper layers of skin

The natural pigment in skin is yellow, dark brown, or black in color. The amount of the melanin in one's body determines the color of the skin, hair, and iris of the eye. Sun exposure, hormonal changes, and genetics determine the level of melanin in an individual. Sunbathing also causes the body to extensively produce more melanin, thus the tanned look.

Albinism, melasma, pigment loss after skin damage, and vitiligo are all considered pigment disorders. Albinism is an extremely rare, inherited disorder in which the skin contains no melanin at all. The body appears pale, with white hair and pink eyes. People with albinism should avoid direct sunlight, since their skin and eyes have little or no protection against the damaging effects of sunlight.

Melasma, also called "mask of pregnancy" appears as brown, symmetrical areas of dark pigment on the face. Most common during pregnancy, melasma can be treated with prescription creams to lighten the dark patches. Wearing sunscreen and limiting sun exposure can stop melasma from getting worse.

A skin injury often produces a blister, burn, or infection. After the area heals, sometimes the skin loses some of its pigment. This condition is not usually treated. Cosmetics may be used to cover the area.

Vitiligo is a disorder that causes smooth, white patches to form on the skin. These patches result as a loss of melanin in the skin and are extremely sensitive to sunlight. Physical injury and illnesses such as diabetes and Addison's disease also cause vitiligo. There is no known cure for vitiligo. Treatments to alleviate symptoms may include dyes to cover over the white spots, light-sensitive drugs, light therapy, and corticosteroid creams. *See also* ADDISON'S DISEASE; ALBINISM; MELANIN; MELASMA; PHOTOSENSITIVITY; SKIN; *and* VITILIGO.

Piles

Also known as Hemorrhoids

Enlarged (varicose) veins in the lower portion of the rectum or anus.

Piles are caused by increased pressure in the veins of the anus. The most common cause of this pressure is straining during bowel movements, but piles can also be caused by fits of coughing, vomiting, sneezing, constipation, prolonged sitting, and anal infection.

Symptoms. Symptoms of piles include rectal bleeding, rectal bleeding following bowel movements, bloody stools, pain during bowel movements, and anal itching. Piles are very common, especially during pregnancy and after childbirth. Treatments for piles include corticosteroid creams, rubber band ligation, cryosurgery, or hemorrhoidectomy. Eating a high-fiber diet and drinking plenty of caffeine free fluids may help prevent the development of piles. *See also* CRYOSURGERY; DIET AND DISEASE; EXERCISE; HEMORRHOIDECTOMY; VARICOSE VEINS *and* VEIN.

Pimple

Also called Pustule

A superficial skin eruption, caused by plugged skin pores.

Pimples result from the clogging of the hair follicle or pore. Sebaceous glands, which secrete an oily substance called sebum, empty into the hair follicle. When the plugged pore breaks open, materials inside the pore, such as bacteria, can enter and cause an inflammation. Treatment includes topical medications, antibiotics, cortisone injections, and surgical intervention. *See also* ACNE; CHAPPED SKIN; FOLLICLE; SEBACEOUS CYST; *and* SKIN.

Pineal Gland

The gland at the back of the hypothalamus that regulates the hormone called melatonin.

The word pineal means pine-cone shaped, and describes this gland rather well. It regulates the hormone, melatonin, which affects the body's sleeping and waking cycles and is involved with mood regulation. *See also* BRAIN; CIRCADIAN RHYTHM; HORMONE REPLACEMENT THERAPY; *and* HORMONES.

Pinguecula

Also known as Conjunctiva

A raised yellow-white growth on the white of either eye due to excessive sunlight exposure.

The cause of these growths is unknown, but researchers generally agree that it comes from exposure to sunlight and chronic irritation of the eye. The spot does not usually grow and the condition normally disappears without treatment. In rare cases, the growth continues until it covers the cornea, causing a pterygium, which may interfere with vision. In such cases, surgical removal is possible and the ophthalmologist will conduct tests to determine if the growth is malignant. *See also* BLURRED VISION; CONJUNCTIVA; CORNEA: *and* EYE.

Pink Puffer

Informal medical term for an emphysema patient whose skin retains its normal appearance.

Pink puffer's skin remains the normal pink color because it is getting an adequate oxygen supply, even though the sufferer has emphysema. Some emphysema patients' skin turns blueish due to inadequate oxygen; these people are informally called blue bloaters. In both pink puffers and blue bloaters, the damage that emphysema does to the lungs creates a persistent shortage of breath; treated consists of bronchodilating medications. *See also* BRONCHODILATOR DRUGS; EMPHYSEMA; LUNGS; *and* TOBACCO SMOKING.

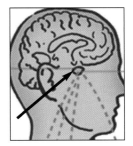

The Position of the Pineal Gland. Above, the pineal gland is located at the bottom of the brain, towards the middle. It is right behind the pituitary gland; and both of these glands are linked via the endocrine system.

Pinta

Chronic skin infection caused by the spiral-shaped bacterium *Treponema carateum*.

Pinta is caused by a bacterium similar to the causative agent of syphilis and yaws. It occurs in remote areas of tropical Latin America, and is acquired through physical contact. After the bacterium incubates for one to three weeks, a small nodule appears on the skin's surface. This gradually enlarges, becoming surrounded with other nodules. The lymph nodes in the affected area also may swell. Subsequently, bluish patches develop over several months, generally on the face and the limbs. These patches gradually subside, often leaving scars. Pinta can usually be cured with penicillin. *See also* SYPHILIS *and* YAWS.

Pituitary Gland

Gland that directs other glands and controls several major bodily functions.

Although only the size of a pea, the pituitary gland is one of the most important glands in the body. It not only controls its own series of organs and bodily processes, but it also releases hormones that regulate the activities of many other glands.

This tiny gland lies deep in the folds of the brain; it is in a cavity in the skull where it hangs from the base of the brain just beneath the optic nerve. A short stem of nerves connects the pituitary gland to the hypothalamus, which directs the gland's activities. The hypothalamus has two ways of sending messages to the pituitary gland: through stimulation from its nerve connections, or through hormones released directly into the pituitary's blood supply.

HORMONES AND LOBES

The pituitary gland is composed of two lobes, each of which secretes its own set of hormones.

The hormones secreted by the anterior pituitary lobe are:

- Growth hormone: The growth hormone is secreted by the pituitary gland, at the command of the hypothalamus. This hormone instructs cells to divide and begins the manufacture of proteins, leading to growth in areas such as bones and cartilage.
- Prolactin: This hormone is responsible both for milk production from the breast during and after pregnancy.
- ACTH: Adrenocorticotropic hormone regulates the release of cortisol and other steroid hormones from the adrenal glands, which are responsible for various aspects of the metabolism of nutrients, and sodium levels in the blood. The pituitary gland produces ACTH based on direction from the hypothalamus, as well as hydrocortisone levels in the blood.
- TSH: Thyroid stimulating hormone activates the thyroid gland, which produces hormones that help maintain normal body metabolism. The pituitary glands release of TSH is regulated by the hypothalamus, which sends TRH, thyroid releasing hormone, to the pituitary when levels of thyroid hormone in the blood are low.
- FSH and LH: Follicle-stimulating hormone (FSH) and luteinizing hormone (LH) are two of the most important of the gonadotropin hormones. They help to regulate sexual development and fertility by activating the gonads, or sex glands.

The hormones released by the posterior pituitary gland are:

- ADH: Antidiuretic hormone helps to maintain fluid levels in the blood. The hypothalamus monitors blood concentration and volume; when the blood does not contain enough water, it directs the pituitary to release ADH. The kidneys then decrease the amount of urine produced. When there is too much water in the blood stream, ADH release is decreased.
- Oxytocin: This hormone helps with the release of milk from the mammary glands, and also induces uterine contractions during labor.

Resources on Endocrine Disorders

Greenspan, Francis S., et al., Basic & Clinical Endocrinology (2000); Krimsky, Sheldon and Lynn Goldman, *Hormonal Chaos: The Scientific and Social Origins of the Environmental Endocrine Hypothesis* (1999); Shin, Linda M., et al., *Endocrine and Metabolic Disorders Sourcebook* (1998); American Thyroid Association, Tel. (718) 882-6047, Online: www.thyroid.org; www.nycornell.org/medicine/edm/index.html.

DISORDERS OF THE PITUITARY GLAND

A problem in the pituitary gland, because of its influence over so many bodily activities, both directly, and indirectly through the regulation of other glands' hormones, can seriously affect any number of bodily processes. Most of the disorders that affect the pituitary gland lead to either too little or too much production of any of the pituitary hormones.

TUMORS

Most tumors in the pituitary gland are benign, but they still can do a great deal of damage. A tumor may destroy some of the hormone producing cells, which causes underproduction of that hormone. Other types of tumors can cause overproduction of the hormone. This in turn can cause over or underproduction of another hormone that is controlled by the pituitary gland. Pituitary tumors can cause further damage by either pressing on the optic nerve, or the hypothalamus.

ALERT

Tumor Related Pituitary Disorders

Some of the disorders caused by tumors of the pituitary gland are:

- Acromegaly: enlargement of facial features, hands and feet, because of the overproduction of human growth hormone.
- Galactorrhea: milk production when there is neither pregnancy or childbirth, caused by excess prolactin production.
- Gigantism: excess production of the growth hormone during childhood can lead to unusually rapid growth and height.
- Hypergonadism: overproduction of the gonadotropin hormones can cause early sexual development.
- Cushing's disease: characterized by swelling in the face and trunk, this condition may be caused by oversecretion of ACTH, which leads to overproduction of the corticosteroid hormones.
- Hypothyroidism: weight gain, lethargy, and weakness are some of the symptoms of this condition, which may be caused by a pituitary tumor's interference in the production of TSH (thyroid-stimulating hormone).

CONGENITAL OR GENETIC DISORDERS

A person may be born without a specific hormone, or an inability to produce certain hormones if the pituitary gland is underdeveloped or damaged during birth. In the absence of the growth hormone, for example, an individual will exhibit a short stature; missing gonadotropin hormones can cause lack of or underdevelopment of sexual characteristics; ACTH deficiency can cause various metabolic and electrolyte disorders.

Radiation or partial removal of the pituitry gland-while attempting to remove a tumor will affect the rest of the gland, leading to the loss of hormone production and of the gland's capabilities other than those which had already been disrupted by the tumor.

For background information about pituitary disorders see ENDOCRINE SYSTEM and HORMONES. Information on hormone related disorders can be found in PITUITARY TUMORS; GIGANTISM; HYPERGONADISM; CUSHING'S DISEASE; and HYPOTHYROIDISM. Specific hormones are discussed in GROWTH HORMONE; LUTEINIZING HORMONE; and THYROID HORMONES. See also HYPOTHALAMUS.

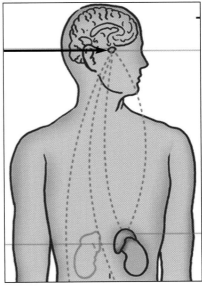

The Pituitary Gland. Above, tucked under the front of the brain is the pituitary gland. Via the pathways of the endocrine system, it sends messages that regulate the body's organs and functions.

Pituitary Tumors

Growths arising in the pituitary gland.

The pituitary gland is the most fundamental of the endocrine glands, which release hormones into the bloodstream. The gland is approximately the size of a pea and it is attached to the base of the brain.

Pituitary tumors are not uncommon. While almost all of them are benign, they can cause problems, usually because they grow large enough to press on other important cranial structures controlling functions of the brain or eye nerves. The resulting symptoms can include headache, loss of peripheral vision, numbness of the face, and drooping eyelids.

The output of one hormone or another may be increased or decreased abnormally by the presence of the tumor, causing problems. For example, overproduction of adrenocorticotropic hormone may cause Cushing's disease, which results in changes in body, fat levels, hair growth, and skin health. Overproduction of prolactin in a woman can stop the menstrual cycle and can make a man impotent. Overproduction of growth hormones cause acromegaly, which results in abnormal bone growth and coarseness of facial features.

Treatment includes surgical removal of the tumor, often followed by radiation therapy and sometimes by chemotherapy. *See also* CANCER; ENDOCRINE DISORDERS; PITUITARY GLAND.

Pityriasis Alba

A common skin problem, caused by mild eczema, resulting in round, colorless, scaly patches of skin, usually on the cheeks.

The rashes caused by pityriasis alba occur most often in children and adolescents. The cause of the disorder is unknown. The most common symptoms are round, white, flat patches. These patches are lighter than the surrounding skin, and they may be on the face, arms, neck, and upper trunk. The lesions don't tan in the summer and usually redden quickly in sunshine. Treatment with analgesics almost always clears up the condition. *See also* SKIN.

Pityriasis Rosea

A skin disorder causing a characteristic rash.

Pityriasis rosea is common in young adults, and is 50 percent more common in females than in males. Attacks usually last from four to eight weeks. Although the condition usually resolves itself over time, a health care practitioner should be consulted to rule out the possibility of syphilis, a serious sexually transmitted disease that causes similar symptoms.

Symptoms of pityriasis rosea include a Christmas tree pattern rash, itching, skin redness, and inflammation. A virus is sus-

Pityriasis Rosea.
Below, a man's chest is affected by pityriasis rosea, which is characterized by salmon colored patches with scaling (which is technically known as palmoplantar keratoderma). This condition is quite rare and it usually resolves itself.

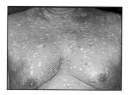

pected as the cause of the condition.

Treatment for pityriasis rosea includes gentle bathing and the use of anti-itching creams and ultraviolet light treatment. Scratching should be avoided, as it may cause the rash to spread. *See also* RASH *and* SYPHILIS.

Placebo

A pill or medication that contains no actual drug, but is given to test patients in order to determine whether the active medication really works.

When researchers test a drug's effectiveness, they need to be able to determine what effects are actually a result of the drug, rather than a result of the patient's state of mind or other factors. To help with this process, placebos, often simple sugar pills, are given to test subjects instead of the actual medication being tested. The researchers then compare the response of those given the medication to that of those given the placebo.

Studies indicate that 30 percent of those receiving a placebo do improve. Further, a percentage of those given the placebo have adverse reactions like nausea, vomiting, hives, diarrhea, and headache. All this speaks to the power of the mind to affect the body, its diseases and its cures. *See also* DRUGS *and* PSYCHOSOMATIC MEDICINES.

Placenta

Tissues that connect with a pregnant mother's blood supply and provide oxygen and nutrients to the fetus while also removing waste.

Everything taken in by the mother's body is transferred to the fetus via the placenta. There is no actual mixing between the mother's bloodstream and that of the fetus; the exchange of materials occurs across the thin membranes that separate fetal capillaries from small pools of maternal blood.

In addition to facilitating the exchange between maternal and fetal blood, the placenta also produces hormones to maintain the pregnancy. The placenta is fully

How The Placenta Develops

The placenta forms during the early stages of development, shortly after the blastocyst, the hollow ball of cells formed from the fertilized egg, implants in the uterine wall. Inner cells of the blastocyst develop into the embryo, and the outer cells form the embryonic membranes which burrow into the uterine wall and eventually become the placenta. These membranes include the chorion, the outer layer of cells responsible for gas exchange, and the amnion, the inner layer of cells which form the amniotic sac. As the placenta grows, tendrils (villi) from its surface extend into the uterine wall and branch out, increasing contact.

formed 18 to 20 weeks into a pregnancy, at about the midway point. By the time of delivery, the placenta usually weighs about one pound. The placenta is also called the afterbirth, because it is expelled from the body during the third stage of labor.

Problems with the placenta during pregnancy include placenta previa, in which the placenta is located in the lower portion of the uterus near or covering the cervix, and abruptio placentae, when the placenta prematurely detaches from the uterine wall. *See also* PLACENTA PREVIA.

Placenta Previa

A condition in which the placenta is located in the lower part of the uterus, either close to or covering the cervix.

Placenta previa occurs in about one of 200 deliveries; it is most common among women who have had several previous pregnancies, multiple pregnancies or have uterine abnormalities such as fibroids.

The only recognizable symptom for placenta previa is painless vaginal bleeding in late pregnancy. The amount of blood may vary. As with any bleeding during pregnancy, the doctor should be notified at once. Often ultrasound is used to distinguish placenta previa from another condition, abruptio placentae, in which the placenta has begun to detach prematurely from the uterine wall.

If the bleeding is minor and premature

delivery is not a threat, a woman may be put on bed rest. If a great deal of blood was lost, she may require a blood transfusion. Once labor is imminent, a Cesarean section is usually performed, as the placenta will detach very early in labor. This will result in an insufficient amount of oxygen for baby and may also result in heavy maternal bleeding. *See also* ABRUPTIO PLACENTAE.

Plague

An infectious disease among wild rodents and rats that may be passed on to humans by fleas.

Yersina pestis, the bacterium that causes plague, circulates among rodents and rats and their fleas. The most common form of plague in humans is the bubonic plague. Fleas feed on the infected blood of rodents and subsequently pass on the disease when they bite humans. Two to eight days later, a person experiences fever, chills, fatigue, and headaches. Hours later lymph nodes in the groin, armpit, or neck swell into bulging ovals up to ten centimeters in length. These are buboes caused by the bacteria in the bloodstream arriving in the lymph nodes.

Three Pandemics of Plague

The first plague pandemic occurred in Egypt or Ethiopia from 540 to 600 A.D and left a hundred million people dead. The 14th century saw the second pandemic, or "Black Death," that first infected central Asia and was then transmitted into Europe. In it more than one-third of Europe's population succumbed. The third and most current, though less severe, pandemic began in China in the 1890s and has so far spread to America, Africa, and Asia when infected rats were accidentally transported on ships. The World Health Organization records about a thousand cases of plague each year, most of which occur in Tanzania and Vietnam. New Mexico and Arizona are home to most of the 20 to 25 cases per year reported in the United States. American Indians have been particularly vulnerable to the disease.

The bacteria are identified upon microscopic examination of blood from a bubo, phlegm, or spinal fluid. Methods

The Plague Bacteria. Below, a photomicrograph of the plague bacteria, *Yersina pestis.* Although the plague is caused by a bacteria that can be treated with antibiotics, cases still appear from time to time in developing nations as well as in the United States. Recent reports indicate that strains of the plague are showing a resistance to antibiotics.

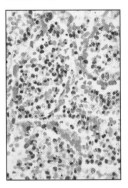

Placenta Previa. Below, top normal placental attachment; bottom placenta previa The placenta (a) should be attach directly to the uterus (b) and it should not cover the cervix (c). If it covers the cervix, there could be bleeding. If there is too much blood loss a transfusion may be required.

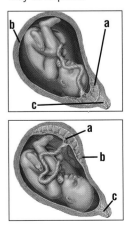

used to control plague include quarantine, rat extermination, and spraying insecticide. Due to the number of rodent species that carry it, sylvatic plague is the most resilient cycle.

THREE CYCLES THAT PERPETUATE PLAGUE

Sylvatic or wild plague spreads among ground and rock squirrels, prairie dogs, and other wild rodents. Urban rat plague infects rats in the seaports and urban centers of poor countries, and infects up to 10 percent of the rat population during epidemics. Pneumonic plague, found solely in humans, spreads when a healthy person inhales the moist breath expelled, as by a cough, from someone with a lung infection. Pneumonic plague may accompany bubonic plague as a secondary infection.

There is also septicemic plague, in which bacteria in the bloodstream increase so rapidly that the patient nearly succumbs prior to the appearance of any swelling. Rarely, plague manifests itself as pharyngitis appearing to be severe tonsillitis or meningitis.

TREATMENT

Along with pneumonic plague, septicemic plague can prove fatal, particularly if antibiotic treatment, in the form of streptomycin, chloramphenicol or tetracycline, is delayed. Diagnosed patients are also quarantined regularly. There is also a plague vaccine; travelers who go to Africa, Asia, Latin America, and the southwestern United States should be inoculated before departing. Preventive measures such as bug repellent and long sleeves and pants are also highly recommended. Travelers should avoid contact with wild animals; contact with domestic animals should be limited, as it is not entirely unlikely that these animals are vectors for plague. When plague is left untreated, the mortality rate is well over 50 percent.

See BACTEREMIA; BACTERIA; *and* EPIDEMIC *for a discussion of the foundations of plague. Treatment is discussed in* ANTIBIOTIC DRUGS *and* VACCINE. *Related material can be found in* INFECTIOUS DISEASE.

Resources on Plague
Biddle, Wayne, *Field Guide to Germs* (1995); Braude, Abraham, *Medical Microbiology and Infectious Diseases* (1981); Cantor, Norman, *In the Wake of the Plague: The Black Death and the World It Made* (2001); Grist, Norman R., et al., *Diseases of Infection: An Illustrated Textbook* (1992); Centers for Disease Contol and Prevention, Tel. (800) 311-3435, Online: www.cdc. gov; Infectious Disease Society of America, Tel. (703) 299-0200, Online: www.idsociety.org; National Institute of Allergy and Infectious Disease, Tel. (301) 496-5717, Online: www.niaid. nih.org; Office of Rare Diseases, Tel. (301) 402-4336, Online: rarediseases .info.nih.gov/ord.

Plantar Wart

A benign skin growth on the sole of the foot that is caused by a virus on the outer layer of skin.

A small, raised bump on the sole of the foot that has a rough surface and clearly defined edges is a plantar wart. Plantar warts are usually painless and do not itch; they are also not cancerous.

A wart is caused by the papilloma virus, which makes some cells grow more rapidly than normal. About 90 percent of adults have had a wart, as they are extremely common. Treatment for plantar warts includes cryotherapy (freezing cells to kill them), or electrosurgery (using heat to kill cells) among other means. *See* CRYOTHERAPY; ELECTROTHERAPY; PAPILLOMA; *and* WART.

Plants, Poisonous

Plants that become harmful through ingestion or mere contact.

Many plants that are kept in the home or in the garden are toxic. These should be avoided by households with small children or pets. All plants in the home and garden should be identified.

ALERT

Poisonous Household Plants

Some plants that people bring into their homes for decoration and color have poisonous properties. If there are small children in the house, these plants should either be removed or kept in a high place—out of reach of small hands. Common poisonous plants include, but are not limited to:

oleander	philodendron
daffodils	hyacinths
narcissus	lily-of-the-valley
lantana	poinsettia
English ivy	jimsonweed
azaleas	rhododendrons
Devil's ivy	caladium
holly	dieffenbachia or dumbcane
may apple	mistletoe
morning glory	schefflera or umbrella tree
iris	yew
peace lily	mountain laurel

Various popular house plants are poisonous, affecting the stomach, intestines, lungs or heart, However, the toxic parts of plants and their toxicity vary widely among different species. Jewelry and other ornaments made from seeds of poisonous plants like castor beans and rosary peas can be extremely toxic if chewed.

If someone has eaten part of a plant that is or may be poisonous, call a poison control center immediately. If symptoms are present, such as difficulty breathing, mouth or throat pain, signs of gastrointestinal distress, hallucinations, convulsions, or unconsciousness, first call EMS. If possible, have a sample of the plant that was ingested on hand. *See also* POISONING *and* TOXIN.

Plaque

Fatty deposits that form on the inner linings of blood vessels.

Plaque starts as clusters of white blood cells that collect cholesterol, calcium deposits, and fibrin, a protein. All of these materials stick to the blood vessel wall and impede the otherwise smooth progress of fluids. The buildup of plaque causes atherosclerosis, the process by which arteries become narrower as their walls become thicker, rougher and less flexible. The blood-carrying capacity of the arteries substantially diminishes as plaque accumulates, and the risk that a clot will form increases.

Even before a person enters their adolescent years, plaque build-up begins. As a person gets older, it merely continues to accumulate. The amount of accumulated plaque is exacerbated by risk factors such as smoking, blood cholesterol levels, blood pressure levels, diabetes, an inconsistent exercise regime, obesity, and stress factors brought about by lifestyle choices.

Plaque comes in different sizes and different shapes. If plaque residue hardens on the outside but not the inside, platelets will collect at the plaque deposit, further narrowing arteries and increasing the likelihood of a major blood clot.

When plaque narrows the arteries enough to reduce the amount of oxygen-carrying blood to the heart, symptoms such as angina pectoris result. The body may also build bypass arteries to restore blood flow, but this can decrease the amount of oxygenated blood that the heart muscle receives or, worse, a clot may form in these collateral arteries completely blocking the blood flow to the heart. Complete blockage of an artery causes a myocardial infarction or a stroke. *See also* ANGINA PECTORIS; ATHEROSCLEROSIS; HEART DISEASE; ISCHEMIA; *and* MYOCARDIAL INFARCTION.

Plaque, Dental

Oral and intradental accumulation of saliva, food debris and bacteria.

Plaque is one of the most damaging substances to mouth, teeth, and gums. It is impossible to avoid plaque, but proper dental care can minimize its harmful effects and perhaps induce some pleasant ones.

Essentially, plaque is the residue that comes from food; it sticks to the teeth and forms a layer that provides fertile ground for the bacteria that are a natural component of everyone's mouth. When plaque becomes hardened, it is called calculus. The bacteria that thrive in plaque and calculus wreak havoc on teeth and gums; unchecked, they can do enough damage to cause tooth decay and loss.

Control. The best way to control plaque is to brush regularly and to use dental floss. Flossing and brushing help remove food particles and other debris or residue that can damage teeth. Cleaning between the teeth and the gums with a dental stimulator removes plaque that a simple toothbrush might miss.

A critical step in plaque control is visiting the dentist for routine check-ups. The dentist or hygienist will use special tools to remove plaque and calculus that may have accumulated on the teeth. Dental professionals can reach plaque that ordinary home dental care may not remove as well. *See also* DENTISTRY *and* TEETH.

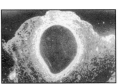
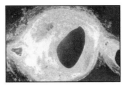

Plaque. Fatty deposits that form on the inner linings of arteries. Above top, a normal unblocked artery. Above bottom, an artery with build up.

Plasmapheresis

A process of mechanically taking an individual's blood and replacing damaged or diseased plasma with healthy plasma.

Medications that treat autoimmune diseases have many unpleasant side effects, so the possibility of mechanically removing the antibodies that cause the problems has become an increasingly popular alternative or supplement to drugs.

The procedure consists of first removing some of a person's blood. Blood cells are filtered out and saved, the plasma is discarded and new plasma is mixed with the blood cells and returned to the patient. The process can take several hours and is done on an outpatient basis. It is a circulating process; that is, blood removed from a vein in the arm is sent to the separator and returned to another vein in the opposite hand or foot, so only a small amount of blood is actually outside the patient at any single moment. The full course of treatment may take six to ten sessions performed once a week, though it may be more frequent in certain instances.

The substances removed include toxins, metabolic substances, and other antibodies, particularly when autoimmunity is involved. Plasmapheresis has been used to treat myasthenia gravis, Lambert-Eaton syndrome, Guillain-Barre syndrome, and other disorders. *See also* GAMMA GLOBULIN; GUILLAIN-BARRE SYNDROME; MYASTHENIA GRAVIS; *and* TOXINS.

Plastic Surgery

A branch of surgery that deals with the repair, reconstruction or replacement of damaged, deformed, lost or imperfect body parts.

The word 'plastic' comes from the Greek plastikos which means "to shape" or "to form." Plastic surgery includes cosmetic surgery, which is performed primarily to improve appearance, and reconstructive surgery, which is done to repair a damaged body part and restore function. Skin, tissue, cartilage, bone, and so on may all be obtained from other areas of the body or, in some cases, from donors. Artificial parts such as prosthetic devices, fixation plates, and wires are used increasingly.

After receiving a doctor of medicine degree, a plastic surgeon must complete three years in an approved residency program in general surgery, spend two additional years' residency in an approved plastic surgery program, and must pass a test administered by the American Board of Plastic Surgery.

Cosmetic Surgery includes procedures such as liposuction, breast augmentation, eyelid surgery, tretinoin treatment, facelift or rhytidoplasty, nose reshaping or rhinoplasty, laser skin resurfacing, tummy tucks or abdominoplasty, collagen injections, forehead lifts, breast lifts, fat injections, dermabrasion, breast reduction (both female and male), chin augmentation, thigh lifts, cheek implants, male-pattern baldness, upper arm lifts, wrinkle injections, and buttock lifts.

Reconstructive Surgery includes procedures such as breast implant removal, some types of ear surgery (otoplasty), cleft lips, cleft palates, club feet, skin grafts, skin cancer removals, keloids and port wine nevi removals, hypospadias, imperforate anus, and physical damage from accidents. Other skin techniques (Z-plasty) are often performed instead of grafts in body areas with loose, available skin.

Liposuction is the most common procedure performed in the States. A plastic surgeon suctions out pockets of fat with a tube and vacuum device to improve the contour of the body, face, neck, arms and legs.

Breast Surgery accounts for many procedures. Breast enlargement (augmentation mammoplasty) is achieved by the surgeon's placing saline implants behind the breasts. Reconstructive breast reduction, reduction mammoplasty, is performed usually to relieve discomfort (especially in the back) caused by over-sized breasts and to improve a woman's figure. Breasts are shaped to be more proportional to the rest of the patient's body. Breast reconstruction usually

Resources on Plastic Surgery

Converse, J.M., *Reconstructive Plastic Surgery* (1977); Engler, Alan, *Body Sculpture: Plastic Surgery of the Body for Men and Women* (2000); Grazer, F.M. and J.R. Klingbeil, *Body Image: A Surgical Perspective* (1980); Henry, Kimberly A., et al., *The Plastic Surgery Sourcebook: Everything You Need to Know* (1999); Rudolph, Ross, et al., *Skin Grafting* (1979); American Society of Plastic Surgeons, Tel. (888) 475-2784, Online: www.plasticsurgery.org; American Society for Aesthetic Plastic Surgery, Tel. (800) 364-2147, Online: surgery.org; www.nycornell.org/ent/.

Common Plastic Surgery

The total number of of procedures for plastic surgery, including both cosmetic and reconstructive surgery procedures, have been increasing in few years. According to the American Society of Plastic Surgeons some of the most common procedures have been:

Tumor Removal	521,678
Liposuction	230,865
Hand Surgery	171,510
Breast Augmentation	167,318
Eyelid Surgery (Blepharoplasty)	142,033
Breast reconstruction	82,975
Breast Reduction	78,169
Facelift (Rhytidectomy)	69,729
Tummy Tuck (Abdominoplasty)	54,977
Collagen Injections	53,197
Chemical Peel	51,589
Laser Skin Resurfacing	50.505
Nose-Reshaping (Rhinoplasty)	46,596
Scar Revision	46,242
Forehead Lift	40,969
Breast Lift (Mastopexy)	38,276
Birth Defect Reconstruction	30,702
Microsurgery	23,200
Burn Care	22,202
Fat Injections	20,503
Breast Implant Removals*	13,009

* INCLUDES IMPLANTS ORIGINALLY INSERTED FOR RECONSTRUCTIVE PURPOSES ONLY. (1999 NATIONAL PLASTIC SURGERY STATISTICS)

follows breast removal, mastectomy, to create a natural looking replacement.

Eyelid surgery, blepharoplasty, corrects drooping eyelids or puffy "bags" under the eyes. The surgeon makes several small incisions hidden within the folds of the eyelids and removes excess fat, skin, and muscle.

For a facelift, rhytidectomy, the surgeon makes incisions hidden behind the hairline, tightens the skin of the face, chin and neck, and removes excess fat to improve the patient's appearance.

In nose surgery, rhinoplasty, the nose is reshaped, usually by removing cartilage and bumps or hooks, in order to achieve a straighter look, to reduce the overall size, to change the shape of the tip or bridge, to narrow the nostrils or change the angle between the nose and the upper lip.

Laser facial resurfacing removes lines and wrinkles from the face, especially around the forehead, eyes and mouth, and minimizes small scars and pigmentations.

POST-ACCIDENT HEAD INJURIES WITH SUBSEQUENT SURGICAL REPAIRS

The surgeon uses a carbon dioxide laser device to precisely remove damaged outer layers of skin, allowing a fresh layer to become the new surface.

In conjunction with or in place of surgery, Retin-A, tretinoin, may be used as a topical treatment of acne vulgaris, for aging facial skin, or as a topical treatment to help the effects of minoxidil in the treatment of hair loss, alopecia. *See also* BODY CONTOUR SURGERY; COSMETIC SURGERY; MAMMOPLASTY; MASTECTOMY; and Z-PLASTY.

Plethora

Plethora is a general term to describe a red, highly flushed condition due to an excess of blood.

A bodily condition characterized by the expansion or excess of blood cells (polycythemia) and marked by a slightly swollen or flushed complexion. Facial features exhibit a ruddyness. This condition is quite rare, occurring in less than one percent of neonatal infants; it is more common among those too large for their gestational age, and it is more likely to happen if a mother has diabetes. *See also* POLYCYTHEMIA.

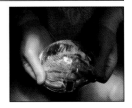

Massive Head Wounds. Above, top, after massive head wounds, plastic surgery is sometimes required to improve the appearance of the head.
Breast Implant. Above bottom, a breast implant before insertion.

Plethysmography

A diagnostic test to measure changes in blood volume in various organs and tissues.

Plethysmography is used to evaluate changes in blood volume in organs, limbs, or other body parts using a device known as a plethysmograph, which can measure the flow of blood through veins. The technique is useful for the diagnosis of blood vessel obstruction or insufficiency of blood flow. Changes in limb volume are typically measured with each pulse of an artery of the limb and during restriction (occlusion) of the venous flow using a pressure cuff. The test may be used to identify blood clots (deep vein thrombosis) that occur in the deep veins of the legs or lower abdomen. Such thromboses sometimes detach themselves and travel to the lung.

Plethysmography of the whole body is used to measure gas volume within the lungs, a key diagnostic indicator for obstructive pulmonary disease and emphysema. Plethysmography is painless and safe. *See also* BLOOD CLOTTING; EMPHYSEMA; PULMONARY INSUFFICIENCY; *and* THROMBOSIS.

Pleural Effusion

An accumulation of fluid between the layers of pleura, which surround the lungs.

A thin layer of fluid lies between the two pleura (the two-layered membrane that lines the upper and lower parts of the abdominal cavity) to allow the lungs to expand and contract against the ribs and chest without rubbing. Tuberculosis, a lung abscess or lung infection, cirrhosis of the liver, and congestive heart failure may all cause an accumulation of fluid between the pleura (pleural effusion). Cancer, tuberculosis, drug reactions, and severe reactions to asbestos can also cause pleural effusion. In addition, traumatic injury to the chest that causes a blood vessel to rupture and pour blood into the pleural cavity, a condition that requires emergency treatment, is the most severe form of pleural effusion.

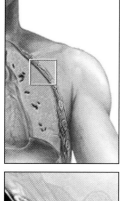
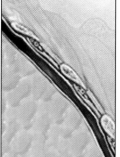

Pleural Effusion. A thin layer of fluid that lies between the upper and lower parts of the abdominal cavity.

Symptoms of pleural effusion include a shortness of breath, dry coughing, fever, and chest pains (from minor to severe), though patients may have no symptoms at all if the accumulation of fluid is small. Pleural effusion is diagnosed by a chest x-ray, computed tomography (CT) scan, or an ultrasound scan. A sample of the fluid will be drawn from the body with a needle to determine the nature and source of the fluid and whether or not either bacteria or cancerous cells are present. In an appreciable number of cases, no source for pleural effusion can be determined despite extensive testing.

Treatment. Untreated, severe pleural effusion can result in the collapse of a lung. Treatment is aimed at controlling the source of the fluid. If the source is a bacterial infection, antibiotics will be administered. Surgical drainage can control the amount of fluid, though the fluid may accumulate again if the underlying problem is not addressed. *See also* CIRRHOSIS; INFECTION; LUNG; PNEUMONIA; *and* TUBERCULOSIS.

Pleurisy

An inflammation of the pleura, a two-layered membrane lining the lungs, diaphragm, and rib cage.

The pleura are the membranes that surround the lungs. They consist of two membranous layers with a thin coating of fluid between them to allow the lungs to slide, as they expand and contract with the effort of breathing, without friction.

When the pleura become inflamed, the lungs do not slide freely, causing shortness of breath, a dry cough, and a sharp, stabbing pain that can be either severe or not. If the cause of pleurisy is a bacterial infection, it will be with treated antibiotics. If the cause is viral, only anti-inflammatory and pain relieving drugs can be given, and the situation needs to be allowed to resolve itself, however, fluid from the pleura can be drained (also with a needle) in order to maintain an individual's comfort. *See also* ANTIBIOTIC DRUGS; LUNG; PLEURAL EFFUSION; PNEUMONIA; *and* TUBERCULOSIS.

Pleurodynia

Also known as Bornholm disease

An influenza-like, epidemic muscle disease, characterized by inflammation and pain in the chest.

Coxsackie Virus B, an epidemic disease that has an incubation period between two and four days, causes pleurodynia. Symptoms generally include fever, severe chest pain, strong upper abdominal (diaphragm musculature) discomfort, lower back pain, sore throat, and headaches. In addition, deep breathing and movement can be painful. The disease usually fades in three to four days without treatment, however, it can recur several times within a few weeks. The disease is most commonly found in children, although it can occur at any age.

In the case of pleurodynia, aspirin can be helpful to reduce pain and fever, otherwise, the condition will usually treat itself in time. Sometimes pleurodynia is accompanied by an inflammation of the heart (pericarditis) or an inflammation of the brain and spinal cord (meningitis). *See also* FEVER; MENINGITIS; *and* PERICARDITIS.

Plication

A surgical procedure in which the size of a hollow organ is reduced by creating folds and tucks and stitching them to the wall of the organ.

In fundoplication—used to treat gastroesophageal reflux disease and hiatal hernias—the fundus, the upper part, of the stomach is wrapped around the lower end of the esophagus to create a valve that prevents gastric acid reflux. Acute perforated duodenal ulcer is usually treated by open Graham patch plication, in which the tongue of omentum (the tissue that holds the stomach in place) is sutured in place. Laparoscopic Graham plication and Nissen fundoplication have become alternative procedures. Plication of the tunica albuginea (the tissue that covers internal sex organs in both males an females) is one of the treatments used for Peyronie's disease. *See also* SURGERY.

Plummer-Vinson Syndrome

Also known as Paterson-Kelly syndrome

Webs of tissue that run across the upper edge of the esophagus.

Individuals with this condition have webs of tissue that have formed across the top of the esophagus, causing rather extreme swallowing difficulties. This condition is most often found in women between the ages of 40 and 65, and appears to be the result of anemia (iron deficiency).

The diagnosis is usually made with an endoscope, a a small flexible tool with an attached viewing instrument that is placed in the esophagus; this also usually breaks the tissue formation causing, or exacerbating, the problem; when the web breaks, which it does easily, there may be some bleeding. Treatment of the anemia, with iron supplements, will usually resolve the condition. *See also* ANEMIA; ENDOSCOPE; ENDOSCOPY; *and* ESOPHAGUS.

Plutonium

A radioactive chemical element derived from uranium.

Plutonium (symbol Pu, atomic number 94) is chemically similar to uranium and is formed through the radioactive decay of another element, neptunium. This element is found in tiny quantities in pitchblende, where it undergoes slow disintegration through the emission of alpha particles, forming uranium 235 (this uranium is fissionable and is often used as fuel for atomic energy); non-isotopic plutonium's normal atomic mass is 244, with 94 protons and 150 neutrons. Plutonium is a highly toxic substance, posing severe risks to human health. Those working with atomic energy or exposed to plutonium through environmental contamination are at particular risk for radiation poisoning. *See also* ENVIRONMENTAL MEDICINE; RADIATION; RADIATION HAZARDS; *and* RADIATION SICKNESS.

Pneumaturia

The passage of gas or air in the urine.

Gas is sometimes present in the urine when infectious bacteria causes the urine to chemically decompose. Most often, it is an indication of an abnormal channel, a fistula, that has developed between the intestine and the bladder that stores the urine. The formation of this abnormal passageway can be the consequence of a variety of conditions, including cancer, Crohn's disease or diverticular disease. *See also* CANCER; CROHN'S DISEASE; DIVERTICULAR DISEASE; *and* FISTULA.

Pneumocystis Pneumonia

Infection of the lungs caused by a bacterium, *Pneumocystis carinii*.

Pneumocystic pneumonia is caused by *Pneumocystis carinii,* a microorganism that is found in normal human lungs, but may become pathogenic in those with impaired immune systems, including premature infants, those taking immunosuppressive medications (used in some transplant operations and cancer treatments), and patients with acquired immune deficiency disorder (AIDS).

Symptoms include high fever, rapid and shallow breathing, coughing, and discoloration of the skin due to lack of oxygen intake. Some drugs, including pentamidine, trimethoprim-sulfamethoxazole, and dapsone have proven effective. Patients at high risk for the disease may be given various prophylactic regimens to prevent or delay the development of Pneumocystis pneumonia. *See also* AIDS *and* HIV.

Pneumoconiosis

Lung disease specifically associated with the inhalation of particular mineral dust.

Pneumoconiosis is primarily an occupational disease. Certain mineral dust can accumulate in the lungs, eventually bringing about lung tissue scarring (fibrosis) and inhibiting adequate breathing. The risk of developing the disease is directly related to the amount of dust inhaled, so that it may take years for symptoms such as breathlessness, chest tightness, and a persistent cough to develop. But exposure to very large concentrations of such dust can develop an acute form of the condition that leads to adult respiratory distress syndrome, in which fluid accumulates in the lung to such an extent that breathing becomes almost impossible.

TYPES

The most common type of pneumoconiosis is called black lung disease or coal miner's pneumonconiosis, occurs primarily in the profession wherein incidence of this disorder is highest. This is due to the inhalation of coal dust—usually that of anthracite rather than bituminous coal.

Another common form, silicosis, is caused by inhalation of silica, also called crystalline quartz. It is seen in sandblasters, drillers, stonecutters, tunnelers, and others working with sand and rock. Pneumonconiosis can also result from inhaling dust containing beryllium, hematite (found in iron ore) or kaolin, a fine clay used in ceramics.

Exacerbating Pneumoconiosis
The risk of developing pneumoconiosis and the severity of the condition are made worse by smoking. The pollutants in tobacco smoke add to the damage done by industrial dust and also increase the risk of lung cancer and respiratory distress emergencies, which are associated with inhalation of hematite. Avoiding, or quitting, smoking can be important to those whose workplace has air containing even small concentrations of industrial dust.

Another condition that can develop in severe cases of pneumoconiosis is cor pulmonale, the impaired function of the right side of the heart resulting from damage to the lung. An episode of asthma in someone with severe pneumoconiosis can result in a potentially fatal respiratory attack and must be treated promptly.

TREATMENT

There is no treatment for pneumoconiosis itself, but measures can be taken against complications caused by this condition, such as an increased risk of lung infections, emphysema, and other breathing problems. Early detection of the condition, by means of chest x-rays and pulmonary function examinations among workers exposed to industrial dust on the job, can prevent damage from becoming severe enough to cause any major problems. Preventive measures, such as improved ventilation of mines and other workplaces, along with enforcement of regulations that limit dust concentrations in the air, and the wearing of protective gear, have reduced the incidence of the condition over the last few decades. However, more than 1,000 cases a year still occur in the United States.

See FIBROSIS; LUNG; LUNG DISEASE, CHRONIC OBSTRUCTIVE; *and* RESPIRATORY SYSTEM *for more information on pneumonconiosis. Related material is found in* RESPIRATORY DISTRESS SYNDROME; RESPIRATORY TRACT INFECTION; COR PULMONALE; *and* EMPHYSEMA.

Pneumonectomy

A surgical operation to remove an entire lung, usually to treat lung cancer.

The operation was once used to treat tuberculosis and other serious lung ailments that can now be remedied by drugs or by partial lung tissue removal, also known as wedge resections and lobectomies.

Before a pneumonectomy is to be performed, the other lung is tested for forced expiratory volume in one second (FEV1) to ensure that it can handle the increased post-operative demand.

With the patient under general anesthesia, the surgeon makes an incision from beneath the armpit to the back of the rib cage, separates the ribs, sometimes removing one, ties off the blood vessels and bronchi leading to the diseased lung, and removes it. A temporary drainage tube is inserted in the chest cavity to drain air, fluid and blood out of the area, the incision is sutured, and the stitches are removed just before the patient leaves the hospital in seven to ten days. *See also* ANESTHESIA, GENERAL *and* LUNG CANCER.

Pneumonia

Lung inflammation caused by an infection.

An infection leading to pneumonia can be due to a variety of agents, including fungi, yeasts, protozoa or mycoplasma, bacteria or viruses. Until the 1930s, pneumonia was a leading cause of death in the United States. The arrival of antibiotics and other treatments has reduced its toll, but pneumonia, with influenza, still ranks as the sixth leading cause of death in this country; influenza can lead to pneumonia in a matter of hours. While mild pneumonia is generally not a major problem for younger people in good health, it can be life-threatening for older people and those with chronic disorders that weaken the body's defenses. About 15 of every 1,000 Americans will have pneumonia each year.

In pneumonia, the infection causes the air sacs (alveoli) of the lung, where oxygen passes into the blood, to become clogged with pus and other secretions, so that the supply of oxygen to the body is reduced. The resulting symptoms include shortness of breath, fever, chills, and a persistent cough that brings up phlegm discolored by pus and sometimes by blood. Chest pain can be caused by pleurisy, inflammation of the lining of the lungs and chest cavity.

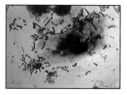

Pneumorcal Pneumonia. Pneumonia is a very common, serious illness. It is caused by many different organisms and can range in seriousness from mild to life-threatening illness.

> ## Legionnaires' Disease
>
> One newer form of pneumonia is Legionnaires' disease, so called because it was first identified in an outbreak that occurred at the Pennsylvania state convention of the American Legion in 1976. Legionnaires' disease is caused by a bacterium that had previously been unknown, which has been named *Legionella pneumonophila*. Legionnaires' disease causes the usual symptoms of pneumonia, but it also may cause diarrhea, nausea, and vomiting. There is no vaccine for the bacterium, but the infection can be treated successfully by antibiotics.

TYPES

Cases of pneumonia can be divided into two primary categories: bronchopneumonia and lobar pneumonia. Bronchopneumonia begins in the airways (bronchi) of the lung, the bronchi that successively branch into smaller bronchioles, and spreads to affect sections of one or both lungs. In lobar pneumonia, the effects of the infection are initially concentrated in a single lobe of one lung.

> **ALERT**
> ### Pneumonia Prevention
>
> Older people and others vulnerable to pneumonia, such as those with impaired immune systems due to advanced HIV infection and some cancer treatments, are advised to take protective measures and to be alert for the first earliest signs of the condition. Protection starts with lifestyle measures, such as an adequate diet, exercise, proper protection in the winter, and avoidance of smoking.
>
> Vaccination is also a basic, and vital, protective measure. Vaccination against influenza is recommended for vulnerable individuals at the beginning of each winter. An influenza vaccine against the strain of the virus that is most likely to be prevalent for the season is developed according to studies done by the federal Centers for Disease Control and Prevention and is widely available each year. The vaccine may cause some side effects, such as muscle aches and a low-grade fever, but generally they last only a few days. A vaccine against pneumonococcal bacteria is also available, and its use is recommended every five years.

DIAGNOSIS

Diagnosis of pneumonia begins with a physical examination. The doctor uses a stethoscope to listen for chest sounds that may indicate a breathing obstruction. A chest x-ray should be done to determine the exact nature and extent of the lung problem, and a blood test may be done to identify the exact infectious agent.

CAUSE

The bacteria that can cause pneumonia include *Streptococcus pneumoniae*, also called pneumococcus; *Haeomophilus influenzae*; *Staphylococcus aureus*; *Pseudomonas aerugi-*

nosa; and *Escherichia coli* (the infamous E. Coli bacteria) These infections can usually be treated with antibiotics.

In addition to the influenza virus, viral pneumonia can be caused by adenovirus, respiratory syncytial virus, or coxsackie virus. Some cases of viral pneumonia may be treated by an antiviral drug such as amantadine or rimantadine.

VIRAL TREATMENT

Viral pneumonia does not respond to antibiotic treatment, but antibiotics may be given if there is a secondary bacterial infection. Other treatments given for all cases of pneumonia include medications to ease a cough and reduce pain. In serious cases, patients my be hospitalized so that they can receive oxygen therapy and assisted mechanical ventilation. Respiratory treatment to help clear the lungs of the deposits clogging the alveoli may also be necessary.

INCIDENCE AND PROGNOSIS

Younger people and those in good general health may need only bed rest and medications for cough and pain. The recovery period for such patients may be two to three weeks. Older patients, those with chronic conditions and those whose immune defenses have been weakened by poor lifestyles or serious health conditions, generally require more intensive treatment, face a longer recovery period, and a higher risk of mortality. In such individuals, pneumonia may last for six to eight weeks, with a recovery period of several months.

The possible complications of pneumonia include the accumulation of fluid in and around the lung (plural effusion); an accumulation of pus in the pleural cavity (empyema); or the formation of a pocket filled with pus (abscess) in the lung. Surgery sometimes becomes necessary in such cases.

> *Background material may be found in* LUNG; RESPIRATORY SYSTEM; *and* RESPIRATORY TRACT INFECTION. *Symptoms of pneumonia are discussed in* ABSCESS; EMPYEMA; *and* PLEURIS. *Related material is found in* LEGIONNAIRES' DISEASE *and* INFLUENZA.

Resources on Infectious Diseases

Austrian, Robert, *Life with the Pneumcoccus* (1985); Grist, Norman R., et al., *Diseases of Infection: An Illustrated Textbook* (1992); Karetzky, Monroe, Burke A. Cunha, and Robert D. Brand-stetter, *The Pneumonias* (1993); Pennington, James E., *Respiratory Infections* (1994); Shaw, Michael, ed., *Everything You Need to Know About Diseases* (1996); Centers for Disease Contol and Prevention, Tel. (800) 311-3435, Online: www.cdc.gov; Infectious Disease Society of America, Tel. (703) 299-0200, Online: www.idsociety.org; Nat. Institute of Allergy and Infectious Disease, Tel. (301) 496-5717, Online: www.niaid.nih.gov; www.nycornell.org/medicine/infectious/index.html

Pneumonitis

Inflammation of the lungs.

Pneumonitis can by caused by a number of conditions, including lung infections, radiation exposure, and the inhalation of dust containing animal or plant matter that stimulates an immune response. This hypersensitivity has many forms, such as farmer's lung, which occurs due to inhaling spores from moldy hay; bird fancier's lung, due to bird droppings; air conditioner lung, from particles in air conditioners and humidifiers; and sequoisis, caused by moldy dust from redwood trees. The condition causes breathing difficulties, coughing, and wheezing. *See also* LUNGS.

Pneumothorax

The presence of air between the two layers of tissue lining the lungs.

Pneumothorax is much more common in men than women. It also has a high incidence rate among young adults who do not have lung disease. In many cases, there is no apparent reason for the condition, but sometimes it is caused by the rupture of a blister (bleb) at the top of a lung. It can also result from a piercing injury to the lung or as a complication of asthma or emphysema. Whatever the cause, it results in the entry of air into the space between the layers of tissue that line the lungs and the inner wall of the chest (pleural cavity) .

The most notable symptoms are chest pain and shortness of breath, which increase as the amount of air in the pleural cavity increases. If leakage of air into the pleural cavity does not stop, it can compress the heart enough to be life-threatening. Pneumothorax is diagnosed by a chest x-ray. In many cases, it will go away without treatment in a matter of days. If the pneumothorax is large or is caused by an underlying lung condition, it is treated by removing the air through a syringe or a suction tube. Surgery may be performed in severe cases. *See also* BLEB; BLISTER; *and* LUNG.

Podiatry

Branch of medicine that treats foot disorders and injuries.

Podiatrists handle a wide variety of foot-related problems. They examine, diagnose, treat, and work on preventing foot problems as well as conditions that may arise due to foot disorders. Podiatrists may deal with walking disorders, fractures, and sprains. They can remove bunions, correct hammer toes or ingrown toenails, and provide aids to alleviate pain and movement disorders due to flat feet or high arches. Podiatrists also treat infections: fungi, foot ulcers, and some infections related to diabetes. *See also* FLATFOOT *and* PRONATION.

Podophyllin

A chemical used to treat genital warts and human papilloma virus.

Podophyllin is derived from the plants *Podophyllin peltatum* and *Podophyllin emodi*, which are grown in North America and the Himalayas, respectively. It is used in the treatment of genital warts and the human papilloma virus. In the past, this chemical has also been used as an antidote for snakebites and as an antifungal treatment. *See also* FUNGI; PAPILLOMA; SEXUALLY TRANSMITTED DISEASES; *and* WARTS, GENITAL.

Poison

Any substance that impairs the body's ability to function normally.

All non-food matter is potentially poisonous in large enough doses. Potentially poisonous items include those things that are known for toxicity, such as household cleansers and pesticides, and less obvious threats such as certain plants, medications, vitamins, and alcohol.

All potentially toxic substances, including house plants, should be stored where children do not have access to them. They should be kept in their original packaging so that, should poisoning occur, the toxin can be readily identified. In the case of poisoning, a local poison control center can give first-aid advice. Treatment varies depending on the nature of the poison; an action, such as inducing vomiting, that may be helpful in some cases may be vitally harmful in others.

See Poisoning; Toxicity; *and* Toxin *for a discussion on the foundations of poison. Details on specific types of poison will be found in* Drug Poisoning; Food Poisoning; Lead Poisoning; Pesticides; Phosphorus Poisoning; Poisonous Plants; Ptomaine Poisoning; *and* Strychnine Poisoning.

Poison Ivy, Oak, & Sumac

Three plants that cause contact dermatitis, or an itchy rash, due to an allergic reaction to their oils.

In and of themselves, these three plants are relatively harmless, however, more than 50 percent of all people are allergic to the oils that they produce. These oils produce a rash that usually takes the form of patches or streaks spread out across the skin that has been exposed. A rash may take a matter of some time to appear, or be recognized, so affected areas are often unknowingly scratched, spreading the oils and the rash all over the body. The longest time a dermatitis may take to become evident is a day or two. About a week later, the rash is at its worst, and may require hospitalization for a short period of time.

Poison ivy is found all over the continental United States; poison oak is generally indigenous to the west coast, and poison sumac tends to grow around the Mississippi river bed. Symptoms for all three are nearly indistinguishable.

Treatment. First scrub the exposed skin with soap and water to remove any remaining oils; wash hands and nails frequently because itching spreads the rash. Do not scratch the rash. Calamine lotion and commercial hydrocortisone creams may relieve itching. If the rash is severe, covering most of the body or areas around the eyes or genitals, consult a doctor. *See also* Dermatitis *and* Poisonous Plants.

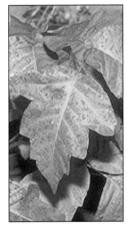

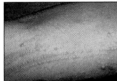

Poisonous Plants. Above top, poison sumac a relatively harmless plant that produces an oil that most people are allergic to. The Allergy is manifested in a red rash, above bottom, on the area of the body that has been affected.

Poisoning

The introduction of a poisonous substance into the body.

Poisoning results from any of a variety of substances entering the body. These substances may enter the body through various means, such as inhalation, skin absorption (merely by touching the substance), ingestion, or injection.

Almost 95 percent of poisoning deaths occur in adults, a large number of whom poison themselves or overdose intentionally. However, over half of all poisoning cases, involve small children, usually under the age of six. If poisoning is suspected, immediately call for emergency medical help. A regional poison control center can provide vital information.

Indications that poisoning has occured, in both children and adults, may include burns around the mouth and on clothing, chemical stains in the area near the victim, chemical odor on the victim's breath or open medicine bottles. Symptoms may include vomiting, convulsions, breathing difficulties, and unconsciousness.

If poisoning is suspected, the following procedures are recommended:

- Call for emergency medical help, and/or consult and a poison control center. The number of your poison control center should be kept by the telephone at all times. The poison control center will provide you with detailed first aid instructions.
- If the poisonous substance is known, check for any first aid instructions written on the label. Folow these instructions if the poison control center cannot be reached quickly. trol center cannot be reached quickly,
- Never induce vomiting unless instructed by a poison control center or a physician. If so instructed, vomiting may be induced with syrup of ipecac.
- Carefully remove any clothing that may have poison on it and flush affected eyes and skin with cool or lukewarm water.

See POISON *and* TOXICITY *for a discussion on the foundations of poisoning. Details on specific types of poison will be found in* DRUG OVERDOSE; DRUG POISONING; FOOD POISONING; LEAD POISONING; PESTICIDES; PHOSPHORUS POISONING; POISONOUS PLANTS; PTOMAINE POISONING; STRYCHNINE POISONING; *and* TOXIC SHOCK SYNDROME.

Poliomyelitis

A viral infection that affects the central nervous system, the brain and spinal cord.

In the first half of the twentieth century more than 50,000 cases of poliomyelitis (more commonly known as polio) were reported each year. Today fewer than ten cases are reported each year, because of the excellent effectiveness of the vaccination program. Today, adults and young girls have a higher poliomyelitis incidence rate, but when young boys contract the virus, they are more likely to suffer more severe effects including paralysis.

Cause. The three viruses that cause polio can each enter the body through infected water or food. Polio is a highly communicable disease and it spreads rather quickly. Direct contact is the most regular means of transmission; the virus enters through the mouth and nose, it breeds inside of the throat, and is then spread through the body in the blood. It takes about five days to a month to incubate.

Symptoms. Children under five years of age are the most vulnerable to polio, however, young children tend to exhibit only very mild cases, with symptoms such as a low-grade fever, headache, sore throat, and vomiting, and the disease can run its course in just a few hours. It is when older children or adults contract the disease that the consequences are much more serious. A week or two after exposure the sufferer will have a severe headache, a high fever, a stiff neck, and back aches resulting from deep muscle pain. If areas of the skin tingle or burn, the virus has moved into the spinal cord or the brain.

If the polio virus reaches the brain, the infection may produce muscle paralysis of the arms, legs, chest, or throat. If it attacks the throat, the infection may interfere with swallowing to the point where the victim may choke on food or liquids. Sometimes complications are delayed for years after the onset of the disease; muscle weakness that results in severe disability may show up many years after the infection. The longer the symptoms of polio last and the more severe the symptoms get, the more likely a person is to become paralyzed.

The Iron Lung. If the polio virus attacks the muscles of the chest, the patient will have difficulty breathing. Patients spend hours each day recuperating in these machines. A person is placed in the iron lung, and the body is surrounded by a tube of steel. Firmly sealed, the neck and head are outside the tube. Air is pumped rhythmically into and out of the machine to raise and lower the air pressure, forcing the chest to expand and contract and thereby enabling the person to breathe. The iron lung is occasionally still used today.

Treatment. There is no cure for poliomyelitis, and antiviral drugs have no effect on this virus. Treatment consists of easing the symptoms. Lifesaving measures are often instituted in the most severe cases. If the spinal chord and brain remain unaffected, then full recovery occurs in over 90 percent of all cases, however, when these organs do get involved, the virus may result in paralysis, disability or even death.

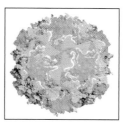

Polio. A disorder caused by a viral infection (poliovirus) that affects the whole body including muscles and nerves. Severe cases may cause permanent paralysis or death.

See BACTEREMIA *and* CENTRAL NERVOUS SYSTEM *for details on the foundations of poliomyelitis. Symptoms of poliomyelitis may be further explained in* BREATHING DIFFICULTY; HEADACHE; PARALYSIS; *and* SPASTIC PARALYSIS. *Treatment is discussed in* RESPIRATORY THERAPY.

Pollution

Environmental contamination by poisons, microorganisms, or radioactive substances.

Pollutants and toxins cause about three percent of all deaths—more than firearms, motor vehicle accidents, and illicit drug use. Concern about pollution grew in the 1950s, when researchers discovered that pesticides were poisoning wildlife and the food chain. At the same time, the public believed that nuclear tests were showering radioactive fallout over broad areas. Concern intensified as a result of several incidents of industrial pollution, including oil tanker spills, acid rain, and fallout from the 1986 explosion of the Chernobyl nuclear reactor in the Ukraine, then part of the former Soviet Union.

The potential harm from the greenhouse effect, a general warming of the Earth caused by increased amounts of carbon dioxide in the atmosphere, is of greatest concern. A byproduct of burning fossil fuels, carbon dioxide traps heat, thereby increasing temperatures. If the amount of carbon dioxide continues to increase, it could cause devastating climatic changes within the next fifty years. The depletion of the ozone layer is of equal concern. Ozone blocks the sun's harmful ultraviolet radiation, but the widespread use of aerosols has eaten it away. Other harmful pollutants are mercury, lead, cadmium, and agricultural pesticides such as DDT and parathion. *See also* ENVIRONMENTAL MEDICINE *and* TOXIN.

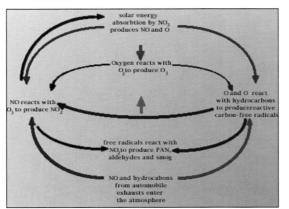

Air Pollution. The urban system that results in the formation of smog. The cycle begins when very small amounts of nitrous oxide in automobile exhaust combine with oxygen to form nitrous dioxide, which then provides the oxygen that combines with hydrocarbons in the air to produce smog.

Polycystic Ovary

Also known as Stein-Leventhal syndrome

A rare disorder in young women in which, when ovulation would normally occur, developing follicles produces cysts instead of eggs.

Women with polycystic ovary are infertile and tend to have irregular menstrual cycles or not menstruate at all, a condition known as oligomenorrhea. Other symptoms of this disorder include the growth of an unusual amount of facial hair, being overweight, infertility, and small breast size.

Treatment varies depending on whether a woman wishes to conceive or not. If she does not want to become a mother, birth control pills or a drug called medroxyprogesterone are given to suppress ovulation and prevent any possible precancerous changes in the uterine lining.

Women who wish to conceive are given clomiphene, a drug which induces ovulation. Approximately 35 percent of women who take clomiphene eventually become pregnant. Gonadotropins are used if clomiphene is unsuccessful. A surgical option is to remove a wedge-shaped section of the ovary. *See also* FERTILITY *and* OVARIES.

Polycythemia

A bone marrow disease in which an overabundance of red blood cells is produced; its cause is not known.

If there are too many red blood cells in the blood, it becomes thick and does not flow easily through the blood vessels. When blood circulation is inhibited, the cells and tissues of the body will not receive enough oxygen, and the immune system is immediately compromised.

Symptoms include fatigue, headache, dizziness, shortness of breath, visual problems, angina pectoris, bleeding of the gums, and bleeding in the gastrointestinal tract. The face and hands may appear reddened because of the higher concentration of red blood cells.

The disease usually develops slowly and, in some cases, it may progress to full-

Polycythemia After 50

Polycythemia occurs most often between the ages of fifty and seventy. To control the possibility of blood clots, a blood thinning agent may be prescribed along with a phlebotomy. Those who undergo the blood-letting and subsequent medication have an average survival rate that is significantly, by about 600 percent, longer than those who do not.

fledged leukemia; since blood clotting is enhanced there is also the danger of pulmonary thrombosis, heart attack, or stroke. Polycythemia may also be diagnosed as a complication of thrombocythemia in elderly persons. Patients live many years after diagnosis, although death by leukemia can occur from thrombosis.

Treatment for many years has been phlebotomy—drainage of some of the blood to reduce the volume in the system. Chemotherapy or interferon A are also regularly used treatments. *See* BLOOD; BLOOD CELLS; BLOOD CLOTTING; LEUKEMIA; THROMBOSIS; *and* THROMBOPHLEBITIS.

Polydactyly

The presence of an extra digit on the hands or feet.

Polydactyly is more commonly found on the hands, as a sixth finger or extra thumb. Usually the extra digit consists entirely of skin and soft tissue; occasionally, it contains bone or cartilage. Surgical removal can be performed when the infant is a few months old. *See also* HAND *and* TRIGGER FINGER.

Polymyalgia Rheumatica

Painful inflammation of the muscles in the neck, shoulder and hips, occurring mostly among the middle-aged and elderly.

Polymyalgia rheumatica is a disease that comes on quite abruptly, with its highest incidence levels among women over fifty. While the cause of the disease is unknown, it is often associated with temporal arteritis, rheumatoid arthritis, systematic lupus erythematosus, and cancer. Symptoms include fatigue, malaise, weight loss, depression,

and anemia. Pain usually occurs as the result of stiffness more than weakness. In some cases it can attack the shoulders, making it difficult to put on a jacket or get out of bed. If it attacks the pelvic muscles, simple tasks like climbing stairs or getting out of a bathtub may become difficult.

Treatment involves staying active since inactivity seems to increase the stiffness, which tends to be at its worst in the morning. If fever, general malaise, weight loss or depression accompany the muscle aches, a muscle biopsy may be in order so that malignancy can be either diagnosed or ruled out. Blood tests for other forms of diseases may indicate anemia, high erythrocyte sedimentation rates, and high levels of C-reactive protein. *See* PROTEIN.

Low doses of prednisone, a corticosteroid, often produce dramatic and lasting results, though it may require two or more doses of medication before the disease is completely controlled. *See also* ANEMIA; CORTICOSTEROID DRUGS; DEPRESSION; EXERCISE; LUPUS; *and* TEMPORAL ARTERITIS.

Polymyositis

A rare inflammatory muscle disease that causes varying amounts of decreased muscular ability.

Polymyositis most often affects teenagers, usually under the age of 18. The disease begins gradually. The most pronounced symptom is a decline in muscle power, especially those muscles closest to the trunk area. In the advanced stages, the patient will have trouble climbing stairs, lifting objects from the floor, getting up out of a chair, or reaching to get something from a top shelf. Some patients experience difficulty in swallowing (dysphagia). The muscles may be tender to the touch. Other side effects include fatigue, a low-grade fever, and significant weight loss.

The symptoms of polymyositis are most commonly treated with the corticosteroid drug prednisone or other immunosuppressants, such as azathioprine. Physical therapy is suggested to prevent muscle atrophy. *See also* ABDOMEN AND MUSCLE.

Polyp

A nonmalignant growth on a mucous membrane.

Polyps are mushroom-shaped growths that tend to arise in the intestine, the cervix, the nose, the vocal cords and elsewhere in the body. Most of them are harmless, but some of them may become cancerous.

When polyps are detected in the intestine, they are examined to determine whether they are benign or in the class called adenomatous polyps, which are premalignant. Many polyps cause no symptoms, but polyps of the vocal cord can cause hoarseness and pain while swallowing or speaking. Simply speaking less can provide relief in most cases, but surgery to remove the polyps from the vocal cords is sometimes necessary. The standard surgical treatment for polyps is simple removal.

An inherited condition, familial adenomatous polyposis, causes the growth of hundreds and sometimes thousands of such polyps in the intestine, making cancer virtually inevitable. In such cases, the entire colon can be removed as a preventive measure. *See also* POLYPOSIS, FAMILIAL.

Polyposis, Familial

A genetic disorder in which hundreds of polyps appear in the colon and rectum.

Familial polyposis follows a dominant inheritance pattern, which means that a child of an affected parent has about a 50 percent chance of inheriting the disorder. The name familial polyposis actually encompasses three different disorders: familial polyposis coli, Gardner's syndrome, and Turcot's syndrome. Each of them involve polyp formation, but differ in symptoms that occur outside the colon. Familial polyposis is also related to Peutz-Jeghers syndrome, in which polyps form in the stomach, small intestine, and colon.

Familial polyposis occurs in approximately one in 8,000 individuals. The average age of onset is during childhood or adolescence. A malignancy develops before age 40 in nearly all untreated patients. Removal of the affected areas eliminates the risk of cancer.

The gene responsible for this condition has been identified and is located on chromosome number five. Symptoms accompanying the disorder may include:

- rectal prolapse;
- obstruction of the large intestine;
- perforation of the large intestine;
- painless bleeding;
- abdominal cramps; and
- bloody diarrhea.

Colonscopy is recommended for all patients past the age of eight every two years. Surgical removal of the affected area may need to be performed as well. *See also* INTESTINE *and* PEUTZ-JEGHERS SYNDROME.

Pomeray Technique

Also known as tubal ligation

Removal of part of the fallopian tubes as a sterilizing method of birth control.

Often done within a few days of a vaginal delivery or with a Cesarean section, this sort of birth control is for women who are sure they do not want to have any future children. This is performed under local anesthetic, and there is little likelihood that the procedure can be reversed. *See also* BARRIER METHODS *and* CONTRACEPTION.

Pompholyx

Also known as dyshidrosis or dyshidrotic eczema

A blistering disease that affects the palms of the hands, the sides of the fingers, and the foot soles.

Pompholyx manifests itself as multiple dense blisters on the palms, soles, and fingers. As the blisters go away, they may cause scaling of the skin. Some patients have also reported increased sweating. A history of asthma and nickel allergy has also been noted in some patients with pompholyx.

Treatment for pompholyx includes the use of steroids and ultraviolet light therapy with topical PUVA, a combination of drugs that make the skin more sensitive to ultraviolet light. *See also* BLISTER *and* PUVA.

Porphyria

An inherited disorder in which the body accumulates too much of the chemical porphyrin.

Porphyrin is used to make heme, the part of blood that carries oxygen. Excess porphyrin is excreted in the urine and feces. In porphyria, an enzyme deficiency disrupts the normal process of heme production. As a result, porphyrin accumulates in the body, resulting in nervous system and skin abnormalities. There are six types of porphyria, varying in specific cause, severity, and age of onset.

Symptoms affecting the nervous system include:
- pain in the chest or abdomen;
- muscle cramps;
- weakness;
- hallucinations;
- seizures;
- purplish-red urine;
- depression;
- anxiety; and
- paranoia.

Porphyria affects the skin, causing blisters, itching, swelling, and hypersensitivity to the sun.

Symptoms appear after exposure to triggers such as certain foods, sun exposure, and various drugs like barbiturates, tranquilizers, birth control pills, and sedatives.

Porphyria cannot be cured. Treatment is geared toward preventing attacks of the disease and alleviating symptoms through medications and a high-carbohydrate diet. *See also* BLISTER; DEPRESSION; *and* SKIN.

Port-Wine Stain

Also known as nevus flammeus

A birthmark consisting of superficial and deep dilated capillaries in the skin, which cause a reddish or purplish discoloration.

Port-wine stains are present at birth, and exist in approximately three out of every 1,000 babies. They are flat, and most often occur on or very near to the face. Over time, port-wine stains may become raised, nodular (consisting of solid bumps), or grape-like, and may distort facial features. Port-wine stains on the eyelids may be associated with glaucoma.

The most effective treatment for port-wine stains is laser surgery. Freezing, non-laser surgery, radiation, and tattooing have all been used in the past, but these procedures were never particularly successful in the treatment of port-wine stains. *See also* GLAUCOMA *and* SKIN.

Portal Hypertension

Abnormally high blood pressure in the portal vein, a major blood vessel carrying blood from the stomach, intestines and spleen through the liver.

The most common cause of portal hypertension in adults is cirrhosis—the scarring and deterioration of the liver—a condition that is almost always related to heavy drinking. It sometimes occurs in children, either because of congenital narrowing of the portal vein, or formation of a blood clot that interferes with blood flow. Sometimes, enlargement of the spleen caused by an infection can induce portal hypertension. In rare cases, it can be caused by an injury that creates an abnormal connection between the portal vein and an artery.

Whatever the cause, portal hypertension results in a buildup of pressure in the veins of the upper stomach and in the esophagus, which makes these organs grow larger than usual and can even cause them to rupture. There is also a buildup of fluid in the abdomen, a condition called ascites. Varices, new veins that bypass the liver, can come into existence, but are often weak and prone to rupture.

SYMPTOMS AND DIAGNOSIS

The immediate symptoms of postal hypertension are the abdominal swelling, discomfort, and breathing difficulties caused by ascites. Rupture of a blood vessel can cause massive bleeding that results in passage of blackened feces and persistent vomiting of blood. This is a life-threatening condition that requires immediate medical care. Portal hypertension can be diagnosed by a patient's signs and symptoms. The diagnosis can be confirmed by ultrasound scanning and angiography, which show the condition of the liver and the portal vein. In case of bleeding varices, endoscopy can determine if the cause is portal hypertension, which is the cause in half of all cases.

> ### Preventing Portal Hypertension
> The key to prevention and treatment of portal hypertension in most patients is to keep alcohol intake at a moderate level to prevent cirrhosis. Heavy drinking is a threat to health in several ways, and cirrhosis is among the leading dangers.

TREATMENT

Ascites can be treated by diuretic drugs that lower blood pressure by increasing the body's elimination of fluid, and by a low-salt diet. Treatment of bleeding varices can start with medications to lower blood pressure and reduce blood flow to the gastrointestinal tract. A ruptured vein can be treated by banding, in which a rubber band is used to tie off the varices, or with sclerotherapy, injection of a chemical solution that causes the broken vein to form a clot and wither. Several sessions of banding and/or sclerotherapy usually are needed. Surgery can be done to create a shunt, a new pathway for blood flow, and some patients are treated with a Sengstaken-Blakemore tube, an inflated balloon that compresses the varices. *See also* ASCITES; CIRRHOSIS; ENDOSCOPY; *and* SCLEROTHERAPY.

Post-Coital Test

A cervical mucus exam to explain infertility.

Post-Coital Tests (PCT) are usually done after other infertility tests are performed. Cervical mucus is collected shortly after intercourse, near ovulation, and examined to test how it interacts with sperm. PCT can reveal infections, antibodies that reject sperm, mucus thickness and density or poor coital technique. These problems can then be assessed and treated as necessary. *See also* ANTIBODY *and* INFERTILITY.

Post-Menopausal Bleeding

Ovulation-like bleeding episodes that occur after menopause.

Post menopausal bleeding (PMB) includes any and all vaginal bleeding that occurs 12 months following the onset of menopause; this is not an uncommon condition, but it is one that must be diagnosed and treated. PMB is often accompanied by abdominal pains and cramps.

Skin disease, infection, atrophic vaginitis, cervix erosion, uterine polyps, and tumors affecting the ovaries, fallopian tubes, uterus, or cervix can all cause PMB. Such bleeding may also come from hormone replacement therapies, including those involving estrogen and progesterone.

Because so many conditions cause PMB, several diagnostic tests may be performed, including cervical smears, uterine tissue samples, endoscopic examinations, and ultrasound scans. The test results will determine the treatment for the disorder. *See also* MENOPAUSE *and* PERIMENOPAUSE.

Postmaturity

A pregnancy which extends beyond the 42nd week.

Forty weeks is considered the average length of pregnancy, dating from the last menstrual period; for a postmature diagnosis the pregnancy must be significantly longer than the usual. One of the biggest problems associated with postmaturity is that the placenta becomes senile and no longer provides the fetus with sufficient oxygen. Fetal growth may stop because the uterine environment has become dangerous. The baby may lose weight. The rate of stillbirths for postmature babies is twice that of those born after normal pregnancy. Additionally, if the baby continues to grow, it may become too large to fit through the vaginal canal. Treatment of postmaturity is a simple matter; once the dates are determined to be correct, labor is induced. *See also* CHILDBIRTH, COMPLICATIONS; INDUCTION OF LABOR; *and* PREGNANCY.

Postnasal Drip

Discharge from the nose into the throat.

Infections that cause inflammation of the mucous membranes in the nose, such as rhinitis, can cause the mucous membranes to produce excess fluid. The fluid then drips from the nose into the nasopharynx, or upper part of the throat. The result is a feeling of hoarseness, or that something is lodged in the throat. There may also be a cough that results as well. The condition usually resolves with the dissipation of the infection. *See also* NASAL CONGESTION; NOSE; PHARYNX; *and* THROAT.

Postnatal Care

Specialized care given to maximize the proper development of a newborn.

In the months following birth, babies learn constantly from the stimuli and people around them. Newborns have certain emotional and physical needs. From the time of birth, a newborn baby will eat every two to five hours. Breast milk is the preferred method of feeding, but formula may also be used. Babies need to be burped after every feeding to expel the excess air they swallow. Newborns should be given sponge baths until the remainder of the umbilical cord has fallen off. Afterwards, babies should be kept clean and bathed regularly, although it is not necessary to bathe the child every day. A baby needs to be kept in a dry, clean diaper. Parents can choose between disposable and cloth diapers.

Research shows that children who are carried in a "snugli" type carrier, close to the parent's body, exhibit greater security and are able to form strong attachments later in life. In addition, it is wise to pick up a baby right away when it cries. This teaches the baby that its needs will be provided. Letting a baby cry for long periods teaches the child that one must cry long and hard to get what one wants, and will cause the baby to cry louder and more often. *See* APGAR SCORE; CHILD DEVELOPMENT; *and* MILK.

Postpartum Depression

Also known as the baby blues

The emotional letdown felt by many women after giving birth.

Postpartum depression may be accompanied by a feeling of being overwhelmed by becoming a mother and taking on the responsibility of a baby. This depression, which can range from mild to severe, most commonly begins within a few days of delivery and can last for several weeks.

Causes. There is no one specific cause for postpartum depression, but rather a variety of contributing factors. These include the tremendous hormonal changes that take place before, during, and after childbirth, as well as an emotional reaction to the end of pregnancy combined with the exhaustion of caring for a newborn. Added to this is feeling overwhelmed and dealing with a negative body image. The vast majority of cases usually clear up within a few weeks. However, some develop into major bouts of depression and require some form of medical intervention.

Treatment. For mild cases, it is important that a new mother get adequate rest. She should concentrate on regaining her physical strength and not on trying to do too much too fast. A supportive partner and family, willing to help with household and caretaking duties, are crucial to her recovery. She should not remain sequestered in the house but should schedule time to go out, with or without the baby. *See also* CHILDBIRTH; DELIVERY; *and* PREGNANCY.

Postpartum Hemorrhage

Continued heavy bleeding after delivery, resulting in the excessive loss of blood.

The majority of bleeding during pregnancy occurs when the placenta separates from the uterine wall. Postpartum hemorrhaging occurs when the uterus, for whatever reason, is unable to contract firmly enough to control the bleeding. The muscles may be tired or weak after a prolonged labor.

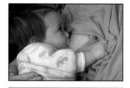
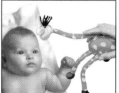

Breast Feeding. Above top, a hungry, eight month old nurses calmly from her mother. **Infant Fixing Vision.** Above bottom, this baby is learning one its earliest motor skills focusing in on an object, in this case a plush giraffe.

Hemorrhage can also be due to damage incurred by the vagina from lacerations or rupture. Occasionally it is caused by a retained placenta. The amount of blood varies greatly. Sometimes blood collects in the uterus instead of being expelled.

The risk of hemorrhage increases with any of the following:

- a large baby;
- multiple fetuses;
- a forceps delivery;
- a vaginal birth after a previous Cesarean section (VBAC);
- several previous deliveries;
- induced labor; and
- hydramnios.

Various drugs are administered to make the uterus contract more strongly. Torn tissue is always repaired. The patient may also need to be given medication to promote blood clotting. If the hemorrhage is still severe, doctors will tie off the major blood vessels of the uterus. A hysterectomy is the absolute last resort. In the case of a retained placenta (one which does not emerge within 30 minutes), the doctor may manually extract it and administer drugs to keep the uterus contracting. *See also* CHILD-BIRTH; HEMORRHAGE; LABOR; PREGNANCY; *and* UTERUS.

Post-Traumatic Stress Disorder

An anxiety reaction in which a traumatic event or series of events is replayed over and over in the victim's mind, causing problems with relationships, and interfering with sleep, work or school.

It is only natural that a person exposed to a traumatic event will experience a powerful emotional reaction. When someone has been the victim or witness of a violent, life-threatening situation such as a fire, a flood, a rape or a shooting, it would be surprising if that person did not become considerably upset by the event. In fact, there is an adaptive quality to reviewing and reliving the incident in that we attempt, at least mentally, to achieve some control over the experience and to learn from it in some way.

CAUSES

The cause for this disorder could be one catastrophic event or a continuing series of events such as child abuse, torture, or being exposed to continuous killing during a war. What all these events have in common is that they are out of the individual's control and induce feelings of helplessness and terror.

SYMPTOMS

An individual should be treated for post-traumatic stress disorder: when replaying the events continues for over a month, causing persistent feelings of fear and helplessness; when the continuous replay causes nightmares and sleep disturbances; when even a mild reminder of the event sets off a reaction; and when one experiences unexplained outbursts of anger. While there may be little or no apparent emotional impact after a traumatic event or series of events, it is possible for the disorder to take hold of a person's emotions months, or even years later when a seemingly incidental event, related in the sufferer's mind sets of the symptoms.

Another symptom of this disorder is a deadening of feelings. One way people survive catastrophes perpetuated by other people is dissociation, which involves separating oneself emotionally from what is happening. If this behavior pattern continues throughout life and becomes a way for the victim to relate in general, it will have a devastating effect on all relationships.

TREATMENT

There are a number of variables that determine whether someone will be affected by post-traumatic stress disorder. A combination of the person's age, emotional fragility, prior tragic experiences, proximity to the event, and the nature of the precipitating event itself will all bear influence. One precaution that can be taken is to seek emotional help immediately after experiencing a trauma. In any case, it is better to face the disaster with help and to deal with it rather than to avoid thinking about it. When the event causes an individual to avoid situations he or she must deal with on a daily basis, it is best to approach the feared situation cautiously. This may be done with the help of a therapist specializing in trauma treatment. If it is necessary to testify in court against a perpetrator, this may be an opportunity to gain control over the event, however, such a decision should be made in consultation with an expert in trauma recovery.

Support Groups. Talking about the event with a supportive and empathetic person, is more helpful than trying to ignore it and pretend the event didn't happen. In the case of severe and acute symptoms that need immediate attention, anti anxiety and anti depressant drugs can be prescribed in combination with psychotherapy. While one may never get over a traumatic experience, it is vital to address the problem head-on in order to attempt to end the debilitating effects of post-traumatic stress disorder.

For details on treatment for this disorder, see ACTING OUT; GROUP THERAPY; *and* PSYCHOTHERAPY. *For details on symptoms, see* INSOMNIA; NIGHT TERROR; NIGHTMARE; SLEEP DEPRIVATION. *Related material may be found in* AVOIDANT PERSONALITY DISORDER; PANIC DISORDER; *and* STRESS.

Postural Drainage

Treatment to remove excess fluids from the lungs.

A number of lung conditions, including bronchitis and cystic fibrosis, cause phlegm and other secretions to accumulate in the lungs, increasing the risk of respiratory infection. Postural drainage is performed to help eliminate these deposits.

Lying in certain positions encourages troublesome secretions to move out of the lungs and into the windpipe (trachea), where they trigger the coughing reflex and are expelled. Further drainage may be supplied by another person clapping the chest wall repeatedly with a cupped hand.

The patient lies on a bed and assumes a number of different positions, each of which is intended for deposits in a different part of the lungs. It is suggested that

forcible breathing and elbow flapping then be repeated while the patient sits up. The same regimen is repeated in a different position. In some cases, a mechanical vibrator may be used to increase the movement of the deposits. *See also* BRONCHITIS; CYSTIC FIBROSIS; *and* LUNG.

Posture

The alignment of various body parts while at rest or in motion.

The word posture makes most people remember growing up and being told to stand up straight and not to slouch. But posture is really about aligning the vertebrae to create a solid column that is able to support the entire body. Most people develop bad posture from slouching habits or by sitting improperly. Though it may seem easier, slouching actually requires more muscles to work than standing up straight.

Good posture prevents neck and back pain. For correct posture, focus on the spine, imagining each vertebra stacked one on top of the other all the way through the neck. The head should pull the body up and be an active part of the line created by the spine, creating a straight column that reaches to the feet. The shoulders should not pull back or droop, and the lower back should not hyperextend.

Exercises for the back and abdomen help to strengthen and improve posture. Dance classes, yoga, and Pilates (methods of balance) are excellent ways to learn about the body. Maintaining good posture also helps to alleviate back pain and stress. *See also* BACK PAIN *and* EXERCISE.

Potassium

A metallic element necessary to the proper functioning of all living cells.

Along with sodium and calcium, potassium regulates the balance in the body's cells and is essential to heart, kidney, and muscle function, the transmission of nerve impulses, and the secretion of digestive fluids.

Resources on Post-Traumatic Stress Disorder
American Psychiatric Association, *Diagnostic and Statistical Manual of Mental Disorders, 4th Edition* (1994); Greist, John H. and James W. Jefferson, *Depression and Its Treatment* (1992); Solomon, Andrew, *The Noonday Demon: An Atlas of Depression* (2001); Herman, Judith L., Trauma and Recovery (1997); Levine, Peter A., and Ann Frederick, *Waking the Tiger: Healing Trauma: The Innate Capacity to Transform Overwhelming Experiences* (1997); National Depressive & Manic-Depressive Association, Tel. (800) 82-NDMDA, Online: www.ndmda.org; National Mental Health Association, Tel. (800) 969-NMHA, Online: www.nmha.org; www.ny-cornell.org/psychiatry/.

> **ALERT**
>
> ### Hyperkalemia
>
> Excesses of potassium in the blood (hyperkalemia) can endanger health. Most of the body's potassium is found in the cells—about 96 percent—and the balance between cellular potassium and blood potassium is vital. Potassium affects cell membranes, the heart, and pathways between the brain and body. Therefore, use of potassium supplements should only occur under the supervision of a doctor. Very high doses can cause irregular heartbeat and, in severe cases, death may occur from heart failure.

A dietary deficiency of potassium is unusual, as potassium is found in most foods. It generally occurs in people who have severe kidney disease, diabetes mellitus, or severe burns, as well as those who suffer from dehydration and loss of fluids from diarrhea, vomiting, fasting, or continuous use of diuretics or laxatives. Symptoms include thirst, dry mouth, lethargy, anxiety, irregular heartbeat, muscle weakness and paralysis, and pain throughout the body.

A balanced diet will generally provide sufficient potassium for those who are not in a risk group for deficiency. Good plant sources of potassium include a variety of fruit and vegetable sources, particularly apricots, avocados, bananas, bran, dried beans and peas, oranges, peanuts, and potatoes.

See BLOOD DISORDERS; HYPERKALEMIA; *and* HYPOKALEMIA *for details on disorders concerning potassium. Related information is contained in* DEHYDRATION; DIET AND DISEASE; DIURETIC DRUGS; LAXATIVES; *and* SODIUM. *Other blood disorders are discussed in* ANEMIA *and* DIABETES.

Potency

In pharmacology, a drug's strength, or ability to produce a desired result. Otherwise, a man's ability to father children.

In order for a man to father children, he must produce healthy sperm that are capable of fertilizing an egg. He must also be able to maintain an erection for penetration to occur during sexual intercourse, and ejaculate to release the sperm into the female reproductive tract. Impotence is an older term for erectile dysfunction (ED), which affects about 30 million men in America. New medications and treatments, such as sildenafil citrate (Viagra), show promising results. If there is a problem with the amount, viability, or motility of the sperm, the term used is infertility. *See also* ERECTION, DISORDERS OF *and* INFERTILITY.

Pott's Fracture

A simultaneous fracture and dislocation of the ankle.

An extreme twisting action can cause the fibula, one of the lower leg bones, to break just above the ankle. The same action can break or tear ligaments in the tibia, or shin, causing the ankle to dislocate.

The first step of treatment is the manipulation of the bones back to their correct position. The foot, ankle and lower leg must then be immobilized in a cast. Screws may also be inserted to increase stability. The injury may take eight to ten weeks to heal. Physical therapy may be required to restore the foot and ankle to full strength. *See also* DISLOCATION; FRACTURE; JOINT; PHYSICAL THERAPY; *and* REDUCTION.

Pox

A disease characterized by small eruptions on the skin.

Pox is a term that is used to refer to a symptom of various viral infections. Chicken pox is caused by the *Varicella zoster* virus. It produces a rash composed of small red spots that soon turn into raised bumps, which blister and itch. The spots open, drain, and crust over. Smallpox has symptoms similar to, but more severe than, those of chickenpox, and is caused by the variola virus. Edward Jenner used cowpox to create the first vaccine against disease, the smallpox vaccine. In 1977, the World Health Organization announced that smallpox had been fully eradicated. *See also* CHICKENPOX; SMALLPOX; *and* SYPHILIS.

Precancerous

Cells or tissue that tends to become malignant.

The development of some cancers is preceded by the presence of cells that are abnormal but do not spread uncontrollably (malignant). The term precancerous is used to describe such growths and any other health condition that may indicate that a person is predisposed to developing a type of cancer.

One example is adenomatous polyps found in the intestine. These polyps are usually removed because they can become cancerous. Other examples include the growths seen in leukoplakia of the mouth, bladder papillomas, and the multiple tumors that appear on the nerves in the condition called neurofibromatosis, or von Recklinghausen's disease.

Persons with Down's syndrome are known to have an increased risk of developing leukemia; the intestinal condition called ulcerative colitis increases the risk of colorectal cancer. A person suffering from such conditions requires regular monitoring for early detection of any cancer that may develop.

Precancerous growths often are removed surgically, but a number of clinical trials are now under way to determine whether treatment with certain drugs or antioxidants, such as vitamin E, can prevent malignancy. *See* CANCER *and* TUMOR.

Precocious Puberty

Premature development of body characteristics that are associated with puberty

Puberty normally occurs between the ages of 13 and 15 in boys and the ages of nine and 16 in girls. Male sexual development before the age of ten and female development before the age of nine is generally considered precocious puberty. The condition is more common in girls.

The condition may cause adverse psychological effects and limit growth. The most common treatment for precocious puberty is hormone therapy. *See* PUBERTY.

Predisposing Factors

Characteristics which make an individual more or less susceptible to certain diseases and disorders.

Predisposing factors can include aspects of a person's lifestyle, physical condition, and genetic makeup. For example, smoking is a predisposing factor for lung cancer and heart disease; obesity is a predisposing factor for diabetes mellitus; and a family history of heart disease is a predisposing factor for heart disease.

Having a predisposing factor does not mean that a person will necessarily develop a disease. It does mean that the chances of developing the disease are greater. If a person has a known predisposing factor—such as a family history of heart disease—he or she is advised to take appropriate precautions in terms of diet and related matters, as well as screen for early signs of disease so that treatment can be pursued promptly.

> *Background material on Predisposing Factors can be found in* DIABETES AND GENETICS. *Related information is contained in* DIET; LUNG CANCER; OBESITY; PREVENTATIVE MEASURES; *and* PREVENTATVE TESTING AND SCREENING;

Prednisolone

An anti-inflammatory drug used to treat arthritis and swelling caused by allergies.

Prednisolone, a corticosteroid, is prescribed to treat the swelling involved in a number of disorders, including arthritis and allergies. This drug, which comes in an ophthalmic solution for the eyes, reduces swelling, itching, and discomfort. The eyedrops can be applied up to six times a day ,and should not be used indefinitely. Patients who use prednisolone for more than a few weeks should consult a physician.

Prednisolone and the Eyes. Any one who uses an opthalmic corticosteroid drug for more than a few weeks should have their eyes examined regularly by an opthalmologist to avoid negative side effects. If the eye condition does not improve within one week, consult a physician. *See also* ARTHRITIS; ASTHMA; *and* CORTICOSTEROID

Preeclampsia

The earlier, less severe form of the serious pregnancy complication eclampsia, characterized by high blood pressure and swelling (edema) of the face and hands and protein in the urine.

Symptoms of preeclampsia include swelling (edema) in the face and hands, headache, nausea, and vision disturbances. Further indications include high blood pressure and protein in the urine.

Incidence and Causes. Preeclampsia occurs in five percent of all pregnancies, with eclampsia developing in 1 in every 1,500 pregnancies. It is most common in first pregnancies, pregnancies with a new father, and multiple pregnancies. Both preeclampsia and eclampsia are called toxemias of pregnancy; however, no toxic substance has been identified. The cause remains largely unknown.

Risk Factors and Complications. Women at higher risk for developing either pre-eclampsia or eclampsia are either very young (teen-age years) or older than 40. Also more predisposed to the condition are women with a history of high blood pressure or women carrying multiple fetuses. A family history of preeclampsia appears to increase the risk.

Eclampsia occurs when preeclampsia is not brought under control. As it progresses there is increased facial puffiness, sudden excessive weight gain, and severe headaches. These are followed by pain in the upper right side of the abdomen, vision disturbances such as seeing flashing lights, severe convulsions, and loss of consciousness. This condition can be fatal for both mother and baby.

Treatment. Mild preeclampsia is treated by bringing the blood pressure under control with diet and medication. Bed rest will be prescribed, with the mother resting on her left side to take the pressure off the great vessels. Sometimes hospitalization is necessary to administer medications for high blood pressure, in order to keep the condition from progressing. If preeclampsia progresses to eclampsia, immediate delivery is needed. Sometimes after an early delivery due to preeclampsia, the mother will develop eclampsia within 24 hours.

In recent years, better prenatal care has helped lower the number of cases of preeclampsia that progress into eclampsia. *See also* Eclampsia *and* Pregnancy.

Pregnancy

The nine-month period during which a fertilized egg develops inside the uterus into a baby capable of existence outside the womb.

Pregnancy can be a very exciting and challenging time for a woman, whether or not she is already a mother. An unborn baby is known as an embryo for the first 8 weeks, and then as a fetus until birth. While in the womb, the fetus experiences many stages of change and growth.

Pregnancy is dated from the last menstrual period. A full term pregnancy lasts between 38 and 42 weeks. The due date is calculated by subtracting 3 months from the beginning of the last menstrual period and adding seven days. Most women deliver within 2 weeks of their due date.

Trimesters. Pregnancy can be divided into 3 trimesters, each lasting approximately 3 months. There are certain key events that are characteristic of each trimester.

The first trimester is the time when the developing embryo is most vulnerable. Every organ is being formed, and the baby is particularly susceptible to the effects of drugs and toxins. Miscarriage is more likely to occur during this time as well. Often miscarried embryos have some abnormality that would prevent them from surviving outside the uterus.

Early symptoms of pregnancy include:
- Missed menstrual period;
- Breast tenderness;
- Morning sickness;
- Fatigue;
- Increased frequency of urination.

During the second trimester, most of these symptoms and discomforts subside. Most pregnant women feel their best at this time. During this middle period of pregnancy, most women begin to "show," mean-

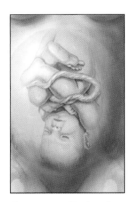

Pregnancy. During the nine–month gestation period for humans, the soon to be born child goes through development from a miniscule cluster of cells (zygote) to a life form able to sustain life outside of the womb.

ing that the abdomen has grown large enough to be noticeable. As the fetus continues to grow in the uterus, the abdomen of the pregnant woman similarly continues to become larger.

Around the twelfth week the baby's heartbeat may be detected. The fetal heart rate is between 140 and 160 beats a minute, much more rapid than an adult's, and may sound like a herd of galloping horses.

About midway through the fifth month, the mother feels the baby's movements. The baby has been active all along, but until now was not large enough for it's movements to be noticeable. The first movements feel like a light fluttering, but within a few weeks it progress to kicks and pokes. Some babies are more active than others.

By the third trimester, the pregnancy has advanced to the point where the mother experiences some of the same discomforts of the early months, caused by the increased size of the uterus and its exerting pressure on all of the neighboring organs. These include increased urination and heartburn, as well as backache. The baby is large enough that its kicking and other activities may interfere with the mother's rest.

What to Expect. Physical changes that the mother can expect during the course of pregnancy, other than a rapidly expanding abdomen, include enlarged breasts, darker nipples and prominent veins. From the fourth month on, a yellowish fluid called colostrum, which is the forerunner to breast milk, may be secreted from the nipples. The normal amount of vaginal discharge will increase. The mother may notice reddish brown streaks (stretch marks) appearing on her abdomen or legs. Their color will fade in time after giving birth but they will never entirely disappear. Some women, particularly those with brown hair, notice a darkening of their facial skin, sometimes refered to as the mask of pregnancy. Other changes include hemorrhoids, varicose veins, and some swelling of the hands and feet, particularly during hot and humid weather.

The physical changes of pregnancy are often accompanied by emotional ones as well. Many women may find they are more emotional, or excitable during pregnancy. Some women experience food cravings.

Background material on Pregnancy can be found in CHILDBIRTH. *. Related information is contained in* ADOLESENCE; ABORTION; PLACENTA; PREECLAMPSIA; PREGNANCY COUNSELLING; PREGNANCY TESTS; PREGNANCY, DRUGS IN; PREGNANCY, FALSE; PREGNANCY, MULTIPLE; PREMATURE BIRTH, PRENATAL CARE; *and* PREVENTATIVE MEASURES. *See also* LAMAZE METHOD *AND* NATURAL CHILDBIRTH *for more on Pregnancy.*

Highlights of Fetal Development by Month:

1st: The embryo has a head, trunk, and limb buds. The heart begins beating around the third week, and the liver and digestive system are developing. The placenta is being formed. At the end of this month the embryo is 1/4 inch long.

2nd: The nervous system develops, as well as the facial features, fingers, and toes. By the end of this month the fetus has a more human appearance. It weighs less than an ounce and is between one–half and one inch long.

3rd: All the major organs are at least partially formed, including the sexual organs. The baby is about four inches long at the end of this month and is opening and closing its fists and mouth.

4th: Nails, hair, eyebrows, eyelids, and eyelashes are forming. The fetus has regular periods of sleep and wakefulness. At the end of this month it is about 6 inches long.

5th: Up till now the skeleton mostly consisted of cartilage, but it is being replaced with bone. Rapid growth occurs. By the end of this month the fetus is 10 inches long and weighs one pound.

6th: More rapid growth. All of the essential organs are formed by the end of this month, and the baby has a chance of independent survival if born at this point. It weighs about two pounds and is one foot long.

7th: The eyes can open and close. Many babies assume a head downward position in the uterus. By the end of the month the baby is 14 inches long and weighs between two and three pounds.

8th: The baby's size results in constricted, forceful movements. The baby weighs between four and five pounds and is 18 inches long.

9th: The baby gains approximately half a pound a week. The average baby weighs seven pounds and is between 18 and 20 inches long at birth. Before labor commences, the baby will settle lower in the mother's abdomen, preparatory to descending into the birth canal.

Pregnancy Counseling

Advice or services given to pregnant women so that they may plan for the arrival of their child.

Pregnancy counseling may include reproductive and complementary health care services, educational programs to help the woman make informed decisions about her health and her child's health, and sessions with a therapist or other medical professional. Services are offered in diverse settings, including public health facilities, private physicians' offices, and community-based outreach centers. *See also* PREGNANCY.

PREGNANT PATIENTS' RIGHTS
Before any treatment plan is undertaken, either to protect the pregnant woman's health or the health of her baby, it is important that she give informed consent. A pregnant patient is considered "informed" if she consents to treatment after being informed about the various steps in the treatment contemplated by the physician, including whether the treatment is new or unusual; the risks and hazards of the treatment; the chances for recovery; the necessity of the treatment; and the feasibility of alternative methods of treatment.

Pregnancy Tests

Clinical or at-home tests to confirm pregnancy.

A variety of simple and painless tests may be administered to confirm pregnancy. Clinical examinations for pregnancy are carried out on a sample of the patient's blood, while home testing kits evaluate urine. In both cases, such tests are designed to detect human chorionic gonadotropin or HCG. This hormone, which is a positive marker for pregnancy, is produced by the developing tissue (placenta) that nourishes the growing baby. HGC is detectable in the urine or blood within 6 days after fertilization of the egg.

Home pregnancy tests rely on a principle known as agglutination. Antibody/antigen complexes will tend to clump together,

or agglutinate, a feature such tests are sensitive to. When agglutination fails to occur, the test results are positive. Laboratory tests carried out on urine or blood serum are somewhat more sensitive and involve a more sophisticated process known as an enzyme immunoassay. ELISA, or enzyme linked immunosorbent assay, can detect even low levels of human chorionic gonadotropin present in a urine sample.

Elevated levels of HCG during pregnancy may indicate disease or multiple pregnancy. In non-pregnant women and in men, increased HCG may be diagnostic sign of ovarian or testicular tumors, melanoma, multiple myeloma, or gastric, hepatic, pancreatic, or breast cancer. Decreased levels in pregnant women may indicate the threat of spontaneous abortion or ectopic pregnancy. During normal pregnancy, the level of HCG roughly doubles every two days in the first two months.

Effectiveness. While positive results from home tests are very reliable, negative results in the presence of symptoms of pregnancy may not be. A follow-up lab test is recommended and provides 95 percent accuracy within three weeks of conception for the urine test or 95 percent accuracy within eight to 10 days for the blood serum analysis. The latter test is 100 percent accurate after six weeks.

Types. While detection of human chorionic gonadotropin is the simplest and most common test for pregnancy, other means exist. Detection of the fetal heartbeat using a specialized stethoscope can confirm pregnancy as early as 18 weeks after conception. Ultrasound studies may be used earlier, from 6 to 8 weeks, to detect fetal heartbeat or enlargement of the uterus, another indicator of pregnancy. Between 16 and 20 weeks following fertilization, the mother may detect pregnancy through the movements of the fetus.

Background material on Pregnancy Tests can be found in CHILDBIRTH AND PRENATAL CARE.. Related information is contained in ABORTION; MISCARRIAGE; PREECLAMPSIA; PREGNANCY COUNSELLING; PREGNANCY, DRUGS IN; PREGNANCY, FALSE; PREGNANCY, MULTIPLE; and PREVENTATIVE MEASURES.

Resources on Pregnancy
Creasy, Robert K. and Robert Resnik, eds., *Maternal-Fetal Medicine: Principles and Practice* (1994); Gonik, Bernard and Renee A. Bobrowski, *Medical Complications in Labor and Delivery* (1996); Sears, William, et al., *The Pregnancy Book: Month-by-Month, Everything You Need to Know From America's Baby Experts* (1997); International Childbirth Education Association, Inc., Tel. (612) 854-8660, Online: www.icea.org; Maternity Center Association, Tel. (212) 777-5000, Online: www.maternity.org; Universe of Women's Health, Tel. (512) 418-2922, Online: www.obgyn.net; www.nycornell.org/obgyn

Pregnancy, Drugs in

Any drug taken during pregnancy carries the risk of causing birth defects or miscarriage, especially during the first trimester. This warning applies even to so-called "safe" or over-the-counter drugs. Women who are pregnant or think they may be should check with a doctor before taking any medication—whether prescription or over-the-counter—to find out if it can be taken during pregnancy.

Drugs can either act directly on a fetus or affect how the placenta functions. Additionally, some drugs affect the uterus, causing it to contract. The effect of a particular drug on a fetus depends on the dosage and the stage of fetal development.

Most drugs taken before the seventeenth day of pregnancy seem to have an "all or nothing" effect—they either cause a miscarriage or have no effect whatsoever. The embryo at this stage seems to be highly resistant to birth defects.

Between the seventeenth and fifty-seventh day of pregnancy, the fetus' susceptibility is much higher, as this is a key stage in organ development. Once organ development is completed, drugs can alter the growth and function of the various tissues.

Sometimes a doctor must weigh the potential damage caused by a drug against the patient's welfare if she is unable to take necessary medication. Various neurological medications fall into this category. Pregnant cancer patients should consult their physician.

DRUGS AND BIRTH DEFECTS

The drugs most commonly associated with birth defects include: alcohol, phenytoin, lithium, streptomycin, tetracycline, thalidomide, warfarin, and anything that interferes with the action of folic acid, such as triameterene and trimethoprim. Nicotine should be avoided during pregnancy.

Illegal drugs can also lead to birth defects. The active ingredient in marijuana, THC, can cross the placenta; and there is a suggested link between heavy use and later abnormal behavior in infants.

Cocaine constricts the blood flow to the fetus, thereby reducing the oxygen supply. This in turn causes abnormal growth and defects in the skeleton and intestines. Additionally, the child may be born with nervous system damage, behavioral problems, or learning problems, which may persist for years. Cocaine can also increase the chances of miscarriage, stillbirth, or premature labor. *See also* PREGNANCY.

Pregnancy, False

Also known as pseudocyesis.

When a woman exhibits some or all of the signs of pregnancy but is not pregnant.

A missed menstrual period, fatigue, morning sickness, bloating, and increased urination are not always a result of pregnancy. They may be caused by other conditions, including cancer, hydatidform moles, ovarian cysts, and thyroid disorders, whose symptoms are similar to those of pregnancy. A psychological disorder can also result in a false pregnancy.

A positive result from a pregnancy test is not always accurate. Tests used for determining pregnancy detect levels of human chorionic gonadotropin (HCG) in the urine or blood. False positives can be caused by the presence of another hormone, leutenizing hormone (LH), which is chemically similar to HCG. Levels of LH are higher during ovulation. Also, women entering menopause have high levels of LH in their urine. Newer tests are significantly more accurate in distinguishing between LH and HCG.

Other causes of false positive results for a pregnancy test include the use of marijuana, methadone, some blood pressure drugs, tranquilizers, and antidepressants. Because it takes time for HCG levels to decrease, a pregnancy test taken up to 10 days after a miscarriage or abortion may still come out positive.

More on False Pregnancy can be found in CHILDBIRTH AND PREGNANCY. *.Related information is contained in* ABORTION; MISCARRIAGE; *and* PREGNANCY COUNSELING.

Pregnancy, Multiple

A pregnancy in which more than one fetus develop at the same time.

A multiple pregnancy may result from a single egg that splits into two or more parts after fertilization, in which case all fetuses carry the same genetic material and are of the same sex. Multiple fetuses can also result when two or more eggs are released at the same time, either naturally or because of fertility drug treatments.

Twins. Most cases of multiple pregnancy result in twins. However, multiple births of more than two are becoming increasingly more common in recent years due to the process of in vitro fertilization. Sometimes multiple embryos are implanted in the uterus in the hope that at least one or two will survive and result in a viable pregnancy. Occasionally, several or all of the embryos survive, and the result is a multiple pregnancy.

The more fetuses there are, the less chance each has of survival, as the uterus is stretched beyond its limits. A multiple pregnancy is harder physically for the mother, and the usual problems and health risks are much more severe.

The majority of multiple pregnancies end with an early delivery by Cesarean section. As with other premature infants, there may be associated health risks for the babies. Because of their prematurity, these babies may experience long-term developmental problems as well.

Parents facing a multiple pregnancy have the option of undergoing selective reduction to increase the chances of survival for the remaining fetus or fetuses.

To date, the largest number of fetuses that have survived are septuplets. In all documented cases of octuplets, at least one of the babies did not survive.

Early diagnosis of multiple pregnancy depends on frequent prenatal visits to a doctor. Early diagnosis is also the most important factor in preventing complications multiple births. *See also* CHILDBIRTH; PREGNANCY *and* PREGNANCY COUNSELING.

Premature Birth

The birth of a baby before the 37th week of pregnancy

The average pregnancy lasts 40 weeks as dated from the last menstrual period. What causes a pregnant woman to go into preterm labor is not well understood. Various medications are used in an attempt to halt, slow, or delay labor, so that the baby can benefit from an additional period of time in utero.

IMMEDIATE PROGNOSIS
The later a premature baby is born, the better its chances of survival and good health. Currently, the earliest a baby can be born and have a fair chance of survival is about 24 weeks. The survival rate is about 40 percent for babies born at 24 weeks, 50 percent at 25 weeks, 60 percent at 26 weeks, 70 percent at 27 weeks, and 80 percent at 28 weeks. Weight is an important determining factor. Babies whose birth weight is less than 1,000 grams (2.2 pounds) do not have as good a chance of survival as babies heavier at birth.

For an individual baby, the prognosis can change with time. The first "milestone" is to survive birth and resuscitation, and then to live through the first few hours.

LONG-TERM COMPLICATIONS
As postnatal technology and care improve, babies can survive being born at earlier gestational ages. However, prematurity can lead to associated health problems.

The most common health concerns are underdevelopment of the lungs and the nervous system. The lungs are among the last organs to develop, since they are not needed for oxygen in utero. Most, if not all, premature babies are not capable of breathing on their own and must spend time on a respirator or ventilator. These machines inflate the babies' lungs and provide crucial oxygen. In recent years, a synthetic form of surfactant has been developed. Surfactant is a naturally occurring substance that lubricates and prevents lung tissue from sticking to itself. The drug has helped to cut down on scarring and the amount of time premature babies need to be on respirators.

Nervous and Immune Systems. Some premature babies are born with an immature nervous system and may suffer from seizures or have an episode of bleeding in the brain. Some develop cerebral palsy, brain damage, or developmental delays. Similarly, the immune system and kidneys of some babies may be underdeveloped, resulting in serious infection and blood poisoning.

During the ninth month of pregnancy, a layer of subcutaneous fat is deposited under the skin, which acts as insulation. Babies born before then may be unable to regulate their body temperature and may need to spend time in an incubator. The specially designed chamber keeps a baby at a safe and healthy temperature.

Feeding. Many premature babies have not yet developed the sucking reflex, and must be fed through a tube. As the infants get older, they gradually learn how to suck and swallow and can be fed with a bottle and then breast fed. In severe cases, the infant is initially fed intravenously.

Brain Disorders. Extremely premature babies who have normal brain scans may still develop cognitive, motor, sensory, emotional and health deficits later on. In early stages of prematurity, such deficits may put infants at risk of "forgetting" to breathe and regulate temperature and blood sugar levels.

Cerebral Palsy

Cerebral palsy (CP) is one of the most common causes of chronic childhood disability worldwide, occurring in 1.4 to 2.7 percent of all births. While the improved survival of extremely preterm infants in many developed countries may result in an increasing number of children with CP, premature babies constitute a minority of the overall number of CP-disabled children. About 10 percent of babies born weighing less than 1,000 grams will eventually be diagnosed with cerebral palsy. However, between 17 percent and 60 percent of CP cases, including babies of normal weight, have no known cause.

DEVELOPMENTAL CHALLENGES

Babies who are born prematurely are developmentally younger than their actual age, and reach many of the milestones of infancy—such as sitting up, crawling, walking, and talking—later than babies born full-term. It may take years for children born prematurely to "catch up" with their peers.

Background material on Premature Birth can be found in CHILDBIRTH. *. Related information is contained in* CEREBRAL PALSY; EMBRYO; PLACENTA; PREGNANCY COUNSELLING; PREGNANCY TESTS; PREGNANCY, DRUGS IN; PREGNANCY, MULTIPLE; PRENATAL CARE; RESPIRATOR *and* VENTILATOR.

Premedication

Drugs administered to a patient in advance of an operation to reduce anxiety or pain, or to reduce the amount of anesthesia subsequently needed.

An anticholinergic drug such as atropine is sometimes administered to dry up secretions in the airways that might otherwise be inhaled during anesthesia.

Types of analgesic painkillers, including meperidine hydrochloride (Demerol), butorphanol tartrate (Stadol), codeine, morphine and other opiate derivatives.

Anxiety reducers and sedatives include: diazepam (Valium), barbiturates, promethazine hydrochloride (Phenergan), and midazolam (Versed).

Premedicating children with a short-acting sedative, such as midazolam, has been shown to be very effective in reducing preoperative anxiety when they are separated from their parents before entering the operating room.

Premedication with propofol, onadsetron, and even simple ginger ale may also be effective in reducing postoperative nausea and vomiting.

Background material on Premedication can be found in ANXIETY AND PREVENTATIVE MEASSURES. *. Related information is contained in* ANESTHESIA; COUNSELING; HOSPITAL; NAUSEA; PREVENTATIVE MEDICINE; PREVENTATIVE SCREENING AND COUNSELING; PSYCHSOMATIC DISORDERS; PSYCHOSOMATIC ILLNESS *and* VOMITING.

Premenstrual Syndrome

Collection of symptoms associated with the onset of each menstrual cycle.

In the week or two before the beginning of a monthly period, many women undergo a series of physical and emotional changes that have become known as premenstrual syndrome. It occurs at the start of ovulation (the development and release of an egg from the ovary), and the symptoms continue until the actual beginning of the menstrual period. Up to 90 percent of all women experience premenstrual syndrome, or PMS, at some time in their lives, with about one–third having it regularly; 10 percent feel that the symptoms interrupt normal daily activities.

Symptoms. The most common symptoms of PMS include cramps, bloating from fluid retention, weight gain, tenderness and swelling in the breasts, skin breakouts, irritability, depression, aggression, feelings of fatigue, and food cravings.

Causes. No actual cause is known. Although undoubtedly due to some kind of hormonal shift during the menstrual cycle, the specific change has not been detected or understood. There has been a suggestion of a link with a lack of vitamins E and B, magnesium, and prostaglandins, but this has not been proven to any degree. Until recently, PMS was actually dismissed as psychosomatic, or a woman's delusion.

Just as there is no single, understood cause for PMS, there is also no foolproof remedy. Drugs such as danazol, and the natural hormone progesterone have been administered to those suffering from PMS, but no conclusions have been reached about either their safety or effectiveness. There are however, some steps a woman can take to alleviate the symptoms.

Ibuprofen, naproxen, or aspirin can help to relieve cramps, as can magnesium and pyridoxine supplements.

Over-the-counter diuretics can help with water retention and bloating, as can reducing salt intake. Reducing sugar and salt, and increasing protein intake allevi-

ates some symptoms.

Cutting back on caffinated products, such as coffee, tea, chocolate, and soft drinks, can help with irritability. Avoiding alcohol can reduce feelings of depression and anxiety, as can exercise.

Natural herbal supplements, such as evening primrose oil and shepherd's purse, claim to ease symptoms such as breast pain and tenderness. *See also* MENSTRUATION.

Premolar

Teeth located between the canines and the molars.

There are eight permanent premolars in the human mouth. The shape of these teeth resemble two cones that have been fused together. Premolars are used primarily for tearing, crushing, and grinding food. *See also* TEETH.

Prenatal Care

Medical care and lifestyle changes that maximize the health of an expectant mother and her developing child.

A woman's health concerns during pregnancy are unique, as the mother has not only her own well-being to be concerned with, but also that of the child.

Medical Care. When pregnancy is confirmed by a doctor, the mother's age, weight, and childbearing history are recorded. The doctor also asks the mother for a history of infectious diseases, such as measles or hepatitis, as well as if she has any chronic conditions, such as high blood pressure, diabetes, or heart disease.

The doctor conducts a physical exam. A Pap test is administered, and samples of blood and urine are taken. The blood is tested to determine if the mother is anemic and also whether or not she is immune to rubella, which can cause severe birth defects if contracted during pregnancy.

The schedule for future prenatal visits is usually once a month until the seventh month, then biweekly until the ninth month. During the last month visits are

Resources on Premenstrual Syndrome
Adashi, Eli Y., John A. Rock and Zev Rosenwaks, *Reproductive Endocrinology, Surgery and Technology* (1987); Glass, Leon, and Michael C. Mackey, *From Clocks to Chaos: The Rhythms of Life* (1988); Golub, Sharon, *Periods: From Menarche to Menopause* (1992); Schafer, Walt, *Stress Mangement for Wellness* (1987); Vliet, Elizabeth Lee, *Women Weight, and Hormones* (2001); Endocrine Web, Online: www.endocrineweb.com; www.nycornell.org/medicine/edm/index.html.

often weekly. If there are any health concerns, the doctor may request more frequent visits.

Weight. One feature of the follow-up visits is measuring weight. An expectant mother must gain an adequate amount of weight to ensure her own good health and the proper development of her baby. The American College of Obstetricians and Gynecologists recommends a weight gain of 22–26 pounds. A woman who is underweight may be told to gain 30 pounds, whereas one who is overweight should confine her weight gain to 22 pounds.

Pregnancy is no time to start a diet, and the primary emphasis should be nutrition. It is extremely important for the mother to consume adequate calories to meet both her own and the baby's needs. Her diet should contain sufficient amounts of protein, vitamins, and minerals. Pregnant women are advised to take supplemental amounts of iron, calcium, and folic acid. If an expectant mother's calorie or nutritional intake is inadequate, the baby will dip into the mother's own reserves.

The mother's blood pressure and urine are tested at each visit as well. The early warning signs of preeclampsia, a serious condition that can develop into life-threatening eclampsia, include high blood pressure and protein in the urine.

Regular visits also provide an opportunity for the mother to discuss any concerns she may have with her health care provider.

Lifestyle Concerns. A pregnant woman is not an invalid, and in the absence of any health concerns, is encouraged to exercise. Moderation is key, however; she should be careful not to exercise to the point of exhaustion. In addition, during pregnancy the joints are much more flexible and "looser" than normal, and she should be aware of the increased possibility for injury.

A common feature of pregnancy is fatigue, and part of good prenatal care means getting an adequate amount of sleep and rest during the day, if possible.

Most women can continue working as long as their health is good and their jobs don't involve working with hazardous materials or in jobs that may endanger their health and safety.

Drugs. Many drugs can cross the placenta, so during pregnancy a woman should avoid taking any drugs, whether prescription or over-the-counter, without her doctor's knowledge and approval.

Background material on Prenatal Care can be found in PREGNANCY COUNSELING *and* PREVENTATIVE SCREENINGS *and* TESTING. *Related information is contained in* ADOLESENCE; DIET; LAMAZE METHOD; PREECLAMPSIA; PREGNANCY TESTS; PREGNANCY, DRUGS IN; PREGNANCY, FALSE; PREGNANCY, MULTIPLE; PREMATURE BIRTH, *and* TOBACCO SMOKING.

Prepared Childbirth

Also known as natural childbirth

Various classes used to teach women and their partners what to expect during the course of labor and delivery.

Prepared childbirth classes usually include learning breathing, imagery, and other relaxation techniques. Lamaze and Bradley are two such classes. The techniques help reduce the need for anesthesia, forceps, and other medical interventions. The less intervention necessary, the better it is for both mother and baby.

Regardless of the different courses and philosophies available, a common theme is the emphasis on childbirth as a natural process. Rather than being simply a passive patient, the pregnant mother is encouraged to be an active participant in the process and to be able to make informed decisions about her care.

In addition to discussing the actual events of labor and delivery, many classes also teach infant care, breastfeeding, and other postpartum issues.

A well-prepared patient—a patient who has consulted with her physician and investigated the subject of pregnancy and fetal health—has a significantly better chance of seeing a pregnancy through to a successful completion than a woman who has not prepared herself for the pregnancy. *See also* LAMAZE METHOD; PREGNANCY; *and* PREGNANCY, DRUGS IN.

Presbycusis

Hearing loss of the higher frequencies, brought on by age.

Just as the eyes lose the ability to focus on near objects as the body ages, one's gradual loss of hearing makes certain higher frequencies less audible. Men tend to experience this hearing loss more than women but even within the male population there is much variation in the degree of severity. Some men are nearly deaf by the age of fifty; others retain excellent hearing into their nineties. The disorder is caused by the deterioration of the nerve fibers and hair cells in the inner ear. The primary symptoms include impaired hearing and difficulty distinguishing between certain speech sounds.

There is no treatment to reverse this process or even slow its progress. Sufferers become more adept at interpreting body language, and eventually learn to read lips. Smaller, more powerful hearing aids can improve hearing significantly. *See* HEARING.

Presbyopia

An age-associated deterioration of the eye, resulting in a gradual loss of the eye's ability to focus on near objects.

Presbyopia usually begins to affect people after the age of 40. A difficulty reading small print is often the first noticeable sign of the condition. In a person with normal eyesight, the lens thickens and becomes more curved when focusing on near objects. Light rays from close objects are then brought into sharp focus and projected onto the retina by the thicker lens. This process is called accommodation. As we age, the lens loses some of its elasticity and the power of accommodation is reduced.

Presbyopia can be corrected by wearing prescription glasses with convex lenses. Because the condition worsens, regular presciption updates are recommended. Usually almost all of one's natural focusing ability is lost by the mid-60s. *See also* BIFOCALS; VISION; *and* VISION, LOSS OF.

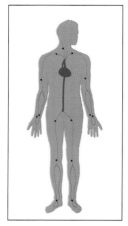

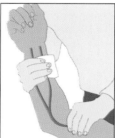

Pressure Points. Locations in the body where a major artery passes close enough to the surface, that the blood flow can be stopped or slowed. Above top, a diagram of the major pressure points in the body. Above bottom, in the cases of major injuries the injured body part should be raised above heart level and pressure should be applied to slow down blood loss.

Pressure Points

Locations on the body where pressure can be applied to bring about a change in body function.

The term pressure points can be used to describe locations on the body where a major artery passes close to the surface and can be used to limit the flow of blood to the area it serves. These points include the carotid artery in the neck, the inside of the arm near the armpit, the wrist, the groin, the ankle, and behind the knee. If a person is bleeding in an area fed by one of these arteries, a caregiver locates the point by feeling for the pulse and then firmly presses the artery to the underlying bone.

The term is also frequently used in reference to the phenomenon of alternative medicine known as acupressure. This form of therapy involves a system of points on the body that are believed by practitioners to contain chi—internal channels of vital force or energy. The points are massaged in an attempt to relieve pain or induce healing. Practitioners believe these points are located along 14 channels (meridians) that run throughout the body. These meridians resemble the circulatory system, but do not correspond with either it or the nervous system in any way. Studies indicate that acupressure may be effective for particular health problems. *See also* ACUPRESSURE; ACUPUNCTURE; BANDAGE; BLEEDING, TREATMENT OF; *and* FIRST AID.

Preservative

Any ingredient that helps to delay or prevent the spoilage of foods or medications.

Spoiled food and medicine can be harmful to a person's health. Preservatives are used in many processed foods and drugs to ensure prolonged freshness once the product has left the manufacturer. For example, nitrates are preservatives that control the growth of microorganisms, such as bacteria and fungi. Antioxidants, another type of preservative, prevent rancidity in foods that contain fats. *See also* FOOD ADDITIVES.

Preventive Dentistry

Branch of dentistry concerned with avoiding tooth decay and gum disease.

The best way to keep from having dental problems is to take care of the teeth before problems occur. This involves two basic steps. First, it is important to take care of the teeth by brushing at least twice daily and flossing at least once daily. The second step is to visit your dentist at least once a year for a check-up and cleaning (scaling). The dentist will examine the teeth to make sure no changes have taken place since the last visit, such as decay and gathering of decay-inducing material; the teeth will be thoroughly cleaned. *See also* Fluoridation; *and* Oral hygiene;

Preventive Medicine

The branch of medicine devoted to the elimination of the root causes of illness, to the early detection of treatable disease, and to minimizing the adverse effects of disease and disability.

Preventive medicine became an important part of health care in the twentieth century. The immunization of children against disease is now a routine element of health care; screening techniques have helped many begin treatment for a myriad of diseases early enough to allow for treatment and possibly cure; and rehabilitative regimens have helped many cope with the symptoms of diseases that would otherwise have debilitating or lethal effects. The field of preventive medicine has, in fact, been configured into three major areas: primary, secondary, and tertiary prevention.

Primary Prevention refers to efforts to remove the causes of illness or protect people from the agents or causes of disease. This includes immunization, efforts to improve the environment by removing toxins and dangerous elements, and laws and policies aimed at prohibiting and discouraging smoking.

Secondary Prevention refers to the many screening techniques aimed at detecting disease at a stage early enough to

allow for treatment that will eliminate the disease or ameliorate the symptoms. Such screening includes tests of blood, urine, and other body elements for diabetes, hypertension, cancer, glaucoma, and a host of other diseases. In environments where hazards are likely to be found, such as a busy and noisy factory, monitoring of the environment and screening of workers' health are routinely conducted so as to identify unhealthful conditions.

Tertiary Prevention refers to actions directed at easing the effects of diseases that have already begun. Rehabilitation in the wake of an accident or a severe illness are examples of this form of preventive medicine. Also included in this category are coronary bypass operations and angioplasty, because their objective is to prevent the catastrohic consequences of heart failure or heart disease.

The greatest measure of the effectiveness of preventive medicine is a comparison between the leading causes of death today with the leading causes at the end of the nineteenth century. In 1900, among the leading causes of death in the United States were infectious diseases such as pneumonia and influenza; tuberculosis was the second leading cause of death and diptheria was tenth. Many of these diseases have been virtually eradicated as causes of death due to effective preventive measures taken by health agencies and individuals.

Studies have repeatedly shown that the cost of preventive care is between 10 and 15 percent of the cost of health care for the treatment of preventable disease. For example, nearly half of all people in the United States with diabetes mellitus are asymptomatic and unaware that they have the disease. A simple, inexpensive urinalysis would prompt a course of treatment that would allow the sufferer of the disease to live a normal life. Yet, the result of undetected and untreated cases of the disease is usually kidney failure, blindness, or amputation, all involving costly medical care. *See also* Counseling; Environmental Medicine; Preventative Screening; *and* Primary Prevention.

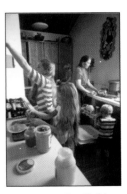

The Prevention Habit. Having the entire family participate in meal preperation is a good way of getting young people to think about the nutrional value of food.

Resources on Preventive Medicine

Anderson, Gaylord, et al., *Communicable Disease Control: A Volume for the Public Health Worker* (1962); Dawson, Deborah, *Breast Cancer Risk Factors and Screening* (1990); Last, John M., et al., Maxcy-Rosenau-Last *Public Health and Preventive Medicine* (1992); Miller, Anthony B., ed., *Screening for Cancer* (1985); U.S. Preventive Services Task Force, Guide to Clinical Preventive Service (1989); American Institute of Preventive Medicine, Tel. (800) 345-2476, Online: www.healthylife.com; American Preventive Medical Associa-tion, Tel. (800) 345-2476, Online: www.apma.net; American Board of Preventive Medicine, Tel. (312) 939-ABPM, Online: www.abprevmed.org;www.med.cornell.edu/public.health/psychiatry/.

Preventive Screening and Counseling

The area of preventive medicine dealing with the early detection of disease or the identification of people with high risk of disease, and the consequent guidance that can be supplied to individuals determined to have a disease or be at high risk of contracting a disease.

Screening. Screening tests are crucial in detecting certain diseases at early stages, thereby enabling doctors to treat or cure the condition. For example, screening tests for cholesterol, may indicate the potential for heart disease and other heart complications. With treatment and counseling, an individual can take the steps necessary in preventing these difficulties. Screening programs can also help protect the public from the spread of infectious disease by identifying infected individuals. Measures can then be taken to help these individuals and limit the spread of the disease. Other screening tests include urinalysis, blood tests, enzyme-linked absorbent assay, or ELISA (to test for HIV), mammogram, and breast self-examination. Some testing is mandatory. For example, many states require those applying for a marriage certificate to be tested for syphilis to protect any children the couple may have in the future from congenital infection.

Screening methods vary in cost and availability. Simple tests, like urinalysis and blood work, are inexpensive, fast, and easy to schedule. Technologically advanced tecniques, such as mammograms and imaging tests, tend to be considerably more expensive and time consuming. However, many insurance companies encourage screening for certain individuals and provide coverage for periodic testing.

Counseling. Sometimes counseling, especially prior to a marriage or planned pregnancy, can help prevent disease, reduce the chances of an unborn child having a disease, and inform future parents of any potential risks. Genetic screening can provide parents with information on their child's chances of being born with genetic disorders or being born with a predisposition to certain diseases or defects.

> *Background material on Preventative Screening and Counseling can be found in* MAMMOGRAM AND URINALYSIS. *Related information is contained in* CANCER; CHOLESTEROL; HEART DISEASE; HIV; *and* PREDISPOSING FACTORS.

Priapism

Continuous, painful penile erection without sexual arousal.

Priapism is a painful erection of the penis that can last for several days. It is not associated with sexual activity. It is a risky condition that requires immediate medical attention. Priapism is caused when the flow of blood into the penis is unable to drain, as it would in a normally flaccid penis. The scarcity of space for the circulating blood causes the blood to become stagnant, acidify and become devoid of oxygen. The deoxygenated red blood cells become hard and are thus unable to drain from the spongy tissue.

Causes. There are several possible causes for priapism, including damage to the nerves that supply the blood to the penis, the existence of a blood disease such as sickle-cell anemia or leukemia, or a blockage of the penis due to an infection such as prostatitis or urethritis. These diseases may cause the blood to thicken or the red blood cells to become rigid. Penile injections to treat impotence can also cause priapism, especially if the dosage is in excess of what is necessary. Psychiatric medications, such as antidepressants, may cause the condition as well.

Treatment. In the case of priapism, immediate treatment is required to prevent scarring of the penis and impotence. The most common procedure involves draining the penis and administering medication to shrink the blood vessels, effectively decreasing the blood flow to the affected area. Another procedure requires the physician to administer a local anesthetic in order to withdraw the trapped blood from the penis. *See* ERECTION, DISORDERS OF.

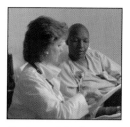

Doctor and Patient. A doctor at the bedside of a bald female chemotherapy patient discussing information in a pamphlet.

Prickly Heat

A skin rash caused by sweat trapped under the skin. The medical term for this condition is rubra miliaria or, in milder cases, miliaria crystallina.

The ducts that sweat travels through to get to the skin's surface are narrow, and sweat can become trapped if these ducts become clogged. People who live in hot and humid climates are more likely to get this condition. Symptoms of prickly heat include skin prickling, itching and irritation, small blisters, and large red areas on the skin. This rash usually develops on sites where sweat accumulates—primarily, the torso, armpits, waist, and thighs, although it can also occur on other areas. The milder form, miliaria crystallina, may produce small blisters filled with fluid as a precursor to rubra miliaria. If the condition does not intensify, these blisters usually dry up on their own. In general, because the symptoms of prickly heat may resemble other skin disorders, a doctor should be consulted.

Prickly heat usually resolves itself if sweating is avoided. Corticosteroid cream and keeping the skin dry may also help alleviate symptoms. *See* RASH *and* SKIN.

Primary

Diagnostic term referring to the first or original occurrence of a disease symptom.

Primary is a general term often used to identify first occurrences. One example includes primary lesion (such as in the initial chancre associated with syphilis). In the case of abnormal growths (tumor), such primary malignancies are to be distinguished from secondary tumors, which spread through a different process from that of the first (metastasis). Primary is also the term for medical professionals with whom a patient has initial contact and an ongoing relationship. This is known as primary health care, and such doctors are known as primary care physicians. *See also* HEALTH INSURANCE; LESION; MALIGNANT; METASTASIS; SYPHILIS; *and* TUMOR.

Primary Prevention

Activities aimed at eliminating disease-causing factors from the environment or harmful activities that cause illness.

Many instances of primary prevention are very cost efficient. Every dollar spent in eradicating toxic or disease-causing elements of the physical or social environment saves over ten times that in terms of medical care that deals with the results of those harmful elements. Campaigns to limit and discourage smoking, for example, represent a minute percentage of the cost to individuals and government of medical care for the victims of smoking. Immunization programs for polio, diphtheria, tetanus, and other diseases, which represent a minimal comparative financial investment, have all but eradicated diseases that wreaked havoc on the population for much of human history.

Other forms of primary prevention are more difficult to implement and more costly. Environmental cleansing, for example, though sometimes critical to the well-being of a population, can often be expensive and have deleterious economic consequences on a region. The same may be said regarding imposing safety regulations in the workplace. The compelling need to create a safe environment in which people can work with safety and some assurance that they are not being exposed to harmful elements must be balanced with the need to get things done.

But the most difficult obstacle to preventive medicine is the human tendency to "leave well enough alone" and to maintain the status quo. The desire to impose preventive measures through legislation must often be balanced against the rights of the individual and the benefit of a population to conduct its many activities unencumbered by restrictive regulatory systems.

Background material on Primary Prevention can be found in ENVIRONMENTAL HEALTH; PREVENTATIVE MEDICINE; PREVENTATIVE SCREENING AND COUNSELING; PUBLIC HEALTH; AND WORK SAFTEY.

Primary Teeth

Temporary first set of teeth that erupt during inf

The primary teeth, also known as the baby teeth, are the first set of teeth that develop in people. Some children may be born with one or two teeth, but primary teeth usually begin to emerge around six months of age. The teeth appear (erupt) in pairs, eventually total 20, and usually are completely in by the toddler years (three to four years old).

The primary teeth begin to fall out, making room for the permanent teeth at age six to seven. The fact that they are temporary does not mean that they require less care than adult teeth. Their care can affect the health of permanent teeth, so proper hygiene and visits to the dentist are essential. *See* ERUPTION OF TEETH *and* TEETH.

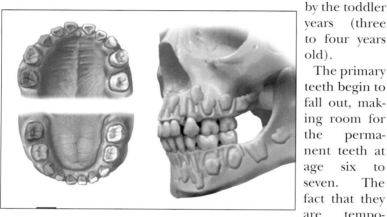

Primary Teeth. Above, left, the twenty deciduous (also called primary, baby or "milk" teeth). The lower molar (green) will be replaced by an adult version of the tooth, which in the normal adult will be the second or middle molar. The first molar (blue) will likewise be replaced by an adult tooth. The cuspid (purple) will be replaced by three teeth: a cuspid and two premolars (or bicuspids). The lateral incisor (orange) and the central incisor (yellow-green) will be replaced by adult versions of those teeth, The illustration at right shows the relative position of the 32 adult teeth relative to the primary teeth in the jaw.

Probucol

A drug used to lower cholesterol level. It works on both the low density lipoproteins (LDL) as well as the high density lipoproteins (HDL).

Probucol (brand name Lorelco) is prescribed for people for whom diet and exercise do not adequately reduce cholesterol levels and who have dangerously high LDL ("bad" cholesterol) levels. A healthy diet and exercise must accompany its use. Side effects may include fainting, chest pain, dizziness, nausea, rapid heart beat, vomiting, abdominal pain, blurred vision, diarrhea, excessive urination, or night sweats. Pregnant women and people taking a diuretic should not take Probucol. *See also* CHOLESTEROL; DIURETIC DRUGS; EXERCISE; LIPID-LOWERING DRUGS; *and* LIPIDS.

Procaine

Local anesthetic used in an injectable saline solution for dental, surgical, and childbirth procedures.

Introduced under the trade name Novocain in 1905, it became the first substitute for cocaine as a local anesthetic because it is not toxic, addictive , or irritating. Its full name is procaine hydrochloride.

Side effects are rare. However, they can include difficulty breathing; shortness of breath; dizziness; drowsiness; lightheadedness; nausea; vomiting; skin rash; itching; hives; slow or irregular heartbeat; palpitations; swelling of the face or mouth; tremors; and seizures.

Procaine has largely been replaced by lidocaine and mepivacaine, which are chemically related drugs that act as a quicker, longer acting anesthesia. *See* ANESTHESIA.

Procidentia

A complete prolapse of the entire rectum.

The protrusion of the rectum through the anus is known as a rectal prolapse. Procidentia is usually not painful, but rectal bleeding can occur. The primary symptom is the noticeable protrusion of the rectum during straining or while walking or standing. A sigmoidoscopy or barium enema x-ray may be necessary to explore for underlying disease. Procidentia can be corrected with surgery. *See also* PROLAPSE.

Proctalgia Fugax

Severe, painful cramps in the rectum with no apparent cause.

The pain of proctalgia fugax can occur at any time, and is usually of short duration. Because it can occur without any signs of disease, the condition is believed to be associated with mental stress or anxiety that results in periodic muscle spasms of the rectum. Treatment generally is aimed at identifying the causes of and relieving anxiety and mental stress. *See also* CRAMP.

Proctitis

Inflammation of the rectum.

Proctitis can be due to ulcerative colitis, a condition that causes inflammation of the colon. It can also result from dysentery, rectal intercourse, gonorrhea or another sexually transmitted disease, and other infections. The symptoms include soreness, bleeding and an emission of pus. It is diagnosed by proctoscopic examination, sometimes accompanied by biopsy. Corticosteroids drugs can relieve the symptoms; treatment of the underlying cause can cure the condition. *See also* DYSENTERY; GONORRHEA; PROCTOSCOPY; RECTUM; *and* ULCERATIVE COLITIS

Prodrome

An early symptom or sign of impending disease.

Prodromes are presymptoms of disorder or disease that usually mark or just precede the onset of characteristic symptoms. Prodrome means literally going before. Migraine headaches are one example of a disorder with a characteristic prodrome—a preheadache known as an aura, during which the patient experiences unusual visual phenomena, including increased sensitivity to bright lights, blank areas within the visual field or various forms of visual distortion. Prodromes are useful diagnostic indicators for physicians as well as early-warning signs for patients with recurring symptoms arising from a given illness. *See also* AURA *and* MIGRAINE

Progeria

An extremely rare disease that causes a child to age at seven times the normal rate.

Progeria is a genetic disease first discovered in 1886 by Jonathan Hutchinson and thus called Hutchinson-Gilford syndrome. Incidence is the same for both men and women and among all races. Characteristics of the disorder include: smallness of stature, wrinkled skin, gray hair, baldness and pinched nose. The face and jaw are usually small relative to the size of the head; tooth formation is delayed; there is atherosclerosis (hardening of the arteries), and cardiovascular problems. Adult progeria, or Werner's Syndrome, begins in early adulthood and follows the same stages as progeria.

CAUSES. The cause seems to be a single mutant gene that becomes dominant because it combines with one normal gene. It is not an inherited gene, since neither parent nor siblings have the gene that seems to mutate spontaneously at conception. The diagnosis is usually made by observation of the child in the first or second year of life.

Researchers have discovered that people with progeria have very low levels of antioxidant enzymes, which is why it is suggested that aging is related to the level of antioxidants in the body.

The presence of antioxidants protect the body from the damage of free radicals. Progeria sufferers offer an invaluable understanding of the aging process. Related studies have offered important breakthroughs for those studying cancer, heart disease and other diseases. *See also* AGING; ATHEROSCLEROSIS; ELDERLY, CARE OF THE; *and* GERONTOLOGY.

Progesterone Drugs

Synthetic or natural forms of the hormone progesterone, a sex hormone that plays a key role in conception.

Progesterone is essential to the metabolism of glucose, the formation of bones, and the human reproductive cycle. There are both natural and synthetic progesterones; the synthetics (called progestins) are much more powerful. Both are used in oral contraceptives, sometimes in combination with estrogen. They are also used to treat the symptoms of menopause and, when taken with estrogen, significantly reduce the incidence of endometrial cancer. *See also* CONTRACEPTION; ESTROGEN DRUGS; HORMONE; *and* MENOPAUSE.

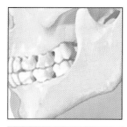

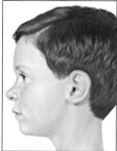

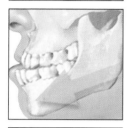

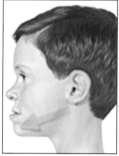

Prognathism. A condition that manifests in the protruding of the lower and sometimes upper jaw. Above first and second from top, the normal structure of the jaw. Above bottom two, shows the jaw already beginning to dislodge itself from its normal spot. In its most extreme cases normal biting and chewing may be interupted.

Progesterone Hormone

Hormone necessary for female reproductive functions.

Progesterone is produced as part of a chain of hormonal signals that begins in the hypothalamus. The hypothalamus secretes luteinizing hormone-releasing hormone, which causes the pituitary gland to release follicle-stimulating hormone (FSH) and luteinizing hormone (LH), two of the gonadotropins. LH causes the ovaries to secrete progesterone, which is also found in small amount in the adrenal glands and testes. Progesterone production occurs during the second half of the menstrual cycle. It is also produced by the placenta during pregnancy.

Progesterone's role during the menstrual cycle is to cause the lining of the uterus to thicken in order to receive a fertilized egg. When fertilization does not occur, hormone production stops and the uterine lining is shed.

DURING PREGNANCY

During pregnancy, progesterone is necessary for the placenta and growth of the fetus. Progesterone is also taken into the fetus's circulatory system and then into the adrenal glands, where it is converted into corticosteroid hormones. Toward the end of pregnancy, a drop in progesterone levels aids in initiating labor.

Synthetic forms of progesterone may be combined with synthetic estrogen or used on their own, as contraceptives or to treat menstrual disorders. They may also treat other conditions, such as endometriosis, and premenstrual syndrome, and to prevent uterine cancer. Progesterone is often used in conjunction with estrogen in hormone replacement therapy to alleviate symptoms of menopause.

> *Background material on Progesterone Hormone can be found in* FEMALE REPRODUCTIVE SYSTEM AND HORMONE *Related information is contained in* ADRENAL GLAND; ESTROGEN; MENSTARTION; OVARIES; OVULATION; PLACENTA *and* PREGANNACY.

Prognathism

The extreme protrusion of the lower jaw.

If the lower jaw or both jaws jut forward to an abnormal degree, it is known as prognathism. This condition, in its most severe examples, may interrupt normal biting and chewing (malocclusion) or cause disfigurement. If the prognathism becomes a problem, orthognathic surgery may be required in order to correct it. This procedure usually involves the removal of a section of bone from both sides of the jaw, then moving the rest of the jaw backward. The jaw may then need to be immobilized during the healing process. *See also* JAW; MALOCCLUSION; ORTHOGNATHIC SURGERY; SKULL; *and* SURGERY

Prognosis

Diagnostician's estimate of the course and outcome of a disease and chance for recovery.

Once a physician has arrived at an identification (diagnosis) of a particular disease or disorder, he or she will evaluate the prognosis—the anticipated course of the disease, its duration, and the patient's likelihood of recovery. The prognosis may be based on the characteristic trajectory of a given illness, statistical probabilities of recovery, or the specifics of a given patient's disease history. Usually a combination of all of these factors, supplemented with the results of various tests, are considered in a thorough prognosis. Prognoses therefore are the physician's best estimate, based on all available information, of the outcome of a disorder, injury, or disease. They should not be seen as inflexible. For example, certain cancers may have a statistically poor prognosis, but mitigating features of a particular case may improve such an estimate for the individual. Simple descriptive terms—such as excellent, good, serious, or grave—may suggest the general nature of a prognosis. In the latter case, the term indicates that the illness typically proves fatal within one year. *See also* DIAGNOSIS.

Prolactin

A hormone that is produced in the frontal lobe of the pituitary gland.

Prolactin—also called lactogenic, luteotropic, or mammotropic hormone—initiates milk secretion in the mammary gland after the mammary tissues have been prepared during pregnancy by the secretion of other pituitary and sex hormones.

After a baby is born, the hormone stimulates milk production in the breast. Initially, the breast produces a thick yellow liquid, which is particularly rich in the disease-fighting substances called antibodies. Within three to five days, the breast produces milk as the suckling infant stimulates the release of another hormone called oxytocin. *See also* BREAST FEEDING; CHILDBIRTH; HORMONES; *and* PREGNANCY.

Prolactinoma

A nonmalignant tumor of the pituitary gland.

Prolactinoma is a benign tumor that can cause troublesome symptoms because of the resulting overprod- uction of the hormone prolactin. In a woman, symptoms can include disturbances of the menstrual cycle that can result in infertility or failure to menstruate. A man with a prolactinoma may become impotent, develop breasts, and even produce milk. Vision can be negatively affected if the tumor grows large enough to press against the optic nerves.

Diagnosis and Treatment. The condition is diagnosed by blood tests for abnormal levels of prolactin and by magnetic resonance imaging (MRI).

Treatment can begin with drug therapy using bromocriptine, pergolide, and cabergoline, which have been found to shrink 50 percent of the tumors to half their size after six months. If drug therapy is not effective, the prolactinoma can be removed surgically in an operation called transphenoidal hypophysectomy. *See also* HORMONE; INFERTILITY; MENSTRUATION, DISORDERS OF; PROLACTIN; *and* TUMOR.

Prolapse

The displacement of an organ or tissue from its correct position.

A prolapse of an organ often occurs because of a weakening in its support structure. Two of the most common examples of this condition are prolapse of the uterus and disk prolapse. The uterus may slip into the vagina as the ligaments that hold it in place become stretched due to childbirth . A disk prolapse occurs when a disk in the spine wears down with age, causing it to protrude and perhaps rupture, exposing its interior. Surgery may be needed to correct the condition. *See also* DISK PROLAPSE *and* UTERUS, PROLAPSE OF.

Prolapsed Cord

Displacement of the umbilical cord before or during labor.

When the umbilical cord passes through the cervix before the baby does, the child is at risk. The cord can become constricted, which may cut off the blood flow. Breech delivery, premature birth, and prematurely ruptured membranes are risks associated with a prolapsed cord. If a prolapse is suspected, a Cesarian section is performed. Vaginal delivery is used in cases where the cervix is fully dilated. *See also* PROLAPSE.

Prolapsed Uterus

Any displacement of the uterus from its normal position.

Uterine prolapse is a fairly common condition, affecting 11 percent of women. Most cases occur in older women. A feeling of fullness and lower back pain are the symptoms. Causes include childbirth, constipation, fibroid tumors, and low estrogen levels. Minor cases can sometimes be corrected with pelvic-floor exercises. In severe cases, where the cervix descends into the vaginal opening, surgery is necessary. *See also* PROLAPSE *and* UTERUS.

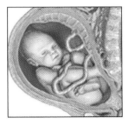

Prolapsed Cord. When the umbilical cord passes through the cervix before the fetus, blood flow may be cut off to the baby. Breech delivery, above, is one of the risks associated with prolapsed cord.

Pronation

Rotation inward of a body part.

Pronation is a general term that may refer to the action of turning a body face down, or reversing a hand so that the palm is facing backward.

Pronation is also commonly used to describe a condition in which the foot has a tendency to roll outward at the heel. Though this requires no treatment in itself, it may cause a predisposition to foot, knee and Achilles' tendon injuries. Shoes, especially those for athletic activity, should be chosen with this in mind. A podiatrist may recommend supports or inserts to help correct the leg's alignment. *See also* PODIATRY.

Prophylactic

Any device used to prevent disease.

Prophylactic refers to any drug, device or procedure used to prevent disease. The term is also used to refer to condoms. The name prophylactic indicates that it is put on prior to sexual intercourse. *See also* CONDOM *and* CONTRACEPTION

Proprioception

Complex, internal system of the body that collects information about the state of muscle contraction and the body's position in the outside world.

Even when the eyes are closed a person has a sense of his or her body position. Proprioception is a process that gathers the spatial information of the body in relation to the external world. The proprioceptors, or stretch receptors, are sensory nerve endings that exist within the hair cells in the balance organ of the inner ear, muscles, tendons, and joints. They relay positional information to the spinal cord and brain. The brain and spinal cord continuously analyze the information and make the necessary adjustments in the way the muscles are contracted so as to always maintain balance and proper movement. While engaging in any kind of physical activity, it is the eyes

and proprioceptors that send information to the brain. This exchange ensures that movement is balanced and coordinated. *See also* BALANCE; BRAIN; *and* SPINAL CORD.

Proptosis

Also known as exopthalmos

Protrusion of the eyeball

A displaced or "bulging" eye is not dangerous in itself, but can be an indication of an underlying disorder. The most common cause of proptosis in adults is Graves' disease. Orbital inflammatory pseudotumor, orbital tumors, and a hemorrhage behind the eye are also causes of proptosis. *See also* GRAVES' DISEASE *and* EYE, DISORDERS OF.

Prostaglandin

Fatty acids that perform like hormones.

Prostaglandins are fatty acids that are manufactured in the body, directly affecting tissues and organs, like hormones. There are different types of prostaglandins, which are categorized according to their chemical makeup. They are found throughout the body, in places such as the uterus, brains, and kidneys. Prostaglandins carry out a variety of activities. They can lower blood pressure and protect against peptic ulcers; they can cause pain and inflammation in damaged tissues, alerting the body to injury; they can widen or narrow airways; they stimulate contractions during labor. Synthetic versions of prostaglandins help stimulate contractions during labor; they may also be used in other disorders, such as peptic ulcers.

Nonsteroidal anti-inflammatory drugs (NSAIDs), aspirin, and corticosteroid drugs can all be used to suppress the prostaglandins that cause pain and inflammation. Because of the prostaglandins' ability to protect the lining of the stomach, long-term use of these drugs can increase the possibility of peptic ulcers. *See also* ASPIRIN; HORMONES; NONSTEROIDAL ANTI-INFLAMMATORY DRUGS; PEPTIC ULCER; PREGNANCY; *and* PROSTAGLANDIN DRUGS.

Prostaglandin Drugs

A family of drugs that mimic the action of the prostaglandin hormones.

Prostaglandins are a large family of hormone-like drugs with widely varying functions. For example, some prostaglandins cause inflammation, while others reduce inflammation. Prostaglandin drugs are usually identified by letter and number. Prostaglandin E1 is injected into the penis to alleviate erectile dysfunction and is used to counteract intestinal bleeding caused when a person takes large amounts of painkillers. Prostaglandin E2 is used to induce abortion and to produce contractions during labor. *See also* PROSTAGLANDIN.

Prostate, Cancer of

Malignant tumor of the prostate gland.

The prostate is a gland, located above the rectum, that surrounds the urethra—the tube through which urine passes from the bladder to the penis.

Almost all prostate cancers are adenocarcinomas, which arise in the glandular tissue. Undetected, the cancer can spread to the seminal vesicles, which carry sperm to the urethra from the testes and to nearby lymph nodes; from there it can spread to the rest of the body. While prostate cancer is highly curable if detected early, it is often not diagnosed until a later stage, because symptoms are ignored. Prostate cancer is the second leading cause of cancer deaths in American men and the second most commonly diagnosed cancer in men .

At Risk. The incidence of prostate cancer is highest in men over the age of 65. A diet high in fats, particularly the saturated fats found in red meat, has been linked to increased risk of prostate cancer. A genetic predisposition also appears to be involved, since a man whose father has had prostate cancer has twice the normal risk; and the risk is tripled for a man whose brother has had prostate cancer. African Americans also are at higher risk, presumably because of some interaction with American lifestyle factors, since the increased incidence is not seen in black Africans.

Symptoms. Most of the symptoms of prostate cancer concern enlargement of the prostate and result from urinary tract malfunctions. There may be difficulty in starting or stopping urination, a weak flow of urine, a frequent urge to urinate, pain during urination, and blood in the urine. The cancer can also affect sexual activity, sometimes causing painful ejaculation. Another possible symptom is general pain in the lower back or upper thighs that results from the compression of a nerve by the enlarged prostate.

Diagnosis. This starts with a test to detect a nodule on the prostate. One such test is a digital rectal examination, in which a lubricated, gloved finger is inserted in the rectum to detect prostate enlargement. A sample of tissue from the nodule is taken for microscopic examination to detect malignant cells. During a specialized ultrasound examination (transrectal ultrasonography), a probe is inserted into the rectum to obtain an image of the gland, resulting in an assessment of its shape and health. X-rays of nearby lymph nodes, computerized tomography (CT), and magnetic resonance (MRI) scans can be done to determine if the cancer has spread beyond the prostate.

Another form of diagnosis is a blood test for prostate-specific antigen, PSA, a substance secreted by the prostate. Benign enlargement of the gland causes a slight increase in PSA levels, but prostate cancer can cause a much greater increase. However, the test is not infallible, since up to 40 percent of men with prostate cancer do not have elevated PSA levels.

Treatment. There is no single routine treatment for prostate cancer. The choice of therapies depends not only on the stage at which the cancer is detected but also on the training of the physicians in different treatments and the age of the patient.

In some cases when a cancer is detected at a very early stage and does not appear to be growing rapidly, the physician may simply monitor the patient carefully, with PSA tests and tissue samples taken every few months. If the cancer appears to become active, treatment begins.

Radical prostatectomy—surgery to remove the prostate and some surrounding tissue—can be a treatment of choice for men in good health and who have a life expectancy of more than ten years. But surgery runs the risk of severing important nerves, causing urinary incontinence and/or impotence.

An alternative to surgery, if the cancer is detected early, is radiation therapy. The radiation may be beamed in from an outside source or come from implanted radioactive sources. Another alternative for early-stage prostate cancer can be hormonal therapy to counteract the tendency of testosterone, the male sex hormone, to stimulate growth of the cancer. Hormonal therapy can have serious side effects, such as impotence and the kind of hot flashes experienced by menopausal women.

Clinical Trials

Therapy for prostate cancer continues to evolve. At any given time, clinical trials of various kinds of chemotherapy, radiation therapy and surgery are under way at major medical centers across the country. Men diagnosed with prostate cancer can consult their physicians about applying for inclusion in such a clinical trial.

Prognosis. Early detection is essential, as it is a decisive factor in the prognosis for prostate cancer. Because of the high incidence of prostate cancer, routine screening tests and examinations are recommended for all men 50 and over, and for younger men in higher-risk categories. Five-year survival rates of nearly 90 percent are possible with the earliest detection. If the cancer has spread significantly, the five-year survival rate can be as low as 20 percent.

Background material on Prostate Cancer can be found in CANCER AND PROSTATE GLAND. *Related information is contained in* AGING; CT SCANNING; MRI; PREVENTATIVE SCREENING AND COUNSELING; PROSTATE ENLARGED; TESTOERONE; TESTES *and* X-RAY.

Resources on Prostate Cancer

Fox, Arnold, and Barry Fox, *The Healthy Prostate: A Doctor's Comprehensive Program for Preventing and Treating Common Problems* (1996); Murphy, G., et al., *Informed Decisions: The Complete Book of Cancer Diagnosis, Treatment, and Recovery* (1997); Renneker, Mark, ed., Understanding Cancer (1988); American Cancer Society, Tel. (800) ACS-2345, Online: www.cancer.org; National Cancer Institue, Tel. (800) 4-CANCER, Online: www.nci. nih.gov; Prostate Cancer Research Institute, Tel. (818) 743-2110, Online: www.prostate-cancer.org/; https:// public1.med.cornell.edu.

Prostate, Enlarged

Enlargement of the prostate gland, which is below the bladder and surrounds the urethra. This gland produces much of the seminal fluid that carries sperm for insemination.

Enlargement of the prostate is called benign prostatic hypertrophy (BPH). It is a condition that starts around 40 years of age and extends to 80 percent of men by age 80. An enlarged prostate can squeeze the urethral tube and cause difficulty in urination. The quantity and force of flow is reduced. BPH is diagnosed by rectal examination and ultrasound.

Symptoms. The person may experience frequent urination at night and sometimes pain. Urination may consistently prove difficult, producing only a weak flow. In some cases, the bladder muscle may become over developed to force urine through the urethra. If the prostate enlarges to the point where it presses on the bladder, the bladder may not empty entirely. Urine trapped in the bladder can become a site for bacterial growth, infection, and the appearance of bladder stones. In addition, the bladder may become enlarged, resulting in a swelling of the abdominal cavity.

Treatment. For mild enlargement, treatment starts with drug therapy. Finasteride may be prescribed; it reduces testosterone but does not affect sexual drive. Alpha blockers relax the muscles of the prostate to improve urinary flow. These drugs are effective in only a small percentage of men, and they are very expensive and must be used indefinitely.

Greater enlargement of the prostate may call for surgery from within the urethra, known as prostate resection surgery, the second most common surgery for men over the age of sixty in the U.S. The surgeon inserts a cystoscope into the urethra and into the area where the obstruction is located. The cystoscope has a lens, a light and a cutting blade so that the surgeon can see to cut through the obstruction and remove tissue for later biopsy, to check for the presence of any cancer. After the surgery has been completed, a catheter will be inserted for a few days to drain the urine while the urethra heals.

In rare cases, this surgery may cause retrograde ejaculation in which the semen flows up to the bladder rather than down through the penis. This is not a harmful effect, but it will make the man incapable of fathering children. In other, rare cases there may also be incontinence and impotence after these surgeries.

More invasive surgical procedures, such as the prostatectomy, approach the prostate from between the scrotum and the rectum or from the abdomen (depending on the size of the prostate). In this procedure, some prostate tissue or the entire prostate gland is removed and the urethra is then reconnected; a catheter is inserted until the urethra heals. While incontinence and impotence are almost inevitable from this procedure, some control may be regained after an extended period of time. *See also* BLADDER; PRO-STATE, CANCER OF; PROSTATE, GLAND; PROSTATISM; URETHRA; URINARY SYSTEM; *and* URINE RETENTION.

Prostate Gland

An organ, found only in men, that surrounds the first part of the urethra.

The prostate gland is located directly under the bladder, in front of the rectum. Ejaculatory ducts from the seminal vessicles pass through the prostate into the urethra. The prostate gland remains small until puberty, at which point androgen hormones cause it to enlarge. When a man reaches the age of 20, the enlargement stops, and the prostate remains at a size of about 20 grams until around age 50, when it usually begins to enlarge again. There are two zones in the prostate, the inner zone and the outer zone. The inner zone produces secretions that moisten the lining of the urethra. The outer zone produces and secretes substances into the semen.

Disorders. Problems affecting the prostate normally occur after the age of 30. The prostate may swell as a result of a bac-

terial infection (prostatitis). In men over the age of 50, the prostate may become enlarged and press on the urethra, interfering with urination. Cancer of the prostate is also common in older men. *See also* PROSTATE, CANCER OF; PROSTATE, ENLARGED; *and* PROSTATECTOMY.

Prostatectomy

The surgical removal of all or part of the prostate gland, usually to treat prostate cancer or enlargement of the prostate.

The major surgical options for prostate disorders that require a prostatectomy include transurethral prostatectomy, radical prostatectomy, and radical retropubic prostatectomy.

The transurethral procedure or resection is usually performed through the urethra using either an endoscope or a resectoscope with a diathermy wire. Transuretheral prostatectomy removes only part of the prostate, so the procedure may have to be repeated in the future.

A radical prostatectomy consists of removal of the entire prostate, seminal vesicles, the neck of the bladder and surrounding tissue, including lymph nodes if necessary. Nerve bundles may also be removed in the process, which can cause erectile dysfunction and incontinence. The operation is performed via an incision on the lower abdomen or through an incision in the perineal area between the scrotum and anus.

The radical retropubic prostatectomy, sometimes referred to as the "nerve-sparing technique," is an improved procedure that minimizes nerve damage. 90 percent of men having the operation in their forties will retain penile function, as will 75 percent of those in their fifties, and 60 percent of those in their sixties.

It is important to note that prostate brachytherapy, or the seeding of radioactive isotopes inside the prostate at precise sites, has been shown to be an effective treatment for early stage prostate cancer. *See also* BRACHYTHERAPY; PROSTATE, CANCER OF; *and* PROSTATITIS.

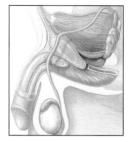

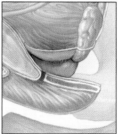

Prostate Gland. The prostate surrounds the urethra just below the bladder. When enlarged it may squeeze the urethra closed, making urination difficult.

Resources on Enlarged Prostate

Bostwick, David G., et al., *The American Cancer Society Book of Prostate Cancer, revised edition* (1999); Fox, Arnold, and Barry Fox, *The Healthy Protate: A Doctor's Comprehensive Program for Preventing and Treating Common Problems* (1996); American Prostate Society, Tel. (410) 859-3735, Online: www.ameripros. org; Prostatitis Foundation, Tel. (888) 891-4200, Online: www. prostatitis. org. Prostate Cancer Research Institute, Tel. (818) 743-2110, Online: www. prostate-cancer.org/; https://public1.med.cornell.edu.

Prostatism

Also known as benign prostatic hypertrophy.

The symptoms of an enlarged prostate gland.

As many as 80 percent of all men experience some enlargement of the prostate gland by the time they are eighty years old. In most cases the condition is benign, and the main symptom involves difficulty with urination. Flow is restricted by the compression of the urethra by the enlarged gland. Most often the bladder compensates by working harder to expel the urine. However, if the prostate gets very large, urination may become very difficult, causing urine trapped in the bladder to become a site for bacterial infection.

Treatment. Many options are available for treatment. Urethral balloon dilation is used with varying success rates. In transurethral resection, a cystoscope is inserted in the urethra with a lens, light, and cutting edge to open the urethra. Finally, the enlarged prostate may be removed entirely. This procedure very often results in incontinence and impotence.

Alpha blockers or hormonal therapies are effective treatments, but they are also expensive and must be continued for life. In addition to these inconveniences, several of these medications have undesirable side effects. *See also* BLADDER; INCONTINENCE; PROSTATE, CANCER OF; PROSTATE GLAND; PROSTATISM; URETHRA; URINARY SYSTEM; AND URINE RETENTION.

Prostatitis

An inflammation of the prostate gland that is usually caused by a bacterial infection.

Enlargement of the prostate gland is very common as men age; however, inflammation of the prostate gland (prostatitis) can also be caused by a bacterial infection that migrates from the bladder or urethra and attacks the prostate gland.

Symptoms of prostatitis include pain in the area between the anus and the scrotum, pain or burning with urination, lower

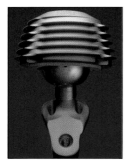

Prosthesis. Prosthetic Titanium Hip.

back discomfort, and fever. If the cause of prostatitis is a bacterial infection the disease will be treated with antibiotics, which will be administered intravenously until the fever returns to normal. If the swollen prostate restricts urine flow, a catheter may be inserted. Oral antibiotics are generally continued for four to six weeks to cure the infection completely. *See also* ANTIBIOTIC DRUGS; BACTERIA; CATHETERIZATION; INFECTION; INFLAMMATION; *and* PROSTATE GLAND.

Prosthesis

Artificial replacement for a body part that is missing, diseased, or deteriorated beyond repair.

If a limb or organ has been amputated, or is no longer useful because of degeneration, it may require a prosthesis. Legs, arms, and hands can be replaced with constructs that not only resemble the limb, but can perform many of its normal functions. Heart valves can be replaced with prostheses in order to keep a diseased heart working. Artificial breasts for mastectomy patients, or glass eyes for those who have lost an eye, may be recommended or desired for cosmetic reasons. *See also* AMPUTATION; HEART VALVE SURGERY; LIMB, ARTIFICIAL; *and* MASTECTOMY.

Prosthodontics

Dentistry that specializes in the creating, fitting and care of artificial teeth.

Prosthodontics is the branch of dentistry that specializes in artificial replacements for teeth. A dentist who specializes in this area is known as a prosthodontist. A prosthodontist specializes in the maintenance and creation of complete and partial dentures, crowns, and bridges. These replacements can be either removable or fixed. Prosthodontists are also typically expert at restoring dental implants and in cosmetic dentistry. The goal of prosthodontics is to preserve the function and appearance of natural teeth. *See also* BRIDGES; CROWNS; *and* DENTURES.

Protein Synthesis

The process during which the body utilizes a combination of essential and nonessential amino acids in order to replenish bodily proteins.

Proteins make up many of the body's structures and are used as enzymes to promote biochemical reactions in the body. They consist of smaller components called amino acids, which are generally divided into two groups: nonessential and essential. Nonessential amino acids can be synthesized by the body. Essential amino acids cannot be made in adequate amounts by the body and must be taken in as food.

In protein synthesis, protein from food is broken down into individual amino acids and then reassembled into configurations that the body can use. DNA contains the information necessary to build proteins from amino acids; different cells create different proteins for different purposes.

When storage of amino acids is unnecessary they are sent to the liver, where nitrogen is stripped from them and excreted, and the remaining protein skeleton is converted into glucose, fat, or glycogen.

Protein synthesis occurs normally unless insufficient amounts of carbohydrate and fat calories are present in the diet (which may occur in extremely reduced calorie diets, as in the case of crash dieting). In such situations, the body begins to break down not only dietary proteins, but also proteins from the blood, pancreas, muscles, liver, and other tissues to use for maintenance of the body's vital functions. *See also* AMINO ACIDS; ENZYME; *and* PROTEINS.

Proteins

Long molecules that are an integral part of the structures and functions of the body.

Proteins are composed of long, folded chains of amino acids. They are essential to all life and to the metabolic activity of every cell. Proteins make up the structure of many tissues in the body, including skin, muscles, and hair. They are also the essential components in enzymes. Enzymes are substances that control the rate of many chemical processes in the body.

Proteins from food supply the body with amino acids, which are then reconfigured to be made into the body's specific proteins. Nonessential amino acids can be synthesized by the body, but essential enzymes must be gotten from food, as the body cannot make them adequately. Both animal and vegetable sources provide proteins; most meat sources provide all the essential amino acids, while many vegetables do not necessarily do so. Certain combinations of vegetables, however, do provide all of the needed amino acids.

Excess Protein. An excess of protein is not beneficial, since the excretion of protein waste products may put a strain on the liver and kidneys and can accelerate loss of calcium from the body. Moreover, much of the protein eaten in the United States is animal protein, which is also typically high in fat, contributing to many cases of obesity and obesity-related illness.

Protein Deficiency. Although a deficiency of protein is unlikely in the average American diet, protein-calorie malnutrition is a grave issue in children in developing countries. Insufficient dietary protein can cause severe and potentially fatal nutritional deficiencies, such as marasmus. *See also* AMINO ACIDS *and* PROTEIN SYNTHESIS.

Proteinuria

Excessive amounts of protein in the urine.

Proteinuria usually occurs as the result of damage that interferes with the normal absorption of protein by the kidneys. The damage may occur to the filtering units of the kidney (glomeruli), causing proteins to leak from the blood into the urine. It can also result from damage done to the tubules, the passageways that carry blood in the kidney. Sometimes proteinuria is a side effect of a condition affecting the whole body, such as myeloma. It usually causes few or no symptoms. Treatment is aimed at the disorder causing the damage. *See also* MULTIPLE MYELOMA *and* URINE.

Protozoa

Single-celled organisms responsible for a wide range of human diseases.

Protozoa belong to the kingdom Protista, and are single-celled organisms, some of which may form colonies. Over 20,000 species are known, including familiar forms such as paramecium and amoeba.

Protozoa are found generally in aquatic habitats, including oceans, lakes, rivers, and ponds. Many protozoa exist parasitically, and are responsible for a broad range of human illnesses. They may be transmitted to humans directly, through the ingestion of contaminated water, or by means of an intermediary vector (i.e mosquito, in the case of plasmodium, the causative agent of malaria; or sand flies, in the case of leishmania protozoa).

Background material on Protozoa can be found in CELL AND WATER. *Related information is contained in* INSECT BITES; LEISHMANIA; *and* WATERBORNE INFECTIONY *See also* ENVIRONMENTAL HELATH AND PUBLIC HEALTH .

Prozac

An antidepressant medication used to treat depression, bulimia, and other similar disorders.

Prozac was originally approved by the FDA (Food and Drug Administration) in 1987. It is also sometimes used to treat panic disorder. Prozac is a selective serotonin-reuptake inhibitor (SSRI), which is a drug that works by blocking the reabsorption of serotonin, a neurotransmitter in the brain. Neurotransmitters are chemicals that help to transmit messages from one neuron (nerve cell) to the other.

Side Effects. The most common side effects of Prozac are anxiety, diarrhea, drowsiness, headache, insomnia, weight loss, changes in appetite, and rash. Decreased sexual drive may also occur. If side effects are severe, they can be treated by reducing the dose, changing the time the medication is taken, or switching to a different antidepressant. *See* ANTIDEPRESSANT DRUGS.

Pruritus

Also called itching; a tingling irritation of the skin that causes a desire to scratch.

Pruritus may be felt all over (generalized) or only in certain areas (localized). It has numerous causes, which can include insect bites, chemical irritation from poison ivy, hives, parasites, infectious disease, allergic reactions, rashes, aging skin, pregnancy, hepatitis, anemia, psoriasis, and a reaction to antibiotics. *See also* ITCHING

Pseudarthrothis

An anatomical "false joint" between long bones caused by deossification.

Pseudarthrosis may form when a fracture fails to unite and the bone ends are separated by fibrous tissue. Congenital hip dislocation may result in the condition, and failed hip replacement surgery may require pseudarthrosis to provide limited mobility.

Pseudarthrosis in the lower tibia (shin) may cause spontaneous fracture and require surgical insertion of a pin or screw through the bone ends and a bone graft. Congenital pseudarthrosis of the ulna (forearm) is very rare but can be treated with a vascularized fibular graft. Pseudarthrosis of the legs can also be treated by the Ilizarov technique, in which new bone is induced between bone surfaces that are very gradually pulled apart by an Ilizarov apparatus, which is a set of a set of external fixators comprising rings, rods, and wires. *See also* FRACTURE.

Pseudodementia

Depression in the elderly, so called because it mimics many of the symptoms of true dementia.

Alzheimer's disease or bacterial or viral infections of the brain can result in the degeneration of brain tissue that leads to dementia. Pseudodementia is the result of depression, however, and elderly sufferers exhibit a series of symptoms that are only some of the symptoms associated with true dementia. There are no language problems; physical reaction time is unchanged; physical coordination is normal. Key symptoms are sleep problems, feelings of guilt and worthlessness, loss of appetite and of sexual drive, and withdrawal.

Treatment for pseudodementia is similar to that for depression. Antidepressant medications are often prescribed with the understanding that the elderly body reacts differently to drugs. For example, many elderly people experience confusion and disorientation in the early evening, particularly if they are in an unfamiliar place, such as a hospital, and have recently undergone surgery. This is called "sundowning" and is a familiar but unexplained phenomenon that may be caused by the slow metabolizing of anesthetics combined with other medications used to control pain. *See also* AGING; DEMENTIA; *and* DEPRESSION.

Pseudogout

Disease of the joints characterized by arthritis-like symptoms.

Gout is a disorder caused by a buildup of uric acid in the blood. The crystals of acid accumulate in areas around joints—typically one joint, such as the big toe. This causes pain and inflammation around the joint, symptoms that fit the definition of arthritis. Pseudogout also exhibits these kinds of symptoms, but is caused by a buildup of calcium pyrophosphate crystals. While gout is generally associated with kidney disease, the cause of pseudogout may be related to hyperparathyroidism, diabetes mellitus, or hemochromatosis.

Pseudogout is diagnosed by an examination of fluid drawn from the affected joint. Discovery of calcium pyrophosphate crystals indicate pseudogout, while uric acid crystals show the presence of gout. Treatment usually begins with joint aspiration, or drawing out the fluid from the joint. Nonsteroidal anti-inflammatory drugs will then reduce inflammation. *See also* CALCIUM *and* GOUT.

Pseudohermaphroditism

A condition in which an affected individual has ambiguous genitalia but either male or female reproductive organs.

True hermaphrodites are children that have both male and female internal reproductive organs, a condition that is extremely rare. Most children with ambiguous genitals are pseudohermaphrodites and have one or the other but not both kinds of reproductive organs.

Female. A female pseudohermaphrodite is genetically female, with the sex chromosomes XX. Her clitoris is larger than normal and resembles a small penis. Her internal organs are those of a female. This condition is caused by prenatal exposure to high levels of male hormones. If the mother took progesterone during pregnancy or has a tumor that produces hormones, her bloodstream may be the source of the male hormones.

Female pseudohermaphrodism can also be due to a condition known as congenital adrenal hyperplasia. With this condition, the female fetus usually has enlarged adrenal glands that overproduce male hormones due to a gene defect in an enzyme that inhibits cortisol production and increases androgen production.

Male. A male pseudohermaphrodite is genetically male, with the sex chromosomes XY. He may be born with a very small or entirely missing penis. This condition is caused by a fetus' inability to produce sufficient quantities of male hormones or by an inability to respond to the hormones produced. The latter is known as androgen resistance syndrome. *See also* CHROMOSOME *and* HERMAPHRODITE.

Psittacosis

Infectious disease spread from birds to humans.

Psittacosis, also known as ornithosis or parrot fever, is an infectious disease usually transmitted to humans from birds belonging to the parrot family, turkeys, ducks, and pigeons. It is caused by *Chlamydia psittaci*,

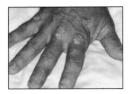

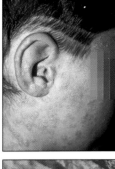

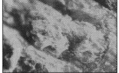

Psoriasis. An inflammatory skin disease, which may be related to the body's immune system. The symptoms include redness on facial skin, middle, and on surfaces like the fingers, top. Bottom, a micrograph of symptomatic skin cells.

Resources on Psoriasis
Cram, David L., et al., *Coping with Psoriasis* (2000); Dvorine, William, *A Dermatologist's Guide to Home Skin Treatment* (1983); Jacknin, Jeanette, *Smart Medicine for Your Skin* (2001); Lamberg, Lynne, *Skin Disorders* (1990); Marks, Ronald, *Psoriasis* (1981); American Academy of Dermatology, Tel. (888) 462-DERM, Online: www.aad.org; American Board of Dermatology, Tel. (313) 874-1088, Online: www.abderm.org; National Psoriasis Foundation, Tel. (800) 723-9166, Online: www.psoriasis.org; www.nycornell.org/dermatology/

an infectious bacterial parasite contained in bird droppings. Those most susceptible to the disease include workers in pet store and slaughterhouses or around domestic fowl. Generally, the disease is acquired by inhaling dust from dried bird droppings or by handling infected birds in poultry processing plants. Human to human transmission is extremely rare.

Symptoms of the disease appear four to fifteen days after exposure and include fever, headache, chills and occasionally pneumonia. The disease responds to antibiotics such as tetracycline, but may prove fatal if left untreated, especially in older individuals. Diagnosis is made through chest x-ray or detection of *Chlamydia psittaci*, in a clinical sample. Psittacosis may be prevented by keeping pet bird cages clean and free of feces that may dry up. Laws require that imported members of the parrot family be kept in quarantine for 30 days prior to sale. *See also* CHLAMYDIA; ORNITHOSIS; PARASITE; *and* PNEUMONIA.

Psoralen Drugs

A group of chemicals that react to ultraviolet light to darken the skin.

Psoralen drugs increase the skin's sensitivity to ultraviolet light. They are used to treat psoriasis, a condition in which the skin grows too quickly and becomes covered with thick, scaly patches. Psoralen drugs are also administered in cases of vitiligo, a condition in which patches of skin, usually on the hands and face, lose their pigmentation and appear white.

A patient takes psoralen orally and is then exposed to ultraviolet light. This alleviates the symptoms of psoriasis. In vitiligo, this causes the skin to darken, although it occurs slowly and treatments may need to be repeated indefinitely.

Side effects of the drug include sunburn, nausea and vomiting, itching, and abnormal hair growth. The ultraviolet exposure may increase the risk of skin cancer. *See also* PSORIASIS; SKIN CANCER; SUNBURN; *and* VITILIGO.

Psoriasis

A common inflammatory skin condition characterized by frequent episodes of skin redness, itching, and thick, dry, silvery scales on the skin surface.

Psoriasis is a very common disorder; eight out of 10,000 people are affected. It affects all ages, but is most common in people aged 15 to 35. This is a condition that recurs frequently. Caucasians commonly affected by psoriasis. The condition seems to be inherited, and seems to be related to the body's immune or inflammatory response. It usually affects the trunk, elbows, knees, scalp, skin folds, and fingernails, but it may affect any area or the entire body.

There are number of factors that may cause psoriasis to recur, including emotional stress, physical illness, and damage to the skin

It normally takes skin a month to move from the bottom layers to the surface. In psoriasis, this process takes only a few days. This causes a build up of dead skin cells. The result is the silvery, thick scales that are characteristic of psoriasis.

Symptoms. Visible signs of this condition include red, dry skin patches, usually covered with silvery scales; skin lesions, including pustules and cracking skin; itching; small scaling dots, especially in children; and joint pain and aching. Nail abnormalities; eye burning, itching and discharge; and increased tearing are symptoms that may be associated with psoriasis.

Treatment. Treatment for mild psoriasis may include prescription shampoos; lotions that contain coal tar, cortisone or corticosteroids; antifungal medications; antibiotics; phenol; and sodium chloride. More severe cases may require intensive treatment and hospitalization. Because the skin barrier function is abnormal, the affected individual becomes susceptible to infections that may lead to septic shock and death. Hospital treatment usually includes analgesic drugs, sedation, intravenous fluids, and antibiotics. *See also* ANALGESIC DRUGS; ANTIBIOTIC DRUGS; DERMATOLOGY; *and* PSORALEN DRUGS.

Psychiatry

A medical specialty concerned with diagnosing and treating mental and emotional ailments.

A psychiatrist is a physician, trained in a four-year medical school, who has completed a four-year residency in psychiatry. Any psychiatrist who wishes to specialize in a field such as child or adolescent psychiatry will continue with additional years of training.

Psychiatrists make diagnoses with the help of the Diagnostic and Statistical Manual, which outlines the current knowledge about psychiatric disorders. They also guide treatment plans. A psychiatrist must be a keen observer of behavior. He or she may use a list of specific questions to help in a diagnosis or combine this method with a free-form conversation to discern the problems from the behavior and expressions of a patient.

Areas of Application. The types of problems a psychiatrist may deal with are varied and wide-ranging. The conditions that psychiatrists address include: substance abuse problems, eating disorders, disorders relating to mood (depression and bipolar disorders), anxiety disorders, sexual difficulties, impulse-control disorders, personality disorders, unexplained physical complaints, problems specific to life-cycle (childhood, adolescence, and aging), cognitive problems, and loss of reality.

Treatments. The treatment plan that a psychiatrist outlines may incorporate several forms of therapy, including the use of medication. A patient may be referred to psychotherapists who specialize in a specific method, such as cognitive or behavioral therapy, or to group or family therapy, or may be treated entirely by the psychiatrist. Only a licensed psychiatrist or physician may prescribe medication.

Recent developments, such as the recognition of the mind–body connection to physical illness and the advent of effective new drugs for mental disorders have improved the public perception of the role of psychiatry. At the same time, however, the increase in managed care and the continuing stigmatization of mental illness have placed limitations on the ability of psychiatry to be used effectively to treat mental and emotional problems.

Background material on Psychiarty can be found in PSY- CHOANALYSIS. *Related information is contained in* ANXIETY; OBSESSIVE COMPLUSIVE DISORDERS; PSYCHOANALYST; PSYCHOMETRY; PSYCHOPATHOLOGY; AND PSYCHOSOMATIC DISORDERS.

Psychoanalysis

A treatment methodology for a range of mental disorders based on the theories developed by Sigmund Freud (1856–1939) and others.

The treatment of the mentally ill or the mentally disturbed through psychoanalysis has become so common that the terms "psychoanalyst" and "psychiatrist" have become virtually synonymous in the contemporary mind. They are not however, as a psychoanalyst need not be a physician to practice, and a psychiatrist, who must be a trained and licensed physician, has the authority to prescribe and dispense medications as a form of treatment not available to all psychoanalysts. Moreover, a psychiatrist may use his or her medical training to discern a physiological cause for behavioral pathologies (such as brain disorders, hormonal imbalance, and even nutritional deficiencies) that would escape the notice of a psychoanalyst without medical training. Yet, psychoanalysis has been used widely by psychoanalysts and psychiatrists alike to treat a wide range of mental disorders.

The Essence of the Theory. Psychoanalytic theory has been developed by several gifted personalities over the past century. Certain central ideas proposed by Sigmund Freud lie at the foundation of the therapeutic method of psychoanalysis and psychoanalytic psychotherapy.

The early psychoanalytic theory postulated that every individual goes through three phases during early life: an oral, anal, and genital phase, corresponding to the parts of the body the child discovers, explores, and comes to terms with. It is only after these early stages of development that the child can direct his or her attention to the outside world and develop relationships with other people.

The first such relationship is with the parents, and this presents the child with a conflict. The child desires the parent of the opposite sex (sexually in the broadest sense, and not in the adult sense, as detractors of the theory believe), and develops a jealousy and elimination fantasy regarding the other parent that stands in the way of

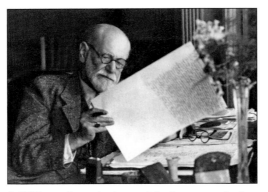

Pioneer of Psychoanalysis. Right, Sigmund Freud in the office of his Vienna home looking at a manuscript.

fulfilling that desire—this is termed the Oedipus complex. In the healthy individual, these feelings become latent by the age of five or six and reemerge in puberty, allowing the individual to pursue healthy sexual relationships with others. If the intervening stages of development have been unhealthy, or the individual's development has been arrested and "fixed" at an early stage, then the individual will have difficulty developing normal and satisfying social and sexual relationships with others.

In the healthy individual, three aspects of the psyche learn to function in the world and deal with one another: the id, which is the instinctive drive of the individual toward the gratification of desires; the ego, which is the conscious, reasoning faculty of the psyche that evaluates the opportunities and challenges presented by the outside world; and the superego, which is the instinctive moral regulator that has been inculcated in the individual from childhood.

Life, in Freud's view, is the drama of the interplay of these forces within the human mind, and the difficulties individuals encounter in dealing with life—from their own self-destructive behavior to the pathologies of their behavior toward others—stem from incidents in an individual's formative years that interfere with the normal development of these mechanisms.

The Essence of the Technique. It was Freud's contention that many of these problems could be resolved and "cured" if the patient relived the episode of trauma and understood the role it played in his or her arrested or unhealthful development. Since people typically resist such self-analysis and self-revelation (often for understandable reasons of personal shame), it is necessary to guide the patient to honestly relate the circumstances of the traumatic incident and confront its reality and impact on his or her life. Freud used hypnosis to treat patients suffering from hysteria. Hypnosis is sometimes used as a psychotherapeutic tool, as is Freud's method for interpreting dreams. Usually, the therapy consists of the patient speaking freely and uninhibitedly about whatever comes to mind. (The therapy is thus sometimes called "the talking cure.") This does not mean that the patient rambles on without guidance. A skilled therapist will be able to direct the patient toward areas of his or her psychic history that will be revealing and helpful in uncovering the trauma that has caused his or her pathological or neurotic behavior. Many psychoanalysts follow Freud and have the patient lie on a couch. This method ensures that the patient is relaxed and unfettered while enabling the analyst to listen and direct the patient in his or her associations without intruding or being a threatening or domineering presence. Others prefer to sit facing the patient; in some cases, such interaction between patient and therapist can be extremely important.

The Seriousness of Psychoanalysis. Psychoanalysis has been used by many individuals seeking to better understand themselves and their place in the world. During the course of psychoanalysis, a close bond may develop between the patient and the analyst, whereby the patient begins to think of the analyst as family or some other important person in the patient's life or past. This process is known as transference. It often gives the analyst a measure of power over the patient and calls for extreme vigilance and propriety on the part of both analyst and patient.

One may wish to discuss with one's personal physician whether one needs psychoanalysis or some other form of psychotherapy. If such treatment is advisable, a referral can be made.

> *Background material on Psychoanalysis can be found in* PSYCHIATRY. *Related information is contained in* ANXIETY; INTELLIGENCE; INTELLIGENCE TESTS; MENTAL ILLNESS; OBSESSIVE COMPLUSIVE DISORDERS; PSYCHOMETRY; PSYCHOSIS; PSYCHOPATHOLOGY; AND PSYCHOSOMATIC DISORDERS.

Psychoanalyst

Anyone who treats mental illness using the techniques of psychoanalysis.

A psychoanalyst is often a physician—a psychiatrist who is trained in the medical treatment of mental disorders as well as in psychoanalysis. A psychoanalyst need not be a physician; however, if the analyst is not licensed to practice medicine, he or she may not prescribe or dispense prescription drugs or any other therapy requiring a medical license. A number of institutes are accredited to train individuals in psychoanalysis. This training includes undergoing psychoanalysis at the hands of another psychoanalyst. These institutes require a medical degree and a residency in psychiatry before admittance. *See* PSYCHOANALYSIS.

Psychometry

Measurement of psychological attributes, including intelligence, aptitude, behavior, and emotion.

Psychometry belongs to the field of clinical, or applied, psychology. It involves a battery of quantitative tests designed to measure various mental variables. Such tests may be used to establish a baseline of psychological attributes in normal patients or as a diagnostic aid for identifying particular pathologies of mental functioning.

Personality tests, for example, may be used to diagnose a range of personality disorders. Similarly, mental deficit in specific psychometric tasks may indicate a pathological disruption of thinking, calculation, visualization, and so forth. Tests for intelligence quotient, or IQ, are the most common form of psychometry, although their accuracy has been a matter of controversy. *See also* INTELLIGENCE; INTELLIGENCE TESTS; MENTAL ILLNESS; PERSONALITY DISORDERS.; *and* PERSONALITY; PERSONALITY TESTS.

Psychopathology

The classification of abnormal and disruptive mental processes and personality-induced behavior.

This term is loosely used to describe any deviance from what is considered normal behavior; as such, it is a highly subjective line of study. But as different disorders show marked similarities in terms of behavioral symptoms and patterns, the term (and hence the discipline) has proven extremely useful in allowing health professionals to know exactly what disorder they are confronting and how they might treat it. *See also* PSYCHIATRY.

Psychosis

A break from reality, involving visual and auditory hallucinations, disordered thoughts, and inappropriate emotional reactions.

Psychosis differs from neurosis (term used for milder mental illnesses) in the respect that sufferers of neurosis generally are aware that they are ill and still have a firm grasp on reality. Psychosis is a general term that encompasses a number of conditions.

Substance-Induced Psychosis. This type of break from reality can be caused by either illegal or prescription drugs used in excess, by using drugs in dangerous combinations, or by abruptly terminating drug use after a long period of ingestion. This includes the excessive use or sudden withdrawal from alcohol. Although some "street" drugs are taken for the express pur-

Resources on Psychoanalysis

American Psychiatric Association, *Diagnostic and Statistical Manual of Mental Disorders, 4th Edition* (1994); Beckham, E. Edward and William R. Leber, eds., *Handbook of Depression: Treatment, Assessment, and Research* (1985); Clark, Ronald, *Freud: The Man and the Cause* (1980); Kaplan, Harold I., and Benjamin J. Saddock, eds., *Comprehensive Textbook of Psychiatry* (1995); Naional. Depressive & Manic-Depressive Association, Tel. (800) 82-NDMDA, Online: www. ndmda.org; National Mental Health Association, Tel. (800) 969-NMHA, Online: www.nmha.org; www.ny-cornell.org/psychiatry/.

pose of creating hallucinations, the unexpected shattering of reality that may be triggered by these drugs can be terrifying. Such psychotic episodes tend to be self-limited and will end after the substance abuse stops or has been successfully treated.

Brief Psychotic Disorder. When the symptoms of psychosis last for up to a month, they are usually the result of one's exposure to a traumatic event. The individual may take on a strange appearance in dress and in movements, will not make sense when speaking or may be mute, and will have rapidly fluctuating and inappropriate emotional responses. Bizarre ideas may be expressed, as well as visual and auditory hallucinations. This temporary disorder usually occurs before the age of 30 and may be treated with psychotherapy and antipsychotic medications.

MEDICAL CONDITIONS. Any brain disease, injury, or illness that affects the brain may cause psychotic symptoms. These include stroke, epilepsy, brain cancer, hydrocephalus, and kidney failure. This type of psychosis is usually found in older adults, but a complete medical examination and appropriate tests should be performed to determine the underlying cause of the break with reality. The psychotic symptoms may be a precursor to a condition such as dementia, which may not otherwise become apparent until much later.

Psychosis Associated with Depression or Mania. In the case of major depression, an individual may suffer from delusions of complete worthlessness or a sense of responsibility for events that were totally out of the person's control, coupled with a desire to be punished for them. A manic psychosis typically takes the form of a delusion related to an overinflated sense of accomplishment. The psychotic events coincide with the incidence of the depression or mania and do not extend to periods when the person's mood is stabilized. A physician's treatment may address the depression, the mania, or the psychosis in combination with psychotherapy to treat this type of psychosis.

Schizophrenia. This is a highly disabling, chronic brain disorder, which typically strikes young adults. The psychosis is accompanied by delusions (bizarre beliefs and paranoid ideas) and/or hallucinations where one hears voices that seem to come from outside the individual, making accusations against the person or directing his or her behavior. Thoughts and speech are disorganized and do not make sense to others. Schizophrenia can be treated with anti-psychotic medications accompanied by psychotherapy, support, and rehabilitation.

Other Causes of Psychosis. A loss of reality may occur in those suffering from delusions alone without other symptoms, from a shared psychotic disorder (where an individual is powerfully influenced and controlled by one or more others, as in a cult), or from a schizoaffective disorder, which has characteristics of both the depressive and manic forms, as well as the schizophrenic forms of psychosis.

Background material on Psychosis can be found in PSYCHOANALYSIS. *Related information is contained in* ANXIETY; MENTAL ILLNESS; OBSESSIVE COMPULSIVE DISORDERS; PSYCHOMETRY; PSYCHOSIS; AND PSYCHOSOMATIC DISORDERS.

Psychosomatic Disorders

Disorders and symptoms that result from conscious and unconscious psychological factors and not from underlying medical conditions.

A number of changes have taken place in the medical community during the past 50 years in attitudes toward this category of illness. Possibly because hypochondriac patients have often tried the patience of physicians, medical practitioners have been reluctant to acknowledge that purely psychological factors may influence the pathology and progress of physical disorders and symptoms. It is now accepted that psychological factors, conscious and unconscious, can trigger disease mechanisms; compromise immune defenses that keep diseases at bay; and aggravate symptoms of a disease or bodily dysfunction. One factor in this revised attitude has been an appreciation of the role stress plays in disease onset, symptoms, progress, and intensity.

Stress and the Immune System. Possibly the most dramatic area of medicine where psychological factors play an important role is in the area of immunity and autoimmune diseases. Virtually every human being alive carries the varicella-zoster virus; it is the organism responsible for chickenpox. During a bout of chickenpox, the body's immune system destroys most of the virus, and an immunity to chickenpox is conferred for life. Yet, some of the virus survives and remains dormant in tissues (mainly in sensory nerves) for years. In ways that are not understood, but which seem almost certainly triggered by compromise of the immune system by stress (among other factors), the virus will suddenly become active and an infection known as shingles will erupt with serious rash symptoms. The disease often inflicts considerable pain, sometimes for many years, and has been known to be life-threatening. Yet, how stress and other psychological factors weaken the immune system and trigger the outbreak of shingles is unclear; and the same may be said regarding a host of other viral disease, including AIDS. In many instances, a virus will remain dormant in its host, sometimes for many years, until some psychobiological event or development will shut down whatever in the immune system is suppressing the virus.

Stress and Autoimmune Disease. A number of diseases involve the immune system of the body losing the ability to distinguish "self" from "non-self," so that the lymphocytes of the immune system, instead of confining their activity to attacking and repelling foreign invaders of the body, attack and destroy vital portions of the body itself. Included in this category is lupus—either the more common (and less dangerous) discoid lupus erythematosus, or the potentially fatal systemic lupus erythematosus—in which the immune system attacks connective tissues (the skin, in the former case, and throughout the body, in the latter); rheumatoid arthritis, in which the immune system attacks tissues of the joints;

and diabetes mellitus, in which the immune system attacks the cells of the pancreas that produce insulin. In the first two disorders, the incidence is significantly higher among women, suggesting that a hormonal imbalance combines with stress factors (a frequently observed combination) to compromise or misdirect the body's immune system. No such imbalance has been observed for diabetes.

Somatoform Disorders. This category of psychosomatic illness includes disorders that are most like the traditional characterization of psychosomatic illnesses, insofar as real symptoms are reported and observed with no medical or physiological cause identifiable. An example of a somatoform disorder is conversion disorder, in which physical functions are lost or curtailed. Sufferers complain of paralysis, impaired vision, and seizures; and exhaustive diagnostic testing reveals no definitive physical cause. Psychiatric analysis of such cases often indicates that the sufferer is unable to cope with stresses or traumatic events and expresses that inability in physical symptoms. This does not mean the symptoms are imaginary or invented; they are real and, since they tend to run in families, may have genetic components. These disorders frequently occur in adolescence and in early adulthood and are often disruptive to the sufferer's life.

Treatment. The treatment for psychosomatic illnesses relies heavily on individual, group, and family psychotherapy and regimens of stress management. The lack of clear protocols for the treatment of psychosomatic illnesses indicates how little is understood about the mind–body connection. Antidepressants have been prescribed for somatoform disorders, but usually the strategy involves supportive psychotherapy and adjusting the work and personal environment of the sufferer with the involvement of his or her family and friends.

Background material on Psychosomatic Disorders can be found in PSYCHIATRY. Related information is contained in ANXIETY; MENTAL ILLNESS; OBSESSIVE COMPULSIVE DISORDERS; PSYCHOSIS; AND PSYCHOSOMATIC DISORDERS.

Psychosurgery

A surgical intervention used to treat an acute mental disorder.

Psychosurgery involves treating mental disorders with brain surgery. The modern application of psychosurgery began with various surgeries that severed nerve tracts in the prefrontal cortex as treatment for acute symptoms of severe psychiatric disorders. Four newer techniques are commonly applied, generally with caution and as a last resort, to patients suffering severe and persistent mental illness that has been unresponsive to conventional therapy.

TYPES

Subcaudate tractotomy has been used to treat major depressive illness, obsessive compulsive disorder, and anxiety states, as well as a variety of other psychiatric diagnoses. The surgery involves two incisions that are made on a skin crease in the forehead so that a stereotactic frame can be attached. Then the procedure requires lesioning an area of the frontal lobe with radio-frequency, heat, before the incisions are stitched.

Anterior cingulotomy utilizes thermocoagulation, which is the term for tissue destruction using high-frequency currents, and has been used to treat depression and obsessive-compulsive disorder.

Limbic leucotomy combines the previous two techniques, using a cryogenic method or thermocoagulation to make multiple lesions in the cingulum. It is used to treat obsessional neurosis, anxiety states, and depression

Anterior capsulotomy was initially applied to people who were suffering from schizophrenia, depression, chronic anxiety states, and obsessional neurosis. Lesioning is conducted using radio frequency thermocoagulation or a gamma knife.

In general, psychosurgery is most productively applied to those with major affective disorder, chronic anxiety states, and obsessive-compulsive disorder. *See also* DE-PRESSION *and* SCHIZOPHRENIA.

Psychotherapy

The practice of using psychoanalysis and other psychological methods to treat certain psychological disorders.

Varieties of psychotherapeutic treatments are wide-ranging, and several may be used in combination to produce positive results. It is dificult for a patient to choose a method of therapy, as it is possible that any one of several different treatments may work for a given problem. Successful treatments are often those that apply a combination of several approaches.

There are a number of different practitioners who may administer psychotherapy: a counselor, social worker, psychologist, or psychiatrist. When deciding on a practitioner, consider training, referrals, the compatibility of the therapist, and experience in treating the illness at issue. Only a psychiatrist, who is a medical doctor, however, can prescribe medication.

The change that results from psychotherapy is a complex process that includes a variety of experiences that occur between the therapist and patient. The activity of self-examination itself, with a supportive and attentive guide, is designed to have a therapeutic effect. The examination is also a learning process, whereby the patient is challenged to give up entrenched beliefs and behaviors that have been counterproductive to his or her relationships and ability to perform in life. In addition, the simple act of sharing a burden—of releasing a secret or confessing to guilty thoughts and behaviors—can help to heal emotional pain.

Psychoanalytically Oriented Psychotherapy. As with many forms of psychotherapy, an important tool for this type of therapist is listening. It is not just the kind of listening that attends to content; it also takes note of tone, facial expressions, body language, and emotional expression. The therapist is trained to pay attention to the signals that a patient is communicating, both verbal and nonverbal. By attending to all of the communication, the therapist can tell a great deal about the individual: education, background, and the extent to which a person is self-aware, trusting, or guarded. This type of listening also attends to what is not being said. During the course of therapy, the therapist notes which emotions are expressed, which are hidden, and what defense mechanisms are used. The therapist also analyzes the transference, which represents the way that a patient transfers his or her feelings and beliefs about a person onto the therapist, relating to the therapist as if they were that person.

It is the relationship between the therapist and patient that is part of the healing process. Through the course of therapy, a patient will come to understand his or her conflicts and motives and develop adaptive ways of behaving to replace ways that have not worked well in the past or have been counterproductive.

Cognitive Therapy. This form of therapy directs its attention to the distorted thinking and misperceptions that cause problems with mood and behavior. For example, a depressed person will be preoccupied with serious doubts about self-worth and beliefs about the hopelessness of any undertaking. Cognitive therapy attempts to change this negative overview. A patient will be taught to pay close attention to thoughts and feelings as they arise and to modify them so they are more realistic and put in perspective.

For example, an individual who feels like a failure for getting a lower grade than expected on a test believes that this is just one more example of how she will never be able to achieve any measure of success. She will be taught that it is more correct to say that she did not do as well as expected, perhaps due to the depression or an extenuating circumstance, and that this test grade will not determine an entire future.

Behavioral Therapy. This form of therapy focuses on changing patterns of behavior, particularly modes of communication and social interactions, by closely monitoring these activities to identify those that are counterproductive. Behavioral therapy for a depressed person will attempt to modify

the immobility typical of depression by encouraging small pleasures, like inviting a friend for tea or taking a walk to the store to buy a magazine. These activities may begin to effect a slight improvement in mood and diminish the feelings of helplessness that result from feeling trapped by the weight of a depression.

Insight-Oriented Psychotherapy. This form of therapy guides a person struggling with emotional illness to understand the unconscious conflicts that have led to the problem, thereby reducing the anxiety. Freud was the first person to theorize that we relive and repeat our unconscious conflicts in an attempt to work them out. The goal of insight-oriented psychotherapy is to bring these conflicts into awareness and find effective ways of responding to them. It happens, however, that knowing why we are behaving a certain way does not make the behavior disappear.

Family Therapy. This form of therapy is appropriate when the problems of one person have a profound affect on the entire family or when the dynamics of the family seem to magnify the difficulties suffered by any individual. Family therapy is one mode of treatment for problems pertaining to alcohol and substance abuse, particularly when the abuse is inflicted by a parent. Family therapy is also considered an important adjunct in treating problems in child psychiatry.

Group Psychotherapy. This form of therapy is used alone or in conjunction with individual psychotherapy and/or medication to help remedy a variety of ailments, including eating disorders and substance abuse. Group therapy may be useful as a means of support to those suffering from a particular illness or major life change such as divorce or bereavement. In addition to providing support, the group comes together, with a therapist as a leader, to instill hope in each other, share pain, impart information, and provide corrective lessons in functioning.

Background material on Psychotherapy can be found in PSYCHOLOGICAL DISORDERS *and* PSYCHOANALYSIS.

Pterygium

A raised growth of the conjunctiva

Pterygium first appears as a wedge-shaped spot in the white of the affected eye. Symptoms include redness, irritation, and tearing. In some cases, the growth may spread over the cornea, severely affecting vision.

Sun exposure is the most common cause of pterygium. It is a good idea to protect the eyes from sun, dust, and wind. Artificial tears relieve some of the symptoms, and nonsteroidal drops are often prescribed to reduce inflammation. If vision is affected, surgical removal of the growth may be necessary. *See also* EYE, DISORDERS OF.

Ptosis

A drooping of the upper eyelid.

Ptosis is usually an indication of muscle weakness in the eyelid. The condition often develops as a result of aging, but can also be caused by nerve or muscle damage brought about by injury or disease. Diabetes, mysthenia gravis, strokes, and aneurysms are examples of diseases that sometimes result in ptosis.

Treatment depends on the underlying cause. Surgery is sometimes necessary to strengthen the eyelid muscle. *See also* ANEURYSM; DIABETES MELLITUS; *and* EYE.

Ptyalsim

Excessive salivary flow.

Many people know the unpleasant feeling associated with dry mouth, in which there is inadequate saliva. With ptyalism, there is often so much saliva flowing that it becomes difficult to swallow.

Most often, ptyalism indicates a digestive tract disorder, irritation of the mouth by ill-fitting dental work, or damage to the nervous system. It can also indicate illness or inflammation of the salivary glands. Ptyalism is also not uncommon in women during the early stages of their pregnancy. Often, ptyalism is accompanied by an excess production of gastric juices as well.

Puberty

The onset of sexual maturation in boys and girls.

Puberty is the stage of growth when a child experiences the physical, hormonal, and sexual changes that make a youth capable of reproduction. During puberty, children experience rapid growth and begin to develop secondary sexual characteristics. This can be an emotionally difficult stage in child development.

The hypothalamus and pituitary glands produce hormones that trigger increases in height and weight, as well as physical changes in the body.

A healthy child will enter puberty between the ages of nine and 16. The exact age is different for everyone, and is determined by heredity, nutrition, and the gender of the child. Girls usually enter puberty about two years earlier than boys.

In both males and females, changes include increased sexual interest, development of secondary sexual characteristics, and increases in height and weight. The sweat glands become more active, and the adolescent may decide to use an underarm deodorant for the first time. The oil glands in the face are triggered, and acne may appear, often resulting in emotional distress. Males and females also go through several different stages of puberty.

Girls. Puberty in girls typically begins between the ages of nine and 16. Before a girl has her first period, she will normally experience the following stages: breast enlargement, rapid growth in height, clear or whitish vaginal discharge, increased hip width, and the growth of pubic, armpit, and leg hair. The ovaries increase their production of estrogen, triggering the menstrual cycle. The average age for first menarche is between 12.3 and 12.7 years of age. After a period of one year, a girl is usually fertile and can carry a baby to term, although her periods may be irregular for quite some time. Girls are usually completely physically mature by the age of 17. Emotional maturity requires many more years than physical maturity.

Boys. Puberty in boys usually begins between the ages of 13 and 15. A typical boy will experience the following stages: rapid growth, increased shoulder width, growth of the penis and testicles, a deepening of the voice, nocturnal emissions (also known as "wet dreams"), and pubic, facial, and armpit hair growth.

There are five stages of development for boys in puberty. Stage one is the prepubertal period, and is characterized by downy pubic hair, similar to the hair on the chest. Stage two involves the enlargement of the scrotum and testes, and a reddening and folding of the skin. The first pubic hair is also seen in stage two. The enlargement of the penis, in both length and width, takes place during the third stage of development. The pubic hair becomes curlier and more coarse in this stage as well. Stage four involves enlargement of the penile glands and the continuing growth of pubic hair. In the last stage, sexual maturation is complete. The penis and scrotum are adult-sized. Pubic hair extends onto the surface of the thighs and onto the abdomen. Nocturnal emissions take place, which allow room for newly manufactured sperm. These "wet dreams" are a normal physiological process.

The Challenge for Parents

Puberty is a time of great change for young people, and with it comes new concerns for parents. The teenage years and the changes that occur during this time can be emotionally taxing. Accidental injuries result in 70 percent of teenage deaths, and homicide is the second leading cause of death for teenagers. Depression in teenagers can lead to suicide, the third leading cause of death. Alcohol and drug abuse are involved in many accidental teenage deaths. In adolescence especially, girls often develop eating disorders such as bulimia and anorexia. It is important that adolescents communicate with their parents and seek help with any of the problems or new emotions that they encounter.

Background material on Pubery can be found in ADOLESCENCE AND DRUGS *Related information is contained in* ABORTION; PREGNANCY; PENIS; TOBACCO SMOKING; RAPE SEXUAL INTERCOURSE; *and* VAGINA.

Pubic Lice

Small parasites that live in pubic hair and feed on human blood.

Pubic lice, also known as crab lice due to their crablike appearance, are tiny ectoparasites that attach themselves to human hairs. They are found in the pubic hair, but may also appear in armpit hair, facial hair, or even eyelashes. The condition of lice infestation, called pediculosis, occurs when adult lice lay eggs on the hair shafts close to the skin. The white and shiny eggs require seven to 10 days to hatch. A typical infestation is by less than a dozen lice.

While the infestation may be asymptomatic, pubic lice typically result in intense itching, usually worsening at night. Lice are difficult to see, as their grayish-white appearance blends in with the skin. Faint bluish spots or, occasionally, an inflamed rash may appear at the location of bites in the skin. Eyes may show inflammation in the case of infestation of the eyebrows.

Pubic lice generally are transmitted through direct physical contact, particularly of the genital areas. Infestation may also occur through contact with an infested person's bedding, towels, or clothing, as lice are able to survive without a human host for one or two days. They are rarely transmitted from bathrooms, toilet seats, or furniture, because the lice that fall from their host are usually injured or dying. Lice do not jump from person to person, and are not transmitted to or by animals. The onset of symptoms may be immediate or delayed 2–4 weeks if eggs have not hatched.

Treatment

Treatment for pubic or crab lice involves application of a pediculocide, used to destroy lice and their eggs. A one precent cream rinse permethrin is commonly used in a shampoo form. It is lathered and left on the hair for 10 minutes, then thoroughly rinsed. A fine comb can be used to comb the eggs from the hair shafts. Furthermore, all bedding, clothing, towels, and other personal items should be immediately machine laundered to avoid reinfestation.

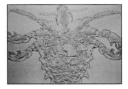

Pubic Lice. This breed of louse is tinier than other lice.Their rounded, broader appearance makes them resemble crabs, from which they derive the popular name crab lice. They end to cause more intense itching, the latter around the penis, vagina, or anus.

Resources on Puberty and Adolescence

Burg, Fredric D., ed., *The Treatment of Infants, Children, and Adolescents* (1990); Chan, Paul D., *Family Medicine* (2001); Goldstein, Mark A., and Myrna Chandler Goldstein, *Boys into Men: Staying Healthy through the Teen Years* (2000); Kimmel, Douglas C., and Irving B. Weiner, *Adolscence: A Developmental Transition* (1995); www.nycornell. org/medicine/edm/index.html.

Infestation with pubic lice requires medication to destroy lice and their eggs. Permethrin one percent cream rinse is most commonly used. Following application, nits may be removed from the hair shafts using a fine-toothed comb. It is critically important that all clothing, towels, and bedding be machine laundered at the same time to prevent reinfestation. Intimate contact should be avoided until the infestation has been definitely eradicated.

Background material on Public Lice can be found in LICE AN D SEXUALLY TRANSMITTED DISEASE. Related information is contained in ANTIBIOTICS; ANUS; HAIR; HEREPES; HYGIENE; PENIS; PUBLIC HEALTH AND ENVIRONMENTAL HEALTH, PREVENTATIVE MEDICINES; SKIN and VAGINA.

Public Health

A branch of medicine that focuses on the collective health of a population.

Public health is a broad field that seeks to address the health problems of a given population. The goal of public health programs is the resolution of health problems and the cultivation of conditions and environments in which people can work safely and lead healthy lives. Toward that end, public health organizations identify health problems and priorities through assessment and monitoring of a population's health and the risks it faces; create policies designed to solve health problems and address health priorities; ensure that all communities have access to appropriate and affordable care, including services that promote health and disease prevention; and evaluate the quality of health care.

The public health and clinical health fields differ in several ways, the most obvious of which is public health's emphasis on the health of a population as a whole, as opposed to clinical health's emphasis on the health of individuals. Usually, clinical physicians consult one patient at a time to treat a specific disease or injury. Public health professionals, however, diagnose and track the diseases and injuries of entire communities and promote curative and preventive health practices and protocols that will keep populations healthy and safe.

Of vital concern to public health is the allocation of resources within a hospital or health care facility. This often requires making difficult economic choices, such as deciding whether to purchase a new machine, hire more staff, or specialize in a way that turns away one type of patient in order to serve another. Another crucial concern to public health is the identification and establishment of the constituency of a particular healthcare facility, which determines whom a hospital aims to serve and how.

BRANCHES OF THE DISCIPLINE
Many professional disciplines fall under the rubric of public health: internal medicine; preventive medicine; pulmonary medicine; nursing; nutrition; dentistry; optometry; social work; health education; occupational health; environmental health; environmental sciences; psychology; psychiatry; and health services administration. All are part of the discipline of public health by virtue of the role each plays in the collective health of human beings.

Occupational Health. Given the importance of work in modern societies and the increased amount of time individuals spend at the workplace, occupational health has become one of the most challenging specialties in modern medicine. Practitioners of occupational health are concerned with the health of employees and the safety of their workplaces. The field calls for the application of knowledge and skills across a wide range of medicine, technology, and workplace design. The

Preventative Messures. This construction worker is wearing a helmet at his job site to prevent any head injuries.

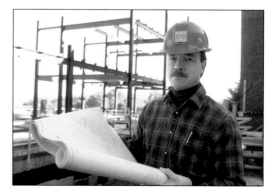

problem may be as simple as insufficient lighting or as insidious as exposure to unnoticed or innocuous-seeming chemicals that may be detected either by using skills in toxicology or epidemiology or by enlisting the aid of specialists. Given the rapid rate of modernization, occupational health pra-ctitioners have taken on more responsibility and must concern themselves with pre- venting health problems that may not become evident for decades. Asbestos, for example, is an insulation material that releases airborne fibers that, when inhaled over time, may cause cancer decades later.

Epidemiology. Epidemiology is the study of the causes, effects, and distribution of disease in the human population. Epidemics of disease, such as the plague, have influenced public health so drastically as to have a profound effect on the course of human history.

Environmental Health. This branch studies the role of the environment, especially changes in the environment caused by humans, in human injuries and disease.

Internal Medicine. Internal medicine focuses on disease of the inner organs, which requires an understanding of the basic chemistry of life. As scientists learn more about what happens at the molecular level of physical processes, they learn more about how the body works. Their discoveries result in new treatments. For example, once the molecular activity behind the physical symptoms of hypertension was understood, scientists were able to create drug treatments for the millions of people who suffer from high blood pressure.

Preventive Medicine. Preventive medicine, as it relates to public health, seeks to protect, promote, and maintain the health of a community or population by emphasizing practices and treatments that prevent disease and death. Primary prevention aims to maintain health by eliminating the causes of disease or by protecting the community from those causes. Immunization against disease, physical exercise to stay fit, and the reduction of pollution are all examples of primary prevention. Secondary prevention is the detection and reversal of

conditions that would otherwise cause disease. Examples are health screening and hearing tests to prevent noise-induced loss of hearing. Tertiary prevention, such as treatment of incapacitating mental illness, is an attempt to reduce the negative effects of disease.

Psychiatry. Psychiatry focuses on mental and emotional illness; and psychiatrists involved with public health are trained in, among other disciplines, community mental health and the social sciences, providing a good example of how disciplines may overlap within the category of public health. For example, a public health psychiatrist may study how aspects of a particular environment, such as a teeming and noisy metropolis, affects the psyches of its residents. It also demonstrates the training required of an employer to effect change in the workplace to minimize adverse conditions and increase positive supports that optimize the mental health of employees, with the end goal being increased productivity and a healthy work force.

HISTORICAL IMPORTANCE

Achievements, discoveries, and events throughout history demonstrate the breadth and importance of public health activities in society. In the 18th century, it was discovered that chimney sweeps were prone to testicular cancer. In the 19th century, widely held as the dawn of the public health, physicians made the connection between certain diseases and the open sewage and contaminated water that caused them. In the early 20th century, the combined ill effects of dust and poor ventilation that caused pneumoconiosis (black lung) and silicosis led to changes that reduced the risks to coal miners.

In the modern era, public health initiatives have accomplished the following:

Vaccination. In various parts of the world, long-term programs of vaccination have eliminated smallpox and poliomyelitis; and they have limited the spread of measles, rubella, tetanus, diphtheria, influenza, and other infectious diseases, particularly among children.

Resources on Public Health

Basch, Paul F., *Textbook of International Health* (1999); Fletcher, Robert H., et al., *Clinical Epidemiology: The Essentials* (1996); Moeller, D.W., *Environmental Health*, revised edition (1997); National Research Council, Committee on Environmental Epidemiology, *Public Health and Hazardous Wastes* (1991); Turnock, Bernard, *Public Health: What It Is and How It Works* (2000); Mothers and Others for Pesticide Limits, Tel. (212) 727-2700, Online: www.mothers.org; U.S. Public Health Service, Tel. (202) 619-0257, Online: phs.os. dhhs.gov/phs/phs.html; www.med.cornell.edu/public.health/

Motor-Vehicle Safety. Advances in engineering have led to the safer design cars and roads. Laws and awareness campaigns have successfully influenced increased use of motorcycle helmets, safety belts, and child safety seats, and decreased drinking and driving. Overall, motor-vehicle-related de-aths have decreased.

Workplaces. Since 1980, the rate of fatal occupational injuries has dropped 40 percent due in large part to safer workplaces. Deaths and injuries related to mining, manufacturing, construction, and transportation have decreased.

Healthier Mothers and Infants. Over the course of the 20th century, improved hygiene and nutrition, antibiotics, better access to healthcare, and advances in maternal and neonatal medicine have made mothers and infants healthier. Since 1900, infant mortality has dropped 90 percent, and maternal mortality has decreased 99 percent.

Family Planning. The social and economic position of women has changed , owing to the availability of family planning and contraceptive services that encourage smaller family size, a longer interval between births, and the use of contraceptives.

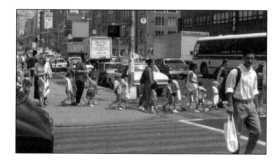

Infectious Diseases. In the early 20th century, contaminated water was a major cause of death and illness. Improved sanitation and clean water have dramatically reduced the incidence of infectious diseases such as typhoid and cholera. Antimicrobial therapy has been crucial to the control of tuberculosis and STDs.

Heart Disease and Stroke. Encouraging people to quit smoking and control their blood pressure, along with improved treat-

ments and swifter detection, contributed to the decreased number of deaths by stroke or heart disease. Death rates for heart disease have dropped 51 percent since 1972.

Food. In the United States major nutritional deficiency diseases such as rickets, goiter, and pellagra have been nearly eradicated by discovering crucial micronutrients and creating food-fortification programs. Since 1900 increased nutritional content and decreased microbial contamination have rendered food safer and more healthful.

Fluoridation. Fluoridation of drinking water by public water supply agencies—an inexpensive process that began in 1945 and in 1999 reached an estimated 144 million people in the United States—helps teeth resist tooth decay. Regardless of socioeconomic status or access to care, fluoridation has played a key role in reducing tooth decay (an estimated 40 to 70 percent in children) and of tooth loss in adults (40 to 60 percent).

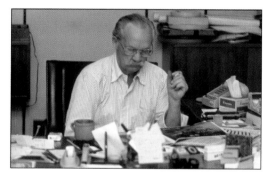

Smoking and Tobacco Use. The 1964 Surgeon General's report on the health risks of smoking resulted in a decrease in smoking among adults and the prevention of millions of smoking-related deaths. Public health antismoking campaigns have shifted social norms toward the cessation of tobacco use and the elimination of secondhand smoke.

GOVERNMENT INVOLVEMENT
Several federal agencies address public health concerns through research and the dissemination of information to those in the medical profession and the general

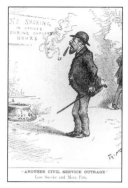

Smoking. Above, this is a cartoon from Harper's Weekly, circa 1890. It shows an office worker, whose smoking cigar is drooping from his mouth, reading a sign on the wall: "No Smoking In Offices During Office Hours". The caption reads: "another civic-service outrage. Less smoke and more fire". Right, a older man is showing the effects of smoking, on a long-term basis. His skin is wrinkled and his complexion pallid.

public. The Centers for Disease Control (CDC) comprises the National Chronic Disease Prevention and Health Promotion; the National Center for Environmental Health; National Center for Health Statistics; the National Center for Infectious Diseases; the National Center for Injury Prevention and Control; the National Center for Prevention Services; and the National Institute for Occupational Safety and Health. The National Institutes of Health (NIH) include 13 institutes, each of which addresses a specific subject or area of medicine, including: aging; allergy and infectious diseases; arthritis and musculoskeletal and skin diseases; cancer; child heatlh and human development; deafness and other communication disorders; dental research; diabetes and digestive and kidney diseases; environmental health sciences; blindness; general medical sciences; heart, lung, and blood; neurological disorders and stroke.

Healthy People 2010

"Healthy People 2010" is a national prevention agenda drafted by the Department of Health and Human Services. It includes a statement of national health objectives designed to identify the most significant preventable threats to health and to establish goals to reduce these threats. The evaluation of managed care providers is a growing component. Individuals, groups, and organizations are encouraged to integrate Healthy People 2010 into current programs, special events, publications, and meetings. Businesses can use the framework to guide worksite health promotion activities as well as community-based initiatives. Schools, colleges, and civic and faith-based organizations can undertake activities to improve the health of all members of their communities. Health-care providers can encourage their patients to pursue healthier lifestyles and to participate in community-based programs. By selecting from among the objectives, individuals and organizations can build an agenda for community health improvement and monitor results over time.

Background material on Public Health can be found in Saftey. *Related information is contained in* Anthrax; Environmental Health; Infectious Diseases, Oncology; Terrorism *and* Tobacco Smoking.. *See also* Accidents and Rabbies *for more on Public Health.*

Public Health Dentistry

Also known as community dentistry.

Concerned with the dental health of the general public rather than of the individual.

Public health dentistry includes identifying trends, such as the incidence of tooth disorders and decay, encouraging proper oral hygiene and the transfer of scientific knowledge to appropriate target groups, checking fluoridation of water supplies, ensuring that the supply of qualified dentists meets the demand for care, adapting dental treatment facilities for those with disabilities, approving new products as safe and effective, assisting the resolution of disputes between dentists and patients, and providing insurance-related information. The American Dental Association, for example, is not only an organization for dental professionals, but also the public's major source of dental information. *See also* PUBLIC HEALTH.

Pudendal Block

A local anesthetic, such as Novocain, which is injected into either side of the birth canal at the time of delivery.

The mother's perineum is numbed during delivery in case of a need for forceps delivery or episiotomy and its repair. This method of anesthesia presents no adverse effects for either mother or baby and is the safest anesthetic in use today. However, increasing evidence supporting the safety of an anesthetic injection in the lower back (epidural anesthesia) in these situations has contributed to a diminished use of pudendal nerve blocks. *See also* CHILDBIRTH.

Puerperal Sepsis

An infection of the vaginal tract occuring within the first two weeks after childbirth.

Puerperal sepsis, also known as childbed fever, was once one of the leading causes of maternal mortality. Thousands of women died of it each year. With the improvement of hygiene, as well as the development of antibiotics, postpartum infections have become much less of a problem. Better prenatal care has also improved the overall health of women prior to giving birth.

In the past, this infection was caused by streptococcus bacteria and transmitted to patients by doctors who went straight from performing autopsies to delivering babies. In 1844, I.P. Semmelweis, a Hungarian physician, became the first to observe this problem and to note that midwives did not transmit this disease to their patients. The simple precaution of washing hands was enough to reduce the transmission of the disease—doctors used soap and water between patients and dipped their hands into a chloride and lime solution after autopsies. Within one month of adopting these measures, mortality dropped significantly. *See also* INFECTION *and* VAGINA.

Puerperium

The period of time following childbirth.

The word puerperium comes from the Latin word for childbirth; it once referred to a period of confinement during and immediately after giving birth. Today this time after birth is more commonly known as the postpartum period, and women are not confined but free to resume their normal daily activities as soon as they feel capable of doing so. *See also* CHILDBIRTH.

Pulmonary Embolism

Blockage of the pulmonary artery or one of its branches by an embolus, a clot or other substance.

A pulmonary embolism usually originates from a blood clot that forms in a deep vein of a leg or the pelvis. This clot, or embolus, can travel through the right side of the heart and then into the pulmonary artery, which carries blood to the lungs. In the same way that an embolism blocking flow to the brain can cause a stroke (the death of brain cells), a pulmonary embolism can cause the death of lung tissue that is deprived of its oxygen supply. Pulmonary embolisms occur in 500,000 Americans every

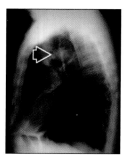

Pulmonary Embolism. A possibly life threatening condition, this mass can cause breathlessness, chest pain and spitting up blood. If it is blocking an artery, dizziness, high pulse rate or severe chest pain can occur. Embolisms can be found with chest x-ray..

year, and 50,000 of those cases are fatal.

Several conditions increase the risk of pulmonary embolism. One is phlebitis, an inflammation of a vein, usually in the leg. Damage to the lining of a vein by infection or injury can also lead to formation of blood clots. Sometimes the underlying cause is the presence of abnormal clotting factors that increase the tendency of blood clots to form. Oral contraceptives also increase the risk of clot formation, a risk that increases with age.

Dangers of Sitting

Older people should be aware that inactivity is a major risk factor for pulmonary embolism. A lack of physical activity makes it easier for blood clots to form in leg veins, so daily exercise is recommended. On a long airplane flight, getting up and moving around the cabin rather than remaining motionless is a basic preventive measure.

SYMPTOMS AND DIAGNOSIS
Pulmonary embolisms cause breathlessness, chest pain, and spitting up of blood. If a very large embolus is blocking an artery, there can be dizziness, a very rapid pulse and severe chest pain. Since pulmonary embolisms can be life-threatening, emergency care should be sought immediately. A pulmonary embolism can be detected through the use of various tests, including a chest x-ray, pulmonary angiography, and a radionuclide lung scan.

TREATMENT
If the embolus is very large, surgery can be performed to remove it. For less life-threatening emboli, clot-dissolving drugs, such as tissue plasminogen activator or streptokinase, can be administered. Blood-thinning medications like heparin can be infused for 10 days or longer to prevent more clots from forming. Patients can then be prescribed warfarin, an anticoagulant drug, for weeks, months, or even indefinitely. If there is a condition that increases the risk of clotting, such as pulmonary hypertension, that condition will be treated. *See also* EMBOLISM; PULMONARY HYPERTENSION.

Pulmonary Fibrosis

Inflammation and stiffening of lung tissue.

Pulmonary fibrosis can affect part or all of the lung. It can be the result of inhalation of pollutants such as asbestos, metal and rock dusts, gases, or fumes. It is most often a case of inflammation resulting from earlier lung inflammation, such as pneumonia, tuberculosis, or sarcoidosis. Pulmonary fibrosis can also be passed from a parent to a child or have no known cause.

The prominent symptom of pulmonary fibrosis is shortness of breath, often accompanied by a persistent cough and chest pain. Treatment consists of high doses of corticosteroids or immunosuppressant agents. In some cases, a lung transplant is necessary. The loss of function caused by pulmonary fibrosis is irreversible, so persons with the condition must have vaccinations and take other preventive measures to avoid additional lung damage. *See* LUNG.

Pulmonary Function Tests

Tests designed to measure the capacity of the lungs to exchange oxygen and carbon dioxide and to diagnose pulmonary disorders.

Many kinds of tests are used to evaluate aspects of pulmonary function, including spirometry, measurements of lung volume, carbon monoxide diffusion, ventilation and perfusion scanning, and airway resistance tests. When combined with diagnostic imaging techniques such as x-ray and CT scanning, pulmonary function tests can help identify abnormal growths as well as functional abnormalities such as asthma and emphysema.

Spirometry uses a device consisting of a breathing tube attached to a measuring gauge. The patient is asked to deeply inhale and exhale into the tube as rapidly and forcefully as possible. The test measures lung volume, and is sometimes performed after a drug is administered to open the respiratory passage (bronchodilatora drug). A peak flow meter is a similar, though simpler, hand-held device for measuring the strength of exhalation. It may be used by asthmatics to monitor the severity of their disease.

Additional pulmonary function tests include measurements of the respiratory muscles, diffusion capacity (the lungs' ability to transfer oxygen into the bloodstream), and evaluations of blood gases (used to assess oxygen transfer to the blood and carbon dioxide elimination). Pulmonary fibrosis, disorders affecting the pulmonary blood vessels, and emphysema may be diagnosed using such procedures. *See also* BLOOD GASES; CT SCAN; EMPHYSEMA; MRI; PEAK FLOW METER; RESPIRATION; RESPIRATORY SYSTEM; SPIROMETRY; VENTILATION; *and* X-RAY.

Pulmonary Hypertension

Abnormally high pressure in the arteries that carry blood from the heart to the lungs.

Most cases of pulmonary hypertension are caused by other cardiovascular conditions that reduce the oxygen supply to lung tissue. The arteries in the lung become thicker, and the heart must work harder to pump blood. Sometimes, the condition is classified as primary pulmonary hypertension, because no cause can be identified.

Symptoms include shortness of breath, chest pains, dizziness, and swelling due to accumulation of fluid in the body. Diagnosis can be based on a patient's symptoms, with confirmation from a chest X-ray and echocardiogram.

If there is an underlying condition, treatment is aimed at that disorder. A diuretic may be prescribed to help remove excess fluid. Primary pulmonary hypertension is more difficult to treat. Drugs that widen the arteries can help, but they must be used with care, because they can cause serious side effects in some patients. Bed rest and supplemental oxygen can relieve symptoms, but most patients will not live for much more than a few years. A lung or heart-lung transplant may be performed if all else fails. *See also* HYPERTENSION.

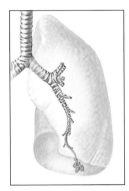

Lungs. The primary organ of the respiratory system.

Pulmonary Insufficiency

An often harmless failure of the pulmonary valve to function properly.

The pulmonary valve controls the flow of blood out of the lower right chamber (ventricle) of the heart. Normally, it closes after the ventricle contracts so that blood does not leak back into the heart. If the valve does not close properly, leakage occurs This is known as pulmonary insufficiency.

Pulmonary insufficiency can result from abnormally high pressure in the pulmonary artery, rheumatic fever, or inflammation of heart tissue (endocarditis). The disorder is sometimes detected as a heart murmur through a stethoscope. However, in most cases, pulmonary insufficiency is not dangerous. If the underlying cause is pulmonary hypertension, heart failure can result. In such cases, the treatment is aimed at reducing pulmonary hypertension.

Background material on Pulmonary Insufficiency can be found in HEART AND HEART, DISORDERS OF. *Related information is contained in* HYPERTENSION; PULMONARY EMBOLISM; PULMONARY FUNCTION TESTS; PULMONARY HYPERTENSION; PULMONARY STENOSIS *and* VENTRICLE.

Pulmonary Stenosis

Abnormal narrowing of the pulmonary valve, the pulmonary artery, or the upper section of the right ventricle that reduces the flow of blood from the heart to the lungs.

Pulmonary stenosis is most often caused by a congenital heart defect, although some cases occur in adults as a complication of rheumatic fever. It occurs in about one child of every 8,000 born in the United States, sometimes as part of a four-part set of heart defects called the tetralogy of Fallot. Pulmonary stenosis makes the heart work harder, causing it to become enlarged, with abnormally stiff, thickened walls. Blood can pool behind the pulmonary valve, causing the abdomen to swell.

SYMPTOMS

In severe cases of pulmonary stenosis, a newborn baby can have difficulty breathing and will often refuse to take nutrition, from breast or bottle. If pulmonary stenosis is accompanied by another congenital condition, such as a septal defect, a hole in the heart, the skin can have a bluish tint, because the blood has not flowed through the heart to pick up adequate oxygen. Mild pulmonary stenosis may not cause symptoms for years, and may be detected only when a doctor hears a heart murmur. Symptoms such as repeated bouts of breathlessness during activity and reddish-purple swollen regions of the skin can appear with age.

TREATMENT

Severe cases of pulmonary stenosis at birth are treated with prostaglandin E1, a hormone-like drug that allows more blood to reach the lungs. If the condition is caused by a narrowed pulmonary valve, the opening can be widened by balloon dilation valvuloplasty. A catheter with a balloon at its tip is directed through an artery or a vein into the heart. When it reaches the pulmonary valve, the balloon is inflated to expand the opening of the valve. The valve can also be repaired surgically. If the defect causing pulmonary stenosis is accompanied by other defects, such as the tetralogy of Fallot, immediate surgery is done. A mild case of pulmonary stenosis detected at or soon after birth may require no more than careful monitoring of the child. When symptoms that impair the quality of life begin to appear, surgery can be done to repair or replace the faulty pulmonary valve.

Risks of Infection
Older people who have pulmonary stenosis because of a previous attack of rheumatic fever should be aware that they are vulnerable to infective carditis. They should take antibiotics before every visit to the dentist and before any minor surgical procedure to prevent this heart infection.

Background material on Pulmonary Stenosis can be found in HEART AND HEART, DISORDERS OF. *Related information is contained in* HYPERTENSION; PULMONARY EMBOLISM; PULMONARY FUNCTION TESTS; PULMONARY HYPERTENSION; PULMONARY INSUFFICIENCY *and* VENTRICLE.

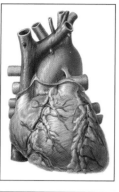

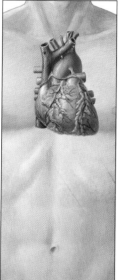

Pulmonary Artery. Above top, indicated in blue. Controls the flow of blood out of the right ventricle, and to the rest of the body, above bottom.

Pulp, Dental

Nerve and blood supply of a tooth.

The dental pulp is the fleshy part inside the tooth that contains the nerves and blood vessels. Essentially, the pulp is what gives the tooth its life; it supplies blood and also gives the tooth sensation. *See also* TEETH.

Unfortunately, when the tooth is diseased or damaged, the pulp becomes inflamed or infected. That sensation is often painful. When the tooth becomes severely decayed, the pulp must be partially or completely removed. A complete removal of the pulp is known as root canal treatment.

Pulpectomy

Complete removal of the pulp of a tooth before doing a root-canal treatment.

The core of a tooth is soft. This fleshy area is known as the pulp and is composed of blood vessels and nerves. Pulpectomy completely removes this soft center and is done in cases of extreme decay. It is part of the procedure known as root-canal treatment.

Even when a tooth is badly decayed, the dentist will try to salvage it by performing root canal. When the dental pulp is severely inflamed, infected or necrotic (dead and no longer vital), it is removed as the first step of a root-canal treatment. This will relieve the pain and discomfort present. The treatment is finished by thoroughly cleaning and filling, as well as supporting, the inside of the tooth. *See* TEETH.

Pulpotomy

Partial removal of the pulp of a tooth.

Within the hard structure of a tooth, the core is soft. The area that houses this soft center is called the pulp chamber. The center itself is known as the pulp and is composed of blood vessels and nerves. A pulpotomy is the partial removal of the pulp of a tooth. When a tooth is extremely decayed, the bacteria can infect the pulp,

inflaming it. The dentist's goal is always to keep as much of the tooth intact as possible. If he or she can save part of the pulp, then a pulpotomy will be performed instead of a complete pulp removal, known as a pulpectomy.

The procedure is normally done with a local anesthetic, which numbs only the part of the mouth being worked on. The damaged part of the tooth and pulp are removed. The healing process of the wound is stimulated by applying a special covering (dressing). The opening of the wound is then repaired by packing it with metallic materials that preserve the tooth's function and appearance. Occasionally, this last step fails and needs to be followed up with the multiple stages of root-canal treatment, which involves pulpectomy. *See* TEETH.

Pulse

The rhythmic expansion and contraction of the arteries as blood is pumped by the heart.

Taking the pulse rate, a routine part of any physical examination, is usually done by pressing a finger against an artery in the wrist. It can also be felt in the neck, inside the elbow, in the groin, and in other places.

Three characteristics of the pulse are important: its rate, rhythm, and strength. Most healthy resting adults will have a pulse rate between 65 and 75 beats per minute. The rhythm will be regular, and the strength will increase on breathing in and decrease on exhaling.

Alterations in any of these characteristics can be symptoms of a cardiovascular condition. For example, a weak pulse of varying strength can be caused by poor pumping action of the heart or a valve disorder. A weak but regular pulse can be a symptom of heart failure. Alternatively strong and weak beats, a condition called pulsus alternans, indicate a late stage of congestive heart failure. An abnormally strong pulse can result from fever, an overactive thyroid gland, or other conditions. An irregular pulse can be a sign of an arrhythmia caused by a problem with the hear's electrical control system. *See* HEART.

Punchdrunk

A condition in which the patient exhibits uncoordinated movement, speech or disorientation.

Punchdrunk is characterized by slurred speech, an impaired ability to concentrate, and awkward, clumsy movements. While the condition is unrelated to alcohol consumption, it is often compared to a state of drunkenness. It is caused by repeated brain injury or concussions in which there is a loss of consciousness. The name is indicative of the fact that there is a high incidence among boxers. *See also* CONCUSSION.

Pupil

Opening responsible for regulating the amount of light that enters the eye.

Muscles in the iris either relax or contract to automatically adjust the size of the pupil, which functions much like the aperture of a camera. In poor lighting, the dilator muscle will respond by enlarging the pupil, allowing as much light as possible to enter the eye. Dilated pupils can also occur in cases of drug use and as a symptom of various disorders. In bright light, and when the eye looks at a nearby object, the sphincter muscle acts to make the pupil smaller, preventing too much light from entering. *See also* DRUG DEPENDENCE *and* EYE.

Pupil. The device in the eye that regulates the amount of light that enters. A muscle contracts or relaxes, making the pupil larger or smaller, to control the amount of light admitted to the eye.

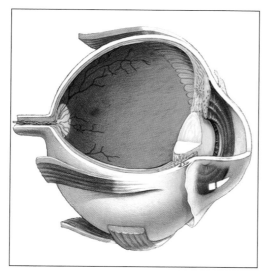

Purpura

Also called blood spots or skin hemorrhages

Purplish discolorations of the skin produced by small, bleeding vessels located near the surface of the skin.

The term pupura refers to discolored patches on the skin, or any one of a number of disorders that result in the occurrence of purplish spots due to bleeding into the skin. Purpura may also occur in the mucous membranes, such as the lining of the mouth, and also in the internal organs. Small purpura are called petechiae, and larger purpura are called ecchymoses. The condition is usually the sign of an underlying illness.

Purpuras are grouped into two categories: nonthrombocytopenic, which indicates normal platelet counts, and thrombocytopenic, which indicates decreased platelet counts. Platelets help maintain the strength of the capillary lining and are important in helping blood clot properly.

Purpuras found in those with normal platelet counts can usually be attributed to any one of the following disorders: pressure changes associated with the vaginal birth of a baby; congenital cytomegalovirus; congenital rubella syndrome; drug-induced platelet dysfunction; and senile purpura. Purpuras found in those with decreased platelet counts usually indicate the presence of one of the following disorders: immune neonatal thrombocytopenia; platelet consumption in cavernous hemangioma; drug-induced thrombocytopenia; and meningococcemia.

Henoch-Schonlein purpura is a type of hypersensitivity and inflammatory response within the blood vessels. It is caused by abnormal responses by the immune system. The condition is usually seen in children, but people of any age may be affected. Symptoms may include purple spots on the skin, hives, joint pain, abdominal pain, nausea, vomiting, diarrhea, bloody stools, and painful menstruation in women. The condition usually resolves itself, and is not normally treated.

Idiopathic thrombocytopenic purpura (ITP) is a bleeding disorder resulting from a shortage of platelets. It causes bleeding under the skin. This condition is caused when the spleen and lymph tissue produce antibodies against the blood's platelets.

These antibodies destroy the platelets in the spleen. Hemorrhage, bruising, sudden or severe loss of blood, and abnormal menstrual bleeding may occur. In children, the condition usually resolves without treatment. In adults, treatment usually involves the steroid prednisone and, in severe cases, spleen removal. *See also* HEMORRHAGE.

Pus

A yellowish-white fluid, consisting of white blood cells, dead tissue, and bacteria.

Pus is produced when the body fights an infection. White blood cells attack and kill bacteria, which they identify as foreign and possibly dangerous. These white blood cells die in the process. Dead white blood cells, other tissue debris, and bacteria combine into a thick, yellow-white fluid, which is pus. The pus may drain out of a sore or it may collect, either under the skin as a boil or elsewhere in the body as an abscess. *See also* ABSCESS *and* BLOOD CELLS.

Pustule

A raised bump on the skin, usually filled with pus.

Under the outermost layers of the skin are glands (which produce sweat to help cool the body and oil to protect and lubricate the surface of the skin), hair follicles (which grow hair), and blood vessels. When the openings to the surface of the skin are clogged with debris or when hormonal changes produce an excess of oil, the trapped fluid can become infected. If an infection occurs, pus forms and collects in small lumps under the skin called pustules. Often pustules come to a head and rupture naturally, or they may be opened with a sterile needle. *See also* ABSCESS; INFECTION; PUS; *and* SKIN.

PUVA

Acronym for Psoralen Ultra-Violet A

A type of therapy that is used in the treatment of psoriasis.

Psoriasis is an inflammation of the skin in which increased numbers of multiplying cells appear in the upper layer of the skin. In PUVA treatment, a drug known as psoralen is taken by the patient, and subsequent exposure to an ultraviolet A lamp causes a photochemical change in quickly dividing cells to reduce the rate of cell growth.

PUVA treatment is 55 to 65 percent effective on the face, trunk, and upper arms. *See also* PSORALEN DRUGS; PSORIASIS; *and* ULTRAVIOLET LIGHT.

Pyelography

Examination by x-ray of the urinary system following injection of a radiopaque medium.

Pyelography (also known as intravenous urography) is a technique used to visualize the shape of the kidneys as well as the urinary pathways from the kidney to the bladder. A radiopaque dye (one visible on x-ray) is injected intravenously. After reaching the kidney (about five minutes), the radiopaque medium is taken up and filtered by the urinary system, with the distribution of dye made visible on x-ray film. The test lasts about 30 minutes and is generally carried out without anesthesia. Some discomfort may accompany the transport of the dye through the vein. The x-ray images are then examined by a physician. Pyelography is a useful means of detecting and diagnosing urinary tract disorders.

Retrograde urography introduces the radiopaque substance directly into the ureter by means of a tube (catheter) or specialized scope.

RISKS AND COMPLICATIONS
Poor kidney functioning undermines the usefulness of the test, as the kidneys are unable to efficiently concentrate the ra-

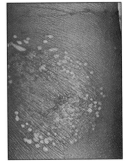

Pustule. When the pores of the skin are clogged, they may become infected and start forming small pus filled pockets on the skin, called pustules.

diopaque substance. Additionally, some danger exists of kidney failure following injection. While the causes of this are not well understood, the risks are increased in elderly patients, those with diabetes, dehydration, prior kidney insufficiency, or multiple myeloma.

BEFORE THE TEST

In either test, it is recommended that the patient avoid eating for 8 hours prior to examination and consume plenty of fluids. A laxative may be prescribed the night before the test to remove feces or gas that might interfere with the x-ray.

ABNORMAL RESULTS

Abnormal results of pyelography may be diagnostic of any of the following ailments: tumors, kidney stones, polycystic kidney disease, renal tuberculosis, or pyelonephritis, as well as irregularities of size, shape or kidney function, ureters, or bladder. *See also* BLADDER; CALCULUS, HYPERTENSION; KIDNEY; KIDNEY FUNCTION TEST; KIDNEY, POLYCYSTIC; TUBERCULOSIS; *and* URINARY TRACT.

Testing

Pyelography involves x-raying the kidneys, ureter and bladder following injection of a radiopaque substance. The procedure is relatively painless and carried out without anesthesia. Pyelography requires about 30 minutes and is used to diagnose a range of diseases and abnormalities of the urinary system. Subsequent testing may confirm or extend diagnosis by pyelography.

Pyelolithotomy

Surgical removal of a kidney stone, which is a nephrolith, or calculi through an incision made in the pelvis.

The surgeon makes a longitudinal incision on the relevant flank, and usually cuts into the posterior surface of the kidney to reach the stone, and then removes it with forceps. Pyelolithotomys are highly successful and carry low risk.

Coagulum pyelolithotomy is a procedure that is used to remove multiple stones in the kidney by injecting a liquid containing calcium chloride, cryoprecipitate, thrombin, and indigo carmine into the kidney. After a few minutes, a jelly-like clot is formed, and the stones become trapped inside the clot. The surgeon then removes the clot with the stones. *See also* BLOOD CELLS; CALCULUS; KIDNEY; LITHOTRIPSY; *and* LITHOTRIPTOR.

Pyelonephritis

Inflammation of the kidney caused by a bacterial infection.

Pyelonephritis usually occurs when an infection of the urinary bladder (cystitis) reaches the kidney by traveling up the ureter (the tubes that carry urine from the bladder to the kidneys). The condition can be chronic, with repeated infections, or acute, with a sudden onset of symptoms such as fevers as high as 102°F or more, chills, pain in the side or back, bloody urine, frequent and uncomfortable urination, weakness, and sometimes diarrhea. Chronic pyelonephritis can begin in childhood, the result of a back flow of urine due to the malformation of the valve regulating flow into the bladder.

The resulting periodic infections can cause permanent kidney damage and hypertension unless the malformation is corrected surgically. Chronic pyelonephritis is treated with antibiotics that are chosen to attack the specific infectious agent, which most often is *Escherechia coli.* Antibiotic treatment usually must be continued for two weeks.

In more severe cases, the patient must be hospitalized so that the antibiotic can be given intravenously. More than one round of antibiotic therapy may be necessary in 10 to 20 percent of all cases. Pyelonephritis is more common in women than men, and tends to be more severe in older women. *See also* ANTIBIOTIC DRUGS; BLADDER; CYSTITIS; HYPERTENSION; KIDNEY; URINARY SYSTEM; *and* URINARY TRACT.

Pyloric Stenosis

Narrowing or blockage of the pylorus, the lower part of the stomach, which leads into the small intestine.

Pyloric stenosis occurs in approximately one in 150 male newborns and one in 750 female newborns. While the exact cause of the disorder is unknown, soon after birth newborns experience a thickening of the pyloric muscle which blocks the passage of food flowing into the small intestine. In adults the condition usually occurs as the result of remaining scar tissue from a peptic ulcer or a malignant stomach tumor.

Symptoms. The symptoms, which include regurgitation and mild vomiting, appear during the first few weeks following birth and gradually grow more severe with frequent bouts of vomiting, dehydration, and eventual weight loss.

Treatment. While medication may treat some cases of infant pyloric stenosis, a surgical procedure known as a pyloromyotomy is necessary to either enlarge the opening between the stomach and the intestine or to remove any obstructions. With the onset of dehydration, replacement fluids should be given. *See* STENOSIS.

Pyloroplasty

Also known as pyloric stenosis repair.

A surgical procedure that widens a narrowed pylorus ensuring that food easily passes from the stomach to the duodenum, in the small intestine.

The operation was often performed along with a vagotomy, a "P & V", as treatment for peptic ulcers, but acid blockers and antibiotics have greatly decreased the need for both operations. This treatment is now also used to relieve pyloric stenosis; which causes vomiting in infants and small children as an acquired defect.

With the patient under general anesthesia, the surgeon makes a lengthwise incision across the pylorus, pushes the two ends of the incision together, and, in stitching them and the rest of the incision together, creates a wider passage to allow food to move along to the duodenum. Balloon pyloroplasty has been used for delayed gastric emptying in children. *See also* ANTIBIOTIC DRUGS; INTESTINE; STOMACH; ULCER; *and* VAGOTOMY.

Pyrogen

A chemical signal that raises the temperature of the body.

The body has its own thermostat in the hypothalamus region of the brain, which controls the temperature of the body to within a degree or two. When the body is under attack by a pathogen (disease-causing agent), when there is an inflammation, or when there is an allergic reaction, pyrogens are released and cause the hypothalamus to reset to a higher temperature. At this higher temperature, the flow of blood to the skin is reduced and the blood is retained in the internal organs so there is less heat lost from the skin. When the danger is past the hypothalamus resets to a lower temperature, and the blood supply to the outer layers of the skin is reestablished. *See also* FEVER *and* TEMPERATURE.

Pyuria

Presence of pus in the urine.

Pus consists largely of white blood cells and tissue debris. Its presence in the urine usually indicates an infection of the kidneys or urinary tract.

The patient's urine is tested (urinalysis), and a microscopic examination of the pus is done to identify the microorganism causing the infection. Antibiotic therapy is then administered as treatment.

Pyuria without an infection can be caused by an inflamed kidney, resulting from a condition such as interstitial nephritis; treatment then is aimed at that condition.

Pyuria, in association with a negative urine culture for bacteria, can be due to tuberculosis, trichomonas, or chlamydia. *See also* NEPHRITIS *and* URINALYSIS .

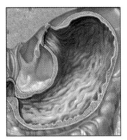

Pyloric Stenosis. A narrowing of the outlet (called the pylorus) from the stomach to the small intestine that occurs in infants.

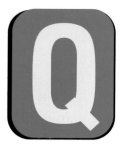

Q Fever

A bacterial disease transmitted from animals to humans.

The bacterium that causes Q fever is *Coxiella burnetii,* and it is transmitted to people who drink milk infected with the bacteria or who inhale contaminated dust. Symptoms include severe headache, fever, chills, sweating, muscle aches, and nausea. Some people who contract Q fever will develop pneumonia, gastrointestinal infections, or infections of the heart valves. The disease is treated with antibiotics, which are effective if the infection is diagnosed early.

Qigong

Pronounced "chee-gong," a combination of visualization, breathing, and gentle movements designed to stimulate the flow of "qi".

In ancient Chinese medicine, qi is the elemental life force. Disease is caused by a malfunction in the flow of qi, and therapies such as acupuncture, acupressure, and qigong attempt to improve the flow of qi and thus maintain health and treat disease.

In qigong, movements are combined with breathing and visualization exercises to stimulate qi to flow more freely. The movements are gentle and can be adapted to any level of physical ability or health. Qigong is known to aid in relaxation and overall fitness. *See* ALTERNATIVE MEDICINE.

Quarantine

Isolation of one or more persons infected by a contagious disease.

Quarantine procedures prevent the spread of an insidious disease by isolating the individuals that carry it. Once a contagious disease has been detected, those infected are confined to a particular room, floor, building, or geographic area, and the objects they come in contact with are consistently cleaned or sterilized. Those quarantined are not permitted to leave until they recover and are no longer a threat. In the case of past plagues, entire regions or cities have been quarantined to prevent the disease from spreading abroad or overseas: all those present, including tourists and visitors, were not permitted to leave until the disease had run its course.

Owing to the increased number and availability of immunizations and the dwindling number of cases of severely infectious disease, quarantine procedures today are rarely needed. Many countries, however, require yellow fever and other vaccinations for all incoming travelers and may restrict the travel of incoming tourists infected with a highly contagious disease.

Quickening

Feeling life; refers to the first noticeable movement of a fetus during pregnancy.

Quickening usually happens sometime during the 5th month. Thinner women tend to feel movement earlier than women who are overweight. The baby's initial movements are most often felt as light tentative touches or tiny pokes. Early in the pregnancy, the baby is not large enough to make its movements noticeable to the mother. As a fetus gets bigger, it moves around more, and the movements feel stronger. By the end of the pregnancy, the mother's sleep may suffer due to the constant poking and kicking. In the later stages of pregnancy, any absence or reduction of movement should be reported immediately to a doctor. *See also* PREGNANCY.

Quinsy

Also known as peritonsillar abscess.

An acute infection of the area behind the tonsils.

Quinsy is an infection that causes the tonsils to become inflamed. This inflammation results in pus-filled abscesses at the back of the throat, chills, a fever, painful swallowing, and a swollen throat and tongue. It is most often caused by streptococcal bacteria but can also be caused by other bacteria. Antibiotics are prescribed to treat quinsy and should be taken for a month even though the symptoms may have disappeared. *See also* TONSILS.

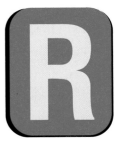

Rabies

Also known as hydrophobia.

A viral infection, transmitted from many animals to humans, which attacks the central nervous system (the brain and spinal cord).

The virus that causes rabies is transmitted to humans from the saliva of infected animals, usually by a bite but also by contamination of an open cut. Worldwide, there are an estimated 15,000 cases of human rabies each year. Less than five cases are reported in the United States annually. Raccoons, bats, foxes, skunks, dogs, and cats are all potential sources of the virus. The virus remains dormant for a period of from ten days to as long as a year. This incubation period gives the victim plenty of time to get a preventive vaccination after a bite. The incubation period will be shortest if the bite is on the head or neck.

Symptoms. The virus that causes rabies travels up the spinal column to the brain and then back down to the salivary glands. Symptoms include pain at the site of infection, followed by numbness or tingling. There is also mental depression and restlessness, changing to irritability and uncontrollable excitement. In advanced stages of the disease, the patient will start to produce copious quantities of saliva. There may be spasms in the throat, which make swallowing extremely painful.

Treatment. Once the symptoms appear, the rabies vaccination will have no effect. Treatment should begin before any symptoms appear. The disease was once considered to be 100 percent fatal, but there have been some survivors when the lung, heart, and brain symptoms were treated promptly. Death is usually caused by asphyxiation due to blocked air passages or from convulsions, exhaustion, or paralysis.

Prevention. People in professions at high risk for contracting rabies (veterinarians, laboratory workers, etc.) should be vaccinated, as should travelers to poorer countries overseas. Since the efficacy of the rabies vaccine declines over time, revaccination is needed every two years. *See* BITES.

After a Bite

• Even if the victim has been vaccinated, clean a bite wound as quickly as possible with soap and water. Deep punctures should be flushed with soapy water.

• Get the victim to an emergency room where he or she can be inoculated with rabies immunoglobulin and injected with rabies vaccine.

• Report the bite to animal control authorities. Usually the animal will be killed to determine if it has rabies; however, a veterinarian may confine the animal for ten days and keep it under observation. If it does not develop symptoms of rabies, the veterinarian may conclude that it did not have the disease at the time of the bite.

Rachitic

A term used to refer to the symptoms of rickets.

Rachitis is a synonym for rickets. The term rachitic is used to describe abnormalities in bone formation and the resulting symptoms of rachitic rosary, and rachitic deformities to the cartilage of the joints in the legs due to insufficient calcification of the bones. Rachitic rosary occurs in children who have rickets, and describes the bead-like expansions and fraying that appear at the cartilaginous growth ends of the ribs along the breastbone. *See also* RICKETS.

RAD

Acronym for radiiation absorbed dose

A standardized unit of measurement for absorbed radiation.

A RAD is defined as the amount of ionizing radiation that is absorbed by a material per unit of mass. Radiation, in the form of x-rays, is of constant concern for patients and health care workers in medical surroundings and must be closely monitored. Effects of radiation overdose include radiation poisoning, damage to cellular structure and function, and disruption of cellular genetics, which can transform cells into malignant ones. A film badge is a simple device worn by medical personnel to evaluate their cumulative exposure to radiation.

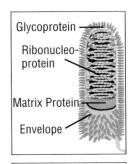

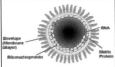

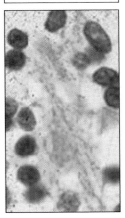

Rabies. Above top, the bullet shaped rabis virus, *rhabdovirus*. The virus is known to reproduce in the salivary glands of the host. Above middle, a cross section of the rabies virus and a microscopic view of the virus, above bottom.

Radiation

Term for the emission of radiant energy from a luminous body, x-ray tube, or fluorescent material.

Most radiation used by medical professionals is in the form of electromagnetic radiation, or EM. Such radiation propagates at the speed of light in straight lines when unaffected by external matter. When EM radiation collides with objects it either scatters or is absorbed, depending on the type of EM and the characteristics of the material it is striking. Radiant heat; radio, TV, and microwaves; infrared, visible, and ultraviolet light; and x-rays and gamma rays, make up the electromagnetic spectrum. The more highly energetic forms of EM, particularly x-ray, have proven invaluable to medicine.

Electromagnetic radiation capable of changing the structure in the atoms that it strikes is called ionizing radiation. By far, the most common form of EM radiation used diagnostically is x-rays. They are produced by bombarding a target made of tungsten (a metallic element that has a high melting point) with high-speed electrons. X-ray imaging relies on the fact that such radiation is absorbed by dense material such as bone, while passing through less dense soft tissue. Typically, a localized x-ray beam is passed through the part of the body under examination. A still image, known as a radiograph, is produced, revealing bone as white and soft tissue as gray.

MEDICAL USE

Through x-rays, soft tissue as well as bone may be analyzed for fracture, malignancy or other abnormality. The refinement of x-ray techniques now allows the subtle differences in tissues to be seen, and the diagnosis of different diseases to be made. Tuberculosis, for example, may be diagnosed through the differential absorption of x-rays by the air spaces of the lungs. Other cavities of the body, such as the gastrointestinal tract, may be filled with opaque fluid, allowing them to be visualized on x-rays.

Radiopaque compounds may also be administered by mouth or by injection into the bloodstream in order to examine the kidneys. The injection of contrast fluid into joints (arthrogram), the spinal canal (myelogram), or an artery, vein or lymph vessel (angiogram) increases the versatility of the x-ray, as do more sophisticated imaging techniques such as computerized axial tomography (CT or CAT), which offers an increase in clarity over conventional x-rays.

Risk Factors

Most cancer deaths from radiation are from skin cancer, which is triggered by too much sun exposure. Sun protection should be worn, particularly by those most vulnerable to the harmful effects of ultraviolet rays, including children and those with naturally fair skin. A lead apron should always be worn during x-ray procedures, to prevent radiation damage to the reproductive system. While nonionizing radiation is emitted by power lines, radar, cellular phones, and microwave ovens, such radiation currently appears to produce no risk to health.

RADIATION HAZARDS

While extremely useful for diagnostic imaging, ionizing radiation carries significant risk to health. Sunlight, for instance, which contains two forms of ultraviolet radiation (UV-A and UV-B), can cause sunburn and skin cancer as well as premature wrinkling and aging of the skin. Ionizing radiation is capable of disrupting cellular function or, if it is of sufficient intensity and duration, destroying cells. The severity of the effect on cells and tissues depends on the particular form of radiation, the quantity and rate of absorption, and the specific radiosensitivity of the exposed tissues. Rapid exposure to high-level radiation generally results in cell death, whereas prolonged exposure to lower levels is associated with cell damage and mutation. Late effects of radiation exposure include an increased incidence of leukemia, as well as cancers of the thyroid, the lung, and the female breast.

The ability of ionizing radiation to kill cells is also employed medically in radiation therapy to treat many forms of cancer.

Symptoms of Radiation Poisoning

When the body is exposed to high-level radiation, a characteristic pattern of injury results. Severe radiation exposure damages the vascular system, causing cerebral edema. This type of injury produces shock and generally leads to death within 48 hours. Somewhat less severe whole-body radiation causes a loss of fluids and electrolytes, severe bone-marrow damage, and terminal infection leading to death within ten days. Still lower absorbed doses cause destruction of bone marrow and may prove fatal within five weeks of exposure. Localized radiation exposure is more common and usually involves localized tissue damage. Delayed effects of ionizing radiation may be detected in various organs, particularly bone marrow, kidneys, lungs, and the lens of the eye. Degeneration and impaired function may be observed as well as damage to blood vessels. Hair loss is a common byproduct of radiation therapy as well as acute radiation overexposure as from nuclear accidents.

This branch of cancer treatment uses finely directed x-ray radiation to destroy malignant cells and tissue. Radiation therapy is often used before or shortly after surgical removal of cancerous tumors to destroy any malignant cells that may linger following the opperation.

Background material on Radiation can be found in CANCER AND ENERGY. *Related information is contained in* ANTHROGRAM; BENIGN; CT SCAN; GALLBLADDER; MALIGNANT; MRI; PUBLIC HEALTH; RADIATION HAZARDS; RADIATION SICKNESS; RADIATION THERAPY; RAIOACTIVIN; RAD *and* X-RAY. *See also* CANCER AND WORK RELATED INJURIES *for more information on Radiation.*

Radiation Hazards

Negative effects caused by external or internal exposure to radiation.

Treatments and imaging machines that use radiation may cause damaging side effects to a patient or his descendants. The incidence or amount of damage depends upon dosage and duration of exposure.

Currently, three basic units are used in the internationally agreed system of measuring radiation levels. The "becquerel," defined as one nuclear disintegration or other transformation per second, measures the radioactivity of a particular source. The "gray" measures the absorbed dose of ionizing radiation. These first two units measure x-rays or gamma rays. The "sievert" is a unit of measure that accounts for all of the other different kinds of radiation and for the resulting effects on tissue associated with each one. Thus, the sievert is the most useful to the medical field.

The risk of damage caused by radiation increases when the dose of radiation exceeds the "threshold," usually measured by one sievert. Doses greater than one sievert may result in radiation sickness, which at its most severe is characterized by fatigue, nausea, vomiting, anxiety, disorientation, and, in a matter of hours, loss of consciousness. Shortly thereafter, the patient may die from the radiation's damage to the nervous system, including edema, increased fluid in the brain. Other effects may be radiation dermatitis (blistering of the skin), hair loss, cataracts, or, several years after the treatment, the failure of certain organs.

The chance that damage will occur also increases as dosages are increased, even if the individual dosages remain below the threshold. Treatment for cancer, which uses x-rays, is the best example, though the damage is not detected until many years afterward: five to fifteen years for leukemia, and 40 or more years for skin, lung, and breast cancers. At the time of treatment, however, the patient feels nothing.

The odds of dying from cancer caused by radiation is about one in 100 per sievert of absorbed radiation, according to the International Commission on Radiological Protection. The same odds are applied to the possibility of a genetic disorder in the victim's subsequent generations.

One way to maximize the effect of radiation therapy and minimize the hazards is by aiming several sources at low power toward the cancerous area. Rays penetrate healthy tissue harmlessly, and their cumulative effect destroys the tumor. Another way is to implant radioactive pellets inside the tumor. A victim of cancer of the thyroid may need to drink radioactive iodine.

Resources on Radiation Hazards

Basch, Paul F., *Textbook of International Health* (1999); Frigerio, Norman, *Your Body and Radiation* (1996); Hall, Eric J., *Radiation and Life* (1984); Moeller, D.W., *Environmental Health* (1997); Prasard, Kedar, N., Handbook o Radiobiology (1995); National Research Council, Committee on Environmental Epidemiology, *Public Health and Hazardous Wastes* (1991); U.S. Public Health Service, Tel. (202) 619-0257, Online: phs.os. dhhs.gov/phs/phs.html; www.med.cornell.edu/public.health/.

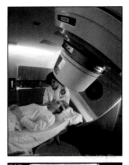

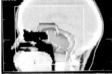

Radiation Therapy. Above top, a female patient is lying on a bed with a technician positioning the patient's head in preparation for radiotherapy. Above bottom, a computer generated image displays focused, positively charged atomic particles.

Boron Neutron CaptBure Therapy. Below, an illustration of a type of treatment for cancer. 1) Boron compound (b) is selectively absorbed by cancer cell(s). 2) Boron beam (n) is aimed at cancer site. 3) Boron absorbs neutron. 4) Boron disintegrates emitting cancer-killing radiation.

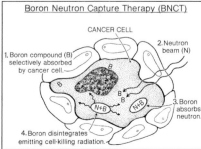

Radiation Sickness

An illness caused by exposure to radiation.

Radiation sickness is caused by radiation poisoning. The condition may be acute or chronic, and may occur as a result of cumulative exposure to small doses of radiation, undue exposure to solar radiation, or exposure to a nuclear explosion or other single large dose of radiation.

Symptoms. The symptoms of radiation sickness vary from mild and temporary to severe, depending on the type of radiation, the dose, and the rate at which exposure was experienced. The symptoms include weakness, loss of appetite, vomiting, diarrhea, a tendency to bleed, increased susceptibility to infection, and increased risk of cancer. Radiation sickness can be fatal.

Treatment. If exposure to radiation occurs, emergency medical assistance is needed immediately. All infected clothes and skin should be washed vigorously with water and a special solution, if available.

It is always advisable to avoid unnecessary exposure to radiation. When exposed to x-rays, individuals should wear shields over the parts of the body not being treated or studied. *See also* MRI *and* RADIOPAQUE.

Radiation Therapy

Use of ionizing radiation for the treatment of cell and tissue malignancy.

Radiation in the x-ray range of the electromagnetic spectrum is capable of producing changes in the atoms of cells and, if of sufficient energy, destroying cells. Such ionizing radiation is used clinically to eliminate and destroy (or at least slow and diminish) the aggressiveness of a variety of malignant tumors. This therapy is commonly used in the treatment of cancer and, provided the correct dosage of radiation is given, should cause little or no damage to normal cells.

This branch of cancer treatment, known as radiation therapy (or radiation oncology), uses finely directed x-ray radiation to destroy cancerous cells and tissue. The dosage of radiation used for cancer therapy is typically about one thousand times that of a diagnostic x-ray. The technique is often used before surgery, to reduce the size of the tumor to be excised, and following surgery, to remove residual cancerous cells from the region under treatment. Radiation therapy is used to treat roughly half of all cancer patients.

Such therapy relies on the fact that radiation is more destructive to rapidly dividing cancerous cells than to normal cells bordering the tumor. Further, cells with sufficient blood supply are more readily destroyed by radiation therapy. As the outer margins of a tumor are killed, areas closer to the center of the tumor begin receiving greater blood supply, making them more susceptible to destruction. This is one reason that radiation doses are typically spread out over a prolonged period, rather than delivered all at once. Such staged cancer treatment maximizes the destructive potential of the radiation to malignant cells while minimizing the effect to healthy cells, which over time are often able to repair radiation damage.

Ionizing radiation may be directed at cancerous tissue from outside the body, a process known as teletherapy (external beam radiotherapy) or from within (brachytherapy). The latter technique uses a radioactive source that is surgically implanted. In teletherapy, the intensity of radiation used depends on the extent and location of cancer. For example, cancers near the surface, including skin cancer are treated with low-energy radiation, while more deep lying tumors may require high energy radiation, capable of penetrating though the body.

The adverse effect to normal tissue depends on the size of the area exposed to radiation, the intensity of radiation and the proximity of cancer to healthy tissues and organs. Where metastasis of cancers exist (that is when cancerous cells are transferred to other parts of the body by way of blood vessels, lymphatic vessels or other membranes) whole-body radiation may be required.

The cycle of radiation therapy will be tailored to each case, and it usually involves five days of therapy followed by two days of rest, lasting up to 8 weeks. Radioactive implants deliver radiation continuously until the desired dose is achieved. Radiation therapy is the treatment of choice for many cancers, providing a cure in many cases, particularly in early stage cancers including medulloblastoma (a tumor of the brain or spinal cord), early breast cancer, Hodgkin's disease and early-stage Hodgkin's lymphoma, squamous cell cancer of the head and neck, prostate cancer, testicular cancer, and cancer of the larynx. Where a cure is not possible, (as with multiple myeloma, or advanced lung, esophogeal, head, neck or stomach cancers) radiation therapy may provide relief from associated symptoms.

Side effects of treatment range from mild to severe. External radiation commonly results in tiredness and lethargy. Nausea and vomiting may occur, but they are generally controlled with medication. Itching or discoloration of the skin, as well as skin rashes are sometimes observed, as is hair loss following radiation. Treatment of tumors of the head and neck may result in inflammation of mucous membranes in the nose and mouth, whereas treatment of the abdominal region can lead to stomach inflammation (gastritis) and inflammation of the lower intestine (enteritis) causing diarrhea. More severe side effects include disruption of normal bone marrow processes,

Treatment Options

Radiation therapy is used to treat half of all cancer patients. It may be combined with chemotherapy (treatment of the cancer with specific chemicals) and sometimes surgery. Beyond eradicating diseased tissue, radiation therapy may relieve symptoms of cancer or may be part of an ongoing process for the prevention of cancer recurrence. The procedure directs ionizing radiation at the area of concern, either by external radiographic beams, or internally, through the implantation of a radioactive source.

Risk factors

Radiation used to destroy cancerous tissue can be lethal to healthy cells. The amount of destruction to normal tissue must be carefully weighed by the physician against the benefits of cancer cell destruction. Ionizing radiation is also capable of producing changes or mutations in healthy cells, altering or disabling their normal function. Radiation poses the risk of genetic damage. Additionally, side effects to radiation therapy are not uncommon and may include tissue ulcers in areas exposed to radiation, nausea and vomiting, weight and hair loss, diarrhea, rashes and irritations of the skin, and, in rare cases, the production of secondary malignancies. The precise amount of exposure to ionizing radiation producing a significant health risk remains, after much study, a matter of fierce debate.

tissue or organ scarring, and, rarely, secondary cancers.

Background material on Radiation can be found in RADIATION AND PREVENTATIVE SCREENING AND COUNSELING. *Related information is contained in* PUBLIC HEALTH; RADIATION HAZARDS; RADIATION SICKNESS; RAIOACTIVIN; *and* RAD.

Radical Surgery

Extended surgical procedures often used to effect a cure rather than merely treat a disorder.

Radical surgeries may be used in nearly any part of the body for a variety of reasons. Many radical surgery procedures treat aggressive forms of cancer, or as a preventative measure for those at high risk.

A radical mastectomy, in which all of the breast tissue, the nipple, lymph nodes in the armpit, and chest wall muscles under the breast are removed, is an example. In the modified radical mastectomy, the chest wall muscles are not removed.

Prostate cancer may be treated by a radical prostatectomy involving removal of the prostate and some of the tissue around it.

Patients suffering from life-threatening epileptic seizures may undergo a radical surgery that severs the corpus callosum, a bundle of nerve tissue connecting the right and left hemispheres of the brain. *See also* MASTECTOMY *and* PROSTATE CANCER.

Radiculopathy

A diseased condition of the roots of the spinal nerves.

Radiculopathy, is a form of nerve root damage in which compression is produced by tumors or injury affecting the root of the nerve and the spinal cord. The squeezing of nerve roots (meninges) that cover the spinal cord often results in intense neck or back pain. Although back pain may seem to be an ordinary symptom, it can be indicative of a more severe condition.

Causes and Symptoms. The peripheral nervous system originates at the nerve roots. Both sides of the spinal cord have either a ventral (anterior motor) or a dorsal (posterior sensory) nerve root. Spinal nerve roots may become damaged anywhere along the spinal vertebral canal and are at a greater risk at the point in which the ventral and dorsal spinal roots connect to form the spinal nerves.

Radiculopathy can be caused by disk prolapse, spinal arthritis, diabetes mellitus, or the ingestion of certain metals, such as lead. A lumbosacral radiculopathy causes the painful condition known as sciatica. Common symptoms include pain, weakness, paralysis, and muscle atrophy.

Treatment. Therapy should begin with treatment of the underlying cause of the radiculopathy. Diagnosis is often complicated by the fact that neck and back pain are symptoms of many illnesses. The symptoms of radiculopathy can be relieved by the use of analgesics, physical therapy, or in extreme cases, surgery. *See also* SPINE.

Radioactivity

The ability of a substance to emit alpha, beta, or gamma particles from its nucleus.

Radioactivity involves the spontaneous disintegration of atomic nuclei through the emission of subatomic particles, (alpha particles and beta particles), or through the emission of electromagnetic rays, x-rays, and gamma rays.

A number of natural elements (such as radium) are naturally radioactive, as the result of a process of constant disintegration known as radioactive decay. Other elements may be made artificially radioactive, through the bombardment of the element's atoms with high-energy particles. Radioactive substances, either naturally or artificially occurring, play important roles in medicine, particularly as radioactive tracers. Their course may be tracked through the body following injection or inhalation, by monitoring the radioactive emission of the substance. This technique is at the core of diagnostic imaging techniques, including radionuclide scanning and positron emission tomography (PET). *See also* COMPUTER-AIDED DIAGNOSIS; RADIATION; RADIONUCLIDE SCANNING; RADIUM; *and* X-RAYS.

Radiology

Medical field concerned with the use of radioactivity including radioisotopes, x-rays, and other radiation for the purpose of diagnosis and treatment.

Radiant energy is used by the radiologist for both diagnosis and treatment. The most common form of diagnostic imaging is the x-ray. Imaging by x-rays relies on the fact that high-energy electromagnetic radiation is absorbed by bone, while passing through less dense, soft tissue. A beam of x-ray radiation is passed through a part of the body under examination. A still image (radiograph) is recorded on film, allowing the radiologist to assess injury or abnormality to bone, or evaluate disorders involving soft tissue, which will appear in varying degrees of grayness on the x-ray image, depending on tissue density. Other sophisticated imaging techniques involving radiation include the use of radionuclides (taken orally or injected into the bloodstream, the radionuclides collect in a "target organ," where they emit radiation) and computer-aided imaging systems such as computed tomography (CT or CAT scanning). Still other techniques use sound waves (ultrasound) or radio waves (MRI).

The ability of high-frequency radiation such as x-rays, to penetrate tissues allows for its use in cancer therapy. In this case, malignant tissue is exposed to radiation by a thin beam of x-rays of sufficient intensity to destroy cancerous cells. A dosage approximately a thousand times as great as that used in diagnostic imaging is directed at the tumor over a cycle of treatment. The repeated, limited use of this radiation will allow healthy neighboring tissue to recover during periods of rest, while malignant tissue is gradually eradicated. While extremely useful for both imaging and treatment, ionizing radiation carries significant risk to on's health. Absorbed dosages (measured in rads) by both health care workers and patients must be carefully monitored and controlled. *See also* CAT SCAN; COMPUTER-AIDED DIAGNOSIS; RAD; RADIATION; RADIATION HAZARDS, RADIATION SICKNESS; RADIATION THERAPY; SCANNING TECHNIQUES; *and* X-RAY.

Radium

A rare, highly radioactive metal element.

An atom of radium has a nucleus that contains 88 protons (its atomic number). There are 13 isotopes of radium, each with a different number of neutrons. Many of these isotopes have been created artificially. The most common naturally occurring isotopes are radium-223, radium-224, radium-228, and radium-226, which is the most abundant. Radium-226 is radioactive. Its half-life is 1,622 years, meaning that half of the atoms in a sample will decay during that period, emitting alpha and beta particles and gamma rays and forming the gas radon. Uranium does not occur in its pure form in nature. Radium ores such as pitchblende and carnotite must be processed chemically to obtain pure radium. Radium's most notorious use is in atomic weapons. It is also used as an energy source to generate electricity. The radiation from radium is a potent carcinogen, capable of causing leukemia and other cancers. Radium-226 was used in radiation therapy,

but it now has been replaced by other radioactive isotopes. *See also* CANCER; ELEMENTS; RADIATION; *and* TUMORS.

Radon

Radon is a colorless, odorless gas created by the natural radioactive decay of uranium-238 found in some soil and rocks, and a carcinogen responsible for thousands of lung cancer deaths each year.

Radon can seep into houses through cracks in foundations, floors, and basements, and accumulate to dangerous levels. Through radioactive decay, the gas forms products which attach to dust particles that are inhaled, and decay in the lungs, damaging cells lining the airways. *See* AVEOLI; CARCINOGEN; GAS; LUNGS; RADIUM; *and* RESPIRTORY SYSTEM.

Rape

Sexual intercourse that is forced on a nonconsenting individual.

In the United States, a rape is reported every six to seven minutes. In addition, it is estimated that 80 to 90 percent of rapes go unreported. Almost half of all rapists are between the ages of 15 and 25. These individuals often feel hatred or violent emotions towards their victims, and may also feel insecure about their own sexual performance. Rape is most often perpetrated by a male upon a female, but many cases of rape in which the woman is the rapist have also been reported. Rape may also occur between individuals of the same sex.

Incidence. The highest incidence of rape is found among women between the ages of ten and 19. However, the incidence of rape among victims over the age of 65 has increased by 800 percent over the last 15 years.

Effects. Emotional reactions to rape vary among victims. These may include-withdrawal, crying, hostility, anxiety, or inappropriate laughter. Physical symptoms other than from the rape itself may also be present, as physical abuse of the victim often occurs along with rape.

Resources on Radiology

Cullinan, John Edward, *Illustrated Guide to X-Ray Techniques* (1980); Kee, Joyce LeFever, *Handbook of Laboratory and Diagnostic Tests with Nursing Implications* (1994); Nuland, Sherwin, *Doctors: The Biography of Medicine* (1995); Ravin, Carl E., ed., *Imaging and Invasive Radiology in the Intensive Care Unit* (1993); Segen, Joseph C., and Joseph Stauffer, *The Patient's Guide to Medical Tests* (1998); American Hospital Association, Tel. (800) 242-2626, Online: www.aha.org; The American Board of Radiology, Tel. (520) 790-2900, Online: www.theabr.org; American Healthcare Radiology Administrators, Online: www.ahra.org; www.ny-cornell.org/radiology/.

Treatment. In general, treatment of rape victims focuses on the emotional effects of the rape on the victim, while attempting to obtain enough physical evidence to verify the rape and prosecute the offender. The potential of pregnancy or sexually transmitted diseases must also be addressed. The victim may be referred to a rape crisis center to receive support from other victims and psychotherapy. *See* Adolcence; Intercourse; *and* Preventative Meassures.

Rash

Also called Rubor or Erythema

An eruption of changes in color or texture of skin, characterized by any one of the following: redness or pinkishness, irritation, itchiness, spots and small bumps.

The cause of most rashes can usually be determined from its visible manifestations and other symptoms. There are numerous possible causes for this condition. Some possibilities include contact dermatitis following exposure to: dyes and other chemicals in clothing, chemicals in elastic and rubber products, cosmetics, deodorants, poison ivy and poison oak, medications that cause allergic reactions, insect bites, and diseases such as measles and lupus erythematosus.

Prevention and Treatment. Preventing rashes is preferred to treating them after they occur. Avoid contact with offending agents, which may include clothing, cosmetics, deodorants, rubber products, and poison ivy and oak. Always wash thoroughly with soap and water to remove chemicals that may be on the skin; this is especially important with materials like cement dust. Rubbing alcohol can remove oily substances from the skin. To treat poison ivy at home, use Domeboro powder or tablets, hot water, and hydrocortisone cream to relieve itching. Calamine lotion may also reduce itching. If home treatment is ineffective, or if the rash gets worse, a health-care provider should be contacted. If other symptoms are experienced, contact a health-care provider. *See also* Skin.

Raynaud's Disease

Reduced blood flow to the fingers and toes on exposure to cold.

Raynaud's disease results from constriction of the small arteries of the fingers and toes, which causes blueness, numbness, tingling and sometimes pain. It affects the fingers more than the toes and is more common in young women.

If there is an underlying cause, such as rheumatoid arthritis or systemic lupus erythematosus, the condition is called Raynaud's phenomenon. The condition can also be triggered by stress, smoking or physical activity. In severe cases, the blood supply can be reduced enough to give the fingers a shiny appearance and lead to ulceration or gangrene. Persons with Raynaud's syndrome are advised to avoid exposure to low temperatures. Smokers are told to give up cigarettes. *See also* Cirrculation *and* Tobacco Smoking.

Raynaud's Phenomenon

A circulatory disorder that constricts blood flow to fingers and toes.

Raynaud's phenomenon, unlike Raynaud's disease, has a known cause, which can be any of the following primary conditions: arterial diseases, connective tissue diseases, the drugs ergotamine and methysergide, and beta blockers. Symptoms include tingling, numbness, or burning in fingers or toes, which turn white; then blue when blood flow slowly returns; then red when normal flow is restored. In the worst, and rarest, incidences, the artery walls expand and stop blood flow altogether, resulting in lacerations or gangrene. To treat it, hands and feet must be kept warm; patients who smoke should quit, as smoking further constricts arteries. Artery walls may relax in response to vasodilator drugs. Sympathectomy, the surgical severing of nerves that effect the thickness of the arteries, is also an option. *See* Carpel Tunnell Syndrome *and* Circulatory System.

Recombinant DNA

DNA that has been artificially engineered to include segments that were not originally part of the sequence.

Since the early 1970s, scientists have been able to splice genes from one cell into another. The most common use of this technology has been to splice a gene for producing a chemical found in the human body, such as insulin or human growth hormone, into bacteria. The bacteria then multiply rapidly and produce large amounts of the hormone. Genetically engineered crops, into which genes have been introduced to make them more resistant to disease or rot, can already be found in supermarkets. Gene therapy, which is still in its infancy, attempts to cure genetic diseases by inserting normal genes into cells that have defective genes. *See also* GENE THERAPY *and* GENETIC ENGINEERING.

Recovery Position

First aid position designed to allow free breathing.

If a person has been in an accident or is unconscious but shows no obvious injury, it is safest to put the individual in the recovery position until emergency medical assistance arrives.

The recovery position is designed to allow free breathing and vomiting without clogging air passages. It assists in blood circulation and allows the victim to rest comfortably. A victim suspected to have suffered head, neck, or spinal injury should never be moved. The recovery position should not be utilized, and individuals should wait until medical personnel arrive.

Placing the Victim in the Recovery Position. Assuming the victim is on his or her back, the caregiver should kneel beside the body, turning the victim's face toward the caregiver. The victim's head should be tilted back to open the airway, and false teeth or any other obstructions should be removed from the mouth. The arm of the victim that is closest to the caregiver should

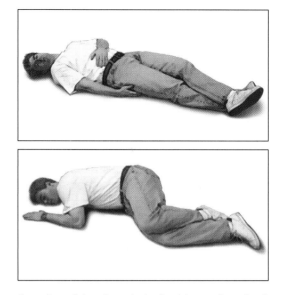

be placed by the victim's side and tucked under the buttock. The other arm should lay across the victim's chest. The far leg is then lifted over the near leg so that the legs cross at the ankle. Supporting the head and grasping the clothing at the hip, the victim should be rolled toward the caregiver until the individual is on his or her stomach. However, the head should be controlled so that the face is clear of foreign objects and turned in the same direction as the body. The near arm and leg should be adjusted so that they form a right angle to the body, preventing the victim from rolling onto his or her face. Lastly, the far arm and leg should be adjusted so that they are straight and parallel to the body. *See also* EMERGENCY FIRST STEPS.

Rectal Bleeding

Bleeding from the anal canal (rectum).

Rectal bleeding can have a number of different causes, including colorectal cancer, polyps of the colon, diverticular disease, and hemorrhoids. The nature of the bleeding can indicate the cause. The presence of bright red blood on toilet paper or feces is usually the result of hemorrhoids, but can also be a symptom of anal fissure, proctitis, or rectal prolapse. Rectal bleeding requires the immediate attention of a physician.

Rectal bleeding due to diverticular disease can result in feces that are darkened by the presence of blood. Blackened, tarry feces may be the result of a peptic ulcer, which causes bleeding high in the digestive tract. An infection such as amebiasis can cause diarrhea that is bloody. Most dangerously, rectal bleeding can be a symptom of a polyp or cancer of the colorectal tract. Since a polyp can turn cancerous, rectal bleeding is a signal for careful examination of the colorectal tract by proctoscopy, sigmoidoscopy, colonoscopy, or a barium x-ray examination, so that potentially cancerous polyps can be detected and removed, and the presence of any other cancer may be diagnosed and treated.

For background material on rectal bleeding, see COLON CANCER; RECTUM; AND RECTUM, CANCER OF. *Further reading can be found in* ANAL FISSURE; DIVERTICULAR DISEASE; HEMORRHOIDS; PROCTITIS; AND RECTAL PROLAPSE. *See also* COLONOSCOPY; PROCTOSCOPY; AND SIGMOIDOSCOPY.

Rectal Examination

Examination of the prostate gland and the mucous linings of the rectum.

Examination of the prostate gland and the mucous layers (mucosa) of the rectum is a common and relatively painless diagnostic test that can help identify abnormalities in the structure of the prostate, benign hypertrophy (enlargement of the prostate gland), and any tumors that might be present. The technique (also known as digital rectal examination) involves inserting a finger that has been coated with lubricating gel into the rectum, rotating the finger in order to test the firmness of the prostate, and carefully feeling for rectal tumors. Rectal examination is a common component of physical examinations, particularly for men over the age of 50.

After the age of 50, the risk of lesions and malignancies of the prostate and rectum increase, as does the incidence of noncancerous growths of the prostate gland (benign prostatic hyperplasia). The reasons for these growths are still poorly un-

Rectal Pain and Itching

Occasional rectal pain and itching, especially when accompanied by an unusually difficult bowel movement, is not serious. However, if the pain persists and there is bleeding or a change in bowel habits, a physician should be consulted. Rectal pain may be the result of various medical conditions, such as inflammatory bowel disease, diverticulitis, food poisoning, proctitis, anal fissure or fistula, hemorrhoids, dermatitis, eczema, a parasitic or yeast infection, a sexually transmitted disease, or even colon cancer.

derstood, but they may result from the hormonal changes associated with aging. The effect of this increase in prostate volume may be to narrow the urethra, occasionally constricting the flow of urine. The condition may make urination difficult and may also prevent the bladder from adequately draining. This can lead to infection and the formation of bladder stones, and sometimes kidney damage. Early detection of benign growths through regular rectal examinations offers a good defense against later complications.

Digital rectal examination is the most common screening technique for the early detection of prostate cancer, the second leading cause of cancer death among men. Rectal examination is often accompanied by a blood test to measure PSA (prostate specific antigen), a blood factor that is usually elevated in patients with prostate cancer. The efficacy of routine PSA tests, however, is a matter of debate.

Detection of a nodule during palpation of the prostate may be followed up by ultrasound scanning and subsequent tissue sampling (biopsy) to determine the nature of the cancer. Most prostate cancers spread slowly; however, some are more aggressive, requiring more immediate intervention to limit their growth and their potential to spread to other tissues, organs, and bone.

Background information on rectal examination can be found in DIAGNOSIS; PROSTATE; AND RECTUM. *For related material, see* ANAL FISSURE; BIOPSY; COLON CANCER; HEMORRHOIDS; PROCTITIS; PROSTATE, ENLARGED; RECTUM, CANCER OF; AND SEXUALLY TRANSMITTED DISEASE.

Rectal Prolapse

Protrusion of the lining of the rectum through the anus.

Rectal prolapse occurs when the lining of the rectum falls, or protrudes, usually as the result of undue straining during defecation. This usually creates discomfort and may cause rectal bleeding. Rectal prolapse may also accompany the presence of hemorrhoids. It is more often found in older women than in men. For younger patients, a diet rich in fiber is usually an effective form of treatment. Some older patients may require surgery. *See also* HEMORRHOIDS.

Rectocele

Protrusion of the rectum into the vagina.

Rectocele occurs when the tissues in the wall of the vagina become weakened. It often is accompanied by cystocele, the protrusion of the bladder into the front of the vagina, or by a prolapsed (fallen) uterus. A rectocele can cause constipation by preventing the rectal muscles from contracting. The condition can be alleviated in many cases by an exercise program to strengthen the pelvic muscles, but surgery may be necessary for some patients. *See also* CYSTOCELE *and* UTERUS, PROLAPSE OF.

Rectum

The end of the large intestine, leading outside the body.

The rectum is the final twenty inches of the large intestine; it is located in front of the bottom two vertebrae, the sacrum and the coccyx. The final two inches of the rectum are the anal canal, lined with a mucous membrane rich in blood vessels. The opening from the anal canal outside the body is the anus, ringed by two circular (sphincter) muscles: an internal, involuntary muscle and an external, voluntary muscle. These keep the anus closed except during elimination. *See also* RECTUM, CANCER OF.

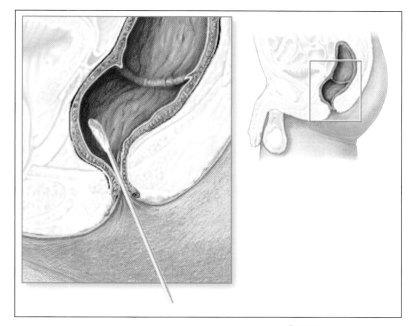

Rectum.
Above, is a diagram of the rectum, the end of the large intestine.

Rectum, Cancer of

Malignant tumor in the lowest part of the large intestine.

Colorectal cancer is responsible for about 20 percent of all cancer deaths in the U.S. The incidence of rectal cancer is highest in people over the age of 65 and in those who eat a high-fat diet. A diet rich in fiber from fruits and vegetables had once been thought to help prevent colorectal cancer; however, large-scale studies have found no beneficial effect in such a diet. Yet, dietary modifica- tions are still recommended because they can reduce the risk of heart attack and stroke. Most cancers of the rectum are adenocarcinomas, arising from the layer of cells that line the muscular wall of the intestine. Many originate from benign growths called adenomas, which can become cancerous if not removed. Periodic screening tests such as annual examination of the stools for blood, or sigmoidoscopy or colonoscopy, are recommended after the age of 40 to detect growths of the colon and rectum. While cancers of the rectum tend to be slow-growing, they can spread to nearby organs in the pelvis, such as the prostate, the ovaries, or the liver.

Symptoms. A major symptom of rectal

Rectal Cancer.
Below, is a barium enema in a patient with cancer of the rectum.

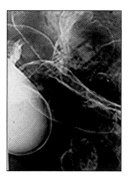

Colostomy

If the anal sphincter must be removed, normal bowel movements are not possible. In that case, an opening in the abdomen through which waste can be removed, called a colostomy, will be created. Special- ized technicians train patients in the care of a colostomy, and support groups exist in many communities to share information on the subject.

cancer is blood in the stool. Other symptoms include diarrhea, a sense of urgency when defecating, excessive straining during bowel movements, and a feeling that bowel movements have not completely emptied the bowel.

Diagnosis. A primary diagnostic test to detect rectal cancer is a manual test, in which the physician inserts a gloved finger into the rectum to feel for growths. Another diagnostic measure that may be used is a computerized tomography (CT) scan. The diagnosis of rectal cancer can be confirmed by visual examination of the rectum, such as in a colonoscopy or sigmoidoscopy, in which a flexible tube is inserted into the rectum. A barium enema air-contrast x-ray test, in which a special solution is inserted into the rectum in enema form, may also be conducted.

Treatment. Surgical removal of the cancer is the first line of treatment. If the cancer is noninvasive and has not spread, surgery alone is curative in a large percentage of cases. If the tumor has spread to the upper part of the rectum, that part of the rectum and the adjacent part of the colon will be removed. If the tumor is in the lower part of the rectum, the rectum and the anus will be removed. Radiation therapy may be done before or after surgery, and chemotherapy may be given in some cases. Prognosis depends on the stage at which the rectal cancer is detected.

For background reading on cancer of the rectum, see CANCER *and* COLON CANCER. *Further information can be found in* ADENOMA; COLONOSCOPY; CT SCAN; DIARRHEA; DIET AND DISEASE; ENEMA; RADIATION THERAPY; RECTAL EXAMINATION. *See also* COLOSTOMY *for more material.*

Reduction

Procedure in which a displaced body part is moved back into position.

Reduction is the term that describes the manipulation of a body part back to its correct place. Most commonly used as the first step in the treatment of fractures or dislocations, reduction also covers such procedures as pushing a displaced intestine back through the abdominal wall to treat a hernia. *See also* DISLOCATION; FRACTURES; HERNIA; *and* JOINT.

Referred Pain

Pain that is felt in an area of the body other than the source of the pain.

Referred pain is felt in a section of the body that is at a distance from the cause of the pain. This phenomenon occurs because the two sites are served by the same nerve or nerve root, the group of nerves that join at the spinal cord at the same location. Referred pain occurs when the nerve impulses from one part of the body are misconstrued by the brain as coming from the other.

When internal organs are injured or inflamed, the pain is normally sensed in the skin. This is possible because the neurons traveling to the brain from the superficial area, such as the skin, and the neurons from the deeper, affected area travel along the identical spinal nerves. The shared nerves stimulate the identical section of the cerebral cortex, which cannot distinguish between the two sources. Pain is perceived in the more superficial of the two areas.

By properly diagnosing referred pain, the physician can better locate the origin of its stimulation, that is, the source of the injury or disease. Common examples of referred pain include pain traveling down the left arm felt by a heart attack victim, pain felt in the tip of the shoulder indicating an irritation of the diaphragm, and the pang felt in the foot from increasing pressure on the spine (such as in disk prolapse). *See also* NERVOUS SYSTEM.

Reflex

An involuntary or instinctive movement in direct response to a stimulus.

A reflex response is an activity that is unplanned and performed automatically. Each reflex is predictable and repeatable in response to an identical sensory stimulus. Reflexes enable the body to adjust to constant changes. Each reflex action involves a particular stimulus, which produces a defined response. The nervous system is responsible for recognizing the stimulus and initiating the reflex action that is to be produced.

Types. Reflex actions can be divided into two categories: unconditioned and conditioned. Unconditioned reflexes occur naturally and involuntarily, without learning or experience. They always occur when the stimulus is displayed. For example, for every occasion in which a light is shined in a person's eye, the pupil becomes smaller. Immediately upon the removal of the light, the pupil enlarges.

Many unconditioned reflex actions are evaluated as part of neurological examinations. The knee jerk (patellar reflex) is elicited by tapping the tendon just beneath the kneecap with a rubber hammer. The knee jerk reflex causes the leg to jolt forward. The reflex indicates that the sensory nerve connected to the spinal cord, the motor nerve connected to the leg muscles, and all the nerve connections are operating properly. The reflex arc proceeds from the knee to the spinal cord and directly back to the leg. The brain is not included in the circuit.

A conditioned reflex, on the other hand, works by associating a particular stimulus with an event. Such reflexes are acquired and are not genetically programmed; in other words, they are a learned response. Conditioned reflexes are the consequences of new pathways formed in the nervous system as a direct result of a person's experiences. Such conditioning can be described as established habits or formed patterns.

Inborn Reflexes

Some reflexes are important for survival, and are termed "inborn." They appear in infants and then disappear later in life. A hungry infant will turn his cheek toward the direction that it is touched, thus turning its head in the direction of the stimulus. If the infant's lips are touched, he will attempt to suck. If a finger is placed in an infant's palm, he will grasp the finger, forming a fist. These inborn reflexes gradually disappear as the child grows.

In an example of a conditioned reflex, the well-known behavioral scientist Pavlov trained a dog to salivate at the sound of a bell. Each time the dog was fed meat, Pavlov rang the bell. Eventually, the dog began to salivate at the ring of the bell even without the presence of the meat. The dog was "conditioned" to salivate without the meat because it associated the sound of the bell with the sensation of the taste of the meat. The bell thus replaced the meat as an appetite stimulus.

How the Reflex Action Works. A sensory nerve cell reacts to a stimulus, such as heat, by transmitting a signal along the nerve fiber to the central nervous system, consisting of the brain and spinal cord. The nerve signal is received by receptors in the eyes, ears, nose, tongue, or skin. Electrical activity is changed into nerve impulses and conducted from the receptor to the central nervous system. The end of the fiber joins another neuron, which in turn becomes stimulated. The electrical activity in the newly excited muscle produces a response, which is the contraction of the muscle.

The completed cycle, known as the "reflex arc," consists of reception, conduction, transmission, and response. The loop is independent of the central nervous system. The reflex arc helps to better explain why people's pupils expand if they turn on a bright lamp or walk into a bright room.

Background information on reflex can be found in AUTNOMIC NERVOUS SYSTEM; INVOLUNTARY MOVEMENTS; AND NERVOUS SYSTEM. *For related material, see* EXAMINATION; NERVE; SPINAL CORD; AND STIMULUS. *See also* CHILD DEVELOPMENT *for more on inborn reflexes.*

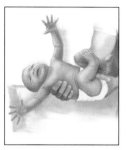

Reflex.
The Moro reflex is a normal reflex for an infant when he or she is startled or feels like they are falling. The infant will have a startled look and the arms will fling out sideways with the palms up and the thumbs flexed. Absence of the Moro reflex in newborns is abnormal and may indicate injury or disease.

Resources on Reflexes and the Nervous System

Germain, Blandine C., *Anatomy of Movement* (1993); Kandel, Eric R., et al., *Principles of Neural Science* (1991); Sanes, Dan Harvey, et al., *Development of the Nervous System* (2000); Sife, Wallace, *After Stroke, Enhancing Quality of Life* (1998); Epilepsy Foundation, Tel. (800) EFA-1000, Online: www.efa.org; Muscular Dystrophy Association of America, Tel. (800) 572-1717, Online: www.mda-usa.org; American Academy of Neurology, Tel. (651) 695-1940, Online: www.aan.com; American Board of Neurological Surgery, Tel. (713) 790-6015, www.abns.org; www.nycornell.org/medicine/neuro/index.html.

Reflexology

A method of healing that involves stimulating the appropriate area in the hands or feet in order to relieve tension and stress.

A technique believed to have its origins in ancient Egypt, Greece, and China, reflexology is a unique form of foot and hand massage designed to treat ailments in the body.

Theory. In its contemporary variations, reflexology is largely based on the European system known as zone therapy, introduced to America by the physician William Fitzgerald. Dr. Fitzgerald found that pressure applied to certain points on the hands and mouth alleviated symptoms in other parts of the body. Yet, it was the work of the physiotherapist Eunice Ingham that brought reflexology into its present form. Ingham mapped organ reflexes onto the feet, creating a "body chart" with specific organs corresponding to different parts of the foot. In addition, she developed a number of techniques for applying pressure and stimulation to the foot to heal individual parts of the body.

Technique. Reflexology sessions begin with an initial examination of the client's medical history and daily habits by the reflexologist. After the feet have been washed and dried, the practitioner will begin by massaging the feet to relax them, avoiding any sore or swollen areas. By applying pressure initially to the toes and working down the length of the foot, the reflexologist aims to stimulate the internal organs and glands. This pressure directly applied to the foot is believed to catalyze the breakdown of lactic acid and calcium crystals surrounding the thousands of nerve endings in the feet. It is the connection between these nerve endings, the spinal cord, and the brain that many proponents of reflexology believe affects the functioning of the internal organs in the body.

For background material on reflexology, see ALTERNATIVE MEDICINE. *Further information can be found in* CALCIUM; CHINESE MEDICINE; LACTIC ACID; NERVE; NERVOUS SYSTEM; AND SPINAL CORD. *See also* MASSAGE.

Regression

A term that describes the process of returning to a child-like state of behavior.

In Freud's psychonalalytic framework, all individuals go through successive stages of development. In some cases, individuals are "fixated" at a particular stage due to conflicts. When under stress, these individuals "regress" to the earlier stage and adopt immature patterns of behavior, which, in their most dramatic forms, may include thumb-sucking, exposing the genitals, or withdrawing into a fetal position. *See also* PSYCHOANALYSIS *and* PSYCHOTHERAPY.

Regurgitation

Return of partially digested fluid or food from the stomach to the mouth.

Regurgitation is common among infants after feeding and often is brought up with gas. This action is sometimes referred to as "spitting up." Regurgitation should not be confused with projectile vomiting, which is far more violent. Another form of regurgitation, the regurgitation of acid from the stomach back into the mouth, is called acid reflux. In addition, the backward flow of blood through a heart valve occurring in the case of mitral or aortic insufficiency is also called regurgitation. *See also* VOMITING.

Rehabilitation

Treatment that retrains a person for life after an illness, injury, or addiction.

After an injury or illness, rehabilitation can teach a patient to function independently with a permanent disability or to recover skills temporarily lost during illness. Rehabilitation may include physical therapy, which focuses on body movements below the waist, or occupational therapy, which focuses on functions of the upper body and hands. Rehabilitation may take place in a specialized center after a hospital stay, or it may be carried out at home.

Rehabilitation from drug or alcohol dependency includes support during and after withdrawal to reduce the chance of a relapse.

Rehydration Therapy

Also known as fluid therapy

Therapy given in order to replace fluids lost through dehydration related to diarrhea, vomiting, and fever.

Oral rehydration solutions, available at pharmacies, contain electrolytes to replace those that have been lost through dehydration. Oral therapy should always be used first, but if dehydration is severe, and even small amounts of fluids are not tolerated, intravenous rehydration may be necessary. In such cases, a saline solution carrying the essential minerals will be administered by injection. Rehydration therapy may be necessary following surgery, and to treat food poisoning, Crohn's disease, ulcerative colitis, traveler's diarrhea, gastroenteritis, and urinary tract infections. *See also* GASTROENTERITIS.

Reimplantation, Dental

The replacement of a dislodged tooth back into its socket.

Dental reimplantation is the replacement of a tooth that has been loosened or knocked out back into its socket. Such a tooth, known as an avulsed tooth, can often be replaced if the ligament connecting the tooth to the alveolar bone has been left intact. An avulsed tooth should ideally be reimplanted within 30 minutes. Even if the nerve has died, the tooth can still sometimes be replaced and reattached up to two hours later. *See also* SPLINT, DENTAL.

Reiter's Syndrome

Condition displaying symptoms of both urethritis and arthritis.

The exact cause of Reiter's syndrome is not known, but is most commonly found in men under the age of 40. There seems to be a genetic tendency to develop the disease, which is believed to be triggered by bacterial infections ranging from dysentery to sexually transmitted diseases.

The first symptoms of Reiter's syndrome are usually similar to those of urethritis, including urethral discharge, urinary urgency, and a burning sensation during urination. A low-grade fever and conjunctivitis (reddened, runny eyes) follow. Symptoms similar to those of arthritis, such as pain, stiffness, and swelling in the joints, will then set in. There may be skin lesions as well. Diagnosis is often delayed, because the symptoms occur far enough apart that the patient may not realize they are related.

The goal of treatment of Reiter's syndrome is to find the underlying bacterial infection that is causing the condition and to administer antibiotics to cure that problem. The symptoms can be treated with analgesics and anti-inflammatory drugs,

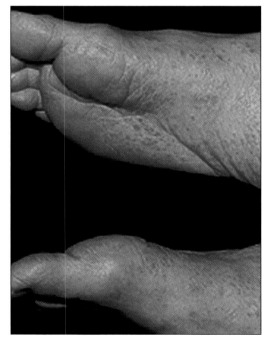

Reiter's Syndrome.
Reiter's syndrome, left, is a disease that consists of inflammation of the joints (arthritis), uretha (urethritis), and the eye. Reiter's frequently includes skin manifestations and is thought to be triggered by an infection. This is a fairly typical rash on the feet associated with Reiter's This type of rash may also appear on the hands.

while physical therapy can help to relieve the pain and stiffness from the arthritis-like symptoms. The condition usually clears up in three to four months, but recurs in half of patients. *See also* ARTHRITIS; SEXUALLY TRANSMITTED DISEASES; *and* URETHRITIS.

Rejection

A situation in which the body's immune system attacks transplanted tissue as if it were a foreign invader.

Rejection is the major complication following transplant surgery. The immune system is programmed to distinguish between "self" and "non-self" cells by means of antigens, or protein markers, on the surface of cell membranes. Any donated organ or tissue is therefore at risk of attack.

Symptoms. In addition to destroying the donated tissue, rejection can also cause symptoms in the patient, such as chills, fever, nausea, fatigue, and a precipitous drop in blood pressure.

Treatment. The majority of transplants are allografts, between two genetically unrelated individuals. Although doctors attempt to find compatible donors, the risk of rejection is still quite high. Various immunosuppressant drugs have been developed, to prevent the immune system's automatic rejection response to the foreign tissue. The major risk of these drugs is that by suppressing the body's reaction to the transplant, they also compromise its ability to fight infection. Immunosuppressant drugs must be taken indefinitely.

Prevention. The best possible donor is an identical twin. However, not many individuals are in this situation. Parents or siblings share many of the same genetic markers; therefore, the chances of rejection are minimized but not eliminated entirely. *See also* GRAFT-VERSUS-HOST DISEASE.

Relapse

The recurrence of disease or particular symptoms following improvement or recovery.

The recurrence or relapsing of a disease or its symptoms may be due to a variety of causes. Some diseases are by their nature recurrent, particularly certain cancers and viral disorders, which may reappear periodically throughout the patient's life. Degenerative disorders often follow a trajectory of temporary improvement, when the disease is said to be in remission, followed by a sudden or gradual worsening or relapse. The patient's behavior is also a critical factor in relapse, particularly relapsing associated with drug use following a period of abstinence. *See also* ALZHEIMER'S DISEASE; DEGENERATIVE DISORDERS; REMISSION; *and* VIRUSES.

Relapsing Fever

Bacterial infection transmitted by ticks.

Relapsing fever is caused by a spirochete, a bacterium of the Borrelia family that is carried by ticks native to the western United States and Canada. Ticks infected with the bacteria carry it for life and may pass it on to the next generation of ticks.

Symptoms. These begin five to 15 days after bacterial transmission with a sudden high fever (103° to 104°F), often accompanied by a rash, lasting two to nine days with periods of remission. The fever may relapse one to ten times. Other symptoms of relapsing fever include headache, vomiting, blood in the urine, muscle and joint aches, chest pain, and blood in the vomit. Low blood pressure and body temperature may follow fever episodes. Relapsing fever may be fatal if left untreated.

Diagnosis and Treatment. A blood test will reveal the presence of spirochetes. Once relapsing fever has been diagnosed, it is treated with antibiotic drugs, such as tetracycline or erythromycin.

Prevention. It is critical to remove ticks from the skin promptly and carefully with tweezers, applying gentle steady traction. Crushing the tick may leave mouth parts in the skin, which can still transmit the disease. Hands should be protected with gloves, cloth, or tissue while the tick is being removed. Means of preventing relapsing fever include the use of insect repellents containing DEET or permethrin on clothing and the avoidance of tick-infested areas, especially in the warmer months. *See also* ANTIBIOTIC DRUGS; SPIROCHETE; TETRACYCLINE DRUGS; *and* TICKS AND DISEASE.

Relaxation Techniques

Methods of reducing anxiety and stress.

Relaxation techniques consist of any method that an individual finds useful for reducing the physiological and emotional effects of stress on the body.

The effects of psychological and emotional stress on the body include increased heart rate, blood pressure, and breathing rate. Digestive system and eating habits change, sexual drive decreases, and sexual dysfunction can become a problem. The long-term effects of stress on the body can be devastating. Since most people face stressors every day that cannot be solved by the body's response, it would be valuable for almost everyone to develop a routine of relaxation techniques to alleviate stress.

Relaxation techniques are also used as treatment for people suffering from anxiety, phobias, post-traumatic stress disorder, sleep disorders, and panic disorder.

The appropriate relaxation technique for any one individual will depend upon that person's interests and lifestyle. The most effective stress-reducing techniques are those that can be employed regularly to lessen the effects of stress in the body.

Exercise. Various forms of exercise reduce stress, because they utilize the energy that builds up to battle stress. As little as 15–20 minutes of aerobic exercise a day may be useful in managing the effects of mild to moderate stress levels.

The Relaxation Response. Relaxation techniques are often used in conjunction with psychotherapy to alleviate anxiety and panic. This method, popularized by Herbert Benson, helps to reduce the physical symptoms of racing heartbeat and rapid breathing. To practice this technique, the person takes purposefully slow, long breaths, while repeating a word or phrase to concentrate the mind away from the thoughts causing the stress.

Meditation. Stress is often caused by worrying about the future or reliving the past. Meditation is an activity that retrains attention on the here and now. There are a variety of types of meditation, but most methods focus on breathing as a means of centering the mind. Instead of getting caught up in a spiraling course of thoughts, the meditator, through practice, learns to become aware of the thoughts without getting caught up in them. Meditation requires practice and discipline, but has been found to have beneficial effects, particularly when used in combination with medical interventions in many ailments that are exacerbated by stress, including heart disease, chronic pain, and diabetes.

Yoga. This is a physical activity that requires concentration to maintain a series of poses. Yoga can be practiced at varying levels of difficulty and is appropriate for healthy individuals of all ages. The meditative quality of yoga, combined with the physical movement, results in a feeling of calm.

Other Relaxation Techniques. A number of other activities have a meditative quality: the mind focuses on a repetitive or consuming activity, providing a release from an onslaught of emotions caused by constant worry. *See also* ALTERNATIVE MEDICINE *and* AROMATHERAPY.

Remission

The period during which the symptoms of a disease lessen or abate.

Remission is a common feature of many diseases. During this phase, the symptoms of an ailment are lessened and sometimes disappear altogether. The term is most often applied to cancer, especially following treatment with radiation and chemotherapy. When treatment has been completely successful, a cure may follow. With many diseases, the extension of remission provides the best hope for complete recovery. In AIDS, for example, drug therapy is used to try to bring the quantity of the HIV virus to undetectable levels. This is believed to impede the virus's ability to replicate, producing remission in the patient. In other cases, the patient may relapse, and symptoms of the disease will recur. *See also* AIDS; CANCER; HIV; RELAPSE; *and* VIRUSES.

Resources on Relaxation and Stress Management
Davis, Martha, Martha Elizabeth Eshelman and Matthew McKay, *The Relaxation and Stress Reduction Workbook* (1988); Humphrey, James H., *Stress Among Older Adults: Understanding and Coping* (1992); Newton, Tim, *Managing Stress: Emotion and Power at Work* (19995); Swenson, David, Ashtanga Yoga (1999); National Center for Complementary and Alternative Medicine, Tel. (888)644-6226, Online: nccam.nih.gov; American Chiropractic Association, Tel. (703) 276-8800, Online: www.amerchi-ro.org; Association for Applied Psychophysiology and Biofeedback, Tel. (303) 442-8892, Online: www.aapb.org. http://www.nycornell.org/medicine/gim/index.html.

Renal Biopsy

Surgical removal of tissue from the kidney for diagnosis of disease or abnormality.

Renal biopsy involves the removal of a small cylindrical core of tissue from the kidney by means of a special needle, which may be guided by feel or with the aid of ultrasonography. The extracted tissue is examined by a pathologist for signs of disease or abnormality. Renal biopsy is used following transplantation (to assess kidney function), after a decrease in kidney function, or of blood or protein in the urine.

For eight hours prior to the test, the patient should abstain from fluids and food. Blood and urine samples will be taken, in order to supplement the information gained from tissue sampling. Following the application of a local anesthetic, a long, thin needle will be carefully inserted into a marked region, generally on the patient's right side. A small incision is made in the skin to allow the locating needle to be inserted into the kidney. As the patient takes repeated deep breaths, the physician detects the position of the needle, guiding it toward the biopsy location. This needle is then removed and the depth of penetration measured. The biopsy needle follows the path made by the locating needle. Generally the patient will remain in the hospital for rest and observation for 24 hours following the test. *See also* KIDNEY CANCER.

Renal Colic

Severe spasms of pain originating in the urinary tract and felt on one side of the back.

The pain of renal colic occurs when a kidney stone obstructs the normal function of the kidney. The pain often is excruciating, radiating across the abdomen, and can be part of a group of symptoms including chills, fever, frequent urination, nausea, and vomiting. An attack may last a few minutes. The condition can be treated by removal of the stones that are causing the pain. *See also* CALCULUS.

Renal Failure

Partial or total loss of kidney function.

The two kidneys of the body filter waste products from the blood, control the levels of water and salt in the body, and help regulate blood pressure. The kidneys also play a vital role in the production of a hormone called erythropoietin and in the production of the active form of vitamin D. Erythropoietin is critical for the production of normal numbers of blood cells, thereby preventing anemia (a low red blood cell count). Vitamin D is responsible for the absorption of calcium from food, and for the maintenance of healthy bones. When the kidneys fail to do their job, the result is a buildup of waste products, accompanied by other abnormalities that can cause a variety of symptoms.

Causes. Acute (sudden) renal failure can be caused by a number of medical problems. These include conditions that block the flow of urine, such as bladder tumors, bladder stones, or an enlarged prostate gland in men. Major bleeding or burns can reduce blood flow to the kidneys enough to cause acute renal failure; a heart attack can have the same effect. Chronic (over time) renal failure can result from untreated high blood pressure (hypertension), diabetes, polycystic kidney disease, or amyloidosis. Overuse of painkillers for a number of years can also result in chronic kidney failure.

Symptoms. If renal failure is acute, symptoms can include a severe decrease in urine production, drowsiness, nausea, vomiting, muscle cramps, headache, and breathlessness. Chronic renal failure brings about all the symptoms of acute failure, as well as a growing sense of weakness, lethargy, anemia, and paleness of the skin. If progressive renal failure cannot be reversed, it can be fatal.

The complications caused by acute kidney failure include an increased risk of infection and internal bleeding. Chronic renal failure can cause anemia, nerve damage, and degeneration of muscle tissue.

Treatment. The treatment of acute kidney failure is aimed at diagnosing the underlying condition and correcting it—for example, by removing a stone that is blocking urine flow. Diuretic drugs may be given to increase the production of urine. In severe cases, artificial kidney treatment (dialysis) may be given until a crisis is over. Treatment of chronic kidney failure can start with dietary changes and include drugs to remove excess fluid from the body and reduce high blood pressure. When these measures cannot prevent end-stage renal failure, continuing dialysis or a kidney transplant can prolong life.

> *Background information on renal failure can be found in* kidney *and* urinary system. *For related material, see* ANEMIA; BLADDER TUMORS; BURNS; DIABETES MELLITUS; HEART ATTACK; *AND* VITAMIN D. *See also* DIALYSIS *AND* DIURETIC DRUGS *for more treatment options.*

Renal Tubular Acidosis

> **Failure of the kidneys to remove acid from the blood.**

Acid is a normal by-product of metabolism that is removed from the blood by the kidneys. When the kidneys do not remove enough acid, the blood becomes abnormally acidic. The result can be weakening of the bones, formation of kidney stones, and calcification of the kidneys. Tubular acidosis can result from kidney damage due to disease, the side effects of medications, or a genetic disorder. Sodium bicarbonate can help to reduce the acidity of the blood. *See also* KIDNEY.

Renin

> **A hormone, produced in the kidneys, that regulates blood pressure.**

The release of renin starts a complex series of changes that constricts blood vessels, raising blood pressure. This hormone also encourages the kidneys to retain fluid and salts, which further increases blood pressure. *See also* HYPERTENSION.

Renography

> **The technique of imaging the kidney by x-ray methods for the purpose of diagnosis.**

Renography is a general term applying to a variety of x-ray imaging studies of the kidney. Renal scanning usually requires the administration of a radiopaque substance —a dye injected intravenously that helps illuminate specific organs and tissues on the x-ray. Several procedures make use of radiopaque or radiocontrast substances; intravenous urography (intravenous pyelography), for example, is used to highlight the kidneys and lower urinary tract. During this test, the passage of the radiopaque substance through the ureters into the bladder is seen and an image of the bladder (cystogram) is produced. Another procedure, retrograde urography, introduces the radiopaque solution directly into the ureters by means of a catheter, and has the potential to offer improved clarity (though the procedure is more dangerous and requires anesthesia). *See also* KIDNEY.

Reportable Diseases

> **Conditions of patients that physicians must report to local health authorities.**

The mandatory reporting of certain diseases helps public health officials take appropriate action to prevent the spread of disease through isolation or immunization, and provides incidence and prevalence statistics that will determine health programs and facilities improvements.

Once informed, local authorities may pass on such reports to the Centers for Disease Control. AIDS, chickenpox, malaria, tetanus, hepatitis, syphilis, gonorrhea, birth defects, and certain occupational diseases are examples of reportable diseases.

> *For background information on reportable diseases. see* public health. *Further reading can be found in* AIDS; BIRTH DEFECTS; CHICKENPOX; GONORRHEA; HEPATITIS; IMMUNIZATION; MALARIA; QUARANTINE; SYPHILIS; *AND* TETANUS. *See also* OCCUPATIONAL MEDICINE *AND* HEALTH.

Resources on Kidneys and Renal Failure

Cameron, Stewart, *Kidney Disease: The Facts* (1986); Legrain, Marcel, et al., *Nephrology* (1987); Campbell, Meredith F., & E. Darracott Vaughan, *Campbell's Urology* (2002); Hinman, Frank, *Atlas of Urologic Surgery* (1989); Tanagho, Emil A. and Jack W. McAninch, eds., *Smith's General Urology* (1995); National Kidney Foundation, Tel. (800) 622-9010, Online: www.kidney.org; American Association of Kidney Patients, Tel. (800) 749-2257, Online: www.aakp.org; American Foundation for Urologic Disease, Tel. (800) 242-AFUD, Online: www.af-ud.org; National Institute of Diabetes and Digestive and Kidney Diseases, Tel. (301) 496-3583, Online: www.niddk.nih.gov;www.nycornell.org/medicine/nephrology/index.html; www.cornellurology.com/.

Reproduction, Sexual

Reproduction that requires two parents—one to provide sperm, the other to provide eggs.

In sexual reproduction, each parent contributes half of the genetic material, resulting in variation among the offspring. Sexual reproduction is the normal method of reproduction among many plant and animal species. *See also* SEXUAL INTERCOURSE.

Reproductive System, Female

The organs in a female that are responsible for the production of ova and, in the event of conception and pregnancy, the development of a fetus until birth.

The female reproductive system consists of the external vulva and the internal ovaries, fallopian tubes, uterus, and vagina. In order for reproduction to occur, a sperm cell from the male must fuse with a mature ovum, which then implants in the uterus and develops into a fetus.

Female Reproductive System.
The diagram at right outlines the female reproductive system and the location of the ovaries, fallopian tubes, uterus, cervix, and vagina. These organs are involved in conception, pregnancy, and fetal development.

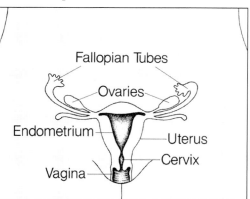

External Organs. The external reproductive organs consist of the mon veneris, the clitoris, and the outer and inner labia. The mons veneris is an area just above the pubic bone that is padded by a layer of fatty tissue; this provides protection from the impact of intercourse. The clitoris, located below the mons veneris and above the opening to the vagina, is a small oval of erectile tissue that contains many nerve endings and is highly sensitive. It is covered by the clitoral hood (prepuce). The outer and inner labia are two sets of folds of skin that cover the opening to the vagina.

Internal Organs. The ovaries are the glands that produce mature egg cells (ova). At birth, the ovaries contain nearly 400,000 potential ova, or follicles. Starting at puberty, the follicles develop into mature ova approximately once every 28 days; these are then released into the fallopian tubes.

The ovaries also produce the hormones estrogen and progesterone, which are responsible for regulating the female reproductive cycle, as well as for the development of secondary sex characteristics.

The fallopian tubes connect the ovaries to the uterus. When a mature egg is released from the ovaries, it travels down a fallopian tube for three or four days. During this time, conception may occur.

The uterus is the primary organ in pregnancy. If an ovum is fertilized, it implants in the uterus, where it is nourished and protected for the following nine months until birth. If the egg is not fertilized, then the egg, tissues lining the inside of the uterus, and blood are discharged in menstruation.

Where the uterus meets the vagina is the cervix. Usually a lining of mucus covers the opening of the cervix, so that the uterus is protected from infection. During ovulation, the mucus lining thins so that sperm cells can enter.

The vagina is the organ through which sperm cells enter the reproductive system, introduced by the penis during coitus. At either side of the vaginal opening are the Bartholin's glands, which produce small amounts of lubricating fluid during sexual arousal. Further in are the hymen glands, which secrete lubricant for the length of the vaginal canal, facilitating penetration.

During birth, the infant passes through the vagina, or birth canal; the vagina is able to stretch to accommodate the infant's size.

Background material on female reproductive system can be found in GYNECOLOGY. *For related material, see* CERVIX; CLITORIS; CONCEPTION; ESTROGEN; MENSTURATION; OVARY; OVULATION; UTERUS; AND VAGINA. *See also childbirth and pregnancy for more on sexual reproduction.*

Reproductive System, Male

System of organs that produces sperm and releases it from the body.

The male reproductive system consists of the external testes, scrotum, and penis, and an internal system of glands and ducts. For reproduction to occur, sperm cells from the male reproductive system must enter the female reproductive system, where one sperm cell eventually fuses with an ovum, resulting in conception.

External Organs. The testes produce and store sperm cells until ejaculation. They also produce testosterone, which regulates the growth and functioning of the male reproductive system and stimulates the development of male secondary sex characteristics. The testes are connected internally to the spermatic cord.

The scrotum is a pouch of skin and connective tissue that holds the testes. One of the scrotum's primary functions is to regulate the temperature at which the testes are kept (usually about 5°F below body temperature). It contracts and relaxes in response to temperature changes and sexual stimuli, drawing the testes closer to the body during sexual arousal and on exposure to cold, and letting the testes relax away from the body on exposure to heat.

The penis introduces semen into the vagina during coitus. The urethra passes through the center of the penis; surrounding the urethra are cylindrical masses of tissue, primarily composed of erectile tissue —spongy tissue that becomes engorged with blood during arousal, causing the penis to become erect. During orgasm, which can occur from sexual activity, masturbation, or dreams, semen is ejaculated from the head of the penis.

Internal Organs. A number of internal glands and ducts produce the components of semen and carry it to the urethra as part of ejaculation.

Semen is the thick, milky fluid that is ejaculated from the penis during orgasm. It carries the sperm cells and contains fluids from the seminal vesicles and bulbourethral, or Cowper's, glands.

Before semen is ejaculated, a thin, clear, slightly basic fluid is secreted by the prostate gland, located just below the urinary bladder and entirely surrounding the urethra. This fluid neutralizes the acidic environment of the urethra and enables the sperm cells to pass through unharmed.

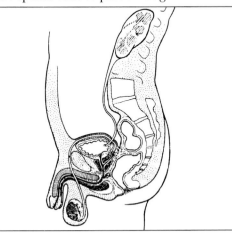

Male Reproductive System.
The diagram at left shows the male reproductive system consisting of the testes, scrotum, and penis, along with the internal system of glands and ducts.

The bulk of semen consists of a fluid produced by the seminal vesicles, located just above and behind the prostate. In addition, a clear, sticky fluid is produced by the bulbourethral glands, located internally just behind the penis. This fluid serves as lubrication and enables semen to pass more easily through the urethra.

For ejaculation to occur, sperm cells travel from the testes through a series of ducts, where they mix with other fluids and are expelled from the urethra. Sperm cells first are carried to the epididymis, a convoluted tube connected to the testes, and then to the vas deferens, a part of the spermatic cord that joins with ducts leading from seminal vesicles, forming the ejaculatory duct. At this point, the sperm mixes with the rest of the semen and then passes through the prostate and through the urethra.

For background information on the male reproductive system, see REPRODUCTION SEXUAL. *Further reading may be found in* CONCEPTION; EJACULATION; ERECTION; GLAND; PENIS; SEMEN; SPERM; TESTES; TESTOTERONE; *AND* URETHA. *See also reproductive system, female for more information.*

Resources on Reproductive System
Adashi, Eli Y, Jouh A. Rock and Zev Rosenwaks, *Reproductive Endocrinology, Surgery, and Technology* (1992); Boston Wo-men's Health Book Collective, *The New Our Bodies, Ourselves: A Book By and For Women* (1992); Hamilton, David, and Frederick Naftolin, *Repro-ductive Function in Men* (1992); Rosenwaks, Zev, et al., *Gynecology: Principles and Practice* (1987); Tyler, Sandra L., et al., *Female Health and Gynecology: Across the Lifespan* (1982); American Board of Obstetrics and Gynecology, Tel. (212) 871-1619, Online: www.abog.org; American Society for Reproductive Medicine, Tel. (205) 978-5000, Online: www.asrm.org; Planned Parenthood Federation of America, Inc., Tel. (800) 829-7732, Online: www.plannedparenthood.org; www.ivf.org/ home.html; www.nycornell.org/obgyn / www.nycornell.org/medicine/womenshealth/html.

Resection

A partial excision of bone or other tissue by surgery.

Resection surgery involves the cutting away of diseased or damaged tissue. Resection of the colon, for example, is the primary treatment for colorectal cancer. Such surgery aims to remove the cancer, restore bowel functioning, and protect neighboring tissue. In addition, colorectal resection may be used to treat gangrene or a narrowing or obstruction of the small intestine.

During a colorectal resection, the small intestine is clamped above and below the diseased area, which is then surgically removed. The resultant open ends of the intestine are then attached with the use of sutures or staples. Rectal tumors may also be resectioned by laser, particularly if they are large. *See also* CANCER *and* GANGRENE.

Resistance

The condition in which a disease no longer responds to treatment with medication.

After exposure to antibiotic, antiviral, or antifungal drugs, some bacteria, viruses, and fungi mutate, and are thus able to survive exposure to the drugs. This process generally occurs over many years and results in resistant strains of pathogens (disease-causing agents). If a person has a disease that is not responding to treatment, the physician has to either increase the dosage of the medication or switch to another drug, if an alternate drug is available. Resistant strains of the bacteria staphylococcus and streptococcus have been identified, and many of the drugs that showed initial promise in combating HIV are becoming less effective, as the virus continues to mutate into drug-resistant forms.

Background material on resistance can be found in BACTERIA; FUNGI; INFECTIOUS DISEASE; AND VIRUSES. *For further reading see* ANTIBIOTIC DRUGS; ANTIBIOTIC RESISTANCE; ANTIFUNGAL DRUGS; AND PATHOGEN. *See also* AIDS; HIV; STAPHYLOCOCCAL INFECTION; AND STREPTOCOCCAL INFECTION.

Resorption, Dental

The loss of substance from a tooth, either external (from the surface of the tooth root) or internal (from the inside of the pulp cavity).

External dental resorption occurs in children as part of the process by which the primary teeth are lost. The pressure from the permanent teeth in the gums causes the resorption of the roots of the primary teeth. The primary teeth become loose and eventually fall out. External resorption of the adult teeth is a harmful process that slowly destroys the tooth. Root-canal treatment may sometimes slow or stop the process.

Internal resorption is a rarer form of resorption, and the cause is unknown. Internal resorption may spread from the pulp cavity outward into the rest of the tooth, resulting in a pink spot that can be seen through the tooth crown. As with external resorption, root-canal treatment may slow or stop the process. *See also* TOOTH DECAY.

Respiratory Arrest

Sudden, life-threatening stoppage of breathing.

Respiratory arrest can be the result of a number of conditions that cause major reduction in the function of the brain center that controls breathing. These causes include cardiac arrest, in which the heart stops beating; overdose of narcotic drugs; stroke; serious injury to the head; or severe seizures that affect the electrical activity of the brain. It can also be the result of a lung disorder, such as emphysema or chronic bronchitis, that is severe enough to stop the normal process of breathing. Respiratory arrest is a medical emergency that requires immediate treatment, because it stops the flow of oxygen to the vital organs of the body. If the flow is not restored within minutes, the patient can suffer brain damage or cardiac arrest, leading to coma and death. If breathing stops, emergency medical assistance should be called. Until it arrives, artificial respiration should be administered. *See also* EMERGENCY FIRST STEPS.

Respiratory Distress Syndrome

A lung disorder that makes breathing increasingly difficult.

Respiratory distress syndrome can occur in adults or in newborn babies.

Adult Respiratory Distress Syndrome. This is a form of pulmonary edema, a condition in which excess fluid accumulates in the bronchioles, the small airways of the lung, and the alveoli, the sacs in the lung where gas exchange occurs. As fluid accumulates, the lung tissue becomes stiffer, the lungs can no longer expand normally, and breathing becomes difficult. The condition can be caused by shock, pneumonia, a blood infection, inhalation of a toxic gas, or a near-drowning experience.

The resulting symptoms include rapid, shallow breathing and shortness of breath. The condition can worsen quickly, producing mental confusion, weakness, and an abnormally fast heart rate. The lack of oxygen supply to the body often affects the ability of other organs to function properly, so that the risk of death is high, even with prompt treatment.

The basic treatment for adult respiratory distress syndrome consists of removing the liquid that affects lung function while maintaining the body's oxygen supply with mechanical ventilation. Any underlying cause should also be treated. Prompt treatment can result in survival with little or no permanent lung damage.

Infant Respiratory Distress Syndrome. This occurs in low-weight and premature babies, because their lungs are not fully developed or are otherwise unable to supply the body with oxygen. The condition, also called hyaline membrane disorder, is a major cause of death for premature infants.

Infant respiratory distress syndrome can be recognized by the grunting noises and involuntary movements made by the babies as their breathing becomes more rapid and more labored. The diagnosis is confirmed by blood tests and an x-ray examination.

Treatment for infant respiratory distress syndrome starts with a supply of adequate oxygen to the patient through continuous positive airway pressure, in which oxygen-rich air is blown under pressure into the nose. The child may also be placed on a ventilator to maintain the oxygen supply. Treatment must be done with delicacy to avoid damaging the fragile lungs. Treated properly, most children can recover after a week, but some suffer permanent lung damage. *See also* LUNG.

Respiratory Failure

A decrease in the oxygen level and increase in the carbon dioxide level of the blood.

Respiratory failure can result from a condition that interferes with the normal transfer of gases between blood and tissues of the body, such as emphysema, bronchitis, or severe asthma. It can also be caused by damage to the brain center that controls respiration or by a drug overdose. Symptoms of the condition include a cough, breathlessness, bluish skin (resulting from a lack of oxygen), and an increase in breathing rate. The symptoms can be relieved by types of treatment that supply more oxygen to the blood, such as placing the patient on a ventilator. Treatment is also aimed at the underlying condition causing the problem. *See also* HYPOXIA *and* OXYGEN THERAPY.

Respiratory System

The organs involved in taking oxygen in from the environment, transferring it to the blood, and expelling waste gases.

The respiratory system is made up of the lungs, bronchi, trachea, larynx, pharynx, mouth, and nose, as well as the muscles that support the process of breathing. The lungs are located in the chest (thoracic) cavity and are protected by the rib cage. The pharynx, larynx, trachea, and bronchi are tubes that lead from the mouth and nose through the throat to the lungs.

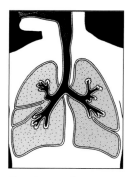

Respiratory System.
The diagrams above and below show the respiratory system, which is made up of the lungs, bronchi, trachea, larynx, pharynx, mouth, and nose. Air is breathed through the nasal passageways, and travels through the trachea and bronchi to the lungs.

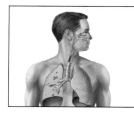

Resources on Lungs and Respiratory System

Crystal, Ronald G., *The Lung: Scientific Foundations* (1997); Crystal, Ronald G., and John B. West *Lung Injury* (1998); Parker, Steve, *The Lungs and Breathiung* (1989); Kittredge, Mary, *The Respiratory System* (1989); Parker, Steve, The Lungs and Breathing (1989); Perry, Angela R., *Essential Guide to Asthma* by American Medical Association (1998); *Lung Cancer: A Guide to Diagnosis and Treatment* (1999); American Lung Association, Tel. (800) LUNG-USA, Online: www.lungusa.org; Lung Line Information Service, Tel. (800) 222-5864, Online: www.nationaljewish.org; Second Wind Lung Transplant Association, Tel. (888) 222-2690, Online: www.2ndwind.org, www.nycornell.org/medicine/pulmonary/index.html.

The respiratory system is reponsible for respiration—both the mechanical act of breathing and the transfer of oxygen to the blood. It also helps in speech formation.

Breathing. There are two phases to breathing: inhalation (inspiration) and exhalation (expiration). Breathing is an involuntary process, although it is possible to consciously control the rate of breathing for a time. Infants breathe between 30 and

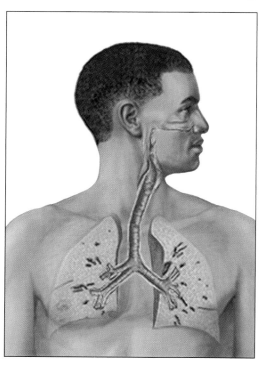

50 times a minute; children, between 20 and 30 times a minute; and adults, between 16 and 20 times a minute.

The external tissue of the lungs is elastic, allowing them to inflate and deflate. The muscles that control breathing are the diaphragm and the intercostal muscles. During inhalation, the diaphragm contracts downward, enlarging the thoracic cavity, and the intercostal muscles pull the ribs upward and outward. The lungs expand, and air flows in. During exhalation, the muscles relax, reducing the size of the thoracic cavity, and the lungs deflate.

Respiration and the Lungs. During inhalation (inspiration), air travels from the nose or mouth through the pharynx, larynx, trachea, and bronchi to the lungs. The

air must travel through this long series of tubes in order to ensure that the air is at body temperature by the time it reaches the lungs, and to filter out foreign particles and microorganisms. The primary mechanism for removing particles from the air is the mucus that lines the mouth and throat. Particles bump against and attach to this sticky substance; cilia, or small hairs, then move the mucus farther up the throat, where it is eventually swallowed.

The mouth and the upper throat carry both food and air; the trachea branches off from the digestive tract and carries air into the chest cavity, where it splits into two bronchi, one leading into each lung. A membrane closes the trachea during swallowing, so that food is not able to enter and clog the airways.

In the lungs, the bronchi branch into smaller tubes known as bronchioles, which in turn split into clusters of tiny sacs known as alveoli. The membranes of the alveoli contain a network of capillaries, which carry blood that is low in oxygen and high in carbon dioxide. Carbon dioxide diffuses out of the cells, and oxygen diffuses into them. There are 750 million alveoli in the lungs, with a surface area approximately equal to that of a tennis court. This ensures that enough gases diffuse for respiration to be efficient.

After passing through the lungs, the oxygenated blood travels to the heart, where it is pumped throughout the body. This blood provides oxygen to cells and picks up carbon dioxide as a waste product, at which point it returns to the lungs to repeat the process.

Speech. The respiratory system is also integral in the formation of speech. When air is exhaled, the larynx can vibrate, creating noise. This noise is shaped by the lips, teeth, and tongue to form the various sounds that we use for comunication.

For background information on respiratory system see AIR AND OXYGEN. *Related material can be found in* LARYNX; LUNG; MOUTH; NOSE; AND TRACHEA. *See also* ASTHMA; BREATHING DIFFICULTY; EMPHYSEMA; AND PNEUMONIA *for more information on respiratory disorders.*

Respiratory Therapy

Maintenance of proper breathing in patients with respiratory problems.

Respiratory therapists work under the supervision of doctors and are required to pass the examination of the National Board for Respiratory Care. Respiratory therapy is necessary for patients with conditions that interfere with normal breathing, such as emphysema or bronchitis, and is also used to promote recovery in patients who have had major surgery. The patient may be placed on a ventilator, which supplies air to the lungs, or on a nebulizer, which administers medicine in the form of an aerosol through a face mask. Breathing exercises may also be performed. *See also* BRONCHITIS *and* EMPHYSEMA.

Respiratory Tract Infection

Infection of the passages carrying air to the lungs.

The respiratory tract runs from the nose all the way down to the alveoli (air sacs) in the lungs, where the exchange of oxygen and carbon dioxide occurs. An infection caused by viruses or bacteria can occur at any point in the respiratory tract. Upper respiratory infections occur in the nose, throat, sinuses, and trachea (the upper part of the main airway to the lungs). They include the common cold, tonsillitis, sinusitis, laryngitis, and croup. Lower respiratory tract infections affect the lower part of the trachea, the bronchi (two branches of the trachea that lead to the two halves of the lungs), and the lungs. Lower respiratory tract infections include pneumonia, bronchitis, and bronchiolitis. All respiratory tract infections are treated with the appropriate antibiotic and antiviral medications, depending on the cause of the individual infection. *See also* BREATHING; BRONCHIOLITIS; BRONCHITIS; COMMON COLD; CROUP; LARYNGITIS; LUNGS; PNEUMONIA; SINUSITIS; *and* TONSILLITIS.

Restless Leg Syndrome

Uncomfortable stinging, crawling or throbbing sensations in the leg muscles.

Restless leg syndrome is characterized by crawling sensations in the limbs, most commonly in the calves, but occasionally in the arms and trunk.

Incidence and Cause. Restless leg syndrome often affects middle-aged women, pregnant women, smokers, heavy coffee drinkers, and anemia and arthritis patients. The cause of the condition is not known, although family history is an important factor.

Symptoms. Symptoms of restless leg syndrome occur during periods of inactivity, and are often more severe at night. Due to this pattern, falling asleep and staying asleep can become difficult because of discomfort due to involuntary jerking of the legs during the night. This may also cause daytime fatigue.

Treatment. For some sufferers, symptoms may be alleviated by decreasing caffeine intake or, for anemic patients, increasing iron intake. Alternative therapy such as massage, exercise, heating pads, or ice packs can alleviate symptoms as well. *See also* GENETICS.

Restoration, Dental

Procedures that artificially rebuild diseased or injured teeth.

People whose teeth have become diseased or damaged often need to have restorative work done. In minor cases of damage, the damaged area of the tooth is removed and the created space is packed with a metallic or composite material (filling). Similarly, chipped teeth are repaired with a protective material. For major damage, a covering may need to be placed over an entire surface of a tooth (onlay, inlay, or crown). In each of these procedures the goal is to remove the damaged area, preserve the remaining tooth structure and function, and maintain a natural appearance. *See also* DENTAL, FILLING *and* ONLAY, DENTAL.

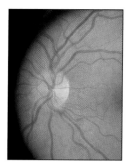

Retina.
Above is a magnification of the retina, the part of the eye responsible for forming images. The retina is divided into two layers, as shown by the diagram below—an outer, non-visual layer and an inner layer of nerve cells.

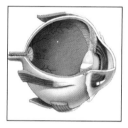

Retina

The portion of the eye responsible for forming images.

The eye is divided into three layers (tunics); the retina is the innermost layer. It surrounds the inner chamber of the eye (vitreous body) and covers only the back portion of the eye. The retina is further divided into two layers: an outer, nonvisual layer made of pigmented tissue; and an inner, visual layer of nerve cells.

The retina's primary purpose is image capture. Light enters the eye through the pupil and lens and reaches nerve cells inside the retina. Light is first detected by photoreceptor cells, which consist of cone and rod cells. Cone cells, primarily located in the central portion of the retina, detect color and work best in bright light. Rod cells, located on the periphery, detect black-and-white vision and are sensitive to dim light. Nerve signals from both types of cells are passed through two types of neurons in the retina (bipolar and ganglion) to the optic nerve, which transmits the signals to the brain. *See also* OPTIC NERVE.

Disorders of the Retina

Retinal disorders may occur as a result of degeneration or as a complication of disorders such as high blood pressure, kidney disease, and diabetes mellitus. They generally disrupt vision and may lead to blindness. Some retinal disorders include:

- color blindness: an inherited inability to differentiate between certain colors;
- diabetic retinopathy: small hemorrhages in the retina that occur in diabetes mellitus;
- detached retina: tearing or separation of the inner layer of the retina;
- glaucoma: increased fluid pressure in the eye;
- retinal hemorrhage: bleeding into the retina, seen in hypertension and diabetes;
- macular degeneration: age-related degeneration of the eye;
- retinal vessel occlusion: a blockage in a retinal artery or vein;
- retinitis pigmentosa: rare disorder of the retina in which the rod cells progressively deteriorate;
- retinoblastoma: rare tumor of the retina, generally found in children under five.

Retinal Artery Occlusion

Blockage of an artery in the retina, leading to vision loss.

An artery in the retina may become blocked by a blood clot, fat deposit, or plaque that has broken free from the inside of a blood vessel. This may occur as a complication of high blood pressure, atherosclerosis, glaucoma, or blood disorders.

Symptoms. The major symptom of retinal artery occlusion is a sudden blurring or loss of vision in one eye.

Treatment. Anticoagulant drugs can prevent further clot formation. Carbon dioxide can dilate retinal vessels, causing the clot to be dislodged. Depending on the cause and severity of the occlusion, vision loss may range from nonexistent to severe. *See also* ATHEROSCLEROSIS; BLOOD, DISORDERS OF; GLAUCOMA; HYPERTENSION; *and* VISION, LOSS OF.

Retinal Detachment

When the inner layer of the retina separates from the outer layer, resulting in vision disruption.

Causes. Retinal detachment is usually a result of degeneration in the eye. Over time, tears may form in the retina; they may be microscopic or extensive. Detachment may also be caused by injury to the eyeball, inflammation, or surgery on the eye. About two-thirds of people with retinal detachment are nearsighted.

Symptoms include flashes of light or moving spots in the field of vision, followed by cloudiness or loss of a portion of vision. Symptoms may appear gradually or suddenly and may vary in severity; in extreme cases, there may be total loss of vision.

Treatment involves one of several types of surgery in which the goal is to properly position the inner layer of the retina and induce the creation of scar tissue, which seals the tear. The latter is usually done with the use of a laser (photocoagulation) or a freezing probe (cryosurgery). *See also* VISION, LOSS OF.

Retinal Hemorrhage

Rupture and bleeding of the blood vessels that lie on the surface of the retina.

Retinal hemorrhage has a number of causes, including severe head injury and complications from diabetes, hypertension, and some clotting disorders.

Retinal hemorrhage in children is often an indication of physical abuse. Over 50 percent of abused infants have retinal hemorrhaging. Common injuries, such as falling, are not severe enough to cause retinal hemorrhaging. *See also* BLOOD, DISORDERS OF; CHILD ABUSE; DIABETES MELLITUS; HEAD INJURY; *and* HYPERTENSION.

Retinal Tear

A rip in the retina, the back portion of the eye responsible for vision.

The retina may tear spontaneously or as a natural result of aging. A tear may be caused by injury or an inflammatory disorder. If fluid from the eye leaks through the tear, that portion of the retina may separate from the rest of the eye, resulting in retinal detachment and disruption or loss of vision. Retinal tears are usually treated with laser (photocoagulation), freezing probe (cryotherapy), scleral buckle, or vitrectomy. *See also* RETINAL DETACHMENT.

Retinal Vein Occlusion

Blockage of an artery in the retina, leading to vision loss.

As in retinal artery occlusion, a vein in the retina may become blocked by a blood clot. High blood pressure, atherosclerosis, or glaucoma may be a risk factor for occlusion.

The main symptom is a sudden blurring or loss of vision in one eye. Treatment involves the prevention of further clot formation; the prognosis varies, depending on the success of treatment. *See also* ATHEROSCLEROSIS; GLAUCOMA; HYPERTENSION; THROMBOSIS; *and* VISION, LOSS OF.

Retinitis Pigmentosa

Rare disorder of the retina in which night and peripheral vision are gradually lost.

In retinitis pigmentosa, rods—nerve cells in the eye that are sensitive to light but not color—gradually deteriorate. This results first in a loss of peripheral and night vision, and eventually the disease progresses until the central field of vision is lost as well.

The cause of retinitis pigmentosa is unknown, but it may be inherited. There is no known prevention and no treatment, although protecting the eyes from ultraviolet light with sunglasses may slow the progression, as may treatment with antioxidants such as vitamin E. *See also* VISION, LOSS OF.

Retinoblastoma

A rare, malignant tumor of the the retina that appears in young children.

Retinoblastoma appears in early childhood, with 80 percent of cases occurring before the age of five. Retinoblastoma may be inherited or arise from an unknown cause. In the hereditary form, a gene that suppresses the formation of tumors is missing. Untreated, retinoblastoma may spread to the optic nerve and the brain.

Symptoms. Retinoblastoma may appear in one or both eyes. The pupil may appear white, the eyes may be crossed, and the irises may be of different colors. The eye may be red and painful, and vision may be impaired, even to the point of blindness.

Treatment is aimed at removing the tumor and maintaining as much vision as possible. A small tumor may be removed with laser surgery or cryotherapy. Larger tumors may require removal of the entire eye. If the tumor has spread, radiation therapy or chemotherapy may be needed.

Prognosis. Most cases of retinoblastoma respond to treatment, with a survival rate of 82 percent. Patients are at an increased risk for developing cancer later in life, especially in cases of hereditary retinoblastoma. *See also* CANCER *and* CROSS-EYE.

Retractor

Surgical instrument that keeps the edges of an operating site (especially an incision) open, including skin, muscle, and other tissue, in order to give the surgeon open access during an operation.

Types of retractors include abdominal retractors, anal retractors used for hemorrhoidectomies, and iris retractors used for vitrectomies and other eye operations. For large operating areas such as the abdomen, retractors feature many blades, prongs, clamps, and rods to keep the area open. Retractors may be self-retaining or held in place by nurses. *See also* SURGERY.

Retrobulbar Neuritis

Inflammation of the optic nerve behind the eyeball.

Retrobulbar neuritis is swelling and deterioration of the myelin sheath covering the optic nerve, resulting in pain and impaired functioning of the nerve. It may be caused by a viral infection, an autoimmune disease, or multiple sclerosis.

Symptoms include sudden vision or color vision loss in one eye and pain upon movement of the eye.

Treatment may include corticosteroids to reduce inflammatory damage. Autoimmune diseases, such as systemic lupus erythematosus, are associated with a poorer prognosis. *See also* AUTOIMMUNE DISORDERS; CORTICOSTEROID DRUGS; VIRUSES; *and* VISION, LOSS OF.

Retrolental Fibroplasia

Nonperfusion of the retina in the eye of a premature infant.

The most severe form of retrolental fibroplasia can cause complications, such as scarring and retinal detachment.

The causes of the disease are not fully understood. Contributing factors include prematurity, illness, too much or too little oxygen, respiratory distress, infection, and congenital heart disease.

Treatment for the condition may include cryotherapy, laser surgery, and surgery to reattach the retina.

The majority of infants with a mild form of the disorder recover completely. Severe cases may cause blindness, progressive myopia, and cataracts. *See also* RETINA.

Retroperitoneal Fibrosis

Fibrous mass of inflamed tissue that grows behind the abdominal wall.

In retroperitoneal fibrosis, a benign growth puts pressure on the ureters (the tubes that conduct urine from the kidneys to the bladder). This pressure may cause eventual obstruction of the ureters, blocking the urine flow and potentially causing kidney failure. This condition occurs primarily in middle-aged men, and the cause is unknown.

Symptoms include abdominal pain, back pain, nausea, vomiting, loss of appetite, weakness, fatigue, and decreased urine output. Men may experience tenderness in the testicles, and women may experience painful menstruation.

Treatment requires the surgical removal of the growth in order to free the ureters. Short-term relief is possible by placing drains in the ureter. Corticosteroids may be effective in reducing the swelling, and thus the pressure, if surgery is impractical. *See also* CORTICOSTEROID DRUGS; KIDNEY; *and* URETER.

Retroverted Uterus

When the uterus is angled backward in the body rather than forward.

A retroverted uterus is usually a normal variation in anatomy. It is found in about 20 percent of women and sometimes occurs naturally with age, as the supporting ligaments in the pelvis become lax. The uterus may also become retroverted during pregnancy. In some cases, however, a retroverted uterus may be associated with an underlying disorder. Some disorders that may cause a tipped uterus include a uterine tumor; endometriosis, in which endometrial tissue forms outside the uterus; salpingitis, or inflammation of a fallopian tube; and pelvic inflammatory disease, or infection of the upper genital tract.

Symptoms. There are usually no symptoms, but backache, pelvis pain, heavy or prolonged menstrual bleeding, and prolonged bleeding after childbirth may occur. Fertility may also be decreased.

Treatment. Usually, no treatment is necessary. If symptoms are severe, a device to support the uterus (vaginal pessary) may be used. Women with symptoms should be examined for any underlying disorders. *See also* REPRODUCTIVE SYSTEM, FEMALE.

Rett's Syndrome

A genetic neurological disorder with symptoms similar to those of autism.

Rett's syndrome affects only females. Children afflicted with this disorder often exhibit behaviors similar to those of autistic children, such as repetitive hand movements, prolonged toe walking, body rocking, and sleep problems. The prevalence of Rett's syndrome is similar to that of autism: one in 10,000–15,000 births.

Cause. Rett's syndrome is an X-linked disorder, meaning that the gene responsible for the condition is located on one of the two X chromosomes. The particular gene that causes Rett's syndrome is involved in the production of methyl cytosine–binding protein. As a result of the disorder, excessive amounts of this protein are produced.

Symptoms. The first symptoms of Rett's syndrome do not appear until an affected child is between the ages of six and 18 months. Common characteristics of affected children include:

- shakiness of the torso and the limbs;
- unsteady, stiff-legged gait;
- breathing difficulties;
- seizures (approximately 80 percent of patients with Rett's syndrome also have epilepsy);

- teeth grinding and difficulty chewing;
- retarded growth and small head;
- mental retardation.

Prognosis. In most cases of Rett's syndrome, there is a regression in cognition, behavior, and social and motor skills. Affected individuals will need intensive care throughout their lifetime. *See also* AUTISM.

Reye's Syndrome

A syndrome of encephalopathy of unknown cause, and the associated liver degeneration.

Reye's syndrome has been associated with certain viruses and viral agents, such as influenza, varicella, toxins, and metabolic defects. It affects children of all ages and may produce changes in mental state, including coma. The syndrome usually follows an upper respiratory infection or chickenpox by one week.

Cause and Symptoms. The cause of Reye's syndrome is unknown, but there is believed to be an association between the condition and the administration of aspirin to children during a viral illness. The disease affects children of all ages. Symptoms include nausea, vomiting, mental changes, lethargy, confusion, loss of consciousness, and seizures. Other symptoms that occur include weakness in the arms and legs, paralysis, double vision, speech difficulty, and hearing loss. Vomiting is generally the first symptom to appear, followed by irritable and combative behavior, semiconsciousness, seizures and coma, and sometimes death.

Treatment. Methods used to treat Reye's syndrome include supportive care and the measures usually employed to reduce brain swelling. Intravenous fluids are usually given to keep the patient hydrated. Monitoring and support during a time of coma are necessary.

Prognosis. The average death rate from Reye's syndrome is 20 percent. The outcome for those who survive the acute period is good. There may be neurological complications, related to the severity of the coma. *See also* COMA *and* INFLUENZA.

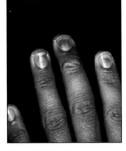

Reye's Syndrome. Nail discoloration, as shown above, is one of the symptons of Reye's Syndrome, a condition that usually follows an upper respiratory infection.

Rhabdomyolosis

An acute disease of skeletal muscle.

Rhabdomyolosis is most often caused by an injury that crushes muscle, although it can also be caused by polymyositis, a viral infection, and sometimes by excessive exercise. The result is progressive destruction of muscle tissue, during which myoglobin, the pigment that carries oxygen, is released into the bloodstream. Rhabdomyolosis leads to weakness or even paralysis of the muscle, but in most cases the muscle regenerates itself without the need for treatment. One kind of rhabdomyolosis is genetically linked. *See also* GENETICS; MUSCLE; *and* POLYMYOSITIS.

Rhabdomyosarcoma

Malignant tumor of skeletal muscle.

One kind of rhabdomyosarcoma occurs in young children and can affect many parts of the body, including the bladder, throat, or vagina, as well as the muscles. Another type of the disease occurs late in life, most often arising in a muscle of an arm or leg. Microscopic examination of the diseased area shows poorly differentiated cells with abnormally large nuclei. Untreated, the cancer can spread rapidly to nearby tissues. Rhabdomyosarcoma is treated with surgery to remove the tumor, radiation therapy, and chemotherapy. *See also* CANCER.

Rheumatic Fever

Allergic reaction to an untreated streptococcus infection, causing an autoimmune attack on the joints and heart.

Rheumatic fever is an allergic reaction in which the body's immune system attacks the heart valve, the joints, and the skin. If the streptococcus infection causing the reaction is treated promptly with antibiotics, there is less likelihood of the development of rheumatic fever. The most vulnerable age group is children from five to 15 years of age. Rheumatic fever is much less common in the United States than it is in developing countries.

Symptoms of rheumatic fever typically do not develop until several weeks after the patient has recovered from a sore throat. The patient's joints become hot and painful with swelling, and the pain may move from joint to joint. There may be a recurrence of fever, chest pain, heart palpitations, jerky movements, and a rash. The pain and fever usually subside after two weeks to a month. Shortness of breath, nausea, vomiting, stomachache, and cough are other symptoms. If the victim survives, he or she may have permanent heart valve damage, which can be exacerbated later in life. *See also* ANTIBIOTIC DRUGS; HEART, DISORDERS OF; *and* HEART VALVE.

Rheumatism

Term describing pain and stiffness in the joints and muscles.

More of a colloquialism than an actual medical condition, rheumatism is a term often used to describe any kind of pain or stiffness in the muscles or joints, from minor aches to pain that is actually related to disorders such as rheumatoid arthritis or arthritis. *See also* ARTHRITIS; OSTEOARTHRITIS; *and* RHEUMATOID ARTHRITIS.

Rheumatoid Arthritis

Form of arthritis that causes joints to become swollen and painful.

Rheumatoid arthritis is the result of an autoimmune disease which attacks the body's own tissues and systems. Overproduction of white blood cells, which usually fight disease, can cause an area of the body, in this case a joint, to become inflamed. The joint becomes swollen, painful, and stiff, and the cartilage is slowly destroyed.

Incidence. Rheumatoid arthritis affects approximately 2.5 million Americans per year, and 60 percent of those diagnosed are women. The risk in women, however, is

Resources on Arthritis
Lorig, Kate, and James F. Fries, Maureen R. Gecht, *The Arthritis Helpbook: A Tested Self-Management Program for Coping with Arthritis and Fibromyalgia* (2000); Costill, David L., *Inside Running: Basics of Sports Physiology* (1986); Shlotzhauer, Tammi L., *Living with Rheumatoid Arthritis* (1993); American Physical Therapy Association, Tel. (800) 999-APTA, Online: www. apta.org; Arthritis Foundation, Tel. (800) 283-7800, Online: www.arthritis.org; Nat. Osteoporosis Found., Tel. (800) 223-9994, On-line: www.nof. org; https:// public1.med. cornell.edu/ cgi; www.nycornell.org/ medicine/cp/index.html.

slightly lower among those who have become pregnant. Rheumatoid arthritis usually begins in young adulthood, with the onset in the majority of cases between the ages of 20 and 45.

Causes. There is no known cause of rheumatoid arthritis, but there does seem to be some indication that genetics, and possibly certain types of infections, may be involved. It is possible that certain genes instigate an attack on the collagen that makes up protein in the joints, because they mistake it for a virus. The intestinal bacteria, *Escherichia coli,* has also been linked to attacks of rheumatoid arthritis.

Symptoms. Rheumatoid arthritis can affect any joint, but the most commonly affected areas are the fingers, wrists, shoulders, hips, and knees. The severity of the disease varies; some patients experience only mild stiffness and swelling, while in others the joints swell to the point of deformity and loss of mobility. The onset of rheumatoid arthritis is gradual and may begin with nonspecific aches and pains; the feeling has been compared with the body aches that precede common flu viruses. Rheumatoid arthritis differs from osteoarthritis in that morning stiffness can last over an hour, and stiffness can set in for any length of time during which a body part is immobile. The condition is suspected if this type of pain persists for over six weeks. The swollen joints may feel warm to the touch; and in some cases, small blood vessels may swell, forming nodules or tiny bumps that can be felt right under the skin. A person may also experience excessive fatigue due to anemia, which is a common side affect of rheumatoid arthritis.

Diagnosis. If these symptoms occur for more than six weeks, x-rays will be taken to confirm the presence of rheumatoid arthritis. Blood tests can also check for the presence of rheumatoid factor antibodies.

Treatment. There is currently no cure for rheumatoid arthritis, but there are ways to manage the pain and live with the disease. The first course of action is generally a combination of drugs that reduce the inflammation around the joints, decreasing pain and improving mobility. These drugs tend to lose their effectiveness over time, so there is a progression from the use of non-steroidal anti-inflammatory drugs (NSAIDs) to the use of slow-acting antirheumatic drugs (SAARDs). Some experts are now urging an approach that begins directly with the antirheumatic drugs, sometimes in combination with the NSAIDs, but there are dangerous side effects with this approach. The combination can be overly toxic for some patients, and there is a danger in overtreating what may be a mild case of rheumatoid arthritis. For more extreme cases of rheumatoid arthritis, a doctor might use immunosuppressants, which suppress the immune system, or corticosteroids, which halt inflammation. Drug therapy is best determined by a physician who knows the patient's individual case.

Occupational therapy is another form of treatment to help the patient learn how to handle everyday tasks performed with the arms and hands. Physical therapy can help a patient relearn how to move around more easily.

For severe cases of rheumatoid arthritis, a joint that has become deformed or immobile may be surgically replaced with an artificial joint. *See also* ARTHRITIS *and* JOINT.

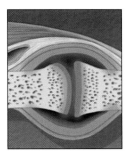
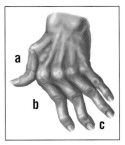

Rheumatoid Arthritis. The effects of rheumatoid arthritis (top) can progress to a degree that is crippling. Deformities distinctive to late stage rheumatoid arthritis (bottom), are exhibited by the hand: (a) boutonniere deviation of the thumb; (b) ulnar deviation of the bones or hand; (c) swan-neck deviation of the fingers. Some of these deformities occur because muscles and tendons on one side of the joint overpower those on the other side, pulling the bones out of alignment.

For background information on rheumatoid arthritis, see ARTHRITIS AND JOINT. *Related material can be found in* ANEMIA; ANTIRHEUMATIC DRUGS; AUTOIMMUNE DISORDERS; GENE; GENETICS; AND NONSTEROIDAL ANTIINFLAMMATORY DRUGS. *See also* ALTERNATIVE MEDICINE AND MASSAGE.

Rheumatoid Arthritis, Juvenile

Also known as juvenile chronic polyarthritis, or JRA

Chronic inflammatory disease with an onset beginning before age 16, causing joint or connective tissue damage.

Juvenile rheumatoid arthritis (JRA) is a complicated disease that is usually broken down into five groups based on the symptoms of patients. In the first group, many joints are involved and there is a positive rheumatoid factor. In the second, many joints are involved and there is a negative rheumatoid factor. In the third, few joints are involved and there is a positive antinuclear antibody. In the fourth group, few joints are involved and there is a positive HLA B27 surface antigen. The fifth group is systemic JRA (JRA throughout the whole body). Systemic JRA affects 20 percent of those with juvenile arthritis.

Incidence. A family history of JRA is a risk factor in developing the disorder. A recent rubella infection or vaccination may also trigger JRA.

Symptoms. General symptoms of JRA include joint stiffness upon waking, limited range of motion, slow growth rate, swelling or pain in the joints, fever, rash, and nodules just below the skin. In the two types of JRA in which only a few joints are involved, eye problems also occur. These include eye pain, red eyes, photophobia (sensitivity to light), and visual changes. Other symptoms of JRA may include chest and abdominal pain and shortness of breath.

Treatment. Because JRA is a long-term, chronic disease, treatment is designed to preserve mobility. Affected patients may take aspirin, nonsteroidal anti-inflammatory agents (NSAIDS), corticosteroids, topical ophthalmic corticosteroids, mydriatics, gold therapy, or chloroquine agents. Physical therapy and exercise may also help patients learn how to move more easily and with less pain. In the most severe cases of JRA, surgical joint replacement may be necessary. *See also* ARTHRITIS; RHEUMATOID ARTHRITIS; *and* THERAPY.

Rheumatology

Field of medicine concerned with diseases of the joints, muscles, and connective tissues.

Rheumatologists work to understand causes, development, and treatment for rheumatological disorders. Their work may include the use of x-rays, blood tests, and examination of muscle and joint functionality. Once a rheumatological disorder has been diagnosed, treatment will vary according to the disease. Such treatment ranges from simple rest to drug therapy or surgery. *See also* RHEUMATOID ARTHRITIS.

Rh Immune Globulin

Also known as RhoGam reflux

Vaccine that attacks red blood cells that are Rh positive.

This vaccine is administered to Rh negative women bearing children of Rh positive fathers after the birth of a child, in order to prevent the mother's body from developing antibodies against an Rh positive child's blood in subsequent pregnancies. The globulin is produced by injecting Rh negative volunteers with Rh positive blood. They develop antibodies to the Rh positive blood, and their blood is concentrated into a serum for injection into an unsensitized mother. The antibodies destroy the child's red blood cells in the mother's blood supply, so the mother won't develop antibodies of her own. *See also* GAMMA GLOBULIN.

Rh Incompatibility

When an Rh negative mother produces antibodies that attack the blood of an Rh positive fetus.

The Rh factor refers to a protein on the surface of red blood cells. If present, the blood is typed Rh positive; if absent, it is typed Rh negative. Fifteen to twenty percent of the general population does not carry the Rh protein and is therefore typed Rh negative. Except for potential transfusion problems, the Rh factor has relatively little effect on a person's general health.

Causes. However, when an Rh positive father and an Rh negative mother conceive an Rh positive child, an incompatibility between the mother and the child may develop. During the first pregnancy, the child's circulatory system is kept separate from the mother's; the mother doesn't develop antibodies against the child, and all is well. But if the mother's blood is exposed to the child's blood—as may occur during amniocentesis, miscarriage, or childbirth—the mother may become sensitized and produce antibodies against the child's blood. The first child is safe, since the sensitization takes place too late to do any damage. But once the mother is sensitized, there is always the chance that the mother's antibodies will cross into the placenta and attack the fetus's red blood cells in later pregnancies with Rh positive children.

Symptons. If Rh incompatibility is suspected, the mother's blood can be tested to see if she has produced antibodies to the Rh positive blood. If she has, the danger to the child is very real. The fetus or newborn child may be jaundiced or suffer heart failure, anemia, brain damage, or death.

If the mother has been sensitized by an earlier birth, the fetus must be monitored carefully. If he or she shows serious evidence of blood disease, a transfusion may be prescribed for the fetus while still in the womb. The transfusions will be repeated every couple of weeks until about the 33rd week of pregnancy, at which time labor is induced or the child is delivered by Caesarean section. One last transfusion is administered to the child after birth. Even if no transfusions were given before birth, the newborn will be transfused with fresh blood to ensure that no damage is inflicted on the child's red blood cells.

If the mother has not been sensitized, she will probably be given an injection of a globulin called RhoGam, which contains antibodies to the Rh factor. The antibodies will destroy any of the child's red blood cells that have migrated to the mother, so the mother won't need to develop antibodies of her own. Sensitivity will have been prevented, and this child and possible later Rh positive children will be safe. RhoGam injections are normally given 28 weeks into a pregnancy and shortly after delivery. Statistics indicate that this treatment is almost 100 percent successful in preventing sensitization. However, RhoGam offers no help if the mother is already sensitized, either from an earlier pregnancy or from a blood transfusion. In addition, in one to two percent of cases in which RhoGam was administered, the mother still becomes sensitized to the Rh positive blood. In these cases the sensitization probably preceded the injection.

Treatment. The 28-week injection of RhoGam to the Rh negative mother when the father is Rh positive has become standard practice in the United States even when the Rh status of the child is not known. The RhoGam is a protection for future children, not the current pregnancy; so if this child is the last one planned by the mother, the injection serves no purpose. Further, there is a small chance that the vaccine may be injurious to the fetus or the mother because of AIDS or another contamination. Thus, the administration of RhoGam to Rh negative mothers impregnated by Rh positive fathers should not be accepted without careful consideration of the risks and potential rewards.

Background material in Rh Incompatibility can be found in Blood Type and Pregnancy. For further information, see AMNICENTESIS; ANEMIA; ANTIBODY; CHILDBIRTH; CIRCULATORY SYSTEM; GAMMA GLOBULIN; HEART FAILURE; AND TRANSFUSION, AUTOLOGOUS. *See also birth defects for more on consequences of untreated Rh Incompatibility.*

Rhinitis

Inflammation of nasal passages.

The nasal passages allow air to enter the body and travel to the lungs. These passages are lined with mucous membranes that help to filter, warm, and moisten the air entering the body. When an infection or irritation is present, the nasal passages can become inflamed. This can cause nasal congestion due to fluid build-up or nasal discharge when the fluid flows out.

TYPES

There are three common types of rhinitis:

Allergic Rhinitis. One of the most common causes of rhinitis, allergies affect many people every year. Dust, molds, pollens, animal hair, and animal dander are common triggers of allergies. A person with allergic rhinitis will develop an overreaction to these substances; when they enter the body, the immune system produces extra antibodies, causing inflammation of the mucous membranes and excess fluid production.

Vasomotor Rhinitis. This form of rhinitis is an oversensitivity to a variety of stimuli. The nose may react and become inflamed by such diverse triggers as smoke, certain smells, temperature changes, or even emotions.

Viral Rhinitis. Colds, flu, and many other viral infections that affect the nose and throat can also lead to inflammation of the nasal passages.

TREATMENT

Avoidance of the irritant is the best prevention against allergic rhinitis. Severe cases may require regular medication. Viral rhinitis will clear up on its own, although symptoms can be relieved with over-the-counter medications. *See also* ALLERGY.

For background material on rhinitis, see Nose and Respiratory Tract Infection. Further information can be found in ALLERGY; ANTIBODY; IMMUNE RESPONSE; INFECTIOUS DISEASE; NASAL CONGESTION; *and* NASAL DISCHARGE. *See also Rhinitis, Allergic for more on that type of rhinitis.*

Rhinitis, Allergic

Also known as hay fever

A common respiratory allergy.

As in other allergies, in allergic rhinitis (also called hay fever), the immune system reacts to a relatively innocuous substance, such as pollen, as if it were a foreign invader. When pollen is inhaled, a sensitized type of white blood cells called B cells (also known as plasma cells), release a type of antibodies called IgE. These antibodies combine with mast cell receptors in the nasal passages. The mast cells trigger the release of histamine, which causes the blood vessels to dilate and become more permeable. This produces the congestion, increased fluid output, and itchy feelings in the respiratory pathways, and often eyes and ears, commonly associated with hay fever.

Symptoms of hay fever include nasal congestion, itchy eyes and throat (and sometimes ears), sneezing, and coughing.

Treatment. Mild cases of hay fever can be treated with antihistamines. For more severe cases, nasal sprays and eye drops can provide relief, although it is important to avoid chronic use of these substances. Immunotherapy, better known as allergy shots, may also be recommended.

Prevention. Avoidance of all known allergens is the best way to prevent hay fever. This involves limiting the amount of time spent outdoors when the specific plant is in bloom. Air conditioning is useful for preventing hay fever as well. *See also* ALLERGY.

Rhinophyma

Enlarged or bulbous red nose once thought to be caused by excessive alcohol consumption, occurring primarily in middle-aged and elderly men.

It is now known that rhinophyma is totally unrelated to alcohol consumption. Instead, it is classified as a form of advanced rosacea (a skin disorder affecting the nose and cheeks).

Symptoms. Rhinophyma results in an inflammation of the nose, thickening of the skin, enlargement of the blood vessels, and an overproduction of oil by the sebaceous glands.

Treatment. The only effective treatment for advanced stages of rhinophyma is a surgical procedure in which the excess tissue is removed from the nose, allowing the skin to heal normally. In early stages, rhinophyma may respond to topical and oral antibiotics, specifically tetracyclines. Persons suffering from this condition should avoid spicy foods, alcohol, sun exposure, heat exposure, and caffeine. *See also* ANTIBIOTIC DRUGS *and* ROSACEA.

Rhinoplasty

Also known as a "nose job"

Surgical procedure that enhances the appearance of the nose by reshaping the cartilage and bone beneath the skin.

Getting the nose "fixed" is usually done for cosmetic reasons or to correct an injury or defect such as a deviated septum.

During the operation, the plastic surgeon breaks the patient's nose and resets it. The aim is usually to make the nose smaller, straighter, and narrower.

Using a local or general anesthetic, the doctor enters through the nostrils and makes incisions inside the nose to avoid creating visible scars. The doctor shaves and shapes cartilage and bone, sometimes using grafts, and alters the septum, which is the vertical wall that divides the nose, if it is necessary or if the patient's breathing ability is impaired by a deviated septum.

After the operation, the nostrils are packed to absorb blood, and the nose is bandaged for about a week. The procedure causes considerable bruising, so it will take weeks for the new appearance to be fully appreciated. *See also* ANESTHESIA, GENERAL; ANESTHESIA, LOCAL; *and* COSMETIC SURGERY.

Rib, Fractured

A break in one or more of the ribs.

The most common causes of a fractured rib are a direct blow or fall. Rib fractures are extremely painful, with swelling and tenderness in the area of the break.

Most rib fractures are clean breaks, where the ends of the broken bone remain in alignment and can heal on their own without complications. Patients may simply be given painkillers and instructed to hold the injured side when breathing deeply. If the bone end splinters or is displaced, there is a chance that it can pierce a lung or the spleen. These cases may require an operation in which the ribs are wired into place to avoid damage to the organs. *See also* FRACTURE.

Riboflavin

Also known as vitamin B$_2$

A vitamin compound essential to the body's metabolism in oxidation-reduction reactions and energy production.

In addition to its key role in metabolism, riboflavin is also necessary to the maintenance of nerve sheaths, the cornea, mucous membranes, and the skin. A deficiency of riboflavin can cause disorders of the skin and mucous membranes, can make the eyes sensitive to light, and can cause cataracts and anemia. Good sources of riboflavin include dairy products, meat, liver, fish, leafy green vegetables, and whole or enriched grains. *See also* NUTRITION.

Rickets

Disease caused by inadequate calcification of the bones, occurring primarily in children.

There are several types of rickets. Nutritional rickets, caused by a diet deficient in vitamin D, is rare in the United States. However, incidence increases in children who are fed a strict vegetarian diet or have been breast-fed long after birth without nutritional supplementation. Nutritional rickets is more common in developing countries, particularly in places where children are kept indoors for protection from sun, so that sufficient vitamin D from sunlight is not synthesized.

The other two forms of rickets, vitamin D–dependent rickets and vitamin D–resistant rickets, are rarer and are thought to have a genetic basis.

Symptoms include enlarged ends of the joints, bowed legs or knock-knees, and curved spines. Infants may demonstrate restlessness and soft skulls with fontanelles ("soft spots") that are slow to close.

Treatment. Vitamin D therapy can improve the condition of most children with rickets, except for those with vitamin D–resistant rickets, who are treated with large doses of calcitriol and phosphate. *See also* FONTANELLE.

Resources on Riboflafin and Nutrition

Groff, James L. and Sareen S. Gropper, *Advanced Nutrition and Human Metabolism* (1999); Heimburger, Douglas C. and R. L. Weinsier, *Handbook of Clinical Nutrition* (1997); Hendler, Sheldon Saul, *The Doctor's Vitamin and Mineral Encyclopedia* (1990); Machlin, Lawrence J., *Handbook of Vitamins* (1991); Rivlin, Richard S. *Riboflavin* (1992); Shils, Maurice E., et al., *Modern Nutrition in Health and Disease* (1999); American Dietetic Association, Tel. (800) 366-1655, Online: www.eatright.org; Center for Nutrition Policy and Promotion, Tel. (202) 418-2312, Online: www.usda.gov/cnpp; Food and Drug Admin., Tel. (888) INFOFDA, Online: www.fda.gov; www.nycornell.org/medicine/nutrition/index.html.

Rickettsia

Genus of bacteria responsible for a range of human illnesses.

Rickettsia are a type of parasitic microorganism that resemble both bacteria and viruses. Rickettsia cause many diseases and are usually transmitted by exoparasites: fleas, lice, mites, and ticks. Illnesses caused by Rickettsia tend to be sudden and have varying symptoms, though the symptom they have in common is the blockage of blood vessels.

Among the diseases caused by rickettsia bacteria are epidemic typhus (transmitted by lice), endemic typhus (transmitted by rodent-borne fleas), Rocky Mountain spotted fever (transmitted by ticks), scrub typhus (transmitted by rodent-borne mites), and trench fever (transmitted by lice). Diagnosis is usually made through blood antibody tests. Illnesses caused by rickettsia are treated with broad-spectrum antibiotics, such as tetracycline drugs or chloramphenicol, which specifically targets rickettsia. Such diseases are best prevented through the use of insecticides or eradication of vectors (the animals that transmit the illnesses). *See also* INSECTS AND DISEASE; RATS AND DISEASE; ROCKY MOUNTAIN SPOTTED FEVER; TRENCH FEVER; *and* TYPHUS.

Rigidity

Increased tone or inflexibility in one or more of the muscles.

Rigidity describes the condition in which the muscles become exceedingly tight and resist bending. This causes the part of the body that these muscles serve to become stiff and unyielding. Causes of rigidity include an injured or diseased muscle, arthritic attack to a nearby joint, a neurological disorder (such as Parkinson's disease) or the constriction of the overlying abdominal muscle in the instance of an inflamed peritoneum. Fibromyalgia, a musculoskeletal disorder, can result in muscle stiffness and pain. *See also* MUSCLE.

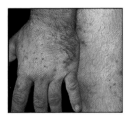

Ringworm.
This is a picture of ringworm, *tinea corporis,* on the hand and leg. *Tinea corporis* is a fungal infection of the skin. Ringworm is not seen as frequently in adults as in children, but when conditions are conducive to growth, the fungus can flourish.

Rigor

Condition of hardness or stiffening in muscles and joints.

Stiffening of the muscles and joints may have several causes. The process occurs as the result of the depletion of ATP, a constituent of all living cells that provides energy. This results in the formation of links between the proteins actin and myosin.

The most common form of rigor occurs shortly after death. Known as rigor mortis, this stiffening of the body continues for hours after death. The pace of the stiffening is characteristic and may be used by forensic scientists, along with other factors, to accurately estimate the time of death. *See also* FORENSIC MEDICINE.

Ringworm

Fungal infection of the skin.

Ringworm is a highly contagious fungal infection that appears most often on the scalp, arms, chest, legs, and back. It is marked by red, ring-shaped patches with clear areas in the center. Ringworm is transmitted by contact with infected people or their possessions, such as combs, brushes, clothing, or towels. The condition is treated with over-the-counter antifungal creams that are rubbed on the skin. If the fungus attacks the scalp, a special shampoo and a prescription oral antifungal medication, such as griseofulvin, may be used to treat the infection. *See also* FUNGAL INFECTIONS.

Ritodrine

Muscle relaxant used to delay preterm labor.

Ritodrine must be administered in the hospital, and the patient should be carefully monitored for side effects. The drug can cause an increased heart rate if administered intravenously. Other side effects of this drug include tremors, palpitations, nausea, vomiting, chest pain, and breathlessness. *See also* PREMATURITY.

Rocky Mountain Spotted Fever

Acute bacterial disease transmitted by ticks.

Rocky Mountain spotted fever is caused by *Rickettsia rickettsii* bacteria, transmitted by the wood tick and the dog tick. The illness usually occurs in the spring and summer months, with an incubation period of two to sixteen days. Once a victim has been bitten, the bacteria spread through the bloodstream and lymphatic system.

Symptoms. Early symptoms of the disease include headache and fever. After two or three days, a blotchy, rose-colored rash appears on the wrists and ankles, changing to dark red and brown as it spreads over the rest of the body.

Thrombosis (blood clot) in the blood vessels also occurs, produced by the invasion of blood vessel cells by the rickettsial organisms. The rickettsia severely damage the lining of the blood vessels, causing the injured vessels to leak, producing potentially lethal hemorrhaging (rupturing of the blood vessels). Loss of fluid from damaged blood vessels may lead to a significant drop in blood pressure, and decreasing blood flow to the kidneys sometimes results in renal (kidney) failure. Untreated, the disease may affect the brain, causing encephalitis or meningoencephalitis.

Diagnosis is usually based on the presence of a rash and probability of tick bite, confirmed through blood testing.

Treatment and Prevention. Rocky Mountain spotted fever is treated with antibiotics, usually tetracycline or chloramphenicol. The disease may be prevented by avoiding tick-infested areas, wearing protective clothing, and using insect repellent. *See also* ENCEPHALITIS; RICKETTSIA; TETRACYCLINE DRUGS; *and* TICKS AND DISEASE.

> *Background information on rocky mountain spotted fever can be found in* BACTERIA; INFECTIOUS DISEASE; AND TICKS AMD DISEASES. *For related material, see* ENCEPHALITIS; FEVER; HEADACHE; HEMORRHAGE; RENAL FAILURE; AND RICKETTSIA. *See also Antibiotic Drugs.*

Rolfing

Also known as structural integration

Form of bodywork that aims to realign the body to improve the flow of energy and balance.

Rolfing was developed by the American biochemist Ida Rolf, whose own respiratory condition was remedied by an osteopath who repositioned her rib, improving the functioning of her respiratory system. This incident and Rolf's exposure to hatha yoga led her to the idea that would form the basis of her bodywork technique: the structure of the body is essential to the overall functioning and well-being of the person.

Rolfing involves stretching, manipulating, and applying pressure to the fascial tissues—connective tissue covering the muscles—to realign the body and restore balance. Rolfing usually consists of ten sessions, each session focusing on a different body part. Movement exercises and counseling have also been integrated into the therapy. *See also* ALTERNATIVE MEDICINE.

Root-Canal Treatment

Dental procedure that saves the outer tooth when the inside is irreparably diseased.

The goal of dentistry is to save natural teeth whenever possible. In the case of a tooth whose fleshy inside (pulp) has been badly diseased, root-canal treatment is necessary to save the tooth.

Most people who have never had a root-canal procedure think that it is very uncomfortable. In fact, with proper anesthetics, there is little discomfort during the treatment, although the mouth may be sore for a brief time afterward. However, root-canal treatment is a lengthy process, which is why it is often divided into several visits to the dentist.

FIRST VISIT
Once a dentist has determined that the procedure is appropriate, the first step is to remove the diseased dental pulp and root of the tooth and fill the resulting cavity. All

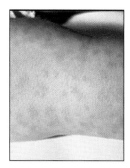

Rocky Mountain Spotted Fever.
This is the appearance of Rocky Mountain spotted fever on the hands and forearms. The rash starts on the wrists and ankles and later spreads to the trunk. It is caused by a bacteria transmitted to humans by a tick bite.

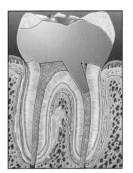

Root Canal.
Above is a diagram of a root canal. In this dental procedure the diseased dental pulp is removed, and the resulting cavity is filled.

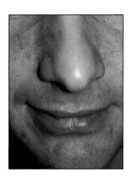

Rosacea.
Rosacea has multiple phases, beginning with flushing of the skin followed by redness, followed by the development of small blood vessels visible in the skin. This is the second stage and is exhibited by this individual's red blisters located on the cheeks, nose, and chin. Underlying redness (erythema) and small blood vessels are also seen.

> ### Rubber Dam
>
> When a dentist works on a patient's teeth, some of the material used is minuscule and could be inhaled or swallowed if it were not for the rubber sheet that is inserted before work begins. Rubber dams are commonly used during intricate procedures such as root-canal treatment.

of the dental pulp must be emptied, otherwise germs or bacteria may be left behind. The dentist cleans out the dental pulp and disinfects the space that is left in the tooth. A temporary filling is then placed in the cavity, and the dentist observes whether any infection remains.

SECOND VISIT
At the next visit, the temporary filling is removed. Assuming there is no further infection, the area to be filled is cleaned once again, and a permanent filling material is inserted. This filling is sealed to prevent the entry of bacteria.

THIRD VISIT
The remaining tooth may appear perfectly normal, but it has been weakened by the removal of the original pulp. Left alone, it is likely to break. Thus, the restorative dentist or prosthodontist will prepare the tooth for a jacket, or crown. A mold of the remaining tooth structure is used to make a crown that will fit securely over the tooth. A temporary crown is used while the permanent crown is made.

FOURTH VISIT
During the fourth and final visit, the dentist fits the crown over the remaining tooth structure, checking for fit and shaping the crown if necessary. Once a good fit has been established, the crown is cemented into place and functions like a natural tooth. Crowns are usually made of porcelain to match the other teeth, but if the tooth is not particularly visible, gold is an equally durable alternative. Assuming the infection has been completely cleared out, the crown can last for many years. *See also* CARIES, DENTAL.

Rorschach Test

Test in which a subject is asked to interpret inkblots. These interpretations are then used to analyze the patient's emotions, attitudes, and inner conflicts.

The Rorschach test was first devised by the Swiss psychiatrist Hermann Rorschach in the early 20th century. It was one of the earliest forms of personality tests, but is only of value in the hands of a trained practitioner. Even then, the highly subjective aspects of the test and the analysis makes this a test of questionable validity. *See also* PSYCHIATRY.

Rosacea

Skin disorder that causes recurrent inflammation of the cheeks, nose, chin, or forehead.

Rosacea may cause skin redness, swelling, increased prominence of blood vessels, and skin eruptions with an appearance similar to that of acne. It involves enlargement of the blood vessels just under the skin. The condition occurs most frequently in fair-skinned people, and men are usually more severely affected than women.

Symptoms of rosacea usually begin between the ages of 30 and 50, and may include a rash or red areas on the face, a tendency to blush easily, a red nose, acne-like skin eruptions, and a burning or stinging feeling on the face.

Treatment involves controlling redness and inflammation. Patients should avoid agents that cause them to flush (commonly alcohol, hot foods and beverages, caffeine, and sunlight), Treatment with topical or oral agents may be necessary. *See also* ACNE.

Roseola Infantum

Also known as exanthem subitum

Acute disease of infants and children, characterized by fever and skin rash.

Roseola infantum is most commonly found in children between the ages of six months and two years. It is a frequent cause of febrile seizures in children of this age.

Cause. Recently, the cause of roseola has been found to be human herpesvirus 6. The incubation period is from five to 15 days, and the disease is most commonly found in the spring and fall.

Symptoms. The disease begins with a high fever. Between the second and fourth day after infection, the fever falls dramatically and a rash appears on the limbs, trunk, and face.

Treatment. There is no determined treatment for roseola, as the disease usually resolves itself. Acetaminophen may be given for fever, and sedatives may be given to control convulsions. Physical activity should be restricted until the rash develops and the fever drops. *See also* HERPES; INFECTIOUS DISEASE.

Roundworm

Parasitic nematode worm causing a variety of human illnesses.

Roundworm infections are common in warm and temperate areas of the world. Most roundworms are found in soil and may be transmitted through the soil to humans. Generally, roundworms reside in, or migrate to, the intestine. Among the more common roundworms are *Enterobius vermicularis*, the pinworm that causes enterobiasis; *Ascaris lumbridoides*, a large intestinal roundworm causing ascariasis; *Necator* and *Ancylostoma*, two types of hookworms that cause ancylostomiasis; *Trichuris trichiura*, the whipworm that causes trichuriasis; *Strongyloides stercoralis*, which causes strongyloidiasis; and *Trichinella spiralis*, which causes trichinosis.

Roundworm infestations vary in nature, severity, mode of transmission, and treatments, depending on the specific roundworm involved.

• **Pinworm** infestation primarily affects children and causes itching in the rectal area and restless sleep.

• **Ascaria** infestations are usually the result of contact with human fecal matter. Larvae of this roundworm may invade the lungs and cause pneumonia, or (rarely) the large adult worms can clump together in large numbers and cause partial or total intestinal obstruction.

• **Hookworm** eggs are also passed in human feces, developing into infective larvae in the soil. When significant numbers of hookworms have reached the intestine, they may produce anemia.

• **Trichinosis** is an infection of tissues by the larvae of the roundworm *Trichinella spiralis*. The disease is produced by ingesting *T. spiralis* larvae in infected pork that has been insufficiently cooked.

Most roundworm infestations are detected in stool samples and are treated with antihelminthic drugs. *See also* PARASITE.

Rubella

Also known as German measles

Mild viral childhood infection.

A disease that is less contagious than measles, rubella is usually very mild and recovery is generally quick. However, the disease is dangerous for pregnant women who if infected during the first trimester of pregnancy, may miscarry, have a stillbirth, or give birth to a baby with birth defects. Once a person has recovered from rubella he or she is immune to the disease for life.

Symptoms. Rubella is transmitted by breathing in the small water droplets coughed or sneezed by an infected person. The disease can also be transmitted through close personal contact with an infected person. The incubation period (a period during which there are no symptoms) is two to three weeks after infection. For the first few days, the victim will feel mildly ill, with a low fever and swollen lymph nodes, followed by a rash of small pink spots that do not itch. The rash begins on the neck and face and quickly spreads to the rest of the body. It lasts for about three days. Adults may also experience joint pain, headache, loss of appetite, and a sore throat. The sufferer is contagious from five days before the rash appears until seven days after it is gone. Infected children should not be sent to school, nor

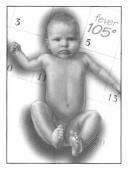

Roseola.
Roseola is an acute disease of infants and young children that is characterized by high fever followed by a rash that appears on the trunk, limbs, neck, and face.

Resources on Roundworm and Parasites
Despommier, Dickson D., et al., *Parasitic Disease* (1995); Donaldson, Raymond Joseph, ed., *Parasites and Western Man* (1979); Huff, Clay B., *A Manual of Medical Parasitology* (1943); Klein, Aaron E., *The Parasites We Humans Harbor* (1981); Nauss, Ralph Welty, *Medical Parasitology and Zoology* (1944); Grist, Norman R., et al., *Diseases of Infection: An Illustrated Textbook* (1992); Shaw, Michael, ed., *Everything You Need to Know About Diseases* (1996); Centers for Disease Contol and Prevention, Tel. (800) 311-3435, Online: www.cdc. gov; Infectious Disease Society of America, Tel. (703) 299-0200, Online: www.idsociety.org; www.nycornell.org/medicine/infectious/index.html.

Resources on Rubella and Infectious Diseases

Grist, Norman R., et al., *Diseases of Infection: An Illustrated Textbook* (1992);Shaw, Michael, ed., *Everything You Need to Know About Diseases* (1996); Silverstein, Alvin, *Measles and Rubella* (1997);* Centers for Disease Contol and Prevention, Tel. (800) 311-3435, Online: www.cdc.gov; Infectious Disease Society of America, Tel. (703) 299-0200, Online: www.idsociety.org; Nat. Institute of Allergy and Infectious Disease, Tel. (301) 496-5717, Online: www.niaid.nih.gov; Birth Defects Reseach for Children, Tel. (407) 895-0802, Online: www.birthdefects.org; www.nycornell.org/medicine/infectious/index.html

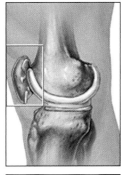

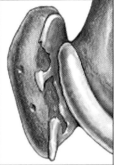

Runner's Knee.
The diagrams above show the rubbing of the kneecap (patella) against the end of the thigh bone. The friction caused by these bones can be very painful.

should they join in other play groups until they are no longer contagious.

Treatment. There is no medication that can treat rubella, as it is a viral disease. In addition, the symptoms of the disease are so mild that treatment is not generally necessary. Instead, treatment deals with the symptoms of rubella. Aspirin or acetaminophen may be given for headache and joint pain. It is important to remember not to give aspirin to children infected with rubella (or any other viral disease) as they may suffer Reye's syndrome, a disease caused by the interaction of aspirin with a virus in children. *See also* VIRUSES.

Rubin Test

A diagnostic procedure to determine whether or not the fallopian tubes are blocked.

When a couple cannot conceive a child, there may be any of a number of underlying causes, each of which may be treated differently. In some cases, a blockage in the fallopian tubes prevents the ova from reaching the uterus. To determine if this is the case, a Rubin test may be performed.

In a Rubin test, carbon dioxide is introduced into the uterus and fallopian tubes at fairly low pressure (less than 120 mm of mercury). If the fallopian tubes are not blocked, carbon dioxide passes through the fallopian tubes into the abdominal cavity, where it causes shoulder pain and may be seen with x-ray or fluoroscopy. If the fallopian tubes are blocked, the pressure in the uterus rises; a pressure of 200 or more indicates complete blockage, while a pressure between 120 and 130 indicates partial obstruction. *See also* INFERTILITY.

Running Injuries

Injuries commonly associated with jogging and running as regular exercise.

Enormous pressure is placed on feet and legs during running. The type and location of the resulting pain can identify the injury. Often, such injuries are preventable.

Preventing Running Injuries

To prevent running injuries, runners should wear footwear that complements the unique characteristics of their feet (flatfoot or inward-tilting ankles, for example). Footwear should be snug and provide adequate support and stability. Shoes should be replaced before the insole cushioning becomes exceedingly worn down. Long periods of running on an uneven surface increases stress on the ankles and knees. A proper running regimen includes warm-up exercises, preparing the body for strenuous activity. Both beginning and advanced runners should keep their routine and distance within reasonable limits.

TYPES

Stress Fractures. The metatarsal bones of the foot are particularly vulnerable to stress fractures, since they take the brunt of the push-off pressure during running. These fractures can be so fine that they are not visible in x-rays, but they can produce pain in the front of the foot during running.

Shin splints is a term used to refer to damage to the muscles that lie parallel to the shin (tibia). These muscles are located in the front and inner leg.

Tendinitis is a tear or inflammation in one of the tendons that control the movement of joints. The tendons most vulnerable to tendinitis are those that run from the calf to the back of the heel and those that run diagonally across the back of the knees.

Runner's knee is pain caused by the rubbing of the kneecap (patella) against the end of the thigh bone.

TREATMENT

Most running injuries will heal without treatment if the patient stops running for a given period of time, often weeks. If the patient does not stop running, the pain may subside quickly at first but will become intense and unremitting with time, signalling worsening of the condition.

For background reading on running injuries, see EXERCISE. *Related material can be found in* AEROBICS; ANAEROBIC; SHIN SPLINTS; STRESS FRACTURE; TENDONITIS; AND X-RAY. *See also* SPORTS INJURIES *and* SPORTS MEDICINE *for more on related injuries and treatment.*

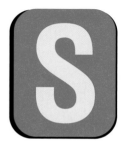

Saccharin

Artificial sweetener derived from petroleum.

Saccharin does not contain any calories and is safe for diabetics, since it does not affect their blood sugar. While it is heat stable, it lacks the texture of sugar and has a bitter aftertaste for some individuals.

Large quantities were once thought to increase the likelihood of bladder tumors in rats. This link was never proven, however, and in 2000 saccharin was removed from the FDA's list of carcinogens (cancer-causing agents). *See also* ARTIFICIAL SWEETENER.

Sacralgia

Discomfort in the sacrum, the triangular bone positioned at the bottom of the spine.

The sacrum is located below the lumbar vertebrae. It is formed by the union of five vertebrae and sits in the back of the pelvis. Sacralgia (pain in the sacrum) may be the result of the compression of a nearby spinal nerve. Generally, sacralgia is the consequence of a disk prolapse, the displacement of a disk from its normal position. In rare cases, the pain appears as a side effect of bone cancer. *See also* SPINAL CORD.

Sacralization

Fusion of the lowest lumbar vertebrae with the sacrum.

The sacrum is a large, triangular bone located at the bottom of the spine. The broad top of the triangle meets and moves with the last of the five bones of the spine (lumbar vertebrae) in the lower back.

Sacralization is usually present at birth. There are no symptoms, and the condition may be discovered only when x-rays are taken for an unrelated back problem. The sacrum and lumbar vertebrae may be fused together surgically to stabilize a displaced area, which occurs in spondylolisthesis or from disk prolapse. *See also* SPINAL CORD.

Sacroiliitis

Inflammation of the sacroiliac joint (located in the lower spine).

The sacrum is a fusion of the five lower vertebrae of the spine. It connects on either side to the right and left ilia. The sacroiliac joint provides a small amount of flexibility to the hips. If the joint is inflamed or the surfaces of the connected bones are roughened, considerable pain in the lower back, thigh, buttocks, and groin can result. If the cause of sacroiliitis is a bacterial infection, fever and malaise (a generalized feeling of sickness) can accompany the pain.

Treatment. Since the pain of sacroiliitis sometimes appears to derive from the spine in general, rather than from the sacroiliac joint itself, oftentimes surgery or other treatments are directed at the wrong area. Sacroiliitis may be treated with anti-inflammatory medications, corticosteroid injections, or, if the joint is infected by bacteria, antibiotic drugs. *See also* SPINAL CORD.

Sadism

Disorder in which the individual seeks and enjoys inflicting pain and abuse on others.

Sadism is often associated with the sexual pleasure experienced when inflicting pain on others. In such cases, the partner may be a masochist (a person who is sexually aroused by being the subject of abuse). If both receiving and inflicting pain causes arousal, the term sadomasochism applies. In almost all instances of sadism, aggression and control play an important role. Sadism is most often encountered in males and is accompanied by other sexual deviations and fetishistic behavior. Sadistic activities include beating, whipping, bond-age, and verbal abuse. Sadistic sexual behavior often results in physical harm, and sometimes in death. The act of rape, for instance, has a sadistic element at its core.

The term sadism is derived from the name of the French novelist the Marquis de Sade. *See also* MASOCHISM.

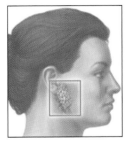

Salivary Gland.
The image above shows an exocrine gland in the mouth which produces saliva at the sight, smell, or taste of food.

Salivary Glands

Exocrine glands in the mouth that produce saliva.

The salivary glands are stimulated to produce saliva by the sight, smell, or taste of food. They normally respond within two to three seconds of such a stimulus, and over the course of a day they produce around three pints of saliva. There are three major pairs of salivary glands: the parotids, located in front of each ear; the submaxillary, located inside the lower jaw; and the sublingual, located under the tongue. There are also smaller salivary glands in the cheeks and the tongue.

Salivary glands may produce too much saliva when irritated by orthodontic appliances or if the digestive or nervous systems are disturbed. They may produce too little saliva as a result of certain drugs or a vitamin B deficiency. *See also* DIGESTIVE SYSTEM.

Salivation

Secretion of saliva by the salivary glands.

Salivary glands are exocrine glands—glands that secrete fluids into ducts that lead directly to an organ or the surface of the body. There are three pairs of salivary glands, one below the ears, one in the floor of the front of the mouth, and one toward the back of the mouth. These glands secrete saliva into ducts that lead into the mouth, a process known as salivation.

Function of Saliva. Saliva is composed mostly of water, but it also contains the enzyme amylase, which aids in digestion by helping to break down carbohydrates. In addition to its role in breaking down food, saliva makes swallowing possible by lubricating particles of food in the mouth. Saliva also keeps the mouth moist and allows the taste buds, which can be activated only by liquid substances, to operate.

Disorders. The salivary glands are operated by the parasympathetic nervous system, which, along with the sympathetic nervous system, makes up the autonomic nervous system. The sympathetic nervous

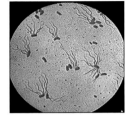

Salmonella.
The causative agent of typhoid fever is the bacterium *salmonella typhi,* shown above.

system slows down saliva production, while the parasympathetic nervous system activates the salivary glands. Thus, any disorder that affects the parasympathetic nervous system can affect the salivary glands.

Other factors that may cause the salivary glands to oversalivate are irritations in the mouth itself, such as mouth ulcers, inflammation of the esophagus (esophagitis), or dental problems, such as gingivitis (inflamed gums) or tooth decay (dental caries). Treatment of these disorders should be aimed at the underlying cause. *See also* AUTONOMIC NERVOUS SYSTEM; CANKER SORE; ESOPHAGITIS; GINGIVITIS; SALIVARY GLANDS; *and* TOOTH DECAY.

Salmonella

Toxic genus of bacteria that causes more cases of food poisoning than any other bacteria.

Salmonella tends to be found in food that is undercooked or prepared in unsanitary conditions. It can also be transmitted by pet turtles and lizards. All strains of salmonella are pathogenic to humans, although their toxicity varies. One form, *Salmonella typhi,* is responsible for typhoid fever.

Most frequently, salmonella infection occurs as a result of exposure to infected eggs or poultry, although other foods can harbor the bacteria. Animal and human feces also contain salmonella, which can be transmitted to humans through improper food handling.

Symptoms. Onset of symptoms occurs less than 24 hours after exposure. Symptoms may include abdominal pain, diarrhea, vomiting, and chills. The potential for severe dehydration exists.

Treatment of salmonella infection is aimed at replacing fluids lost through diarrhea. Antibiotic drugs are usually not necessary unless symptoms are severe.

Prevention. Salmonella thrives between 44° and 115°F, but cannot survive above 140°F for more than ten minutes. Proper food storage and preparation can thus prevent salmonella infection. *See also* BACTERIA; HYGIENE; *and* INFECTIOUS DISEASE.

Salpingectomy

Surgical removal of one or both fallopian tubes.

A salpingectomy may be performed to treat an infection of the fallopian tubes, to remove tumors or cysts, or to treat an ectopic pregnancy that has ruptured or is bleeding. A salpingectomy is also performed as a method of contraception, resulting in permanent sterilization, because it prevents passage of egg cells from the ovary to the uterus. Salpingectomy is also performed in conjunction with the removal of the ovaries and uterus. *See also* CONTRACEPTION; ECTOPIC PREGNANCY; *and* FALLOPIAN TUBE.

Salpingitis

Inflammation of the fallopian tubes, related to pelvic inflammatory disease (PID).

Salpingitis is caused by bacteria that enter the reproductive tract. Women most at risk for developing the condition are between the ages of 20 and 31 and have multiple sexual partners.

Symptoms include pain and tenderness in the lower abdomen, a foul-smelling vaginal discharge, fever, and heavy or irregular menstrual periods with severe cramps.

Complications. Left untreated, salpingitis may lead to the formation of adhesions, possibly resulting in infertility. It also increases the likelihood of an ectopic pregnancy. Very rarely, the infection can result in an abscess.

Treatment. Any sexually transmitted diseases causing salpingitis are treated with antibiotics. Surgery is sometimes performed to remove some of the adhesions. Very severe cases may require the removal of the fallopian tubes.

Prevention. Safer sexual practices reduce the risk of sexually transmitted diseases (STDs) and thus of salpingitis. Prompt treatment of STDs can reduce the risk of salpingitis. Regular gynecological screenings can catch the disease at an early stage, minimizing complications. *See also* SEXUALLY TRANSMITTED DISEASE.

Salpingo-oophorectomy

Surgical removal of one or both fallopian tubes.

Salpingo-oophorectomy may be performed to treat ovarian germ cell cancer; endometriosis; ovarian cysts; cancer of the ovaries, uterus, and placental tissue (choriocarcinoma); and infection and inflammation of the fallopian tubes (salpingitis). The operation is often performed at the same time as removal of the uterus and cervix (hysterectomy).

The procedure for salpingo-oophorectomy is simple and has few complications. The patient is put under general anesthesia, and the surgery is performed through an abdominal incision. Many gynecologists now utilize laparoscopic surgery, which minimizes surgical damage and decreases recovery time. *See also* FALLOPIAN TUBE; HYSTERECTOMY; *and* LAPAROSCOPY.

Salt

Also known as sodium chloride

Mineral compound composed of sodium and chloride ions.

Both sodium and chloride ions are necessary for the maintenance of the fluid balance in the body, and sodium plays a variety of regulatory roles. However, excess salt in the diet should be avoided by individuals who are predisposed to hypertension, or who suffer from heart disease or other conditions that cause fluid retention.

Table salt provides the major portion of sodium in the average American diet. Minimizing the use of salt during cooking and eating is an effective approach to limiting salt consumption. Many canned, packaged, pickled, cured, and fast foods contain high amounts of sodium, as do baked goods, which are made with leavening agents that contain sodium. Reducing consumption of these foods will also reduce the level of salt in the diet.

Consumers should be aware that any ingredient with sodium, salt, or soda in its name contains salt. *See also* ELECTROLYTES; HYPERTENSION; *and* SODIUM.

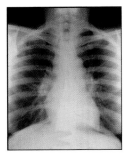

Sarcoidosis.
Sarcoidosis is a lung (pulmonary) disease. In the early stages, a chest x-ray, above, may show enlargement of lymph nodes in the center of the chest, near the heart.

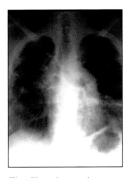

The film above shows advanced sarcoidosis, scarring of the lungs (the light streaking), and cavity formation (the dark areas in the upper right side of picture.

Sand Fly Bites

Bites from species of flies responsible for a number of diseases.

Sand flies can be found worldwide and possess long mouth parts adapted for sucking blood from a host. Many such insects can transmit human disease.

Phlebotomus fever is a viral ailment transmitted by a female *Phlebotomus papatasii* sand fly. Symptoms appear one to five days after exposure and include abdominal distress and dizziness, followed by chills and a rapid rise in body temperature.

Bartonellosis (caused by the *Bartonella bacilliformis* bacteria) is transmitted by several species of lutzomyia flies. Two forms of the illness exist. Oroya fever causes fever, weakness, headache, and bone and joint pain, followed by severe anemia and lymph node damage. Veruga peruana produces nodules on the face and limbs.

Visceral and cutaneous leishmaniasis are common diseases caused by a protozoan parasite transmitted by sand fly bite. The cutaneous form produces ulcers that resemble skin cancer or leprosy. Visceral leishmaniasis degrades the immune system and is potentially fatal.

Prevention. Use of insecticides, protective clothing, and netting in sleeping areas may offer defense against sand flies in endemic regions. Treatment is symptom- and disease-dependent. *See also* VECTOR.

Sanitary Napkin

Absorbent pad used to soak up blood during menstruation.

Sanitary napkins are made of layers of cotton or synthetic materials, with adhesive linings on the bottom that allow them to stick to the inside of underwear. They are made in various sizes and thicknesses for heavier or lighter blood flow. Sanitary napkins should be wrapped and disposed of properly. An alternative to the sanitary napkin is the tampon, which is inserted into the vagina. *See also* TAMPON.

Sarcoidosis

Granulomatous disease in which inflammation occurs in the lymph nodes, lungs, liver, eyes, skin, and other areas.

Sarcoidosis is rare in young children; it occurs more likely in adolescence. The disease mainly affects adults between the ages of 30 and 50.

Cause. The specific cause of sarcoidosis is not known. Some people may be genetically predisposed to the condition.

Incidence. The highest incidence of sarcoidosis is found among African Americans and Caucasians. Among African Americans, women are affected more often than men. Two out of every ten thousand people will contract the disease.

Symptoms. Sarcoidosis is characterized by fever, shortness of breath, cough, skin lesions, rash, headache, visual and neurological changes, swollen glands, enlarged liver and spleen, and dry mouth. Two other symptoms, fatigue and weight loss, are the most common symptoms among children with the disease. Other possible symptoms include decreased tearing, seizures, nosebleed, hair loss, and joint stiffness. Complications may include respiratory problems, glaucoma, and cardiac arrhythmia.

Treatment. Sarcoidosis is treated with corticosteroids, for up to two years if necessary. *See also* GENETICS.

Sarcoma

Malignant tumor of connective tissue.

A sarcoma is a type of cancer that arises in bone, cartilage, fibrous tissue, fat, or muscle. About one quarter of sarcomas arise in the bones, most often in an arm or leg. Sarcomas of soft tissues occur in many parts of the body. Sarcomas are named for the cells in which they originate. For example, a sarcoma arising in cartilage is called a chondrosarcoma, a sarcoma arising in fibrous connective tissue is referred to as a fibrosarcoma, and a sarcoma arising in fat cells is called a liposarcoma. *See also* CANCER.

Scab

Crusty formation of dried blood, pus, or other fluid over a break in the skin.

After the skin is damaged, a wound releases blood and pus. This combination of fluid dries and forms a crusty, protective layer over the damaged area. A scab will generally fall off in about ten days. The scab protects the wound or blister from infection while the injury heals. *See also* WOUND.

Scabies

Skin disease caused by a mite, characterized by an itchy rash.

Scabies is a disease produced by a parasite known as the itch mite. Mites infest the outer layers of the skin, and irritation is caused by a reaction to the mites' waste products. Infestations are usually found in folds of skin, such as between the fingers, under the arms, and in the lower buttock, nipple, breast, waist, thigh, and genital areas. Itching typically worsens at night.

Scabies is highly contagious, and is transmitted through contact with an infected person or object. Crowded or unsanitary conditions can help to spread the disease. Infested clothing may also transmit scabies. Institutions, including child care centers and nursing homes, are sometimes subject to outbreaks of scabies.

Symptoms of scabies include intense itching, commencing two to four weeks after initial infestation, and raised red bumps, which are the mites' burrows in the skin. Secondary bacterial infections may follow due to scratching of irritated skin.

Treatment. Scabies is treated with a lotion containing permethrin or lindane, which is applied over the entire body. A second application seven to ten days later is recommended. The disease produces a heightened sensitivity to the mite, and re-infestation may cause more severe symptoms, with onset occurring one to four days following re-exposure. *See also* ECTOPARA-SITES *and* MITES AND DISEASE.

Scaling, Dental

Professional removal of plaque from the surface of the teeth and gums.

Dental scaling is usually part of a dental examination and involves scraping plaque (a sticky coating made of saliva, bacteria, and food debris) off the teeth with specially designed instruments. After this is done, the teeth are cleaned and polished.

Periodic scaling is important because even the most thorough brushing and flossing cannot remove all plaque. Ideally, people should have their teeth cleaned professionally at least twice a year. *See also* PLAQUE, DENTAL.

Scalp

The skin and flesh of the head, usually covered with hair.

The scalp is distinctly different from other areas of skin in that it is directly connected to muscle. It is with this layer of muscle, running from the forehead to the top of the neck, that many human facial expressions are possible.

The scalp can be affected by a variety of disorders. These range from dandruff to hair loss, abnormal growths, and infections. *See also* DANDRUFF *and* HAIR GROWTH.

Scalpel

Surgical knife used in operations.

Scalpels are usually made of stainless steel or carbon steel. Hospitals are often supplied with disposable, sterile scalpels with preassembled stainless steel surgical blades mounted on plastic handles.

"Bloodless surgery" is increasingly being used instead of scalpels. Stanford University's computer-mediated stereotaxis radio-surgery system ("cyberknife") can destroy brain and spinal tumors without scalpels. The cyberknife is a robotic x-ray gun that shoots highly targeted radiation into tumors. *See also* SURGERY.

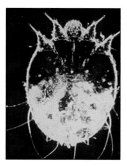

Scabies mite.
This is a highly magnified micrograph of the mite that causes scabies.

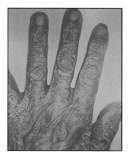

Scabies.
This is a photo of the rash and excoriation (rawness) from a scabies infection.

Scanning Techniques

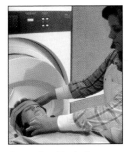

Scanning Techniques. Above, a woman's head is being prepared by a technician for a magnetic resonance imaging (MRI) test.

Diagnostic imaging of tissue, usually with the aid of radioactive substances.

Scanning techniques allow the physician to visualize the body's internal structures, as well as its metabolic processes, for the purpose of diagnosis. A sophisticated array of methods include noninvasive nonradioactive techniques, such as ultrasound scanning and magnetic resonance imaging (MRI), as well as techniques that use ionizing radiation (such as CT scans or PET scans).

Radionuclide Scanning. Radionuclide scanning makes use of radioactive tracers that are injected intravenously (or sometimes inhaled) and follow the blood flow though the body. Particular tracers have an affinity for particular organs or structures. The radioactive emission from the tracer is detected using a gamma camera or scintillation detector. Some cameras are able to produce computer-enhanced cross-sectional images through a process known as single photon emission computed tomography (SPECT).

Other Scanning Techniques. A more refined method, known as positron emission tomography, or PET, relies on a metabolite labeled with a positron-emitting radioisotope. This technique has been particularly useful in studies of the heart and brain metabolism. High-resolution scanning methods that avoid the use of radiation, particularly MRI, are becoming widely favored for their safety, painlessness, and image clarity. *See also* MRI; NONINVASIVE; PET SCANNING; *and* TRACER.

Scar

Tissue that forms as a healing response to injury to the skin.

Scars form after skin injuries, such those that occur after surgical incisions, wounds, vaccinations, burns, chickenpox, or acne. Most scars become less apparent after a few years. *See also* SCAB.

Scarlet Fever

Also known as scarlatina

Infection caused by group AB-hemolytic streptococcal bacteria.

Scarlet fever was once a deadly disease, but it is now easily treated. It occurs in a small percentage of people who contract strep throat. The bacteria responsible for scarlet fever produces a toxin that causes a rash on the neck and chest, and later on the rest of the body as well. The rash lasts for about three days, and peeling may occur around the fingertips, toes, and groin.

Symptoms. Sore throat, fever, and vomiting are symptoms of the disease. The tongue may become red and swollen, and the patient may experience headache, discomfort, and chills, as well as peeling and redness in the underarm and groin areas.

Treatment. Antibiotics are given to treat scarlet fever. Analgesics may help to alleviate symptoms, as will rest and extra fluids. Although complications are rare, the bacteria may spread to other body parts and cause ear infections, sinusitis, and rheumatic fever. *See also* BACTERIA.

Schistosome

Parasitic worms causing a variety of diseases.

Some schistosomes cause schistosomiasis, a group of diseases affecting people who live in tropical and subtropical climates. Schistosome infections are transmitted through contact with contaminated water. The infective stage of the parasite is known as the cercariae, a free-swimming organism that burrows into the skin of a human host. The larva then migrates to the lungs and liver, where it develops into an adult. Adult worms next migrate to their preferred location, depending on the specific species involved. The adults then lay eggs, which are excreted from the human host back into the environment. Newly hatched larvae live in freshwater snails, within which they develop into the infective stage and then return to the water. *See also* PARASITE.

Schistosomiasis

Range of diseases caused by infestation by parasitic schistosome worms.

Schistosomiasis is a disease caused by parasitic worms called schistosomes, which are common to tropical and subtropical regions. Approximately 150 to 200 million people worldwide are afflicted with some form of schistosomiasis. A number of species of schistosomes are found in the United States, causing irritations of the skin known as swimmer's itch.

Schistosomes exist in two primary life cycles: adult and larva. Their adult form survives in mammalian hosts, particularly humans. Their larval stages develop in certain species of freshwater snails.

Schistosome eggs are discharged from the mammalian host into the water, where they hatch. The larvae then infect aquatic snails, which serve as intermediate hosts. Within the snail, the larvae undergo partial maturation, and once they have matured they escape back into the water as mature larvae. They are then able to penetrate human skin from the water, migrating to the capillaries as maturation continues. There they remain and lay eggs.

Incidence. People who walk barefoot through water harboring the parasites or who perform agricultural labor in rice paddies or other water-logged areas are particularly vulnerable to schistosome infestation.

Types. Three main types of schistosome are responsible for serious diseases in humans: *Schistosoma mansoni, S. haematobium,* and *S. japonicum.*

S. haematobium, also known as the Egyptian blood fluke, pierces the skin or mucous membranes of humans in infested water. Developing into a fluke, the parasite migrates through the circulatory system to the capillaries of the bladder, where it mates and deposits eggs, producing a severe inflammatory reaction in the walls of the bladder. Hemorrhaging results, leading to painful urination and blood in the urine. Diagnosis of *S. haematobium* infestation is made after eggs are detected in the urine.

Two other common flukes, *S. mansoni* and *S. japonicum* (the Japanese blood fluke), infest the blood vessels of the large intestine and liver. They may be carried via the portal veins to the liver, causing inflammation and scarring, and resulting in enlargement of the liver and spleen. Serious internal bleeding, due to obstruction of blood flow through the liver and enlargement of veins, often follows.

Symptoms. A rash or other skin irritation is often the first sign of schistosome infestation, appearing a few days after parasites enter the system. Subsequent symptoms begin after a month and include fever, chills, cough, and muscle aches, although many forms remain asymptomatic until much later. Repeated infection can damage the liver, intestines, lungs, or bladder, and may also cause blindness.

Treatment. For schistosomiasis, oral administration of praziquantel, a highly effective antihelminthic drug, is used as treatment. *See* ANTIHELMINTHIC DRUGS; SCHISTOSOME; SNAILS AND DISEASE; TROPICAL DISEASES; *and* WORM INFESTATION.

Schizoid Personality Disorder

Personality disorder characterized by social isolation and diminished desire for human contact.

A person with schizoid personality disorder is not able to enjoy relationships with others, selects activities that can be participated in alone, and has little interest in friends or family. Such individuals never attained mutually gratifying relationships in their lives, thus, as relationships are not experienced as a potential source of gratification, but still pose the threat of frustration, they are avoided, except in their most superficial form. The patterns of behavior characteristic of schizoid personality disorder begin in childhood, when the isolation becomes apparent at an early age. For those with this disorder, social contacts are awkward and uncomfortable, and emotional expression is minimal. *See also* CHILD ABUSE *and* PSYCHIATRY.

Schizophrenia

Inability to distinguish reality from fantasy, or to control emotions, as well as problems with perception and communication.

Schizophrenia is a chronic brain disorder that typically strikes in young adulthood and affects about one percent of the population. Sufferers are severely disabled at some point in their lives. Individuals with schizophrenia are susceptible to suicide, with a mortality rate of about 10 percent.

Unlike other mental illnesses that involve problems in thinking and communicating, such as Alzheimer's disease, schizophrenia is not a degenerative disease and can actually stabilize and possibly improve with treatment after the initial onset.

CAUSES

While understanding of the causes of schizophrenia has improved, the definitive cause is still unknown. Schizophrenia probably occurs as the result of a number of variables, including genetic and environmental factors. Based on observable characteristics, it is believed that schizophrenia is actually a problem in the brain whereby neural activity is "short-circuited." Other possible causes beyond genetic predisposition include poor prenatal nutrition or prenatal damage.

SYMPTOMS

Schizophrenia is diagnosed when an individual has two or more of the following symptoms lasting for six months or more:

Delusions. Delusions are unfounded beliefs and fantasies. In schizophrenia, the most common types of delusions are paranoid, which include the belief that a person is being conspired against or followed. Another common type of delusion is one where the sufferer believes that all unrelated comments and events are directly related to him or her, even to the extent that people on television are communicating directly with him or her.

Hallucinations. Hallucinations are voices, sounds, and sights that are experienced, but which do not exist. The images are usually negative, and the voices are threatening and aggressive.

Disorganized Thought or Speech. Schizophrenic patients are often not able to maintain a logical train of thought in conversation. In the most severe forms, the words make no sense at all.

Disorganized Behavior. Patients with schizophrenia often display behavior that is out of character with their environment, including meaningless gestures or inappropriate verbalizations. Catatonic behavior, which also falls into this category, involves behavior that shows no emotional response and little or no physical movement.

TREATMENT

Schizophrenia requires lifelong treatment since it is a chronic illness. There are two phases of the disease that are treated differently: the acute psychotic phase, where there is a complete loss of reality, and the maintenance phase between relapses.

Antipsychotic medications are used to treat disorganized thought, delusions, and hallucinations. As important as it is to stay on antipsychotic medications, many patients find this difficult due to side effects, such as restlessness, fluctuations in weight, and sexual dysfunction. If side effects are limiting a patient's compliance, a physician should be alerted, since the dosage may be adjusted or the drug changed. Newer antipsychotics with fewer side effects, known as atypical antipsychotic drugs, have recently become available.

In addition to medication, some form of psychotherapy for the patient (either individual or group), as well as family therapy, is necessary. Coping skills and rehabilitation after a psychotic episode may help the sufferer live a more mainstream life. For the family of an individual with schizophrenia, group therapy may be helpful.

Background material on schizophrenia can be found in MENTAL ILLNESS *and* PSYCHIATRY*. For further information, see* ALZHEIMER'S DISEASE; ANTIPSYCHOTIC DRUGS; FAMILY THERAPY; GROUP THERAPY; HALLUCINATION; SEXUAL DYSFUNCTION; AND WEIGHT. *See also Physcotherapy.*

Resources on Schizophrenia

American Psychiatric Association, *Diagnostic and Statistical Manual of Mental Disorders, 4th Edition* (1994); Barchas, Jack D., *Psychopharmacology: From Theory to Practice* (1977); Gottesman, Irving I., *Schizophrenia Genesis: The Origins of Madness* (1991); Beckham, E. Edward and William R. Leber, eds., *Handbook of Depression: Treatment, Assessment, and Research* (1985); Wender, P.H. and D.F. Klein, *Mind, Mood, and Medicine: A Guide to the New Biopsychiatry* (1981); Nat. Depressive & Manic-Depressive Association, Tel. (800) 82-NDMDA, Online: www.ndmda.org; National Mental Health Association, Tel. (800) 969-NMHA; www.nmha.org; www.ny-cornell.org/psychiatry/.

Schonlein-Henoch Purpura

Inflammation of the knees or ankles caused by bleeding into the skin or mucous membranes.

Schonlein-Henoch purpura is an unusual affliction found in children or young adults, usually following an upper respiratory infection, such as a cold or flu.

Symptoms of Schonlein-Henoch purpura include swelling or discoloration around the knees or ankles, accompanied by pain in the abdomen. The joints may be warm and tender, but there is usually no damage to the bone structure or to the ligaments in the joints. Affected individuals may also have blood and excess protein in the urine.

Treatment. Most cases of Schonlein-Henoch purpura resolve spontaneously and do not need treatment. Severe cases may be treated with corticosteroids, a group of anti-inflammatory drugs that mimic the effect of specific hormones produced by the adrenal glands. *See also* CORTICOSTEROID HORMONES.

School Phobia

A child's inordinate and persistent fear of school, despite reassurance.

Most children are anxious about first going to school, because they must leave the security of home and parents and enter a new and uncertain social environment. Usually, they soon learn to adapt, develop relationships, and feel comfortable and safe. Sometimes the fear persists, and a child may avoid active participation when in school or even refuse to go to school. Supportive reassurance is often sufficient, but sometimes the distress continues to be a problem. It is important to understand, perhaps with professional assistance, how separation anxiety, socialization difficulties, learning problems, or other factors may contribute to school phobia in order to develop treatment. *See also* PSYCHOTHERAPY.

Sciatica

Pain along the sciatic nerve and its branches in the buttock, thigh, and leg.

The sciatic nerve travels from the pelvis down the back of each leg to the foot. It is responsible for sensation in the leg and foot. Sciatica is a form of neuralgia, a pain that is caused by a damaged nerve. In the case of sciatica, the sciatic nerve is damaged.

Cause. Sciatica is usually caused by damage to the nerve caused by pressure on one of the nerve roots that form the sciatic nerve. The most common cause of sciatica is a prolapsed intervertebral disk, a disk from the vertebrae that is displaced from its normal position and presses on the nerve root. Less frequently, sciatica can also be caused by excess pressure on the nerve due to a blood clot, abscess, or tumor. In addition, conditions that affect the nerves, such as diabetes mellitus, may produce sciatica.

Treatment. Most cases of sciatica will improve with bed rest. Analgesic drugs are often prescribed to relieve the pain; however, the condition often recurs. In severe cases, surgery can relieve the pressure on the sciatic nerve. *See also* NEURALGIA.

SCID

Severe combined immunodeficiency disorder

Genetic disorder in which the body cannot fight infection due to an immune system deficiency.

SCID is caused by a number of genetic defects that result in an immune deficiency of antibodies, as well as white blood cells known as B and T cells. The most common early infections of SCID patients are pneumonia and a fungal infection called thrush. Without treatment, patients with SCID will die before they reach the age of two.

Individual infections can usually be treated with antibiotics and injections of immune globulin to stimulate the immune system. To cure the condition itself, bone marrow or umbilical cord blood transplants have proved effective. *See also* AUTOIMMUNE DISORDERS.

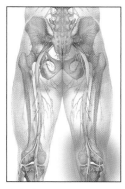

Sciatica.
The diagram above shows a damaged sciatic nerve that travels from the pelvis down to the back of each leg causing sciatica, a form of neuralgia.

Scleritis

Inflammation of the sclera, the white outer coating of the eyeball.

Scleritis is a painful swelling of the sclera, the white of the eye. It generally occurs in conjunction with collagen diseases, such as rheumatoid arthritis. The condition also accompanies the virus *Herpes zoster ophthalmicus*. Scleritis may cause thinning or perforation of the sclera. In severe cases, it can lead to the loss of the eye.

Treatment. Scleritis is treated with anti-inflammatory drugs and corticosteroids. If the sclera continues to swell, drugs that suppress the immune system, such as cyclophosphamide or azathioprine, may be prescribed. *See also* EYE, DISORDERS OF.

Scleroderma

Also known as progressive systemic sclerosis

Connective-tissue disorder in which excessive amounts of the protein collagen are produced, causing the skin to harden.

Incidence. Scleroderma usually develops in individuals between the ages of 20 and 40. Women are four times as likely to have the condition as men.

Symptoms. Symptoms of scleroderma include thickening and tightening of the skin, a loss of flexibility in joints, joint pain and stiffness, scarring, and, in some cases, damage to internal organs.

Scleroderma can also affect the lower end of the esophagus, making it difficult to propel food into the stomach. Swallowing difficulties and heartburn may develop as well. Barrett's syndrome, the growth of abnormal cells in the esophagus, may occur, increasing the risk of esophageal blockage or cancer. The intestines may also be affected, interfering with their ability to absorb nutrients. The kidneys and lungs may be affected as well.

Raynaud's syndrome, in which the fingers become numb in response to cold, commonly occurs together with scleroderma and may be seen as an early symptom of the condition.

Treatment. Scleroderma is treated with medication to alleviate individual symptoms. The disease cannot be cured nor its progress halted, but nonsteroidal anti-inflammatory drugs and corticosteroids can relieve pain. Organ damage can be reduced by penicillamine, but this drug has harmful side effects. Immunosuppressive drugs may also be administered. Physical therapy can help maintain muscle strength, but it cannot prevent joint immobility. *See also* RAYNAUD'S SYNDROME.

Scleromalacia

Softening or thinning of the sclera (the white of the eye).

Scleromalacia is generally a complication of scleritis (an inflammation of the sclera), particularly scleritis caused by rheumatoid arthritis. If the condition spreads to the entire sclera, it is specified as scleromalacia perforans, which is especially severe. Symptoms of scleromalacia perforans include the distention and ballooning of the choroid, which is located underneath the sclera. Perforation of the sclera may eventually result. *See also* SCLERITIS.

Sclerotherapy

Treatment of varicose veins by injection of an irritating solution that causes inflammation to block the veins completely, obliterating them.

Sclerotherapy can be done when the usual method of treating varicose veins—wearing support stockings—is not effective. The first step is to empty the vein of blood as much as possible. Then a solution, formulated to irritate the lining of the vein, is injected, while the leg with the varicose veins is kept elevated. Rubber pads are applied to the injected veins to compress them as much as possible. The bandages are kept on for three weeks, during which the patient can continue normal daily activities, while maintaining pressure against the veins. As they are shut down completely, other veins take over their function.

Women who undergo sclerotherapy should not take oral contraceptives for at least six weeks before treatment to prevent blood clot formation. The treated areas may turn brown, but this color usually fades with time.

Sclerotherapy is also used to treat hemorrhoids (varicose veins in the anus) and esophageal varices (swollen veins in the esophagus). *See also* VARICOSE VEINS.

Scoliosis

Bend or curve in the spine.

Viewed from behind, the spine should be a straight column that supports the body. However, during growth, the spine may begin to curve to one side or another, the curvature becoming more and more pronounced, until growth stops. Meanwhile, another part of the spine may begin to compensate by curving in the opposite direction. The result of this abnormal growth is an S-shaped spine, which can affect balance, posture, and, in severe cases, produce visible deformity.

Most of the curves resulting from scoliosis are located in the chest (thoracic) or lower back (lumbar) areas. The cause of juvenile scoliosis, which begins in childhood and becomes more pronounced during adolescence, is unknown. Scoliosis may occasionally be present at birth, or the condition may develop after polio causes weakness in the muscles of the spine on one side of the body.

Treatment. Scoliosis may progress undetected if the curvature is minor, and treatment is often not required. If it is noticed at a young age, however, the progression of the curve should be carefully tracked so as to medically intervene as soon as possible. This treatment may include stabilization with a brace, or surgery to fuse the bones together in the correct alignment. Another option is to insert a metal rod to hold the spine straight until the bones finish growing and fuse together. *See also* BACK; BACK PAIN; BRACE; KYPHOSIS; LORDOSIS; ORTHOPEDIC; POLIOMYELITIS; *and* VERTEBRA.

Scorpion Stings

Potentially venomous stings from the tail of a scorpion.

Scorpions are arthropods whose venom is used to capture prey and for self-defense. They are most active at night in warm weather, are not aggressive, and sting only when threatened. Their stings can range from the transiently painful, much like a bee or wasp sting, to the potentially deadly.

Of all of the species of scorpion native to the United States, only one is considered life-threatening. The bark scorpion (*Centruroides exilicauda*), between one-half and an inch-and-a-half in size, is found mainly in Arizona and adjacent areas. The venom of this species can cause severe swelling and pain at the sting site, numbness, breathing difficulties, muscle twitching, and convulsions. Death rarely occurs, however, and an antivenin does exist.

In most cases, scorpion stings cause localized pain, hypersensitivity, numbness, and tingling; bites to healthy adults can be treated at home by applying ice packs and elevating the sting area to heart level. However, a poison control center should be contacted in any case where a scorpion sting is suspected. Children, the elderly, and those with respiratory problems are most at risk. *See also* POISONING.

Screening

Diagnostic testing for potential disease or abnormality in the absence of obvious symptoms.

It is possible to screen for many diseases using a vast array of diagnostic tests. During pregnancy, for example, prenatal screening techniques (including ultrasound, chorionic villus sampling, and amniocentesis) can determine the health of the fetus. The use of screening tests may be based on the individual patient's medical history or on statistics indicating the risk factors for a particular disease in the general population. A combination of both of these criteria may also be used. *See also* DIAGNOSTICS.

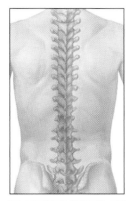
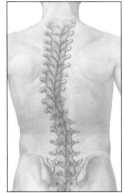

Scoliosis.
The image at the top shows a normal straight spine. Lateral curvature of the spine, scoliosis, above bottom, is a relatively common condition. The majority of individuals with scoliosis don't require surgery or braces because their condition is self-limiting. Progressive scoliosis requires therapy. The S-shaped curve is usually more apparent in an x-ray.

Scrofula

Inflammation of the lymph nodes caused by the bacterium *Mycobacterium tuberculosis*.

The term scrofula refers to a tuberculosis infection of the lymph nodes. In the past, scrofula was sometimes called "the king's evil," because it was believed the disease could be cured by the touch of a king. Scrofula is marked by abscesses in the lymph nodes. It is a very rare disease in most countries. Antituberculous agents have proved successful in the treatment of scrofula. *See also* ANTIBIOTIC DRUGS *and* TUBERCULOSIS.

Scuba-Diving Medicine

Small branch of medicine that studies the physiological effects of diving with SCUBA (self-contained underwater breathing apparatus).

Scuba-diving medicine is an umbrella term for the medical study of the effects of scuba diving on the body. Scuba-diving medicine studies the physiology of deep-sea diving, the psychological and physical effects of diving on the human body, and the treatment and prevention of diving-related illnesses.

Scuba divers use a piece of special equipment called a self-contained underwater breathing apparatus (SCUBA). This equipment allows them to dive to greater depths below the surface than would be possible without it.

EFFECTS OF DIVING ON THE BODY

Changes in the environment during scuba diving affect the human body. Divers face the physiological stress of pressurized air and the psychological trauma of being deep below the water's surface.

As divers descend, they experience an increasingly hyperbaric (high-pressure) environment. The increased pressure has multiple effects on the body. Divers must descend slowly enough to avoid creating a dramatic difference between the pressure in their head cavities and the pressure in the hyperbaric deep-sea environment. The lower the divers are planning to dive, the more slowly they must descend, since the percentage change in pressure is greater at greater depths. In addition, under hyperbaric conditions the effect of oxygen on the body changes. It becomes a toxic gas below a certain depth or during a dive of longer than twenty minutes. Thus, divers must monitor their depth and the length of their dive, factoring in the type of breathing apparatus they are using, to avoid experiencing the toxic effects of oxygen.

During ascent, divers face a risk of developing the bends, also called decompression sickness, in which the rapid reduction in air pressure causes nitrogen bubbles to form in the blood vessels and body tissues. These bubbles can block small blood vessels, leading to a serious disruption of circulation. Divers can also develop pressure-related trauma (barotrauma) of the lungs if they hold their breath during ascent. As the ambient pressure decreases, the air in the lungs expands, rupturing lung tissue.

The need to breathe from a special apparatus also presents multiple health risks. The use of pure oxygen can lead to serious health risks if the oxygen tank is mishandled. The amount of oxygen consumed by the diver may fall below safe levels, causing loss of consciousness. Using compressed gas mixtures, however, can lead to dangerous disorders of the central nervous system at extreme depths.

Psychologically, divers sometimes experience a feeling of panic while they are underwater. This can lead to hyperventilation or cessation of breathing (brought on by spasms that cause the vocal cords to block the passage of air).

SYMPTOMS OF DIVING-RELATED ILLNESS

Flaws in breathing equipment can lead to a disruption in oxygen flow to the diver, causing symptoms such as dizziness, loss of consciousness, memory problems, shortness of breath, nausea, headache, or even death. Below a depth of 80 meters, divers may also experience nitrogen narcosis, a depressed mental state due to the pressure of inhaled nitrogen.

Symptoms of decompression sickness include cough, itching, reddened skin, and extreme pain. Barotrauma of the lungs can lead to strong pain in the chest, cough, leakage of blood from the mouth and nose, shortness of breath, fatigue, limb paralysis, and loss of consciousness.

As scuba diving grows in popularity, scientists are beginning to evaluate its potential long-term health consequences. For every successfully treated case of decompression illness, there are many divers who are not treated soon enough because they do not experience symptoms right away. There is also statistical evidence that diving has permanent neurological effects (as a result of lack of oxygen to the brain).

TREATMENT

Appropriate treatment depends on the disorder. In general, breathing-related problems during descent can be treated by returning to the surface to breathe fresh air. Conversely, decompression sickness is alleviated if the diver descends to a depth of greater pressure. A recompression chamber, in which the air pressure is changed slowly to allow the lungs to adjust, can be used to treat both decompression sickness and barotrauma of the lungs.

PREVENTION

The best way to prevent diving-related mishaps is to learn proper diving procedure. Divers should be aware of the health risks they face at varying depths with different types of equipment. Certain innovations in scuba equipment also help prevent illness. "Heads up" displays show dive data inside a diver's mask, instead of on the wrist in the traditional fashion, ensuring that the diver pays attention to critical information. In addition, recompression chambers near diving sites help divers avoid the bends and other ascent-related disorders.

For background information on scuba diving medicine, see AVIATION MEDICINE AND WATER SAFETY. R*elated material can be found in* AIR; BREATHING DIFFICULTY; DECOMPRESSION SICKNESS; LUNG; MEMORY; NAUSEA; OXYGEN AND PANIC ATTACK. *See also Respiratory System.*

Scurvy

Disease caused by a deficiency of vitamin C.

Vitamin C functions in the production of collagen, or cellular connective tissue, thus aiding in the maintenance of teeth, bones, cartilage, and capillaries. Symptoms of scurvy result from diminished collagen production and include loose teeth, swollen and bleeding gums, joint problems, bruising, poor healing of wounds, and muscle wasting.

Since even minimal vitamin C intake will prevent scurvy, it is extremely rare in the United States. It tends to occur generally only among alcoholics whose primary source of calories is alcohol, people who already have another underlying illness, or those on fad diets.

Very little vitamin C, between five and ten milligrams, is needed to prevent scurvy. In contrast, most Americans exceed this amount, consuming approximately 72 milligrams—120 percent of the Recommended Dietary Allowance. Fresh fruits and vegetables are the best source of vitamin C. Vitamin C is fragile and easily destroyed by overcooking, soaking in water, exposure to air, handling and cutting, yet a sufficient amount generally survives the cooking process. *See also* NUTRITION *and* VITAMIN C.

Sealants, Dental

Protective synthetic materials applied to the grinding surfaces of the teeth.

Dental sealants are sometimes used to add protection to teeth against decay-causing substances such as plaque. The sealant material is durable and is bonded directly to the tooth, where it keeps harmful bacteria from reaching the tooth's surface.

Sealant treatment has become increasingly popular for children. Sealants are also occasionally used on adult teeth, particularly on the back molars. Sealants are preventive; however, they do not take the place of proper dental care. *See also* BONDING, DENTAL *and* CARIES, DENTAL.

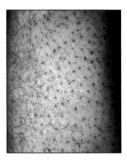

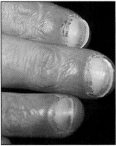

Scurvy.
Scurvy is a nutritional disease caused by deficiency of vitamin C. Common symptons include pinpoint bleeding around hair follicles, along the gums, and under the nails as seen in the photos above. This disease rarely occurs in the U.S.

Sebaceous Cyst

Abnormal whitish-yellow, painless growth under the skin.

A sebaceous cyst usually appears as a rounded, nontender swelling of varying size. As skin grows, matures, and sheds, a quantity of skin will sometimes become trapped under a layer of growing skin. Sebaceous cysts are common and are not serious, although the jelly-like material in the cysts is foul-smelling. These cysts usually occur on the head, the back of the neck, and the upper chest and back.

Symptoms indicating the presence of a sebaceous cyst include a small lump, redness, increased temperature of the skin, and sometimes discharge of a grayish-white material from the cyst. Sebaceous cysts are usually not treated unless they become infected. If this is the case, the area will redden, swell, and hurt. Antibiotics and warm compresses are generally used to treat infected sebaceous cysts, although in severe cases, surgical drainage of the cyst may be necessary. *See also* ACNE *and* CYST.

Seborrhea

Oily, flaky skin that results from overproduction of oil on the skin.

Normally, glands in the skin (sebaceous glands) produce an oily discharge (sebum), which protects and moisturizes the skin. When the sebaceous glands produce too much sebum, seborrhea may result. The skin becomes red and oily, and yellowish scales flake off; often the affected skin itches or burns. This may occur on the face, scalp (in which case it is referred to as dandruff), under the breasts, and in the folds of skin in the genital area.

Treatment. Commercial products, such as shampoos containing selenium sulfide, zinc pyrithione, or tar, may lessen symptoms. If seborrhea is severe, a physician may be able to prescribe more effective medication. There is no known prevention for seborrhea. *See also* ACNE *and* SEBUM.

Sebum

Oily and waxy secretion produced by the sebaceous glands onto the skin.

Sebum is a complex mixture of triglycerides (fats), waxes, and cholesterol, as well as remnants of dying and dead skin cells. The function of sebum is to lubricate and protect the epidermis (skin) and hair. *See also* ACNE; CHOLESTEROL; *and* SKIN.

Seizure

Repeated and abnormal electrical discharges from the brain that results in a lack of body control.

A seizure or convulsion can be caused by any event that disturbs the brain's electrical activity. Patients who experience seizures are characterized as suffering from a form of epilepsy.

CAUSE
Seizures can be the result of a severe head injury, brain damage at birth, a stroke, an infection, a tumor in the brain, or alcohol withdrawal. Seizures may consist of abnormal electrical activity in a small confined area of the brain, or it can spread to other parts of the brain. A very small percentage of patients with seizures experience sensations (auras) prior to the onset of a seizure.

SYMPTOMS
Neuromuscular signs and symptoms of a seizure include tingling of the skin, uncontrollable twitching of the face or limbs, spasms, and tremors. Other potential signs and symptoms include hallucinations, phobias, or a sense of deja vú, which is a feeling of familiarity. Abnormal electrical activity spread throughout the brain, produces a generalized seizure, referred to as grand mal. A grand mal seizure which continues for more than a few minutes is referred to as "status epilepticus." In these cases, consciousness is typically lost.

TREATMENT
It is very important that anyone suffering a

seizure receive medical help immediately. The most important thing to do for any seizure victim is to move any dangerous objects—that could be used for striking—away from the patient to prevent them from injuring themselves. Under no circumstances should any object be placed in the victim's mouth. It may obstruct the airway, or cause injury. *See also* EPILEPSY.

> *Background reading on seizures can be found in brain and central nervous system. For further information, see* AURA; BIRTH DEFECTS; BRAIN DISORDERS; BRAIN TUMOR; EPILEPSY; HALLUCINATION; PHOBIA; AND STROKE. *See also Anticonvulsant Drugs for more on treatment on epileptic seizures.*

Seizure, Febrile

> **Jerking of the limbs accompanied by loss of consciousness, occurring mainly in children.**

A febrile seizure usually occurs in young children between the ages of three months and five years. This type of seizure tends to run in families. It is estimated that as many as five percent of all children will experience a febrile seizure. The seizures are short in duration and usually occur only once.

Cause and Symptoms. Febrile seizures may be the result of abnormal electrical activity in the brain, brought on by a high fever. This type of seizure generally occurs early on in the course of the fever. Febrile seizures are usually not the result of a brain abnormality. They frequently stem from the high fevers that accompany acute infectious diseases such as tonsillitis (infection of the tonsils) or otitis media (middle ear infection). The seizures include a short period (lasting from a few seconds to up to a few minutes) of wrenching and jerking movements. The child may be exhausted upon regaining consciousness. Even though a particular child has experienced one febrile seizure, the child will not necessarily experience a febrile seizure every time he or she has a fever. However, children who have febrile seizures regularly have a greater chance of developing epilepsy in the future.

Treatment. It is very important to move any dangerous objects out of reach of a child who is having a febrile seizure. If the seizure continues for longer than five minutes, emergency medical attention should be sought. In all cases, a doctor should be consulted. Single seizures are generally not treated with anticonvulsant drugs.

Prevention. The most effective method of preventing febrile seizures is to treat the high fever with acetaminophen or ibuprofen, given every four hours. It is especially important not to give aspirin to a child who may have a viral infection, due to the risk of developing Reye's syndrome. *See also* EPILEPSY *and* REYE'S SYNDROME.

Selenium

> **Trace mineral and powerful antioxidant that works with vitamin E to prevent the degradation of fats and the formation of free radicals.**

The selenium content of various foods is highly contingent on the selenium levels present in the soil in which the food was grown. Therefore, a varied food supply is likely to provide sufficient amounts of selenium. Many water supplies also contain selenium.

A deficiency of selenium is extremely rare, and has been found only in areas of the world in which the food supply has been grown in soil that lacks selenium. This was the case in China, where selenium deficiency led to white muscle disease with skeletal muscle weakness, degeneration of the heart muscle, heart failure, and death in both humans and cattle.

Good sources of selenium include egg yolks, chicken, garlic, onions, mushrooms, and whole grain products. Supplementation in those who do not have a deficiency is unnecessary, and an excess of selenium can be highly toxic.

Symptoms of an overdose can include lethargy, irritability, abdominal pain, diarrhea, nausea, and death. Individuals should be wary of dietary supplements containing large amounts of selenium. *See also* HEART FAILURE *and* VITAMIN E.

Self-Mutilation

Deliberate attempt to cause injury to oneself without the conscious intent to commit suicide.

Self-mutilation often begins in adolescence. It is three times more common in women than in men. Self-mutilation may take many forms, including cutting of the skin with a sharp knife or needles, intentionally burning the skin, or pulling out the hair (known as trichotillomania). Other forms of self-mutilation include substance abuse and neglecting to take medication that is necessary for sustaining life.

Causes. The physical wounds that are visible in self-mutilation are symptomatic of an emotional problem and can often be seen as a cry for help. Many teens who harm themselves say that they feel empty inside and that self-mutilation is a way of experiencing any sort of feeling. Self-harm begins when a person experiences painful emotions and feels driven to inflict pain on his or her own body, thereby reducing these feelings. In fact, there is probably a great deal of pain that the person who is self-injuring has bottled up and is afraid to experience. Sometimes individuals who self-mutilate have a history of childhood abuse (physical, emotional, or sexual) or neglect. The lack of ability to tolerate the painful emotions may result from the fact that the pain feels unbearably intense, or from having grown up in an environment in which expressing anger or distress was seen as unacceptable.

An unhealthy environment that might cause a person to self-mutilate could consist of parents who neglect the feelings of their child, or it could involve parents who could not accept uncomfortable emotions. Such parents would typically invalidate the child's feelings by insisting on positive expressions of thought, and emotion. Harming oneself is an alternative way of communicating negative feelings. The self-injurer usually suffers from low self-esteem and feelings of shame. *See also* CHILD ABUSE; PSYCHIATRY; PSYCHOANALYSIS; PSYCHOTHERAPY; *and* SHAME.

Semen Analysis

Clinical testing designed to evaluate the condition and number of sperm.

Sperm are released from the penis within a secretion known as semen. Produced primarily by the prostate gland and the seminal vesicles, semen provides nourishment for the sperm, as well as a liquid medium though which they can swim. The amount of semen released per ejaculation is equivalent to one or two tablespoons and contains between 400 and 600 million sperm.

Semen analysis is generally used to diagnose possible causes of infertility. Testing of the semen may be conducted after a couple has been unable to conceive for one year.

Collection. The sperm sample to be analyzed is collected either during sexual intercourse using a special condom supplied by the physician, or through masturbation into a sterile container. In either case, the sperm must be delivered for analysis within two hours of ejaculation. Ejaculation should be avoided for five to seven days prior to testing.

Analysis. After collection, the volume of the semen sample is measured, and several drops of ejaculate are examined under a microscope. The researcher will examine the motion of the sperm, the sperm count, and the structure of the sperm, comparing these values with standardized ranges. A sperm count of less than 20×106 /mL, a volume of less than 1.0 mL, and a level of fewer than 60 percent of mature sperm or 50 percent of actively motile sperm are abnormal values that may be associated with infertility. Lowered sperm count or damaged sperm may be the result of medications, alcohol, recreational drugs, or the use of saunas and hot tubs. Couples may be advised to avoid these activities to improve their chances of conceiving. Semen analysis is also used in cases of rape and to evaluate the success of vasectomy surgery. *See also* CONCEPTION; CONDOM; EJACULATION; EJACULATION, DISORDERS OF; FERTILITY; FERTILITY DRUGS; FERTILIZATION; INFERTILITY; RAPE; SPERM; *and* VASECTOMY.

Semen, Blood in the

The appearance of blood in ejaculate fluid.

Blood in the semen is not an unusual event, and the cause usually remains unknown. It may appear after a long period of abstinence or after frequent sexual activity. Men who do not have a good clotting response or who suffer from hemophilia should not be surprised to see blood in their semen. Episodes can be repetitive or they can occur only once. Although blood in the semen is usually harmless, it may indicate an underlying problem or infection.

There is no specific recommended treatment for blood in the semen. Some urologists prescribe the antibiotic drug tetracycline (in case there is a bacterial infection) and massage, but there is no evidence that these treatments have any effect. *See also* ANTIBIOTIC DRUGS; BLOOD CLOTTING; HEMOPHILIA; *and* REPRODUCTIVE SYSTEM, MALE.

Senility

Term used to describe the mental degeneration caused by old age.

Many people retain full intellectual capacity throughout their entire lives. There may be some short-term memory loss, and the capacity to learn new things may be reduced; but dementia or senility in any of its many forms is not an inevitable consequence of aging. It is currently estimated that fewer than ten percent of all people will become senile during their lifetime. In contrast, however, by the time a person reaches 85, almost one out of every two will exhibit symptoms of senility.

Causes. A general loss of intellectual capacity was originally thought to be the result of brain cell loss, which was viewed as a normal result of aging. But recent research suggests that senility is symptom of Alzheimer's disease and is not present in all elderly people. Thus, it is now believed that senility is not an inevitability for every aging person.

High blood pressure may also be a contributing factor to senility. It is now suspected that over time this condition may cause the tiny blood vessels in the brain to leak, resulting in a series of minor strokes that interfere with cognitive function.

Symptoms. Senility takes many forms. Memory loss is most common, and is one of the first symptoms of Alzheimer's disease. Forgetting small details, like where a person last put his or her keys, is not a sign of senility; forgetting where a person lives, however, may indicate early signs of mental deterioration. The senile person may clearly remember events of the distant past but be unable to tell you the current date or who the president is. He or she may appear confused and may be unable to recognize friends or family.

Occasional irritability is common to all humans, and periods of irritability are not uncommon. When the irritability becomes universal and continuous, causing noticeable personality changes, in many causes this behavior is the consequence of senility. Depression often follows as the person becomes aware of his or her lost intellectual and physical strength and impatient with his or her diminished capacity. *See also* AGE; AGING; ALZHEIMER'S DISEASE; BLOOD PRESSURE; GERONTOLOGY; *and* HYPERTENSION.

Resources on Senility
Damasio, Antonio R., *Descartes' Error: Emotion Reason and the Human Brain* (1994); Restak, Richard, *The Secret Life of the Brain* (2001); Schach-ter, Daniel L., *Searching for Memory: The Brain, The Mind, and the Past* (1996); Terry, Robet D., ed., *Aging and the Brain* (1988); West, Robin L. and Jan D. Sinnott, eds., *Everyday Memory and Aging* (1992); National Mental Health Association, Tel. (800) 969-NMHA, On-line: www.nmha.org; Alzheimer's Disease Education and Referral Center, Tel. (800) 438-4380, On-line: www.alzheimers.org; www.nycornell.org/medicine/neurology/index.html;www.nyp.org/css/.

Sensate Focus Technique

A therapy technique designed to treat sexual disorders.

Sensate focus technique is used to treat the inability to reach orgasm. The underlying idea is that a couple may be having sexual difficulties because they have become overly concerned with reaching orgasm.

Partners begin by touching each other without trying to induce arousal. Over a period of several days or weeks, touching becomes more explicitly sexual, but the focus remains on sharing sensation and giving pleasure, rather than achieving orgasm. Through this technique, couples learn new ways to interact sexually without focusing on orgasm. *See also* SEX THERAPY.

Sensation

Experience of the sense organs, such as sight, smell, hearing, taste, or touch.

The senses are responsible for collecting information about the outside world and transmitting it to the central nervous system (CNS), which consists of the brain and the spinal cord.

SENSORY RECEPTORS

Sensory receptors are specialized cells that are sensitive to stimuli and are responsible for gathering information. They are present throughout the body. These receptors are specialized; each group is sensitive to a specific stimulus. Sensory receptors can be divided into external or internal receptors.

External Senses. External receptors transfer information that occurs outside the body. Only a small amount of the sensation actually reaches the receptor. The receptor cells for the senses are neatly packed together, and most sensory information is transmitted directly to the cerebral cortex of the brain.

Internal or Touch Senses. Internal receptors detect chemical and physical changes that take place inside the body. Internal receptors respond to the body's movement, position, hunger, thirst, pain, and fatigue.

ABNORMAL SENSATIONS

Abnormal sensations are caused by injury to or excess pressure on a sensory nerve. The senses can be disabled or modified by an injury to a sensory organ or nerve tract.

Common examples of abnormal sensations include feelings of numbness, pins and needles, numbing, pain, burning, and coldness. A disorder called neuralgia is exemplified by intermittent, piercing pain.

Dietary changes may eliminate abnormal sensations. When other methods of treatment fail, the affected sensory nerve fibers may be surgically severed, or chemicals may be injected to block pain signals. *See also* BRAIN; NEURALGIA; NEUROPATHY; PROPRIOCEPTION; *and* SENSORY CORTEX.

Separation Anxiety

A child's feelings of anxiety brought on by the prospect of leaving the immediate company of his or her parent or parents.

Infants are completely dependent on adult caregivers for physical and emotional support. Even brief separation can lead to distress and the need for reassurance. By age three or four, this normal separation anxiety fades. However, some children may have persistent separation anxiety beyond early childhood. Children may verbalize their fear of separation, or demonstrate it with complaints of emotional or physical distress, such as nightmares, dizziness, stomach cramps, or headaches.

Parental illness, death in the family, or a traumatic event can trigger or worsen separation anxiety. Children with persistent separation anxiety should have professional consultation to determine any contributing factors, such as a socialization or learning difficulty. *See also* PSYCHOTHERAPY.

Sepsis

Bacterial infection of the body.

Bacteria may enter the body during surgery of the intestines, from the insertion of a catheter, or through a wound. Bacterial infection in the body leads to the formation of pus and the multiplication of the bacteria in the blood.

Sepsis is more likely to affect people with compromised immune systems. The immune systems of these people have difficulty controlling the spread of the infecting bacteria.

Symptoms of sepsis include fever, chills, shivering, confusion, and tachycardia (a rapid heartbeat). There may also be a rash, hyperventilation (fast breathing), joint pain, and hallucinations.

Once sepsis is diagnosed, hospitalization is usually necessary. The condition is normally treated with intravenous antibiotic drugs. *See also* ANTIBIOTIC DRUGS; INFECTIOUS DISEASES; *and* SEPTIC SHOCK.

Septal Defect

Congenital heart defect in which there is a hole in the wall of the septum separating the left and right sides of the heart.

A septal defect can occur in either the septum separating the ventricles, the lower chambers of the heart, or the septum separating the atria, the upper chambers of the heart. These defects occur in about one of every 400 births in the United States, with ventricular defects four times more common than atrial defects.

Symptoms depend on the size and location of the hole. If the hole is small, there may be few or no symptoms. A larger opening between the ventricles causes some of the oxygen-rich blood in the left ventricle to go back to the lungs, rather than out to the body. The result can be shortness of breath, as the lungs become congested, and failure of the patient to grow properly. The left ventricle must work harder to pump blood to the body, so it can become abnormally enlarged. These symptoms may develop days or weeks after birth.

A major atrial septal defect usually does not cause either breathing problems or affect growth in the first years of life. The right atrium and ventricle can become enlarged in later years, resulting in atrial fibrillation and heart failure.

Diagnosis. A first sign of a septal defect can be a heart murmur. Existence of a defect can be confirmed by tests such as a chest x-ray, electrocardiogram, and echocardiogram, which will identify the location and size of the opening.

Treatment. Some septal defects close without treatment. In other cases, the hole is small enough to require only careful monitoring in the first years of childhood. The symptoms of a ventricular septal defect can be treated with medications including diuretics, vasodilators, and digitalis drugs. The ultimate treatment for a septal defect is open-heart surgery to close the hole in the septum. The operation usually is done when the patient is between the ages of two and six, but in the case of atrial septal defects, it can be performed during adulthood. Surgery for a ventricular septal defect that is causing severe symptoms is done in the first two years after birth. Some defects are small enough to be sewn shut. Open-heart surgery for septal defects is usually successful in restoring normal heart function. *See also* CONGENITAL.

Septic Shock

Condition in which the blood pressure drops precipitously as a result of septicemia (the infection of the blood with bacteria) or toxemia (the presence of the toxins produced by bacteria in the blood).

Septicemia is an infection of the blood by bacteria that are introduced into the bloodstream during surgery of the intestines, by insertion of a contaminated needle, after a serious burn, from bedsores, from a wound, or through other means. The bacteria produce toxins in the blood, causing toxemia, and a sudden drop in blood pressure, called septic shock, is the body's response to these toxins.

Incidence. Septic shock is most common in infants, the elderly, and people with compromised immune systems.

Symptoms. In a patient with septic shock, the blood vessels dilate and the blood pressure falls suddenly. The heart rate goes up in an effort to compensate for the drop in blood pressure, but flow to the organs is reduced, which is particularly dangerous for the brain and the kidneys. Early symptoms of septic shock include shaking and chills, fever, and flushed skin tones. Breathing is also rapid and shallow. Even with medical intervention, septic shock is an extremely serious condition. Almost 50 percent of people who experience septic shock do not survive.

Treatment. Treatment for septic shock must be provided promptly. The patient is moved to an intensive care unit, where fluids are injected to increase blood pressure. Drugs to constrict the blood vessels may also be administered. Antibiotics will be prescribed to fight the infection. If the lungs are affected, the patient may be put on a ventilator. *See also* SEPTICEMIA.

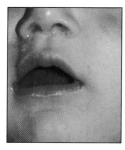

Septicemia.
The red, slightly elevated lesion on this infant's left cheek resulted from septicemia caused by pseudomonas. This is a skin manifestation of widespread infection. The discharge from the nose contains pus.

Septicemia

Also known as blood poisoning

Invasion of the blood stream by pathogenic (disease-causing) bacteria.

Septicemia often arises following a localized infection elsewhere in the body. Septicemia can quickly lead to septic shock (a sudden drop in blood pressure) and death.

Incidence. Those at greatest risk for septicemia are infants, the elderly, and those with compromised immune systems, such as people with AIDS, people taking chemotherapy for cancer, or people who are recovering from an organ transplant.

Symptoms. Early symptoms of septicemia include: a sudden spiking fever; chills; rapid shallow breathing; and an increased heart rate. The sufferer may also progress into septic shock, with lowered body temperature, lowered blood pressure, confusion, and other mental changes, such as irritability, anxiety, unresponsiveness, and lethargy.

Treatment. Septicemia is treated with immediate administration of intravenous fluids to kill the bacteria. Broad-spectrum antibiotics will be administered until the specific source of the bacterial infection can be identified by laboratory tests. If the infection can be recognized and treated as soon as possible, the survival rate from septicemia is high. *See also* ANTIBIOTIC DRUGS; BLOOD PRESSURE; SEPSIS; *and* SEPTIC SHOCK.

Sequela

Term referring to a condition, sign, or symptom appearing after a disease and resulting from it.

Visible or detectable symptoms or conditions that follow the occurrence of a disease are called sequela. Indications may include lesions, scarring, various forms of tissue damage, or organ dysfunction, and range from mild and benign to severe and life-threatening. Sequela also vary in duration. Sequela may be intermittent or chronic, depending on the disease that produces them. *See also* SYMPTOM.

Sequestration

Separation or abnormal fusion of dead tissue to healthy tissue.

Tissue that is diseased or has died may pull away from the surrounding healthy area. The most common instance of sequestration is in the case of osteomyelitis (a bone infection). In this situation, the segment of bone that is diseased eventually dies and separates from the live bone. The term is also used to refer to a rare abnormality of the lungs, present at birth, in which part of a lung connects to surrounding air sacs rather than the airway. *See also* OS-TEOMYELITIS.

Serology

Diagnostic testing of the blood to evaluate the body's immune response to disease-causing organisms (pathogens).

A variety of clinical laboratory tests may be performed on the blood in order to evaluate the condition of the immune response to pathogens, particularly viruses. During such tests, blood is drawn from a vein, often from the back of the hand or the elbow. An elastic band is secured over the arm to restrict the blood flow through the punctured vein into the collecting syringe.

Infection by microorganisms produces distinct, disease-specific antibodies that may be measured in the blood. These antibodies react with antigens (substances that stimulate the production of antibodies) presented during serological testing, allowing diagnosis of the pathogen causing the infection. Depending on the suspected antigen, one of several blood tests may be performed, including agglutination, complement-fixation, precipitation, and fluorescent antibody testing. Those at risk for certain diseases, particularly viral diseases, may undergo serologic testing as a screening method, even in the absence of obvious symptoms. For example, serology is used to test for exposure to HIV, the virus that causes AIDS. *See also* DIAGNOSTICS.

Serotonin

Protein instrumental in controlling the transmission of signals through the synapses of human brain cells.

Neurotransmission of signals in the brain is facilitated by serotonin. It is also involved in controlling appetite and sleep. Drugs that inhibit the brain's ability to process serotonin (called selective serotonin reuptake inhibitors) control human mood disorders, such as depression, violence, and other aggressive behaviors. The precise way these drugs control the levels of serotonin is not completely understood, but antidepressants like fluoxetine and paroxetine and others have proved effective with few side effects. *See also* ANTIDEPRESSANT DRUGS *and* NEUROTRANSMITTERS.

Serum Sickness

Allergic reaction to a transfusion of serum, an administered drug (antithymocyte globulin), or an injection of certain antitoxins used to treat diphtheria, tetanus, or poisonous snake or spider bites.

If a sample of blood has been allowed to clot for a period of time, a clear yellowish fluid called serum remains. This fluid carries the antibodies that function in the immune system.

Symptoms of serum sickness appear one to three weeks after the introduction of a drug or other foreign substance. It is not a life-threatening disease, and patients normally recover after a week to ten days. Fever and hives are common symptoms of serum sickness. There may be swelling of the face, neck, and lymph nodes, flushing, and muscle pain. The wrist, ankle, elbow, and knee joints may be painful. There may be abdominal cramps, diarrhea, and nausea. In rare cases, there is inflammation of the heart or kidneys.

Treatment. Aspirin is prescribed to relieve the discomfort, and antihistamines to reduce the allergic reaction. If the symptoms are severe, steroids or plasma cleansing may be prescribed. *See also* ALLERGY; ANTIHISTAMINE DRUGS; *and* ASPIRIN.

Sex

Biological gender.

The two sexes (male and female) are distinguished from each other not only by internal reproductive organs and external genitalia, but also by body size, muscle mass, and body fat—both as a percentage of body mass and its distribution. Recent research indicates that various body systems, including the cardiovascular system, react differently in males and females.

Intersex refers to an individual born with ambiguous genitals. These individuals are, however, genetically normal males or females in terms of their internal organs. *See also* REPRODUCTIVE SYSTEM, FEMALE *and* REPRODUCTIVE SYSTEM, MALE.

Sex Change

Also known as sex reassignment surgery

Surgical procedure designed to alter the external genitalia to resemble those of the opposite sex, or performed on infants with ambiguous genitalia in order to assign them an anatomical sex.

For those who wish to change their gender, surgery is only the final step in a long process. Hormone treatments are first administered over the course of a year, starting the transformation of secondary sex characteristics. After the surgery, hormone treatments continue to maintain the appearance of the new gender.

Sex change surgery does not alter the genetic signature of an individual—a male who undergoes a sex change operation still has the male chromosomes XY, and a female who undergoes the procedure still has the female chromosomes XX.

Male-to-female surgery is ten times more common than female-to-male surgery. The penis and testicles are removed, and an artificial vagina is constructed. Female-to-male surgery is more difficult. The internal reproductive organs are removed, and skin grafts are used to create a penis. Individuals who have had sex change surgery are unable to reproduce. *See also* TRANSVESTISM.

Sex Chromosomes

Genetic material that determines whether an individual is male or female.

Every human body cell contains 46 chromosomes, arranged in 23 pairs. Of these, 22 pairs are autosomes, or regular chromosomes, and one pair consists of the sex chromosomes. The sex chromosomes are referred to as X and Y chromosomes. A female has two X chromosomes, and a male has one X and one Y.

Sperm and eggs are produced by meiosis, which results in germ cells, that contain only half the number of chromosomes as a regular body cell—one from each pair. Thus, all egg cells contain an X chromosome. Half of the sperm cells carry an X chromosome, the other half a Y chromosome. During fertilization, the chromosomes carried by the sperm combine with those of the egg to form the zygote, which develops into a new organism. If an X sperm fertilizes the egg, the zygote will have XX chromosomes and will be female. If a Y sperm fertilizes the egg, the zygote will be XY and male. *See also* CONCEPTION.

Sex Determination

Process by which an organism develops into a male or a female.

The sex of a fetus depends on which sperm fertilizes the egg. Half of all sperm carry an X chromosome, the other half carry a Y. All eggs carry an X chromosome. If a Y-bearing sperm fertilizes an egg, the resulting embryo will be XY and male. If an X-bearing sperm fertilizes an egg, the resulting embryo will be XX and female.

The primitive sex organs of the embryo secrete male or female hormones, and the fetus develops either a male or female urogenital system. Sometimes there is a problem with hormone production or reception of hormones by target cells. As a result, a child can be born with sexually ambiguous genitals or missing some or all internal reproductive organs. *See also* INTERSEX.

Sex Hormones

Hormones responsible for sexual development and functions.

The three types of sex hormones are: androgen hormones, which aid in male sexual development; estrogen hormones, which are for female sex characteristics at puberty; and progesterone hormones, which help the body prepare for pregnancy. Sex hormones are responsible for pubertal development of males and females. They also carry out functions such as menstruation and the production of eggs in females and the manufacture of sperm in males. Estrogen is present in small amounts in males, and, similarly, testosterone is found in small quantities in females. *See also* ANDROGEN HORMONES; ESTROGEN HORMONES; *and* GONADOTROPINS.

Sex-Linked

Characteristic caused by a gene located on the X chromosome; its expression is affected by whether an individual is male or female.

Sex linked characteristics are caused by recessive genes on the X chromosome. Color-blindness is a sex-linked condition. These traits are expressed only if there is no matching dominant gene to mask their effects. In females, who have two X chromosomes, it is likely that a recessive gene on one chromosome will be masked by a dominant gene on the other chromosome. In males, the Y chromosome contains many fewer genes than the X chromosome, and the recessive trait is expressed.

A female who has one dominant and one recessive gene is a carrier; that is, she does not have the disease, but may pass it on to her offspring. A male inherits his X chromosome from his mother. If she is a carrier, her son has a 50 percent chance of inheriting the disorder. If she has the condition, he has a 100 percent chance of having it as well. For a female child to have a sex-linked trait, she must inherit the recessive gene from both parents. *See also* CARRIER.

Sex Therapy

Course of treatment for sexual dysfunction that is due in part or entirely to psychological factors.

It is estimated that over half of married couples experience the inability to have or to enjoy sexual relations at some point in their marriage. In some instances, the problems may be caused by physical factors, possibly unrecognized by either partner. In many instances, however, the cause is psychological. Few people pass through their formative years completely unscathed emotionally in ways that affect their attitudes about sex. This can adversely impact their ability to enjoy sex and to function sexually. When such problems threaten the integrity of a marriage or partnership, it is often helpful for the couple to engage in a course of sex therapy counseling. Among the problems that may be addressed by sex therapy are the following:

Loss of Desire. Loss of sexual desire by one or both partners may be caused by anxieties over performance or confusion about how to give and receive sexual pleasure. One technique often taught to address this problem is the sensate focus technique, in which partners are encouraged to place themselves in relaxed surroundings and concentrate on giving a partner sensual (as opposed to sexual) pleasure by massaging the body.

Both partners are required to abstain from intercourse during the period of time that they are engaged in this technique. They are instructed to take turns at giving and receiving sensual massage on any part of the body, at first excluding the breasts and genitals. The recipient instructs the giver about the type of massage that is most enjoyable. After engaging in several successful massages, the couple progresses to the next stage, which includes breast and genital massage short of orgasm. The couple's response to the exercises are discussed in therapy sessions. The couple then attempts vaginal containment without vigorous movement, and, when both partners are ready, unrestricted intercourse.

Premature Ejaculation. A common difficulty in men, premature ejaculation can be addressed in two ways. One method is by pausing in the thrusting that accompanies sexual intercourse just before ejaculation. Practicing this a number of times results over the course of time in the man obtaining increased control over the ejaculatory response. Another method is the squeeze technique, in which either partner squeezes the penis by gripping the organ beneath the glans (head) and applying pressure with thumb and forefingers.

Failure to Achieve Vaginal Penetration or Orgasm. Women whose vaginal muscles spasm during attempts at intercourse (vaginismus), making penetration difficult if not impossible, may be treated by learning to progressively relax and to explore their sexual anatomy. After receiving some basic educational information, the woman is advised to view her genitals with a handheld mirror and to penetrate her vagina with her fingers or with vaginal dilators of increasing size. The use of a topical lubricant is recommended.

Women who have never achieved orgasm on their own are also educated about relaxation and exploration of their genitals. They are instructed to self-stimulate in a way that is most pleasurable to them. They report back to the therapist regarding their observations and reactions, in a technique referred to as directed masturbation. *See also* SENSATE FOCUS TECHNIQUE.

Sexual Abuse

Sexual activity that causes physical or psychological damage.

Sexually oriented child abuse, sexual harassment among adults, and rape are examples of sexual abuse. Rape is the act of forcing someone into sexual intercourse against his or her will. In most cases the rapist and the victim know each other, either as acquaintances, lovers, or family members. Rape is not specific to gender or sexual orientation, nor is it ever "provoked." *See also* CHILD ABUSE *and* RAPE.

Sexual Characteristics, Secondary

Physical features, such as body shape and amount and pattern of body hair, that appear at puberty.

Hormones responsible for the onset of puberty also cause the development of secondary sexual characteristics.

Male secondary sexual characteristics include the growth of hair in the genital area and under the arms, on the face, and sometimes on the chest. The penis and testicles grow in size, the shoulders broaden, the Adam's apple becomes more prominent, and the voice deepens.

Female secondary sexual characteristics include the growth of hair in the pubic area and under the arms. The first visible change is breast development. The voice deepens, but not as much as in males. Body fat increases around the hips, stomach, and thighs. Menarche, the first menstrual period, usually occurs within a year of the start of development. *See also* PUBERTY.

Sexual Desire, Inhibited

Prolonged lack of sexual desire and inability to become aroused during sexual activity.

Persistent problems an individual may experience becoming sexually aroused have many causes and may or may not be indicative of an underlying physical abnormality.

Causes. Some antidepressants, sleeping pills, antihypertensive drugs, and contraceptives can cause reduced sexual desire, as can alcohol. Victims of rape and incest, or of violent attack, may experience loss of sexual desire for an extended period. People under severe stress may experience loss of sexual desire. Sufferers of depression, anxiety disorders, or more severe disorders are likely to experience sexual inhibition. An underlying problem regarding the relationship with the partner may also be causing the lack of desire, and can be addressed in marital counseling or individual psychotherapy. *See also* PSYCHOTHERAPY.

Sexual Dysfunction

Problems relating to sexual performance.

Sexual dysfunction may occur at one or more of the stages of sexual activity—desire, arousal, and orgasm. When sexual functioning causes problems in a relationship, it is important to determine the cause.

Sexual dysfunction relating to desire results in a lack of interest in sexual relations, the most serious problem being a complete aversion to sexual activity or even to touching another person. However, sometimes the problem is not a true lack of sexual desire, but actually a disparity in the levels of sexual interest between the two partners.

Physical arousal involves engorgement of the genitals leading (in men) to an erection and (in women) to engorgement of the clitoris and labia, and vaginal widening and lubrication. When physical causes are ruled out, dysfunction at this stage is usually related to performance anxiety or feelings of shame or guilt.

Problems reaching orgasm, the third stage of sexual activity, may be temporary or lifelong. The affected person may experience normal levels of sexual desire and arousal. A small percentage of women experience a lifelong inability to achieve an orgasm. When a woman who was once able to achieve an orgasm loses the ability to do so, physical, emotional or relationship problems may be responsible. The decline in hormones that accompanies menopause is a common cause of sexual dysfunction, affecting all phases of the sexual response cycle. In men, orgasm may occur too rapidly, as in the case of premature ejaculation, or too slowly, only after prolonged, sometimes vigorous stimulation.

Causes. The problems relating to sexual functioning may be physical, such as with diabetes, hormone deficiencies, surgery, or the use of certain medications or substances of abuse. Antidepressant medications, such as Zoloft and Prozac, that fall into the category of drugs referred to as SSRIs are commonly associated with diminished sexual desire, arousal, and orgasm.

Similar side effects occur with certain drugs used to treat hypertension. Together, a patient and doctor can weigh the impact of a medication's side effects and consider alternatives when available.

When a sexual problem occurs only under certain circumstances, it is said to be situational, and is likely to have a psychological basis. Difficulty at any stage of sexual activity may be related to psychological factors such as restrictive upbringing, fear of failure, intimacy concerns, feelings of shame or guilt, or a preference for a different type of sexual activity. Inexperience may also play a part in sexual dysfunction, particularly in cases of premature ejaculation and female orgasm disorder.

Treatment. The form of treatment will depend upon the cause of the sexual dysfunction. For those with problems resulting from psychological or situational causes, cognitive-behavioral sex therapy is most effective. One well-known cognitive-behavioral technique that shifts the focus from performance to giving and receiving pleasure is the sensate focus technique. Engaging in a course of sex therapy often benefits the couple's overall relationship, in addition to the specific sexual problem.

If the sexual problem appears to have a physical cause, the underlying medical issue must be addressed.

Sex and Aging. Over the course of a lifetime, most men will find that they cannot achieve or maintain an erection every time they want to. The chance of having this difficulty increases with age. At 50, the problem affects only about 5 percent of men, but up to half of men over 75 are affected. The introduction of Viagra to treat erectile dysfunction has significantly improved the ability of men with this problem to enjoy a more active sex life. Some older couples have difficulty adjusting to differences in levels of sexual desire when the man uses Viagra. Psychosexual therapy is effective in helping couples adjust. The benefit of this drug to women has yet to be established. *See also* ANTIDEPRESSANT DRUGS; DEPRESSION; DIABETES; SENSATE FOCUS TEHCNIQUE; *and* SEX THERAPY.

Sexual Intercourse

The act of an erect penis being inserted into a female vagina.

The penis becomes erect when sexually stimulated. In response to the stimulation, which can be physical or psychological, blood flow to the penis increases. The erectile tissue and sinuses of the penis accommodate the increased blood volume. The erection is usually maintained for a short while after ejaculation has occurred. Afterward there is a refractory period, ranging from a few minutes to half a day, until the penis can become erect once more.

During sexual excitement, erectile tissue elsewhere in the body is similarly affected. In women, the clitoris, a small structure located above the urethra and roughly analogous to the male penis, becomes erect, as may the nipples of both sexes. Females also experience an increase in vaginal discharge and lubrication when sexually stimulated.

Sexual response consists of four phases: arousal, plateau, orgasm, and resolution. Lack of communication between partners or an underlying physical problem may interfere with any one of these phases.

Once ejaculation occurs, the sperm are released into the female reproductive tract and swim through the uterus and fallopian tubes. If a healthy egg is present, a single sperm will penetrate the outer membrane and combine its genetic material with that of the egg in conception.

Sexual intercourse is performed for reasons other than procreation. Vaginal intercourse is not the only type of intercourse. Many couples also enjoy manual, oral, and anal sex.

Sexual intercourse is also an efficient method of transmitting many different diseases. "Safe sex" measures involve the use of condoms, either the male and female variety, as well as latex dental dams during oral sex to avoid contracting or spreading disease. *See also* SEX HORMONES; SEX THERAPY; SEXUAL ABUSE; SEXUAL DESIRE, INHIBITED; *and* SEXUAL DYSFUNCTION.

Resources on Sexual Dysfunction
Adashi, Eli Y, Jouh A. Rock and Zev Rosenwaks, *Reproductive Endocrinology, Surgery, and Technology* (1992); Boston Women's Health Book Collective, *The New Our Bodies, Ourselves: A Book By and For Women* (1992); Hamilton, David, and Frederick Naftolin, *Reproductive Function in Men* (1992); Kaplan, Helen Singer, *The Sexual Desire Disorders: Dysfunctional Regulation of Sexual Motivation* (1995); Tyler, Sandra L., et al., *Female Health and Gynecology: Across the Lifespan* (1982); American Board of Obstetrics and Gynecology, Tel. (212) 871-1619, Online: www.abog.org; American Society for Reproductive Medicine, Tel. (205) 978-5000, Online: www.asrm.org; www.ivf.org/ home.html; www.nycornell.org/obgyn / www.nycornell.org/medicine/womenshealth/html.

Sexual Obsession

A preoccupation with sex that interferes with participation in and enjoyment of personal, social, and job-related activities.

Generally, sexual activity that takes place between consenting adults, does not cause physical harm, and when incorporated into an otherwise normal lifestyle is considered healthy sexual activity. In some cases, an individual may become so preoccupied with sex that it prevents him or her from forming healthy relationships, maintaining employment, or enjoying other activities.

Symptoms. Individuals with sexual obsession may cheat on monogamous partners; spend inordinate amounts of time and money pursuing sex or sex-related activites, such as pornography or sex-related phone lines or chat rooms; or have sex in nonconsensual situations. Such sexual behavior does not cause lasting fulfillment and limits the ability to function in day-to-day life.

Treatment of sexual obsession may include psychotherapy, marriage counseling, or antidepressant drugs. Underlying problems, such as depression, anxiety, or impulse control disorders, must be diagnosed and treated first to combat out-of-control sexual behavior. *See also* PSYCHOTHERAPY.

Sexual Response

The cycle of physical changes that occur during sexual activity.

The four-stage model of sexual activity proposed by Masters and Johnson in the 1950s is the most widely accepted. The stages are excitement, in which a person first responds to sexual stimuli; plateau, in which heart rate and breathing increase, and blood engorges genital tissue; orgasm, in which sexual excitement peaks and is released; and resolution, in which the body returns to its original state. The progression of sexual response is basically the same in men and women, although men tend to respond and reach orgasm more quickly than women. *See also* SEXUAL INTERCOURSE.

Sexuality

Behavior connected with reproduction and the use of the reproductive organs.

Human sexuality means different things at different times of life. For children, sexuality involves learning about their bodies and the world around them, and often about learning expectations by observing adult behavior. From early childhood, children typically identify with a particular gender and the expectations that go along with it.

For adolescents, sexuality involves the many changes arising from the development of sexual maturity. Adolescents develop a sexual identity in the physical sense and begin to learn the role of a mature male or female. At this time they also develop attractions to others and may often experiment sexually. The years of adolescence and early adulthood are marked by a growing awareness of the implications of sexual behavior and the necessity of taking responsibility for actions.

Sexuality in the 20s and 30s is often wrapped up in family and parenting responsibilities. Parents' images of themselves and each other as sexual beings may be temporarily overshadowed by the demands of raising a family.

The definition of sexuality changes again in middle age. For women going through menopause, this time period marks the end of the reproductive years. Men of this age also have to make readjustments. This time period, however, does not mark an end to sexuality. Provided there is no underlying physical problem, sexual behavior can continue into old age.

In general, sexuality is expressed through both behavior and a sense of self. Physically, sexuality may be expressed through activities ranging from masturbation to sexual intercourse. Sexual attraction may be toward the opposite or same sex—the current theory is that sexual preference ranges from exclusively heterosexual to exclusively homosexual, with most people falling somewhere in between the two extremes. *See also* SEX.

Sexually Transmitted Disease

Also known as STD or venereal disease

Disease that is usually transmitted during sexual activity.

Sexually transmitted diseases (STDs) are spread through the exchange of bodily fluids like semen, vaginal secretions, or blood. If someone has an STD, there is a good chance that the disease will be transmitted to any sexual partner. Most of these diseases are very contagious; it can take only one encounter with an infected individual for a person to catch the disease. Vaginal intercourse is the usual transfer event; however, anal or oral intercourse will also spread an STD, and a mother may also transfer such an infection to her child during childbirth.

TYPES

Herpes is believed to affect one-sixth of the population of the United States. Herpes is a viral disease for which there is no cure. Antiviral drugs may reduce the severity and duration of an acute bout of herpes, but they cannot completely eradicate the virus from the body. There are several different types of herpes. Cytomegalovirus attacks the eyes of people with acquired immunodeficiency syndrome (AIDS). Herpes simplex type 1 produces fever blisters around the mouth, fever, fatigue, and swollen glands. Herpes simplex type 2 produces painful sores on the genitals or anus.

Chlamydia is the most widespread STD, because in over one-half of people infected with the disease it is asymptomatic (without symptoms). It is estimated that 45 percent of sexually active teenagers have been exposed to chlamydia. Infected men may display symptoms such as a white, puslike discharge from the penis, swollen testicles, and painful urination. Infected women may bleed during intercourse or between periods. Some women with chlamydia may also suffer cervicitis, an inflammation of the cervix. A women who has chlamydia and gets pregnant is at risk for an ectopic

pregnancy (in which a fetus grows outside the uterus). Even if the child is born normally, it may be born with a birth defect, such as blindness, or suffering from a disease, such as pneumonia.

Gonorrhea is caused by a bacterium that prefers warm, moist places in the body, such as the cervix, urethra, mouth, or rectum. The initial symptoms of gonorrhea are mild to nonexistent. Two to ten days after exposure, a man will notice a yellowgreen discharge from his penis and will experience a burning sensation during urination. Women will also experience a burning sensation during urination and may also have an abnormal vaginal discharge. Women may also experience a rash on the palms and a mild sore throat. An infected pregnant woman can pass gonorrhea to her child during birth, which can cause blindness in the child.

Syphilis is one of the oldest reported STDs. The bacterium that causes the disease is called *Treponema pallidum*, and looks like a coiled spring under a microscope. In the early stages of syphilis, canker sores (ulcers located on the genitals and around the mouth) will appear, and the lymph nodes in the groin will become swollen. These symptoms then subside, and the canker sores heal leaving no scars. If the disease is left untreated, in a few months the second stage of the disease begins. Symptoms of this stage include a rash on the palms of the hands and the soles of the feet. There may also be weight loss, fatigue, and hair loss. After the second stage, there may be a long latency period when there are no symptoms and no sense of sickness. Without treatment, the third stage may be delayed for years, but eventually this stage can lead to irreversible heart and central nervous system problems.

Acquired Immunodeficiency Syndrome (AIDS) is one of the most virulent diseases to attack humans. Once the virus enters the body, it penetrates a healthy cell (often one of the white blood cells that are critical to the immune system) and incorporates itself into the DNA of the infected cell. The cell is then destroyed and releases new

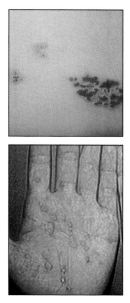

Sexually Transmitted Disease.
Above top is a photo of the herpes lesion; the photo below is of the syphilis virus. Secondary syphilis is one of the few infectious diseases that produces rashes on the palms and soles, as well as a generalized rash. If an ulcer on the penis is followed several weeks later by a rash, the person should be evaluated for syphilis.

copies of the virus to attack other cells. The process is slow, and it may take years until the damage is so serious that the sufferer becomes vulnerable to any one of a number of other diseases, including the STDs mentioned above.

Other STDs include chancroid, granuloma inguinale, lymphogranuloma venerium, crabs (body lice), genital and anal warts, and trichomoniasis.

SYMPTOMS

Symptoms of STDs are more obvious in men than in women, and STDs can often be misdiagnosed because of the similarity of their symptoms to those of other diseases. Furthermore, women infected with an STD may have no symptoms at all and therefore may unknowingly transmit the disease to others. Like most infections, STDs weaken the immune system, so that an individual with one of these diseases is vulnerable not only to other STDs but to other secondary infections as well. Unlike some bacterial infections, recovery from a bout with one of these diseases confers no immunity against that disease, and a person is just as likely to get infected with the same disease again if he or she has unprotected sexual contact.

PREVENTION

The prevalence and intractability of AIDS has made most people a lot more careful in their choice of sexual partners. There is much to be said for the value of abstinence or monogamy, with or without marriage, in the prevention of STDs. If an individual is planning on having sexual relations with multiple partners, it is important to practice "safe sex" in order to avoid contracting an STD. "Safe sex" practices entail the proper use of a new condom before every sexual encounter, whether vaginal, oral, or anal sex is practiced.

> *For background material on sexually transmitted disease, see* INFECTIOUS DISEASE AND SEXUAL INTERCOURSE. *Further information can be found in* AIDS; BACTERIA; CHILDBIRTH; CHLAMYDIA; CYTOMEGALOVIRUS; GONORRHEA; HERPES; PENIS; PREGNANCY; SYPHILIS; AND VIRUSES.

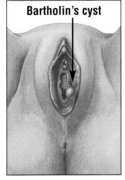

Bartholin's cyst

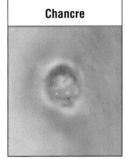

Chancre

Sexually Transmitted Diseases.
Sores or lesions on the female genitalia, in the photos above, are often the result of infections caused by sexually transmitted diseases.

Sezary Syndrome

Cancer of the lymph nodes, liver, spleen, and skin, occurring mostly among the middle-aged and the elderly.

In its early stages, sezary syndrome is called mycosis fungoides. It is most often found in elderly men.

Symptoms. Sezary syndrome is characterized by redness of the skin, fever, chills, weight loss, and malaise (a generalized feeling of illness). In advanced stages, an itchy rash on the skin may develop. Sezary syndrome may arise spontaneously, or it may develop following the cancer called cutaneous T-cell lymphoma.

Diagnosis and Treatment. Sezary syndrome is diagnosed after biopsies of the skin rash reveal cancerous tumors. There may also be involvement of the lymph nodes. If the spread of the disease is limited, it may be treated with topical chemotherapy, sometimes in combination with exposure to ultraviolet light. If the disease has spread throughout the skin, treatment may include total skin electron beam radiation, which destroys the abnormal cells and can cure the condition if applied early enough in the course of the disease. *See also* CHEMOTHERAPY; CUTANEOUS; GERONTOLOGY; *and* ULTRAVIOLET LIGHT.

Shame

A strong feeling of unworthiness, guilt, embarrassment, or disgrace.

Shame can play a role in developing normal feelings of self-esteem, identity, and conscience, or it can be an overwhelming emotion that inhibits a person's enjoyment of and engagement in life. Physical indications of shame include a lowered head, down-turned eyes, and blushing.

Characteristics and disorders that may have shame as a component include depression, anger, shyness, and paranoia. On a healthy level, shame can be useful in determining and responding to social norms. On an unhealthy level, a person may be prone to feelings of shame that are out of proportion to actual events, or a person may feel shame as a result of abuse, addiction, or other traumatic experiences. Often feelings of shame must be dealt with in the process of recovering from such experiences. *See also* DEPRESSION *and* PARANOIA.

Sheehan's Disease

Also known as postpartum hypopituitarism

Death of pituitary gland tissue resulting from postpartum bleeding (hemorrhage) in the uterus.

Sheehan's syndrome can occur if uterine hemorrhage during childbirth leads to a collapse of the circulatory system, resulting in loss of nourishment to and subsequent death of pituitary tissue. Because of improved prenatal and obstetrical care, this syndrome is very rare. *See also* CHILDBIRTH.

The pituitary gland produces a number of hormones, including hormones that stimulate reproductive functions, production of breast milk, and the thyroid and adrenal glands. Loss of pituitary function can result in symptoms including cessation of menstruation (amenorrhea), lack of milk production, and fatigue. Symptoms vary depending on the extent of damage to the pituitary gland. Sheehan's syndrome can be effectively treated with lifelong use of replacement hormones, with an excellent prognosis. *See also* PITUITARY GLAND.

Shiatsu

A form of stress-relieving bodywork involving finger pressure along the meridians of the body.

An ancient form of massage developed in China and later brought to Japan. The technique is based on the principles of acupressure, and combines many healing techniques including physiotherapy and osteopathy.

The primary aim of shiatsu sessions is to restore the flow of chi, or ki in Japanese, an energy force present throughout the entire body. Treatment involves the application of sustained pressure to specific meridians for three to ten seconds in an effort to relax the muscles and tissues. The practitioner will encourage a style of breathing and will also partake in the breathing alongside the client while he or she applies pressure with the fingers, palms, knuckles, and elbows. The sessions usually last between 60 and 90 minutes. *See also* ACUPRESSURE *and* YOGA.

Shigellosis

Also known as bacillary dysentery

Type of bacterial infection in the intestine, caused by the shigella organism.

Outbreaks of shigellosis are most common in developing countries. The disorder is sometimes contracted by travelers visiting those areas. On occasion, there have been outbreaks of shigellosis in the United States (it affects about 15,000 people annually). Affected individuals typically are between the ages of 1 and 3 years years old.

Causes. Shigella is transmitted from person to person by the the feces of infected people. A person who has not washed his or her hands after defecation may spread the disease by handling food thereby contaminating it. Flies also carry the disease. Although it is still uncommon, day-care centers, nursing homes, and mental institutions are the most regular sites for shigellosis outbreaks.

Diagnosis and Symptoms. Stool cultures are used to diagnose the condition. Symptoms include watery diarrhea, cramps, nausea, vomiting, and fever. As the condition becomes worse, the need to defecate becomes more severe, and a person may pass small, watery stools containing pus and blood. Dehydration is common among young children and the elderly who experience persistent diarrhea. The presence of bacterial poisons in the blood can cause a high fever and occasionally delirium.

Treatment. Antibiotics such as ampicillin help shorten the course of the disease and eliminate the infectious organism. In most cases the illness lasts only a week, although for some it may last several weeks. In rare instances, shigellosis has proved fatal, although only in cases of severe dehydration. *See also* BACTERIA; DEHYDRATION; DIARRHEA; FEVER; *and* VOMITING.

Shin Splints

Pain in the front and along the sides of the lower leg that increases with activity or stress.

The pain from shin splints may be the result of a compartment fracture, or pressure on a muscle, myositis (muscle inflammation), tendinitis (tendon inflammation), or periostitis, the inflammation of an outer layer of bone. A muscle tear in the area of the shin may also cause pain and swelling.

Shin splints are most common in those who repeatedly put stress or pounding on the leg, most notably runners. A week or two of rest usually relieves the pain and inflammation, as will anti-inflammatory drugs. Proper stretching and motion mechanics can help reduce the chance of reoccurrence. *See also* BONE; INFLAMMATION; MYOSITIS; *and* STRESS FRACTURES.

Shock

Dangerous drop in blood pressure that results in inadequate flow to the tissues of the body.

Although sometimes used to refer to states of mental or emotional distress, medical shock is the result of decreased blood flow to the brain and vital organs. Shock is a secondary effect of severe injury or illness.

CAUSES

Shock may be caused by massive blood loss, blood vessel blockage or widening, or the inability of the heart to pump blood. These conditions are produced by heart attack, injury, allergic reaction, bacterial infection, electric shock, poisoning, heat stroke, extensive burns, some metabolic disorders, drug overdose, and spinal cord injury. Shock is life-threatening.

ALERT

The Shock Position

Lay the person on his or her back and cover him or her with a blanket to keep warm. Elevate the legs slightly (but not if the person has had a venomous bite). If there is absoluetly no possibility of a neck injury, turn the head to the side so that vomiting will not block air passages. Do not offer beverages or any other food. Loosen clothing that may inhibit breathing. Seek professional medical help immediately.

SYMPTOMS

In early stages a person may be tired, dizzy upon standing, easily fatigued, nauseated, and thirsty. In later stages the skin pales, and lips and fingernails may show a bluish coloration (cyanosis). The skin is cool and sweaty; the pulse becomes weak and rapid; breathing may be shallow or fast. Blood pressure can be unmeasurably low.

TREATMENT

A person administering first aid should check to see that there has been no damage to the person's neck or spine, and that the individual is breathing. If necessary, cardiopulmonary resuscitation (CPR) should

ALERT

Anaphylactic Shock

If a person is allergic to food (especially in the case of nuts), he or she may go into anaphylactic shock. Symptoms include swelling of tongue and face, gasping and choking, hives, a weak and rapid pulse, dizziness, nausea, vomiting, and unconsciousness. A serious case of anaphylactic shock can kill within fifteen minutes. People who known that they are sensitive to certain substances, will often wear a medical ID bracelet or tag so that the proper treatment can be administered quickly.

ALERT

Septic Shock

A bacterial invasion of the bloodstream (septicemia and toxemia) can be so severe that a person goes into shock. Only blood tests can reveal the presence of septic shock. In this case, circulation may be preserved until relatively late in the course, and then become severely compromised causing shock. If there is reason to believe a person is suffering from septic shock, he or she should be put in the shock position until emergency medical assistance arrives.

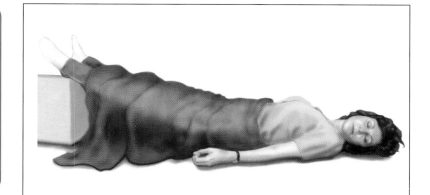

be administered. any bleeding that may be evident must be controlled with direct pressure. The patient should be kept warm and in a supine position (the shock position). Medical assistance from a trained professionals (emergency medical technicians) should be alerted immediately.

SHOCK and related issues are discussed in ANAPHYLACTIC SHOCK; CARDIOPULMONARY RESUSCITATION; EMERGENCY MEDICINE; FIRST AID; and SEPTICEMIA. Symptoms are clearly covered in BACTERIA; BLOOD PRESSURE; CYANOSIS; DIZZINESS; DOUBLE VISION; and PULSE. See also BLEEDING TREATMENT for more information about pressure points and the treatment of conditions that may lead to shock.

Short Stature

Term describing those who fall below the smallest five percent of the average height for those of the same age and sex.

Short but otherwise normal parents are likely to have a child who is also short. If a child appears to be growing too slowly, or if his or her limbs are disproportionate, that may indicate a problem. One simple cause of slow growth or short height in children is poor nutrition. Some medications may slow growth. Hypothyroidism, a disorder in which the body does not produce enough thyroid hormone, can also slow growth in children unless it is treated.

A lack of production of the growth hormone can cause pituitary dwarfism. With this condition, the child is small, but proportionate. Currently, hormone treatment (GH) is used; it improves growth rate, but this may slow over the long-term.

A true solution has not yet been found. Achondroplasia, in which the long ends of the bone stop growing too early causes disproportionately short limbs, and thus short stature. This is an inherited, permanent disorder. *See ACHONDROPLASIA; DNA; HERITABILITY; HYPOTHYROIDISM; and PITUITARY.*

Shoulder Dislocation

Irregular movement of the head of the upper arm bone (humerus) out of the shoulder joint.

The humerus has a round head that rolls into the shoulder joint, giving it a wide range of movement. If the hand takes the weight of the body during a fall, for example, the humerus can be jarred out of place. This is known as an anterior (forward) dislocation, because the head of the humerus slides in front of the joint. Posterior (backward) dislocations, in which the humerus is jarred back behind the joint, are more rare; it would take an extremely sharp direct blow, or violent twisting to send the bone backward.

The main symptom of a dislocated shoulder is pain, worsened by movement. Anterior dislocations are visible to the eye, but posterior ones may not be noticed. X-rays can confirm the diagnosis.

Treatment consists of moving the bone back into place, followed by immobilization in a sling during healing. Severe dislocations may also damage surrounding muscles and nerves, which may require further surgery. *See also DIAGNOSIS; DISLOCATION, JOINT; SHOULDER; and X-RAY.*

The Shock Position. One of the first steps in many emergency first aid treatments is to put an individual in the shock position, as pictured above. In the shock position, a person's feet should be elevated and the body kept somewhat warm. Only turn the head if there is absolutely no chance that the injury is affecting the head or neck.

Resources on Shoulder

Costill, David L., *Inside Running: Basics of Sports Physiology* (1986); Jordan, Barry, and Russell F. Warren, et al., *Sports Neurology* (1998); McArdle, William D., et al., *Exercise Physiology: Energy, Nutrition, and Human Performance* (1996); Warren, Russell F., *The Unstable Shoulder* (1998); American Physical Therapy Association, Tel. (800) 999-APTA, Online: www.apta.org; National Osteoporosis Foundation, Tel. (800) 223-9994, Online: www.nof.org; President's Council on Physical Fitness and Sports, Tel. (202) 690-9000, Online: www.fitness.gov; Women's Sports Foundation, Tel. (800) 227-3988, Online: www.lifetimetv.com/WoSport; https://public1.med.cornell.edu/orthopedics/index.html.

Shoulder-Hand Syndrome

Also known as reflex sympathetic dystrophy

Pain and stiffness in a shoulder and hand.

In shoulder-hand syndrome, one shoulder is painful and stiff, often with restricted movement, and the hand of the same arm is painful and swollen. Usually the elbow is not affected. This may occur after a heart attack, trauma, with specific medications or as a result of other causes. Shoulder-hand syndrome can be treated with corticosteroids. *See also* HEART ATTACK *and* TRAUMA.

Shunt

Procedure or device that reroutes body fluid from one area to another.

The device usually consists of a tube (catheter), which is inserted into a body part or cavity to redirect body fluid and to reduce pressure in the area. The two major types of shunts are used in the treatment of hydrocephalus and for hypertension in the portal system. *See also* HYDROCEPHALUS.

Hydrocephalus (literally "water brain") —a condition in which excess cerebrospinal fluid accumulates in the brain—may be treated with either a ventriculoatrial shunt, in which a catheter is led from the cerebral ventricles to the right atrium of the heart, or a ventriculoperitoneal shunt, which goes from the cerebral ventricles to the abdomen. The excess fluid is safely absorbed into the new body area. With a hydrocephalic newborn, a ventriculopleural shunt diverts cerebrospinal fluid into the chest area. *See also* BRAIN *and* HEART.

In a portacaval shunt, the hepatic portal vein is connected to the inferior vena cava (the largest vein the body) to release pressure in the veins from the digestive organs and spleen to the liver. A portacaval shunt is usually performed to prevent bleeding of esophageal varixes (veins in the lower esophagus) or to improve blood flow to the liver in cases of cirrhosis. Other shunts are used in heart bypass surgery, in hemodialysis, and in eye surgery to drain aqueous fluid.

Shy-Drager Syndrome

Also known as multiple system atrophy

A swelling of the optic nerve that causes increased intracranial pressure.

This rare disease is characterized by a general progressive failure of the central and autonomic nervous systems. The disease is frequently confused with Parkinson's disease, but the damage to the nervous system is much more extensive in Shy-Drager syndrome. It is most often found among men over the age of 60. The cause of this disease is not known, nor is there a cure.

Symptoms. This syndrome causes the failure of essential involuntary body functions like regulation of the blood pressure, heart rate, sweating, focus, bowel, and urinary control. Symptoms usually include very low blood pressure when standing up, constipation, and incontinence. Other symptoms include generalized weakness, double vision, speech impairment, and difficulties breathing and swallowing as well as an irregular heart rate. *See also* VISION.

Treatment. Treatment is limited to managing the blood pressure with beta blockers or vasoconstrictors or other blood pressure medications. Muscular tremors may be treated with amantadine or anticholinergic medication. *See also* TREMOR.

SIADH

Also known as dilutional hyponatremia

Excessive production of ADH, the antidiuretic hormone.

Syndrome of inappropriate antidiuretic hormone, or SIADH, means that the pituitary gland is producing too much antidiuretic hormone (ADH), the hormone that helps to control the balance of fluids in the body. If the blood contains too little water and too much sodium, the hypothalamus signals the pituitary gland to release ADH, which instructs the kidneys to retain water. When there is too much water, the pituitary slows down its production of ADH, which lets water pass through the body. SIADH is not a condition that occurs by itself, but is usually related to other disorders; it has been connected to certain cancers, Hodgkin's disease, lung diseases (such as pneumonia), and brain disorders such as hemorrhages or encephalitis. Any condition that affects the brain, hypothalamus, or pituitary gland may also result in SIADH. Symptoms include weight gain, water retention, loss of appetite, weakness, nausea, and vomiting. Treatment should cure the underlying disorder. *See also* ADH.

Siamese Twins

Also known as conjoined twins

Identical twins from an incompletely separated egg who are born physically attached to each other.

Siamese twins come from the same egg. Shortly after fertilization, the egg undergoes several rapid rounds of cell division. It is not uncommon for it to split into two completely separate entities at this point. This is the origin of identical twins. However, sometimes the separation is incomplete, and the two embryos remain partly joined together. *See also* CONCEPTION.

The twins may share only some layers of skin or muscle, or they may share entire blood vessels, organs, or systems. They may be joined at any point of the body. The most common connection sites are the head, chest, and pelvis. Surgical separation depends on how many tissues the twins share and if both can live independently.

The degree of organ sharing also determines wether the twins can survive in a joined or separated state. The surgery involved is quite intricate, particularly if many vessels and organs are shared. *See also* DELIVERY *and* PREGNANCY, MULTIPLE.

Sibling Rivalry

Intense competition between siblings.

Feelings of rivalry or jealousy between children are normal. After the birth of a sibling, an older child may feel neglected in light of the care paid to the newborn. Even if dealt with carefully, this resentment and hostility may last into adult life. Parents are wise to make the older child feel important in the life of the now larger family and in the life of the newborn. Two messages should be imparted unequivocally to the older child: that the parents are no less loving and caring of the welfare of the older child; and that no harm inflicted on the newborn by the older child (no matter how playful) will be tolerated. *See also* FAMILY THERAPY.

Sick Building Syndrome

A disorder in which many people in the same office building complain of similar symptoms.

Breathing in asbestos, widely used as insulation in public buildings, increases the chance of developing lung cancer later in life. Shipyard workers were the first affected by this. Today, aging buildings expose millions to airborne particles that make them ill. Symptoms include respiratory problems, fatigue, headaches, and dry eyes, nose, and throat. Air conditioning, fluorescent light, and an absence of natural light and air have all been blamed for this disorder, but the cause is unknown. Those who suffer from multiple chemical sensitivities were found to have more psychological disorders but no real connection has been established. If psychology does not play a role then, the only possible solution may be altering buildings. *See* ASBESTOSIS.

Sickle Cell Anemia

An inherited disease in which red blood cells in the presence of oxygen become sticky and rigid and assume a crescent shape.

This is an inherited disease that affects mostly individuals whose ancestors came from Africa, the Middle East, the Mediterranean, and India. The hemoglobin S gene, the cause of the disease, is recessive. A carrier (who has only one S gene) will have no symptoms, though he or she may have some percentage of deformed red blood cells. A child who inherits the

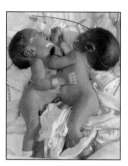

Siamese Twins. The term "Siamese twins" is rarely used today; the term "conjoined twins" describes the condition, pictured above, more accurately. The older term is derived from regular usage to describe Chang and Eng, probably the most famous of conjoined twins (who happened to be of Siamese descent). They were born in 1811 and were joined at the chest so they shared a liver. They were successful businessmen and, after they were wed to Adelaide and Sarah Anne Yates (sisters) they had a total of 21 children during their lifetime.

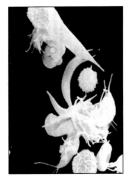

Cell Sickling. Normal red blood cells undergo sickling after delivering oxygen to the furthest (in the extremities, farthest from the heart) and most remote sections of the body. Individuals who live with sickle cell anemia have an amino acid substitution in the hemoglobin of their red blood cells. This causes cells to sickle too quickly, thus altering the shape of the blood cell and making it appear like those pictured above.

Resources on Sickle Cell Anemia
Harris, Jacqueline L., *Sickle Cell Disease* (2001); Mazza, Joseph J., *Manual of Clinical Hematology* (1998); Seeman, Bernard, *The River of Life: The Story of Man's Blood from Magic to Science* (1961); Starr, Douglas, *Blood: An Epic History of Medicine and Commerce* (1998); The Sickle Cell Founda-tion, Tel. 404-616-3572, Online: http://www. emory. edu/PEDS/SICK-LE The National Hemophilia Foundation, Tel. (800) 42-HANDI, On line: www.hemophi-lia.org; www.nycornell. org/medicine/hema tology/index.html;www.nyp. org/css/.

hemoglobin S gene from both parents will exhibit the symptoms of sickle cell anemia. It is a chronic condition; there is no cure other than bone marrow transplantation.

Sickle cell anemia becomes symptomatic late in a baby's first year; blood tests reveal the condition shortly after birth. The problem is in the bone marrow, which produces red blood cells that carry defective hemoglobin. This results in a condition called hemolytic anemia. The affected person may have periods of good health but will experience episodes of severe illness. The defective blood cells become rigid and cannot move through the smaller capillaries, and tissues are starved for oxygen. The spleen, kidneys, bones, and other organs are particularly vulnerable; they often malfunction and cause pain. The red blood cells are fragile and break easily. The bone marrow tries to make up for the lost red blood cells, but it can not produce enough healthy red blood cells to compensate. Those that it does produce are often deformed. *See also* Blood Groups.

Symptoms

Anemic crises are signaled by fatigue, rapid heart beat, and lightheadedness. The affected individual is extremely susceptible to infection and skin ulcers on the lower legs that do not heal, or heal very slowly. Inadequate blood flow to the organs results in acute pain and fever. Children may experience chest pain and difficulty breathing, possibly because of small blood clots in their lungs. They may also have vision problems in general, as well as slowed growth and development.

Any experience that reduces available oxygen will stress the sickle cell anemia sufferer. High altitudes, aircraft flight without pressurization, and even vigorous exercise can exacerbate symptoms. Most people who live with sickle cell anemia develop an enlarged spleen during childhood; by the time they reach puberty, the spleen will be completely dysfunctional. The liver will be enlarged, and gallstones will develop. The heart is often enlarged, and heart murmurs are common.

ALERT

Sickle Cell Anemia and Pregnancy
Women who have sickle cell anemia must be careful to avoid infection during their pregnancy. An affected pregnant woman is vulnerable to pneumonia, urinary infection, and uterus infection. A large percentage of women who have sickle cell anemia develop high blood pressure during their pregnancies and have a higher potential for heart attack. They may also develop small blood clots in the lungs.

Treatment

The most significant treatments include lifestyle changes that assist in dealing with the disorder. A child will be treated with penicillin for the first six years of life to control infections. Adults should also be wary of exposure, since their immune system is compromised; pneumonia and flu vaccinations are advisable. If a person with sickle cell anemia must undergo surgery or becomes pregnant, the doctors should be kept fully informed about the disease.

Traditional treatments may call for blood transfusions, dietary folic acid supplements, and antibiotics to control susceptibility to infection. In crisis situations, pain relief medication will be administered, and intravenous salt solutions will help control dehydration. If blood oxygen is low, a person may be given oxygen.

For more severe situations, new drugs have become available recently. These reduce the severity of the crises and may alleviate some of the pain and discomfort. A medication called hydroxyurea (Hydrea) has been used in cancer and AIDS therapy, and recently, it has been successfully prescribed for sickle cell anemia. There are some dangers in this treatment, since the drug is toxic to cells. As a last resort, bone marrow transplants have proven successful for children under 14 years of age. The Sickle Cell Disease Association is headquartered in Los Angeles; it has chapters in many cities that offer advice and assistance.

Articles about related forms of Anemia *include* Anemia, Aplastic; Anemia, Hemolytic; Anemia, Iron-Deficiency; Anemia, Megaloblastic; *and* Blood. *Issues regarding treatment options include* Blood Transfusion *and* Nutrition.

Sick Sinus Syndrome

Abnormal function of the sinoatrial node, the heart's natural pacemaker.

If the sinoatrial node is damaged by disease or the wear and tear of aging, the result is alternating episodes of bradycardia (abnormally slow heartbeat) and tachycardia (abnormally fast heartbeat). The symptoms include dizziness, fatigue, fainting, and palpitations. Sick sinus syndrome can also be a side effect of some drugs. It can be diagnosed by a 24-hour electrocardiogram recording, in which the patient wears a Holter monitor in exercise testing. Medication can help control the condition, but most patients are helped by having a pacemaker implanted. *See also* BRADYCARDIA; HEART; HOLTER MONITOR; PACEMAKER; SINOATRIAL NODE; *and* TACHYCARDIA.

Side Effect

A reaction, usually negative, to a drug other than the intended reaction.

Because most drugs affect the entire body rather than just the diseased part of the body, they often cause reactions that are unintended and unwanted; these may range from mild to life-threatening. For example, aspirin can cause a minor stomach irritation; drugs used in chemotherapy may cause severe side effects, such as nausea and hair loss, and anticoagulants may cause internal bleeding. Side effects vary from person to person; one person may experience no side effects from a drug, while another may have a severe reaction. The dosage of a drug also affects the severity of side effects. Today, most drugs are taken orally, so common side effects are stomach and intestinal problems, including nausea, vomiting, and diarrhea. *See* PREMEDICATION.

Siderosis

A lung condition caused by the chronic inhalation of iron particles, particularly iron oxide fumes, which results in iron deposits in the lungs.

In the majority of cases, siderosis is a benign and asymptomatic condition; but in some cases, symptoms may include shortness of breath, wheezing, and coughing.

Siderosis is also used to refer to any condition in which an excess of iron accumulates in the body's tissues. Iron overload can cause damage to organs, tissues, and glandular systems. Rarely, siderosis is an indicator of the existence of a disease such as thalassemia. *See also* IRON *and* THALASSEMIA.

Sight, Partial

Visual impairment in which an individual has some vision.

A person may be born partially sighted or may become so due to disease or injury. The most common causes for loss of eyesight in the U.S. are accidents, diabetes, and macular degeneration. Worldwide, the lead- ing cause of sight loss is vitamin A deficiency. Depending on the severity of vision loss, people with partial sight may utilize a variety of aids in order to help them to live independently. A cane may be useful to navigate unfamiliar areas. Children with partial sight may benefit from large-print books or from brightly colored or high-contrast visual aids. *See also* VISION.

Sigmoidoscopy

A means of colon study involving a fiberoptic instrument called a sigmoidoscope.

Sigmoidoscopy allows a physician to directly observe the colon, by means of a flexible instrument known as a sigmoidoscope. The procedure is commonly used to diagnose colon cancer as well as to detect bleeding, submucosal air pockets, polyps, or small sacs that arise as the result of protrusions from the inner lining of the intestine (diverticula). *See also* COLON.

The sigmoidoscopy specialized endoscope, consists of a flexible tube approximately 2 feet long. A tiny lighted video camera at the front of the device allows the doctor to see into the sigmoid and proximal colon, following insertion of the sigmoidoscope into the rectum. About 65 percent of all colorectal cancers may be detected with sigmoidoscopy. Many such cancers are not seen in a standard x-ray. Additionally, sigmoidoscopy may be used to diagnose inflammatory bowel disease, obstruction of the bowel, and diverticulosis (small pouches in the intestine), as well as the source of unexplained abdominal pain and diarrhea. *See also* DIVERTICULOSIS.

During the procedure, a person lies on the left side with his or her knees drawn up toward the chest. The gastroenterologist inserts the lubricated sigmoidoscope into the rectum and guides it toward the colon. Air is forced into the colon to improve the visibility of structure. The device is able to photograph the colon for analysis and also, where appropriate, remove a small tissue sample, or biopsy, through a hollow channel in the flexible tube. Such tissue may be evaluated by a pathologist for the presence of abnormalities. Detection of a potentially malignant polyp may be followed by colonoscopy, as the colonoscope has a longer reach into the colon.

What to Expect. Sigmoidoscopy is completed without anesthesia in about 30 minutes. Prior to the test, an enema is required to thoroughly clean the bowel and provide a clear view. Anyone undergoing this procedure should avoid eating after midnight, before the procedure. The examination is safe and though somewhat uncomfortable, it is relatively painless. Potential complications include minute perforations in the colon lining, bleeding (in the case of biopsy), and some risk of infection, though generally slight. The test is useful for older individuals as well as those displaying signs of lower gastrointestinal abnormality or disease (including chronic diarrhea, blood in the stool, weight loss or lower abdominal pain). Sigmoidoscopy is the primary diagnostic test for colorectal cancer.

Further information can be found in BIOPSY; CANCER; COLON; COLONOSCOPY; DIVERTICULAR DISEASE; ENDOSCOPE; GASTROENTEROLOGY; INFLAMMATORY BOWEL DISEASE; *and* RECTUM CANCER OF. *Information about the primary techniques for diagnosis can be found in* DIAGNOSIS.

Silicone

Any one of a number of organic compounds in which all or part of the carbon is replaced by silicon, a nonmetallic element.

Silicone, which can be fluid, resinous, or rubbery, is used in oils, greases, lubricants, adhesives, plastics, synthetic rubber, and resins. It is water-repellent and highly stable at high temperatures.

Silicone gel breast implants became popular in cosmetic and reconstructive surgery in the 1980s because of their favorable properties, but were banned by the Food and Drug Administration (FDA) in early 1992 because of pressure by lawsuits and unfavorable press coverage. In July 1998 the Institute of Medicine, National Academy of Sciences in Washington, D.C., determined that silicone implants posed no large risk for the development of breast cancer and connective-tissue disease (CTD). Regardless of this development, saline implants have replaced silicone, for the most part, in current breast enlargement procedures, though the FDA still permits unapproved silicone gel implants to be sold. *See also* MAMMOPLASTY *and* TISSUE.

Silicosis

Lung disease resulting from inhalation of crystalline quartz.

Silica (crystalline quartz) is a mineral found in sandrock, chert, diatomite, granite, and other kinds of rock. Persons who work with rock, such as tunnelers, sandblasters, stonecutters, and drillers, can inhale tiny particles of silica if ventilation in the workplace is poor, or if they work without respiratory masks. As silica accumulates in the lung, it can cause fibrosis, a stiffening and scarring of lung tissue that lessens breathing ability. This damage usually occurs over a period of years, but very large concentrations of silica in the air can cause a more rapidly developing form of the condition that can be immediately life-threatening. *See also* PNEUMOCONIOSIS.

Singer's Nodes

Lumps on the vocal cords due to overuse.

Excess strain or overworking the voice can lead to the formation of white-gray lumps on the vocal cords, causing the loss of voice. The condition commonly affects those who use their voices constantly, especially professional singers, teachers, and campaigning politicians.

Loss of voice should first be investigated to rule out cancer of the larynx. The nodes should then be removed. Reoccurrence can be prevented with proper vocal training. *See also* LARYNGITIS; LARYNX, CANCER OF *and* VOICE, LOSS OF.

Sinoatrial Node

The natural pacemaker of the heart.

Also called the sinus node, the sinoatrial node consists of a specialized group of cells in the wall of the right atrium, one of the upper chambers of the heart, near the vena cava. These cells generate regular electrical impulses that control the contractions of the myocardium, the heart muscle. These pulses travel through the heart from top to bottom, causing the regular rhythmic muscular contractions that are felt as the heartbeat. The activity of the sinoatrial node is measured by an electrocardiogram, which records the electrical activity of the heart. Disorders of the sinoatrial node can cause arrhythmias, abnormal heartbeats. *See also* ARRHYTHMIA; ELECTROCARDIOGRAM; *and* SICK SINUS SYNDROME.

Sinus Bradycardia

A slow heart rhythm, less than 60 beats per minute, that originates in the sinoatrial node.

A very slow heartbeat need not be caused by a heart problem. Trained athletes and individuals who eat a balanced diet and exercise on a regular basis can have a heart rate of less than 60 beats per minute during the day, and the rate may be as low as 40 beats per minute during sleep, with a normally functioning sinoatrial node. Sinus bradycardia becomes a problem when the cardiac output does not meet the body's demand for oxygen during normal activity, which can be caused by sick sinus syndrome. This condition is, however, quite rare, affecting less than 3 of every 10,000 people. *See also* BRADYCARDIA; SICK SINUS SYNDROME; *and* SINOATRIAL NODE.

Sinus, Facial

Air-filled cavities in the bone of the face.

Sinus is a general term for any air-filled cavity in the body, but the facial sinuses are the best known, the most easily recognized and the most easily infected. The sinuses in the face serve to reduce the total weight of the head, provide insulation for the skull, and help to add resonance to the voice. There are four sets of sinuses in the face: in the bone of the forehead, behind the cheekbones, between the eyes, and behind the eyes. These cavities are lined with mucous membranes which, if infected, can become inflamed, causing sinusitis. *See also* FLU; SINUSITIS; *and* SKULL.

Sinus Tachycardia

A rapid but regular heart rate, more than 100 beats a minute, originating in the sinoatrial node.

Sinus tachycardia is a normal response to stress, unusual emotional responses, or exercise as the sinoatrial node (which is often described as the heart's natural pacemaker) increases its rate temporarily. It can be a problem if it occurs regularly, which can result from a fever, an overactive thyroid gland, and some heart conditions, such as congestive heart failure; it will often result in breathlessness, lightheadedness, and palpitations that can interfere with a person's routine. The treatment of persistent sinus tachycardia is aimed at the underlying condition, including medication to manage the thyroid or heart failure. *See also* SINOATRIAL NODE *and* TACHYCARDIA.

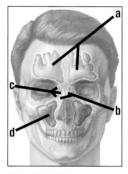

The Facial Sinuses Above, a diagram exhibiting the major facial sinuses, including: (a) the frontal sinus; (b) the sphenoid sinus; (c) the ethmoid sinus; and (d) the maxillary sinus. According to the American Academy of Otolaryngology: Head and Neck Surgery, more than 37 million Americans suffer from at least one incident of sinusitis (an inflammation of the membrane lining the sinuses) each year. Elevated resistance to antibiotics, pollution, and the increasing population density are major contributing factors to such disorders.

Sinusitis

Inflammation of the facial sinuses.

The sinuses in the face receive the most attention because they are the most often affected. Sinuses include all air-filled cavities in the bone. There are four sets of facial sinuses, found in the forehead, behind the cheekbones, between the eyes, and behind the eyes. All of these cavities are lined with mucous membranes; the mucous drains into a channel that empties into the nose.

If the fluid cannot drain properly, it will build up in the sinus cavities. This build up will cause bacteria to grow, leading to further blockage or inflammation. This is sinusitis. Attacks that last less than eight weeks, or that occur less than four times a year, are called acute sinusitis; more frequent attacks that cause no significant damage are known as recurrent acute sinusitis; and episodes that last more than eight weeks, or occur more than four times a year, that cause damage to the mucous membranes are called chronic sinusitis.

CAUSES

Sinusitis is usually related to another infection in the body.

Viral Infections. Colds and flu are the most common causes of acute sinusitis. These infections will block the upper respiratory tract, which then prevents proper sinus drainage. *See* VIRUS.

Fungal Infections. Although this is rather uncommon, acute sinusitis can come from a fungal infection that causes nasal passage blockage. Most people have a natural resistance to the fungi in the environment, but those whose immune system does not function properly may be susceptible to sinusitis-causing fungal infections.

Allergies. Substances that cause regular allergic reactions can also lead to sinusitis, due to the continual inflammation of the nasal passages.

Asthma. Up to 30 percent of people with asthma may develop sinusitis. Those who have chronic sinusitis, however, are also at a higher risk for developing asthma.

SYMPTOMS

The typical, and most prominent symptoms of sinusitis include headaches and facial pain. The location of the pain will vary, depending on which sinus is affected. Usually there is also nasal congestion and heavy sinus discharge.

DIAGNOSIS AND TREATMENT

Sinusitis needs to be diagnosed by a physician, who, based on an examination and the patient's medical history, can determine whether the symptoms are those of sinusitis or just a lingering cold. A physician will also be able to tell if the condition is acute or chronic.

Acute sinusitis often resolves on its own, but in some cases, antibiotics may be prescribed to bring down the inflammation that is causing blockage. For chronic sinusitis, the treatment may range from oral steroid medications to surgery to widen the sinuses, and allow drainage to occur easily. *See also* ALLERGY; ASTHMA; COLD; INFLUENZA; SINUS, FACIAL; *and* SINUS, FACIAL.

Sjögren Syndrome

A chronic disorder characterized by excessive inflammation and dryness of the eyes, nose, throat, mouth, and other mucous membranes, including the vulva and vagina.

Sjögren syndrome is thought to be an autoimmune disease, in which the body attacks its own tissues. The cause is as yet unknown. Sjögren syndrome is more common in women than in men. Different organs and systems are affected in different people; and affected areas may include the trachea, lungs, liver, pancreas, spleen, kidneys, and lymph nodes. Approximately a third of the sufferers develop rheumatoid arthritis, although the symptoms may be milder than in conventional cases of arthritis. Lymphoma is 44 times more common among patients with Sjögren's syndrome. No cure is known for Sjögren's syndrome. Treatment is generally limited to alleviating the symptoms and trying to make the patient comfortable. *See also* AUTOIMMUNE DISORDERS; INFLAMMATION; *and* LYMPHOMA.

Skeleton

The system of bones that provides the body's supporting framework, protects internal organs, and helps make movement possible.

The word "skeleton," which comes from Greek origins, means dried-out body or mummy; an ignoble description for one of the human body's many masterpieces of functional design. Responsible for protection and movement, the bones in the skeleton are quite light and are still very strong.

PARTS OF THE SKELETON

The adult human skeleton contains 206 bones, and it is divided into two main parts: axial and appendicular.

The axial skeleton consists of 80 bones of the head and the trunk. The skull contains 28 bones, only one of which—the mandible—can move. The spine contains 26 bones (vertebrae): seven in the neck (cervical bones); 12 in the chest region (thoracic vertebrae), which attach to ribs that in turn attach to the sternum; and seven in the lower back (lumbar vertebrae, sacrum, and coccyx).

The appendicular skeleton consists of 126 bones in the shoulders, hips, and extremities (arms and legs). The shoulders consist of the collarbones (clavicles) and shoulder blades (scapulae), which connect to the sternum. The arm contains the upper arm bone (humerus) and two lower arm bones (ulna and radius). The wrist contains eight small carpal bones, and each hand contains five metacarpals and 14 finger bones (phalanges).

The hip (pelvis) consists of the pelvic bone and the sacrum and coccyx from the spine. The upper leg bone (femur) connects to the lower leg bones (tibia and fibula). The knee is covered by the kneecap (patella). Each ankle consists of 7 tarsal bones, and each foot of 5 metatarsals and 14 toe bones (phalanges).

FUNCTIONS OF THE SKELETON

One of the primary functions of the skeleton is to help the body maintain its shape

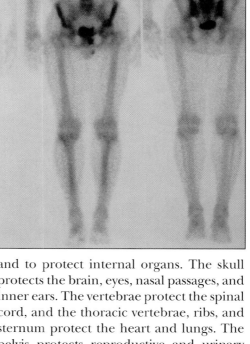

and to protect internal organs. The skull protects the brain, eyes, nasal passages, and inner ears. The vertebrae protect the spinal cord, and the thoracic vertebrae, ribs, and sternum protect the heart and lungs. The pelvis protects reproductive and urinary system organs.

The skeleton is also integral to movement. Muscles are connected to bones with tendons, and force from the muscles causes the skeleton to bend at one or more joints. Thus, the skeleton provides the body with its locomotive function.

In addition, stem cells in the bone marrow produce new blood cells, and the bones store and help maintain an appropriate level of calcium and other minerals in the body.

Background information about the SKELETON can be found in ANATOMY; BONE; FEMUR; MOVEMENT; and SKULL. Information related to bone problems can be found in BONE CANCER; BONE, DISORDERS OF; BONE GRAFT; BRITTLE BONES; FEMUR; and FINGER, JOINT REPLACEMENT OF.

The Human Skeletal System. The human skeleton is an amazing piece of biological construction. Left, a full-body x-ray, anterior (front) view; at right a posterior (back) view. Below, the foot bone groups, showing the tarsals; the metatarsals; and the phalanges (toe bones). The foot and hand have strikingly similar structural features. .

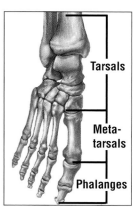

Tarsals

Metatarsals

Phalanges

Resources on Skin
Dvorine, William, *A Dermatologist's Guide to Home Skin Treatment* (1983); Jacknin, Jeanette, *Smart Medicine for Your Skin: A Comprehensive Guide to Understanding Conventional and Alternative Therapies to Heal Common Skin Problems* (2001); Turkington, Carol A. and Jeffrey S. Dover, *Skin Deep : An A-Z of Skin Disorders, Treatments and Health* (1998); American Academy of Dermatology, Tel. (888) 462-DERM, Online: www.aad.org; American Board of Dermatology, Tel. (313) 874-1088, Online: www.abderm.org; National Psoriasis Foundation, Tel. (800) 723-9166, Online: www.psoriasis.org;www.nycornell.org/dermatology/

The Skin and its Layers. To the right is a detailed illustration of the layers of the skin. At the top of the skin, colored in red, is the epidermis; this layer provides much of the body's protection against foreign substances. In the middle, in pink, is the dermis; the dermis supplies blood to the epidermis as it is well-supplied with blood vessels. The roots of the hair follicles and pores also reside here (and in the hypodermis) . At the bottom, in yellow, is the hypodermis; this layer is made primarily of fat so it helps to insulate the body.

Skene's Glands

Also known as the paraurethral glands

A small gland, or set of glands, on each side of the urethra contained by the urethral sponge.

The exact quantity, size and placement of the Skene's glands varies among women. There may be as many as 30 in some individuals, and drastically fewer in others. During arousal, these glands fill with an alkaline fluid similar to that found in the male prostate; this fluid is sometimes referred to as the female ejaculate fluid. The Skene's glands, (and breast tissue) produce prostate-specific antigen (PSA), an important marker for prostate cancer, although the function of the PSA remains unknown. There has been little research done on the Skene's glands, especially in relation to the amount of research done on the prostate. *See also* ANTIGEN *and* PROSTATE.

Skin

Also known at cutaneous membrane

The organ that covers the outer surface of the body.

The skin is one of the largest of the organs, with an adult surface area of about two square miles. It is made of two main layers: the outer epidermis, which is made of epithelial tissue; and the inner dermis, made of connective tissue. Attached to and underlying these layers is a subcutaneous layer of connective and fatty tissues; this layer, known as the hypodermis in turn

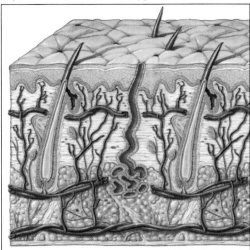

connects to the body's internal organs. The hypodermis is not usually considered part of the skin, although it is composed of similar tissues and serves a parallel function—to protect the body's organs.

The skin serves several key purposes. It protects the body from injury and from the introduction of pathogens. It also is important in maintaining body temperature; the body is cooled through sweat released from the glands in the skin, and changes in blood flow can alter the skin's insulating ability. Nerves in the skin allow for reception of stimuli. Vitamin D is synthesized in the skin upon exposure to ultraviolet radiation; some cells in the epidermis form part of the immune system.

SKIN COLOR

Skin color is a function of three different kinds pigment cells made in the skin and elsewhere in the body; these are carotene, hemoglobin, and melanin. Of these, only melanin is produced in the skin. Carotene is a yellow-orange pigment that accumulates in the hypodermis, and its color is most apparent on the palms of the hands and the soles of the feet. Red blood cells circulating through capillaries in the epidermal skin layer contain the hemoglobin that makes some people's skin appear as though it has a pinkish hue.

Perhaps the most important of the skin pigments is melanin—its color ranges from yellow, to brown and reddish brown, to black. Skin color variations are caused by the kind and amount of melanin that a body produces. Individuals with black or brown skin produce more melanin than those with pale yellow or pink skin. Freckles are close collections of melanin. Melanin is produced by cells called malanocyes; production increases when they are exposed to sunlight, thus leading to sunburn.

Relevant related anatomical articles include ANATOMY; FORESKIN; NERVE; VITAMIN D; WART; *and* WRINKLE. *Information related to skin color can be found in* BLOOD; FRECKLE; HEMOGLOBIN; *and* MELANIN. *Skin problems are discussed in* ACNE; CARCINOMA; CHAPPED SKIN; CHERRY ANGIOMA; MELANOMA; NEUROCUTANEOUS DISORDERS; SKIN ALLERGY; *and* SKIN CANCER. *See also* POISON IVY, OAK, AND SUMAC.

Skin Allergy

An adverse and marked reaction to allergens, which cause burning sensations, stinging, itching, or redness of the skin.

Skin allergies are known as irritant or allergic contact dermatitis. Irritant contact dermatitis is the result of a product irritating the skin. Bath soap, detergents, antiperspirants, cosmetics, moisturizers, and shampoos are common causes of allergies, as is poison ivy. Allergic contact dermatitis is a reaction to a certain ingredient in a product, which may take days to appear. Symptoms include redness, swelling, and clear blisters. Itching is usually a prominent symptom, and it can be difficult to determine if a reaction is allergic or irritant.

There are several causes of reactions but fragrances are the most common. Products that are labeled "unscented" may actually contain a fragrance, designed to cover over chemical scents. Products labeled "fragrance-free" or "without perfume" cannot have any fragrances. Preservatives in cosmetics and skin-care products also cause skin allergies. Cosmetics that contain water must also contain a preservative to prevent bacteria and fungi from developing. Many people are also allergic to lanolin, found in cosmetics and skin cleansers. Products that use the term "hypoallergenic" sometimes contain lanolin. *See also* ALLERGEN.

Metals such as nickel, chrome, and cobalt also cause allergies. Costume jewelry made of alloys usually contain these metals. Body-piercing is frequently a cause of allergic reactions. Piercing locations such as the ears, lips, nose, septum, tongue, navel, and genitalia may produce skin reactions. Latex, used in surgical gloves and condoms, is also a common source of allergy for many people. Dermatologists believe that about two of every 1,000 people have severe reactions to chemicals and metals. *See* SKIN.

To prevent allergic skin reactions, rinse clothes twice after washing. Choose clothes that are pure cotton, and avoid blends. Avoid all perfumes and dyes, and do not use nail polish or hair spray. *See* DERMATOLOGY.

Skin and Muscle Flap

Sections of skin and associated muscle used in grafting and transplant procedures.

Skin and muscle flaps may be surgically harvested from many areas of the body and grafted to new areas of damaged skin. Such grafts may be split thickness (that is, including more layers of ski), or full thickness, which include all the layers of skin. Thinner grafts may be used to replace contaminated surfaces of skin, areas damaged by burns, or surfaces lacking adequate blood supply. Full thickness grafts, including muscle, are more difficult to transplant but more durable and trauma-resistant.

Skin and muscle flap surgery is especially effective in reconstructing the breast after a mastectomy. An oval section of skin, fat, and muscle is removed from the lower portion of the abdomen or back. It is then slid through a tunnel under the skin to the breast area. The tissue is shaped into a natural looking breast and sutured into place. *See also* MASTECTOMY; SKIN; *and* SKIN GRAFT.

Skin Biopsy

Removal of a small section of skin tissue for diagnostic laboratory analysis.

There are three methods of obtaining skin samples with a biopsy: a shave biopsy is performed by applying a local anesthetic, removing a thin outer layer of skin, and cutting the protruding tissue growth with a scalpel. The second method is known as a punch biopsy; with this, a cylindrical section of tissue is extracted by means of a hollow punch instrument pushed into the skin and rotated. Generally, a small piece of skin is removed by this method, though larger punch wounds may be sealed with stitches; these are used when a larger skin biopsy is required. An excision biopsy is more extensive and involves removing the entire area (sore, spot, lump) of suspect tissue. Depending on the extent of tissue involved, the region affected by the biopsy may require a skin transplant. *See* BIOPSY.

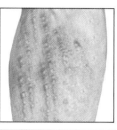

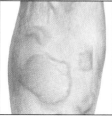

Tests for Skin Allergies. Above, various types of skin reactions can be caused by allergic reactions. At the very top is an illustration of a rash, and the lower image above shows hives. Allergists (physicians who treat allergies) will try to elicit such a skin reaction in order to determine exactly what a person is allergic to. Other examples are shown below. At the very bottom is a positive reaction to a PDD, which tests for tuberculosis. Below, at the top, is an arm that tests positive for a reaction to Candida. This test is used to ensure an individual's immune system is working properly.

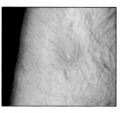

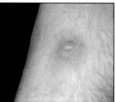

Resources on Skin Cancer

Jacknin, Jeanette, *Smart Medicine for Your Skin* (2001); Kenet, Barney J., et al., *Saving Your Skin: Prevention, Early Detection, and Treatment of Melanoma and Other Skin Cancers* (1998); American Academy of Dermatology, Tel. (888) 462-DERM, Online: www.aad.org; American Cancer Society, Tel. (800) ACS-2345, Online: www.cancer.org; National Cancer Institue, Tel. (800) 4-CANCER, Online: www. nci.nih.gov; www.nycornell.org/dermatology/

Skin Cancer. At the very bottom is a picture of malignant melanoma. This is perhaps the most deadly form of skin cancer. Characteristically, it has an irregular border, and the sore displays multiple colors; it is also highly prone to bleeding. Below, at the top, is a picture of another melanoma lesion. This sort of lesion is sometimes referred to as a "patriotic" lesion because it displays elements of red, white and blue (black and blue).

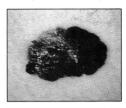

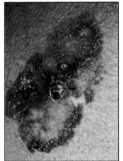

Skin biopsy is relatively painless, though a brief stinging may occur when the anesthetic is injected, and some tenderness may follow the procedure. The technique may be used in order to diagnose benign abnormal growths, chronic fungal or bacterial infections, and melanoma. Where a viral or bacterial infection is suspected, cells from the biopsy tissue will often be sent to a laboratory for culturing and diagnosis. Certain abnormalities of the skin suggest system-wide diseases, for example the skin rash common to sufferers of systemic lupus erythematosus. *See also* FUNGAL INFECTIONS; LUPUS; MELANOMA, JUVENILE; MELANOMA, MALIGNANT; *and* SKIN TUMORS.

Skin Cancer

A malignant tumor of the skin

Skin cancer is the most common form of cancer in the United States, and its incidence has been increasing steadily in recent years. One reason for the increased incidence of skin cancer is the erosion of the Earth's ozone layer, which absorbs ultraviolet radiation, by industrial chemicals released into the atmosphere. A much more important reason is the tendency of Americans to ignore the dangers of sun exposure in their desire to show off a tan.

Melanin, the coloring element of the skin, provides some protection against ultraviolet radiation, and so individuals with darker skin have a substantially lower rate of skin cancer. Hats, protective clothing, and sunscreens offer protection to everyone.

Geography also plays an important role in skin cancer incidence. The incidence is highest in tropical or sunny regions, where daily exposure to sunlight is greatest. Age is another major factor, since the extent of exposure to sunlight increases with age. Fairer-skinned individuals are at higher risk at any age.

A small percentage of skin cancers are caused by exposure to industrial chemicals such as arsenic, coal, paraffin, tars, or oils containing the carcinogens called polycyclic aromatic hydrocarbons.

TYPES

There are three major forms of skin cancer. The most common types are basal cell carcinoma and squamous cell carcinoma. Squamous cell carcinomas arise in the layer of cells that lies just below the thin coating of dead cells on the skin's surface. Basal cell carcinomas arise in the cell layer below the squamous cells. The third, least common but deadliest form of skin cancer is melanoma, which arises in the melanocytes, the cells that produce melanin.

New Therapies

New treatments for skin cancer are constantly being tested. One newer method is photodynamic therapy, in which a medication is taken orally to increase the sensitivity of cancer cells to laser light. Another is use of drugs called retinoids, which are derived from vitamin A, and these are either taken by mouth or applied to the skin. Immunotherapy, arousing the body's defenses with injections of interferon, can be effective, but it causes side effects, including fever, chills, itching, and general malaise.

SYMPTOMS

The American Cancer Society has an ABCD formula for melanoma: a skin lesion that is Asymmetric, whose Border is irregular, whose Color is unusual and whose Diameter is greater than six millimeters (that is about the size of a small pencil eraser) could be a melanoma.

Basal cell carcinomas can be flesh-colored, translucent nodes; red, scaly patches that resemble psoriasis; lesions that resemble scar tissue, or dark-pigmented lesions.

Squamous cell carcinomas usually are reddish, scaly lesions with raised edges. Any sore or skin mark that is associated with pain, ulceration, scabbing, or erosion can be a symptom of this kind of skin cancer.

DIAGNOSIS

A basic method of diagnosing skin cancer is through a microscopic examination of a tissue sample (biopsy) taken from a suspicious lesion to detect cancerous cells. Chest x-rays and blood tests may be done if the cancer is advanced enough to have spread beyond the skin. *See* SKIN TUMORS.

TREATMENT

Skin cancer removal is enough of a curative if it is diagnosed early. Surgery is the treatment of choice; it involves removing the cancer and enough surrounding tissue to be safe while impacting appearance minimally. The cancer may be cut away or removed by curettage, which consists of scraping the malignant area followed by application of an electronic probe to ensure destruction of all cancer cells.

Cryosurgery, in which a liquid nitrogen spray or probe kills the cancerous cells, is also used. Laser-light therapy is a new procedure. If the cancer is at a conspicuous site, such as the face, radiation therapy is preferred; this involves small doses of radiation over a period of weeks.

Chemotherapy, using drugs applied directly to the skin, can be performed when there are many small cancers or precancerous lesions. If the cancer is detected at a later stage when it has spread beyond the skin, chemotherapy and radiation therapy may be required. In all cases, treatment for a first skin cancer calls for periodic follow-ups, with regular self-inspections, examinations by a physician, and sometimes regular magnetic resonance imaging (MRI) and computerized tomography (CT) scans.

PREVENTION AND PROGNOSIS

Skin cancer is the one of the most preventable cancers and one of the most treatable, with long-term survival rates close to 100 percent for cancers that are detected and treated early. Skin cancer is preventable because almost all cases are caused by prolonged, unprotected to sunlight—specifically, to the damage done by the ultraviolet radiation in sunlight, which causes mutations in skin cells that can result in uncontrolled growth. Using sunscreens and wearing garments that protect the skin from direct sunlight—especially the face, neck, and arms—greatly reduces the chances of developing skin cancers.

> *Skin Cancer and related topics are further discussed in* BASAL CELL CARCINOMA; CANCER; CARCINOMA; MELANOMA; *and* SQUAMOUS CELL CARCINOMA. *Related anatomical information is included in* MELANIN *and* SKIN. *See also* BIOPSY.

Skin Graft

Also known as skin transplant

A surgical procedure in which a cross-section of skin from one area of the body is transplanted to another part of the body.

Skin grafts may be used in some surgical procedures (including a biopsy) or to treat extensive wounds or burns. A flap of healthy skin is removed from the patient's body and placed on the area to be covered. This grafted skin can be either split thickness (containing only some layers of skin) or full thickness (containing all skin layers). An individual who undergoes this treatment will be placed under anaesthesia, either local or total. The graft may be sutured or held in place with a sterile bandage. New blood vessels begin to grow into the transplanted skin in less than two days; about six weeks are needed for complete recovery. *See also* BURN; SKIN; SKIN BIOPSY; SKIN CANCER; SURGERY; *and* Z-PLASTY.

Skin Peeling, Chemical

Also known as dermabrasion

A procedure in plastic surgery in which the top layer of skin is removed using a wire disc, steel wool, or chemicals.

Skin peeling may be performed in order to to treat acne, age spots, sun damage, wrinkling, unevenly pigmented skin, superficial scarring, or for the removal precancerous growths. There are 2 primary types of chemicals commonly used: alpha hydroxy acids (AHA), for superficial peels, and trichloroacetic acid (TCA), for deeper peels. There are various advantages to each type of peel; whereas anesthesia is often required for TCA peels, it is rarely used for AHA peels; however, TCA peels tend to be more beneficial for individuals with darker skin tones. A doctor should be consulted in order to decide which treatment method will be most beneficial. The procedure is often quite painful. Depending on the type of skin peel, results can persist for one month to six months. *See also* ACNE; DERMABRASION; PLASTIC SURGERY; *and* WRINKLE.

Images of Skin Cancer. Below, bottom, is a picture of squamous cell carcinoma on the hands; this will have to be surgically removed. Middle is a picture of a man with skin cancer behind his ear; it commonly appears as a nodule one to one and a half centimeters across; in this case blood vessels are also visible. Below, top, is a picture of basal cell carcinoma on the nose. Its classic appearance is as a small, dome-shaped lesion with visible blood vessels.

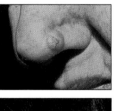

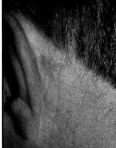

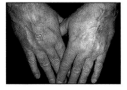

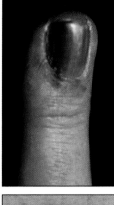

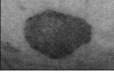

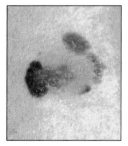

Skin Test and Skin Tumor. At the very top is a malignant melanoma under the fingernail; this type of melanoma spreads quickly. It appears as a black or blueish discoloration. In the middle is a picture of basal cell carcinoma that is between five and six centimeters across. It exhibits a characteristic well-defined border of brownish pigment. At the bottom is an image of malignant lentigo melanoma. This sort of tumor is more common among the elderly population, as it may grow for years before developing its most aggressive patterns.

Skin Tag

Also known as acrochordons or cutaneous tags

A condition involving a small, benign skin growth.

Skin tags are common, usually painless skin protrusions that occur most commonly after the age of 50. They do not grow or change, and their cause is unknown. Skin tags are often found on the neck, under the arms, on the abdomen, and in body folds. They may have a small stalk and are usually the same color as the rest of the skin. Treatment for skin tags is unnecessary, unless they cause irritation. *See* SKIN.

Skin Tests

Any one of a variety of tests on skin to identify and diagnose infection, disease or abnormality.

Most skin tests exploit the human body's allergic defense system, which involves the formation of antibodies or the release of histamine, a chemical that is released in cells during an allergic reaction.

Scratch Testing. With the scratch test method, the allergen is placed on the skin of the forearm, upper arm, or back. The area is then scratched or lightly pricked in order to introduce the allergen under the skin surface. Positive results including redness, itchiness, or swelling may appear after 20 minutes. The person being tested may also exhibit watery eyes, nasal discharge, sneezing, and other symptoms associated with common colds.

Intradermal Testing. Allergens may also be injected directly between skin layers; this diagnostic method is known as intradermal testing. Such testing may be used to diagnose respiratory allergies, allergic reactions to drugs, or to insect bites; patch testing involves applying an adhesive patch containing one or more suspected allergens directly to an area of skin. This test is the most common means of diagnosing the source of contact dermatitis (skin allergies). The tuberculin skin test likewise relies on the body's immune response, in this case to a protein derived from *Mycobac-*

terium tuberculosis, the causa-tive agent of tuberculosis. A small quantity of the protein is injected between skin layers and the reaction noted after a period of two days. *See also* ALLERGY; ANTIBODY; DERMATITIS; DIAGNOSIS; HISTAMINE; IMMUNITY; SKIN; SKIN ALLERGY; *and* TUBERCULOSIS.

Skin Tumors

Benign and malignant growths on or in the skin.

The abnormal and uncontrolled multiplication of skin cells that indicates the presence of skin tumors begins to appear in people over the age of 20. Most of these tumors do not pose any serious health problems—these tumors can be benign or not—although they may be unattractive.

Types. One common benign skin tumor is a seborrheic keratosis, which is a wart-like growth whose color ranges from tan to dark brown and whose sizes range from a fraction of an inch to more than an inch. They are not dangerous but they should be examined, because some of them resemble malignant melanomas.

Cutaneous tags are another kind of benign skin tumor. They are protrusions that appear most often under the arms, under the breasts, or on the neck or groin. They can be painful when irritated by clothing or jewelry. They can be cut off or removed by heating or freezing, but often recur.

Squamous papillomas are flesh-colored, wartlike growths that originate in the skin and in the epithelium, the tissue that lines the hollow organs of the body.

Sebaceous cysts are whitish-yellow or skin colored growths that appear under the surface of the skin. Most sebaceous cysts are small, but some can grow to several inches in diameter. A sebaceous cyst can rupture or become infected, requiring surgical removal.

All skin tumors should be examined for indications that they may be malignant, especially if they have suddenly changed size, shape, or color. *See also* SKIN; SKIN CANCER; SKIN GRAFT; SKIN PEELING, CHEMICAL; SKIN TESTS; *and* SUNBURN.

Skull

The bones of the head.

The two main portions of the skull are the cranium, which is made of several immobile bones that form the front, back, and sides of the head, and the 14 facial bones, which include the mandible (the moveable jawbone). Although it is quite thin, the rounded shape of the cranial bones render it quite strong and light. Facial bones ensure that the face is framed, facial muscles and the teeth are secured, and cavities are provided for three of the sense organs (sight, taste and smell) as well as for the passage of air and food.

The skull has approximately 85 openings, including the orbits that house the eyeballs, the ear cavities, the nasal cavity, as well as cavities for the spinal cord and blood vessels. Skull bones also contain air filled sinuses. Surrounding the nasal cavity are the paranasal sinuses; these get "stuffed up" when a person is suffering from a cold or the flu.

The primary purpose of the skull is to protect the brain; the skull's rounded structure is strong and tends to deflect blows. At birth, the joints of the skull are flexible, allowing the infant's head to change shape as it passes through the birth canal. *See also* BRAIN; EYE; SINUS, FACIAL; *and* SKELETON.

Skull, Fractured

A fracture in any of the bones that make up the skull (cranium).

Eight bones make up the cranium, surrounding and protecting the brain and facial bones. As with other bones, a direct or heavy blow can cause a fracture. The bones of the skull are relatively strong and most fractures are closed; that is, they are clean fractures in which the bones remain beneath the skin, and there is little serious tissue damage. There may be few symptoms, so a person who has suffered any kind of direct blow to the head should have it x-

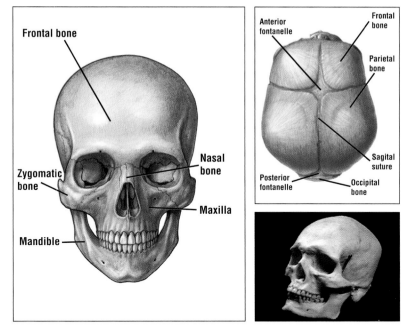

The Skull. Above, three views of the skull and the bones that make up the skull. As is apparent from the image on the right, it resides just beneath the skin and contains sockets for the mouth, nose, and eyes. Top, right, a view of an newborn's skull; the bones are separate at birth, but they fuse over time. Bottom, right, a picture of the full-grown adult skull with bones fused.

rayed as soon as possible to check for fractures, and, if necessary, she or he will be monitored for complications. Even if the fracture is minor, or if there is no break, there still may be damage to the brain, such as internal bleeding (hemorrhage). A CAT scan can detect these injuries. Otherwise, a closed skull fracture may require little treatment besides rest.

Open fractures, when the skin is broken and bones or blood vessels are damaged, can be much more dangerous and may be life-threatening. These injuries often require surgery, especially if bone fragments have to be removed and tissue repaired. Hemorrhages may need to be drained, or the membrane that covers the skull (meninges) may require repair. As with all open fractures, antibiotics are necessary to

A fractured skull is a type of TRAUMA *that usually requires immediate* FIRST AID. *The* SKULL *is a* BONE *that protects the* BRAIN *which is subject to* FRACTURE *that can be diagnosed with* BRAIN IMAGING *techniques including* CAT SCAN *and* X-RAY. *See also* HEMORRHAGE *and* MEMORY.

Skull X-Ray

Radiographic imaging of the skull for the purposes of diagnosis.

X-rays are a form of high-energy electromagnetic wave, capable of penetrating soft tissue and being absorbed by denser materials, including the cranial bones. They are produced by bombarding tungsten, an elemental metal, with high-speed electrons. Their differential absorption is used to create an image on photographic film that may be used for diagnosis. Bone appears whitish in such images, while less dense tissue will be seen in varying shades of gray.

Conventional x-ray is used to visualize skull fractures, concussions, and other trauma to the braincase, as well as the presence of gross tumors or bleeding. Skull shape, particularly in children, may be evaluated for its relevance to possible disease. The more detailed radiographic images provided by CAT or MRI scanning can provide a doctor with cross-sectional images through the cranium.

An x-ray of the skull will be used as a precautionary measure in cases of significant trauma or injury to the head, even in the absence of obvious symptoms. Skull x-rays, whether conventional or more sophisticated, is a painless procedure, generally conducted in a hospital's radiology department. *See also* SKULL *and* X-RAY.

Sleep

A naturally recurring state of rest and slumber that is accompanied by unconsciousness.

Sleep is a period of rest in which the nervous system is inactive, muscles are relaxed, and metabolism is reduced. Sleep can be differentiated from a coma because a loud noise or strong light can easily awaken the sleeper, while a person in a coma will not awaken. A minimum of seven hours of sleep is necessary for an adult to maintain proper health; it has been estimated that people spend approximately one-third to one-quarter of their lives asleep.

Physiology. The brain emits impulses or waves whether it is asleep or awake. There are two distinct types of sleep that can be recorded by an EEG (electroencephalograph): REM, or rapid eye movement sleep and NREM, or nonrapid eye movement sleep. The two patterns alternate every 90 minutes throughout the sleep period. REM sleep is a period of fast, small waves, similar to those of an awake individual. REM sleep is characterized by rapidly moving eyes and is recognized as the time in which people dream. Each eight hours of sleep contains approximately four periods of REM sleep. Each period persists for about five to 30 minutes for every 100 minutes of sleep time. The slower and larger waves of NREM sleep account for most sleep. Dreams usually do not occur during this period.

Functions. Sleep is necessary for humans. It allows the body to rest and rejuvenate, as well as dream. Scientists suggest that dreaming may be advantageous for the brain, permitting it to separate the information that has been col- lected during the day. Sleep deprivation causes individuals to become irritable and unable to concentrate or be productive. It is not certain why some people can exist with very little sleep and do not manifest the usual sleep-deprivation symptoms. *See also* SLEEP APNEA.

Sleep Requirements. Sleep requirements vary according to the age of a person. People require less sleep with age. Babies require a minimum of 14 hours of sleep per day; children may require 10 hours; adults may need seven to eight hours per night. As people age, they have difficulty sleeping through the night. They may also have a tendency to doze off throughout the day.

Sleep Disorders. There are many forms of sleep disorders. They can be classified as difficulties falling asleep (insomnias), difficulties staying awake, difficulties sticking to a sleep-wake schedule, and sleep-disruptive lifestyles. Stress, illness, and psychological factors often cause insomnia. Individuals who exhibit sleep irregularities may find relief at sleep disorder centers, which specialize in the treatment of sleep-related conditions. *See also* BRAIN *and* INSOMNIA.

Resources on Sleep

Carskadon, Mary A., ed., *Encyclopedia of Sleep and Dreaming* (1993); Coren, Stanley, *Sleep Thieves* (1996); Dement, William C., and Christopher Vaughan, *The Promise of Sleep* (1999); Hobson, J. Allen, *Sleep* (1995); Lam-berg, Lynne, *Bodyrhythms*, (1994); National Sleep Foundation, Tel. (202) 347-3471, Online: http://www. sleepfoundation.org/; www.nycornell.org/psychiatry; www.nycornell. org/neurology/

Sleep Apnea

Brief interruptions of breathing during sleep.

A person with sleep apnea experiences frequent episodes of breathing pauses, lasting about 10 seconds, that can occur 30 or more times an hour, usually accompanied by snoring. Sleep apnea occurs at all ages and to both sexes, but it appears to be more common in men. Contributing factors include weight, blood pressure, and obstructions in the nose and throat. Heavy drinking or use of sleeping pills can also play a serious role.

ALERT

Sleep Apnea and Children

Sleep apnea also regularly occurs in children aged three to 12, and it is usually caused by enlarged tonsils or adenoids. Some research has found that ethnicity plays a role in the incidence of sleep apnea, as children of African descent are affected two to three times more often than Caucasian children. If a child snores, is restless during sleep, gasps for breath and sleeps with his or her mouth open, apnea may be the cause. Morning headaches, crankiness, and daytime sleepiness are also common in affected children.

TYPES

There are two forms of sleep apnea. The less common form, central sleep apnea, occurs when the brain does not send the periodic signals that control breathing. The more common form, obstructive sleep apnea, usually occurs when the tongue and the muscles of the throat relax during sleep, partially blocking the airway. Obstructive sleep apnea also results from enlargement of the tonsils or adenoids.

In many cases, the interruptions caused by sleep apnea go unnoticed during the night, but the loss of steady sleep shows up during the daytime, in the form of excessive sleepiness, and regular morning headaches. A higher risk of heart disease has been noted in persons with sleep apnea, but it is not clear whether heart disease is associated with the weight issues that increase with the incidence of sleep apnea, or with the condition itself.

TREATMENT

Treatment for sleep apnea starts with lifestyle changes such as weight loss, reduced alcohol intake, and ending sleeping-pill use. If the condition occurs only when a person sleeps on her or his back, a position-changing device may help.

When lifestyle changes are not effective, continuous positive airway pressure, usually referred to as CPAP, can be used. A person wears a mask over her or his nose, and a blower forces air through the mask into the airway. Some people may undergo surgery to remove tonsils, adenoids, or other tissue that blocks the airway. If sleep apnea is severe enough to pose a major danger to life, it can be relieved by tracheostomy—a surgery in which a small hole is cut in the windpipe. The hole is opened only at night, so that air can enter the respiratory tract without obstruction.

Sleep Apnea is a condition affecting the RESPIRATORY SYSTEM *that can be related to* TONSILLITIS, *which can be treated with a* TONSILLECTOMY. HEADACHES *and* SNORING *are two articles that discuss the symptoms. See* SLEEP.

Sleep Deprivation

An inadequate amount of sleep, often less than three hours per night.

Sleep-deprived individuals are generally irritable, disagreeable, and unable to concentrate. These individuals lack sufficient energy to get through the day and to accomplish complicated tasks. At work, they are able to perform and focus only for a short period of time, and they will make many mistakes. Sleep-deprived individuals may doze off and nap at lectures, in meetings, at the desk, or at the wheel of a vehicle.

Individuals who are deprived of sleep for more than three days have difficulty reasoning, hearing, and observing. They may also hallucinate, become paranoid, or confuse daydreams with reality. Individuals who suffer from epilepsy are more prone to attacks when they are deprived of an adequate amount of sleep. *See also* INSOMNIA; SLEEP; SLEEP APNEA; *and* SLEEPING DRUGS.

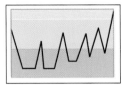

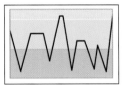

Sleeping Patterns. Above, two graphs of the amount of time spent awake, in green; in REM (rapid eye motion, this is when a person dreams) sleep; and deep sleep, in blue. The top graph displays sleep patterns for younger individuals who spend more time in periods of deep sleep; and below that is the graph of older individuals who tend to spend more time in REM sleep. Sleep patterns change over time due to anxiety and changes in the body's chemistry.

Sleeping Drugs

Drugs used to induce sleep, primarily barbiturates and benzodiazepines. Neither type should be used on a regular basis.

Barbiturates and benzodiazepines are sedatives and tranquilizers. They promote sleep by calming and reducing anxiety. However, they may be addictive—either physically or psychologically. Sudden cessation of these medications can produce some rather serious withdrawal symptoms that have the potential to be life-threatening. Further, these sedatives do not mix well with alcohol. The elderly should be especially careful when taking these medications. They can produce severe dizziness when rising from bed, and, as the body become more sensitive to medications as a person ages, what seems like a normal dosage may actually be an overdose. *See also* BARBITURATE DRUGS.

Sleeping Sickness

Also known as African trypanosomiasis

An infectious parasitic disease spread by the tsetse fly that causes characteristic sleep disturbances.

Sleeping sickness is a tropical disease that causes inflammation to the brain and surrounding tissue. Two distinct organisms are responsible for two forms of the disease: *Trypanosoma brucei rhodesiense* and *Trypanosoma brucei gambiense*. The rhodesiense organism causes a more severe form of the illness. Sleeping sickness is transmitted by the bite of the infected tsetse fly, which injects parasites that multiply in the blood, lymph, or spinal fluid. They then invade the central nervous system.

A swollen, red area first appears at the location of the bite. Soon after, the lymph nodes become enlarged. After invasion of the brain, behavioral and sleep changes will follow, accompanied by headache, fever and weakness. Sufferers are often drowsy during the day and unable to sleep at night. Diagnosis is based on symptoms and confirmed by the presence of trypanosoma in sampled blood, lymph, or spinal fluid.

Drug treatment should begin as soon as possible, as the disease is more difficult to treat once inflammation of the brain and meninges develops. Rhodesiense may cause death within six months if left untreated, while gambiense infection may take up to two years before symptoms appear. Both forms respond well if treatment begins early. *See also* CHAGAS' DISEASE; INSECTS AND DISEASE; SLEEP; *and* TRYPANOSOMIASIS.

Sleep Paralysis

A sensation of the inability to execute voluntary movements, occurring at the onset of sleep or upon awakening.

Sleep paralysis is a condition in which a person feels quite incapable of movement. There is no known explanation for sleep paralysis, but it is not harmful. It appears as an episode of muscle paralysis. Symptoms of sleep paralysis include the inability to move the trunk or limbs and the condition may be associated with hallucinations. The experience is common in small children but also appears in healthy adults. Sleep paralysis is often a complication of a sleep disorder called narcolepsy, in which the affected person falls asleep throughout the day. Sleep paralysis can be prevented by getting sufficient sleep, reducing stress, exercising regularly, and retiring at the same time each night. Medication is prescribed only for those who experience episodes at least once a week for six months. *See* SLEEP *and* STRESS.

Sleepwalking

Also known as somnambulism

Walking while asleep.

Sleepwalking is more common in children—about 75 percent of children will have walked in their sleep at least once—and in the elderly. Sleepwalking takes place during the nonrapid eye movement (NREM) part of sleep, and thus does not represent dreams acted out. Also rare is the popular image of the sleepwalker walking with arms stretched out before him or her and stepping with closed eyes. In most instances, the sleepwalker will get out of bed and wander around for a few minutes, eyes open but unaware of his or her surroundings and unresponsive to others who may talk to him or her. In the case of children, the sleepwalking may be a symptom of night terror, in which case the wandering will be more frantic, and may be accompanied by shrieking, flailing of arms, the utterance of words (usually making no sense), and possibly urinating in inappropriate places. The episode usually lasts just a few minutes, and the child may then get into the wrong bed.

It is not necessary to wake the sleepwalker (it is also usually difficult); the best strategy is to steer the sleepwalker wordlessly back to his or her bed. If sleepwalking persists, it may be an indication that the sleepwalker is under unusual stress or is experiencing anxiety about something taking place in his or her waking life. Children who sleepwalk generally do not continue doing so in adolescence; only about 5 percent of the adult population sleepwalks.

> *Background information regarding this topic can be found in* Dreaming; Family Medicine; Sleep; Sleep Deprivation; *and* Urinary System. Anxiety; Stress; *and* Psychoanalysis *are all related topics available for review.*

Sling

A type of bandage used to immobilize, support, or elevate an arm.

Slings are often an important part of first aid for fractures, sprains or other injuries in which the arm or hand needs some form of stabilization until help is reached. Slings also are used to elevate arms or hands in emergency situations, as they can help to stop or slow blood flow and reduce attendant swelling. A person may need to keep an arm or hand in a sling throughout the healing process in order to support and immobilize the injured area. Slings are usually made of a triangular bandage, but in emergencies, just about anything will do. *See also* First Aid; Fracture; *and* Splint.

Slit Lamp

An instrument used for studying the eye, consisting of a beam of light emitted through a narrow slit.

The slit lamp projects a concentrated beam of light on structures within the eye, allowing the ophthalmologist to clearly observe anterior regions including the conjunctiva, sclera, lids, iris, cornea, and anterior chamber of the eye. As the name implies, the slit lamp is capable of focusing a narrow slit of light upon these structures, while the examiner studies them under magnification.

Prior to examination, a solution will be applied to dilate the pupils and numb the eyes. The test is painless, and may help the ophthalmologist diagnose a range of disorders, including, foreign bodies within the eye, conjunctivitis, herpes, corneal ulcer, cataracts, glaucoma, and others. *See also* Cataract; Conjunctivitis; Cornea, Disorders of; Corneal Ulcer; Eye; Eye, Disorders of; Eye Drop; Eye, Examination of; Eye, Foreign Bodies in; Eye Injuries; Eye Tumors; Eyelid; *and* Glaucoma.

Slow Virus Disease

A newly discovered family of diseases that produces symptoms long after the original exposure.

Slow virus diseases are usually caused by viruses, or what are now considered near-viruses because of their unique structure; near-viruses are also referred to as prions. A prion is a kind of virus (or near-virus) that multiplies by inducing normal protein molecules to change their shape. Prions are responsible for mad cow disease, kuru, and Creutzfeld-Jacob syndrome. A brain disorder that occurs in individuals with AIDS (progressive multifocal leukoencephalopathy, or PML) is also considered a slow virus disease, because affected individuals may go without symptoms for months or even years after exposure. Slow virus diseases are all fatal at the present time, and research into their causes and treatment continues. *See also* AIDS; Cell; Creutzfeld-Jacob Syndrome; HIV; Kuru; *and* Virus.

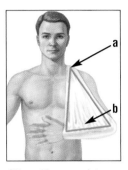

Sling. Above, a picture of a sling. The sling should be placed over the shoulder (a); and the injured arm should lie level within the bandage (b). The shoulder, elbow and wrist should make a fairly even-sided triangle. Slings are temporary measures and a cast should be put on by a physician in order to immobilize the affected arm.

Small-Cell Carcinoma

Rapidly growing form of lung cancer.

About one of every four lung cancers is a small-cell carcinoma. They grow more rapidly than other lung cancers, doubling in size every 30 days, and they spread more rapidly to the lymph nodes and other tissues, so that they often are untreatable when they are detected. Small-cell carcinomas are classified as either limited, meaning that only one lung and its associated lymph nodes are involved, or extensive, meaning that they have spread to other lymph nodes and tissues. About two thirds of small-cell carcinomas are extensive.

Treatment of small-cell carcinoma consists of using a variety of drugs in different combinations (chemotherapy). Patients with limited small-cell carcinoma may also receive radiation therapy aimed at the cancer and lymph nodes. While up to 80 percent of patients with small-cell carcinoma respond to chemotherapy, 90 percent of them will have a recurrence of the cancer within two or three years. Surgery usually is not an option for small-cell carcinoma, because it generally has spread too much by the time it is detected, making it impossible to remove by operation. *See also* CANCER; CANCER, LUNG; CARCINOMA; *and* LUNG.

Smallpox

A disease caused by the variola virus; the first disease for which humans were made immune by vaccination procedures.

Smallpox starts with a fever that may spike to 106°F, followed by the chills, a backache, and a headache. In four days the fever will drop, but a characteristic rash appears covering the entire body. Over the next few days the rash changes from small pimples to pustules. In a few more days the pustules come to a head and rupture, drain, and scab over. The scabs eventually fall off leaving depressed pockmarks. If the virus attacks the eyes, lungs, throat, heart, or liver, it can be fatal.

There is no cure for smallpox, which was disastrous from the Middle Ages into the late nineteenth century, when thousands died of the disease. Inoculation for small pox was first attempted in China in the seventeenth century. Dust scraped from smallpox scabs was blown into the nose. The person got the disease and, if she or he lived, became immune. Edward Jenner cultured the cowpox virus, a much milder form of smallpox, to create the first vaccine against disease. In 1977 the World Health Organization announced that smallpox had been virtually eradicated.

> *Background information about Smallpox can be found in* IMMUNITY; VACCINATIONS; *and* VIRUS. *Symptoms are expanded upon in* FEVER; PUSTULE; RASH; *and* SCAB. *See also* CENTERS FOR DISEASE CONTROL *and* PUBLIC HEALTH.

Smegma

A buildup of secretions from the sebaceous glands found under the foreskin of uncircumcised males.

Sebum, the lubricating substance secreted by the sebaceous glands, becomes susceptible to bacteria when left on the skin. Smegma, the accumulation of sebum under the penis's foreskin, may develop bacterial or fungal infections, which can cause inflammation of the glans (balanitis). If a child has a tight foreskin, smegma may harden into a stone, or smegma pearl. Good hygiene and regular washing of the penis and foreskin can prevent smegma buildup. *See also* BALANITIS *and* FORESKIN.

Smell

One of the five senses (the others are hearing, sight, touch, and taste).

The human sense of smell, or the olfactory system, can distinguish thousands of odors and aromas. Researchers have identified genes that they believe are responsible for the coding of specific odor binding sites (receptors), which are located in the olfactory lining of the nose. The receptors gather information in the olfactory bulbs, located at the end of olfactory nerves, and interpret their patterns as distinct odors.

PHYSIOLOGY

The nose contains specialized sensory neurons, with hair-like fibers (cilia) on one end. Each neuron sends an axon nerve fiber to the olfactory bulb that is located in the brain. Studies suggest that specialized olfactory neurons respond to distinct odors that stimulate precise patterns of activity in the olfactory bulb. Brain-mapping techniques indicate that odors create distinct patterns that are encoded in the brain.

DISORDERS

Olfactory disorders result from changes in the nerves that travel from the nose to the brain. Partial or total loss of smell (anosmia) and abnormal perception of smell (dysomia) can result from illnesses that causes the nasal mucous membranes to become inflamed. The common cold, influenza, allergic rhinitis (hay fever), and tobacco usage may cause anosmia. In cancer radiation patients or head trauma victims, anosmia can linger for months. Schizophrenics, epileptics, and alcoholic patients sometimes experience dysomia, the imagining of offensive smells that do not exist. Some patients experience hypersensitivity to smell (hypersomia), in which ordinary odors are perceived as noxious.

DIAGNOSIS

Medical care for olfactory disorders depends on the cause of the disorder. To determine the cause, a patient's sense of smell is examined through testing with fragrant spices, oils, and soaps.

TREATMENT

To treat olfactory disorders, zinc supplements are sometimes prescribed. These supplements speed up the healing process if the disorder is caused by a nasal infection or a sore throat.

> *Articles related to the sense of Smell can be found in* ANATOMY; COLD, COMMON; GENE; *and* NASAL OBSTRUCTION. *It may also be informative to see* BRAIN IMAGING.

Smoking, Passive

Inhaling cigarette smoke from nearby smokers.

Among the people most at risk from passive smoking are children of parents who smoke. It is estimated that approximately four million children a year become ill from second-hand smoke. Smoking during pregnancy increases a child's risk for disorders such as attention deficit hyperactivity disorder (ADHD), conduct disorder, depression, and substance abuse. Prenatal and infant exposure to smoke is linked to sudden infant death syndrome. Exposure to cigarette smoke in childhood increases the risk for diseases such as asthma, bronchitis, pneumonia, meningococcal disease, lung defects, ear infections, and eczema. *See also* ASTHMA *and* TOBACCO SMOKING.

Snails and Disease

Illnesses caused by parasites associated with aquatic snails.

A number of serious diseases are caused by blood flukes (including schistosomes, also known as bilharzia), a class of parasitic worm that inhabits freshwater snails as an intermediary host. Eggs, which are discharged into a human host, hatch in the water, forming a larval stage organism (miracidia), which then infects an aquatic snail. When the larval stage has sufficiently matured within the snail, it escapes back into water as a cercariae, which subsequently penetrates the human skin, producing the characteristic symptoms of schistosomiasis.

In the United States, transportation of snails that carry pathogens requires a permit from the Centers for Disease Control. Snail eradication programs are also being mounted throughout the world. Endod (*Phytolacca dodecandra*) is a shrub from which an effective molluscicide is extracted. This extract is regularly used in parts of Africa and America to reduce incidence of diseases caused by snails. *See also* FLUKE; LIVER FLUKE; PUBLIC HEALTH; SCHISTOSOMIASIS; *and* WORM INFESTATION.

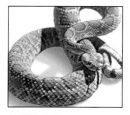

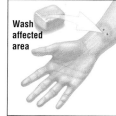

Wash affected area

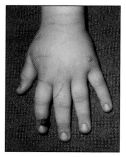

Snakebites. At the top, an illustration of a snake. The first and most important thing to do when any snake bites is to wash out the wound with warm soapy water, as pictured in the middle. At the bottom, a finger has been bitten by a snake. Such bites can cause tissue death; this bite has caused swelling and some characteristic tissue death on the first finger.

Snakebites

The bite of a snake, which may or may not be venomous.

Only two families of the hundreds of kinds of snakes native to the United States are venomous. The pit vipers—which include copperheads, rattlesnakes, and water moccasins—are characterized by triangular, wedge-shaped heads, small pits under the eyes, and large fangs; consequently, they leave visible bite marks. They are responsible for close to 99 percent of snakebites in this country. Coral snakes, which are fairly small and thin, have a highly neurotoxic venom that will cause respiratory paralysis. The coral snake's fangs are much smaller than those of pit vipers, and their bites are therefore less obvious. Bites of both types of native venomous snakes can be treated effectively with antivenin. Since antivenin is made with horse serum, people sensitive to horse products may experience a severe reaction. *See also* TOXIN.

Symptoms of venomous snakebites include weakness, dizziness, nausea, headache, difficulty breathing, tissue damage, shock, and tingling lips and tongue.

Treatment. A bite from any snake must be treated as an emergency; since many snakebite victims cannot positively identify the species that bit them, physicians insist that all snakebites receive prompt attention. Bites incurred from nonpoisonous species may cause an allergic reactions in some people. Most frequently, doctors treat venomous snakebites by administering antivenin, an antidote to snake venom.

Before medical care arrives, some simple first aid can be applied to the individual who has been bitten. First, wash the area with soap and water. Keep the bite still, and below the heart. Then go to the hospital or call an ambulance. Never treat snakebites with any of the following: ice, ice packs, or any other cooling substance, tourniquets, incisions, or electric shock. Never try to orally suck the venom from the bite. If the victim is unable to reach the hospital within 30 minutes, a bandage (loose enough to slip a finger underneath) may be wrapped two to four inches above the bite. A suction device available in commercial snakebite kits may be used to draw venom from the wound. *See* VENOMOUS BITES AND STINGS.

Prevention. The majority of snakebites that occur could be prevented, since most snakes bite humans only to protect themselves. Give any snake that you pass plenty of space—snakes can often strike the distance of half their length. Do not walk in tall grasses unless you are wearing leather hiking boots and long pants. If you see a snake do not try to catch or kill it—this is how many preventable bites occur. *See also* BITES.

Sneezing

Involuntary expulsion of air from the nose and mouth.

Sneezing is a reflex that is usually a reaction to irritation of the inner lining (mucous membrane) of the nose and upper part of the respiratory system, or sometimes to a bright light striking the eye. The muscles of the respiratory system contract involuntarily to expel air and anything that may be causing the irritation. Sneezing can be caused by an allergy, the common cold, influenza, or other respiratory disorders, or by inhaling any irritating substance, such as dust or pollen. In cases of viral or bacterial infection, the droplets that are expelled with the sneeze contain the infecting agent. A handkerchief over the nose and mouth prevents spreading infection. *See also* INFECTION; *and* INFLUENZA.

Snellen's Chart

A diagnostic test for visual acuity, consisting of printed letters ranging in size from the smallest (at the bottom) to the largest (at the top).

Tests for visual acuity measure the eye's ability to recognize visual shapes and details. The Snellen's chart is a calibrated test that measures the patient's ability to read letters at a distance, relative to a recognized standard for normal vision.

The subject is asked to read the smallest letters on the chart that can be resolved from a distance of 20 feet. The result is a measurement of distance acuity. A reading of small print held close to the eyes then yields the near visual acuity. The eyes are tested in this way individually, with a score rating the acuity of each eye. 20/20 vision is considered normal, meaning the eye can read a 3/8 inch letter from a distance of 20 feet. 20/40 vision means that the eye can see at 20 feet what a normal eye is able to make out at 40 feet. 20/200 vision qualifies the test subject as legally blind.

The Snellen's chart may be read through a device known as a phoropter, which interposes lenses of varying strength in order to help prescribe corrective lenses. Abnormal results on the Snellen's chart may indicate nearsightedness, farsightedness, astigmatism or presbyopia age-related diminishment of the lenses' ability to focus on close objects. *See also* ASTIGMATISM; BLINDNESS; EYE; EYE, DISORDERS OF; EYE, EXAMINATION OF; GLASSES; LENS; PRESBYOPIA; VISION, VOSS OF; *and* VISUAL ACUITY.

Snoring

Breathing loudly, with harsh sounds, when asleep.

In most cases, snoring is a normal phenomenon and is not a cause for alarm. It may occur for no known reason, follow overuse of alcohol or sedatives, or result from congestion or enlarged adenoids or tonsils (which may require treatment). In some cases, however, snoring may be a symptom of sleep apnea, a breathing disorder in which breathing is disturbed or stops entirely during sleep. A physician should be consulted if snoring is accompanied by excessive sleepiness during the day or actual cessation of breathing during sleep. Weight loss can also help in some cases, and other people may benefit from time spent at a sleep clinic, where they may undergo a polysomnogram, which tests REM sleep, as well as heart and breathing rate. *See also* BARBITURATE DRUGS; SLEEP; SLEEP APNEA; WEIGHT LOSS; *and* WEIGHT REDUCTION.

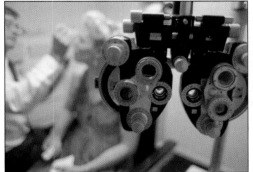

Sodium

An electrolyte and positively charged ion; a mineral essential for proper health.

Working with positively charged potassium ions, sodium functions to regulate the amount of water in the body's cells, controlling blood volume, maintaining the body's acid-base balance, and transporting nutrients across cell membranes; it is also instrumental in the transmission of nerve impulses and muscle contractions.

An excess of dietary sodium, however, has the potential to cause harm in certain individuals with hypertension. People who have kidney failure, cirrhosis with complications, and other conditions involving fluid retention should also restrict sodium intake at a balanced level.

Individuals who are monitoring sodium consumption should, in addition to limiting the amount of salt used in cooking, carefully read labels of packaged and processed foods, since sodium and its compounds are regularly used preservatives.

A deficiency of sodium is quite unusual in the United States, since the American diet tends to be high in salt; however, it may occur from extreme, profuse sweating, vomiting, diarrhea, and from some medications. Symptoms of sodium depletion may include headaches, nausea, vomiting, dehydration, absence of an appetite, acidosis, and muscle weakness. *See also* ACIDOSIS; CIRRHOSIS; DEHYDRATION; DIARRHEA; ELECTROLYTE; FOOD ADDITIVES; HYPERTENSION; ION; LOSS OF APPETITE; NAUSEA; POTASSIUM; PRESERVATIVES; *and* VOMITING.

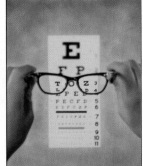

An Eye Examinatio and a Snellen's Chart. At the right is a Snellen's chart, invented by the Dutch ophthalmologist Hermann Snellen. A person stands 20 feet from the chart in order to test for distance vision. Average eyesight is 20/20 (the number is always expressed as a ratio). 20/10 vision is exceptional; it means that a person can see at 20 feet what a person with normal eyesight can see only at 10 feet. A person with 20/200 vision is legally blind. To the left, is a more sophisticated apparatus for testing vision; these are optometry lenses. An optometrist uses these to test an individual in order to gauge what strength glasses or contact lenses he or she will need in order to have 20/20 vision.

Soft-Tissue Injury

Injuries that affect the tissues that surround and support the joints and bones.

Ligaments, tendons, and muscles are all tissues that connect and operate the bones and joints. Activity that stretches these tissues beyond their normal range of motion can result in a complete or partial tear. Ligament injuries are called sprains; muscle tears are known as strains, inflammation of the tendon is called tendinitis, and a complete tear of a tendon is a rupture.

Soft-tissue injuries usually exhibit symptoms such as pain, tenderness, and some swelling. The typical treatment is to rest the injured area, apply ice to the affected site, and elevate the damaged part in order to reduce the swelling. *See also* ICE PACKS; SPRAIN; STRAIN; *and* TENDINITIS.

Solvent Abuse

The practice of inhaling intoxicating fumes from solvent or other volatile liquids.

Sniffing glue is the most common form of this type of substance abuse, but other liquids are also used, particularly those containing acetone and toluene. The practice is most common among boys in poor urban areas, possibly also in schools where boys first encounter glues and other solvents.

Abusers generally tire of the practice once it loses its novelty and cease inhalation after a few months. Prolonged abuse can result in headaches, vomiting, stupor, confusion, and, in extreme cases, coma and death. Occasionally, coma or death may result from a toxic effect directly on the heart or from a fall, when the inhaler chokes on his or her own vomit, or asphyxiation from the clinging plastic bag used to facilitate inhalation. *See also* MARIJUANA.

Long-term damage to the kidneys, nasal membranes, liver, and the central nervous system has been reported. Parents and teachers should be particularly attentive to some of the signs of abuse—ulcers around the mouth; the aroma of solvent; a flushed face; mood and personality changes—and seek immediate counseling for the abuser. Acute symptoms from solvent abuse, namely, coma and vomiting, require immediate and urgent medical attention. *See also* COMA; SUBSTANCE ABUSE; *and* VOMITING.

Somatization Disorder

A neurotic disorder in which the sufferer complains of symptoms that have no physical cause.

People often experience pains of uncertain origin, but somatization disorder is characterized by prolonged complaints (over a period of many years), and accompanied by many tests, physician attention, and, frequently, hospitalization coupled with unnecessary tests and surgery. The disorder usually first appears before the age of thirty and is slightly more prevalent in women, particularly where there is a history of antisocial personality disorder in male relatives. Common symptoms include visual abnormalities (double vision and blurr-ed vision), neurological symptoms (dizziness; seizures; weakness; fatigue), gyneco- logical pain (painful menstruation; pain during intercourse), and gastrointestinal complaints (nausea; abdominal pain).

Generally, the disorder is a result of deep-seated emotional problems, such as depression, anxieties, or trauma-induced neuroses that the sufferer has found too painful to confront and has unconsciously displaced onto the body. Treatment may entail psychotherapy or may simply require prolonged counseling. The danger in approaching the disorder is that it may be applied by health practitioners to a patient simply because current medical diagnostics are not able to determine the cause of a person's legitimate and accurately perceived symptoms. *See also* HYPOCHONDRIASIS.

Somatization disorder may be distinguished from hypochondriasis in that in the former, there are physical symptoms perceived by the sufferer, and in the latter, the sufferer experiences anxieties over possible illness in the virtual absence of any confirmable symptoms. *See also* ANXIETY.

Sore

A painful lesion on the skin or on a mucous membrane.

A sore is a patch of open, reddened, painful skin. Types of sores include cold sores, canker sores, and sores typical of genital herpes. Sores may range from benign, such as canker sores or sores from minor injury, to severe, such as leukoplakia, a precancerous sore that appears on the mouth after repeated irritation, or lesions from autoimmune disorders. A sore that does not heal may be an indication of skin cancer and should be examined by a physician. *See also* BEDSORES; BENIGN; CANKER SORE; COLD SORE; LESION; SKIN; *and* SORE THROAT.

Sore Throat

A rough irritated feeling in the throat.

Sore throats are a symptom of a variety of conditions; they are often a signal of such viral infections as colds, influenza, chicken pox, mumps, or measles. It may indicate an inflamed pharynx (pharyngitis) or swollen tonsils (tonsillitis). Bacterial infections, such as strep throat, are also signaled by a sore throat. Disorders of the esophagus, such as acid reflux (acid from the stomach washing into the esophagus), and pharyngoesophageal diverticulum (an infected pouch in the pharynx), may also cause a sore throat and swallowing problems.

A sore throat is a rough, raw, painful feeling in the throat that may also cause swallowing and speaking difficulties. Examination of a sore throat may reveal a red inflamed area, or in the cases of pharyngitis and tonsillitis, there may be white spots or pus in the infected area.

Viral infections will usually clear up on their own, but in cases of bacterial infections, antibiotics may be necessary to treat the infection. *See also* ACID REFLUX; ANTIBIOTICS; COLD; ESOPHAGUS; FLU; PHARYNGOESOPHAGEAL DIVERTICULUM; PHARYNX; PHARYNGITIS; TONSILLITIS; STREP THROAT; STREPTOCOCCAL INFECTIONS; *and* THROAT.

Sounding of the Uterus

A procedure to measure the depth and position of the uterus.

Sounding of the uterus is usually performed prior to the insertion of an intrauterine device (IUD), a form of birth control. Before the device can be inserted, it is important that the physician know the exact size and position of the uterus so that the IUD can be placed correctly.

Procedure. The physician first opens the vagina with a speculum and washes the cervix with disinfectant. He or she then grasps the cervix with a long clamp (tenaculum) to stabilize the uterus, and inserts a blunt plastic rod (uterine sound) through the cervical canal to measure the depth of the uterus. *See also* BIRTH CONTROL; INTRAUTERINE DEVICE (IUD); *and* UTERUS.

Space Medicine

A small area of medicine concerned with the health and safety of humans in space.

The goal of space medicine is to promote the safety and well-being of people while they are exposed to the stresses and unusual environmental conditions of space travel. These conditions include extreme changes in air pressure and gravitational force, the weightlessness of zero gravity, motion sickness, and the psychological disturbances of confinement and isolation, among others. The study of space medicine attempts to determine how well and for how long human beings can withstand the conditions encountered in space. It also endeavors to assess the ability of human beings to readapt to the Earth's environment after travel in space.

Astronauts perform special exercises to limit the loss of muscle mass while in space. To avoid disruption of the internal biological clock due to lack of night and day cycles, astronauts adopt a regular schedule that prevents disruption of the internal rhythms of the body. *See also* AVIATION MEDICINE; CIRCADIAN RHYTHM; *and* MUSCLE.

Spasm

A sudden, abnormal, or involuntary muscular contraction.

A spasm is an intense muscle contraction that can affect one or more muscles and can occur once or several times. Pain is not always associated with spasms. Spasms can be either clonic, characterized by alternate contraction and relaxation of muscles, or tonic, characterized by prolonged contraction without an extended period of relaxation. *See also* MUSCLE.

Spasms can be the result of a central nervous system (CNS) disorder or a muscle disorder. Common examples of spasms include muscle cramps, hiccups, and tics. Muscle cramps affect the muscles in the calves, hiccups affect the diaphragm, and tics involve facial muscles. Less commonly experienced, hemifacial spasm is a neuromuscular disorder characterized by frequent involuntary contractions of the muscles on one side of the face. Rarely, violent spasms can be caused by rabies or by the bite of a black widow spider.

Spastic Paralysis

A condition in which a person cannot move specific muscles, accompanied by their tightness.

Spastic paralysis is characterized by an inability to move part of the body due to stiffness that occurs as muscles become tight or lock in position. It results from a stroke, cerebral palsy, or multiple sclerosis.

Spasticity

A condition in which particular muscles are continually contracted, causing tightness.

Spasticity is an increased stiffness in the muscles and can occur independent of spastic paralysis, the inability to move the affected muscles. Cerebral palsy is an example of spasticity accompanying paralysis, while Parkinson's disease involves spasticity without paralysis. *See also* MUSCLE.

The muscle contraction that characterizes spasticity may interfere with gait, movement, and speech. Spasticity results from damage to the part of the central nervous system that controls voluntary movement. Symptoms of the condition include excess muscle tone, rapid muscle contractions, muscle spasms, scissoring (involuntary leg crossing), and fixed joints. Spasticity may be treated with medications such as baclofen and diazepam. Muscle stretching and physical therapy can prevent the shrinkage or shortening of muscles. *See also* MUSCLE.

Specimen

A representative sample of tissue or fluid taken by a physician for analysis.

Specimens are taken to provide information useful to diagnosis. Such samples may be of blood, sputum, semen, urine, pus, stool, or other fluid, or they may be tissue samples extracted through biopsy or other means. Specimens are sent to a laboratory for analysis and further testing. This may include a microscopic analysis of cell number, size, shape, range of motion, genetic qualities, or other features. Fluids are often evaluated for the presence of microorganisms that signal bacterial or viral infection. Even hair specimens may be used, for example in the diagnosis of arsenic or other poisoning. *See also* BLOOD TESTS.

Speculum

An instrument designed to dilate and keep an orifice open so a doctor may examine the inside.

Speculums are used to examine the ear, eye, rectum, nose, and vagina. The ear speculum is critical to an otoscope as it aids inner ear viewing. Its funnel shape straightens the ear canal for a better sight-line; these are used in check-ups. Vaginal speculums, often made of metal or plastic, are used in pelvic examinations and I.U.D. insertions; they include the most common "duckbill" design and a more recent one, a speculum with four polymer blades.

Speech

A person's ability to use words to communicate.

Speech is the verbal medium of communication of language and of culture. It includes an audible code of sounds produced by the speaker and a visible code that includes gestures, hand motions, grimaces and facial expressions. Language, on the other hand, is the use of signs or symbols to convey information or to form words that represent objects or ideas. The symbols can be either spoken, written, or compose a set of of hand motions (as in sign language). Adequate language ability is based on one's ability to comprehend and use words in a grammatical sequence in order to produce a sensible thought. All forms of language employ patterns of muscle movements. The muscles associated with speech are related to breathing; these include: the voice box (larynx), tongue, soft palate, lips, lower jaw, and face.

LANGUAGE CENTERS IN THE BRAIN

The cerebral cortex, located in the left hemisphere, is the language center of the brain. The left posterior lobe of the cerebral cortex is responsible for speech, and the right lobe is responsible for musical ability. The anterior region of the cerebral cortex, adjacent to the area of the motor cortex, controls muscle movement of the lips, tongue, jaw, and vocal cords. Damage to this area results in slow and labored speech; however, it does not affect comprehension. Wernicke's area is the center that processes and gives significance to incoming messages. Damage to the posterior cortex results in fluent, but meaningless speech and comprehension of spoken and written words is also impaired.

SPEECH PRODUCTION

Speech is produced as a result of signals traveling from the nerves to the muscles controlling the larynx and tongue. Air travels from the nostrils to the pharynx and continues to the larynx, located in the upper front section of the neck. The vocal cords are stretched across the triangle-shaped larynx. Vibration of the vocal cords upon expiration of air produces the sounds associated with speech. The vocal cords become longer and thicker in teenage boys creating new and sometimes, awkward sounds. If the vocal cords become inflamed, they are unable to vibrate, producing the illness known as laryngitis.

Articulation is a term used to describe the movements necessary to modify the airflow in the larynx and to emit sounds. Sounds are classified according to their place and method of enunciation. Different sounds of air are emitted from different parts of the mouth.

PHONOLOGICAL DEVELOPMENT

A child gradually acquires language and speech. This process involves three significant aspects: the manner in which a sound is stored in the child's mind, the manner in which the sound is uttered by a child, and the rules that connect the former. Children make pronunciation errors when they are beginning to speak, and by the time a child has reached the age of five, most speech difficulties should solve themselves; ones that have not can be treated.

Speech Developments in Children

A child's speech develops along a recognized pattern of milestones coming at fairly regular, although never exact, intervals.

- **3 months:** Babies babble. It is essential for the development of patterns that later produce speech.
- **9 months:** Children mimic the speech that they hear, discovering that groups of sounds have meaning.
- **12 to 18 months:** Children utter easy words with simple meanings, for example, "bye-bye."
- **18 to 24 months:** A child forms two-word sentences, such as "Hi, Mom."
- **2 to 3 years:** The child's sentences involve the use of adjectives and verbs.

For background information about Speech see VOCAL CORDS, *Directly related areas of interest include* SPEECH DISORDERS *and* SPEECH THERAPY. *Other, indirectly related articles available for review include* BRAIN; CHILD DEVELOPMENT; LIPREADING; SORE THROAT; *and* STREP THROAT.

Speech Disorders

Language defects that may originate in the nervous system, in the muscles, or in the mouth.

Speech disorders impede and obstruct an individual's ability to efficiently and clearly communicate thoughts and ideas. Speech disorders deserve significant attention, because speech is the primary medium through which humans communicate.

DISORDERS OF LANGUAGE

In most people, the center of language is in the left temporal and frontal lobe. Aphasia occurs when this area of the brain is damaged, as the result of a stroke, head injury, or brain tumor. Such brain injuries impair one's ability to speak, write or understand spoken or written forms of language. Aphasia can occur in both children and adults, and there are many possible variations: Alexia is the inability to understand written words, anomia is the inability to recall the names of objects or general terms, and dysarthia is the inability to articulate the words correctly.

A lag in a child's development of language is manifested by slow comprehension, a below grade-level vocabulary, and immature sentence structure. A hearing test must be performed. Developmental delays can result from insufficient stimulation or emotional disorders.

ARTICULATION DISORDERS

Articulation refers to the ability to produce the sounds essential for speech, form the words of language, and express the words clearly. The articulating structures include the lips, tongue, teeth, jaw, and palate. Speech is articulated by impeding or shaping both the vocalized and unvocalized streams of air flowing past the tongue, lips, lower jaw, and soft palate. The teeth generate specific speech sounds. Dysarthia is the term used to denote a defect in articulation. Damage anywhere along the nerve route from the brain to the larynx muscles (voice box), mouth, or lips, may cause speech to be delayed and slurred. Parkin-

son's disease, multiple sclerosis, brain tumors, and strokes can cause dysarthia. Structural abnormalities, such as a cleft palate or a poorly aligned tooth, can cause a reduced level of articulation.

Stuttering

Stuttering is a form of nonfluent speech in which sounds, syllables, and words are repeated. Stuttering is largely a childhood disorder. Its early forms often appear as seemingly effortless repetitions of sounds, syllables, or words at the beginnings of phrases or sentences. The cause of stuttering has yet to be determined, although it does tend to run in families. Some researchers believe that stuttering may be a slight form of brain damage; others claim that it is predominately a psychological disorder.

DISORDERS OF VOICE PRODUCTION

Voice disorders occur as the result of disease or accidents affecting the larynx. They may also be caused by such physical anomalies as incomplete development or other congenital defects of the vocal cords. The most frequent cause, however, is chronic abuse of the vocal apparatus, either by overuse or by improper production of the voice; this may result in such pathological changes as a thickening and swelling of the vocal cords, or the outbreak of small growths. Larynx disorders can result in a voice that has a high, hoarse, or nasal pitch. Abnormal nasal resonance occurs as the result of too much air (hypernasality) or too little air (hyponasality) flowing through the nasal cavity while speaking. Hyponasality may also develop as the result of blocked nasal passages due to excess mucus. *See also* ANXIETY; APHASIA; BRAIN; BRAIN DAMAGE; CLEFT PALATE; HEARING; LIPREADING; PSYCHIATRY; SPEECH; SPEECH THERAPY; STUTTERING; TONGUE; *and* TUMOR.

Speech Therapy

Treatment to improve a stammer or other speech disorders.

Speech-language therapists work with both children and adults to evaluate and correct their speech problem. Speech therapy is important for improving a person's sense of self-esteem and also to allow listeners to be able to comprehend what is said.

There are five main categories of speech defects: articulation problems, or the inability to produce certain sounds, stuttering or slurred speech, voice disorders (including pitch, quality, and volume), delayed speech in children, and aphasia or the partial or total loss of the ability to speak or comprehend language.

Articulation therapy stresses behavioral techniques that focus on teaching children new sounds, in place of incorrect sounds or omitted sounds. Slowly they are introduced to longer sentences. Children with difficulties such as lisping (saying 'th' in place of 's' and 'z'), or problems saying 'r,' 'l' or 'th' are usually described as having functional speech disorders. For example, the word "super" may be pronounced as "thooper."

Stuttering is a speech problem that involves repeating syllables and stammering. If the stutter is produced as the result of a specific pattern of nerve impulses from the vocal cords, then treatment will aim to prevent this particular pattern from ever reaching the brain.

Treatment. The speech therapist is responsible for analyzing the patient's speech disorder. The method when training young children is to develop good speech habits. When working with teenagers or adults, the therapist must use corrective measures. The first step is to help the person differentiate between his or her speech and normal speech. The therapist may record the patient's speech, allowing the person to listen to his or her voice, with the hope that he or she will gradually be able to differentiate between correct and incorrect speech. Videos are also an effective tool for helping a person identify pronunciation errors.

Generally the therapist will instruct patients as to where to place their tongues in order to improve their speech. She or he may test language comprehension by displaying pictures of items that the patients must identify. Usually the therapist devises a program consisting of exercises for patients to practice. If the patient is younger,

the therapist will involve the parents and teachers in the particular forms of treatment. The goal of speech therapy is to enable the patient to communicate effectively in society. *See also* ANXIETY *and* LISP.

Sperm

Male germ cells.

Sperm are produced in the testicles and stored in the seminal vesicles. At the climax of sexual intercourse, they are released from the penis in a fluid called semen.

Sperm production begins at puberty and, barring any major health problems, continues into old age. Each sperm contains half the chromosomes of a regular body cell. During fertilization, the chromosomes of the sperm combine with those of an egg to produce the zygote, which will develop into a new organism. A sperm cell consists of a head, collar, and tail. The head contains the chromosomes. The collar has hundreds of mitochondria, structures that are responsible for energy production. The tail is for locomotion. *See also* TESTES.

The sex of a baby depends solely on the sperm. Unlike the egg, half of the sperm produced carry the sex chromosome X, and the other half Y. If an X sperm fertilizes the egg, the resulting baby will be a `female; Y sperm produce baby males. Sperm are viable for approximately two to four days after being released into the female. If they are released into any other environment, they are viable only for a few moments. *See* BIRTH *and* REPRODUCTION.

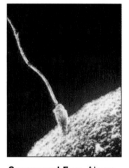

Sperm and Egg. Above, the moment when a sperm meets and fertilizes the egg. Once it penetrates the egg, a chemical response is triggered, and no other sperm can enter. Whether this is done inside the body or out, this is how conception begins.

Spermicides

Chemicals that kill sperm.

One of the best-known spermicides is nonoxynol-9. Many condoms use this spermicide. It is also found in various contraceptive foams, creams, and jellies that can be used alone or with a diaphragm or cervical cap. While spermicides can help prevent conception, alone they are not an effective protection against sexually transmitted diseases. *See also* CONTRACEPTION.

Spherocytosis, Hereditary

An abnormality in the shape of the red blood cells in which the cells are small, spherical, and rigid, rather than disk-shaped and flexible.

A rare cause of hemolytic anemia, spherocytosis is a disease almost exclusively limited to Caucasians of European descent. Red blood cells are normally disk-shaped with concave top and bottom surfaces. They are strong and flexible enough to pass through tiny capillaries to carry oxygen to the tissues. Spherocytosis is a condition in which the red blood cells are smaller, spherical in shape, and fragile, so that they break easily. The damaged cells are filtered out in the spleen, which becomes engorged.

Symptoms. The disease is usually diagnosed early in life, though milder cases may not be discovered until much later in life. When the disease is severe, a newborn child may exhibit jaundice and other common effects of anemia, including fatigue, shortness of breath, dizziness, rapid heartbeat and a sharply increased sensitivity to high altitudes. A child may exhibit retarded growth and a marked vulnerability to even the most minor infections. An aplastic crisis (when the bone marrow temporarily stops producing healthy red blood cells to replace the damaged ones) may be induced by infection or appear spontaneously. Leg ulcers are not entirely uncommon, due to poor circulation of the blood to the lower extremities.

Treatment. Folic acid supplements are usually prescribed. In a crisis, a transfusion or multiple transfusions of healthy red blood cells may be necessary. Surgical removal of the spleen is often performed and usually results in the normalization of red blood cell count.

> *Hereditary Spherocytosis is discussed further in the entries detailing* ANEMIA; ANEMIA, HEMOLYTIC; BLOOD; *and* JAUNDICE. *For information about the hereditary aspect of this disorder see* GENETIC CODE *and* HERITABILITY.

Sphincter, Artificial

A device composed of a fluid-filled system that surrounds the urethra or anus with a silicone cuff, whicj functions like a sphincter.

The sphincter is a contractile muscle allowing for fine control of both urinary and bowel function. When either becomes damaged due to injury, disease, or other disorder, it may be replaced with a device called an artificial sphincter. A urinary sphincter is a cuff that is placed around the bladder neck to ensure its closure; a control pump is situated in either the labia or the scrotum and a fluid reservoir balloon is placed in the lower abdominal cavity. During urination, the pump's release valve is squeezed, allowing the fluid to leave the cuff and return to the reservoir. After urination is complete, the pump is squeezed and the fluid returns to the cuff to occlude the urethra. Artificial rectal sphincters are a more recent advance, and they operate on the same principle. *See also* ANUS CANCER OF; BLADDER; RECTUM; *and* URETHRA.

Spherocytosis and the Family

Inherited spherocytosis is in most instances caused by a dominant gene that is not sex-specific. When either parent has the disease, about 50 percent of his or her children are likely to be born with the disease. However, there may be a recessive form as well, since about 10 to 25 percent of children with the disease have parents neither of whom will ever experience any of the common symptoms. If both parents have the recessive gene, about 25 percent of their children are likely to inherit the condition.

Sphincterotomy

Procedure in which the sphincter muscle is surgically opened to allow the passage of gallstones.

Stones in the bile duct are a fairly common occurrence, particularly in patients undergoing cholecystectomy, (gallbladder removal surgery). *See also* GALLBLADDER.

In endoscopic sphincterotomy, which is also called papillotomy, small incisions are made to widen the junction between the common bile duct, the pancreas, and part of the intestine. This junction is known as the ampulla of Vater. A catheter is passed into the common bile duct, and the stones are captured in a microbasket so they can be pulled back into the intestine. This is the preferred procedure when stones remain after gallbladder surgery.

Spider Bites

Potentially venomous bites from spiders.

The bites of most spiders are not particularly dangerous. However, the bites of certain species can be poisonous and deadly.

Bites of some species of tarantulas, black widows (*Lactrodectus mactans*—a black spider identified by a red hourglass-shaped mark on its underside), and brown recluses (*Loxosceles reclusa*—brown spiders with a violin-shaped marking on top), in particular, are known for their toxicity. These species thrive in dark places in warm, dry climates. The venom of these spiders causes a localized skin reaction at the site of the bite and a systemic reaction that will include intense pain, nausea, and fever. *See also* TOXIN.

The bite itself may feel like a slight pinprick and thus go unnoticed. However, in a matter of hours, the bite will swell and become tender. Breathing difficulties will also ensue. If these symptoms are exhibited, a health care professional must be sought as soon as possible. An accurate description of the spider will help emergency medical technicians properly treat the bite. If the bite is on a limb, keep it still and apply a snug bandage between the bite and the heart to retard the spread of the venom. Do not elevate the limb—allow it to hang down. Also, apply an ice-filled towel to the bite and wait for help to arrive. *See also* ANTIVENIN+ *and* VENOMOUS BITES AND STINGS.

Spider Nevus

Plural, spider nevi: a bright red group of abnormal blood vessels that produces the appearance of a spiderweb on the skin.

A spider nevus has a reddish central spot where all its other projections come together. It appears as a red dot in the center of the nevus with a reddish blush extending out for a distance from it. In children, spider nevi are common and are not associated with other diseases. In adults, they may be associated with other conditions, such as liver failure. Treatment for spider nevi is not usually necessary, as the lesions may resolve on their own. Facial spider nevi can be corrected with electronic cauterization or laser treatment. *See* SKIN *and* LIVER.

Spina Bifida

Birth defect in which a segment of vertebrae does not cover the spinal cord.

One of the most common defects of the brain and spinal cord, spina bifida may be found anywhere along the spine, although it is most often located in the lower back (at the lumbar or sacral areas). When the vertebrae do not grow to the correct size, the spinal cord and the membrane that covers it protrude at the back. Severity of the condition ranges from mild weakness in the legs to extreme physical challenge affecting the entire body. *See also* BIRTH DEFECTS.

There is no exact known cause as of this time, although there is some research that relates the incidence of spina bifida to folic acid deficiencies. The incidence of spina bifida also drastically increases once it appears in a family. Having one child with spina bifida increases the chances tenfold that the mother will give birth to another child with this condition. *See* DNA.

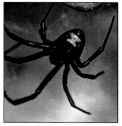

Spider Bites. Above, the characteristic black widow spider with the small hourglass marking; they are usually about one and a half inches long. These spiders infest the warmer regions of the United States and much of Mexico. When they are hatched, they are usually white or light yellow—they take on their distinctive color later in life.

Types. There are four primary types of spina bifida:

Myelocele accounts for 75 percent of all cases of spina bifida. The spinal cord protrudes through the back and is covered with a raw swelling instead of skin. The exposed site is susceptible to infections, such as meningitis, and often results in paralysis. Complications such as hip dislocation, and hydrocephalus, in which spinal fluid accumulates in the brain, are common. It may be accompanied by cerebral palsy, vision problems, epilepsy, and incontinence.

Meningocele is less severe. The spinal cord remains in place, and the protrusion is covered by skin. With early repair, it may not affect any functions.

Encephalocele is a very rare and strikingly severe type of spina bifida in which the protrusion is located in the skull. It causes severe brain damage.

Spina bifida occulta is the least serious spina bifida. The spinal cord remains in place and the only visible evidence of the condition may be a dimple or small tuft of hair over the affected area of the spine. Although it may go completely unnoticed in infants, it may cause problems later in life, including leg weakness or incontinence.

Diagnosis. The spine should fully form in the first four weeks of pregnancy, so spina bifida can often be detected with ultrasound or amniocentesis. The extent of the damage can be determined after birth.

Treatment. Surgery should be performed as soon as possible on the newborn to correct the condition and limit brain damage. Draining of any accumulated spinal fluid may be necessary. Fetal surgery is a possibility that may prevent some of the complications of the condition (abnormally small head growth for example).

Physical therapy or walking aids can increase mobility as the child grows. Other treatment depends on the type and severity of accompanying disorders.

Resources on Spina Bifida and Birth Defects

Apgar, Virginia and Joan Beck, *Is My Baby All Right?* (1972); Behrman, Richard E., *Nelson Textbook of Pediatrics* (1996); Moore, Harold, and Barry O'Donnel, *The Developing Human* (1992); American Academy of Pediatrics, Tel. (847) 228-5005, Online: www.aap.org; Fed. for Children with Special Needs, Tel. (800) 331-0688, Online: www.fcsn.org; Birth Defects Reseach for Children, Tel. (407) 895-0802, Online: www.birthdefects.org; Spina Bifida Association of America, Tel. (800) 621-3141, On line: http://sbaa@sbaa.org; www.ny-cornell.org/pediatrics/.

Background information about Spina Bifida can be found in AMNIOCENTESIS; BIRTH DEFECTS; SPINE; *and* VERTEBRA. *Related disorders include* CEREBRAL PALSY; EPILEPSY; *and* MENINGITIS. *Also see* PHYSICAL THERAPY.

Spinal Anesthesia

A specific type of regional anesthesia in which a local anesthetic is injected into the cerebrospinal fluid around the spinal cord.

Spinal anesthesias provide pain relief during surgery on the lower extremities and abdomen. It is sometimes referred to as intrathecal anesthesia. *See also* ANESTHESIA.

Spinal anesthesia is prescribed for patients whose condition makes them unsuitable for a general anesthetic (for example, if they suffer from a respiratory disease), and for procedures below the ribcage, such as hip, obstetric, gynecologic, and urologic operations. Spinals are also intended for older patients and those with diabetes or sickle cell disease. Spinals are relatively easy to employ, and are sometimes used when a skilled anesthetist is not available to administer general anesthesia. *See* SPINAL CORD.

The procedure is performed by inserting a fine needle between two vertebrae in the lower part (lumbar region) of the spine, and injecting the anesthetic into the cerebrospinal fluid (CSF) around the spinal cord. The nerves of the spinal cord absorb the anesthetic and block transmission of pain impulses to the brain.

The most common anesthetics used in spinals are hyperbaric bupivacaine, lignocaine, cinchocaine, amethocaine, and mepivacaine. Spinals take effect quicker than general anesthesia. They may cause a rapid drop in blood pressure in some patients. After spinal anesthesia, which can last up to six hours, about one to five percent of patients develop headaches. *See also* VERTEBRA.

Spinal Cord

Long column of nerve cells running through the center of the spine.

The spinal cord is the main pathway connecting the brain to the other nerves in the body. It is about 18 inches long and less than three-quarters of an inch thick. It passes through the center of the vertebrae to the lower back, where it branches off into a number of nerve endings. Thirty one pairs of spinal nerves branch off along the length of the spinal cord and transmit signals to various parts of the body. There are 26 bones in the spine protecting the spinal cord. These bones are attached to each other in such a way as to maintain their protective function while still being able to move and stretch with an amazing amount of flexibility. *See also* VERTEBRA.

Function. The spinal cord is a pathway for nerve impulses traveling both to and from the brain. Some reflexes are controlled from the spinal cord. Central pattern generators (a self-sustaining pattern produced by a neural unit) in the spine can initiate and control complex forms of body movement; however, these are controlled by the brain. *See also* BRAIN.

Spinal Damage. Damage to the spinal cord may result from trauma; from weakening or disease of the vertebrae; or from nervous system disorders. Impairment of the spinal cord often results in symptoms in other parts of the body, such as numbness or paralysis in the arms or the legs. *See also* NERVOUS SYSTEM *and* TRAUMA.

Spinal Fusion

A surgical process in which two or more vertebrae are fused together.

When the spinal motion between vertebrae causes severe pain, two (or more) vertebrae may be surgically fused together. This sort of treatment limits some amount of motion, but because the fusion surgery affects such small bones, the limitation is generaly minor. Between the affected vertebra, bone (usually from the patient him- or herself) is placed for fusion. Kyphosis, scoliosis, and spinal injuries (including slipped disks) can all be effectively treated with spinal fusion surgery. According to the American Academy of Orthopedic Surgeons, about 258,000 spinal fusion operations were performed in 1999, the last year for which data were available at press time. *See also* KYPHOSIS; SCOLIOSIS; SPINAL CORD; SPINAL INJURY; SURGERY; *and* VERTEBRA.

Spinal Injury

Damage to the spine and possibly to the spinal cord, resulting in a loss of sensation and muscle weakness.

The spinal cord resembles an interstate highway with its many connecting nerves; it is responsible for the communication between the brain and the rest of the body. The spinal cord nerves that are situated on the front side of the body contain motor nerves that transmit information to the muscles. The spinal cord nerves situated on the back side of the body contain sensory nerves that transmit sensory information regarding touch, smell, heat, and cold. Damage to the spine can affect parts of the body below the point of injury and can cause permanent disability.

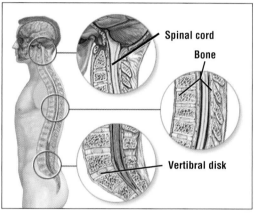

Spinal cord

Bone

Vertibral disk

Causes and Types. The spinal cord can be severed in a car accident or it can be damaged by an infection, disease, or reduced blood supply. Spinal cord compression injuries can be classified as longitudinal, hinging, or shearing. Longitudinal compression is caused by a fall, producing a longitudinal crack in the vertebrae. Hinging is caused by a whiplash injury from an automobile accident, twisting the spine. Shearing occurs when an individual is run over by an automobile. It combines hinging with additional rotational torque.

Symptoms. Spinal cord injuries produce swelling and severe pain. Damage to the spinal cord results in paralysis and the loss of motor capabilities below the affected area. Damage below the neck often causes a weakness or paralysis of the legs and trunk (paraplegia). Damage to the neck may produce weakness or paralysis in the arms and legs (quadriplegia). Other symptoms include bladder and bowel incontinence. Spinal cord injury can be fatal.

Spinal Injury. Above, there are many places and ways in which the spine can be injured. The bottom bones in the vertebra (near the lumbar region of the back) in many people fuse together; although not entirely serious, this can cause severe back pain. Any damage to the spinal cord can cause paralysis in varying degrees. Damage to disks can cause paralysis too, in some cases. Exercise that strengthens the back often helps prevent these problems.

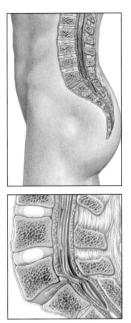

Spinal Stenosis.
Above, one injury that may occur in the back is spinal stenosis (at the top) due to disk herniation—which is a bulging or protrusion of a disk (at the bottom). Spinal stenosis is a narrowing of the spinal cord that can cause some measure of pain. Surgery is not recommended, except in the most sever cases. Treatments for this include exercise on a stationary bike or daily walking, as well as resting when pain occurs. To the far right, an illustration of a boy using a spirometer. Spirometry tests lung function. It is usually expressed in two numbers: air flow and air volume.

Diagnosis and Treatment. It is important to avoid further impairment of the spine in spinal cord injury patients. It is therefore crucial that the spinal injury victim be moved only by a professional trained in first aid. To evaluate the extent of the spinal damage, x-rays are taken. The injury is first treated with corticosteroid medications (prednisone) to limit the swelling. Muscle relaxants and pain relievers are administered to reduce spasms. Spinal cord compression caused by infection is treated with antibiotics. A neurosurgeon may drain accumulated fluid or blood aggregating near the spinal cord. Physical therapists and nurses are necessary to prevent development of bedsores and the locking of the joints, and it is necessary to establish a general rehabilitation program.

Prevention. Spinal cord injuries can be serious. The best method of treatment is always prevention. Seat belts should always be worn in automobiles. Helmets should always be worn when riding motorcycles or bicycles, skateboarding, or inline skating. *See also* NSAIDs; Paralysis Spinal Cord; *and* Spinal Fusion.

Spirituality

Belief in a religious system or a higher power or powers.

Spirituality can play an important role in a person's health. On a basic level, people's spiritual beliefs affect what health care decisions they make: such as how they react to illness, what treatment options they pursue (or do not pursue), and what decisions they make in the event of terminal illness.

People who participate in some form of spirituality, whether through attending church or other religious meetings, reading spiritual texts, or otherwise engaging in a spiritual community, often have a lower incidence of depression, heart disease, stroke, and similar illnesses. Spirituality often plays a role in recovery from addiction, especially in twelve-step programs. *See also* Alternative Medicine; Aromatherapy; Meditation; *and* Mind/Body Therapy.

Spirochete

A spiral-shaped bacterium.

There are six basic categories of spirochetes, with only slightly different determining factors for each—some have an outer sheath, some do not. Spirochetes cause a number of diseases in humans, including syphilis, Lyme disease, relapsing fever, leptospirosis, and rat bite fever. Most of these diseases are transmitted to humans by ticks or body lice, though some are transmitted through direct contact with dogs, cats, rats, or farm animals. Spirochetes are successfully treated with antibiotics. *See also* Antibiotic Drugs; Bacteria; Lyme Disease; Pathogen; *and* Syphilis.

Spirometry

Technique to measure the volume of air inhaled or exhaled by the lung.

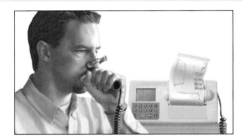

An instrument known as a spirometer is used to test pulmonary function. The spirometer measures the volume and rate of air inhaled or exhaled during a specified period. Spirometry is used to diagnose asthma. A physician will compare the person's normal airflow with airflow during an attack and airflow following medication, to assess severity of asthma and success of treatment. A spirometer consists of a mouthpiece attached to a length of tubing. This is connected to a recording device that measures airflow. The person will be asked to inhale deeply, then exhale as forcefully as possible. A bronchodilator, a drug used to dilate the air passageways, may be used during the test. *See also* Breathing; Breathing Difficulty; Breathlessness; Peak Flow Meter; *and* Pulmonary Insufficiency.

Spleen

Small organ in the upper abdominal cavity that serves primarily to filter out old and damaged blood cells.

Found on the lower left side of the abdomen, the spleen is about five to six inches long and it becomes enlarged after digestion or when it is diseased. It is surrounded by a thin tissue layer for protection. If this capsule is ruptured, by trauma or due to a pathogen, then the spleen will have to be removed.

The spleen's primary function is as a filtering organ. Blood passes through the spleen, where cells known as phagocytes remove old blood cells, damaged cells, platelets, parasites, and foreign or toxic substances. The spleen stores the blood's platelets and also saves the iron contained in the old red blood cells for storage and reuse. *See also* TOXIN.

Prior to birth, the spleen and the liver produce red blood cells, a function that is later taken over by the bone marrow. *See also* ABDOMEN; BLOOD; HYPERSPLENISM; IRON; PARASITE; *and* SPLENECTOMY.

Splenectomy

Surgical removal of the spleen.

A splenectomy is often required in the emergency treatment of severe bleeding from a ruptured spleen, the causes of which may be physical trauma from automobile accidents or body contact sports, or, more rarely, from rapid enlargement of the spleen in aggressive Epstein-Barr viral disease as well as for an enlarged spleen in conjunction with cirrhosis. Splenectomy also may be needed to treat varicose veins in the esophagus that cause internal bleeding; HIV splenomegaly; some blood diseases such as leukemia, and lymphoma.

Removal of the spleen is a common consideration because the organ is difficult to repair, and its absence produces no ill effects because other organs (the liver and lymphatic system) seem to take over its functions—namely, to remove bacteria and to filter, make, and store blood.

The operation may be performed by traditional or laparoscopic surgery. The patient is given a general anesthetic, and the surgeon makes either a vertical or horizontal incision in the upper left abdomen to expose the spleen; or she makes three or four small incisions and uses a laparoscope. All the securing tissues are cut, and blood vessels to and from the spleen are tied and severed; and the spleen is then removed.

The operation takes about an hour. Patients who undergo the laparoscopic procedure will have to stay at the hospital for two to three days, and some patients will require several more days of recovery. *See also* EPSTEIN-BARR SYNDROME *and* SPLEEN.

Splint

Appliance used for immobilization of an injured body part.

Splints are often applied as part of first aid for a fracture. A splint is important if a victim needs to be moved from an accident scene, as jarring may cause more damage. A splint may also be applied to keep a body part stable during the healing process. Bones begin to repair themselves rapidly, so the sooner bone ends are reunited the better the chance there is of the fracture healing without any further complications.

A splint is usually made from lightweight material (acrylic, polyethylene foam, plaster of Paris, or aluminum). Ambulances or emergency workers carry portable, inflatable splints. In emergencies, a splint may be made from any non-bending material (such as wood, metal, or stiff corrugated cardboard). A person's injured leg can be splinted to the uninjured one. To apply an emergency splint, gently support the injured limb while sliding the splint material underneath the fractured area. Secure it firmly with tape or string, but make sure it is not so tight as to cut off circulation. Try to move the limb as little as possible while waiting for or traveling to a physician. *See also* FIRST AID *and* FRACTURE.

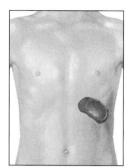
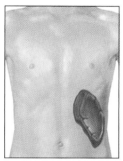

The Spleen. At the top is an image of a normal spleen. This organ, which is about the size of a fist, is a filtering device. Above, at the bottom, is an enlarged spleen (which is sometimes known as splenomegaly), that will probably have to be removed. Disorders such as brucellosis, Hand-Schüller-Christian disease, hepatitis, hypersplenism, kala-azar, thalassemia, and tuberculosis can all cause the spleen to enlarge.

Splinting, Dental

Application of a device that immobilizes and supports teeth during the healing process.

Dental splints are commonly implemented in the reimplantation of dislodged teeth; when a tooth is knocked out of its socket and replaced, it is necessary to hold it in place. Dentists have a variety of devices, including wire, quick-setting plastic, and crowns bonded together, that can act as a splint to allow the tooth to heal and reattach to nerves and blood supply. Dental splints can also be used to secure fractured or loosened teeth. They are sometimes used to aid maintenance teeth alignment after corrective jaw surgery. *See also* DENTISTRY; LUXATED TOOTH; ORTHOGNATHIC SURGERY; *and* REIMPLANTATION, DENTAL

Spondylitis

Joint inflammation located between the vertebrae of the spine.

Rheumatic disorders, such as rheumatoid arthritis or ankylosing spondylitis, or occasionally a bacterial infection located elsewhere in the body, may cause the joints between the vertebrae to become inflamed. Diagnosis of the underlying cause of the problem should dictate what course of treatment will follow. *See also* ANKYLOSING SPONDYLITIS *and* RHEUMATOID ARTHRITIS.

Spondylolisthesis

Forward slippage of a vertebrae onto the one below it.

The vertebrae are generally divided into three parts—the neck section (cervical), the rib cage area (thoracic), and the lower back (lumbar). The most common place for spondylolisthesis to occur is in the lumbar region, between the last (fifth) lumbar vertebra and the sacrum, which rests on the pelvis. Occasionally it may occur between the fourth and fifth lumbar vertebrae, or between the cervical vertebrae. Spondylolis-

thesis is often the result of stress fractures, traumatic fractures, or deterioration from osteoarthritis. Spondylolysis, a condition in which the bone of the lumbar vertebra fractures, may cause the slippage.

Symptoms include lower back pain, sciatica due to pressure from the slipped vertebra, and noticeably significant lordosis, or inward curving of the lower spine.

Spondylolisthesis is best diagnosed with x-rays. Treatment depends on the severity. It may include traction to immobilize the area, physical therapy to strengthen it, or, in extreme cases, surgery to fuse the slipping vertebra. *See also* BACK PAIN; LORDOSIS OSTEOARTHRITIS; *and* SPONDYLOLYSIS.

Spondylolysis

Condition where arch of the fifth lumbar vertebra is made of a soft, fibrous tissue instead of bone.

Spondylolysis itself rarely displays any symptoms. Its real danger lies in the fact that the fracture of the affected vertebra makes it vulnerable to slippage over a nearby vertebra (spondylolisthesis). The relatively weak vertebra also causes the whole area of the arch to be more easily damaged by stress or injury. Spondylolysis may also occur in the fourth vertebra of the lumbar area, although that is much less common. *See* BACK PAIN; LORDOSIS; OSTEOTOMY; SPONDYLOLISTHESIS; *and* VERTEBRA.

Sponge, Contraceptive

A barrier contraceptive consisting of a small synthetic sponge, prefilled with spermicide, that is inserted into the vagina and placed against the cervix prior to sexual intercourse.

Unlike the diaphragm or cervical cap, a contraceptive sponge can be purchased over the counter and does not need to be fitted by a medical practitioner. Each sponge is effective for 24 hours. No additional spermicide needs to be added for repeated acts of sexual intercourse. The sponge must be left in place for six hours after the last act of intercourse.

In addition to blocking the cervix, the sponge also absorbs and kills sperm, making it a very effective means of contraception. However, in recent years the only American company to make contraceptive sponges ceased production. There have been reports that soon contraceptive sponges will be available once again in the United States. *See* BARRIER METHODS; CONTRACEPTION; *and* NATURAL CONTRACEPTION.

Sporotrichosis

An skin infection caused by the fungus *Sporothrix schenckii*, which is acquired from roses and other thorny plants as well as from moss and hay.

Sporothrix schenckii, the fungus that causes sporotrichosis, usually enters the body through a skin break, producing a small lump on a finger or hand. The lump slowly enlarges and then opens into a suppurating (pus-filled) sore. The infection spreads through the lymph system, forming nodules and sores. Unless the fungus attacks the lungs, there are no other symptoms. If the lungs are attacked (usually in someone who already has another upper respiratory infection), the disease takes the form of pneumonia, with symptoms that include a dry cough and chest pain. On rare occasions, the disease attacks other tissues, the joints, the bones, the muscles, or the eyes. Iodides and antifungal agents are useful in the treatment of sporotrichosis. *See also* ANTIFUNGAL DRUGS *and* LYMPHATIC SYSTEM.

Sports Injuries

Injuries directly related to participation in a sport or other athletic activity.

Sports injuries fall into two categories. Traumatic, or acute, injuries result from a single instance of extreme trauma (though risk factors make some individuals particularly vulnerable to acute injury). The cause of the injury might be direct force to the body, such as when a football player suffers a concussion from a blow to the head, or it might be more subtle, such as when a run-ner pulls a hamstring during a race. The second type of sports injury, called an overuse injury, is due to overuse or repetitive strain. Over time, for example, a runner might develop swelling in the knees from the repeated stress of running.

TYPES

Approximately 95 percent of sports injuries involve minor trauma to soft tissue, affecting muscles, ligaments, or tendons. These injuries fall into three categories: contusions, sprains, and strains. A contusion (bruise) is an injury to soft tissue, often produced by a blunt force, such as kick, fall, or blow. It results in pain, swelling, and discoloration in the injured area. Sprains, which account for one-third of all sports injuries, result from a partial or complete tear of a ligament, a strong band of tissue that connects bones to one another and stabilizes joints. A sprain is most often caused by a forced or awkward twisting of the ligament, and usually affects the ankles, knees, or wrists. A strain is an injury to a muscle or tendon. In most cases, strains are caused by overuse of the affected muscle or tendon. Repeated stress on a tendon can cause inflammation of the tendon (tendinitis) or inflammation of the fluid-filled sacs that allow tendons to move easily over bones (bursitis). Tendinitis and bursitis often occur at the same time.

Fractures (bone breaks) account for nearly all of the remaining five percent of sports injuries. They are usually caused by a blow to the bone or a fall. The bones of the arms and legs are the most vulnerable to fracture, while the bones of the spine and skull are the least likely to be affected by sports-related fractures. The bones of the legs and feet are the most susceptible to stress fractures, which occur when muscle strains or contractions make bones bend. Stress fractures are especially common in ballet dancers, in long-distance runners, and in people whose bones are thin.

The most common type of fatal sports injury is a brain injury, or brain concussion. A concussion is a brain injury that can result from even a minor blow to the head.

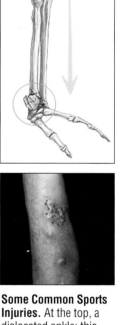

Some Common Sports Injuries. At the top, a dislocated ankle; this sort of injury happens to runners, and to those whose sports involve running, somewhat frequently. In the middle is an image of a Colles' fracture in the wrist. This may happen when a person attempts to break a fall (perhaps in order to prevent a more serious injury) with the hands. At the bottom is a case of sporotrichosis on the forearm; this fungal infection has a higher incidence among farmers and gardners than among others.

Concussions can be minor injuries, or they can even be fatal. More than 8 million sports injuries occur each year in the U.S. Young children are most likely to suffer from sports-related injuries. Each year, about 3.2 million children between the ages of 5 and 14 are injured while participating in athletic activities. Annually, more than 775,000 boys and girls under the age of 14 are treated in hospital emergency rooms for sports-related injuries.

SYMPTOMS

Symptoms of sports injuries depend on the type of injury. Soft-tissue injuries commonly cause swelling, pain or tenderness in the area of the injury, discoloration, or weakness in an affected joint. Fractures may cause, among others, symptoms including: mild to severe pain, bruising, swelling, paleness, weakness or immobility of the affected bone, or numbness. Concussions can result in disturbed balance, impaired speech, hearing or vision loss, or even loss of consciousness.

TREATMENT

Immediate treatment for almost all acute athletic injuries is rest, ice, compression (pressure on the injured area), and elevation. These four treatments are commonly referred to by the acronym RICE. Rest helps the injured person avoid hemorrhaging or swelling. Ice limits inflammation and reduces the pain. Compression and elevation help reduce edema (that is, the accumulation of fluids in tissue spaces or body cavities). To reduce pain, especially in fracture cases, the injured area is regularly immobilized in a medically appropriate manner using supportive bandaging and splinting techniques.

The best treatment for injuries due to overuse is to abstain from the activity that is causing the problem. Medication or ice might also be used to limit swelling. The injured can often prevent recurrence by identifying the motion or set of motions that is putting physical stress on the affected site. Tennis players, golfers, and others often consult a trained professional to identify the source of an injury.

PREVENTION

The best way to avoid acute injuries is to check that the environment is safe and that all appropriate protective equipment is being used. Appropriate safety gear, such as helmets, mouth guards, and shin guards, should be worn at all times. Stretching before a game or workout also reduces the chance of injury. Individuals can also avoid overuse injuries by paying close attention to the stress their activities place on the body. Any pain or discomfort that occurs during athletic exertion should be investigated by a doctor or a trainer. Overuse injuries develop gradually, and it is often possible to avoid a serious injury by catching the problem at an early stage. In general, individuals are more resistant to injury when they are physically fit, and when they avoid engaging in physical activity if they are tired, sick, or in pain.

Background information about this topic can be found in BRUISE; CONCUSSION; FRACTURES; *and* SPORTS MEDICINE. *Related topics include* EXERCISE *and* PHYSICAL TRAINING. *For information about treatment see* PHYSICAL THERAPY.

Sports Medicine

An area of medicine that prepares athletes for competition and treats sports-related injuries.

Sports medicine is a broad term encompassing a wide range of specialists who apply medical knowledge to the care and treatment of athletes and sports-related injuries. It is an interdisciplinary field that incorporates physiology, biomechanics, psychology, and various other areas. As participation in athletic activities has increased, the

---

ALERT

Kids and Sports Injuries

Injuries to children between five and 14 years of age account for 40 percent of all sports-related injuries. There are many reasons that children are most vulnerable to injury during an athletic activity. Immature coordination and poor nutrition are two of the most basic health-related risk factors that regularly result in injury. There are also many environmental causes for sports-related injury to children. Professional sporting arenas are cared for diligently by crews of grounds keepers; kids will participate in sports wherever they can, regardless of the condition of the land or their playing surface. Children may lack protective gear or they may wear poorly fitting safety equipment. Unless instructed properly by a coach, they may not perform necessary preparatory exercises, such as stretching, and they may not respond appropriately to pain by resting.

need for doctors who can treat sports-related health problems has grown. Sports physicians supervise athletes during training and treat injuries that occur as a result of athletic activities.

Exercise and Aging

Sports doctors often supervise the athletic training of middle-aged and elderly individuals. Exercise, particularly weight training, benefits elderly individuals, since people begin to lose muscle mass between the ages of 20 and 30 at a rate of about one percent a year, a process that often goes unnoticed until it has already begun causing health problems. Elderly people can increase the strength of their muscles and bones through a well-designed exercise regime.

There are four essential components to sports medicine: preparation (proper training), prevention of illness or injury, diagnosis and treatment of sports-related health problems, and rehabilitation for injured athletes. Sports physicians often work with physical therapists in the diagnosis and treatment of sports injuries. *See also* EXERCISE; NUTRITION; *and* SPORTS INJURIES.

Sports, Unlawful Drugs and

The use of drugs to enhance athletic ability.

Athletes sometimes use unlawful or illegal drugs or improperly use prescription drugs in order to enhance performance in their sport. Drugs that are used and that are prohibited by a number of sports regulatory agencies, such as the International and U.S. Olympic Committees, the National Collegiate Athletic Association (NCAA), and the U.S. Anti-Doping Agency (USADA), include stimulants, narcotics, diuretics, anabolic steroids, masking agents, and other hormones. Some over-the-counter diet pills and dietary supplements are prohibited under these rules. There are also many drugs that may be illegal in themselves; many of these are prohibited because they may give an athlete an unfair advantage in competition, and often have severe and even life-threatening side effects. *See also* STEROIDS, ANABOLIC *and* STIMULANT DRUGS.

Sprain

Tearing or overstretching of ligaments caused by a sudden pull.

The bone ends that meet in a joint are held together by strands of ligaments, tough fibrous tissue that allow the bones to move but prevent the joint from moving too much or in an incorrect way. When that does occur, the ligaments may be torn or overstretched. All of the ligaments in an area may tear, or, in less severe cases, only a few may be damaged. Some of the most common sprains happen to the knee and the ankle, which may twist abnormally while changing direction rapidly (as in a sporting activity) or falling awkwardly. A severe sprain may lead to joint dislocation.

Symptoms of a sprain include pain and swelling. X-rays can ensure there is no fracture. Initial treatment usually consists of ice and elevation of the injured area to reduce pain and swelling. Analgesics or mild painkillers may be prescribed. A cast is usually not necessary, although sometimes a light brace or support may be recommended. Rest is helpful at first, but normal, weight-bearing activity seems to be more successful than keeping weight off the injury during the entire healing process. For the most severe cases, physical therapy may be needed to strengthen or retrain an area where there has been nerve damage. *See also* FRACTURES *and* PHYSICAL THERAPY.

Sprue, Tropical

A malabsorption syndrome from the tropics that causes gastroenterological dysfunction.

Tropical sprue may be the result of an infectious organism, vitamin deficiency, food toxin, or parasite infestation. It is probably transmitted by drinking contaminated water or eating contaminated food. Sprue causes malabsorption. Tropical sprue is distinct from celiac sprue, which is caused by a sensitivity to gluten, the protein found in wheat and wheat products. Tropical sprue is most prevalent in areas where polished

Resources on Sports Medicine

Costill, David L., *Inside Running: Basics of Sports Physiology* (1986); Jordan, Barry, and Russell F. Warren, et al., *Sports Neurology* (1998); McArdle, William D., et al., *Exercise Physiology: Energy, Nutrition, and Human Performance* (1996); Warren, Russell F., *The Unstable Shoulder* (1998); American Physical Therapy Association, Tel. (800) 999-APTA, Online: www.apta.org; National Osteoporosis Foundation, Tel. (800) 223-9994, Online: www.nof.org; President's Council on Physical Fitness and Sports, Tel. (202) 690-9000, Online: www.fitness.gov; Women's Sports Foundation, Tel. (800) 227-3988, Online: www.lifetimetv.com/WoSport; https://public1.med.cornell.edu/orthopedics/index.html.

rice is the staple food, as well as in the Caribbean, southeast Asia, and India.

Symptoms. Both residents and visitors to endemic areas may be affected by this illness, which causes severe diarrhea, upset stomach, weight loss, pallor, muscle spasms, tingling in the extremities, severe vomiting, fatigue, flatus, cramps weight loss, and pale clay-colored stool. Inflammation of the small intestine due to the illness results in decreased fat digestion and absorption and may lead to symptoms of vitamin deficiencies. If left untreated, lesions of the mouth and fissures of the tongue develop. In children, the disease often leads to delayed skeletal maturation.

Diagnosis. Diagnosis may be made through a biopsy of the small bowel, indicating malabsorption or infection, a stool sample indicating increased fecal fat content; a positive CBC (complete blood-cell count) test for anemia; and blood tests for serum cholesterol, albumin, serum phosphorus, and serum calcium.

Treatment. Tropical sprue is treated with antibiotics such as tetracycline, which is not used with children; as well as folic acid to correct anemia, weight loss, and diarrhea. Vitamin supplements are also given to replace those lost through removal. The antibiotic treatment may need to be administered for an extended period of time, depending on the severity of the disease. *See also* BLOOD COUNT; TETRACYCLINE DRUGS; *and* TROPICAL DISEASES.

Sputum

Liquid material made in the respiratory tract.

Sputum is produced by the cells that line the walls of the airways, nose, and sinuses. Also known as phlegm, sputum normally is almost colorless. It lubricates and protects the sensitive skinlike lining (mucous membrane) of the respiratory tract.

A change in color, the presence of other matter in sputum, or an increase in the amount of sputum often is an indication of medical conditions that range from trivial to life-threatening. For example, a large in-

crease in the amount of sputum can result from an allergic reaction, asthma, or an infection of the respiratory tract.

Irritation of the respiratory track by pollutants can also increase sputum production; one example of this phenomenon is smokers' cough. *See also* COUGH, SMOKERS'.

Blood in the sputum can be a sign of lung cancer or another life-threatening condition. Yellowish or green sputum is an indicator of a bacterial infection, while pinkish, frothy sputum can be due to excess fluid accumulation in the lungs. If an infection is suspected, the infectious agent can be determined by microscopic examination of sputum or a laboratory culture to grow bacteria. Any drastic change in the color of the sputum warrants consultation with a physician. *See also* MUCUS.

Squamous Cell Carcinoma

Malignant tumor of the skin or similar tissue.

Squamous cell carcinoma is a common cancer of the skin, but it can also arise in the tissue lining many organs, including the bladder, the esophagus, the lung, and the vagina. In the skin, squamous cell carcinoma originates in the layer of tissue just below the epidermis, the outermost layer.

As with other skin cancers, the incidence of squamous cell carcinoma is directly related to exposure to sunlight. Those at highest risk are fair-skinned individuals over the age of 60 who have spent a lot of time outdoors with minimal protection from sunlight. Occupational exposure to chemicals such as arsenic, heavy oils, tar, and paraffin also increases the risk of squamous cell carcinoma.

Risk factors differ for other areas of the body. For example, squamous cell carcinoma of the vagina is believed to be associated with a sexually transmitted virus, human papilloma virus (HPV). Squamous cell carcinoma of the lung, like other lung cancers, is caused by cigarette smoking.

Symptoms. On the skin, squamous cell carcinoma first appears as a small patch or lump that usually resembles a wart; it is

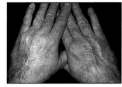

Squamous Cell Carcinoma. Above, an image of squamous cell carcinoma affecting the skin on the hands. These discolorations should be removed as soon as they are diagnosed, as they have a tendency to metastasize rather quickly. The case above has spread to a dangerous extent.

painless and it grows rather slowly. Symptoms of squamous cell carcinoma in other parts of the body depend on the affected organ; in the lung, for example, the symptoms include persistent coughing that may produce: blood, hoarseness, recurrent pneumonia, and bronchitis.

Diagnosis. Squamous cell carcinoma of the skin is diagnosed primarily by microscopic examination of a tissue sample (biopsy). X-ray examinations and blood tests may be done if the cancer has developed enough for a health care professional to worry that it has spread to tissue beyond the skin. Magnetic resonance imaging (MRI) may be used to assess the size and shape of a carcinoma within the body.

Immunotherapy Treatment

One new treatment for squamous cell carcinoma of the skin is immunotherapy, in which interferon, a biologically active molecule produced through bioengineering, is injected into the cancer two or three times a week for several weeks. Immunotherapy is effective in more than 80 percent of cases, but its side effects include fever, aches and pains, general malaise, and itching at the site of injection.

Treatment. The object in treating squamous cell carcinoma is complete destruction of the cancer. If the carcinoma has not spread, simple surgery usually is sufficient. Removal may also be accomplished by using a specialized instrument (curettage) to scrape away the cancer; by freezing (cryotherapy); or by laser surgery. Radiation therapy or chemotherapy may be done if the cancer is in an area such as the nose, where surgery can be disfiguring. The prognosis depends on the stage at which the cancer is diagnosed and treated.

Background information about Squamous Cell Carcinoma can be found in CANCER; SKIN; SKIN CANCER; *and* SMALL-CELL CARCINOMA. *Treatment is discussed in* CURETTAGE; LASER TREATMENT; *and* SURGERY. *See* BIOPSY *and* MRI.

Stable

A term describing a symptom or condition that has reached a temporary equilibrium.

A stable condition is one in which improvement is shown and deterioration of the patient's condition or the progress of her or his injury or disease has been arrested. In emergency situations, stabilization of the patient is the most immediate goal. Once vital life signs have been restored to a stable baseline, treatments for a cure may begin, though a stable condition can take a sudden turn for the worse. Many measurements of the body's vital signs may be evaluated relative to the stability or instability of a person, including evaluation of his or her electroencephalogram, heart rate, and characteristics (measured by electrocardiogram), breathing, pulse, blood loss, and circulation, state of infection, etc. *See also* CIRCULATORY SYSTEM; ECHOCARDIOGRAPHY; ELECTROCARDIOGRAM; *and* VITAL SIGN.

Stage

Term denoting a particular, recognizable period in the course of a disease or characteristic phase of development in the life history of an organism.

Stage may be used as a general description in the course of an illness—late stage, latent stage, asymptomatic stage—providing an overall sense of the progress. It may also be used with greater specificity. The trajectory of cancer, for example, is often described in discrete stages from 1(I) to 5 (V). Increasing stages indicate the severity and spread of the disease. Cancer staging is crucial to designing appropriate therapy. Stage may also be used to define discrete phases of development in the life of an organism; for example, the larval stage of certain microorganisms. *See also* ASYMPTOMATIC; CANCER; *and* MICROORGANISM.

Stapedectomy

Surgical removal and prosthetic replacement of a bone in the ear to treat hearing loss.

The stapes (stirrup) is one of the ossicles in the middle ear, all of which are critical to hearing. The other bones are the incus (anvil) and malleus (hammer). *See also* EAR.

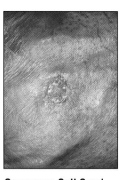

Squamous Cell Carcinoma. This is the second most common form of skin cancer in the United States, afflicting over 200,000 individuals each year, according to The Skin Cancer Foundation. Wherever it occurs on the skin, it will always make a nasty-looking mark that may bleed for weeks; sometimes it looks like a mere wart, but it should not be mistaken for one. All individuals at risk for this sort of skin damage, should have such sores examined by a physician.

Normally, the stapes transmits sound to the inner ear; but with otosclerosis, the base of the stapes (the innermost of the three sound-conducting bones) acquires a growth of spongy or calcified bone. This prevents the stapes from moving freely enough to transmit sound.

To correct the condition, the affected individual is given a local or general anesthetic, and the surgeon removes all or most of the stapes and an artificial bone is placed properly and attached to the incus (the middle bone or anvil). The prosthesis is made of plastic and stainless steel wire. In an alternate version of the surgery, the doctor saves part of the foot-plate of the stapes and attaches the prosthesis to a hole in it. The latter procedure is simpler and safer than the traditional surgery.

Better than 90 percent of all patients recover the ability to hear but one to two percent lose all hearing in the ear. It is therefore general practice that only one ear be operated upon at a time, even if both ears are affected by otosclerosis. *See* EAR, EXAMINATION OF *and* OTOSCLEROSIS.

Staphylococcal Infections

Infections caused by a bacteria of the staphylococcus group.

Staphylococcus bacteria can enter the body through a break in the skin. They can then move almost anywhere in the body to produce serious disease. People most vulnerable to staphylococcal infections are the very young, the elderly, people with compromised immune systems, and people who are suffering from a chronic disease, such as AIDS, diabetes, or cancer.

Staphylococcal infections usually produce pus-filled abscesses. If they are near the skin, they are called boils and can be drained and cleaned by a health care professional. If they are attached to an internal organ like the bones (osteomyelitis) or the heart (endocarditis), they may be life-threatening. Staphylococcal pneumonia is often an opportunistic infection (an infection that strikes people with compromised

immune systems). This form of pneumonia affects people with AIDS, cancer, bronchitis, emphysema, or influenza. Staphylococcal bacteremia (an infection of the blood with staphylococci) is often fatal in people who have suffered traumatic burns. There is always a risk of staphylococcal infection introduced during surgery, since the bacteria is often found in hospitals.

Staphylococcal infections are treated with antibiotics; oral if the infection is in the skin; intravenous if the infection is in the blood or a deep organ. Strains resistant to methicillin and some of the other standard antibiotics are becoming increasingly evident, particularly in hospitals. See also AIDS; ANTIBIOTIC DRUGS; BACTERIA; CANCER; IMMUNE SYSTEM; *and* PNEUMONIA.

Starvation

The most severe form of malnutrition.

Worldwide, one person dies of starvation every second; three out of four of those people are children under the age of five.

Starvation can result from lack of food, a diet that lacks essential nutrients, or disorders in which the body is unable to properly digest or utilize certain foods. It may also be the result of prolonged fasting, anorexia nervosa, or coma.

As malnutrition progresses, many of the bodys systems become impaired. The stomach reduces acid production, breathing slows, the number of blood cells drops (anemia), body temperature drops, as does the heart rate, and the immune system and thyroid system becomes less effective.

Organs such as the heart, muscles, and reproductive organs shrink in size. A person who is starving may have frequent, severe bouts of diarrhea and feel listless and irritable. Over time, starvation can lead to heart and respiratory failure and, ultimately, death. Treatment of starvation involves reversing the malnutrition—which must be done gradually, either by the slow introduction of proper foods or by treating any underlying disorders. *See also* DEATH; FASTING; MALABSORPTION; *and* NUTRITION.

Inflammation and Staphylococcal Infections. Staphylococcal infections regularly cause inflammation of the lymph system; more specifically, the condition is known as staphylococcal lymphangitis. Below, the smallest finger affected by such an inflammation, has become swollen and its movement range has become limited.

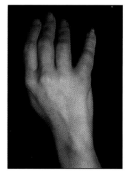

Statistics and Indicators, Medical

The science of medical statistics.

Medical statistics are the basis upon which insurance companies and the public make sense of the increasing number of medical treatments. Statisticians have become as common as physicians in medical research institutions. Statisticians advise researchers on how to design medical trials for optimum accuracy, analyze and interpret results, and come to valid conclusions. Specifically, a statistician determines the number of subjects in a trial, how to divide them into different treatment groups, how often to administer treatments and measure outcomes, and how to examine the results. Statisticians play a role in the compilation of other medical data, from rates of incidence and prevalence of disease to post-surgery infection rates to how long patients have to wait for appointments at clinics to the assessment of vital statistics, which depends on birth and death rates.

Indicators. Health status indicators are used to determine the health status of a particular group or population. Indicators provide an overview of a populations health and precise statistics that are used by government, social, and health organizations to address particular areas of the populations health. Introduced by the Centers for Disease Control and Prevention in 1990, the indicators include 18 measures of health status, factors that increase the risk of disease or early death (per 100,000 population unless otherwise noted): race or ethnicity-specific infant mortality as measured by the rate (per 1,000 live births) of deaths among infants under one year old; total deaths; motor vehicle crash deaths; work-related injury deaths; suicides; homicides; lung cancer deaths; female breast cancer deaths; cardiovascular disease deaths; reported incidence of AIDS; reported incidence of measles; reported incidence of tuberculosis; reported incidence of primary and secondary syphilis; preva-

lence of low birth weight as measured by the percentage of live born infants weighing under 2,500 grams at birth; births to adolescents (ages ten to 17 years) as a percentage of total live births; prenatal care as measured by the percentage of mothers delivering live infants who did not receive care during the first trimester; childhood poverty, measured by the proportion of children under 15 living in families at or below the poverty level; proportion of persons living in counties exceeding U.S. Environmental Protectional Agency standards for air quality. *See also* PUBLIC HEALTH.

Statistics, Vital

Statistics describing incidence of birth, disease, mortality, longevity, and other quantitative indicators relating to public health.

Vital statistics are a numerical analysis of primary social events, including those relating to birth, disease, mortality, marriage and other major indicators. Social and population trends are deduced through demographic reports concerning public health. Such information is especially vital to policy-making and epidemiology. These statistics are published by the National Center for Health Statistics of the Department of Health and Human Services.

Vital statistics are organized into crude rates that pertain to the general population, and refined rates that refer only to specific segments of the population. Thus, the overall infant mortality is a crude rate, but infant mortality among African Americans, for example, is a refined rate. Such information is compiled by census gathering services worldwide and may be used to track the success of public health programs, alert governments to environmental hazards, inform doctors of the prevalence of various conditions, monitor the spread of disease, locate unhygenic conditions, track emerging threats to society, evaluate and plan for population growth, urban development and so forth. *See also* EPIDEMIC; INFANT MORTALITY; MORTALITY; *and* STATISTICS AND INDICATORS, MEDICAL.

Resources on Medical Statistics and Public Health

Basch, Paul F., *Textbook of International Health* (1999); Fletcher, Robert H., et al., *Clinical Epidemiology: The Essentials* (1996); Moeller, D.W., *Environmental Health,* revised edition (1997); National Research Council, Committee on Environmental Epidemiology, *Public Health and Hazardous Wastes* (1991); Turnock, Bernard, *Public Health: What It Is and How It Works (2000);* Mothers and Others for Pesticide Limits, Tel. (212) 727-2700, Online: www. mothers.org; U.S. Public Health Service, Tel. (202) 619-0257, Online: phs.os. dhhs.gov/phs/phs.html; www.med.cornell.edu/public.health/

Status Asthmaticus

A severe, prolonged asthma attack.

The key symptoms of status asthmaticus are extreme difficulty in breathing, a bluish tinge to the lips and face, extreme anxiety, heavy perspiration, and an abnormally rapid pulse. It is potentially life-threatening. Persons prone to status asthmaticus can use a breathing (peak flow) meter to detect changes in breathing ability. There are warning signs that accompany episodes, and these can be useful in prevention. Depending on the details of the attack, the person can be brought to the emergency room or temporarily treated on the spot if friends and associates are informed of the condition, the warning signs, and the administration of medication. Prolonged hospitalization is often necessary.

Steatorrhea

Excess fat in the feces.

Steatorrhea occurs when the intestines' ability to break down and remove dietary fat is impaired. Causes of steatorrhea include disorders such as celiac sprue and pancreatitis, although the condition can be a side effect of medications taken to lower lipid (fat) levels. The resulting symptoms include unusually odorous, bulky feces that are lighter than normal and thus more difficult to flush away. Treatment must be aimed at alleviating the underlying condition. *See also* PANCREATITIS *and* SPRUE.

Stenosis

Narrowing of a blood vessel, valve, or any other passage in the body.

Stenosis is a significant cause of many disorders of the cardiovascular system. Aortic stenosis, which affects the valve controlling blood flow from the left ventricle of the heart to the aorta, can lead to congestive heart failure. Stenosis can also affect the mitral valve, which controls flow between the left atrium and the left ventricle; the tricuspid valve, which controls flow between the right atrium and the right ventricle; the pulmonic valve, which controls blood flow from the heart to the lungs; and the carotid arteries, which supply blood to the brain.

Stereotaxic Surgery

Method of locating precise areas of the body for surgical procedures.

Stereotaxic surgery uses three-dimensional coordinates to pinpoint regions of the body for treatment. The basic coordinates x, y, and z allow positions to be exactly localized anywhere on, or in, the body. Such surgery is used to remove brain and breast tumors. Stereotaxic surgery is often used for neurosurgical procedures that require a supreme level of accuracy; for example, the placement of electrodes in the brain to lesion an exact region is guided by a doctor trained in the stereotaxic technique.

Usually the patient's head is placed in a rigid frame to prevent movement, and exact coordinates are noted prior to surgery using MRI, angiography, or CT scanning. Stereotaxic lesioning may be used to treat movement disorders, including those produced by Parkinson's disease. This is also a minimally invasive method of surgery, because tumors and areas to be lesioned can be localized with precision, and any necessary skull openings are tiny. *See also* ANGIOGRAPHY; BRAIN, DISORDERS OF; BRAIN IMAGING; BRAIN TUMOR; CAT SCANNING; PARKINSON'S DISEASE; *and* SURGERY.

Sterility

The inability to produce children.

Sterility is almost synonymous with infertility. However, infertility implies the presence of a problem that once corrected, will allow the individual to be fertile. Sterility is a permanent condition.

A sterile man is one whose semen contains no viable sperm, either because he is not capable of producing such sperm, or because something is preventing the passage of sperm into the semen. A vasectomy is a surgical procedure in which the vas deferens, the tube through with the sperm travel from the testes, is severed. This surgically imposed sterility is usually a permanent method of contraception.

A sterile female is a person who has no viable eggs. She is considered to be infertile if her fallopian tubes are blocked, thereby preventing fertilization, as she still has viable eggs and can become pregnant by other means. With donor eggs and in vitro fertilization, a sterile woman can still experience pregnancy, provided her uterus is normal. However, she will not be genetically related to her child. *See also* IN VITRO FERTILIZATION; PREGNANCY; *and* VASECTOMY.

Sterilization, Female

A permanent form of contraception.

A tubal ligation involves surgically cutting and tying off a woman's Fallopian tubes in order to prevent the sperm from having access to the egg. Its effectiveness rate is close to 100 percent. Possible side effects include scarring and an increased chance of ectopic pregnancy. Tubal ligation is rarely reversible, and then only with great difficulty.

A hysterectomy is performed for medical reasons having nothing to do with contraceptive purposes. However, a woman who undergoes this operation will no longer be able to become pregnant and give birth. *See also* CONTRACEPTION.

Sterilization, Male

A permanent form of contraception.

A vasectomy is an operation that involves severing the vas deferens, preventing sperm from being released in the semen. This operation is close to 100 percent effective. After surgery, there may be sperm present in the semen for a few weeks; during that time another method of contraception should be used. A vasectomy is rarely reversible, and then only with great difficulty.

Steroids, Anabolic

A family of synthetic substances that promote the growth of skeletal muscles and development of other male sex characteristics.

Anabolic steroids were developed to treat testosterone deficiency, which inhibits normal growth and sexual development. They were soon taken up by athletes and body builders to enhance their strength and stamina. Steroids are taken orally, by injection, or as creams rubbed into the skin.

Health consequences of steroid abuse are quite serious. Men can suffer infertility, breast development, and shrinking of the testes. Women can experience enlargement of the clitoris and growth of body hair. Both sexes may develop mood swings, male pattern baldness, acne, and cysts on the face and body. *See also* TESTOSTERONE.

Stethoscope

A Y-shaped diagnostic instrument used to listen to sounds from the body.

A stethoscope is used to monitor various sounds produced by the body, for diagnostic purposes. Sounds produced by the stomach, heart, and lungs are monitored with a stethoscope in a process known as auscultation. The stethoscope consists of a bell or receiving head, which amplifies sound and conveys it through a length of tubing, attached to two earpieces.

Using the stethoscope, with the receiving bell resting on the patient's chest, the doctor will listen for the characteristic sounds produced by the opening and closing of the heart valves, as well as the overall heart rate, timing, strength of pulse and other remarkable characteristics. A physician may detect irregularities that includes fluttering, arrhythmias, and a turbulent flow through narrowed valves, which cause specific kinds of heartbeats. Another class of sounds produced by turbulent blood flow, known as bruits, may be heard by placing the stethoscope over arteries and veins in the patient's arms or legs. *See* DIAGNOSIS.

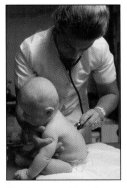

Stethoscope Examination. Above, the symbol of a physician, recognized throughout the world, is probably the stethoscope. It is the most common of the diagnostic instruments and one of the oldest. It was invented by the French Doctor R.T.H. Laënnec, in 1781.

Respiratory and pulmonary irregularities also produce diagnostic noises audible to the stethoscope. Auscultation using the stethoscope is a standard component of a general physical checkup.

> *For further information about disorders that the Stethoscope is used to diagnose see* Arrhythmia, Cardiac; Auscultation; *and* Heart, Disorders of. *For related anatomical information, see* Heart; Heart Beat; Heart Rate; Heart Sounds; Heart Valve; *and* Pulmonary Insufficiency.

Stiff Neck

Also known as torticollis and wryneck

A symptom caused by an involuntary contraction or a muscle spasm in the side or back of the neck, making it nearly impossible and quite painful to lower the chin to the chest.

Stiff neck is a common symptom that usually surfaces in the morning. It appears suddenly for no apparent reason. Closer study suggests that a stiff neck is actually the result of a minor neck impairment. A sprained ligament in the neck or a partial dislocation (subluxation) of any of the cervical neck joints irritates the cervical spinal nerves, which generates a muscle spasm. A stiff neck can also be a symptom produced by a disk prolapse, the displacement of a disk from its normal position, or by a whiplash injury, which often accompanies motor vehicle accidents.

A stiff neck can be risky if it is caused by meningitis, an infection of the brain and spinal cord. In addition to neck pain, meningitis is accompanied by fever, headache, a sore throat, and vomiting. It often follows a respiratory illness. If there is a suspicion of meningitis, immediate medical supervision is necessary. *See also* Meningitis.

Stillbirth

The death of a fetus after the 20th week of pregnancy.

The risk of stillbirth doubles for women in their late 30s and quadruples by age 45. This is possibly because older mothers have a greater incidence of preexisting condi-

tions, such as hypertension and diabetes, that can cause abnormal fetal growth and increase the chances of death just prior to birth (intrauterine death). The eggs of older women also have a greater chance of carrying chromosomal abnormalities. Prenatal diagnosis of family genetic disorders often prove helpful.

Causes. Contributing factors for intrauterine death include:

- preeclampsia;
- eclampsia;
- maternal diabetes;
- antepartum hemorrhage;
- postmaturity;
- Rh disease; and
- severe congenital abnormalities.

Treatment. Usually labor begins within two weeks of fetal death. If it does not occur on its own, it may be induced, as the mother can rarely develop blood-clotting abnormalities, which may lead to hemorrhaging. However, this condition is rare.

Many women find counseling to be valuable in dealing with the accompanying feelings of grief and loss.

> *Important background information can be found in the articles that deal with* Antepartum Hemorrhage; Diabetic Pregnancy; Eclampsia; Postmaturity; Preeclampsia; Rh incompatibility; *and* Severe Congenital Abnormalities. *Articles on* Counseling *and* Grieving *may also be helpful*.

Stimulant Drugs

Medications that create a sensation of alertness and euphoria.

Mild stimulants, such as caffeine, are commonly available, commonly used, and sometimes abused. More potent stimulants, such as dextroamphetamines and cocaine, are illegal in the U.S. Stimulants affect the brain's synapses and constrict blood vessels, producing a feeling of alertness.

Amphetamine drugs were originally developed to control narcolepsy and hyperactivity in children. However, they became popular as recreational drugs for the euphoria and "high" experienced by users. These drugs are highly addictive and put excessive demands on the heart. They produce deep mood swings and irritability. Low doses produce appetite loss, rapid breathing and heartbeat, high blood pressure, and dilated pupils. Symptoms of overdose include agitation, fever, sweating, headache, heart palpitations, and blurred vision. *See also* AMPHETAMINE DRUGS; CAFFEINE; COCAINE; *and* SUBSTANCE ABUSE.

Stimulus

Anything that excites a part of the body to a specific response.

A stimulus is something that evokes a response from the body, such as the transmission of a signal along a nerve, the moving of a muscle, or a changed state of consciousness. An illustration of a stimuli-produced response is when the sight or smell of food produces salivation. Nerve receptors are specialized to respond to particular stimuli. For example, the rods and cones of the eyes respond to changing light.

Stings

Lesions caused by stinging insects.

Stings from bees, yellow jackets, wasps, hornets, tarantulas, and fire ants may be painful; but for those who are allergic they can prove extremely dangerous. Since bees' stingers contain venom, remove them by sweeping a stiff, flat object such as a credit card against the sting; fingernails also work. If a severe reaction occurs, which may include hives, swelling of the mouth, face and hands, difficulty breathing, confusion, anxiety, nausea, vomiting, or loss of consciousness; immediately call EMS. Do so as well if the victim has been stung many times, as can occur with fire ants and bees. Monitor the victim's airway, breathing, and circulation, and give an antihistamine while waiting for medical personnel.

If stings in the mouth cause swelling and obstruct the airway, call EMS immediately, then administer artificial respiration. Also, those who know that they are allergic to

ALERT

Stings from Marine Wildlife

Insects such as bees, yellow jackets, hornets (with the most potent sting), and fire ants are not the only creatures that people are regularly stung by. Jellyfish, men-of-war, stone fish, stingrays and a number of other sorts of marine wildlife will also sting unsuspecting bathers. Stings from these animals generally have symptoms similar to those of insects; however, treatment options are more delicate: Never remove stingers from animal wildlife with your bare hands. This could be potentially harmful. Also, do not raise the stung body part; the poison should not be allowed to move throughout the body.

stings should carry around a sting kit for emergencies. These kits include epinephrine or adrenaline to inject immediately after what would otherwise be a possibly fatal sting. If there is no allergic reaction, wash the sting with soap and water, then treat with hydrocortisone cream, calamine lotion, or a paste of baking soda and water. Ice will reduce swelling.

Stings and related issues are discussed further in FIRST AID; SCORPION STINGS; *and* VENOMOUS BITES AND STINGS. *Related topics include* ALLERGY; ANAPHYLACTIC SHOCK; NONSTEROIDAL ANTI-INFLAMMATORY DRUGS; *and* SPIDER BITES.

Stitch

A sudden, brief pain in the abdomen.

Although no one knows exactly what causes stitches, they are thought to be spasms in the diaphragm muscle. They usually occur during exercise and are more common in people who are less physically fit. They may be exacerbated by a large intake of fluid just before exercise. When a stitch occurs, slow the pace of exercise or walk until the pain dissipates, and then resume normal activity. *See also* EXERCISE.

Medically, the term stitch can also refer to a knotted loop made during suturing. An open wound will need to be sutured and closed tightly with a specific sort of knot that will hold tightly. Staples, instead of stitches, are also being used in some cases when the cut is straight. *See* TRAUMA.

Stokes-Adams Syndrome

Fainting spells caused by deficient blood flow to the brain.

The blood supply to the brain can be interrupted by an arrhythmia, either an abnormally fast or slow heartbeat, or by heart block, a temporary stoppage of the heartbeat. The result is a sudden faint, with a very slow pulse and a bluish skin due to reduced blood flow. If unconsciousness lasts a long time, cardiopulmonary resuscitation should be performed to prevent brain damage. Stokes-Adams syndrome can be treated with a pacemaker. *See also* PACEMAKER.

Stomach

The body's storage tank for food where chemical break down continues.

After food passes through the esophagus, the stomach absorbs nutrients and breaks the food down into chyme, which is then digested by the small and large intestines. The stomach is about 10 inches long, but its size varies depending on the amount of food in it. Serotonin, histamine, and gastrin are just a few of the enzymes released when there is food in the stomach. These hormones aide in the digestive process.

The Stomach. The anatomy of the stomach involves the (a) adventitia; (b) esophagus; (c) body; (d) circular muscle; (e) oblique muscle; (f) greater curvature; (g) submucosa; (h) pyloric sphincter; (i) duodenum (which is both the last part of the stomach and the first part of the intestinal tract); (j) gastric rugae; and (k) longitudinal muscle. This is a highly useful organ, but it is actually quite dispensable. The digestive process could get along even without this all-but-vital organ.

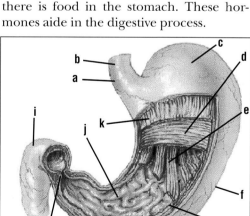

For background information see ANATOMY; BILE; BILIARY SYSTEM; *and* DIGESTIVE SYSTEM. *A minor stomach problem is detailed in* INDIGESTION *but this may be a sign of a more serious disorder such as* DUODENAL ULCER; PEPTIC ULCER; STOMACH CANCER; *and* STRESS ULCER.

Stomach Cancer

Also known as gastric cancer

A malignant tumor of the stomach; one of the most common forms of cancer.

Stomach cancers most often are adenocarcinomas, which arise in the glands that secrete digestive enzymes and natural stomach acids used in digestion. Fewer than 10 percent are lymphomas. About half of the adenocarcinomas arise in the lower part of the stomach; the prognosis is better for them than for cancers arising in the upper part of the stomach.

SYMPTOMS
The early symptoms of stomach cancer resemble those of an ulcer or other stomach disorder, and they include: discomfort, indigestion, excess belching, and a feeling of fullness after eating even a small amount of food. There may be weakness and weight loss. As the cancer advances, it can cause severe abdominal pain, bloody stools, severe weight loss, vomiting, and swelling due to an accumulation of fluid in the abdomen.

AT RISK: INCIDENCE
Stomach cancer usually occurs in the middle and later years of life; people between the ages of 50 and 70 are most at risk. The incidence is about two out of 10,000 people, and twice as high in men as in women, for unknown reasons. The risk is increased by any condition that reduces the production of stomach acids, which break down bacteria as well as food; in persons who have experienced an infection with the *Helicobacter pylori* bacteria; and in persons who have had stomach surgery. Risk factors also include a family history of gastric cancer and various gastric disorders, and having blood type A.

DIAGNOSIS
Because symptoms of early stage stomach cancer are often confused with minor stomach ailments—and thus are regularly treated as such or ignored—physicians are usually not sought out until late-stage de-

velopment. Tests for stomach cancer include x-ray scans that are specialized for the gastrointestinal system by having the patient swallow barium prior to imaging. Other diagnostic techniques consist of computerized tomography (CT) and ultrasound scans, and examination of the stomach done through a tube (endoscope) inserted into the digestive tract.

TREATMENT

Surgery is used to remove the cancer as well as either all or part of the stomach. Chemotherapy and radiation therapy, alone or in combination, may be used before or after surgery. In some cases, if the cancer is detected at an early stage, radiation therapy and chemotherapy may be done without surgery. Most often, however, the cancer is well advanced when it is diagnosed, and so the prognosis for most patients is not good. Stomach surgery usually requires a major change in eating habits, with smaller and more frequent meals to reduce the possibility of nausea, vomiting, dizziness, and sweating that can occur when the digestive capacity is reduced.

ABDOMEN; ANTICANCER DRUGS; CANCER; CANCER SCREENING; GASTROSTOMY; GASTROENTEROLOGY; MRI; SURGERY; *and* X-RAY *are all vital to the understanding of this condition.* INDIGESTION; VOMITING; *and* WEIGHT LOSS *are all symptoms.*

Stomach Ulcer

A loss of tissue in the stomach lining.

Stomach ulcers involve the loss of tissue in the stomach lining, and, contrary to popular belief, most ulcers are not associated with excessive acid levels, stress, or spicy foods. According to the Centers for Disease Control and Prevention, about 80 percent of all stomach ulcers are caused by the *Helicobacter pylori* bacterium. This bacterium weakens the protective mucous coating of the stomach so that acids can get to the sensitive lining underneath.

Symptoms. The primary symptom is a burning pain in the stomach that is most severe before meals and at bedtime. The pain diminishes after meals when food is present. Other symptoms include nausea, indigestion, fatigue, loss of appetite, vomiting, and sometimes weight loss.

Treatment. Antacids and similar medications can reduce or prevent acid production. Proton pump inhibitors may also be used, as they limit stomach acids. Antibiotics such as metronidazole, tetracycline, and amoxicillin can clear up the infection but in cases with complications, surgery may be necessary. *See also* BACTERIA.

Stomatitis

Inflammation of the mouth.

Stomatitis is the general term for any inflammation or ulceration located in the mouth. Examples include cold sores, mouth ulcers, fungal infections (candidiasis), or Vincent's disease, which is a bacterial infection of the gums. *See also* COLD SORES; CANDIDIASIS; *and* VINCENT'S DISEASE.

Strain

A tearing or overstretching of a muscle.

Although they may seem to be similar, a strain is actually quite different from a sprain. A strain occurs when a muscle has been stretched too far or torn, while a sprain is an injury to a ligament. Symptoms of a strain include pain, swelling, and sometimes bruising. The usual treatment for a strain is rest of the injured area, application of ice, and elevation of the limb to reduce swelling. Stretching exercises during healing will reduce the chance of the buildup of scar tissue. Stretching well be-

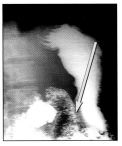

Upper GI Series. A barium mixture is used to show the passage of food or a radiopaque substance through the gastrointestinal tract in these x-rays. The stomach ulceration is present on the right side. Barium x-rays are a common diagnostic tool for such disorders.

fore exercise, in order to warm up the muscles, may help to prevent reoccurrence in the future. *See also* FIRST AID; ICE PACKS; SOFT-TISSUE INJURIES; *and* SPRAIN.

Strangulation

Twisting or compression of a tube or vessel in the body.

Strangulation disrupts the flow of blood or air, or the ability of an organ to function. Commonly, the term refers to the cessation of air flow through the windpipe by pressure on the neck. Compression of the jugular veins stops the flow of blood to and from the head, leading to a loss of consciousness, brain damage, and finally death. Medically, the term often refers to a pinched or twisted part of the intestine. Accidental strangulation is a risk especially for children. In order to prevent this, avoid toys, furniture, and clothes with dangling strings, cords, or ropes be avoided. *See also* DEATH *and* INTESTINAL STRANGULATION.

Strangury

Frequent, painful, and sparse urination.

Strangury causes an urge to urinate frequently. The process of urination is painful, and the urine passes drop by drop. It is sometimes accompanied by tenesmus, comparably frequent urges to defecate with the painful production of only small amounts of feces. Causes of strangury include inflammation of the prostate, bladder cancer, and cystitis. *See also* CYSTITIS.

Strapping

The use of adhesive tape to put pressure on a part of the body and to secure the structure in place.

Strapping is a procedure that is used to ease pain, inflammation, and bruising. Such injury can be caused by soft-tissue damage, such as sprains and tears in the muscle tendon. Thick adhesive tape is used to bind the arm or leg. This procedure

strengthens torn joints or ligaments by securing them in place, impeding further movement and a possible recurrence. *See also* JOINT; SPLINT; SPRAIN; *and* STRAIN.

Strep Throat

An infection of the throat caused by bacteria of the streptococcus family.

Like staphylococci, streptococci live on the skin and in the mouths, throats, urethras, and vaginas of most people without causing disease. These bacteria are grouped into four major types, depending on their specific characteristics and the specific diseases they produce. The most common site of streptococcal infection is in the throat. A throat infection with streptococci bacteria is known as strep throat.

Symptoms. Strep throat produces symptoms of a sore throat, a fever, a headache, nausea, vomiting, and a rapid heart rate. The tonsils will be swollen and crimson, and the lymph nodes of the neck will be enlarged and tender. The symptoms of strep throat are similar to those of many other diseases, and so the choice of which medication to use depends upon quick identification of the cause. A new in-office rapid test for strep throat takes less than 30 minutes and allows doctors to make quick and accurate diagnoses and to prescribe the correct antibiotic.

Treatment. People normally recover from strep throat in two weeks whether or not they receive antibiotics, but these medications will shorten the time of infection and prevent complications. Patients are advised to gargle with warm salt water, to drink tea with lemon and honey, to drink cool liquids, and to use acetaminophen to reduce fever and ease muscle aches. Possible complications of strep throat include scarlet fever, rheumatic fever, and glomerulonephritis, a severe kidney infection.

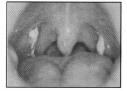

Strep Throat. As seen in the image above, strep throat causes the throat to appear bright red; the whitish material on the tonsils (exudate) can clearly be seen. Mononucleosis and streptococcal tonsillitis appear quite similar, so a throat culture will have to be taken in order to determine the exact nature of the disorder.

More information about related causes are in BACTERIA; INFECTIOUS DISEASES; PNEUMONIA; *and* SCARLET FEVER. FEVER; NAUSEA; VOMITING; *and an affected* LYMPHATIC SYSTEM *often accompany a* SORE THROAT. *See also* ANTIBIOTIC DRUGS.

Streptococcal Infections

Infections of the body caused by bacteria of the streptococcus family.

Streptococci live on the skin and in the respiratory tract, the nose, the mouth, the urethra, and the vagina. Most of the time these bacteria are harmless; however, when permitted to enter the bloodstream, such as from a cut, bruise, or contaminated needle, they can cause life-threatening disease.

Streptococci can invade almost any organ of the body to produce a number of diseases. They attack the throat, causing strep throat; the lungs, causing pneumonia; and the heart, causing endocarditis. These bacteria are responsible for rheumatic fever, scarlet fever, septic arthritis, skin infections, wound infections, kidney infections, bladder infections, and septicemia (blood poisoning).

Treatment. Antibiotics are generally prescribed to treat streptococcal infections. The course of antibiotics lasts for ten days, although the symptoms will begin to disappear in as few as 2 days. The entire course of the antibiotic should be taken to kill the bacteria completely. *See also* ANTIBIOTIC DRUGS; PNEUMONIA; *and* STREP THROAT.

Strabismus

A condition in which the eyes focus in different directions.

In strabismus, instead of tracking together and focusing on the same point, the eyes move out of alignment and send different images to the brain. Generally, one eye becomes dominant, and the brain ignores signals from the weaker, misaligned eye. Strabismus can lead to amblyopia (lazy eye), Guillain-Barré syndrome, rubella, and cerebral palsy. If untreated, this may lead to a permanent loss of vision in that eye. Treatment of strabismus may include putting a patch over the stronger eye, the use of corrective lenses, and possibly surgery on the muscles of the eye. *See also* CROSS-EYE; EYE; SIGHT, PARTIAL; *and* VISION.

Streptokinase

A drug that dissolves newly formed blood clots.

This medication is administered in emergency rooms to admitted individuals who are experiencing heart attacks. It has a short effective life and should be injected within six hours of the onset of the attack in an effort to dissolve the clot. It is not appropriate for persons whose blood has poor clotting factors or who have had recent surgery, have high blood pressure, have severe kidney or liver disease, or are over 70 years of age. *See also* BLOOD; BLOOD CLOTTING; CARDIAC AND RESPIRATORY ARREST; EMERGENCY MEDICINE; *and* LIVER.

Stress

Environmental events and internal physical and mental conditions that have the potential to disrupt a person's health or ability to function.

One of the great advances of medicine in the past century has been the recognition that stress—the pressures of life that we perceive and encounter day in and day out—can have an enormous impact on our health and long-term well-being. All living things respond to external stimuli, and all sentient animals depend on their bodily responses to perceived danger to act in a manner that allows them to survive, but humans are virtually unique in that they respond to intellectual dangers and social pressures—the possibility of a business reversal; the consequences of being late for an appointment; the centrality of family demands; or the importance of a job interview. A person sitting at a desk will typically experience the same increase in his or her heart rate and the attendant hormonal changes during an "important" business call as during a five-mile jog. From this alone, one may reasonably conclude that a life in which there are many intellectual pressures and urgencies will be subjecting the physical body to a great deal of turmoil and activity, possibly to a degree for which the body is not conditioned or prepared.

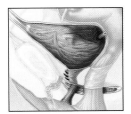

Urinary Stress Incontinence: Treatment. Above, the bladder neck is elevated by stitching it and the urethra to another pubic bone. There are multiple causes of urinary stress incontinence, but strenuous physical activity is chief among them. Pelvic-floor strengthening is a preferred treatment after the condition has been properly diagnosed.

THE BIOCHEMISTRY OF STRESS

The increase of heart rate when the body is under stress is a small part of the total picture. The body is a complex system in which nerve impulses and hormonal secretions regulate the performance of specialized cells so the body can respond to dangers, real and imagined. The sudden increase of electrical activity in millions of nerve cells throughout the body will activate systems everywhere: the skeletal muscles will tense and be poised for action; the muscles of the heart will accelerate and intensify their action, so that the heart will beat faster and provide more oxygen and nutrients to the rest of the body. Respiration will increase, so that the blood will receive more oxygen, and the blood vessels will constrict so that blood will flow faster to remote portions of the body. In addition, metabolic hormones (including cortisol and adrenaline) are released to increase mobilization of energy stores.

THE EFFECTS OF STRESS

To enhance blood supply to the muscles and brain, blood flow is directed away from the stomach and other gastrointestinal organs. This change in blood flow decreases the activity of the glands that produce mucus to protect the stomach lining from digestive acids.

As important as these changes in the body's various functions are, even more devastating is the attendant disruption of the body's balance—its homeostasis. The various systems of the body operate in harmony with one another, moving out of that balance in emergencies. Prolonged stress can disrupt that balance, and it produces a cascading effect in which the various systems of the body behave chaotically. For example, the balance between the production of insulin in the beta cells of the pancreas in response to elevated glucose levels in the blood, and the production of glycogen in the alpha cells of the same organ in response to low glucose levels, is influenced by subtle changes in the physiochemical environment. Similarly, the body maintains a constant blood temperature and a constant pH (acid-base balance), again in a way that is very sensitive to slight variations in the chemical environment. When stress-induced changes are allowed to persist, the result can be a shattering of this harmony and the body responds chaotically and often disastrously.

The undersecretion of mucus in the stomach can result in ulcers on the stomach lining. The changes in heart rate and the constriction of the blood vessels can lead to heart disease and high blood pressure. Evidence indicates that the hormonal imbalance creates abnormal tissue functioning as hormones trigger inappropriate cellular genetic expression, and this may result in a cancerous mutation of the cells. In fact, a wide variety of diseases and disorders have been attributed to stress-related fact- ors, including: heart disease; cancer; stroke; mental illness; allergies; autoimmune disease; substance abuse; asthma; diabetes—the list continues to grow.

Stress and Personality

Psychologists have determined that there are two stress-descriptive personality types, labeled Type A and Type B, that describe patterns in two lifestyles. Type A behavior is typified by time-consciousness, anxiousness, and a drive toward accomplishment and task-fulfillment. Type B behavior is more relaxed and less time-conscious. Type A behavior has been demonstrated to be more prone to the ravages of stress-related disorders. While it has become commonplace to refer to individuals as either Type A or Type B, in fact each person is a mixture of the two types of behavior. The critical factor in managing stress is to determine the contexts in which Type A behavior is most exemplified and learn to control and manage the stress that behavior engenders.

TREATMENT

The treatment of stress has taken two distinct roads: one has been to teach individuals how to relax and control their environment so that they experience minimal physiological disruption as a result of stress. Prolonged exposure to stress can lead to heart irregularities, depression, dyspepsia, and a host of mental disorders. Exposure to extreme trauma can result in post-traumatic stress disorder, a wide-ranging and varied number of symptoms that requires counseling and extended therapy. *See also* RELAXATION TECHNIQUES

The second approach to stress has been to promote the reduction of stress in society. It may not be possible (or even advisable) to eliminate stress in society at large. But it may be possible to teach people (preferably in childhood) how best to cope with stress and how to minimize its deleterious effects. To that end, programs that promote socialization (the arts, sports, and communally oriented volunteer programs), once thought of as activities that the modern competitive economy could ill afford, are now seen as vital to effective, functioning, and healthy adults. Similarly, teaching time management, strengthening family bonds, involving young people in projects that improve their self-esteem and promote peer interaction, physical exercise, and an appreciation of the value of relaxation will all result in an adult population less prone to disease, less inclined to crime and violence, more productive, happier and more content, and better able to rise to the challenge of whatever the future has in store.

> *Stress and similar topics are discussed in* ALTERNATIVE MEDICINE *categories such as* BIOFEEDBACK/BIOFEEDBACK TRAINING; CHINESE MEDICINE; HERBAL MEDICINE; *and* MASSAGE. *Also see* BLOOD PRESSURE; HEART RATE; *and* PERSONALITY.

Stress Fracture

A bone fracture caused by repeated stress at a single site.

Most fractures are caused by a sudden direct blow or extreme pressure on a bone. Stress fractures, however, happen when a bone that is subjected to repeated jarring over a period of time develops a series of minute breaks. Common areas for stress fractures include the foot, leg, and the lumbar area of the spine. Runners, gymnasts, skaters, basketball players, or any other athlete who runs and jumps frequently, especially on hard surfaces, are also likely candidates for stress fractures.

Pain, tenderness, and swelling are all symptomatic of stress fractures. Treatment usually consists of rest for about four to six weeks, and in some cases immobilization in a cast. *See also* FRACTURE; IMMOBILITY; SHIN SPLINTS; *and* SPORTS MEDICINE.

Stress Ulcer

Small bruises in the stomach lining that may bleed if left untreated.

Stress ulcers form in the lining of the stomach or duodenum following severe injury, infection, or shock. Small bruises may appear in the lining within hours of the injury and rapidly develop into ulcers. If recovery is prolonged, the ulcers may enlarge and begin to bleed. *See also* PEPTIC ULCER.

There may initially be mild discomfort in the upper abdomen. As the ulcers enlarge and begin to bleed, stools may turn tarry black. In severe cases, bleeding can be massive and cause blood pressure to drop precipitously. Complications that may affect the treatment of a stress ulcer include severe bleeding and gastrointestinal perforations. *See also* GASTRIC ULCER.

Prophylactic medications such as histamine-2 antagonists, sucralfate, or proton pump inhibitors may be administered to reduce the gravest bleeding. To prevent stress ulcers from developing after an injury, antacids and antiulcer drugs are regularly administered. With the recent widespread use of such prevention measures in critically ill patients, the incidence of stress ulcers has declined. *See also* STOMACH.

Striae

Also known as stretch marks

Skin defects that appear as bands and are associated with rapid growth or with certain conditions.

Striae, or stretch marks, are associated with rapid skin stretching. They look like parallel streaks of red, glossy skin that later become white and take on the appearance of a scar. They may be slightly depressed and have an abnormal texture. S*ee* PREGNANCY.

Resources on Stress and Stress Management

Davis, Martha, Martha Elizabeth Eshelman and Matthew McKay, *The Relaxation and Stress Reduction Workbook* (1988); Humphrey, James H., *Stress Among Older Adults: Understanding and Coping* (1992); Newton, Tim, *Managing Stress: Emotion and Power at Work* (19995); Swenson, David, Ashtanga Yoga (1999); National Center for Complementary and Alternative Medicine, Tel. (888)644-6226, Online: nccam.nih.gov; American Chiropractic Association, Tel. (703) 276-8800, Online: www.amerchiro.org; Association for Applied Psychophysiology and Biofeedback, Tel. (303) 442-8892, Online: www.aapb.org. http://www.nycornell.org/medicine/gim/index.html.

Common causes of stretch marks include pregnancy, puberty, obesity, Cushing's syndrome, overuse of topical corticosteroids, Prader-Willi syndrome, Laurance-Moon-Biedel syndrome, and Ehler-Danlos syndrome. Stria may also be associated with diabetes. *See also* PUBERTY.

There is no effective treatment for stretch marks, but they often become less noticeable when the source of the skin stretching is gone. *See also* EHLER-DANLOS SYNDROME; OBESITY; *and* SKIN.

Stridor

High-pitched breathing caused by a narrowing of the airways.

Stridor is most often heard in young children, especially those experiencing croup, the inflammation and narrowing of the airways caused by a common cold or other viral infection of the upper respiratory tract (larynx or trachea). The same kind of narrowing can be caused by epiglottiditis, a bacterial infection of the flap of cartilage at the entrance of the larynx. Infection can cause the epiglottis to block the normal passage of air. An inhaled foreign body or a tumor of the larynx can also cause stridor.

Stroke

A disruption in brain function caused by a sudden obstruction or the rupture of an artery leading to the brain.

The brain, which consists of just two percent of the body's mass, uses 25 percent of the body's oxygen supply. A brief interruption of the flow of oxygen-carrying blood to any part of the brain has an immediate effect on the functions controlled by that region; an interruption that lasts as little as four minutes can cause the death of brain cells in that region. Until recently, researchers believed that new brain cells are not produced after maturity, so the damage caused by a stroke was believed to be permanent.

That belief has been challenged by recent biomedical discoveries, but those find-ings have not yet been put to widespread medical use, and a stroke's immediate threat to life has not yet changed. If the interruption of blood flow affects a region of the brain that controls a basic function of life, death can occur in minutes. About a third of all major strokes are fatal.

Strokes are classified by the mechanism of the blood vessel blockage that causes them. There are two major categories of stroke, ischemic and hemorrhagic. A hemorrhagic stroke results from rupture of a blood vessel in or near the brain. About a quarter of all strokes are hemorrhagic. Ischemic strokes can be classified as those caused by a thrombus, a clot that has formed on the wall of a brain artery, and those caused by an embolism, a clot that has traveled to the brain from another part of the body. Cerebral thrombosis causes about half of all strokes, and cerebral embolism causes about a quarter of them.

Further divisions are possible. For example, hemorrhagic strokes can be classified as either intracerebral or subarachnoid. An intracerebral hemorrhage is the rupture of a small blood vessel within the brain. In a subarachnoid hemorrhage, the bleeding occurs in the space between the arachnoid (the middle of the three meninges that cover the brain) and the pia mater (the innermost of the meninges).

ALERT

Transient Ischemic Attack

An interruption of blood flow to the brain may be temporary, lasting a few minutes or several hours. Such a transient ischemic attack (TIA) can be caused by a clot that is carried away after blocking an artery or by atherosclerosis, the chronic narrowing of an artery. The symptoms of a TIA are the same as those of a stroke, except that they disappear after a while. While TIAs do not cause permanent damage, with full recovery after the episode, they are warning signs that should not be ignored. Anyone who suffers a TIA is at high risk for both stroke and heart attack. The symptoms of a TIA—numbness or weakness of one side of the body, temporary loss of speech, loss of coordination—are signals that medical attention should be sought and the exact cause diagnosed so appropriate masures can be taken.

Carotid Artery. Below, an image of the carotid artery. This is the main artery that supplies blood to the brain. Individuals of East Asian and Pacific Island lineage have a higher incidence of carotid artery disease. This condition, which is a major indicator for stroke, especially when it is coupled with transient ischemic attacks, has a hereditary element.

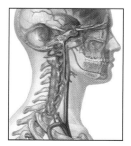

SYMPTOMS

The symptoms of a stroke depend on its cause and the part of the brain that is damaged; however, there are features common to all strokes. The major symptoms of a stroke include: a sudden feeling of weakness or numbness in the face or an arm or leg on one side of the body; a sudden loss of speech abilities, feeling, or vision in one or both eyes; fainting, near-fainting or light headedness; confusion; a severe headache; sudden loss of either short-term or long-term memory; and unexplained dizziness.

In the case of a stroke caused by cerebral thrombosis, the symptoms may occur gradually, sometimes fading and progressing over several days as blood flow through the artery decreases. The symptoms of a stroke caused by an embolism usually come on quickly, as a clot blocks the artery suddenly. A stroke caused by a subarachnoid hemorrhage usually is signaled by sudden onset of an extremely painful headache, with nausea, vomiting, and mental confusion, sometimes accompanied by seizures.

These symptoms require an immediate call for medical help, since permanent brain damage can be prevented or severely reduced if treatment begins quickly. A physician or emergency medical service should be called, or the patient should be taken to the nearest hospital emergency room as quickly as possible.

DIAGNOSIS

Diagnosis of a stroke starts with taking a medical history and doing a physical examination of the patient. The medical history can come from an individual who accompanies the patient to the hospital and who can describe risk factors such as hypertension, diabetes, smoking, and high cholesterol levels. The physical examination can identify the severity and nature of the stroke and the part of the brain that is affected. For example, weakness and numbness on the right side of the body indicates damage to the left side of the brain. The examining physician will test a number of brain functions, such as the ability to walk and exercise other motor skills; reading, speaking, and writing abilities; and memory. The physical examination can also look for evidence of hypertension, cardiovascular disease, and other associated conditions.

The tests done after this initial evaluation usually start with an electrocardiogram to record the electrical activity of the heart. Images of the brain may be obtained by a computerized tomography (CAT) scan, which uses computer analysis of x-ray pictures, or magnetic resonance imaging (MRI), in which images are produced by strong magnetic fields. Immediately, these scans can tell whether the stroke is ischemic or hemorrhagic. They usually are repeated several days later to determine the size and location of the brain region affected by the stroke.

Images of blood flow to and within the brain can be obtained by techniques such as positron emission tomography (PET), computerized tomography and single-photon-emission tomography, which will show which regions are not receiving the normal supply of blood. Ultrasound tests may also be done to measure blood flow in the carotid arteries, which run through the neck to the brain, and blood flow in the arteries within the brain.

RISK FACTORS

Most of the risk factors for stroke are the same as or similar to those for myocardial infarction, but there are some vital differences. Lifestyle factors—notably smoking but also lack of physical exercise, a diet high in fats and cholesterol, and being overweight—are all associated with increased risk. So are medical conditions such as hypertension, transient ischemic attacks, and sickle cell disease. Age is an unavoidable factor; the risk goes up as one grows older. After 55, it doubles every 10 years. Stroke risk is also be inherited; it is higher when there is a family history—although family tendencies such as overeating and underexercising can be as important as genetic factors. The weather may also play a role, since deaths from stroke are reported to be more common when it is very hot or very cold.

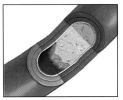

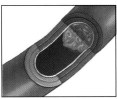

Clots. Above, top, an atherosclerotic clot is caused by an aggregation of platelets, low-density lipoprotiens (LDL—the "bad" form of cholesterol), and calcium to form a clot that can lead to a stroke. Above, bottom, a blood clot has fewer elements than an atherosclerotic clot, but leads to similar ends; a stroke-causing clot in the brain will cause the death of brain tissue due to a shortage in the blood supply.

Resources on Stroke
Frye-Pierson, Janice, and James F. Toole, *Stroke: A Guide for the Patient and Family* (1987); Hess, Lucille J., and Robert E. Bahr, *What Every Family Should Know About Strokes* (1981); Sife, Wallace, *After Stroke, Enhancing Quality of Life* (1998); Wiebers, David O., Valery L. Feigin and Robert D. Brown, *Handbook of Stroke* (1997); National Institute of Neurological Disorders and Stroke, Tel. (800) 352-9424, Online: www.ninds.nih.org/; American Board of Neurological Surgery, Tel. (713) 790-6015, Online: www.abns.org; www.nycornell.org/neuro

TREATMENT

If a stroke patient is unconscious, steps will be taken to maintain breathing, often by inserting an endotracheal tube. For an ischemic stroke, anticoagulant medications such as heparin can be given, not so much to dissolve the clot causing the stroke but to prevent the formation of new clots. The clot-dissolving medication—tissue plasmin-ogen activator (tPa)—has been shown to limit brain damage if it is infused within the first hours after a stroke occurs. The treatments aimed at ischemic stroke cannot be used for hemorrhagic strokes, since the need in those cases is to limit the amount of bleeding. Surgery may be done in some cases of hemorrhagic stroke to repair the damaged blood vessel that is causing the bleeding.

Over a longer term, treatment is aimed at physical rehabilitation and the prevention of future strokes. Rehabilitation can begin in the first few days after the stroke occurs, with physicians, nurses, and even family members moving the affected arms or legs to maintain proper blood flow, joint flexibility, and muscle tone. After the acute phase of treatment, rehabilitation can include several types of therapy, designed around individual cases, and carried out for prolonged periods of time.

The Outlook for Stroke Therapy

Laboratory studies showing that new nerve cells can grow in the adult brains of animals have changed the long-term outlook for stroke therapy. And while these findings have not yet moved into medical practice, a training technique has been reported to restore function for stroke patients.

The technique, called constraint-induced movement therapy, apparently "rewires" the brain so that nerve cells are recruited to take over the work of cells killed by the stroke. The therapy starts by immobilizing an arm that has been affected by the stroke for 90 percent of waking hours over two or three weeks. The patient then goes into training, doing simple things such as raising a glass to his or her mouth or throwing a ball, again and again for seven hours a day, five days a week. Tests have shown an expansion of the cortex, the part of the brain that controls movement, in the area damaged by the stroke. A large-scale test of the new technique is being funded by the National Institutes of Health.

Physical Therapy. Physical therapy is designed to help patients walk again if they are left partially paralyzed. It starts with a set of simple exercises to increase the function ability of the affected limbs and goes on to get patients up and about, using such aids as a cane with a four-footed base or a walker. Studies have found that more than 75 percent of stroke patients can be taught to walk by themselves.

If a stroke has caused speech difficulties, therapy will be targeted at the specific problem. Aphasia, a specific sort of difficulty with language comprehension, is caused by damage to the left side of the brain. Some patients may not be able to understand speech or writing, while others have trouble making themselves understood by others. Dysarthria is a difficulty in speaking, resulting from damage to the muscles in the face, mouth, throat, or neck.

Speech therapists have a number of techniques, all involving repetition and all applied over a long period, to help stroke patients recover the ability to understand and to communicate. The help of family members usually is an essential element in rehabilitation programs. They often are trained to help carry out physical therapy and to help recovering patients understand speech and writing and make themselves understood. These therapies are often successful in the long run.

Background information can be found in ANEURYSM; ARTERIES, DISORDERS OF; BRAIN; BRAIN HEMORRHAGE, CAROTID ARTERY; EMBOLISM; *and* INTRACEREBRAL HEMORRHAGE. *Related information is in* CHOLESTEROL; DIET AND DISEASE; *and* STRESS. *See also* PHYSICAL THERAPY *and* SURGERY.

Strongyloidiasis

Infectious disease caused by the parasitic roundworm *Strongyloides stercoralis*.

Strongyloidiasis is caused by a parasitic roundworm prevalent in warm, moist areas worldwide, including parts of North America. It is acquired through direct contact with contaminated soil and generally invades the body through bare feet. The worm responsible for the illness is barely visible to the naked eye. The worm's life cycle displays three distinct phases. In larval form, the parasite pierces the skin, after which it develops into a secondary stage and migrates through the bloodstream to the lungs. It is then coughed up in mucus and swallowed, reaching the intestine. The parasite then burrows into the intestinal wall and matures to adult form and begins producing larvae.

Larvae expelled in feces are immediately infective. They may therefore penetrate the tissue of the anus as they are expelled and reinfect the human host. Areas around the anus where reinfection occurs become reddened and irritated.

Symptoms of strongyloidiasis include vomiting, diarrhea, and abdominal pain. If left untreated, the disease causes malabsorption, weight loss, and damage to the intestinal mucosa. Antihelminthic drugs such as thiabendazole are used in treatment, which usually results in full recovery. *See also* HOOKWORM INFESTATION; MALABSORPTION; *and* WORM INFESTATION.

Strontium

A reactive, metallic chemical element whose radioactive isotope (strontium-89) is used in disease therapy.

Several radioactive isotopes of strontium exist, including strontium-90, a dangerous byproduct of nuclear fallout, with a half-life of 28 years. Strontium chloride-89 is used as a radiopharmaceutical and is effective in cancer treatment, particularly for relieving bone pain. Strontium is taken up by the bone and the natural radiation offers pain relief. The toxicity and radiation hazard of strontium-89 therapy must be carefully weighed by the physician against the benefits of treatment. Such treatment is not advised for pregnant women; and breastfeeding must be avoided, as strontium may be passed through the breast milk. Side effects of treatment include a lowered white blood cell count. *See also* BONE; CANCER; NUCLEAR MEDICINE; *and* RADIATION THERAPY.

Strychnine Poisoning

Poisoning from the toxic alkaloid strychnine.

Strychnine has been used as a rodenticide for hundreds of years. It causes violent convulsions shortly following ingestion, due to the extreme stimulation of the central nervous system, particularly the spinal cord. Death can result not from these convulsions, but from the paralysis of the brain's central respiratory center. *See also* BRAIN.

Strychnine can be fatal if ingested, inhaled, or absorbed through the skin. Exposure to lesser amounts can cause anxiety or restlessness, cramps, stiffness, or twitching. It may also cause kidney damage.

If you suspect that someone you know has been exposed to strychnine, immediately call EMS. If possible, keep her or him in a dark and quiet place until help arrives—stimuli such as loud noises, abrupt movements, and bright lights can bring on seizures. Inducing vomiting is dangerous because convulsions may cause the victim to aspirate and choke. *See also* CHOKING.

While no longer frequently used to control vermin, strychnine may still be found in quite a few households. All pesticides should be used with extreme caution, and if possible, particularly when there are children or pets in the home, use alternative methods of vermin control. *See also* POISONING; POISON; SEIZURE; *and* SPINAL CHORD.

Sturge-Weber Syndrome

A congenital disorder characterized by a birthmark on the face and neurological abnormalities.

Sturge-Weber syndrome is a congenital disorder of unknown cause. Blood vessels develop abnormally, resulting in overgrowths (angiomas) on the face and on the membranes around the brain (meninges). The angiomas on the meninges are typically located near the back of the brain and may cause seizures and mental impairment.

Symptoms. The most prominent feature of Sturge-Weber syndrome is a large birthmark (port-wine stain) that is present at birth and usually involves at least one upper eyelid and the forehead. The mark, which may vary in color from light pink to deep purple, is caused by an overabundance of capillaries beneath the surface of the skin.

Neurological symptoms include seizures, which often start before one year of age and may become more severe as the child grows older. The convulsions usually appear on the side of the body opposite the port-wine stain and vary in severity. A weakening or loss of use of the side of the body opposite the port-wine stain may also develop. Other symptoms, which vary widely among patients, include developmental delay, glaucoma, and enlargement of the coatings of the eye (buphthalmos).

Treatment. Treatment is geared toward alleviating the symptoms. Physical therapy can help with weakness, and educational intervention may be necessary for learning disabilities. Laser treatment may be used to lighten or remove port-wine stains. Medications are prescribed for seizures, and in some cases surgery may be performed to prevent them. In most cases the disorder is not severe and does not affect life expectancy.

This condition and related disorders are discussed in Birthmark; Port-Wine Stain; Learning Disabilities; Glaucoma; *and* Seizure. *Treatment options are included in the entries on* Laser Therapy; Physical Therapy; *and* Surgery. *See also* Neurocutaneous Disorders.

Stuttering

A speech disorder characterized by stammering or repetition of the same sound.

Stuttering is a speech disorder characterized by repetition of sounds and syllables, delaying, or by total verbal blocks in which no tone is produced. There is a higher incidence of stuttering among boys, sets of twins, and left-handed individuals, and it is more prevalent in Western societies than in developing countries. In 90 percent of the cases, the onset begins before the age of eight. This type of stuttering is not to be confused with the stuttering that is common in children under the age of four, which disappears with maturity.

The cause of stuttering is not known; however, the condition runs in families. Some speculate that it is the result of a minor brain injury or a psychological problem. People who stutter have difficulty vocalizing specific sounds or words. In addition, the affected person may also manifest odd movements that include tremors or tics, such as eye blinks, neck and facial contortions, or head jerks; these vary in severity. Frequently, the severity of the stutter intensifies with the level of anxiety the affected person feels. An individual may shy away from using the telephone or speaking in public. Some individuals experience the opposite, an increased incidence of stuttering when they are calm.

Speech pathologists use different methods to improve the condition of stutterers. These methods include reading aloud in a group, speaking, singing in a welcoming environment, or articulating to a pet. Therapists also employ electronic aids and headphones to teach the patient to properly enunciate each syllable. *See also* Pathology; Speech; Speech Disorders; Speech Therapy; Tics; *and* Voice, Loss of.

Stye

A bacterial infection at the root of an eyelash.

A stye usually appears as a painful, reddish bump on the lining of the eyelid and it causes increased tearing. More than one stye may appear if the infection spreads. Styes often disappear on their own but may recur. Applying warm compresses for 10 to 15 minutes every few hours may promote drainage and prevent the spread of infection, which is often caused by a bacteria from the staphylococcus family. If a stye does not go away with simple treatment, a small surgical incision may be needed to drain it. If styes recur, antibiotic cream may help prevent further outbreaks. *See also* Antibiotic Drugs; Bacteria; Dacryocystitis; Eye; Eyelid; Ice Packs; *and* Infection.

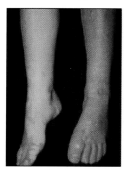

The Effects of Sturge-Weber Syndrome on the Leg. The apparent red vascular markings on the legs are port-wine stains that are regularly associated with Sturge-Weber syndrome. The case pictured below is quite unusual due to the extensive size of the marking. This can be treated with laser therapy.

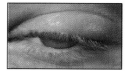

A Stye on the Eyelid. Below, the red bump on the eyelid near the lashes is a stye. Often, these are caused by staph (staphylococci) bacteria. These often cause an increased sensitivity to bright light but are easily treated.

Subarachnoid Hemorrhage

Bleeding from a ruptured blood vessel in the space between the arachnoid, the middle of the three membranes that cover the brain, and the pia mater, the innermost membrane.

Subarachnoid hemorrhage usually is caused by a burst aneurysm, a weakened place in an artery, but may also result from breakage of an angioma, a tangle of blood vessels within the brain. The result is sudden onset of an extremely painful headache, often with loss of consciousness. If the person suffering the hemorrhage does not faint, there may be nausea, vomiting, drowsiness, a stiff neck, and photophobia, a reaction to bright light. The diagnosis is based on those symptoms and confirmed by computerized tomography (CT) or magnetic resonance imaging (MRI), which can be followed by a spinal tap to detect evidence of bleeding. In some cases, surgery will be done to repair a burst aneurysm or angioma, and drugs to reduce blood pressure can be used, but generally the patient is given life support measures and is monitored carefully for signs of a second hemorrhage. Half of all patients do not survive the hemorrhage. Of those that do survive, about one in three will suffer lasting damage to physical or mental function. *See also* ANEURYSM *and* BRAIN HEMORRHAGE.

Subclavian Steal Syndrome

A number of symptoms associated with blockage or constriction of the arteries.

Subclavian steal syndrome is generally an indication of an underlying disorder of the arteries. Disorders that can lead to this syndrome include trauma, blood clots, atherosclerosis, and inborn abnormalities of the blood vessels. Symptoms include an increase or decrease in blood pressure; a reduced heart rate; and blurred vision, dizziness, or weakness. Treatment is aimed at the underlying cause. *See also* ARTERY.

Subconjunctival Hemorrhage

Bleeding of one or more capillaries in an eye, leading to a bright red patch.

Although it looks alarming, a subconjunctival hemorrhage is usually harmless. The red patch, caused by pooling of blood as in a bruise, may affect only a small area or nearly all of the white of the eye. Capillaries in the eye can be ruptured as a result of severe pressure changes, as may occur with violent sneezing or coughing, vomiting, or injury. It seems to be more common in people with diabetes or high blood pressure, but is also common in newborns, possibly because of stress during delivery.

A subconjunctival hemorrhage requires no treatment and will fade in two to three weeks, first becoming brown or green and then disappearing entirely. If a bright red patch is accompanied by pain, affects vision, or does not disappear within three weeks, consult a physician. *See also* BLEEDING; BRUISE; *and* EYE.

Subconscious

The thoughts, emotions, and ideas that one has, but of which one is temporarily unaware.

Ideas lodged in the subconscious can be brought to consciousness under the right circumstances. The existence of the subconscious is perhaps the key discovery (or principle) of psychoanalytic theory, and the one concept that Freud defended most vigorously during his career. *See also* CONSCIOUS; PSYCHOANALYSIS; *and* UNCONSCIOUS.

Subcutaneous

Beneath the skin.

"Cutaneous" means of or in the skin, and the prefix "sub-" means under. Thus anything that occurs underneath the skin is considered subcutaneous. For example, a cyst that is below the skin's surface is considered subcutaneous. *See* CYST *and* SKIN.

Subdural Hemorrhage

Bleeding under one of the tissue layers that surround the brain.

The dura is one of two tissue layers that surround the brain. Bleeding under the dura puts pressure on the brain, with extremely dangerous consequences.

A stroke occurs when a blood vessel is blocked by a clot or when there is intracranial bleeding. Because there is nowhere for the blood to flow when such bleeding occurs, it collects into clots and puts pressure on delicate brain tissues. The bleeding may occur soon after a head injury or it may be delayed and slowly accumulate into a hematoma (swelling filled with blood).

Causes. Most often intracranial bleeding is the result of a blow or other injury to the head. Less frequently there may be a deformation in the blood vessels that serve the brain or a weak spot may develop in a vessel, which may break open and release blood. This is known as an aneurysm and may be caused by high blood pressure. If the opening is small, the blood leaks out slowly; symptoms may not develop for days or even weeks. If the opening in the vessel is large and the breakage sudden, the person may collapse and even die very quickly.

A person in his or her 70s is 12 times more likely to suffer a stroke than a person in his or her late 50s. Hardening of the arteries is the most probable cause of strokes in the elderly, whether ischemic or from hemorrhage. In addition, tumors may develop in the skull and put pressure on the brain, causing many of the same symptoms as those of a stroke.

Symptoms. Headaches, partial paralysis, slurred speech, mental confusion, vision problems, numbness, and coma are all possible. Since these symptoms may have a number of different causes, the physician will require an MRI (magnetic resonance imaging) scan, which will distinguish between ischemia—a blockage in the blood vessel—or a hemorrhage. This MRI scan will indicate where in the brain the damage is and how extensive it is.

Treatment. Blood thinners are avoided when the cause of bleeding is subdural hemorrhage. If the location of the break is accessible, the surgeon will drill a hole in the skull to drain the accumulated blood and to relieve the pressure. However, permanent brain damage is likely, with some neurological symptoms almost inevitable. If the person has high blood pressure, the dangers are multiplied and if the loss of blood is substantial, death is likely. *See also* ANEURYSM; HEMORRHAGE; *and* STROKE.

Subluxation

Partial dislocation of a joint.

A complete dislocation of joint means that the bones are not in contact at all. An incomplete dislocation of a joint, or subluxation, refers to bones that are turned away from each other, but still have some level of contact. A subluxation is less severe than a dislocation, but the symptoms are often the same—pain, bruising, and loss of mobility. Treatment is not usually required, as the bones will often move back into place on their own. *See also* DISLOCATION *and* JOINT.

Submucous Resection

Surgical removal of tissue underneath the mucous membranes.

Submucous resection is used in a number of procedures, including correction of a deviated nasal septum (the cartilage and bone that divide the nostrils). Once the deformed cartilage and bone have been repaired, this procedure is designed to allow the two layers of mucous membrane dividing the nose to align themselves vertically along the horizontal center.

Hysteroscopic submucous resection is carried out on the interior of the uterine wall and is used to treat submucous fibroids, noncancerous growths composed of smooth muscle and connective tissue. Using a special viewing instrument, the surgeon looks inside the uterus and shaves off protruding fibroids. *See also* FIBROID.

Subphrenic Abscess

An abscess under the diaphragm.

The diaphragm is the muscular structure below the lungs that aids in the breathing process. The subphrenic space lies under the diaphragm (below the ribcage) and above the colon. A collection of pus (an abscess) in this region can be caused by bacterial infection due to disease or injury, but most often is a complication of surgery on the duodenum, stomach, or biliary tract.

Symptoms, which may not appear for months, include fever, pain, loss of appetite, and weight loss. Patients often have chest pain, shoulder pain, and difficulty breathing, because the abscess affects the diaphragm. Untreated, a subphrenic abscess can be life-threatening. Treatment involves undergoing surgery to remove the abscess, accompanied by antibiotic therapy. *See also* ABSCESS *and* DIAPHRAGM.

Substance Abuse

A general term for excessive consumption of a substance, endangering a person's health.

Substance abuse is a broad term used in reference to a number of different types of behavior. Any person who consumes a substance in excess or beyond the prescribed amount, may be said to have a substance abuse problem. Substance abuse includes, but is not limited to, alcohol, food, recreational drugs, hard drugs, prescription medications, and diet medications. Dependence on any one of these substances over time may occur as the result of genetic predisposition, peer influence, or a social or psychological disorder.

Alcohol Abuse. For more information regarding alcohol abuse and dependence, *see also* ALCOHOL DEPENDENCE; ALCOHOLICS ANONYMOUS; ALCOHOL INTOXICATION; *and* ALCOHOL-RELATED DISORDERS.

Drug Abuse. For more information concerning drug abuse and dependence, *see* DRUG; DRUG DEPENDENCE; DRUG OVERDOSE; *and* DRUG POISONING.

Eating Disorders. For more information on food-related abuse, *see* DIET AND DISEASE; DIURETICS; EATING DISORDER; *and* LAXATIVE DRUGS.

Addictive Substances. For additional information on addictive substances, *see* CAFFEINE *and* NICOTINE.

Substrate

The molecule with which an enzyme interacts.

A substrate is a molecule that is changed by an enzyme. An enzyme is a protein that acts within the body to carry out one of the many chemical reactions of life. For example, the enzyme amylase operates within the digestive system. Its substrate is starch, a molecule made up of many sugar, or saccharide, units. Amylase acts to break a starch molecule down into saccharides.

Substrates have highly specific structures that allow enzymes to dock with them and carry out the necessary chemical reaction. The substrate emerges from the reaction changed in some way, but the enzyme retains its original form and function so that it can operate on other substrate molecules. *See also* ENZYME *and* PROTEIN.

Subunit Vaccine

A vaccine containing only part of an antigen (a foreign protein), or a sequence from the viral coat, instead of the whole microorganism.

A vaccine can be created from a part (subunit) of an organism by means of genetic engineering. Subunit vaccines result in the formation of antibodies that are specific to the organisms that the vaccines work against. They may also reduce the number of adverse effects caused by vaccines. Another advantage of subunit vacci-nes is seen in the case of a rapidly mutating pathogen (disease-causing organism), such as the HIV virus. In these circumstances, the subunit vaccine can be made to target an unchanging portion of the pathogen, and thus may be very effective. *See also* ANTIGEN *and* PATHOGEN.

Resources on Substance Abuse

Barchas, Jack D., *Biological Basis for Substance Abuse* (1993); Dupont, Robert L., *The Selfish Brain: Learning from Addiction* (1997); Ketcham, Katherine, *Be-yond the Influence: Understanding and Defeating Alcoholism* (2000); Alcoholics Anonymous (local chapters in the phone book); Al-Anon: (800) 356-9996, On-line: www.alanon.alateen.org; Mothers Against Drunk Driving: (800) 438-MADD, National Council on Alcoholism and Drug Dependence, (800) 622-2255, www.-ncadd. org/-problems.html National Mental Health Association, Tel. (800) 969-NMHA, Online: www.nmha.org; www.ny-cornell.org/psychiatry/.

Sucking Wound

Wound that penetrates the lung, causing breathlessness and partial collapse of the organ.

A sucking wound leads to the collapse of a lung on the injured side. Occasionally, the injury will cause the lung contents to shift, leading to a partial collapse of the other lung as well. Respiration is not possible if the lung has collapsed and blood cannot be oxygenated. For emergency first aid, a sealing bandage made of any air-proof material (preferably plastic) should be applied to the wound so that air does not enter during the victim's respiration. The dressing is tightly sealed until professional help arrives. *See also* LUNG *and* SHOCK.

Sucralfate

A drug containing a sucrose-aluminum complex that is used to treat peptic ulcer.

The drug sucralfate works locally, rather than systemically, to form a barrier over the ulcer base to protect it from the effects of acid, pepsin, and bile salts of the stomach and intestine. Sucralfate has also been used to treat gastroesophageal reflux disease (GERD), in which liquids and food in the stomach back up into the throat.

Constipation is a side effect that occurs in three to five percent of patients. Other side effects can be, to a lesser degree, diarrhea, nausea, vomiting, gastric discomfort, indigestion, flatulence, dry mouth, dizziness, insomnia, sleepiness, vertigo, back pain, and headache. *See also* ACID REFLUX *and* GASTROESOPHAGEAL REFLUX.

Suction

Technique for removing fluid, tissue, or other matter by reduction of air pressure.

Suction is used in a variety of medical procedures. During surgery, blood or other body fluid, as well as loose tissue, may be suctioned to clear the way for instruments and provide a clear view to the surgeon.

The technique is used during surgery within the body cavity as well as during oral surgery. Suction is applied to remove the fetus from the vaginal opening during abortion procedures. Cosmetic surgeons make use of suction for a variety of operations, including liposuction to remove excess body fat, and surgical breast reduction. *See also* ABORTION, ELECTIVE; BREAST SURGERY; *and* COSMETIC SURGERY.

Sudden Death

Sudden and unexpected death, following minutes or hours, from a nonviolent cause.

Sudden death results from a variety of causes. Most commonly, it may occur when the pumping of the heart abruptly stops and respiration ceases (cardiac arrest). The most common cause for this condition is a heart attack, or myocardial infarction, in which a portion of heart tissue dies.

Other causes of cardiac arrest include excessive blood loss (hemorrhage), cessation of breathing, dislodged blood clot (embolus), severe electrical injury, drug overdose, or profound allergic reaction (anaphylactic shock).

Some cases of sudden death remain speculative; for example, SIDS (sudden infant death syndrome) occurs during sleep in infants under one year. *See also* SIDS.

Sudden Infant Death Syndrome

Also known as crib death or SIDS

The sudden, unexpected death of an infant, usually under one year old, in which an autopsy does not reveal any explainable cause of death.

Nearly all SIDS deaths occur when the infant is sleeping, without any warning signs or symptoms. Babies who die of SIDS do not seem to have struggled or suffered.

The cause of SIDS is unknown; however, there are many theories as to why it occurs. It is commonly believed among researchers that babies who die of SIDS are born with any number of conditions that make them particularly susceptible to the stresses occurring in the life of an infant. In fact, most researchers believe that SIDS does not have one cause, but several. These may include problems with sleep arousal and an inability to sense the build-up of carbon dioxide in the blood.

Incidences of SIDS have decreased over 40 percent since 1992, when parents were first cautioned to place babies on their backs or sides to sleep, instead of on their stomachs. The National Center for Health Statistics reported a rate of 69 SIDS deaths per 1,000 infants in 1997. Still SIDS is the most common cause of death in infants from one month to one year of age. Ninety percent of deaths occur by six months of age. Native Americans and African Americans have a higher incidence.

National Foundation for Sudden Infant Death Syndrome

Parents who have lost a child because of SIDS are encouraged to join a SIDS support group. Since there is no logical cause of death, many parents suffer feelings of guilt. These feelings are made worse by police investigations regarding cause of death. The National Foundation for Sudden Infant Death Syndrome can suggest counseling and give reassurance to parents affected by the syndrome.

There are no symptoms of SIDS. The single most important way to prevent SIDS is to place a child on its back when sleeping. Also, babies should sleep on firm mattresses, and all soft bedding, plush toys and comforters should be removed. The use of home ap-nea monitors has not lessened the incidence of SIDS. Other recommendations include: ensure good prenatal care, if possible breast-feed the baby, do not let the baby become too warm especially if a cold or infection is suspected (i.e., avoid too much clothing, heavy bedding, or a warm room), and always keep the baby in a smoke-free environment.

Background material on SIDS may be found in POSTNATAL CARE. *For additional information see* BREATHING; CARBON DIOXIDE; *and* SLEEP. *Related information contained in* INFANT MORTALITY *and* PUBLIC HEALTH.

Sudeck's Atrophy

Swelling and inability to use a hand or foot normally following an injury.

After a cast has been removed from an injured area, such as a fracture, swelling, stiffness and pain may develop. At this point, despite attempts to return to normal use, the symptoms may still persist. The nails may stop growing, and there may be a loss of body hair in the area.

Treatment will include elevation of the injured area in order to reduce swelling, and exercise and heat treatment. Full recovery can be expected in about four months; if there is no improvement at that point, a nerve block, or sympathectomy, may be performed to improve the blood supply. *See also* FRACTURE; NERVE BLOCK; *and* SYMPATHECTOMY.

Suffocation

Obstruction of the flow of air into the lungs.

Suffocation can be caused by an obstruction anywhere in the major airways leading to the lungs—the nose and mouth, the pharynx or larynx, or the main airway (trachea) to the lungs; or by noxious gases, such as carbon monoxide, that inhibit the function of the lungs. Unattended to, suffocation can be fatal within minutes. Treatment starts with removal of whatever is blocking respiration—taking a foreign object out of the body or moving the person into open air. Artificial respiration may be necessary to restore normal breathing. Infants are especially at risk of suffocation during sleeping as the result of bedding, pillows, or bed-sharing with parents. Children are at possible risk of strangulation from clothing, scarves, and mittens. Parents should inspect all beds, clothing, and toys to ensure against such accidents.

See AIRWAY OBSTRUCTION *and* BREATHING *for a discussion of the foundations of suffocation. For further information, see* CARBON MONOXIDE; LARYNX; *and* POISONING. *Related information is contained in* ARTIFICIAL RESPIRATION.

Resources on SIDS
Berger, Edward C., *SIDS and Sleep Disorders* (1996); Apgar, Virginia and Joan Beck, *Is My Baby All Right?* (1972); Behrman, Richard E., *Nelson Textbook of Pediatrics* (1996); Taubman, Bruce, *Your Child's Symptoms* (1992); American Academy of Pediatrics, Tel. (847) 228-5005, Online: www. aap.org; www.nycornell. org/pediatrics/index.html.

Suicide

Act of intentionally taking one's own life.

Suicide is the eighth leading cause of death in the United States, resulting in over 30,500 fatalities a year. More Americans have died over the last five years as a result of suicide than from AIDS, and over five million Americans have attempted to kill themselves at least once. Notably, suicide is the third leading cause of death among adolescents and young adults, and the elderly have the highest suicide rates. Suicide can be prevented, if warning signs are identified and treated.

Many people experience periods when life's problems seem overwhelming. During those phases, a person might feel depressed, use drugs or alcohol, and have fleeting thoughts of taking his or her own life. People are at a higher risk of suicide throughout periods of significant change, adolescence, after a break-up, when failing to achieve a cherished goal, or when seriously ill. Those suffering from depression or psychosis are at the highest risk. Although suicide can be based on a sudden impulse, it usually involves energy and planning. As a result, ironically, the riskiest time for a potential suicide is when depression is beginning to subside.

How to Help. Threats of suicide and warning signs should be taken seriously. Whether or not a person is at a high risk for suicide at the time he or she exhibits the warning signs or not, the risk can easily increase if there is no treatment. Do not be afraid to address the issue directly by asking, "Are you feeling so badly that you are thinking of suicide?" Contrary to popular belief, mentioning suicide does not give a person the idea to do it; it helps to get the issue out in the open and allows it to be dealt with. The risk for suicide is increased if the person has thought about how he or she would carry out the plan and if a time has been set to commit suicide. People who exhibit this type of planning should be taken for mental health assessment by a mental health care provider.

Depression can be treated and the risk for suicide reduced. A friend or family member can be helpful to someone suffering from depression simply by listening attentively and openly to that person. When someone you care about is depressed, the natural inclination may be to cheer the person up, to deny that the situation is really so bad, or to give advice. In all of these cases, what the sufferer will hear is a negation of feelings and a lack of faith in the individual's ability to make a decision. Allowing the person to express the feelings associated with depression is important and does not mean that you will encourage harm or that you agree with the individual; rather it allows the sufferer to feel soothed and understood.

Professional Care. Anyone exhibiting the warning signs below should be seen by a physician, who will most likely offer a referral for treatment by a psychiatrist. Such a person should have treatment which may include therapy and medication.

ALERT
Warning Signs

The following are a list of warning signs a person may exhibit if he or she is contemplating suicide:

- Behavior that is sad, withdrawn, anxious, exhausted, apathetic, and indecisive;
- Difficulty concentrating on school or work;
- Changes in sleep patterns, sleeping excessively or suffering from insomnia or nightmares;
- Changes in eating habits;
- Loss of interest in friends, sex or any activity that was previously enjoyed;
- Feeling out of control, like one is "going crazy";
- Statements of helplessness, hopelessness or worthlessness;
- Substance abuse problems;
- Recent losses including death, divorce, broken relationships, etc.;
- Giving away important possessions;
- Expression of a wish for it to be "all over" or verbally expressing a desire for death.

Background material on suicide may be found in ACCIDENTS. *For additional information see* ANXIETY; BIPOLAR DISORDER; DEPRESSION; DRUGS; MENTAL ILLNESS; *and* PSYCHIATRY. *Related information is contained in* EMERGENCY, FIRST STEPS; GROUP THERAPY; *and* PSYCHOTHERAPY.

Resources on Suicide

Greist, John H. and James W. Jefferson, *Depression and Its Treatment* (1992); Hafen, Brent Q., and Kathryn J. Frandsen, *Youth Suicide: Depression and Loneliness* (1986); Lester, David, *Making Sense of Suicide: An In-Depth Look at Why People Kill Themselves* (1997); Wender, P.H., and D.F. Klein, *Mind, Mood, and Medicine: A Guide to the New Biopsychiatry* (1981); American Foundation for Suicide Prevention, Tel. (888) 333-AFSP, Online: www.afsp. org [Suicide Hotlines operate in most major cities: see local telephone listings.]; National Alliance for the Mentally Ill, Tel. (800) 950-6264, Online: www. nami.org; Nat. Depressive & Manic-Depressive Association, Tel. (800) 82-NDMDA, Online: www. ndmda.org; National Mental Health Association, Tel. (800) 969-NMHA, Online: www.nmha.org; www.ny-cornell.org/psychiatryin-dex.html.

Sulfinpyrazone

A drug used for the treatment of gout.

Gout is a painful disease of the joints caused by high levels of uric acid in the blood. Sulfinpyrazone helps the body secrete uric acid. It is used as a long-term preventive measure rather than to treat acute attacks; it may take months of dosage before the results are noticed. Side effects are rare, but may include nausea, vomiting, abdominal pain, lower back pain, and painful or difficult urination. *See also* GOUT.

Sulfamethoxazole

An antibiotic, one of a number of drugs given to people with HIV.

Sulfamethoxazole was originally used to treat urinary tract infections, but today it is one of the cocktail of drugs given to people with HIV. Pneumocystis pneumonia (PCP) was a rare disease before the advent of AIDS, but today it is the leading cause of death resulting from HIV infection. Sulfamethoxazole is used as a preventive measure to control PCP.

Side effects include skin rashes, hives, itching, localized swelling, reddened eyes, headache, nausea, ringing in the ears, and loss of appetite. To counteract these side effects, it is recommended that the drug be taken with high caloric fluids in sufficient quantity to avoid dehydration. *See also* AIDS *and* PNEUMOCYSTIS PNEUMONIA.

Sulfisoxazole

A sulfa antibiotic used to treat severe and long-lasting urinary tract and kidney infections.

Sulfisoxazole is also used to treat bacterial meningitis and as a preventive measure for those who have been exposed to the disease. It is used to treat middle-ear infections in combination with penicillin, and malaria when chloroquine is not effective. Sulfisoxazole and trimethoprin are used together in Bactrin, used for ear and other infections. The most serious side effects are skin rash, sore throat, fever, joint pain, shortness of breath, and cough. Like other sulfa drugs, sulfisoxazole may induce severe and even fatal allergic reactions. Pregnant and breastfeeding women should not take it. *See also* SULFONAMIDE DRUGS.

Sulfonamide Drugs

Also called sulfa drugs, synthetic antibiotics were developed in the early 1930s and first used to treat humans in 1935.

Today sulfa drugs are mostly used in combination with trimethoprim, making a very effective antibiotic against pneumonia, meningitis, and urinary infections. They are used in HIV patients to treat pneumocystis pneumonia. Sulfadoxine and pyrimethamine are used to treat cases of malaria that are resistant to chloroquine.

Sulfa drugs may induce allergic reactions. Side effects include nausea, vomiting, diarrhea, rashes, and headache. Pregnant or nursing mothers should not take any sulfa drugs. *See* AIDS; ALLERGY; ANTIBIOTIC DRUGS; *and* ANTIBIOTIC RESISTANCE.

Sulfur

A chemical element which is an essential component of proteins.

Foods rich in protein, such as meats, fish, peas, and beans, contain sulfur. Therefore, any diet that contains high quality protein should contain adequate amounts of sulfur. However, certain sulfur compounds may pose problems. These include the sulfites added to some foods and wines, which can cause asthma attacks in those with sulfite-sensitive asthma. Sulfur dioxide is an air pollutant produced by paper nabufacture; it is an irritant that affects the eyes, bronchial tubes, and mucous membranes of the nose and throat; exposure can aggravate existing pulmonary conditions. *See also* AMINO ACID; ASTHMA; FOOD ADDITIVES; PROTEIN; *and* PROTEIN SYNTHESIS.

Sunburn

Skin burned by overexposure to the sun or another source of ultraviolet light.

Sunburn develops when the amount of sun exposure or exposure to another ultraviolet light source exceeds the ability of melanin, the body's protective pigment, to protect the skin. A light-skinned person may become sunburned after as little as 15 minutes of midday sun exposure, while a dark-skinned person may not burn nearly as quickly.

Symptoms. Sunburn pain tends to be worst between six and 48 hours after excessive sun exposure. Severe sunburn may cause painful skin blistering. Because inflammatory substances are released with sunburn, fever can accompany the pain of severe sunburn. The skin will usually start to peel and flake sometime between three and eight days after exposure.

Long-term effects of sunburn are serious. Statistically, a history of blistering sunburn significantly increases the chances of developing malignant melanoma, the most serious form of skin cancer. Basal cell and squamous cell cancers, two other common forms of skin cancer, are directly related to the amount of sun exposure and individual skin pigmentation. Prolonged exposure to sunlight in childhood is especially associated with an increased risk of developing skin cancer later in life. Sun exposure and ultraviolet light have also been implicated in the development of cataracts.

Prevention of sunburn is important in order to avoid its painful symptoms and the resultant damage to the skin. To prevent sunburn, a sunscreen with an SPF of 15 or above should be used. Wearing protective clothing and UV-protected sunglasses are also recommended to prevent excessive exposure to the sun.

Background material on burns may be found in SUNLIGHT, ADVERSE EFFECTS OF. *For additional information see* BASAL CELL CARCINOMA; BURNS; MELANOMA; SKIN CANCER; *and* SQUAMOUS CELL CARCINOMA. *Related information contained in* SUNTAN *and* ULTRAVIOLET LIGHT.

Resources on Harmful Effects of Sunlight
Walker, Mary-Ellen, Safe in the Sun (1990); Jacknin, Jeanette, *Smart Medicine for Your Skin: A Comprehensive Guide to Understanding Conventional and Alternative Therapies to Heal Common Skin Problems* (2001); Kenet, Barney J., *Saving Your Skin: Prevention, Early Detection, and Treatment of Melanoma and Other Skin Cancers* (1998); American Academy of Dermatology, Tel. (888) 462-DERM, Online: www.aad.org; American Board of Dermatology, Tel. (313) 874-1088, Online: www.abderm.org; Nat. Psoriasis Foundation, Tel. (800) 723-9166, Online: www.nycornell.org/dermatology/index.html.

Sunlight, Adverse Effects of

Major health problems that are linked to overexposure to sunlight. They may include skin cancer (melanoma and nonmelanoma), premature aging of the skin and other skin problems, cataracts, and immune system suppression.

Skin Cancer. One in five Americans will develop skin cancer in his or her lifetime. Melanoma, the most serious form of skin cancer, is also one of the fastest spreading types of cancer. Cases of melanoma have more than doubled between 1980 and 2000. There may be a link between childhood sunburn and melanoma later in life. Nonmelanoma skin cancers include basal cell carcinoma and squamous cell carcinoma. About 95 percent of nonmelanoma skin cancers can be cured if detected early. Basal cell carcinoma is the most common type of skin cancer. It appears as small, fleshy bumps or nodules, and can occur anywhere on the body. This type of cancer grows slowly, but can penetrate to the bone and cause severe damage. Squamous cell carcinoma appears as nodules or as red, scaly, or rough patches, and can spread to other body areas. *See also* SKIN CANCER.

Premature Skin Aging. Sunlight also causes actinic keratoses and premature skin aging. Actinic keratoses are raised, reddish skin growths that are considered precancerous. Excessive exposure to the sun causes the skin to become thick, wrinkled, and leathery. *See also* KERATOSIS.

Cataracts. Overexposure to sunlight can cause cataracts. Cataracts develop when a loss of transparency in the lens of the eye clouds vision. If untreated, cataracts can lead to blindness. *See also* EYE, DISORDERS OF.

Immune System Suppression. Overexposure to ultraviolet (UV) light may cause suppression of the body's immune system. Effects of this suppression play a role in susceptibility to skin cancer. Some scientists believe that UV light-induced immunosuppression impairs the body's response to immunizations and increases its vulnerability to infectious disease. *See* IMMUNE SYSTEM.

Suntan

Darkening of the skin color caused by exposure to the sun, tanning beds, and sun lamps.

With exposure to sunlight, the skin of most people darkens though increased production of melanin in the skin. Although the sun provides the body with a small amount of vitamin D, its effects on the skin can be extremely damaging. The sun can cause pro-blems ranging from premature skin aging to potentially deadly skin cancer.

In response to the harmful rays of the sun, especially ultraviolet rays, the outer layer of skin produces more protective skin coloration (melanin pigment). Melanin absorbs the ultraviolet light as a means of protecting important structures and molecules in the skin. People who spend significant time in the sun become temporarily darker-skinned as a result of the increased production of the melanin pigment.

The skin's sensitivity to sunlight is described by six skin types. The lightest skin, type I or Celtic-like skin, always burns and never tans. Type II burns very easily and tans minimally. The average Caucasian burns moderately and tans to light brown; this is type III. Type IV is described as olive skin, and burns minimally and tans well. Skin that rarely ever burns and tans profusely is type V, and appears brown. Type VI, which appears black, never burns and is extremely pigmented.

Regular and long periods of time in the sun cause premature aging and wrinkling of the skin. Sunburns, in addition to suntans, increase the risk of skin cancer. The Food and Drug Administration (FDA) and Centers for Disease Control and Prevention (CDC) recommend avoiding the use of tanning beds and sun lamps. Malignant melanoma, a severe type of skin cancer, has been linked to sun exposure. It is often fatal, and the number of cases is increasing. About one million cases of malignat melanoma are diagnosed each year in the United States. *See also* MELANIN; MELANOMA; SKIN CANCER; SUNBURN: SUNLIGHT, ADVERSE EFFECTS OF; *and* VITAMIN D.

Superfecundation

The fertilization, through separate acts of intercourse, of two or more ova.

Generally when a woman ovulates, only one ovum is released. At times, however, two or more ova may be released at once, which can, in rare instances, result in multiple births. In superfecundation, multiple ova are fertilized at slightly different times. If the different acts of intercourse are with different men, this can result in the development of twins who have different fathers. *See also* CONCEPTION; FERTILIZATION; MULTIPLE BIRTHS; OVUM; PREGNANCY; *and* SUPERFETATION.

Superfetation

Fertilization and implantation of an ovum when another fetus is already present in the uterus.

In superfetation, a woman who is already pregnant ovulates and successfully conceives. This can result in the birth of twins whose ages differ slightly. This phenomenon is very rare. *See also* CONCEPTION; FERTILIZATION; MULTIPLE BIRTHS; OVUM; PREGNANCY; *and* SUPERFECUNDATION.

Superficial

On or near the surface.

Superficial is often used as an adjective, identifying structures, traits, or processes lying on or near the surface. Superficial blood vessels are those near the skin surface while the superficial fascia are a thin layer of loose connective tissue just below the skin, attaching to the so-called deep fascia beneath. The term may also be used to describe a mild injury. A superficial wound is distinct from one that has penetrated deeply into the tissue, and is generally non-threatening, for example, a superficial cut or abrasion. Superficial wounds do not usually constitute an emergency situation. *See also* BLOOD VESSELS; FASCIA; FIRST AID; *and* WOUND.

Superinfection

An infection that occurs during the course of an already existing infection.

Superinfections can be resistant strains of a prior infection, or they can be invasions by a new pathogenic (disease-causing) organism. When antibiotics are used to control an infection, they also kill a number of other bacteria that are helpful to the body. When these helpful bacteria are destroyed, fungi and other resistant bacteria are then free to multiply and cause secondary infections. These infections are called opportunistic because they would not be allowed to thrive in the body normally. *See also* ANTIBIOTIC DRUGS *and* INFECTION.

Superiority Complex

An exaggerated sense of one's worth and the feeling that one is superior to other people.

Superiority complexes result from feelings of inferiority and inadequacy. Both the superiority and the inferiority complexes are, in modern psychoanalytic theory, two sides of the same coin. When feelings of low self-esteem result in a sense of self-loathing and an unwillingness to overcome obstacles, the person may be said to be suffering from an inferiority complex. When the same feelings lead a person to have an unrealistic estimation of his or her worth and abilities, the person is said to be suffering from a superiority complex. In both cases, the source of the complex is the person's own feelings of inadequacy and unworthiness. *See also* INFERIORITY COMPLEX.

Supernumerary

Greater than the normal number, as of teeth, fingers, etc.

Many human mutations can produce extra anatomical features. Such additional structures or components are called supernumerary, though specific conditions may bear distinct medical names. Polymastia, for example, is a term for the presence of nipples, including areolas, or breast tissue beyond the usual number of two. The condition is fairly common, with the supernumerary nipples generally smaller and less distinct. Supernumerary digits are any beyond the normal ten fingers and ten toes. The condition is known as polydactyly, and may be the result of genetic disease or abnormality. The size and morphology of supernumerary digits varies. They are often surgically removed without future complication. Other supernumerary features include teeth and ribs. *See also* POLYDACTYL.

Support Group

Organization of people with a common health, personal, or social concern who share experiences and offer advice with the goal of aiding in treatment and in helping each other cope with their difficulties.

Support groups exist for countless issues, ranging from diseases such as cancer or muscular dystrophy; to psychological issues, such as addiction or coping with abuse; to social concerns, such as living as a member of a sexual minority or advancing in a particular career field. They may be based out of a professional organization or may be run on a grass-roots level by people who share a relevant concern.

Support groups give people a chance to learn from each other's experiences, offer encouragement and support in times of difficulty, and connect members to potentially helpful resources. Groups may also participate in public education, provide material aid to members, and engage in social advocacy.

With the flourishing of the Internet, the number and accessibility of support groups has greatly increased. People with rare concerns can now often find others around the world who share similar experiences.

See PSYCHIATRY *for background material on support group. For additional information see* GROUP THERAPY; *and* PSYCHOTHERAPY. *Related information contained in* ALCOHOL DEPENDENCE; DRUG DEPENDENCE; PSYCHOANALYSIS; *and* PUBLIC HEALTH.

Suppository

A small, solid object that carries medication into an opening of the body.

Suppositories carry not only medication but also ingredients to promote the absorption of the medication by the body. These cone-shaped objects are usually inserted into the anal or vaginal canal where the temperature of the body causes the suppository to melt and release the medicinal substance.

Vaginal suppositories are used to treat disorders, such as candidiasis (fungal infection), and they can also be used as contraceptives that contain spermicides. Rectal suppositories may be used to soften feces and aid in bowel movements, in addition to treating hemorrhoids and other intestinal disorders. Suppositories that carry corticosteroids, antifungal drugs, antibiotics and other medications are used against a large variety of disorders. *See also* ANTIBIOTIC DRUGS; ANTIFUNGAL DRUGS; CANDIDIASIS; CONTRACEPTION; CORTICOSTEROID DRUGS; *and* HEMORRHOIDS.

Suppuration

The formation and discharge of pus.

Pus is a yellowish-white fluid, consisting of white blood cells, dead tissue, and bacteria. Suppuration is the process by which pus is formed and discharged. The fluid is produced by the body in response to infection. Pus usually collects at the site of an inflammation and may collect in a pocket called an abscess in body tissue and a boil or a pustule on the skin. Abscesses may appear anywhere in the body, such as in the lungs or attached to infected organs or bones. Often, the body is capable of reabsorbing the pus and excreting it in the feces or urine. Sometimes the pus must be drained surgically or removed by other means, such as drains placed under radiologic guidance. *See also* ABSCESS; BACTERIA; BLOOD CELLS; INFECTIOUS DISEASES; PUS; URINE; *and* WHITE BLOOD CELLS.

Supraventricular Tachycardia

An abnormally fast heart rate that originates in the electrical pathway of the heart, specifically above the ventricles.

Supraventricular tachycardia can cause the heart to beat 140 to 240 times a minute—in some cases, even faster—for hours or days. It results from electrical impulses that originate in the atria, the chambers of the heart above the ventricles, and that override the normal signals that control the heartbeat. Symptoms include lightheadedness, breathlessness, palpitations, chest pain, shortness of breath, and fainting spells. The condition is diagnosed by an electrocardiogram taken while symptoms are occurring. This tachycardia usually is not life-threatening, and treatment is aimed at controlling the symptoms. Something as simple as drinking a glass of cold water can terminate an attack. Patients may also be told to breathe out forcefully while pinching the nose and holding the mouth shut, a tactic called the Valsalvaí maneuver. If these actions are not effective, recurrent attacks can be treated by antiarrythmic medications. Sometimes the condition requires an electric shock to the heart to restore normal heart rhythm, or radiofrequency ablation, in which the abnormal electric pathways in the heart are located and destroyed, a technique that is effective in more than 90 percent of cases. *See* HEART.

Surfers' Nodules

Bony outgrowths on the foot or top of the shin.

Small bumps of bone (exostoses) may develop in an area that is subject to frequent jarring. The name comes from the tendency for surfers to develop this condition. They spend a great deal of time in positions in which their board bangs against their knees or feet repeatedly while paddling out into the surf. To avoid this, it is recommended that surfers paddle while lying facedown on the board.

Resources on Surgery

Cottrell, James E. and Stephanie Golden, *Under the Mask: A Guide to Feeling Secure and Comfortable During Anesthesia and Surgery* (2001); Rutkow, Ira M., *Surgery: An Illustrated History* (1993); Youngson, Robert M., *The Surgery Book : An Illustrated Guide to 73 of the Most Common Operations* (1997); American College of Surgeons, Tel. (312) 202-5000, Online: www. facs.org; American Medi-cal Association, Tel. (312) 464-5000, Online: www. amaassn.org; American College of Physicians–American Society of Internal Medicine, Tel. (800) 523-1546, Online: www. acponline.org; www. med.cornell.edu/surgery/; www.nycornell.org/medicine/gim/index.html; www.nycornell.org/medicine/emergency/html.

Operating Room. Major surgeries are usually performed in an operating room (below). The room is a clean, sterile environment that contains all the tools that will be needed during the procedure. The surgeon, nurses, an anesthesiologist, and other specialists may be present during the operation.

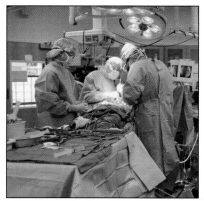

Surgeon

A physician who has been specially trained to perform operations that involve cutting into body tissue and organs, primarily to correct a health problem or to alter the body.

Surgery may involve diagnostic probes and the removal or repair of diseased or malfunctioning organs and body parts.

Top surgeons are board certified, namely by a national surgical board approved by the American Board of Medical Specialties. Most respected surgeons are also Fellows in the American College of Surgeons (F.A.C.S.) and maintain a practice with an accredited health care facility, especially a hospital that is accredited by the Joint Commission on Accreditation of Health Care Organizations (JCAHO).

Surgery

Medical treatment that involves direct manipulation of the body and its organs, usually (but not always) requiring piercing of the skin.

Surgery involves the application of medical techniques directly to parts of the body; it is, arguably, the branch of medicine that requires the deftest control and the most care. Surgery often involves encroaching through the skin and manipulating, removing, adjusting, or enhancing some internal organ or portion of the body. The body has many mechanisms for resisting such encroachment, and in any case it will react to such procedures in a variety of untoward and unpredictable ways. As a result, surgeons have come to specialize in ever narrower fields of surgery, so that an orthopedic surgeon, for example, who once may have dealt with many areas of the body will today typically specialize in hands, or in hips.

Why Have Surgery? Surgery may be performed for a variety of reasons. Some operations are necessary as emergency procedures, as in the case of a Ce-

sarean section childbirth to save the life of the mother or the fetus. Other operations may provide a patient with the only means of surviving a disease such as cancer. Still other surgical procedures are "exploratory," insofar as they provide a physician a means of evaluating the condition of internal organs. Surgery may also be performed to substantially improve a patient's quality of life, such as the replacement of a hip or the correction of an eye problem. When the surgery is performed for purely cosmetic purposes, it is deemed "elective." Surgery can be characterized as "major," indicating that it requires general anesthesia; or "minor," which usually indicates that it requires only local anesthesia.

The tools of surgery have advanced considerably since the beginning of the 20th century, yet most surgery still depends on incision with a sharp instrument and the sewing of tissues with sutures. Even this requires careful monitoring and control of bodily functions. Surgeons are continually developing new tools to improve their control and effectiveness. Advanced tools include: microscopes; computer-enhanced imaging; fiberoptics; incison enhancers such as laser beams and robot-controlled scalpels; and machines that assist in the surgical process by relieving the body of some of its functions, such as a heart-lung machine or a kidney-dialysis machine.

Surgery places demands on a patient's blood supply, and today more careful management of the patient's blood is practiced through the use of storage of a patient's own blood (autologous blood storage) before surgery or by stimulating the blood production as a preparatory step for surgery. Another important area of study connected with surgery is pain management —accomplished during surgery through the use of anesthesia, but also important in the postoperative recovery period.

See Operating Room *and* Surgeon *for background information on surgery. For additional information see* Anesthesia; Cauterizing; Dressing; Scalpal; *and* Suture. *Related information contained in* Blood Transfusion; Imaging Techniques; Laser Surgery *and* Plastic Surgery.

Surrogate Mother

A woman who is hired to carry a baby to term for a couple who cannot cannot conceive together.

Surrogate motherhood is an option for couples in which the female partner is infertile. Surrogate motherhood usually takes one of two forms. If the female partner is completely infertile, then the male partner can artificially inseminate the surrogate mother; the resulting child will be the genetic offspring of the father and the surrogate mother. If the female partner is able to produce a fetus but cannot carry a baby to term, a fertilized egg can be implanted into the surrogate mother; the child will be the genetic offspring of both partners.

Surrogate mothers may be found through a fertility program. A couple may also choose a surrogate on their own and write up a contract with the aid of a lawyer who specializes in family care and adoption. In choosing a surrogate mother, a couple may wish to consider a number of health and personal factors. Generally, a potential surrogate mother is screened for sexually transmitted diseases and genetic disorders. If the surrogate mother is going to be the genetic mother of the child, the couple may wish to find a woman who is genetically similar to the female partner. In some cases, a couple may choose a sibling or other close relative to be the surrogate, especially if they want to share as much as possible in the experience of pregnancy. In a surrogacy contract, issues to be considered include how involved the surrogate mother will be in parenting the child (if at all), what to do in the event of a miscarriage, and related issues. A clear contract can be invaluable in preventing custody battles after the birth of the child. Generally, a surrogate mother is paid a fee ranging from $10,000 to $100,000.

Background material on surrogate mother can be found in INFERTILITY and PREGNANCY. Additional information can be found in ARTIFICIAL INSEMINATION; IN VITRO FERTILIZATION; and IMPLANTATION, EGG. See also REPRODUCTIVE SYSTEM, FEMALE AND MALE for related information.

Suturing

The surgical closing of a wound, cut, or incision through the use of sterile stitches to facilitate the healing process.

Suturing involves the surgeon or physician sewing the wound together with thread made of any of a variety of materials: catgut, silk, synthetic fibers made from nylon or polymers, linen, and stainless steel wire. The thickness of sutures will vary depending on the body area. For instance, the thinnest (0.004 inch) type is used in eye and blood vessel surgery.

Some sutures are absorbable, such as catgut, and others are removed after the area has sufficiently healed, usually in one to two weeks. Types of stitching techniques include blanket, continuous, vertical mattress, interrupted, and purse string sutures. The needles are generally curved and held by a tweezer-like instrument. *See* SURGERY.

Swab

A wad or piece of absorbent material used to obtain a sample of a patient's mucus, pus, or other bodily fluid for bacteriological analysis or used in surgery to apply antiseptic solutions, ointments, and medications to wounds and incisions.

A common type of swab is a twist of cotton on a wooden stick. For clinical use they are usually larger and sterilized. A doctor or nurse may use a swab to get throat cultures for strep analysis, nasal mucus samples, vaginal swabs, pap test and sample cells from the cervix, rectal swabs, and skin lesion samples. This type of swab is also used to apply tinctures, ointments, and medications, for example, to cauterize capillaries inside the nose to stop bleeding.

The other type of swab, a folded piece of cotton gauze, acts as a surgical sponge and is held in the hand or in a clamp. It is used either to apply antiseptic solution before an incision is made or to soak up blood and body fluids during or after an operation.

A swab may also contain material that an x-ray will detect to ensure that it is not accidentally left inside a patient. *See* GAUZE.

Swallowing

The process that takes food from the mouth into the stomach.

Swallowing is a body function that uses both voluntary and involuntary actions. A person directs the food that is broken down by chewing and enzymes in the saliva, then unconsciously instructs the tongue and palate to push it back into the throat and into the pharynx. At that point, a series of a involuntary reflexes take over. Once food is in the pharynx, the epiglottis (a flap of skin over the larynx) closes to prevent food from entering that area and the windpipe. The sphincter, a round muscle at the top of the esophagus, relaxes to allow the entry of the food. The pharynx then takes the food and squeezes it into a lump called a bolus. It then pushes the bolus into the esophagus, and from there contractions in the esophagus forces it down to the stomach. Muscles at the top of the stomach then open, and the bolus enters the stomach.

Any disorders that affect the esophagus, pharynx, or involuntary nervous system may also affect swallowing. *See also* ENZYME; ESOPHAGUS; PHARYNX; SALIVA: STOMACH; THROAT; *and* TONGUE.

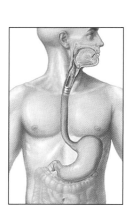

Upper G.I. System. The upper gastro-intestinal system (above) contains the esophagus, pharynx, and mouth.

Swallowing Difficulties

Inability to swallow normally.

Swallowing is the action that brings food or liquid from the mouth into the esophagus, then to the stomach. Food is broken down by chewing and by enzymes in saliva. The tongue pushes the food towards the back of the mouth, where muscles in the palate bring it into the pharynx. Then a series of reflexes sends the food from the pharynx into the esophagus. Therefore, conditions that affect any of these parts can result in swallowing difficulties.

There are numerous causes that may result in swallowing difficulties.

Obstruction. A foreign object that is lodged in the esophagus will prevent the passage of food.

Esophageal Stricture. Narrowing of the esophagus prevents food from passing easily into the stomach. This can be caused by a variety of conditions. Acid reflux is one such cause. Stomach acid that washes back into the esophagus is another cause of this condition; it results in the esophagus becoming inflamed and swollen, culminating in a build-up of scar tissue. Swallowing corrosive substances, or persistent viral or bacterial infections that cause inflammation can also lead to a swollen esophagus, leaving a narrow passageway.

Esophageal Spasm. Spasms in the esophagus disrupt the series of reflexes that allow food to pass into the stomach. The spasms may be caused by acid reflux, or a malfunction in the lower esophagus. This malfunction is often caused by a hiatal hernia (a condition in which the upper portion of the stomach moves around between the chest and abdomen).

Esophageal Cancer. Swallowing difficulties may be the result of a tumor in the esophagus. Because of this possibility, problems with swallowing should be taken seriously and investigated to rule out the possibility of cancer.

Pharyngoesophageal Diverticulum. This is a pouch that forms at the entrance of the pharynx. If the sphincter muscle (located at the top of the esophagus) is not functioning properly, it can cause food particles to become trapped in the pouch. It will enlarge and cause swallowing problems. The pouch usually needs to be removed in a surgical procedure.

Other causes of swallowing difficulties are goiters (swollen thyroid glands) or nerve disorders such as a stroke, which can affect the muscles that permit swallowing. A swollen or enlarged tongue will also prevent normal swallowing.

Treatment of swallowing difficulties should be based on the underlying cause.

Background material on swallowing difficulties is found in SWALLOWING. *For further reading, see* ENZYME; ESOPHAGUS; MOUTH; PHARYNX; SALIVA; *and* TONGUE. *For related diseases, see* ESOPHAGEAL CANCER; ESOPHAGEAL DIVERTICULUM; ESOPHAGEAL SPASM; ESOPHAGEAL STRICTURE; *and*

Sweat

Fluid secreted by the sweat glands.

Sweat is a fluid composed mostly of water and salt that is secreted by the sweat glands. There are two types of sweat gland. Eccrine glands are located throughout the body, notably in places such as the palms of the hands and soles of the feet; apocrine glands are found in places where there is hair, such as the armpits and pubic area. The apocrine glands differ from the eccrine glands in that the fluid they secrete contains not only water and salt, but also cellular material. If left on the skin, this material decomposes, resulting in body odor.

Sweat Glands

Glands that produce sweat.

Located throughout the body, the sweat glands are tiny tubes that lead directly to the surface of the skin. The majority are eccrine glands, which are found in places like the palms of the hands and soles of the feet. Apocrine glands are located in hairy places, such as the armpits and pubic area; they develop after puberty. While sweat is primarily composed of water and salt, the fluid released by apocrine glands also contains cellular material. When left upon the surface of the skin, this material becomes vulnerable to bacteria and may produce body odor.

The sweat glands are controlled by the autonomic nervous system, or the part of the nervous system that runs seemingly involuntary bodily activities. The main activity of the sweat glands is to cool the body. When the body senses that its temperature has risen too high, due to a warm atmosphere, heightened activity, or fever, the glands release sweat, usually on the forehead, or above the lip, neck, and chest. Sweating may also occur as a reaction to stress or fear; in these cases, the sweat will usually first appear on the palms of the hands, soles of the feet, and armpits. *See also* APOCRINE GLANDS *and* BODY ODOR.

Swelling

Build-up of fluid or tissue growth.

Swelling (edema) is the result of an imbalance between the amount of water that is forced out of the capillaries and pumped throughout the body by blood and the rate at which it is taken back into the capillaries. When these processes are not synchronized, fluid builds up, and the area becomes swollen. Swelling may occur in an isolated area or throughout the body.

Causes. Swelling of a specific area often occurs after an injury from a direct blow, such as a fracture or sprain. Other types of swelling that afflict individual areas are joint swelling due to arthritis, insect bites, swollen gums (gingivitis), muscle tears, and many other traumas or infections. Swelling of the legs, feet, and hands is not uncommon during hot weather, and it also often occurs during pregnancy.

Swelling throughout the body may be caused by a variety of serious conditions. Massive edema may be caused by a lack of albumin, a protein that regulates the movement of fluid in the body. Heart failure can cause a build up of blood in the veins. Pressure caused by a tumor may cause the same effect. Nephritis can interrupt the flow of fluid into the tissues, while renal failure and cirrhosis of the liver can cause retention of salt and therefore of water. A high salt intake, therefore, can also cause a general bloating or swelling. Corticosteroids, androgen drugs, and some contraceptives can affect the kidneys, leading to salt retention.

Diagnosis. Generalized swelling may be difficult to detect, as it can be interpreted as weight gain. If the swelling is sudden, or there seems to be identifiable causes such as injury, a physician should be consulted. A doctor may ask some of the following questions:

How long has the swelling been noticeable? Is it always present or does it come and go?

Is it in one particular area or throughout the body?

Sweat Glands.
Sweat glands, top, are tiny tubes that lead directly to the surface of the skin. Their primary function is to cool the body. Bottom, an illustration of the epithelial cells that line sweat glands. The epithelium makes up the entire surface of the body and lines many structures contained within it.

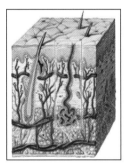

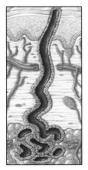

How much is it swollen? Does a dent remain in the area if you press on it?

Does it hurt? Does anything make it better, or worse?

Treatment. Once the cause of the swelling has been diagnosed, the underlying condition must be remedied. This should bring down the swelling; but if it does not, diuretic drugs meant to increase the flow of urine and restricted salt intake may be prescribed. If related to injuries, ice packs and keeping the affected area raised may bring down the swelling. *See also* ALBUMIN; ARTHRITIS; CIRRHOSIS; DIURETIC DRUGS; GINGEVITIS; HEART FAILURE; NEPHRITIS; RENAL FAILURE; *and* SALT.

Sycosis Vulgaris

Inflammatory disease of facial hair follicles.

Sycosis vulgaris is a subacute or chronic infection in hair follicles caused by the bacteria *Staphylococcus aureus.* In lupoid sycosis, hair follicles are destroyed by scarring. Although the condition usually affects the beard area (sycosis barbae), sycosis can also affect the scalp and other areas that are covered by hair. Treatment of the condition involves antibiotics and careful attention to hygiene. *See also* FOLLICLE.

Sympathectomy

Chemical or surgical removal of sympathetic nerves, usually in the hands.

Sympathetic nerves, part of the involuntary nervous system, are responsible for bodily changes associated with stress and excitement. In some disorders, the body exhibits evidence of stress—such as narrowing of peripheral blood vessels or sweating excessively and without appropriate cause. In such cases, severing the appropriate sympathetic nerves may result in relief of symptoms. Sympathectomy may be performed using drugs, open surgery, or endoscopic surgery, depending on the type and location of the disorder. Sympathectomy may be used to treat excessive sweating (hyper-

hidrosis) of the face, hands, armpits, or feet; Raynaud's phenomenon in the hands or feet; Buerger's disease; and severe causalgia. Generally, sympathectomies affecting the lower limbs are more effective than those affecting the hands. *See also* HYPERHIDROSIS *and* NERVOUS SYSTEM.

Synapse

The junction between two neurons (nerve cells) across which nerve impulses and signals pass.

Neurons may have many synapses with neighboring neurons. Transmission of nerve impulses is a two-step process. The arrival of the electrical signal at the nerve end causes the cell to produce chemicals called neurotansmitters. These chemicals then travel from the membrane of the cell at which the impulse originates to the membrane of the cell receiving the impulse.

In some instances, the neurotransmitter increases the likelihood that the synapse will "fire," that is, allow a nerve impulse to pass from neuron to neuron, in which case it is said to be an "excitatory" synapse. In other instances, the neurotransmitter will decrease the likelihood that the synapse will fire, in which case it is an "inhibitory" synapse. *See* NERVOUS SYSTEM *and* NEURON.

Syndactyly

A birth defect in which two or more digits of the hands or feet are joined.

Syndactyly is often inherited and sometimes may be associated with other birth defects. Severity can range from a flap of connecting skin to fusion of the bones.

Syndactyly of the hands can cause problems with movement, as the bones of the fingers are of different lengths and the joints of the fused fingers do not line up properly. In order to gain full use of the digits, they must be surgically separated.

Webbed toes are more of a cosmetic problem than one of functionality. Surgical separation may result in scars more unsightly than the defect. *See* BIRTH DEFECTS.

Synovectomy

The surgical removal of the synovial tissue that lines a movable bone joint, in order to treat recurring inflammation, synovitis, common among patients with severe rheumatoid arthritis.

The procedure is employed when corticosteroid drugs, non-steroidal anti-inflammatory drugs, or anti-rheumatic drugs no longer satisfactorily treat the problem. The operation may be performed via traditional open surgery or by a less invasive arthroscopic surgery. *See also* SYNOVITIS.

A promising new technique called boron neutron capture synovectomy is now being tested. Drops of boron are injected into the arthritic joint and exposed to a beam of neutrons for several minutes. The newly created radioactivity kills the inflamed tissue, which quickly decays away.

Synovitis

The inflammation of synovium, the connective tissue that lines the moving surfaces of the joints.

The synovial membrane is a thin, smooth membrane that lines the surfaces of the joints where free movement is necessary. The membrane secretes a transparent, thick fluid that lubricates the joints. The synovial membrane may inflame as a result of an infection elsewhere in the body or as a consequence of a sports injury. Synovitis is also suspected to precede rheumatoid arthritis.

Transient synovitis of the hip is a swelling of the tissues of the hip joint reported in children between three and ten years of age. It is more common in boys than girls. The cause is unknown, though a virus or an allergic reaction is suspected. The onset of the condition may be rapid or delayed, but eventually the child may limp or even refuse to stand because of the pain. There will be no fever, indicating that the cause is not bacterial, and blood tests and x-rays will eventually rule out any other cause. Transient synovitis resolves completely in three or four days with bed rest and ibuprofen. *See* SYNOVECTOMY.

Syphilis

A sexually transmitted disease caused by a bacterium called *Treponema pallidum*.

Syphilis is an extremely contagious sexually transmitted disease. The bacteria enter the body through the mucous membranes of the vagina or mouth, or even through tiny abrasions of the skin. Within hours the bacteria reach the adjacent lymph nodes and move throughout the body with the blood stream. Syphilis sores offer an easy way for AIDS to be transferred from person to person. Pregnant women with the disease pass it to their children, causing abnormalities.

STAGES OF SYPHIILS

Primary Stage. The incubation period (during which no symptoms appear) may be as short as a week or as long as three months. After the incubation period, a single chancre (a small, red, painless ulcer) appears at the site of original infection. This site is often the penis in men or the vulva in women. Chancres can also appear on the anus, lips, tongue, throat, cervix, or fingers. The chancre will rupture, draining a clear fluid that is highly contagious. The lymph nodes may swell. The chancre heals in a few weeks and, since it is painless, it is often ignored.

Secondary Stage. A copper-colored rash may appear before the chancre has completely healed, or the rash may not appear until several weeks later. The most characteristic symptom is when the rash appears on the palms of the hands or the soles of the feet. It may also look like prickly heat (small blotches or scales) all over the body or whitish patches in the mouth. These patches can develop into small pus-filled abscesses. The rash lasts for from one to three months. Mouth sores are common in this stage, as are inflamed lymph nodes and sore eyes. There may be patchy hair loss, a general feeling of malaise (illness), fatigue, a fever, and anemia.

Latency. After the secondary stage is completed, syphilis seems to go into remission (latency). There are no symptoms at

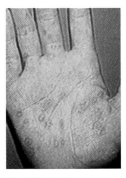

Syphilis Rash. When syphilis reaches its secondary stage, rashes tend to appear all over the body, particularly on the hands (above) and soles. Mouth sores and hair loss are other visible symptoms of the disease.

The Mathematics of Contagion

It is important to consider how syphilis cannot be transmitted. Syphilis cannot be transmitted from a toilet seat, a door knob, a swimming pool, a hot tub, a bathtub, or through shared clothing or towels. However, because early symptoms of syphilis can be mild or even nonexistent, it is easy for people to unknowingly transmit the disease to sexual partners. Washing the genitals, douching, or urinating after sex does not prevent infection. A person in primary stage syphilis is contagious for a period of three months from their first exposure to the bacteria. A person in secondary stage syphilis is contagious for a period of twelve months after the initial exposure. Tertiary syphilis is not contagious. It makes sense, therefore to:

• Know your sexual partners.

• Use a condom.

• Insist that your sexual partners take laboratory tests to confirm that they are free of sexually transmitted disease.

toms, including headache, a stiff neck, irritability, confusion, disorientation, visual disturbances, abnormal reflexes, incontinence, weakness, muscle atrophy, and uncoordinated movement.

Tabes Dorsalis

Tabes dorsalis is a complication of syphilis. The condition may be described as a progressive destruction of the nerves in the spinal cord. Tabes dorsalis may appear in the third (tertiary) stage of syphilis. The condition produces an intense stabbing pain and a numbness of the limbs. Balance and motor control problems make walking unsteady and the patient walks with a characteristic high-stepping gait. Long-term administration of antibiotics may kill the syphilis-causing bacteria, but permanent nerve damage is likely and cannot be reversed.

Resources on Syphilis and Sexually Transmitted Diseases

Grist, Norman R., et al., *Diseases of Infection: An Illustrated Textbook* (1992); Shaw, Michael, ed., *Everything You Need to Know About Diseases* (1996); Rosenwaks, Zev, *Gynecology: Principles and Practice* (1987); Centers for Disease Control and Prevention, Tel. (800) 311-3435, Online: www.cdc.gov, STD hotline: (800) 227-8922; Infectious Disease Society of America, Tel. (703) 299-0200, Online: www.idsociety.org; National Institute of Allergy and Infectious Disease, Tel. (301) 496-5717, Online: www.niaid. nih.org; https://public1. med.cornell.edu/cgi-.

all, and the latent condition may last for many years or even for the rest of the person's life. During the latent period, the bacteria remain in the body and begin to attack the other organs, such as the brain, the nerves, the eyes, the heart, the liver, the bones, and the joints.

Tertiary Stage. In the tertiary stage, syphilis is not contagious. However, if it has still been left untreated, the disease will take one of three possible paths. In benign tertiary syphilis, gummas (lumps) begin to appear anywhere in or on the body. These gummas are painful nodules that enlarge slowly and heal very gradually. Cardiovascular syphilis usually appears ten or more years after the original exposure. The bacteria attack the main artery, leaving the heart or the valve that controls flow to this aretry damaged. Symptoms of cardiovascular syphilis are chest pain and heart failure. The heart damage caused by cardiovascular syphilis can prove fatal. In a small percentage of the sufferers who reach the tertiary stage of untreated syphilis, the bacteria infect the spinal cord and brain. This rare condition is called neurosyphilis. The sufferer experiences a number of symp-

Diagnosis and Treatment. Shortly after initial exposure to syphilis, the body normally produces antibodies to the disease that can be detected with blood tests. Alternatively the bacteria themselves, taken with a swab from the vagina or from a suppurating (pus-filled) sore, can be identified through a microscope. Treatment of primary stage syphilis is with a single injection of penicillin. For secondary or latency stage syphilis, the penicillin will be given weekly over a period of three weeks. In tertiary stage syphilis, the penicillin will be administered intravenously. As in the earlier stages, in tertiary stage syphilis, the bacteria will almost certainly be destroyed; however, damage already done to the organs is irrevers- ible. If the sufferer has reached the tertiary stage of syphilis without treatment, death is almost inevitable.

People treated with penicillin often have a severe reaction within a few hours of the initial treatment. They may develop a fever, a headache, chills, and excessive sweating. It is believed that this is a reaction to the destruction of millions of bacteria. The reaction is treated with antihistamines.

Background material may be found in BACTERIA *and* SEXUALLY TRANSMITTED DISEASES. *More on syphilis is contained in* AIDS; CHANCRE; LYMPH NODES; NEUROSYPHILIS; *and* RASH. *For information on treatment and prevention, see* CONDOM; MEDICAL TESTS *and* PENICILIN.

Syringe

A device for delivering fluids to or removing fluids from the body.

A syringe is a glass or plastic tube with a piston that moves in the cylinder. The piston seals tightly against the inner surface of the tube with rubber seals. If the piston is pushed forward, it forces fluid in the cylinder out through a hollow needle. If the piston is withdrawn it draws fluid (blood, for example) out.

Some people do not like needles because they hurt when the skin is penetrated. New syringes are being made with needles so small they can hardly be felt as they penetrate the skin. Alternatives to syringes include a device that uses pressurized helium to throw dry powder medications through the skin. *See also* BLOOD TESTS; DIAGNOSIS; IMMUNIZATION; INOCULATION; *and* VACCINIATION.

Syringing of the Ear

Method of removing excess wax or foreign matter from the ear.

The outer ear contains glands that secrete a waxy substance known as cerumen, which keeps the ear lubricated and prevents foreign particles from entering the ear canal. Most people only produce as much as is needed for these responsibilities; some people, however, secrete too much, causing the wax to build up and block the ear canal. When this occurs, it must be removed. Easy cases may be handled at home with gentle cleaning, or over-the-counter solutions to dissolve the wax. Syringing of the ear may be necessary in tougher cases.

Ear syringing should be done by a physician or health professional, in order to minimize the possibility of damage to the eardrum. A physician will also be able to conduct an initial examination of the ear to check for other types of damage; if the examination reveals any initial rupture in the eardrum, then the ear should not be syringed.

How it is Done. Before proceeding with syringing, the physician may put some oil, or drops that contain a softening agent, into the ear, in order to soften and dislodge the wax. Next, a bulb syringe is filled with warm or room temperature water; sometimes, solutions of water and peroxide, or water with a few drops of a dissolving agent may be used as well. The syringe is then gently placed in the ear canal; pulling the outside of the ear (the pinna) up will straighten the ear canal and maintain the force of the water. The water is then launched into the ear, which should dislodge the softened wax.

Afterwards, the ear must be completely dried. If water remains in the ear canal, bacteria may grow and infect the area, causing the condition known as swimmers' ear (otitis externa). Alcohol drops can help to dry the ear. *See also* EAR; EAR, FOREIGN MATTER IN; EARDRUM; EARDRUM, PERFORATION OF; EARWAX; *and* OTITIS EXTERNA.

Syringomyelia

A rare condition in which a fluid-filled sac forms within the brain stem or spinal cord.

Syringomyelia is a congenital condition in which a cavity or cyst forms in the brain stem or spinal cord. The cyst enlarges, expands, and fills with cerebrospinal fluid that harms the nerve fibers.

Causes/Symptoms. Cysts caused by syringomyelia are often present at birth and enlarge during the teenage years. Babies who are born with syringomyelia frequently have additional birth defects. Most forms of syringomyelia are caused by an injury or tumor. An early symptom of the condition is the inability to sense pain or changes in temperature in the neck, shoulder, arms, or hands. This can frequently lead to a catastrophe, permitting patients to sustain burns and other bodily harm without their awareness. Syringomyelia causes the muscles in the neck, shoulders, and arms to atrophy. Patients with advanced stages of syringomyelia may manifest symptoms such as rigidness or spasticity in the legs, nasal speech, and difficulty swallowing. In the advanced stages of the disease, the patient is wheelchair-bound.

DIAGNOSIS AND TREATMENT.

Syringomyelia is suspected in individuals with severely cut or burnt fingers that, due to the nerve damage caused by the condition, can no longer perceive the pain caused by their injuries. Magnetic resonance imaging (MRI) is used to identify the cyst caused by syringomyelia. No drug therapy for the condition is available. A neurosurgeon may drain the fluid from the cyst in order to relieve the pressure, but this can only momentarily halt the progression of the disease.

> *Basic anatomical information on syringomyelia may be found in* BRAIN STEM *and* SPINAL CORD. *For additional information see* ATROPHY; BIRTH DEFECTS; CYST; NERVE; NERVE INJURY; *and* SPASTICITY. *For information on diagnosis and treatment, see* MRI *and* SURGERY.

Systemic

> **Disease or disorder affecting the entire body.**

Systemic diseases (also known as somatic diseases) are those affecting the whole body, rather than a specific organ or body part. Often such illness are the result of immune malfunction. Autoimmune diseases are those caused by the body's hostile immune reaction to its own cells and tissues. Disorders such as systemic lupus erythematosus (SLE) and others are the result of an autoimmune assault on the body's blood cells and tissues, affecting the skin, joints, and internal organs. Suppressed immune systems can cause other generalized, systemic diseases. Such illnesses vary widely in severity from mild to life-threatening, and they may be chronic, cyclic, or disappear altogether. The term systemic may also be applied to remedies affecting the entire body. *See also* AUTOIMMUNE DISORDERS; IMMUNITY; *and* LUPUS ERYTHEMATOSUS.

Systole

> **The phase of the heart beat cycle in which the ventricles pump blood.**

In systole, the heart muscle contracts and the tricuspid and mitral valves close, so that the ventricles, the lower chambers of the heart, can pump blood to the lungs and the rest of the body. Systole is followed by diastole, in which the tricuspid and mitral valves are open and the atria, the upper chambers of the heart, contract, moving blood into the ventricles. Systole is the shorter phase of the heartbeat, taking up a third of the cycle. In a reading of blood pressure, say 120/80, the higher number measures pressure during systole. *See* DIASTOLE *and* HEARTBEAT.

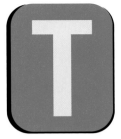

T'ai Chi

A martial art that may have healing properties.

Dating back to 1000 ce, T'ai Chi combined the Taoist study of Chi Kung, which dealt with physical health and spiritual growth, with the need of the monks to protect themselves from bandits and warlords. The result was a unique blend of exercises that could be used for healing and defense.

T'ai Chi emphasizes concentration and being "centered," both physically and mentally. The lower abdomen is considered the center of the being; and once awareness of that area is achieved, it can send energy throughout the rest of the body. T'ai Chi is considered a "movement art," not just in the physical sense, but in the way the whole body and mind adapts to change around it. The idea of T'ai Chi is to willingly participate in change. *See* ALTERNATIVE MEDICINE.

Aside from developing mental abilities such as concentration and relaxation, T'ai Chi has many physical benefits. It can help patients with arthritis by strengthening the joints, especially in the hips and ankles, and seniors who are losing their sense of balance by improving body awareness and posture. Athletes can develop better coordination and learn to use their whole body more efficiently in their particular sport.

Tachycardia

An abnormally rapid heartbeat.

Tachycardia is usually defined as a resting heart rate of over 100 beats per minute, compared to the average adult heart rate of about 75 beats per minute. There are many types and causes of tachycardia, which can affect different regions of the heart. Causes range from heart disease to the side effects of some medications. Symptoms include breathlessness, lightheadedness, and palpitations. Treatment depends on the cause of the tachycardia and the region of the heart that it affects. The most serious tachycardias are those that affect the ventricles, the two lower chambers of the heart. *See* HEART.

Tachypnea

Abnormally fast rate of breathing.

In adults, tachypnea can be caused by strenuous activity, simple anxiety, lung disorders such as emphysema, or heart problems such as heart failure.

One form of the condition, transient tachypnea, is seen in newborn babies, often in those delivered by Caesarean section. They have rapid, shallow breathing resulting from accumulation of fluid in the lungs. Infants with the condition may be given oxygen for hours or days, and may require special feeding, intravenously or through a tube, for several days. *See also* BREATHING DIFFICULTIES.

Tacrolimus

A drug administered to transplant recipients to prevent rejection the new organ or tissue.

As with any immunosuppressant, tacrolimus must be taken indefinitely. A major risk of immunosuppressant drugs is that by suppressing the body's reaction to the transplant, the ability to fight infection is compromised. *See also* REJECTION.

Talipes

Also known as clubfoot

Any of several congenital disorders in which the foot is twisted out of shape or position.

Talipes occurs in one in 1,000 births. In the majority of cases, the forefoot is twisted down and in, with the heel turned inward.

Treatment. Treatment must begin shortly after birth in order to be effective. The feet are manipulated into the normal position and kept in place by means of casts or other orthopedic devices. The process must be repeated every few days during the first two weeks of treatment, and then at regular one to two week intervals. Afterwards, corrective shoes are used. If this method is unsuccessful, surgery is performed by age two or three months. *See also* FOOT *and* ORTHOPEDICS.

Tampon

A plug, usually of cotton, inserted in a body cavity to absorb blood, mucous, or other discharges.

Tampons are inserted by women into their vaginas during their menstrual cycle to absorb the discharge. When superabsorbent tampons were introduced in 1980, there was a rash of reports of toxic shock syndrome. This is a staphlococcus infection caused by a bacterium that is normally relatively harmless but can turn toxic and produce a life-threatening disease. These superabsorbent tampons were discontinued. Women are cautioned to change tampons every eight hours. *See also* VAGINA.

Tamponade

Compression of the heart caused by accumulation of fluid under its membrane, the pericardium.

Tamponade can be the result of pericarditis, an inflammation of the pericardium. It can also be caused by a penetrating injury to the chest or cancer of the breast or lung. It can cause extreme breathlessness and fainting, as the heart does not pump enough blood to the brain. Tamponade can be diagnosed by a chest x-ray or echocardiogram. It is treated by removing the excess fluid under the pericardium through a hollow needle. Surgery is sometimes necessary to remove any blood clots that have formed. *See also* HEART.

Tannin

A substance found in many plants, including tree bark, coffee, and tea. It is an essential ingredient of wine and is used to preserve leather. Tannin is used medicinally for its astringent qualities.

In leather making, tannin is impregnated into animal skins to help them resist decomposition and retain their soft pliability. Tannin also gives wine its dry taste.

Compresses of tea leaves applied to the skin serve to tighten the tissues and shrink mucous membranes, reducing the discharge of blood or mucous.

Tantrum

An angry outburst of violent (usually self-directed) common in toddlers, especially in 2 year olds.

Tantrums are the result of a child's inability to deal with frustration at constraints imposed by parents during a period when the child first experiences a degree of independence and self-reliance. The child will frequently associate the failure to have a desire gratified with abandonment, and thus tantrums are more common following the birth of a younger sibling. In time, the child will learn to verbalize the frustration and deal with the constraint, realizing that it is not equivalent to a lack of parental love and concern.

A tantrum can be a trying experience for a parent. It is often accompanied by crying, kicking and screaming, rolling and stomping on the floor, spitting, and biting (sometimes himself or herself). It is common for a child to hold his or her breath until his or her face turns blue, sometimes for a period long enough to cause the child to lose consciousness momentarily.

What to Do. The best solution for parents is to try to divert the child's attention to a game or something interesting in the environment. It is important not to scold or argue with the child; expressing anger only aggravates the underlying cause of the behavior. Firm and consistent behavior by the parent is essential; it is particularly counter-productive to punish the child and then give in to the child's demands. In time, most children learn to verbalize their frustration. Encouraging a child to verbalize wants and disappointments will thus help him or her to pass through this phase more easily and quickly—and no longer resort to this behavior. If tantrums continue past the age of four, counseling and some professional help may be advisable.

Background material on tantrum may be found in CHILD DEVELOPMENT *and* PSYCHIATRY. *For additional information treatment, see* BEHAVIOR THERAPY; ELECTRICAL INJURY; *and* FAMILY THERAPY. *Related information contained in* SIBLING RIVALRY.

Tapeworm Infestation

Invasion of the body by parasitic flatworms of the class *Cestoda*.

Tapeworms are slender, flattened worms also known as cestodes. Many varieties exist, some reaching lengths of 15 to 20 feet. They are equipped with a hooked head (scolex) that attaches to the intestinal wall of their host, and hundreds of egg carrying segments follow the head. These segments break off, pass out of the host in fecal matter, and are subsequently consumed by the primary host—either pigs, cattle, or fish. Humans become infected with tapeworms by eating undercooked, contaminated fish or meat. Eggs hatch into larvae, which penetrate the intestinal wall and migrate through the blood circulation.

TYPES OF TAPEWORM

Three main kinds of tapeworm are responsible for disease in humans: *Taenia saginata* (beef tapeworm); *Taenia solium* (pork tapeworm); and *Diphyllobothrium latum* (fish tapeworm). Another species, *Echinococcus granulosus*, is also known to occasionally infest people, causing the formation of cysts in the liver.

• *Taenia solium* is acquired through eating the larval form of the parasite in undercooked pork. These larva then develop in the intestine into adult egg-laying worms. Eggs are passed with the feces and go on to infect pigs, beginning the cycle anew. If eggs are eaten, the larvae may infect the central nervous system and brain, causing seizures and a neurological condition known as cysticercosis.

• *Taenia saginata* tapeworms spread to humans by meat from infected cattle. They may reach a length of more than 12 feet. The segments are able to crawl and may be seen moving in the feces. While the pork tapeworm may infest humans through either larvae or eggs, only the encysted larvae can infect humans.

• Some freshwater fish and salmon may also carry a tapeworm called *Diphyllobothrium latum*, which can grow to 25 feet.

Symptoms. Infestation may cause no immediate symptoms. Heavy infestation may produce symptoms that include abdominal pain, diarrhea, and weight loss.

Diagnosis. Stool may be examined for the presence of eggs and mature parasites. In the case of pork tapeworms, moving segments may be observed.

Treatment. Oral antihelmintic drugs such as niclosamide are used to destroy the tapeworm. Supportive therapy may be required if complications, including anemia or neurological involvement, are present.

Prevention. Fish, pork, and beef must be properly cooked to avoid tapeworm infestation. In the case of those already infected, good hygiene will help prevent reinfection during treatment. *See* PARASITE.

Tarsalgia

Foot pain at the joint of the ankle.

Foot pain located in this area is usually associated with the condition flatfoot. Therefore, it may be assumed that the pain is caused by the incorrect mechanics of foot movement and stance due to the lack of an arch in the foot. In order to relieve tarsalgia, the problem of flatfoot must first be addressed. A podiatrist may recommend orthotics or other inserts designed to give the foot a shape that can take the stresses of every day activity. *See also* FLATFOOT.

Tarsorrhaphy

A surgical procedure in which the upper and lower eyelids are partially sewn together to narrow the opening. It is usually performed to promote healing of the cornea or to protect the eye from drying.

Among the conditions that may require tarsorrhaphy are Sjögren's syndrome, a systemic disorder in which inflammation suppresses tear, and salivary, duct production and may damage the glands; Bell's palsy, in which one side of the face is paralyzed with one eye unable to close; and myasthenia gravis, which causes droopy upper eyelids—ptosis. A stroke can jeopardize a patient's cornea health.

Other conditions that may call for tarsorrhaphy include:

- exophthalmos, bulging eyes, which is associated with Graves' disease;
- enophthalmos, sunken eyes, dendritic ulcers of the cornea, in which the eyelids function as a bandage;
- keratoconjunctivitis sicca, which is a drying of the conjunctiva and cornea due to inadequate tear volume or evaporation.

The ophthalmologist puts stitches at the corners of the eyelid openings, the palpebral fissures, to narrow the area and to lessen corneal exposure to air. This outpatient procedure is done under local anesthetic. If the condition improves, the eyelids can be surgically separated.

Taste

Sensation involving the perception of flavors.

Taste is one of the five senses and is characterized by the ability to respond to molecules that dissolve in the mouth cavity. Smell is the sense that detects airborne molecules. People identify taste with taste receptor cells that combine inside the taste buds. Each taste bud has a pore that is exposed to the surface of the tongue, allowing molecules entering the mouth to make contact with receptor cells. The four primary tastes are sweet, salty, sour, and bitter. Many different flavors are identified through the blending of both the sense of taste and smell. It is because of the blending of the senses of taste and smell that individuals with stuffed noses are not only unable to smell, but in addition, are unable to taste. Furthermore, a food's appearance and temperature can affect its taste.

How Taste Works. There are 10,000 taste buds on the tongue, palate, and throat, whose function is to determine taste. The taste buds are grouped together into papillae. Each taste bud contains taste cells representing all four taste sensations (bitter, salty, sour, and sweet). Chemicals in the food dissolve in the saliva and permeate the papillae on the surface of the tongue. The chemicals stimulate the hairs

on the receptor cell, which transmit a signal along the sensory nerves to the brain.

Different nerves may respond differently to the same foods. The nerves that serve the taste buds join at the back part of the brain stem. The taste signals are separated according to the nerve and taste. Taste signals travel to the thalamus then to the cerebral cortex of the brain. After the brain interprets the information, taste is perceived. The taste bud receptor cells are continuously replaced. They develop from the skin encompassing the taste buds. Approximately fifty percent of the receptor cells are replaced every ten days.

The taste system, though not highly developed, does allow an individual to recognize food and choose what one likes and dislikes. Often, the ability to taste deteriorates with age; in some cases, this can result in malnourishment.

LOSS OF TASTE

The most common cause of loss of taste is a cold, sinus infection, or other infection affecting the nose and throat, which blocks the sense of smell. Eating something hot can temporarily damage the taste buds, and the taste buds gradually decrease in number as a person ages.

Anything that dries out the mouth, such as damage to the salivary glands or use of drugs that have dry mouth as a side effect, can also cause a loss of taste, as saliva is necessary for the taste buds to work. Mouth cancer and radiation treatment for mouth cancer often damage the taste buds or salivary glands. Damage to the nerves from the tongue to the brain, such as from brain injury, or can also cause a loss of taste. A related condition, dysgeusia, is a distortion of taste. In some psychiatric disorders there may be a hallucination of taste.

If the loss of taste is caused by a cold or infection, treatment of that condition should restore taste. If a drug side effect is the cause, removal of the drug should restore the sensation. If the mouth is chronically dry, sucking on hard candy may help the mouth maintain a necessary amount of saliva. *See also* SMELL *and* TONGUE.

Tattooing

The practice of creating designs on the body by introducing pigment through a break in the skin.

Tattooing is the practice of drawing permanent designs, symbols, or marks on the body by inserting pigment under the skin. The designs range from simple, monochromatic marks to complex, multicolored marks that may cover large areas of the body surface.

Incidence. Tattooing has long been practiced in societies throughout the world. The oldest tattoos date from 3300 bce, in the form of simple marks discovered on a mummified human body. Today, tattooing is practiced by people from all cultures and in countless styles.

Methods. The implement used to tattoo the body varies from a needle coated with soot used in Siberia to a rack-like utensil used in Malaysia to prick the skin. In the United States, tattooing is performed with a small machine consisting of one or more needles connected to tubes filled with dye. The needles inject dye between the layers of the skin. The procedure is sometimes very painful, and usually takes about seven to ten days to heal.

Health Risks. Some people have an allergic reaction to the pigments used in tattooing. Also, if unsanitary equipment is used, the tattoo recipient risks contracting an infection from a blood-borne virus, such as hepatitis B or HIV. Under sterile conditions, however, the risk of blood-borne viral infection is extremely low.

Tattoo Removal. Years ago, tattoo removal could leave a disfiguring scar. The methods of removal included an abrasive chemical peel, freezing, or a skin graft. Today, however, lasers are used that leave no bleeding, blisters, or scars when applied carefully.

> *Background material on tattooing may be found in* SKIN. *For further reading, see* NEEDLE *and* SCAR. *Related information on complications of tattooing is contained in* ALLERGY; BLEEDING; BLISTERING; HEPATITIS; HIV; INFECTION; LASER SURGERY; SKIN GRAFT; *and* SKIN PEELING.

Tay-Sachs Disease

An inherited disorder that results in progressive mental and motor deterioration.

Tay-Sachs disease affects Ashkenazic (Eastern European) Jews 100 times more often than the general population. It is caused by an autosomal recessive gene; thus, if both parents are carriers, each child has a 25 percent chance of having the disease.

Tay-Sachs is caused by an enzyme deficiency for hexosaminidase A. This results in poor responsiveness and low muscle tone, as well as atrophy of the optic nerve.

Symptoms. The first symptoms begin to appear by age six to 12 months. They include apathy, poor responsiveness, muscle weakness and atrophy, loss of vision, and eventual paralysis. Children with the disorder usually die by age five.

Treatment. There is no way of halting the progression of the disease. Couples of Ashkenazic descent are urged to undergo genetic screening. *See also* INHERITANCE.

T-Cell

A type of lymphocyte, or white blood cell, that is produced in the bone marrow and matures in the thymus gland.

When an antigen (foreign protein) is detected in the body, specific lymphocytes (a type of white blood cell) become activated, or sensitized. They increase in size and then divide rapidly to form hundreds of cells. T- cells are one type of cell that is produced. Each variety of T-cell is capable of responding to a particular type of antigen.

T-cells are involved in immune response. There many different types of T- cells. Killer T-cells destroy host-cells that are infected by viruses. Helper T-cells enhance immune responses. Suppressor T-cells inhibit defenses several weeks after the infection is over. After the antigen is destroyed, a few T-cells will remain in the lymph nodes as memory cells in the event that the antigen is discovered again. This is called acquired immunity. *See also* IMMUNITY.

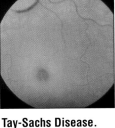

Tay-Sachs Disease. Tay-Sachs disease is a recessive disorder that affects the nervous system. A cherry-red spot appears in the eye (above), usually resulting in a loss of vision.

Tears

Secretion of the lacrimal glands.

Tears are the fluid produced by the lacrimal glands, in order to keep the eye moist, wash away debris, and express emotion. There are three layers of tears over the eyes: mucous film produced by the conjunctiva, which is the covering over the white of the eye and inside of the eyelid; a layer of salty water produced by the lacrimal glands, and an exterior, more oily layer produced by the meibomian glands.

An excessive amount of tears is known as watery eye; lack of tears is called keratoconjunctivitis sicca. *See also* EYE; LACRIMAL APPARATUS; TEARS; *and* WATERY EYE .

Tears, Artificial

Sterile solutions of water and other compounds, possibly with a preservative, that put a film of lubrication on the surface of the eyes.

Dry-eye syndrome can be caused by low humidity in the environment, by certain medications or as a result of hormone changes during menopause. Artificial tears are available without a prescription and work very well in most situations. They come in small compressible plastic bottles. To apply, the lower lid of the eye is pulled down, forming a pocket, and one or two drops are squeezed out of the bottle. *See* EYE DROPS.

Technetium

A gamma-emitting radionuclide used in medical imaging.

Radionuclides are radioactive agents used for diagnostic imaging. Technetium is a metallic element. It has a radioactive isotope technetium-99 that is used in a variety of radionuclide scanning techniques. It may be given by mouth, injected, or placed in the eye or bladder. Technetium then follows the course of the blood flow, becoming absorbed by bone or tissue under study. The emission of gamma particles is moni-

tored with a device known as a gamma camera. These radio emissions are converted into a detailed image, used for diagnosis.

Technetium may be used to diagnose cancerous tissue (malignancy), image the gallbladder for inflammation, assess the functioning of biliary ducts, image and visualize the heart, examine disorders of the digestive tract, and for bone and heart imaging. *See also* BILIARY SYSTEM; BILIARY DUCTS; BONE; BONE IMAGING; GALLBLADDER; GALLBLADDER, DISORDERS OF, GASTROINTESTINAL TRACT; HEART; HEART IMAGING; LIVER; LIVER IMAGING; RADIONUCLIDE SCANNING; *and* SPLEEN.

Teeth

Plural of tooth

The hard, bone-like structures in the mouth that are used for biting and chewing.

Adults normally have about 32 teeth—16 in each jaw—that are used to bite, chew, and grind food, marking the beginning of the digestive process. Teeth also play an important role in maintaining the contour of the face and in the appearance of a person, so that good care of teeth is an important personal health activity that must be impressed upon and taught to people from early childhood.

Teeth.
The adult mouth (right) usually contains 32 teeth. There are four types of teeth: incisors, to cut food; canines, to tear food; premolars, to begin the chewing and grinding of food; and molars, to complete the chewing of food, thus preparing it for digestion.

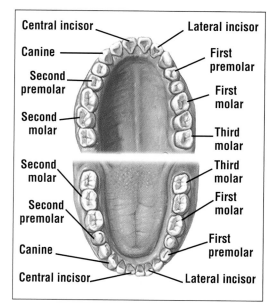

Central incisor — Lateral incisor
Canine — First premolar
Second premolar — First molar
Second molar — Third molar
Second molar — Third molar
Second premolar — First molar
Canine — First premolar
Central incisor — Lateral incisor

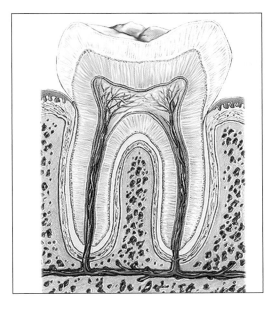

Types of Teeth. There are four basic types of teeth in the adult mouth. At the front of the mouth are the incisors—sharp, chisel-like teeth (four upper and four lower) that cut food and hold it in place. In the normal mouth, the upper incisors overlap the lower incisors slightly when the jaws are closed. Behind the incisors are the canine teeth—larger, pointed teeth (two upper and two lower, on either side of the mouth) with deep roots that tear food and reduce it to manageable size for chewing. The upper canines are known as eye teeth. Behind the canines are eight premolars (two upper, on either side of the mouth and the same in the lower jaw); also known as bicuspids because of their distinctive double edges (cusps), these teeth begin the grinding and chewing process. Babies do not have premolar teeth. In the back of each side of the mouth are the molars— wide, strong teeth that chew and grind food, preparing it for digestion further along the digestive tract. Most people have eight molars, though a set of four additional molar teeth "erupt" (emerge) at the back of the mouth in some people during adulthood, and are thus known as wisdom teeth.

Tooth Structure. The part of the tooth that rises above the gums (the gingiva) is called the crown and is covered by a thick layer of non-living tissue called enamel. Beneath the enamel is living ivory-like tissue known as dentin; this is supplied with blood from below and has nerve endings in it. The tooth narrows at the gumline in a portion of the tooth known as the neck; below is the root of the tooth, which anchors the tooth into the jawbone. Beneath the dentin is the pulp, the heart of the tooth, containing blood vessels and nerves. The root of the tooth is surrounded by a hard, sensitive tissue called the cementum, which protects the root and connects with the periodontal ligament, the tissue that anchors the tooth to the jawbone.

Tooth Care. The basic elements of tooth care (oral hygiene) involve cleaning teeth and between teeth to remove food particles that cause tooth decay, inflammation of the gums (gingivitis), and bad breath (halitosis); brushing teeth and flossing to remove plaque, the sticky substance that contains bacteria that eat away at teeth and infect the gums; regulating the consumption of foods that are heavy in sugar, which feeds the bacteria that attack teeth; and establishing a regimen of visits to a dentist or dental hygienist for regular cleaning and care of the teeth.

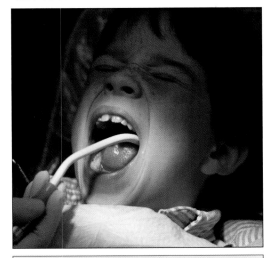

Basis anatomical information on teeth may be found in Cusp, Dental; Primary Teeth; *and* Pulp, Dental. *For additional information on tooth complications, see* Abrasion, Dental; Calculus, Dental; Fracture, Dental; *and* Gingivitis. *Related information is contained in* Flossing; Oral Hygiene; Root-Canal Treatment; *and* Toothbrushing.

Tooth.
A tooth (left) consists of enamel, dentin, pulp, and a root. A tooth can decay and become quite painful. Because of this, it is important to practice good oral hygiene and have regular dental checkups (below).

Teething

Pain children experience as teeth grow in.

Teething accompanies the normal growth of teeth through an infant's gums and is caused by pressure on the tissue in the mouth as the teeth come in. The first teeth usually come in fairly easily, and pain may be minimal. But when the molars begin to appear, at about one year of age, the teething becomes much more painful.

Most babies get their first tooth around six to eight months of age; but possibly as late as 12 to 14 months. Teething infants may have a small, pale bump under their gum. They may have increased drooling, bouts of chewing, a runny nose with clear mucus, red cheeks, some diarrhea, and they may be more fussy than usual. A baby who is teething may also have trouble sleeping, may refuse food, and may bite down on hard objects.

Remedies. To ease a baby's pain while teething, there are many conventional and unconventional methods of treatment. Doctors recommend that parents should give a teething baby hard objects to chew on, such as teething rings, cookies, or zwieback biscuits. Acetaminophen may help relieve symptoms, but a pediatrician should be consulted first. Cool or frozen objects, such as a teething ring, chilled apple, or an ice cold washcloth may relieve pain. Over-the-counter teething medications that contain a topical anesthetic may also help a teething baby feel better.

There are several homeopathic remedies and herbs that may help a teething baby. Clove oil may be applied to a baby's gums a few times a day in order to numb them. A few teaspoonfuls of chamomile tea every few hours may calm the baby. The tea can also be poured on a clean washcloth and put in the refrigerator, then given to a baby to suck on. Chamomile pellets (Chamomile 6c), placed under a baby's tongue or dissolved in water, may provide relief. Belladonna and alcohol preparations should be avoided. *See also* CHILD DEVELOPMENT *and* TEETH.

Telangiecstasia

A condition of enlarged capillaries most often noticed in the skin but also occasionally in internal organs, including the eyes, brain, and lungs.

Telangiectasia may be a sign of several diseases, most of them inherited as recessive genes. It may also have no known cause. Ataxia-telangiectasia is usually diagnosed in the second year of life. The signs are dizziness and lack of muscle coordination. Spiders of tiny red veins develop in the eyes and on the ears and cheeks. The child has frequent respiratory problems. The disease may include development of cancers of the blood and lymph system and leukemia. Most patients die in their teens or twenties.

Hereditary hemorrhagic telangiectasia is a circulatory abnormality in which arteries connect directly to veins rather than through the capillary system. The location of this short circuit is usually fragile and bleeds easily. It is most often found in the nose, face, hands, and mouth, but it is also seen in the stomach, intestines, brain, and lungs. Minor bleeding from the nose may be stopped if the mucous membranes are kept moist. Laser coagulation is recommended for more serious cases. Bleeding in the stomach or intestines may produce anemia. Lung telangiectasia may respond to embolization, in which a small balloon or coil is inserted to block the artery leading to the malformed blood vessel. *See also* ANEMIA *and* MUCOUS MEMBRANE.

Temperature

Measured through the use of a thermometer, body temperature is important in diagnosing various ailments. The average normal body temperature is 98.6° Fahrenheit.

When normal body temperature is elevated or depressed, illness of some type is usually present. For medical purposes, body temperature is generally measured using the Fahrenheit scale, a temperature system that assigns the freezing point of water a value of 32° and the boiling point, 212°. In this system, normal body temperature varies by a degree or two around 98.6˚. In non-English countries, the Celsius system is commonly used. On the Celsius scale, the freezing point of water is assigned the value 0˚, with the boiling point at 100˚. Normal body temperature is estimated to be around 37˚.

Testing

Taking temperature using a thermometer, is a simple, painless procedure, carried out in a matter of minutes. The thermometer, after sterilization, is placed in the mouth or alternately inserted into the rectum. Normal body temperature hovers around 98.6 degrees Fahrenheit. Temperature measurement may be used to diagnose illness as well as chart the progress of recovery. Common illnesses, particularly influenza, typically produce elevated temperature or fever. Should this fever rise above 102 degrees, it is advised that steps be taken to reduce it, often with aspirin and ice packs. Subnormal values are also symptomatic of disease; and in severe cases, the body temperature must be artificially raised through hot baths or other methods.

Traditional thermometers consist of a fine glass tube filled with liquid, usually mercury. Such thermometers work on the principle that changing temperatures proportionally effect the volume of liquids. Hence, mercury will expand with rising temperature, along the length of the glass tubing that has been calibrated so that precise temperature may be read. The thermometer should always be thoroughly cleaned before use and disinfected by wiping the surface with alcohol. It may then be placed under the tongue for several minutes, in order to register correctly. An alternate technique is to measure body temperature rectally, a procedure often used with children.

Elevation of normal body temperature indicates that the natural defense mechanism used by the body to combat illness is in effect. In extreme cases of acute infection such as pneumonia, meningitis, scarlet fever, typhoid, typhus, or small pox, temperature may rise to 106˚ Fahrenheit. Subnormal temperatures may be due to hypothermia, though they may also be pro-

duced by disease, as in the case of cholera, where temperature may plummet to between 80 and 90˚. Seriously elevated or subnormal temperature must be treated to prevent brain damage and nervous system failure.

See DIAGNOSIS *and* TESTS, MEDICAL *for background information on temperature. For additional information, see* CELSIUS SCALE; FEVER; FAHRENHEIT SCALE; MERCURY; *and* THERMOMETER. *For further information on conditions mentioned in this article, see* HYPOTHERMIA; INFECTION; INFLUENZA; *and* PNEUMONIA.

Temporal Arteritis

Also called giant cell arteritis

Inflammation of the walls of the arteries that cross over the temple and scalp.

Temporal arteritis is considered an autoimmune reaction. It most often occurs in men over the age of 50, though only in rare instances. Often this disease appears with polymyalgia rheumatica, an inflammation of muscles in the neck, shoulders, and jaw muscles.

Symptoms. Symptoms include stiffness, muscle pain, fever, severe headaches, vision loss, fatigue, malaise, weight loss, depression, anemia, shaking, and sweating.

Treatment. Recommended medications include the corticosteroids and cytotoxic drugs. Treatment may also involve the removal and replacement of blood plasma, intravenous gamma globulin, and cyclosporin. Corticosteroids are usually prescribed at the first sign of this disease, as the risk of blindness exists. Medication may slowly be reduced over the course of one to two years.

While temporal arteritis is a chronic disorder, medications can successfully treat the symptoms and are effective in prevent serious vision problems. Mild cases are usually not life-threatening, however, severe cases can be permanently disabling. *See also* ARTERITIS; ARTERY; AUTOIMMUNE DISORDERS; BLINDNESS; CORTICOSTEROID DRUGS; GAMMA GLOBULIN; INFLAMMATION; *and* POLYMYALGIA RHEUMATICA.

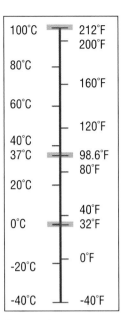

Temperature.
Above, the Celsius and Fahrenheit scales.

Temporal Lobe Epilepsy

A form of epilepsy in which seizures are limited to the temporal lobe of the brain.

Temporal lobe epilepsy usually occurs in adults. The seizures that are caused by the condition are typified by abnormal electrical discharges that are localized in the temporal lobe of the brain. These seizures are different from general epileptic seizures, such as the grand mal or the petite mal types, which are not localized seizures but are generalized throughout the brain. Most temporal lobe seizures are brief, but they can last anywhere from a few minutes to an hour.

Cause. Temporal lobe seizures are the consequence of an injury to the temporal lobe of the brain. The impairment may be caused by a brain or head injury, a brain tumor, a brain abscess, or a stroke. Temporal lobe seizures may adversely affect the senses of hearing, vision, smell, and taste; and they may affect the patient's memory.

Symptoms. Patients with temporal lobe seizures suffer from a reduced degree of consciousness. Most other seizures have muscular side effects. Temporal lobe seizures, on the other hand, create an unreal or illusionary experience. The patient encounters offensive hallucinations of smell or taste, as well as a sense of deja vú, a feeling of familiarity. These feelings are usually intense and specific, and seem real to the patient. Seizures may include grimacing, repetitive circling of head and eyes, and slurping or chewing movements. Temporal lobe seizures can later develop into a generalized grand mal seizure.

Treatment. Temporal lobe seizures are only brought to the attention of a medical professional if the condition becomes painful. Drug treatment for temporal lobe epilepsy is similar to that for general epilepsy, and consists of anticonvulsant medications. A surgical procedure to remove a section of the temporal lobe (lobectomy) is performed only if drug therapy fails. *See also* Anticonvulsant Drugs; Brain; Epilepsy; *and* Seizures.

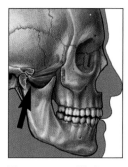

Temporomandibular Joint Syndrome. TMJ is a pain or discomfort in the temporomandibular joint (above). The condition is usually caused by spasms and tension in the muscle surrounding the joint.

Resources on Epilepsy
Berkow, Robert, and Andrew J. Fletcher, *Living Well with Epilepsy* (1992); Kandel, Eric R., et al., Principles of Neural Science (1991); Sanes, Dan Harvey, et al., Development of the Nervous System (2000); Epilepsy Foundation, Tel. (800) EFA-1000, Online: www.efa.org; Muscular Dystrophy Association of America, Tel. (800) 572-1717, Online: www.md-ausa.org; American Academy of Neurology, Tel. (651) 695-1940, Online: www.aan.com; Epilepsy Foundation, Tel. (800) EFA-1000, Online: www.efa.org; Epilepsy Institute, Tel. (212) 677-8550; American Board of Neurological Surgery, Tel. (713) 790-6015, Online: www.abns.org; www.med.cornell.edu/neuro/.

Temporomandibular Joint Syndrome

Discomfort affecting the head, jaw, and face, resulting from improperly functioning jaw joints.

Pain in the jaw area is referred to as temporomandibular joint syndrome, or myofascial pain dysfunction. The temporomandibular joints are the points where the temporal bone of the skull connects to the lower jaw or mandible. The ligaments, tendons, and muscles support the movement of the jaw. Since human beings eat and speak with a moving jaw, they require a sophisticated lower jaw that is connected to the temporal bones of the skull.

Incidence. The greatest incidence of temporomandibular joint syndrome is among women between the ages of 20 and 40. Men are four times less likely than women to complain of TMJ, and the condition is very seldom found in children.

Cause. Spasms of the chewing muscles are the most frequent cause of temporomandibular joint syndrome. The condition is often caused by a combination of muscle tension and jaw-related joint problems. In some instances, there can be a psychological aspect to the condition as well.

Symptoms of temporomandibular joint syndrome include persistent headaches; pain in the area near the ears, experienced particularly upon awakening; and continuous pain in the muscles on one or both sides of the face. Other symptoms of the condition may include a cracking or popping sensation when opening the mouth to chew or to yawn, a locking or sticking of the jaws, or trouble opening the mouth.

Diagnosis. Dentists can diagnose the syndrome based upon either a physical examination or an x-ray after dye is injected into the joint (an arthogram). They may also use electromyography, a test that measures muscle activity with electrodes, in order to study the facial muscles.

Treatment. Temporomandibular joint syndrome is usually a temporary condition that rectifies itself without treatment. Symptoms can be eased with over-the-counter remedies. The condition usually improves quickly with rest and painkillers. In some cases, individuals perceive chronic pain that radiates through the face and around the neck and shoulders; this pain may result from other disorders. If there is constant pain, medical attention is necessary. Although the syndrome begins as a functional disorder, it can develop into a condition in which there are changes in the joints or muscles used for chewing. *See* JAW.

Tenderness

A pain or hypersensitivity in an area of the body.

Tenderness can be experienced when pressure is applied to an area of the body, either during a routine physical examination (medical palpation) or in the course of daily interactions. Tenderness is most often accompanied by swelling, redness, and warmth of the affected area. Tenderness is usually a result of an underlying inflammation in the body. For example, arthritis, an inflammation of the joints, produces tenderness and sensitivity of the affected joints. Similarly, appendicitis, an inflammation of the appendix, produces tenderness and soreness in the abdominal cavity.

Tendolysis

Surgery to free a tendon from adhesions.

Fibrous bands known as adhesions may develop around tendons, inhibiting their free movement. Adhesions often result from a condition known as tenosynovitis, an inflammation of the tendon sheath's inner lining. Tendolysis is a surgical procedure that frees tendons of these fibrous bands. The surgeon makes an incision through the skin and into the tendon, parting the tendon's outer sheath. The adhesions are cut away from the surface of the tendon. The incisions in the tendon sheath and the skin are then stitched closed. Adhesions sometimes re-form following tendolysis, causing symptoms of tenosynovitis to recur.

Tendon

Flexible cords, consisting of collagen, that join muscle to bone or muscle to muscle.

Tendons consist of clusters of a fibrous protein, called collagen. Larger tendons may contain nerves and some may even be bundled with blood vessels. Tendons in the hands, feet, and wrists are aided by fluid that acts as a lubricant and prevents friction. Tendons are very durable, strong, and flexible. Damage to them, however, can seriously affect the ability to move and function properly.

Tendonitis, an inflammation of a tendon that often follows an injury, is the most common tendon disorder. A rupture of the Achilles tendon, located at the calf, is a particularly devastating sports injury. Such an injury greatly affects a person's mobility and requires a lengthy period of recovery. Severe injuries may require tendon repair surgery to reconnect torn tendons. In some cases, this operation includes a tendon transfer, in which a tendon from one part of the body is transferred to an injured part in an effort to restore function.

Background information on the structure of a tendon is contained in COLLAGEN *and* NERVE. *For information on disorders, see* SOFT-TISSUE INJURY *and* TENDONITIS. *Related topics include* TENDON REPAIR *and* TENDON TRANSFER.

Tendon Repair

Surgery to repair damaged tendons.

Tendon repair surgery may be performed either to rejoin the cut or torn ends of an injured tendon, or to replace one that has suffered extensive damage. Ends can often be easily connected with simple suturing, just like mending a piece of cloth that has ripped. If, however, the ends are so widely separated that they cannot reach each other easily, a graft of a piece of another tendon may be necessary. Tendons for a graft are often taken from the foot. *See also* SOFT-TISSUE INJURIES; SUTURE; TENDON; TENDONITIS; *and* TENDON TRANSFER.

Tendon Transfer

Surgery in which tendons from one part of the body are transferred to another part in order to restore function.

Tendon transfer surgery involves the use of a healthy tendon of muscle to replace tendons of other muscles disabled by injury or disease. Frequently, tendons from the lower extremities will be transferred to replace upper extremity tendons required for fine control. Tendon transfer to treat hand disorders is common. Spinal cord injuries may leave victims quadriplegic, in which case tendon-transfer techniques are used to restore various degrees of upper-body functioning by removing tendons from paralyzed legs and spare arm muscles and transferring them to improve arm and hand function. *See also* TENDON.

Tendonitis

Condition in which a tendon becomes inflamed, usually because of injury.

Tendons are strands of fibrous tissue made of collagen and a few blood vessels. These strands connect muscles to bones. They are strong and flexible, but not elastic. Therefore, overstretching or small, repeated stresses on a tendon may cause it to become inflamed. Swimmers, golfers, baseball players, and tennis players may be prone to tendonitis in the arms or shoulders, while runners and soccer, football, and basketball players are more likely to have it in their legs or feet.

Symptoms of tendonitis usually include pain, tenderness, and in more extreme cases, restricted function of the muscle to which the affected tendon is attached. When an area is affected by tendonitis, the tendon also becomes more likely to rupture, so tendinitis should not be taken lightly. Treatment includes resting the affected area, application of ice, and anti-inflammatory drugs. Working to correct improper movement or motion mechanics may prevent reccurrence. *See* TENDON.

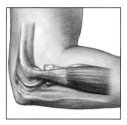

Tennis Elbow.
Tennis elbow is the term commonly used to describe an inflammation of the epicondyle (above), which often results from repetitive activities, such as tennis.

Tennis Elbow

Inflammation of the epicondyle.

The epicondyles are the two bony prominences at the end of the humerus, or upper arm bone. Tendons connect various muscles to either of the epicondyles, so repeated tugging at the point where the tendons attach can cause them to become inflamed. The muscles that attach to the outer epicondyle are responsible for straightening the fingers and wrist, so people who participate in activities such as tennis or other racket sports, in which this action constantly occurs, are likely to suffer from tennis elbow, the common term for epicondylitis. The muscles attached to the inner epicondyle bend the fingers and wrist; inflammation of that area is known as golfer's elbow. Of course many other non-tennis activities, such as gardening or painting, may cause the condition as well.

Symptoms of tennis elbow include pain and tenderness on the inner part of the forearm from the elbow to the wrist. Treatment usually consists of rest for the arm, the application of ice packs, and either painkillers or anti-inflammatory drugs. Re-evaluating and correcting faulty motion or mechanics may prevent the condition from occurring in the future. *See* INFLAMMATION.

Tenosynovitis

Inflammation of the synovial sheath of a tendon.

Tendons are the tissues that connect muscle to muscle, or bone to muscle. The tendons in the hands, wrists, and feet are covered by a fibrous capsule, known as the synovial sheath. These body parts require extra protection because of their ability to move in many directions, so the synovial sheath produces a fluid that keeps the area lubricated and prevents friction. Overuse of the tendon, or repetitive motions, however, can cause the synovial lining to become inflamed. Bacterial infection may also lead to inflammation. Tenosynovitis usually affects the hands and wrists.

Symptoms of tenosynovitis are pain, swelling, and tenderness over the affected tendons. The sound of the tendon moving (crepitus) may be audible. Treatment may include anti-inflammatory drugs or, in severe cases, an injection of a corticosteroid. The hand and wrist may be immobilized in a splint to prevent excessive movement. Antibiotics may be prescribed for tenosynovitis caused by infection. If untreated, or if it reoccurs frequently, tenosynovitis may lead to the buildup of adhesions between the tendon and sheath, which can restrict movement. In these cases, surgery may be required to remove the adhesions. *See also* INFECTION *and* TENDON.

Tenovaginitis

Condition in which the tendon's sheath becomes inflamed.

The tendons are fibrous cords that connect bone to muscle or muscle to muscle. Those that help to operate the hands, wrists, and feet require extra protection, due to their ability to move in a wide range of directions. Therefore, they are covered with a fibrous capsule known as the synovial sheath that works to keep the area lubricated, so as to prevent friction. When this sheath becomes inflamed, or thickened, it is known as tenovaginitis. The cause of tenovaginitis is currently unknown. *See also* TENDON.

Terminal Health Care

Medical or nursing care that is given to patients in the terminal, or final, stages of an illness.

Terminal health care is medical care given to people who are dying. Instead of trying to cure the patient's illness or prolong life, the aim of terminal health care is to make the patient as comfortable as possible and to sustain the quality of life. Terminal care may be given in the home, in a homelike setting, in a nursing home, or in a hospital. *See* AIDS; ALZHEIMER'S DISEASES; DEATH; DEPRESSION; ETHICS, MEDICAL; NURSING HOME; HOSPICE CARE; *and* HOSPITAL, TYPES OF.

Terrorism

The use of explosives or chemical or biological weapons against civilians for political ends.

The threat of terrorism, especially of bioterrorism—the use of biological or chemical agents as a terrorist weapon—has created a new set of health issues for the twenty-first century. Though the responsibility of dealing with acts of terrorism rests with public officials and agencies of government, there are still cautionary measures that individuals can take to protect themselves when terrorism is expected:

1. Be alert. Be aware of surroundings and note and report suspicious behavior or unattended packages. It is also important, however, that one does not become paranoid or unmindful of the rights and dignity of others. *See* EMERGENCY, FIRST STEPS.

2. Be prepared. When public agencies advise a medical procedure—taking antibiotics; being vaccinated; etc.—follow those instructions and note how members of your family will contact one another or meet in the event of an emergency. *See* ANTHRAX; INFECTIOUS DISEASE.

3. Be calm. Much of the harm terrorists seek to inflict is psychological, so it is important to stay calm in the face of terrorist acts and be mindful of the need to treat members of one's family and one's neighbors with particular consideration. *See* DEPRESSION; STRESS.

4. Be cooperative. During periods of alert, normal functions are curtailed in the interest of security, which will often create inconvenience: traffic will be more congested because of checkpoints; large buildings will be more difficult to enter; areas will be designated as off-limits. Cooperate with law-enforcement and emergency personnel and patiently follw their directives .

5. Be supportive. The agencies responsible for protecting the public will be under great pressure during periods of heightened terrorist activity. In the interest of health and safety, criticism and complaining should be tempered with consideration and patience. *See* PUBLIC HEALTH.

Testicular Feminization Syndrome

Also known as androgen resistance syndrome

Syndrome occuring when a male does not respond to male sex hormones and develops as a female.

Testicular feminization syndrome is caused by abnormal androgen receptors, meaning the organs were unable to properly receive the signals from the male hormones directing them during development.

A child with testicular feminization syndrome is genetically male, with the sex chromosomes XY, and undescended testes within the body. The external genitals appear female, however, and the child develops as a girl. At puberty, the child develops female secondary sex characteristics but does not menstruate. Generally, the condition is diagnosed after an adolescent fails to menstruate. *See also* CHROMOSOME.

Treatment. The testes are surgically removed, as they are at risk for developing cancer. The individual is sterile but can otherwise live normally as a woman.

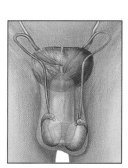

Testicles.
The testicles, above, are situated in the scrotum, outside the body. They are responsible for the production of sperm and testosterone.

Testis

One of the two male sex organs responsible for the production of sperm and testosterone.

When the male child is in the womb, the testes begin to form in the abdominal cavity. Prompted by hormones, the testes then begin to make their way through the inguinal canal before finally ending up in a pouch of skin called the scrotum shortly before birth. If this process fails to take place, the child is said to have undescended testes and must have the testes surgically lowered. Each one of the testes contains seminiferous tubules, which are responsible for sperm production. These tubes are connected to the vas deferens, which carry the sperm to the epididymis, where the sperm mature. The testes also contain cells that produce the male sex hormone, testosterone. *See also* REPRODUCTIVE SYSTEM, MALE; TESTOSTERONE.

Testis, Cancer of

Malignant tumor of the testis.

Cancer of the testis is the second most common malignancy among men ages 15 to 35, but it is usually curable. In more than 95 percent of cases, the cancer occurs in just one testis. The men at highest risk are those with a history of undescended testes (cryptorchidism), failure of one or both of the testes to descend from the pelvis. Men born with extra nipples also are at higher risk, as are those who have had hernias. Almost all cancers of the testis are seminomas, germinal tumors, which arise in the sperm-forming cells, but a few develop from other testicular tissue.

Symptoms. The most obvious symptom of cancer of the testis is a swelling of the testis, which is usually painless but sometimes causes pain or inflammation. There may be a feeling of heaviness in the lower abdomen. If the cancer is not diagnosed until it has spread beyond the testis, there may be pain in the abdomen and a persistent cough that brings up bloody sputum.

Diagnosis can include one or more tests to rule out other causes of testicular swelling. Among these tests are computerized tomography scans, magnetic resonance imaging scans, and ultrasound. Blood tests to determine the levels of hormones such as alpha fetoprotein, lactate-dehydrogenase, and human chorionic gonadotrophin may be performed, and a tissue sample may be taken for microscopic examination.

Treatment. Testicular cancers that are seminomas are highly curable if detected at an early stage. Orchiectomy, surgery to remove the affected testis, is often enough to affect a cure. Nearby lymph nodes may also be removed or will be given radiation therapy, and the surviving testis will also be given radiation therapy, even if there are no indications that the cancer has spread. Surgery for nonseminomas almost always involves removal of lymph nodes. If the cancer has progressed, removal of the testis will be followed by combination chemotherapy, which can involve several drugs given in different combinations. A follow-up is done even if the cancer is detected early, with periodic x-rays, blood tests, and perhaps computerized tomography scans over the following two years, when relapses are most common. *See also* TESTIS.

Testicular Cancer and Infertility

For younger men with cancer of the testis, maintenance of fertility is an important issue. Surgery can affect sexual performance, as can platinum-containing cancer drugs. Men about to undergo treatment are advised to consult their physicians about banking sperm for future attempts at fatherhood.

Testis, Pain in the

Injury or damage to the testis, causing discomfort.

The testis can become painful even if only a mild jolt or bruise is sustained. Although there is usually no permanent damage, a direct blow to the testis can produce a laceration along the testicular wall. If this is the case, the pain may be excruciating and a procedure may be required to drain the blood that has collected in the testis.

Pain in the testis can be caused by injury to the genital area or by inflammation (orchitis) that is caused by infection. Torsion, the rotation or twisting of the testis, causes the blood vessels to become kinked, cutting off all blood flow to the testis and causing permanent damage if left untreated. On occasion, pain that seems to come from the testis is actually the result of a kidney stone situated in the ureter.

Physicians cannot always determine the cause of pain in the testis. In many of these cases, the pain passes without formal treatment. *See also* CALCULUS *and* TESTIS.

Testis, Retractile

A phenomenon, seen most often in young boys, in which the testes are drawn into the abdominal cavity, usually for protective purposes.

Testes form in the abdomen and do not descend into the scrotum until shortly before birth. Undescended testes occur in a small percentage of boys. They may eventually descend on their own, but, in some cases, may require medical or surgical intervention. In order to produce viable sperm, the testes require a slightly lower temperature and therefore must be situated outside of the abdominal cavity.

Once permanently positioned in the scrotum, the testes are still capable of movement. When the outside temperature is lowered, the spermatic cords on which the testes are suspended move them upward, nearer the body where it is warmer. When the outside temperature is increased, the testes are lowered so they are further away.

For protective purposes, the testes may even be drawn up into the abdominal cavity, a condition known as retractile testis. This is normal in young boys but usually does not occur after puberty. Parents may be concerned that their son's testes are undescended because one or both appear to be temporarily "missing;" if the testes have previously been observed in the scrotum, they are not undescended. *See also* TESTIS.

Testis, Swollen

Swelling in the scrotum.

Swollen testes result from a number of conditions, including epidymitis, a scrotal tumor, hydrocele, variocele, and orchitis.

Epidymitis is an inflammation of the epididymis, the coiled tube that transports sperm from the testicles to the vas deferens. It is usually caused by a bacterial infection and is treated with antibiotics.

Scrotal mass is the term for swelling in the scrotum. It may be due to injury, a cyst, or a tumor. Growths within the testicles are usually malignant, whereas elsewhere in the scrotum they are often benign. Surgery is required to remove a tumor.

Hydrocele. A hydrocele is an accumulation of fluid in the sheath surrounding the testis. Normally, only a small amount of fluid is located there for the purposes of lubrication. An excess amount may accumulate if too much fluid is being produced or if it is not being absorbed properly. Hydroceles are relatively common and may occur at any age, though they are more likely to develop in older men. Treatment is usually not required unless the patient is experiencing a great deal of discomfort. In that event, excess fluid may be removed with a needle. However, the condition may recur.

Varioceles are basically varicose veins in the scrotum. It is not serious but may be a cause of infertility. Corrective surgery can be done on an outpatient basis.

Orchitis, an inflammation of the testis, is most commonly caused by mumps, but may also be a result of a prostate infection. Orchitis can permanently damage the testes and result in infertility. Antibiotics are prescribed if bacterial infection has caused the condition. For a viral cause, medication is prescribed to relieve the pain. *See* TESTIS.

Testis, Torsion of

A painful condition in which the testis twists, cutting off its blood supply.

Within the scrotum, each testis or testicle is attached to a spermatic cord, which contains the blood vessels that supply the testicle. Sometimes the testicle twists upon its cord, cutting off the blood supply and producing sudden severe pain, a condition known as testicular torsion.

Causes. Testicular torsion can occur after strenuous physical activity, but often there is no apparent cause. It is a relatively uncommon condition. It can occur at any age, although it is most often seen in young children or those nearing puberty.

Symptoms of testicular torsion also include nausea, faintness, and vomiting. These same symptoms can be caused by an inflammation in the scrotum. To distinguish between them, the doctor lifts the painful testicle. In the event of testicular torsion, the pain will increase.

Treatment. The twisted cord may spontaneously right itself without any intervention. However, prompt surgical correction is recommended, as the lack of blood supply may cause the testicle to atrophy. The

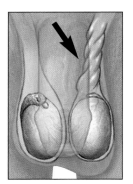

Torsion of Testicles. Testicular torsion is relatively rare condition which sometimes occurs following strenuous activities. It is the term used to describe a twisting of the testis, causing the blood supply to be cut off.

surgeon untwists the cord and anchors the testicles in their normal position to prevent recurrence of the problem. *See* TESTIS.

Testis, Undescended

Also known as cryptorchidism

A condition in which one or both testes remain inside the abdomen after birth.

During pregnancy, the testes of a male fetus develop inside the abdomen. Shortly before birth, they descend into their permanent place in the scrotum, a small sac located below the penis. Viable sperm require a cooler temperature, which is why the testes do not remain in the abdomen. However, a small number of males are born with one or both testes undescended. Usually, the testes will move into the scrotum on their own; sometimes, medical intervention is necessary. Any testes that remain in the abdomen by age five may be infertile.

Treatment. Hormone therapy is administered to cause the testis to descend. If necessary, the testis can be moved surgically. This operation is usually performed when a boy is a year old. A child with undescended testes is more likely to develop cancer later in life. *See* TESTIS *and* TESTIS, RETRACTILE.

Testosterone

Primary male sex hormone.

The androgen hormones provide the male with secondary sexual characteristics during puberty, such as a deepened voice, increased muscle mass, and body hair. Testosterone is the most important of these. It may be found in the testes in males, and is produced in very small amounts in the ovaries of the female. *See also* HORMONE.

Synthetic forms of testosterone may be used in cases where a boy is not experiencing puberty at the normal age, usually because of a disorder in the testes or pituitary gland. Females who use it may experience virilism, such as increased facial and body hair, muscle mass, acne and increased libido. *See* SPORTS, UNLAWFULL DRUGS AND.

Tests, Medical

Any diagnostic procedures designed to confirm or negate the presence of disorder or disease.

Medical tests help the physician to properly analyze the patient's state of health, diagnose illness, or chart the progress of therapy. Such tests range from very simple, requiring no special equipment, to extremely sophisticated. Further, tests may be used when symptoms are present and a particular illness is suspected or may be used to screen for possible disorders where no symptoms exist. Test results may be inconclusive or unequivocal, and testing can involve widely varying degrees of risk to the patient, depending on the procedure and patient's age, sex, and medical history. Medical testing continues to undergo expansion and refinement. It remains a cornerstone of modern diagnosis.

Testing

A thorough understanding of the medical tests requested by a physician often reduces the anxiety that patients experience. The doctor should explain the procedure in detail, as well as the information provided by the test. It is essential for the doctor to be fully acquainted with the patient's medical history before testing. New techniques in all phases of testing have greatly served to decrease risk and discomfort, while improving the accuracy of results.

General Physical Exam. Many medical tests are carried out routinely, for example as part of a physical examination. Here, the purpose will be to assess overall health as well as check for obvious signs of illness or abnormality. In addition to examining the patient's medical history, and listening to any specific medical complaints, the physician will carry out a number of standard tests, which will vary somewhat in number and kind depending on the doctor and patient specifics. The doctor will begin by visually inspecting the patient, first generally, then by specific systems of the body. In addition to measurements of height, weight, body temperature, blood pressure, pulse and respiration, a standard physical will involve auscultation—listening to the activity of the heart, blood vessels, lungs, and abdomen through a stethoscope. The doctor may also test various reflexes, hearing, and eyesight. A sample of blood will often be taken and subjected to a standard workup.

Blood Workup. A complete blood count (CBC) will test for the number of red blood cells, white blood cells, and platelets in a given unit of blood. Blood supplies a wealth of information concerning health, and disease. The CBC, one of innumerable blood tests, may be used to diagnose anemias and some cancers, including leukemia and lymphomas, and evaluate blood loss and response to infection. Today, high-speed automation allows clinical laboratories to perform thousands of tests per minute on blood. Hematologists—those who study blood—will also examine samples microscopically, identifying abnormal blood cells and possible blood disorders, infections, and antibodies to pathogens, including viruses. Blood tests may be used to identify genetic disorders, which can lead to disease or be passed to offspring.

Other body fluids are also the focus of medical tests. Urinalysis is used to test the acidity, glucose level, blood, protein, and white blood cell count of urine. Other features of urine may suggest infection, as well as diabetes or liver abnormality. Pleural fluid from the lungs may be used to diagnose tuberculosis, lung abscess, pancreatitis, bacterial or fungal infection, and other pulmonary conditions. Sputum, another fluid produced in the lungs—commonly called phlegm, is also used to diagnose tuberculosis (TB) and monitor ongoing progress in TB patients. Cerebrospinal fluid (CSF) is fluid in the spine that is sampled through a procedure known as a lumbar puncture, or spinal tap. A number of serious infectious diseases may be diagnosed by this method, including various forms of bacterial meningitis. Vaginal fluids may be swabbed and tested for bacterial and viral infection, and semen examined for sperm count and other features useful in fertility analysis. Amniotic fluid, originating in the cushioned sac around a developing fetus, is extracted during a test known as amniocentesis and allows for diagnosis of abnormality in the fetus.

Diagnostic Imaging. A number of techniques allow the physician to directly observe the body's interior, often with enormous clarity and precision. The specific imaging technique requested by the physician will be the one posing the least risk while providing the most useful information for diagnosis. The most common imaging technique is the x-ray. It is used to diagnose conditions as varied as bone fractures, abnormal tissue in the lungs, or dental caries and abscesses. X-rays rely on the differing absorption rates of the high speed x-radiation into differing bone or tissue density (as well as depicting fat, water, muscle, and air). Bone will appear as white in the image, with grayer areas showing soft tissue. Diseased tissue may appear different than its normal counterpart, a fact useful in the x-ray diagnoses of pneumonia, emphysema, lung cancer, and other diseases.

CAT scan (also known as computerized axial tomography or CT scan) is a more recent and sophisticated x-ray technique. It uses computers to compose an image from repeated x-ray samplings gathered from an apparatus that rotates 180 degrees around the body. A fine radiographic beam scans between 100 and 1,200 points to compose an image. Radiation is recorded by detectors opposite the x-ray source, which along with the detectors, rotates as it scans. The resultant x-ray data is processed by computer into a thin slice, or tomogram, of stunning clarity. CAT scanning provides a thousandfold increase in resolution over conventional x-ray, and is capable of identifying lesions of less than two mm diameter.

Ultrasound or ultrasonography uses high frequency sound to image organs or tissues in the body. The echo of sound waves from structures of differing densities and depths is translated into an image. Two of the most common uses of ultrasound are for studies of the heart and during pregnancy. Echocardiography is used to visualize the size, shape, condition, and press-

ures associated with the heart and to study cardiac metabolism. Several forms of ultrasonography enable the cardiologist to see all cardiac valves, dimensions of each ventricle, and the left atrium.

Like x-ray and CAT, ultrasound scanning is a nonsurgical (noninvasive) technique. But unlike x-ray and CAT, it is free of the potentially harmful effects of ionizing radiation, which is capable of damaging or destroying healthy cells and tissues. This makes ultrasound a particularly desirable form of imaging, especially for studies of the developing fetus.

Risk Factors

Many medical tests involve some risk, although, for many of the most common (blood tests, noninvasive imaging, and standard physical tests), the risk is insignificant. It has long been recognized that ionizing radiation, such as x-ray, is hazardous to cells and tissues. As imaging techniques have evolved, steps have been taken to reduce the patient's dose of radiation. Of the techniques described above, CAT scanning—with its multiple x-rays—often delivers the largest dose. MRI and ultrasound, by contrast, are completely free of such dangers.

MRI, or magnetic resonance imaging, is a recent and powerful advance in imaging technology, using radiofrequency magnetic fields that act on the hydrogen ions (protons) contained in human cells. Cell nuclei placed in a magnetic field are induced to "resonate," emitting a signal, which a computer reassembles into an extremely high resolution picture. Like ultrasound, MRI is free of harmful radiation and thoroughly noninvasive. The technique, though expensive, has proven invaluable, particularly in brain imaging, allowing the physician to precisely diagnose small tumors, abscesses, nerve damage, swelling, bleeding, and tissue lesions.

Radionuclide scanning involves the injection of a radioactive tracer substance. The course of this radioactive isotope is followed by means of a gamma camera, which detects and records the particle emissions from the tracer substance. These emissions in turn, are translated into an image. Different tracers are taken up selectively by different tissues and structures, and are used to image different areas of the body.

PET, or positron emission tomography, combines radionuclide and computerized tomography techniques, though it is considerably more sensitive than either. The radionuclide tracer carries a very short-lived radioactive particle known as a positron. The radioactivity follows the course of the blood flow, and is recorded by a detector. Metabolism, particularly cerebral and cardiac, may be visualized in real time. Abnormal portraits of cerebral metabolism recorded by PET may be diagnostic of AIDS, dementia, epilepsy, Parkinson's disease, and other disorders.

Tissue testing. Where noninvasive techniques are inadequate, the physician may need to sample living tissue for the presence of disease. This is accomplished through some form of biopsy. Tissue may be extracted from the surface or interior of the body. Generally only a small portion of tissue is required, and may be extracted using a slender biopsy needle, before being sent for laboratory analysis. Tissue may also be sampled during exploratory surgery.

Screening Tests

A number of tests are recommended to ensure good health later in life. Women over 50 are especially vulnerable to various cancers. A yearly mammogram and pap smear are strongly advised. Routine measurements of cardiac health for men and women are also encouraged. Men over the age of 50 are at increased risk for prostate cancer. Colon cancer may affect both men and women and is best detected by colonoscopy. They should be examined by a physician who specializes in disorders of the anus and rectum (proctologist) and who may recommend special viewing scopes, or such tests as sigmoidoscopy, to aid in diagnosis.

Screening tests are used to monitor disease rates in the general population as well as in the individual. Such tests may be recommended for a specific group, for example, those exposed to an environmental disease-causing substance (pathogen), or who engage in high risk behaviors, i.e., smoking or promiscuous, unprotected sexual activity. Screening may be more generally recommended, particularly for those of a certain age. Screening tests include the mammogram for women between the ages of 50 and 79, prostate tests for men over 50, and eye examinations for drivers. Screening is also carried out on a widespread basis to test a population for the prevalence of disease. Such tests have contributed invaluable data to the study of widespread, contagious disease (epidemiology).

Alternatives

In selecting medical tests, the doctor hopes to strike a balance between the least painful, invasive, and expensive test and the greatest amount of useful diagnostic information gleaned from testing. When the results of a particular medical test prove inconclusive, the doctor may combine results of other tests, always considering the margin of error and specifics of each case. Home tests have proven a useful alternative in some cases, often providing early warning for disorders requiring further medical attention.

Home Tests. While most medical testing is performed either in a doctor's office or hospital, many tests may now be performed by the patient at home. Though the accuracy of such tests is usually lower than the accuracy of those performed in a medical setting by a physician, high rates of accuracy and simple procedures, coupled with convenience, have made many such tests, particularly for pregnancy, routine. Controversy surrounds home tests such as those for AIDS, as the possibility of mistakes and lack of personal follow-up after results diminish their safety and effectiveness.

For types of medical tests see BLOOD TESTS; CULTURE; IMAGING TECHNIQUES; PREGNANCY TESTS; SCREENING TESTS AND URINALYSIS. *For further reading on specific tests see* AMNIOCENTISIS; BIOPSY; BLOOD COUNT; BLOOD PRESSURE; BLOOD SMEAR; BONE IMAGING; BRONCHOSCOPY; CALORIMETRY; CAT SCAN; CYSTOSCOPY; ECHOCARDIOGRAPHY; ELECTROCARDIOGRAM; EMG; ELISA TEST; ENDOSCOPY MRI; MAMMOGRAM; PET SCAN; RADIATION; RADIONUCLIDE SCANNING; SIGMOIDOSCOPY; SEMEN ANALYSIS; SPUTUM; STETHOSCOPE; THYROID SCANNING; *and* X-RAY.

Resources on Medical Tests and Diagnostics
Cullinan, John Edward, *Illustrated Guide to X-Ray Techniques* (1980); Kee, Joyce LeFever, *Handbook of Laboratory and Diagnostic Tests with Nursing Implications* (1994); Nuland, Sherwin, *Doctors: The Biography of Medicine* (1995); Ravin, Carl E., ed., *Imaging and Invasive Radiology in the Intensive Care Unit* (1993); Segen, Joseph C., and Joseph Stauffer, *The Patient's Guide to Medical Tests* (1998); American Hospital Association, Tel. (800) 242-2626, Online: www.aha.org; The American Board of Radiology, Tel. (520) 790-2900, Online: www.theabr.org; American Healthcare Radiology Administrators, Online: www.ahra.org; www.ny-cornell.org/radiology/.

Tetanus

An infection of a wound with the spores of the bacterium *Clostridium tetani*.

Tetanus is caused by the bacterium *Clostridium tetani,* which has spores that can remain dormant for many years in the soil or the feces of animals. These spores can reactivate when they are lodged in an open wound.

Symptoms. As the *Clostridium tetani* bacteria multiply, they excrete a toxin that produces tight muscles in the jaw, face, neck, and back, as well as difficulty in breathing and swallowing. Muscle spasms are also a common symptom of tetanus. Because tense facial muscles are characteristic of tetanus, the disease is also called lockjaw. Tetanus can be fatal in the very young or very old. People who suffer severe burns are also at risk for contracting tetanus.

Prevention and Treatment. The tetanus vaccination is included in a series that also protects against diphtheria and pertussis (whooping cough). A booster shot is recommended every five to ten years and is especially recommended for anyone who has a wound and has not had a booster in the last five years. Thorough and deep cleansing of all wounds with soap and warm water is recommended. If the disease is contracted, tetanus immunoglobulin is administered to neutralize the toxin, combined with antibiotics to control the infection. *See also* ANTIBIOTIC DRUGS; IMMUNOGLOBULINS; INFECTIOUS DISEASES; *and* LOCKJAW.

Tetany

Spasms and contortions of the muscles, usually those in the hands and feet.

Tetany is a condition characterized by convulsive and seizure-like movements in the hands and feet. Occasionally, the face, the voice box (larynx), or the spinal muscles may be affected. At the onset of the disease the spasms are painless, but as the disease progresses they become increasingly agonizing and painful. *See also* SPASM.

Tetany is an indication of a biochemical irregularity in the body. It is usually caused by a reduction in the calcium level in the blood (hypocalcemia), due to an insufficient intake of vitamin D. It can also be the result of hyperventilation, or of a decrease in blood potassium levels (hypokalemia).

Tetracycline Drugs

Broad spectrum antibiotics prescribed for a number of bacterial infections.

A good alternative for people allergic to penicillin, the tetracyclines are given for upper respiratory infections, typhus fever, tick fevers, pneumonia, gonorrhea, and urinary tract infections. They should not be used during the last four months of pregnancy nor for children younger than eight. The full course of treatment must be followed when taking this drug, or relapse is likely. Tetracycline that is not fresh is toxic to the kidneys. Side effects include blood disorders, blurred vision, and headache. They should not be taken with antacids, calcium or iron supplements, or dairy products. *See also* ANTIBIOTIC DRUGS.

Tetrahydroaminoacridine

The first drug approved by the FDA to treat Alzheimer's disease.

In Alzheimer's disease, certain brain cells degenerate for unknown reasons. Normally, acetylcholine is generated by the nerve cells, released, and then broken down in a continuing process. In sufferers of Alzheimer's disease, the breakdown is more rapid than normal, and this is believed to account for the loss of memory.

Tetrahydroaminoacridine (trade name Tacrine) retards the breakdown of acetylcholine and, in some patients, improves memory. It does not stop the degeneration of brain cells, nor does it regenerate brain cells. Side effects include an increase in a liver enzyme, nausea, vomiting, diarrhea, abdominal pain, indigestion, and skin rash. *See also* ALZHEIMER'S DISEASE.

Tetralogy of Fallot

A congenital heart disease in which there are four structural defects of the heart.

The two most serious abnormalities occurring in tetralogy of Fallot are ventricular septal defect, in which there is an opening in the wall between the two ventricles, and pulmonary stenosis, an obstruction of blood flow from the right atrium to the lungs caused by a narrowing of the pulmonary valve. The other two are displacement of the aorta, the main artery from the heart, and right ventricular hypertrophy, enlargement of the right ventricle. This constellation of defects is seen in about 50 of every 100,000 newborns.

Because their blood is poorly supplied with oxygen, these are "blue babies." The condition is treated by surgery to repair the defects. Depending on the severity of the defects, surgery can be done shortly after birth or in the early childhood years, before the child begins school. Often, the first operation is done to improve blood flow to the lungs. Surgical repair of ventricular septal defect and pulmonary stenosis may be done in a single operation. While children born with tetralogy of Fallot require lifetime monitoring, long-term studies after surgery have found that more than 90 percent achieve good heart function into the adult years. *See also* CONGENITAL; HEART DISEASE; *and* SEPTAL DEFECT.

Thalamus

A mass of nerve cells located directly above the brain stem.

The thalamus appears as two walnut-sized bundles of nerve tissue. It functions as a relay center for sensory information from the various sense organs, such as the eyes, ears, and touch receptors. The thalamus then acts as a neurological filter, allowing only important information to enter the consciousness. It is also believed to play some role in the storage of long-term memory. *See also* BRAIN.

Thalassemia

Also known as cooley's anemia

An inherited abnormality of hemoglobin with life-threatening potential in severe cases.

Thalassemia is found most frequently among people of Italian, Greek, Middle Eastern, Southern Asian, and African descent. The condition is caused by an abnormality in hemoglobin molecules. The hemoglobin molecule is made up of two copies, each containing two proteins, hemoglobin A and hemoglobin B. A gene abnormality of hemoglobin A is referred to as alpha thalassemia; an abnormality of hemoglobin B is called beta thalassemia.

Symptoms. The symptoms are typical of anemia. They include dizziness, fatigue, shortness of breath, and jaundice. The symptoms are exacerbated by exertion or the lower oxygen content at high altitudes.

Beta thalassemia is by far the more severe form of this disease. The symptoms will become evident in the first year of life. The child will be listless and irritable, develop slowly, and often suffer from jaundice. If untreated, the child will have an enlarged spleen, liver, and heart. The bones may be thin and easily broken. The facial bones are distorted. Death can be caused by heart failure or infection.

Treatment. Frequent blood transfusions will help restore normal oxygen levels to the blood, and antibiotics help the immune system resist infection. Most of the anemia and other growth malformations can be prevented in this way. However, the frequent blood transfusions ultimately produce an excess of iron in the body that collects in the heart and liver. To counteract this problem, drugs that remove iron from the system are administered daily with a pump that forces the drug under the skin while the child is asleep. Bone marrow transplantation offers some hope as a potential cure for this disease; however, it requires a suitable donor and the procedure has risks. *See also* ANEMIA; BONE MARROW TRANSPLANT; HEMOGLOBIN; INHERITANCE; JAUNDICE; *and* TRANSPLANT SURGERY.

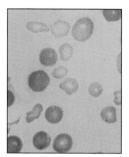

Thalassemia Cells. Thalassemia is a severe form of anemia, which is potentially fatal and extremely dangerous. Small, pale, and deformed red blood cells (above) are characteristic of the disease.

Thallium

An element whose radioisotope thallium-201 is used medically for radionuclide imaging of the heart muscle.

Thallium is a rare metallic element. An artificial radioactive isotope of the element, called thallium 201, is often used medically to evaluate blood flow through the heart muscle (which is also called the myocardium). The technique, also known as a myocardial perfusion scan or thallium stress test, requires injection of thallium and detection of radio emissions with a gamma or scintillation camera. Thallium follows the course of the blood flow and allows the diagnosing physician to observe the heart's response to stress produced by blood flow reduction owing to clotting or narrowing of a heart artery (stenosis).

MEDICAL USE

Thallium stress testing is used to diagnose a patient's risk of heart attack. Technetium is also used for this purpose. If the patient is found to be at an increased risk, the physician will prescribe the proper course of treatment. *See also* ANGINA; BLOOD; BLOOD CLOTTING BLOOD, DISORDERS OF; HEART ATTACK; HEART, DISORDERS OF; HEART IMAGING; MEDICAL TESTS; NUCLEAR MEDICINE; RADIONUCLIDE SCANNING; *and* STENOSIS.

Therapeutic Community

Psychotherapeutic technique that emphasizes social influences in the rehabilitation of patients.

The therapeutic community is a method of treating antisocial behavior, such as alcohol and drug dependence or personality disorders. In this psychotherapeutic technique, patients live together as a group with professional medical staff in a nonhospital environment. Staff and patients meet in a group to make all decisions, emphasizing interpersonal relationships and helping the patients to learn social skills. *See also* ALCOHOL DEPENDENCE; DRUG DEPENDENCE *and* GROUP THERAPY.

Therapeutic Touch

An interpretation of several healing practices that involves transmitting positive healing energies through hand motion.

The theory of therapeutic touch is based on the idea that every individual possesses an energy field that radiates beyond the skin. The treatment itself does not actually involve touch, rather the practitioner will place his or her hands two to six inches from the body in an attempt to detect "blockages" in the person's energy field. Because it is believed that these blockages cause health problems, the practitioner will consciously try to transmit energy to the receiver to catalyze energy flows.

Proponents of therapeutic touch claim the technique alleviates pain and brings about a state of relaxation. Although the technique is popular among many nurses, it has been received with a degree of skepticism from the medical community. *See also* ALTERNATIVE MEDICINE.

Thermography

A technique using infrared sensing devices to measure the temperature of the body or organ.

Long wavelength electromagnetic radiation (between 750 and 1,000,000 nanometers) is known as infrared radiation or, more commonly, heat energy. Differences in heat in different parts of the body body indicate different rates of processing energy (metabolism)—a characteristic that is useful for diagnosis. The most common use of thermography has been for breast examination, as an aid to the diagnosis of breast cancer, fibrocystic disease, or infection, all of which produce increased, localized metabolic activity. The procedure is painless and takes only 15 minutes.

During the thermograph, a special camera capable of detecting heat radiation in the body is used. The process is nonsurgical (noninvasive) and completely safe. It has, however, largely fallen into disfavor, and has been almost thoroughly displaced by ultrasound studies and other diagnostic methods. Diagnosis of breast disease, including cancer, by thermography, ultrasound, or other means will often be confirmed through tissue sampling (biopsy). *See also* BIOPSY; BREAST; BREAST CANCER; BREAST DISORDERS; COMPUTER-AIDED DIAGNOSIS; DIAGNOSIS; DIAGNOSTICS IN WOMEN'S HEALTH; FIBROCYSTIC DISEASE; IMAGING TECHNIQUES; METABOLISM; NUCLEAR MEDICINE; *and* TEMPERATURE.

Thermometer

An instrument for measuring temperature, used medically to test for fever or low body temperature—indicators of infection or other illness.

The thermometer is one of the most commonly used diagnostic aids. When normal body temperature is elevated or depressed, illness of some type is usually present. Traditional thermometers consist of a fine glass tube filled with liquid, usually mercury. Such thermometers work on the principle that changing temperatures proportionally affect the volume of liquids. Mercury, hence, will expand with rising temperature along the length of the glass tubing, which has been calibrated so that a precise temperature may be read.

Thirst

The body's natural desire for fluid, particularly water to replenish and rehydrate the system.

Thirst is a common and natural response to bodily depletion of water. Thirst may also be symptomatic of dehydration due to illness. Water is a central component of the body, essential to tissues, cells and blood. Two-thirds of the human body is composed of water. The body requires additional water to replace what is lost through evaporation, sweating, and urination. If the intake of water falls short of output dehydration occurs, producing thirst.

Symptoms of thirst include dry mouth and throat. These are usually relieved immediately on consumption of water or a water-containing drink. Consuming fluid by drinking is the primary means of replenishing the body's supply of water, though some water is also acquired through foods and as a byproduct of cellular respiration.

The mechanisms producing thirst are not completely understood, though a hydration center located in the hypothalamus—a portion of the brain also concerned with temperature regulation and hunger—appears to be involved. A sensitivity to salts helps the hydration center to evaluate the water levels in the body, stimulating the thirst response when a certain limit is reached.

Depending on the cause, however, thirst may not always follow dehydration, which may be the result of sweating, diarrhea, vomiting, heat exhaustion, or fluid loss through wounds or other injuries. Urine production, frequency of urination, and urine color are often better indicators of water balance in the body.

While thirst is a common experience in normal individuals, it can also indicate disease, particularly if the thirst sensation is chronic. Extreme or excessive thirst may be symptomatic of diabetes. This is due to the oversaturation of a form of sugar (glucose) in the blood, which has the effect of inducing frequent urination and therefore dehydration and chronic thirst.

Symptoms

Excessive or prolonged thirst may be symptomatic of disease and should receive immediate medical attention, particularly when accompanied by weight loss, lethargy, passing of over five quarts of urine per day, or blurred vision. Such conditions may be symptomatic of diabetes. Furthermore, a chronic lack of thirst may also suggest disease or disorder in the hypothalamus, liver, or throat. When thirst-related disorders are suspected, the physician will often begin the diagnostic process with an analysis of blood serum and urine.

Background material on thirst may be found in WATER. *For additional information treatment, see* DEHYDRATION; DEHYDRATION IN INFANTS; SWEAT; *and* URINATION. *Related information is contained in* DIABETES; DIARRHEA; HYPOTHALAMUS; *and* URINATION, FREQUENT.*.*

Thoracic Outlet Syndrome

A condition caused by the compression of the brachial plexus, the roots of the nerves that pass into the arms from the neck.

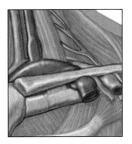

Thoracic Outlet.
Thoracic outlet syndrome results in pain in the shoulder, arm, or hand. The condition is caused by pressure on the brachial plexus (above), the nerves that pass through the arms, from the neck.

Symptoms of thoracic outlet syndrome include pain in the shoulder, arm, or hand. In some cases, pain is experienced in all three of these places. The pain in the hand is most acute in the fourth and fifth digit. Moving the arm can be excruciating and the arm may feel weak.

The first goal of treatment for thoracic outlet syndrome is to straighten the postural abnormalities that lead to the nerve root compression. The second aim is to establish and maintain an exercise program to strengthen the shoulder muscles. Most individuals who are treated by physical therapists recover significantly from the condition. If vascular or extensive neurological impairment exists, surgical decompression of the brachial plexus may be necessary. *See also* BRACHIAL PLEXUS.

Thought Disorders

A general term for behavioral abnormalities that are caused by dysfunctions in an individual's thought processes.

Many thought disorders are symptomatic of deeper-seated and more clearly defined psychological disorders. For example, thought disorders frequently accompany schizophrenia—associations made by schizophrenics are often illogical and unrelated, or are based on sound similarities or incidental and obscure comparisons. Schizophrenia is also characterized by frequent inventing of new or nonsense words (neologism); interruptions of the train of thought; delusional thinking, in which the sufferer is certain that propositions with little basis are true; and the sense that thoughts are being inserted or withdrawn from the mind of the sufferer by an outside force, or by voices that the sufferer hears that communicate to the sufferer or repeat words or thoughts.

Other thought disorders include:

Hypomania is the inability to maintain a train of thought because thoughts are coming too quickly to be analyzed or expressed, resulting in confusion and anxiety;

Depression results in slow thought processes in which trains of thought are lost and incomplete, or in which undue attention is given to trivialities or incidentals;

Obsessive-compulsive behavior is characterized by ideas that occur to the sufferer repeatedly and obscure further clear thought, arresting the sufferer's attention and thought processes.

Treatment is required for the underlying disorder if the thought disorder is to be improved. *See also* DEPRESSION; HYPOMANIA; *and* OBSESSIVE-COMPULSIVE DISORDER.

Thrill

A vibrating sensation in the chest caused by abnormal blood flow.

Thrill can be felt by holding a hand against the front of the chest. It is accompanied by a murmur, another sound caused by abnormal bloodflow. Thrill can be the result of a faulty heart valve, an aneurysm, or some form of congenital heart disease. There are different forms of thrill. Purring thrill is felt over the center of the heart and results from a valve condition or aneurysm. Presystolic thrill is felt over the apex of the heart and occurs just before systole, the stage of the heartbeat when the ventricles contract. *See also* ANEURYSM *and* HEART VALVE.

Thrombectomy

Removal of a clot that is blocking a blood vessel.

A thrombus, or blood clot, that blocks a coronary artery can cause a heart attack. One that blocks an artery supplying the brain can cause a stroke. Thrombectomy is often done as an emergency measure to prevent such major damage. It can also be done to prevent a clot from breaking away to block a blood vessel. Before surgery, anticoagulant drugs are given to reduce the tendency of blood to clot. The site of the blockage is then opened and the thrombus is sucked out. The procedure requires general anesthesia. *See also* BLOOD CLOTTING.

Thrombocytopenia

A condition in which the blood platelet counts are low and, therefore, blood clotting is impaired.

Low platelet counts can be the result of a number of different problems. The bone marrow may not be producing its normal quota of platelets, platelets may be trapped as they flow through the spleen, or the survival rate of existing platelets may have dropped. When the platelet count is low, blood does not clot normally even at small ruptures of blood vessels.

Thrombocytopenia can occur during pregnancy, which is considered relatively benign. However, it can also result from radiation or chemotherapy used to control cancer, or after exposure to certain chemicals like benzene and insecticides. It can be a complication of the immune system or cancers that attack the bone marrow.

The first signs of the condition are bleeding under the skin, dark purple stains, and bruises. Severe cases result in bleeding from the nose and mucous membranes and into the stomach and intestines.

Treatment usually consists of intravenous gamma globulin, if the cause is immune-related. Transfusions of platelets are used if the cause is impaired production of platelets in the bone marrow. The patient is advised to avoid blood thinning medications, such as aspirin. *See* BLOOD CLOTTING.

Thromboembolism

Blockage of a blood vessel.

Embolisms are caused by the migration of tissue, pieces of blood clot, and foreign material. In the case of the thromboembolism, the blockage is caused by a part of a blood clot that has broken off from its original site and moved through the circulatory system. Embolisms are often associa\ted

with pregnancy, childbirth, and recovery from surgery. However, they may occur at any time. If the embolism moves into the lungs, heart, or brain it can be life-threatening. It is treated with anticoagulants.

THROMBOLYTIC DRUGS

Anticoagulants, such as heparin and warfarin, are medications prescribed for people in danger of blood clot formation in the circulatory systems. They function by interfering with the blood clotting process. People confined to bed for long periods of time or who have artificial heart valves may be particularly vulnerable to the formation of blood clots and may be given these drugs as a preventive measure. *See also* EMBOLISM.

Thrombophlebitis

An inflammation of a vein caused by a blood clot.

Superficial thrombophlebitis may be caused by a physical trauma such as a blow. It swells quickly and is red and warm to the touch. The blood clots and clings tightly to the vein and so is unlikely to break loose and travel through the circulatory system. When the phlebitis is in a deeper vein, there is not much swelling since the tissues and muscles compress the break. However, adjacent muscles may squeeze and dislodge the clot so that it travels through the bloodstream and becomes an embolus.

Symptoms of thrombophlebitis are pain and redness of the skin near the break. The clotted blood in the vein makes it feel hard, perhaps for the vein's entire length. Deep vein thrombosis (DVT) can also cause pain and swelling in the leg.

Treatment. There is not much that needs to be done for superficial phlebitis. Aspirin or ibuprofen may relieve the pain. The discomfort will usually subside within a few days. If acute, the thrombus may be removed by surgery. DVT is treated with anticoagulation drugs. Phlebitis often attacks the elderly, who have varicose veins that may be fragile and prone to rupture. Compression stockings and pressure bandages are good preventive measures. *See* VEIN.

Thrombosis

A blood clot formed in an artery or vein that obstructs the flow of blood.

Thrombosis.
Thrombosis occurs most commonly in the lower leg and thigh and obstructs bloodflow. It is caused by a clot in an artery or vein.

When a blood clot forms in an artery or vein, it blocks the free flow of blood to or from the tissues served by that blood vessel. If blood cannot get to an organ, the tissues of the organ die. If the blood cannot leave an organ, pressure builds up, the organ swells, and tissues are destroyed.

A thrombus can form anywhere in the circulatory system. It may be caused by physical trauma from an external source, disease, or surgery. The thrombus normally stays attached to the vein or artery. If it breaks loose and starts to travel through the bloodstream, it is called an embolus. A deep vein thrombosis usually occurs in the pelvis or legs. People with prostate, ovary, or breast cancer are especially susceptible.

The seriousness of the problem depends on where the thrombosis occurs. If the thrombosis forms in the carotid artery that provides the blood supply to the brain, brain cells will die and the person is said to have suffered a stroke. If the thrombosis is in one of the arteries providing oxygen to the heart, the heart muscle dies and the person is said to have suffered a coronary thrombosis or heart attack. If the thrombosis is in the lungs, the person is said to suffer a pulmonary thrombosis. The lung may be unable to function properly and may even collapse.

Heparin is the drug of choice for thrombosis. The goal is to reduce the blood clotting ability of the blood so that further clots will not develop and progress to life-threatening sites in the body. The heparin is provided by intravenous infusion on an inpatient basis. Low molecular weight heparin is now available and is simpler to use than regular heparin. It is injected two times a day for a week to ten days.

Warfarin is an oral anticoagulant that is started at the same time as the heparin and continued for three to six months on an outpatient basis.

Neither heparin nor warfarin actually reduce an existing clot. If there is danger of pulmonary thrombosis, heart embolism, or stroke, streptokinase or tissue plasminogen activator may be administered in an effort to dissolve the clot.

DEEP VEIN THROMBOSIS

Deep vein thrombosis often follows surgery, accident, stroke, or when a person is inactive for a long period of time. It usually occurs in the pelvis or legs. People with prostate, ovary, or breast cancer are especially vulnerable. The danger is for the clot to break free and travel to the lungs, brain, or heart, where it becomes life-threatening.

Diagnosis of this problem is often difficult, since there may be few symptoms. Doppler ultrasound is the best and least intrusive test for deep vein thrombosis.

If the patient is bedridden, he or she should be encouraged to move the arms and legs and breathe deeply. If the patient is unconscious, a therapist or caregiver must move the limbs for him or her.

Women who smoke and are taking birth control pills may wish to discuss the likelihood of thrombosis with their gynecologists. The elderly in particular should avoid situations in which there are long periods of inactivity, such as car or airplane trips. If they are unavoidable, change positions frequently. Stop the car and take a short walk. Get up from the seat and walk up and down the aisle for a few minutes every hour. Support hose or compression band-ages may help keep the blood from pooling in the lower extremities. *See also* ANTI-COAGULANT DRUGS; BLOOD; BLOOD CLOTTING BLOOD DISORDERS; CIRCULATORY SYSTEM; EMERGENCY FIRST STEPS; HEART; *and* TRAUMA.

ALERT

Health Alert to Avoid Thrombosis

- If you are taking birth control pills and smoke, immediately stop smoking.
- Avoid long periods of inactivity, as on airplanes or auto trips.
- Lie flat with the legs above the heart level.
- Wear support stockings.

Thumb-Sucking

Sucking the thumb, and sometimes the hand, is one way an infant comforts him- or herself.

Thumb-sucking usually increases when a baby is weaned from the breast or bottle. Doctors believe the behavior is a baby's way of coping with emotional challenges.

The peak of thumb-sucking usually occurs around age one-and-a-half. Most children will give it up themselves by age four.

The best approach to help an infant give up thumb-sucking is to substitute something else for the thumb. Nursing the infant longer may help, and a pacifier may be another possibility. Scolding and criticizing the child do not work, and may make the thumb-sucking worse.

If a child persists in thumb-sucking past age four, he or she should see a dentist to make sure tooth alignment has not been compromised. If it has, an oral appliance may be necessary to correct the problem.

Thymoma

Tumor arising in the thymus gland.

The thymus, located in the upper chest, is a gland that creates lymphocytes, cells of the immune system, which attack viruses and other infectious invaders. Thymomas are usually benign tumors and can occur in the varying thymus tissue types. *See* THYMUS.

Epithelial thymomas arise in the tissue that covers the surface of the gland. They generally do not spread to other parts of the body. A lymphoid thymoma that arises in the lymphoid tissue of the gland generally evolves to result in a cancer—non-Hodgkin's lymphoma. Another thymoma is a teratoma, which contains cells that are not normally found in thymus tissue. Thymic teratomas tend to be benign in women but malignant in men.

About 15 percent of patients with myasthenia gravis, a disease of the immune system, have a tumor of the thymus, but the relationship of the tumor to this neuromuscular condition is unclear.

Thymus

A gland, located in the upper chest, that forms an important part of the immune system.

The thymus is located directly behind the breastbone and is split into two halves that connect directly in front of the trachea. The gland consists of compact clusters of lymphocytes, epithelium, and lipids. The main function of the thymus is that it transforms lymphocytes (a type of white blood cell) into T-cells, a specific type of white blood cell that is crucial in combatting infection and cancer.

The thymus develops and grows until a child reaches puberty, at which point the gland begins to shrink. Abnormal development of the thymus may result in immunodeficiency disorders. An enlarged thymus may lead to several disorders, including Addison's disease, thyrotoxicosis, and acromegaly. *See also* ACROMEGALY; ADDISON'S DISEASE; IMMUNE SYSTEM; IMMUNODEFICIENY DISORDERS; LIPID; LYMPHOCYTE; T-CELL; *and* THYROTOXICOSIS.

Thyroglossal Disorders

A condition in which the thyroglossal duct (and a cyst) is present following embryonic development.

The thyroglossal duct is functional in human embryos and runs from the end of the tongue to the thyroid gland in the neck. A defect may cause this duct to remain (completely or partially) well after the child is born. The duct remains as a cyst, which becomes swollen and almost always results in an infection. If this infection becomes severe, a thyroglossal fistula may form, resulting in an improper pathway between the cyst and the neck.

This condition must be treated by surgically by removing the cyst or fistula and completely ridding the child of any remaining portions of the thryoglossal duct. If this procedure is not completed, the child is placed at risk of repeated infection of the region. *See also* CYST; EMBRYO; FISTULA; THYROID; *and* TONGUE.

Thyroid Gland.
The thyroid gland,
right, is made up of
two lobes and located
in the front of the neck.
The gland regulates
metabolism, the release
of energy from nutri-
ents, and blood calci-
um levels.

Thyroid

Gland that aids in metabolism and maintenance of calcium levels.

One of the most important glands in the endocrine system, the thyroid gland is made up of two lobes that are located just beneath the larynx, in front of the neck. Each lobe lies on either side of the larynx, and they are connected by a band of tissue called the isthmus. The hormones secreted by the gland, T_4, some T_3, and calcitonin, affect almost all of the tissue in the body at any given moment because of their roles in such ongoing processes as the storage and release of energy from nutrients and the monitoring of blood calcium levels.

The thyroid gland is built from two types of cells; follicular and parafollicular. Follicular cells are responsible for the hormones and thyroxine (T_4) and some T_3 both of which contain iodine. Most T_3 comes from peripheral conversion from some T_4. These hormones control such basic functions as the building and breakdown of proteins, production of cholesterol, breakdown of fatty tissues, heart rhythms, menstrual cycles, and even the speed at which all cell activity happens. The parafollicular cells, also known as C-cells, are found in between the follicular cells. Their main job is to secrete the hormone calcitonin, which helps regulate the levels of calcium in the body by directing the rate of absorption from the bones.

The production of thyroid hormones is directed by the hypothalamus and pituitary gland. The hypothalamus monitors the rate of activity in the body, and, when levels of thyroid hormones are low, releases thyrotopin-releasing hormone (TRH). The pituitary gland receives this signal, and secretes thyroid-stimulating hormone. This then directs the thyroid to release T_4. If levels of thyroid hormones are too high, the process is reversed.

Disorders. Because the thyroid gland affects so many basic bodily processes, any disruption or variation in levels of thyroid hormones can cause serious problems.

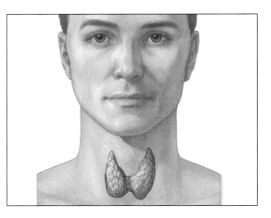

Thyroid gland disorders can be due either to a problem in the thyroid itself, or, because of its dependence on the hypothalamus and pituitary gland, diseases in those organs can also affect thyroid hormone production. Thyroid disorders usually fall into one of several categories:

Autoimmune Disorders. In these disorders, antibodies, which are meant to attack diseases in tissue, instead are generated for no apparent reason, and attack healthy organs. In this case, the thyroid may respond by overproducing and or underproducing the thyroid hormone.

Congenital Disorders. The thyroid may either be completely missing at birth, thus producing little or no thyroid hormone. Some children can develop cretinism, which is characterized by mental retardation, lack of growth, and coarsened facial features.

Genetic Disorders. Thyroid disorders may be caused by inherited deficiencies in the enzymes necessary to make thyroid hormone; as a result, the gland does not produce enough thyroid hormone. Attempts by the pituitary gland to increase production by secreting more thyroid-stimulating hormone (TSH) may result in thyroid swelling, or goiter, as it tries to increase the hormone production.

Hormonal Disorders. Puberty or pregnancy can lead to changes in hormone levels that can increase thyroid production; this may result in a slight goiter that will usually return to normal.

Infections in the thyroid itself, or in other parts of the body, can inflame the thyroid gland, leading to excessive production of the thyroid hormones.

Nutritional Deficiencies. Since thyroid hormones contain iodine, a lack of iodine in the diet can cause the gland to swell, producing a goiter. Although rare, this may occur in areas in which the water and soil are low in iodine.

Tumors. Benign or (rarely) malignant tumors in the thyroid gland can lead to excessive production of the thyroid hormone.

In rare instances, the source of a thyroid problem, however, may lie in the pituitary gland.

Common Thyroid Disorders:

• **Hyperthyroidism due to Graves' disease:** Autoimmune disorder that leads to excessive production of the thyroid hormone. Symptoms include unexplained weight loss, weakness, heart palpitations, weakness, sweating, and bulging of the eyes. Treatment may involve antithyroid medication, radiation treatment to reduce the thyroid, or surgical removal of all or part of the thyroid gland.

• **Hypothyroidism:** Often, the result of a genetic or congenital defect, causing little or no production of the thyroid hormone. Symptoms include weight gain and fluid retention, sensitivity to cold, muscle and joint pain, and coarse hair. Dry, thickened skin and coarsened facial features are known as myxedema, a condition associated with hypothyroidism. Treatment includes thyroid replacement drugs.

• **Hashimoto's thyroiditis:** Chronic autoimmune disorder, most common among middle age women, that leads to underproduction of the thyroid hormones. Symptoms include goiter, weight gain and fluid retention, sensitivity to cold, muscle and joint pain, coarse hair, and dry skin. Treatment may include thyroid replacement medication.

• **Goiter:** Swelling of the thyroid, caused by an overactive thyroid gland; any condition, such as a tumor or autoimmune disorder, that forces the thyroid to overwork may lead to a goiter. A lack of iodine in the diet may also cause a goiter. Treatment depends on the root of the cause.

See CALCITONIN; CALCIUM *and* GLAND *for background information on thyroid gland. For additional information, see* THYROID, DISORDERS OF; THYROID FUNCTION TESTS; *and* THYROID SCANNING. *For further information on thyroid disorders, see* GOITER; HYPERTHYROIDISM; HYPOTHYROIDISM; HASHIMOTO'S SYNDROME; *and* THYROID CANCER.

Thyroid, Cancer of the

Malignant tumor of the thyroid gland.

Thyroid cancer is the most common cancer of the endocrine glands, which secrete hormones, but it is uncommon among all cancers, causing about one percent of cases. A major risk factor for thyroid cancer is exposure to radioactivity.

The thyroid is a located in the front of the neck, just below the Adam's apple. It secretes hormones that help regulate a number of bodily functions. The thyroid contains two main tissue types: follicular cells, which make up most of the gland and form hollow spheres called follicles, and parafollicular cells, which are found between the follicles. The most common kind of thyroid cancer is papillary cancer, followed by follicular cancer, medullary cancer, Hurthale-cell carcinoma, and undifferentiated thyroid cancer. All can spread from the thyroid to neighboring tissues and the rest of the body if not detected and treated early.

SYMPTOMS

The first symptom of thyroid cancer usually is a painless, firm lump in the neck. There can be enlarged lymph nodes in the neck, pain in the neck, difficulty swallowing, and hoarseness as the cancer progresses.

DIAGNOSIS

A physical examination usually cannot distinguish between a cancer and a nonmalignant growth. Ultrasound examination may be done, and a tissue sample of a suspicious lump can be taken for microscopic examination (biopsy). A thyroid scan, in which a trace of a radioactive substance is injected, can help distinguish between a malignant and a benign tumor.

TREATMENT

Treatment of a thyroid cancer is based not only on the type of cancer and the stage at which it is diagnosed, but also on the age and sex of the patient. The cancer is more aggressive in patients over the age of 50

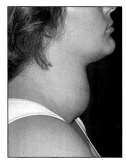

Thyroid Cancer.
The thyroid gland is located in the front of the neck. Because of this, tumors of the thyroid will usually become evident through the appearance of a lump in the throat (above). Hoarseness, difficulty swallowing, and pain in the neck may follow.

Resources on Thyroid Disorders

Nuland, Sherwin B., *The Wisdom of the Body* (1997); Greenspan, Francis S., et al., *Basic & Clinical Endocrinology* (2000); Shin, Linda M., et al., *Endocrine and Metabolic Disorders Sourcebook* (1998); Arem, Ridha, *The Thyroid Solution* (2000); Rosenthal, M. Sara, *The Thyroid Sourcebook for Women* (1999); Hypoglycemia Support Foundation, Tel. (518) 272-7154, Online: www.hypoglycemia.org; Thyroid Foundation of America, Tel. (800) 832-8321, Online: www.tsh.org; American Thyroid Association, Tel. (718) 882-6047, Online: www.thyroid.org; www.nycornell.org/medicine/edm/index.html.

and in men. Lobectomy or subtotal thyroidectomy, surgery to remove only part of the gland is sometimes possible, but removal of the entire thyroid, and perhaps neighboring tissue, may be necessary, depending on the extent of the disease; thyroid hormone supplements are given after such surgery. Radiation therapy often is given after surgery using radioactive iodine. Radioactive iodine-131 can destroy cancer cells located in the thyroid and elsewhere without major affects on the rest of the body. The prognosis is best for younger patients whose cancer is detected at an early stage, with a five-year survival rate of about 95 percent in these cases.

Genetic Disorders

Fewer than a third of the cases of thyroid cancer results from an inherited genetic condition. Two such genetic conditions are familial medullary thyroid carcinoma and multiple endocrine neoplasia, in which tumors can occur in several hormone-secreting glands. Screening tests for early detection of any cancer are recommended in such families.

See Thyroid Gland *for background information on thyroid cancer. Further information can be found in* Cancer; Genetic Disorders; *and* Tumor. *For information on diagnosis and treatment, see* Radiation Therapy; Thyroidectomy; Thyroid Function Test; *and* Thyroid Scanning.

Thyroidectomy

A surgical procedure that involves the removal of the thyroid gland.

A thyroidectomy is performed to treat thyroid cancer, symptomatic thyroid enlargement (also known as a non-toxic goiter), hyperthyroidism (overactivity of the thyroid), hypothyroidism (sometimes called underactivity of the thyroid).

Types of Thyroid Tumors.

The general types of thyroid cancer are:
- papillary, which is the most common;
- follicular;
- medullary;

- undifferentiated or anaplastic, which is a particularly virulent type.

In papillary carcinoma, tumors larger than 1.5 cm usually require total thyroidectomy and possibly subsequent radioiodine treatment. Follicular carcinoma usually requires removal and radioiodine treatment. Total thyroidectomy is necessary for medullary carcinoma and probable removal of the neck lymph nodes if the cancer has spread. Anaplastic thyroid cancer spreads quickly and requires the full treatment of thyroidectomy, external beam radiation therapy, and radiation therapy. Sometimes, a tracheostomy is ne-eded to keep the patient breathing. Of the four types of thyroid cancer, anaplastic has the lowest survival rate.

After a partial or total thyroidectom or radiation, depending on the type of thyroid cancer being treated and the extent of the disease, the patient is put on a synthetic thyroid hormone (levothyroxine) replacement therapy for life. The road to recovery is slow, but patients generally begin to see steady improvement in skin, hair, and voice after several weeks. *See also* Thyroid *and* Thyroid, Cancer of.

Thyroid Function Test

Diagnostic exams used to evaluate the health and performance of the thyroid gland.

The thyroid gland is a butterfly-shaped endocrine gland located in the neck, found on either side of windpipe (trachea). Responsible for the control of processing energy in the body (metabolism), the thyroid gland secretes a number of critical natural chemicals (hormones), including thyroxine. A variety of tests allow the functioning of the thyroid and production of thyroxine to be measured and evaluated.

Another hormone of interest in evaluating the thyroid is thyroid-stimulating hormone (TSH), which is released by the pituitary gland. When blood levels of TSH are high, an underactive thyroid is indicated, while low TSH suggests an overactive thyroid—conditions referred to as hypothyroidism and hyperthyroidism, respectively. When hypothyroidism is suspected, blood may also be tested for antithyroid antibodies, as an infection-fighting (autoimmune) reaction against the thyroid is the most common cause of the disease—also known as Hashimoto's thyroiditis.

Symptoms and Treatment. In hyperthyroidism, the body's metabolic functions speed up. Symptoms include rapid heart rate, high blood pressure, sweating, moist skin, shakiness, increased appetite and weight loss, weakness, diarrhea, swollen and reddened eyes that may bulge, and confusion. Hypothyroidism, by contrast, slows the pulse. Facial features may become puffy, speech is slowed, eyebrow hair is lost, eyelids droop, constipation and weight gain may occur, and depression and confusion may result. Hyperthyroidism may be treated with medication, surgical removal of the thyroid gland, or treatment with radioactive iodine. Hypothyroidism is usually treated with synthetic thyroid hormone to counteract the deficit. *See also* THYROID.

Thyroiditis

An inflammation of the thyroid gland, which controls production of the thyroid hormone.

The most common form of thyroiditis is called Hashimoto's thyroiditis. In this form of thyroiditis, the autoimmune system produces antibodies that attack the thyroid gland. Hashimoto's thyroiditis is reported eight times as often among women as among men. It is also more common among the elderly. Hashimoto's thyroiditis starts with a painless inflammation of the thyroid gland. As the disease progresses, the gland produces too little thyroid hormone (hypothyroidism). *See also* THYROID.

Subacute granulomatous thyroiditis is a less common, but more severe, form of thyroiditis. Symptoms of subacute granulomatous thyroiditis include neck pain, low grade fever, and weight loss. The thyroid overproduces thyroid hormones (hyperthyroidism) followed by a transient underproduction, creating a seesaw effect. Most people recover from subacute granulomatous thyroiditis in a matter of months without treatment, though permanent hypothyroidism is reported in some cases.

Silent lymphocytic thyroiditis frequently follows childbirth in women. The thyroid is overactive for a time, after which it is underactive before returning to normal. Permanent hypothyroidism is reported in some cases of silent lymphocytic thyroiditis.

Thyroid Scanning

Technique used for diagnostic imaging of the thyroid gland.

A thyroid scan involves taking a picture of the thyroid—a butterfly-shaped endocrine gland located in the neck, after the administration of radioactive iodine. The iodine may be given in pill form or to drink, and is absorbed by the thyroid. A special camera, able to detect the emission of high speed radiation (gamma rays) emitted from the ingested radioactive iodine, is used. Scanning will begin from four to six hours following ingestion of the iodine, after the compound has been absorbed by the thyroid. The detector or scintillation camera sends the emission data to a computer, which assembles the information into a two-dimensional diagnostic image. This technique—also known as radionuclide scanning has many other medical applications. It is based on characteristic times and patterns of absorption of radionuclide by the organ or tissue under study. Deviation from normal absorption rates are indicative of disorder.

What to Expect. The procedure is completely painless. Usually the patient will be required to fast overnight before the test. The doctor should be informed of any medication taken, and will ask the patient to abstain from using iodine-containing drugs or thyroid medicine. Thyroid scanning is used in the diagnosis of thyroid cancer as well as to inspect thyroid nodules, which excrete important natural hormones. The procedure is somewhat faster when done with Technetium. *See* THYROID.

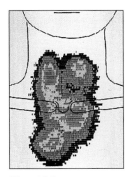

Thyroid Scan.
A thyroid scan involves taking a picture of the thyroid, following the ingestion of a radioactive tracer fluid. This is used to diagnose thyroid disorders. The scan above indicates an enlargement of the thyroid and an extension behind the breastbone.

Thyrotoxicosis

A toxic condition caused by an overactive thyroid.

The thyroid gland, responsible for energy storage and release and maintenance of calcium levels, can become overactive because of conditions such as tumors or autoimmune disorders. This is known as a hyperthyroid, or in the case of autoimmune disorders, Graves' disease. Thyrotoxicosis is the term used to describe any toxic condition that is the result of hyperthyroidism. It is used as another name for Graves' disease. *See* Graves' Disease *and* Thyroid.

Tic

A repetitive and involuntary jerking movement.

Tics are chronic and random. Most tics develop before the age of seven, and are an indication of a minor psychological problem. They are more pronounced when the patient experiences fatigue or tension.

Tics may consist of eye blinking or twitching muscle contractions of the head, neck, shoulders, and mouth. They can also be exhibited as vocal tics, which include coughing, grunting, and spastic breathing. Tics may also include hitting, kicking, snorting, and humming.

A more severe form of tic is called Tourette's syndrome. The patient grunts and vocalizes repeatedly, and may involuntarily say swear words. Tourette's syndrome is especially prevalent in boys. The situation is complex, because parents and teachers are usually unaware that the patient is not deliberately making noises or using curse words. Tourette's syndrome demands an accurate diagnosis and a strong support system consisting of teachers and friends.

Tics are harmless and usually disappear with time. Mild tics tend not to require treatment. If tics manifest over a period of more than a few years, a physician should be consulted. Benzodiazepine and antipsychotic drugs, such as haloperidol, are used to suppress tics. *See* Antipsychotic Drugs.

Ticks and Disease

Various human diseases transmitted to humans by tick bite.

There are over 800 species of tick, many of which are disease-carriers. In the United States, three primary genera of ticks can transmit bacteria, viruses, rickettsiae, and protozoa—all of which can produce disease in humans.

Babesiosis is caused by the protozoan *Babesia,* which produces an illness similar to malaria. It is transmitted by the black-legged tick or through contaminated blood. Symptoms include fever, chills, fatigue, headache, muscle and joint pain, and destruction of red blood cells (hemolytic anemia). The disease is endemic in the Northeastern United States.

Colorado tick fever is a viral disease found in the mountainous regions of the western United States.

The disease, transmitted by the Rocky Mountain wood tick, is usually of short duration and is rarely fatal. Symptoms include fever, chills, severe headache, muscle aches, and sometimes a faint rash, lasting about a week. Following a short period of remission, symptoms often recur, accompanied by a drop in white blood cells.

Lyme disease has become prevalent in wooded regions of the American Northeast. It is caused by the bacterium *Borrelia burgdorferi* and produces flu-like symptoms in its earlier stages. It often produces a characteristic spreading rash with a cleared center (bullseye rash) around the site of the bite. Later, multiple rashes, joint swelling or pain, loss of coordination, facial paralysis, cognitive or behavioral changes, peripheral nerve damage, heart conduction defects, and eye inflammation may be seen. Lyme disease is transmitted by the black-legged tick and the western black-legged tick.

Rocky Mountain spotted fever (RMSF) is caused by *Rickettsia rickettsii,* a pathogen transmitted by the Lone-Star tick, American dog tick, Rocky Mountain wood tick, black-legged tick, western black-legged tick, and brown dog tick. Symptoms of RMSF include flu-like aches and pain, headache, chills, confusion, light sensitivity, and high fever. A measles-like rash begins on the extremities and may continue to spread over the entire body. If symptoms of this disease appear, seek emergency medical attention immediately.

Tick-borne relapsing fever is caused by three species of spiral-shaped bacteria. Symptoms include repeating bouts of fever lasting two to nine days, with periods of intermediate remission. Fever is accompanied by flu-like symptoms. The infection is transmitted by *Ornithodoros hermsi* and the relapsing fever tick.

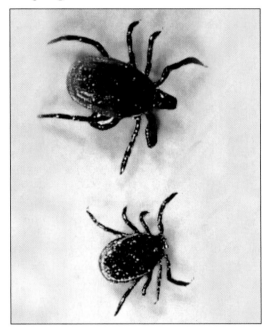

Diagnosis of tick-borne disease is based on physical examination, particularly where rashes or skin disorders accompany the bite, likelihood of tick presence, and disease-specific symptoms. Such diseases are usually confirmed by the presence of the tick-borne pathogen in the blood, or through appropriate antibody tests.

> *Background information on* TICKS AND DISEASE *can be found in* PARASITE *and* PROTOZOA. *For additional information see* BABESIOSIS; BACTERIA; ECTOPARASITE; LYME DISEASE; ROCKY MOUNTAIN SPOTTED FEVER; *and* VIRUS. *For related information see* MITES AND DISEASE *and* RASH.

Tietze's Syndrome

An inflammation of the cartilage of the ribcage.

Tietze's syndrome is characterized by chest pain that is confined to the front of the chest cavity. The pain becomes increasingly severe when patients move their arms or trunk. Tietze's syndrome is caused by the swelling of one or more of the interior edges of the rib cartilage, either at the point where it meets the breastbone (sternum) or at the point where it connects with the bony section of the rib. Uncomfortable and painful symptoms can persist for a few months. Tietze's syndrome can usually be treated easily with a combination of analgesic drugs and nonsteroidal anti-inflammatory drugs. *See also* ANALGESIC DRUGS *and* ANTI-INFLAMMATORY DRUGS.

Timolol

A drug used in different forms to treat heart conditions and glaucoma.

Timolol is a member of the beta-blocker family of drugs. It acts by blocking the activity of norepinephrine and adrenaline, hormones that make the heart beat faster and with greater force. By reducing heart activity, timolol and other beta-blockers reduce blood pressure. Timolol in pill form is given to treat hypertension and angina pectoris. Timolol eye drops are used to treat glaucoma, a condition in which increased pressure of fluid inside the eye damages vision. Because of its side effects, timolol is not recommended for persons with diabetes or asthma. *See* ASTHMA.

> ## Risks of Combining Drugs
>
> The combination of beta-blockers and injections of epinephrine can be extremely dangerous, since it may raise the blood pressure to very high levels. Also, nonsteroidal anti-inflammatory drugs like aspirin or Tylenol can negate the effects of beta-blockers. Do not stop taking beta-blockers abruptly, since that can cause the blood pressure to spike and result in heart attack or stroke.

Ticks.
Ticks are ectoparasites, meaning that they live on the skin of other animals. Many species of ticks can transmit the disease. The dog tick (left) is the most common vector for Rocky Mountain spotted fever (RMSF).

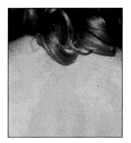

Tinea.
Tinea is a general term used to describe fungal infections of the skin. Tinea Versicolor (above) causes areas of skin discoloration on the back, chest, neck and upper arms.

Tinea

One of a group of fungal infections of the skin.

Athlete's foot (Tinea pedis) prefers the damp warm areas between the toes. It can produce mild scaling or an itchy, raw, and painful blistering rash on the feet. The tendency for the skin to crack leaves the sufferer open to bacterial infection. The fungus that is responsible for athlete's foot is often acquired in communal showers and bathtubs.

Jock itch (Tinea cruris) causes an itchy, red rash in the groin area. Tight, damp underwear encourages this infection.

Scalp or body ringworm (Tinea capitis) are highly contagious fungal infections that are found most often among children. Ringworm is transmitted by personal contact, and through the sharing of combs, brushes, clothing, or towels. It produces a red, scaly rash and, in some people, hair loss. The rash takes the form of circles of red with clear centers. If the fungus attacks the scalp, it may require treatment with selenium sulfide shampoo and oral antifungal medications.

Tinea versicolor produces areas of skin discoloration on the back, chest, neck, and upper arms.

Treatment. All tinea infections will respond to over-the-counter antifungal drugs. The affected areas should be kept cool, clean, and dry. *See also* ANTIFUNGAL DRUGS; ATHLETE'S FOOT; RINGWORM; *and* TINEA VERSICOLOR.

Tinea Versicolor

A chronic fungal infection of the skin, which causes white to light brown skin patches and scaling.

Tinea versicolor is caused by the yeast *Pityrosporum orbiculare*. This fungus is normally found in the skin, which becomes infected only under certain circumstances. The most commonly affected areas are the underarms, upper arms, chest, and neck.

Symptoms. Lesions associated with tinea versicolor appear flat, scaly, and discolored, with a clearly defined border. Itching may or may not accompany the lesions. Other symptoms may include persistent areas of reddish-tan skin, scales, increased sweating, and itching.

Tinea versicolor is most prevalent in hot climates, and is associated with increased sweating. Adolescents and young men are the groups most affected by the disorder.

Diagnosis. A healthcare provider will diagnose the condition using a Woods lamp, a device that uses ultraviolet light to cause skin lesions to glow and be identified. A skin scraping is sometimes also performed.

Treatment may include antifungal agents, such as clotrimazole, ketoconazole, and miconazole. *See also* ANTIFUNGAL DRUGS; FUNGAL INFECTION; FUNGI; ITCHING; LESION; *and* TINEA.

Tinnitus

A ringing, buzzing, or other noise heard in the ear that is not environmental in origin.

Tinnitus is a condition in which the patient experiences unwanted background noise in the ear. The condition is caused by the transmission of nerve impulses to the brain that are not in response to vibrations created by external sound waves. It is estimated that one out of every five adults experience some degree of tinnitus.

There are two types of tinnitus, objective or subjective. Objective tinnitus is a rarer form in which the patient emits head noise that is also audible to other people. It is caused by repetitive muscle contractions or structural defects of the inner ear. Objective tinnitus can also be an early sign of increased intracranial pressure (pressure in the head) due to abnormalities of the blood vessels. Subjective tinnitus is more common than objective tinnitus, but is less understood. In subjective tinnitus, only the sufferer can hear specific sounds. The sounds can range from a metallic ringing to a buzzing, humming, or popping noise. Subjective tinnitus may be accompanied by deafness. *See also* HEARING.

Tiredness

Fatigue or the desire to sleep or rest.

Tiredness is a feeling of lethargy, weakness, or exhaustion. Factors that can cause fatigue include anemia; an accumulation of waste products in the body; a lack of protein, calories, vitamins or minerals; a disruption of sleep; boredom; stress; anxiety; and depression. Fatigue may also be experienced as a side effect in patients undergoing radiation therapy.

Tiredness can be caused by serious conditions, such as anemia or cancer. If the heart does not pump with maximum efficiency, the individual experiences fatigue during exercise. This is common in people over 50. Tiredness can also be caused by chronic fatigue syndrome, a condition characterized by debilitating fatigue accompanied by swollen lymph nodes.

To minimize tiredness, it is necessary to get enough rest, to exercise each day, to drink three quarts of fluid each day to minimize the build-up of cellular waste, and to consume enough iron to prevent anemia. Depression-related disorders should be treated, and alcoholic beverages should be avoided. *See* ENERGY *and* FATIGUE.

Tissue Fluid

Also known as interstitial fluid

The watery medium that fills the spaces between living cells in organs and throughout the body.

The living cells of the body are suspended in a watery substance that serves as the conduit between the cells and the pulmonary system of blood vessels and the lymphatic system. Oxygen and nutrients must pass from the blood to the tissue fluid and then into the cell, and waste products must pass out of the cell into the tissue fluid and from there back into the blood to be eliminated.

The movement of these elements is controlled by the chemical makeup of the tissue fluid as it interacts with the blood, lymph and with the walls and internal components of the cells. This is accomplished by controlling the ions contained in the fluid. Tissue fluid contains higher concentrations of sodium ions than cellular fluid and lower concentration of potassium ions. This difference causes water and material dissolved in that water to flow through the cell wall in a process known as diffusion.

The ion levels in the tissue fluid also play an important role in the transmission of nerve impulses to muscles. It is thus vital that the tissue fluid be of the right constituents and volume if living cells and the body as a whole are to function properly. The flow of tissue fluid is controlled by the major organs of the body responding to the hormonal cues sent out by the endocrine system in a complex feedback system. When there is a need to lower the amount of fluid in the body or to alter the concentration of ions in the tissue fluid, the glands prompt the kidneys to increase their operation and remove excess fluid from the bloodstream. This may cause the heart to pump faster to increase the flow of blood through the kidneys.

Care of Tissue Fluid. There are various ways in which the delicate balance of the amount and content of the tissue fluid can be disrupted, putting the living cells of the body and the organs in which they are located at risk.

If the heart is functioning inefficiently, blood will not be pumped through the body at a rate sufficient to carry away fluids and these fluid will build up in tissues. This disease, known as congestive heart failure, often has symptoms such as edema—puffy, fluid-filled areas, particularly in the feet, that, when pressed, remain indented for a few minutes. Congestive heart failure is treated with vasodilator drugs, diuretic drugs (to remove excess fluid), and, in extreme case, heart transplant surgery. People of all ages may develop congestive heart failure.

Background material on tissue fluidcan be found in CELL. *Additional information is contained in* BLOOD; CIRCULATORY SYSTEM; CONGESTIVE HEART FAILURE; GLAND; ION; LYMPHATIC SYSTEM; OXYGEN *and* TRANSPLANT SURGERY. *Detailed information can be found in* EDEMA; HEART; HORMONE; KIDNEY; POTASSIUM; SODIUM *and* WATER.

Tissue Plasminogen Activator

A clot-dissolving drug used when persons are experiencing a thrombosis.

In 1995, this drug was approved by the Food and Drug Administration for use in the early stages of heart attack, stroke, pulmonary embolism, or deep vein thrombosis. It must be given within three hours of the onset of symptoms to be effective and preclude damage to heart muscles or brain tissue. Depending on the exact formulation, it is administered by injection or intravenous infusion into the artery. The major disadvantages of this medication are the increased risk of bleeding and the narrow window of opportunity for its use.

Symptoms of a Heart Attack

Symptoms of heart attack include pain in the center of the chest that lasts more than a few minutes or returns and spreads to the neck or arms. Sweating, nausea, and shortness of breath may also be experienced, sometimes without pain.

Symptoms of a Stroke

Symptoms of stroke include sudden weakness in an arm or leg, numbness of the face, confusion and aphasia, vision problems, dizziness, problems keeping balance, and sudden severe headache.

Tissue Typing

Analysis of tissue to determine compatibility with donor tissue prior to transplantation.

Tissue typing, also known as histocompatibility testing, is used to identify surface groups of proteins called human leukocyte antigens (HLAs or MHC for major histocompatibility complex). Tissue compatibility or histocompatibility is identified through analysis of HLAs, which are unique to each individual. Histocompatibility molecules occur on the surfaces of cells known as lymphocytes and allow the body to distinguish itself from foreign matter, a feature of central importance to the body's infection-fighting (immune) system. Matching of histocompatibility antigens between donor and recipient tissue helps reduce the risk of tissue or organ rejection. Such graft-host rejection, a common hazard of transplantation and tissue grafting, is caused by the body's immune response to the donor tissue. Matching of HLA systems may also be used to establish parentage (paternity), as these surface antigens, substances that induce the formation of specific antibodies, are inherited.

HLAs are detected and analyzed through a test (immunoassay) designed to measure the antigen-antibody response. Where organ transplantation is to be carried out, donor and recipient histocompatibility antigens will be compared to assess suitability. Similarly, father and child HLAs may be compared to confirm paternity. Certain human leukocyte agents are also used as diagnostic indicators for particular diseases, such as ankylosing spondylitis, Hashimoto's thyroiditis, Graves' disease, and multiple sclerosis.

See Donor *and* Transplant *for background information on tissue typing. For additional information, see* Graft Versus Host Disease; Histocompatability Antigens; Infection; Lymphocytes; *and* Rejection. *Related information is available in* Graves' Disease; Hashimoto's Thyroiditis; Immunoassay; *and* Multiple Sclerosis.

Titanium Dental Implants

Alternative to dentures and bridgework as a replacement for teeth.

When titanium dental implants are needed, an oral surgeon, periodontist, or other dental specialist prepares tiny holes in the jaw top or bottom and inserts titanium or synthetic implant screws or dowels. The implants are allowed to heal and fuse to the bone over a period of three to six months. They are then used like new tooth roots to support bridges or dentures. Properly cared for, titanium dental implants can last for decades. *See* Denture.

Tobacco Smoking

Tobacco smoking is one of the primary causes of death in the U.S.—about one in every six deaths is tobacco-related, and about half of all lifelong smokers will die of smoking-related illness.

Tobacco smoke is composed of many carcinogenic substances and it can cause cancers of the lungs, esophagus, throat, mouth, stomach, bladder, kidneys, and pancreas. Smokeless tobacco products can also cause cancer of the stomach and esophagus, throat, gums, and tongue.

Smoking can cause noncancerous forms of pulmonary disease, such as emphysema. It also exacerbates the symptoms of asthma, causes bronchitis, and increases the likelihood of contracting pneumonia.

Although the public often associates smoking with pulmonary disease, the mortality rate from cardiovascular disease aggravated by smoking is greater. Nicotine and carbon monoxide, when combined stresses the heart. Nicotine, a stimulant, increases the heart rate, while carbon monoxide, an asphyxiant, replaces the oxygen necessary for increased activity. Smoking also increases the likelihood of stroke and atherosclerosis—artery hardening.

Smoking affects the health of those who are in contact with them. Some believe that secondhand smoke is responsible for more fatalities than AIDS. While smokers often inhale filtered smoke, the smoke from the lit end of a cigarette is unfiltered, and contains higher concentrations of nicotine, tar, and other gases. Children in households with one or more smokers are more likely to suffer from asthma, bronchitis, and pneumonia, illnesses that can all be fatal.

People who smoke should pay particular attention to nutrition, especially to calcium intake, since smokers use more calcium than non-smokers and are at greater risk for osteoporosis, and they should emphasize exercise for cardiovascular and pulmonary health. Smokers should also have thorough annual checkups, focusing on cardiovascular and pulmonary health and including tests to detect the presence of cancers.

Articles with basic information about this include ANXIETY; CARBON MONOXIDE; CARCINOGEN; *and* STRESS. *Information about the effects of* TOBACCO SMOKING *can be found in* ASTHMA; ATHEROSCLEROSIS; EMPHYSEMA; BRONCHITIS; PNEUMONIA; *and* STROKE. *Also see* MARIJUANA.

Tocography

An obstetric procedure to record uterine muscle contractions during childbirth.

Tocography is performed together with fetal heart monitoring to assess the progress of labor and the frequency of contractions.

Toilet-Training

The ability to control the bowels is a milestone in a child's life. Children learn toilet-training gradually.

Toddlers tend to begin toilet-training around the age of 18 to 24 months. However, all children develop differently and should not be rushed. Some children do not have the necessary cognitive and physical skills until they are three or four.

A child may be ready to start toilet training if she or he has regular, soft bowel movements. Children may imitate the habits of their parents. Making grunting noises or squatting is common when the child feels the need to have a bowel movement. A child who uses words specifying stool and urine may be ready to start toilet-training. Children who can pull down their pants, sit down and follow simple instructions may be ready to begin using a toilet or potty seat.

Quitting Smoking

Nicotine is a highly addictive substance and, consequently, quitting smoking is extremely difficult. For many people, it takes multiple attempts to quit successfully. Rather than regarding them as failures, understand these attempts are part of a complex learning process. Your doctor can help you select different approaches such as nicotine patches, gums, nasal sprays, and therapy groups. Certain antidepressants have also been used to help quit the habit.

Quitting Smoking: The Patch. Below, a number of drug companies have begun producing "The Patch." This is a nicotine delivery system that does not involve cigarette smoking or tobacco chewing, which both have well documented cancer-causing side-effects.

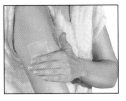

Before beginning the toilet training process, parents should make sure they have the right equipment. A child-sized potty seat or seat that attaches to the toilet is essential. *See also* CHILD DEVELOPMENT.

Seat the child, fully clothed, on the potty a few times a day. This will make the process familiar and spark interest in doing it. If the child does not want to sit on the potty, do not force it. Put the potty away for a while and try again later.

Seat your child on the potty without pants after you are sure the toilet routine is understood and accepted. Explain that this is the way other people use the toilet. The next time you child soils a diaper, let him or her flush away the waste. This can help a child connect going into the bathroom with the concept of using the toilet. Children should be encouraged to use the toilet whenever they want. *See also* CHILD DEVELOPMENT; DIARRHEA; FAMILY PRACTITIONER; INCONTINENCE; NUTRITION; PEDIATRICS; *and* PLAY THERAPY.

Tomography

Imaging method that shows a tissue plane; a "slice" of tissue.

Tomography uses a radioactive beam to sweep over sections of tissue. The resulting data is processed by a computer to form a detailed 3-dimensional tissue slice (tomogram), based on analysis of the different rates of absorption of radiation by the tissue. The imaging technique typically shows a "slice" or section of tissue, and offers a thousandfold increase in clarity over conventional x-rays. Tomography is particularly valuable for imaging soft tissue, blood vessels, muscles, and organs. Such imaging can detect growths, bleeding, and other abnormalities not seen on standard x-rays.

Other forms of tomography include emission tomography, in which a radioactive substance is injected and its course through the bloodstream monitored by a gamma or scintillation camera. As in the case of CAT scanning, such radionuclide imaging, uses a computer to reassemble the data into a tomogram. SPECT (single photon emission computed tomography) is a special form of radionuclide tomography as is positron emission tomography (PET) in which positrons are the radiation source. PET scans offer tremendous resolution and are especially useful in brain studies. *See* CAT SCAN *and* IMAGING TECHNIQUES.

Tone, Muscle

The tension of a muscle at rest.

Muscle tone determines how the body is able to carry out the actions. Too much tension makes the muscles rigid or stiff; too little causes the body to be weak and flabby. Weight bearing and aerobic activities will increase the muscle tone. *See also* EXERCISE; MUSCLE; PHYSICAL THERAPY; *and* POSTURE.

Tongue Cancer

A malignant tumor of the tongue.

Tongue cancer is a malignancy caused by tobacco use. It is also associated with the intake of alcohol; poor oral hygiene increases risk too. Tongue cancer usually occurs after the age of 40 and is more common in men than in women. Tongue cancers are dangerous as they can spread rapidly.

Symptoms. A first sign of a tongue cancer can be leukoplakia, one or more persistent white patches in the mouth. Such a patch usually is painless and often is discovered by a dentist during routine treatment. While many of these patches are not malignant, some can turn cancerous. If a cancer develops, the symptoms include tongue stiffening, difficulty swallowing, excessive saliva production, and bad breath. In its late stages, tongue cancer can be painful. In extreme cases, it can grow large enough to interfere with swallowing and breathing.

Diagnosis. Tongue cancer is diagnosed by taking a tissue sample of a suspected lesion for microscopic examination. Such a tissue sample is recommended as a general rule for leukoplakia, especially for smokers and other tobacco users.

Tomography. Below, a physician examines a Computerized axial tomography for abnormalities. CAT scans are becoming more and more popular for the resolution they provide which makes diagnosis more accurate than they have ever been before.

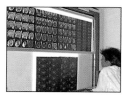

Treatment. The basic treatment for tongue cancer is tumor removal. Surgery can often effect a cure, if the cancer is detected early. If the cancer has spread to nearby lymph nodes, the entire tongue, the effected lymph nodes and part of the jaw may be removed. In such cases, radiation therapy and chemotherapy may follow surgery. Rehabilitation therapy is often necessary; plastic and reconstructive surgery can be done to restore normal appearance. The prognosis depends on the stage at which the cancer is diagnosed and treated. Because many tongue cancers are not detected early, the five-year survival rate tends to be low. *See also* CANCER *and* TUMOR.

Tonometry

A test to measure intraocular pressure using a device known as a tonometer.

Tonometry is used to measure pressure of fluid within the eyes—between its transparent lenses. The test is a useful diagnostic tool for detecting glaucoma, a disease caused by excessive pressure within the eye, causing impaired vision.

In the Schiotz method of tonometry, a drop of anesthetic is placed in the eye. The person then looks at a spot on the ceiling while the indentation tonometer is lowered onto the eye surface to measure pressure.

The applanation method uses a special dye to stain the eye for examination. With this, the pressure required to depress an area of the cornea is measured. An instrument supports the head, while the tonometer is brought into contact with the cornea.

The physician looks through an eyepiece and carefully adjusts the tonometer's pressure on the eye.

The noncontact or air puff method uses an instrument to blow a brief puff of air into the eye. Pressure is then calculated from the change in light reflected off the cornea as the puff of air touches it.

The tests, conducted for both eyes, are painless and low risk though with the two contact methods, there is some danger of damage to the lens. Pressure readings are in millimeters (mm) of mercury (Hg), with 20 mm Hg or lower a normal reading. Higher readings indicate either glaucoma or abnormal eye pressure. *See also* CORNEA; EYE; EYE, DISORDERS OF THE; EYE DROPS; EYE, EXAMINATION OF; GLAUCOMA; *and* LENS.

Tonsillectomy

The surgical removal of the tonsils of the throat.

The tonsils, two masses of tissue on either side of the back of the throat, assist the body's immune system by producing antibodies that resist infection. While tonsil infections may be treated with antibiotics, repeated or chronic infections may require tonsillectomy. Such infections, which may be either bacterial or viral, also affect the ear, causing earaches and hearing loss. If left untreated, tonsillitis can lead to a severe condition called a peritonsillar abscess, in which the swollen tonsils cause difficulty in breathing, requiring removal.

A tonsillectomy is carried out under general anesthesia. Patients may remain in the hospital one or two days, though the surgery is often completed on an outpatient basis. The mouth is held open and the tongue pulled forward to reveal the tonsils. The tonsils are pulled away from the back of the throat and carefully cut away. Recovery requires about three weeks, and the wound usually needs no further attention. Ice packs and analgesics like acetaminophen help with swelling and pain. Soft foods should be eaten and spicy foods avoided until healing is complete. *See also* BACTERIA; SURGERY; *and* TONSILLITIS.

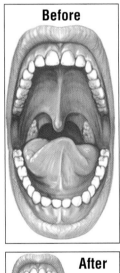

Before

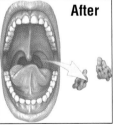

After

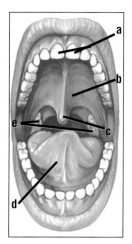

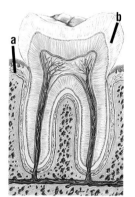

Dentistry and the Mouth. Top, an image of the mouth, wherein the tonsils may become inflamed and, in some cases, need to be removed. In the mouth there are the (a) teeth; (b) soft palate; (c) uvula; (d)tongue; and (e) tonsils. Above, bottom an illustration of how gingivitis happens. Gingivitis is an inflammatory condition of the gums which results in plaque, bacteria, and enzyme build up. These damage the gums and can affect the tooth root. Pictured is (a) the inflamed—and receding—gums; and (b) the plaque that causes the inflammation.

Tonsillitis

An inflammation of the tonsils caused by a bacterial or viral infection.

The tonsils are accumulations of lymph tissue at the back of the throat. They are part of the immune system. When infected, the tonsils swell and turn red. A common cause of tonsillitis is the *Streptococcus* bacterium that also causes strep throat.

The person affected with tonsillitis has a fever, sore throat, and a general feeling of sickness. The lymph nodes in the neck will swell and be tender. A doctor will see pus and a white membrane on the tonsils that can be pulled away without pain.

Whether the tonsillitis is viral or bacterial in origin, it is treated with pain-relieving medications, throat lozenges, warm salt water gargles, and hot tea. Do not give aspirin to children; they may develop Reye's syndrome, a serious disorder of the brain, liver, and blood that can occur if children with viral infections are given aspirin. If the cause of the tonsillitis is bacterial, a doctor will prescribe antibiotics.

Many years ago, tonsillectomy was almost a standard procedure for children, since the function of the tonsils was unknown and tonsillitis seemed an unnecessary childhood sickness. Today the surgery is only recommended if the child suffers from repeated infections and responds poorly to antibiotic treatment. *See also* ANTIBIOTIC DRUGS *and* STREPTOCOCCAL INFECTION.

Toothache

Pain in or around a tooth or teeth.

There are many causes for toothaches, but they all have one thing in common; they are the result of inflamation or injury to dental pulp. The most common cause of a toothache is simple tooth decay (caries) that irritates and can possibly affect the pulp of the teeth. As infection sets in, the pain increases. *See also* INFECTION.

The infection can progress to become an abscess. An abscess occurs a pus-filled sac forms around the root. This can be painful and dangerous; the abscess infection can spread into the bloodstream. Interestingly, a burst abscess is often mistakenly thought to be a good sign, since it relieves the pain because there is no longer pressure.

Toothache always warrants the attention of a dentist. Sometimes the pain will go away for a while; this may be a sign of a dead nerve, which needs to be addressed promptly if the tooth can be saved. *See also* CARRIES, DENTAL; DENTISTRY; FLOSSING, DENTAL; PREVENTIVE DENTISTRY; PUBLIC HEALTH DENTISTRY; *and* TOOTHBRUSHING.

Toothbrushing

Removal of food particles and plaque from teeth.

Proper tooth care includes brushing the teeth at least twice a day. Food particles can stick to the teeth and begin to decay; bacteria in the mouth can cause bad breath (halitosis) and gum disease (gingivitis or periodontitis). Tooth care should include brushing, flossing, and gum stimulation.

Correct toothbrushing requires a soft-bristled brush. It is not how hard people brush but how thoroughly that matters. Working from the gums toward the tooth and brushing in a circular motion works best. Brushing in a haphazard fashion merely moves the food particles and bacteria around; it does not eliminate them. Brushing should begin in the front and then work toward the back of the mouth, taking extra care when brushing the rearmost teeth where the most food particles get trapped. Two to three minutes should be spent brushing teeth, finishing with a thorough rinse of the mouth.

Some dentists advise using an automatic toothbrush, which is a cross between a regular brush and the professional electric brush used by dental hygienists. These brushes can sometimes do a better job of eliminating food particles than a regular brush, and there are several models available. *See also* FLOSSING, DENTAL; GINGIVITIS; PERIODONTITIS; *and* PREVENTIVE DENTISTRY.

Torticollis

Abnormal head rotation or tilt, due to neck twisting.

An injury to the neck that irritates the cervical nerves may cause the neck muscles to spasm. The spasm may then pull the head over to one side; this is torticollis. The muscle spasms that lead to torticollis can also be caused by sleeping with the neck placed at an awkward angle, or if a person holds tension from anxiety in his or her neck. In some cases, torticollis is the result of a birth injury that affects the neck muscles. Burns or other conditions that cause heavy scarring can also pull down the head.

Heat treatment, ultrasound, or wearing an orthopedic collar are the usual recommendations for torticollis. In severe cases, physical therapy may be necessary to restore movement. For head tilting from scar tissue, plastic surgery may be required to release the tension. When torticollis is caused by a birth injury, muscle stretching may help relieve the condition, although surgery may be necessary to cut and release the muscle. *See also* MUSCLE SPASM; PHYSICAL THERAPY; *and* ULTRASOUND TREATMENT.

Touch

The sense of tactility.

Touch is the sense by which data such as size, shape, temperature, and density is learned through physical contact with an object. Touching an object can produce feelings of warmth, cold, pressure, or pain.

There are numerous types of touch receptors in the skin that detect information. Some of these receptors (sensory nerve endings) are found in hairy areas, others in nonhairy areas, and a third group are found embedded deep within tissue. In hairy areas, webs of sensory nerve cell endings cloak the hair. Movement of the hair triggers the receptor cells. In smooth areas—the lips or fingertips—the cell endings are not web-like; they are free standing. In these smooth areas, pain is detected by free nerve endings in the skin tissue.

Physiology. Touch sensation is perceived when an object makes contact with a sense organ and moves it or touches an adjacent hair. Touch receptors transmit the signals they receive along the sensory nerves to the spinal cord. These impulses continue from the spinal cord to the brain, where the sensations are interpreted.

Sensitivity. The distribution of touch receptors in the body varies. Certain areas have more receptors and are more sensitive. The cornea of the eye is highly sensitive to pain. The fingertips are highly sensitive to touch. The back is the least sensitive to pressure. *See also* PAIN *and* SKIN.

Tourette's Syndrome

Also known as Gilles de la Tourette Syndrome

A brain disorder characterized by facial, muscular, and vocal tics.

Tourette's syndrome involves motor and vocal tics, which are involuntary, repetitive movements or utterances. It is more common in males than in females and is a chronic illness. Facial tics may include sniffing, blinking or grimacing. Vocal tics include grunts, barks, shrieks, throat clearing, or hisses. Coprolalia, a particular type of vocal tic, involves uttering socially unacceptable or curse words. Although this type of tic has received a great deal of attention, it affects less than 10 percent of those who suffer from this disorder. Tourette's syndrome may be diagnosed if tics occur daily, last for at least a year, and begin before the age of 21. Motor tics may involve jumping, grooming, or foot stomping.

Symptoms. The symptoms vary and can be temporarily suppressed. The tics tend to be exacerbated by stress or fatigue, and when they occur they appear to relieve stress. In some cases, they may be reduced with stress management and relaxation techniques. Support from family and friends and a structured and predictable schedule are also helpful in providing a comforting environment that helps relieve symptoms. An individual suffering from Tourette's may be able to resist the urge to express tics for a period of time or during a specific activity, but will most likely experience an eruption of tics that are more violent later.

Cause. Based on twin studies, Tourette's is probably an inherited disease. When one member of a family has Tourette's, others are often found to have some tics or related symptoms. A parent with the disease has a 50 percent chance of passing it on to a child. Although research is not conclusive, abnormal metabolism of neurotransmitters are believed to be related to Tourette's.

Treatment. Tourette's syndrome may be treated with antipsychotic medications such as halperidol, fluphenazine, risperidone, or pimozide. These drugs often cause side effects that patients find unacceptable including, a feeling of being slowed down and dull, or weight gain. Other drugs that may have fewer side effects, but also tend to be less effective, include klonopin, which is used to treat anxiety and seizure; or clonidine, which is used to treat attention-deficit hyperactivity disorder.

Complementary techniques including various methods of stress reduction or behavioral treatments that train a person to use an opposite movement to counteract the tic.

Related Illnesses. Several disorders have been associated with Tourette's syndrome, including obsessive-compulsive disorder, and about 60 percent of patients are affected by attention deficit hyperactivity disorder, and impulse control disorders.

> *Background information about* TOURETTE'S SYNDROME *can be found in* METABOLISM *and* OBSESSIVE-COMPULSIVE BEHAVIOR. *For information concerning the genetic aspects of this see* DNA; GENE; HERITABILITY; *and* INHERITANCE.

Tourniquet

A band of fabric wrapped tightly around a limb at a pressure point until blood flow is stopped.

Tourniquets are considered a very dangerous way to stop bleeding. They are not used unless an extremity has been amputated. If a tourniquet must be used, the band should be at least two inches wide so as not to cut into the skin. Wrap the strip tightly just above the wound, and knot it directly above the pressure point so that the artery is compressed. Release the knot every five minutes to restore circulation. *See* BLEEDING, TREATMENT OF *and* PRESSURE POINTS.

Toxemia

A condition in pregnancy characterized by high blood pressure, swelling, and protein in the urine.

Toxemia develops any time between the 20th week of pregnancy and the first week after giving birth. Preeclampsia is a milder form of toxemia. If left untreated, it will develop into eclampsia, which is a life-threatening condition for both mother and baby.

As preeclampsia develops into eclampsia, there is increased facial puffiness, sudden weight gain, and severe headaches. These are followed by pain in the upper right side of the abdomen, vision disturbances such as seeing flashing lights, severe convulsions, and loss of consciousness.

Mild preeclampsia is treated by bringing blood pressure under control with diet and medication. Bed rest is often prescribed. Sometimes hospitalization is necessary to administer medications for high blood pressure. Once eclampsia sets in, prompt delivery is required. In recent years, better prenatal care has helped lower the number of cases of preeclampsia that progress into eclampsia. *See also* ECLAMPSIA; PREECLAMPSIA; *and* TOXIN.

Toxic Shock Syndrome

A severe systemic illness which is a complication of an infection.

Toxic shock syndrome is caused not by the bacteria itself, but by toxins produced by the bacteria. Although toxic shock syndrome has been associated primarily with tampon use, it can affect people of both sexes and all ages, and is often linked to postoperative situations, when bacteria infiltrate wounds and enter the bloodstream, causing blood poisoning.

Researchers theorize that tampons of the highest absorbencies provide a fertile environment in which normally harmless bacteria can multiply. Therefore, women who use tampons should change them frequently, never leaving one in place for longer than eight hours.

Symptoms include sudden onset of a high fever (over 102°F), diarrhea, vomiting, headache, muscle ache, weakness, fainting, and a rash on the extremities that resembles a severe sunburn. Toxic shock syndrome can be fatal. Treatment involves fluid replacement to counter dehydration from fever, diarrhea, or vomiting; antibiotics; and, if relevant, removal of the cause of the toxin buildup. *See also* BLOOD POISONING; ENDOTOXIN: *and* INFECTIONS.

Toxicity

Potential for a poisonous substance to cause harm to a particular living organism.

Tiny amounts of poisonous substances will cause toxicity symptoms, while it takes much larger doses of other substances (such as vitamins A and D and iron) to do the same. Toxicity can apply to chemicals such as pesticides, pollutants, or drugs, as well as to naturally occurring toxins such as venom and the toxins found in plants or fungi. Toxicity may vary, particularly in regards to naturally occurring toxins. However, in toxicological tests, scientists aim to understand what level of a particular toxin is capable of causing a specific level of harm. Toxins can affect various body systems, including the nervous system, the blood, the respiratory system, or the skin. *See also* PESTICIDE; POISON; *and* TOXIN.

Toxicology

The study of how chemicals affect organisms.

Toxicology addresses and examines aspects of poisons on biological systems, including the physiological, social, and legal effects of these substances. Toxicological research provides information on potentially toxic substances to regulatory organizations and to the public. Such research often gives rise to regulations affecting occupational or other public exposure to toxic chemicals, as well as regulations for drugs and medications. *See also* POISON *and* TOXIN.

Toxin

Any chemical substance that is harmful to humans.

The majority, though not all, of these substances are neurotoxins affecting the nervous system and brain. Other types of toxins include hemotoxins that affect the blood and circulation; and enterotoxins produced by pathogenic bacteria in the digestive tract that cause gastrointestinal symptoms. Toxins may occur naturally or be produced synthetically. Some scientists differentiate between toxins that occur naturally and toxicants that are synthetic. Toxins can be produced either by living organisms such as bacteria and fungi, or they may be organic or inorganic substances that produce symptoms of toxicity. *See also* DRUG POISONING; LEAD POISONING; SALMONELLA; TOXIC SHOCK SYNDROME; *and* TOXICOLOGY.

Toxoid

An inactivated bacterial product or a single specific component of bacteria used in making vaccines.

Toxoids stimulate the immune system to act against a specific pathogen (disease-causing agent). However, toxoids do not actually cause illness. Examples of vaccines made with toxoids include those for tetanus and meningitis. *See also* IMMUNE SYSTEM.

Toxoplasmosis

Infectious disease caused by a parasite found in feline excrement or undercooked meat.

Toxoplasmosis is caused by ingesting soil contaminated with parasites, consuming undercooked meat, or handling cat litter. It can also be passed through the placenta of a pregnant woman carrying the disease,

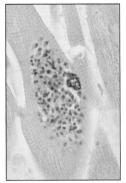

Toxoplasmosis. Below, a micrograph of a cell containing the parasite that causes toxoplasmosis; it is called Toxoplasma gondii. This parasite is found all over the planet; in the United States, it affects over 60 million individuals. Of those millions, only a few will ever show symptoms. Pregnant women can pass this infection to their baby.

in which case the infant runs the risk of complications, including nervous system disorders, enlargement of the liver and spleen, blindness, and mental retardation. Those with suppressed immune systems are also vulnerable to the disease, which may affect the brain, lung, heart, eyes, or liver.

Symptoms. In otherwise healthy people, symptoms are similar to influenza and include swollen lymph nodes, headache, sore throat, and aches. Those taking immune suppressants may experience brain lesions, confusion, seizures, and blurred vision.

Diagnosis. The disease may be diagnosed with a blood test, MRI or CT scans, or brain biopsy. Treatment depends on specifics, and may include medications.

Preventive measures include avoiding undercooked meat and soil contaminated with animal feces. Hands should be washed frequently and thoroughly after handling cat litter or contaminated soil. *See also* BLOOD TESTS; MONONUCLEOSIS; *and* MRI.

Trabeculectomy

Also known as glacumo filtration surgery

An operation that reduces pressure in the eyes by draining aqueous humor, eye fluid.

Trabeculectomy is the most common surgery for glaucoma. The operation is required when medications do not alleviate the pressure that will injure the optic nerve and lead to visual field loss. The surgeon removes a small piece of the sclera—the white part of the eye—enabling aqueous humor to escape from the eye's front chamber, reducing pressure.

Research from the National Institutes of Health confirms that laser therapy is significantly more effective than incisional trabeculectomy for African Americans who suffer the advanced stages of glaucoma. White patients respond better to incisional trabeculectomy. African Americans are especially at risk for glaucoma: one in 13 has it, and incidence is four to six times greater than in the white population. African Americans are also more likely to go blind as a result of glaucoma. *See also* GLAUCOMA.

Trace Elements

Minerals essential to health, which typically work in many of the body's metabolic processes.

The body needs trace elements in minute quantities; in large quantities they can be toxic. Fluoride, iodine, iron, and zinc are the best known of the trace elements. Other trace elements that are instrumental in a variety of vital metabolic processes, but whose functions are less well understood, include arsenic, boron, cobalt, copper, manganese, nickel, selenium, silicon, tin, and vanadium. A varied and balanced diet will supply sufficient amounts of trace minerals. *See also* ARSENIC; IRON; MINERALS; *and* ZINC.

Tracer

A radioactive solution used so that its course through the body may be followed.

Tracer substances with an affinity for a particular organ may be radioactively tagged (labeled) with a radioisotope—an element that has the same atomic number but different atomic mass than its non-radioactive counterpart. After the tracer is given by injection or by mouth, particle decay is monitored by a counter or gamma camera. This information is relayed to a computer and assembled into an image of the site under study. Tracers may be used to study blood flow, as in PET scanning, or to examine specific structures, as in radionuclide imaging of the gallbladder. *See* NUCLEAR MEDICINE.

Tracheitis

Also known as acute bacterial tracheitis

A bacterial infection of the trachea that may produce airway obstruction.

Young children are primarily affected by tracheitis. When a child rapidly develops a cough, difficulty breathing, and a high fever, hospitalization is necessary.

Symptoms of tracheitis include a cough following an upper-respiratory infection, a crowing sound when the child breathes, high fever, labored breathing, and a general look of sickness. A breathing tube is usually inserted into the child's throat to help her or him breathe. Oxygen and penicillin are given, and oxygen levels are monitored. *See also* BACTERIA *and* LUNG.

Tracheoesophageal Fistula

An abnormal connection between the esophagus and the trachea.

Tracheoesophogeal fistula is a condition that usually occurs with esophageal atresia—the incomplete development of the esophagus. Symptoms include excessive saliva, coughing after attempts to swallow, and the skin will have a bluish cast. Saliva may enter the lungs, putting the infant at risk for aspiration pneumonia. Surgery is performed to close the fistula. Until then, the infant must be fed intravenously. Continuous suction must also be applied to prevent saliva from entering the lungs.

The term tracheoesophageal fistula also applies to a valve surgically inserted between the trachea and esophagus to enable an individual to speak after removal of the vocal cords. The valve forces air into the esophagus while the person inhales, producing a sound. However, food and liquids may enter the trachea through the valve if it is not working properly. *See* ESOPHAGUS.

Tracheostomy

Surgical incision of the trachea to permit airflow in the case of obstruction.

Tracheotomy is a surgical procedure carried out in the operating room under general anesthesia. An incision in the throat is made, and forms a temporary or permanent opening in the windpipe known as a tracheostomy. The incision is usually vertical and runs from the second to fourth rings of cartilage that make up the outer wall of the trachea. Two of these rings are severed and a tube is inserted into the resulting opening to allow the passage of air and the removal of secretions.

The individual is then able to breathe through his or her tracheostomy tube, rather than through the nose and mouth, thus bypassing the upper airway. Tracheostomy is used to treat tumors and infections. Vocal cord injury and laryngeal spasm or injury may also be treated through tracheostomy surgery. Additionally, congenital abnormality of the larynx or trachea, severe neck or mouth injuries, occlusion of the airway by a large foreign object, or long term unconsciousness or coma may require tracheostomy.

The tracheostomy tube has three parts: the outer cannula, the inner cannula, and the obturator, which is used for inserting the tube. The outer cannula remains permanently in the windpipe, except during cleaning. The inner cannula provides a safety valve to keep the airway open. It is removed only for cleaning.

Often the surgery is performed on an emergency basis. The technique bypasses the upper airway and glottis, to avoid complications. Patients are able to eat and, with careful practice, speak. Sometimes the patient will be discharged with the tracheostomy tube in place; the patient will not be able to speak and suctioning of the device may be necessary to remove secretions. *See* CROUP *and* LARYNGECTOMY.

Tracheotomy

Creating an opening in the trachea in the front of the neck below the pharynx.

Tracheotomies are performed almost exclusively in emergency situations to bypass a throat obstruction to prevent suffocation. Less often, they may be used to get a biopsy specimen or to get at a lesion.

A tracheotomy may be performed before major surgery on the throat because postoperative swelling can obstruct breathing. In emergency situations a tracheotomy

> **ALERT**
>
> ## Mediastinal Emphysema
>
> In addition to the risk of infection and scarring of the trachea characteristic of such surgery, tracheostomy can induce a condition known as mediastinal emphysema, in which the tracheostomy tube is ejected when the patient coughs. This may be prevented by thoroughly securing the tracheostomy tube in place.

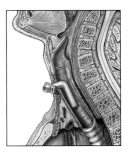

Tracheotomy. Tracheotomy should only be done in the most dire emergency situations. Above, an image of where the tracheotomy tube (often a mere pen barrel) should go. The tracheotomy is one of the oldest proceedures know to humankind. There are images of the proceedure dating back to 3000 years b.c.e., although the first surgery is often attributed to Asclepiades around 100 b.c.e.

may be performed with a pen knife or a letter opener. The hole will heal by itself. This is the same procedure as a tracheotomy except that the suffix -stomy refers to the opening and the suffix -otomy refers to the incision. *See also* SURGERY.

Trachoma

A bacterial disease of the conjunctiva and cornea.

Trachoma is a disease common among people dwelling in overcrowded conditions, with limited access to water and poor health care. It causes repeated infections throughout childhood. Mothers of children with this disease are extremely susceptible to trachoma.

A *Chlamydia trachomatis* infection produces acute conjunctivitis, pain, and tearing. The eyes become swollen and inflamed. Trachoma is often accompanied by damage to the mucus-secreting cells and to tear-producing cells (the lacrimal glands). The cornea becomes opaque because of an abnormal growth. As the disease progresses, the eyelashes roll in and may rub the cornea. Increased corneal scarring leads to vision loss or blindness.

As with all infectious disease, prevention is the best treatment for trachoma. The easiest method of prevention is to increase the frequency of face washing among children at risk for the disease. Antibiotic drugs can destroy the bacteria in the early stages of disease. A surgical procedure can prevent irritation of the eyelashes and can remove the scar tissue. *See also* EYE.

Traction

Tension applied to an injury in order to correct alignment during healing.

Traction is used for fractures where healing is disrupted by the surrounding muscles that pull the bones out of the correct position; spinal and leg injuries are the most typical examples. Traction for a leg injury usually involves elevating the leg with an overhead frame. For a spinal injury, a per-

son will lie flat and weighted tongs will be inserted into either side of the skull. The patient will have to remain in traction as long as is necessary for the bones to correctly heal. *See also* FRACTURE.

Trager Psychophysical Integration

A form of bodywork designed to release tension and loosen the muscles and joints.

Having suffered from a severe back ailment, Dr. Milton Trager developed a system of healing that emphasizes the relationship between mind and body. It is used primarily to treat people with neuromuscular disorders, however, athletes also use it to enhance their output and gain stamina. Trager worked with a number of people with various disorders to develop this approach to healing.

The objective of the Trager method is to help the client learn to recognize how his or her body holds tension. By working with a practitioner, the individual, through relaxation techniques, learns to release tension and, in doing so, will achieve greater flexibility and range of motion. To work towards these ends, the client must learn to surrender conscious muscular control, thereby enabling the unconscious mind to adopt—with the help of the practitioner—a freer range of motion.

Dr. Trager believes that certain movement can produce pleasurable feelings and the mind will then learn to "mimic" such movements. For this reason, his technique does not focus on isolated muscle movement, rather it focuses on the feelings created by motion and the relaxation that results. *See also* BODYWORK.

Most Trager sessions require the client to lie on a flat table while a practitioner manipulates his or her limbs. These sessions will also include ongoing instruction in Trager "Mentastics." These exercises, performed at home, consist of a combination of mind-directed dance-like movements that encourage relaxation and free-flowing motion. *See also* ALTERNATIVE MEDICINE.

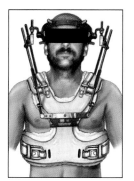

Traction. Below, a picture of the a man in traction. Traction keeps a person in the optimal position for a quick recovery. Although, often, it is uncomfortable, it is always best to augment the healing process in this fashion. The proper amount of tension and stabilization can be put on joints and bones so that they can be immobilized with for optimal results.

Trait

A genetically inherited characteristic.

A trait may be physical, such as height or blood type, or it may be mental, such as spatial ability. Usually there are two genes responsible for a trait, one from each parent. For some traits, however, more than one set of genes are involved. Gene expression also depends upon the environment. Certain factors can interfere with the expression. For example, with height, an individual may have the genes for being tall, but if he or she is deprived of nutrients this trait will not express itself. *See also* GENETICS.

Transfusion, Autologous

When a person is transfused with his or her own previously donated blood.

The safest blood to receive by transfusion is one's own; since there is no question about incompatibility. Sometimes blood is collected during surgery for replacement. More often a person anticipating surgery donates blood before the scheduled procedure, which is then available for transfusion if necessary. *See also* BLOOD GROUPS.

Transient Ischemic Attack

A brain function irregularity caused by a deficiency in the quantity of blood supplied to the brain.

A transient ischemic attack (TIA) is similar to a stroke, except that it lasts for a shorter period of time. If the attack continues for more than 24 hours, it is referred to as a stroke. A TIA occurs when the blood supply to part of the brain decreases momentarily. It is often a precursor to a stroke.

Incidence. The risk of experiencing a transient ischemic attack increases in individuals with high blood pressure, heart disease, diabetes, or an excess of red blood cells; incidence also increases among the elderly. A small percentage of young adults who suffer from heart disease or blood disorders also experience such attacks.

Causes. In a TIA, the walls of the arteries that lead to the brain become blocked because of a build-up of fat and calcium deposits. Also, small masses of platelets and blood clots may block the arteries, cutting off the blood supply to the brain.

Symptoms. TIAs usually occur without warning. The symptoms are similar to those of a stroke but have a shorter duration; these include numbness, weakness in the face, arm, or leg, confusion, difficulty speaking and understanding speech, an inability to recognize body parts, blurred vision, a partial hearing loss, difficulty walking, dizziness, balance and coordination loss, and loss of bladder control. TIAs often recur or develop into a stroke; this happens in about 33 percent of patients.

Treatment. Since there is there is no way to be certain whether the symptoms are the result of a TIA or an acute stroke, patients should regard all stroke-like symptoms as an emergency. After an examination, the physician may prescribe medication, surgery or both to prevent a recurrence and to reduce the possibility of a stroke. Antiplatelet agents, specifically aspirin, may be prescribed. Anticoagulants may be prescribed for patients with an irregular heart beat (atrial fibrillation). *See also* Stroke.

Transillumination

A means of examining an organ or tissue by passing light through it.

Transillumination is a diagnostic technique that involves directing light through a cavity or organ—often the head, breast, scrotum, or, with infants, the chest. Transillumination is used to diagnose excess fluid in a newborn's brain, excess fluid around the testicles, and breast lesions or cysts. The technique relies on the fact that abnormal air or fluid in a region under study will increase light transmission, while other abnormalities block light transmission. Lesions and bleeding within the breast for example appear dark, as blood fails to transilluminate. Transillumination is completely safe, and pain-free. *See* DIAGNOSIS.

Transient Ischemic Attack: TIA. The brain (a) receives blood from the carotid arteries (b). During a Transient ischemic attack, the blood flow to the brain decreases. The heavy white arrows on the left represent the normal blood flow to the brain; the lighter white arrows on the right represent the decreased blood flow to the brain that happens during a TIA.

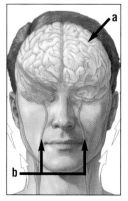

Transmissible

An infectious disease or a genetic trait that can be passed from one person to another.

How transmissible an infectious disease is depends on the disease's cause and how it is spread. A disease such as the common cold is highly transmissible, whereas HIV can be transmitted only by exposure to an affected person's body fluids.

Genetics. In genetics, several factors affect a trait's transmission, including how a trait is influenced by genetic or environmental factors, and whether the gene or genes causing a trait are dominant, recessive, or sex-linked. In general, serious diseases and disorders are less transmissible than more benign disorders. *See also* INHERITANCE.

Transplant Surgery

The grafting of tissue from one area to another, or transfer of an organ from one person to another.

Transplant surgery is used to transfer tissue from one area of the body to another in order to restore function, or to graft whole organs from a donor to a recipient. When whole organs are transplanted from a donor, the transplantation is often life-saving. Hearts, livers, kidneys, pancreas, cornea, as well as many types of tissue have been successfully transplanted.

The main obstacle to transplantation is the rejection of tissue by the recipient's immune system; this is known as graft-host disease. Blood and tissue cells carry identifying proteins recognized by the immune system; when another person's blood or tissue is introduced, the immune system treats it as a foreign intruder and rejects the donor organ. In some cases, such as kidney transplantation, careful tissue matching is carried out to ensure compatibility. Immunosuppressant drugs are often administered during and following transplant surgery to limit tissue rejection caused by tissue incompatibility. Close family members offer the best prospects for successful organ donation. *See also* HEART TRANSPLANT.

Resources on Transplant Surgery

Cottrell, James E. and Stephanie Golden, *Under the Mask: A Guide to Feeling Secure and Comfortable During Anesthesia and Surgery* (2001); Finn, Robert, et al., *Organ Transplants: Making the Most of Your Gift of Life* (2000); Rutkow, Ira M., *Surgery: An Illustrated History* (1993); Silber, Irwin and Eugene Wolf, *A Patient's Guide to Knee and Hip Replacement* (1999); American College of Surgeons, Tel. (312) 202-5000, Online: www.facs.org; American College of Physicians–American Society of Internal Medicine, Tel. (800) 523-1546, Online: www.acponline.org; www.med.cornell.edu/surgery/; www.nycornell.org/medicine/emergency/html.

Transposition of the Great Vessels

A heart disease in which the arteries carrying blood from the heart are in each other's position.

In unaffected hearts, the pulmonary artery carries blood to the lungs for oxygenation, and the aorta carries oxygenated blood to the rest of the body. If these vessels are transposed, blood that is already oxygenated is returned to the lungs, while oxygen-poor blood is circulated to the body. Unless the defect is corrected quickly, there is a 90 percent chance that the baby will die within his or her first year. Balloon septostomy is an emergency measure that allows blood to move between heart chambers; this is like a ventricular septal defect. Prolonged survival can be achieved if surgery is done to move the arteries so that they occupy the normal positions. The best results have been achieved when the operation is performed in the first two weeks of life. *See also* HEART DISEASE, CONGENITAL.

Transsexualism

A condition in which a person feels incompatible with the gender in which he or she was born.

Although transsexualism is fairly rare, it tends to be more common among men. It also often follows a period of cross-dressing. Transsexuals often have a sense since childhood that he or she is "in the wrong body" and that he or she would be better adjusted in the body of a member of the opposite sex. *See also* TRANSVESTISM.

Transsexualism should not be confused with the behavior of homosexual men or masculine females, who have no desire to change their anatomy or sexuality. Transsexuals will often seek to change their gender surgically and through the use of hormone therapy.

A series of surgical and hormonal treatments are possible. Transsexuals often experience bouts of depression, anxiety, drug and alcohol abuse, and work dysfunction;

some however, are able to function normally and productively. Transsexuals often experience low sex drive, although, some people have been able to lead active sexual lives. While nearly all women who seek sex reassignment are homosexual, about 25 percent of male transsexual individuals are sexually attracted to women. *See also* HETEROSEXUALITY *and* HOMOSEXUALITY.

Transvestism

Also known as cross-dressing

A persistent desire to dress in the clothing regularly worn by members of the opposite sex.

In most cases of transvestism, a male wears female clothing, often wearing female underwear as a means of heightening arousal. In rare instances, transvestism is linked to transsexualism. Many transvestites have heterosexual partners and function normally in society. Though society has stigmatized radical forms of this behavior (and has ignored the prevalence of transvestite behavior throughout society), the behavior is not deemed a reason to seek treatment. *See also* TRANSSEXUALISM.

Trauma

Any injury to the body and its effects on the mind.

Physical trauma has a number of causes, from a fall to an automobile accident to a gun shot. A sprain, a broken bone, and a bleeding wound, are examples of trauma. Emotional trauma is a term applied to a person's reaction to a serious physical trauma. Physical trauma is treated with first aid and emergency medical personnel. The psycological conditon that often follows any type of trauma is referred to as post-traumatic stress disorder. *See* FIRST AID.

Traumatology

The study and treatment of trauma.

Traumatology involves the study and treatment of all trauma—it is the science of in-

jury, what leads to it, and how it is prevented, and treated. Many specializations are involved with traumatology including sports, surgical, orthopedic, and geriatric medicines. *See also* CRISIS INTERVENTION.

Travel Immunizations

Vaccinations against infectious diseases for which travelers are at risk.

Travel immunizations are given to protect against infectious diseases found in the specific region of the world that the traveler plans to visit. Travelers should visit the doctor four to six months prior to traveling to give the vaccines time to take effect and to reduce the likelihood of side effects. The Centers for Disease Control (CDC) recommends certain vaccinations for travelers.

Recommended Vaccinations. In general, the CDC recommends that people have up-to-date vaccinations for hepatitis A, typhoid, polio, measles, mumps, rubella, diphtheria, tetanus, and pertussis. The exact requirements, however, vary. Travelers to tropical climates, for example, should also receive a vaccination for yellow fever or malaria, as needed.

Travel Vaccinations for Children

Children under the age of two often need more vaccines than adults, since they are less likely to have already received the complete course of standard vaccines. Several vaccinations require multiple injections over a period of time to be effective. For that reason, it is vitally important that individuals traveling with children under the age of two consult a doctor as far in advance of the travel date as possible.

Some people have special vaccination requirements. Travelers who will work with animals should receive the rabies vaccine; health care workers who anticipate coming into contact with blood should receive the hepatitis B vaccine. Travelers with weak immune systems should consult their doctor before receiving vaccines, as the risk of infection from the vaccine may outweigh the benefits of vaccination. *See also* HEPATITIS; TRAVEL MEDICINE; *and* VACCINATION .

Travel Medicine

An area of medicine that covers health risks faced by travelers and suggests precautions to avoid illness while traveling.

Travel medicine identifies the health risks a traveler faces in a particular area of the world, offers suggestions as to how to stay healthy, and prescribes treatments for travel-related illnesses. The ease with which people can travel from one place to another has resulted in a dramatic increase in the number of people who travel internationally. As a result, travelers encounter many potential health risks abroad, ranging from the innocuous but annoying experience of diarrhea to more serious illness like hepatitis and malaria.

Incidence. Travelers face an increased risk of contracting a disease while abroad. The greatest risk is for traveler's diarrhea, which afflicts almost half of all tourists who go to developing countries. Malaria poses a a very serious threat to a traveler's health; for every one million travelers staying abroad for a month, 24,000 develop malaria; of that same group, 3,000 will contract hepatitis A, and an equal number will be infected with a sexually transmitted disease. Yellow fever or cholera infections are much rarer.

Prevention. All travelers should ensure that they are up-to-date on the appropriate immunizations. In addition, travelers should avoid tap water, eat only thoroughly cooked meat, and avoid fruits and vegetables that may have been washed with tap water. Where malaria is a risk, travelers should use insect repellent. Doctors advise travelers to take essential first-aid remedies, such as pain-relievers, anti-diarrheal medication, and band-aids, with them on trips, particularly to developing areas of the world.

Treatment. The treatment for travel-related illnesses depends on the illness. A range of antidiarrheal medications are available. Antibiotics and medications to reduce intestinal spasms may also be used. Several medications are available for malaria, yellow fever, and cholera. For most types of hepatitis, however, no effective treatment is available.

Other important related articles include DIARRHEA; FEVER; INFECTIOUS DISEASE; MALARIA; TRAVELER'S DIARRHEA; TRAVEL IMMUNIZATION; *and* YELLOW FEVER. *It is also vital to have an understanding of the* SAND FLY BITES *and* TSETSE FLY BITES. *See also* ANTIBIOTIC DRUGS *and* PARASITE.

Traveler's Diarrhea

Also known as Montezuma's revenge

Diarrhea that attacks those visiting foreign regions; it is caused by different infectious agents.

Traveler's diarrhea can be caused by several factors: unfamiliar food, a shift in the bacteria that normally inhabit the intestines or exposure to pathogenic bacteria, and, rarely, viral infections. In case precautions fail, medications can be taken to stop diarrhea. It is important to drink plenty of liquids in order to prevent dehydration. A light, bland diet should suffice for the first day or two when the appetite returns. To prevent diarrhea, only boiled or bottled water should be used. Foods that have been cooked thoroughly and refrigerated afterwards should not cause any digestive upsets. Avoid raw foods, such as fruits and vegetables, unless they can be peeled immediately prior to eating. *See also* MALARIA.

Tremor

An involuntary, rhythmic, muscular contraction.

Tremors are characterized by rhythmic oscillations in the body. They often affect the hands, the head, the face, the vocal cords, the trunk, and the legs. The majority of tremors occur in the hands.

ALERT

Malaria

Each year, about 30,000 Americans and Europeans contract malaria when they travel. A mosquito-borne parasite, malaria causes fever, sweats, malaise, and headaches. Symptoms can reappear months or even years after exposure to the parasite.

The standard preventive drug for malaria is chloroquine, though the rise in resistant strains of the parasite limits its use. Doxycycline can prevent malaria, but it cannot be taken by pregnant women or by children under the age of 8. Mefloquine prevents malaria; however, its side effects include seizures, psychosis, and anxiety. No medication is 100 percent effective, and symptoms can develop even in people who have taken the above medications. Travelers who show symptoms of malaria should see a doctor immediately. If symptoms of malaria develop and medical care is not available, the drug Fansidar should be taken until medical help arrives.

Types. Tremors can be classified according to behavior or position. A static tremor occurs when the muscle is at rest. People with Parkinson's disease experience this type of tremor. A postural tremor occurs when a person tries to maintain posture; it is seen in those with basal ganglia disease. A task-specific tremor appears when the patient is executing goal-oriented tasks such as handwriting or standing. Hysterical tremors are common and are experienced at times of increased emotion. They occur in both older and younger patients.

Causes. Tremors may accompany disorders associated with aging. Although tremors are not hazardous, it can be accountable for functional disability and social awkwardness. Healthy people may experience tremors when afraid. These tremors are caused by the body's reaction to an increase in the production of the hormone epinephrine.

Treatment. The underlying condition causing tremors must first be identified to treat tremors. Symptomatic drug therapy is used to treat tremors related to disease. For example, levodopa, the drug used to treat Parkinson's patients, helps to eradicate tremors. For the cases of tremor in which there is no effective drug treatment, measures such as bracing the affected limb during the tremor are helpful. Surgical intervention may be necessary in extreme cases. *See* AGING *and* PARKINSON'S DISEASE.

Trench Fever

The disease caused by the Bartonella quintana organism; it was prevalent during World War I.

Trench fever nearly disappeared after the end of the first World War. Today it is being reported among the homeless it is caused by a louse that carries a ricketsial organism, *Bartonella quintana*. Rickettsiae have characteristics that are both viral and bacterial. The incubation period for trench fever can be as short as five days. After this period the victim experiences backaches and headaches. The site of infection may become ulcerous; there is a rash on the chest, ab-

domen, and limbs, as well as a fever. The victim is listless and confused if not delirious. Before the availability of antibiotics, trench fever was often fatal, as it was left untreate . Today some antibiotics are effective against the organism that causes the disease. *See* ANTIBIOTIC DRUGS *and* RICKETTSIAE.

Trial, Clinical

A series of tests supervised by the Food and Drug Administration to determine if a new medication is safe and effective.

Clinical trials involve a three-phase procedure. In Phase I the new drug is given to a small group of people to determine if it is toxic. This phase establishes how to deliver the drug to the patient and how much is safe. In Phase II people who have not been helped by other treatments are given the tested drug. Subjects are carefully monitored for efficacy and side effects. In Phase III the number of subjects is increased, and time is extended to discover long-term side effects. *See* FOOD AND DRUG ADMINISTRATION.

Trichiasis

A condition in which the eyelashes are directed toward the eye and scratch the cornea's surface.

In trichiasis, the position of the lower lid is normal, but the lashes point in the wrong direction. This may lead to infection and scarring of the cornea. The most common cause is inflammation with lower lid scarring. Treatment involves either removal of the offending lashes, which is only a temporary measure, or destruction of the lash follicle. In approximately one third of cases, the lashes re-grow and treatment must be repeated. *See also* DACROCYSTITIS.

Trichinosis

Infectious disease caused by a parasitic worm and transmitted through undercooked meat.

Trichinosis (trichinellosis) is caused by eating poorly cooked or raw meat that is infect-

Trichinella Spiralis. Below, photomicrographs of the parasites that cause trichinosis. Pork and other uncooked meats carry these worms that will hatch in the intestines before migrating to muscle tissue where they will cause rather severe pain and swelling.

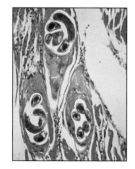

ed with the *Trichinella spiralis* parasite, a roundworm. Despite inspection of meat, trichinosis may pass examination; the parasites are difficult to detect. Digestive juices break down cysts, freeing the larvae and causing intestinal tract irritation. Larvae develop in the digestive tract, where adult male and female worms mate. Female worms burrow into the intestinal wall and in six days begin producing larvae.

Seven days after contaminated meat has been consumed, newly hatched larvae migrate into the lymph channels of the intestine, where they enter the bloodstream. After two weeks, the hatched larvae penetrate muscle tissue, developing until they are 16 days old. Larval development then ceases, and the larvae form a capsule around themselves, using the host's skeletal muscle. This capsule becomes a calcified cyst.

Symptoms. Often, infection occurs without symptoms. When symptoms exist, they occur within the first week and may include stomach ache, nausea, vomiting, and diarrhea. During the migration through the tissues, fever, muscle aches, rash, eye swelling or hemorrhages, and puffiness of the face may result. If left untreated, complications may involve the heart, central nervous system and lungs. Damage to muscle tissue is also common.

Diagnosis. Trichinosis is diagnosed with a blood test to detect trichinella antibodies. Muscle tissue may also be examined microscopically for the presence of *T. spiralis* parasites following biopsy.

Treatment. Trichinosis may be effectively treated with thiabendazole during the intestinal phase. Drug treatment may prove ineffective once the larvae have migrated, and no treatment exists once the parasites have become encysted in muscle. The disease is usually self-limiting after six months. While trichinosis is rarely fatal, the disease can cause permanent heart or eye damage. *See also* CYST; FEVER; INFECTION; INTESTINE; MUSCLE; *and* PARASITE.

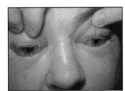
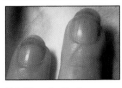

Trichinosis Cysts. Above, top, trichinosis, a tiny roundworm affecting the eyes. Although trichinosis usually causes facial swelling and edema at the eyes, this is a particularly severe case in which the eyes are deeply affected. Above, bottom, a trichinosis worm affecting the finger. Although the hand is often less affected by trichinosis, it is how the parasite most commonly spreads. The hands should always be washed after handling any kind of meat and especially after handling pork.

Preventing Trichinosis

Trichina cysts in pork are destroyed by freezing the meat at 5º F for 21 days or -22º F for about 25 hours. Unencysted trichina larvae are destroyed when the meat is heated to 150º F. It is important to note that ordinary curing and smoking processes do not render pork suitable for consumption.

Trichomoniasis

Sexually transmitted infection caused by a protozoan parasite.

Trichomoniasis is caused by *Trichomonas vaginalis*, a single cell parasite that propels itself through vaginal and urethral mucus. The disease exists worldwide and is transmitted sexually or, more rarely, through contact with contaminated surfaces, such as washcloths or toilet seats. The protozoan must be transmitted directly to the penis or vagina; it cannot survive contact with the mouth or rectum. While men acquire the disease only from women, infected women can pass the disease either to other women or to men.

The disease produces different symptoms in men and women. Men often remain asymptomatic, and the illness is usually self-limiting after a few weeks. Male symptoms may include urethral discomfort during or after urination or ejaculation, sometimes developing into inflammation of the prostate or epididymis. Women develop a foul-smelling vaginal discharge that may be yellowish or greenish in color, accompanied by labial itching or swelling and discomfort during intercourse. *See also* PAP SMEAR *and* SEXUALLY TRANSMITTED DISEASE.

Tricuspid Insufficiency

Failure of the tricuspid valve to close, causing blood to leak on the heart's right side.

The tricuspid valve controls the flow of blood from the right ventricle (the lower chamber on the heart's right side), to the right atrium (the upper chamber on the right side). If the valve does not close properly and blood leaks back to the ventricle, the right ventricle can become enlarged as it works harder. The result can be right-sided heart failure, causing edema (excess collection of fluid in the abdomen and ankles), as well as congestion of the liver.

Tricuspid insufficiency can be caused by pulmonary hypertension and rheumatic fever or a bacterial infection. The symptoms can often be managed by drug therapy with angiotensin-converting enzyme (ACE) inhibitors and diuretics. If drug treatment is not successful, open-heart surgery can be done to repair a valve or replace it with a mechanical valve. *See also* HEART VALVE SURGERY *and* VALVULOPLASTY.

Trigeminal Neuralgia

Also known as tic douloureux

A malfunction of the trigeminal nerve (fifth cranial nerve) producing brief, excruciating pain in different areas of the face.

The trigeminal nerve begins in the brain stem and divides into nerve networks. It carries sensation from the face to the brain, so damage along the nerve route disrupts sensations along the pathway. In addition, a disease in one area supplied by the trigeminal nerve can produce a domino effect, causing referred pain in other areas along its route.

The cause of trigeminal neuralgia is uncertain; it is sometimes the result of an artery that has drifted out of place and presses on a nerve adjacent to the brain. It can also be related to multiple sclerosis or a herpes zoster infection. Trigeminal neuralgia produces a burning pain on the side of the face. Trigeminal neuralgia can be triggered by an everyday activity such as eating, drinking, talking, or face washing.

Drug treatment is difficult because many people develop a resistance to the antiseizure drug normally used in treatment. Carbmazepine is prescribed to curb the pain. Some patients require, but are unable to tolerate, a high dosage of the drug. Surgical options are a last resort. *See also* HERPES; MULTIPLE SCLEROSIS; *and* REFERRED PAIN.

Trigger Finger

Also known as stenosing tenosynovitis

The locking of a finger or fingers in a bent position.

Characteristic of this condition is a snapping or clicking sound when the locked finger is straightened or closed. Usually the digit is locked into an abnormally bent po-

sition. Trigger finger is caused by local swelling, inflammation, or scarring of the tendons that pull the affected digit inward toward the palm. This condition usually appears alone but it can also be a side effect of illnesses that produce tissue inflammation in the hand, such as rheumatoid arthritis.

Treatment includes the application of ice, stretching techniques, and anti-inflammatory medicines. Injections of corticosteroid into the affected tendon can provide relief. If the condition persists, surgery can correct the condition. *See* INFLAMMATION.

Trismus

More commonly known as lockjaw

Involuntary contraction of the jaw muscles.

Trismus is a condition in which jaw movement is restricted. It becomes difficult to open the mouth wide enough for swallowing, chewing, or tooth brushing. It may result in impaired speech and nutrition.

Trismus is the result of shrinking and breakdown of the connective tissue in the postmandibular region. It is often caused by trauma, such as a burn or gunshot wound, infection, surgery, or radiation treatment. It can also be symptomatic of tetanus, tonsillitis, mumps, tooth abscess, head and neck cancer, or Parkinson's disease as well as anorexia nervosa. Trismus treatment begins with an accurate diagnosis of the underlying cause. Rehabilitation appliances and exercises can increase the mouth's ability to open. *See also* ANOREXIA NERVOSA *and* PARKINSON'S DISEASE.

Trisomy

The presence of three copies of a chromosome.

Normally, there are 23 pairs of chromosomes with one pair consisting of the two sex chromosomes. Trisomy refers to the presence of an extra chromosome.

Autosomal trisomies, the presence of an extra nonsex chromosome, are usually fatal. The exception is Down's syndrome, which is caused by an extra copy of chromo-

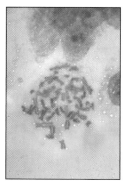

Mitosis. Below, a picture of the chromosomes of a human cell undergoing mitosis (the process of cell division by which it divides). This is not always the most orderly process that a cell undergoes, and sometimes, during the first few moments after conception a third copy of a chromosome (there are only supposed to be two) may accidently form.

some 21. Down's syndrome results in characteristic facial anomalies, mental retardation, and heart defects. Most affected individuals live into middle age.

Trisomy 18, known as Edward's syndrome, is due to the presence of an extra copy of chromosome 18. Children with this have facial abnormalities as well as severe retardation and usually only survive for a few months. Trisomy 13, known as Patau's syndrome, involves the presence of an extra chromosome 13. Infants born with this syndrome have severe brain and eye defects and rarely survive past one year.

Sex chromosome trisomies are not fatal, but have a range of effects. Triple X syndrome, which occurs in one in 1000 female births, results in low intelligence. "Triple" X is a misnomer, as there can be more than one additional chromosome. As the number increases, so does the chance of mental retardation and physical abnormalities.

Boys born with Klinefelter's syndrome have an extra X chromosome, resulting in a pattern of XXY. This occurs in approximately one in 700 male births. The physical characteristics can vary, but these males are tall, with feminized bodies including breast development. Their testes are small and they are usually sterile. Boys with this syndrome have normal intelligence but usually exhibit speech and reading disabilities.

Sometimes a male has an extra Y chromosome, resulting in a pattern of XYY. These males are usually tall and experience language difficulties. *See also* DOWN'S SYNDROME *and* KLINEFELTER'S SYNDROME.

Tropical Diseases

Diseases found primarily in tropical and subtropical regions.

Few tropical diseases are confined solely to tropical areas, though most cases of these illnesses are found in these regions due to the climate, poor sanitation, and a lack of resources to combat them. Thousands of tropical diseases exist, though few are widespread; and they are often transmitted through animal hosts.

Mosquitoes transmit a number of tropical diseases. Malaria, for example, is transmitted by mosquitoes. The disease affects the red blood cells, causing them to first swell and burst. Certain strains can produce cerebral malaria, a potentially fatal disease. Other mosquito-borne diseases include dengue fever and encephalitis, both carried by the asian tiger mosquito, as well as yellow fever and infestation by filarial worms (filariasis).

Flies also carry and transmit tropical diseases such as river blindness (onchocerciasis). It is caused by a parasitic worm and transmitted by a black fly common to fast rivers in Africa and South America. The tsetse fly causes African sleeping sickness (trypanosomiasis), a disease affecting the brain and surrounding tissues. Sand-flies can carry leishmania protozoa, which cause leishmaniasis, an infectious disease affecting the skin, nasal passages, and pharynx.

A parasitic worm (schistosome) causes a variety of tropical diseases, known collectively as schistosomiasis. Schistosomes complete a part of their lifecycle in the bodies of freshwater snails. Schistosome infection can damage the liver, intestines, lungs, or urinary bladder.

> *For foundational information about* TROPICAL DISEASES *see* INSECT BITES; INSECTS AND DISEASE; MOSQUITO BITES; PARASITE; PROTOZOA; SNAILS AND DISEASE; *and* WORM INFESTATION. *Articles detailing examples of* TROPICAL DISEASES *include* DENGUE; ENCEPHALITIS; FILARIASIS; KALA-AZAR; LEISHMANIASIS; MALARIA; ONCHOCERCIASIS; SCHISTOSOMIASIS; SLEEPING SICKNESS; *and* YELLOW FEVER. *See also* LIVER FLUKE; SAND-FLY BITES; SNAILS AND DISEASE; *and* TSETSE FLY BITES.

Tropical Ulcer

Open sore of the skin caused by parasitic infection.

Ulcers of the skin due to various infections are common among children and young adults who live in tropical regions. Tropical ulcers are often found on the lower extremities and may be the result of bacterial, environmental or nutritional factors, or a combination of these.

Tropical ulcers are easily acquired in moist, humid regions through minor trauma to the skin followed by secondary infection. A localized region usually develops a pustule within five to six days and then ruptures, producing a bloody, foul-smell-ing discharge. When deeper tissues are involved, the ulcer can destroy tendons, muscles, joints, and bone.

The term tropical ulcer is also sometimes used specifically for sores produced by cutaneous leishmaniasis, a parasitic disease transmitted by sand-flies. Such infections affect the mucous membranes and may produce severe ulcers resembling leprosy, skin cancer or fungal infection. *See* KALA-AZAR; LEISHMANIASIS; *and* PROTOZOA.

Trypanosomiasis

Also known as African sleeping sickness

Infectious disease spread by the African tsetse fly.

Trypanosomiasis causes inflammation to the brain and to its surrounding tissue (meninges). The disease is caused by two different organisms, *Trypanosoma brucei rhodesiense* and *Trypanosoma brucei gambiense*. Both types of trypanosomiasis are transmitted by the tsetse fly. If left untreated, trypanosomiasis causes headache, fever, weakness, and sleep disorders, followed, in the case of the rhodesiense variety, by death in about six months. *See* CHAGAS' DISEASE; INSECTS AND DISEASE; *and* TROPICAL DISEASES.

Tsetse Fly Bites

Bites from African flies that transmit disease.

Tsetse flies, native to sub-Saharan Africa, feed on the blood of humans and other animals. They are somewhat larger than a housefly, have sparse hairs and are yellowish to dark brown in color. Two species of tsetse flies transmit the protozoan parasites that cause sleeping sickness. The fly *Glossina palpalis* carries *Trypanosoma brucei gambiense*, common to western and central Africa. The fly, *G. morsitans* is the carrier of *T. brucei rhodesiense*, which causes a more severe form of the disease endemic in eastern Africa. *See also* CHAGAS' DISEASE; MENINGITIS; PROTOZOA; SLEEPING SICKNESS; *and* TRYPANOSOMIASIS.

Tubal Ligation

A surgical form of sterilization for women.

During ovulation, an egg travels to a fallopian tube, where it may become fertilized, and then to the uterus. In tubal ligation, the fallopian tubes are surgically cut apart. This prevents ova from reaching the uterus and sperm from reaching ova, but does not interfere with normal ovulation and menstruation. Tubal ligation is 95 to 99 percent effective. While it is sometimes possible to surgically reverse tubal ligation, results are usually poor; and thus tubal ligation is considered a permanent form of sterilization.

Advantages and Disadvantages. Women who are comfortable with permanent sterilization may prefer tubal ligation; since, in the long run, it is simpler than temporary forms of contraception, has no hormonal side effects, and is more cost effective. However, it does require minor surgery, which may not be covered under insurance. Furthermore, there is no simple way to determine if surgery was successful; if a woman suspects that she may be pregnant after having a tubal ligation, she should see a physician immediately, as the chance of ectopic pregnancy is higher. Also, if a woman later decides she does want to give birth, the procedure may not be reversible.

Procedure. Tubal ligation is performed under general anesthesia. It takes about half an hour and can be performed on an outpatient basis. First, the abdomen is filled with carbon dioxide gas so that the abdominal wall separates from the uterus and fallopian tubes. The surgeon makes two small incisions above the pubic hairline. A laparoscope, a long, flexible viewing instrument, is inserted through one incision, and surgical instruments are manipulated through the other incision. The fallopians tubes are cut, and then each end is either sewn up or sealed through the application of heat.

For further information on TUBAL LIGATION **see** FERTILIZATION **and** STERILIZATION, FEMALE. **See also** BIRTH CONTROL; CONTRACEPTION; FAMILY PLANNING; **and** INFERTILITY.

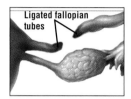

Tubal Ligation.
Above, with a tubal ligation, the fallopian tubes are sealed shut. Surgical sterilization which permanently prevents the transport of the egg to the uterus by means of sealing the fallopian tubes is called tubal ligation, commonly called having one's tubes tied. This operation can be performed laparoscopically or in conjunction with a cesarean section after the baby is delivered. Tubal ligation is considered permanent but in some rare cases, surgical reversal can be done sucessfully.

Resources on Tuberculosis

Daniel, Thomas, *Captain of Death: The Story of Tuberculosis* (1997); Lutwick, Larry I., *Tuberculosis: A Clinical Handbook* (19955); Rom, William, and Stuart. M. Garay, *Tuberculosis* (1996); Taylor, Robert, *Saranac: America's Magic Mountain* (1988); Centers for Disease Contol and Prevention, Tel. (800) 311-3435, Online: www.cdc.gov; www.nycornell.org/medicine/infectious/html.

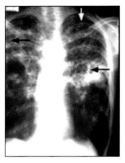

Tuberculosis.
Tuberculosis is an infectious disease that causes inflammation, the formation of tubercules and other growths within tissue, as above, and can cause tissue death. This chest x-ray shows advanced pulmonary tuberculosis. There are multiple light areas (opacities) of varying size that run together (coalesce). Arrows indicate cavities within these light areas.

Tubercule

A small prominence that appears in areas infected by the tuberculosis bacterium.

Tubercules may be morbid growths; the lesions found in tuberculosis are made up of a packed mass of white blood cells along with the destroyed products of the immune system. The term tubercule is also used to refer to natural and healthy protrusions, such as the locations on bones where ligaments are attached. *See also* TUBERCULOSIS.

Tuberculin Tests

Diagnostic testing to detect a previous infection with *Mycobacterium tuberculosis*.

Initial diagnosis of tuberculosis infection is carried out through one of several tests. Tuberculin—a solution that stimulates the body to fight infection —is injected into the skin. Exposure to tuberculosis will produce an infection-fighting reaction, causing redness and swelling at the injection site after two or three days. Such tests only indicate exposure to *Mycobacterium tuberculosis* and the development of infection-fighting matter. This alone does not confirm active tuberculosis. This is carried out through chest x-ray and saliva analysis.

Three types of tuberculin skin tests exist, differing only in the method of introducing the antigen. In the Mantoux test, tuberculin PPD (purified protein derivative) is injected through the skin. The Heaf test uses an instrument to repeatedly prick the skin, introducing the tuberculin antigen into the skin (dermis). Finally, the tuberculin tine test makes use of a different type of needle and introduces the tuberculin more superficially into the skin. Current infection is diagnosed with sputum inspection. *See also* TUBERCULOSIS.

The Tuberculosis Skin Test

A doctor will be able to do an in-office skin test for those who have been exposed to tuberculosis.She or he will inject a protein, derived from the tuberculosis bacteria, under the skin. Within two or three days a person who has the bacteria in their system will show a swelling and redness at the site of injection. False positive and false negative reactions to this test are possible, so the diagnosis should be confirmed by microscopic examination of the sputum.

Tuberculosis

A bacterial infection of the lungs that may spread to other parts of the body.

Tuberculosis was once a common illness throughout the world. It accounted for almost 30 percent of all deaths during the industrial revolution. In developed countries, tuberculosis now effects mainly the elderly, and those who live with AIDS.

The bacterium that causes tuberculosis, *Mycobacterium tuberculosis*, is carried in the air when an infected person sneezes or coughs. In 95 percent of cases the immune system will protect against infection when the bacteria are inhaled. In the remaining five percent, the disease may take years to incubate. When the immune system is compromised by some other infection or by advanced age, the bacteria can reactivate.

Symptoms. Tuberculosis is initially experienced as a feeling of malaise and a mild cough, which may produce green or yellow mucous. As the disease progresses, the quantity of sputum increases; and there may be blood in it. A characteristic symptom of tuberculosis is waking at night covered with sweat. Fluid in the pleural space may make the sufferer short of breath.

Occasionally the infection will spread to other parts of the body, including the kidneys, the bladder, the prostate, or the ovaries. The tuberculosis bacterium can attack the skin, heart, brain, or bones.

Diagnosis of tuberculosis begins with an x-ray that shows irregular white areas in the lungs or a pleural effusion. A patient is also given a skin test and an examination of the sputum for bacterial identification.

Treatment. Antibiotics are usually successful even if the disease is relatively advanced. Two or more antibiotics may be necessary to eliminate all the bacteria, and treatment will continue long after the person feels completely cured. Surgery may be necessary to drain abscesses.

For background reading on TUBERCULOSIS *see* IMMUNE SYSTEM; PLEURAL EFFUSION; *and* SPUTUM. *Further information can be found in* ANTIBIOTIC DRUGS; *and* BACTERIA. *See also* ABSCESS; INFECTIOUS DISEASE; *and* SURGERY.

Tuberous Sclerosis

A genetic disorder that affects the nervous system and the skin.

Tuberous sclerosis derives its name from tuber-like growths located on the brain which calcify and become hard (scleroses) as a person ages.

Symptoms which vary greatly in severity, include epileptic seizures, mental retardation, developmental delay, motor difficulties, and behavior abnormalities. Other symptoms include tumors of the brain, kidneys, eyes, or other organs. Acne-like skin sores are also prominent.

Tuberous sclerosis is inherited as a dominant disorder; thus a child of an affected parent has a 50 percent chance of contracting the disease. Once considered to be an extremely rare disease, the number of cases has been rising recently, due to better diagnostic techniques and the inclusion of patients with less severe manifestations of the disorder. A recent study estimates that one in 6,000 newborns is affected by tuberous sclerosis to some degree.

Treatment. There is no known cure for the disorder. Treatment is geared toward controlling and suppressing many of the symptoms. *See also* NERVOUS SYSTEM.

Tuboplasty

Surgery to repair a damaged fallopian tube.

Tuboplasty is usually performed as a treatment for infertility. Microsurgery is usually used to unblock the tubes. Balloon tuboplasty, in which a catheter is inserted into the fallopian tubes and a balloon at the end is inflated to expand the tubes, has also been recently introduced.

Following tuboplasty, the fertility rate ranges from five to 50 percent, depending on the extent of the damage and whether there are other factors present affecting fertility. Women who undergo tuboplasty have an increased risk for ectopic pregnancy. *See also* FERTILITY; FERTILITY DRUGS; IN VITRO FERTILIZATION; *and* UTERUS.

Tularemia

Also known as rabbit fever

A bacterial infection transmitted to humans from animals or ticks.

The bacterium that causes tularemia, *Francisella tularensis*, can penetrate unbroken skin. Therefore, this disease is easily transmitted to butchers, hunters, farmers, and laboratory workers. The bacteria that cause tularemia can also be inhaled into the lungs or they can enter the blood stream from an open wound.

Symptoms. The incubation period lasts from two to four days. After this incubation period, the affected individual will experience headaches, nausea, vomiting, muscle aches, extreme weakness, and fatigue. The fever may spike as high as 104°F and there may be copious sweating. The patient will have a cough and chest pain if the bacteria were inhaled. If the bacteria entered the body through the skin, a red blister will appear at the site of infection. This blister generally fills with pus, ruptures, and turns into an ulcer. The lymph nodes near the infection site may swell and drain pus as well.

Treatment. Tularemia is treated with antibiotics. If an ulcer is present, it should be covered with a moist bandage that is changed frequently. A small percentage of people with tularemia will develop pneumonia or an infection of the meninges, the heart, the bones, or the peritoneal cavity. A person who recovers from tularemia will be immune from the disease for life. *See* ANTIBIOTIC DRUGS; BACTERIA; IMMUNITY; INFECTION; LUNG; PNEUMONIA; SKIN; *and* ULCER.

Tumor

A swelling or growth of tissue.

"Tumor" was originally defined as "swelling." That definition has been expanded so that the term refers to growths. A tumor results from abnormal multiplication of the cells of a tissue in the body. Many tumors are benign, with their growth limited, they will not spread to neighboring tissues

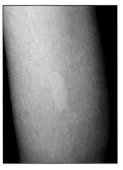

Tuberous Sclerosis. This area of decreased pigment (hypopigmentation) is referred to as "ash leaf macule," and is seen with the inherited disorder; tuberous sclerosis. Another finding "confetti hypopigmentation" is evident as scattered white spots around the ash leaf spot, as seen above.

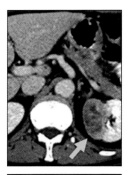

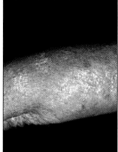

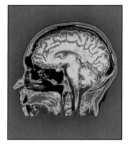

Tumor.
At top, the CT scan of the abdomen shows a tumor in the left kidney (hypernephroma) located on the lower right side of the picture. Middle: For people with actinic keratosis, accumulative skin damage is caused by repeated exposure to all ultraviolet light, including that found in sunshine. Over the years the genetic material of the cell becomes irreparably damaged and produces lesions. The lesions like those seen on the arm may later become cancerous. At the bottom is a MRI scan of the brain. MRI imagery is often the best diagnostic tool.

or other parts of the body. Some tumors are malignant, or cancerous, multiplying uncontrollably, spreading to nearby tissue and sending metastases, or colonies throughout the body.

Many benign tumors are surrounded by a fibrous capsule and cause few or no problems. But the growth of a benign tumor, even when it is limited, can cause problems as the mass of the tumor pushes against healthy tissue, disrupting their function. For example, a meningioma, a benign tumor of the brain, can affect physical and mental function.

Cancerous tumors differ widely in their rates of growth and spread. Some grow aggressively, posing an immediate threat to well-being and life. One example is small-cell carcinoma, a form of lung cancer. A common feature of malignant tumors is that their cells can differ greatly from the normal cells of the tissue in which they arose. The difference can be due to the mutation, or change in the genetic material, of a cell, which causes the loss of the normal controls on cell division and multiplication.

> *Background material about* TUMORS *can be found in* BE-NIGN; BIOPSY; CANCER; CELL; MALIGNANT; METASTASIS; *and* RA-DIATION. *Articles detailing examples of* TUMORS *include* BRAIN TUMOR; DESMOID; FIBROID; GERM CELL TUMOR; KIDNEY TUMORS; LUNG TUMORS; *and* TROPHOBLASTIC TUMOR.

Tumor-Specific Antigen

Natural chemical (hormone) that stimulates resistance to infection (antigen) and surround the surfaces of cancerous cells, triggering an attack by the body's immune system.

Antigens are identifying proteins on the surfaces of cells that help the body distinguish itself from foreign substances and defend against invasion. When certain cells become cancerous, they produce tumor-specific antigens alerting the body to disorder. The body's response to these unfamiliar cell markers is to mount an infection-fighting (immune) response, producing infection-fighting substances (anti-

bodies) to attempt to destroy diseased cells and tissue, a process known as cell-mediated immunity. Bone cancer (osteosarcoma), malignant melanoma, and certain digestive system (gastrointestinal) cancers are among those producing recognized tumor-specific antigens. Though the body mounts an immune response, producing antibodies to the tumor antigens, the response is generally inadequate in retarding or eliminating the cancer and may in some cases actually facilitate its growth.

Some tumor antigens may be detected in the bloodstream, and may be symptomatic of future infection in patients who don't currently have symptoms. Such tumor markers as they are called, are used currently to evaluate the effectiveness of cancer treatment. Two such markers are carcinoembryonic antigen (CEA)—found in patients with cancer of the colon, breast, cervix, pancreas or bladder, as well as in heavy cigarette smokers and those with ulcerative colitis or liver cirrhosis. PSA or prostate-specific antigen is found at elevated levels in those with enlarged prostates and high levels in those with prostate cancer.

> *For basic information on* TUMOR-SPECIFIC ANTIGEN *see also* ANTIGEN; ANTIBODY; ASYMPTOMATIC CANCER; CANCER SCREEN-ING; MALIGNANT; *and* MELANOMA. *See also* BONE CANCER; IM-MUNE RESPONSE; IMMUNE SYSTEM; IMMUNOLOGY; IMMUNO-THERAPY; OSTEOSARCOMA; PROSTATE; *and* TUMOR.

Tunnel Vision

A loss of peripheral vision.

In cases of tunnel vision, an individual's central field of vision is clear, but his or her peripheral vision is impaired, so that it seems as if a person is viewing the world through a tube or tunnel. A person with tunnel vision may also have night blindness, an inability to see well when light levels get below a certain level. This occurs because the peripheral field of vision is highly sensitive to low levels of light, while the central field of vision functions better in bright light.

Causes of tunnel vision may include glaucoma, in which pressure inside the eyeball becomes too high, leading to a loss of peripheral and, in very advanced cases, central vision; and retinitis pigmentosa, an inherited disease in which the pigmented cells in the retina responsible for collecting images progressively break down. Tunnel vision is treated by determining and treating the underlying cause, if possible.

In psychology—where the term is less frequently used—tunnel vision refers to an individual who has a narrow emotional or intellectual range. It may occur due to various forms of emotional or psychological trauma. *See also* GLAUCOMA *and* VISION TESTS.

Turner's Syndrome

A type of chromosomal abnormality in which a girl has only a single X chromosome instead of two.

Individuals with Turner's syndrome tend to have short stature and limbs, and wide chests with broad-spaced nipples. Their breasts and genitals remain undeveloped past puberty. The ovaries do not produce eggs and menstruation does not occur. Mental retardation is rare, although affected individuals may experience difficulties with spatial relationships and mathematics. Turner's syndrome occurs in approximately one in 3000 births. *See also* BIRTH; DOWN'S SYNDROME; DNA; GENE; GENETICS; HERITABILITY; *and* TRISOMY.

Twins

Two children who develop and are born at the same time, from the same mother.

Twins can be either fraternal or identical. If they began as two separately released and fertilized eggs, they are fraternal and are not necessarily the same sex. In fact, other than being "womb mates," fraternal twins are no more genetically (and often physically and emotionally) alike than any other two siblings that share both parents.

Identical twins come from a single fertilized egg that separates into two separate entities during the rapid rounds of cell division that take place in early development. (Sometimes the division is incomplete, resulting in conjoined or Siamese twins.) Consequently, they share all of their genetic material and must be the same sex. They may even share a single placenta.

Regardless of whether they are identical or not, twins are subjected to the same environment in utero but may experience different effects nonetheless. One twin may get more nutrients or oxygen, and as a result may be a pound or so larger than the other. Babies may even be born with bruises from their interactions with each other in their cramped environment.

INCIDENCE

An increased incidence of twins runs in families, and the likelihood of giving birth to twins also increases with age. In the vast majority of cases, the presence of two babies is known well ahead of birth. With ultrasound imaging techniques, the location and presence of the twins can be determined exactly.

HEALTH CONCERNS AND COMPLICATIONS

Women who are pregnant with twins have a greater chance of premature delivery. They are more likely to experience high blood pressure, varicose veins, backaches, and many of the other common discomforts that come along with pregnancy. These discomforts, plus the greater demands on the uterus, usually trigger early labor. Therefore, twins have a greater likelihood of being born before the 37th week, with the accompanying problems of prematurity, including low birth-weight.

Twins have a higher rate of Cesarean section than single births; due to early delivery, they are more likely to be breech, which usually warrants a Cesarean section.

Further material on TWINS *can be found in* FERTILIZATION; GENETICS; PREGNANCY; *and* PREGNANCY, MULTIPLE. *It is also vital to be familiar with* FERTILITY DRUGS; FETAL HEART MONITORING; PREGNANCY TESTS; PREMATURITY; *and* ULTRASOUND. *Information about the specifics relating to birth can be found in* ALTERNATIVE BIRTH METHODS; BIRTH; DELIVERY; *and* EMERGENCY CHILDBIRTH. *See also* SIAMESE TWINS.

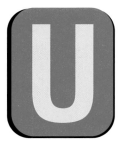

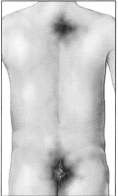

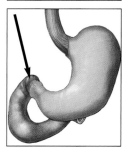

Ulcer. Aphthous ulcers or canker sores are very common. Typically they are a shallow with a white or yellowish base surrounded by a red border. The ulcer, at top, is located in front and below the bottom teeth. The middle image shows pressure ulcers or bedsores caused by lying too long on one side of the body. The bottom image, a duodenal ulcer, is found below the stomach.

Ulcer

A crater-like lesion on the skin or mucous membrane caused by an inflammatory or infectious condition, or life-threatening (malignant) abnormal growths (tumors).

As a general term that describes abnormal openings in the skin or mucous membrane, there are various specific types of ulcers: eye ulcer, gastric ulcer, herpes, mouth ulcers, and inflammation of the colon (ulcerative colitis). Three common forms are canker and bed sores, and leg ulcers.

Aphthous ulcers also known as canker sores are mild and benign, open sores in the mouth. They appear as painful white or yellow sores, surrounded by a bright red area. Canker sores are quite common. Symptoms include a burning sensation, skin lesion on mucous membrane of the mouth, the formation of a small ulcer, a single lesion or clusters of lesions, and a gray membrane just prior to healing. There seems to be an inherited predisposition to the development of canker sores. There are numerous triggers for the development of the condition, including dental injury, aggressive tooth cleaning, biting the inside cheek, stress, dietary insufficiencies, menstrual periods, hormonal changes, and food allergies. There are numerous other types of mouth ulcers, including leukoplakia, gingivostomatitis, oral cancer, oral lichen planus, and oral thrush.

Pressure ulcers also known as bedsores are abnormal openings in the skin caused by lying too long on one side of the body. Bedsores are common among the elderly, incontinent, and those confined to their beds. Three out of four cases develop in nursing homes. On average, patients in nursing homes who are not able to change position in bed themselves need to be turned every two hours. Bedsores are uncomfortable, and they can be serious.

Leg ulcers. An ulcer can occur on the ankle, due to venous stasis disease (a vein disorder involving varicose veins and poor circulation in the legs). This type of ulcer produces significant inflammation surrounding the ulcer. An ischemic ulcer on the leg is caused by lack of circulation to areas of tissue. This can cause localized tissue death (necrosis). Any condition that stops or interrupts blood flow can cause this type of ulcer. *See* BENIGN *and* BEDSORE.

Ulcer-Healing Drugs

Drugs used to heal sores (ulcers) in the stomach.

Stomach ulcers were originally thought to be caused by stress; however, it is now known that they are caused by the bacteria *Helicobacter pylori*, which thrive in the acidic environment of the stomach. Treatment begins with substances that reduce the acidity of the stomach, such as antacids. If these do not work well, sulcralfate is used to coat the ulcer and promote healing, as well as H_2 blockers including cimetidine, ranitidine and famotidine. New alternatives to antacid medications are omeprazole and lansoprazole, which inhibit the production of stomach acids. The treatment is followed up with antibiotics like clarithromycin or tetracycline to actually kill the bacteria that cause the ulcer. *See also* GASTRIC ULCER; PEPTIC ULCER; *and* ULCER.

Ulcerative Colitis

An intestinal disease that is marked by an inflammatory disorder of the bowels.

Ulcerative colitis and Crohn's disease are both types of inflammatory bowel disease. Their cause is unknown. Ulcerative colitis affects the large intestine exclusively. The condition is characterized by the development of small ulcers and inflammation in the lining of the colon. The disease is known as ulcerative proctitis if the inflammation is limited to the rectum.

Ulcerative colitis tends to run in families. The average age of onset is between the ages of 15 and 35.

Symptoms. The symptoms of ulcerative colitis include:
• abdominal and joint pain;
• non-bloody or bloody diarrhea;

- eye pain under bright lights;
- oral canker sores;
- painful bowel movements;
- fever; and
- weight loss.

Diagnosis. A barium enema may be performed, although the diagnosis is most often made through the use of flexible proctosigmoidoscopy or colonoscopy.

Complications. The degree of inflammation varies among patients. In its most severe form, there is a risk of toxic megacolon or perforation of the colon. When ulcerative colitis is limited to the rectum, it is called ulcerative proctitis. Other parts of the body may be affected as well. Some individuals develop joint pain, skin lesions, eye inflammation, or cholestasis. Patients with severe ulcerative colitis also have an increased risk of developing cancer of the colon. *See also* INFLAMMATORY BOWEL DISEASE.

Treatment is aimed at alleviating the inflammation. Anti-inflammatory drugs are used as well as antibiotics. In the most severe cases, corticosteroids (prednisone) or other immune system suppressing drugs are prescribed. In addition, severe diarrhea may lead to dehydration and nutritional deficiencies. A liquid diet is often prescribed in the most severe cases to offer the bowels a chance to rest for a few weeks.

Approximately 25 percent of all patients with ulcerative colitis require surgery at some point. The most common operation performed is an ileoanal anastomosis, sometimes referred to as the "J-pouch" operation, in which the damaged colon is removed and the ileum, the last segment of the small intestine, is connected directly to the anus. *See also* COLON *and* MEGACOLON.

Ultrasound

An imaging technique using high-frequency sound waves, often used for diagnostic purposes.

Ultrasound scanning is a nonsurgical (non-invasive) technique for visualizing different parts of the body. Using a very high frequency sound wave (2.25 to 10 megahertz; MHz) the ultrasound apparatus sends a penetrating sound wave into the tissue under study, by means of a transducer. A portion of the sound wave is reflected back to the transducer, the rate and magnitude of this reflection owing to the density of tissue and bone encountered by the sound wave. The resulting information is relayed to a computer, which will either compose a graphic representation, showing ultrasound peaks representing tissue depth, or a two-dimensional tissue slice, (tomogram) displayed on a screen. Ultrasound finds wide diagnostic applicability due to its nonsurgical nature and lack of potentially harmful ionizing radiation. *See also* ECHOCARDIOGRAPHY; HEART IMAGING; *and* IMAGING TECHNIQUES.

Ultrasound Scanning

Diagnostic imaging technique using high-frequency sound waves.

Ultrasound scanning has many diagnostic applications. It is used to image the kidneys, uterus, prostate, breast, liver, and gallbladder. Heart structures may be visualized in fine detail enabling the physician to see all valves of the heart, dimensions of its chambers, as well as observe the contractions and function of the heart. Diagnosis of cardiomyopathies, atrial tumors or pericardial effusions (abnormal fluid collection around the heart), may be made; and the motion of the cardiac wall following a heart attack may be evaluated. Other uses for ultrasound include screening for ovarian cancer, evaluating the liver, and gallstone (calculi) identification.

One of the most useful applications of ultrasound scanning is in the area of obstetrics, allowing the physician to observe the developing fetus through real-time two-dimensional images displayed in rapid succession, somewhat like a cinematic film. Measurements of the head (cephalometry), chest (thorax), and abdomen are readily made as well as estimates of growth and maturation, and overall health. A range of abnormalities including retardation of growth, hydrocephaly, meningocele,

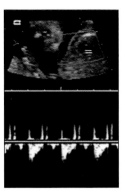

Ultrasound. This a normal fetal ultrasound showing one pattern of the fetal heartbeat. Some ultrasound machines have the ability to focus on different areas of the heart and evaluate the heartbeat. This is useful in the early diagnosis of congenital heart abnormalities.

congenital heart disease, fetal tumors, polycystic kidney illness and gastrointestinal obstruction may be identified. Ultrasound scanning allows the quantity of amniotic fluid to be evaluated, and during the third trimester of pregnancy, the sex of the fetus may be determined. Ultrasound is also used visually to guide surgical operations, and aid in the proper placement of the needle used in procedures such as amniocentesis. *See also* HEART; *and* HEART DISEASE.

More articles related to ULTRASOUND SCANNING *can be found in* COMPUTER-AIDED DIAGNOSIS; IMAGING TECHNIQUES; *and* ULTRASOUND. *Related information is contained in* AMNIOCENTESIS; HYDROCELE; *and* ULTRASOUND TREATMENT.. *See also* HEART; HEART DISEASE; HEART DISORDERS OF; KIDNEY; KIDNEY IMAGING: *and* LIVER IMAGING.

Ultrasound Treatment

Use of high frequency sound waves for the treatment of illness or as therapy following injury.

In addition to its usefulness for diagnostic imaging, ultrasound finds a number of applications as a treatment. Physical therapy using ultrasound sends high frequency sound waves through inflamed, scarred, sore or stiffened tissues in the body in order to relieve inflammation and pain, and restore movement, generally through the heating effects of the ultrasound.

The sound waves in therapeutic ultrasound are usually transmitted through a conductive gel, to the site of disease or injury. Once the sound waves penetrate the tissue they are converted into deep heat, increasing the circulation in the area and helping to carry away the energy and waste processing products of inflammation. The level of penetration may be adjusted, depending on specific needs, with the greatest penetration reaching to the bone.

In addition to wound healing and relief from arthritic and inflammatory conditions, ultrasound treatment has been applied as a healing therapy for bone fractures, particularly acute radius and tibia fractures. Ongoing research into this versatile technology includes experimental

treatment for prostate cancer using high intensity focused ultrasound (HIFU), destruction of tumors in the uterus, and as a breakthrough technology to help the profoundly deaf to hear. *See* DEAFNESS; HEARING; INFLAMMATION; *and* PHYSICAL THERAPY.

Ultraviolet Light

Also known as UV light

Also called UV light, the short frequency component of sunlight, which can damage the skin.

Too much UV light can cause immediate effects, such as sunburn, and long-term problems, such as skin cancer and cataracts. The UV index, which was developed by the Environmental Protection Agency and the National Weather Service, provides information in order to help prevent overexposure. The index predicts UV intensity levels on a scale of 0 to 10+, where 0 indicates minimal risk and 10+ indicates very high risk. The local UV index takes into account clouds and other local conditions that affect the amount of UV radiation that reaches the ground. The range zero to two is considered minimal, three to four is low, five to six is moderate, seven to nine is high, and over 10 is very high risk.

To avoid overexposure to ultraviolet light, time spent in the sun should be limited. A sunscreen with a sun protection factor of at least 15 should be used. UV protective sunglasses should be worn to protect the eyes and prevent cataracts. Sun lamps and tanning salons should be avoided. *See* SUNLIGHT, ADVERSE EFFECTS OF.

Umbilical Cord

A long semi-transparent jelly-like rope, is attached at the fetal navel, that is the connection between the baby and the placenta.

The umbilical cord is basically a continuation of the blood vessels that extend into the placenta, through which the exchange of nutrients and wastes takes place. After delivery, the cord serves no further function. It is clamped in two places, one close

Resources on Diagnostics

Chervenak, Frank A., *Ultrasound in Obstetrics and Gynecology* (1997); Kee, Joyce LeFever, *Handbook of Laboratory and Diagnostic Tests with Nursing Implications* (1994); Nuland, Sherwin, *Doctors: The Biography of Medicine* (1995); Ravin, Carl E., ed., *Imaging and Invasive Radiology in the Intensive Care Unit* (1993); Segen, Joseph C., and Joseph Stauffer, *The Patient's Guide to Medical Tests* (1998); American Hospital Association, Tel. (800) 242-2626, Online: www.aha.org; The American Board of Radiology, Tel. (520) 790-2900, Online: www.theabr.org; American Healthcare Radiology Administrators, Online: www.ahra.org; www.ny-cornell.org/radiology/.

to the baby's abdomen, and then cut. The stump takes about a week or two to slough off. This is the origin of the navel.

Until it falls off, the cord should be kept clean and dry. Redness or oozing is an indication of an infection; bleeding should be brought to a doctor's attention.

Complications. During pregnancy, the cord may be a source of problems. Active babies can get tangled in their cords. A prolapsed cord, in which the cord precedes the baby through the birth canal, occurs in one in every 1,000 births. The cord becomes compressed and interferes with the baby's oxygen supply from the placenta.

An overt prolapsed cord occurs when the membranes surrounding the baby have already ruptured, and the cord protrudes into the vagina before the baby. This usually happens during a breech birth, but, it can also occur when the baby is in the normal head first position if the water breaks too early or if the fetus has not yet descended into the mother's pelvis. The rush of fluid sweeps the cord down. This is why a doctor will not rupture the membranes until the baby's head has descended. A prolapsed cord requires an emergency Cesarean section, because the baby's placental blood supply is cut off. The doctor may have to literally hold the baby off of the cord in order to avoid compression.

In an occult prolapse, the membranes are still intact, and the cord is trapped in front of the baby's head or shoulder. This condition is identified by a sudden change in the fetal heart rate. It is usually cor-rectable by changing the mother's position or raising the baby's head to take pressure off the cord. Sometimes, a case of occult prolapse requires a Cesarean section delivery.

Diagnostic Use. Percutaneous umbilical blood sampling is a form of prenatal testing. A sample of cord blood can be obtained for chromosomal analysis (which is rarely indicated and should only be performed by a maternal-fetal specialist), Rh determination or other tests. *See also* BIRTH; DELIVERY; *and* PREGNANCY.

Unconsciousness

Being unable to respond to external stimuli.

Unconsciousness can be described as a condition in which affected patients are confused and lack awareness of their own state and environment. Reduced brain stem activity causes unconsciousness. Unconsciousness can emerge from a brief fainting spell or from an extended concussion or coma. Unconsciousness can result from injuries to the head, shock, stroke, a loss of blood to the brain, a decrease in the level of oxygen in the blood (as in the case of a drowning victim), chemical changes (for example, insulin in a diabetic), or from recreational drugs. *See also* FAINTING.

Underbite

An abnormal protrusion of the lower jaw beyond the upper.

An underbite occurs when the lower teeth extend past the upper teeth. This is the opposite of the condition known as overbite and both are forms of improperly aligned teeth (malocclusion). Sometimes the underbite is not pronounced enough to have any serious effect, but a severe underbite can cause pain and discomfort and ultimately damage to the teeth. For many people, even a mild underbite can be a cosmetic issue as well. Dentists treat an underbite the same way they treat an overbite—through orthodontics and occasional surgery. *See also* DENTISTRY *and* MALOCCLUSION.

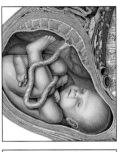

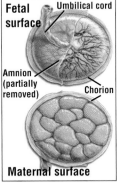

Umbilical Cord. The placenta provides the fetus with oxygen and nutrients and takes away wastes through the umbilical cord. Above, top, the placement of the umbilical cord; coming form the fetal navel, it attaches to the placenta. Above, bottom, the anatomy of the umbilical cord attachment sites on the mother and fetus. Somewhat surprisingly, they are different.

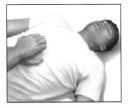

Unconscious. Above, the first aid procedure for an unconscious person who is choking is to administer the heimlich maneuver while the person is lying on their back until the object is dislodged or until help arrives.

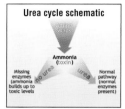

Urea. The buildup of ammonia in the body is toxic and can cause brain damage, seizures, and coma. Above, the urea cycle and how toxins are removed from the body.

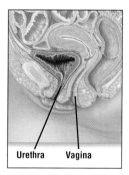

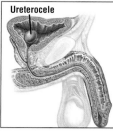

Urethra. The diagram at top shows the female uretha, which is the tube that carries urine to the bladder. The bottom diagram shows aureterocele which occurs in males, It is located at the base of the bladder and reduces or prevents the flow of urine into the urethra.

Urea

A waste product occurring as a product of protein metabolism.

Urea is produced in the liver, where proteins in food and from the body's cells are broken down into amino acids. While the body needs a certain amount of these amino acids, what it does not use is converted into urea. From the liver, the urea is transported to the kidneys, where it is excreted in the urine.

The kidneys are responsible for eliminating urea from the body. When they malfunction, urea may not be efficiently eliminated, resulting in a condition known as uremia. Blood urea is a standard diagnostic tests for this and for kidney function in general. In cases of liver damage, or during pregnancy, the level of urea drops.

Urea also has a number of medical uses. It is sometimes used as a medication to treat skin disorders, or it may act as a diuretic, especially in cases when pressure must be reduced, such as with cerebral edema or glaucoma. *See also* UREMIA.

Ureter

One of the two tubes carrying urine from the kidneys to the bladder.

In an adult, each ureter is 10 to 12 inches long and consists of three tissue layers. The innermost layer is a thin membrane, surrounded by muscular tissue, which is surrounded by a fibrous outer layer. The point of entry of each ureter into the bladder is set at an angle to prevent urine from flowing backward out of the bladder when its muscles contract.

Problems that can affect the ureters include complete or partial blockage by a kidney stone that can cause renal colic, ureteral cancer, or blockage by a disease outside the ureter such as colon, uterine or bladder cancer. Double ureter is a congenital condition in which there are two ureters on one or both sides. While double ureter can cause no symptoms, it some-

times results in back flow of the urine and requires surgical repair. *See also* URETHRITIS.

Ureterolithotomy

Surgery to remove a stone (calculi) from a ureter.

The ureters carry urine from the kidneys to the bladder. Blockage of a ureter due to stones can cause renal colic, severe spasms of pain, and can result in kidney damage. A ureterolithotomy is performed under general anesthesia, after the location of the stone causing the blockage is determined. The stone is removed through an incision in the abdomen, and a tube is inserted to drain urine that may leak from the affected ureter. A hospital stay of four or five days is required for the procedure, which is rarely performed; because most urethral stones are broken in pieces within the ureter during ureteroscopy or broken by focused shock waves (extracorporeal shockwave lithotripsy). *See also* CALCULUS *and* RENAL COLIC.

Urethra

The tube carrying urine from the bladder.

A woman's urethra is shorter than that of men, running to the front of the vagina. In men, the urethra runs the length of the penis, with the prostate gland around its upper end. Urethra disorders including infections, injuries, and congenital defects are more common in men. Inflammation of the urethra can come from infection, a minor injury, or irritation and can result in scarring that results in a stricture that impedes urine flow. A stone that lodges in the urethra can block urine flow. An accident that injures the pelvic region in men can cause urethral damage that may require surgery. Hypospadias is a disorder in which the opening of the urethra is not at the end of the penis but to the side. A urethral valve is an abnormal flap of tissue that interferes with the urine flow. The resulting back flow of urine can result in kidney damage. These can all be corrected by surgery. *See also* HYPOSPADIAS *and* STONES.

Urethral Dilation

Widening of an abnormally narrow urethra.

The urethra is the tube that carries urine from the bladder. In a man, the urethra runs through the penis. It can be narrowed or shortened by injury, inflammation, or a condition called urethral stricture that causes difficulty in urination and ejaculation. A urethral dilation is performed to treat the stricture by inserting a slim instrument at the end of the urethra. A first insertion widens the urethra, then successively wider instruments make the opening even wider. It is done under local or general anesthesia, and can be repeated if necessary. If urethral dilation fails, the urethra can be widened by an instrument that cuts through the blockage or by plastic surgery. *See also* PENIS *and* URETHRAL STRICTURE.

Urethral Discharge

Abnormal fluid flow from the urethra.

An infection of the urethra, the tube that carries urine from the bladder, can cause this outflow. In most cases, the fluid flow has no color due to an infection, often chlamydia or trichomona. If the outflow is caused by gonorrhea, the fluid is yellow, because it contains pus. Urethral discharge is treated by curing the underlying infection that causes the discharge. *See* GONORRHEA.

Urethral Stricture

Blockage that limits the ability of the urethra to transport urine.

The urethra can be blocked by scarring due to a defect existing at birth, an infection, injury, or other causes such as radiation therapy for cancer. The resulting stricture can cause difficulty in ejaculating for men and may result in kidney damage due to fluid buildup. A urethral structure can be treated with urethral dilation, in which a thin instrument is inserted to widen the urethra, and progressively wider instruments are inserted to gradually enlarge the opening. In severe cases, surgery may be required. *See* URETHRAL DILATION.

Urethral Syndrome, Acute

A disorder of the urethra causing abdominal pain and frequent urination.

Acute urethral syndrome occurs most often in women. Its cause is generally unknown, although it is sometimes due to inflammation of the vulva in postmenopausal women. In these cases, estrogen medications or corticosteroid ointments can relieve symptoms. There is no accepted treatment for these cases, with careful attention to personal hygiene and a high intake of fluid recommended. *See also* MENOPAUSE; PERIMENOPAUSE; *and* VULVA.

Urethritis

Inflammation of the urethra.

Urethritis can be caused by injury to the urethra, the tube that carries urine from the bladder, but the most common cause is an infection. Often, the infectious agent is the bacterium that causes gonorrhea or chlamydia. Because urethritis often produces no symptoms in women, it can be spread to a man by sexual intercourse. In men, the principal symptoms are discharge, pain, and a burning sensation when urinating, sometimes accompanied by fever. The urine may be discolored by blood or pus. Untreated, urethritis can lead to scarring and the formation of a urethral stricture that limits the flow of urine.

Urethritis is treated by determining the infectious agent and curing the infection, by antibiotic drugs for a bacterial infection or other agents for a yeast or chlamydial infection. Because the infection is so often incurred during sexual intercourse, the sexual partner of a person with urethritis should be checked for the infection. A basic preventive measure is the use of a condom during intercourse. *See* CHLAMYDIA; GONORRHEA; *and* URETHRAL STRICTURE.

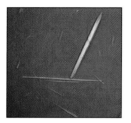

Uric Acid. Above, uric acid crystals that have been photographed under polarized light. When such crystals collect in the joints, the attendant disorder is called gout.

Uric Acid

A waste product resulting from the breakdown of nucleic acids in cells.

Uric acid is produced not only when the cells of the body die but also from foods rich in nucleic acids, the genetic material in the nucleus of all cells. The liver and kidney organs are especially rich in nucleic acids. In the body, most uric acid is removed from the blood in the kidney and is excreted in the urine, with a small percentage broken down by bacteria in the intestines. If uric acid excretion is below normal because of poor kidney function or another disorder, abnormally high levels of uric acid in the blood can lead to gout or the formation of kidney stones. *See also* BACTERIA; GOUT; KIDNEY; STONES; *and* URINE.

Urinalysis

Any tests performed on a sample of urine for the purposes of diagnosis.

Analysis of urine can provide a wealth of diagnostic information and may be used as a standard screening test or an attempt to detect specific ailments. The procedure often used for these routine tests is the dipstick method, wherein a strip of plastic is dipped into the urine sample. Chemicals on the pretreated strip react with substances in the urine, indicating their presence with a color change.

The dipstick method allows the physician to assess the content of protein, nitrates, and various enzymes—findings used to diagnose a variety of illnesses. Protein in the urine may be symptomatic of kidney disease, though further testing of blood and urine is required to confirm this. Sugar (glucose) in the urine (glucosuria) is often symptomatic of diabetes, though when accompanying blood glucose is normal, kidney disease may be indicated. Ketones are byproducts of the processing (metabolism) of fat in the body. Their presence in urine may be due to alcohol intoxication or unchecked diabetes. Nitrates in urine are

diagnostic of infection. Urine concentration is important in evaluating the functioning of the kidneys. The urine sample may be taken randomly, or following a hormone injection, or water consumption; and the kidneys ability to concentrate urine (one of their primary functions) will be evaluated.

Urine Testing

Urinalysis is a safe and—in most cases—painless diagnostic exam. A sample of urine will be analyzed using plastic strips or dipsticks to detect the presence and concentrations of various factors that may be relate to a disease. The urine may also undergo microscopic analysis and bacterial culturing in the laboratory if a urinary tract infection is suspected. Urinalysis is useful for the diagnosis of renal disease (glomerulonephritis), kidney disease, diabetes, and other metabolic diseases.

Sometimes, a physician will need a "clean" sample, that is, a sample that does not include any skin cells or bacteria. Men will have to wipe off the tip of their penis with an antiseptic cloth and women will be asked to hold open their labia. The initial urine stream should not be caught; this stream is used to clean the urethra. The middle and end of the stream are the cleanest parts of the sample.

Bacteria found in urine may be grown in a lab to diagnose urinary tract infections. Generally, urine is sampled directly during normal urination using the clean catch method. The person will begin filling a sample vial after some urine has been expelled into the toilet, ensuring it will be sterile. In addition to dipstick analysis, urine samples may be cultured in a laboratory to detect and identify bacteria when urinary tract infection is suspected. The sample may be acquired through the "clean catch" method or by direct extraction from the bladder, following the insertion of a tube through the urethra or a needle passed through the abdominal wall and into the bladder. Microscopic analysis of urine is used to detect bacteria, fungi or parasites, crystals, and cell structures as well as to study urine sediment.

For more information on urinalysis see GLOMERULONEPHRITIS; GLUCOSE; GLYCOSURIA; UREA; URIC ACID; URINARY TRACT INFECTION; URINATION, PAINFUL; URINE; *and* URINE RETENTION. *See also* KIDNEY *and* URINARY SYSTEM.

Urinary Diversion

Surgery to restore normal flow of urine caused by a medical condition or an operation.

Urinary diversion can be a temporary measure when urine flow is blocked by an enlarged prostate gland or an urethral stricture, or by surgery performed on the urinary tract. The procedure requires a tube to be implanted through the abdominal wall connecting it to the bladder. Permanent urinary diversion is done when the bladder must be removed because of the existence of cancer or when the nerves controlling bladder activity are severely injured. In such cases, a substitute bladder is created, with a dowel passing through the wall of the abdomen to a bag outside of the abdomen where urine is retained. Most patients are thus required to wear this bag attached to the skin at all times.

Currently, the bowel can be reconstructed to form a continent diversion when a bag is not used and the patient drains the pouch with a catheter. Another technique is to create a new bladder from bowel (neo-bladder) which is connected to the patient's urethra; this allows normal urination in most cases. *See also* BALLOON CATHETER; BLADDER; CATHETER; KIDNEY; PROSTATE, ENLARGED; URETHRAL STRICTURE; URINARY TRACT INFECTION; *and* VAGINA.

Urinary System

The organs responsible for production and excretion of urine: the kidneys, ureters, urinary bladder, and urethra.

The urinary system removes wastes from the blood in the form of urine, which is made up of water and dissolved waste products such as urea. By controlling the amount and composition of urine, the urinary system helps control the volume and composition of the blood. Increased production of urine can lower the blood pressure and raise the pH of blood, while decreased production of urine raises blood pressure and decreases pH.

The urinary system consists of the two kidneys, the ureters, the urinary bladder, and the urethra. The ureters lead from each kidney to the urinary bladder, and the urethra leads from the bladder to the exterior of the body.

The kidneys are four to five inches long and shaped like kidney beans. They are located in the top and back of the abdomen, just inside the lowest part of the rib cage. Blood travels to the kidneys through the renal artery and away from the kidneys through the renal vein. The primary functioning part of the kidney is the nephron, a system of tubes consisting of the glomerulus, Bowman's capsule, and a tubule. The nephrons filter water and small dissolved substances out of the blood to create ur-ine; normally, larger solutes such as plasma proteins do not pass into the kidneys and thus remain in the blood. The presence of some substances in urine, such as proteins or glucose, is often indicative of a disorder.

After urine has been created in the kidneys, it passes through the ureters to the urinary bladder. The ureters are narrow tubes approximately 10 to 12 inches long. A valve between the ureters and the bladder prevents urine from traveling back toward the kidneys. The urinary bladder stores urine until it is excreted, at which time it passes through the urethra to the outside of the body.

Male Urinary Tract

Kidney · Ureteropelvic junction (UPJ) · Renal pelvis · Ureter · Urinary bladder · Prostate · Urethra

Female Urinary Tract

Kidney · Uretero-pelvic junction (UPJ) · Renal pelvis · Ureter · Urinary bladder · Urethra

The Urinary System. Above, top, the male urinary tract. Above, bottom, the female urinary tract. The female and male urinary tracts are quite similar (they process wastes with the same organs, which function the same way, in the same order, except that the male urethra is somewhat longer than the female.

For anatomical information on the URINARY ΑΥSTEM, *see* BLADDER *and* KIDNEY. *Related information can also be found in* BLOOD PRESSURE; PROTEINS; UREA; URIC ACID; URINARY TRACT INFECTION; URINATION, PAINFUL; URINE; URINE, ABNORMAL; *and* URINE RETENTION. *See also* SALT.

Urinary Tract Infection

Infection in the bladder, urethra, or another part of the urinary tract

Urinary tract infections are caused by a number of bacteria (*Escherichia Coli* being the most common), including gonorrhea and chlamydia. They can result in cystitis, which is the inflammation of the bladder; urethritis, inflammation of the urethra; pyelonephritis, inflammation of kidneys; and other problems. In women, the incidence of infections of the bladder (the organ that holds urine) is more common than in men, because the female urethra, while short, is more exposed to outside effects due to the fact that it runs to the vagina. In addition, pregnancy also increases the risk of developing a urinary tract infection. Many factors can increase the risk in both men and women, including birth defects, such as the condition spina bifida (which affects the emptying of urine from the bladder), and injuries to the spinal cord. A stone in the urinary tract or a bladder tumor can also lead to urinary tract infections. However, in many cases, urinary tract infections occur without any clear underlying cause.

The symptoms of urinary tract infections depend on the region of the tract that is affected. For urethritis, a burning sensation is felt during urination. For cystitis, there is pain in the abdomen, an urge to urinate frequently, with urine that can be discolored by the presence of blood, and an overall feeling of weakness. A kidney infection results in pain in the loins, accompanied by a fever.

Any urinary tract infection must be treated to prevent permanent damage; untreated infections will cause severe damage to the urinary tract that may require surgery. Kidney infections can cause permanent loss of kidney function; if the infection spreads to the rest of the body through the blood, the patient can go into shock rather quickly.

Treatment of an infection starts with a urine specimen that is examined to determine the specific agent causing the infection. In some severe cases, a pyelogram, an x-ray examination, or an ultrasound scan can be done to determine whether a stone, a tumor or a congenital abnormality is responsible. If such a cause is identified, surgery may be needed to correct the defect or remove a tumor. In most cases, however, antibiotic treatment is enough to cure an infection; the antibiotic given to the patient depends on the agent responsible for the infection.

> *For more information on urinary tract infection, see* URINARY SYSTEM. *Related material can be found in* CYSTITIS; POLYNEPHRITIS; SPINA BIFIDA; STONES; TUMOR; ULTRASOUND SCANNING; *and* URETHRITIS.

ALERT

Simple Prevention

The risk of urinary tract infections can be reduced by simple lifestyle measures, which are important for anyone who is especially vulnerable to an infection (such as pregnant women and those with compromised immune systems due to cancer treatment or the advanced stages of HIV or AIDS). Careful attention to personal hygiene is perhaps the most important preventive measure. Ample intake of fluids and urinating on a regular schedule to empty the bladder are also important if not essentially vital.

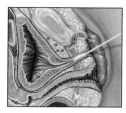

Urinary Tract Infection. A urethral tissue culture, above, is used to test for the cause of a urinary tract infection. A cotton swab is gently inserted about three-quarters of an inch into the urethra and rotated to obtain a sample for testing.

Urination, Excessive

Production of abnormally large quantities of urine.

A normal adult typically produces approximately five pints of urine each and every day. Excessive urination above that amount, (polyuria), usually indicates the presence of a physical illness, although it can also be an early sign of pregnancy, continuing until the mother brings the child to term.

One unusual cause of excessive urination is a specific type of mental illness that impels an individual to drink an excessive amount of water or other fluids. This condition is called polydipsia.

Excessive urination can also be caused by diabetes mellitus, the most common form of diabetes in which there is little or no production of insulin. Diabetes insipidus, a much less common disorder of the pituitary gland in which there is an insufficient production of ADH (an antidiuretic hormone that acts to concentrate urine in the kidneys), also causes excessive urination. Other disorders that may affect the ability of the kidneys to limit loss of water or to respond to normal levels of ADH can also result in this disorder, including nephrogenic diabetes insipidus.

Treatment of the condition is aimed at the underlying cause. Some patients are merely required to reduce water intake; however, for those with diabetes or another disease affecting the output of urine, more complex treatment is usually necessary. *See also* DIABETES INSIPIDUS; DIABETES MELLITUS; HORMONES; INSULIN; KIDNEY; POLYDIPSIA; URINE; *and* WATER.

Urination, Frequent

Abnormally frequent passage of urine.

An adult normally passes urine four to six times during the day and rarely at night. The frequency of urination can be increased by a number of factors, the most obvious of which is an increased intake of fluid. The amount of urine produced by the kidneys can be increased by a number of diseases, including diabetes mellitus and diabetes insipidus.

One common cause of frequent urination in middle-aged and older men is enlargement of the prostate gland. Enlargement of the prostate is common for men over the age of 50, and the resulting blockage of urine flow can cause the bladder to become overactive; this can usually be treated with medicine to shrink or relax the prostate. In severe cases, enlargement of the prostate may require surgery.

Bladder stones can also lead to a similar result, as can a bladder tumor. Overactivity of the bladder can also be due to an inflammation in the lining of the bladder that often is caused by an infection (cystitis). Many patients with cystitis reduce their fluid intake, which results in a more concentrated urine that irritates the bladder and increases the urge to urinate. An increase in fluid intake is advisable. In some cases, anxiety can increase the frequency of urination. *See also* CYSTITIS; DIABETES INSIPIDUS; DIABETES MELLITUS; KIDNEY; STONES; TUMOR; *and* URINATION, EXCESSIVE.

Urination, Painful

Discomfort or pain when passing urine.

Painful urination (dysuria) can be caused by a number of conditions that affect the bladder, the urethra, the prostate gland or other parts of the urinary or genital tracts. The burning pain of dysuria is often accompanied by difficulty in beginning urination. Sometimes the pain persists after the flow of urine stops, a condition called strangury. This may be a result of one of the common conditions that cause dysuria: inflammation of the bladder, most often due to an infection (cystitis), or a bladder stone. Strangury can result from spasms of the wall of the irritated bladder. Other causes of painful urination in men include inflammation of the prostate gland (prostatitis), and gonorrhea; this infection usually does not cause painful urination in women. Inflammation of the tip (glans) of the penis, called balanitis, can also cause painful urination in men. In women, causes include the vaginal infection vaginitis, candidiasis (a fungal infection), and an allergic reaction to a vaginal deodorant. Painful urination is treated after performing tests such as urinalysis and urine culture to detect an underlying condition determining necessary treatment. *See also* BALANITIS; CANDIDIASIS; CYSTITIS; GONORRHEA; PROSTATITIS; URINALYSIS; *and* URINE.

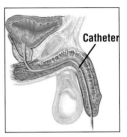

Urinary Tract Catheterization. Many urinary tract disorders, including incontinence, painful urination, and retention of urine, can be treated by catheterization (above). In catheterization, a catheter is passed up the urethra and into the bladder, and urine is collected.

Urine

A yellow fluid produced as the kidneys filter wastes from the blood.

Every minute, almost two pints of blood that have collected waste products in their passage through the body, pass into the two kidneys of a normal adult. The blood arrives through the two renal arteries, which divide into smaller and smaller arteries within the kidney. There it comes into contact with millions of nephrons, the filtering units of the kidney, which consist of two subunits: the glomerulus, which filters both waste and fluid from the blood; and

and the tubule, which concentrates the waste products and puts useful substances such as minerals, nutrients, and essential salts back into the blood that flows out of the kidney.

The major ingredient of urine is urea, a nitrogen-containing substance produced by the breakdown of proteins. Urine also contains uric acid; chloride, sodium, potassium, phosphate, and sulfate ions; and other chemicals. *See also* BLADDER *and* UREA.

Urine, Abnormal

Production of urine in abnormal quantities or composition.

An average adult normally produces about five pints of urine every 24 hours. A number of conditions can affect both the amount of urine produced and its composition. For example, excess urine production, polyuria, can be due to excessive intake of fluids or to a hormonal imbalance. Unusually low urine production, oliguria, can result from kidney failure or from dehydration. In extreme cases of kidney failure, no urine may be produced at all.

Sometimes the appearance of urine is enough to indicate a medical problem. An infection of the urinary tract can result in cloudy, smelly urine. Cloudy urine may also be due to stones in the urinary tract. Reddish urine may be caused by the presence of blood. Urinalysis is done to help diagnose such conditions. *See also* OLIGURIA; POLYURIA; PORPHYRIA; *and* URINALYSIS.

Urine Retention

Failure to empty the bladder when urinating.

Urine retention is more common in men than women, and the cause most often is an enlargement of the prostate gland, which obstructs the flow of urine from the bladder through the urethra. A tumor of the bladder can also obstruct the flow of urine, as can bladder stones. Other causes, in men and women, include urethral stricture, scarring or narrowing of the urethra

or treatment such as x-ray therapy for cancer, a birth defect, or narrowing of the opening of the urethra. Urine retention can also be caused by a malfunctioning nervous system that controls the need to urinate and the emptying of the bladder.

Urine retention can be partial or complete. Temporary urine retention can be a side effect of some medications, including decongestant drugs, calcium channel blockers for hypertension, and narcotic painkillers. Complete retention is treated by implanting a catheter to drain the bladder to relieve the pain and other symptoms of the problem. Surgery may also be a solution to removing the blockage permanently. If abnormal nerve function is the cause, a permanent catheter can be implanted to prevent kidney damage due to the backup or urine. *See also* PROSTATE, ENLARGED; STONES; TUMOR; *and* URETHRAL STRICTURE.

Urology

The branch of medicine that deals with the urinary tract.

Urology is concerned with the functioning, structure, and disorders of the adrenals, kidneys, ureters, bladder, and urethra—the structures in which urine is created, processed, transported, and excreted. In men, the field also includes the structures of the reproductive tract—the testes, epididymis, prostate gland, seminal vesicles and penis. *See also* URINARY TRACT.

Uterus

Also known as the womb

A pear shaped organ in the lower female abdomen. During pregnancy, the fetus develops in the uterus.

The fallopian tubes are located above and on either side of the uterus. The base or neck of the uterus is called the cervix and is the point where the vagina is attached.

Within seven days of conception, a fertilized egg finishes its journey through the fallopian tube, reaches the uterus, and then implants itself in the uterine wall.

Resources on Urology
Campbell, Meredith F., E. Derracott Vaughan, et al., *Campbell's Urology* (2002); Cameron Stewart, *Kidney Disease: The Facts* (1986); Hinman, Frank, *Atlas of Urologic Surgery* (1989); Smith, Homer W., *From Fish to Philosopher: The Story of Our Internal Environment* (1959); Tanagho, Emil A. and Jack W. McAninch, eds., *Smith's General Urology* (1995); National Kidney Foundation, Tel. (800) 622-9010, Online: www.kidney.org; American Association of Kidney Patients, Tel. (800) 749-2257, Online: www.aakp.org; American Foundation for Urologic Disease, Tel. (800) 242-AFUD, Online: www.afud.org; National Institute of Diabetes and Digestive and Kidney Diseases, Tel. (301) 496-3583, Online: www.niddk.nih.gov; www.ny-cornell.org/medicine/nephrology/index.html; www.cornellurology.com/

There it continues to develop for approximately the next nine months.

In preparation for pregnancy, a special lining (called the endometrium), consisting of blood vessels and other tissues, builds up in the uterus in response to the hormone progesterone, produced by the corpus luteum. If no pregnancy occurs, the endometrium begins to break down approximately 14 days after ovulation and is shed in the process known as menstruation. As soon as the lining has been completely expelled, new endometrial tissue begins to develop in response to the hormonal signals that begin the next cycle.

The uterus is an extremely muscular organ, yet a surprisingly flexible one as well. Over the course of pregnancy it can expand to 400 times its original volume, in order to accommodate the growing fetus. The enlarging uterus pushes the other abdominal organs out of the way to make room for itself. Many of the symptoms of late pregnancy, such as heartburn, shortness of breath, and increased frequency of urination, are due to the expanding uterus pressing against other organs.

Labor consists of a series of powerful uterine contractions, in which the uterus squeezes together to push the baby out. As labor progresses, the contractions become more powerful and occur at shorter intervals. Approximately four to six weeks after giving birth, the uterus should be close to its prepregnancy size. *See also* DELIVERY; DIAGNOSTICS IN WOMEN'S HEALTH; PREGNANCY; *and* UTERUS, CANCER OF.

Uterus, Cancer of

Malignant tumor of the uterus.

The most common cancer in American women is endometrial cancer, which arises in the tissue that lines the uterus (endometrium). The incidence is highest in women who have had prolonged exposure to the hormone estrogen without a counterbalancing exposure to the hormone, progesterone. Women at highest risk include those who have never had a preg-

nancy (since progesterone is produced during pregnancy), obese women, and those in whom menopause occurred after the age of 52. Use of birth control pills decreases the risk of uterine cancer, but estrogen replacement therapy without accompanying progesterone increases the risk.

INCIDENCE

Incidence is elevated slightly among women who have taken tamoxifen, a drug prescribed to prevent breast cancer or its recurrence. Most endometrial cancers are endometrial adenocarcinomas, which arise in glands in the tissue lining the uterus; however, some arise from both gland cells and squamous cells of the endometrium. Another type of endometrial cancer is stromal sarcoma, which arises in the smooth muscle of the uterus.

Hysterectomy and Menopause

Women who undergo hysterectomy because of uterine cancer must be prepared for the sudden onset of the symptoms of menopause, such as hot flashes and night sweats, which are more severe than in natural menopause. The estrogen therapy that can be prescribed for such symptoms is not advised for these women, but other treatments, such as progesterone therapy, can ease some symptoms.

SYMPTOMS

The most common symptom of uterine cancer is abnormal bleeding, which may be heavy. There may be changes in bowel or bladder function, weight loss, weakness and pain in the back, pelvis, or legs.

DIAGNOSIS

Tests for cancer of the uterus include transvaginal ultrasound, computerized tomography, and magnetic resonance imaging scans; blood tests to detect chemical markers of cancer; and x-rays, if the cancer is believed to have spread. A tissue sample of the endometrium may be taken for microscopic analysis. In some cases when the sample is equivocal, a dilation and curettage may be done, in which tissue is scraped from the surface of the uterus in a procedure that requires general anesthesia.

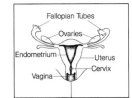

Uterus. Above, the place of the uterus in the female reproductive system. During pregnancy, the fetus develops in the uterus for approximately nine months.

TREATMENT

Uterine cancer generally requires surgery, either a hysterectomy to remove the uterus or a more extensive procedure in which both the uterus and the fallopian tubes are removed, since they are likely sites for spread of the cancer. Adjoining lymph nodes, another potential site of spread, are often removed. Radiation therapy usually follows surgery, and chemotherapy may be needed if the cancer has spread out of the uterus. Surgery may not be performed in some cases, because it may be too extreme for the patient; or radiation therapy alone may be administered when the cancer is detected at a very early stage in a younger woman who want to have children. The prognosis depends on the stage at which the cancer is detected, and survival rates are generally better for carcinoma than for sarcoma.

> **For background material on cancer of the uterus, see** CANCER **and** REPRODUCTIVE SYSTEM, FEMALE. **Further information can be found in** BREAST CANCER; ESTROGEN HORMONES; MENOPAUSE; OBESITY; ORAL CONTRACEPTIVES; PREGNANCY; **and** PROGESTERONE. See also TUBAL LIGATION.

Resources on Uterine Cancer

Dahm, Nancy Hassett, *Mind, Body, and Soul: A Guide to Living with Cancer* (2001); Murphy, G., et al., *Informed Deci-sions: The Complete Book of Cancer Diagnosis, Treatment, and Recovery* (1997); Renneker, Mark, ed., *Understanding Cancer* (1988); Steen, R. Grant, *A Conspiracy of Cells: The Basic Science of Cancer* (1993); Steward, Clifford T., ed., *Cancer: Prevention, Detection, Causes, Treatment* (1988); American Cancer Society, Tel. (800) ACS-2345, Online: www.cancer.org; National Cancer Institue, Tel. (800) 4-CANCER, Online: www.nci.nih.gov.

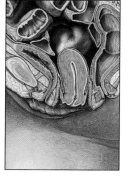

Prolapsed Uterus. Prolapse of the uterus (above) is common in women who have had complicated deliveries or in postmenopausal women. It occurs when the muscles that normally support the uterus are weakened by age or injury.

Uterus, Prolapse of

Also known as procideentia

A disorder in which the uterus drops into the vagina.

Prolapse of the uterus is caused by a weakening of the muscles that normally prop up the uterus. A prolapsed uterus can also be accompanied by other organs, such as the bladder, rectum, or part of the intestine, bulging into the vagina as well.

Causes. The muscles that normally support the uterus can become weakened by age or injury to the vaginal tissues. Women who have had children or difficult labor and deliveries commonly develop this condition. However, a prolapsed uterus usually does not occur until after menopause, when the decreased levels of estrogen cause further weakening of the muscles and result in a decreased blood supply.

Uterine prolapse tends to run in families. In addition, it can be caused by anything that exerts excessive pressure on the abdomen and weakens pelvic support, such as heavy lifting, tight girdles, or obesity.

Symptoms. The main symptom of a prolapsed uterus is a feeling of heaviness in the pelvic region. Other women may experience backaches or stress incontinence. In a case of severe prolapse, the uterus and cervix can actually protrude through the vaginal opening. Symptoms usually are worse when a woman is standing up and can be relieved by lying down. The symptoms will also get worse during the course of the day. See also STRESS and UTERUS.

Treatment. Treatment depends on the severity of the uterine prolapse. A mild case can be helped by exercises that strengthen the pelvic muscles, such as Kegel exercises. A pessary is a rubber device that can be worn to support the uterus. Estrogen replacement therapy can help restore some elasticity to the vaginal tissues. Surgery to repair damaged tissues is also an option. Sometimes a hysterectomy is recommended for very severe cases. See also ESTROGEN DRUGS and KEGEL EXERCISES.

Uterus, Tipped

Also referred to as retroverted uterus

A condition in which in which the uterus is tilted backward and down instead of the normal forward-tilted position.

A tipped uterus occurs in about 20 percent of all women. It does not usually cause any symptoms or result in any problems.

Occasionally, a tipped uterus can be the source of backaches, especially during a menstrual period. Very rarely, deep penetration during sexual intercourse can be painful for women whose uterus is tipped.

During pregnancy the uterus generally tilts forward in the normal position, although it may revert after giving birth.

Treatment. No treatment is usually necessary. If intercourse is painful, a woman can be fitted with a pessary that covers the cervix and props up the uterus. A surgical option also exists, in which the uterus is sutured into the forward tilting position. See also CERVIX; PREGNANCY; and UTERUS.

Uveitis

Inflammation of the uvea, the layer of the eye that includes the iris, ciliary body, and choroid.

The uvea is the layer of the eye between the white of the eye and the retina. The uvea includes the iris, the pigmented area surrounding the pupil; the ciliary body, a part of the eye that produces the fluid inside the eye; and the choroid, a lining of the eye behind the retina that is rich in blood vessels and supplies blood to the retina.

CAUSES

The uvea may become inflamed as a result of injury, infection, exposure to chemicals, an allergic reaction, or an autoimmune response. It may also become inflamed for no known reason.

TYPES

Anterior uveitis accounts for 75 percent of all cases; it affects the iris and ciliary body at the front of the uvea. It often is caused by autoimmune diseases such as rheumatoid arthritis, ankylosing spondilitis, or inflammatory bowel disease. It may affect only one eye and is common among young and middle-aged people.

Posterior uveitis affects the back portion of the uvea; it may also affect the retina. This condition is caused by a number of diseases including toxoplasmosis, sarcoidosis, tuberculosis, ulcerative colitis, multiple sclerosis, and syphilis. It may also be caused by injury, particularly in young children.

SYMPTOMS

Symptoms of uveitis often appear suddenly. They may include redness, pain, burning, and itching in the eye; eye discharge; blurred vision, dark spots (floaters) in vision, or sensitivity to light; and constricted pupils. Posterior uveitis is more likely to be painless, and floaters are more common.

TREATMENT

Anterior uveitis can be treated with warm compresses on the eyes, pain relief (analgesic) medication, dark glasses to protect the eyes from light sensitivity, and eye drops to paralyze the iris and dilate the pupils. Corticosteroids or nonsteroidal anti-inflammatory drugs (NSAIDs) are often used to reduce inflammation.

Posterior uveitis is generally treated by determining and treating the underlying cause. Corticosteroid drugs may also be used to reduce inflammation.

PROGNOSIS

Anterior uveitis usually goes away after a few days to a few weeks, but it often recurs. Persistent uveitis may eventually result in vision loss. Posterior uveitis may last for months or years, even with treatment, and may result in scarring that permanently interferes with vision. Other possible complications of uveitis include an increase in pressure inside the eye (glaucoma), clouding of the lens of the eye (cataracts), the presence of fluid in the retina, and retinal detachment. Inflammation may also spread to other parts of the eye. *See also* EYE; NSAIDs; RETINA; *and* SYPHILIS.

Uvula

The small, tongue-shaped portion of tissue that hangs from the top of the back of the mouth.

The uvula is the pendulous piece of fleshy tissue that hangs down at the back of the throat. This tissue acts as a barrier between the respiratory and digestive functions of the mouth.

When a person is not swallowing, the uvula hangs down, allowing air from the nose to pass down into the lungs. This ensures that respiration is possible.

During swallowing, the uvula pushes on a ridge of muscle at the back of the throat, isolating the nasal passages from the mouth and allowing food or drink to pass from the mouth down the esophagus and into the stomach. If the nasal passages are not closed off from the mouth sufficiently, food may pass into the lungs, and choking is possible. *See also* CHOKING; DIGESTIVE SYSTEM; EMERGENCY FIRST STEPS; HEIMLICH MANEUVER; *and* RESPIRATORY SYSTEM.

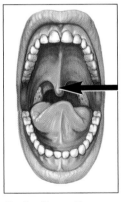

Uvula. Above, the uvula is a small flap of tissue located at the back of the throat. Its main function is to prevent food from entering the airways during swallowing.

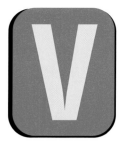

Vaccination

The administration of a substance that triggers immunity to a virus or other infectious disease.

A vaccine contains a small amount of a weakened disease-causing substance (antigen). While the antigen in the vaccine is not strong enough to cause disease, it triggers the body to create memory cells and thus provide immunity. In effect, the body learns to recognize the disease without having to suffer illness.

The antigen in a vaccine may consist of a weakened version of a virus; a killed virus or bacterium; a toxin produced by a virus or bacterium; or a synthetic substance that can trigger antibodies. A weakened virus can provide longer-lasting protection; but it may cause infection in people with weakened immune systems.

Vaccination is also called active immunization, and it provides long-term immunity from a particular disease. This is contrasted with passive immunization, in which antibodies against a particular pathogen are injected directly, providing only short-term immunity from a specific disease. See also IMMUNITY and VACCINE.

Common Vaccinations

In addition to being routinely administered in infancy and early childhood, vaccinations may be administered to older children and adults, especially travelers, who are at risk for contracting a disease and have not been previously vaccinated.

Vaccine	When it is Administered
Chicken pox	Two doses between 18 months and adolescence.
Diphtheria, tetanus, and pertussis (DTP)	Four shots at two, four, six and 15 to 18 months. Booster shot between ages four and six.
Haemophilus influenza type B (HIB)	Four doses at two, four, six, and 12 to 15 months.
Hepatitis B	As early as infancy; preferably before adolescence.
Influenza	Administered in the autumn to people at risk.
Measles, mumps, and rubella (MMR)	Two doses, between 12 and 15 months and between four and six years.
Pneumococcal pneumonia	No specific time. Often if at high risk or if the immune system is compromised.
Poliomyelitis	Four doses at two, four, and six to 18 months, and between four and six years.
Rotavirus	Three doses at two, four, and six months. Should not be started in children over six months old.
Tetanus and diphtheria (Td)	Between ages 11 and 15, and once every ten years afterward. Possibly also after a severe wound.

Vaccine

A harmless substance that stimulates the immune system to produce antibodies against a disease.

After a vaccine is administered, the body's immune systems responds against the antigens contained in the vaccine. The immune system also develops memory cells in case the same antigens should return.

When a vaccine is introduced into the body, a person becomes immune to the particular disease. A virus may be weakened by passing it through cells of non-human hosts. Mutations then occur that adapt the pathogen to the nonhuman host so it can no longer cause disease in humans. The vaccines for polio, smallpox, and measles are produced in this way. Other vaccines, such as those for typhoid fever and whooping cough, were made from dead pathogens that still had the necessary antigens to stimulate an immune response. The vaccines for tetanus and botulism are made from toxins secreted by the pathogens. The toxin is inactivated so that it can no longer destroy tissues, but its antigens are still intact. See also VACCINATIONS.

Vacuum Extraction

A method used in vaginal deliveries to help move a baby's head through the birth canal.

Vacuum extraction uses a plastic cup which fits over the baby's head and a vacuum pump to gently pull the baby out of the vagina. Vacuum extraction may cause some swelling or bruising to the baby's head.

Use of vacuum extraction may be indicated under the following circumstances:
- the baby is too large to move through the birth canal;
- there are indications the baby is being deprived of oxygen;
- there are other signs of fetal distress;
- the mother does not have the energy or ability to push to push the baby out.

See also BIRTH; BREECH DELIVERY; CESAREAN SECTION; CONCEPTION; DELIVERY; FORCEPS DELIVERY; and PREGNANCY COUNSELING.

Vagina

The passageway leading from the vulva to the uterus.

The vagina is a tubular organ surrounded by highly elastic smooth muscle tissue. It is about four inches long; a recess known as the fornix surrounds the cervix. The lining of the vagina, a mucous membrane, produces lubrication when a woman is aroused. Semen, which is basic, neutralizes the acidity, which deters bacterial growth, in the vagina. At birth, the opening to the vagina is covered with a thin membrane known as the hymen. It is usually thought to be broken at first sexual intercourse, although other activities, such as exercise, may also tear it. *See also* VAGINAL ATROPHY.

Vaginal Atrophy

Also known as atrophic vaginitis

Lack of lubrication and thinning of the vaginal wall in response to a lack of estrogen.

Vaginal atrophy may occur when estrogen levels decline, such as after menopause, following a hysterectomy, or it may occur temporarily while nursing. Following menopause, about 20 to 40 percent of women experience vaginal atrophy. Although this condition is not life-threatening, it can cause a range of emotional stresses.

Symptoms include dryness and loss of elasticity in the vaginal area as well as a measure of pain during sexual intercourse. Over time, the vaginal area becomes thinner and may bleed easily.

Treatment may involve the use of estrogen creams or suppositories, which increase estrogen levels in the vaginal area. These should not be used by women who are taking hormone replacement therapy or who had or have breast cancer. Another option is the use of petroleum- or water-based lubricants during intercourse. The latter can be safely used with latex prophylactics. In some cases, increased sexual activity can reduce symptoms of atrophic vaginitis. *See also* MENOPAUSE *and* VAGINA.

Vaginal Bleeding

Normal and abnormal bleeding from the vagina.

Normal vaginal bleeding occurs approximately once a month for women in their reproductive years; regular menstrual cycles end at menopause. Abnormal vaginal bleeding can occur for a variety of reasons. The bleeding categories are quite broad and include spotting or full bleeding midcycle, unusually heavy periods, staining in postmenopausal women or irregular menstrual periods in teenagers.

Sometimes different medications, such as anticoagulants, can cause bleeding. It is not uncommon to have midcycle staining for the first few months of taking birth control pills. This is known as "breakthrough bleeding." The pill is also responsible for withdrawal bleeding, which is bleeding that occurs when the body's levels of progesterone or estrogen drops suddenly. Postmenopausal women undergoing hormone replacement therapy may also experience irregular bleeding for three to six months, particularly if the dosage is too low.

Vaginal bleeding can be a warning sign of cancer to the reproductive tract, including the vagina, cervix, and ovaries. The presence of an IUD can cause heavier than normal periods. Bleeding is also caused by:

- laceration or other physical injury to the reproductive tract;
- cervical polyps;
- endometrial polyps;
- ovarian cysts;
- pelvic inflammatory disease;
- endometriosis; and
- fibroids.

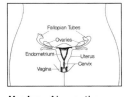

Vagina. Above, the vagina is part of the female reproductive system. It is a canal made of highly elastic muscle that can stretch to accommodate the delivery of a baby.

ALERT
Vaginal Bleeding During Pregnancy

Vaginal bleeding during pregnancy is different from the other kinds of bleeding described above. Some spotting may occur around the time the egg implants in the uterine wall. In early pregnancy, bleeding is often a sign of a miscarriage, ectopic pregnancy, or molar pregnancy. Sometimes bleeding occurs that is unrelated to the pregnancy but due to problems such as polyps, inflammation of the cervix, or cervical cancer. Bleeding late in pregnancy may be due to placenta previa, placenta abruptio or premature labor. Any such bleeding requires a physician's examination.

Irregular periods are common in adolescents for the first few years, however, frequent ovulation rarely occurs. If the corpus luteum is absent, the lack of progesterone and the constant estrogen secretions will cause the endometrium to become thicker and then eventually be discharged, resulting in irregular bleeding.

As a woman approaches menopause, her hormone levels fluctuate, which results in irregular bleeding. Postmenopausal women may experience vaginal atrophy, which can result in bleeding after sexual intercourse. Medical conditions such as hypothyroidism and hyperprolactinemia can increase the frequency of menstruation.

> *Background material on* VAGINAL BLEEDING *can be found in* MENSTRUATION, VAGINA, *AND* VAGINAL DISCHARGE. *Related information is contained in* BLOOD, FEMALE REPRODUCTIVE SYSTEM, *AND* HORMONES. *Finally, see also* CERVIX.

Vaginal Discharge

Normal and abnormal discharge from the vagina.

Normal vaginal discharge is odorless and clear to whitish in color. The amount, as well as the consistency, varies at different points of the monthly cycle. Shortly before ovulation occurs, the discharge becomes thinner and more copious. As menstruation approaches, it becomes thicker and dryer. The amount of discharge also increases during sexual arousal, periods of stress, and pregnancy.

A change in the color or odor of the discharge usually signifies an infection. It may be gray or greenish and have a frothy consistency with a strong odor.

Douching is sometimes used as a hygienic measure to wash away irritating discharge. This practice is neither necessary nor advisable. Regular bathing is sufficient. Any unusually heavy or irritating discharge should be brought to a doctor's attention as it may signify an infection or other more serious condition. Douching may also force bacteria or other microorganisms further up the vagina, where they can promote infection. *See also* VAGINA *and* VAGINITIS.

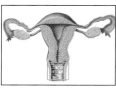

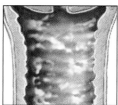

Yeast Infection. A yeast infection caused by the fungal organism Candida albicans. Above bottom, a close-up of the Candida albicans on the vaginal walls.

Vaginal Itching

Irritation of the vagina or surrounding area usually due to infection.

Bacterial vaginosis, yeast infection, trichomonas, atrophic vaginitis, and cytolytic vaginosis all cause some degree of vaginal itching. Sometimes itching is caused by an increase in vaginal discharge, such as occurs around the time of ovulation or during pregnancy. Treating the underlying cause, such as is the case with an infection, will usually eliminate the itching. Simple changes in hygienic practices will also help. Other measures include always wiping from front to back after a bowel movement and not leaving tampons or other objects in for too long. *See also* VAGINITIS.

Vaginal Repair

Repair for tissue damage to the lining of the vagina.

Vaginal tears and lacerations may occur due to trauma, ranging from accidents that result in pelvic fractures or accidental penetration injuries, rape or other sexual abuse, or difficult and prolonged labor and delivery. Uncomplicated tears can be repaired as an outpatient procedure. Tears that are accompanied by a significant bleeding or swelling may require more serious surgery. Antibiotics are usually administered in the latter cases to prevent infection. *See also* SURGERY *and* VAGINA.

Vaginismus

Disorder in which biological processes in the vagina do not function for facilitating intercourse.

Vaginismus occurs when the vagina does not become lubricated during arousal and the muscles surrounding the vaginal entrance contract, making penetration difficult or impossible. It may have a psychological origin. This disorder is distinct from dyspareunia (painful intercourse), although the two conditions may be related.

Any underlying gynecological problem is treated first. A water-soluble lubricant may be helpful. Behavioral modification therapy is also recommended in which the vaginal muscles are "conditioned" to accept penetration. *See also* GYNECOLOGY.

Vaginitis

An inflammation of the vagina or the nearby area.

The primary symptoms include vaginal irritation accompanied by unusual discharge. The vagina and vulva may itch or have a burning sensation. Pain during urination is usually due to urine irritating the sore tissue. Discharge may be gray or greenish, and appear frothy. The amount of vaginal discharge may be heavier than usual and have an intense odor. *See also* GYNECOLOGY.

Usually the vagina has an acidic pH and is populated by certain "good" bacteria that prevent infections by other bacteria, fungi or protozoa. When something affects the vagina's natural environmental balance, it is left open to infection by other microorganisms. *See also* BACTERIA *and* INFECTION.

Bacterial vaginosis is caused by several different types of bacteria, all of which cause similar symptoms of gray discharge with a strong odor. This is the most common cause of vaginitis.

Yeast infections are caused by the *Candida* fungus. The symptoms include itching and burning, accompanied by a thick discharge that may have a yeast odor. Some women are more susceptible than others.

Trichomonas are single-celled parasites which cause a sexually transmitted disease that results in vaginitis. The chief symptoms include itching and a foul smelling frothy green or gray discharge. Occasionally a retained foreign object, such as a tampon, can result in vaginitis.

Vaginal infections are treated by various medications, designed to combat the microorganism that is causing the infection. Some of these treatments are available over the counter, but for first time infections, a woman should seek medical attention to rule out other conditions. *See also* YEASTS.

Vagotomy

A surgery for peptic ulcers that severs the branches of the nerve that controls digestive acid production.

Once a common surgical response for peptic ulcers, the number of vagotomies declined in the mid-1970s when H^2 histamine blockers began their marketing runs and declined even further when ranitidine HCl (Zantac) was introduced. With a vagotomy, a surgeon makes an incision on the upper abdomen and cuts both branches of the vagus nerve near the esophagus where they pass through the diaphragm muscle, and ties up the nerve endings.

This procedure reduces the secretion of hydrochloric acid by the stomach. Vagotomies were often performed with a pyloroplasty, a surgery performed on the pyloric channel, and was known as a P&V because it caused the pylorus muscles, at the lower end of the stomach, to relax.

Subsequently, researchers learned that a stomach bacteria named *Helicobacter pylori* caused peptic ulcers, and antibiotics became part of ulcer treatment. Although medication reduces the need for vagotomies, the surgery is still performed in the most dire cases. *See also* ANTIBIOTIC DRUGS; BACTERIA; *and* PEPTIC ULCER.

Valsalva's Maneuver

A forced effort to expel breath.

Valsalva's maneuver, named for an eighteenth-century Italian anatomist, consists of taking a deep breath and holding it in while holding the vocal cords tightly together, (pinching the nose and keeping the mouth closed), an effort similar to that done during a difficult bowel movement. It is often done naturally, during a bowel movement, while straining to lift a heavy object or when sneezing. As a medical procedure, Valsalva's maneuver can be done to restore a normal heartbeat that has become too rapid because of a disturbance of the center controlling the rhythm of the heart. *See also* ECTOPIC HEART BEAT.

Valvuloplasty

A procedure to repair a defective heart valve.

Repairing a clogged or narrowed valve once required open-heart surgery. Now it is usually done by threading a catheter through a blood vessel to the valve and then opening a balloon at the end of the catheter. Balloon valvuloplasty is sometimes done as a temporary measure for a severely damaged valve, to improve performance of the valve until it can be repaired or replaced. *See also* BALLOON CATHETER *and* HEART VALVE SURGERY.

Varicose Veins

Twisted, swollen veins below the skin of the legs.

Blood flowing upward in the legs must fight gravity to return to the heart. To prevent the blood from flowing downward, the leg veins have a series of one-way valves that allow blood to pass upward and then shut tightly to keep it from flowing down. In some people, these valves do not work right. If one valve malfunctions, the resulting backflow can cause a section of a vein to enlarge; this puts extra pressure on the valve below it. That valve can then malfunction, which puts pressure on another section of the vein, and so on. Because leg veins have little structural support, they can develop bulges (varicosities). About 15 percent of adult Americans will develop varicose veins at some time in their lives. They are more common among women. Varicose veins are not dangerous, but they can be painful. The major medical danger is an increased risk of deep vein thrombosis, clots that can block blood flow and can break away to travel to the lung and cause pulmonary embolism.

SYMPTOMS

In many cases, varicose veins cause no symptoms. Some people can experience a chronic ache in the affected area of the leg, with a persistent itch and swelling of the feet and ankles. The skin above the ankles can become thin, leading to bleeding episodes that can be severe. Even a slight injury can cause damaged veins to bleed. In severe cases of varicose veins, the backflow of blood can lead to a lack of oxygen in the skin, which can become dry, discolored and scaly, with the formation of ulcers. Someone with varicose veins who experiences shortness of breath or another symptom of a pulmonary embolism should seek medical care at once.

TREATMENT

For many people, the only treatment for varicose veins is to wear elastic support stockings, which provide support for the veins. These stockings are available in all sizes and in many colors for both men and women. Elastic stockings can also be worn as a preventive measure for anyone who does not have varicose veins but is at high risk of developing them. The pain caused by varicose veins can be relieved by keeping the legs elevated when sitting down.

Varicosities in smaller veins can be treated by sclerotherapy. An irritating solution is injected into the vein to cause scarring that shuts down blood flow through the vein. This interruption of blood flow does not cause a problem, because most of the flow in the legs goes through larger, deeper veins.

In severe cases, such as when ulcers have formed and other symptoms are persistent, a procedure called stripping can be done. One or more incisions are made along the affected section of the vein. A suture can

---

Risk Factors For Varicose Veins

Varicose veins do not always occur in the legs; a person's family history is a major determining factor in understanding where they are likely to occur. When the affected veins are in the anus, the result is hemorrhoids. When they are in scrotum, they are called varicocoele. Esophageal varices occur in the lower part of the esophagus, which leads from the mouth to the stomach, and sometimes in the upper part of the stomach. They are associated with chronic liver disease and can cause episodes of vomiting of blood.

Other factors can also increase the potential for developing varicose veins. Anyone whose job calls for prolonged standing or heavy lifting also is at higher risk, because that puts extra pressure on the veins of the lower legs. Being overweight or being pregnant also increases the pressure on leg veins and thus increases the risk of varicose veins.

then be tied in to stop blood flow through that section, or the vein can be tied off in multiple places, so that the sections of the vein between the tied sites can be clipped out. As with sclerotherapy, adequate blood flow upward in the leg will be maintained by deeper veins.

These treatments, accompanied by preventive measures—such as wearing elastic stocking and losing weight—are sufficient for dealing with most varicose veins. But because the disorder is chronic, there is always the risk of a recurrence.

> *Background material on* Varicose Veins *can be found in* Blood; Leg; *and* Oxygen. *Related information is contained in* Esposhageal Varices; Obesity; Pregnancy, Preventative Measures; Pulmonary Embolism; Scrotum; Thrombosis; Vein; *and* Vomiting. *See also* Weight Loss.

Vasectomy

A type of contraceptive surgery that makes males sterile by severing the vas deferens (sperm ducts).

Vasectomy is a highly effective contraceptive and family planning technique; it is almost 100 percent effective and it does not affect sexual desire or erectile function. The operation is quick, easy, and can usually be done under a local anesthetic as an outpatient procedure. After shaving the scrotum, a surgeon makes an incision in it then cuts the two sperm ducts. The sperm ducts are then stitched, clipped, or cauterized closed; it takes less than half an hour.

After surgery, cold packs are applied to decrease swelling and pain, and the man may wear a protective supporter. The patient will suffer discomfort for several days.

No-scalpel vasectomy is a new procedure that provides an option that reduces the amount of bleeding and decreases the possibility of infection, bruising, and other complications. With this method, the urologist does not cut the skin of the scrotum, but makes one tiny puncture to reach both sperm ducts so that they can be pulled out through the puncture and then sealed off using the methods mentioned earlier. The operation is quick, the puncture heals

quickly, no stitches are needed, and no scarring occurs. The method only takes about 10 minutes to complete.

The patient can be fertile for about two months—approximately 15–20 ejaculations—after the operation, because it takes a while for all the sperm to die or be ejaculated from the seminal vesicles. A man still produces an ejaculate during orgasm, but it no longer contains sperm.

Some men may have anxieties about the procedure, but the quick return of the sex drive usually assuages any doubts about masculinity or potency. Individuals who intend to bank their sperm for possible future use should be cautioned that some sperm do not survive the freezing process, and they may lose their ability to fertilize an egg due to immotility. *See* Family Planning.

Vasoconstriction

A narrowing of the blood vessels.

Vasoconstriction is caused by constrictor nerve fibers that are part of the sympathetic nervous system, which controls involuntary activity of the glands, organs, and other body parts. These nerve fibers release adrenaline and noradrenaline, which cause arterial constriction in the smallest arteries. Thromboxane A2, produced by the platelets, also contributes to constriction, as do natural chemicals that release calcium or move calcium from smooth muscle cells. A high degree of vasoconstriction causes hypertension, which is a major risk factor for cardiovascular disease if it persists for a long time. *See* Hypertension.

Vasodilation

A widening of the blood vessels.

Vasodilation can occur naturally, as the body responds to hot weather. It can also be induced as a treatment for a number of cardiovascular conditions, including hypertension, heart failure, and coronary artery disease. A number of different drugs can be prescribed as vasodilators. They in clude nitroglycerin and related nitrate compounds; calcium channel blockers; beta blockers; and angiotensin-converting enzyme (ACE) inhibitors, each working in a different way and often prescribed as part of combination therapy. All vasodilator drugs cause similar side effects, such as headaches, flushed skin, dizziness and swelling of the ankles. *See* Coronary Heart Disease; Heart Failure; *and* Hypertension.

Vasodilator Drugs

Drugs that dilate the blood vessels to lower blood pressure, reduce angina, and protect against heart attack. They are often taken in combination with diuretics to reduce blood volume.

Among the families of drugs that enlarge the blood vessels are:

Alpha blockers (prazosin, terazosin, doxazosin) relax the thin muscular layer of the arteries. They also raise the level of HDL (good cholesterol). Side effects include low blood pressure, fainting, heart palpitations, headache, and nervousness. They are usually prescribed in combination with other drugs.

Nitrates (amyl nitrate, isosorbide dinitrate, nitroglycerin and pentaerythritol tetranitrate) relax the smooth muscles of arteries and veins. Side effects include headache, dizziness, and flushing,.

Angiotensin-converting enzyme (ACE) inhibitors (captopril, enalapril, lisonopril, quinapril, ramipil) reduce salt and water retention and enhance blood flow. Negative side effects include low blood pressure, dizziness, cough, and rash.

Direct vasodilators (hydralazine, minoxidil) relax the artery smooth muscles and increase the heart rate. Negative side effects include headache, palpitations, nausea, vomiting, increased heart rate, fluid retention, and low blood pressure.

Calcium channel blockers (diltiazem, verapamil, amlodipine, felodipine, isradipine, nicardipine, nifedipine) interfere with the migration of calcium so the blood vessel muscles cannot spasm or constrict as strongly. Side effects include slow heart rate, dizziness, fluid retention, flushing, headache, nausea, rash, and weakness.

All of these drugs are essentially stopgap methods to control the pain of angina or to forestall an actual heart attack. They do not address the basic problems of high blood pressure or artherosclerosis. For these, lifestyle changes involving diet and exercise, stopping smoking, and perhaps cholesterol-lowering drugs may be prescribed. *See also* Arteries; Atherosclerosis; Blood Pressure; *and* Heart, Disorders of.

Vector

An insect or animal that transmits a pathogen from one organism to another.

Mosquitoes, fleas, ticks, and lice are the most common vectors, that carry disease from animals and humans to other humans. There are numerous examples of diseases for which insects act as vectors, from lyme disease and malaria to plague and encephalitis. Yellow fever is transmitted by mosquitoes, as are dengue fever, the West Nile virus, and typhus. When the infectious agent is bacterial, antibiotics can control the disease. When the agent is viral, the immune system will have to kill the infectious agent on its own. *See also* Bacteria; Infectious Diseases; *and* Viruses.

Vegetarianism

Practice of restricting the diet to nonmeat sources.

Various forms and degrees of vegetarianism exist. Some vegetarians eat eggs and dairy products. Strict vegetarians (vegans) eat no animal products at all. It is possible to eat a nutritious and balanced vegetarian diet. In fact, a balanced vegetarian diet can provide a variety of health benefits—reduced incidence of heart disease, high blood pressure, obesity, and some cancers.

Vegetarians have to be certain to eat a variety of foods to provide the same nutrients that nonvegetarians get from animal foods, particularly proteins, essential amino acids, calcium, iron, zinc, and vitamins B_{12}

and D. Most of these nutrients can be provided even by a vegan diet, yet it is essential to eat foods that will provide sufficient amounts of these nutrients, and to emphasize a variety of types of vegetable proteins. Vitamin B_{12}, however, occurs only in animal foods. A supplement may be necessary, although other possible sources include fortified soy products and enriched cereals.

It is critical that a vegetarian diet be well planned and balanced, especially in those whose nutrient needs are high, such as infants and children, and pregnant or lactating women. *See also* AMINO ACIDS; CALCIUM; HYPERTENSION; *and* VITAMIN SUPPLEMENTS.

Vegetative State

A state, such as unconsciousness or a coma, in which a patient experiences a lack of awareness.

A vegetative state is one in which a person does not have the capacity for conscious behavior and so is unaware of the external environment. The person maintains involuntary functions, such as sleep cycles, heart rate, and breathing; head and limb movement along with eye opening have been observed in patients in a vegetative state.

A vegetative state is produced when the upper part of the brain, which is responsible for controlling mental function, is destroyed, while the brain stem and thalamus, responsible for involuntary actions, remains intact; often due to severe trauma. The longer the vegetative state persists, the less likely it is that the victim will recover. *See also* COMA *and* UNCONSCIOUSNESS.

Vein

The blood vessels that carry blood back to the heart from the rest of the body.

Blood carried through the veins is unaerated—there is less oxygen in it than in arteries—because it has been used by the body's muscles and tissues. If the veins are not functioning properly (due to increased pressure), they may grow thinner and weaker (varicose veins). *See* VARICOSE VEINS.

Veins, Disorders of

Conditions affecting the health of the vessels carrying blood to the right side of the heart.

The most common disorder of the veins is venous thrombosis, the formation of blood clots in the veins. It can also be the most dangerous, since a thrombus (clot) that forms in the deep veins of the legs or the abdomen can break away and float to the lungs, where it will cause complete or partial blockage of blood vessel. The resulting pulmonary embolus can be life-threatening. Thrombosis can be treated with anticoagulant or blood-thinning medication. Venous thrombosis can also lead to chronic venous insufficiency, in which a clot blocks a vessel in a leg. It causes swelling and discoloration of the affected leg.

Varicose veins, swelling of the blood vessels, usually occurs in veins just below the skin of the legs but can also affect veins of the anus, esophagus and scrotum. *See also* THROMBOSIS *and* VARICOSE VEINS.

Vena Cava

The two large veins that collect blood flowing from the body to the heart.

There are two vena cavae, superior and inferior, each nearly one inch in diameter. Blood from the upper part of the body flows through the superior vena cava into the right atrium, one of the upper chambers of the heart, while blood from the lower part of the body enters the right atrium through the inferior vena cava. The blood then enters the right ventricle and is pumped through the pulmonary artery to the lungs, where it loses carbon dioxide and picks up oxygen.

The superior vena cava originates at the top of the right side of the chest, close to the breastbone and behind the first rib. It is the end of one venous tree which starts with the subclavian veins, which drain blood from the arms; the jugular vein, which receives blood from the brain; and some minor veins, and which then from the

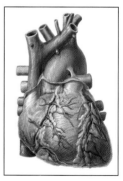

The Vena Cava. Below, the vena cava are the two veins (in blue) that circulate blood from the body to the heart.

right and left brachiocephalic veins. They lead into the superior vena cava, which connects with the right atrium.

The inferior vena cava begins in the lower abdomen, in front of the fifth lumbar vertebra. It is longer than the superior vena cava, coming from the front of the spine before entering the right atrium. It is also the end of a venous tree, forming from the two common iliac veins, through which blood flows from the legs and pelvis. The inferior vena cava also sends blood to the heart from the renal veins, which receive blood from the kidneys, and the hepatic vein, which receives blood from the liver. *See also* BLOOD *and* CIRCULATORY SYSTEM.

Venerology

The study of diseases that are transmitted during sexual acts.

Venereal diseases are spread through the interchange of bodily fluids, such as vaginal secretions, semen, and blood. Symptoms of venereal diseases are more obvious among men than women, but these diseases can often be misdiagnosed because of the similarity of their symptoms to those of other disorders. Further, women infected with venereal diseases may not exhibit symptoms and, therefore, may unknowingly carry these diseases. The most common venereal diseases are herpes, chlamydia, gonorrhea, syphilis, and AIDS. *See also* AIDS; CHLAMYDIA; GONORRHEA; HERPES; *and* SEXUALLY TRANSMITTED DISEASES.

Venipuncture

Puncturing of a vein using a hollow bore needle in order to extract a specimen of blood for analysis.

Sampling blood is a key diagnostic technique, used to test for an enormous range of diseases and abnormalities. The most common means of obtaining a blood sample is through venipuncture, a technique using a sterile needle to pierce a vein, typically in the upper arm. An elastic band is secured as a tourniquet around the arm to

increase pressure to the venipuncture area and to restrict the blood flow through the vein. Veins below the tourniquet will expand with blood. The venipuncture needle is then inserted into the vein and the blood sample drawn into a syringe. The tourniquet is removed during the drawing of blood, restoring normal circulation.

Blood sampling by venipuncture is safe and relatively painless—only a brief prick is felt as the needle is inserted. Occasionally some blood may collect under the site of the venipuncture (hematoma), and some soreness may persist for a day or two. There is some risk of infection, though it is minimal, providing proper methods of sterilization are observed. *See also* BLOOD; BLOOD CELLS; BLOOD TESTS; HEMATOMA; *and* VEIN.

Venography

Also known as phlebography or venogram

Radiographic study of the veins following injection of a radiocontrast medium.

Venography is used to diagnose accumulations of blood factors known as thrombi, blood clots, and other obstructive abnormalities of the veins.

A radiocontrast medium is injected intravenously. The solution outlines the location and structure of veins, when exposed to x-ray. The technique is particularly useful for the lower extremities, to diagnose a condition known as deep venous thrombosis. If thrombosis is an issue, then a regimen of anticoagulation medicine may be prescribed, depending on the needs of the patient.

Allergic Reactions to the Radiocontrast Medium

There is always a chance of discovering an allergy to any form of treatment; even a diagnostic procedure such as venography. Since the procedure is performed less often, as new diagnostic tools gain favor, fewer and fewer people know whether or not they are allergic to the radiocontrast medium. This is an issue that should be discussed with the health care provider before undergoing such treatment. He or she may have a alternate option if there is any concern about the possibility of an allergic reaction.

Pregnant women are often advised against undergoing any sort of x-ray examination, including a venogram, as are the elderly. Ultrasound is being used more often instead of this procedure as the use of venography continues to be replaced by other, more effective, procedures throughout hospitals across the country. *See also* BLOOD; BLOOD CELLS; BLOOD TESTS; DIAGNOSIS; MRI; NUCLEAR MEDICINE; PET SCAN; RADIOPAQUE; THROMBOSIS; THROMBUS; VEIN; VEINS, DISORDERS OF; *and* X-RAY.

Venomous Bites and Stings

Any attack by animal or insect that results in poisons or irritants getting into the tissue or blood.

While insect bites are often nothing more than an annoyance, the bites and stings of some types of bees, ants, wasps, scorpions, and spiders are venomous—some highly toxic, even deadly. Among these are tarantulas, black widow spiders, and brown recluse spiders. Certain marine animals, particularly jellyfish, can produce painful and potentially dangerous stings as well. Even the stings of less venomous insects like honey bees can provoke a life-threatening allergic reaction in some people. *See* ANAPHYLACTIC SHOCK; FIRST AID; JELLYFISH STINGS; SAND FLY BITES; SCORPION STINGS; SNAKEBITES; SPIDER BITES; *and* STINGS.

ALERT
In Case of an Emergency
If the victim experiences a sudden and severe reaction, or has been bitten or stung multiple times, immediately contact EMS. If the offending creature can safely be killed or captured, do so for accurate identification. Carefully monitor the victim's airway, breathing, and circulation until help arrives. If the bite is on an extremity, apply a snug-fitting bandage (not a tourniquet) between the bite and the heart to slow diffusion of the venom. Do not elevate the bite area above the heart level. After approximately five minutes, or if the bandage causes a loss of sensation, remove it and put an ice pack on the bite.

Ventilation

Mechanically assisted breathing during a respiratory crisis or surgery.

Ventilation becomes necessary when a person has lost the ability to breathe normally. Normal breathing is controlled by the brain stem. If it is damaged by head injury, disease, or drug overdose, regular respiration can be lost. Alternately, the problem may originate in the respiratory system, caused by a chest injury, respiratory disease, complication of surgery, or a disorder of the nerves or muscles. Newborn babies may require ventilation when their breathing mechanism is not fully developed.

Procedure. Ventilation is done mechanically using a ventilator, which consists of a motor that expands and contracts rhythmically to pump air into a tube. This tube is put into the nose or mouth so that air is delivered to the lungs. In some cases where ventilation must be carried out for a long period, an opening is made in the airway leading to the lungs, and the tube is inserted in that opening.

The amount of air that is delivered to the patient and the oxygen content of the air can be controlled depending on his or her needs. A patient cannot eat during ventilation, and so nourishment is provided by intravenous infusion of appropriate liquid nutrition. In many cases, secretions may accumulate in the lungs because the patient cannot expel them by coughing. They can be removed by suction, with therapy to prevent further fluid accumulations.

Ventilation is ended gradually, with the patient being disconnected from the ventilator for a brief period. These periods of normal breathing become longer until normal respiration is achieved. Blood tests to measure oxygen levels determine when ventilation is no longer necessary.

Background material on VENTILATION *can be found in* RESPIRATION. *Related information is contained in* AIRWAY OBSTRUCTION; AMBULANCE; BLOOD; CHILDBIRTH; LUNGS; PREMATURE BIRTH; *and* SURGERY. *See also* BREATHING DIFFICULTY.

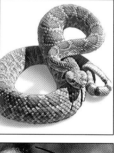
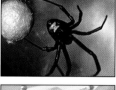
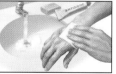

Venomous Bites.
Above, top, the rattlesnake, one of the deadliest poisonous snakes found in North America. Above, center, the black widow spider. If one is bitten by a potentially poisonous creature, the first step is to wash the bite area, above, bottom.

Ventilator

Also known as a respirator

A machine that maintains respiration when normal breathing fails.

A ventilator consists of a bellows that is expanded by an electric pump and contracted by a weight, connected to a humidifier, so that a normal supply of air can be delivered to a person who has lost the ability to breathe due to an injury or illness. The air is first pumped through a humidifier, which adds moisture so that the lungs will not become dry, and is then pumped into a tube placed in the main airway (trachea) leading to the lungs. The air is expelled from the lungs by a natural force of their contraction, so that the natural cycle of inhaling and exhaling is carried out. The amount of air pumped and the oxygen content of the air can be adjusted according to the patient's needs. *See also* BREATHING DIFFICULTY; LUNGS; *and* VENTILATION.

Ventricle

One of the two bottom chambers of the heart; also: one of four cavities in the brain.

In the heart. The ventricles are the cavities that form the bottom of the heart. Blood flows into the two top chambers (the atria) and into the ventricles, where it is pumped out of the heart. The right ventricle pumps blood from the heart to the lungs, and the left ventricle pumps blood to the rest of the body. The left ventricle is the strongest chamber of the heart and contracts the most forcefully. *See also* HEART.

In the brain. The ventricles are cavities in the interior of the brain that produce cerebrospinal fluid, a fluid that cushions the brain and spinal cord. The first two (lateral) ventricles are located in each side of the cerebrum. The third ventricle is in the center of the brain; its walls consist of the thalamus and hypothalamus. The fourth ventricle is lower in the brain; cerebrospinal fluid flows from the fourth ventricle to surround the spinal cord. *See also* BRAIN.

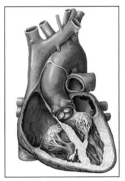

Ventricles. Blood that flows into the heart via the atria is pumped out by the ventricles, the lower two chambers of the heart. From the right ventricle, blood goes to the lungs for oxygen; from the left atria, blood goes to the rest of the body.

Ventricular Ectopic Beat

An abnormal heart beat caused by an electric impulse generated in the ventricles.

When an electric impulse that causes the heart muscle to contract originates in the ventricles, the lower chambers of the heart, it causes premature contractions of those chambers. These premature beats are usually not dangerous and often do not cause any symptoms.

Older people with healthy hearts are more likely to experience these abnormal beats. They may also be caused by heart damage due to a myocardial infarction (heart attack) or a fever, or by extreme fatigue, smoking, heavy consumption of coffee, or other caffeine-containing beverages, or emotional stress. These ectopic beats can also occur after heart surgery or during heart catheterization, and they can be a side effect of digitalis drugs.

Ventricular ectopic beats can be diagnosed by the distinctive patterns they produce on an electrocardiogram. If there is no underlying cause, ventricular ectopic beats can often be managed by changes in lifestyle, such as more rest, ceasing smoking, and reduced caffeine intake. If the cause is a myocardial infarction or if the ectopic beats occur often enough to cause discomfort, an antiarrhythmic drug may be prescribed. *See also* CAFFEINE; ECTOPIC HEART BEAT; HEART; *and* HEART ATTACK.

Ventricular Fibrillation

Rapid, uncoordinated contractions of the heart that eliminate its ability to pump blood.

Ventricular fibrillation results from uncoordinated electrical impulses that arise in the ventricles and that override the normal system of impulses that cause the heart to beat normally. The heart begins to twitch uselessly, and death can result in a few short minutes unless the normal heartbeat is restored. Ventricular fibrillation can be preceded by ventricular tachycardia, abnormally fast beating of the ventricles.

A myocardial infarction (heart attack) that causes heart tissue scarring is a major risk factor for ventricular fibrillation. Implantation of a defibrillator that monitors the heart rhythm and can deliver electrical pulses when fibrillation occurs is done for many people at high risk. Studies have found a major reduction in deaths among patients given implantable defibrillators. Antiarrhythmic drugs such as beta blockers may be prescribed for some patients.

If ventricular fibrillation does occur, cardiopulmonary resuscitation (CPR) must be started within four to six minutes to prevent death. CPR involves breathing air into the victim's lungs and applying external heart massage. External defibrillators are now available in some public places to be used if a cardiac emergency occurs. *See* ARRHYTHMIA, CARDIAC; DEFIBRILLATION; HEART; *and* VENTRICULAR TACHYCARDIA.

Ventricular Tachycardia

An abnormally fast heart beat originating in the ventricles.

Ventricular tachycardia is a potentially life-threatening arrhythmia that does not arise in the sinoatrial node—the center in the right atrium that controls the heart beat—but in the ventricles, the lower chambers that pump blood to the lungs and the rest of the body. The heart rate can increase to more than 200 beats per minute, and there is a danger that this tachycardia can lead to ventricular fibrillation.

Ventricular tachycardia can result from a myocardial infarction that damages the heart muscle enough to create scarred regions that block the passage of the electrical impulses from the sinoatrial node.

Persons at high risk of ventricular tachycardia can be given an implantable defibrillator, which is programmed to detect arrhythmias and delivers electric pulses to restore the normal heart beat. Another treatment is radiofrequency catheter ablation, which uses an electric current to destroy the region of the ventricle where the abnormal rhythm originates. Beta blockers

and other medications may be prescribed for some patients. *See also* ARRHYTHMIA; CARDIAC; *and* VENTRICULAR FIBRILLATION.

Vernix

A white greasy material which coats a baby's body at and just before birth.

Vernix covers a baby in the twentieth week in order to protect it from the watery amniotic fluid. There is usually less vernix on the body of a baby born at 40 or more weeks. *See also* AMNIOSCOPY *and* BIRTH.

Version

The obstetric procedure used to change a baby's position in the uterus.

Most babies are born head first and are oriented that way in the uterus from the seventh month onwards. Breech babies are positioned so that their feet or buttocks will emerge first; these babys need to be repositioned before birth.

Between the thirty-fourth and thirty-seventh week, the obstetrician may be able to manipulate a breech baby into the proper presentation (the position that faces outwards) by a procedure called external version. With one hand on the new mother's abdomen just over the baby's head and the other hand over the baby's buttocks, the obstetrician gently attempts to rotate the baby, bringing its head down into the mother's pelvis. This procedure has a high success rate.

External version may be done with general anesthesia; drugs may also be administered to relax the uterus, making the procedure easier for the obstetrician. The procedure carries a small risk of inducing premature labor, rupture of the membranes, or antepartum hemorrhage, or of twisting the umbilical cord.

Background material on VERSION *can be found in* CAESAREAN SECTION *and* CHILDBIRTH. *Related information is contained in* NATURAL CHILDBIRTH; PROLAPSED CORD; UMBILICAL CORD; *and* UTERUS, PROLAPSE OF. *See also* CONCEPTION.

Vertebra

The small bones that join together to form the backbone and protect the spine.

The spinal column is composed of five major segments containing a total of 31 bones; eight cervical, 12 thoracic, five lumbar, five sacral, and one coccygeal. These bones form a system that is quite flexible, the bones at the bottom may become fused. This is rarely a problem, although it may cause some complications if a bone that is damaged is fused to a healthy bone.

These bones pass from the base of the skull to the bottom of the lumbar region of the back. Inside of the vertebra, which are shaped somewhat like a butterfly, is the spinal chord. The spinal chord is an essential part of the central nervous system. It is composed of sensory and motor neurons that control the body's motion and provides the brain with sensory information.

The spine should be perfectly straight, without any sideways curves (which would otherwise indicate scoliosis) and it should bend in slightly at the bottom and out, slightly at the top. Damage to the vertebra can cause musculoskeletal disorders. *See also* SPINAL INJURY; *and* SPINE.

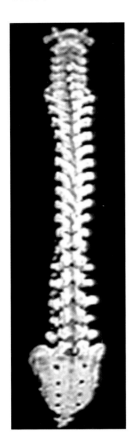

Vertebra. Above, an image of the individual bones that make up the backbone that protect the spinal cord. There are 31 separate vertebra that compose the spinal column. Sometimes, the bones at the bottom become fused; this may require surgery.

Vertebrobasilar Insufficiency

Episodes of dizziness, speech difficulties, and general weakness caused by insufficient blood flow to the brain stem and the cerebellum.

Vertebrobasilar insufficiency is typified by double vision, faintness, and speech irregularities. These symptoms are a reaction to an obstruction of blood flow that is caused by a narrowing of the basilar and vertebral arteries in the brain. In general, the arterial constriction is a result of a build-up of fat deposits (atherosclerosis).

Fat-containing plaque deposits on the arterial walls of the vertebral and basilar arteries are the most common causes of vertebrobasilar insufficiency. Other possible causes include cervical arthrosis of the cer-

vical spine, aneurysm, trauma, and extrinsic compressions. *See also* ANEURYSM; ATHEROSCLEROSIS; BLINDNESS; *and* VISION.

Vertigo

Also known as Benign Paroxysmal Postural Vertigo

A sensation of dizziness or moving that is accompanied by a feeling of losing one's balance.

Vertigo is an illusionary sense that a person or his or her surroundings are spinning. It is a common complaint and rarely is it linked to an underlying illness. The condition is often referred to as lightheadedness or dizziness. Vertigo can last for a few minutes or it can continue for days.

Types. Motion-sickness is the most prevalent form of vertigo; it is the side effect of a bumpy car ride or sitting in a swaying boat. Motion-sickness vertigo is common among young children with sensitive inner ears. Meniere's disease is a serious condition that combines vertigo with ringing in the ears (tinnitus).

Causes. The body perceives position and maintains balance through the organs in the inner ear that are responsible for transmitting nerve connections to the brain. If there is a disorder in the canals in the inner ear (labyrinthitis) or its connecting nerves, it results in vertigo followed by nausea. Vertigo can be a side effect of abrupt changes in blood pressure, vision-related illnesses, bacteria or viral infections, tumors, nerve inflammation, or exposure to toxins.

Treatment. The method of treatment depends on the underlying cause; however, bed rest without head motion can generally minimize the spinning sensation and associated nausea. Sudden vertigo can be treated with antihistamines or anticholinergic drugs. A scopolamine patch can prevent motion sickness if it is worn a few days before a long trip.

> *Background material on* VERTIGO *can be found in* DIZZINESS *and* MENIERE'S DISEASE. *Related information is contained in* BACTERIAL INFECTIONS; BLOOD PRESSURE; EAR, INNER EAR; MOTION SICKNESS; *and* TINNITUS. *See also* BALANCE.

Viability

The ability to survive, grow, and develop.

Viability is a general term used to indicate the potential for growth, development, or survival. It is used in areas as diverse as grafting and transplantation (where tissues or organs may be said to be viable when the prognosis of acceptance by the patient is high), studies where the proportion of living cells in a sample is evaluated, and reproductive testing of sperm and egg for viability in fertilization. Viability tests are often performed to determine the efficacy of treatment options; the health of cells, tissues, or organs under study; or the reproductive potential for tissues, organs, and cells. *See also* GRAFTING; GRAFT-VERSUS-HOST DISEASE; *and* TRANSPLANT SURGERY.

Viagra

A drug introduced in 1998 to treat men with erectile dysfunction.

Millions of men suffer from episodes of erectile dysfunction, often as the natural result of aging. Viagra was introduced as a drug that can correct this problem. Within a little more than an hour of taking a dose of the drug, a man will respond to sexual stimulation with a natural erection.

Viagra is dangerous for men taking nitrate drugs (such as nitroglycerine) and may interact with other medications as well. It is important that men notify their physician of preexisting conditions or medications prior to taking Viagra. Side effects include headaches, facial flushing, upset stomach, blurred vision, and sensitivity to light. *See also* ERECTION, DISORDERS OF.

Vincent's Disease

Also known as trench mouth

A bacterial infection of the gums that was epidemic during World War I, when soldiers could not practice good oral hygiene.

Vincent's disease is a noncontagious disease in which the gums become inflamed, painful, and bleed easily. The breath of the patient is foul and there is usually a fever. The lymph nodes under the jaw swell and are tender. Vincent's disease usually attacks people who are already in poor health, those with poor oral hygiene, those with throat infections, or those who are under severe physical or emotional stress.

Vincent's disease is first treated with a gentle cleaning in which dead tissue and tartar are removed from the gums and teeth. The patient will be advised to rinse with a warm hydrogen peroxide solution three times a day, as this will be less painful than attempting to brush the teeth. Professional cleaning by a dental hygienist every day or two is recommended for the first few weeks. Antibiotics may also be prescribed to destroy the bacteria that cause Vincent's disease. The patient will also be advised to get plenty of rest, to eat a well-balanced diet, and to avoid spicy foods and irritants like smoking. *See also* ANTIBIOTIC DRUGS.

Viremia

The presence of a virus in the blood stream.

When a virus invades the body, it finds its way to the bloodstream and travels through the blood to the organs of the body. Viral diseases do not respond to antibiotics, but are controlled by the body's natural immune system. Gamma globulin is a prepared substance that contains human antibodies and that can be injected intravenously to assist the body in the fight against viral intruders.

Viruses differ from bacteria in that they are smaller; so much smaller, in fact, that it is unclear whether they are very simple microorganisms or very complex molecules. They survive by penetrating healthy cells and multiplying within the cells, which finally break open and discharge millions of new viruses into the organism.

Viruses are responsible for a host of diseases, from the common cold and influenza to hepatitis, herpes, and AIDS. *See also* AIDS; COLD, COMMON; GAMMA GLOBULIN; HIV; *and* VIRUSES.

Virginity

The state of not having had sexual intercourse.

The term "virgin" is used to refer to an individual, male or female, who has not yet experienced sexual intercourse. In females, the term specifically refers to a young girl whose hymen remains intact. *See also* SEXUAL INTERCOURSE.

Virilism

A hormonal disorder that causes a woman to develop masculine sexual characteristics.

The hormones that cause development of sexual characteristics are present in both sexes. Women have estrogen in their ovaries for reproductive purposes, but men also have a small amount in their bodies. Similarly, the androgen hormones that cause men to develop masculine sexual characteristics are also present in small amounts in the adrenal glands and ovaries of women. Virilism occurs when a woman produces excess amounts of androgen hormones. Women with this condition experience such traits as excess body hair, male pattern baldness, irregular periods or a total lack of menstruation, an enlarged clitoris, overdevelopment of muscles in the arms and shoulders, and a deepened voice.

Virilism is usually the result of a disorder that affects the adrenal glands or ovaries, such as polycystic ovary (cysts in the ovary), tumors of the ovaries or adrenal glands, or congenital adrenal hyperplasia. Congenital adrenal hyperplasia is a condition in which an infant female is born with what appears to be an intersex condition or male genitalia. In less severe cases, affected females may develop the signs of virilism during puberty. Treatment for virilism depends upon the cause.

> *Background information on virilism can be found in* SEXUAL CHARACTERISTICS, SECONDARY. *For related material, see* ANDROGEN HORMONES; CLITORIS; ESTROGEN; HAIR LOSS; MENSTRUATION; PROGESTERONE; PUBERTY; *and* TESTOSTERONE. *See also* ADRENAL HYPERPLASIA *and* ADRENAL TUMORS.

Virility

The ability to procreate.

In the biological sense, the term virility can be used interchangeably with male fertility, which is dependent on a few factors. A male must produce healthy normal sperm capable of fertilizing an egg. He must be able to maintain an erection in order for penetration to occur during sexual intercourse; and he must achieve orgasm and ejaculate so that the sperm can swim up the female reproductive tract to the waiting egg. *See also* FERTILITY.

Virilization

Development of male sexual characteristics in a female.

The androgen hormones help men develop secondary sexual characteristics during puberty, such as a deepened voice, increased muscle mass, and body hair. Androgen hormones are also present in small amounts in a woman's adrenal glands and ovaries. When a disorder causes overproduction of these hormones in a woman, the condition known as virilism results; it is the actual process that leads to this condition that is called virilization.

Disorders that cause virilization include adrenal tumors, ovarian cysts or tumors, or congenital adrenal hyperplasia. Treatment usually includes hormone therapy. *See also* ADRENAL GLANDS; ADRENAL HYPERPLASIA, CONGENITAL; ANDROGEN HORMONES; CONGENITAL; OVARIAN CYSTS; *and* VIRILISM.

Virology

The study of viruses, the diseases they produce, and the cures for these diseases.

The virus is much smaller than the fungus and the bacterium. It is so small, in fact, that it cannot be seen with an ordinary microscope. In order to multiply, the virus attacks and penetrates a living cell and takes control of that cell, using the cell's metabolism to replicate itself and then releasing copies of itself into the surrounding tissue or bloodstream to attack other cells.

Viral infections are spread by person-to-person contact or on droplets of water that are coughed or sneezed by an infected person. The lifespan of viruses without a host organism is very short.

The skin and mucous membranes are the body's first line of defense against viral infection. The second line of defense is the immune system, consisting of the white blood cells that engulf infected cells and the antibodies that limit the reproductive ability of the virus.

Vaccination can stimulate immunity to specific viruses by inducing the production of antibodies to these viruses. Resistance to viral infection is also raised by injections of gamma globulin, which contains antibodies produced in another person or in an animal. There are far fewer antiviral drugs than antibiotics; most viral infections are curtailed by the body's own immune system. *See also* ANTIBIOTIC DRUGS; ANTIVIRAL DRUGS; *and* VACCINATION.

Virulence

Disease-causing potential of a given pathogen.

Virulence is a qualitative measure of the aggressiveness of a particular disease-causing pathogen. The term implies rapidity of infection and reproduction of the pathogens; in the case of viral assault, it is the relative lack of ability of cells, tissues, or systems to combat the pathogen and the pathogen's destructive effect.

Diseases vary enormously in virulence, from the fairly benign, with weak properties of communicability, to highly contagious, often lethal, strains. Virulence is often applied to distinguish among related disease manifestations (for example, different forms of cancer), and to rank lethality of viral disease strains, including HIV (the causative agent of AIDS) and viruses of even greater virulence, such as the Ebola virus. *See also* AIDS; HIV; PATHOGEN; VIROLOGY; *and* VIRUSES.

Viruses

Microscopic infectious agents.

Viruses are up to 100 times smaller than bacteria, and their structure differs from that of bacteria as well. They are only active when they are inside the cells of a host organism and cannot live on their own. The number of different kinds of viruses greatly exceeds the number of types of any other organisms. Many viruses cause disease, though some viruses do not.

Structure and Replication. All viruses contain a core of nucleic acid surrounded by protective shells (capsids) made of protein. The nucleic acid contains genes with instructions for replication of the virus. To replicate, the virus must invade a living cell of a host organism. It lands on the host cell and injects nucleic acid inside the cell. The nucleic acid then replicates itself in the host cell in large numbers, and each new nucleic acid stimulates the growth of its own capsid. The new virus particles are then released from the host cell, which is sometimes destroyed.

Viruses and Disease. Viruses cause disease in many ways. First, the activities of the host cells are disrupted, causing serious consequences if the host cells are located in a major organ. Second, the body's immune system response to a viral invasion may also cause symptoms, such as fever, inflammation, or fatigue. Third, viruses may interfere with the function of the immune system itself, leaving the body vulnerable to secondary infections. Fourth, the viruses may cause mutations in the chromosomes of the host cells, and these cells may become cancerous.

Treatment of Viral Diseases. Viral diseases are harder to cure than bacterial diseases, because viral drugs must target the virus and not the host cell. In contrast, immunization has been very effective against viral diseases. Successful vaccines are available to treat many serious viral diseases, including hepatitis B, measles, mumps, rabies, and many others. *See also* AIDS; ANTIVIRAL DRUGS; VACCINATION; *and* VACCINE.

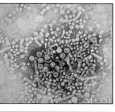
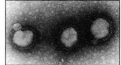

Viruses.
Viruses are extremely small organisms that can infect humans and cause disease. There are billions of different types of viruses, including the hepatitis B virus (top), the influenza virus (bottom).

Resources on Viruses
Fettner, Ann Guidici, *The Science of Viruses* (1990); Fields, Bernard, et al., *Fields' Virology* (1996); Garrett, Laurie, *The Coming Plague* (1994); Grist, Norman R., et al., *Diseases of Infection: An Illustrated Textbook* (1992); Radetsky, Peter, *The Invisible Invaders* (1991); Centers for Disease Contol and Prevention, Tel. (800) 311-3435, Online: www.cdc.gov; Infectious Disease Society of America, Tel. (703) 299-0200, Online: www.idsociety.org; National Institute of Allergy and Infectious Disease, Tel. (301) 496-5717, Online: www.niaid.nih.org; Office of Rare Diseases, Tel. (301) 402-4336, Online: rarediseases.info.nih.gov/ordg; www.nycornell.org/infectious/index.html.

Viscosity

The thickness of a liquid.

When the oxygen content of the air is low, as it is at high altitudes, the body tries to compensate by producing additional red blood cells. As a result, the blood becomes thick, and more pressure from the heart is needed in order to pump the blood through the blood vessels.

The viscosity of the blood is also high when the bone marrow produces too many blood cells. This disorder is called primary polycythemia; symptoms include weakness, vision abnormalities, tinnitus (ringing in the ears), and headaches. *See also* BLOOD *and* POLYCYTHEMIA.

Vision

The ability to see.

The organs that are most involved with vision are the eyes and the brain. Vision starts in the retina, which is located at the back of the eye and contains special cells called rods and cones. Rods are low light-sensitive and cones are color-sensitive.

The function of the majority of the rest of the eye is to properly focus the correct quantities of light onto the retina. The majority of the focusing is done by the cornea, however, fine focusing (called accommodation) is accomplished through changes in the curvature of the lens.

Resources on Vision and the Eyes
Davson, *The Eye* (1984); Peninsula Center for the Blind, *The First Steps: How to Help People Who are Losing Their Sight* (1982); Schmidt, Robert F., *Fundamentals of Sensory Physiology* (1986); Wolf, K.P., *Eyewise: Eye Disorders and Their Treatment* (1982); American Foundation for the Blind, Tel. (800) 232-5463 (AFB-LINE), Online: www.afb.org; National Fed. of the Blind, Tel., (410) 659-9314, Online: www.nfb.org; Prevent Blindness America, Tel. (800) 331-2020, Online: www.pba.org; www.nycornell.org/op/.

Vision, Disorders of. At right, periorbital cellulitis is an infection of the tissues surrounding the eye. As a result, the orbit of the eye may become infected and the eye may protrude.

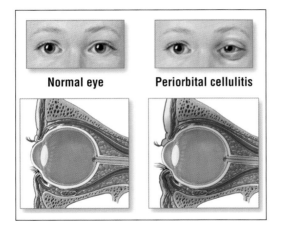

Normal eye   **Periorbital cellulitis**

Once the light reaches the rods and cones, it is converted into nerve impulses that pass through the optic nerve behind the eye into the brain. Alignment of the eyes allows the brain to fuse the slightly different images that are received from each eye. This also allows the brain to calculate depth and is important in the judgment of distance. *See also* COLOR VISION; VISION, DISORDERS OF; *and* VISION, LOSS OF.

Vision, Disorders of

Conditions affecting the eye, the nerves, or the brain, and influencing the vision.

The most common disorders of vision involve disorders of refraction (the focusing of light onto the retina by the curved lens). Problems with the curvature of the cornea result in visual disorders, such as nearsightedness (myopia), farsightedness (hyperopia), and astigmatism. Refractive disorders can almost always be successfully treated with corrective lenses, either glasses or contact lenses. Visual disorders that are not refractive may result from problems with the eye or optic nerve, disorders of the nerve pathways from the eyes to the brain, and brain disorders.

Eye and Optic Nerve Disorders. Disorders of the eye or optic nerve generally only affect the vision on the side that is affected. Loss of eye transparency, which occurs from corneal ulceration or injury, cataracts, or vitreous hemorrhage (bleeding into the fluid of the eye), can result in cloudy vision. Defects in the center of the retina, such as degeneration, can cause problems in the center of the visual field; defects on the sides of the retina, which occur in the early stage of glaucoma, can affect peripheral vision. Optic nerve defects may cause a scotoma (blind spot), and may be the result of optic neuritis, which is at times a sign of multiple sclerosis.

Nerve Pathway Disorders. Disorders of one of the nerve pathways to the brain affect vision in both eyes, because half of the fibers from each optic nerve cross before entering the brain.

Brain Disorders. Damage to the visual area of the brain, which may occur from stroke, causes loss of vision. Other brain disorders affecting vision include agnosia (failure to recognize objects) and hallucinations. *See also* AGNOSIA; CATARACT; CORNEAL ULCER; GLAUCOMA; *and* STROKE.

Vision, Loss of

The inability to see, which may develop gradually or suddenly.

Vision loss may be total or partial, and may affect one or both eyes. It may affect the center or the periphery of the visual field, and may be temporary or permanent.

Gradual Loss of Vision. Chronic and progressive vision loss is common with age, and may be the result of a loss of transparency of the lenses in the eye caused by the development of cataracts. Other possible causes of gradual vision loss include diabetes mellitus, glaucoma, retinitis pigmentosa, and macular degeneration.

Sudden Loss of Vision. Bleeding in the eye, which can be caused by injury, may cause sudden vision loss. Retinal disorders, such as detachment and hemorrhage, may also cause sudden vision loss, as may tumors or inflammation. *See also* BLINDNESS; CATARACT; DIABETES MELLITUS; GLAUCOMA; MACULAR DEGENERATION; RETINAL DETACHMENT; *and* RETINITIS PIGMENTOSA.

Vision Tests

Examinations carried out to assess eyesight and diagnose any vision deficits.

Vision tests may be administered as part of a routine exam used for employment, to obtain a driver's license, or to diagnose vision problems and prescribe treatment. Such tests are carried out by a trained ophthalmologist or optometrist. Ophthalmologists test the eyes for diseases and irregularities that may require surgical correction, while optometrists diagnose visual deficits that are treatable without surgery. Specific vision tests will depend on the particular

physician, as well as the history and needs of the patient.

Tests for visual acuity commonly employ a chart known as a Snellen's chart, consisting of letters of decreasing size, which the subject is asked to read. Visual acuity is measured at varying distances and the eyes are tested separately. With normal vision, the subject should be able to read letters three-eighths of an inch in height from 20 feet away; this is called 20/20 vision. Visual acuity testing is used to diagnose nearsightedness, farsightedness, astigmatism, or presbyopia (an age-related inability to focus on objects). Diagnosis of visual problems may be followed by a prescription for corrective lenses.

Central and peripheral vision are evaluated using a visual field test, during which the patient is asked to track a moving object across a visual field. Such tests are useful in the diagnosis of glaucoma, retinitis pigmentosa, or brain tumors. Glaucoma may also be diagnosed using a device known as a tonometer to measure pressure within the eye. Some tonometers are placed on the eye surface to directly measure pressure, while others deliver a tiny puff of air to the eye surface, measuring changes in light reflection off the cornea.

A test of color vision is carried out using plates composed of dot patterns in primary colors superimposed on a background of randomly mixed colors. Normal color vision allows the subject to identify the dot figure or pattern from the background. *See also* COLOR VISION; GLAUCOMA; RETINITIS PIGMENTOSA; VISION; VISION, DISORDERS OF; *and* VISION, LOSS OF.

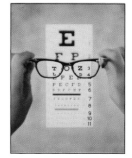

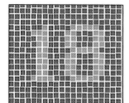

Vision Tests. Vision deficits of any kind can be discovered by the use of vision tests. Above, top, abnormal results from a color vision test may lead to a diagnosis of color blindness. Above, bottom, a Snellen's chart is used to test visual acuity.

Visual Acuity

Preciseness of vision.

Visual acuity is not the sharpness of peripheral vision; it is only the clarity of central vision. Visual acuity is measured during vision tests.

The most common causes of problems with visual acuity are refractive problems (errors of the curvature of the cornea). Refractive errors include myopia (nearsightedness), hyperopia (farsightedness), and astigmatism, and can almost always be treated successfully with corrective lenses, either glasses or contact lenses. *See also* ASTIGMATISM; HYPEROPIA; MYOPIA; VISION; *and* VISION, DISORDERS OF.

Visual Field

The total region in which sight is possible while looking straight ahead.

The normal visual field extends for 90° in either direction from the middle of the face, although it may be more limited above and below the center if the eyes are deep-set or the eyebrows are prominent.

The visual fields of each eye overlap at the center to produce binocular vision. This allows the brain to interpret distance and depth. Visual acuity is much lower at the periphery of the visual field than at the center. *See also* VISUAL ACUITY.

Vital Signs

Indicators of life, including heart and breathing rates, body temperature, and blood pressure.

Vital signs may be any signs of life displayed by a patient. However, the term is generally used for a few readily measured variables. These include body temperature, pulse (heart rate), respiratory rate, and blood pressure. Vital signs are not fixed values but fluctuate continuously, depending on the degree of exertion, time of day, patterns of sleep, overall health of the body, state of mind, and other factors.

Changes in Vital Signs. Some vital signs change over the course of a lifetime. For example, resting heart rate tends to become slower with age, requiring more time to speed up during exercise and a longer period to return to baseline. Maximum heart rate also falls as a person gets older.

Normal body temperature remains consistent through life, though temperature regulation becomes more difficult for older people, particularly during extremes of hot or cold weather, because of the loss of subcutaneous (under the skin) fat. As a result, heat stroke (hyperthermia) and exposure (hypothermia) are a greater risk for aging individuals. Blood pressure is raised over time, as blood vessels lose some of their elasticity. Normal breathing remains constant through life, though the functioning of the lungs decreases. Heart rate and rhythm problems are not uncommon among elderly patients. These include slowed pulse (bradycardia) and various rhythm irregularities, including atrial fibrillation. *See also* ATRIAL FIBRILLATION; BLOOD PRESSURE; BRADYCARDIA; BREATHING; HEART RATE; HYPERTHERMIA; HYPOTHERMIA; PULSE; *and* TEMPERATURE.

Vitamin A

Organic solution that plays a role in reproduction and the maintenance of tissue, bones, teeth, and vision.

Vitamin A is one of the four fat-soluble vitamins; it is absorbed by the body with the aid of bile and is stored in fat and in the liver. It plays an important role in reproduction and in maintenance of the mucous membranes, skin, teeth, bones, and vision.

Good sources of vitamin A include deep yellow and orange vegetables and fruits, green vegetables, dairy products, fortified cereals, and organ meats. Since fat-soluble vitamins are stored in the body, daily consumption of them is not necessary. However, deficiency can occur in individuals on extremely low-fat diets, even if sufficient amounts of the vitamin are consumed.

Signs of vitamin A deficiency include diminished resistance to infection, dry skin, night blindness, dry eyes, and, in children, stunted growth.

Megadoses of vitamin A supplements can result in a build-up of dangerous levels of the vitamin in the body, causing loss of appetite, fatigue, headaches, diarrhea, pain in joints and bones, hair loss, rashes, dry and itchy skin, irregular menstruation, liver damage, and, if taken during early pregnancy, birth defects. Consumption of toxic doses from dietary sources is not likely, although large doses of cod-liver and other fish oils can be dangerous. *See also* COD LIVER OIL *and* VITAMIN SUPPLEMENTS.

Vitamin B$_{12}$

Organic substance important for blood cell and nerve maintenance.

Vitamin B$_{12}$ is essential to the creation of nerve sheaths, to proper nerve function, blood cell formation, and normal DNA and fatty acid synthesis. It is the only water-soluble vitamin stored in the body for significant periods of time. Therefore, symptoms of deficiency can take time to emerge.

Vitamin B$_{12}$ Deficiency in the Elderly

Those over the age of 50 are most at risk for developing a vitamin B$_{12}$ deficiency, since the incidence of this condition increases with age. Levels of vitamin B$_{12}$ should be tested at age 60 and then periodically. If B$_{12}$ levels are found to be low, a doctor may determine that injections of the vitamin are necessary.

Vitamin B$_{12}$ is found only in animal proteins including eggs, dairy products, seafood, meats, and poultry. Therefore, strict vegetarians, or vegans, need to take supplements or to eat sufficient amounts of fortified foods like soy milk to ensure that they do not become deficient. People with malabsorption syndromes are also at risk for deficiency.

Vitamin B$_{12}$ interacts with folate, or folic acid, in DNA synthesis and in the creation of cells, particularly blood cells. Symptoms of deficiency are severe anemia and nerve damage. Folic acid deficiency also results in severe anemia, but does not cause similar neurological abnormalities. *See also* ANEMIA; COBALAMIN; FATTY ACIDS; FOLIC ACID; MALABSORPTION; NERVE; NUCLEIC ACIDS; PROTEIN; VEGETARIANISM; VITAMIN B COMPLEX; *and* VITAMIN SUPPLEMENTS.

Vitamin B Complex

Combination of vitamins critical to energy processing (metabolism) and several body functions.

Vitamin B complex refers to eight vitamins: thiamine (B$_1$), riboflavin (B$_2$), niacin (B$_3$), pyroxidine (B$_6$), cobalamin (B$_{12}$), folic acid, pantothenic acid, and biotin. A balanced diet contains all eight B vitamins.

Thiamine (B$_1$) is important to carbohydrate metabolism and nervous system function. Good sources are whole grains, legumes, seafood, and pork. Severe deficiency causes beriberi.

Riboflavin (B$_2$) is essential to metabolism, vision, and the maintenance of mucous membranes. Symptoms of deficiency include a sore, swollen mouth, and psychological problems. Excessive amounts can reduce metabolism of vitamins B$_1$ and B$_6$. Good sources are green vegetables, meats, poultry, dairy products, and whole grains.

Niacin (B$_3$) is essential to appetite, digestion, and nerve function; and it is found in poultry, meats, fish, nuts, yeast, and whole grains. High therapeutic doses in the form of nicotinic acid are used to lower cholesterol under medical supervision, since potentially dangerous side effects may occur. Deficiency manifests itself in mouth sores and diarrhea. Overdose can cause hot flashes, itching, elevated blood sugar and uric acid levels, arrhythmias, liver damage, and ulcers.

Pantothenic acid (B$_5$) is produced by intestinal bacteria and can be found in nearly all plant and animal foods. Deficiency is rare. Excess may increase the need for B$_1$.

Pyroxidine (B$_6$) plays an important role in protein and carbohydrate metabolism; and it is found in meats, poultry, fish, grains, dark green leafy vegetables, pota-

Resources on Vitamins
Groff, James L. and Sareen S. Gropper, *Advanced Nutrition and Human Metabolism* (1999); Heimburger, Douglas C. and R. L. Weinsier, *Handbook of Clinical Nutrition* (1997); Hendler, Sheldon Saul, *The Doctor's Vitamin and Mineral Encyclopedia* (1990); Machlin, Lawrence J., *Handbook of Vitamins* (1991); Shils, Maurice E., et al., *Modern Nutrition in Health and Disease* (1999); American Dietetic Association, Tel. (800) 366-1655, Online: www.eatright.org; Center for Nutrition Policy and Promotion, Tel. (202) 418-2312, Online: www.usda. gov/cnpp; Food and Drug Admin., Tel. (888) INFOFDA, Online: www.fda.gov; www.nycornell.org/medicine/nutrition/index.html.

toes, prunes, and bananas. Deficiency can cause confusion, depression, itchy scaly skin, and, in infants, convulsions. Overdose destroys the sensory nerves.

Cobalamin (B$_{12}$) is essential to the creation of genetic material and cell formation. It is present only in animal products, thus vegans need supplementation.

Biotin is needed for metabolic processes. It is produced by digestive tract bacteria and found in vegetables, legumes, nuts, seeds, eggs, meats, poultry, and fish.

Folic acid, found in fresh fruits and vegetables. It is necessary for the creation of RNA, DNA, and red blood cells, and is essential to proper fetal health. Deficiency can cause anemia. Supplementation is recommended for all women of childbearing age to prevent malformation of the fetal nervous system. *See also* COBALA-MIN; BERI-BERI; FOLIC ACID; NUTRITION; VITAMIN B$_{12}$; *and* VITAMIN SUPPLEMENTS.

Vitamin C

Also known as ascorbic acid

Organic substance important to the maintenance of circulation and tissue.

Vitamin C plays an important role in the maintenance of capillaries, cartilage, teeth, and bones; in the production of collagen; in increasing the absorption of iron; and in preventing the oxidation of fatty acids.

Signs of vitamin C deficiency include a propensity to bruise, a slow healing response, dry skin, loss of appetite, loose teeth, and bleeding gums. Extreme cases of vitamin C deficiency can result in scurvy.

High doses of vitamin C are usually excreted (as they are water soluble); however, they may cause diarrhea, irritation of the urinary tract from an increase in acidity of the urine, kidney stones, deposits in the heart and other tissues, blood damage, and excessive iron binding.

Sources of Vitamin C. Good sources of vitamin C include: citrus fruits; melons; berries; kiwis; green vegetables; sweet potatoes; peppers; and plantains. *See also* ANTI-HISTAMINE; COLLAGEN; IRON; SCURVY; *and* VITAMIN SUPPLEMENTS.

Vitamin D

Organic substance essential to the building and maintenance of bones and teeth, and the absorption of calcium.

As a fat-soluble vitamin, excess vitamin D is stored in the body and can be highly toxic. Vitamin D supplementation should occur only under a doctor's supervision, since toxicity can occur at fairly low doses, particularly in children. An excess of vitamin D can result in calcium deposits in the heart, blood vessels, kidneys and elsewhere. Other consequences are hypertension, elevated cholesterol levels, brittle bones, headache, lethargy, and loss of appetite.

A deficiency of vitamin D will result in skeletal disorders, such as rickets, deformities, dental abnormalities in children, and osteomalacia and osteoporosis in adults. Other symptoms of deficiency include cramps, muscle twitching, and convulsions.

Vitamin D is found in liver, egg yolks, fortified milk and milk products, fish oils, and cold water fish, such as tuna. It is also produced by the body following exposure to sunlight. Ten to fifteen minutes of exposure to the summer sun in the middle of the day twice or three times weekly should provide sufficient amounts of vitamin D. Elderly people, who are less efficient at synthesizing vitamin D, may need up to 30 minutes of sun exposure. *See also* CALCIF-EROL; CHOLECALCIFEROL; OSTEOMALACIA; OSTEOPOROSIS; RACHITIC; *and* RICKETS.

Vitamin E

Organic substance important in tissue maintenance, and especially against cell deterioration.

Vitamin E is a fat-soluble vitamin composed of a group of compounds known as tocopherols. The full extent of the vitamin's functions is not completely known. However, it is understood that it has antioxidant properties, protecting tissues and other substances, such as polyunsaturated fatty acids and vitamin A, from activated oxygen; and it is important to the formation and maintenance of muscles, cell membranes, and other tissues.

Individuals with malabsorption syndromes often develop deficiencies of vitamin E, as well as other fat-soluble vitamins. Newborn infants, particularly those that are premature, may suffer from severe anemia because of damaged red blood cells. Vitamin E supplementation can treat this potentially fatal form of anemia.

Good sources of vitamin E include dark green leafy vegetables, legumes, nuts and seeds, whole grains, enriched cereals, wheat germ, safflower and other vegetable oils, seafood, poultry, and eggs.

As is the case with all fat-soluble vitamins, the potential for vitamin E toxicity exists. Symptoms of overdose are rare, but may include excessive bleeding due to interference with vitamin K metabolism. *See also* ANEMIA; FATTY ACIDS; MALABSORPTION SYNDROMES; PREMATURITY; VITAMIN A; *and* VITAMIN C.

Vitamin K

Organic fat-soluble substance essential to normal blood clotting and bone nutrient processing (metabolism).

Vitamin K is normally synthesized by bacteria in the gastrointestinal tract. Therefore, deficiency of this vitamin is rare, although patients with malabsorption syndromes, certain types of kidney disease or cancer, and those who are taking antibiotics for a prolonged periodmay be at risk. Newborn infants may be in danger of vitamin K deficiency before bacterial flora is established in the intestines. For this reason, some hospitals give vitamin K injections to newborn infants following delivery. Symptoms of vitamin K deficiency include severe bleeding and liver damage. An overdose of the vitamin in infants can cause jaundice.

Dietary sources of vitamin K include leafy green vegetables; avocados; kiwis; soybeans; lentils; pistachios; whole grains and cereals; cabbage; cauliflower; potatoes; organ meats; and soybean, canola, and fish oils. *See also* ANTICOAGULANT DRUGS; JAUNDICE; MALABSORPTION; *and* WARFARIN.

Vitamin Supplements

Natural or artificial substances added to the diet in order to better fulfill nutritional needs.

Vitamin supplements have often been touted as safe and effective promoters of good health. Supplementation, however, should be undertaken with care—vitamins in supplement form should be viewed as medications, and regarded with the same level of caution as other medications. Supplements should not be taken in doses greater than 100 percent of the Recommended Daily Allowance unless prescribed by a physician.

Vitamins are classified into two types: water-soluble and fat-soluble. The fat-soluble vitamins, A, D, E, and K, are stored by the liver for months. Deficiency is therefore fairly rare, and excessive supplementation, particularly of vitamins A and D, can cause symptoms of toxicity. The water-soluble vitamins pose less of a risk of overdose, since excess amounts are excreted, but excesses may still result in side effects.

Vitamin supplements are appropriate for some people. Those who have food allergies, and therefore are on a limited diet, may not receive the same range of nutrients as those who are able to consume a variety of foods. Vegans, strict vegetarians who do not eat any animal products, may require a vitamin B_{12} supplement if they do not eat sufficient amounts of fortified foods such as soy milk. People who regularly consume excessive amounts of alcohol, which impairs the body's ability to absorb and metabolize certain vitamins, may benefit from supplements. Women of child bearing age may require folic acid. The bodies of older people are less efficient at absorbing the vitamins B_6, B_{12}, and D, thus, individuals over the age of 65 may require a supplement of these vitamins.

For background information on vitamin supplements, see NUTRITION *and* NUTRITIONAL DISORDERS. *Further reading material can be found in* AGING; DIET AND DISEASE; TOXICITY; VITAMIN A; VITAMIN B COMPLEX; VITAMIN D; VITAMIN E; *and* VITAMIN K. *See also* VEGETARIANISM.

Vitiligo

A skin condition that causes milky-white patches of skin to develop.

Vitiligo occurs most often on the face, lips, hands, arms, legs, and genitals, although it can occur anywhere on the body. There is a considerable amount of evidence that this is an autoimmune disease in which the immune system attacks the pigment-producing cells in the skin. The process involves the loss of melanocytes (the cells that produce skin color). The resulting white patches are sensitive to sunlight.

The amount of pigment lost varies from person to person. White patches develop on most light-skinned individuals only during the summer, while the patches appear year-round on dark-skinned individuals.

Treatment. There is no cure for vitiligo. However, the various methods that reduce the effect of vitiligo include covering small patches of skin with long-lasting dyes in combination with light-sensitive drugs and ultraviolet light A (UV-A) therapy. In general, these treatments restore pigment (repigmentation). In rare cases, the use of agents to eliminate remaining pigment (depigmentation) may be considered.

Children under the age of 12 are usually not treated. It is recommended that affected children stay covered and use sunscreen when outdoors. *See also* ADDISON'S DISEASE *and* DIABETES.

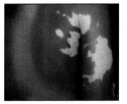

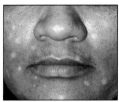

Vitiligo.
Vitiligo is a condition marked by patches of white skin on different areas of the body, such as an arm (above, top) or the face (above, bottom). It is an immune system disorder.

Vocal Cords

Two sheets of fibrous tissue located in the larynx (voice box) and responsible for voice production.

For the majority of the time, the vocal cords lie apart in the shape of a "V," allowing air to get to the lungs. Sounds are produced when the cords close and vibrate as air from the lungs is expelled between them. Slight differences in the tension of the vocal cords produce different pitches of sound, which are then modulated by the tongue, palate, and lips into speech. *See also* LARYNX *and* SPEECH DISORDERS.

Voice, Loss of

Also known as dysphonia

Inability to create sound with the vocal cords.

Loss of voice, or dysphonia, is usually a temporary condition. The most common cause is straining of the muscles in the voice box (larynx), which are then unable to operate the vocal cords. Viral or bacterial infections that cause inflammation in the throat can also affect the vocal cords. Benign growths on the vocal cords, known as polyps, can also cause loss of voice, as can injury to the vocal cords or nerves.

Loss of voice can also be an indication of a more serious condition. An underactive thyroid gland can cause the vocal cords to thicken, leading to a husky voice, which can progress to an inability to speak. In addition, loss of voice can be an indicator of cancer of the larynx, thyroid, or esophagus. *See also* APHONIA; DYSPHONIA; ESOPHAGUS; HYPOTHYROIDISM; LARYNX; *and* THYROID.

Volkmann's Contracture

Condition in which the fingers and wrist become fixed in a bent position.

The most common cause of a Volkmann's contracture is ischemia (a reduction in the blood supply to the muscles) of the forearm. This may be brought on by an injury to the brachial artery, usually from a fractured humerus or a dislocation of the elbow. Edema (fluid retention) may also cause swelling that constricts the blood vessels, hindering bloodflow.

Symptoms. Volkmann's contracture sets in quickly. The fingers become cold and numb, and movement is difficult and painful. Within a few hours, the fingers and wrist become fixed in a bent position.

Treatment. If a misplaced bone is affecting the blood supply, a physician will move the bone back into the correct position. Tissue may also be cut to reduce pressure. In extreme cases, a graft from another vein may replace the damaged artery. *See also* CONTRACTURE *and* WRISTDROP.

Volvulus

The twisting of a loop of the intestine that causes an obstruction.

When the intestine twists into a loop, intestinal strangulation may occur, resulting in obstruction of the blood supply.

Symptoms. Patients with volvulus may experience abdominal cramps and pain, distention, bloating, and sometimes vomiting. A fever may result if the intestinal wall is perforated. Some people may experience shock due to dehydration, bowel ischemia, or peritonitis.

Complications. Intestinal strangulation occurs in approximately 25 percent of cases of volvulus. Gangrene can develop within six hours, and can lead to perforation, peritonitis, and further infection.

Treatment. Surgery, including various decompression techniques, is usually performed as soon as possible to alleviate volvulus. *See also* ISCHEMIA *and* PERITONITIS.

Vomiting

The forceful ejection of the contents of the stomach through the esophagus and out of the mouth.

Nausea and vomiting are common symptoms of a variety of diseases and conditions affecting the gastrointestinal system. They may also be accompanied by diarrhea.

CAUSES
Some of the many possible causes of vomiting include alcoholism, bulimia, chemotherapy, food poisoning, food allergies, gastritis, intestinal obstruction, migraine headaches, morning sickness, certain medications, motion sickness, unpleasant smells, and viral infections.

In infants less than six months of age, vomiting may be caused by congenital pyloric stenosis (a narrowing in the lower portion of the stomach). Vomiting may also occur from a disturbed equilibrium when the baby is bounced immediately after feeding. Projectile vomiting should not be confused with regurgitation or "spit-

ting up," which is commonly seen in many infants and is not cause for concern.

Induced vomiting is seen in individuals with eating disorders, such as bulimia. As part of the "binge and purge" cycle, individuals, usually young girls, force themselves to vomit after eating. The frequency of the vomiting increases over time. Severe complications may result from bulimia, including malnutrition, dehydration, major systemic organ failure, and even death.

COMPLICATIONS
Dehydration is the biggest concern in most vomiting episodes. The rate with which dehydration takes place depends on the size of the person, the frequency of the vomiting, and if diarrhea is also present. Infants with frequent vomiting and diarrhea are at the greatest risk for dehydration and need immediate medical attention. Signs of dehydration include increased thirst, infrequent urination or dark yellow urine, dry mouth, eyes that appear sunken, and skin that has lost its normal elasticity.

DIAGNOSIS
The cause of vomiting may be diagnosed with various tests. Blood tests, such as the CBC or blood differential; urinalysis; and x-rays of the abdomen may all be necessary.

TREATMENT
If the underlying condition causing the vomiting is diagnosed, it will be treated. A person experiencing prolonged or copious vomiting is in serious danger of becoming dehydrated. It is important to take in as much fluid as possible without upsetting the stomach any further. Clear fluids should be ingested slowly over time. A normal diet should be resumed gradually if it can be tolerated. In severe cases, antiemetic drugs can be administered to prevent nausea and vomiting.

Background information on vomiting can be found in DIGESTIVE SYSTEM *and* GASTROINTESTINAL TRACT. *For related material, see* ALCOHOL DEPENDENCE; BULIMIA; CHEMOTHERAPY; DEHYDRATION; DIARRHEA; GASTRITIS; HEADACHE; MORNING SICKNESS; NAUSEA; *and* PYLORIC STENOSIS.

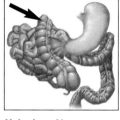

Volvulus. Above, volvulus is a twisting of the intestine into a loop. Volvulus is one cause of intestinal obstruction, and it may also cause intestinal strangulation.

Vomiting Blood

Also known as hematemesis

The regurgitation of blood from the stomach or esophagus.

Causes. Prolonged or vigorous vomiting may cause a tear in the small blood vessels of the throat or esophagus, producing streaks of blood in the vomit. This is related to Mallory-Weiss syndrome, which is a laceration or tear of the lower esophagus and the upper part of the stomach. The amount of blood present in the vomit depends on the extent of the damage.

Bleeding ulcers located in the stomach or duodenum are also a source of vomited blood, as are certain types of esophageal irritation or the erosion of the lining of the esophagus or stomach.

Other sources of blood in the vomit include bleeding esophageal varices; ingested blood, for example, blood swallowed after a nosebleed; severe gastritis or gastroenteritis; severe injury or electrical shock; tumors of the stomach or esophagus; and vascular malformations in the gastrointestinal tract.

Treatment. Treatments for vomiting blood vary, because they depend upon the specific cause. In general, it is a good idea to drink small amounts of water regularly to prevent dehydration. It is very important to seek medical help. *See also* GASTROENTERITIS; *and* MALLORY-WEISS SYNDROME.

Vomiting in Pregnancy

Pregnant women most commonly experience short waves of nausea a few mornings a week. This nausea, which is not limited to the morning, is generally worse among those who have sensitive digestive systems. Upset stomach is believed to be related to the hormones estrogen and human chorionic gonadotropin (hCG), which are elevated in early pregnancy. The nausea and vomiting is usually a temporary condition and disappears by the fourth month.

Prevention and Treatment. There are currently no antiemetic (antinausea) drugs that are approved for use during pregnancy. However, the condition can be alleviated by keeping meals small and simple, and by avoiding fried or greasy food. Lying down for a short time after meals may also be beneficial. By the time a woman discovers the remedy that works best for her, the period of morning sickness is usually over.

Severe nausea and vomiting, defined as vomiting several times within an hour, can be an indication of a serious problem, and a doctor should be notified as soon as possible. Excessive vomiting, known as hyperemsesis gravidarum, can result in severe dehydration and malnutrition, and may warrant hospitalization. *See also* PREGNANCY *and* VOMITING.

Von Willebrand's Disease

A chronic bleeding condition caused by an abnormality of one of the blood's clotting factors.

Healthy clotting following injury or surgery involves a complex sequence of events to properly stop bleeding and promote healing. More than a dozen factors in the blood that perform important functions in this sequence have been identified. The von Willebrand factor and factor VIII work together to stimulate platelets to clot. If the von Willebrand factor is defective or absent, the bleeding is not controlled as quickly as it should be. Von Willebrand's disease is usually an inherited deficiency.

Symptoms. Easy bruising, nosebleeds, heavy menstrual bleeding, and bleeding in the digestive system are symptoms of von Willebrand's disease.

Treatment. People who suffer from this disease must treat any bleeding as serious. Aspirin or other blood thinners should not be taken. A doctor should be informed of the condition before the patient undergoes surgery. Transfusion of platelets and plasma containing the necessary clotting factors may be necessary if the condition is serious. Usually, however, the condition is mild, and appropriate treatment can prevent major complications. *See also* BLEEDING DISORDERS *and* BLOOD CLOTTING.

Vulva, Cancer of

Malignant tumor of the external female genitalia.

Cancer of the vulva is uncommon. It almost always occurs in women over the age of 50, and its incidence increases with age. Factors that increase the risk of vulvar cancer include a history of cervical cancer, having multiple sex partners, and a history of sexually transmitted diseases, such as syphilis, herpes simplex, and the human papilloma virus. Periodic self-examination to detect the early signs of vulvar cancer is recommended for women with these risk factors. Most cancers of the vulva are squamous cell carcinomas, which can arise in the labia, the lips of the vulva, or the clitoris. There are rare cases of melanoma, adenocarcinoma, and other forms of cancer.

Symptoms. Symptoms of vulvar cancer include a visible lump; a change in color or appearance of the vulva; bleeding that is not menstrual; and itching, burning, or pain. These symptoms usually appear months before the cancer is diagnosed.

Diagnosis. Diagnostic tests for cancer of the vulva include inspection of a tissue sample to determine if a tumor is malignant and visual examination by cystoscopy, sigmoidoscopy, or another means.

Treatment. The basic treatment for cancer of the vulva is surgery, the extent of which varies depending on the stage at which the cancer is diagnosed. For early-stage cancers, the tumor and some surrounding tissue may be removed. For advanced cancers, surgery to remove the entire vulva, or the vulva and other pelvic organs, such as the uterus and ovaries, may be necessary. Chemotherapy or radiation therapy may follow surgery. The prognosis depends on the stage at which the cancer is diagnosed. The five-year survival rate for cancer of the vulva detected at the earliest stage is nearly 100 percent.

> *For background reading on cancer of the vulva, see* CANCER *and* REPRODUCTIVE SYSTEM, FEMALE. *Related material can be found in* CERVIX, CANCER OF THE; CLITORIS; CYSTOSCOPY; SIGMOIDOSCOPY; *and* SQUAMOUS CELL CARCINOMA.

Vulvitis

An inflammation of the external part of the female genitals (the vulva).

Inflammation of the vulva may be caused by bacterial, viral, or fungal infection; radiation; drugs; changes in hormones; or irritation from chemicals.

Symptoms. Symptoms of vulvitis include redness of the skin, burning or itching, small cracks in the skin, and an abnormal vaginal discharge.

Treatment. Vulvitis is first treated by removing any potential irritants. Topical corticosteroids may reduce the inflammation associated with the condition. If there is a bacterial, fungal, or viral infection, a physician will prescribe antibiotics, antifungal medications, or antiviral medications.

Prevention. Vulvitis can be prevented by avoiding tight clothes that rub against the skin or restrict air circulation. To avoid a recurrence, patients should promptly change out of damp exercise clothing. The use of feminine hygiene sprays, fragrances, or powders should be avoided. Daily cleansing of the area with a mild soap and thorough drying of the area is also an excellent way to prevent vulvitis. *See also* SEXUALLY TRANSMITTED DISEASES *and* VULVOVAGINITIS.

Vulvovaginitis

An inflammation of the vulva and vaginal areas.

Vulvovaginitis can be caused by bacterial, viral, or fungal infection, or it can be an allergic reaction to chemical substances, such as soaps or perfumes. The condition is often reported in young girls, whose vaginal secretions are less acidic than they are after puberty. Tight clothing can also produce irritation in the genital area.

Treatment. To treat vulvovaginitis, the irritating factor should be removed from the area. If a sexually transmitted disease is involved, antibiotic, antifungal, or antiviral medications are prescribed as required. A corticosteroid cream may control itching. *See also* ANTIBIOTIC DRUGS *and* VULVITIS.

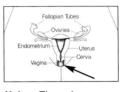

Vulva. The vulva (marked with an arrow above) is the external part of the female genitalia. Conditions affecting the vulva may include cancer, infection, and inflammation.

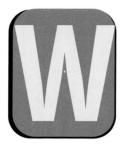

Walking

Movement in one direction, as propelled by the legs and feet.

The impulse to walk is relayed from the basal ganglia and the cerebellum (located at the back of the brain) to the spinal cord, which then sends the signal to the muscles. As the body's position changes, the brain constantly gathers information from other parts of the body, such as the eye, the inner-ear, and the surrounding muscles and joints. A new set of signals are then sent to these areas to ensure smooth movement and coordination.

Most babies begin to walk by the age of 15 months. If a child is not walking by 18 months, this may be evidence of a muscular or neurological disorder.

WALKING DISORDERS

The normal walking pattern (gait) can be disrupted by a variety of disorders.

Muscular dysfunction occurs when the muscles in the legs and feet are injured or diseased. Muscular dystrophy is one example of a disease that causes muscular dysfunction; poliomyelitis (polio) is another. In mild cases, polio may cause weakness in the muscles, and thus an imbalance in gait. Severe cases of polio can lead to paralysis.

Skeletal deformities, such as clubfoot or a congenital dislocation of the hip, can lead to an abnormal gait. Bowed legs that have not been corrected in childhood can also cause walking problems.

Neurological disorders are those in which the brain has been damaged, impairing its ability to send or understand nerve impulses. A stroke can cause paralysis on one side of the body. Parkinson's disease may lead to a lack of muscle control. Other neurological disorders, such as myelitis, neuritis, or multiple sclerosis, affect the gait by damaging the spinal cord.

Background information on walking can be found in CENTRAL NERVOUS SYSTEM *and* MOVEMENT. *For further reading, see* BASAL GANGLIA; CEREBELLUM; MULTIPLE SCLEROSIS; MUSCULAR DYSTROPHY; NEURITIS; *and* POLIOMYELITIS.

Scissors Gait

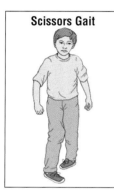

Spastic Gait

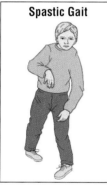

Walking Disorders. There are many disorders that affect the ability to walk. Above, top, in a scissors gait, the legs cross over each other. Above, bottom, in a spastic gait, the toes usually drag on the ground. Both of these disorders are usually caused by neurological problems.

Walking Aids

Any device that helps a person walk, either permanently or temporarily.

Individuals recovering from fractures or sprains, or suffering from the effects of a stroke, arthritis, or polio, may need a walking aid to help them regain mobility.

Walkers are an excellent way to provide support for people who are suffering from muscle weakness, pain, and stiffness. Walkers can also help patients whose balance is impaired because of injury or disease. Walkers are usually made of light-weight metal and have rubber-tipped legs. The main drawback of walkers is that they only allow for slow movement.

Crutches are best suited for injuries in which a person has to avoid putting weight on one leg. The other leg may still have strength and mobility, and the upper body needs to be strong in order to use crutches.

Full-length crutches extend to the ground from underneath the arms. The weight of the body is supported by the hands. They are appropriate for people suffering from bone fractures, or sprains of muscles, joints, ligaments, or tendons.

Elbow crutches only reach to the elbow. The arms slide into a cuff, and the hands rest on bars that extend below. This allows the elbows to support the weight of the body. These are particularly good for those recovering from strokes, as it allows for a more natural movement than a walker. Elbow crutches can be difficult for those who suffer from arthritis in the upper body because of the additional stress placed on the joints.

Canes are best for people who have stiffness or weakness only on one side. A cane may be the last walking aid needed by someone recovering from injury; rehabilitation is often started with crutches, but once the leg or foot can bear some weight, a cane may be recommended. Canes are usually made of wood, with handles that are designed to accommodate different kinds of grips. *See also* PHYSICAL THERAPY *and* WALKING.

Warfarin

One of a number of anticoagulant drugs used to reduce or dissolve blood clots.

Warfarin acts by interfering with the action of vitamin K, a critical step in the clotting process. Unlike heparin, another anticoagulant drug, warfarin is administered by pills rather than injection. It is often used in conjunction with heparin.

The problem with all anticoagulant drugs is that, in addition to dissolving clots or controlling clot formation, they allow for easy bleeding. The physician must carefully monitor the dosage to maintain a delicate balance between protection against thrombosis (blood clots) and protection against uncontrolled bleeding. *See also* ANTICOAGULANT DRUGS; BLOOD CLOTTING; HEPARIN; *and* THROMBOSIS.

Wart

A benign skin growth caused by a virus.

Warts are caused by an infectious viruses and may occur anywhere on the body, but are most commonly seen on the hands, feet, and face. Warts are named by their location and appearance. Warts on the soles of the feet are called plantar warts. Warts that are located around and under the fingernails are called periungual and subungual warts, respectively. Warts on the hands, arms, legs, and other body areas are called verrucae vulgaris or common warts.

A wart is usually a rough, round, or oval protruding lump on the surface of the skin, and it may be lighter or darker than the surrounding skin. Since plantar warts are on the sole of the foot, they can be painful due to pressure. Periungual and subungual warts are much more difficult to cure than common warts because of their location.

Treatment is not always necessary, but is often desired by the patient. Over-the-counter medications, which contain salicylic and lactic acid, can be effective in treating warts if applied every day for several weeks. Prescription medicines may be necessary for stubborn warts. Removal by freezing (cryotherapy), burning (electrocautery), or laser treatment may also be necessary in rare cases. Even with treatment, warts recur 25 percent of the time. *See also* PLANTAR WART.

Warts, Genital

A relatively common symptom of sexually transmitted disease.

Genital warts appear in warm, moist areas, such as the vulva, vagina, cervix, penis, or rectum. The presence of genital warts may also be an indication of an impaired immune system.

Cause. Genital warts are caused by human papilloma viruses. The viruses may also be responsible for cancers of the vagina, vulva, anus, penis, mouth, throat, and esophagus.

Symptoms. The warts appear one to six months after infection. They begin as tiny, soft, moist, pink or red swellings that grow rapidly and develop stalks. Multiple warts may appear in the same area, with rough surfaces that give them a cauliflower-like appearance. In pregnant women or those with an impaired immune system, the warts grow very rapidly.

Any unusual warts or sores in the genital region should be examined by a medical practitioner. A woman who has cervical warts should undergo regular pap tests to detect any early signs of cervical cancer.

Treatment. External warts can be removed by laser, freezing (cryotherapy), or conventional surgery. Chemical treatments, applied directly to the warts, may also be effective, although this method requires repeat applications and can harm the surrounding skin.

Prognosis. Genital warts tend to recur and require repeated treatment.

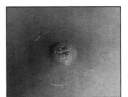
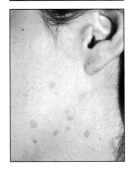

Warts.
Warts are harmless skin growths that are caused by a viral infection. They may appear anywhere on the body, but are most often seen on the hands (above, top), feet, and face (above, bottom).

> *For background reading on genital warts, see* INFECTIOUS DISEASE *and* SEXUALLY TRANSMITTED DISEASE. *Related material can be found in* CANCER; CERVIX; PAPILLOMA, INTRODUCTAL; PENIS; RECTUM; *and* VAGINA. *See also* CRYOTHERAPY; LASER TREATMENT; *and* SURGERY *for more on treatment.*

Water

Essential and often overlooked element that is crucial to good health.

All of the body's systems require water to function. In fact, water makes up about two-thirds of the human body. Water is instrumental in regulating body temperature, removing wastes and toxins, cushioning joints, transporting oxygen and nutrients to the cells, and dissolving nutrients so that they can be utilized.

The consumption of sufficient amounts of water helps to prevent constipation. One study has shown that women who drank five or more glasses of water daily reduced their risk of colon cancer by 45 percent compared to those who drank fewer than two glasses daily.

Recommended water consumption is often given as eight glasses a day, but each individual is likely to have a personal requirement of water intake. The requirement is greater in heat, high altitudes, and when undertaking any activity that causes perspiration. Older people should drink regularly, even when not thirsty.

Beverages containing alcohol or caffeine are dehydrating, so it is important to drink more water to compensate if these beverages are consumed regularly. *See also* CAFFEINE; DEHYDRATION; PERSPIRATION; REHYDRATION THERAPY; *and* WATER SAFETY.

Waterborne Infection

Any infection transmitted through water.

Bacterial, viral, and parasitic infections can spread through contaminated water. The pathogenic (disease-causing) organisms are present in excretory products that are discharged into the water.

City water supplies in the United States are always in danger of contamination, despite vigilant testing and purifying. Oceans and lakes used by swimmers are often dumps for chemicals or sewage and carry a host of disease-causing organisms. The water supply is even more dangerous in developing countries, as the water may carry strains of bacteria to which the traveler has no immunity.

There are many examples of infectious outbreaks that have occurred as a result of contaminated water. In 1993, the Milwaukee water supply was contaminated with the intestinal parasite *Cryptosporidium parvum*, causing an epidemic of diarrhea, nausea, fever, and abdominal cramping in over 400,000 people. For many years bottled fruit drinks were considered safe, but in 1996, several children became ill from drinking unpasteurized apple juice contaminated with *Escherichia coli* bacteria. The United States government now requires juice producers to label unpasteurized juices. *See also* BACTERIA.

Waterhouse-Friderichsen Syndrome

Infection of bacterial meningitis that moves to the adrenal glands.

Meningitis is inflammation of the covering of the spinal cord that is caused by a bacterial infection, usually with meningococci bacteria. Waterhouse-Friderichsen syndrome develops when the progress of the infection is very rapid, leading to diarrhea, vomiting, seizure, internal bleeding, shock, and even death.

Antibiotic and corticosteroid drugs are prescribed immediately to patients suffering from Waterhouse-Friderichsen syndrome to kill the bacteria and to control inflammation. *See also* MENINGITIS.

Watering Eye

Excessive tear production by the eye.

Tears, the watery, salty secretion of the lacrimal apparatus, are usually produced to keep the cornea moist, to wash away irritation, or for psychological reasons. Watering eyes is an overflow of tears, caused by corneal irritation, sadness, or a blockage of the ducts that drain the tears. *See also* EYE; LACRIMAL APPARATUS; *and* TEARS.

Water Intoxication

Excess water in the brain, which causes neurological problems.

The underlying cause of water intoxication is excessively low levels of sodium ions in the blood (hyponatremia). A number of disorders can disrupt the normal balance of blood sodium, resulting in the retention of excess water in all body tissues, including the brain. Kidney failure, cirrhosis of the liver, heart failure, and conditions affecting the adrenal glands may result in water intoxication. Surgery can increase the risk of water intoxication, as the stress it causes can stimulate excess absorption of water by the kidneys. Water intoxication can also occur in childbirth, when the hormone oxytocin is given to induce labor.

Symptoms. The major symptoms of water intoxication include lethargy, dizziness, headache, confusion, and nausea. Severe water intoxication can cause seizures, loss of consciousness, and death.

Treatment. Treatment of water intoxication is aimed at restoring the normal balance of sodium in the blood. *See also* CIRRHOSIS; OXYTOCIN; *and* TUMORS.

Water-on-the-Knee

Fluid accumulation around the knee joint.

Water-on-the-knee is a general term that is applied to conditions in which there is swelling, pain, and lack of mobility of the knee due to a build-up of fluid. Causes of these symptoms may include osteoarthritis, inflammation from rheumatoid arthritis, swelling as a result of a cartilage injury, or infection. The most typical cause, however, is bursitis, an inflammation of the bursa sacs located at the knee joint.

Ice, elevation of the leg, and antiinflammatory drugs can bring down swelling of the knee. Strengthening the rest of the leg can reduce the chance of recurrence by taking some of the burden off the knee joint. *See also* BURSITIS; EFFUSION, JOINT; OSTEOARTHRITIS; *and* RHEUMATOID ARTHRITIS.

Water Safety

Practices that reduce the possibility of accident or illness related to water.

Water safety practices are the various lifesaving skills that can prevent drownings or water-related disease. These skills are important to learn to reduce the possibility of water-related injury or illness.

Drownings. Liquid in the airways disrupts the breathing process. Without air sufficiently passing into the lungs, the brain and body become starved of oxygen. Victims of drowning can suffer unconsciousness, brain damage, and death.

After motor vehicle accidents and falls, drownings are the third leading cause of fatal accidents. A small number of drownings occur to practitioners of extreme water sports such as scuba and skin diving, surfing, and water skiing. These cases are often related to poor equipment maintenance or judgment, or disabling physical trauma. Two-thirds of drowning victims are nonswimmers who fall from docks, pool sides, or boats.

Many drownings could be prevented with the implementation of basic skills of life saving, first aid, and vehicle and equipment handling. Organizations like the American Red Cross, the YMCA and YWCA, and the U.S. Coast Guard Auxiliary provide courses in life-saving techniques.

Lifesaving. Lifesaving refers to the various methods of rescuing potential drowning victims. In general, aid can be given from land, by boat, or in water.

Reaching the victim from land is the safest and simplest form of rescue. The rescuer can extend an arm or leg to a person in need of help. In cases where a person is just beyond reach, an article of clothing, pole, or board can be used to pull someone to shore. Even when someone is out of the reach of these attempts, ropes and ringbouys can be thrown within the grasp of the victim, who can then be drawn to safety.

Rescue by boat involves putting a portion of the boat within the reach of the victim. Sometimes it is easier to do this if there

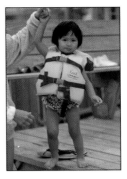

Water Safety.
Water safety practices reduce the chance of drownings or other water-related accidents. Above, a life jacket is worn to keep a person afloat if the person cannot swim or is fatigued.

are two people in the boat—one to navigate and one to keep sight of the victim or the place where the victim was last seen. As in land rescues, extending a limb or object is a means of drawing the person in. Since a small boat can be capsized if a sudden and large weight is sustained on one of its sides, the rear and front are the preferred areas from which to perform a boat rescue.

Water rescues should only be made by persons trained in lifesaving. This is because of the high risk of the rescuer becoming a potential victim of drowning. Lifesaving skills emphasize approaching victims from various angles and being prepared to be seized by panicking persons. A variety of methods are used to retrieve submerged persons, tow these individuals to shore, and administer artificial respiration.

Water Pollution. The majority of Americans receive their water from large municipal water agencies, which are regulated by the Environmental Protection Agency and are monitored and tested on a regular basis. This water undergoes a variety of treatment procedures to remove potentially dangerous contaminants, such as heavy metals, chemical pollutants, and microorganisms. While treatment measures do kill or remove the majority of contaminants, some may remain and multiply to unacceptable levels if water treatment facilities malfunction.

Most groundwater is tapped by private wells in rural areas. Even though surface water may be easily polluted by dumped or leaking industrial waste, runoff from fertilizers or pesticides, motor vehicle leakage, and acid rain and storm runoff, chemicals often seep into groundwater in concentrations that can be hundreds of times higher than those found in surface water.

Unexplained diarrhea and nausea in healthy adults can be the result of contaminated water. Such contaminations usually pose a far greater risk to those with compromised immune systems, the very young, and the very old.

Lead may enter the water supply between the treatment center and the faucet. Regardless of the source of drinking water,

it is a good idea to test the water for lead if there are children under the age of six in the home, if a member of the household is pregnant, if the house is either newly built or was built more than thirty years ago, or if lead solder has been used in the pipes.

Unhealthily high levels of nitrates can leak into the water supply from sewage, fertilizers, and feedlots, and can also occur naturally in the soil. Nitrates can cause methemoglobinemia, or "blue baby syndrome," in infants younger than six months. Methemoglobinemia can also occasionally affect pregnant women and other adults.

Waterborne Infection. Contaminated drinking water can cause viral, bacterial, and parasitic infection. In developed countries, the risk of waterborne infection is minimal because of extensive water filtration and sewage management processes. Tap water from public supply, bottled water, and spring water in these countries are generally safe for drinking. In developing countries, these sources can be suspect, especially if the water has an unpleasant appearance or odor, or is from rivers, lakes, and canals. It should be noted that swimming in contaminated water or the eating of fish or shellfish from such areas can also result in infection.

In areas of potentially contaminated water, using bottled water of well-known brand names for all drinking and food preparation is the best way to prevent water-related illnesses. Though rainwater may be a source of other pollutants, it is not a source of infective organisms as long as it is not left to stand for long periods of time.

In addition, there are several commercial systems for filtering and chemical sterilization of water. Boiling water is always a reliable way to sterilize water that is suspected to contain infective organisms.

Background material on water safety can be found in INFECTIOUS DISEASE; POLLUTION; and WATER. For further reading, see AIR; BLUE BABY; BRAIN DISORDERS; COMA; DIARRHEA; DROWNING; NAUSEA; SCUBA-DIVING MEDICINE; and WATERBORNE INFECTION. See also AGING for more on populations at higher risk for the effects of water pollution.

Wax Bath

A soothing heat therapy used by rheumatoid arthritis sufferers for relief from chronic joint pain and inflammation.

A paraffin wax bath is a method of treatment in which hot liquid wax is brushed on painful joints or muscles to provide relief. Paraffin wax heat soothes the pain and stiffness of arthritis, as well as sports injuries, muscle spasms, and muscle stiffness. The affected body parts are dipped into the bath for approximately 15 minutes. Paraffin wax therapy penetrates deeply. The treatment is effective, because heat is administered directly to the affected area. *See also* RHEUMATOID ARTHRITIS.

Weakness

A reduction in strength or tone of the muscles.

Weakness is an important symptom that can be either subjective or objective, localized or general. Weakness often follows a stroke or trauma to a motor nerve root or peripheral nerve. Muscle weakness can be accompanied by changes in spasticity, tone, and muscle reflexes.

Causes. Measurable weakness may result from a variety of conditions. These conditions include cerebellar degeneration, disorders in nerve transmission (such as myasthenia gravis), neurologic disorders (such as stroke, multiple sclerosis, or cerebral palsy), muscular diseases, and metabolic disorders (such as diabetes). *See also* CEREBRAL PALSY; DIABETES; MULTIPLE SCLEROSIS; MYASTHENIA GRAVIS; *and* STROKE.

Webbing

A congenital (present at birth) condition in which there is a flap of skin located between adjacent fingers or toes.

Webbing is a common congenital (present at birth) abnormality that may affect two or more fingers or toes. It is often inherited, appearing in more than one generation of the same family.

Mild cases of webbing are harmless and only affect the appearance of the hands or feet. The digits may be surgically corrected for cosmetic reasons if the patient desires. More severe cases of webbing may be accompanied by complete fusion of the affected fingers or toes, called syndactyly. Syndactyly of the hands usually causes problems with movement, and the fingers are surgically separated. Syndactyly of the toes does not affect movement, although separation may be performed for cosmetic reasons. *See also* GENETICS *and* SYNDACTYLY.

Wegener's Granulomatosis

Inflammation of blood vessels of the sinuses, lungs, and kidneys.

Wegener's granulomatosis is a rare form of vasculitis, an inflammatory process that attacks blood vessels. The condition most often occurs in patients 40 years of age and older. It is believed to be an autoimmune disease, in which the body's defense system against infection attacks its own tissue. Wegener's granulomatosis gets its name from the presence of nodules of abnormal cells (granulomas) in the affected areas.

Symptoms. The first signs of the condition are chronic sinusitis, nasal crusting, nosebleeds, a chronic cough, coughing up blood, chest pain while breathing, and breathlessness. Many patients also have arthritis and fever.

Diagnosis. Diagnosis is made by blood tests to detect the presence of abnormal antibodies, and by performing a chest x-ray or computed tomography (CT) scan. A lung biopsy may also be needed.

Treatment. Treatment with cyclophosphamide, an anticancer drug, and with immunosuppressant drugs can usually control Wegener's granulomatosis, although the condition may recur. Without treatment, serious complications, such as perforation of the nasal septum, skin rash or ulceration, or heart damage, can also occur. *See also* AUTOIMMUNE DISORDERS *and* GRANULOMA.

Weight

The measurable heaviness of a person or object.

Weight plays many roles in human development. When a person reaches his or her full height, weight should stabilize. However, cultural and lifestyle influences can disturb this balance, and many people gain and lose weight throughout their lives.

Weight and Growth. When a baby is born, weight is the most important indicator of health. As a child grows, weight increases proportionately. The body must take in enough fuel during these years to support not only normal activity, but the energy required for the body to grow. If a child is underweight or overweight, this may be an indication of poor nutrition, inadequate exercise, or illness.

By adulthood, the body only needs enough calories to perform everyday tasks. If the amount of fuel, or calories from food, equals the amount of energy expended, the weight remains stable. If this balance is disturbed, however, either in the amount of calories taken in or energy output, the result is weight gain or loss.

Normal Body Weight. The brain regulates eating patterns through the hypothalamus and pituitary gland. These areas control feelings of hunger by interpreting information from chemicals that indicate the amount of sugar and fat stores in the body. If these signals are obeyed, a person eats the correct amount; ignoring them can result in eating too much or too little.

Another part of the brain that affects a person's weight is the adipostat, which maintains a set body weight. The brain regulates its output of energy to maintain fat stores at a level set by the adipostat. Sometimes the adipostat may set an unhealthy weight, perhaps based on childhood needs or steady weight gain during adulthood. In this case, weight loss can be extremely difficult, as dieting can be undermined as the body works against all efforts to lose weight. Long periods of consistent healthy eating and exercise can, however, cause the adipostat to reset at a more desirable weight.

Weight Measurement. There are a variety of ways to check if a person is of a healthy weight. Certain charts corroborate heights with general weight ranges. A more precise indicator of health is to calculate the body's fat percentage. The amount of fat a person has compared to the amount of muscle is important. Muscles are responsible for movement, and they help to support and protect bones and joints. The less muscle a person has, the more difficult these functions become. However, muscle weighs more than fat; therefore, in a case of two people who are the same height, but of different weights, the larger individual may actually weigh less. *See also* NUTRITION; WEIGHT LOSS; *and* WEIGHT REDUCTION.

Weight Loss

Loss of body mass.

Loss of body weight without a voluntary decrease in food or increase in activity may indicate disease.

Causes. Unintentional weight loss can be caused by diseases that either affect the appetite or cause metabolic disorders.

Loss of Appetite. Appetite may be lost due to diseases that make eating painful or cause a lack of interest in eating. Peptic ulcers can cause a person to avoid food rather than endure the pain associated with eating. Kidney disorders can raise the level of urea in the blood, resulting in loss of appetite. Gastroenteritis can lead to vomiting and a loss of appetite. Depression may also cause a loss of appetite; 0anorexia nervosa, an eating disorder, can cause a person to willfully stop eating.

Metabolic Disorders. Metabolism may be affected by some diseases, leading to an increase in expenditure of calories. Hyperthyroidism, in which the thyroid becomes overactive, increases metabolism, as does the autoimmune disorder Graves' disease. When diabetes mellitus is left untreated, weight loss may occur due to an increase in fluid loss from excessive urination.

Many types of cancers, especially cancer of the esophagus or stomach, can cause weight loss. Radiation treatment and chemotherapy for cancer can also cause vomiting or loss of appetite.

Treatment. Any kind of unexplained weight loss should be taken seriously, and a physician should be consulted. The physician will be able to diagnose and treat the disorder accordingly. *See also* APPETITE; DIABETES; GASTROENTERITIS; GRAVES' DISEASE; HYPERTHYROIDISM; METABOLISM; WEIGHT; *and* WEIGHT REDUCTION.

Weight Reduction

Purposeful weight loss in order to improve health or appearance.

Maintaining a healthy weight can play an important part in preventing diabetes, hypertension, and heart disease. Healthful weight loss should occur slowly from a combination of diet and exercise. Excess fat and sugar should be eliminated from the diet and replaced with a balance of fruits, vegetables, whole grains, lean meats, and fish. Exercise plays a crucial part in losing weight and maintaining weight loss, as it can help to speed up metabolism.

Fad diets are never a long-term solution to a weight problem. A physician, nutritionist, or fitness professional can help an overweight individual find the program that will be most successful. *See also* EXERCISE; NUTRITION; *and* WEIGHT.

Werdnig-Hoffman Disease

Also known as spinal muscular atrophy or SMA

A group of inherited diseases that cause progressive muscle weakness and degeneration.

Werdnig-Hoffman disease, or SMA, is the second leading cause of neuromuscular disease (the first is Duchenne muscular dystrophy). Spinal muscular atrophy is an inherited disease.

Incidence. The tendency to develop SMA is an inherited recessive trait. About three or four out of every 100,000 people develop the disease. A family history of SMA increases the likelihood of being born with the illness.

Types. There are three types of the disease. SMA I, the most serious form of the illness, causes infants to be born floppy and weak, with thin muscles and feeding and breathing problems. Infants with SMA II are born with less severe symptoms, but they become weaker with time. The least severe form of the disease, SMA III, may not be diagnosed until the affected child is two years old. Progressive weakness is usually the first symptom, and the child may survive into young adulthood.

Treatment. There is no treatment for SMA. Physiotherapy is usually necessary to prevent contractures and scoliosis in affected children. *See also* CONTRACTURE; MUSCULAR DYSTROPHY; *and* SCOLIOSIS.

Wernicke-Korsakoff Syndrome

A brain disease resembling amnesia that develops in individuals who do not meet the daily nutritional requirements for thiamine.

Wernicke-Korsakoff syndrome is marked by an intense state of confusion and a prolonged period of amnesia. It is caused by a brain dysfunction that results from thiamine deficiency.

Causes and Symptoms. Wernicke-Korsakoff syndrome often appears in alcoholics. It has also been found in malnourished individuals and in AIDS patients. The syndrome can result when excess fluid is administered intravenously to poorly nourished individuals. Affected individuals may stagger, develop visual problems, experience memory loss, and develop a loss of sensation or a feeling of "pins and needles" (neuropathy).

Treatment. If left untreated, Wernicke-Korsakoff syndrome can cause permanent memory loss, coma, or even death. Thiamine reserves may need to be replenished at a rate of up to 100 times the recommended daily allowance. Since this dosage is so high, the patient should be monitored closely. *See also* AMNESIA *and* NEUROPATHY.

Resources on Weight Loss

Groff, James L. and Sareen S. Gropper, *Advanced Nutrition and Human Metabolism* (1999); Heimburger, Douglas C. and R. L. Weinsier, *Handbook of Clinical Nutrition* (1997); Vliet, Elizabeth Lee, *Women, Weight and Hormones* (2001); Wardlaw, George M., and Paul M. Insel, *Perspectives in Nutrition* (1992); American Dietetic Association, Tel. (800) 366-1655, Online: www.eatright.org; Center for Nutrition Policy and Promotion, Tel. (202) 418-2312, Online: www.usda. gov/cnpp; Food and Drug Admin., Tel. (888) INFOFDA, Online: www.fda.gov; President's Council on Physical Fitness and Sports, Tel. (202) 690-9000, Online: www.fitness.gov; www.nycornell.org/medicine/nutrition/index.html.

West Nile Virus

Mosquito-borne virus causing inflammation of the brain (West Nile encephalitis).

West Nile virus, originally confined to Africa, Eastern Europe, and West Asia, is transmitted by the Northern house mosquito. The virus produces West Nile encephalitis, a brain infection that causes inflammation, impairing nervous system functioning. In North America, the disease spreads primarily in the late summer and early fall. Those over the age of 50 are at greater risk for West Nile virus.

Birds are the carriers for West Nile virus; mosquitoes acquire the virus and pass it to humans after consuming blood from infected birds. West Nile virus multiplies in the bloodstream following infection, crossing the blood-brain barrier to reach the brain, usually within 15 days of infection.

Symptoms include fever, headache, and body aches. More severe infections produce a high fever, stupor, disorientation, coma, tremors, convulsions, and paralysis.

Treatment. No specific treatment exists for West Nile virus.

Prevention efforts are aimed at mosquito control and eradication. Reducing the amount of standing water available for mosquito breeding and using insecticides can help reduce the risk of infection. *See also* ENCEPHALITIS; INSECTS AND DISEASE; MOSQUITOES AND DISEASE; *and* VIRUSES.

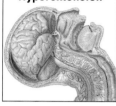

Hyperextension

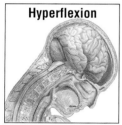

Hyperflexion

Whiplash Injury. Whiplash is a violent injury to the neck, which causes a sprain or strain of the tissues and muscles in that area. Hyperextension (above, top) is when the head and neck are bent too far backward, while hyperflexion (above, bottom) is when they are bent too far forward.

Wheelchair

A chair on wheels for a person who is unable to walk.

Manual wheelchairs may be propelled by the person in the chair, who rotates the wheels by hand. Other wheelchairs may be battery powered; they are operated by pushing buttons or other devices that can accommodate people who cannot use their arms or hands. Wheelchairs are usually made of light metals, and are often foldable and portable for easy travel. *See also* DISABLED, AIDS FOR.

Wheeze

A rasping or whistling sound related to some breathing disorders.

A wheeze is caused by narrowing of the airways in the lung. Breathing disorders that result in wheezing include asthma, bronchitis, and bronchiolitis. Wheezing can also be caused by excess fluid in the lungs (pulmonary edema) or inhalation of a foreign body that blocks the flow of air. Treatment relies on the resolution of the underlying cause. *See also* ASTHMA; BRONCHITIS; BRONCHIOLITIS; *and* PULMONARY EDEMA.

Whiplash Injury

Trauma to the neck caused by violent jerking.

Whiplash usually results in a minor sprain or a joint dislocation. In extreme cases, a vertebra may fracture or a ligament may be torn. Symptoms are pain and stiffness that begin after the trauma. Painkillers or muscle relaxants may be prescribed. In some cases, the area may need to be immobilized with an orthopedic collar. Physical therapy can help to restore movement. *See also* FRACTURES AND DISLOCATIONS; INJURY; PHYSICAL THERAPY; SPRAIN; *and* SUBLUXATION.

Whipple's Disease

A rare intestinal disease, caused by the bacterium *Trophyrema whippelii*.

Trophyrema whippelii, the bacteria that cause Whipple's disease, reside in the soil. As a result, most sufferers of this disorder are middle-aged men and farmers. The bacteria attack the small intestine, but the infection can also spread to the brain, heart, lungs, and eyes. Symptoms of Whipple's disease include fever, joint pain, cough, and abdominal pain. Untreated, the disease is fatal; but antibiotic drugs can reduce the symptoms within a couple of weeks. Long-term administration of antibiotics is necessary for a complete cure. *See also* ANTIBIOTIC DRUGS *and* PENICILLIN.

Whipworm Infestation

Infection of a human host by parasitic whipworms (trichurid worms).

Whipworms, named for their whiplike shape, can infest the body after ingestion of food, water, or soil contaminated with whipworm eggs that have been expelled in fecal matter. Ingested eggs hatch internally, and the whipworm embeds in the mucus membrane. Whipworms live in the large intestine of infected individuals.

Symptoms. Symptoms include abdominal pain, diarrhea, vomiting, and weight loss. Severe whipworm infestation can result in bloody diarrhea.

Diagnosis and Treatment. A stool sample to check for parasites and eggs can confirm a diagnosis. Whipworm infestations are treated with antihelmintic drugs, especially mebendazole. Proper hygiene can reduce risk of infection. *See also* ANTIHELMINTIC DRUGS; MEBENDAZOLE; NEMATODE; *and* WORM INFESTATION.

Whooping Cough

Also known as pertussis

A highly contagious bacterial respiratory disease, which causes spasms of coughing that usually end with a high-pitched whooping sound.

The *Bordetella pertussis* bacteria invade the throat, trachea, and bronchial tubes. Heavy coughing and whooping may cause an infected person to vomit or lose consciousness. Whooping cough is spread through the air by respiratory droplets that are expelled by diseased individuals.

Symptoms. Symptoms of whooping cough include a runny nose, a severe and sudden cough, loss of consciousness, difficulty breathing, and vomiting.

Infants need constant supervision if they develop whooping cough, due to the possibility that they may stop breathing during a coughing episode. If the case is severe, an infant may need to be in an oxygen tent, and therefore should be hospitalized.

Diagnosis. Tests that may indicate whooping cough include a nasopharyngial swab culture, a complete blood count (CBC), and serologic tests for *Bordetella pertussis* bacteria.

Treatment. If untreated, whooping cough is a severe disease with a poor prognosis. The death rate from whooping cough is between one and two percent, and is higher for infants with the disease. Complications of the disease may include pneumonia, convulsions, nosebleeds, ear infections, encephalopathy, cerebral hemorrhage, permanent seizure disorder, and developmental retardation.

Prevention. The whooping cough vaccine, DTP, is given to most children at six months of age. If an epidemic breaks out, unimmunized children under the age of seven should be kept away from school for two weeks after the last reported exposure. Booster immunizations may also help prevent whooping cough.

For background information on whooping cough, see INFECTIOUS DISEASE *and* RESPIRATORY SYSTEM. *Related material can be found in* BACTERIA; BREATHING DIFFICULTY; COUGH; IMMUNIZATION; OXYGEN; *and* VOMITING. *See also* EPIDEMIC *for more on a definition of a situation that can be defined as an epidemic.*

Wilson's Disease

A hereditary disorder in which copper accumulates in various organs of the body, particularly the liver, kidneys, brain, and eyes.

Incidence. Wilson's disease occurs in one out of every 30,000 people.

Symptoms. Symptoms of Wilson's disease include tremors, changes in eye pigmentation, mental impairment, and liver disease that may develop into cirrhosis.

Treatment. Treatment involves removing the excess copper from the body with chelation therapy, or using the drug penicillamine to bind to the copper so it can be excreted. The treatment can halt the progression of the disease; or if the disease is diagnosed before symptoms appear, treatment may prevent the development of symptoms altogether. The treatment must be continued throughout life, or the symptoms will return. *See also* GENETICS.

Wiring of the Jaw

The application of wires to hold the jaws in place.

A fractured jaw may have to be immobilized with wires or rubber bands, so that the broken bones are able to heal in the correct position.

Fractured jaws are immobilized for a period of six to eight weeks in order to allow the bones to heal correctly. Occasionally, the fractured bones need to be secured together with devices such as small screws or plates in order to permit proper healing. *See also* FRACTURES; JAW, DISLOCATED; *and* JAW, FRACTURED.

Wisdom Tooth

One of the four late appearing molars in the rear corners of the mouth.

The wisdom teeth are the third set of molars, and erupt in late adolescence. Occasionally, these molars become infected or inflamed because they do not or cannot fully erupt. In these cases, the affected teeth must be removed. *See also* DENTISTRY.

Witches' Milk

Discharge from an infant's nipple.

Witches' milk is a temporary response to maternal hormones that enter the circulation of a newborn infant in the womb. The condition will disappear within weeks, once the level of maternal hormones falls. *See also* CHILDBIRTH; CHILD DEVELOPMENT; *and* GYNECOMASTIA.

Withdrawal, Emotional

Behavior in which an individual severely curtails contact with other members of society.

A degree of solitude that impinges on an individual's ability to function may be an indication of a psychological disorder.

Diagnosis. Emotional withdrawal is a difficult disorder to diagnose, but there are some types of behavior that may indicate that treatment is advisable. If, following a personally traumatic incident, an individual cuts off communication from family and friends, or experiences difficulty communicating with coworkers, there is reason to suspect that this person is experiencing symptoms of emotional withdrawal. Emotional withdrawal may also be indicated in cases where the individual is preoccupied with his or her own work, hobbies, or concerns in ways that preclude the participation of other people.

Emotional withdrawal may be masking feelings of shame, guilt, or inadequacy over past events, as well as depression, anxiety, or other psychological disorders. Psychotherapy or other treatment may be necessary. *See also* ANXIETY *and* DEPRESSION.

World Health Organization

Also known as WHO

A specialized agency of the United Nations that is responsible for public health and the coordination of international health activities.

Founded in 1948 and headquartered in Geneva, Switzerland, the World Health Organization (WHO) helps governments improve health services.

Some of the responsibilities of the WHO are to provide information and counsel to national governments in the field of health, to promote and conduct health research, and to establish international standards for food and other biological products. *See also* PUBLIC HEALTH.

Worm Infestation

Infection by any of a number of disease-causing parasitic worms.

Worm infestation poses a major health risk in tropical and subtropical regions. It can cause anemia, malnutrition, and serious pathological and surgical conditions. Three major groups of parasitic worms responsible for disease in humans are round-

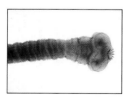

Tapeworm.
Worm infestation is a major problem in tropical regions. One of the most common disease-causing parasitic worms is the tapeworm, shown above.

worms (nematodes), tapeworms (cestodes) and flukes (trematodes).

Diagnosis of worm infestation is based on symptoms, coupled with blood and stool samples to identify the specific parasite. Such infestations are treated with antihelmintic drugs. *See also* ANTIHELMINTIC DRUGS *and* HELMINTH INFESTATION.

Wound

Damage to the skin or tissues beneath the skin.

Wounds are usually caused by accidents, violent attacks, or during surgery. Open wounds occur when the skin is broken; closed wounds occur underneath the skin.

Types. Incisions are clean cuts, such as an incision made by a surgeon. Abrasions scrape away only surface tissue. Lacerations tear the skin, as from a bite. Penetrating wounds travel into the skin, as from a stab or gunshot. Contusions are from a blunt instrument, and cause damage to underlying tissue and sometimes organs.

Treatment. Open wounds should be cleaned of dirt or foreign material, and an antiseptic should be applied to prevent infection. Surface wounds, such as abrasions, may require only a protective bandage during the healing process, but lacerations or incisions may need to be stitched together. Penetrating wounds and contusions should be attended to by a physician because of the possibility of trauma to the underlying tissue and organs. *See also* FIRST AID.

Wound Infection

Infection by bacteria, which enter through a break in the skin.

Wounds may be the result of an accident or they may be deliberate, such as those that are made by a surgeon. Whatever the cause of the wound, the danger of bacterial infection is present. If the wound is suffered as a result of an accident, it should be cleaned and treated with antiseptics. A patient may be given anticipatory antibiotics before surgery to prevent infection.

Symptoms. Symptoms of a wound infection include redness, swelling, and tenderness of the area; throbbing pain; red streaks leading away from the wound; pus or a watery discharge; swollen glands; a foul odor; chills; or fever.

Treatment. If fluids or pus collect under the wound, it may have to be reopened and drained. Antibiotics are usually prescribed to kill the bacteria causing the infection. *See also* ANTIBIOTIC DRUGS *and* BACTERIA.

Wrinkle

Visible crease in the skin.

Although wrinkles are often associated with aging, sunlight exposure causes the most noticeable changes. Many environmental factors can increase the rate at which the skin ages. Frequent sun exposure increases wrinkling, as does cigarette smoking.

Treatment. Isotretinoin topical agents, such as Retin-A and Renova, are sometimes prescribed to treat wrinkles, and they can produce some modest improvements. Plastic procedures may also be performed for cosmetic purposes. To delay facial wrinkling, sun exposure should be avoided as much as possible. Protective clothing should be worn and sunscreen should be used if exposure to the sun cannot be avoided. *See also* AGING *and* SKIN.

Wristdrop

Inability to straighten the wrist.

Wristdrop causes the hand to remain in a dropped position. This weakens the grip, as the hand muscles work best when the wrist is straight.

Cause and Treatment. Wristdrop is usually the result of damage to the radial nerve, a nerve in the inner arm. Pressure in the armpit or a fracture of the humerus can damage the nerve. Treatment may include straightening the wrist with a splint. If the nerve is irreparably damaged, however, surgical fusion of the bones in the wrist may be required. *See also* GRIP *and* RADIAL NERVE.

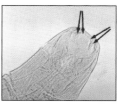
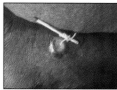

Worm Infestation. Above, top, another common parasitic worm is the hookworm. Worms may have to be removed surgically if the patient is not treated early with antihelmintic drugs. Above, bottom, a guinea worm being surgically removed.

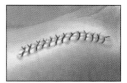
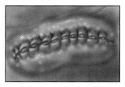

Wound Infection. Wounds (surgical or otherwise) may be infected by bacteria. Above, top, a clean wound. Above, bottom, an infected wound, in which gangrene has developed.

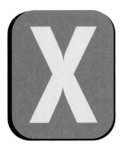

Xanthomatosis

A rare genetic disorder caused by accumulation of cholestanol, a product of cholesterol metabolism.

Symptoms of xanthomatosis include uncoordinated movements, cataracts, a decline in mental ability (dementia), and fatty growths (xanthomas) on the tendons. The symptoms often appear after a patient is over the age of 30.

The progression of xanthomatosis can be prevented by the drug chenodiol. However, this drug cannot repair the damage previously done by the disease. *See also* DEMENTIA *and* METABOLISM.

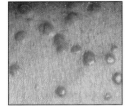

Xanthoma. Xanthomas are raised pink or yellow growths that may appear on the trunk, arms, and legs. Xanthomas are associated with high levels of fats in the blood.

Xenotransplantation

The transplantation of organs or tissues between members of different species.

Since the 1990s, the demand for donor organs for organ transplants has increased sharply, while the number of organs available has remained insufficient. The waiting time varies according to organ type, but the range is approximately one to three years. Because of the scarcity of human donors, xenotransplantation has become a popular field of research.

History. Experiments with xenotransplants were first conducted in the early 1960s. In 1964, a woman received the kidney of a chimpanzee and lived for nine months. In October 1984, doctors in California transplanted a heart from a seven-month-old baboon into a newborn human. The baby, named Fae, died 20 days later.

In June 1992, doctors at the University of Pittsburgh Medical Center performed a liver transplant from a baboon. The patient died from a brain hemorrhage 71 days later, but the liver was still functioning properly. In January 1993, another patient with hepatitis, a 62-year-old man, received a baboon liver at the University of Pittsburgh, but died a short time later.

Sources for Organs. Pigs are considered to be a more compatible source of xenotransplants than baboons or other primates, in terms of physiology as well as availability. Recent developments with techniques of genetic engineering and new antirejection drugs are beginning to solve some of the problems associated with xenotransplants. However, concern still remains about the possibility of cross-species infection, in which an unknown virus present in the donated organ could infect the patient.

Background material on xenotransplantation can be found in ORGAN DONATION *and* TRANSPLANT SURGERY. *For further information, see* GENETIC ENGINEERING; HEART-LUNG TRANSPLANT; KIDNEY TRANSPLANT; LIVER TRANSPLANT; *and* VIRUSES. *See also* HEPATITIS.

Xeroderma Pigmentosum

A rare genetic disorder characterized by changes in pigment, premature skin aging, and the early development of malignant skin tumors.

The symptoms of xeroderma pigmentosum are caused by a hypersensitivity to ultraviolet radiation, resulting from a genetic defect. The condition is recessive; genes for the disorder must be inherited from both parents for it to be expressed.

Incidence. Approximately one in every 250,000 individuals in the United States and Europe is affected by xeroderma pigmentosum. It is higher in Japan, with one in every 40,000 individuals affected.

Symptoms. A history of severe persistent sunburn can be found in many cases. Other symptoms include scaling and atrophy of the skin, areas of uneven pigmentation, malignant skin tumors, eye problems, and neurological abnormalities. Symptoms begin to appear when the affected individual is between one and two years old.

Complications. Patients have a thousand-fold increase in the incidence of skin cancer. The mean age at the time skin cancer develops is eight in these individuals, compared to 60 in the general population.

Prognosis. Less than 40 percent of affected individuals survive beyond age 20. However, individuals with a milder form of the disease may survive beyond middle age. *See also* SKIN CANCER.

X-Linked Disorders

Disorders caused by genes on the X chromosome.

X-linked disorders are usually recessive; they must be inherited from both parents. Examples of recessively inherited disorders include color blindness and hemophilia.

Recessive Patterns of Inheritance. X-linked recessive disorders are more common among men than women. For women (who have two X chromosomes), the presence of a dominant, normal gene on the other X chromosome prevents the disorder from being expressed. For men (who have only one X chromosome), the abnormal gene cannot be masked.

A man inherits his X chromosome from his mother, while a woman inherits an X from each parent. Thus, a mother can pass the gene for an X-linked disorder to either child, while a father can only pass a gene on the X chromosome to a daughter, as the son will not inherit his X chromosome.

A woman who has one gene for an X-linked disorder but has one normal, dominant gene is known as a carrier. She does not have the disease but may pass the abnormal gene to her offspring. A carrier has a 50 percent chance of passing on the condition to a son. If a woman has two genes for an X-linked disorder, she will have the disease and will pass it on to her son.

For a woman to have an X-linked disorder, she must inherit the recessive gene from both parents. If her mother is a carrier and her father is normal, she has a 50 percent chance of also being a carrier, but she will not have the disorder. If her mother is a carrier and her father has the condition, she has a 50/50 chance of being a carrier or inheriting the disorder. If her mother has the condition and her father is normal, she will only be a carrier.

Dominant Patterns of Inheritance. Some X-linked disorders are dominant, which means that a person can inherit the disorder from only one parent. A woman may inherit a dominant disease from either her mother or her father, and a man can inherit the disease only from his mother (as

his X chromosome only comes from his mother). X-linked dominant disorders include familial rickets and hereditary nephritis. *See also* GENETICS; HEMOPHILIA; NEPHRITIS; *and* RICKETS.

X-Ray

A high-energy electromagnetic wave used for imaging and treatment.

X-rays are a high-energy form of radiation that are very useful to medicine. As a diagnostic tool, x-rays are used to visualize the skeleton and evaluate bone fractures, abnormal tissue in the heart and lungs, dental caries and abscesses, and for many other applications. The technique relies on differing absorption rates of the radiation by air, tissue, bone, and muscle, based on their respective density. A black and white photographic image is made as the bone or tissue under study is exposed to x-rays. The resulting image can clearly indicate hairline bone fractures, and it is also capable of revealing diseased tissue; for example, in standard x-rays of the lung, abnormalities appear lighter than normal tissue. Pneumonia, emphysema, lung cancer, and other abnormalties and diseases are often diagnosed in this way.

Related Technologies. The use of x-rays in diagnostic imaging has undergone considerable evolution, with new techniques greatly enhancing the precision and clarity of the image. One of the more powerful forms is known as computerized axial tomography or CAT. Rather than a single x-ray exposure, CAT surveys a slice of tissue with a fine radiographic beam. The result-

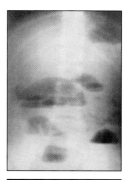
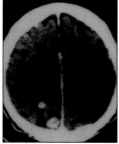

X-Ray.
X-ray technology is important in diagnosing various disorders throughout the body. Above, top, an x-ray of the abdomen can reveal an obstruction of the bowel. Above, bottom, a CAT scan of the head showing a cerebral hemorrhage (bleeding in the brain).

X-Ray Treatment

In addition to their use in diagnostic imaging, x-rays have been applied to the treatment of disease. External radiation therapy uses a concentrated beam of focused x-rays directed at diseased tissue and tumors. The procedure may be combined with chemotherapy or may be used to reduce tumor size prior to surgery. Radiation therapy may also be used after surgery to destroy residual cancer cells.

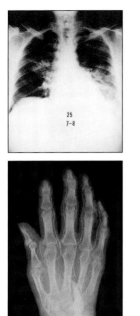

X-Ray.
Above, top, an x-ray of the lungs of a person with Legionnaires' disease. Above, bottom, an x-ray of a hand that reveals a broken bone.

Resources on Diagnostics

Cullinan, John Edward, *Illustrated Guide to X-Ray Techniques* (1980); Kee, Joyce LeFever, *Handbook of Laboratory and Diagnostic Tests with Nursing Implications* (1994); Nuland, Sherwin, *Doctors: The Biography of Medicine* (1995); Ravin, Carl E., ed., *Imaging and Invasive Radiology in the Intensive Care Unit* (1993); Segen, Joseph C., and Joseph Stauffer, *The Patient's Guide to Medical Tests* (1998); American Hospital Association, Tel. (800) 242-2626, Online: www.aha.org; The American Board of Radiology, Tel. (520) 790-2900, Online: www.theabr.org; American Healthcare Radiology Administrators, Online: www.ahra.org; www.ny-cornell.org/radiology/.

Alternatives to X-Rays

While x-rays remain a central method for diagnostic imaging, a number of highly sophisticated alternatives have been developed. These include various forms of radionuclide imaging, in which a radioactive substance is injected into the body and its location is imaged from the gamma emissions produced. Positron emission tomography (PET) and single photon emission computed tomography (SPECT) are two variants of this technique. Increasingly, noninvasive imaging techniques that avoid harmful radiation are coming into common usage. These include ultrasound scanning, in which a high frequency sound wave is directed at tissue, and the reflected waves are used to create an image; and magnetic resonance imaging (MRI), a technique using radio frequency signals emitted from cells placed under a powerful magnetic field.

ing image or tomogram is composed when the 100 to 1200 x-ray projections are translated by computer into the thin slice visible on a monitor. CAT produces images of startling quality, offering a thousand-fold increase in image resolution over conventional x-rays.

The CAT scanning machine consists of a donut-shaped apparatus surrounding a moveable table on which the patient lies. After a section of the body has been scanned by the rotating beam, the table slides to allow data from the next slice of tissue to be acquired. The procedure generally takes about 15 minutes. The computer is also capable of assembling three-dimensional images from the sequential x-ray data. CAT scanning has proven particularly useful for high-resolution imaging of the brain, allowing detection of lesions less than two millimeters in diameter, which are invisible to standard x-rays.

Additional enhancements to x-ray methods include the use of radiocontrast or radiopaque substances. Radiopaque compounds are injected and circulate to organs, tissues, and body structures. The substance, usually some form of dye, blocks the penetration of x-rays and allows these areas to appear clearly on the x-ray image. For example, a solution of barium sulfate is used for x-ray studies of the digestive tract.

Precautions. While x-rays have revolutionized diagnostic imaging, such radiation, which produces changes in the nuclei of cells, can also present a serious risk to health. X-ray radiation has the potential to damage or kill healthy cells and tissue, depending on the intensity of the radiation and the duration of exposure. Due to possible danger to reproductive cells and tissues, it is advisable to shield these areas with a lead apron during an x-ray scan. In addition, exposure to x-rays should always be avoided in pregnant women.

X-Rays as Treatment. The ability of x-ray radiation to kill cells has also been used to medical advantage in the treatment of certain cancers. In this procedure, known as radiation therapy, a powerful focused beam of radiation (roughly a thousand times the intensity used for diagnostic imaging) is directed at tumors and other cancerous areas to irradiate and destroy the diseased tissue.

Radiation therapy is often used before surgery to reduce the size of the tumor to be removed, as well as following surgery to remove residual cancerous cells from the region under treatment. Roughly half of all cancer patients receive some form of radiation therapy. The intensity of the radiation depends on the extent and location of the cancer; low-intensity radiation is used for cancers near the surface, including skin cancers, while high-energy radiation capable of penetration is used for cancers deeper within the body. If the cancer has spread, whole-body radiation may be required. Side effects of radiation therapy range from mild to severe, and typically include nausea, lethargy, weight and hair loss, diarrhea, and rashes and other irritations of the skin There is also a low risk of producing additional cancerous cells, due to the mutating properties of x-rays.

Background material on X-Ray can be found in IMAGING TECHNIQUES. *Related information is contained in* CAT SCAN; COMPUTER-AIDED DIAGNOSIS; MRI, PET SCANNING; RADIONUCLIDE SCANNING; RADIOPAQUE; SPECT; *and* TOMOGRAPHY. *See also* RADIATION *and* RADIATION THERAPY *for more on specific therapies.*

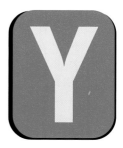

Yawning

An involuntarily opening of the mouth and drawing in of a deep breath, usually occurring when an individual is tired or bored.

Yawns produce a temporary increase in blood flow and heart rate, causing the capillaries to constrict.

Yawns are often accompanied by watering of the eyes, due to pressure on the tear glands because of exaggerated facial movements. Yawning is usually caused by drowsiness and by daytime sleepiness. Excessive yawning may be an indicator of cardiac problems or a low level of oxygen in the brain or lungs. *See also* HYPOXIA.

Yaws

An infectious tropical disease characterized by skin lesions and subsequent bone damage.

Yaws is spread through direct contact with infected individuals and often occurs in children. The illness is caused by a bacterium related to syphilis.

Symptoms. The first symptom of yaws is an itchy lesion. Scratching spreads the infection to other areas of the body. If the disease is not treated, crippling deformities of the legs, nose, palate, and upper jaw may eventually result. Like syphilis, yaws undergoes periods of remission followed by destructive external and internal lesions.

Diagnosis and Treatment. Yaws can be diagnosed with a blood test. It is treated with intramuscular penicillin. *See also* SYPHILIS *and* TROPICAL DISEASES.

Yeast

A type of fungal organism.

Some yeasts can infect the body and cause disease. Candidiasis (popularly called a yeast infection) is a common infection of the *Candida albicans* fungus.

Symptoms of a yeast infection include itchiness, soreness, a rash on the vagina, and a burning sensation when urinating.

Over-the-counter drugs for the treatment of yeast infections are readily available. If these drugs do not clear up the infection within two or three days, or if the infection returns, a physician should be consulted. *See also* ANTIFUNGAL DRUGS.

Yellow Fever

A viral disease carried by mosquitoes in tropical and subtropical regions.

After an individual is infected with yellow fever once, he or she will be immune from the disease for life.

Symptoms. Initial symptoms include jaundice (from which the disease gets its name), fever, severe headache, vomiting, backache, chills, muscle aches, nausea, and diarrhea. In more severe cases, there may be bleeding from the gums, a high fever, and blood in the urine. Symptoms usually subside after two to three days.

Diagnosis. Blood tests and antibody tests can be used to identify the virus.

Treatment. There is no specific treatment for yellow fever. Those traveling to areas where yellow fever is common should be immunized.

Prognosis. In mild cases, the prognosis is good, although a full recovery can take several weeks. In more severe cases, the mortality rate is high. *See also* JAUNDICE *and* MOSQUITOES AND DISEASE.

Yoga

A combination of physical and spiritual exercises to promote relaxation, flexibility, and health.

The foundation for yoga is found in a collection of Indian scriptures, the Upanishads, dating back to the second century BCE. These postures are practiced as part of an overall system of health in which enlightenment is the primary aim. The combination of yoga postures practiced with controlled breathing and meditation has proven an effective means of combating a number of physical ailments. *See also* ALTERNATIVE MEDICINE.

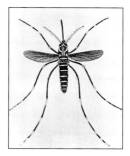

Yellow Fever.
Yellow fever is a viral disease that is transmitted to humans and other animals by mosquitoes, such as the one pictured above. In most cases, the body's immune system is able to fight the disease without treatment.

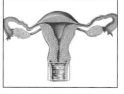

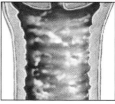

Yeast Infection.
A yeast infection is an infection by the fungus *Candida albicans*. Above, top, the infected area is marked by a square. Above, bottom, the fungus infects the walls of the vagina.

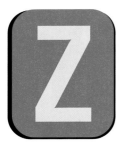

Zidovudine

Also known as AZT

A drug used to control HIV/AIDS, now used in combination with other drugs.

Treatments for HIV are most effective when they are started before symptoms of AIDS appear. Treatment with zidovudine, also called AZT, may slow the progress of the disease. Currently, treatment for HIV consists of a "cocktail" of different drugs, which are more effective than any single drug because of HIV's high mutation rate and adaptability.

Side effects of AZT include abdominal cramps, nausea, and headaches. Extended use of AZT can damage bone marrow, resulting in anemia. *See also* AIDS; ANEMIA; *and* HIV.

Zinc

Mineral that plays an important role in many of the body's biochemical processes, especially as a component of enzymes involved with regulating growth and processing carbohydrates.

A deficiency of zinc can cause appetite loss, changes in smell and taste, poor wound healing, increased susceptibility to infection, hair loss, and dermatitis of the limbs and face. In children and adolescents, deficiency is associated with impaired growth and sexual development.

Sources. Good dietary sources of zinc include meat, poultry, seafood, tofu, miso, dairy products, wheat germ, corn, nuts, dried legumes, and spinach. Whole grain products contain a form of zinc not easily absorbed by the body. A varied, balanced diet will provide sufficient amounts.

Deficiency. Zinc deficiency occurs most often in sufferers of inflammatory bowel disease, malabsorption syndromes, pancreatic or kidney disease, or hemolitic anemia.

Zinc supplements should only be used to treat a documented living-tissue deficiency, as an overdose of zinc may cause symptoms such as nausea, vomiting, and diarrhea. *See also* CHOLESTEROL *and* MALABSORPTION SYNDROMES.

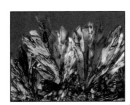

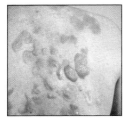

AZT.
Zidovudine, also known as AZT, is a drug that is commonly used to control the progress of HIV and AIDS. Above, top, AZT crystals shown under magnification. AZT is also used to treat the secondary infections that accompany AIDS, such as Kaposi's sarcoma. Second from the top, the back of a person with Kaposi's sarcoma before treatment. At the bottom, the back of the same person after treatment with AZT.

Zoonosis

A disease transmitted from animals to humans.

Zoonoses may be caused by bacteria, viruses, fungi, or parasites. Animals that transmit the diseases may be wild or tame.

One example of a bacterial zoonosis is cat-scratch fever, which may be acquired from infected cats or dogs.

Viral zoonoses include encephalitis, which is acquired from horses and rodents, and rabies, which is transmitted by cats, dogs, raccoons, skunks, bats, and foxes.

Ringworm, which is contracted through close contact with infected cats or cattle, is a fungal zoonosis.

Toxocariasis, also known as viceral larval migrans, is a parasitic zoonosis transmitted by contact with dog, cat, or raccoon feces. *See also* CAT-SCRATCH FEVER; ENCEPHALITIS; RINGWORM; *and* TOXOCARIASIS.

Z-Plasty

Also known as zigzagplasty

A type of surgery used to reposition a scar.

Z-plasty is a surgical technique used to reposition a scar so that it follows natural skin lines and creases. Z-plasty relieves pain from the contracture of the skin that takes place after serious injury.

Z-plasty is often used on facial scars, such as a cleft lip revision; it is also used on fingers or in armpits to restore flexibility. *See also* COSMETIC SURGERY.

Zygote

A fertilized egg, formed by the union of sperm and egg at conception.

Half of a zygote's genetic material comes from the sperm, the other half from the egg. The zygote undergoes several rapid rounds of cell division as it travels through the fallopian tube. By the time implantation in the uterus occurs, the zygote has grown to become a ball of hollow cells called a blastocyst. *See also* CONCEPTION.

Appendix

Emergency Medicine and First Aid

This appendix is provided as a quick reference guide for those immediately in need of information regarding emergency situations. Included below are some of the most frequently occurring disorders that require quick and immediate attention. This section begins with a detailed description of *First Aid* and the *Emergency First Steps* that can be taken in nearly any emergency situation.

These articles are edited, so as to focus on their most important content—the following text deals with the immediate treatment needs of an affected person. For example, the article on *Asthma* has become an article dealing with the specifics of what to do during an *Asthma Attack.* Complete entries can be found in the body of the book; cross references also refer to articles in the body of the book.

These 50 articles were chosen because of their essential importance in emergency situations. As in all emergency situations, it is best to seek immediate help from trained personnel and to see a physician for treatment and an evaluation as soon as possible after the emergency.

If a victim has lost consciousness, it is important to find out if he or she is breathing by checking for a pulse (above, right). If it appears that the victim is not breathing, open the airways (left) and perform mouth to mouth resuscitation or CPR. Middle, if the victim is bleeding it is important to bandage the wound until help arrives.

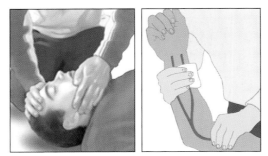

Emergency, First Steps

Critical situation that requires immediate medical attention.

In the United States, there exists a complete network of emergency services, including medical, fire, police, and psychological departments. Emergency vehicles range from helicopters, to ambulances, to boats. Dialing 911 anywhere in the United States activates a connection between a caller and the nearest emergency service dispatcher. However, in an emergency situation, a bystander must often take the first critical steps before emergency medical assistance is available. In such instances, important considerations include:

Breathing. Are the victim's air passages clear, and is he or she breathing? If there is a foreign object lodged in the throat, use the Heimlich maneuver. If the passages are clear but the victim is not breathing, use artificial ventilation.

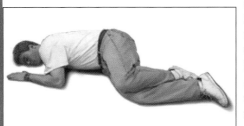

Recovery Position.
An unconscious victim that is still breathing, should be placed in the recovery position until help arrives. The casualty should lie on their stomach with the near arm and top knee bent forward (as pictured).

Bleeding. Use some form pressure to control bleeding. If an artery has been injured, a tourniquet may be required as a last resort, but the use of pressure is far more preferable. A cut artery will spurt or pulse; it is far more serious than a cut vein. In contrast, the blood from the latter will have a tendency to ooze. If a ruptured artery is suspected, treat the wound immediately, as a victim can die in minutes.

Heartbeat. Is there a detectable pulse? If not, the patient will require cardiopulmonary resuscitation (CPR) or artificial ventilation.

Protect Yourself. Avoid exposure to the blood or bodily fluids of a victim, as they may be a major source of infection.

First Aid

Immediate assistance offered during an emergency situation.

When a sudden illness or accident occurs, the first people on the scene will most likely not be medically trained. First aid is the assistance that is offered until trained medical personnel arrive on the scene. The goal of first aid is to preserve a victim's life and to prevent further harm.

Everyone should learn the basics of first aid, because responding to an emergency demands preparation, and almost everyone encounters an emergency sometime during his or her life.

An important first step in an emergency is to remain calm—effective first aid cannot be administered in a state of panic. Another basic step in first aid is assessing the situation—who is hurt, how badly, what sort of help is needed, and what sort of help can be offered. Key concerns in assessing the severity of an emergency include heartbeat, breathing, bleeding, and consciousness. If the victim is not breathing or has no pulse, CPR (cardiopulmonary resuscitation), should be administered while someone else calls for emergency medical help. It is important to know that dialing 911 in the United States accesses the nearest emergency dispatch station. If a person is bleeding profusely, blood loss should be controlled by applying direct pressure to the wound.

Those administering first aid should protect themselves against liability. If the person to be rescued is conscious, they must be asked for permission to be helped. If permission is not obtained, the rescuer may be subject to a lawsuit. More information regarding the rights of rescuers can be found under Good Samaritan Laws at a local library; some web-sites may also contain similar information, but local statutes often apply.

Airway Obstruction

Blockage of the respiratory passages resulting in difficulty or cessation of breathing.

Most deaths caused by a foreign body in the air passages occur in children under the age of five, two-thirds of whom are infants. Adults are acutely aware of a foreign body in the airways, but children may show no symptoms unless the air passages are almost entirely obstructed. The Heimlich maneuver for children over the age of one is the same as that for adults, except that the compression should be gentler. Do not use the Heimlich maneuver for children under the age of one. Lay the infant face down with its chest on one open hand tapping firmly between the shoulder blades with the heel of your other hand. *See also* CARDIOPULMONARY RESUSCITATION (CPR).

Asphyxia

A lack of oxygen or an excess of carbon dioxide in the body.

Every organ in the body depends upon a constant supply of oxygen, taken in by the lungs and carried by the blood to every part of the body. Anything that interferes with this process can lead to asphyxia. Causes of asphyxia include abnormally low levels of oxygen in the air (such as in mines or at very high altitudes), obstruction or closing of the breathing passages (as in asthma), trauma to the chest or lungs, or certain poisons. Sufferers usually breathe more rapidly and deeply to overcome the lack of oxygen. If the problem is not corrected, loss of consciousness and death can result.

If the airway is obstructed, the object causing the obstruction must be cleared. Victims who are in a place that lacks adequate oxygen, such as a mine shaft or an area of high altitude, must be immediately transported to a location with higher oxygen levels, but only if the rescuer's breathing will not be compromised. If poisoning is involved, a trained medical professional should be contacted. *See also* ANOXIA.

Asthma Attack

A respiratory disorder causing attacks of breathlessness and wheezing.

Asthma can occur at any age, but about half of all cases strike children under the age of ten. Childhood cases often become less severe or clear up entirely with age. There appears to be a genetic factor—overall incidence in the American population is about five percent, but someone with a child or parent who has asthma runs a 20 to 25 percent risk of developing the disorder.

Asthma attacks are unpredictable. They can occur often or seldom, with variations in severity, and can happen at any time, although they are slightly more likely to take place at night. In addition to breathlessness and wheezing, asthma attacks can cause coughing and chest tightness.

Emergency Diagnosis. A large part of asthma management relies on early diagnosis and treatment. Diagnosis is based first on the symptoms: breathing difficulty, coughing, and wheezing. Asthma is a congenital condition.

Treatment. Treatment of an asthma attack starts with the earliest possible detection of the onset of the attack. In most cases, warning signs begin hours before the onset of symptoms. Deterioration of breathing that signals an oncoming attack can be monitored by a device called a peak flow meter, which indicates the efficiency of breathing. A reading below 80 percent of maximum effectiveness is an indication that preventive measures should be taken, such as increasing the dose of asthma medications. A reading below 50 percent is a clear sign of trouble needing medical attention. The symptoms of an asthma emergency include severe breathing difficulty, blue-tinted lips and nails because of a shortage of oxygen, and an abnormally fast heartbeat.

Background material on asthma and similar conditions can be found in BREATHING DIFFICULTY. *Related information is contained in* BRONCHODILATOR DRUGS; EMPHYSEMA; INFLAMMATION; STEROIDS, ANABOLIC; *and* X-RAY. *See also* LUNG *for the most vital anatomical information.*

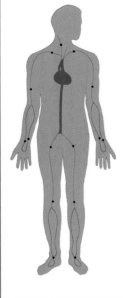

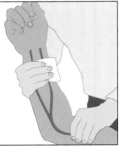

Treating Bleeding.
Pressure points are marked with black dots (top). Pressure should be applied at these points to manage rapid bleeding. Even though these points may be a distance from the bleeding itself, the arteries bringing blood to the wound are supplied from blood vessels at these points, thus, pressure will slow the bleeding. Below, pressure applied directly to the trauma site will also slow bleeding. Whenever possible, the injury should be elevated.

Bites

The wounding, piercing or stinging of the flesh by an animal, insect or another person.

Animal Bites. Depending on the region of the world, some animal bites are more likely than others. In Pacific coastal areas, attacks from sharks, jellyfish, and other aquatic creatures are not uncommon. In regions of Central and South America, crocodile attacks are serious. Bites from cattle, horses, and pigs can also be fatal. However, in totality, dogs are responsible for the greatest number of animal attacks.

Any bite from an animal that breaks the skin presents the danger of infection. The mouth of an animal contains many bacteria and viruses, many of which can cause infections. Rabies, from dogs, cats, bats, and other animals is a major risks. Superficial bites and scratches can be treated the same as minor wounds. In all other cases, professional treatment must be sought.

TREATMENT

Treatment of a severe animal bite begins with cleaning and examination of the wound. Instead of stitching a wound, the physician may choose to bandage it to avoid enclosing bacteria from the bite in the wound. To reduce infection, a course of antibiotics or an antitetanus injection may be administered as a preventive measure. An antirabies vaccine or immunogloublin may also be administered.

Emergency rooms report far more human bites than most expect. The human mouth contains many bacteria and viruses that can infect a wound. Human bites rarely cause significant tissue damage and thus are deceptive in appearing more benign than they are.

Most human bites can be treated by washing the area with soap and warm water and applying a cold compress to reduce swelling and pain. At times infectious antibiotics are necessary to adequately heal a developing bacterial infection. *See also* BACTERIA; BITES; BLEEDING, TREATMENT OF; SPIDER BITES; *and* VENOMOUS BITES.

Bleeding, Treatment of

Measures used to stop bleeding. These vary according to the nature and severity of the wound.

Blood pressure in the veins is lower than that in the arteries. Bleeding from the veins tends to be slow and steady while bleeding from the arteries may be copious and pulsating. Any bleeding should be controlled as quickly as possible, but bleeding from the arteries is particularly dangerous.

Ascertaining the Severity of a Wound. The amount of blood lost is not a good indicator of the seriousness or severity of the trauma. Bleeding from head wounds can be heavy even from minor cuts or scrapes, because the blood vessels are close to the surface. Bleeding from a deeper wound elsewhere on the body might seem less dangerous, while a large share of the bleeding is internal.

It is best not to come into direct contact with the blood, since this is one of the most direct ways of contracting AIDS or other infectious diseases. Immediately after treating a bleeding wound, a person should wash her or his hands in hot, soapy water.

Pregnancy. Some amount of bleeding or spotting is not unusual during pregnancy, particularly in the first trimester. Vaginal bleeding, however can signal the start of a serious problem. A physician should be contacted immediately.

Home Treatment. The first rule in bleeding treatment is to put pressure on the wound and hold it until the bleeding stops or more specific remedies can be applied. However, this is not true if there is a

ALERT
Shock
When the word "shock" is used, very often it is meant to convey a sense of psychological trauma that doses not have medical significance. However, in medical terminology shock results when there is not enough blood flow to the vital organs. If there is a danger of shock, stop any ongoing blood loss by applying direct pressure to the wound. Have the patient lie flat on his or her back. Keep the patient covered and warm and call emergency medical service (EMS) personnel as soon as possible.

possible skull fracture or some other broken bone near the wound or if there is an object embedded in the wound. If the wound is to one or both eyes, a light clean dressing must be applied to both eyes, since any eye movements may damage the wounded eye. If the wound is to the nose and it is unbroken, a cold compress should be applied.

Tourniquets. Once, a common treatment, tourniquets are now considered a dangerous means of stopping bleeding. Wrapped tourniquets can cause gangrene, making an injury worse. The only time a tourniquet can even be considered is when an extremity has been amputated in an accident. Tourniquets are made of straps or fabric folded to about two inches wide; a belt or strap of fabric is best. It should be wrapped just above the wound and knotted at the pressure point. A bandage and properly applied pressure is preferred.

Types of Injuries. Bruises are the result of blows that do not break the skin. They may cause tissue damage appearing as discolorations under the skin, as well as internal bleeding if the blow is severe. Internal bleeding should be treated only by a doctor.

Scrapes or other abrasions should be washed in warm, soapy water. If there are loose foreign objects in the wound, try to rinse or pluck them out. After cleansing, an antibiotic ointment and bandage with sterile gauze can be applied.

Puncture wounds may be as mild as a splinter or as serious as a gunshot wound. Any penetrating wound offers serious danger of infection, since the foreign object carries bacteria through the protective layer of skin. Tetanus shots are usually recommended if the puncture wound is relatively deep, since the bacteria that cause tetanus are likely to have contaminated most puncturing objects. Tetanus prophylaxis may be needed so a medical professional should be contacted to assess the appropriateness of such a treatment.

> *Further information may be found in* BLEEDING DISORDERS; BLOOD TRANSFUSION; *and* INTERNAL BLEEDING. *Details may be found in* ANTICOAGULANT DRUGS; *and* OCCULT BLOOD.

Breathing Difficulty

An abnormal change in depth and rate of breathing.

Breathing difficulty can be a symptom of many different diseases, or it can be a general physical and lifestyle characteristic. It results from any condition that affects airflow into or out of the lungs, the ability of the lungs to infuse the blood with oxygen, or the ability of the brain stem to regulate breathing.

Breathing difficulty can be either labored breathing or pain related to breathing movements. Whether a person is asleep, resting, or exercising, breathing difficulty can occur.

Anxiety. Times of stress or tension can bring on abnormally rapid or deep breathing (hyperventilation) that causes faintness and a feeling of being unable to breathe adequately, sometimes accompanied by muscle spasms or numbness of the hands and feet. These symptoms are caused by an excess loss of carbon dioxide from the blood and can be lessened by breathing into a paper bag, which helps to restore normal carbon dioxide levels.

Altitude Sickness. Breathing difficulty can occur at high altitudes, where the air is thinner and less oxygen is taken in with each inhalation. It is often experienced by individuals who are unaccustomed to high altitudes and can worsen with activity for those who are less physically fit. As the lungs work harder to supply the body with oxygen, there is a feeling of breathlessness. Eventually, the individual's system becomes accustomed to the thinner air. Problems can be lessened by a reduction in physical activity while this change occurs.

Breathlessness is the inability to breathe at the rate required by the body. It is most commonly associated with exertion (intense exercise) and panic attacks. This is normal for those in good health and not a cause for concern. Other more serious causes of breathlessness include heart problems, regular or repeated exposure to poor air quality (as in smoky or dusty workplaces), allergies, and smoking. Treatment of these problems will help to remedy the symptom of breathlessness.

Circulation Disorders. Chronic heart conditions, such as impaired ability of the heart to pump blood—heart failure—can cause breathing difficulty. Other heart con-

ditions that cause breathing difficulty include a blood clot in the lung (pulmonary embolism) and abnormally high blood pressure in the arteries of the lung (pulmonary hypertension).

Lack of Fitness. Many physically inactive people do not have the heart and lung capacity needed to respond to the body's increased demand for oxygen at times of exertion. The increased demand causes discomfort and pain. The remedy is to cease the physical activity. The long-term solution is regular fitness training.

Lung Damage. Conditions that cause temporary or permanent damage to the lungs inevitably result in breathing difficulty. Emphysema (chronic breathing difficulty) damages the lungs by destroying the sensitive tissue where oxygen enters the blood and carbon dioxide is removed from blood. Breathing difficulty can be due to inflammation of the lungs (pneumonia) or inflammation of the airways of the lung (bronchitis). In these cases, breathing difficulty may be temporary, easing when the infection that causes the inflammation yields to treatment. Physical damage, such as a collapsed lung (pneumothorax) or excess fluid around the lung (pleural effusion), also causes breathing difficulty.

Basic anatomical information on BREATHING DIFFICULTIES *is contained in* BLOOD CELLS; HEART; *and* LUNG. *Further information may be found in* ALLERGY; ALTITUDE SICKNESS; ANEMIA; ANXIETY; BRONCHITIS; EMPHYSEMA; HEART, DISORDERS OF; OBESITY; PNEUMONIA; *and* SHOCK.

Bruise

Injury-related skin discoloration.

Everyone experiences bruises—from minor bumps to sprains—in the course of a normal life. The purple discoloration appears when the blood from small ruptured vessels leaks into tissue and under the skin. Bruising typically occurs from a blow, but it can also result from a twisted ankle, a strained muscle, or a scrape that removes parts of the skin. People who have blood clotting problems bruise easily, because the blood continues to leak into the skin.

Other than applying a cold compresses on the bruised site for ten to fifteen minutes every hour to reduce swelling and pain, there is no specific treatment for

Bruises in the Elderly

Because of thinner skin and more fragile blood vessels—particularly if they have been exposed to a lot of sun—the elderly bruise easily even from what might seem normal hand pressure. Often, bruises will appear on the forearms and the backs of the hands. No treatment is necessary, though reabsorption of the blood may take a long time.

bruising. Most bruises will eventually heal on their own as the blood is reabsorbed into the body.

Background material on BRUISE *may be found in* BLOOD; CIRCULATORY SYSTEM; *and* SKIN. *Further information is contained in* COMPRESS; PURPURA; *and* SPRAIN. *Related material can be found in* ELDERLY, CARE OF THE FIRST AID; *and* SWELLING.

Burns

Destruction of the skin or deeper tissues from excessive heat.

Burns result from direct dry heat, fire, and wet heat, as well as from scalding, chemicals such as acids, and electric current. Burns are divided into three categories.

First-degree burns damage only the outer surface of the skin. After a burn, the skin becomes red, extremely sensitive to the touch, wet, and swollen.

Second-degree burns are deeper. Blisters form and are filled with a clear, thick liquid. The area is painfully sensitive to touch and is swollen.

Third-degree burns go deeper still. The immediate surface may be charred and leathery or white and soft, so that observers may not realize that a burn has taken place. There may be blistering. The area may be extremely painful to the touch or, if nerve endings have been destroyed, there may be no pain at all.

Inhalation and Chemical Burns. Inhalation burns occur when hot gases enter the mouth, air passages, or lungs. Chemical burns of the throat and esophagus can be the result of drinking acid, alkalis, mustard gas, or phosphorus.

Treatment depends on the source and depth of the burn. Extensive second-degree burns and all third-degree burns should be treated by a physician.

Doctors will first make sure the victim can breathe properly. Oxygen will be supplied if carbon monoxide poisoning is suspected. Lost fluids will be replaced intravenously; this method also serves as a preliminary response to treating shock.

The site will be carefully cleaned; if necessary, doctors may administer an anesthetic so that the area can be scrubbed with a soft brush. An antibiotic cream may be applied and the area covered with a loose bandage. The burn area will be vulnerable to infection, so it must be kept clean and covered with sterile bandages.

Skin Grafts. More extensive burns often require a section of skin to be taken from an unburned part of the body, from another person or even from a pig, since pig skin most resembles human skin. Grafts from the victim will integrate well with the surrounding skin. Grafts from other sources will serve to protect the area for ten days to two weeks; the grafts are sloughed off as the person heals.

Besides being painful, burns take a long time to heal, can be disfiguring, and require extensive physical therapy.

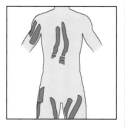

Skin Grafts. Extensive burns may require skin grafts (above), which involve removing skin from an unburned part of the body and using it to replace the skin on the severely burned area.

ALERT

First-Aid Treatment for Burns

FIRST-DEGREE BURNS are red, mildly painful, swollen. If treated properly they will heal in a few days.
- Immerse the affected area in cool water or cover with a cold, wet cloth until pain subsides;
- Clean with warm, soapy water;
- Cover with clean, dry gauze dressing;
- Change dressing frequently.

SECOND-DEGREE BURNS are blistered, rough on the surface, swollen, and extremely painful. If treated properly they will heal in a few weeks. If extensive, they should be treated by trained medical personnel.
- Immerse the affected area in cool water or cover with a cold, wet cloth;
- Clean with warm, soapy water. Do not rub!
- Blot gently;
- Cover with clean, dry gauze dressing;
- Change dressing frequently.

THIRD-DEGREE BURNS have a charred or white appearance. They should be treated by trained medical personnel.
- Do not remove clothing on or near the burn;
- Do not apply cold water or medications to the burn;
- Place a clean, dry cloth over the burned area;
- Check frequently to be sure victim is breathing properly;
- Call 911. The victim must immediately be taken to an emergency department.

CHEMICAL BURNS
- Wash the area thoroughly with large amounts of cool water for at least 20 minutes;
- Cover with a sterile gauze dressing;
- Call 911. The victim must immediately be taken to an emergency department.

ELECTRICAL BURNS
- Make sure victim is free of contact with the electrical power source before you attempt a rescue.
- Check that the victim is breathing and has a pulse; If not, apply CPR;
- Treat as for a third-degree burn;
- Call 911. The victim must immediately be taken to an emergency department.

Background material on burns may be found in ACCIDENTS; EMERGENCY; INJURY; *and* SKIN. *For additional information see* BANDAGE; BLISTERING; ELECTRICAL INJURY; EMERGENCY, FIRST STEPS; FIRST AID; GAUZE; GLIOMA; *and* MENINGIOMA. *Related information contained in* SKIN GRAFT *and* SKIN PEELING.

Cardiac Arrest

The sudden failure of the heart to pump blood.

Cardiac arrest is frequently caused by ventricular fibrillation, a severely irregular rhythm of the heart. Ventricular fibrillation is usually brought on by a heart attack (myocardial infarction). Asystole, which means that the heart has ceased to beat, can cause cardiac arrest. Cardiac arrest can be related to an underlying cardiovascular condition, such as cardiomyopathy, heart failure, or hypertension. It can also occur in people with severe burns, major injuries that result in the massive loss of blood, severe allergic reactions, drug overdoses, or electric shock.

ALERT

In Case of Cardiac Arrest

If cardiac arrest occurs in a home or public place, emergency cardiopulmonary resuscitation must be administered to restore heart function or to maintain viability until more sophisticated measures and rescue personnel arrive. In CPR, the patient's airway is opened, and the person administering CPR breathes into the mouth while compressing the chest at regular intervals. Emergency medical help should be called while CPR is being performed.

Symptoms are swift and devastating and include: failure to breathe, loss of consciousness, physical collapse, and absence of the normal pulse. Symptoms usually occur without warning, although the patient may have felt chest pain, shortness of breath, or severe fatigue in the days before cardiac arrest takes place.

Treatment. Emergency teams are trained in defibrillation—the delivery of a shock to the heart or administration of medication intended to start normal beating rhythms again. In a hospital, more advanced techniques can be used, and drugs such as lidocaine can be given intravenously to stabilize the heartbeat.

Prognosis. When the heart stops beating quick treatment is necessary to prevent major damage to the brain, which can occur from lack of oxygen. Permanent age can take place in as little as three minutes. Even with treatment, the outcome may not be favorable. About two-thirds of cardiac arrest patients die immediately, and the death rate for survivors in the year following the arrest is quite high. People at high risk of cardiac arrest should be on the alert for warning signs. For patients with serious arrhythmia affecting the ventricles, implantation of a defibrillator can reduce the risk of cardiac arrest. *See also* DEFIBRIL-LATION *and* HEART ATTACK.

Choking

Partial or complete obstruction of the airway, resulting in coughing, gagging or wheezing.

Symptoms. A choking victim will not be able to speak. The person who is choking may, occasionally, place both hands around the neck or lean forward in an attempt to dislodge the obstruction. The victim is likely to make wheezing or snorting sounds and may become pale or blue in the face. Sometimes choking victims will faint.

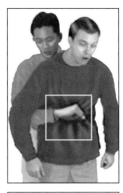

ALERT

Anaphylactic Shock

If a person appears to be choking but there is no obstruction, he or she may actually be suffering from anaphylactic shock. This is a severe allergic reaction to food, medication, or an insect bite, which results in shock and can be fatal in as little as 15 minutes. Accompanying symptoms may include hives, swelling, and redness or blueness of the skin.

Treatment. An object caught in the air passages may be removed by using the Heimlich maneuver (see illustration, top right). The Heimlich maneuver should only be preformed on a conscious person. Once normal breathing resumes, it is important to determine if any part of the object was inhaled into the lungs, since this can cause subsequent medical problems, including pneumonia.

In all cases of blockage, emergency medical help should be sought immediately. If the Heimlich maneuver does not remove a blockage, or if there is no object

ALERT

Preventing Choking in Children
• Keep chunks of meat or cheese, grapes, hard candy, and other foods that children may choke on, out of their reach. Nuts should not be given to any child under the age of seven.
• Teach older children not to offer foods that may cause choking to younger siblings.
• Cut firmer foods into small pieces before feeding to a small child.
• Teach children to be careful with stick foods such as peanut butter and some kinds of cancy.
• Teach children to chew well before swallowing.
• Children should never be allowed to run or play with food or drinking straws in their mouths.
• Always keep small toy parts and other household objects out of the reach of small children.

in the air passages, medical technicians will decide if a surgical procedure on the airway should be used and whether or not the victim should be taken to the hospital. Oxygen deprivation for more than five or six minutes may cause brain damage.

Choking in Children. Children beginning solid food for the first time and children under the age of four who do not chew their food well are at high risk for choking. Nuts, chunks of meat such as hot dogs and cheese, grapes, hard candy, and popcorn are the most dangerous foods for small children. Common household items may also pose a potential hazard to a young child's air passages. Rubber or latex balloons, coins, marbles, small parts of toys, pen caps, and button-type batteries are also frequent causes of airway obstructions.

Concussion

Mild injury to the brain as a result of a blow to or violent motion of the head.

Any blow to the head may force the brain against the bony structure of the skull. Concussion is a form of injury to the brain that is sometimes associated with a brief loss of consciousness.

Symptoms. Beyond a loss of consciousness, symptoms can include loss of memory, dizziness, vomiting, nausea, and headache. Head injury causing unconsciousness

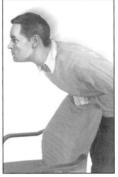

Heimlich Maneuver. A choking victim can be helped by using the Heimlich maneuver. Top, the person helping the victim should go behind the person, wrap their arms around the victims upper abdomen and thrust inward near the bottom of the rib cage. Choking victims who are alone may use the back of a chair to simulate the thrust another person would give them.

ALERT

Children and Head Injury

Children are at particular risk for brain injury because they are more prone to accidental falls. Also, infants and toddlers are, accidentally or intentionally, easily shaken by adults and can suffer severe brain injury. Any vomiting, paleness, drowsiness, or even a very brief period of unconsciousness following a blow to the head is evidence of brain injury, and the child should be checked by a physician as soon as possible.

should be investigated by a doctor. Recovery generally occurs without treatment and is complete within 24 to 48 hours.

Serious symptoms may develop after a period of time, including persistent headaches, amnesia, increasing confusion, and increasing sleepiness and lethargy. Emergency symptoms include persistent unconsciousness, seizures, drowsiness, repeated vomiting, unequal pupil size, confusion, and difficulty walking.

Children and Concussion. Children are particularly at risk for brain injury, because they are more prone to falls. Any fall or blow to the head of a child that results in a loss of consciousness warrants an immediate evaluation by a medical professional. *See also* AMNESIA; BRAIN; BRAIN DAMAGE; CRYING IN INFANTS; *and* TRAUMA.

Coughing Up Blood

Also known as hemoptysis

Blood in the sputum.

Any number of medical conditions can result in the presence of blood in the sputum (hemoptysis), including bacterial infections, lung cancer, bleeding disorders such as hemophilia, inflammation of the trachea, heart failure, mitral stenosis, and congestive heart failure. Any of these conditions can result in broken blood vessels in the airways, nose, throat, or another part of the respiratory system. While a simple persistent cough can cause blood in the sputum; such blood is usually a sign of a serious underlying condition that requires medical attention.

CAUSES

Most often, coughing up blood is the result of a respiratory tract infection such as tuberculosis, bronchitis, or pneumonia. Such an infection can inflame the airways (bronchi) of the lung or the small sacs (alveoli) where air is exchanged in the lung. An infection may also damage a blood vessel of the respiratory tract enough to cause it to rupture.

When the bronchi become enlarged and distorted (bronchiectasis), one of the blood vessels within the bronchi may break open. This can also happen with tracheitis, or inflammation of the windpipe. Within the lung itself, congestion can put enough pressure on blood vessels to cause them to rupture. Congestion can be due to a narrowing of the valve between the upper and lower chambers of the heart (mitral stenosis), or blockage of a lung artery by a clot (pulmonary embolism). Lung cancer can also weaken and eventually rupture a blood vessel, causing hemoptysis.

DIAGNOSIS

The appearance of the blood coughed up can give clues to the underlying disorder. Only rarely is the blood bright red and unmixed with other secretions. It may have a pink, foamy, or streaked appearance, or take the form of clots.

A cough that persists for months, worsens dramatically, and produces blood may be an indication of lung cancer. A high fever and shortness of breath may suggest pneumonia. A chest x-ray can be done to detect abnormalities in the lungs and respiratory tract. In some cases, visual examination of the respiratory tract with a bronchoscope may be performed.

TREATMENT

Treatment may include antibiotic drugs for bacterial infections, diuretics to reduce fluid retention, and anticoagulant drugs to prevent abnormal blood clotting. *See also* ANTIBIOTIC DRUGS; ANTICOAGULANT DRUGS; BACTERIA; BRONCHOSCOPY; HEART FAILURE; HEMOPHILIA; MITRAL STENOSIS; *and* RESPIRATORY TRACT INFECTION.

Cardiopulmonary Resuscitation (CPR)

An emergency method used to restart the heart and initiate breathing when a person's pulse has stopped (cardiac arrest).

Cardiopulmonary resuscitation combines cardiac compression to restart or maintain the heartbeat and if possible mouth to mouth resuscitation to supplement or enhance ventilation and oxygen delivery to the lungs. When the heart stops beating its pumping action ceases and, oxygen-rich blood fails to reach the brain. This can result in permanent brain damage after only three or four minutes and death after eight to ten minutes. It is therefore crucial to begin CPR as quickly as possible.

Ideally, a person performing cardiopulmonary resuscitation should be formally trained. You can locate the nearest CPR class in your area by contacting your local chapter of the American Heart Association or the American Red Cross. Mouth-to-mouth resuscitation can be successfully administered by an untrained individual, but the most effective method of restoring circulation is cardiac compression massage performed by a trained individual. The instructions included here are **not** a substitute for classroom training.

HOW TO PERFORM CPR

First, it is important to verify that the victim has indeed suffered cardiac arrest and is not merely unconscious. Look in the victim's mouth to make sure that no food or foreign material is obstructing the airway, then with your ear over the victims mouth and nostrils listen for signs of breathing. If a spinal injury is suspected, do not move the head or neck, as that may worsen the injury.

Immediately call for emergency medical help. Have a person not performing CPR make the call. If you are alone, call before starting CPR.

Remember to be gentle when applying pressure to the chest, particularly with children. Be sure to press straight down; do not

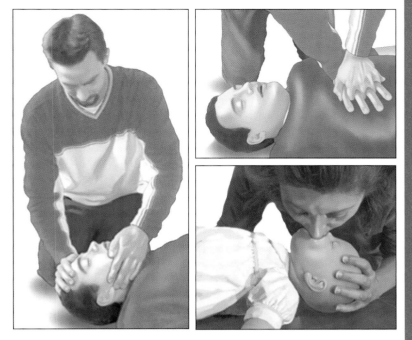

Performing CPR.
Above left, first check for breathing. Right, top, apply chest compressions. Bottom, apply mouth to mouth resuscitation.

rock. Count the compressions so that they are evenly spaced.If the victim vomits while CPR is being administered, roll him over to his left side until he is finished. Clear the air passages, and resume CPR if there is still no heartbeat or breathing.

ADULTS

- Place the person on his back, tilt the head back, and lift the chin.
- Pinch the nose and make an airtight mouth to mouth seal. Give two full breaths. The victim's chest will rise if he is getting enough air.
- If there is no response or pulse, begin chest compressions at about 100 per minute, with two breaths given after every 15 compressions. Place one hand on top of the other and position the hands about two finger-widths above the lowest part of the person's breast bone. Press straight down, about one and one-half to two inches. and release.
- Continue until help arrives, or breathing and pulse begin again, or your fatigue becomes overwhelming.

CHILDREN AGES ONE TO EIGHT

- Place the child on his or her back, tilt the head back, and lift the chin.

- Pinch the nose and make an airtight mouth to mouth seal. Give two full breaths. The victim's chest will rise if he or she is getting enough air.
- If there is no pulse, begin chest compressions at a rate of 100 per minute. Place the heel of the hand about two finger-widths above the lowest part of the child's breastbone. Press gently straight down about one to one and one-half inches and then release. After every five compressions, give one breath.
- Continue until help arrives, breathing and pulse begin again, or your fatigue becomes overwhelming.

INFANTS

- Place the infant on his or her back across your knees, tilt the head back, and lift the chin.
- Create a seal over the mouth and nose of the victim. Give two small puffs. The child's chest will rise if he or she is getting enough air.
- If there is no pulse, begin quick chest compressions at a rate of 100 to 120 per minute; after every five compressions give one puff of breath. Place two fingers in the middle of the breast bone between the nipples. Press gently straight down about a one-half inch to one inch and release.
- Continue until help arrives, breathing and pulse begin again, or your fatigue becomes overwhelming.

Performing CPR on an Infant. First, check the breathing of the infant. Then create a seal over the mouth and nose and give two small puffs (right) . Afterwards, begin quick chest compressions.

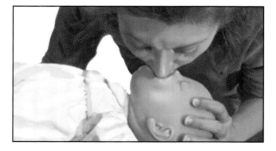

For background material on cardiopulmonary resuscitation, see ANOXIA; ARTIFICIAL RESPIRATION; CHOKING; HEART RATE; *and* HEIMLICH MANEUVER. *Further information can be found in* EMERGENCY FIRST STEPS *and* FIRST AID. *See also* HEART ATTACK.

Dehydration

A loss of water through vomiting, diarrhea or perspiration.

If not restored by fluid intake, dehydration can have many serious consequences, including low blood pressure, loss of consciousness, heart failure, and, in the most extreme cases, even death.

Causes. Dehydration occurs when there is an imbalance between intake and outflow of bodily fluids. This can happen during strenuous exercise or when the person is in hot dry environments. Fluid loss can also be the result of diarrhea and vomiting. Dehydration is also a consequence of many diseases, such as diabetes or virus infections like. In the case of children too young to feed themselves, dehydration may be caused by parental neglect.

Symptoms. In the early stages, a person with dehydration becomes thirsty. An infant may cry without tears. Symptoms include dry mouth and nasal passages; an individual may have a flushed face; experience cramped limbs; he or she will become confused and have; and urinary output may decrease. Severe dehydration can produce low blood pressure leading to a loss of consciousness, a medical emergency.

Treatment. Mild dehydration is easily treated by drinking water. Before, during, and after strenuous exercise, a person should drink plenty of fluids and increase salt intake. People with heart or kidney problems should be especially careful and consult a physician before starting heavy exercise. In emergencies involving severe blood loss, dehydration, or shock, medical personnel will rapidly apply intravenous solutions of salt water.

Dehydration in infants is most often caused by vomiting, diarrhea, or inadequate fluid intake. Treatment regularly includes intravenous fluids and electrolytes. For treatment of slight dehydration, a non-prescription drink, such as Pedialyte, may be used to balance the infant's electrolytes, unless a pediatrician recommends otherwise. *See also* CRYING IN INFANTS.

Dental Emergencies

Situations of injury to or severe pain in the teeth.

Dental emergencies require immediate medical attention either because the pain is debilitating or because a slow response might result in infection, deformity or other complications.

Tooth Avulsion. A tooth that has been knocked out or badly loosened (avulsed) in an accident is treatable. The more immediately tended to, the better the chances are that the tooth or teeth will be reimplanted. The procedure involves attaching the tooth or teeth to surrounding teeth, or dental splinting; this is a process similar to placing a cast on a broken bone.

Fractured Tooth. Another dental emergency is a fractured tooth. Treatment varies, depending on the size and location of the break. A fracture in the lower portion of a tooth (root) is often repaired by dental splinting, but sometimes this is unsuccessful and the tooth is removed. Fractures in the upper part of the tooth (crown) receive fillings that prevent pain and infection. A fracture of this sort, that affects the inner nerve and blood vessels of the tooth, requires a root canal.

Broken jaw. If the jaw breaks, the parts are wired together, immobilizing them in order to heal. *See also* CAST.

Swelling, inflammation, and general pain in the mouth can be caused by toothache, dental abscesses, or gingivitis. Sometimes pain can be relieved simply by brushing and flossing. If these measures are insufficient, a visit to the dentist is usually necessary. *See also* DENTAL EXAMINATION; DENTAL X-RAY; RESTORATION, DENTAL; *and* SPLINTING, DENTAL.

Drowning

Death by suffocation in water or some other fluid.

When a person is subjected to prolonged immersion in water, death can be caused by suffocation and a lack of oxygen. Drowning can occur in two ways. In one instance, a

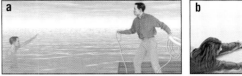
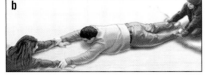

Drowning Assistance. There are several methods one can use when trying to rescue a drowning victim. (a) If available, toss a floating object to the drowning victim to keep them afloat until help arrives. Otherwise, try to offer an object such as a board, pole, or stick (c) to the victim and attempt to pull him or her out of the water. One should not place themselves at risk when rescuing a drowning victim, but as a last resort the human chain method (b) may be attempted.

person inhales liquid into the lungs. In the other, no liquid enters lungs, as the water is instead diverted into the stomach. In these cases, the drowning death is caused by oxygen deprivation; this is referred to as dry drowning. Near-drowning describes an event in which a drowning victim is resuscitated back to life. Drowning is the third leading cause of accidental death in the U.S., following auto accidents and falls.

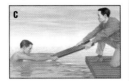

> ### Spinal Cord Damage
>
> Divers rescued from drowning in shallow water or surf might also be victims of spinal cord damage if they slipped and hit their head on a hard surface, or if the strength of the surf tossed them onto the floor of the ocean, resulting in head or neck injury. If a spinal cord injury is suspected, the swimmer should be moved as little as is necessary to restore breathing and should be kept still until medical assistance arrives.

Rescue. The best help for a drowning person comes from a trained lifeguard; a panicking swimmer can pull down an untrained rescuer. The person in danger should be given something—a rope, a large floating object, the end of an oar—to hold onto while the rescuer gets him or her ashore or into a boat.

Once the victim is on a firm surface, the rescuer should immediately check his or her breathing and pulse. It is important to remember that even a swimmer who has suffered cardiac arrest can sometimes be revived. Artificial ventilation or cardiopulmonary resuscitation should be provided as needed. Emergency medical technicians should be called as soon as possible; it is essential that all victims of drowning or near-drowning be taken to an emergency department. *See also* ACCIDENTS.

Drug Overdose

The accidental or deliberate ingestion of an excessive amount of a drug.

Deliberate and unintentional drug overdoses are a leading cause of poisoning and death in the U.S. The Food and Drug Administration decides which drugs are safe to be sold over-the-counter, and which require a prescription. Considerations for a given drug's safety include whether the drug can be harmful when taken by itself and whether it is habit-forming.

Legal drugs are usually safe when a recommended dosage is taken, but they can be dangerous if too much is consumed at once or if they are combined with other drugs. Some accidental medication overdoses occur because a patient believes that increasing the dosage will speed up or enhance the drug's effect. For patients prone to forgetfulness, the dosage should be written and highlighted on the label, so they can check it every time the medication is taken. Sometimes overdose occurs as a complication of kidney or liver malfunction, in which case the medication is not effectively processed and builds up in the bloodstream.

Illegal Drugs. The effects of illegal drugs vary; an overdose can cause unpredictable reactions. Because such drugs do not have to pass any regulations before they are sold, users may expose themselves to illegal drugs that have been mixed together or diluted with harmful substances.

Accidents. Children are at risk of accidental drug overdose, because they may not realize what they are consuming. It is important to keep drugs out of childrens' reach and in the proper containers; also talk to older children about drug safety.

Signs of a Drug Overdose. Indications of a drug overdose vary depending on the drug and the dosage. Symptoms include: abnormal breathing; slurred speech; lack of coordination; abnormal pulse rate; abnormal body temperature; enlarged or constricted pupils; sweating; drowsiness; convulsions; and hallucinations.

Drugs and Age

The elderly are particularly sensitive to drugs like barbiturates and benzodiazepines. Psychoactives and alcohol can lower the body temperature, and nonsteroidal anti-inflammatory drugs can cause gastrointestinal bleeding and kidney malfunction.

IN CASE OF AN EMERGENCY

If the victim is a child, his or her mouth should be checked for pills or other medication, which must be removed at once. If the victim is an adult and unconscious, make sure he or she is breathing. Act immediately if there is any sign of bluish coloring. The air passages should be checked for obstructions. Opening the air passageways to allow the person to breathe is essential. This is done by pushing on the forehead while pulling the jaw upward. This is also good preparation in case the victim is still not breathing and needs mouth-to-mouth resuscitation (artificial respiration). In addition to the air passages, it is important to check breathing, temperature, and pulse. Cardiopulmonary resuscitation (CPR) should be administered if necessary.

A poison control center should be called immediately. Information about the specific drug ingested is vital to determining proper treatment. Vomiting should not be induced unless it is specifically advised by the poison control center or a qualified health professional.

If a victim is conscious and hallucinating, convulsing, or breathing slowly and shallowly, emergency medical help should be called. Do not administer anything by mouth. *See also* ACCIDENTS *and* POISONING.

Ear, Foreign Body in

Matter in the ear that causes an obstruction.

Occasionally objects may become lodged in the outer-ear canal, either accidentally or by intent. Flies or insects may enter and then become trapped in the ear canal. During accidents, an object may be forced into the ear canal. Children frequently insert objects into their ears, such as small toys, beads, buttons, or stones. Small children also often force certain foods, such as peas, into their ears.

Treatment. If an insect has flown or crawled into the ear, a physician may have to remove it. An untrained person should not attempt to remove any type of matter from the ear canal. In these cases, the object should be left alone until a physician can attend to it. Do not attempt to remove foreign objects by flushing the ear with water, as that may cause some objects to swell. A trained physician can safely remove the object with a syringe, tiny forceps, or other specialized suction devices. Occasionally, anesthetic may be required for this procedure. *See also* EAR; EAR, DISORDERS OF;

Electrical Injury

Also Known as electrical shock

Injury to the skin or internal organs resulting from exposure to an electrical current.

The human body is an excellent conductor of electricity. Because of this, direct contact with an electric current is potentially fatal. While some resulting burns look minor, the shock is still capable of inflicting serious damage to internal organs.

An electric current can injure the body in three main ways. Cardiac arrest can result from the effect of an electric current on the heart. Massive muscle destruction can be caused from the current passing through the body. Finally, contact with the electrical source can cause thermal burns.

Incidence. In the U.S., about 1,000 people die annually of electric shock. Statistically, children under two have a slightly higher risk of electrical injury.

Cause. Electrical injury occurs through exposure to an electric current. Accidental contact with the exposed part of an electrical appliance or wiring; lightning; and contact with high-voltage electric lines are the common sources of electrical injury.

Symptoms. Electrical injury causes a diverse range of symptoms. Fatigue, headache, fracture, heart attack, muscle spasms, muscular pain, skin burns, unconsciousness, and loss of vision are some of the signs

that exposure to an electric current may have resulted in bodily injury.

Treatment. The first step in treatment is to insure that you are not at risk for shock. Having done so, if possible, try to remove the source of the electric current. Often, turning off an appliance will not stop the flow of electric current. The appliance must be unplugged, or the fuse removed from the fuse box. The immediate source of the current should not be touched. If the current cannot be turned off, a non-conducting object, such as a broom or rubber doormat, can be used to push the victim away from the source of the current. Call for medical help. Once the source of the electricity has been stopped, check for signs of breathing and a pulse. If either has stopped, CPR is necessary. Clothing should be removed from burned areas. The victim's head and neck should remain immobile in case internal or spinal injuries have been suffered.

Prevention. Simple measures can help to prevent exposure to electric current. Electrical appliances should not be used while showering or while wet. Never touch an electrical appliance while touching a faucet or water. Frayed or exposed wires should also never be touched and should be replaced to prevent fires. *See also* EAR.

Emergency Childbirth

The act of delivering a child without the supervision of a physician or midwife.

NECESSARY ITEMS FOR DELIVERY
- five-inch pieces of clean cloth
- sterilized scissors (boil to make sterile)
- bucket in case of vomiting
- container for afterbirth to be taken to the physician
- towels or sanitary napkins to place over the vagina following thE birth.

PREPARATION FOR DELIVERY
- **First.** Call the mother's obstetrician or gynecologist, or the nearest hospital for assistance. Do not delay the birth. It is important to remain calm and to assist the mother in whatever way possible.

• **Second**. Wash your hands and clean underneath the nails. Wash your hands repeatedly during the birth.

• **Third.** Prepare a clean, flat surface with a towel (use newspaper if necessary). If possible, prop up the mother up with pillows so her legs are bent and her feet flat.

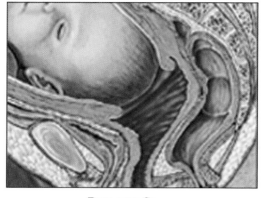

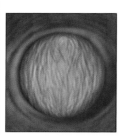

Emergency Childbirth. If the cervix becomes dilated to 10 cm (above), the pregnant woman begins to push out the baby (top left) and childbirth is imminent, whether the mother is in the delivery room or not. The mother may experience the urge to have a bowel movement due to the baby's head pushing against the rectum (far right).

DELIVERY STEPS

• **First.** Encourage the mother to breathe as much as possible. Once the delivery begins, support the baby's head with your hands as it comes into view. Any visible membrane over the face should be torn away and removed. CAUTION: If the umbilical cord is looped around the neck, ease it over the head to prevent breathing problems. DO NOT pull on the baby's head!

• **Second.** Support the shoulders and the head as the baby emerges further. Allow one shoulder to emerge first and the second should follow if you gently raise the baby's head.

• **Third.** Wipe clean any mucus or blood from the baby's mouth so he or she can breathe freely. Continue supporting the body as it emerges.

• **Fourth.** Once the baby is entirely out, check to make sure it is breathing properly. If he or she is unable to breathe, hold the head lower than the body to drain away excess mucus. Blowing onto the chest, or tapping the soles of the feet may also help.

DO NOT slap the baby's back to initiate breathing! If the infant is still unable to breathe, begin CPR and call emergency medical services immediately.

• **Fifth.** Allow the cord to stay connected to the mother. Once it ceases to pulsate, tie the cord four inches from the baby's navel.

• **Sixth.** Wrap the baby and place him or her with the mother.

• **Seventh.** Usually, the afterbirth follows ten minutes after the birth. Gently massaging the mother's abdomen will help control the flow of blood.

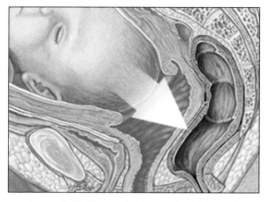

Breech Delivery. If the baby's head does not emerge first, gently press on the mother's abdomen directly above her pubic hair. Support the body of the baby as it emerges, and carefully lift it in the process, exposing the face so as to allow the infant to breathe. DO NOT pull or tug the infant under any circumstances. Clean out the baby's mouth with a towel once the face is outside of the mother. *See also* CHILDBIRTH *and* CHILDBIRTH, COMPLICATIONS.

Emergency Hospitalization

The treatment and care that an individual receives in a medical emergency.

Emergency departments are designed to deal with unexpected, life-threatening situations that require immediate medical attention, although people often go to the emergency room to treat relatively minor problems.

Triage. Once in the emergency department, patients who are the most severely ill or injured will be treated first. As a result of this need-based system of seeing patients (known as triage), someone with a minor problem may have to wait several hours to be examined. In addition to the wait, the cost of treatment in an emergency department can be as much as three times higher than that of a doctor's office. It can also be difficult to convince some HMOs to reimburse a patient for the costs of a visit to an emergency ward.

WHAT TO EXPECT

Upon arrival at the emergency room, unless you are severely ill or injured and require immediate attention, you will be interviewed by a staff member who will obtain personal and medical insurance information and have you sign treatment consent forms. After you are triaged, you will either be treated and released or admitted into the hospital for extensive care, depending on the nature of your injury.

Even if your life is not in immediate danger, there are still a number of symptoms that may require hospitalization. These include: severe bleeding (especially from an artery); loss of consciousness; pain; high fever; convulsions; difficulty breathing; severe headache; shock; weakness; and numbness in the extremities. All of these symptoms require emergency care, especially if the victim's physician is unavailable. *See also* DELIVERY; EMERGENCY CHILDBIRTH; *and* EMERGENCY, FIRST STEPS.

Epilepsy

A chronic nervous system disorder characterized by recurring seizures.

Seizures are characterized by a partial or complete loss of consciousness, generally accompanied by convulsions or uncontrolled movements. Seizures result from a breakdown in orderly communication between nerve cells (neurons). Neurons in the brain communicate by sending electrical signals back and forth in an orderly manner. During a seizure, electrical signals from one group of neurons become excessively strong and overwhelm neighboring neurons, resulting in a chaotic pattern.

In epilepsy, seizures are recurrent and are not caused by a non-neurological disorder, such as a fever. About one million people in the United States have epilepsy.

Causes. Scientists do not know why the brain sometimes misfires or why certain people are more prone to seizures than others. Two-thirds of people with epilepsy do not have a physical abnormality in the brain that appears to cause the seizures. The remaining third can link the seizures to a brain irregularity, brain damage at birth, head injury, stroke, brain tumor, infection such as meningitis or encephalitis, drug intoxication, or a metabolic imbalance. It is speculated that epilepsy may be genetically related.

Symptoms. The primary symptom of epilepsy is a seizure. There are two different classifications of seizures, generalized and partial. Generalized seizures affect most or all of the brain, influence the entire body, and produce a loss of consciousness. In contrast, partial seizures are caused by a misfiring of a smaller area of the brain and do not necessarily result in loss of consciousness. Many epileptics do not exhibit any symptoms between seizures. Some recognize when a seizure is imminent because of an aura, an often unpleasant feeling or hallucination that precedes an attack.

Generalized Seizure consist of grand mal and petit mal, or absence, seizures.

Grand mal seizures affect the entire body. The person may cry out and then fall to the ground. The muscles will first be rigid for a few moments and will then proceed to spasm. Breathing may be irregular or absent; if the seizure lasts for more than one or two minutes, there is danger of brain damage.

Status epilepticus is a type of grand mal seizure in which the convulsions do not cease, producing a medical emergency. It is accompanied by strong muscle contractions, rapid electrical discharge throughout the brain, and difficulty breathing. The patient must get medical help immediately to prevent brain damage or death.

Petit mal seizures are characterized by a temporary loss of consciousness without any abnormal behavior. They generally occur in children, usually before age five, and disappear after adolescence. A child may appear to be daydreaming but in reality loses awareness for a few seconds. Afterwards, the child continues as if nothing has happened. Petit mal seizures can occur countless times during a day and can impede a child's scholastic performance.

Partial seizures can be subdivided into simple seizures, in which the victim maintains consciousness, and complex seizures, in which the person loses consciousness.

Simple seizures occur when a chaotic electrical flow in an area of the brain remains confined. The accompanying symptoms are spasm-like movements, tingling of the skin, and hallucinatory sensations. The sufferer remains conscious. In a Jacksonian seizure, movements begin in a hand or foot and slowly travel up the body but remain on one side of the body. The seizure ends after a few minutes.

Complex seizures are characterized by a lack of awareness of surroundings for an interval of a minute or two. The sufferer may perform repeated movements, such as picking at clothes, wandering aimlessly, or babbling unintelligible sounds without conscious intent (automatism).

Treatment. Treatment begins with addressing abnormal conditions that are easily correctable, such as high or low blood sugar or sodium levels. At times, this is sufficient to eliminate or reduce seizures. If epileptic attacks persist, anticonvulsant drugs are prescribed to control these attacks; however, these drugs can cause marked drowsiness. A combination of more than one drug may be needed. Fifty percent of patients who successfully respond to anticonvulsant drug therapy can eventually suspend the treatment without relapse. Brain surgery is considered if drug therapy has failed and brain damage in the temporal lobe is the cause of the seizures.

Eye Injuries

Trauma to the eye, including foreign objects in the eye, chemical damage, and burns.

Injuries to the eye are almost always accompanied by pain or intense itching; some may impair vision. Bleeding, redness, or fluid discharge may occur. The person may become extremely sensitive to light and develop a headache. The pupils of the eye may appear to be different sizes.

Trauma. All trauma to the eye should receive treatment from trained medical personnel. Both eyes should be lightly covered until medical treatment occurs. Pressure should never be applied to the eye, and the victim should not rub the injured area. An object that has penetrated the eye should not be removed. Contact lenses should not be removed unless medical assistance is delayed.

Chemical Burns. If the eye has come into contact with chemicals, it should be flushed as quickly as possible with large amounts (at least three to five quarts) of saline solution or clean water. If a household chemical is involved, the label should contain emergency instructions. If no instructions are available, water should be used. Contact lenses should be removed after rinsing.

Burns. Eye burns may result from fireworks, gas explosions, or even sunlight or sunlamps. If the skin around the face has peeled or blistered, and sunglasses designed to filter out ultraviolet radiation have not been used, the eyes have probably been damaged. A cool compress gently placed over both eyes may reduce pain.

ALERT

First Aid for an Epileptic Seizure

- Do not restrain the person or attempt to put anything in his or her mouth.
- Do not move the person unless he or she is in danger of injuring himself/herself.
- Loosen the clothing around the neck and, if possible, move the head to one side so saliva can drain out of the mouth.
- When the attack has subsided, place the person in the recovery position.
- Remain with the person until he or she regains consciousness, and help reorient him or her.
- If the seizure lasts more than a couple of minutes or if the person does not regain consciousness, seek emergency medical help.

Emergency medical help should be contacted.

Abrasions. A scratch on the cornea may come from a foreign object in the eye or from rubbing the eye with a finger or fingernail. Contact lenses that trap an object under them or lenses that fit poorly and have been worn for too long may also damage the eye. The eye should be kept closed and should not be rubbed. Because all corneal abrasions carry the risk of deeper injury and infection, they should be examined by a medical professional.

Black Eye. With a black eye, purple bruising appears around the eye and on the eyelid from burst blood vessels. There may be swelling of the eyelid. Over time, the color changes to yellow and green. This is essentially an external injury, though frequently the eye itself is also injured. Cool compresses applied gently but immediately will reduce pain and swelling. Normally, a black eye will not require a doctor's attention unless there is continued pain, double vision, or light sensitivity, or if the discoloration does not subside in a few days.

Eye, Foreign Body in

An object that is touching or has entered the eye.

Any foreign object that has entered the eye can cause tearing, blurred vision, light sensitivity, or swelling of the eyelid. The white of the eye can become red and irritated. The object may scratch the eyeball's transparent tissue (cornea). Scratched eyes may become infected by bacteria.

WASHING THE EYE
Sometimes the eye's own tears are enough to wash away the object. If they do not, the eye should be flushed with clear water or saline solution for fifteen minutes. Contact lenses should be left in place. The head should be held to one side, and the eyelids held open, although the eye itself must not be touched. If both eyes are involved, the person may wish to use a shower, holding the face up to the shower head and allowing a gentle flow of water into the eyes. Alterna-

tively, the person may immerse his or her head in a large bowl of water until the eyes are covered. The eyes should remain open—blinking repeatedly may scratch the cornea.

REMOVING OBJECTS
Sometimes a foreign body can be removed. If the object is visible, it may be possible to remove it with a cotton swab or the corner of a clean cloth. However, too much pressure may cause the object to become more deeply embedded. **Removal of a foreign body should not be attempted if it is on the cornea. Never attempt to remove an object that is embedded in the eye.**

If the object cannot be removed easily, the entire eye should be covered with a light bandage, and medical attention should be sought. The doctor will examine the eye with a microscope and remove the object with a tweezer, needle, or other instrument. An antibiotic ointment will be applied to fight infection, and drops will be put into the eye to relax the muscle. An eye patch may be put in place to protect the eye from further injury and to keep the eyelid closed while it heals. If an object has penetrated the eye, it must be removed by an ophthalmologist.

Occasionally a small irritation, known as a stye, may swell into a bump on the inner surface of the eyelid; this may feel like a foreign object. The doctor will roll the eyelid

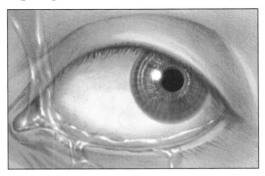

Eye, Foreign Body in. Left, when a foreign body irritates the eye, it generally causes pain, redness, tearing, and blepharospasm (uncontrollable eyelid contractions).

over a thin stick to examine the inner surface of the eyelid to see if a stye is responsible. An antibiotic ointment and rest, with an eye patch in place, usually eliminates this irritation. *See also* EYE, EXAMINATION OF; EYE INJURIES; *and* STYE.

Fever

An elevated body temperature, usually in response to an illness or infection.

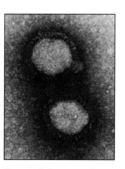

Fever. A fever can be caused by bacterial or viral infections such as influenza (above), or tonsillitis. In such cases, proteins called pyrogens are released when the body's white blood cells fight the microorganisms responsible for the illness. The proteins raise body temperature to try to destroy the invading microorganisms.

Body temperature is controlled by the hypothalamus, which acts as a natural thermostat, keeping temperature within a normal range. Normal body temperature ranges from 97° to 99°F, with an average of 98.6°F. Body temperature follows a 24 hour cycle, reaching its peak at around 4 P.M. and its lowest level in the early morning. During a fever, the hypothalamus works to maintain body temperature a few degrees above normal; after a fever breaks, the range returns to normal.

Causes. Fever is one of the body's generalized responses to infection. Substances that trigger a fever are known as pyrogens; they include bacteria and other microorganisms, as well as the toxins they produce. Body temperature becomes elevated during an illness, because microorganisms do not survive well in an environment that is too hot; the fever helps the body better fight infection. Therefore, it may not be necessary or even wise to try to bring a fever down quickly, unless body temperature rises to a dangerous level.

In addition to infection, fevers may be caused by dehydration, heat stroke, reactions to medication, autoimmune reactions, hormonal disorders, and cancer. They may also have no known cause.

Symptoms. A fever can often be felt as a warmth and flushing of the skin, as blood vessels near the surface of skin dilate to eliminate excess heat. A person with a fever may also experience chills.

A fever may regularly fluctuate, with temperature rising and falling in a regular pattern. This is accompanied by the alternating chills and flushing experienced in many illnesses. A spike occurs when temperature elevates sharply within a very short period of time. In small children, it is not uncommon for a fever to spike suddenly at the beginning of an illness.

When a fever breaks, the patient often sweats profusely, which helps to lower the temperature.

Treatment. Over-the-counter drugs such as aspirin, ibuprofen, and acetaminophen are effective at lowering a fever. Aspirin should not be given to children, because Reye's syndrome, a life-threatening condition, may develop in children with viral infections who have taken aspirin.

Cold compresses and sponging with lukewarm or cool (never cold) water can lower fever and make the patient feel more comfortable. A person with a fever should rest and drink plenty of fluids.

Febrile Seizures. A febrile seizure is a seizure caused by a fever. There is a brief period of unconsciousness and the seizure may be accompanied by convulsions.

Febrile seizures occur in approximately two to five percent of all children under the age of five. The tendency for febrile seizures runs in families. In most cases, a child prone to febrile seizures usually outgrows them.

Febrile seizures usually occur when the temperature is either falling or rising rapidly. If a serious disease such as meningitis or encephalitis has been ruled out and the period of unconsciousness lasts only a few minutes, the seizure should not be a major cause for concern.

Anticonvulsant medication may be prescribed to reduce the likelihood of future occurrences. *See also* DEHYDRATION.

ALERT
Emergency Situations

A fever is considered an emergency if it is accompanied by a severe headache, a stiff neck, severe swelling in the throat, or mental confusion.

A very high fever can also be an emergency. The temperature at which a fever becomes dangerous varies according to age:

- In infants from newborn to six months of age, a fever over 100.5°F is cause for concern, and above 101°F is serious.
- In children and adults, a fever of 103°F is serious, and a fever of 105°F or more is considered dangerous and potentially fatal.

If a fever is 101º F and persists for 3 days or more or if a low-grade fever persists for several weeks, a doctor should be consulted.

Fracture

An injury that causes a break in a bone.

A fracture occurs when more force or pressure is applied to a bone than it can bear. The force may come from a direct blow or torsion applied to the bone. The weight of a person's own body can cause a fracture if the person steps or falls at an angle at which bone must suddenly bear the weight of the whole body.

TYPES

The speed, angle, and weight of the responsible object determines just how the bone will break. Bones usually break at an angle, but they may also split lengthwise from torsion. Fractures are organized into two categories, closed and open. Within these two main categories are many different types of fracture.

Closed (or simple) fractures are fractures in which the broken bone remains below the skin. Because the surface has not been breached, there is little chance of infection.

Open (or compound) fractures occur when the ends of the bones break through the surface of the skin and are exposed. In these cases, there is a great risk of infection, as the bones and tissues are exposed to the typically nonsterile environment.

Spiral fractures are caused by twisting of the bones, such as those that may occur in skiing accidents.

Transverse fractures are horizontal breaks directly across the bone. Stress fractures, which are caused by a repetitive, damaging motion, such as running or jumping, are usually transverse.

Greenstick fractures, usually the result of sudden force, are characterized by a splintering of the top layer of the bone; they resemble a piece of bark peeled from a tree. They are most common in children.

Comminuted fractures are those in which the bone shatters into fragments. Comminuted fractures are caused by severe force, such as that experienced in a car accident.

SYMPTOMS

The following signs suggest a fracture:
- A limb that is visibly deformed or out of place—an open fracture is obvious as the ends of the bone can be seen;
- Limited movement, or movement that intensifies the pain;
- Swelling;
- Tenderness;
- Bruising;
- Inability to bear weight.

Even if a fracture is not immediately obvious, a doctor should be consulted. A break that is not easily detectable can still heal incorrectly and cause problems in the future if it is left to heal on its own.

TREATMENT

Bones begin to heal very rapidly, so it is important that a fracture be treated by a physician in order to ensure that the bones heal in the correct position. Until a physician can be reached, however, the following temporary measures may be taken:
- The injured person should be moved as little as possible;
- If the person must be moved, the affected area should be splinted in order to immobilize it;
- The injured person should not be given food or water; this can impede the function of anesthetia if surgery is deemed necessary.

The first thing a doctor will do to treat a fracture (usually after x-rays) is to move the bone ends back together; this process is called a closed reduction. A splint or cast may be applied after the closed reduction. If an operation is necessary, then it is called an open reduction. After an open reduction, the injured area must be immobilized so that the bones will stay in place as they heal. This may be done with a plaster cast. In more serious cases, pins or screws may have to be inserted to stabilize the bone.

When a bone heals, a blood clot is first formed to seal the ends of the blood vessels. Thus, for a period of time, painkillers that inhibit the clotting of blood should not be given to patients with bone fractures. After the ends of the blood vessels

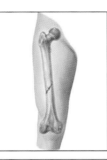
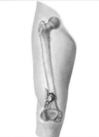
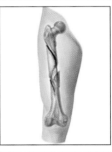
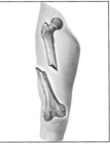

Fracture. Above, a fracture is a break in a bone commonly caused by a fall. A bone is usually broken across its width, but it can also be broken lengthwise, obliquely, or spirally.

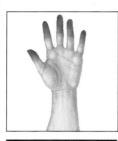

Frostbite. Above, frostbite is damage to the fingers, toes, nose, and ears caused by extremely cold temperatures—below 32°F (0°C).

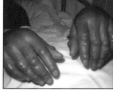

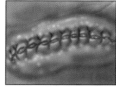

Gangrene. Gangrene is the death of body tissue caused by poor blood supply to the area. Above, top, a normal wound can be contrasted with a gangrenous wound, above, bottom. The first sign of gangrene is generally a reddening of the dying tissue.

are sealed, the body begins to dispose of any debris from the break that is left in the injured area, and a mesh-like layer forms between the bone ends to provide a base for the new bone. A callus of new bone then fills into the fracture and bone ends, and over a period of weeks denser and stronger bone with calcium builds on top.

Bone grafts may be necessary if the bone ends cannot meet adequately. If a bone heals incorrectly, surgery may be needed to rebreak and reset the bone so it can heal properly.

REHABILITATION

A fracture takes a number of weeks to heal. During the healing period, the injured area must remain immobilized. Depending on the severity and location of the break, physical therapy may be necessary to restore strength and movement in the injured area. *See also* AMPUTATION; BONE; SPORTS MEDICINE; PHYSICAL THERAPY; SPRAIN; STRAIN; *and* TRAUMA.

Frostbite

Damage to the skin and underlying tissue caused by exposure to extreme cold.

Symptoms. Frostbite is distinguished by the cold, hard, pale appearance of skin that has been exposed to cold for an extended period of time. The area may feel numb, but there is also usually a sharp, aching pain. Any part of the body may get frostbite, but the hands, feet, nose, and ears are the most commonly affected areas.

The first symptom of frostbite is usually a "pins and needles" sensation, followed by numbness. The skin is hard and has no feeling. As the affected area thaws, the skin will become red and painful. While the area is warming, it is common to feel pain and tingling, a sensation called chilblains or pernio. In severe cases of frostbite, blisters may appear. Frostbite is often found in conjunction with hypothermia, a lowering of the body's core temperature. Symptoms of hypothermia include slurred speech, shivering, and memory loss.

Treatment. Rapid warming of the affected area is recommended. The affected area should not be rubbed with snow, as this may cause further damage to the area. Affected areas should be rested and protected from any trauma. EMTs should be contacted quickly.

Risk Factors. People who take beta-blockers, which decrease blood flow to the skin, are particularly susceptible to frostbite. People with atherosclerosis—thickening and hardening of the arteries—are also at high risk. Other factors that increase the chances of frostbite include smoking, exposure to windy weather, diabetes mellitus, and peripheral neuropathy or Raynaud's phenomenon. *See also* AMPUTATION; ATHEROSCLEROSIS; PERNIO; SKIN; *and* TRAUMA.

Gangrene

Damage or death of body tissue due to poor blood supply.

Any injury, surgical wound, or disease that restricts or stops the flow of blood to tissue can cause the tissue to die. This process is called gangrene. Injuries that occur on the body's surface, such as bedsores, chemical and deep burns, and frostbite, can result in gangrene. Decreased blood-flow within the body can also result in gangrene.

Types. "Dry" gangrene is usually associated with diabetes or arteriosclerosis. Gangrene complicated by bacterial infection is considered "moist" or "wet," and is not as common as dry gangrene.

SYMPTOMS

One of the earliest signs of either type of gangrene is a reddening of the dying tissue. Initially, dry gangrene is painful, but the area becomes increasingly numb. The skin turns purple and then black. Moist gangrene may begin with blisters and swelling. The infection spreads quickly, causing bruise-like discolorations as the tissue dies. The infection may also release a foul smell, and immediate hospitalization is necessary to treat the condition.

Treatment. Antibiotics are administered as soon as gangrene is suspected. Damaged tissue must be removed surgically. Individuals suffering from moist gangrene may be put into a hyperbaric chamber, in which oxygen under pressure helps to kill the bacteria causing the infection.

> *Background material on gangrene can be found in* INFECTION. *For further information, see* ATROPHY; COMPLICATION; *and* DIABETES MELLITUS. *See also* AMPUTATION *and* DEATH *for more on possible consequences if a severe case of gangrene is left untreated.* ANTIBIOTIC DRUGS *and* SURGERY *contains information about treatment of this condition.*

Head Injury

> **Damage to the scalp, skull, or brain as a result of a blow to the head.**

Head injuries may occur as a result of any blow to the head. In minor head injuries, the skull protects the brain from damage. A significant blow to the head may fracture the skull or cause brain damage. In addition, injured blood vessels in the brain can bleed (hemorrhage), and significant brain damage can result.

CONCUSSION

A concussion is a form of injury to the brain that is sometimes associated with a brief loss of consciousness. Symptoms of a concussion may include loss of memory, dizziness, nausea, and headache.

Progressively worsening symptoms may indicate a more serious head injury, and medical attention should be sought.

SKULL FRACTURES

Skull fractures may damage arteries and veins, causing bleeding around the tissue of the brain. The fractures may allow foreign material into the brain, leading to bacterial infection.

SERIOUS INJURIES

More serious injuries result in damage to the brain itself. Bruising or tearing of brain tissue can result in permanent loss of brain function. Pools or clots of blood be-tween the brain and the skull can put pressure on the brain, causing swelling and destruction of brain tissue. Symptoms such as severe headache, dizziness, repeated vomiting, visual changes, pupils of different sizes, and diminished consciousness may indicate serious head injury; anyone who exhibits such symptoms requires immediate medical treatment.

Brain damage may be indicated by an extended loss of consciousness, followed by memory loss (amnesia) of the period before or after the injury . The longer the period of unconsciousness or memory loss, the more severe the damage may be. Damage to the brain may result in symptoms such as muscular weakness (paralysis), speech impairment (aphasia), or changes in mental capabilities or personality.

Treatment. Patients who become dizzy or unconscious should be placed under medical supervision. Blood clots and severe skull fractures, which can be life-threatening, require surgical repair. Serious, progressive brain damage along with loss of consciousness always requires emergency intervention, of-ten involving life support and surgery.

> ## Preventing Vehicular Head Injury
>
> The most effective means of preventing severe head injuries caused by car and motorcycle accidents is by wearing a seatbelt in a car and wearing a helmet when riding a motorcycle or bicycle. These measures can prevent or minimize head injuries in case of an accident. Many states have enacted mandatory seatbelt and helmet laws.

Prognosis. The survival rate of patients who have had major head injury has improved. However, some head injuries cause permanent physical or mental incapacity or personality changes. There is also an increase in the chance of seizures after a head injury. Recovery can be slow; improvement can take years after injury.

> *Background material on head injury can be found in* ACCIDENTS *and* HEADACHE. *For related information, see* APHASIA; BLEEDING; BRAIN, DISORDERS OF; CONCUSSION; CONFUSION; EPILEPSY; PARALYSIS; *and* SKULL, FRACTURED.

Head, Neck, and Back Injuries

Injuries in areas vital to human function.

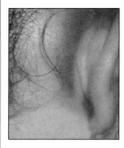

Head Injury. Skull fractures are commonly found in children and are caused by abuse or accidents. At left, Battle's sign appears several days following a fracture at the base of the skull. Blood may have come from the ear soon after the fracture.

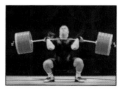

Head, Neck, and Back Injuries. Head, neck, and back injuries can be caused by improper form during heavy lifting. Above, a weight lifter at the 2000 Olympics shows proper form, which can help prevent this type of injury.

The head, neck, and back contain the central nervous system—the brain and spinal cord. Falls, sports injuries, and other traumas can cause damage to these areas.

A severe blow to the head can fracture the skull, causing brain damage and amnesia. Prolonged unconsciousness can cause paralysis and brain damage. The survival rate after major head injury has improved, but recovery is slow.

An injury at birth or skin contracture—shrinkage of scar tissue owing to burns or injuries—can cause wryneck, or torticollis, where the head is permanently twisted to one side. Paralysis or death may result from dislocations, fractures, or whiplash of neck vertebrae. Strangulation can cut off breathing and blood flow, while lacerations to the jugular vein or carotid artery can cause serious blood loss or death.

Severe injury to the spine may cause paralysis. Heavy lifting and carrying, prolonged sitting in the workplace, and obesity can cause muscle pulls and tears, ligament strains, and spinal or nerve damage, mak-

For background information on head, neck, and back injuries, see BRAIN; CENTRAL NERVOUS SYSTEM; *and* SPINAL CORD. *Further information can be found in* FRACTURES AND DISLOCATIONS; OBESITY; PARALYSIS; *and* TORTICOLLIS.

ing life a daily struggle.

Heart Attack

Also known as a myocardial infarction

The death of heart tissue caused by interruption of the supply of oxygen-rich blood to the heart.

The immediate cause of a heart attack is the blockage of a narrowed coronary artery. The section of heart muscle that loses its blood supply can die in minutes. The risk to a person's life depends largely on which part of the heart is affected. Death of tissue that controls the electric impulse system (heartbeat) can precipitate lethal heart rhythm irregularities. If a less vital part of the heart muscle is affected, survival is possible, even if 30 percent or more of the heart muscle dies.

SYMPTOMS

Chest pain is perhaps the most noticeable symptom of a heart attack, but chest pain can occur in different ways: as a severe, crushing feeling in the center of the chest; as a persistent but dull ache; or as pain that spreads from the chest to the shoulders and sometimes to the arms, neck, and jaw. Chest pain is occasionally ignored by patients because it is similar to the symptoms of indigestion. In some cases, a heart attack

ALERT

Heart Attack Warning Signs

Every year thousands of deaths can be prevented by heeding the warning signs of heart attack. Often, people believe discomfort will pass and the waiting costs them their lives. Others either fail to recognize the signs or consider them not severe enough to warrant a visit to the doctor. Know the many forms a heart attack can take. Anyone suffering from any of the following symptoms must receive emergency medical treatment as soon as possible: crushing or squeezing pain in the chest beneath the sternum (breastbone); chest pain and vomiting or nausea; chest pain and a cold sweat or damp, sticky skin; chest pain and pale, blue skin, especially around the lips; chest pain and extreme anxiety—a feeling of imminent death; pain that spreads from the chest into the arm, neck, back, shoulders, or jaw; lightheadedness, dizziness, breathlessness, giddiness, or fainting; and a heartbeat that feels strange or out of sync.

can occur without pain.

Other symptoms of a heart attack include cold sweats, dizziness, or weakness (sometimes enough to cause fainting); nausea and vomiting; shortness of breath; and a shallow, irregular pulse. When these symptoms occur, medical help should be sought at once by calling 911. Prompt treatment can be life-saving and can limit the damage to the heart. While quick treat-

covery, the best source of medical help is a hospital emergency department that is associated with an intensive care unit specializing in cardiovascular crises.

Emergency Balloon Angioplasty

A newer treatment for a heart attack is an emergency balloon angioplasty. In this procedure, a thin tube, called a catheter, with a balloon at its end is threaded through a blood vessel (in a process called cardiac catheterization) to the site of the blockage. Then the balloon is inflated to reopen the blocked artery. Balloon angioplasty is widely used in non-emergency treatment for narrowed coronary arteries, although many medical centers are now using it during the actual heart attack.

DIAGNOSIS AND TREATMENT

The diagnosis of a heart attack may require an electrocardiogram that shows abnormal electrical activity of the heart, as well as blood tests that can detect the molecules secreted by dying heart cells.

In the most severe cases, if the heart is fibrillating, normal rhythm can be restored by transmitting an electrical impulse from a defibrillator to the heart muscle through electrodes held to the chest. If the heart has stopped, emergency department personnel will try to maintain the pumping action by performing cardiopulmonary resuscitation (CPR) and administering various medications. Because most heart attacks are caused by blood clots, patients will often be treated with reperfusion therapy, which may involve the injection of thrombolytic (clot-dissolving) drugs into a vein, or a direct intervention, such as balloon angioplasty performed via cardiac catheterization. Experience has shown that thrombolytic therapy can dissolve clots and salvage heart tissue if it is given in the first few minutes or even hours after a heart attack occurs. In addition to thrombolytic agents, the patient will also be given aspirin and heparin, both of which are drugs that reduce clotting in the body.

PROGNOSIS

After emergency department treatment, patients usually go to a coronary care unit

ALERT

Heart Attack Risk Factors

Each year, 1.5 million Americans suffer heart attacks, and more than 500,000 of these people die. Smoking, an unhealthy diet, obesity, and lack of exercise place people at serious risk for a heart attack. The most important fact about heart attack symptoms is that 60 percent of deaths occur before a patient reaches a hospital. Sometimes this happens because death is sudden, but often treatment is not sought in time because the symptoms of a heart attack are not recognized or are ignored.

(CCU), an area of the hospital staffed by specially trained doctors, nurses, and technicians. A CCU will have electrocardiogram equipment and a variety of devices that allow for a minute-by-minute monitoring of the patient's condition. This equipment will recognize any heart irregularities and sound an alarm. The CCU will also be equipped with defibrillators and other lifesaving equipment will be on hand for immediate use.

Patients typically stay in a CCU for several days, until the heart and other vital organs are functioning regularly. At that point, the patient may be moved to a regular hospital room. The duration of the hospital stay for a heart attack victim depends on the degree of damage detected by electrocardiograms, blood tests, cardiac stress tests, and other diagnostic procedures.

A second heart attack can occur in up to 25 percent of first heart attack patients. If the risk is high, bypass surgery or balloon angioplasty may be performed to maintain blood flow to the heart.

Full recovery from a heart attack usually takes several months. A rehabilitation program to enable restoration of normal or near-normal activity, accompanied by drug treatment that can include aspirin, heparin, and beta-blockers, is successful in a large percentage of cases.

Background material on heart attack can be found in CARDIOLOGY; CIRCULATORY SYSTEM; and HEART. For further information, see CARDIAC ARREST; CARDIAC STRESS TEST; ECG; HEART DISORDERS; HEART FAILURE; HEART IMAGING; THROMBOSIS; and VENTRICLE. See also ANGIOPLASTY, BALLOON and DEFIBRILLATION for more on treatment options.

Heat Exhaustion

Excessive sweating and a drop in blood pressure as a result of exposure to high heat conditions over a period of time.

Heat exhaustion usually follows a period of strenuous exercise in hot weather when fluids in the body are not replaced. Salt lost through sweating is also a factor, upsetting the balance of sodium and potassium in the blood stream and compromising brain function. The elderly are particularly vulnerable to heat exhaustion, as are chronic alcoholics, the obese, and those taking medications such as antihistamines and antipsychotic drugs.

Symptoms of heat exhaustion include: fatigue; weakness; hot, dry, and flushed skin; nausea; dizziness; and headache. The pulse is slow and weak. Breathing is rapid and shallow. The victim may be confused and may faint or act irrationally.

Treatment is aimed at cooling the affected person and replacing lost fluids. Shade, air conditioning, a cool wet towel, and immersion in cool water are all means of treatment. The victim should be given sport drinks, electrolyte beverages, or a small amount of salt dissolved in water. Emergency medical personnel may provide fluids and salt directly into the blood stream (intravenously). Recovery is usually rapid. *See also* FIRST AID *and* HEAT STROKE.

Heat Stroke

A body temperature high enough to incapacitate the body's cooling mechanisms.

Heat stroke is the most severe of the heat-related syndromes. It results from excessive exposure to very high temperatures and is accelerated by heavy exertion and direct sunlight. Especially on very humid days, the victim cannot sweat enough to reduce body temperature. Diabetes, alcoholism, vomiting, and diarrhea add to the risk of heat stroke in hot weather.

Symptoms of heat stroke include a body temperature of above 105°F, headache, ver-

tigo, and fatigue. The affected individual does not sweat. The skin is red, hot, and dry. The pulse is weak and rapid, breathing becomes fast and shallow, and the pupils are often dilated. The victim is likely to be confused and may experience convulsions and lose consciousness. Heat stroke can be fatal if left untreated.

Preventing Heat Stroke

Heat stroke is a potentially dangerous medical situation. The following simple measures can help to prevent heat stroke:

- Do not leave a child or elderly person in a closed, parked car during hot weather.
- Do not leave an elderly person in a closed room or apartment without air conditioning during summer heat waves.
- At the first signs of heat exhaustion, move to a shady area and drink cool liquids.
- Do not exercise during the hottest times of the day (between 12 and 3 PM).
- Wear light, loose-fitting clothing and a hat.
- Drink lots of liquids and monitor urine color. Urine should be clear or light yellow. Sip often; do not drink large quantities at once.
- Limit time in a hot tub or sauna to fifteen minutes during summer months.
- Limit consumption of alcoholic beverages or caffeinated beverages in hot weather.
- Do not wrap an infant in blankets or heavy clothing in hot weather, as the cooling system of infants is not fully developed.

Treatment and Recovery. If the temperature of a victim of heat stroke is not reduced quickly, permanent brain damage may result. The victim should be wrapped in cool wet sheets or immersed in cool water. Emergency medical assistance (911) should be called immediately. The body temperature should be monitored constantly to make sure it is not lowered too far. Drugs may be administered to control convulsions that may occur. The body temperature of the victim may vary erratically for days or even weeks afterward.

For background material on heat stroke, see FEVER; HEAT DISORDERS; *and* HEAT EXHAUSTION. *Further information can be found in* EMERGENCY FIRST STEPS; FIRST AID; HEADACHE; SEIZURE; *and* TEMPERATURE. *See also* ELDERLY, CARE OF THE *and* INFANT *for more on high risk groups.*

Heimlich Maneuver

Method for clearing an obstruction from the air passages.

The Heimlich maneuver is only applied to a conscious adult or child older than one year of age with complete airway obstruction. Patients with complete airway obstructions will be unable to speak and may use the universal sign of choking, placing their hands around their throats. If these signs are present, the victim should be approached from behind and "hugged" be-low the ribs, just above the navel. With one fist grasped by the other hand, five thrusts are delivered in quick succession, pulling inward and slightly upward. The thrusts should be firm and sharp. If the obstruction is not removed, the process is repeated. If the airway is cleared and the victim is not breathing, emergency help must be called and artificial respiration must be administered immediately.

A child victim requires gentler thrusts. If the victim is an infant, he or she should be held face down with one hand supporting the chest, and the head held slightly lower than the body. With the heel of the other hand, the child should be struck between the shoulder blades five times in quick succession. If this does not clear the obstruction, the baby should be turned on his or her back. Using the forefinger and second finger, five thrusts should be made to the breastbone. If the object can be seen, it should be removed. If not, careful attention should be paid not to push the object further down the throat. Emergency help should always be summoned.

Hypothermia

Dangerously low body temperature.

Hypothermia is the condition in which the body is incapable of maintaining a temperature greater than 95˚F. Individuals with poor circulation, such as those with diabetes and the elderly, congenital heart failure, and alcoholics, are especially susceptible. Prolonged exposure to icy water, or exposure to envi-

ronments with cool temperatures and high humidity (especially when coupled with drinking alcoholic beverages in such settings), can cause hypothermia.

Symptoms. The onset of hypothermia is slow and subtle. A person's reaction time slows; the or she may become confused, loose coordination, and may even begin to have hallucinations. The affected person often becomes sleepy and unmotivated. For example, if hypothermia sets in while a person is in icy water, he or she may cease trying to swim or struggle and simply drown. In the most extreme cases, the muscles can become rigid, heartbeat can become irregular, and the person with hypothermia becomes drowsy and has difficulty speaking. If help is not provided, the person soon becomes unconscious, lapses into a coma, and may die.

Treatment. Whenever possible, move the victim to a warm environment; all wet clothing should be removed and replaced with warm, dry clotting. The victim should be wrapped in a blanket. If he or she is awake and alert, warm beverages, without caffeine or alcohol, may be given. If he or she is not breathing and has no pulse, cardiopulmonary resuscitation (CPR) should be administered, and emergency help should be summoned immediately *See also* CARDIOPULMONARY RESUSCITATION (CPR); COLD INJURY; FIRST AID; FROSTBITE TREATMENT; MUSCLE; *and* TRAUMA.

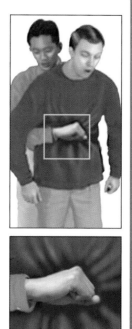

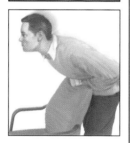

Heimlich Maneuver. Above, top, a choking adult should be firmly grasped around the abdomen from behind. A fist should be placed just under the breast bone, and pulled up and in quickly to dislodge the blockage. If the object is not dislodged, chest compressions should be given. Bottom, if choking when alone, a person should thrust his or her body weight on the back of a chair.

Insect Stings

Perforation of the skin by stinging insects such as wasps, bees, yellow jackets, ants, and hornets.

A small number of stinging insects are known to attack humans. While stings of wasps, ants, bees, yellow jackets, and other insects are often painful, they are by and large not a serious risk to health. It's not the piercing of the skin, but the insect's injection of a swelling and irritation–inducing liquid (venom) that causes pain. This discomfort is usually minor and lasts one to two days. However, some people exhibit severe allergic reactions in addition to the characteristic swelling, redness, and discomfort normally associated with such stings. In cases of allergy, these individuals may experience anaphylactic shock, a potentially life-threatening condition.

Bees and Wasps. In the U.S., bee and wasp stings are common. In general, a person may withstand ten such stings per pound of body weight without risk of serious complication. Attacks involving multiple stings can cause circulatory collapse or cardiac arrest. Those with severe allergy to such stings may lapse into anaphylactic shock from a single sting. Certain aggressive species of bee, such as the Africanized honeybee, or killer bee, pose another threat due to their tendency to attack in swarms with little provocation.

Fire ants produce painful, occasionally fatal stings and are common to the American South. Such stings produce immediate pain, followed by swelling and blistering. When the blister ruptures, often after 30 to 70 hours, a secondary infection may develop and in some cases the entire limb may swell. Fire-ant stings are likewise capable of inducing anaphylactic shock, which acts to constrict the air passages and lower blood pressure, although this reaction occurs in fewer than one percent of cases.

Treatment. Bees, fire ants, and wasps may leave a stinger embedded in the skin following attack. Care must be taken to gently remove the stinger without squeezing it, which will inject more venom into the skin. Scraping with a dull table knife or credit card against the skin next to the embedded stinger will help to remove it. Tweezers should be avoided. Ice may be applied to reduce the pain. Antihistamine or corticosteroid cream is helpful in reducing swelling and for pain relief. It is critical that the area be repeatedly washed during the healing process to avoid infection. Consult a physician if an infection develops.

Allergy Alert. Individuals known to have allergies to stinging insects should carry allergy kits including antihistamines and syringes for injecting epinephrine to improve breathing and circulation. Symptoms of (whole-body) reaction to insect stings include nausea; hives; facial swelling; shortness of breath and wheezing; difficulty swallowing; light-headedness and fainting; chest and throat tightness; and swell- ing or redness over most of the body. The onset of symptoms can occur anywhere from within minutes to several hours later. A doctor should be contacted immediately. *See also* ALLERGY.

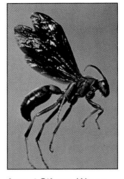

Insect Stings. Wasps, shown above, are not known to carry human diseases, but allergic reactions to their venom and the venom of insects such as yellow jackets, and bees, can cause reactions in humans ranging from mild to fatal.

Loss of Consciousness

A state of being unable to respond to external stimuli resulting from reduced brain activity.

Someone who has lost consciousness may be suffering from something as minor as fainting, or as serious as a stroke. Unconsciousness can result from injuries to the head, shock, a loss of blood to the brain, hypotemia (too little oxygen in the blood), hypoglycemia (too little sugar in the blood), or other chemical changes, or drug overdoses or exposure to toxins.

The first step in dealing with an unconscious victim is to check the victim's airways to make sure he or she is breathing. If the victim is not breathing, remove any obstruction from the airways and begin artificial respiration or CPR if necessary. Call for medical help, but try not to leave the unconscious person unattended. Do not give food or drinks to anyone who is unconscious. *See also* DRUG OVERDOSE; FIRST AID; SHOCK; *and* STROKE.

Nosebleed

Bleeding from inside the nose.

Nosebleeds can occur frequently and without apparent injury. They are usually not an indication of a serious problem, but in rare cases may indicate that there is an urgent disorder.

Causes. Nosebleeds are more likely to occur in the dry winter months when the humidity is low and when mucous membranes are dry and brittle, cracked, or split. Persistent nosebleeds may result from poor blood clotting or a blood disease such as hemophilia.

Treating Nosebleeds at Home

A person with a nosebleed should remain calm and sit with his or her head tiled forward slightly (to prevent the blood from draining back into the throat), breathing from the mouth. If there is nothing caught in the nostrils, they should be held shut, and a cold compress should be applied for five or ten minutes. If there is something caught in the nostril, the clear nostril should be pinched shut, and the person should breathe in through his or her mouth and blow out gently through the nose. Once the obstructing object has been removed, pressure and a cold compress should be applied to the area. If the bleeding continues for more than half an hour, medical attention should be sought.

Nosebleeds frequently result from minor trauma; such as a blow or when a child puts a finger or an object in his or her nose and breaks the fragile blood vessels. Such nosebleeds generally occur in the forward part of the nasal passages and can be treated at home. Nosebleeds originating deeper in the nasal passages can bleed "backwards" down the throat. They are, as a consequence, more serious.

When a person is taking a blood thinning medication, such as coumadin or heparin, or regular doses of aspirin, the blood may not clot properly. To stop a nosebleed, a doctor may apply a blood clotting agent to the bleeding area or apply cauterization. Packing the bleeding nostril with gauze or sponge will generally control the bleeding,

but should only be done by trained medical personnel. *See also* ANTICOAGULANT DRUGS; ASPIRIN; *and* HEMOPHILIA.

Poison Ivy, Oak, & Sumac

Three plants that cause contact dermatitis, or an itchy rash, due to an allergic reaction to their oils.

In and of themselves, these three plants are relatively harmless, however, more than 50 percent of all people are allergic to the oils that they produce. These oils produce a rash that usually takes the form of patches or streaks spread out across the skin that has been exposed. A rash may take a matter of some time to appear, or be recognized, so affected areas are often unknowingly scratched, spreading the oils and the rash all over the body. The longest time a dermatitis may take to become evident is a day or two. About a week later, the rash is at its worst, and may require hospitalization for a short period of time.

Poison ivy is found all over the continental United States; poison oak is generally indigenous to the west coast, and poison sumac tends to grow around the Mississippi river bed. Symptoms for all three are nearly indistinguishable.

Treatment. First scrub the exposed skin with soap and water to remove any remaining oils; wash hands and nails frequently because itching spreads the rash. Do not scratch the rash. Calamine lotion and commercial hydrocortisone creams may relieve itching. If the rash is severe, covering most of the body or areas around the eyes or genitals, consult a doctor. *See* DERMATITIS.

Poisoning

The introduction of a poisonous substance into the body.

Poisoning results from any of a variety of substances entering the body. These substances may enter the body through various means, such as inhalation, skin absorption (merely by touching the substance), ingestion, or injection.

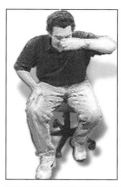

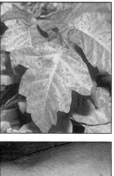

Nosebleed. To treat a nosebleed, sit down and lean forward slightly (above, top). Pinch the nostrils closed and breathe through the mouth (above, bottom) until the bleeding has stopped.

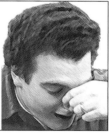

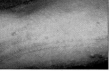

Poisonous Plants. Above top, poison sumac a plant that produces an oil that most people are allergic to. The Allergy is manifested in a red rash, above bottom, on the area of the body that has been affected.

See Poison and Toxicity *for a discussion on the foundations of poisoning. Details on specific types of poison will be found in* Drug Overdose; Drug Poisoning; Food Poisoning; Lead Poisoning; Pesticides; Phosphorus Poisoning; Poisonous Plants; Ptomaine Poisoning; Strychnine Poisoning; *and* Toxic Shock Syndrome.

Keeping Children Safe

There are several measures that parents can take to safeguard against accidental poisoning in the home. Store all cleaners, chemicals, and medicines out of children's reach or in locked cabinets. Some decorative plants that people bring into their homes have poisonous properties. If there are small children in the house, these plants should either be removed or kept in a high place. See Plants, Poisonous for a list of potentially dangerous plants.

Almost 95 percent of poisoning deaths occur in adults, a large number of whom poison themselves or overdose as a means of attempting suicide; incidence is high among young adults. However, over half of all poisoning cases, involve small children, usually under the age of six. If poisoning is suspected, immediately call for emergency medical help. A regional poison control center can provide vital information.

Indications that poisoning has occurred, in both children and adults, may include burns around the mouth and on clothing, chemical stains in the area near the victim, chemical odor on the victim's breath or open medicine bottles. Symptoms may include vomiting, convulsions, breathing difficulties, and unconsciousness.

If poisoning is suspected, the following procedures are recommended:

- Call for emergency medical help, and/or consult and a poison control center. The number of your poison control center should be kept by the telephone at all times. The poison control center will provide you with detailed first aid instructions.
- If the poisonous substance is known, check for any first aid instructions written on the label. Follow these instructions if the poison control center cannot be reached quickly.
- Never induce vomiting unless instructed by a poison control center or a physician. If so instructed, vomiting may be induced with syrup of ipecac.
- Carefully remove any clothing that may have poison on it and flush affected eyes and skin with cool or lukewarm water.

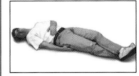

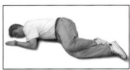

Recovery Position.
The photos at left show the correct recovery position an injured person should be placed in to allow free breathing, blood circulation, and a comfortable rest until medical assistance arrives.

Recovery Position

First aid position designed to allow free breathing.

If a person has been in an accident or is unconscious but shows no obvious injury, it is safest to put the individual in the recovery position until emergency medical assistance arrives.

The recovery position is designed to allow free breathing and vomiting without clogging air passages. It assists in blood circulation and allows the victim to rest comfortably. A victim suspected to have suffered head, neck, or spinal injury should never be moved. The recovery position should not be utilized, and individuals should wait until medical personnel arrive.

Placing the Victim in the Recovery Position. Assuming the victim is on his or her back, the emergency caregiver should kneel beside the body, turning the victim's face toward the him- or herself. The victim's head should be tilted back to open the airway, and false teeth or any other obstructions should be removed from the mouth. The arm of the victim that is closest to the caregiver should be placed by the victim's side and tucked under the buttock. The other arm should lay across the victim's chest. The far leg is then lifted over the near leg so that the legs cross at the ankle. Supporting the head and grasping the clothing at the hip, the victim should be rolled toward the caregiver until the individual is on his or her stomach. However, the head should be controlled so that the face is clear of foreign objects and turned in the same direction as the body. The near arm and leg should be adjusted so that they form a right angle to the body, preventing the victim from rolling onto his or her face. Lastly, the far arm and leg should be adjusted so that they are straight and parallel to the body. *See also* Emergency First Steps.

Seizure

Reaction to uncurbed and abnormal electrical discharges from the brain that results in a lack of body control.

A seizure or convulsion can be caused by any event that disturbs the brain's electrical activity. Patients who experience seizures are often characterized as suffering from a form of epilepsy.

Cause. Seizures can be the result of a severe head injury, brain damage at birth, a stroke, an infection, a tumor in the brain, or alcohol withdrawal. Seizures may consist of abnormal electrical activity in a small confined area of the brain, or it can spread to other parts of the brain. A very small percentage of patients with seizures experience a specific set of sensations (known as auras) prior to the onset of a seizure.

Symptoms. Neuromuscular signs and symptoms of a seizure include tingling (or prickling) of the skin, uncontrollable twitching of the face or limbs, spasms, and tremors. Other potential signs and symptoms include hallucinations, phobias, or a sense of deja vú, which is a feeling of familiarity. Abnormal electrical activity spread throughout the brain, produces a generalized seizure, referred to as grand mal. A grand mal seizure which continues for more than a few minutes is referred to as "status epilepticus." In these cases, consciousness is typically lost.

Treatment. It is very important that anyone suffering a seizure receive medical help immediately. The most important thing to do for any seizure victim is to move any dangerous objects—that could be used for striking— away from the patient to prevent them from injuring themselves. Under no circumstances should any object be placed in the victim's mouth. It may obstruct the airway, or cause injury.

Background reading on seizures can be found in Brain and Central Nervous System. For further information, see Aura; Birth Defects; Brain Disorders; Brain Tumor; Epilepsy; Hallucination; Phobia; and Stroke. *See also* Anticonvulsant Drugs *for more on treatment options.*

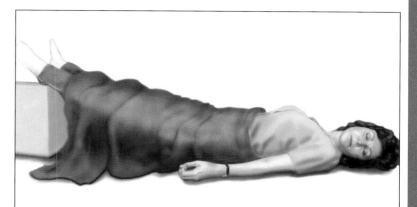

Shock

Dangerous drop in blood pressure that results in inadequate flow to the tissues of the body.

Though sometimes applied to states mental or emotional distress, medical shock is the result of decreased blood flow to the brain and vital organs. Shock is a secondary effect of severe injury or illness.

ALERT

The Shock Position

Lay the person on his or her back and cover him or her with a blanket to keep warm. Elevate the legs slightly (but not if the person has had a venomous bite). If there is absolutely no possibility of a neck injury, turn the head to the side so that vomiting will not block air passages. Do not offer beverages or any other food. Loosen clothing that may inhibit breathing. Seek professional medical help immediately.

Causes. Shock may be caused by massive blood loss, blood vessel blockage or widening, or the ability of the heart to pump blood. These conditions are produced by heart attack, injury, allergic reaction, bacterial infection, electric shock, poisoning, heat stroke, extensive burns, some metabolic disorders, drug overdose, and spinal cord injury. Shock is life-threatening.

Symptoms. In early stages a person may be tired, dizzy upon standing, easily fatigued, nauseated and thirsty. In later stages the skin pales, and lips and fingernails may show a bluish coloration (cyanosis). The skin is cool and sweaty; the pulse becomes weak and rapid; breathing

The Shock Position. One of the first steps in many emergency first aid treatments is to put an individual in the shock position, as pictured above. In the shock position, a person's feet should be elevated and their body kept somewhat warm. Only turn the head if there is *absolutely* no chance that the injury is affecting the head or neck.

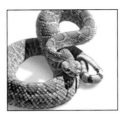

Wash affected area

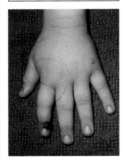

Snakebites. In the U.S., pit vipers, rattlesnakes (top), and coral snakes are venomous, and many different varieties of snakes bite. The first and most important thing to do when any snake bites is to wash out the wound with warm soapy water, as pictured in the middle. At the bottom, a finger has been bitten by a snake. Such bites can cause tissue death, this bite has caused swelling and some characteristic tissue death on the first finger.

> **ALERT**
>
> ### Anaphylactic Shock
>
> If a person is allergic to food (especially in the case of nuts), he or she may go into anaphylactic shock. Symptoms include swelling of tongue and face, gasping and choking, hives, a weak and rapid pulse, dizziness, nausea, vomiting, and unconsciousness. A serious case of anaphylactic shock can kill within fifteen minutes. People who known that they are sensitive to certain substances, will often wear a medical ID bracelet or tag so that the proper treatment can be administered quickly.

may be shallow or fast. Blood pressure can be unmeasurably low.

Treatment. A person administering first aid should check to see that there has been no damage to the person's neck or spine, and that the individual is breathing. If necessary, cardiopulmonary resuscitation (CPR) should be administered. any bleeding that may be evident must be controlled with direct pressure. The patient should be kept in a supine position (the shock position) and kept warm. Medical assistance from a trained professionals (emergency medical technicians) should be alerted immediately. *See also* ANAPHYLACTIC SHOCK; BLOOD PRESSURE; CARDIOPULMONARY RESUSCITATION (CPR); *and* PULSE.

> **ALERT**
>
> ### Septic Shock
>
> A bacterial invasion of the bloodstream (septicemia and toxemia) can be so severe that a person goes into shock. Only blood tests can reveal the presence of septic shock. In this case, circulation may be preserved until relatively late in the course, and then become severely compromised causing shock. If there is reason to believe a person suffering from septic shock should be put in the shock position until emergency medical assistance arrives.

Snakebites

The bite of a snake, which may or may not be venomous.

Only two families of the hundreds of kinds of snakes native to the United States are venomous. The pit vipers—which include copperheads, rattlesnakes, and water moccasins—are characterized by triangular, wedge-shaped heads, small pits under the eyes, and large fangs; consequently, they leave visible bite marks. They are responsible for close to 99 percent of snakebites in this country. Coral snakes, which are fairly small and thin, have a highly neurotoxic venom that will cause respiratory paralysis. The coral snake's fangs are much smaller than those of pit vipers, and their bites are therefore less obvious. Bites of both types of native venomous snakes can be treated effectively with antivenin. Since antivenin is made with horse serum, people sensitive to horse products may experience a severe reaction. *See also* TOXIN.

Symptoms of venomous snakebites include weakness, dizziness, nausea, headache, difficulty breathing, tissue damage, shock, and tingling lips and tongue.

Treatment. A bite from any snake must be treated as an emergency; since many snakebite victims cannot positively identify the species that bit them, physicians insist that all snakebites receive prompt attention. Bites incurred from nonpoisonous species may cause an allergic reactions in some people. Most frequently, doctors treat venomous snakebites by administering antivenin, an antidote to snake venom.

Before medical care arrives, some simple first aid can be applied to the individual who has been bitten. First, wash the area with soap and water. Keep the bite still, and below the heart. Then go to the hospital or call an ambulance. Never treat snakebites with any of the following: ice, ice packs, or any other cooling substance, tourniquets, incisions, or electric shock. Never try to orally suck the venom from the bite. If the victim is unable to reach the hospital within 30 minutes, a bandage (loose enough to slip a finger underneath) may be wrapped two to four inches above the bite. A suction device available in commercial snakebite kits may be used to draw venom from the wound. *See* VENOMOUS BITES AND STINGS.

Prevention. The majority of snakebites that occur could be prevented, since most snakes bite humans only to protect themselves. Give any snake that you pass plenty of space—snakes can often strike the distance of half their length. Do not walk in tall grasses unless you are wearing leather hiking boots and long pants. If you see a snake do not try to catch or kill it—this is how many preventable bites occur. *See also* BITES

Stings

Lesions caused by stinging insects.

Stings from bees, yellow jackets, wasps, hornets, tarantulas, and fire ants may be painful; but for those who are allergic they can prove extremely dangerous. Since bees' stingers contain venom, remove them by sweeping a stiff, flat object such as a credit card against the sting; fingernails also work. If a severe reaction occurs, which may include hives, swelling of the mouth,

---

ALERT

Stings from Marine Wildlife

Insects such as bees, yellow jackets, hornets (with the most potent sting), and fire ants are not the only creatures that people are regularly stung by. Jellyfish, men-of-war, stone fish, stingrays and a number of other sorts of marine wildlife will also sting unsuspecting bathers. Stings from these animals generally have symptoms similar to those of insects; however, treatment options are more delicate: Never remove stingers from animal wildlife with your bare hands. This could be potentially harmful. Also, do not raise the stung body part; the poison should not be allowed to move throughout the body.

---

face and hands, difficulty breathing, confusion, anxiety, nausea, vomiting, or loss of consciousness; immediately call EMS. Do so as well if the victim has been stung many times, as can occur with fire ants and bees. Monitor the victim's airway, breathing, and circulation, and give an antihistamine while waiting for medical personnel.

If stings in the mouth cause swelling and obstruct the airway, call EMS immediately, then administer artificial respiration. Also, those who know that they are allergic to stings should carry around a sting kit for

emergencies. These kits include epinephrine or adrenaline to inject immediately after what would otherwise be a possibly fatal sting. If there is no allergic reaction, wash the sting with soap and water, then treat with hydrocortisone cream, calamine lotion, or a paste of baking soda and water. Ice will reduce swelling.

Stroke

A disruption in brain function caused by a sudden obstruction or the rupture of an artery leading to the brain.

A brief interruption of the flow of oxygen-carrying blood to any part of the brain has an immediate effect on the functions controlled by that region; an interruption that lasts as little as four minutes can cause the death of brain cells in that region. If the interruption of blood flow affects a region of the brain that controls a basic function of life, death can occur in minutes.

Types. There are two major categories of stroke, ischemic and hemorrhagic. A hemorrhagic stroke results from rupture of a blood vessel in or near the brain. Ischemic strokes can be classified as those caused by a thrombus, a clot that has formed on the wall of a brain artery, and those caused by an embolism, a clot that has traveled to the brain from another part of the body. Cerebral thrombosis causes about half of all strokes, and cerebral embolism causes about a quarter of them.

Symptoms. The symptoms of a stroke depend on its cause and the part of the brain that is damaged; however, there are features common to all strokes. The major symptoms of a stroke include: a sudden feeling of weakness or numbness in the face or an arm or leg on one side of the body; a sudden loss of speech abilities, feeling, or vision in one or both eyes; fainting, near-fainting or light headedness; confusion; a severe headache; sudden loss of either short-term or long-term memory; and unexplained dizziness.

In the case of a stroke caused by cerebral thrombosis, the symptoms may occur

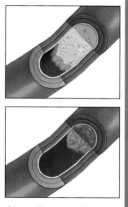

Clots. Top, an atherosclerotic clot is caused by an aggregation of platelets, low-density lipoprotiens and calcium to form a clot which can lead to a stroke. Above, bottom, a blood clot has fewer elements than an atherosclerotic clot, but leads to similar ends; a stroke-causing clot in the brain that will cause the death of brain tissue due to a shortage in the blood supply.

Carotid Artery. Below, an image of the carotid artery. This is the main artery that supplies blood to the brain. Individuals of East Asian and Pacific Island lineage have a higher incidence of carotid artery disease. This condition, which is a major indicator for stroke especially when it is coupled with transient ischemic attacks, has a hereditary element.

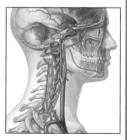

gradually, sometimes fading and progressing over several days as blood flow through the artery decreases. The symptoms of a stroke caused by an embolism usually come on quickly, as a clot blocks the artery suddenly. A stroke caused by a subarachnoid hemorrhage usually is signaled by sudden onset of an extremely painful headache, with nausea, vomiting, and mental confusion, sometimes accompanied by seizures.

These symptoms require an immediate call for medical help, since permanent brain damage can be prevented or severely reduced if treatment begins quickly. A physician or emergency medical service should be called, or the patient should be taken to the nearest hospital emergency room as quickly as possible.

Treatment. If a stroke patient is unconscious, steps will be taken to maintain breathing, often by inserting an endotracheal tube. For an ischemic stroke, anticoagulant medications such as heparin can be given, not so much to dissolve the clot causing the stroke but to prevent the formation of new clots. The clot-dissolving medication—tissue plasminogen activator (tPa)—has been shown to limit brain damage if it is infused within the first hours after a stroke occurs. The treatments aimed at ischemic stroke cannot be used for hemorrhagic strokes, since the need in those cases is to limit the amount of bleeding. Surgery may be done in some cases of hemorrhagic stroke to repair the damaged blood vessel that is causing the bleeding.

Over a longer term, treatment is aimed at physical rehabilitation—mostly through physical therapy—and the prevention of future strokes. Prevention often requires major lifestyle changes. Rehabilitation can begin in the first days after the stroke occurs, with physicians, nurses, and even family members moving the affected arms or legs to maintain proper blood flow, joint flexibility, and muscle tone.

> *Background information can be found in* ANEURYSM; ARTERIES, DISORDERS OF; BRAIN; BRAIN HEMORRHAGE, CAROTID ARTERY; EMBOLISM; *and* INTRACEREBRAL HEMORRHAGE. *Related information is in* CHOLESTEROL; DIET AND DISEASE; *and* STRESS. *See also* PHYSICAL THERAPY *and* SURGERY.

Hyperextension

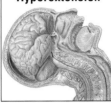

Hyperflexion

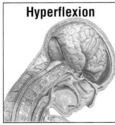

Whiplash Injury. Whiplash is a violent injury to the neck, which causes a sprain or strain of the tissues and muscles in that area. Hyperextension (above, top) is when the head and neck are bent too far backward, while hyperflexion (above, bottom) is when they are bent too far forward.

Vomiting Blood

Also known as hematemesis

The regurgitation of blood from the stomach or esophagus.

Causes. Prolonged or vigorous vomiting may cause a tear in the small blood vessels of the throat or esophagus, producing streaks of blood in the vomit. This is related to Mallory-Weiss syndrome, which is a laceration or tear of the lower esophagus and the upper part of the stomach. The amount of blood present in the vomit depends on the extent of the damage.

Bleeding ulcers located in the stomach or duodenum (the first part of the intestine) are also a source of vomited blood, as are certain types of esophageal irritation or the erosion of the lining of the esophagus or stomach.

Other sources of blood in the vomit include bleeding esophageal varices; ingested blood; blood swallowed following a nosebleed, for example; severe gastritis or gastroenteritis; severe injury or electrical shock; tumors of the stomach or esophagus; and vascular malformations in the gastrointestinal tract.

Treatment. Treatments for vomiting blood vary, because they depend upon the specific cause. In general, it is a good idea to drink small amounts of water regularly to prevent dehydration. It is very important to seek medical help. *See also* GASTROENTERITIS; *and* MALLORY-WEISS SYNDROME.

Whiplash Injury

Trauma to the neck caused by violent jerking.

Whiplash usually results in a minor sprain or a joint dislocation. In extreme cases, a vertebra may fracture or a ligament may be torn. Symptoms are pain and stiffness that begin after the trauma. Painkillers or muscle relaxants may be prescribed. In some cases, the area may need to be immobilized with an orthopedic collar. Physical therapy can help to restore movement. *See also* FRACTURES AND DISLOCATIONS; INJURY; PHYSICAL THERAPY; SPRAIN; *and* SUBLUXATION.

INDEX

A

Abdomen, 21. *see also individual organs and structures*
pain in, 21–22
swelling of, *23*, 23
x-ray, 23
Abducens nerves, *23*, 23
Ablation, 24
Abortifacient, 24
Abortion, 24–25
menstrual extraction, 764
spontaneous, 782
Abrasion, dental, 25
Abrasions, in eyes, 480
Abscesses, 26
Abuse
of children, 276
dates, 40
Acanthosis nigricans, 26
Access to care, 26. *see also* Health insurance
Accidents, 27
Accommodation, 28
Accreditation, 28. *see also* Certification
ACE inhibitors, 101
Acetaminophen
liver damage alert, 726
Acetic acid, 28
Achalasia, 28
Achlorhydria, 28
Achondroplasia, 29
Acid reflux, *29*, 29, 467
drug treatment, 91
Acidosis, 29, 1001
Acne, *30*, 30, 370, *371*
Acoustic nerve, 31
Acoustic neuroma, 31
Acrochordons, 1066
Acrocyanosis, 31
Acrodermatitis enteropathica, 31
Acromegaly, 31–32, 911
Acromioclavicular joint, 32
ACTH (adrenocorticotropic hormone), 32, *32*, 609, *609*, 910
Acting out, 33
Actinic, 33

Actinomycosis, *33*, 33
Acupressure, 33–34
for nausea, *810*
pressure points, 944, *944*
Acupuncture, 34–35, *35*
pressure points, 944, *944*
Addison's disease, 36, 445, 447
Adenitis, 36
Adenoidectomy, *37*, 37
Adenoma, 37
Adenomatosis, 37
Adenosine triphosphate (ATP), 130
ADH (antidiuretic hormone), 37, 375, 609, 910
ADHD. *see* Attention deficit/hyperactivity disorder (ADHD)
Adolescence, 38–40
Adolescents. *see also* Children
breast development, 209
puberty, 968–969
self-mutilation, 1038
Adrenal glands, 40–41. *see also* Addison's disease
Adrenal hyperplasia, 42
Adrenal tumors, 42
Adrenalectomy, laparoscopic, 42
Advance directives, 396
Adynamic ileus, 636
Aerobics, 43
Aerodontalgia, 43
Aerophagia, 43
Aflatoxin, 43
Afterbirth, 43, 912–913
Afterpains, 43
Agent Orange, 44
Aggression, 44
Aging, 44–45, 949
Agnosia, 46
Agoraphobia, 46
AIDS (acquired immune deficiency syndrome), 47–49, 1049
Air, 50
Air conditioning, 50
Airway obstruction, 50, 515
Akinesia, 50
Albinism, 51

Albuminuria, 51
Alcohol dependence, 52–53
alert, 52
Alcohol (drinking)
alert, 774
liver damage alert, 726
Alcohol intoxication, 54, *55*
Alcohol related disorders, 54–55
Alcoholics Anonymous, 53
Aldosterone, 56, 609
Alexander technique, 56
Alkalosis, 56–57
Allergens, *57*, 57
Allergies, 57–59
to cats, 256
drug treatment, 100
erythema multiforme, 464
to food, 510–511
hay fever, 1016
hives, 604
immune function, 640–641
insect stings, 665–666
skin, 1063, *1063*
Allergy shots, 647
Allopurinol, 59
Alopecia areata, 59, 481
Alpha-blocking drugs, 101, 623
Alpha-fetoprotein, 60
Alpha-l antitrypsin (AAT), 441
ALS (amyotrophic lateral sclerosis, Lou Gehrig's disease), 791
Alternative birth methods, 60–61
Alternative medicine
acupressure, 33–34, *810*, 944
acupuncture, 34–35, *35*, 944
aromatherapy, 115
auriculotherapy, 35
Ayurvedic medicine, 139–140, *140*
biofeedback, 154, 162, *162*
Chinese medicine, 282
chiropractic, 283–284
environmental medicine, 454–456
essential oils, 115
Gerson diet, 237
homeopathy, 606–607

macrobiotics, 741
nutrition and diet, 833–834
Alternative medicine, 61–63.
see also Bodywork
Altitude sickness, 63–64, 216
Aluminum, 64
Alveoli, 65, *441*
Alveolitis, 64
Alveoplasty, 65
Alzheimer's disease, 65–67
Amalgam, dental, 67
Amaurosis fugax, 67
Amaurotic familial idiocy, 67
Ambidexterity, 68
Amblyopia, 68, 178
Ambulance, 68–69, *69*
Ambulatory care, 69
Amebiasis, 69
Amelogenesis imperfecta, 70
Amenorrhea, 70
American Board of Medical
Specialties, 397
**American Medical Association,
71**
Amino acids, 71
Amnesia, 71
Amniocentesis, 72
Amnioscopy, 73
Amoebic dysentery, 876
Amphetamine drugs, 73
Amputation, 73–74
phantom limb, 903
Amyloidosis, 74
Amyotrophy, 74
Anabolic reaction, 772
Anaerobic, 75
Anal canal, *107*
Analeptic drugs, 76
Analgesic drugs, *76*, 76
general anesthesia, 83
Anaphylactic shock, 58, 76
alert, *76*, 1052
allergies, 216
Anastomosis, 77
Anatomy, 77
Androgen drugs, 77
Androgen hormones, 78, 609
Androgen resistance syndrome,
1144
Androgenic antagonists, 623
Anemia, *79*
aplastic, 79–80
hemolytic, 80
iron-deficiency, 81
megaloblastic, *81*, 81
signs of, *81*
Anencephaly, 82
Anesthesia, 82
dental, 82
general, 82–84
local, 84–85
spinal, *85*, 85, 1084

Aneurysm, 85–86, *86*
aortic, 23
Angel dust, 86
Angina pectoris, 86–87, *87*, 331
heart disease warning sign,
273, 330, 331
ischemic heart disease, 573
Angioedema, 87
Angiography, 88
abdominal, *23*
Angioma, 88
Angioplasty, balloon, 88–89, *89*,
435, 569
Angiotensin, 89
Angiotensin-converting enzyme
(ACE), 623
Anisometropia, 90
Ankle, fractured, 934
Ankylosing spondylitis, 90
Anorexia nervosa, 419–420
Anorgasmia, 90–91
Anoxia, 91
Antacid drugs, 91
Antepartum hemorrhage, 91
Anterior capsulotomy, 966
Anterior cingulotomy, 966
Anthracosis, 92
Anthrax, 92
Antiarrhythmic drugs, 93
Antibiotic drugs, *93*, 93
sulfonathide drugs, 1117
Antibiotic resistance, 93–94
Antibodies, 94, 639
Anticancer drugs, 94–95
Anticholinergic drugs, 96
Antidepressant drugs, *97*, 97
pain relief, 869
Antidiarrheal drugs, 98
Antidote, 98
Antiemetic drugs, 98
Antifreeze poisoning, 98
Antifungal drugs, 98–99
Antigen capture assay, 643
Antigens, 99
tumor-specific, 1188
Antihelminthic drugs, 99
Antihistamine drugs, 100
Antihypertensive drugs, 101
Anti-inflammatory drugs,
102–103
Antioxidants, 834
Antiperspirant, 103
Antipsychotic drugs, 103
Antirheumatic drugs, 104
Antiseptics, 104
Antisocial personality disorder,
104
Antispasmodic drugs, 105
Antitoxin, 105
Antivenin, 105
Antiviral drugs, 105
Antral irrigation, 106

Anuria, 106–107
Anus
abscess, *26*
anal canal, *107*
cancer, 107
dilation, 75
discharge, 75
disorders of, 107
fissure, 75
fistula, 75–76
imperforate, 107
Anvil, 415
Anxiety, 108, 216, 821
drug treatment, 92
Anxiety disorders, 108–109,
767
Aorta, 21, *109*, 109, 251
aneurysm, 109
coarctation, 304–305
dissection of, 109, 273
Aortic insufficiency, 110
Aortic stenosis, *110*, 110
Aortic valve regurgitation, 273
Aortitis, 110–111
APGAR score, 111
Aphakia, 111
Aphasia, 111, 374
Aphonia, 112
Aphthous ulcers, 1190
Apnea, 112
Appendectomy, 112
Appendicitis, 22, *113*, 113
Appendix, *112*
Appetite, loss of, 113
Appetite stimulants, 113–114
Appetite suppressants, 114. *see*
also Amphetamines
Apraxia, 114
Arachnoiditis, 114–115
Arcus senilis, 115
Aromatherapy, 115
alert, 115
Arrhenoblastoma, 116
Arrhythmia, cardiac, 116–117
drug treatment, 93
Arsenic, 117
Arteries, 118
disorders of, 117
Arteriography, *88*
Arteriosclerosis, *117*, 117, 249
Arteriovenous fistula, 118
Arteritis, 118
Arthralgia, 118
Arthritis, *119*, 119
osteoarthritis, 852–853
rheumatoid, 104, 119, *119*,
1012–1013, *1013*
rheumatoid, juvenile, 1014
Arthrodesis, 120
Arthroplasty, 120
Arthroscopy, 120
Articulation disorders, 1080

Artificial insemination, 121
Artificial sweeteners, 121
Asbestosis, 121–122
Ascariasis, 122, 1021
Ascites, 122
Ascorbic acid, 1224
Ash leaf macule, *1187*
Aspartame, *121*
Aspergillosis, 123
Asphyxia, 123
Aspirin, *76, 123*, 123
Assam fever, 687
Assisted living, 427
Astereognosis, 123
Asthma, 124, *125*
  alert, 124
  inhalers, 662
  nebulizer, 811
  spirometry, 1086
  status asthmaticus, 1096
Astigmatism, 126
Aston patterning, 126
Astrocytoma, 126
Asymptomatic, 126
Ataxia, 127
Atelectasis, 127
Atherosclerosis, 128, *128*, 249,
  573
Atherosclerotic clot, *1107*
Athetosis, 129
Athletes
  androgen abuse, 77
  baseball elbow & finger, 151
  energy requirements, 452
  golfer's elbow, 547
  heart rate, 201
  joggers' nipple, 685
  jumper's knee, 686
  meniscectomy, 762
  mononucleosis alert, 787
  neurapraxia, 818
  performance enhancement,
    1091, 1097
  running injuries, 1022
  shin splints, 1052
  sports injuries, 1089–1090
  steroids, anabolic, 1097
  stitch, 1099
  surfers' nodules, 1121
  tennis elbow, 1142, *1142*
Athlete's foot, *129*, 129, 1164
Atkins diet, 385
Atony, 129
Atopic dermatitis, *369*
ATP (adenosine triphosphate),
  130, 130
Atrial fibrillation, 130
Atrial flutter, 131
Atrial natriuretic peptide, 131
Atrophic vaginitis, 1205
Atrophy, 131
Attention deficit/hyperactivity

disorder (ADHD), 132–133,
  132–133, 709
Audiogram, 566
Audiology, 133
Aura (migraine), 133
Auriculotherapy, 35. *see also*
  Acupressure
Auscultation, *133*, 133–134,
  473
Autism, 134–135, 374
Autoeroticism, 752
Autoimmune disorders, 135,
  641, 965
  thyroid, 1158
Automobile safety, 136
Autonomic nervous system,
  136
Autopsy, 137
Autosomal disorders, 534
Aviation medicine, 137–138
Avoidant personality disorder,
  138
Avulsion, 139
Ayurvedic medicine, 139–140,
  140
AZT (zidovudine), *49*, 1246

B

B cells, 152
Babesiosis, 141, 876
"Baby blues," 931
Bacilli, 141
Bacillus Calmette-Guerin vacci-
  nation, 152
Back pain, *141*, 141–142, *142*
Bacteremia, 142–143
Bacteria, *143*, 143
Bacteriuria, 144
Bad breath, 556
Baker's cyst, 144
Balance, *144*, 144
  dizziness, 395
  inner ear, 415
  labyrinthitis, 699
  Ménière's disease, 760
  vertigo, 1216
Balanitis, 145
Ball-and-socket joint, 686
Balloon angioplasty, 88–89, *89*,
  435, 569
Balloon catheter, 145, *145*
Bandages, *146*, 146
  compresses, 317
  dressings, 402
  Esmarch bandage, 465
Barbiturate drugs, 146
  alert, 146
Barium x-rays, *147*, 147
  abdominal view, 23
  alert, 147
Barotrauma, 148

Barrett's esophagus, 148
Barrier methods of contracep-
  tion, 148–149
Bartholin's glands, 150
Bartonellosis, 1026
Basal cell carcinoma, 150, 371,
  1065, 1066
Basal ganglia, 151
Basal metabolic rate, *151*, 151
Baseball elbow & finger, 151
Basophils, *179*
Battle's sign, *561*
BCG (bacillus Calmette-
  Guerin), 152
Becker's muscular dystrophy,
  799
Bedbugs, *152*, 152
Beds, hospital, 152–153, *153*
Bedsores, *153*, 153, 1190
Bedwetting, 454
Bees, 665–666
Behavior. *see specific conducts,
  such as* Acting out;
  Aggression
Behavior therapy, 153–154, 967
Behçet's syndrome, 154
Belching, 154
Belladonna, 154–155
Bell's palsy, 482–483
Bends, 155, 357, 1034
Benign, 155
Benign prostatic hypertrophy,
  956
Benzodiazepine drugs, 155
Bereavement, 156
Beriberi, 156
Berylliosis, 156
Beta-blocker drugs, 101, 157,
  622
  alert, 157
Betamethasone, 157
Bezoar, 157
Bifocals, 157
Bile, 157
Bile-duct obstruction, 157, 524
Biliary atresia, 158
Biliary cirrhosis, primary, 159
Biliary colic, 159, 524
Biliary system, *160*, 160
Bilirubin, 161
Billing's method, 161
Billroth II procedure, 530
Billroth's operation, 161
Binge-eating disorder, 420
Biofeedback, 62, 154, *162*, 162
Bioflavonoids, 163
Biomechanical engineering,
  163, 163
Biopsy, *164*, 164
Biorhythms, 165
Biotin, 1224
Bipolar disorder, 165–167, 787

alert, 166
Birth, *279*
Birth control, 167. *see also*
  Contraception
Birth defects, 167–168, 169
  alpha-fetoprotein testing, 60
  amniocentesis, 72
  anencephaly, 82
  Down syndrome, *168*, 400,
    769
  fetal alcohol syndrome, 55,
    494
  hearing loss, 564
  heart disease, 572
  limbs, 719
  maternal drugs, 939
  teratogens, 1143
  testing, 294
Birth weight, *169*, 169
Birthmarks, *88*, 170
Bisexuality, 170
Bites, 170–171, *171. see also*
  Stings
  animal, 983
  snakes, 1074, *1074*
  spiders, 1083, *1083*
  ticks, 1162–1163, *1163*
  tsetse flies, 1185
  venomous, 1213, *1213*
Black eye, *171*, 171, 480
Black lung disease, 92, 920
Black tongue, *94*
Blackwater fever, 171
Bladder, 21, 171
  biopsy, *172*
  herniation, 351
  removal, 348
  tumors, 172
Bladder control, 171
Blastocyst transfer, 172
Blastomycosis, 173, 521
Bleaching, dental, 173
Bleb, 173
Bleeding, 173
  alert, 173
  breakthrough, 208
  disorders of, 174–175
  gastrointestinal, 529
  hemophilia, 588–589
  postpartum hemorrhage, 931
  pressure points, 944, *944*
  shock alert, 176
  treatment of, 175
Blepharitis, 481
Blepharoplasty, 176
Blind-loop syndrome, 176
Blind spot, *177*, 177
Blindness, 177
Blisters, 178, 224
Blood, 179. *see also* Bleeding
  coughing of, 336
  discharge, 391

Rh incompatability alert, 179
  vomiting of, 1228
Blood cells, *179*, 180
Blood clots, 1107, *1107*, 1156,
  1166
Blood clotting
  fibrinolysis, 498
  hemostasis, 591
  hypercoagulable state, 618
  photocoagulation, 907
  thrombocytopenia, 1155
  vitamin K, 1225
Blood clotting test, 182
Blood count, 182
Blood disorders, 182–183
Blood donation, 184
Blood flukes, 507
Blood gasses, 184
Blood groups, *184*, 184–185
  crossmatching, 341
Blood poisoning, 185
  alert, 185
Blood pressure, *186*, 186, 300
  alert, 186
Blood products, 187, 189
Blood smear, 187
Blood tests, *188*, 188, 1147
  CBC, 182
Blood transfusion, *189*, 189
Blue babies, *190*, 190, 1151
Blue Cross/Blue Shield, 190
Blurred vision, 190
Blushing, 190
Board certification, 191
Body, regions of, 77
Body contour surgery, 191
  alert, 191
Body lice, 715
Body mass index (BMI), 835,
  836
Body odor, 192
Bodywork, *192*, 192
  Alexander technique, 56
  Aston patterning, 126
  Feldenkrais method, 491
  Hellerwork, 582
  Rolfing, 1019
Boil, 192
Bonding, dental, 193
Bonding, family, 193
  infant feeding, 199
Bone, *193*, 193
Bone, disorders of, 194–195
Bone cancer, *194*, 194
Bone cysts, 194
Bone grafts, 195
Bone imaging, *195*, 195–196
Bone marrow, 196
  biopsy, 164, 196
  registry, 197
  transplant, 196–197
Bone spurs, 856

Bone tumors, 197–198
Bones. *see also* Fractures
  osteoporosis, 857–858
Bones, brittle, 218
Boosters, 198
Borborygmi, 198
**Borderline personality
  disorder,** 198
Bornholm disease, 199, 919
Boron neutron capture
  therapy, *986*
Bottle-feeding, *199*, 199,
  490–491
Botulism, 200
  alert, 200
Bougies, 200
Bovine spongiform
  encephalopathy (BSE), 339
Bowed legs, 200
Bowen's disease, 200
Braces, 200–201
Brachial plexus, 201
Bradycardia, 201
Braille, 201–202, *202, 203*
Brain, *202*, 202–203, *251*
  abscess, 204
  disorders of, 204–205
  hemorrhage, 205
  tumors of, 126, *207*, 207
  ventricles, 1214
Brain damage, from
  Alzheimer's disease, *65, 66*
Brain death, 204, 355
Brain imaging, *206*, 206
Brain stem, 202, 206–207
Branchial disorders, 208
Brandt syndrome, 31
Brash, water, 208
Braxton-Hicks contractions,
  208
Breakbone fever, 363
Breakthrough bleeding, 208
Breast cancer, *210*, 210–211
Breast-feeding, *213*, 213, 490,
  931
  prolactin, 951
Breast implants, *917*
Breast milk, 209
  expressing, 475
  galactorrhea, 523
  mammary ducts, 746
Breast pump, 214
Breast surgery, *215*, 215
Breasts, *209*, 209
  disorders of, *212*, 212
  fibrocystitis, 499
  gynecomastia, 554
  lumps in, 214
  mammography, 747
  mastectomy, 750–751
  mastitis, 751
  nipples, 826

pain, 746
papilloma, intraductal, 873
self-examination, 214–215, *215*
tenderness, 215
Breathing
alert, 216
apnea, 112, 1069
artificial ventilation, 1213
asthma, 124–125
Cheyne-Stokes respiration, 274
hyperventilation, 624
mechanism, 1006
orthopnea, 851
peak flow meter, 883
respiratory arrest, 1004
sleep apnea, 1069
stitch, 1099
stridor, 1106
suffocation, 1115
tachypnea, 1131
Valsalva's maneuver, 1207
wheeze, 1238
Breathing difficulty, 216–217
Breech delivery, *217*, 217
version, 1215
Bridge, dental, 218
Bronchiectasis, 218
Bronchiolitis, 218
Bronchitis, *219*, 219
Bronchoconstrictor, 220
Bronchodilator drugs
alert, 220
Bronchopneumonia, 220–221
Bronchoscopy, *221*, 221
Bronchospasm, 221
Brown fat, 221
Brucellosis, 222
Bruises, 173, 222–223, *223*
Bruits, 223
Bruxism, 223
BSE (bovine spongiform encephalopathy), 339
Buck teeth, 223, 864
Budd-Chiarri syndrome, 224
Buerger's disease, 224
Bulimia, 420
Bullae, 178, 224
Bunions, *224*, 224
Burkitt's lymphoma, 225
Burns, 27, 225–226
alert, 226
electrical injuries, 428–429
in eyes, 480
Burping, 154
Bursitis, *226*, 226
Bypass, 227

C

Cachexia, 228

Cadmium poisoning, 228
Café au lait spots, 228, *819*
Caffeine, 228–229
alert, 220
Calabar swelling, 502
Calcaneus, *229*, 229
Calcification, dental, 229
Calcinosis, 229
Calcitonin, 230, 609
Calcium, 230, 857
Calcium channel blockers, 101, 230, 622
Calculus, dental, 231
Calculus, urinary tract, 231. *see also* Stones
Caliper splints, 232
Calluses, 232
Caloric test, 232
Calories, 233
Calorimetry, 233
Cancer, 234–236. *see also specific body sites*
causes, 242
cell reproduction, *95*
diet therapy for, 236–237
drug treatment, 94–95
enhancers, 243
metastasis, 773
promoters, 243
risk factors, 236
in situ, 649
Cancer screening, *237*, 237–238
Cancer treatment options, *235*
Candida albicans, 381, 521, *1206*
Candidiasis, 238, 1245, *1245*
Canes, 1230
Canker sores, 239, *239*, 1190
Cannula, 239
Capillaries, 239
Capitation, 564
Carbamazepine, 239
Carbohydrates, 240, 832
Carbon dioxide, 240
Carbon monoxide, 241
alert, 241
Carbon tetrachloride, 241
Carbuncles, 241
Carcinogens, 242–243
Cardiac arrest, 244–245
alert, 245
Cardiac catheterization, 255, *255*
Cardiac output, 245
Cardiac stress test, 245
Cardiology, 245
Cardiomegaly, 246
Cardiomyopathy, 246, 574

Cardiopulmonary resuscitation (CPR), *247*, 247–248
Cardiovascular disorders, 248–249
Carditis, 250
Caries, dental, 250
Carotene, 250
Carotid arteries, 250, *251*, 1106
Carpal tunnel syndrome, 250
Carrier, 252
Cast, *252*, 252
CAT scan (computerized axial tomography), *252*, 252
bone imaging, 195
brain, 206
heart, 575
mechanism, 637, 1148
x-ray use, 1243–1244
Cat-scratch fever, 256
Catabolic reaction, 772
Catalepsy, 253
Cataplexy, 253
Cataract surgery, 253–254, *254*
Cataracts, *253*
Catastrophic health insurance, 255
Cats, diseases from, 256
Caudal block, 257
Cauliflower ear, 257
Causalgia, 257
Cauterization, *257*, 257
Cavernous sinus thrombosis, 258
Cavities, dental, 250
CBC (complete blood count), 182, 188
Cecum, *21*
Celcius scale, *1139*
Celebrex, 258
Celiac sprue, 258, 370, 545
Cells, *259*, 259. *see also* specific types such as Lymphocytes; White blood cells
cancerous, *234*
membrane, 758
Celsius scale, 250, 260
Centers for Disease Control, 260
Central nervous system, *260*, 260, 816
Centrifuge, 261
Cephalhematoma, 261
Cephalosporins, 261
Cerebellum, *202*, 202, *261*, 261–262
Cerebral cortex, 202
Cerebral palsy, 262, 374, 941
Cerebrovascular accident, 263
Cerebrovascular disease, 263
Cerebrum, 202, *263*, 263
Certificate of need, 264
Certification, 264. *see also*

Accreditation
Cervical cap, 149, 324
Cervical osteoarthritis,
264–265
Cervical rib, 265
Cervicitis, 265
Cervix, *265,* 265
  cancer alert, 266
  cancer of, *244, 266,* 266–267
  disorders of, 267
  dysplasia, 267
  erosion, 264
  incompetent, 264, 650, 782
  location, 1002
  Pap smear, 872–873
Cesarean section, 268, *268,*
  280
Chagas' disease, 269, 756, 876
Chalazion, 269
Chancre, hard, 269
Chancroid, 269–270, 536
Chapped skin, 270
Charcot-Marie-Tooth disease,
  898
Charcot's joint, 270
Chelating agents, 270
Chelation therapy, 270–271
Chemical burns
  in eyes, 480
Chemical sensitivity. *see*
  Environmental medicine
Chemonucleolysis, 271
Chemotherapy, 271–272, *272.*
  see also Anticancer drugs
Chenodiol, 272
Cherry angioma, 272
Chest pain, 273
  alert, 273
Chest x-ray, 274
Chewing, 751
Cheyne-Stokes respiration, 274
Chickenpox, 274–275
Chigger bite, *275,* 275
Chigoe, 275
Chilblains, 308, 898
Child abuse, 276
Child development, *277,*
  277–278
Child safety seats, *27*
Childbed fever, 973–974
Childbirth, *279,* 279–280
  alternative methods, 60–61
  anesthesia, 84–85
  Braxton-Hicks contractions,
  208
  breech delivery, 217
  caudal block, 257
  Cesarean section, 268
  childbed fever, 973–974
  complications, 280–281
  contractions, 326
  delivery, 362

  emergency, 438
  engagement, 452
  episiotomy, 461
  forceps delivery, 514–515
  labor induction, 652
  Lamaze method, 701–702
  laminaria, 702
  lightening, 719
  lochia, 731
  malpresentation, 746
  midwives, 778
  mortality risk, 752–753
  natural, 943
  oxytocin, 866
  pain management, 280
  pelvimetry, 888
  postpartum depression, 931
  prepared childbirth, 943
  prolapsed cord, 951, *951*
  pudendal block, 973
  puerperal sepsis, 973–974
  stillbirth, 1098
  tocography, 1167
  vacuum extraction, 1204
  version, 1215
Children. *see also* Adolescents;
  Infants; Newborns
  abdominal pain in, 22
  acting out, 33
  adolescence, 38–40
  automobile safety, 136
  baby teeth, 948
  choking alert, 286
  cough, 335
  CPR, *247,* 247–248
  dehydration, 360
  development delay, 373–374
  drug poisoning alert, 408
  early weight patterns, *169*
  electrical shock, *429*
  failure to thrive, 483–484
  growth in, 551–552
  head injury alert, 318
  lisping, 722–723
  mutism, 801
  night terrors, 825
  Oedipus complex, 840
  pediatrics, 883, *883*
  psychological development,
  962
  public health hazard, 562
  Reye's syndrome, 1011, *1011*
  safety measures, 27, *27*
  separation anxiety, 1040
  sleep apnea, 1069
  soiling, 444
  speech development, 1079
  speech therapy, 1081
  sports injury alert, 1090
  tantrums, 1132
  temperature taking, 496
  thumb-sucking, 1157

  toilet-training, 1167–1168
  vaccinations, 642, 655, 1179,
  1204
  vision improvement, 852
  weight and growth, 1236
Chills, 282
Chinese medicine, 282
Chinese restaurant syndrome,
  283
Chiropractic, 283–284
Chlamydia, 284, 1049
Chloasma, 284
Chlorate poisoning alert, 285
Chloroform, 285
Chlorosis, 285
Chlorthalidone, 285
Choking, 286
  alert, 286
  Heimlich maneuver, 582
Cholangiocarcinoma, 286
Cholangiography, 287
Cholangitis, 287
Cholecalciferol, 288
Cholecystectomy, 288
Cholecystitis, 289, 525
Cholecystography, 289
Cholecystokinin, 609
Cholera, 289–290
Cholestasis, 290, 683
Cholesteatoma, 290
Cholesterol, *291,* 291, 619
  lipids, 720–721
Cholesterol-reducing drugs,
  884
Chondritis, 291
Chondrodystrophy, 374
Chondromalacia patellae, 292
Chondromatosis, 292
Chondrosarcoma, 292
Chordee, 292–293
Chorea, 293
Choriocarcinoma, 293–294
Chorionic villus sampling, 72,
  294
Choroiditis, 294
Christmas disease, 295
Chromaffin tumor, 905
Chromium, 295
Chromosomal abnormalities,
  295, 295
Chromosome analysis, 297–298
  alert, 297
Chromosomes, 296, 534. *see*
  also Genetics
Chronic fatigue syndrome, 298
Chronic obstructive pulmonary
  disease (COPD), *441,* 734
Chyme, 386
Circulation
  capillaries, 239
  heartbeat, 570
Circulatory system, *299,*

299–300
Circumcision, female, 301
Circumcision, male, 301
Cirrhosis, 302, 725, 726
Clap, the, 548, 1049
Claustrophobia, 302
Claw foot and hand, 303
Clay, alert, 908
Cleft lip and palate, 167, *303*, 303
Clinical ecology. *see* Environmental medicine
Clinical trials, 326
  lung cancer, 733
Clinics, ambulatory care, 69
Clitoris, 303
Clomiphene, 304
Clones, 304
Clubbing, 304
Clubfoot, 1131
Cluster headaches, *559*
Coarctation of the aorta, 304–305
Cobalamin (vitamin B_{12}), 1224
Cocaine, 305
Coccygodynia, 305
Coccyx, *305*, 305
Cochlear implants, 306, 355
Cod liver oil, 306
Codeine, 307
Cognitive-behavior therapy, 307
Cognitive disorder, 767
Cognitive therapy, 967
Cold, common, 308–309
Cold injury, 308, 519
Cold remedies, 308
Cold sores, 308, 497
Cold therapy, 635
Colectomy, 309
Colic, 310, 343
Colic, infantile, 310
Colitis, 310–311, 1190–1191
Collagen, 311
Collars, orthopedic, 311
Colles' fracture, 311
Colon, *21*, *312*, 312
  cancer of, 312–313, *313*
Colonoscopy, *313*, 314, *1057*
Color vision, *314*, 314–315
Colostomy, 315, 994
Colostrum, 209, 213, 315
Colposcopy, *316*, 316, 873
Coma, 316, 1211
Commensal, 317
Community dentistry, 973
Complement fixation, 643
Complete blood count (CBC), 182, 188
Complex carbohydrates, 240
Compliance, 317, 405
Complications, 317

Compresses, 317
Compression syndrome, 343
Conception, *318*, 318, 493. *see also* Fertility; Infertility
  fertility drugs, 493
  fertilization, 493
  superfecundation, 1119
Concussions, 318, 560
  alert, 318
  sports-related, 1090
Condoms, *148*, 149, 318–319, *319*, 324, *325*
Cone biopsy, 319
Cones, 477
Confabulation, 319
Confetti hypopigmentation, *1187*
Confusion, 319–320
Congenital, 320
Congenital sexually transmitted diseases (STDs), 320
Congestion, 320–321
Congestive heart failure, 321, 1165
Conjoined twins, *168*, 1055
Conjunctivitis, *321*, 321
Conn's syndrome, 322
Consciousness, loss of, 731
Consent, 322
Constipation, 322–323, 489
Contact lenses, *323*, 323
Contact tracing, 324
Continuous positive airway pressure (CPAP), 1069
Contraception, 324–325, *325*
  condoms, 318–319
  estrogen drugs, 469
  IUDs, 677
  morning after pill, 788
  natural, 809
  oral contraceptives, 847
  Pomeray technique, 928
  sponge, 149, 1088–1089
  sterilization, 1097
  tubal ligation, 1185, *1185*
  vasectomy, 1209
Contractions, 326
Contracture, 326
Contrast imaging, 984, 1212, 1244
Controlled trials, 326
Contusions, 326
Convalescence, 327
Cooley's anemia, 1151
Copper, 327
  Wilson's disease, 1239
Cor pulmonale, 327
Cord blood, 1193
Cordotomy, 327
Corneas, *328*, 328
  abrasion, 328
  disorders of, 328

grafts, 329
  ulcers, 329
Corns, 327
Coronary, 329
Coronary artery bypass, 227, 330
Coronary care unit, 330
Coronary heart disease, 330–332, *331*, *332*
  alert, 331
Coronary thrombosis, 332
Corset, 332
Corticosteroid drugs, 102–103, 333, 646
Corticosteroid hormones, 333
Cosmetic dentistry, 333
Cosmetic surgery, 333–334
  blepharoplasty, 176
  body contour surgery, 191
  breast implants, *917*
  dermabrasion, 1065
  examples, 916
  face-lift, 482
  liposuction, 722
  mammoplasty, 747
  otoplasty, 860–861
  rhinoplasty, 1017
  Z-plasty, 1246
Costalgia, 334
Cough, 334–335
  expectorants, 475
Cough, smokers', 336
Coughing up blood, 336
Counseling, 337
  post-abortion, 25
Cowpox, 337
Coxa vara, 337
CPR (cardiopulmonary resuscitation), *247*, 247–248
Crabs (pubic lice), 715–716, *716*, *969*, 969–970
Cradle cap, *337*, 337, 354
Cramps, 338
  menstrual, 765
  muscle, 798
Craniopharyngioma, 338
Craniosynostosis, 338
Craniotomy, 339
Crepitus, 339
Cretinism, 446
Creutzfeldt-Jakob disease (CJD), *339*, 339
Cri du chat syndrome, 296, 339
Crisis intervention, 340
Crohn's disease, *340*, 340–341
  alert, 341
Cromolyn sodium, 341
Cross-dressing, 1179
Cross-eye, 342, 1103
Crossmatching, 341
Croup, 335, 342
Crowding, 342–343

Crush syndrome, 343
Crutch palsy, 343
Crutches, 1230
Crying in infants, 343
Cryopreservation, 344
Cryosurgery, 344
Cryptococcal meningitis, 521
Cryptococcosis, 344–345
Cryptosporidosis, 876
Cultures, 345
Curettage, *345*, 345
Curling's ulcer, 345
Cushing's syndrome, 346, 445, 447, 911
Cusp, dental, 346
Cutaneous membrane, 1062, *1062*
Cutaneous tags, 1066
Cutdown, 347
Cyanide, 347
Cyanosis, 347
Cyclophosphamide, 348
Cyclothymic disorder, 166
Cystectomy, 348
Cystic fibrosis, *349*, 349–350, 500
Cystinuria, 607
Cystitis, 350–351
  frequent urination, 1199
Cystocele, 351
Cystometry, 351
Cystoscopy, 351–352
Cystostomy, 352
Cysts, 348
Cytology, 352
Cytomegalovirus (CMV), 352, *352*
Cytoplasm, 259

D

D and C (dilation and curettage), 353
D-galactose, 701
Dacryocystitis, 353
Dairy foods, 832
Danazol, 353–354
Danbolt-Closs syndrome, 31
Dandruff, 354
Dandy fever, 363
Deafness, 354–355
Death, 355–356
  caution about, in drowning victims, 403
Debridement, 24, 356
Decalcification, dental, 356
Decerebrate, 357
Deciduous teeth, *463*, 948
Decompression, spinal canal or cord, 357
Decompression sickness, 155, 357, 1034

Decongestant drugs, 357–358
Deep vein thrombosis, 1156
Defibrillation, *358*, 358
Defoliate poisoning, 358
Deformity, 358
Degeneration, 358–359
Degenerative disorders, 359
Dehiscence, 359
Dehydration, 359–360
  alert, 360
  in infants, 361
  vomiting, 1227
Delirium, 362
Delivery, 362
  alternative methods, 60–61
  emergency, 438
Delusions, 1030
Dementia, 362
Demyelination, 362
Dengue, 363
Dental abscesses, 26
Dental emergencies, 363–364
Dental examination, 364
Dental x-rays, 364
Dentures, *365*, 365
Dependent personality disorder, 366
Depersonalization, 366
Depilatory, 366
Depot injection, 366
Depressants, 406
Depression, *97*, 367–368
  adolescents, 39
  bipolar disorder, 166
  drug treatment, 97
  in the elderly, 958–959
  neuroses, 821
  postpartum, 931
  suicide, 1116
  symptoms, 787
  thought process, 1154
Dermabrasion, 369, 1065
Dermatitis, *369*, 369
Dermatitis herpetiformis, 370
Dermatology, 370–371
Dermatomyositis, 372
Dermatophyte infections, 372
Dermographia, 369
Dermoid cyst, 372–373
DES (diethylstilbestrol), 386
Desensitization, 153–154
Desmoid tumor, 373
Detergent poisoning, 373
Detoxification, 62–63, 487, 834
  from alcohol, 53
Development delay, *373*, 373–374
Dextrocardia, 375
Dextrose, 375
Diabetes insipidus, 375
Diabetes mellitus, 375–376
  alert, 618

Diagnosis, 378–379
  alert, 378
  screening, 1033
  techniques, *378*
Diagnosis-related group, 379
Diagnostic imaging, 1148
  CAT scan, 252, *252*, 637, 1148
  kidneys, 1001
  MRI (magnetic resonance imaging), 794, *794*
  PET scans, 901, *901*
  pyelography, 979–980
  scanning techniques, 1028, *1028*
  thyroid, 1161
  transillumination, 1177
  X-rays, 1243–1244
Diagnostics in women's health, 379
Dialysis, 380–381
Diaphragm (contraceptive), 149, *149*, 324
Diaphragm (muscle), *21*, 382
Diarrhea, 361, 382–383
  alert, 383
  drug treatment, 98
Diastole, 383
Diathermy, 257, 383
Diet. *see also* Nutrition
  cancer therapy, 236–237
  and disease, 384
Diets
  Atkins, 385
  fads, 384
  metabolism, 772
Dietary fiber, 385, 497
Dietary supplements, 832, 833
  digestive enzymes, 870
  multivitamins, 797
  niacin alert, 884
  vitamins, 1225
Diethylstilbestrol (DES), 386
Differential diagnosis, 379
Differentiation, 386
Digestion, in Parkinson's disease, 879
Digestive enzyme supplements, 870
Digestive system, 386–387, *387*
Digital rectal examination, 953
Digitalis drugs, 387
Digoxin, 388
Dilation and curettage (D and C), 353
Dilutional hyponatremia, 1054–1055
Diminished fertility, 388–389
Diminished ovarian reserve, 388–389
Dioxin, 44
Diphtheria, 389, 400
Diplopia, 399

Emergency childbirth, *438*, 438
Emergency hospitalization, 439
Emetic, 440
EMG (electromyogram), 440
Emphysema, 440–441
  surgical, 442
Empyema, 442
Encephalitis, 442
Encephalitis lethargica, 442–443
Encephalomyelitis, 443
Encephalopathy, 443
Encopresis, 444
Endarterectomy, 444
Endemic illness, 444
Endocarditis, 444–445
Endocrine disorders, 445
Endocrine glands, 474, 541
Endocrine system, *446*, 446–447, *541*
Endodontics, 447
Endometrial cancer, 1201
Endometriosis, 448, 633
Endometritis, 448
Endorphins, 448, 609
Endoscopy, *449*, 449
Endothelium, 450
Endotoxin, 450
Endotracheal tube, 450
Enema, 450
Energy, 451. *see also* Calories
Energy medicine. *see specific modalities, such as* Acupressure; Ayurvedic medicine
Energy requirements, 451–452
Engagement, 452
Enkephalins, 609
Enophthalmos, 452
Enteral nutrition, 490
Enteritis, 452
Enterostomy, 453
Enterotoxin, 453
Entropion, 453, 481
Enuresis, 454
Environmental health, 971
Environmental medicine, 454–456
  sick building syndrome, 1055
Enzymes, *456*, 456
  digestive supplements, 870
Eosinophils, *179*
Ependyoma, 457
Epidemic myalgia, 199
Epidemics, 457
Epidemiology, *457*, 457, 971
Epidermolysis bullosa, 457–458
Epididymis, 458
Epididymitis, 1145
Epididymoorchitis, 458
Epidural anesthesia, 85, *458*, 458
Epiglottis, 342

Epiglottitis, 459
Epilepsy, 459–460, *460*
  alert, 460
  seizure, 1036–1037
  temporal lobe, 1140
Epinephrine, 461, 609
Epiphysis, 461
Episcleritis, 461
Episiotomy, 279, 461
Epispadias, 461
Epithelium, 462
Epstein-Barr virus, *462*, 462
  Hodgkin's disease, 605
  mononucleosis, 786–787
Erectile dysfunction, 462–463
Erection, *462*, 462
  disorders of, 462–463, 1217
Ergometer, 463
Ergonomics, 463
Erosion, dental, 463
Eruption of teeth, *463*, 463
Erysipelas, 464, 883
Erythema, 464, 990
Erythema ab igne, 464
Erythema infectiosum, 501
Erythema multiforme, *464*, 464
Erythema nodosum, *465*, 465
Erythroblastosis neonatorum, 588
Erythrocyte sedimentation rate (ESR), 469
Erythrocytes, *179*, 465
Erythropoietin, 609
Esmarch bandage, 465
Esophageal atresia, 465–466
Esophagitis, 467
Esophagoscopy, *467*, 467
Esophagus, *21*, *468*, 468
  cancer of, 468
  dilatation, 466
  diverticulum, 466
  spasm, 466
  stricture, 466–467
  swallowing difficulties, 1124
  varices, 467
ESR (erythrocyte sedimentation rate), 469
Essential oils, 115
Estimated life expectancy, 538, 717
Estrogen drugs, 469–470
Estrogen hormones, 470, 609
Ethics, medical, 470–471
Etiology, 472
Euphoria, 472
Eustachian tube, 472
Euthanasia, 472
Evoked responses, 472–473
Ewing's sarcoma, 473
Examination, physical, *473*, 473
Excision, 473
Exercise, 474, 999

  aerobic, 43, 474
Exocrine glands, 541
Exomphalos, 474
Exophthalmos, 474, 952
Exotoxin, 475
Expectorants, 475
Exploratory surgery, 475
Expressing milk, 475
Extraction, dental, 476
Extradural hemorrhage, 476
Extrapyramidal system, 476
Exudation, 476
Eye drops, 478
Eye surgery, laser, *706*
Eyelash disorders, 481
Eyelid, 481
Eyes, *477*, 477, *537*. *see also entries relating to* vision, *and those beginning with* oph-; opt-
  accommodation, 28
  artificial, 478
  discharge, 390–391
  ectropion, 424
  enophthalmos, 452
  examination of, *478*, 478
  exophthalmos, 474
  foreign body in, *479*, 479
  injuries to, 479–480
  tumors, 480
Eyestrain, 481
Eyewear, protective, 177, *177*, *837*

F

Face-lift, 482
Facial pain, 482
  trigeminal neuralgia, 1183
Facial palsy, 482–483
Facial spasm, 483
Fad diets, 384
Fahrenheit scale, *483*, 483, *1139*
Failure to thrive, 483–484
Fainting, 484
  hypotension, 629
  Stokes-Adams syndrome, 1100
Falls, preventing, 484–485
Familial Mediterranean fever, 485
Family planning, 324, 485, 972. *see also* Contraception
  Billing's method, 161
Family practitioner, 485
Family therapy, 486, 967
Fanconi's syndrome, 486
Farmer's lung, 486–487
Fascia, 487
Fasciotomy, 487
Fasting, 487, 834
Fat (body), 222. *see also* Adipose tissue

Fatigue, 298, 1165
Fats and oils, 488
Fats (dietary), 832
Fatty acids, 488
Fecal impaction, 489
Feces, 489
  abnormal, 489
Fee for service, 489
Feeding, artificial, *490*, 490,
    531, 617
Feeding, infant, 490–491
Feet, *514*, 514
  flatfoot, 505
  pains in, 774
  podiatry, 923
  pronation, 952
  talipes, 1131
Feldenkrais method, 491
Femoral artery bypass, *227*
Femoral nerve, 491
Femur, 492
  fracture of, 492
Fertility, 492
  diminished, 388
  polycystic ovary, 926
  semen analysis, 1038
Fertility drugs, 493
Fertilization, 493
  in vitro, 649
Fetal alcohol syndrome, 55,
    374, 494
Fetal circulation, 494
Fetal disease, 281
Fetal distress, 494
Fetal heart monitoring, 279,
    495
Fetoscopy, *495*, 495
Fetus, *437*, 495
  development stages, 937
  umbilical cord, 1192–1193
Fever, 495–496, *496*, 639
  alert, 495
  pyrogen, 981
  seizures, 1037
Fever blister, *497*, 497
Fiber, dietary, 385, 497
  alert, 385
Fiber optics, *498*, 498
  endoscopy, 449
Fibrillation, 498
Fibrinolysis, 498
Fibrocystic breast disorder, 214
Fibrocystic disease, 499
Fibroids, 499
Fibroma, 500
Fibrosarcoma, 500
Fibrosis, 500
Fibrositis, 500–501
Fibula, 501
Fifth disease, 501
Fight or flight response, 501
Filariasis, 502, 876

Filling, dental, 502–503
Finger joint replacement, 503
Fingernails, 881
Fire ants, 665–666
First aid, 503
  assessment, 439
  bleeding treatment, 175–176
Fitness, 504
Fitness testing, 504
Fixation, 504
Flail chest, 505
Flatfoot, 505
Flatulence, 505
Flatus, 505
Flatworms, 506
Fleas, 423, *876*
Floaters, 506
Flossing, dental, 506
Flow cytometry, 507
Flu, 550–551, *660*, 660–661
Fluctuation, 507
Fluid therapy, 997
Flukes, 506, 507
Fluorescein, 507–508
Fluoridation, 508, 972
Fluoride, 508
Fluoroscopy, of the heart, 575
Folic acid, 508, 1224
Follicle-stimulating hormone
    (FSH), 509, 609, 910
Follicles, *509*, 509
Folliculitis, 509
Fomites, 509
Fontanelles, 338, 509
Food additives, 510
Food allergies, 510–511
Food and Drug
    Administration, 511
Food contamination, 511–512
Food fads, 512
Food Guide Pyramid, 832
Food intolerance, 512–513
Food poisoning, 513
Food preservatives, 944
Food safety
  irradiation alert, 881
  pasteurization, 881
  trichinosis, 1181–1182, *1182*
Foods, caloric content, 233
Footdrop, 514
Forceps, 514, *514*
Forceps delivery, 514–515
Forebrain, 202
Foreign bodies, 515
  in eyes, 479
Forensic medicine, 515–516
Foreskin, 516, 516
Formaldehyde, 516
Formication, 516
Formulas (infant), 199,
    490–491
Fracture

hips, 601
skull, 1067
Fracture, dental, 518
Fractures, 517, *517*
  ankle, 934
  femur, 492
  jaw, 683
  sports-related, 1089
  stress, 1105
Fragile X syndrome, 296, 518,
    769
Freckle, 519
Freud, Sigmund, 962
Friedreich's ataxia, 262, 519
Frontal lobe, 202
Frostbite, 519, *519*
Frozen section, 520
Frozen shoulder, 520
Fruit, 347
FSH (follicle-stimulating hor-
    mone), 509, 609, 910
Fugue, dissociative, 520
Fulminant, 520–521
Fundoplication, 29
Funduscien, 507–508
Fungal infections, 521, *521*
  athlete's foot, 129
  candidiasis, 238
  drug treatment, 98–99
Fungus, 522, *522*
Furuncles, 192

G

G6PD deficiency (glucose-6-
    phosphate dehydrogenase),
    523
GABA (gamma-amino-butyric
    acid), 523
Galactorrhea, 523, 911
Galactosemia, 524, 773
Gallbladder, 21, 160, 524, *524*
  cancer of, 524
  disorders of, 524–525
  removal, 288
Gallstones, 525, *525*
Gamma-amino-butyric acid
    (GABA), 523
Gamma globulin, 525
Ganglion cyst, 526
Gangrene, 526, *526*
Ganser's syndrome, 526
Garderella vaginalis, 527
Gardner's syndrome, 928
Gas, intestinal, 22, 505
Gastrectomy, 527, *527*
Gastric bypass, 530
Gastric cancer, 1100–1101
Gastric erosion, 528
Gastric lavage, 528
Gastrin, 530, 609
Gastritis, 528

H

Using this Index

Article titles can be found in **bold blue**.
Symptoms are listed in green. Symptoms that are also article
titles are listed in **bold green**.
Emergency medicine-related material is red. Emergency medi-
cine article titles are **bold red**.
Numbers of pages on which images can be found are *italicized*.

---

vomiting, 1227
Infections, *653*, 653
 congenital, 654
 opportunistic, 845
 viral, drug treatment, 105–106
Infectious disease, *655*,
    655–657
Infective arthritis, 119
Inferiority complex, 657
Infertility, 657–658
 Rubin test, 1022
Inflammation, 639, 659
Influenza, 550–551, *660*,
    660–661
Informed consent, 322
Infrared, 661
Ingrown toenails, *661*, 661
Inhalers, 661–662
Inheritance, 662–664
Injury, *664*, 664
Inner ear, 415
Inoculations, 641–643, 665. *see
    also* Vaccinations
 immune system, 640
Inoperable, 665
Insect bites, *665*, 665
 mosquitoes, 789
Insect stings, 665–666, *666*, 667
 alert, 666
Insecticides, 789
Insects and disease, 666–667
Insight psychotherapy, 667, 967
Insomnia, 667–668
Insulin, 376, 610, 668–669, *669*
Insulinoma, 669
Integrative medicine, 61–63
Intelligence, 669–670
 mental retardation, 769–770
Intelligence tests, 670–671
Intensive care, 671
Intercourse, painful, 671
Interferon, 672
Intermittent claudication,
    896–897
Internal bleeding, 672
Internal medicine, 971
Internist, 672
Intersex, 672–673
Interstitial fluid, 1165
Interstitial pulmonary fibrosis,
    673
Interstitial radiation therapy,
    673–674
Intertrigo, 674
Intestinal flukes, 507
Intestines, *674*, 674
 cancer of, 675
 noises in, 198
 obstruction of, 675–676, *676*,
    1227
 tumors of, 676
Intracavitary therapy, 676

Intracerebral hemorrhage,
    676–677, *677*
Intrauterine device (IUD), *325*,
    325
 alert, 677
Intrauterine growth
    retardation, 373, 677–678
Intravenous infusion, *678*, 678
Introitus, 678
Intubation, 678–679
Intussusception, *679*, 679
Involuntary movements, 679
Iodine, 679
Ionizing radiation, 984
Ions, 680
Ipecac, 680
IQ (intelligence quotient),
    670–671
Iridology, 61
Iron, 680
 anemia, 79, 81
 hemochromatosis, 586
 siderosis, 1057
Irradiation alert, 881
Irrigation, wound, 681
Irritable bladder, 681
Irritable bowel disease, 659
Irritable bowel syndrome,
    681–682
Ischemia, 682
Islets of Langerhans, 376, 869
Isolation, 682
Itching, 958
IUD (intrauterine device), *325*,
    325
 alert, 677

J

Jaundice, 161, 683
Jaw
 dislocated, 683
 fractured, 683
 prognathism, *950*, 950
 wiring of the, 1240
Jealousy (delusional), 684
Jejunal biopsy, 684
Jejunum, 21
Jellyfish stings, 684
Jet lag, 685
Jock itch, 1164
Joggers' nipple, 685
Joints, *686*, 686
 dislocation alert, 393
 fingers, 503
 replacement, 120
Journal of the American
    Medical Association, 71
Jumper's knee, 686
Juvenile chronic polyarthritis,
    1014

K

Kala-azar, 687
Kaposi's sarcoma, 48, *687*, 687
Karyotyping, 297
Kawasaki disease, 687
Kegel exercises, 687, 886
Keloids, 311, *688*, 688
Keratin, 688
Keratitis, 688
Keratocanthoma, *688*, 688
Keratoconjunctivits, 688
Keratoconus, 689
Keratomalacia, 689
Keratopathy, 689
Keratosis, actinic, 689
Keratosis pilaris, *689*, 689
Keratotomy, radial, 690
Ketoacidosis, 376
Ketosis, 690
Kidney function test, 693
Kidney stones, 692, 813. *see
    also* Calculus, urinary tract
 renal colic, 1000
 surgical removal, 980
Kidney transplant, 694
Kidneys, *691*, 691, 693, 813. *see
    also entries beginning with*
    nephr-
 cancer of, *692*, 692
 cysts, 692
 glomerulonephritis, 543
 hypertension, *622*, *814*
 pain, 22
 polycystic, 695
 removal, 812
 tumors in, *695*, 695
Kilocalorie, 695
Klinefelter's syndrome,
    295–296, 695, 1184
Klumpke's paralysis, 695
Knee, *696*, 696
Knee joint replacement, 696,
    697
Knock-knee, 697
Koplik's spots, 697, *753*
Kuru, 698
Kwashiorkor, 698
Kyphoscoliosis, 698
Kyphosis, 698

L

Labial adhesions, 699
Labile, 699
Labor. *see* Childbirth
Labyrinthitis, 417
Laceration, 700
Lacrimal apparatus, 700
Lactation, 213
Lactic acid, 701

Lactose intolerance, 701
  alert, 701
Lactulose, 701
Lamaze method, 701–702, *702*
Laminaria, 702
Laminectomy, 702
Lance, 702
Lanugo hair, 702–703
Laparoscopy, 703
Laparotomy, exploratory,
  703–704
Large intestine, 386
Larva migrans, 704
Laryngectomy, 704
Laryngitis, 704, 1226
Laryngoscopy, *704*, 704–705
Larynx, 705
  cancer of, 705
Laser treatment, 706
Lasers, 705
Lassa fever, 706
Latency, 651
Laurence-Moon-Biedl
  syndrome, 707
Laxative drugs, 707
Lead poisoning, 707–708
Learning disabilities, 708–709
Leeches, 709
Leg, shortening of, 710
Leg ulcers, 709, 1190
Legionnaires' disease, *710*, 710,
  921
Leiomyoma, 710
Leishmaniasis, 687, *687*, *710*,
  710–711, 876, 1026
Lens, 477, *711*, 711
Lens dislocation, 711
Lentigo, *1066*
Leprechaunism, 711–712
Leprosy, *712*, 712
Lesion, 712
Leukemia, *183*, 235, *713*, 713
  chronic lymphoid, 714
  chronic myeloid, 714
Leukocytes, 714
Leukodystrophies, 715
Leukoplakia, 715
Liability insurance,
  professional, 715
Liaison Committee on Medical
  Education, 28
Libido, 1045
Lice, 423, *715*, 715–716
Licensure, 716
Lichen planus, *716*, 716
Lichen simplex, 716
Lichenification, 717
Lid lag, 717
Life expectancy, 538, 717
Life jackets, 27
Life support, 471, 717
Ligaments, *718*, 718

abdominal, 21
  sprains, 1091
Ligation, 718
Ligature, 718
Light therapy, 718–719, 907
Lightening, 719
Limb defects, 719
Limbic system, 203, 720
Limbs, artificial, 719
Linear accelerator, 720
Lip cancer, 720
Lip reading, 722
Lipid-lowering drugs, 721
Lipids, *721*, 721
  disorders of, 720–721
  hyperlipidemias, 619
Lipoatrophy, 721
Lipoma, 722
Liposarcoma, 722
Liposuction, 722, 916
Listeriosis, 723
Lithium, 723
Lithotomy, 723
Lithotomy position, 723
Lithotripsy, 723
Lithotriptor, 724
Livedo reticularis, 724
Liver, *21*, *724*, 724–725. *see also*
  entries beginning with
  hepat-
  abscess, 725
  biopsy, 725
  cancer, 726
  cirrhosis, 302
  disease, *592*
  diseases of, alcohol- or drug-
    induced, *726*, 726–727
  alert, 726
  failure, 727–728
  imaging, 728
  transplant, 727, 729–730
Liver flukes, 507, 728
Liver function, 405
Liver function tests, 728
Lobectomy, 730
  lung, *731*, 731
Lochia, 731
Lockjaw, 400, 731, 1150, 1183
Loose bodies, 731
Loss of consciousness, 731
Lou Gehrig's disease, 791
Ludwig's angina, 732
Lumbar puncture, *732*, 732
Lumbosacral spasm, 732
Lumpectomy, 751
Lung disease, chronic
  obstructive, 734
Lung flukes, 507
Lungs, 732, 975
  alveoli, 65
  cancer of, *733*, 733–734, 1072
  collapsed, 127

imaging, 734
in newborns, 940–941
tumors, 735
Lupus erythematosus, *735*, 735
Lupus vulgaris, *735*, 735
Luteal phase defect, 735
Luteinized unruptured follicle
  syndrome, 736
Luteinizing hormone (LH),
  610, 736
Luteinizing hormone releasing
  hormone (LHRH), 736
Luxated tooth, 736
Lyme disease, *737*, 737
Lymph glands
  swollen, 541
Lymph nodes, 738
Lymph vessels, 738
Lymphadenitis, 36
Lymphangiography, 737
Lymphangioma, 615, 738
Lymphangitis, 738
Lymphatic system, 738–739
Lymphedema, 739
Lymphocytes, 180, 183,
  739–740
  T cell, 1136
Lymphogranuloma venereum,
  537
Lymphoma, 235, 740
  non-Hodgkin's, 740

M

Macrobiotics, 741, 833
Macroglossia, 741
Macrophages, *179*
Macular degeneration, *741*,
  741–742
Mad cow disease, *339*
Magnesium, 742
Magnetic resonance imaging.
  see MRI
Magnetic therapy, 742
Malabsorption, 743
  after gastrectomy, 527
  diarrhea, 382
  sprue, tropical, 1091–1092
Malalignment, 743
Malar flush, 743
Malaria, *744*, 744–745
  alert, 1180
Malignant, 745
Mallet toe, 745
Mallory-Weiss syndrome, 745
Malocclusion, 743, 746
Malpractice, 397
Malpresentation, 746
Malta fever, 222
Mammalgia, 746
Mammary duct, 746
Mammography, *238*, *379*, *747*,

747
  schedule recommendations,
    211, *211*, 238
Mammoplasty, 747
Mania, 165–167, 748
Manic-depression, 787
Manometry, 748
Marasmus, 748–749
March fracture, 749
Marfan's syndrome, *749*, 749
Marijuana, 406, 749
Marine animals, sting alert,
    1099
Marital counseling, 749–750
Marsupialization, 750
Masochism, 750
Massage therapy, *62*, 750. *see
    also* Bodywork
  reflexology, 996
Mast cell, 750
Mastectomy, *214*, 750–751
Mastication, 751
Mastitis, 751
Mastocytosis, 752
Mastodynia, 746
Mastoiditis, 417, *752*, 752
Masturbation, 752
Maternal mortality, 752–753
McArdle's disease, 753
Measles, 753, 753
Meat, cancer link, *832*
Mebendazole, 754
Meckel's diverticulum, *754*,
    754
Mediastinoscopy, 754–755
Medicaid, 755
Medical schools, accreditation,
    28
Medicare, 755
Medicine chest, 755
Meditation, 756, 999
Mediterranean fever, 222
Medulla oblongata, *202*
Megacolon, 756
Megalomania, 756–757
Meibomianitis, 757
Meigs' syndrome, 757
Melanin, 757
Melanoma, 371, *371*, 757, *757*,
    1064, 1066
Melanosis, 758
Melasma, 284
Melatonin, 685
Melena, 758
Melioidosis, 758
Membrane, cell, *758*, 758
Memory, 71, 759
Menarche, 760, 764–765
Ménière's disease, 417, *760*,
    760
Meningioma, 761
Meningitis, *761*, 761

Meniscectomy, 762
Menopause, 762–763
  hot flashes, 611
  hysterectomy, 1201
  perimenopause, 894
Menorrhagia, 763, 766
Menstrual extraction, 25, 764
Menstrual pain, 22
Menstruation, 764–765
  amenorrhea, 70
  breakthrough bleeding, 208
  disorders of, 765–766
  dysmenorrhea, 413
  Mittelschmerz, 784
  tampon, 1132
Mental fitness, in the elderly,
    45
Mental health
  adolescents, 39
  DSM IV, 409
Mental hospital, 766
Mental illness, 767–768
  incidence, 766
  mania, 748
  shock therapy, 431
  signs of, 768
  types, 767
Mental retardation, 769–770
Meperidine, 771
Mercury, 771
Mercury poisoning, 771,
    780–781
Mesenteric lymphadenitis, 772
Mesothelioma, 772
Metabolic rate, energy
    requirements, 451
Metabolism, 772
  inborn errors of, 773
Metabolites, *773*, 773
Metaplasia, 773
Metastasis, 234, 244, 773
Metatarsalgia, 774
Methanol, 774
  alert, 774
Methotrexate, 774
Microcephaly, 774
Microorganism, 775
Microscope, 775
Microsurgery, 776
Mid-life crisis, 777
Middle ear, 415
Middle-ear effusion, persistent,
    776–777
Midwifery, 778
Mifepristone, 24, 25
Migraines, 559, *559*, 779
  aura, 133
Milia, 779
Miliaria, 580
Miliaria crystallina, 947
Milk, 780
Milk-alkali syndrome, 780

Milk intolerance, 701
Milk of magnesia, 780
Minamata disease, 780–781
Mind-body medicine, *781*, 781
Mineral oil, 781
Minerals, 781
Miscarriage, 782. *see also*
    Abortion
Mites, 423, 783
Mitosis, *1183*
Mitral insufficiency, 783
  alert, 783
Mitral stenosis, 784
Mitral valve prolapse, 273, 784
Mittelschmerz, 784
Mobilization, 784
Molar pregnancy, 785
Mold, 785
Moles, 785
Molluscum contagiosum, *785*,
    785
Mongolian spot, *786*, 786
Monitors, 786
Monoamine-oxidase inhibitors
    (MAOIs), 97
Monoarthritis, 786
Monocytes, *179*, 180
Mononucleosis, 786–787
  alert, 787
Monosodium glutamate, 283
Monteggia's fracture, 787
Mood disorders, 767, 787
Morbidity, 788
Morning after pill, 788
Morning sickness, 788, 1228
Morphea, 788
Morphine, 788
Mortality, 789
Mosaicism, 664, 789
Mosquito bites, *789*, 789
Motion sickness, 790
Motor neuron disease, 790–791
Mouth, 386, *791*, 791
  cancer of, 791–792
  dry, 792
  ulcers in, *792*, 792–793
Mouthwash, 793
Movement, 793
MRI (magnetic resonance
    imaging), *238*, *794*, 794, *827*
  bone imaging, 195
  brain, 206
  heart, 575
  mechanism, 637, 1148
MSH (melanocyte-stimulating
    hormone), 610
Mucopolysaccharidosis, 311,
    795
Multiple births, 493
Multiple personality disorder,
    795
Multiple sclerosis, *796*, 796

Multivitamins, 797
  alert, 797
  niacin alert, 884
  supplements, 1225
Mumps, *797*, 797
Münchausen syndrome, 797
Murmur, heart, 798
Muscle-relaxant drugs, 799
  general anesthesia, 83
Muscles, *798*, 798
  paralysis, 874–875
  spasm, 798, 1078
  strain, 1101–1102
  surgical removal, 803
  tone, 1168
Muscular dystrophy, 414, 799
Mushroom poisoning, *799*, 799
  alert, 800
Mutagen, 800
Mutation, 800–801
  cancer, 234–235
Mutism, 801
Myalgia, 801
Myasthenia gravis, 802
Mycoplasma, 802
Mycosis fungoides, 803
Myectomy, 803
Myelin, 715
Myelitis, 803
Myelocele, 803
Myelodysplastic syndrome, 803
Myelofibrosis, 500
Myelography, 804
Myelomas, 235
Myelomeningocele, 804
Myelopathy, 804
Myelosclerosis, 804
Myiasis, 805
Myocarditis, *805*, 805
Myoclonus, 806
Myoma, 499
Myomectomy, 806
Myopathy, 806
Myopia, 806
Myotonia congenita, 806
Myringoplasty, 418
Myringotomy, 419
Myxedema, 446–447

N

Nabothian cysts, 267
Nalidixic acid, 807
Narcissism, 807
Narcolepsy, 807
Narcosis, 808
Narcotics, 868
Nasogastric tube, 809
Nasopharynx, cancer of, 809
Natural contraception, 809
Naturopathy, 810
Nausea, *810*, 810

motion sickness, 790
  in pregnancy, 618, 1228
Near-sightedness, 806
Nebulizer, 811
Neck, *811*, 811
  dissection, radical, 811
  rigidity, 811
  stiffness, 1098
  torticollis, 561, 1098, 1171
  whiplash injury, 1238, *1238*
Necrolysis, toxic epidermal, 812
Necrosis, 812
Neonatology, 812
Neoplasia, 812
Nephrectomy, 812
Nephritis, 813
Nephrocalcinosis, 813
Nephrolithotomy, 813
Nephrology, 813–814
Nephropathy, 814
Nephrosclerosis, 814
Nephrostomy, 814
Nephrotic syndrome, 814
Nerve, acoustic, 31
Nerve, trapped, 815
Nerve block, 815
  local anesthesia, 84–85
Nerves, *815*, 815
  abducens, *23*, 23
  brachial plexus, 201
  central nervous system, 260
  injury, 815, 821
Nervous breakdown, 816
Nervous system, 816–817
  autonomic, 136
Network-model HMO, 564
Neural tube defects, 818
Neuralgia, 817
Neurapraxia, 818
Neuritis, 818
Neuroblastoma, 818–819
Neurocutaneous disorders, 819
Neurodermatitis, 716
Neurofibromatosis, *819*, 819
Neuroleptics, 103
Neuroma, 820
Neuropathic joint, 820
Neuropathy, 376, *820*, 820–821, 868
  paralysis, 874
Neurosis, 821
Neurosyphilis, 821
Neurotoxin, 821
Neutrophils, *179*, 180, 183
Nevus flammeus, 583
Nevus (nevi), 785, 821
  alert, 821
Newborns, 822–823. *see also*
  Infants
  hemolytic disease, 588
  postnatal care, 931

premature birth, 940–941
  reflexes, 995
  umbilical cord, 1192–1193
  vernix, 1215
Niacin, 1223
  overdose alert, 884
  pellagra, 884
Nickel, 823
Niclosamide, 823
Nicotine, 823–824
  alert, 824
  smoking cessation aid, 1167
Niemann-Pick disease, 824
Night blindness, 825
Night terror, 825
Nightmare, 825
NIH (National Institutes of Health), 825
Nipples, *826*, 826
Nitrites, 826
Nitrogen, 826
Nocardiosis, 826
Nocturia, 826
Nocturnal emission, 827
Noise, 827
  in the workplace, 839
Noninvasive techniques, 827
Nonspecific urethritis, 828
Nonsteroidal anti-inflammatory drugs (NSAIDs), 102–103, 828
Norepinephrine, 609, 829
Norwalk virus, 382
Nose
  broken, 829–830
  congestion, 808
  discharge, 808
  obstruction, 808–809
Nosebleed, *829*, 829
Nuclear jaundice, 690
Nuclear medicine, 830
Nucleus, 259
Numbness, 830
Nurse, *831*, 831
Nurse, home care, 831
Nurse-midwives, 778
Nursing, 213
Nursing homes, 427–428, 538
Nutrition, 832
  Parkinson's disease, 879
Nutrition and diet, alternative therapies, 833–834
Nutritional disorders, 834
Nutritional supplements
  alert, 797
  multivitamins, 797
  vitamins, 1225
Nycturia, 826
Nystagmus, 433
Nystagmus, 835

O

Obesity, 836
  body mass index (BMI), 835, 836
  cancer risk factor, 242
Obsessive-compulsive disorder, 836, 1154
Occipital lobe, *202*
Occult blood, fecal, 837
Occupational medicine and health, *837,* 837–839
Occupational therapy, 840
Oedipus complex, 840
Oligohydramnios, 840
Oligomennorhea, 765
Oligomenorrhea, 840
Oligospermia, 840
Oliguria, 841
Omentum, *21*
Omphalocele, 474
Onchocerciasis, 502, 841
Oncogene, *841,* 841
Oncology, 842
Onlay, dental, 842
Onychogryphosis, 842
Onycholysis, 842
Oophorectomy, 843
Open heart surgery, 843
Operable conditions, 843
Operant conditioning, 154
Operating room, *844,* 844, *1122*
Operation, 844
Ophthalmology, 844
Ophthalmoscope, *845,* 845
Opiates, 406, 845
Opportunistic infection, 845
Optic atrophy, 846
Optic disk edema, 846
Optic nerve, *846,* 846, 1220
Optometry, 846
Oral and maxillofacial surgery, 847–848
Oral contraceptives, 847
Oral hygiene, 847
Orbit, 848
Orchiectomy, 848
Orchiopexy, 848
Orchitis, 849, 1145
Organ donation, 849
Organelles, 259
Orgasm, 850
Oriental medicine. *see specific modalities, such as* Acupressure; Herbal medicine;
Ornithosis, 850
Oroya fever, 1026
Orthodontic appliances, *850,* 850–851
Orthodonture, 201
Orthognathic surgery, 851

Orthopedics, 851
Orthopnea, 851
Orthoptics, 852
Orthostatic hypotension, 628
Osgood-Schlatter disease, 852
Osteitis, 852
Osteoarthritis, 119, *119,* 852–853, *853*
Osteoarthropathy, 304
Osteochondritis dissecans, 852–853
Osteochondritis juvenilis, 853
Osteochondroma, 854
Osteodystrophy, 854
Osteogenesis imperfecta, 311
Osteogenesis imperfecta, 854
Osteoid osteoma, 854
Osteoma, 854
Osteomyetitis, *855,* 855
Osteopathic medicine, 855–856
Osteopetrosis, 856
Osteophyte, 856
Osteoporosis, 857–858
Osteosarcoma, *858,* 858
Osteosclerosis, 858
Osteotomy, 859
Ostomy
  colostomy, 315, 994
  enterostomy, 453
  ileostomy, 635–636
  nephrostomy, 814
Otitis, 415
Otitis externa, 859
Otitis media, 776–777, *860,* 860
Otoplasty, 860–861
Otorhinolaryngology, 861
Otosclerosis, 417, 861
Otoscope, 861–862, *862*
Ototoxicity, 862
Outpatient treatment, 862
Ovaries, 447, 863, 1002
  cancer of, *863,* 863
  cysts in, *862,* 862
  polycystic, 926
  removal, 843
Overbite and overjet, 864
Overcrowding, dental, 864
Overuse injury, 864
Ovulation, 864
  fertility drugs, 493
  infertility, 658
Ovum, 864
Oxygen, 865
Oxygen storage
  alert, 865
Oxygen therapy, 441, 865–866
Oxytocin, 610, 866, 910
Ozena, 866
Ozone, 866

P

Pacemaker, *116, 867,* 867
Paget's disease, 867
Pain, 867–868
  kidney (*see* Calculus, urinary tract)
  muscular, 801
  neuralgia, 817
  pelvic, 887
  referred, 994
Pain relief, 868
Pain relievers
  morphine, 788
  opiate, 845
Painful arc syndrome, 869
Palpation, 473
Palpitation, 869
Pancreas, *376,* 447, *869,* 869
Pancreas, cancer of, 870
Pancreatectomy, 870–871
Pancreatitis, 871
Pancreatography, 871–872
Panic disorder, 108
Panic disorder, 872
Pantothenic acid, 1223
Pap smear, 872–873, *873*
  recommendations, 237
Papilledema, 873
Papilloma, intraductal, 873
Papule, 873
Paraffin bath, 1235
Paralysis, 874–875
Paralysis, periodic, 875
Paranoid personality disorder, 875
Paraphimosis, 876
Paraplegia, 876
Parasites, 876
  external, 422–423
  flatworms, 506
  lice, *715,* 715–716
  liver flukes, 728
  mites, 783
  pubic lice, *969,* 969–970
  snails, 1073
Parasitic diseases
  alert, 423
  amebiasis, 69
  amoebic dysentery, 876
  Chagas' disease, 269, 756, 876
  drug treatment, 99
  dysentery, 412
  filariasis, 502
  flukes, 507
  giardiasis, 539
  Guinea worm disease, 553
  histoplasmosis, 603
  hydatid disease, 612
  kala-azar, 687
  larva migrans, 704
  malaria, 744–745
  onchocerciasis, 841
  roundworm, 1021

schistosome, 1028
schistosomiasis, 1029
sleeping sickness, African,
    1070
strongyloidiasis, 1108–1109
tapeworm infestation, 1133
toxoplasmosis, 1173–1174
trichomoniasis, 1182
whipworm infestation, 1239
Parasympathetic nervous
    system, 136
Parathesia, 878–879
Parathion, 877
Parathyroid glands, 447, *619,*
    877
  hyperparathyroidism, 617
  hypoparathyroidism, 626–627
Parathyroid hormone, 610
Parathyroid tumor, 878
Parathyroidectomy, 878
Paratyphoid fever, 878
Paraurethral glands, 1062
Parenteral nutrition, 490, 617
Parietal lobe, *202*
Parkinsonism, 880
Parkinson's disease, 793,
    879–880
Paronychia, 881
Parrot fever, 850, 959–960
**Passive-aggressive personality
    trait,** 881
Pasteurization, 881
Patau's syndrome, 295, 1184
Patent ductus arteriosus, 882
Paternity testing, 882
Pathogens, *653,* 655, 882
Pathognomonic, 882
Pathology, 882
PCP (phencyclidine), 86
PCR (polymerase chain reac-
    tion), 345
Peak flow meter, 883
Peau d'orange, 883
Pediatrics, *883,* 883
Pedicle, 884
Pediculosis, 481
Pedophilia, 884
Peer groups
  adolescents, 39
Pellagra, 884
Pelvic floor exercises, 886
Pelvic inflammatory disease,
    886
Pelvimetry, 888
Pelvis, *888,* 888
  examination, *885,* 885
  infection, 886
  pain, chronic, 887
Pemphigoid, bullous, 888
Pemphigus, 888
Penicillin drugs, *93,* 889, 889
Penile implant, *889,* 889

Penis, *890,* 890, 1003
  balanitis, 145
  cancer of, 890
  circumcision, 301, *301*
  foreskin, 516
  Peyronie's disease, 902
  priapism, 946
  smegma, 1072
Peptic ulcer, 22, 890, *891*
Perception, 891
Percussion, 473, *892,* 892
Percutaneous, 892
Perforation, 893
Periarteritis nodosa, 893
Pericarditis, 273, 893–894, *894*
Perimenopause, 762, 894
Perimetry, 895
Periodic abstinence, 325
Periodic fever, 485
Periodontal disease, 895
Periodontics, 895
Periodontitis, 895–896
Periostitis, 896
Peripheral neuropathy, 820
Peripheral smear, 187
Peripheral vascular disease
  alert, 897
Peripheral vascular disease,
    896–897
Peritoneal dialysis, 381
Peritoneum, *21*
Peritonitis, *897,* 897
Peritonsillar abscess, 982
Permanent teeth, *463,* 898, *948*
Pernio, 898
Peroneal muscular atrophy,
    898
Personality, 898
  stress, 1104
Personality disorders, 767, 899
  antisocial, 104
  avoidant, 138
  borderline, 198
  dependent, 366
  histrionic, 603
  multiple, 795
  narcissism, 807
  paranoia, 875
  schizoid, 1029
Personality tests, 900
Perthes disease, 900
Pertussis, 400, 1239
Pessary, 900
Pesticides, 900–901
  alert, 900
  strychnine, 1109
PET scanning (positron emis-
    sion tomography), 637, *901,*
    901, 1149
Petechiae, 902
Peterson-Kelly syndrome, 919
Petit mal seizures, 460

Peutz-Jeghers syndrome, 902
Payronie's disease, 902
PH, *902,* 902. *see also* Acidosis;
    Alkalosis
Phagocyte, 902
Phantom limb, 903
Pharmacology, 903
**Pharyngioesophageal
    diverticulum,** 904
Pharyngitis, *903,* 903
Pharynx, cancer of, 904
Phenacetin, 692
Phenylketonuria, 769, 773, 905
Pheochromocytoma, 905
Philadelphia chromosome, 714
Phlebitis, 249, 905, 1155
Phlebography, 1212–1213
Phlebotomus fever, 1026
Phlegm, 335, 1092
Phobias, 108, 906
Phocomelia, 906
Phosphates, 906
Phosphorus poisoning, 906
Photocoagulation, 907
Photosensitivity, 907
Phototherapy, 907
Phthiriasis, 481
Physical exam, 1147
Physical therapy, 907–908
  after stroke, 1108
Physician-assisted suicide, 471,
    472
Pica, 908
  alert, 908
Pickwickian syndrome, 216
Pigeon toes, 908
Pigmentation, 908–909
  vitiligo, 1226
Piles, 909
Pimples, 909. *see also* Acne
Pineal gland, *909,* 909
Pinel, Phillip, *962*
Pinguecula, 909
Pink puffer, 909
Pins and needles, 878–879
Pinta, 910
Pinworms, 1021
Pituitary gland, 203, 446,
    910–911, *911*
Pituitary tumors, 911–912
Pityriasis alba, 912
Pityriasis rosea, 912, *912*
Pivot joint, 686
Placebo, 912
Placenta, 912–913
Placenta previa, *913,* 913
Plague, *913,* 913
Plantar wart, 914
Plants, poisonous, 914–915,
    924. see also Poison ivy, oak,
    & sumac
  alert, 914

Plaque, dental, *915*, 915. *see also* Calculus, dental
discolored teeth, 391

Plaque, 332, 915
periodontitis, 895–896

Plasma, 179

Plasmapheresis, 916

Plastic surgery, 916–917. *see also* Cosmetic surgery

Platelets, *179*, 180, 183

Plethora, 917

Plethysmography, 918

Pleural effusion, *918*, 918

Pleurisy, 918

Pleurodynia, 199, 919

Plication, 919

Plummer-Vinson syndrome, 919

Plutonium, 919

PMS (premenstrual syndrome), 942

Pneumaturia, 920

Pneumoconiosis, 411, 920–921

Pneumocystis pneumonia, 920

Pneumonectomy, 921

Pneumonia, 921–922
alert, 922

Pneumonitis, 923

Pneumothorax, 923

Podegra, 548

Podiatry, 923

Podophyllin, 923

Poison, 923–924

Poison ivy, oak, & sumac, *924*, 924

Poisoning, 27, 924–925
Agent Orange, 44
cadmium, 228
chlorate alert, 285
defoliates, 358
detergents, 373
drug overdose, 407
drugs (pharmaceutical), 408
food poisoning, 513
lead poisoning, 707–708
mercury poisoning, 771

Poliomyelitis, *925*, 925

Pollen, *57*

Pollution, 926

Polyarteritis nodosa, 893

Polycystic ovary, 926

Polycythemia, 926–927

Polydactyly, *927*, 927

Polymerase chain reaction (PCR), 345

Polymyalgia rheumatica, 927

Polymyositis, 927

Polyp, 928

Polyposis, familial, 928

Pomeray technique, 928

Pompholyx, 928

Pons, *202*

Porphyria, 929

Port-wine stains, 583, *929*, 929

Portal hypertension, 929–930

Post-coital test, 930

Post-menopausal bleeding, 930

Post-traumatic stress disorder, 932–933

Postmaturity, 930

Postnasal drip, 931

Postnatal care, 931

Postpartum depression, 931

Postpartum hemorrhage, 931

Posttraumatic stress disorder, 108–109

Postural drainage, 933

Posture, 933

Potassium, 933–934
alert, 934

Potency, 934

Pott's fracture, 934

Pox, 934

Precancerous, 935

Precocious puberty, 935

Predisposing factors, 935

Prednisolone, 935

Preeclampsia, 422, 936

Pregnancy, 936–937, *937. see also* Fetus
amniocentesis, 72
amnioscopy, 73
antepartum hemorrhage, 91
breast changes, 209
cats, cautions, 256
conception, 318, *318*
counseling, 938
drugs in, 939
eclampsia, 422
ectopic, 423–424
energy requirements, 451–452
false, 939
hyperemesis, 618, 1228
implantation, egg, 648
infant's retardation, 769–770
molar pregnancy, 785
morning sickness, 788
mortality risk, 752–753
multiple, 940
pica alert, 908
postmaturity, 930
preeclampsia, 422, 936
premature birth, 940–941, 1018
prenatal care, 942–943
quickening, 982
Rh incompatibility, 1014–1015
ritodrine, 1018
rubella, 1021–1022
superfetation, 1119
surrogate mother, 1123
tests for, 938
toxemia, 1172
toxoplasmosis, 1173–1174

with twins, 1189
ultrasound scanning, 1191–1192
uterus, 1200–1201
vaginal bleeding alert, 1205
vomiting, 1228

Premature birth, 940–941

Premature ejaculation, 426, 1045

Premedication, 941

Premenstrual syndrome (PMS), 942

Premolar, 942

Prenatal care, 942–943

Prepared childbirth, 943

Prepuce, 516

Presbycusis, 944

Presbyopia, *478*, 478, 944

Prescription drugs, 404

Preservative, 944

Pressure points, 175, 175, *944*, 944

Pressure ulcers, 1190

Preventive dentistry, 945

Preventive medicine, 945, 971

Preventive screening and counseling, 946

Priapism, 463, 946

Prickly heat, 947

Primary, 947

Primary prevention, 947

Primary teeth, 948

Prions, 1071

Probucol, 948

Procaine, 948

Processed foods, 622

Procidentia, 948, 1202, *1202*

Proctalgia fugax, 948

Proctitis, 949

Prodrome, 949

Progeria, 949

Progesterone drugs, 949

Progesterone hormone, 609, 950

Prognathism, *950*, 950

Prognosis, 950

Progressive systemic sclerosis, 1032

Prolactin, 610, 910, 951

Prolactinoma, 951

Prolapse, 951

Prolapsed cord, 281, *951*, 951

Prolapsed uterus, 951

Pronation, 952

Prophylactic, 952

Prophylactics, 149

Proprioception, 952

Proptosis, 952

Prostaglandin, 952

Prostaglandin drugs, 953
abortifacient, 24, 25

Prostate gland, *955*, 955

cancer of, 953–954
digital rectal examination, 992
enlarged, 1199
enlarged, 954–955
hyperplasia, *620*
Prostate-specific antigen, 953
Prostatectomy, *955*, 955
Prostatism, 956
Prostatitis, 956
Prosthesis, *163*, *956*, 956
artificial heart, 300, *300*
finger joint, 503
hip replacement, 601–602
knee joint, 696
limbs, 719
Prosthodontics, 956
Protective clothing, 839, *839*
Protective eyewear, *837*
Protein (dietary)
kwashiorkor, 698
Protein synthesis, 957
Proteins, 832, 957
Proteinuria, 957
Prothrombin time, 182
Protozoa, 958
Prozac, 958
Pruritus, 958
Pseudarthrosis, 958
Pseudocyesis, 939
Pseudodementia, 958–959
Pseudogout, 959
Pseudohermaphrodism, 959
Pseudohermaphrodites, 672–673
Psittacosis, 850, 959–960
Psoralen drugs, 960, 979
Psoriasis, 370, *960*, 960
Psychiatry, 961, 971
Psychoanalysis, 961–963
Psychoanalyst, 963
Psychometry, 963
Psychopath, 104
Psychopathology, 963
Psychosis, 767, 963–964
drug treatment, 103
Psychosomatic disorders, 964–965
somatization disorder, 1076
Psychosurgery, 966
Psychotherapy, 966–967. *see also specific treatments, such as* Cognitive behavior therapy
family therapy, 486
Pterygium, 968
Ptosis, 968
Ptyalsim, 968
Puberty, 968–969
precocious puberty, 935
signs, 38
Pubic lice, 715–716, *716*, *969*,

969–970
Public health, 970–973
disease reporting, 1001
Public health dentistry, 973
Pudendal block, 973
Puerperal sepsis, 973–974
Puerperium, 974
Pulmonary alveolitis, 591
Pulmonary artery, *976*
Pulmonary embolism, *974*, 974
Pulmonary fibrosis, 500, 975
Pulmonary function tests, 975
Pulmonary hypertension, 975
Pulmonary insufficiency, 976
Pulmonary stenosis, 976
Pulp, dental, 977
Pulpectomy, 977
Pulpotomy, 977
Pulse, 977
Punch grafting, 556
Punchdrunk, 978
Pupils, 477, *978*, 978
Purpura, 978–979
Pus, 391, 979
empyema, 442
Pustules, 909, 979
PUVA (psoralen/UV-A therapy), 979
Pyelography, 979
Pyelolithotomy, 980
Pyelonephritis, 813, 980
Pyeloric stenosis, *981*, 981
Pyloroplasty, 981
Pyridoxine (vitamin B_6), 1223
Pyrogen, 981
Pyuria, 981

Q

Q fever, 982
Qi. *see* Acupressure, Acupuncture
Qigong, 982
Quarantine, 982
Quickening, 982
Quinsy, 982

R

Rabbit fever, 1187
Rabies, *983*, 983
Rachitic, 983
RAD, 983
Radiation, 838, 984–985
cancer, 242
poisoning symptoms, 984
workplace hazard, 838
Radiation hazards, 985
Radiation poisoning, 984
Radiation sickness, 986
Radiation therapy, 986,

986–987, 1243, 1244
Radical mastectomy, 751
Radical surgery, 987
Radiculopathy, 988
Radioactivity, 988
Radiology, 988–989
Radionuclide scanning, 195–196, 1148
Radium, 989
Radon, 989
Raloxifene, 470
Rape, 989–990
Rash, 990
RAST test, 58
Raynaud's disease, 990
Raynaud's phenomenon, 249, 990
Rebound headache, 559
Recessive patterns, 1243
Recombinant DNA, 991
Reconstructive surgery, 916
Recovery position, 439, 991, 991
Rectal bleeding, 991–992
Rectal examination, 992
Rectal prolapse, 993
Rectocele, 993
Rectum, 993, *994*
cancer of, *993*, 993
Red blood cells, 180, 182–183
sperocytosis, hereditary, 1082
Reduction, 994
Referred pain, 994
Reflex action, 817
Reflex sympathetic dystrophy, 1054
Reflexes, *995*, 995
newborn, 822
Reflexology, 996
Regional enteritis, 340–341
Regression, 996
Regurgitation, 996
Rehabilitation, 996–997
Rehydration therapy, 997
Reimplantation, dental, 997
Reiter's syndrome, *997*, 997
Rejection, 998
Relapse, 998
Relapsing fever, 998
Relaxation
biofeedback, 162
meditation, 756
Relaxation response, 999
Relaxation techniques, 999
REM sleep, 401, 1068
Remission, 999
Renal biopsy, *1000*, 1000
Renal colic, 1000
Renal failure, 1000–1001
Renal tubular acidosis, 1000–1001
Renin, 610, 1001

Renography, 1001
Repetitive strain injuries
  (RSIs), 838, *838*
Reportable diseases, 1001
Reproduction, sexual, 735,
  1002
 fertility, 492
 infertility, 657–658
 luteinized unruptured follicle
   syndrome, 736
 luteinizing hormone, 736
 luteinizing hormone releasing
   hormone, 736
 menopause, 762–763
 menstruation, 764–765
 ovulation, 864
 sperm, 1081, *1081*
 sterility, 1096–1097
 zygote, 1246
Reproductive system, female,
  1002, 1002
Reproductive system, male,
  1003, 1003
Reproductive technology, 471
Rescue, of drowning victims,
  1233–1234
Resection, 1004
Resistance, 1004
Resorption, dental, 1004
Respiration, 1006
Respirator, 1214
Respiratory arrest, 1004
Respiratory distress syndrome,
  1005
Respiratory failure, 1005
Respiratory system, 1005–1006,
  1006
Respiratory therapy, 1007
Respiratory tract infection,
  1007
Resting Metabolic Rate (RMR),
  772
Restless leg syndrome, 1007
Restoration, dental, 1007
 onlays, 842
Retardation, mental, 769–770
Retinal artery occlusion, 1008
Retinal detachment, 1008
Retinal hemorrhage, 1009
Retinal tear, 1009
Retinal vein occlusion, 1009
Retinas, 477, *477*, *1008*, 1008
Retinitis pigmentosa, 1009
Retinoblastoma, 1009
Retinopathy, 376
Retractor, 1010
Retrobulbar neuritis, 1010
Retrograde ejaculation, 426
Retrolental fibroplasia, 1010
Retroperitoneal fibrosis, 1010
Retroverted uterus, 1010–1011,
  1202

Rett's syndrome, 1011
Reye's syndrome, 275, *1011*,
  1011
Rh (rhesus) factor, 179, 184
Rh immune globulin, 1014
Rh incompatibility, 1014–1015
Rhabdomyolosis, 1012
Rhabdomyosarcoma, 1012
Rheumatic fever, 1012
Rheumatism, 1012
Rheumatoid arthritis, 119, *119*,
  1012–1013, *1013*
 drug treatment, 104
Rheumatoid arthritis, juvenile,
  1014
Rheumatology, 1014
Rhinitis, 1015–1016
 allergic, 1016
Rhinophyma, 1016
Rhinoplasty, 1017
Rhythm method, 325
Rib, fractured, 1017
Riboflavin (vitamin B$_2$), 1017,
  1223
Ribosomes, 259
Ribs
 cervical, 265
Rickets, 1017
Rickettsia, 1018
Rigidity, 1018
Rigor, 1018
Ringing in the ears, 417
Ringworm, 372, *1018*, 1018,
  1164
Ritodrine, 1018
Roberts syndrome, 906
Robotic surgery, 288
Rocky Mountain spotted fever,
  1019, 1019
Rods, 477
Rolfing, 1019
Root-canal treatment, 977,
  1019–1020, *1020. see also*
  Endodontics
Rorschach test, 1020
Rosacea, *1020*, 1020
 rhinophyma, 1016
Roseola, infantum, 1020–1021,
  1021
Rotavirus, 361, 382
Roundworm, 1021
RU-486, 24, 25

Rubber dam, 1020
Rubella, 1021–1022
 congenital, 654
Rubin test, 1022
Rubor test, *117*, 990
Rubra miliaria, 947
Runner's knee, 1022, *1022*
Running injuries, 1022

S

Saccharin, 1023
Sacralgia, 1023
Sacralization, 1023
Sacroiliitis, 1023
Sadism, 1023
Saliva
 dry mouth, 792
Salivary glands, *1024*, 1024
Salivation, 1024
 excess (water thrush), 208
Salmon patches, 170
Salmonella, *1024*, 1024
Salpingectomy, 1025
Salpingitis, 1025
Salpingo-oophorectomy, 1025
Salt, 1025
Sand fleas, 275
Sand fly bites, 1026
Sanitary napkin, 1026
Sarcoid, *1026*
Sarcoidosis, 1026
Sarcomas, 235, 1026
Saturated fats, 488
Scabies, *1027*, 1027
Scabs, 1027
Scaling, dental, 1027
Scalp, 1027
Scalp reduction, 556
Scalpel, 1027
Scanning techniques, *1028*,
  1028
Scarlet fever, 1028
Scarletina, 1028
Scars, 1028
 keloid, 688
Schistosome, 1028
Schistosomiasis, 1029
Schizoid personality disorder,
  1029
Schizophrenia, 767, 964, 1030
Schönlein-Henoch purpura,

Using this Index
Article titles can be found in **bold blue.**
Symptoms are listed in green. Symptoms that are also article
titles are listed in **bold green.**
Emergency medicine-related material is red. Emergency medi-
cine article titles are **bold red.**
Numbers of pages on which images can be found are *italicized.*

Sleep walking, 1070
Sleeping drugs, 1070
Sleeping sickness, African, 442–443, 876, 1070, 1185
Slings, *1071*, 1071
Slit lamp, 1071
Slow virus disease, 1071
Small-cell carcinoma, 1072
Small intestine, 386
Smallpox, 1072
Smegma, 1072
Smell, 1072–1073
Smoking, passive, 1073
Smoking, tobacco, 972, 1167
  breathing, 217
  cancer, 242
  carcinogens, *824*
  cessation, 407, 1167, *1167*
  nicotine, 823–824
  tongue cancer alert, 1169
Snails and disease, 1073
Snakebites, *1074*, 1074
Sneezing, 1074
Snellen chart, 1074–1075, *1075*
Snoring, 1075
Sobriety test, *55*
Social maturity, signs of, 38
Sociopath, 104
Sodium, 1075
Sodium chloride, 1025
Soft palate, 1203, *1203*
Soft spot, 509
Soft-tissue injury, 1076
Solvent abuse, 1076
Somatization, 821
Somatization disorder, 1076
Somatostatin, 610
Somnambulism, 1070
Sore throat, 1077
Sores, 1077
Sounding of the uterus, 1077
Space medicine, 1077
Spasms, 1078
  drug treatment, 105
  tic, 1162
Spastic paralysis, 1078
Spasticity, 1078
Specimens, 1078
Speculum, 1078
Speech, 1079
  mechanism, 1006
Speech disorders, 1080
Speech therapy, 1080–1081
Speech threshold audiometry, 566
Sperm, 318, *1081*, 1081
Sperm count, 658, 840
Spermicide, 1082
Sperocytosis, hereditary, 1082
Sphincter, artificial, 1082
Sphincterotomy, 1083
Spider bites, *170*, *1083*, 1083

Spider nevus, 1083
Spider veins, 583
Spina bifida, 818, 1083–1084
Spinal anesthesia, 1084
Spinal block, 84–85
Spinal cord, 1084–1085
Spinal cord damage
  drowning, 403
Spinal fusion, 1085
Spinal injury, 1085–1086
Spinal muscular atrophy, 1237
Spinal stenosis, *1086*
Spine, *391*, *392*
  disks, 391
  vertebra, 1216, *1216*
Spirituality, 1086
Spirochete, 1086
Spirometry, *1086*, 1086
Spleen, *21*, 620, *1087*, 1087
Splenectomy, 1087
Splint, 1087
Splinting, dental, 1088
Spondylitis, 1088
Spondylolisthesis, 1088
Spondylolysis, 1088
Sporotrichosis, *1089*, 1089
Sports injuries, 1089–1090
Sports medicine, 1090–1091.
  see also Athletes
Sports, unlawful drugs and, 1091
Sprains, 1091
Sprue
  celiac, 258
  Tropical, 1091–1092
Sputum, 1092
Squamous cell carcinoma, 371, *1065*, *1092*, 1092–1093, *1093*
Squamous papillomas, 1066
St. Vitus' dance, 293, 612
Stable, 1093
Staff-model HMO, 564
Stages, 1093
Stapedectomy, 1093–1094
Staphylococcal infections, *1094*, 1094
Starches, 240
Starvation, 1094
Statistics, vital, 717, 1095
Statistics and indicators, medical, 1095
Status asthmaticus, 1096
Status epilepticus, 460
Steatorrhea, 1096
Stein Levanthal syndrome, 926
Steiner's disease, 806
Stem cells, from cord blood, 1193
Stenosing tenosynovitis, 1183
Stenosis, 1096
Stereotaxic surgery, 1096
Sterility, 1096–1097

Sterilization, 325
  female, 1097
  male, 1097
Steroids, anabolic, 1097
Stethoscope, *1097*, 1097–1098
Stevens-Johnson syndrome, 464
Stiff neck, 811, 1098
Stillbirth, 1098
Stimulant drugs, 406, 1098–1099
Stimulus, 1099
Stings, 1099. *see also* Bites
  insect, 665–666
  jellyfish, 684
  marine animal alert, 1099
  scorpion, 1033
  venomous, 1213, *1213*
Stirrup, 415
Stitch, 1099
Stokes-Adams syndrome, 1100
Stomach, *21*, 386
  gastrectomy, 527, *527*
  noises in, 198
Stomach, *1100*, 1100
Stomach cancer, 1100–1101
Stomach ulcer, *1101*, 1101
Stomatitis, 1101
Stones
  kidney, 813
  ureteral, 1194
Strabismus, 342
  abducens nerve, 23
Strabismus, 1103
Strain, 1101–1102
Strangulation, 1102
Strangury, 1102
Strapping, 1102
Strawberry hemangioma, 583
Strep throat, 903, *1102*, 1102
Streptococcal infections, 1103
Streptokinase, 1103
Stress, 1103–1105
  fight or flight response, 501
  immune system, 965
  management, 63
  meditation, 756
  reduction, 999
  in the workplace, 838
Stress fractures, 1022, 1105
Stress response
  norepinephrine, 829
Stress test (cardiac), 245, 430
Stress ulcer, 1105
Stria, 1105–1106
Stridor, 1106
Strip grafting, 556
Stroke, *1106*, 1106–1108
  alert, 205
  hemorrhagic, 677
  mechanism, 435
  paralysis, 874
  symptoms, 1166

therapy after, 1108
transient ischemic attack, 1177, *1177*
Strongyloidiasis, 1108–1109
Strontium, 1109
Strychnine poisoning, 1109
Sturge-Weber syndrome, 1109–1110, *1110*
Stuttering, 1080, 1110
Styes, 192, 481, *1110*, 1110
Subarachnoid hemorrhage, 1111
Subcaudate tractotomy, 966
Subclavian steal syndrome, 1111
Subconjunctival hemorrhage, 1111
Subconscious, 1111
Subcutaneous, 1111
Subdural hemorrhage, 1112
Subluxation, 1112
Submucous resection, 1112
Subphrenic abscess, 1113
Substance abuse, 767, 1113
  alcohol dependence, 52–53
  amphetamines, 73
  cocaine, 305
  drug dependence, 406–407
  marijuana, 749
  psychosis, 963–964
  solvents, 1076
  stimulant drugs, 1098–1099
Substrate, 1113
Subunit vaccine, 1113
Sucking wound, 1114
Sucralfate, 1114
Suction, 1114
Sudden death, 1114
Sudden infant death syndrome, 1114–1115
Sudeck's atrophy, 1115
Suffocation, 1115
Sugar, 240
  hyperactivity myth, 616
Sugar substitutes, 121
Suicide, 1116
  adolescents, 39
  physician-assisted, 471
  poisoning, 924–925
  warning signs alert, 1116
Sulfamethoxazole, 1117
Sulfinpyrazone, 1117
Sulfisoxazole, 1117
Sulfonathide drugs, 1117
Sulfur, 1117
Sunburn, 1118
Sunlight
  adverse effects of, 1118
  cancer, 243
  ultraviolet light, 1192
Suntan, 1119
Superfecundation, 1119

Superfetation, 1119
Superficial, 1119
Superinfection, 1120
Superiority complex, 1120
Supernumerary, 1120
Support groups, 1120
Suppositories, 1121
Suppuration, 1121
Supraventricular tachycardia, 1121
Surfers' nodules, 1121
Surgeons, 1122
Surgery, 1122
  elective, 428. *see also specific procedures, such as* Cosmetic surgery; Liposuction
  exploratory, 475
  microsurgery, 776
  operating room, 844
  premedication, 941
Surrogate mothers, 1123
Suturing, 1123. *see also* Stitches
Swab, 1123
Swallowing, 1124
Swallowing difficulties, 1124
Swallowing of air, 43
Sweat, 1125
Sweat glands, *1125*, 1125
Swelling, 1125–1126
  abdominal, *23*, 23
Swimmer's ear, 859
Sycosis vulgaris, 1126
Sydenham's chorea, 293
Sympathectomy, 1126
Sympathetic nervous system, 136
Synapses, 1126
Syncope. *see* Fainting
Syndactyly, 1126
Synovectomy, 1127
Synovitis, 1127
Syphilis, 1049, *1049*, *1127*, 1127–1128
  congenital, 654
  "general paralysis of the insane," 533
  nerve damage, 821
  ulceration, 536
Syringe, 1129
Syringing of the ear, 1129
Syringomyelia, 1129–1130
Systemic, 1130
Systemic lupus erythematosus, 735, *735*
Systole, 1130

T

T cells, 639, 1136
Tabes dorsalis, 1128

Tachycardia, 1131
Tachypnea, 1131
Tacrolimus, 1131
T'ai chi, 1131
Talipes, 1131
Tamoxifen, 470
Tamponade, 1132
Tampons, 1132
Tannins, 1132
Tantrums, 1132
Tapeworm infestation, 1133
Tapeworms, 506, *876*, *1240*
Tarsalgia, 1133
Tarsorrhaphy, 1133–1134
Tartar. *see* Calculus, dental
Taste, 1134
Tattooing, 1135
Tay-Sachs disease, *534*, *1136*, 1136
Tear sac infection, 353
Tears, 700, 1137
  artificial, 1137
Technetium, 1137
Teeth, *1136*, 1136–1137, *1137*
  abrasion, 25
  abscess, *26*
  calcification, 229
  eruption, 463
  extraction, 476
  fillings, 502
  permanent teeth, 898
  plaque, 230
  premolar, 942
  preventive dentistry, 945
  primary teeth, 948
  reimplantation, 997
Teething, 1138
Telangiecstasia, 1138
Temperature, 1138–1139
  Celsius scale, 260
  Fahrenheit scale, 483
  fever, 495
  thermography, 1152–1153
Temporal arteritis, 1139
Temporal lobe, *202*
Temporal lobe epilepsy, 1140
Temporomandibular joint syndrome, *1140*, 1140–1141
Tenderness, 1141
Tendolysis, 1141
Tendon, 1141
Tendon reflex test, 473
Tendon repair, 1141
Tendon transfer, 1142
Tendonitis, 1022, 1142
Tennis elbow, *1142*, 1142
Tenosynovitis, 1142–1143
Tenovaginitis, 1143
Tension headache, 559, *559*
Terminal health care, 1143
Terrorism, 1143
Testes, 447, 1003, *1144*, 1144

cancer of, 1144–1145
descending, 848
pain in the, 1145
removal, 848
retractile, 1145
swollen, 1145–1146
torsion of, *1146*, 1146
undescended, 1146
Testicular feminization
syndrome, 1144
Testosterone, 610, 1146
Tests, medical, 1147–1148
Tetanus, 400, 1150
Tetany, 1150
Tetracycline drugs, 1150
Tetrahydroaminoacridine,
1150
Tetralogy of Fallot, 1151
Thalamus, 1151
Thalassemia, *1151*, 1151
Thallium, 1152
Thallium stress test, 430
Therapeutic community, 1152
Therapeutic touch, 1152
Thermography, 1152–1153
Thermometer, 1153
Thiamine, 1223, 1237
Thirst, 1153
Thomsen's disease, 806
Thoracic outlet syndrome,
1154, 1154
Thought disorders, 1154
Thrill, 1154
Thrombectomy, 1154–1155
Thrombocytopenia, 174,
978–979, 1155
Thrombocytosis, 174
Thromboembolism, 1155
Thrombophlebitis, 1155
Thrombosis, 249, 1156
alert, 1156
Thumb-sucking, 1157
Thymoma, 1157
Thymus, 1157
Thyroglossal disorders, 1157
Thyroid function test,
1160–1161
Thyroid gland, *1158*,
1158–1159
cancer of, *1159*, 1159–1160
goiter, 546
Grave's disease, 550
Hashimoto's thyroiditis, 558
hyperthyroidism, 623, *623*,
1159
hypothyroidism, 631
underactivity, 631
Thyroid hormone, 610
Thyroid scanning, *1161*, 1161
Thyroidectomy, 1160
Thyroiditis, 1161
Thyrotoxicosis, 445, 1162

Tic douloureux, 1183
Ticks and disease, 1162–1163,
1163
relapsing fever, 998
Rocky Mountain spotted
fever, 1019, *1019*
Tics, 1162
facial, 483
Tourette's syndrome, 540,
1171–1172
Tietze's syndrome, 1163
Timolol, 1163
Tinea, *1164*, 1164
Tinea corporis, *1018*
Tinea pedis, 129
Tinea versicolor, 1164
Tinnitus, 417, 1164
Tiredness, 1165
Tissue fluid, 1165
Tissue plasminogen activator,
1166
Tissue typing, 1166
Titanium dental implants, 1166
Tobacco smoking, 1167
cancer, 242
carcinogens, *824*
nicotine, 823–824
Tocography, 1167
Toilet-training, 1167–1168
Tomography, 1168
Tone, muscle, 1168
Tongue cancer, 1168–1169
smokers' alert, 1169
Tonometry, 1169
Tonsillectomy, *1169*, 1169
Tonsillitis, 1170
Tooth care, 1170, *1171*
Toothache, 1170
Toothbrushes, 25
Toothbrushing, 1170
Tophi, 548
Torticollis, 561, 1098, 1171
Touch, 1171
Touch therapy, 1152
Tourette's syndrome, 540, 793,
1171–1172
Tourniquets, 175, 1172
Toxemia, 1172
Toxic epidermal necrolysis
(TEN), 464
Toxic shock syndrome,
1172–1173
Toxicity, 1173
Toxicology, 1173
Toxins, 1173
Toxocariasis, 704
Toxoids, 1173
Toxoplasma gondii, *1173*
Toxoplasmosis, 1173–1174
congenital, 654
Trabeculectomy, 1174
Trace elements, 1174

Tracers, 1174
Tracheitis, 1174–1175
Tracheoesophageal fistula,
1175
Tracheostomy, 1175
alert, 1175
Tracheotomy, *1175*, 1175–1176
Trachoma, 1176
Traction, *1176*, 1176
Trager psychophysical
integration, 1176
Trait, 1177
Tranquilizers, 155, 1070
Transcendental meditation,
756
Transfusion, autologous, 1177
Transient ischemic attack,
1177, 1177
alert, 1106
Transillumination, 1177
Transmissible, 1178
Transplant surgery, 1178
Transplants
bone marrow, 196
cornea, 329
graft-*versus*-host disease, 549
grafting, 549
hair, 556
heart, 578
heart-lung, 576
histocompatibility antigens,
602–603
immunosuppressants, 646
kidney, 380, 694
liver, 729–730
organ donation, 849
rejection, 998
skin, 1065
tissue typing, 1166
xenotransplantation, 1242
Transposition of the great
vessels, 1178
Transsexualism, 1178–1179
Transvestism, 1179
Trauma, 1179
Traumatology, 1179
Travel immunizations, 1179
Travel medicine, 1180
Traveler's diarrhea, 1180
Tremors, 1180–1181
Parkinson's disease, 879–880
Trench fever, 1181
Trench foot, 638
Trench mouth, 1217
Trials
clinical, 1181
controlled, 326
Trichiasis, 481, 1181
Trichinosis, 1021, 1181–1182,
1182
Trichomonas, 1207
Trichomoniasis, 1182

Tricuspid insufficiency,
1182–1183
Tricyclic antidepressants, 97
Trigeminal neuralgia, 1183
Trigger finger, 1183
Triple X syndrome, 295, 1184
Trismus, 1183
Trisomy, 295, *1183*, 1183–1184
Trisomy 21, 400
Tropical diseases, 1184
Tropical ulcers, 1184–1185
Trypanosomiasis, 1070, 1185
Tsetse fly bites, 1185
TSH (thyroid stimulating
hormone), 610, 910
Tubal ligation, 325, *1185*, 1185
Tube feeding, 531
Tubercle, 1186
Tuberculin tests, 1186
Tuberculosis, *1186*, 1186
congenital, 654
Tuberous sclerosis, *1187*, 1187
Tuboplasty, 1187
Tularemia, 1187
Tumor-specific antigen, 1188
Tumors, 1187–1188
malignant process, 234
Tunics, 477
Tunnel vision, 1188
Turcot's syndrome, 928
Turner's syndrome, 296, 374,
1189
Twins, 940, 1189
Tympanometry, 566

U

Ulcer-healing drugs, 1190
Ulcers, 1190
after burns, 345
corneal, 329
duodenal, 410
genital, 269, 536–537
leg, 709
mouth, 792–793
oral, 239
peptic, 582, 890–891, *891*
possible infection, 1184–1185
skin, 153
stomach, 1101
stress, 890, 1105
sucralfate therapy, 1114
tropical, 1184–1185
Ultrasound, 637, 1148, *1191*,
1191
Ultrasound scanning,
1191–1192
Ultrasound treatment, 1192
Ultraviolet light, 1192
Umbilical cord, 1192–1193,
1193
prolapse, 951

Unconsciousness, *1193*, 1193
Underbite, 1193
Undulant fever, 222
Unsaturated fats, 488
Urea, 1194
Ureter, 1194
Ureterolithotomy, 1194
Urethra, *1194*, 1194
Urethral dilation, 1195
Urethral discharge, 1195
Urethral stricture, 1195
Urethral syndrome, acute,
1195
Urethritis, 1195
nonspecific, 828
Uric acid, *1196*, 1196
Urinalysis, 1196
Urinary catheterization, 255,
1199
Urinary diversion, 1197
Urinary incontinence, 650
Urinary stress incontinence,
1103
Urinary system, *1197*, 1197
Urinary tract infection, 1198
alert, 1198
Urination
excessive, 1198–1199
frequent, 1199
painful, 1199
Urine, 1199–1200
abnormal, 1200
Urine retention, 1200
Urine testing, 1196
Urology, 1200
Urticaria, 604
Urticaria pigmentosa, 752
Uterus, *633*, 1002, 1200–1201,
1201
cancer of, 1201–1202
fibroid, 499
prolapse of, 951, *1202*, 1202
retroverted, 1010–1011
sounding of the, 1077
Uveitis, 1203
Uvula, *1203*, 1203

V

Vaccinations, 641–643, 971,
1204
bacillus Calmette-Guerin, 152
children, 655
immune system, 640
pneumonia, 922
for travel, 1179
Vaccine, 1204
Vacuum extraction, 1204
Vagina, 1002, *1205*, 1205
Vaginal atrophy, 1205
Vaginal bleeding, 1205–1206
pregnancy alert, 1205

Vaginal discharge, 1206
Vaginal dryness, 763
Vaginal itching, 1206
Vaginal repair, 1206
Vaginismus, 1206–1207
Vaginitis, 1207
Vagotomy, 1207
Valsalva's maneuver, 1207
Valvuloplasty, 1208
Varicose veins, 249, 1208–1209
Varioceles, 1145
Variola, 337
Vasectomy, 325, 1097, *1209*,
1209
Vasoconstriction, 1209
Vasodilation, 1209–1210
Vasodilator drugs, 623, 1210
Vectors, 1210
Vegetarianism, 833, 1210–1211
Vegetative state, 1211
Veins, 1211
disorders of, 1211
phlebitis, 905
Vena cava, 21, *1211*, 1211
Venerology, 1212
Venipuncture, 1212
Venography, 1212–1213
Venomous bites and stings,
1213, 1213
alert, 1213
Ventilation, 1213
Ventilators, 1214
Ventricles, 1214
Ventricles (brain), 203
Ventricular ectopic beat, 1214
Ventricular fibrillation,
1214–1215
Ventricular tachycardia, 1215
Vernix, 1215
Version, 1215
Vertebrae, *1216*, 1216
Vertebrobasilar insufficiency,
1216
Vertigo, 699, 1216
Veruga peruana, 1026
Vesicle, 178
Viability, 1217
Viagra, 1217
Vincent's disease, 1217
Vinegar. *see* Acetic acid
Viral infections, drug
treatment, 105–106
Viremia, 1217
Virginity, 1218
Virilism, 1218
Virility, 1218
Virilization, 1218
Virology, 1218–1219
Virulence, 1219
Viruses, 653, *1219*, 1219
Viscosity, 1220
Vision, 1220

double vision, 399
Vision, disorders of, *1220,*
1220–1221
Vision loss, 1221. *see also*
Blindness
alert, 1221
amaurosis fugax, *67*
amblyopia, 68
blurred vision, 190
macular degeneration,
741–742
night blindness, 825
presbyopia, 944
retinal artery occlusion, 1008
retinitis pigmentosa, 1009
tunnel vision, 1188
Vision tests, *1221,* 1221
perimetry, 895
Snellen chart, 1074–1075,
1075
Vison
color, *314,* 314–315
Visual acuity, 1222
Visual field, *1222,* 1222
Vital signs, 1222
Vitamin A, 1222–1223
Vitamin B complex, 1223
Vitamin B$_1$ (thiamine), 443
Vitamin B$_2$ (riboflavin), 1017,
1223
Vitamin B$_3$ (niacin), 1223
overdose alert, 884
pellagra, 884
Vitamin B$_{12}$ (cobalamin),
1223, 1224
Vitamin C, 1224
cancer treatment, 237
Vitamin D, 288, 610, 1224
rickets, 1017
Vitamin E, 1224–1225
Vitamin K, 1225
Vitamin deficiencies
beriberi (thiamine, B$_1$), 156
pellagra, 884
rickets, 1017
scurvy, 1035, *1035*
Vitamin supplements, 1225
Vitiligo, 908–909, 1226
Vocal cords, 1226
Voice
loss of, 1226
speech disorders, 1080
Voice box, 705
Volkmann's contracture, 1226
Volvulus, *1227,* 1227
Vomiting, 1227
drug treatment, 98
hyperemesis in pregnancy,
618, 1228
regurgitation, 996
Vomiting blood, 1227
Vomiting in pregnancy, 1228

Von Recklinghausen's disease,
819
Von Willebrand's disease, 174,
183, 1228
Vulva, *1229*
Vulva, cancer of, 1229
Vulvitis, 1229
Vulvovaginitis, 1229

W

Walkers, 1230
Walking, 1230
disorders, 1230
Walking aids, 1230
Warfarin, 1231
Warts, *1231,* 1231
genital, 1231
plantar warts, 914
Wasps, 665–666
Wasting. *see* Cachexia
Water, 832, 1232
fluoridation, 508
Water cures, 614
Water intoxication, 1233
Water on the brain, 614, 1054
Water on the knee, 1233
Water pills, 101, 393, 622
Water pollution, 1234
Water safety, 1233–1234
Waterborne infection, 1232,
1234
Waterhouse-Friderichsen
syndrome, 1232
Watering eyes, 1232
Wax baths, 1235
Weakness, 1235
Webbing, 1235
Wedge resection, 751
Wegener's granulomatosis,
1235
Weight, 1236
Weight loss, 1236–1237
Weight reduction, 1237
body contour surgery, 191
Werdnig-Hoffman disease,
1237
Werner's encephalopathy, 443
Wernicke-Korsakoff syndrome,
54
West Nile virus, 1238
West syndrome, 653
Western blot test, 643
"Wet dreams," 827
Wheat allergy, 258, 370
Wheelchairs, 1238
Wheeze, 1238
Whiplash injury, *1238,* 1238
Whipple restriction, 870
Whipple's disease, 1238
Whipworm infestation, 1239
White blood cells, 180, 183

phagocytes, 902
White cell count, 639
WHO, 1240
Whooping cough, 400, 1239
Williams syndrome, 711–712
Wilms' tumor, 692
Wilson's disease, 1239
Wiring of the jaw, 1240
Wisdom teeth, 1240
Witches' milk, 1240
Withdrawal
from alcohol, 52
benzodiazepines, 155
Withdrawal, emotional, 1240
Womb, 1200–1201
Workplace health, 837–839
World Health Organization,
1240
Worm infestations, *1240,*
1240–1241, *1241*
drug treatment, 99
Wound infection, *1241,* 1241
Wounds, 1241
irrigation, 681
sucking, 1114
Wrinkles, 1241
Wristdrop, 1241
Writer's cramp, 338
Wryneck, 561, 1098

X

X-linked disorders, 1243
X-rays, *274,* 637, 984, *1243,*
1243–1244
alternatives, 1244
Xanthomatosis, *1242,* 1242
Xenotransplantation, 1242
Xeroderma pigmentosum,
1242

Y

Yawning, 1245
Yaws, 1245
Yeast, *1245,* 1245
Yellow fever, *1245,* 1245
Yew tree, *237*
Yoga, 999, 1245

Z

Z-plasty, 1246
Zidovudine (AZT), 49, 1246
Zinc, 1246
Zollinger-Ellison syndrome,
530
Zoonosis, 1246
Zygote, 318, 1246

Art Credits and Acknowledgments

**T: Top   M: Middle   B: Bottom   TM: Top Middle   BM: Bottom Middle
ICL: In Text Column, Left   ICR: In Text Colum, Right**

21- Lido. 23- T: CDC; IC: CORBIS/Lester V. Bergman; B: Lido. 24- ADAM. 26- T: Lido; B; Lido. 27- T: Corbis/Jennie Woodcock; M: Corbis/Richard Olivier; B: CORBIS/Michael S. Yamashita; IC; Troy Schremmer. 28- Lido. 29- Troy Schremmer. 30- T: CORBIS/ Lester V. Bergman; B: Troy Schremmer. 32- T: Lido; M, B: Troy Schremmer. 33- ADAM. 34- CORBIS. 35- T: CORBIS/Peter Turnley; B: ADAM. 37- ADAM. 38- T: CORBIS/Peter Turnley; B: NCI/Linda Bartlett. 39- T: CORBIS/Laura Dwight; B: NCI. 40- CORBIS/ Dennis Degnan. 43- CDC. 45- CORBIS/Laura Dwight. 48- T:CORBIS/Roger Ressmeyer; IC, M, B: NCI. 49- NCI. 50- Lido. 55- CORBIS/Michael S. Yamashita. 58- Troy Schremmer. 59- ADAM 61- CORBIS/Roger Ressmeyer. 62- B: CORBIS/Roger Ressmeyer. 64- CORBIS/Lester V. Bergman. 69- ICL: CORBIS/Patrick Ward; ICR: CORBIS/Joseph Sohm; TR; Ed Kashi. 77- Troy Schremmer. 79- B: CORBIS/Lester V. Bergman. 80- ADAM. 81- T: ADAM; B: CORBIS/ Lester V. Bergman. 84- CORBIS/Robert Maass. 85- T: CORBIS/Lester V. Bergman; B: Lido. 86- T: CORBIS/Lester V. Bergman; B: Lido. 87- Rachael Soltis. 88- T: CORBIS/Lester V. Bergman; B: ADAM. 92- CDC. 93- B: CORBIS/Rick Price. 94- T: CORBIS/Lester V. Bergman; B: CORBIS/Darrell Gulin. 95- CORBIS/Stanley Coffman. 97- CORBIS/Lawrence Manning. 107- Lido. 109-ADAM. 110- ADAM. 112- Troy Schremmer. 113- Rachael Soltis. 116- CORBIS/Charles O'Rear. 117- B: CORBIS/Lester V. Bergman. 118- T: CORBIS/Jim Zuckerman; B: CORBIS/Ron Boardman. 119- B: CORBIS/Lester V. Bergman. 120- Lido. 125- Rachael Soltis. 129- CORBIS/Lester V. Bergman. 133- CORBIS/Owen Franken. 134- Lido. 136- T: CORBIS/RIchard Olivier. 137- CORBIS/Michael Prince. 141- Lido. 142- Rachael Soltis. 145- Lido. 146 T: CORBIS/Richard Bailey; B; Troy Schremmer. 147- CDC. 149- Troy Schremmer. 150- NCI. 151- Troy Schremmer. 152- ADAM. 153- T: CORBIS/Warren Morgan; B: Lido. 160- ICL- ADAM; ICR- CORBIS/Lester V. Bergman. 161- CORBIS/Christel Gertensberg. 162- CORBIS/Owen Franken. 163- T: CORBIS/Roger Ressmeyer; B: CORBIS/Michael Freeman. 164- T: NCI/Linda Bartlett B: NCI. 167- T: CORBIS; B: Lido. 168- T: CORBIS/Lester V. Bergman; B: CORBIS. 169- Troy Schremmer. 170- ADAM. 171- ADAM. 172- ADAM. 173- CORBIS/Lester V. Bergman. 175- Rachael Soltis. 177- B: CORBIS/Colin Garratt. 178- T: CORBIS; B: CORBIS/Lowell Georgia. 179- IC: ADAM 181- Troy Schremmer. 182- Lido. 183- CDC. 184- ADAM. 186- T: NCI/Linda Bartlett; IC: CORBIS/Bennett Dean. 188- T: ADAM; B: NCI/Bill Branson; IC: CORBIS/Owen Franken. 189- CORBIS/Bob Rowan. 190- CORBIS/David Turnley. 192- CORBIS/Roger Ressmeyer. 194- T: CORBIS/Lester V. Bergman; B: NCI. 195- CORBIS/Charles O'Rear. 196- CORBIS/Lester V.Bergman. 199- T: CORBIS/Laura Dwight; TM: CORBIS/ Laura Dwight; BM: CORBIS/Laura Dwight; B: CORBIS/Richard T. Nowitz. 200- T: CORBIS/ Lester V. Bergman; M: CORBIS/Ed Young; B: CORBIS/Owen Franken. 201- CORBIS/Richard Smith. 202- T: CORBIS/ Lowell Georgia; B; ADAM 203- ICL: NIC/Linda Bartlett; ICR: Lido. 206- T: CORBIS/Roger Ressmeyer; B: NCI. 207- T: CORBIS/Charles O'Rear; B: CORBIS/Leif Skoogfors. 209- IC: ADAM; T: NCI. 210- T: NCI/Linda Bartlett; TM: NCI/Dr. Cecil Fox; BM: NCI; B: NCI/Linda Bartlett. 211- T: NCI/Bill Branson; M, B: NCI. 212- ADAM. 213- CORBIS/ Laura Dwight. 214- NCI/Linda Bartlett. 215- T: CORBIS/ George Lee White; M, B: NCI/ Linda Bartlett. 217- ADAM. 219- Lido. 221- ADAM 224- CORBIS/Lester V. Bergman. 225- T: NCI/ Jane Hurd; B: Lido. 226- T: ADAM; IC: Lido. 227- Lido. 229- Lido. 234- T, M: NCI; 235- NCI. 236- NCI. 237- NCI. 238- NCI. 239. ADAM. 243- NCI. 244- T: ADAM; M, B: NCI. 246- Lido. 247- ADAM. 248- ADAM. 251- IC:

ADAM; T: ADAM; M: Lido. 253- T: ADAM; B: Lido. 254- CORBIS. 255- Lido. 257- Lido. 266- NCI. 267- ADAM. 268- ADAM. 271- NCI. 272- NCI. 275- ADAM. 277- CORBIS. 279- ADAM. 284- CORBIS. 286- ADAM. 295- NCI. 296- B: NCI. 299- ADAM. 200- CORBIS. 301- ADAM. 305- ADAM. 308- CORBIS. 312- ADAM. 313- T, ICT: ADAM; ICB: NCI. 314- ADAM. 316- ADAM. 321- Lido. 323- CORBIS. 325- T, TM: CORBIS; B, BM: ADAM. 332- ADAM. 337- CORBIS. 339- T: CORBIS; B: ADAM. 340- ADAM. 344- ADAM. 352- ADAM. 358- CORBIS. 364- CORBIS. 365- CORBIS. 369- ADAM. 370- ADAM. 371- B: ADAM. 372- ADAM. 373- ADAM. 377- CORBIS. 381- ADAM. 387- ADAM. 390- CDC. 391- ADAM. 392- ADAM. 393- ADAM. 402- B: Lido. 403- ADAM. 410- ADAM. 417- CORBIS. 418- ADAM. 424- T: CDC, B: ADAM. 427- M: CORBIS, B: NCI. 429- ADAM. 432- CORBIS. 434- COR-BIS. 434- Lido. 437- CDC. 438- ADAM. 439- ADAM. 441- ADAM. 448- ADAM. 456- ICR: NCI. 457- CDC. 458- T: Lido. 461- ADAM. 462- CORBIS. 463- ADAM. 464- ADAM. 465- ADAM. 467- ADAM. 468- ADAM. 471- NCI. 473- T: ADAM; B: CDC. 474- CDC. 478- M, B: CORBIS. 479- ADAM. 490- CORBIS. 492- ADAM. 496- CORBIS. 501- ADAM. 503- ADAM. 504- NCI. 509- NCI. 514- T: ADAM. 517- ADAM. 519- ADAM. 521- CORBIS. 522- IC: COR-BIS. 525- ADAM. 526- ADAM. 527- ADAM. 528- CORBIS. 530- ADAM. 531- CORBIS. 537- ADAM. 540- ADAM. 541- CDC. 542- ADAM. 544- CORBIS. 546- ADAM. 548- T: ADAM; B: CORBIS. 549- CORBIS. 550- T, M: ADAM. 555- Lido. 558- ADAM. 559- ADAM. 561- IC: ADAM; B: CORBIS. 562- T, M: CDC; B: NCI. 565- ADAM. 567- ADAM. 569- ADAM. 570- ADAM; 572: ADAM; 573: ADAM; 575: ADAM; 577: ADAM; 584: ADAM; 590: ADAM; 592: CDC; 593: ADAM; 598: Corbis; 599-T: ADAM; M: Corbis; B: ADAM; 601-T: Corbis; 601-B: ADAM; 603: Corbis; 604: NCI; 605: Corbis; 608: CDC; 619: ADAM; 620: ADAM; 621: ADAM; 622: ADAM; 623-B: ADAM; 633: ADAM; 639: ADAM; 640: ADAM; 641-T: NCI; 647: ADAM; 653: CDC; 655: CDC; 661: ADAM; 663: ADAM; 664: NCI; 665: CDC; 666-T: ADAM; B: CDC; 669-B: CDC; 674: ADAM; 676: ADAM; 677: ADAM; 678: ADAM; 679: ADAM; 683: ADAM; 684: ADAM; 685: Corbis; 686: ADAM; 687-T: ADAM; 688: ADAM; 689: ADAM; 691: ADAM; 692: ADAM; 695: ADAM; 696: ADAM; 697: ADAM; 698: CDC; 700: ADAM; 702: Corbis; 704: ADAM; 705: NCI; 710-T: CDC; M/B: ADAM; 713: NCI; 715-T: CDC; B: ADAM; 716: ADAM; 717: CDC; 724: ADAM; 726-T: ADAM; B: CDC; 731: ADAM; 732: ADAM; 733-T: ADAM; 735-T/B: ADAM; 736-M/B ADAM; 738-T: NCI; ICR: ADAM; 740-T: NCI/Dr. Lance Liotta Laboratory; B: Lester V. Bergman/Corbis; 741-T: ADAM; ICR: Stephen P. Smith; 746-ADAM; 747-T:NCI/Dr. Dwight Kaufman. National Cancer Institute; B-NCI/Bill Branson; 749-ADAM; 751: NCI/Linda Barlett; 752: ADAM; 753: ADAM; 754: ADAM; 757: ADAM; 763: ADAM; 773: NCI/Understanding Cancer 8; 781-L: Duomo/Corbis Chris Trotman; 783: ADAM; 786: ADAM; 791: ADAM; 792: ADAM; 796: ADAM; 798: ADAM; 799: CDC; 808: ADAM; 810: ADAM; 811: ADAM; 819: ADAM; 820: ADAM; 822: ADAM; 824: NCI/Linda Bartlett; 826: ADAM; 829: ADAM; 832-T: ADAM B: NCI; 839: CDC; 841-T: NCI/Understanding Cancer 43; B: NCI/Understanding Cancer 45; 842: ADAM; 844: NCI/Linda Bartlett; 845: ADAM; 846: ADAM; 852: ADAM; 853: ADAM; 857: ADAM; 862: ADAM; 863: ADAM; 867: Charles O'Rear/Corbis; 869: ADAM; 873: ADAM; 876: CDC; 885: ADAM; 886: ADAM; 888: ADAM; 889-M: CDC; 889-B: ADAM; 890: ADAM; 892: ADAM; 893: ADAM; 897: ADAM; 905: ADAM; 912: ADAM; 913-T: CDC; M/B: ADAM; 917-T: ADAM; 918: ADAM; 921: ADAM; 924-T: CDC; B: ADAM; 925: CDC; 936: ADAM; 945: NCI; 950: ADAM; 955: ADAM; 960: ADAM; 961: David & Peter Tumley/Corbis; 962-T: Bettmann/Corbis; 962-B: Bettamnn/Corbis; 972-ICL: CDC; ICR: NCI/Linda Bartlett; T: NCI; 974: ADAM; 976: ADAM; 979: ADAM; 981: ADAM; 983: CDC; 986; 986-M: NCI/Dr. Michael Goitein Massachusettes General Hospital; T: NCI/Michael Anderson; B: NCI/Pat Kenny; 991: ADAM; 993: ADAM; 995: ADAM; 997: ADAM; 1000: ADAM; 1006: ADAM; 1011: ADAM; 10013: ADAM; 1018: ADAM; 1019: ADAM; 1020-T: Laura Dwight/Corbis; M/B: ADAM; 1021-T: ADAM; B-CDC; 1022-T: CDC; B-ADAM; 1023: ADAM; 1024: ADAM; 1026: ADAM; 1027: ADAM; 1031: ADAM;

1033: ADAM; 1035: ADAM; 1042: ADAM; 1049: ADAM; 1050: ADAM; 1053: ADAM; 1059: ADAM; 1061: ADAM; 1062: ADAM; 1063: ADAM; 1064: ADAM; 1065: ADAM; 1066: ADAM; 1064: ADAM; 1065: ADAM; 1066: ADAM; 1067: ADAM; 1071: ADAM; 1074: ADAM; 1075-L: Owen Franken/Corbis; R: Nation Wong/Corbis; 1085: ADAM; 1086: ADAM; 1087: ADAM; 1089: ADAM; 1093: ADAM; 1094: ADAM; 1101: ADAM; 1102: ADAM; 1103: ADAM; 1107: ADAM: 1110-T: ADAM; B: Lester V. Bergman/Corbis; 1122: Owen Franken/Corbis; 1124: ADAM; 1125: ADAM; 1127: ADAM; 1136: ADAM; 1137-ICL: ADAM; ICR: Karen Huntt Mason/Corbis; 1140: ADAM; 1142: ADAM; 1144: ADAM; 1146: ADAM; 1151: ADAM; 1154: ADAM; 1156: ADAM; 1158: ADAM; 1161: ADAM; 1164: ADAM; 1176: ADAM; 1169: ADAM; 1170: ADAM; 1173: CDC; 1175: ADAM; 1176: ADAM; 1177: ADAM; 1181: ADAM; 1182: ADAM; 1185: ADAM; 1186: ADAM; 1187: ADAM; 1193: ADAM; 1194: ADAM; 1196: ADAM; 1197: ADAM; 1198: ADAM; 1199: ADAM; 1201: NCI; 1202: ADAM; 1206: ADAM; 1209: ADAM; 1211: ADAM; 1216: ADAM; 1220: ADAM; 1222: ADAM; 1226: ADAM; 1227: ADAM; 1230: ADAM; 1231: ADAM; 1238: ADAM; 1240: CDC: 1241-T: CDC; TM/BM/B: ADAM; 1242: ADAM; 1246: NCI/Larry Ostby.

The editors, publishers, and producers of this book would like to thank the Corbis Archives, the National Cancer Institute and all of its fine photographers, the Centers for Disease Control and Prevention for all of the fine work they do, the staff at ADAM.com, Lido.com, Troy Schremmer, Bob Antler along with his design crew, and Rachel Soltis. Without the assistance of these people, producing this book would have been an impossible task.